MARGULIS AND BURHENNE'S
ALIMENTARY
TRACT RADIOLOGY

VOLUME ONE

MARGULIS AND BURHENNE'S

ALIMENTARY
TRACT
RADIOLOGY

PATRICK C. FREENY, MD

Professor of Radiology
Director of Abdominal Imaging, Department of Radiology
University of Washington Medical Center
Seattle, Washington

GILES W. STEVENSON, FRCP, FRCR, FRCP(C)

Professor and Chairman
Department of Radiology, McMaster University;
Chief, Department of Radiology
Chedoke-McMaster Hospitals
Hamilton, Ontario

FIFTH EDITION

with 4605 illustrations, including 52 in color

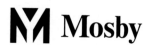

St. Louis Baltimore Boston Chicago London Madrid Philadelphia Sydney Toronto

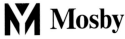

Dedicated to Publishing Excellence

Publisher: George Stamathis
Editor: Robert Farrell
Developmental Editor: Kathryn Falk
Project Manager: Patricia Tannian
Production Editors: John P. Casey, Kathy Teal
Senior Book Designer: Gail Morey Hudson
Manufacturing Supervisor: Karen Lewis

FIFTH EDITION

Printed in the United States of America
Composition by Clarinda Company
Printing/Binding by Maple-Vail Book Mfg. Group

Mosby–Year Book, Inc.
11830 Westline Industrial Drive
St. Louis, Missouri 63146

Library of Congress Cataloging in Publication Data

Margulis and Burhenne's alimentary tract radiology. —5th ed. /
    [edited by] Patrick C. Freeny, Giles W. Stevenson.
        p.   cm.
    Rev. ed. of: Alimentary tract radiology / edited by Alxander R.
Margulis, H. Joachim Burhenne. 4th ed. 1989.
    Includes bibliographical references and index.
    ISBN 0-8016-6707-0 (set)
    1. Alimentary canal—Radiography.   I. Margulis, Alexander R.
II. Burhenne, H. Joachim (Hans Joachim), 1925-   .   III. Freeny,
Patrick C.   IV. Stevenson, Giles W.   V. Title: Alimentary tract
radiology.
    [DNLM: 1. Digestive System—radiography.   WI 141 M3313 1994]
RC804.R6A4   1994
616.3'30757—dc20
DNLM/DLC
for Library of Congress   93-37100
                                                                  CIP

93 94 95 96 97 / 9 8 7 6 5 4 3 2 1

Contributors

MICHAEL M. ABECASSIS, MD

Assistant Professor of Surgery
Director of the Liver Transplantation Program
Division of Organ Transplantation, Department of Surgery
Northwestern University Medical School
Northwestern Memorial Hospital
Chicago, Illinois

MONZER M. ABU-YOUSEF, MD

Professor, Department of Radiology
Director of Ultrasound, Department of Radiology
The University of Iowa Hospitals and Clinics
Iowa City, Iowa

SERGE AGOSTINI, MD

Professor of Radiology, Radiology Department
Sainte Marguerite Hospital
Marseille, France

ABASS ALAVI, MD

Professor of Radiology
Chief, Division of Nuclear Medicine
Department of Radiology
Hospital of the University of Pennsylvania
Philadelphia, Pennsylvania

DAVID J. ALLISON, BSC, MD, MRCP, FRCR

Professor and Chairman, Diagnostic Radiology
Royal Postgraduate Medical School/Hammersmith Hospital
London, England

JOHN R. AMBERG, MD

Professor of Radiology
University of California–San Diego
San Diego, California

MARK E. BAKER, MD

Associate Professor of Radiology
Chief, Section of Abdominal Imaging
Duke University Medical Center
Durham, North Carolina

DENNIS M. BALFE, MD

Professor of Radiology
Chief, GI Radiology and Radiology Residency Program Director
Mallinckrodt Institute of Radiology
St. Louis, Missouri

EMIL J. BALTHAZAR, MD

Professor of Radiology
New York University–Bellevue Medical Center
New York, New York

RICHARD L. BARON, MD

Professor of Radiology
Co-Director of Abdominal Imaging
Department of Radiology
The University of Pittsburgh Medical Center
Pittsburgh, Pennsylvania

RICHARD E. BARTON, MD

Assistant Professor
Dotter Interventional Institute;
Assistant Professor, Diagnostic Radiology
Department of Diagnostic and Interventional Radiology
Oregon Health Sciences University
Portland, Oregon

CLIVE I. BARTRAM, FRCP, FRCR

Consultant Radiologist, St. Mark's Hospital
London, England

DAVID E. BECKLY, MB, FRCP, FRCR

Consultant Radiologist, Department of Radiology
Plymouth General Hospital
Plymouth, England

JOHN BEYNON, MS, FRCS

Consultant Surgeon
Wrexham Maelor Hospital
Wrexham, Clwyd, North Wales

BERNARD A. BIRNBAUM, MD

Chief of Computed Tomography
Assistant Professor, Department of Radiology
Hospital of the University of Pennsylvania
Philadelphia, Pennsylvania

GILES W. BOLAND, MD

Clinical Assistant in Radiology
Massachusetts General Hospital
Boston, Massachusetts

JOSE F. BOTET, MD

Associate Attending, Department of Radiology
Memorial Sloan-Kettering Cancer Center;
Associate Attending, Department of Radiology
Cornell University Medical College
New York, New York

DAVID G. BRAGG, MD

Professor and Chairman, Department of Radiology
University of Utah School of Medicine
Salt Lake City, Utah

H. JOACHIM BURHENNE, MD, FRCP(C), FFR(RSCI) (Hon)

Professor of Radiology
University of British Columbia
Vancouver, British Columbia

WILLIAM L. CAMPBELL, MD

Professor of Radiology
Co-Director of Abdominal Imaging
Department of Radiology
University of Pittsburgh Medical Center
Pittsburgh, Pennsylvania

JAMES C. CARR, MB, BCH, DMRD, FFR(I), FRCR

Consultant Radiologist, Department of Radiology, Beaumont
Hospital
Senior Lecturer in Radiology, Royal College of Surgeons in
Ireland
Dublin, Ireland

GIOVANNA CASOLA, MD

Associate Professor, Department of Radiology
University of California–San Diego Medical Center
San Diego, California

J. WILLIAM CHARBONEAU, MD

Professor of Radiology
Mayo Clinic
Rochester, Minnesota

JUDITH L. CHEZMAR, MD

Department of Radiology
Emory University School of Medicine
Atlanta, Georgia

KEDAR N. CHINTAPALLI, MD

Chief of Body Imaging
Associate Professor of Radiology
University of Texas Health Science Center
San Antonio, Texas

KYUNG J. CHO, MD

Professor of Radiology
Director, Vascular and Interventional Radiology
Radiology Department
University of Michigan Hospitals
Ann Arbor, Michigan

CAROLYN C. COMPTON, MD, PHD

Associate Professor, Department of Pathology
Harvard Medical School;
Director, Gastrointestinal Pathology
Massachusetts General Hospital;
Chief, Shriner's Burns Institute
Shriner's Hospital for Crippled Children
Boston, Massachusetts

PETER L. COOPERBERG, MDCM, FRCP

Professor of Radiology
University of British Columbia;
Chairman, Department of Radiology
St. Paul's Hospital
Vancouver, British Columbia

PETER B. COTTON, MD, FRCP

Professor of Medicine, Duke University
Durham, North Carolina

EMMETT T. CUNNINGHAM, JR., MD, PHD, MPH

Department of Radiology & Radiological Science
Johns Hopkins Swallowing Center
Johns Hopkins Hospital
Baltimore, Maryland

HUGH D. CURTIN, MD

Professor of Radiology and Otolaryngology
Director, Department of Radiology
Eye and Ear Institute Pavilion
Pittsburgh, Pennsylvania

HORACIO D'AGOSTINO, MD

Assistant Professor, Department of Radiology
University of California–San Diego Medical Center
San Diego, California

SIGMUND DAWISKIBA, MD

Senior Lecturer in Cytology
Departments of Pathology and Cytology
Cytology Division
University Hospital
Lund, Sweden

STEVEN L. DAWSON, MD

Associate Professor
Harvard Medical School;
Head GI Interventional Radiology
Associate Director, MGH Center for Innovative Minimally
Invasive Therapy
Massachusetts General Hospital
Boston, Massachusetts

†WYLIE J. DODDS, MD

Department of Radiology
Milwaukee County Medical Complex
Milwaukee, Wisconsin

---

†Deceased.

†MARTIN W. DONNER, MD, FACR

Professor of Radiology
Founder, The Johns Hopkins Swallowing Center
Johns Hopkins University School of Medicine
Baltimore, Maryland

BERTRAND DUVOISIN, MD

Privat Docent et Agrégé
Department of Diagnostic Radiology
University Hospital
Lausanne, Switzerland

OLLE EKBERG, MD

Head, Gastrointestinal Radiology
University of Lund
Malmo General Hospital
Malmo, Sweden

J. STEPHEN FACHE, MD

Head, Division of Abdominal Imaging
Vancouver General Hospital
University of British Columbia
Vancouver, British Columbia

PETER J. FECZKO, MD

Staff Radiologist
William Beaumont Hospital
Royal Oak, Michigan

JOSEPH T. FERRUCCI, MD

Professor and Chairman, Department of Radiology
Boston University School of Medicine
Boston, Massachusetts

STUART FIELD, MA, MB, B CHIR., DMRD, FRCR

Consultant, Department of Diagnostic Radiology
Kent & Canterbury Hospital NHS Trust
Canterbury, Kent, England

W. DENNIS FOLEY, MD

Professor, Department of Radiology
Director, Section of Digital Imaging
Medical College of Wisconsin
Milwaukee, Wisconsin

FRANS-THOMAS FORK, MD, PHD

Associate Professor, Department of Diagnostic Radiology
University of Lund
Malmo General Hospital
Malmo, Sweden

ISAAC R. FRANCIS, MB, BS

Professor, Department of Radiology
University of Michigan
Ann Arbor, Michigan

EDMUND A. FRANKEN, JR., MD

Professor and Head, Department of Radiology
The University of Iowa Hospitals and Clinics
Iowa City, Iowa

PATRICK C. FREENY, MD

Professor of Radiology
Director of Abdominal Imaging
Department of Radiology
University of Washington School of Medicine
Seattle, Washington

BRIGID M. GERETY, MD

Diagnostic Radiologist
Northwest Radiology Consultants
Atlanta, Georgia

GARY M. GLAZER, MD

Professor and Chairman, Department of Radiology
Stanford University School of Medicine
Stanford, California

HENRY I. GOLDBERG, MD

Professor of Radiology, Radiology Department
University of California–San Francisco
San Francisco, California

ROBERT A. HALVORSEN, MD

Professor & Vice Chairman, Department of Radiology
University of California–San Francisco;
Chief, Department of Radiology
San Francisco General Hospital
San Francisco, California

TSUTOMU HAMADA, MD

Chief, Department of Gastroenterology
The Social Health Insurance Medical Center
Tokyo, Japan

KEITH M. HARRIS, BM, FRCS ED., FRCR

Senior Registrar, Department of Radiology Service Centre
University Hospital of Wales
Cardiff, South Glamorgan, Wales

DONALD R. HAWES, MD

Professor of Radiology, Department of Radiology
Wishard Memorial Hospital
Indiana University Medical Center
Indianapolis, Indiana

MICHAEL HENRY, MD

Central Middlesex Hospital NHS Trust
London, England

---

†Deceased.

CHIA-SING HO, MD

Professor, Department of Radiology
University of Toronto;
Pathologist-in-Chief
Department of Radiology
Toronto General Hospital
Toronto, Ontario

KEES HUIBREGTSE, MD, PHD

Department of Gastroenterology and Hepatology
University of Amsterdam
Amsterdam, The Netherlands

EDWARD W. HUMPHREY, MD, PHD

Professor and Interim Chairman
Department of Surgery
University of Minnesota
Minneapolis, Minnesota

YUGI ITAI, MD

Professor and Chairman, Department of Radiology
University of Tsukuba Institute of Clinical Medicine
Tsukuba, Ibaraki, Japan

JAMES E. JACKSON, MRCP, FRCR

Doctor (Consultant)
Diagnostic Radiology Department
Royal Postgraduate Medical School
Hammersmith Hospital
London, England

R. BROOKE JEFFREY, JR., MD

Professor of Radiology
Chief of Abdominal Imaging, Radiology Department
Stanford University School of Medicine
Stanford, California

C. DANIEL JOHNSON, MD

Associate Professor of Radiology
Mayo Medical School;
Department of Diagnostic Radiology
Mayo Clinic and Mayo Foundation
Rochester, Minnesota

BRONWYN JONES, MB, BS, FRACP, FRCR

Professor of Radiology
Director, Johns Hopkins Swallowing Center
Johns Hopkins University School of Medicine
Baltimore, Maryland

MICHAEL D. KATZ, MD

Assistant Professor, Department of Radiology
University of Southern California School of Medicine
Los Angeles, California

KEIICHI KAWAI, PHD, MD

Director, Kyoto Prefectural University of Medicine
Kyota, Japan

ELIAS KAZAM, MD

Professor of Radiology
Head, Division of Ultrasound and Computed Body Tomography
The New York Hospital/Cornell Medical Center
New York, New York

FREDERICK S. KELLER, MD

Cook Professor and Director
Dotter Interventional Institute;
Chairman, Department of Diagnostic Radiology
Oregon Health Sciences University
Portland, Oregon

FREDERICK M. KELVIN, MD

Staff Radiologist, Methodist Hospital of Indiana
Clinical Professor of Radiology
Indiana University School of Medicine;
Department of Radiology
Methodist Hospital of Indiana
Indianapolis, Indiana

THOMAS A. KIM, MD

Department of Diagnostic Radiology
Allegheny General Hospital
Pittsburgh, Pennsylvania

ROBERT E. KOEHLER, MD

Professor and Vice Chairman
Department of Radiology
University of Alabama School of Medicine
Birmingham, Alabama

RICHARD A. KOZAREK, MD

Chief of Gastroenterology
Virginia Mason Clinic;
Clinical Professor of Medicine
University of Washington
Seattle, Washington

YOSHIHISA KUROSAKI, MD

Assistant Professor, Department of Radiology
University of Tsukuba Institute of Clinical Medicine
Tsukuba, Ibaraki, Japan

FAYE C. LAING, MD

Associate Professor, Department of Radiology
Harvard University School of Medicine
Boston, Massachusetts

BRIAN W. LAWRIE, DMRD, FRCR

Consultant Radiologist, Clinical Director, Radiology Department
University Hospital of Wales
Cardiff, Wales

THOMAS L. LAWSON, MD

Professor and Chairman, Department of Radiology
Loyola University—Chicago Stritch School of Medicine
Loyola University Medical Center
Maywood, Illinois

MICHAEL J. LEE, MD

Assistant Professor of Radiology
Harvard Medical School;
Assistant Director of Ultrasound
Massachusetts General Hospital
Boston, Massachusetts

ROBERT A. LEE, MD

Assistant Professor, Department of Radiology
Mayo Clinic
Rochester, Minnesota

GEORGE R. LEOPOLD, MD

Department of Radiology
University of California–San Diego Medical Center
San Diego, California

JOSEPH W.C. LEUNG, MD, FRCP(GLAS) FRCP(EDIN)

Professor of Medicine, Division of Gastroenterology
Department of Medicine
Duke University Medical Center
Durham, North Carolina

CHARLES J. LIGHTDALE, MD

Professor of Clinical Medicine
Director, Clinical Gastroenterology
Columbia-Presbyterian Medical Center
Columbia University College of Physicians and Surgeons
New York, New York

ANDERS LUNDERQUIST, MD, PHD

Professor of Radiology
Central Department of Diagnostic Radiology
University Hospital
Lund, Sweden

DEAN D.T. MAGLINTE, MD

Chief, Section of Gastrointestinal Radiology
Methodist Hospital of Indiana;
Clinical Professor of Radiology
Indiana University School of Medicine
Indianapolis, Indiana

DERMOT E. MALONE, MD

Assistant Professor, Department of Radiology
Chedoke-McMaster Hospitals
Hamilton, Ontario

GUY MARCHAL, MD

Professor of Radiology, Department of Radiology
University Hospital K. U. Leuven
Leuven, Belgium

ALEXANDER R. MARGULIS, MD

Professor of Radiology
University of California–San Francisco
San Francisco, California

JOHN A. MARKISZ, MD

Associate Professor
Department of Radiology
New York Hospital–Cornell Medical Center
New York, New York

MASAKAZU MARUYAMA, MD

Department of Internal Medicine
Cancer Institute Hospital
Tokyo, Japan

DIDIER MATHIEU, MD

Professor of Radiology
Henri Mondor Hospital
Creteil, France

OSAMU MATSUI, MD

Associate Professor, Department of Radiology
Kanazawa University School of Medicine
Kanazawa, Ishikawa, Japan

F.P. MCGRATH, MB, MSC, FFR(RCSI), FRCR, FRCP(C)

Assistant Professor
Department of Radiology
McMaster University Medical Centre
Hamilton, Ontario

ALEC J. MEGIBOW, MD

Professor of Radiology, Department of Radiology
New York University Medical Center
New York, New York

DONALD L. MILLER, MD

Chief, Vascular/Interventional Radiology
Professor of Radiology, Department of Radiology
State University of New York
Health Science Center at Syracuse
Syracuse, New York

PETER R. MUELLER, MD

Associate Professor of Radiology, Harvard Medical School;
Division Head, Abdominal Imaging and
Interventional Radiology, Department of Radiology
Massachusetts General Hospital, Boston, Massachusetts

MASATUGU NAKAJIMA, MD

Kyoto, Japan

RENDON C. NELSON, MD

Associate Professor, Department of Radiology
Director, Frederik Phillips Magnetic Resonance Research Center
Emory University School of Medicine
Atlanta, Georgia

SIDNEY W. NELSON, MD

Clinical Professor, Department of Radiology
University of Washington
Harborview Medical Center
Seattle, Washington

DANIEL J. NOLAN, MD

Consultant Radiologist
John Radcliffe Hospital
Oxford, England

KUNI OHTOMO, MD

Associate Professor, Department of Radiology
Yamanashi Medical College
Tomaho Yamanashi, Japan

GARY M. ONIK, MD

Professor of Neurosurgery
Medical College of Pennsylvania
Allegheny General Hospital
Pittsburgh, Pennsylvania

MARK B. ORRINGER, MD

Professor and Head, Section of Thoracic Surgery
Department of Surgery
University of Michigan Medical Center
Ann Arbor, Michigan

J. ODO OP DEN ORTH, MD

Wapserveen, The Netherlands

PHILIP E.S. PALMER, MD

Professor Emeritus
University of California–Davis School of Medicine
Davis, California

ROBERT S. PERRET, MD

Director of Ultrasound and Computed Tomography
Department of Radiology
St. Joseph's Hospital and Medical Center
Phoenix, Arizona

LESLIE E. QUINT, MD

Associate Professor, Department of Radiology
University of Michigan Medical Center
Ann Arbor, Michigan

ALAIN RAHMOUNI, MD

Assistant Professor, Department of Radiology
Henri Mondor Hospital
Creteil, France

CARL C. READING, MD

Associate Professor of Radiology
Mayo Clinic
Rochester, Minnesota

MAURICE M. REEDER, MD, FACR

Chairman, Department of Radiology
University of Hawaii School of Medicine
Honolulu, Hawaii

JACQUES W.A.J. REEDERS, MD, PHD

Head, Department of GI-Radiology and Hepatopancreato-Biliary
Imaging
Department of Radiology
Academic Medical Center
Amsterdam, The Netherlands

S. RIVERA-MACMURRAY, MD

Division of Gastroenterology and Hepatology
University of Amsterdam
Amsterdam, The Netherlands

GERAINT M. ROBERTS, MD, FRCP, FRCR

Professor, Department of Medical Imaging
University of Wales College of Medicine
Cardiff, South Glamorgan, Wales

CHARLES A. ROHRMANN, JR., MD

Professor and Vice Chairman
Director of Gastrointestinal Radiology
Department of Radiology
University of Washington School of Medicine
Seattle, Washington

PABLO R. ROS, MD

Professor of Radiology
Director, Division of Abdominal Imaging and MRI
Department of Radiology
University of Florida College of Medicine
Gainesville, Florida

JOSEF RÖSCH, MD

Professor of Radiology and Surgery
Research Director, Dotter Interventional Institute
Oregon Health Sciences University
Portland, Oregon

GERD ROSENBUSCH, MD, PHD

Professor of Abdominal Radiology, Department of Radiology
University Hospital Sint Radboud
Nijmegen, The Netherlands

WILLIAM A. RUBENSTEIN, MD

Associate Professor
Department of Radiology
New York Hospital–Cornell University Medical Center
New York, New York

ERNST RUMMENY, MD, DR. MED.

Oberarzt, Institute for Clinical Radiology
Westfaelische Wilhelms-Universitaet
Muenster, Germany

MAX RYAN, FFR (I), FRCR, FACR (Hon)

Professor and Chairman, Department of Radiology
Royal College of Surgeons in Ireland;
Senior Consultant Radiologist
Beaumont Hospital
Dublin, Ireland

SANJAY SAINI, MD

Associate Professor of Radiology
Harvard Medical School;
Director, Computed Tomography
Department of Radiology
Massachusetts General Hospital
Boston, Massachusetts

ROBERT SANCHEZ, MD

Assistant Professor, Department of Radiology
University of California–San Diego Medical Center
San Diego, California

PROFESSOR DR. MED. TILMAN SAUERBRUCH

Chairman of the Unit for General Internal Medicine
Department of Medicine
University Hospital
Bonn, Germany

SALVATORE J.A. SCLAFANI, MD

Professor, Department of Radiology
State University of New York
Downstate Medical School
Brooklyn, New York

PIERRE SCHNYDER, MD

Professor and Chairman, Department of Radiology
University of Lausanne
Lausanne, Switzerland

SCOTT J. SCHULTE, MD

Assistant Professor, Department of Radiology
University of Washington Medical Center
Seattle, Washington

PHILIP J. SHORVON, MD, MBBS, MRCP, FRCR

Director of Radiology
Central Middlesex Hospital NHS Trust
London, England

ALAN SIEGEL, MD

Department of Nuclear Medicine
Philadelphia VA Medical Center
Philadelphia, Pennsylvania

MARILYN J. SIEGEL, MD

Professor of Radiology
Associate Professor of Pediatrics
Mallinckrodt Institute of Radiology
Washington University School of Medicine
St. Louis, Missouri

CLAIRE SMITH, MD

Professor, Rush Medical College
Section Director, Gastrointestinal Radiology
Director, Residency Training Program
Department of Diagnostic Radiology and Nuclear Medicine
Rush-Presbyterian–St. Luke's Medical Center
Chicago, Illinois

SAT SOMERS, MD, FRCP(C)

Professor of Radiology
Head, Gastrointestinal Radiology
McMaster University Medical Centre
Hamilton, Ontario

DAVID H. STEPHENS, MD

Professor of Radiology
Mayo Medical School;
Department of Diagnostic Radiology
Mayo Clinic and Mayo Foundation
Rochester, Minnesota

GILES W. STEVENSON, FRCP, FRCR, FRCP(C)

Professor and Chairman, Department of Radiology
McMaster University;
Chief, Department of Radiology
Chedoke-McMaster Hospitals
Hamilton, Ontario

EDWARD T. STEWART, MD

Professor, Department of Radiology
Chief, Gastrointestinal Radiology
Medical College of Wisconsin
Milwaukee, Wisconsin

DAVID STRINGER, MD

Head, Section of Ultrasound and General Radiology
British Columbia Children's Hospital;
Professor, Department of Radiology
University of British Columbia
Vancouver, British Columbia

GEORGE P. TEITELBAUM, MD

Assistant Professor, Department of Radiology
University of California–San Francisco
San Francisco, California

RUEDI F. THOENI, MD

Professor of Radiology, Department of Radiology
Chief CT/GI-MRI
University of California–San Francisco
San Francisco, California

M. KRISTIN THORSEN, MD

Associate Professor, Department of Radiology
Medical College of Wisconsin
Milwaukee, Wisconsin

WILLIAM M. THOMPSON, MD

Professor and Chairman
Vilhelmina and Eugene Gedgaudas Chair
Department of Radiology
University of Minnesota
Minneapolis, Minnesota

T.L. TIO, MD

Professor of Medicine, Department of Medicine
Division of Gastroenterology
Georgetown University Medical Center
Washington, D.C.

ERIC VANSONNENBERG, MD

Chairman of Radiology
Professor of Radiology, Medicine, and Surgery
The University of Texas Medical Branch
Galveston, Texas

PIERRE-JEAN VALETTE, MD

Professor of Radiology, Department of Radiology
Edouard Herriot Hospital
Lyon, France

WILLIAM C. VEZINA, MD

Associate Professor
Department of Nuclear Medicine
University Hospital
London, Ontario

ELLEN M. WARD, MD

Assistant Professor
Mayo Clinic
Rochester, Minnesota

JOSEPH P. WHALEN, MD

Dean, College of Medicine
State University of New York Health Science Center
Syracuse, New York

E. MAUREEN WHITE, MD

Associate Professor of Radiology
Northwestern University Medical School;
Chief, Body Imaging Section, Department of Radiology
Evanston Hospital, Evanston, Illinois

ROGER WILLÉN, MD, PHD

Associate Professor, Department of Pathology
Pathology Division
University Hospital
Lund, Sweden

STEPHANIE R. WILSON, MD

Head, Division of Ultrasound
The Toronto Hospital;
Professor, Department of Radiology
University of Toronto
Toronto, Ontario

THOMAS C. WINTER III, MD

Assistant Professor, Department of Radiology
University of Washington
Seattle, Washington

TSUNEYOSHI YAO, MD

Professor, Department of Gastroenterology
Fukuoka University, Chikushi Hospital
Chikushino City, Fukuoka, Japan

KENJIRO YASUDA, MD, PHD

Associate Chief, Department of Gastroenterology
Kyota Second Red Cross Hospital
Kamigyo-ku, Kyoto, Japan

EUGENE YIU-CHUNG YEUNG, MBBS (Lond), BSC(Hon), MRCP(UK), FRCR, FRCP(C)

Assistant Professor, Diagnostic Radiology
The Toronto Hospital, General Division
Toronto, Ontario

WILLIAM T.C. YUH, MD, MSEE

Associate Professor, Department of Radiology
Director of MRI Center
Department of Radiology
The University of Iowa Hospitals and Clinics
Iowa City, Iowa

ROBERT K. ZEMAN, MD

Professor and Clinical Director of Diagnostic Radiology
Department of Radiology
Georgetown University Medical Center
Washington, D.C.

KENNETH ZIRINSKY, MD

Director, South Region MRI
Tacoma Specialty Center
Tacoma, Washington

Foreword

It is with pleasure and pride that we welcome and endorse the new edition of *Alimentary Tract Radiology* organized and orchestrated by the new pair of most distinguished editors, Drs. Patrick C. Freeny and Giles W. Stevenson.

During the four editions of *Alimentary Tract Radiology* (including a supplement on new cross-sectional modalities in the second edition), gastrointestinal radiology along with all medical imaging has undergone revolutionary changes. We recognized this by changing the name of the book from *Alimentary Tract Roentgenology* to *Alimentary Tract Radiology* starting with the third edition. Gastrointestinal radiology, as we've always considered it, covers the alimentary tube and its appendages—the liver and pancreas—which are examined by all imaging methods. It covers also interventional radiology as applied to these organs. We have continued to expand our coverage of radiologic techniques, including nuclear medicine ultrasonography, computed tomography, and eventually magnetic resonance imaging. Mosby meticulously adheres to the high standards of superb reproduction of illustrations and refined printing.

We are happy that the new editors share our philosophy of making this book the international cutting edge final word on alimentary tract radiology. This assembly of exquisitely organized and executed chapters written by leading authorities around the world is testimony that this book will endure.

Alexander R. Margulis
H. Joachim Burhenne

Preface

The preface to the 1967 first edition of Alexander Margulis and Joachim Burhenne's *Alimentary Tract Roentgenology* begins "Alimentary tract roentgenology has undergone great expansion in the last two decades." Over 1200 pages then presented in great detail the current status of gastrointestinal radiology, with emphasis on barium radiology and fluoroscopy. Diagnostic angiography, percutaneous splenoportography, and transhepatic cholangiography were the spearhead trio representing the new advances of the 1960s.

Much of what we accept as routine today was not even conceived. There were no cross-sectional imaging techniques, such as transcutaneous or endoscopic ultrasonography, computed tomography, and magnetic resonance imaging; no endoscopy or therapeutic endoscopic procedures, such as retrograde cholangiopancreatography, endoscopic sphincterotomy and biliary tract stone removal, pancreatic or biliary stent placement, and gastroesophageal variceal sclerotherapy; no radiologically guided interventional procedures, such as percutaneous biopsy, catheter drainage of abdominal abscesses and fluid collections, biliary stent placements, and biliary stone dissolution or removal, percutaneous cholecystostomy, gastrostomy and enterostomy; and no therapeutic angiographic procedures, such as embolic or pharmacologic control of gastrointestinal bleeding or abdominal neoplasms, and creation of percutaneous portocaval shunts.

Needless to say, even the above list is incomplete, and new diagnostic and interventional procedures are being developed and introduced as this fifth edition is going to press. The only certainty, and a galling one to all the contributors, is that this fifth edition will be partly out of date by the time it appears and will certainly need major revision within 4 or 5 years.

The explosion in technology that has occurred during the previous four editions of this book has provided GI radiologists with one of the most interesting and challenging careers in medicine. It has also taken them from the isolated, darkened reporting rooms and fluoroscopy suites into the bright new world of computerized and digitized imaging techniques, and back to the mainstream of clinical medicine with ever-closer working relationships with surgeons, gastroenterologists, nurses, and technologists—in the department, in the ward, and even in the operating rooms. GI radiologists have become the directors of new imaging and therapeutic techniques that have revolutionized the diagnosis and treatment of many diseases. With this move has also come a responsibility for defining the proper role of these techniques, evaluating their efficacy against older and more established methods, and providing our referring physicians with guidance through this labyrinth of expensive and amazing technology.

We are delighted to have contributions from three of the original 47 authors from the first edition: Drs. Amberg, Burhenne, and Margulis. There are many more new authors in the fifth edition, and we have included the work of colleagues from around the world, including England, Wales, Ireland, France, Switzerland, Germany, Belgium, Holland, Sweden, Hong Kong, and Japan, in addition to the United States and Canada. As in the first edition, we have deliberately allowed some overlap of material, and readers will find a diversity of opinion in a number of areas. We hope that the breadth of views and practice illustrated in this new edition will encourage radiologists to try different approaches in devising strategies to suit their own patients' needs.

No doubt there are errors, and we are responsible for these. We would like to encourage our readers to write to us with critical comments on the book, especially with suggestions for better coverage of important areas, for different approaches that you feel would be interesting or useful, and with notes of errors that should be corrected.

ACKNOWLEDGMENTS

We particularly thank Anne Patterson, Kathy Falk, John Casey, and Robert Farrell at Mosby in St. Louis for their help and encouragement in getting the manuscripts prepared and edited on time and with minimal difficulty. We also thank our secretaries, Philomena Kedziorski at the University of Washington in Seattle, and Elaine Hewitt at McMaster University in Hamilton, for their help in typing, editing, and mailing the manuscripts around the world.

Patrick C. Freeny
Giles W. Stevenson

Contents

VOLUME ONE

PART I HISTORY

1 History of Alimentary Tract Radiology, 1
H. Joachim Burhenne and Alexander R. Margulis

Gastrointestinal tract, 1
  Upper GI study, 2
  Small bowel, 8
  Colon, 8
Gallbladder and biliary system, 10
  Cholecystography, 11
  Cholangiography, 13
  Scintigraphy, 13
Liver, spleen, and pancreas, 13
Cross-sectional imaging, 16
  Ultrasound, 16
  Computed tomography, 17
  Magnetic resonance, 19
Intervention, 23

PART II ANATOMY AND PHYSIOLOGY

2 Anatomy, 28
Elias Kazam, William A. Rubenstein, John A. Markisz,
Joseph P. Whalen, and Kenneth Zirinsky

Diaphragm, 32
Liver, 32
Hepatic veins, 33
Portal veins, 33
Portacaval space, 34
Gallbladder, 34
Spleen, 34
Stomach, 34
Duodenum, 35
Colon, 35
Intraperitoneal compartments, 35
Pancreas, 47
Adrenal glands, 61
Kidneys, 61
Retroperitoneal compartments, 63
Abdominal great vessels, 65

3 Gastrointestinal Physiology, 67
F.P. McGrath and Giles W. Stevenson

Enteric neuropeptides and enteric hormones, 67
  Anatomy of the gut-endocrine system, 67
  Gastrin, 67
  Cholecystokinin, 69
  Secretion, 69
  Insulin, 69
  Glucagon, 69
  Vasoactive intestinal polypeptide, 69
  Somatostatin, 69

  Distal intestinal peptides, 69
  Clinical implication of gut peptides, 69
  Prostaglandins and the gut, 72
  Proton pump inhibitors, 72
Oropharynx and swallowing, 73
  Esophagus, transit, and acid neutralization, 73
  Physiology of the stomach, 75
  Gastric secretion, 75
Gastric motility, 77
Duodenum and small intestine, 79
  Digestion and absorption, 79
  Malabsorption, 80
  Motility, 81
  Immunology, 82
Biliary system and liver, 83
  Anatomy and function, 83
  Synthesis, 84
  Secretion, 84
  Bile flow, 86
  Physiology of ascites, 87
Pancreas, 87
  Endocrine pancreas, 87
  Exocrine pancreas, 87
  Pancreatic cell function tests, 88
  Pancreatic digestion tests, 88
Colon, 88
  Transit, 88
  Assessment of colonic function, 88
  Absorption, 89
  Diarrhea, 89
  Physiology of bowel preparation, 90
  Defecation, 91

PART III PHARYNX

**4 Normal Anatomy and Techniques of
Examination of the Pharynx, 94**
Emmett T. Cunningham, Jr., Bronwyn Jones, and
Martin W. Donner

General indications, 94
Pharyngeal anatomy, 94
Normal pharyngeal swallow, 98
Neural control of the pharyngeal phase, 98
Techniques of examination, 101
  Choice of studies, 101
  Plain radiography, 101
  Barium studies, 101
  Axial studies, 106
Future directions in imaging, 112

5 Benign Structural Diseases of the Pharynx, 114
Olle Ekberg

Benign neoplasms, 114
Mucosal abnormalities, 114

Foreign bodies, 114
Trauma, 115
Lateral pharyngeal outpouchings, 115
The pharyngoesophageal segment, 118
  Zenker's diverticulum, 118
Killian-Jamieson's diverticulum, 118
  Webs, 118
Branchial cleft anomalies, 120
Enlarged tonsils, 120
Parapharyngeal abnormalities, 120
  Thyroid gland, 120
  Laryngoceles, 120
  Cervical spine osteophytes, spurs, and kyphosis, 120
  Parapharyngeal abscesses, 120
  Tortuous vessels, 120
  Retropharyngeal tendinitis, 126
  Thyroglossal cysts, 126
  Calcified lymph nodes, 126
  Parapharyngeal neoplasms, 126

6 Functional Abnormalities of the Pharynx, 127

Olle Ekberg

Oral stage, 127
Pharyngeal stage, 129
  Hyoid bone, 129
  Epiglottis, 129
  Laryngeal vestibule, 130
  Pharyngeal constrictors, 130
PE segment dysfunction, 133
Cause of dysfunction, 133
Adaptation, compensation, and decompensation, 135
Treatment planning, 137

7 Malignant Diseases of the Pharynx, 139

Hugh D. Curtin and Thomas A. Kim

Pathology, 139
  Squamous cell carcinoma, 139
  Minor salivary gland tumors, 139
  Lymphoma, 139
  Other, 139
Staging, 139
  Imaging, 140
  Tumor spread, 142
Specific anatomic locations, 144
  Oral cavity, 144
  Oropharynx, 150
  Hypopharynx, 157
  Nasopharynx, 160
Reconstruction and postoperative evaluation, 160
Summary, 163

8 A Multidisciplinary Approach to the Patient with Swallowing Impairment, 165

Bronwyn Jones and Martin W. Donner

PART IV ESOPHAGUS

9 Normal Anatomy and Techniques of Examination of the Esophagus: Fluoroscopy, CT, MRI, and Scintigraphy, 168

Olle Ekberg

Normal anatomy, 168
  General radiographic anatomy of the esophagus, 168

Aspects of cross-sectional anatomy, 173
Technique of examination, 176
  Fluoroscopic evaluation, 176
  Cross-sectional techniques, 184
  Other techniques, 184

10 Normal Anatomy and Techniques of Examination of the Esophagus: Endosonography, 186

Jose F. Botet and Charles J. Lightdale

Fundamentals of intraluminal sonography, 186
Evaluation of the gastrointestinal wall, 186
  Ultrasound, 186
  Tissues, 186
  Absorption and scattering, 187
  Frequency and penetration, 187
  Focal zone, 187
  Axial resolution, 187
The gastrointestinal wall, 187
The esophagus, 187
  Normal anatomy, 187
  Examination technique, 190

11 Radiology of the Esophagus, 192

Edward T. Stewart and Wylie J. Dodds

Types of examination, 192
Performance of examination, 192
Normal esophageal anatomy, 193
  Resting conditions, 194
  Peristaltic contractions, 194
  Nonperistaltic contractions, 196
  Radiographic evaluation, 196
Esophageal motility disorders, 198
  Radiographic and manometric features, 198
  Primary motility disorders, 202
  Secondary motility disorders, 206
  Differential diagnosis, 210
Congenital anomalies, 212
  Atresia and tracheoesophageal fistula, 212
  Duplication, 212
  Miscellaneous anomalies, 212
Esophageal diverticula, 214
  Intramural pseudodiverticulosis, 216
Traumatic lesions, 216
  Foreign bodies, 216
  Esophageal perforation, 216
  Miscellaneous lesions, 218
Hiatus hernia, 218
Esophagitis, 220
  Gastroesophageal reflux disease, 220
  Barrett's esophagus, 224
  Infectious esophagitis, 226
  Caustic esophagitis, 229
  Drug-induced esophagitis, 230
  Radiation esophagitis, 232
  Miscellaneous causes, 232
Rings, webs, and strictures, 233
  Esophageal rings, 233
  Esophageal webs, 235
  Esophageal strictures, 236
Esophageal varices, 238
Esophageal tumors, 242
  Malignant tumors, 242
  Metastases, 249
  Benign tumors, 250

Indentations and displacement, 252
  Indentations, 252
    Deviation, 254
Diaphragm, 255
  Anatomy, 255
  Defects, 255
  Movement and location, 256
  Neoplasms, 256

12 Endosonography of the Esophagus, 264

T.L. Tio

Instrumentation, 264
Technique, 264
Image interpretation, 265
Staging of cancer, 265
Assessment of recurrence, 269
Submucosal lesion assessment, 269
  Leiomyoma versus leiomyosarcoma, leiomyoblastoma,
    and other nonepithelial malignancies, 269
Evaluation of the mediastinum, 270
Conclusions, 270

**13 CT and MR Staging of Tumors of the Esophagus
and Gastroesophageal Junction and Detection
of Postoperative Recurrence,** 272

**Leslie E. Quint, Isaac R. Francis, Gary M. Glazer, and
Mark B. Orringer**

Computed tomography, 272
  Normal esophagus, 272
  Esophageal carcinoma, 272
  CT staging of esophageal carcinoma, 273
  Recurrent tumor, 278
Magnetic resonance imaging, 278

PART V STOMACH AND DUODENUM

**14 Normal Anatomy and Techniques of
Examination of the Stomach and
Duodenum,** 282

K.M. Harris, G.M. Roberts, and B.W. Lawrie

Radiologic anatomy of the stomach and duodenum, 282
  Stomach, 282
Normal anatomic variants and indentations that may
  simulate disease, 285
  Stomach, 285
  Duodenum, 285
Barium meal technique, 286
  Historical perspective, 286
  Indications, 286
  Contraindications, 286
  Patient preparation, 286
  Contrast media, 287
  Paralysis of peristalsis, 288
  Gas-producing agents, 288
  Techniques, 289
  Techniques for the examination of the duodenum, 296
  Hypotonic duodenography, 296
Modified barium meal techniques for specific clinical
  situations, 297
  Suspected gastroduodenal perforation, 297
  Studies of the postoperative stomach and
    duodenum, 297
  Upper gastrointestinal bleeding, 298

The roles of barium studies and endoscopy in the
  investigation of the stomach and duodenum, 298
  Clinical diagnosis, 299
  Patient preference, 300
  Safety, 300
  Availability and cost, 300
Upper gastrointestinal endoscopy, 301
  Basic technique, 301
  Patient preparation, 301
  Sedation, 302
  Intubation, 302
  Normal appearances, 304
  Aftercare, 304
  Alternative imaging modalities, 305
  Computed tomography, 305
  Technique, 305
  Normal CT anatomy, 306
  Magnetic resonance imaging, 307

**15 Endosonography: Normal Anatomy and
Techniques of Examination of the Stomach and
Duodenum,** 311

Jose F. Botet and Charles J. Lightdale

The stomach, 311
  Normal anatomy, 311
  Examination technique, 314
The duodenum, 314
  Normal anatomy, 314
  Examination technique, 316

16 Nonneoplastic Diseases of the Stomach, 318

Charles A. Rohrmann, Jr., and Sidney W. Nelson

Congenital lesions, 318
  Gastric duplication, 318
  Gastric diverticulum, 318
  Adenomyosis, 318
  Ectopic pancreas, 318
  Antral diaphragm or web, 320
  Adult pyloric hypertrophy, 322
Inflammatory diseases, 325
  Radiographic signs of gastritis, 327
  Erosive gastritis, 329
  Hemorrhagic gastritis, 330
  Chronic gastritis, 330
  Atrophic gastritis, 330
  Granulomatous gastritis, 330
  Syphilis, 331
  Crohn's disease, 333
  Gastric sarcoidosis, 333
  Infective gastritis, 333
Peptic ulcer disease, 336
  Epidemiology, 336
  Definitions and location, 336
  Ulcer healing, 347
  Complications, 347
Hypertrophic gastropathy, 347
  Hyperrugosity, 351
  Zollinger-Ellison syndrome, 351
  Pseudolymphoma, 354
  Injury gastropathy, 357
  Corrosive gastropathy, 357
  Gastric radiation injury, 359
Miscellaneous gastropathies, 359
  Eosinophilic gastropathy, 359
  Amyloidosis, 360

Abnormalities of function, 361
Varices, 365
Gastric rupture, 369

17 Benign Tumors of the Stomach, 373
E. Maureen White

Radiologic evaluation of benign gastric tumors and
polyps, 373
Benign epithelial polyps and tumors, 373
Hyperplastic (regenerative) polyps, 374
Gastric adenomas, 374
Hamartomatous polyps, 375
Retention polyps (Cronkhite-Canada syndrome), 376
Heterotopic polyps (ectopic pancreas, adenomyomas,
Brunner's gland hyperplasia), 377
Teratoma, 377
Benign nonepithelial tumors, 377
Smooth muscle tumors (spindle cell leiomyoma,
epithelioid variant), 377
Neurogenic tumors (schwannoma, neurofibroma,
paraganglioma, ganglioneuroma), 379
Lipoma, 381
Inflammatory fibroid polyp, 381
Glomus tumor, 383
Vascular tumors (hemangioma, lymphangioma,
hemangiopericytoma, hemangioendothelioma), 383
Carcinoid tumor (benign form), 384
Granular cell tumor (myoblastoma), 384
Lymphoid hyperplasia (pseudolymphoma), 384
Plasmacytoma, 384

18 Diagnosis of Gastric Cancer in Europe, 387
J. Odo Op Den Orth

Barium examination, 387
State-of-the-art-technique, 387
Limitations of barium examination, 387
Cross-sectional techniques, 389
Transabdominal gastric ultrasound, 389
Diagnostic value of barium examination
versus endoscopy, 392
Diagnosis of early and advanced gastric carcinoma, 394
Current role of radiology, 394
Macroscopic types of gastric carcinoma, 394
Protruded type, 394
Superficial type, 395
Excavated lesions, 395
Linitis plastica, 395
Experience in a Dutch general hospital, 397

19 Diagnosis of Gastric Cancer in Japan, 399
Maskazu Maruyama and Tsutomu Hamada

Japanese approach to the radiographic examination of the
stomach, 399
Basic approach, 399
Technical considerations in the initial (routine)
study, 400
Difference in image quality of the initial and detailed
studies, 401
Diagnosis of gastric cancer, 402
General considerations, 402
Application of computed radiography to the
double-contrast examination, 402
Role of endoscopic ultrasonography, 404

Definition and classification of early gastric cancer, 404
Radiographic diagnosis of early gastric cancer and
correlation with endoscopy, 405
Diagnosis of early polypoid cancer, 406
General considerations, 406
Gross appearance of polypoid lesions, 406
Adenoma, 406
Types I and IIa, 407
Types IIa + IIc and IIc + IIa, 407
Radiographic diagnosis of early depressed cancer, 410
General considerations, 410
Correlation of histologic type and depressed early
cancer, 410
Types IIc, IIc + III, and III, 412
Early cancer smaller than 1 cm, 413
Type IIb-like lesion, 414
Superficial spreading carcinoma, 415
Radiographic diagnosis of advanced cancer, 416
General considerations, 416
Classification, 416
Bormann types 1 and 2, 416
Bormann type 3, 416
Bormann type 4, 419
Linitis plastica–type of carcinoma and its early
phase, 420
Advanced cancer simulating type IIc, 421
Esophageal invasion of gastric cancer, 422
Carcinoma of the gastric stump after gastrectomy, 423
General considerations, 423
Carcinoma of the gastric stump after gastrectomy for
benign lesions, 423
Residual and recurrent cancer of the gastric stump, 423
Multiple cancers, 424
Evaluation of a mass screening program for stomach
cancer, 424
Value of mass screening, 424
Method of mass screening, 425
Cost-effectiveness analysis, 427

20 Malignant Tumors of the Stomach, 429
Henry I. Goldberg

Lymphoma, 429
Gross and histologic appearance, 429
Radiographic findings—upper GI barium
examination, 429
Ultrasound findings, 429
CT findings, 429
Leiomyosarcoma, 432
Radiographic features, 432
Ultrasound features, 433
CT features, 433
Metastases, 433
Carcinoid tumors, 434
Kaposi's sarcoma, 435
Villous adenoma, 435
Gastric involvement by leukemia, 435

21 CT and MR Staging of Gastric Carcinoma, 437
Robert A. Halvorsen

Pathology, 437
Anatomic considerations, 438
Staging, 438
Staging systems, 439
Primary site (T), 439

Regional lymph nodes (N), 440
Distant metastases (M), 441
Stage grouping, 441
Histopathologic staging, 441
Computed tomographic staging of gastric carcinoma, 441
Adenopathy, 442
Pancreatic invasion, 443
TNM staging, 443
Magnetic resonance imaging of the stomach, 445
Conclusion, 446
Role of CT, 446
Role of MRI, 446

22 Endoscopic Ultrasound of the Stomach, 448

Jose F. Botet

Benign processes, 448
Inflammatory processes, 448
Large gastric folds, 449
Submucosal tumors, 449
Polyps, 451
Malignant tumors, 451
Gastric cancer, 451
Gastric lymphoma, 453
Others, 453
Anastomotic recurrences, 453
Summary, 454

23 Radiology of the Stomach after Gastric Surgery for Obesity, 455

Claire Smith

General overview, 455
Gastric bypass, 455
Gastroplasty, 458
Weight control, 458
Radiologic studies, 458
Immediate complications, 459
Anastomotic leak and abscess, 459
Pouch perforation, 460
Staple line dehiscence, 460
Channel obstruction, 461
Delayed complications, 461
General principles, 461
Pouch dilatation, 463
Staple line dehiscence, 464
Channel widening, 464
Channel stenosis and obstruction, 464
Ulceration, 464
Summary, 464

24 Radiology of Benign and Malignant Diseases of the Duodenum, 467

Jacques W.A.J. Reeders and G. Rosenbusch

Congenital and miscellaneous abnormalities, 467
Congenital positional anomalies, 467
Congenital diaphragm of the duodenum, 467
Ladd's band, 467
Annular pancreas, 467
Duodenal diverticulum, 468
Intraluminal diverticulum, 469
Wall cysts of the duodenum, 471
Antral mucosal prolapse, 472
Intussusception, 472
Paraduodenal hernias, 473

Inflammation, 473
Nonspecific duodenitis, 473
Erosions, 473
Crohn's duodenitis, 473
Eosinophilic gastroduodenitis, 475
Radiation ischemic duodenitis, 476
Caustic ingestion, 476
Infective duodenitis, 476
Peptic ulcer, 477
General aspects, 477
Radiologic features, 478
Linear ulcer, 484
Giant duodenal ulcer, 484
Postbulbar ulcer, 486
Complications, 486
Differential diagnosis and pitfalls, 487
X ray versus endoscopy, 488
Tumors, 488
Adenoma, 488
Adenocarcinoma, 488
Kaposi's sarcoma, 492
Carcinoid, 492
Nonepithelial tumors, 496
Tumorlike lesions, 497
Vascular abnormalities, 501
Vascular malformation, 501
Duodenal varices, 501
Arterioduodenal fistula, 501
Traumatic changes of duodenum, 502
Intramural hematoma or bleeding, 503
Superior mesenteric artery compression syndrome, 506
Duodenal involvement as part of more extensive disease, 506
Celiac disease, 506
Whipple's disease, 506
Progressive systemic sclerosis (scleroderma), 506
Cystic fibrosis, 506
Amyloidosis, 508
Venous congestion, hypoproteinemia, 508
Zollinger-Ellison syndrome, 508
Metastasis to the duodenum, 508

PART VI   SMALL BOWEL

25 The Small Bowel: Anatomy and Nontube Examinations, 512

Sat Somers and Giles W. Stevenson

Anatomy, 512
Examination techniques, 514
Barium examination, 514
Summary: nontube barium examinations, 525
Ultrasound examination, 526
CT examination, 527
MRI examination, 530

26 Biphasic Enteroclysis with Methylcellulose, 533

Dean D.T. Maglinte

Methylcellulose for double-contrast small bowel radiography, 534
Patient preparation, 534
Contrast materials, 534
Fluoroscopy and filming sequence, 534
Infusion rates, 535
Technique-related problems: avoidance and solution, 539

Modifications of the technique, 542
Biphasic enteroclysis for evaluation of unexplained
gastrointestinal bleeding, 545
Advantages, 546
Complications, 546

27 **Double-Contrast Enteroclysis with Air,** 548

Tsuneyoshi Yao

Technique, 548
Patient preparation, 548
Barium, 548
Radiography, 548
Problems, 550

28 **Percutaneous Fine-Needle Aspiration, Cytology,
and Peroral Biopsy of the Small Bowel,** 552

Sigmund Dawiskiba, Anders Lunderquist, and Roger Willén

Peroral biopsy, 552
Cytologic aspiration technique, 555
Complications of fine-needle aspiration cytology, 562

29 **Idiopathic Inflammatory Disease of the Large
and Small Bowel,** 564

Ruedi F. Thoeni

Techniques and indications for fluoroscopic examinations
in large and small bowel, 564
Plain films of the abdomen, 564
Barium examinations, 565
Indications for barium examinations, 567
Pathology, 568
Ulcerative colitis, 573
Clinical features, 573
Endoscopic findings, 574
Extraintestinal manifestations, 574
Radiographic features, 575
Accuracy of radiographic examination, 580
Complications, 581
Surgical procedures, 584
Crohn's disease, 585
Clinical features, 585
Endoscopic findings, 587
Extraintestinal manifestations, 588
Radiographic features, 589
Differential diagnosis of ulcerative colitis and Crohn's
disease, 603
Role of colonoscopy, 608
Role of radiologic follow-up examinations in evaluation
of therapy, 609
Scintigraphy for inflammatory bowel disease, 609
Computed tomography for inflammatory disease of the
colon, 610
Sonography for inflammatory bowel disease, 615
Magnetic resonance imaging for inflammatory bowel
disease, 616

30 **Small Bowel Neoplasms,** 627

Robert E. Koehler

Radiographic detection, 627
Barium studies, 627
Computed tomography, 627
Benign tumors, 627
Leiomyomas, 627
Lipomas, 628

Adenomas, 629
Hemangiomas, 629
Uncommon tumors, 630
Polyposis syndromes, 631
Peutz-Jeghers syndrome, 631
Cronkhite-Canada syndrome, 632
Syndromes rarely affecting the small bowel, 632
Carcinoid tumors, 632
Clinical features, 632
Carcinoid syndrome, 632
Radiographic features, 633
Lymphomas, 634
Clinical features, 634
Associated conditions, 635
Radiographic features, 635
Lymphoma variants, 639
Differential diagnosis, 639
Adenocarcinomas, 639
Clinical features, 639
Radiographic features, 640
Associated conditions, 640
Sarcomas, 640
Metastatic tumors, 643
General features, 643
Metastatic melanoma, 643
Metastatic carcinoma, 645
Kaposi's sarcoma, 645
Germ cell tumors, 645

31 **Vascular Disorders of the Small Intestine,** 649

Daniel J. Nolan

Mesenteric ischemia and infarction, 649
Ischemic intestinal strictures, 650
Intramural hemorrhage, 650
Chronic radiation enteritis, 651
Systemic sclerosis, 653
Vasculitis, 653
Henoch-Schönlein purpura, 653
Polyarteritis nodosa, 653
Behçet's disease, 655
Rheumatoid arthritis, 655
Ehlers-Danlos syndrome, 655
Thromboangiitis obliterans, 655
Systemic lupus erythematosus, 656
Cogan's syndrome, 656
Cryoglobulinemia, 656
Nonsteroidal antiinflammatory drug–induced
enteritis, 656
Vascular malformations, 657
Intestinal varices, 657

32 **Malabsorption, Immunodeficiency, and
Miscellaneous Disorders of the Small
Bowel,** 659

Max Ryan and James C. Carr

Main radiologic findings in functional disease of the
small bowel, 659
Dilatation, 660
Valvulae conniventes, 660
Increased intestinal fluid, 661
Nodulation, 661
Motility changes, 661
Narrowing, 661
Primary small intestinal disease, 661
Celiac disease (gluten-induced enteropathy), 663

Herpetiform dermatitis, 663
Refractory celiac disease, 663
Unclassified celiac disease, 663
Tropical sprue, 663
Radiology of celiac disease, 663
Dilatation, 663
The valvulae conniventes, 664
Hypersecretion, 664
Flocculation, 664
The moulage sign, 665
Intussusception, 665
Complications of celiac disease, 665
Lymphoma, 665
Chronic ulcerative jejunoileitis, 665
Collagenous sprue, 666
Cow's milk protein and soy protein allergy, 666
Intestinal lymphangiectasia, 666
Abetalipoproteinemia, 667
Stasis, 669
Hollow visceral myopathy (intestinal
pseudoobstruction), 669
Infestations with malabsorption patterns, 669
Giardiasis, 669
Strongyloides stercoralis infection, 670
Enteropathic immunoglobulin deficiency states, 671
Acquired immunodeficiency syndrome, 671
Graft-versus-host disease, 674
Primary immunodeficiency syndromes, 676
Systemic diseases, 677
Mediterranean lymphoma (alpha-chain disease), 677
Mediterranean fever, 678
Scleroderma, 678
Whipple's disease, 679
Amyloidosis, 681
Waldenstrom's macroglobulinemia, 681
Mastocytosis, 682
Histoplasmosis, 682
GI pathology and biochemical changes, 683
Zollinger-Ellison syndrome, 683
Eosinophilic gastroenteritis, 683
Chronic pancreatitis, 684
Cystic fibrosis, 684
Intestinal lactase deficiency, 684
Inflammatory diseases, 684
Secondary changes resulting from other causes, 684
Short bowel syndrome, 684
Small intestinal edema, 684
Drugs, 684
Ischemic enteritis, 685
Radiation enteritis, 685
Irritable bowel syndrome, 686

33   **Small Bowel Examination: Overview,** 689
John R. Amberg

Small bowel follow-through method, 689
Enteroclysis with methylcellulose, 689
Enteroclysis with air contrast, 690
General discussion, 691

PART VII   COLON

34   **Normal Anatomy and Techniques of
Examination of the Colon: Barium, CT, and
MRI,** 692
Giles W. Stevenson

Anatomy, 692
Techniques of examination, 696
Endoscopy of the colon, 715
Integration of endoscopy and radiology, 716
Magnetic resonance scanning, 719
Functional metabolic imaging of the colon, 720

35   **Normal Anatomy and Techniques of
Examination of the Colon and Rectum:
Endosonography,** 725
Jose F. Botet and Charles J. Lightdale

Colon, 725
Normal anatomy, 725
Examination technique, 726
Rectum, 727
Normal anatomy, 727
Examination technique, 729

36   **Diverticular Disease of the Colon: Conventional
Radiology,** 730
Pierre Schnyder and Bertrand DuVoisin

Method of examination, 730
Incidence, 731
Pathogenesis, 732
Diverticula, 733
Significance and radiology of a muscular
abnormality, 737
Diverticulitis, 739
Deformed sacs, 739
Demonstration of abscess, 739
Extravasation of contrast material, 739
Accuracy of diagnosis, 741
Differential diagnosis, 742
Carcinoma, 742
Polyps, 742
Other causes of extrinsic-pressure defects, 743
Ischemic colitis, 744
Complications, 744
Obstructions, 744
Bleeding, 745
Spread of inflammation and fistula formation, 745
Diseases coexisting with diverticula, 745
Diverticular disease with neoplasm, 745
Diverticular disease with Crohn's disease, 747
Diverticular disease with ulcerative colitis, 747
Diverticular disease with angiodysplasia, 747
Classification, 747
Scattered diverticula, 747
Diverticulosis, 747
Diverticular disease without diverticula, 747
Diverticular disease, 747
Diverticulitis, 747

37   **Cross-Sectional Imaging in the Evaluation of
Acute Diverticulitis,** 750
Mark E. Baker

Pathophysiology, 750
Clinical presentation, 750
Treatment, 751
Computed tomography, 753
Technique, 753
CT diagnosis of acute diverticulitis and differential
diagnosis, 754

CT versus the contrast enema study, 757
Right-sided diverticulitis, 759
Sonography in the diagnosis of acute diverticulitis, 760

38   Neoplastic Colonic Lesions, 762

Edward T. Stewart and Wylie J. Dodds

Definitions, 762
Classification, 762
Pathology, 762
   Histology, 762
   Morphology, 763
   Distribution, 763
   Cancer origin, 764
High-risk groups, 765
Clinical symptoms, 765
Detection, 765
   Contrast enema, 765
   Colonoscopy, 767
   Confidence level, 770
Radiologic features, 771
   Differentiation from artifacts, 771
   Morphologic findings, 772
   Potential for malignancy, 774
Specific polypoid lesions, 777
   Adenomas, 777
   Lipomas, 777
   Juvenile polyps, 778
   Carcinoid tumors, 778
   Endometriosis, 778
   Other tumors, 779
Management, 779
   Treatment, 779
   Surveillance, 779
Polyposis syndromes, 779
   Familial multiple polyposis, 780
   Gardner's syndrome, 781
   Peutz-Jeghers syndrome, 783
   Ruvalcaba-Myhre-Smith syndrome, 785
   Turcot syndrome, 786
   Muir-Torre syndrome, 786
   Cowden's disease: multiple hamartoma syndrome, 786
   Cronkhite-Canada syndrome, 787
   Juvenile polyposis, 787
Hereditary nonpolyposis colorectal carcinoma, 788
   Differential diagnosis, 790
Malignancies of the colon, 790
   Complications of carcinoma of the colon, 793
   Caveats pertaining to radiologic examination of
      carcinoma of the colon, 795

**39   Computed Tomography and Magnetic
Resonance Imaging in Colorectal Carcinoma:
Staging and Detection of Postoperative
Recurrence,** 801

Alex J. Megibow

Goals of imaging studies, 801
Computed tomography, 801
   Techniques, 801
   Appearance of primary colorectal carcinoma, 803
   Lymph node metastases, 803
   Distant metastases, 804
   Accuracy of CT staging, 805
   Complications of colorectal cancer, 805

Magnetic resonance imaging, 806
Follow-up imaging of colorectal carcinoma, 809
Other imaging modalities, 810

40   Endosonographic Staging of Rectal Cancer, 813

Clive I. Bartram and John Beynon

Technique and apparatus, 813
Normal endosonographic anatomy of the rectal wall, 814
Assessment of depth of tumor penetration, 815
Lymph node involvement, 818
Local recurrence, 820
The role of endosonography in rectal cancer, 821

41   Colorectal Cancer Screening, 824

F.T. Fork and Giles W. Stevenson

Incidence of colorectal neoplasia, 824
   Colorectal cancer, 824
   Colorectal adenoma, 824
Risk factors for CRC, 824
   Age and sex, 824
   Adenoma patient, 824
   Carcinoma patient, 825
   Cancer family syndromes, 825
   Chronic ulcerative colitis, 827
   Crohn's enterocolitis, 829
Prevention of CRC, 829
   General principles of screening, 829
   Principles in evaluating screening programs, 830
   Screening methodology, 831
   Diagnostic follow-up procedures, 832
   Results of screening programs to date, 833
   Summary and screening guidelines, 835

**42   Defecography: Techniques and Normal
Findings,** 840

Frederick M. Kelvin and Giles W. Stevenson

Anatomic and physiologic considerations, 840
Techniques of defecography, 841
   Defecographic equipment, 841
   Contrast media, 841
   Vaginal opacification, 841
   Special commode, 842
   Recording of rectal evacuation, 842
Variations of defecographic technique, 844
   Balloon proctography, 844
   The balloon expulsion test, 844
   Simplified defecography, 844
   Quantification of rectal evacuation, 844
Examination procedure, 844
   Aiding mechanisms, 845
Normal appearances, 845
   Anal canal, 845
   Anorectal junction level, 845
   Anorectal angle, 845
   Rectovaginal septum, 847
   Changes during defecography, 847

**43   Investigation of Constipation and
Incontinence,** 852

Philip J. Shorvon and Michael Henry

Constipation, 852
   Patient history and definition, 852

Investigation, 852
Symptoms suggestive of onset in childhood, 852
Onset of symptoms in adulthood, 855
Pseudoobstruction, 855
Constipation in the elderly, 856
Chronic idiopathic constipation, 856
Measurement of colonic transit, 857
Slow transit constipation, 858
Outlet obstruction, 858
Incontinence, 858
  Enteric causes, 858
  Physiologic components of the mechanisms of fecal
    continence and their testing, 858
  Physiologic tests of anorectal function, 863
  Neurologic causes, 864
  Radiologic value in investigation of incontinence
    patients, 864
  Role of defecography, 865
Rectal prolapse, 865
  Role of proctography in prolapse, 868
  Magnetic resonance imaging, 870

44 Anal Endosonography, 873

Clive I. Bartram

Technique, 873
Normal anatomy, 873
Internal sphincter abnormalities, 875
External sphincter abnormalities, 875
Incontinence, 877
Constipation, 879
Conclusion and indications, 879

**45 Applications and Limitations of Imaging in
Staging and Follow-up of Gastrointestinal
Neoplasms,** 881

**David G. Bragg, William M. Thompson, and
Edward W. Humphrey**

Esophageal cancer, 881
Gastric cancer, 883
Colorectal cancer, 885

**PART VIII MISCELLANEOUS DISORDERS OF THE
GASTROINTESTINAL TRACT**

46 Infections and Infestations, 888

Maurice M. Reeder and Philip E.S. Palmer

Bacterial infections, 888
  Gastrointestinal tuberculosis, 888
  Salmonella infections, 895
  Typhoid fever, 895
  Bacillary dysentery, 898
  Campylobacter infection, 900
  Pseudomembranous enterocolitis, 901
  Acute gastroenteritis, 903
  Helicobacter pylori, 904
Chlamydia infections, 904
  Lymphogranuloma venereum, 904
Fungal infections, 908
  Gastrointestinal candidiasis, 908
  Gastrointestinal histoplasmosis, 909
Unknown etiology, 910
  Tropical sprue, 910
Parasitic diseases, 913

Parasitic infections, 913
Helminthic infections, 926

**47 Gastrointestinal Manifestations of the Acquired
Immunodeficiency Syndrome,** 952

Peter J. Feczko

Human immunodeficiency virus, 952
Clinical presentation and staging of HIV infection, 952
Epidemiology and natural history, 953
Clinical testing, 953
Imaging of the patient with HIV infection, 954
Opportunistic infections of the GI tract, 954
  Enteric pathogens, 954
  AIDS and HIV enteropathy, 959
  Hepatobiliary abnormalities, 960
Neoplastic disease in AIDS, 961
  Kaposi's sarcoma, 961
  AIDS-related lymphoma, 962
Radiologic practice in an HIV environment, 963

**48 Gastrointestinal Bleeding: Endoscopy and
Diagnostic Approach,** 967

D.E. Beckly

Clinical aspects, 967
Timing of endoscopy, 967
Technique of upper GI endoscopy in acute bleeding, 968
Common conditions and their treatment, 968
  Esophageal varices, 968
  Gastric varices, 969
  Varices and pregnancy, 970
  Bleeding peptic ulcer, 970
  Other common causes of upper GI bleeding, 972
  Uncommon or infrequently recognized causes of upper
    GI bleeding, 974
  Lower GI bleeding, 976
Summary, 979

**49 Scintigraphic Evaluation of Gastrointestinal
Hemorrhage,** 983

Alan Siegel and Abass Alavi

Extent of the problem and causes of bleeding, 983
Surgery for the treatment of GI hemorrhage, 983
Nonscintigraphic modes of evaluation 984
Scintigraphic modes of evaluation, 984
  Sulfur colloid, 984
  Albumin, heat-damaged red blood cells, and
    DTPA, 986
  Labeled red blood cells, 986
  Meckel's scans, 989
Conclusions, 992

**50 Angiographic Diagnosis and Therapy of
Gastrointestinal Tract Bleeding,** 994

Frederick S. Keller, Robert E. Barton, and Josef Rosch

Acute GI hemorrhage, 994
Diagnosis of acute arterial bleeding, 994
Pharmacoangiography, 994
Angiographic control of acute GI hemorrhage, 995
  Vasoconstrictive infusion therapy, 995
  Arterial embolotherapy, 997
  Chronic GI hemorrhage, 999
  Angiodysplasia, 1000

Meckel's diverticulum, 1004
GI bleeding from extraalimentary tract sources, 1004
    Hemobilia, 1004
    Pancreatic hemorrhage, 1004
    Aortoenteric and arterioenteric fistulas, 1005
GI hemorrhage of venous origin, 1006
    Diagnosis of venous bleeding, 1006
    Therapy for variceal hemorrhage, 1006
    Transhepatic embolization of gastroesophageal
        varices, 1006
    Transjugular intrahepatic portosystemic
        shunting, 1007

VOLUME TWO

PART IX   PANCREAS

51 **Radiology of the Pancreas: Diagnostic and
    Interventional Techniques,** 1017
    Patrick C. Freeny

    Diagnostic examinations, 1017
    Interventional procedures, 1017
    Computed tomography, 1017
        Technique, 1018
        Normal anatomy, 1018
    Magnetic resonance imaging, 1018
        Technique, 1018
        Normal anatomy, 1019
    Endoscopic retrograde cholangiopancreatography, 1022
        Technique, 1022
        Normal anatomy, 1022
    Percutaneous transhepatic cholangiography, 1022
        Technique, 1022
    Angiography, 1023
        Technique, 1023
        Normal anatomy, 1023
    Transhepatic pancreatic venography, 1023
        Technique, 1023
        Normal anatomy, 1024
    Fine-needle aspiration biopsy, 1024
        Technique, 1024
    Aspiration of pancreatic fluid collections and
        percutaneous pancreatography, 1025
    Percutaneous catheter drainage, 1025

52 **Ultrasonography,** 1027
    George R. Leopold

    General considerations, 1027
    Patient preparation, 1027
    Conduct of the examination, 1027
        Real-time examination, 1028
        Static gray scale examination, 1028
        Endoscopic sonography, 1028
        Operative sonography, 1029
    Normal anatomy, 1029
        Regional anatomy, 1029
        Pancreatic size, 1031
        Pancreatic texture, 1031
    Pancreatic pathology, 1031
        Pancreatitis, 1031
        Texture, 1031
        Size, 1031
        Other findings, 1031
        Clinical utility, 1032

    Cysts, 1033
        Ordinary pseudocysts, 1033
        Ectopic pseudocyst, 1034
        Temporal relationships, 1034
        False-positive pseudocysts, 1035
        Other cystic lesions, 1035
        Carcinomas, 1036
        Pancreatic biopsy, 1037

53 **Embryology, Normal Variation, and Congenital
    Anomalies of the Pancreas,** 1039
    Scott J. Schulte

    Embryology, 1039
    Variations of duct drainage, 1039
    Fusion anomalies, 1042
        Pancreas divisum, 1042
        Incomplete pancreas divisum, 1044
        Stenosis of main pancreatic duct, 1045
    Agenesis and hypoplasia, 1045
    Annular pancreas, 1046
    Ectopic pancreas, 1048
    Duplication anomalies, 1049
    Anomalous ducts producing pseudomasses, 1049

54 **Inflammatory Disease of the Pancreas,** 1052
    Patrick C. Freeny and Charles A. Rohrmann, Jr.

    Pancreatitis: general considerations, 1052
        Cambridge and Marseille classifications, 1052
        Acute pancreatitis, 1052
        Chronic pancreatitis, 1052
    Radiologic diagnosis of pancreatitis, 1053
        Acute pancreatitis, 1053
        Radiologic diagnosis, 1053
        Contrast studies, 1053
        Cross-sectional imaging studies, 1054
        Chronic pancreatitis, 1056
    Clinical and radiologic staging of pancreatitis, 1062
        Acute pancreatitis, 1062
        Chronic pancreatitis, 1065
    Etiology of pancreatitis: radiologic evaluation, 1066
        Biliary tract disease, 1066
        Stomach and duodenum, 1066
        Pancreas divisum, 1066
        Hereditary pancreatitis, 1067
        Traumatic pancreatitis, 1067
    Complications of pancreatitis: radiologic detection and
        treatment, 1068
        Pancreatic and extrapancreatic fluid collections, 1068
        Radiologic diagnosis, 1068
        Ultrasonography and computed tomography, 1069
        Percutaneous catheter drainage, 1070
        Pancreatic phlegmon, 1074
        Pancreatic abscess, 1074
        Percutaneous catheter drainage, 1076
        Pancreatic necrosis, 1076
        Biliary complications, 1076
        Nonoperative biliary drainage, 1079
        Vascular complications, 1080
        Pancreatic ascites, 1080
        Osseous complications, 1083
        Pulmonary complications, 1084
    Preoperative and postoperative radiologic evaluation of
        pancreatitis, 1086
        Chronic pancreatitis, 1086

55 Endoscopic Therapy of Chronic Pancreatitis, 1091

Richard A. Kozarek

Relapsing pancreatitis and chronic pain, 1091
  Sphincterotomy, 1091
  Calculus extraction, 1091
  Prosthesis placement, 1094
  Pseudocyst drainage, 1097
  Biliary obstruction, 1098
Abandoned endoscopic therapies, 1099

56 Extracorporeal Shock Wave Lithotripsy of Pancreatic Duct Calculi, 1101

Tilman Sauerbruch

Principles of extracorporeal shock wave lithotripsy, 1101
Indications, 1102
Procedure, 1102
Results, 1102
Adverse effects, 1105
Conclusion, 1106

57 Pancreatic Adenocarcinoma: Radiologic Diagnosis and Staging, 1107

David H. Stephens

Clinical manifestations, 1107
Pathologic anatomy and biologic behavior, 1107
Diagnostic imaging: rationale, 1109
  Diagnosis, 1109
  Staging, 1109
  Choice of methods, 1110
Computed tomography, 1110
  Technical considerations, 1110
  Interpretation, 1112
Ultrasonography, 1118
  Technical considerations, 1118
  Interpretation, 1119
  Complementary roles of CT and
    ultrasonography, 1119
Magnetic resonance imaging, 1120
Differential diagnosis, 1120
  Normal variants, 1120
  Extrapancreatic masses, 1121
  Carcinoma versus pancreatitis, 1121
  Other pancreatic tumors, 1121
Endoscopic retrograde cholangiopancreatography, 1122
Percutaneous transhepatic cholangiography, 1123
Angiography, 1123
Gastrointestinal examinations, 1124
Percutaneous biopsy, 1125

58 Endosonography in the Diagnosis and Staging of Pancreatic Cancer, 1127

Kenjiro Yasuda, Masatugu Nakajima, and Keiichi Kawai

Demonstration of the whole pancreas by endoscopic
  ultrasonography, 1127
Detectability of pancreatic tumors by endoscopic
  ultrasonography, 1127
Differentiation of cancer from pancreatitis, 1127
Staging of pancreatic cancer by endoscopic
  ultrasonography, 1129
  Summary, 1130

Role of pancreatic endoscopic ultrasonography, 1131
Summary, 1131

59 Rare Tumors of the Pancreas, 1132

Didier Mathieu, Alain Rahmouni, Serge Agostini, Pierre-Jean Valette, and Pablo R. Ros

Intraductal pancreatic tumors, 1132
  Intraductal papillary neoplasms, 1133
  Intraductal mucin-hypersecreting tumors of the
    pancreatic ducts, 1134
  Ductectatic mucinous cystadenoma and
    cystadenocarcinoma, 1134
  Imaging procedures, 1135
Serous (microcystic) adenomas, 1138
  Pathologic features, 1139
  Imaging procedures, 1141
Mucinous cystic neoplasms, 1141
  Pathologic features, 1144
  Imaging procedures, 1146
Papillary cystic neoplasm, 1149
  Pathologic features, 1150
  Imaging procedures, 1151
Subtypes of ductal adenocarcinoma, 1152
  Mucinous carcinoma, 1152
  Adenosquamous carcinoma, 1152
  Giant cell, or pleomorphic, carcinoma, 1152
  Pancreatic giant cell tumor with osteoclast-type
    cells, 1153
Acinar cell carcinoma, 1153
Acinar cell cystadenocarcinoma, 1155
Sarcomas, 1155
Pancreatoblastoma, 1155
Other rare pancreatic lesions, 1156
  Nontumoral true cysts of the pancreas, 1156
  Adult polycystic kidney disease, 1156
  Von Hippel–Lindau disease, 1156
  Cystic fibrosis, 1157
  Cystic islet cell tumors, 1157
  Pancreatic metastases, 1158
  Primary hydatid disease of the pancreas, 1159
  Cystic teratoma, 1158
  Pancreatic hemangioma, 1158
  Pancreatic lymphangioma, 1160
  Lymphoma, 1162
  Plasmocytoma, 1163

60 Islet Cell Tumors of the Pancreas: Diagnosis and Localization, 1167

Donald L. Miller

Epidemiology, 1167
Pancreatic islet, 1167
Pathology, 1167
Multiple endocrine neoplasia, 1168
Clinical syndromes and diagnosis, 1169
  Insulinoma, 1169
  Gastrinoma, 1170
  Glucagonoma, 1171
  VIPoma, 1171
  Somatostatinoma, 1171
  Other functioning tumors, 1172
  Nonfunctioning tumors, 1172
Localization, 1173
  When is localization required?, 1173
  Specific localization procedures, 1173
  How should localization be done?, 1191

61 Pancreatic Transplant Imaging, 1197

William T.C. Yuh, Donald R. Hawes,
Monzer M. Abu-Yousef, Michael M. Abecassis,
and Edmund A. Franken, Jr.

Complications—etiology and clinical and pathologic
findings, 1197
Parenchymal abnormalities, 1197
Vascular abnormalities, 1198
Abnormal fluid collections, 1198
Radiologic diagnosis of complications, 1198
Imaging techniques and normal imaging
findings, 1199
Imaging of complications, 1206

PART X   BILIARY TRACT

**62 Anatomy and Techniques of Examination of
Biliary Tract and Gallbladder (Oral
Cholecystography, Computed Tomography,
Cholescintigraphy, Magnetic Resonance
Imaging, and Cholangiography),** 1223

Robert K. Zeman

Normal biliary anatomy, 1223
Intrahepatic ductal anatomy, 1223
Porta hepatis, 1224
The distal extrahepatic bile duct and the
gallbladder, 1225
Technical considerations in biliary imaging, 1227
Oral cholecystography, 1227
Computed tomography, 1230
Cholescintigraphy, 1233
Magnetic resonance imaging, 1235
Percutaneous transhepatic cholangiography, 1236
Endoscopic retrograde cholangiopancreatography, 1240

63 Gallbladder Sonography, 1246

Peter L. Cooperberg

Preparation, 1246
Equipment, 1246
Examination, 1246

**64 Embryology, Normal Variation, and Congenital
Anomalies of the Gallbladder and Biliary
Tract,** 1251

Scott J. Schulte

Embryology, 1251
Gallbladder, 1251
Gallbladder number, 1251
Gallbladder position, 1254
Gallbladder shape, 1255
Bile ducts, 1256
Intrahepatic and hepatic ducts, 1256
Anomalous bile ducts, 1256
Common hepatic and common bile ducts, 1258
Cystic duct, 1259
Site of the major papilla, 1262
Pancreaticobiliary duct union, 1262
Choledochal cyst, 1263
Choledochocele, 1268
Caroli's disease, 1270
Bile duct duplications, 1271

**65 Inflammatory and Nonneoplastic Diseases of
the Gallbladder,** 1275

R. Brooke Jeffrey, Jr.

Acute cholecystitis, 1275
Clinical features, 1275
Pathophysiology of acute calculous cholecystitis, 1275
Imaging studies, 1275
Imaging findings for uncomplicated cases, 1276
Acute acalculous cholecystitis, 1279
Complications, 1281

66 Nonneoplastic Diseases of the Bile Ducts, 1294

Richard L. Baron and William L. Campbell

Choledocholithiasis, 1294
Cholangiography, 1294
Ultrasound, 1296
Computed tomography (CT), 1298
Magnetic resonance imaging (MRI), 1300
Overview of imaging approach, 1300
Recurrent pyogenic cholangitis, 1302
Bacterial cholangitis, 1303
Plain radiography, 1304
Cholangiography, 1304
CT and ultrasound, 1305
Nuclear medicine, 1306
Primary sclerosing cholangitis, 1306
Cholangiography, 1307
CT and ultrasound, 1308
Other cholangitides, 1310
Acquired immunodeficiency syndrome, 1310
Chemotherapy-induced, 1311
Rare infections, 1311
Rare cholangitides, 1312
Parasitic diseases, 1312
Benign strictures, 1314
Posttraumatic strictures, 1314
Postinflammatory strictures, 1315
Bile duct fistulas, 1316
Liver diseases affecting the biliary tract, 1318
Other miscellaneous conditions, 1318
Ampullary stenosis, 1318
Hepatic hilar cysts, 1319
Other conditions, 1319

**67 Neoplastic Diseases of the Gallbladder and
Biliary Tract,** 1325

Robert S. Perret, M. Kristin Thorsen, and
Thomas L. Lawson

Gallbladder carcinoma, 1325
Pathogenesis, 1325
Presentation, 1325
Pathology, 1325
Mode of spread, 1326
Staging, 1327
Diagnostic imaging, 1327
Prognosis and treatment, 1333
Cholangiocarcinoma, 1333
History, 1333
Pathology, 1333
Location, 1334
Presentation, 1334
Diagnostic imaging, 1334
Differential diagnosis, 1336
Management, 1340

68 Endoscopic Intervention in Calculus Disease, 1344

Joseph W.C. Leung and Peter B. Cotton

Diagnostic ERCP, 1344
Endoscopic management of duct stones, 1345
  Technique, 1345
  Success rates and complications, 1346
  Indications, 1347
  Technical difficulties of sphincterotomy and stone
    extraction, 1348
Choledochoscopy, 1350
Endoscopic management of gallbladder stones, 1351

69 Interventional Techniques in the Gallbladder and Biliary Tract: Extracorporeal Shock Wave Lithotripsy, 1355

Dermot E. Malone and Joseph T. Ferrucci

Physical principles, 1355
Treatment of gallbladder stones, 1355
  Patient selection, 1355
  Results, 1359
  Contraindications, 1359
  Oral bile acids, 1359
  Preliminary investigations, 1359
  Procedure, 1359
  Symptoms and complications after biliary
    lithotripsy, 1360
  Follow-up, 1360
  Long-term risks of gallbladder conservation, 1360
  Biliary lithotripsy and transcatheter stone
    dissolution, 1361
  Summary, 1361
Treatment of bile duct stones, 1361
  Patient selection, 1361
  Results, 1361
  Contraindications, 1364
  Preliminary investigations, 1364
  Procedure, 1364
  Follow-up and repeat sessions, 1364
  Complications, 1364
Summary, 1364
Postmortem, 1365

70 Percutaneous Intervention in Benign Disease of the Gallbladder and Biliary Ducts, 1367

Giles Boland, Steven L. Dawson, Michael J. Lee,
Peter R. Mueller, and H. Joachim Burhenne

Bile ducts, 1367
  Biliary duct stone disease, 1367
  Percutaneous choledocholithotomy, 1367
  Shock wave lithotripsy, 1373
  Transcholecystic extraction, 1373
Combined radiologic and surgical techniques, 1374
  Minicholecystostomy, 1374
  Percutaneous cholecystolithotomy, 1375
  Dissolution of common bile duct stones, 1375
  Fragmentation, 1375
Gallbladder, 1375
  Gallbladder stones, 1375
  Percutaneous cholecystolithotomy: large tract, 1376
  Percutaneous cholecystolithotomy: small tract, 1378
  Percutaneous dissolution, 1378
Interventional procedures for acute cholecystitis, 1380

Fine-needle aspiration, 1380
Percutaneous cholecystostomy, 1381
Pericholecystic abscess drainage, 1381
Gallbladder biopsy, 1382
Gallbladder and cystic duct ablation, 1382
Percutaneous balloon dilation of benign biliary
  strictures, 1383
  Patient selection, 1383
  Imaging, 1383
  Technique, 1385
  Access, 1386
  Analgesia, 1386
  Antibiotic coverage, 1386
  Number of dilations, 1386
  Role of stenting, 1389
  Results, 1390
  Metallic stents, 1396
  Morbidity and mortality, 1396

71 Percutaneous Intervention in Malignant Biliary Tract Disease, 1399

J. Stephen Fache

Indications, 1399
Contraindications, 1400
Technique, 1400
  General considerations, 1400
  Equipment, 1401
  Anesthetic and analgesic administration, 1401
  Technical approach: right and left biliary duct
    entry, 1401
  Predrainage cholangiography, 1403
  Catheter insertion, 1405
  Catheter selection, 1407
  Combined transhepatic-endoscopic approach
    (rendezvous procedure), 1411
  Alternate access routes, 1414
Management of the catheter and patient after
  drainage, 1417
Complications of biliary drainage, 1418
Results of biliary drainage, 1420

72 Percutaneous Endoscopy of the Biliary Tract, 1423

Chia-Sing Ho and Eugene Y. Yeung

Endoscopes, 1423
Technique, 1424
Indications, 1425
  Stones in the biliary tract, 1425
  Bile duct obstruction, 1426
  Percutaneous biliary interventions, 1426
Results and complications, 1426
  Gallstones, 1426
  Common bile duct and intrahepatic stones, 1427
Conclusion, 1429

73 Endoscopic Intervention in Biliary Duct Neoplasm, 1430

Kees Huibregtse and S. Rivera-MacMurray

Techniques, 1430
  Stent exchange, 1431
  Rendezvous procedure, 1431
Indications for biliary stent placement, 1432
  Preoperative biliary drainage, 1432
  Palliative biliary drainage, 1432

Complications, 1434
    Early, 1434
    Late, 1436
Metallic expanding stents, 1436
Comparison of endoscopic stents to other palliative
    treatment modalities, 1437
    Percutaneous versus endoscopic stent placement,
    Surgical bypass versus endoscopic stent, 1437
Conclusion, 1438

PART XI   LIVER

74   Normal Segmental Anatomy of the Liver, 1440
    Rendon C. Nelson

Historical background, 1440
Segmental anatomy of the liver, 1440
    Segment I, 1441
    Segment II, 1441
    Segment III, 1442
    Segment IV, 1442
    Segment V, 1442
    Segment VI, 1444
    Segment VII, 1444
    Segment VII, 1444
Portal veins, 1444
Hepatic veins, 1444
Hepatic arteries and bile ducts, 1446
Diagnostic imaging and segmental anatomy, 1446
    Dynamic computed tomography, 1446
    Delayed computed tomography, 1447
    Computed tomography during arterial
        portography, 1447
    Three-dimensional computed tomography during
        arterial portography, 1448
    Ultrasound, 1449
    Magnetic resonance imaging, 1449
Surgical implications of segmental anatomy, 1451

75   Hepatic Computed Tomography, 1453
    Patrick C. Freeny

CT scanner technology, 1453
    Rotating gantry scanners, 1453
    Spiral scanners, 1453
    Electron-beam scanners (ultrafast CT), 1453
Contrast administration, 1453
    Noncontrast CT, 1453
    Incremental dynamic bolus CT, 1455
    Delayed iodine scan, 1458
    CT angiography and CT portography, 1459
Applications of IDBCT, DIS, and CT-A/CT-AP, 1463
    Abdominal survey, 1463
    Liver survey, 1463
    Lesion detection, 1464
Conclusions, 1464

76   Hepatic Ultrasound, 1466
    Thomas C. Winter III and Faye C. Laing

Technical considerations, 1466
Anatomic considerations, 1468
Diffuse parenchymal disease, 1469
Hepatic vascular system, 1469
Focal hepatic lesions, 1473
    General concepts, 1473
    Cysts, 1474

Abscesses, 1475
Trauma, 1475
Primary benign hepatic neoplasms, 1476
Primary malignant hepatic lesions, 1477
Metastases to the liver, 1478
Rare focal liver lesions, 1480
Doppler analysis of focal hepatic lesions, 1480
Intraoperative sonography, 1481

77   Hepatic Magnetic Resonance Imaging, 1486
    Guy Marchal

General aspects, 1486
Technical considerations, 1486
    Imaging strategies, 1487
    Spatial resolution, 1487
    Contract-to-noise ratio, 1487
    Motion-induced artifacts, 1487
    Techniques to reduce motion artifacts, 1487
    Influence of magnetic field, 1489
Tissue characterization, 1490
    Focal liver lesions, 1491
    Diffuse liver disease, 1496
Contrast-enhanced MRI, 1496
Vascular imaging, 1503

78   Liver and Spleen Scintigraphy, 1508
    William C. Vezina

Technetium 99m sulfur colloid, 1508
    Imaging, 1508
    Primary tumor, 1508
    Secondary tumor, 1514
    Nontumor, 1514
Tc 99m–IDA hepatic parenchymal imaging, 1522
    Primary tumor, 1523
    Nontumor, 1523
Tc 99m–red blood cell imaging, 1527
    Hemangioma, 1527
Tc 99m heat-damaged RBC, 1528
Indium 111/Tc 99m WBC, 1529
    Indium 111–white blood cell imaging, 1529
    Tc 99m WBC, 1531
Ga 67, 1531
    Hepatocellular carcinoma (hepatoma), 1531
    Abscess, 1531
Miscellaneous, 1531
    Tc 99m microspheres, 1531
    Tc 99m phosphate, 1531
    Xe 133, 1531
    Indium 111 platelets, 1532

79   Hepatic Cirrhosis, 1534
    Yugi Itai and Yoshihisa Kurosaki

General considerations, 1534
Classifications of cirrhosis, 1534
Clinical aspects of cirrhosis, 1534
Diagnosis of cirrhosis, 1534
    Imaging diagnosis, 1535
    Cirrhotic findings on individual modalities, 1537

80   Fatty Infiltration, 1547
    Kuni Ohtomo

Pathophysiology, 1547
    Classification, 1547

Kwashiorkor, 1547
Prolonged parenteral nutrition, 1548
Alcoholic liver diseases, 1548
Acute fatty liver of pregnancy, 1549
Reye's syndrome, 1549
Radiology of the fatty liver, 1549
Radiologic classification of the fatty liver, 1549
Fatty infiltration in hepatitis and cirrhosis, 1553
Differential diagnosis of focal fatty infiltration from
hepatic masses, 1553
Round fatty infiltration, 1554
Focally spared liver, 1554
Pitfalls in the evaluation of fatty liver, 1556

81 Hemochromatosis, 1560

Brigid M. Gerety

Classification, 1560
Primary hemochromatosis, 1560
Secondary hemochromatosis, 1560
Parenteral iron overload, 1560
Clinical presentation, 1561
Hepatic complications, 1561
Diagnosis, 1561
Serologic tests, 1561
HLA typing, 1562
Liver biopsy, 1562
Noninvasive evaluation of the liver, 1562
Single-energy computed tomography, 1563
Dual-energy computed tomography, 1563
Magnetic resonance imaging, 1563
Superconducting quantum-interference device, 1564
Treatment, 1564

82 Portal Venous System, 1566

Patrick C. Freeny and Yugi Itai

Portal venous system anatomy, 1566
Portal venography, 1566
Splenoportography, 1566
Transhepatic portography, 1566
Transjugular portography, 1567
Arterial portography, 1567
Umbilical portography, 1572
Portal hypertension, 1572
Hyperkinetic portal hypertension, 1572
Increased portal venous resistance, 1574
Radiologic evaluation of intrahepatic portal
hypertension, 1574
Preoperative and postoperative portosystemic shunt
evaluation, 1584
Extrahepatic portal hypertension, 1591
Prehepatic, 1592
Direct tumor invasion of the portal vein, 1592
Pancreatitis and pancreatic carcinoma, 1593
Splenic vein obstruction, 1593
Radiologic evaluation of prehepatic portal
hypertension, 1594
Sonography, computed tomography, and magnetic
resonance imaging, 1594
Angiography and venography, 1596
Gastrointestinal tract: mesenteric venous
diseases, 1596

83 Vascular Diseases of the Liver, 1604

Kyung J. Cho

Technical considerations, 1604
Equipment and radiographic technique, 1604
Contrast medium, 1604
Catheterization technique, 1604
Contraindications to angiography, 1605
Complications, 1605
Angiographic technique, 1605
Arteriography, 1606
Arterial portography, 1606
Hepatic vein catheterization, 1607
Portal vein catheterization, 1608
Vascular anatomy, 1608
Hepatic artery, 1608
Portal vein, 1610
Hepatic veins, 1610
Hepatic sinusoids, 1611
Hepatic physiology and circulation, 1611
Diseases of the hepatic artery, 1611
Hepatic artery spasm and dissection, 1611
Arteriosclerosis, 1615
Hepatic artery aneurysm, 1615
Arteritis, 1616
Hepatic infarction, 1616
Arteriovenous fistulas, 1617
Hereditary hemorrhagic telangiectasia, 1618
Peliosis hepatis, 1618
Hepatic sinusoidal and arterial changes in
cirrhosis, 1619
Diseases of the portal vein, 1619
Congenital anomalies of the portal vein, 1622
Portal vein thrombosis, 1622
Neoplastic portal venous occlusion, 1623
Portal vein aneurysm, 1623
Intrahepatic portohepatic venous shunt, 1625
Diseases of the hepatic veins, 1625
Hepatic vein obstruction (Budd-Chiari
syndrome), 1626
Intrahepatic vascular changes in cirrhosis, 1628
Transcatheter therapy, 1628

**84 Benign Tumors of the Liver: Hepatic
Hemangiomas,** 1630

Bernard A. Birnbaum

Imaging features of cavernous hemangiomas, 1630
Plain film findings, 1630
Ultrasound, 1631
Computed tomography, 1632
Magnetic resonance imaging, 1635
Red blood cell scintigraphy, 1639
Angiography, 1640
Role of percutaneous biopsy, 1642
Approach to imaging of suspected hemangiomas, 1642

**85 Benign Tumors of the Liver: Hepatocellular
Adenoma, Focal Nodular Hyperplasia, and
Others,** 1645

Ernst Rummeny, Sanjay Saini, and Carolyn C. Compton

Hepatocellular adenoma, 1645
Clinical background, 1645
Pathology, 1645
Radiology, 1645
Conclusion, 1649
Focal nodular hyperplasia, 1651
Clinical background, 1651
Pathology, 1651

Radiology, 1651
Conclusion, 1654
Macroregenerative nodule and nodular regenerative
    hyperplasia, 1655
    Clinical background, 1655
    Pathology, 1655
    Radiology, 1656
Hepatic cysts, 1656
    Clinical background and pathology, 1656
    Radiology, 1657
    Conclusion, 1658
Polycystic liver disease, 1658
    Clinical background and pathology, 1658
    Radiology, 1658
Mesenchymal tumors and heterotopic rests, 1658
    Clinical background and pathology, 1658
    Radiology, 1659

**86   Primary Malignant Neoplasms of the
      Liver, 1662**
David H. Stephens and C. Daniel Johnson

Hepatocellular carcinoma, 1662
    Epidemiology, 1662
    Risk factors, 1662
    Clinical presentation, 1663
    Morbid anatomy, 1665
    Radiologic imaging: rationale and general
        considerations, 1666
    Ultrasonography, 1667
    Computed tomography, 1669
    Magnetic resonance imaging, 1674
    Differential diagnosis, 1676
    Angiography, 1677
    Combined CT and angiography, 1678
Fibrolamellar carcinoma, 1678
Sclerosing hepatic carcinoma, 1680
Intrahepatic cholangiocarcinoma, 1680
Biliary cystadenocarcinoma, 1681
Epithelioid hemangioendothelioma, 1682
Angiosarcoma, 1684
Other sarcomas, 1684
Lymphoma, 1684

**87   Hepatocellular Carcinoma: Japanese
      Experience, 1688**
Osamu Matsui and Yugi Itai

Imaging methods for detection and diagnosis of small
    HCCs, 1688
Screening for small (early stage) HCCs, 1688
Histologic aspects of various types of hepatic nodular
    lesions associated with liver cirrhosis, 1692
Imaging findings and differential diagnosis of classical
    small HCCs, 1692
    Ultrasound, 1692
    Computed tomography, 1692
    Magnetic resonance, 1692
    Angiography, 1692
Imaging findings and differential diagnosis of classical
    HCCs with atypical histologic features, 1698
    Fatty metamorphosis, 1698
    Necrosis, 1700
Differential diagnosis of various types of hepatic nodular
    lesions associated with liver cirrhosis, 1701
Interventional radiology for the treatment of small
    HCCs, 1702

88   Hepatic Metastases, 1706
Judith L. Chezmar

Imaging methods used for detection of hepatic
    metastases, 1706
    Computed tomography, 1706
    Magnetic resonance imaging, 1707
    Sonography, 1708
    Scintigraphy, 1708
Tumor-related factors in metastasis detection, 1708
    Histology, 1708
    Size of vascular and interstitial compartments, 1709
    Tumor vascularity, 1710
    Necrosis, 1713
    Calcification, 1714
    Size, 1714
Surgical resection, 1715
    Candidates for resection, 1715
    Radiologic evaluation of the surgical patient, 1715

**89   Radiologically Guided Percutaneous and
      Intraoperative Treatment of Hepatic
      Tumors, 1717**
Gary M. Onik

Percutaneous procedures, 1717
    Transcatheter embolization, 1717
    Ethanol injections, 1718
    Laser heat ablation, 1719
Intraoperative procedures, 1719
    Resection, 1719
    Cryosurgery, 1720
Conclusions, 1721

**90   Transcatheter Embolization of Hepatic
      Neoplasms, 1722**
James E. Jackson and David J. Allison

Vascular anatomy of hepatic tumors, 1722
Hepatic arterial embolization, 1723
    Indications, 1723
    Contraindications, 1724
    Technique, 1724
    Adjuvant therapy, 1728
    Complications, 1729
Portal vein embolization, 1729
    Technique, 1731
Results, 1732
    Hepatocellular carcinoma, 1732
    Carcinoid metastases, 1732
Conclusion, 1732

91   Radiology of Liver Transplantation, 1735
Ellen M. Ward

Pretransplant imaging, 1735
    Duplex ultrasound, 1735
    Computed tomography, 1736
    Cholangiography, 1736
    Angiography, 1736
Hepatic transplant, 1736
Postoperative imaging of the normal liver
    transplant, 1737
    Duplex ultrasound, 1737
    Computed tomography, 1737
    Cholangiography, 1738

Imaging of postoperative complications of liver
 transplantation, 1738
 Biliary complications, 1738
 Biliary obstruction, 1740
 Vascular complications, 1744
 Rejection, 1747
 Abdominal complications, 1747
 Malignancy after transplantation, 1748

PART XII **SPLEEN**

92 **Radiographic Techniques and Normal Anatomy
 of the Spleen,** 1751
 Kedar N. Chintapalli

 Radiographic evaluation of the spleen: techniques, 1751
  Plain radiographs, 1751
  Sonography, 1751
  Radionuclide studies, 1753
  Computed tomography, 1757
  Magnetic resonance imaging, 1757
  Angiography, 1759
 Normal anatomy, 1760
  Gross anatomy, 1760
  Histology, 1760
  Embryology, 1761
 Functions of the spleen, 1762

93 **Diseases of the Spleen,** 1763
 Kedar N. Chintapalli

 Anatomic variants, 1763
  Accessory spleen, 1763
  Splenic lobulation and clefts, 1765
  Splenorenal and splenogonadal fusion, 1765
  Asplenia and polysplenia syndromes, 1766
  Functional asplenia, 1766
  Ectopic spleen, 1769
  Wandering spleen, 1769
 Splenomegaly, 1771
  Hypersplenism, 1772
 Splenic calcifications, 1772
 Focal mass lesions of the spleen, 1774
  Splenic cysts, 1774
  Splenic infarcts, 1776
  Splenic hematoma, 1777
  Splenic infections and abscess, 1780
  Tumors of the spleen, 1780
 Parasplenic abnormalities, 1788
  Splenic vein thrombosis, 1789
 Splenectomy, 1789
 Interventional procedures, 1791
  Splenic artery embolization, 1791

PART XIII **PERITONEUM AND RETROPERITONEUM**

94 **Diseases of the Peritoneum,** 1795
 Dennis M. Balfe

 Anatomy of the peritoneal cavity, 1795
  Embryology, 1795
  Adult anatomy, 1797
 Pathology of the peritoneal cavity, 1801
  Fluid collections, 1801
  Peritonitis, 1802
  Primary tumors, 1803
  Secondary tumors, 1803

95 **Diseases of the Retroperitoneum and
 Mesentery,** 1807
 Dennis M. Balfe

 Retroperitoneal anatomy, 1807
  The laminar retroperitoneum, 1807
  Psoas muscle, 1809
  Posterior pararenal space, 1809
  Perirenal space, 1810
  Anterior pararenal space, 1810
  Great vessel space, 1811
 Specific retroperitoneal pathology, 1812
  Primary neoplasms, 1812
  Metastatic neoplasms, 1815
  Retroperitoneal fibrosis, 1815
  Fluid collections, 1816
  Primary inflammation, 1818
  Vascular conditions, 1819
 Mesenteric anatomy, 1820
 Pathologic conditions of the small bowel
  mesentery, 1822
  Diseases arising in the bowel, 1822
  Diseases of retroperitoneal origin, 1823
  Diseases of peritoneal origin, 1823
  Diseases of systemic origin, 1823
  Diseases primary to the mesenteries, 1824

PART XIV **PEDIATRIC GASTROINTESTINAL
 RADIOLOGY**

96 **Pediatric Pharynx and Esophagus,** 1826
 Marilyn J. Siegel

 Techniques, 1826
 Pharynx, 1826
  Normal anatomy, 1826
  Motility disturbances, 1828
  Congenital anomalies, 1829
  Diverticula and webs, 1831
  Masses, 1832
  Inflammatory lesions, 1834
  Trauma, 1835
 Esophagus, 1836
  Normal anatomy, 1836
  Motility, 1838
  Congenital abnormalities, 1839
  Neoplasms, 1844
  Esophagitis, 1846
  Esophageal varices, 1848
  Trauma, 1850

97 **Pediatric Diaphragm and Esophagogastric
 Junction,** 1853
 David Stringer

 Congenital and developmental anomalies of the
  diaphragm, 1853
  Bochdalek's (pleuroperitoneal) hernia, 1853
  Diaphragmatic eventration, 1856
  Morgagni's (retrosternal) hernia, 1856
  Miscellaneous congenital hernial defects, 1858
  Traumatic hernia, 1858
 Diaphragm paralysis, 1858
 Gastroesophageal reflux and hiatus hernia, 1859
  Imaging and other investigations for hiatus hernia and
   gastroesophageal reflux, 1859
  Gastroesophageal reflux complications, 1861

98   Pediatric Stomach, 1865

David Stringer

Developmental and congenital gastric anomalies, 1865
  Situs, 1865
  Duplication of the stomach, 1865
  Microgastria and agastria, 1865
  Gastric atresia or web, 1865
Acquired outlet obstruction of the stomach, 1866
  Hypertrophic pyloric stenosis, 1868
  Conditions that mimic hypertrophic pyloric
    stenosis, 1869
Acquired abnormalities of the stomach, 1869
  Gastritis, 1869
  Gastric ulcer, 1872
  Gastric neoplasms, 1873
  Miscellaneous disorders of the stomach, 1873

99   Pediatric Small Bowel, 1878

David Stringer

General considerations and normal rotation, 1878
Congenital anomalies, 1878
  Abnormal rotation and fixation of the midgut
    (malrotation and malfixation), 1878
  Duodenal atresia and stenosis, 1884
  Annular pancreas, 1884
  Preduodenal portal vein, 1885
  Jejunal or ileal atresia or stenosis, 1885
  Meconium ileus, 1886
  Omental and mesenteric cysts, 1888
  Omphalomesenteric duct anomalies, 1889
  Anterior abdominal wall defects, 1890
Infection and inflammation, 1891
  Gastroenteritis, 1891
  Meconium peritonitis, 1891
  Idiopathic inflammatory bowel disease, 1892
Small bowel neoplasms, 1894
  Benign tumors, 1894
  Malignant tumors, 1895
Trauma and hemorrhage, 1896
  Trauma, 1896
  Henoch-Schönlein purpura, 1896
Malabsorption and mucosal disease, 1896
  Cystic fibrosis, 1896
  Distal intestinal obstruction syndrome (meconium ileus
    equivalent), 1897
  Shwachman syndrome, 1897
  Celiac disease, 1898
  Intestinal lymphangiectasis, 1898
  Immunoglobulin deficiency syndromes, 1898
  Graft-versus-host disease, 1898
Short gut syndrome, 1898
Intestinal obstruction, 1899
  Intussusception, 1899
Pseudoobstruction, 1902
Miscellaneous disorders, 1903
  Superior mesenteric artery and cast syndromes, 1903
  Duodenal ulcer, 1903
  Dermatomyositis, 1904

100   Pediatric Large Bowel, 1907

David Stringer

Embryology, 1907
Anatomy, 1907
  Normal appearance, 1907
  Lymphoid follicular pattern and lymphoid
    hyperplasia, 1907
Developmental and congenital anomalies, 1909
  Large bowel atresia, 1909
  Anorectal malformations, 1909
Functional motility disorders, 1912
  Abnormal myenteric plexus, 1913
  Normal myenteric plexus, 1915
  Inspissated milk or milk curd syndrome, 1915
Infection and inflammation, 1916
  Neonatal necrotizing enterocolitis, 1916
  Neutropenic colitis (necrotizing enteropathy or
    typhlitis), 1919
  Idiopathic inflammatory bowel disease, 1919
  Appendicitis, 1925
Neoplasms, 1926
  Benign tumors, 1926
  Malignant tumors, 1927
Trauma, 1927
  Miscellaneous disorders, 1930
  Cystic fibrosis, 1930

101   Pediatric Spleen, 1932

Marilyn J. Siegel

Normal anatomy, 1932
Normal variants and congenital anomalies, 1932
  Wandering spleen, 1933
  Accessory spleen, 1933
  Visceroatrial anomalies, 1933
Splenomegaly, 1935
Inflammatory disease, 1936
  Pyogenic abscess, 1936
  Fungal abscess, 1937
  Granulomatous infection, 1937
Neoplasm, 1937
  Benign tumors, 1937
  Malignant tumors, 1937
  Secondary tumors, 1937
  Cysts, 1938
Trauma, 1939
Infarction, 1941

102   Pediatric Pancreas, 1944

Marilyn J. Siegel

Anatomy, 1944
Imaging technique, 1944
Imaging features, 1944
Developmental variants and anomalies, 1946
  Annular pancreas, 1946
  Dorsal pancreas agenesis, 1946
  Ectopic pancreas, 1947
Congenital diseases, 1947
  Cystic fibrosis, 1947
  Shwachman-Diamond syndrome, 1948
  Von Hippel–Lindau disease, 1949
  Nesidioblastosis, 1950
Pancreatitis, 1950
  Acute pancreatitis, 1950
  Chronic pancreatitis, 1952
Neoplasms, 1952
  Endocrine tumors, 1952
  Exocrine tumors, 1954
  Cystic neoplasms, 1954
Trauma, 1054

103 Pediatric Liver and Biliary Tract, 1958

Marilyn J. Siegel

Technique, 1958
Liver, 1958
  Normal anatomy, 1958
  Inflammatory lesions, 1958
Neoplasms, 1961
  Primary malignant neoplasms, 1961
  Fibrolamellar hepatocarcinoma, 1964
  Hepatic metastases, 1964
  Benign neoplasms, 1966
  Diffuse diseases, 1969
  Disorders of hepatic vessels, 1971
  Trauma, 1974
  Other hepatic lesions, 1975
Diseases of the biliary tract, 1975
  Congenital anomalies of the biliary tree, 1976
  Spontaneous perforation of the common bile
    duct, 1977
  Biliary tract obstruction, 1978
Gallbladder, 1980
  Hydrops, 1980
  Inflammatory conditions, 1980
  Cholelithiasis, 1981
  Sludge, 1981
Biliary atresia and neonatal hepatitis, 1981

**PART XV   INTERVENTIONAL ABDOMINAL
RADIOLOGY**

**104 Percutaneous Biopsy of Abdominal
Masses,** 1987

Robert A. Lee, Carl C. Reading, and
J. William Charboneau

Indications and contraindications, 1987
Needle selection, 1987
Patient preparation, 1988
Guidance systems, 1988
  Fluoroscopy, 1989
  Computed tomography, 1989
  Ultrasonography, 1989
Selected biopsy sites, 1991
  Liver, 1991
  Pancreas, 1992
  Adrenal gland and kidney, 1992
  Retroperitoneum and pelvis, 1994
Complications, 1995
Summary, 1996

**105 Percutaneous Abscess Drainage for
Gastrointestinal Diseases,** 1998

Eric vanSonnenberg, Horacio D'Agostino, Giovanna Casola,
and Robert Sanchez

Fundamentals of PAD, 1998
  Imaging for PAD, 1998
  Diagnostic aspiration, 1999
  Technique and materials, 1999
  Follow-up care, 2000
Specific gastrointestinal abscesses, 2001
  Hepatic, 2001
  Pancreatic abscesses and fluid collections, 2002
  Splenic abscess, cysts, and tumors, 2004
  Crohn's abscess, 2005
  Peridiverticular abscess, 2005

  Periappendiceal abscess, 2006
  Enteric tumors, 2007
  Anastomotic leaks, 2007

**106 Percutaneous Fluoroscopically Guided
Gastrostomy,** 2011

Chia-Sing Ho and Eugene Y. Yeung

Historical review, 2011
Indications, 2011
  Nutritional support, 2011
  Decompression of the stomach and small
    intestine, 2011
Contraindications, 2011
Technique, 2012
  Patient preparation and preprocedural
    assessment, 2012
  Choice of puncture site and needle, 2012
  Gastrostomy insertion, 2013
  Placement of the gastrostomy catheter, 2013
  Placement of the transgastric jejunostomy
    catheter, 2013
  Choice of gastrostomy catheter, 2014
Modifications to the technique, 2015
  Aftercare, 2016
Long-term management of gastrostomy catheters, 2016
Results and complications, 2016
Gastrostomy insertion in infants, 2018
Comparison of fluoroscopically guided, surgical, and
  endoscopic gastrostomy, 2018
Conclusion, 2018

PART XVI   ACUTE ABDOMEN

**107 The Acute Abdomen: Plain Films and Contrast
Studies,** 2020

Stuart Field

Radiographic techniques, 2020
  Chest radiographs, 2020
  Abdominal radiographs, 2021
Normal appearances, 2022
Abdominal calcification, 2023
Pneumoperitoneum, 2023
Use of contrast media in suspected perforation, 2026
Pneumoperitoneum without peritonitis, 2026
Conditions simulating a pneumoperitoneum—
  pseudopneumoperitoneum, 2027
Postoperative abdomen, 2028
Intraperitoneal fluid collections—ascites, 2028
Inflammatory conditions, 2029
  Acute appendicitis, 2029
  Acute cholecystitis, 2031
  Mucocele and empyema of the gallbladder, 2032
  Acute bile duct obstruction, 2032
  Emphysematous cholecystitis, 2032
Acute pancreatitis, 2032
  Acute diverticulitis, 2034
  Intraabdominal abscesses, 2035
  Subphrenic and subhepatic abscesses, 2036
  Lesser sac abscess, 2037
  Paracolic abscesses, 2039
  Pelvic abscesses, 2039
  Retroperitoneal abscesses, 2039
Intestinal obstruction, 2042
  Gastric dilation, 2042
  Duodenal obstruction, 2044

The distinction between small and large bowel
   dilatation, 2044
Small bowel obstruction, 2045
Large bowel obstruction, 2057
Postoperative abdomen, 2063
Acute colitis, 2065
   Acute inflammatory colitis, 2965
   Toxic megacolon, 2065
   Pseudomembranous colitis (*Clostridium*
       difficile–associated colitis), 2067
   Amebic colitis, 2067
   Ischemic colitis, 2068
   Intramural gas, 2068
      Cystic pneumatosis (pneumatosis intestinalis), 2068
      Interstitial emphysema, 2069
      Gas-forming infections, 2070
      Emphysematous gastritis, 2070
      Emphysematous cholecystitis, 2070
      Emphysematous enterocolitis, 2070
      Emphysematous cystitis, 2070
   Renal colic, 2070
   Leaking abdominal aortic aneurysm, 2071
   Acute gynecologic disorders, 2073
   Calcification associated with acute abdominal
       conditions, 2073

108 Computed Tomography of the Acute Abdomen, 2076

Emil J. Balthazar and Alec J. Megibow

Technical considerations, 2076
Gastrointestinal perforation and peritonitis, 2077
   Intraperitoneal air, 2077
   Extraperitoneal air, 2078
   Site and etiology of perforation, 2079
   Peritonitis, 2080
   Sealed-off performations, 2080
   Limitations to the CT diagnosis, 2080
   Intraperitoneal abscess, 2081
   Solid organ abscess, 2082
Acute inflammatory gastrointestinal lesions, 2084
   Acute appendicitis, 2084
   Acute diverticulitis, 2085
   Acute necrotizing enteritis and colitis, 2086
   Gangrenous cholecystitis, 2087
Intraabdominal hemorrhage, 2087
Intestinal ischemia and intramural hemorrhage, 2089
Strangulating small bowel obstruction, 2091
Abdominal trauma, 2094

109 The Acute Abdomen of Gastrointestinal Tract Origin: Sonographic Evaluation, 2099

Stephanie R. Wilson

Sonographic approach, 2099
Acute abdomen originating from the hollow
   viscera, 2101
   Extraintestinal manifestations of hollow gut
       disease, 2101
   Acute appendicitis, 2102
   Acute terminal ileitis, 2104
   Acute typhlitis, 2104
   Acute diverticulitis, 2104
   Mechanical bowel obstruction, 2106
   Ischemic bowel, 2108
   Peptic ulcer, 2108

Acute abdomen of biliary origin, 2108
   Acute cholecystitis, 2109
   Biliary colic, 2111
Acute abdomen of pancreatic origin, 2112
   Acute pancreatitis, 2112
Acute abdomen of hepatic origin, 2114
   Acute hepatitis, 2114
   Complications of preexisting liver masses, 2114
Acute abdomen of splenic origin, 2115
   Epidermoid cysts of the spleen, 2115
   Splenic infarction, 2115
   Splenic rupture, 2115
   Splenic torsion, 2115

110 Overview: The Acute Abdomen, 2118

John R. Amberg

The plain films, 2118
Ultrasonography, 2119
Computed tomography, 2119
Other methods, 2119
Conclusion, 2119

PART XVII ABDOMINAL TRAUMA

111 Imaging in Abdominal Trauma, 2120

W. Dennis Foley

Blunt injury: mechanism and pattern of injury, 2120
Intraperitoneal fluid: CT and diagnostic peritoneal
   lavage, 2120
CT: logistics and technique, 2121
CT and patient management, 2122
Liver, 2123
Spleen, 2130
Pancreas, 2133
Duodenum, 2133
Kidney, 2135
Bladder, 2135
Mesentery and bowel, 2138
Vascular injury, 2139
Spinal fracture, 2139
Pelvis, 2140
Penetrating injuries, 2140
Diaphragmatic rupture, 2141
Summary, 2141

112 Arteriography and Therapeutic Embolization in Abdominal Trauma, 2143

George P. Teitelbaum, Michael D. Katz, and Salvatore J.A. Sclafani

Initial evaluation of the polytrauma patient, 2143
Diagnostic arteriography in trauma, 2143
Materials and techniques for transcatheter
   embolization, 2144
Arteriography and interventions in the spleen, 2146
Arteriography and interventions in hepatic vascular
   injuries, 2147
Arteriography and interventions in the renal vascular
   injuries, 2149
Arteriography and interventions in the pelvis, 2150
Miscellaneous injuries, 2153
Conclusion, 2153

MARGULIS AND BURHENNE'S
ALIMENTARY
TRACT RADIOLOGY

PART I

HISTORY

1 *History of Alimentary Tract Radiology*

H. JOACHIM BURHENNE
ALEXANDER R. MARGULIS

. . . The world is ever ready to erect monuments in stone and sculptured bronze for the heros of martial deeds, but the heroes of Roentgenology have their names perpetuated in the minds of students of medical history.

Dr. Preston M. Hickey

The discovery of a new type of radiation by Wilhelm Conrad Roentgen (Fig. 1-1) in 1895 had a profound impact on medicine. Within the first year over 1000 articles related to Roentgen's new rays were published.[1] X rays were to have a revolutionary effect in the investigation and diagnosis of the alimentary tract.

Radiologists studying the history of alimentary tract radiology may be grateful to Dr. Preston M. Hickey for coining the term *roentgenology*. He was the founding editor of the *American Quarterly of Roentgenology* in 1906, which was succeeded in 1913 by the monthly *American Journal of Roentgenology* with Hickey as editor until 1916. The early issues of the journal provide fascinating reading. One of Hickey's contributions was an article titled "The First Decade of Roentgenology."[2]

GASTROINTESTINAL TRACT

Radiologic studies of the gastrointestinal (GI) tract began early in 1986, within months after Roentgen had discovered almost simultaneously both the fluorescent effects of x-rays on a screen coated with crystals and the photographic effect on a sensitive emulsion. The third required element for GI examination, contrast media, was already being investigated. The first stomach examination was published by Becher[3]: "One needs only to introduce into a hollow organ a solution of the metal salt in such an amount that the walls of the organ are somewhat distended." Publications in radiology of the alimentary tract had started. As Rigler and Weiner[4] wrote in 1983: "The writing on the first pages may have been hesitant and irregular, but here

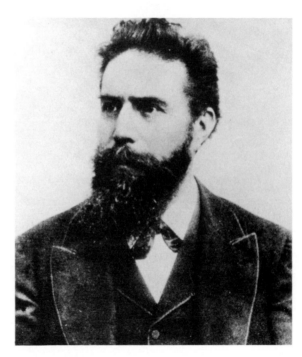

Fig. 1-1 Wilhelm Conrad Roentgen (1845-1923). Roentgen was already a noted physicist when at the age of 50 he discovered x rays. A modest man, he never referred to his discovery as Roentgen rays but always used the prefix *x*, borrowed from the traditional algebraic term for the unknown. In 1901 he received the first Nobel Prize for physics.
From Klickstein HS: *Mallinckrodt classics of radiology,* vol 1, St Louis, 1966, Mallinckrodt Chemical Works.

and there even during these first years can be observed bold strokes that were prophetic of the advances to come."

It is remarkable that the possibilities of roentgenographic diagnosis were so quickly perceived. It would be hard to find anywhere in the annals of medical science so rapid an acceptance of such a revolutionary discovery. In the practice of medicine a new horizon had been discovered. The possibility of visual observation, in the living subject, of structures that heretofore could be seen only in surgery or at autopsy was so attractive that the impulse toward investigation and experimentation was well-nigh irresistible. Confined to the lesser senses of perception, touch, and sound, with the visual senses restricted to limited use in an indirect way, diagnosticians had always labored under great difficulty; their results were not inconsistent with such handicaps, as any comparison of clinical diagnosis with autopsy findings, even during the second decade of this century, will abundantly attest. The opportunity of performing a veritable *autopsia in vivo* must have been dazzling to the physician who appreciated fully the limitations of his own methods and the possibilities of the new procedure. Many were literally searching for light in dark places.

Upper GI study

Radiographic equipment in the first years of the x ray did permit good reproduction of a motionless human hand placed on the x-ray plate (Fig. 1-2), but the exposure of the stomach through the thick portions of the body was quite a different challenge and required about a 30-minute exposure. The GI tract as a moving organ could therefore not be recorded on a photographic plate at that time. Early investigations were done with the fluoroscope. Thomas Edison had noted that Roentgen used barium platinocyanide to detect the presence of x rays. His laboratory tested many different substances for fluorescence, and in March of 1896 Edison announced that he found calcium tungstate to give splendid fluorescence with roentgen rays[5] (Fig. 1-3). Edison and his assistants gave memorable fluoroscopic demonstrations at the Annual Exposition of the National Electric Association held in New York City. This was the first large public exhibition in the United States of the roentgen

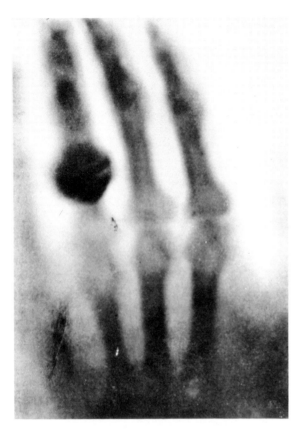

Fig. 1-2 Frau Roentgen's hand. This demonstration of the newly discovered ray's ability to penetrate the human body laid groundwork for future medical applications.
From Klickstein HS: *Mallinckrodt classics of radiology,* vol 1, St Louis, 1966, Mallinckrodt Chemical Works.

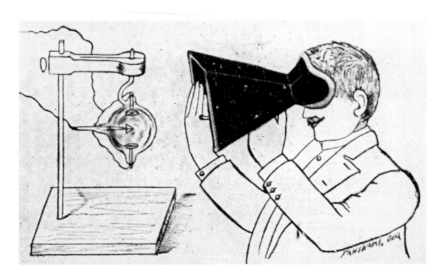

Fig. 1-3 Edison and MacIntyre's fluoroscope, a term coined by Edison.
From Thompson EP: *Röntgen rays and phenomena of the anode and cathode,* New York, 1896, D. van Nostrand.

rays made visible by means of their effect on fluorescent substances. Clarence Dally was an indispensible member of the team of highly trained men that conducted the demonstration. By 1900 it was becoming apparent that skin changes were occurring in Dally's hands and face with increasing severity. Also, at the base of his little finger there was evidence of carcinoma, and his left hand was amputated. All further efforts were in vain, however, and death followed for this first American martyr to science through the roentgen rays in October 1904.[6] Edison immediately discontinued experimenting with x rays when he realized what was happening to his unfortunate assistant.

Fluoroscopy was the examination of choice until the radiographic power source was sufficiently improved and intensifying screens were developed, reducing the exposure times to seconds. The debate over the respective merits of fluoroscopy and radiography for gastrointestinal examination, however, continued until both techniques were perfected and gastrointestinal radiologists agreed that fluoroscopy, spot filming, and overhead radiographs were part of a quality upper gastrointestinal study. In 1903 the group of Viennese radiologists headed by Guido Holzknecht (Fig. 1-4) and other distinguished European radiologists of the time such as Rieder (Fig. 1-5), Albers-Schönberg and Haenisch made numerous presentations dealing with fluoroscopy of the upper GI tract. The radiologist drew diagrams of his fluoroscopic observations. The same group in Vienna had developed a wooden spoon for manipulating the stomach to avoid the dangerous manual manipulation.

In the United States, Pfahler (Fig. 1-6), Hulst, Skinner, Pancoast, and Case were some of the physicians adopting this new speciality. Case (Fig. 1-7) is credited with the first report of the demonstration of a diverticulum. He used an upright fluoroscope. Horizontally arranged fluoroscopes were not manufactured until described by Haenisch in 1910.[7]

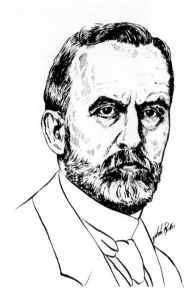

Fig. 1-5 Hermann Rieder (1885-1932). Rieder's rapid serial filming of the GI tract following bismuth ingestion became a popular technique. This preparation for GI tract examination soon became internationally known as the "Rieder meal."

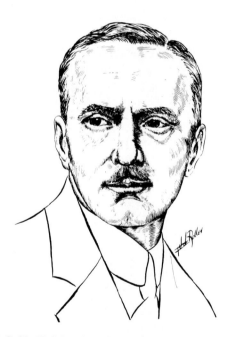

Fig. 1-4 Guido Holzknecht (1872-1931). As a leader of the Vienna school of radiology, Holzknecht was an influential, internationally recognized radiologist and a proponent of fluoroscopy for investigation of the GI tract. He died of complications caused by excessive radiation exposure.

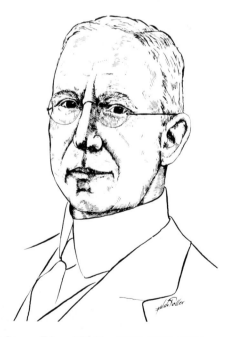

Fig. 1-6 George Edward Pfahler (1874-1957). Pfahler was one of several influential radiologists who practiced in Philadelphia. He received many honors during his career and in 1924 became the first president of the American College of Radiology.

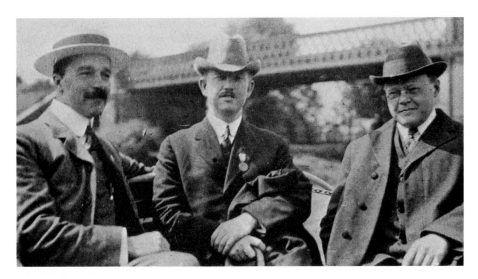

Fig. 1-7 A group of unusually distinguished radiologists, shown in 1913. On the left is Dr. A.E. Barclay of England, whose book on gastrointestinal radiology was one of the first in the English language. In the center is Dr. James T. Case, whose work is commented on extensively in the text, and on the right is Dr. Henry K. Pancoast of Philadelphia, who was likewise one of the pioneers in gastrointestinal radiology.
Courtesy Dr. Ross Golden.

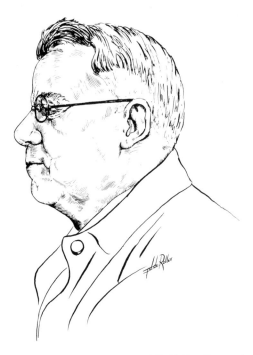

Fig. 1-8 Walter Bradford Cannon (1871-1945). Cannon initiated his x-ray investigation of the GI tract while a Harvard medical student. His early use of bismuth as a contrast agent paved the way for future developments in the field. His interest was soon drawn to physiology of the GI tract, then the adrenal gland. Cannon became best known for his subsequent work in endocrinology.

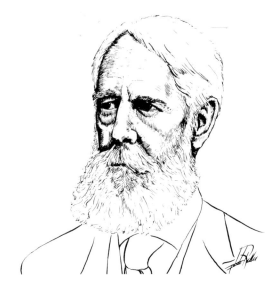

Fig. 1-9 Francis Henry Williams (1852-1936). Williams was one of the first to use the new x rays in a variety of clinical situations. His textbook, *The Roentgen Rays in Medicine and Surgery,* published in 1901, provided a lengthy and thorough discussion of x-ray technique and diagnostic findings. A small portion of the book concerns GI tract problems.

With the availability of radiography and fluoroscopy, the need was now apparent for a method of making hollow viscera visible on film and screen. Many radiologists must have had the opportunity to discover accidentally the value of bismuth as a contrast medium, since bismuth was used at that time as a gastric ulcer remedy.[8] At about the same time, in April of 1897, Rumpel[9] used a 5% suspension of bismuth subnitrate to observe a dilated esophagus fluoroscopically. Also in April of 1897, the great pioneer, Walter B. Cannon (Fig. 1-8) fed bread soaked in warm water and mixed with bismuth subnitrate to a cat and noted with fascination the series of wavelike contractions known as peristalsis passing along the mucosal coating of the stomach.[8] The results were reported in *Science* in June 1897. Cannon had already reported in December 1896 at the American Physiological Society in Boston his observation of the phenomena of deglutition as exhibited in a goose when swallowing capsules containing bismuth subnitrate.

Cannon and Moser extended their work in 1897, examining a 7-year-old girl with gelatin capsules containing bismuth. Williams (Fig. 1-9) of Harvard Medical School, often called the first radiologist in North America, joined forces with Cannon and Moser. Tracings were made of digestion, outlining the shape and position of the stomach (Fig. 1-10). These drawings were published by Williams in 1903.[10] Leonard in the United States and Holzknecht in Vienna, among others, used bismuth before the turn of the century, but the bismuth meal was popularized by Rieder in Germany. His descriptions of a standard meal with standard positions, timing for fluoroscopic observation, and multiple plates to observe peristalsis were published in 1904 and 1905.[11,12] He also described early observations on follow through into small bowel and colon after ingesting bismuth. Pfahler, Hulst, Crane, Leonard (Fig. 1-11) and Pancoast adopted the Rieder meal and reported in 1908 on its use for studying the physiology and abnormalities of upper GI tract motion. They concluded that x-ray examination of the GI tract was of equal importance to that of the bones and joints. Hulst, in his presidential address to the American Roentgen Ray Society, said: "No gastroenterologist, I dare say, ever looked for the first time at good roentgenographs of the stomach without being profoundly impressed by their diagnostic value, if not positively shocked by the striking inadequacy of the older methods which the pictures served to reveal."[13]

Barium sulfate gradually replaced bismuth as the contrast medium for upper GI studies after 1910. Barium was many times cheaper than bismuth, it was more easily purified, and it did not have the toxic effects occasionally observed with bismuth preparations. It was again Cannon who first suggested barium as a candidate for contrast medium to be used in the GI tract. Credit for the initial use of barium is usually given to European radiologists, but it was Cannon who first tried barium sulfate mixed with food and showed that it "was quite as satisfactory as bismuth subnitrate." He re-

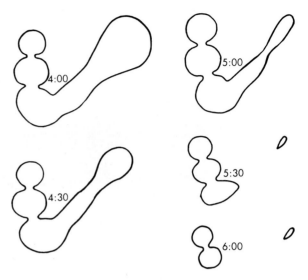

Fig. 1-10 Line drawings of the stomach. This series of drawings is taken from one of Cannon's first papers on the use of x rays to study stomach motion. Outlines of the stomach were traced onto toilet paper applied directly to the fluoroscope.
From Bruwer AJ: *Classic descriptions in diagnostic roentgenology,* Springfield, Ill, 1964, Charles C Thomas.

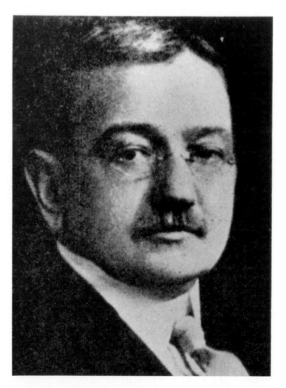

Fig. 1-11 Charles Lester Leonard (1861-1913). Leonard was one of the Philadelphia pioneers in the new field of radiology. He was one of the first to use orally administered bismuth to radiograph the stomach but was even better known for his influence in urologic radiology. He served as President of the American Roentgen Ray Society in 1904 and 1905. He died of complications resulting from excessive exposure to x rays.
From *The American Roentgen Ray Society 1900-1950,* Springfield, Ill, 1950, Charles C Thomas.

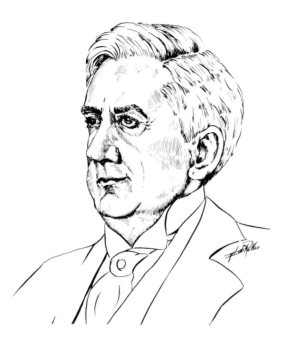

Fig. 1-12 Gösta Forssell, whose work on radiographic anatomy and the coating of the mucous membrane of the gastrointestinal tract contributed fundamentally to x-ray diagnosis.

ported on the virtues of barium sulfate in the *American Journal of Physiology* in 1904, 6 years before it was introduced in Europe.[8] Barium sulfate was mixed with buttermilk in the early 1920s, followed by colloid suspension of barium, and more recently, organic iodines. Gases were added by means of carbonated drinks or the use of chemicals to achieve air-barium contrast examinations.

The requirement for dark-out adaptation for fluoroscopy was first correctly described by Béclère in 1899.[14] Red lights in the fluoroscopic examining room were used to preserve the operator's dark adaptation. Red adaptation goggles were introduced by Trendelenburg in 1916.[15] The next great step forward was to substantially improve the brightness of fluoroscopic screens and to develop image intensification. The industry accomplished these advances in response to brilliant work by Chamberlain in 1942[16] and Morgan in 1956.[17] Image intensifiers coming on the market proved the principles outlined by Chamberlain[8]:

1. The fluoroscopic images were so bright that they could be viewed in an undarkened room without prior dark adaptation—a notable saving in the valuable time of the radiologist.
2. Details could be seen which were invisible using conventional fluoroscopy.
3. The recording of the image on moving picture film or on magnetic tape became feasible. Many earlier systems of cinefluoroscopy, dating back to 1896, had been proposed and even tried, but the inherent dimness of the fluoroscopic screen made them of little value prior to the development of image amplification.

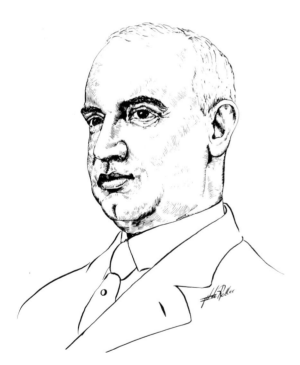

Fig. 1-13 Martin Haudek (1880-1931). Haudek is pictured at an executive committee meeting of the second International Congress of Radiology. He was influential in the Austrian Roentgen Society and is credited as being the first to describe the ulcer niche.

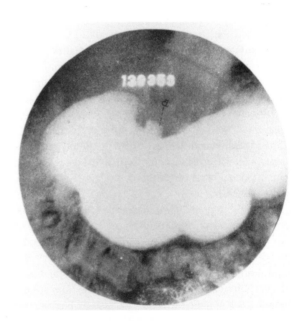

Fig. 1-14 Ulcer niche, a term coined by Haudek.
From Carman RD: *The Roentgen diagnosis of the alimentary canal*, ed 1, Philadelphia, 1917, WB Saunders.

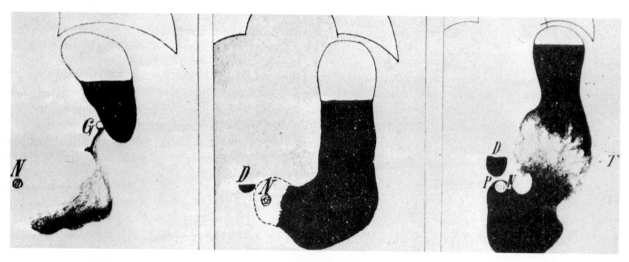

Fig. 1-15 Illustrations from the book by Clairmont and Haudek, published in 1911, with fluoroscopic observations on stomach ulcer and stomach cancer.

4. Stereoscopic fluoroscopy also became feasible.
5. The x-ray exposure of the examining physician was reduced almost to zero.
6. The x-ray dosage to the patient was also notably reduced, making possible types of examination previously impossible.

Forssell in Sweden (Fig. 1-12) developed early in the century fluoroscopic attachments for what he called *focus roentgenograms,* today's *spot films.* His terminology for radiographic anatomy of the stomach is still used today. The first diagnostic advances in the upper GI tract occurred at about the same time when Haudek (Fig. 1-13) in Vienna described the gastric ulcer niche (Fig. 1-14). Radiologists have been using this sign ever since to make a conclusive morphologic diagnosis of gastric ulcer when they saw the niche. Haudek, together with his surgical colleague Clairmont, was already differentiating roentgen signs of benign ulcer disease and malignant ulceration of the stomach[18] (Fig. 1-15). Cole (Fig. 1-16) and Carman[19] (Fig. 1-17) in the United States made great contributions in the diagnosis of gastrointestinal lesions in the 1920s. Carman's book was to have a great influence on the further development of radiology of the alimentary tract. In the fall of 1925 Carman was returning from a trip to Europe and had just been elected president of the American Roentgen Ray Society when he had a gastric upset on his return to the Mayo Clinic. He received a radiologic upper GI study, and when he was shown the radiographs, he made his own diagnosis of "inoperable cancer of the stomach." He died 8 months later in June 1926. Fortunately, Carman had by this time published the second edition of his book, another milestone in alimentary tract radiology with descriptions of the hourglass stomach, the ulcer niche, cancer, duodenal scarring,

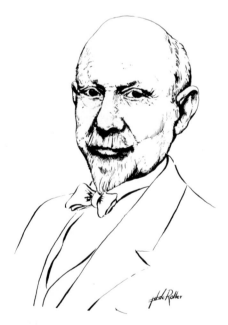

Fig. 1-16 Lewis Gregory Cole (1874-1954). This innovative New York radiologist developed many early radiologic devices, including the golden flame coil (one of the first radiographic and fluoroscopic tables) and the Cole floor push. In 1913 the first Coolidge hot cathode x-ray tube was installed in Cole's private radiology office. He served as president of the American Roentgen Ray Society in 1917.

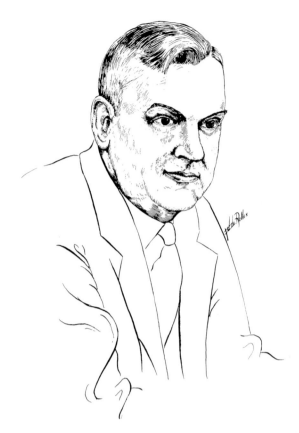

Fig. 1-17 Russell D. Carman of the Mayo Clinic, a pioneer in both the technique of fluoroscopy of the gastrointestinal tract and the diagnosis of its various diseases, and the author in 1917 of the first important American book on this subject.

and characteristic features of major lesions of the upper GI tract. He contributed further signs to the differentiation between benign and malignant stomach involvement. Serial representations of the stomach (Fig. 1-18) constituted Cole's approach to upper GI diagnosis. He was one of the first to delineate the mucous membrane of the stomach.[20]

The limitations of conventional single-contrast examination of the stomach were alleviated by the double-contrast technique. The combination of bismuth and effervescent agents was first used by Holzknecht in 1906. The mixture of ingested air plus barium to demonstrate ulcers was reported by Hampton in 1937.[21] Shirakabe[22] and other Japanese investigators used double-contrast techniques extensively in the 1950s. Improved barium suspensions and effervescent agents are now used routinely for high-quality double-contrast studies of the upper GI tract. It can be combined with pharmacoradiology to produce intestinal atony and distention. Porcher in Hamburg in 1944 used morphine to relax the duodenum. Miller[23] reported on the use of glucagon in 1974, and Simpkins[24] on buscopan in 1976.

Small bowel

The development of roentgenologic examination of the small bowel lagged behind the interest paid to the esopha-

gus, stomach, and colon, no doubt because the small bowel was less accessible to contrast application. The pylorus of the stomach presented a relative obstacle to the outflow of contrast. Carman in the second edition of his textbook *The Roentgen Diagnosis of Diseases of the Alimentary Canal* in 1920 noted that "the small intestine may be studied as a supplement to examination of the stomach. With the patient in the right lateral decubitus position, the duodenum is occasionally more completely filled. Visualization can often be assisted by manual expression of the gastric contents."[25] The shortest chapter in Carman's textbook is the one on the small bowel. He gives credit to Cannon[26] for studying the small intestine in animals, and to Béclère[27] for examining the small bowel in humans. Further work on radiology of the small bowel followed in the next decade by Morse and Cole[28] and Pendergrass.[29] Schwarz[30] in Vienna described small bowel obstruction as early as 1911. Pesquera[31] in New York recommended the use of an intestinal tube for the first time. It would overcome the delay of pyloric emptying and would permit controlled filling of the small intestine. Ten years after Pesquera's publication, Gershon-Cohen and Shay[32] in Philadelphia published use of the same direct examination of the small intestine by intubation, calling it *barium enteroclysis*. It permitted single- and double-contrast examination. Schatzki[33] also used a small intestinal enema in 1943. Trickey and his group[34] modified the small bowel enema by the effect of double contrast with hydroxymethylcellulose and barium instillation.

Enteroclysis is becoming more widely used today, since it permits better visualization of the entire small bowel and interval spot filming of any loop of small bowel suspect for abnormality. The usual small bowel study, however, remains the follow-through after upper GI application of contrast. Ice water or meglumine diatrizoate (Gastrografin) is added for more rapid transit through the small bowel. Golden[35] contributed greatly to our understanding of normal and abnormal physiology of the small bowel and its disease states.

When radiologists learned that barium sulfate caused granulomatous reactions in the peritoneal cavity after leakage through a perforation, water-soluble contrast agents were introduced as agents of choice if leakage from the GI tract was suspected and in cases of stab wounds, sinuses, and fistulas to the peritoneal cavity. Credit for the original work goes to Canada[36] in 1955.

Colon

Schüle[37] is credited with probing the rectum and instilling contrast medium for the first opaque enema in 1904. He used oil suspension of bismuth subnitrate with the patient in the knee-chest position. This examination technique was not practical until the horizontal fluoroscopy table became available. Haenisch[38] (Fig. 1-19) is considered the father of the roentgen examination of the large intestine. Holzknecht[39] and Schwarz[40] also played an important role

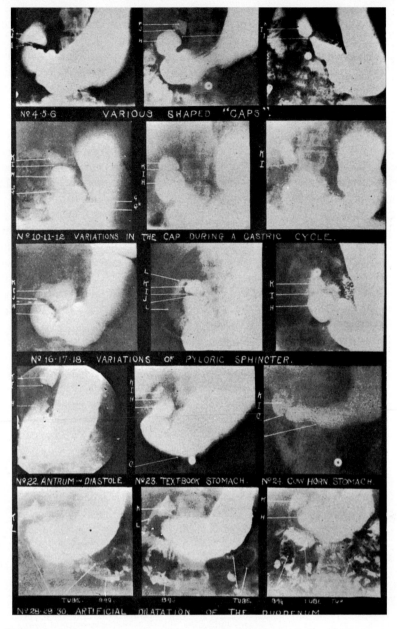

Fig. 1-18 Serialographic representation of the stomach, as presented in Dr. Cole's book, a method of gastric radiography that he practiced as early as 1910.

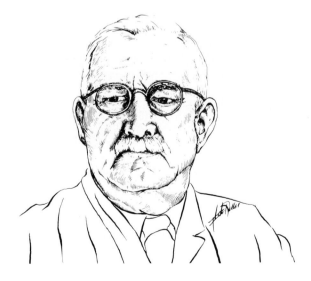

Fig. 1-19 George Fedor Haenisch (1874-1952). Haenisch was an influential German radiologist perhaps best known for developing the fluoroscopic barium enema. In the early 1900s he was made an honorary member of the New York and American Roentgen Ray Societies.
From Bruwer AJ: *Classic descriptions in diagnostic roentgenology,* Springfield, Ill, 1964, Charles C Thomas.

in publicizing the importance of colon examination. Carman[24] used for the "clysma" 250 mg barium sulfate and 500 ml of mucilage of acacia, adding to this the contents of two or three cans of condensed milk to make a total of 2 liters. "The patient, stripped to his hips, lies on his back on the screen-table. The tip of the inflow tube, anointed with Vaseline, is introduced into the rectum. When all is ready, the roomlights are turned out and the spring-clip is released."[24] Haenisch withdrew the enema through the tube at the end of the examination, permitting the patient to "go to a closet and empty the bowel."

Haenisch stressed the importance of the fluoroscopic observation of the opaque material as it filled the colon to detect any interruption in flow. This of course was made possible by the horizontal table equipped with fluoroscopy, which was his invention. Haenisch also stressed the importance of cleansing the colon with cathartics and enemas. Overhead films were obtained after the colon was filled (see Fig. 1-12). Double-contrast examination of the colon presented the next step forward. Although air alone had been considered as a colon contrast early on, it was not practiced until Laurell in Sweden in 1921,[4] and Fischer[41] in Frankfurt in 1923, first performed double-contrast colon ex-

amination. Fischer popularized this method, and it became the state of the art for colon examination. When combined with multiple radiographs in various patient positions, refinements of his technique were contributed by radiologists at the Mayo Clinic and by Welin[42] in Sweden.

Evacuation is an important part of bowel function, and although radiologic studies of the filling phase of the gut are routine, the process of emptying through ostomies and the rectum was not examined until Burhenne described the intestinal evacuation study in 1964.[43] Cinefluorographic recording was used for examining patients with such problems as Hirschsprung's disease and ileostomy dysfunction. Brown and colleagues[44] initiated the term *defecography* for large bowel evacuation examination. The main indications for defecography today are terminal constipation, prolapse, incomplete evacuation, tenesmus, and functional evaluation before and after rectopexy and after anal repair.[45]

GALLBLADDER AND BILIARY SYSTEM

Radiographs of gallstones in situ with the invisible rays of professor Roentgen were published in *Lancet* in 1896.[46] Williams[10] published on the radiology of gallstones in 1903, and the first report on milk of calcium bile appeared

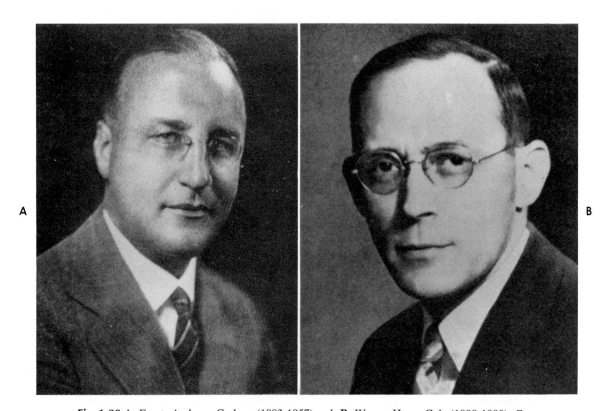

Fig. 1-20 A, Evarts Ambrose Graham (1883-1957) and, **B,** Warren Henry Cole (1898-1990). Graham, a professor of surgery, and Cole, a surgical resident at Washington University in St. Louis, collaborated on the first successful cholecystogram in 1924. Graham was the first chairman of the American Board of Surgery, and Cole served as president of the American College of Surgeons in 1955.
From Bruwer AJ: *Classic descriptions in diagnostic roentgenology,* Springfield, Ill, 1964. Charles C Thomas.

in 1911 by Churchman[47]; but the majority of stones in the gallbladder could not be detected without the help of a contrast medium.

Cholecystography

In 1923 Graham (Fig. 1-20, *A*), a professor of surgery in St. Louis, asked Cole (Fig. 1-20, *B*), a second year resident in surgery, to come to his office to discuss his activities for the following year.[48] Graham was aware that earlier publications had recognized that the tetrachlor derivative of phenolphthalein was excreted in the conjugated form in the bile.[8] The project was to radiograph the gallbladder after intravenous administration of halogenated phenolphthaleins. After injecting as many as 200 dogs and rabbits without obtaining a single gallbladder shadow, they learned that it would require 6 to 10 hours after injection of the solution for the gallbladder to concentrate it. In November 1923 Dr. Cole succeeded in securing a single film on which he could clearly see the dog's gallbladder. Better

gallbladder opacification was obtained in fasting animals. Continued studies resulted in selecting tetrabromophenolphthalein for use in human experimentation. In 1924, news of the successful Graham-Cole test for gallbladder visualization (Fig. 1-21) was published widely and successfully repeated in other countries.[49,50]

The inconvenience of intravenous injection for cholecystography was soon to be remedied. Sosman (Fig. 1-22) in Boston noticed that the gallbladder image disappeared 1 day after intravenous cholecystography but reappeared 3 days later on films done for an upper GI study. He reasoned that some of the contrast expelled from a gallbladder must have been absorbed from the small bowel. Oral administration of iodinated phenolphthalein resulted in successful opacification of the gallbladder in humans[51] (Fig. 1-23). Improved contrast media for cholecystography were introduced since 1925. Today, ultrasonography is more convenient and less expensive for the diagnosis of cholecystolithiasis, but oral cholecystography is still in use in many parts of the world

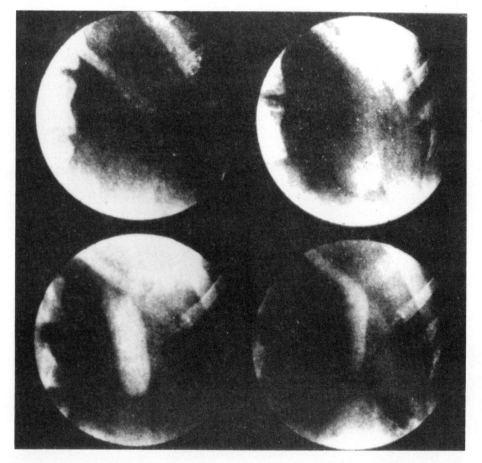

Fig. 1-21 First human cholecystogram. This study, performed on February 21, 1924, demonstrates filling of the gallbladder with tetrabromphenolphthalein. The successful demonstration of a normal gallbladder renewed the efforts by Graham and Cole to pursue cholecystography. Within a short time this study became the standard for diagnosis of gallbladder disease.
From Bruwer AJ: *Classic descriptions in diagnostic roentgenology*, Springfield, Ill, 1964, Charles C Thomas.

Fig. 1-22 Merrill Clary Sosman (1890-1959). In 1925 while working at Peter Bent Brigham Hospital in Boston, Sosman made an observation that led to oral cholecystography. He served as president of the American Roentgen Ray Society in 1940.
From *American Roentgen Ray Society 1900-1950,* Springfield, Ill, 1950, Charles C Thomas.

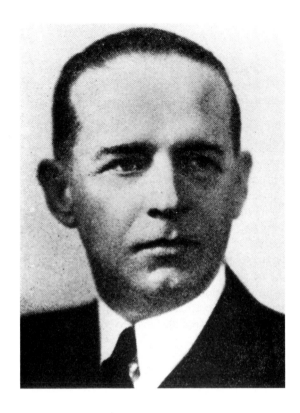

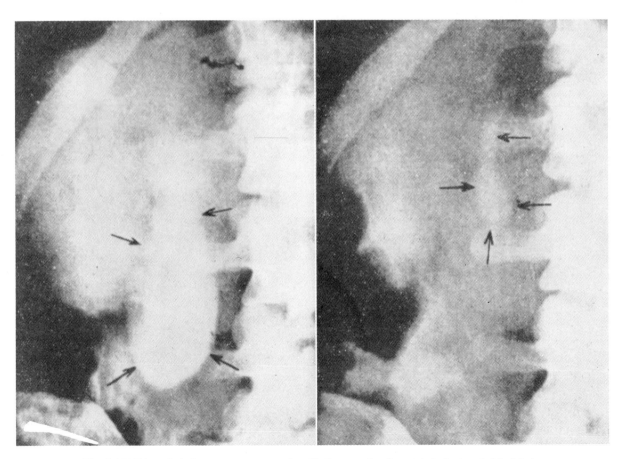

Fig. 1-23 This oral cholecystogram was made with the use of sodium tetraiodophenolphthalein by Whitaker shortly after Sosman observed a contrast-filled gallbladder in a patient 3 days after intravenous cholecystography. In 1925 oral cholecystography became the method of choice for diagnosing diseases of the gallbladder.

where ultrasound is not available or when characterization of gallstones is needed such as in oral systemic chemolitholysis.

The first radiographic demonstration of nonopaque gallstones was actually reported in 1921 by Burckhardt and Muller.[52] They succeeded by percutaneous transhepatic needle puncture injection of a silver-containing contrast agent and air into the gallbladder. Their work also resulted in the first in vivo roentgen demonstration of the bile ducts, the beginning of cholangiography.

Cholangiography

Unintentional cholangiograms resulted from contrast escaping through a fistula into the bile ducts during upper GI study, and intentional cholangiograms resulted from fistula injection. Cotte[53] obtained a high quality cholangiogram by injecting Lipiodol into a fistula (Fig. 1-24). Cotte's anticipated use of operative cholangiography was realized and perfected in 1931 by Mirizzi and Losada of Argentina.[54] Nonoperative percutaneous transhepatic direct cholangiography followed in 1937 by Huard and Do-Xuan-Hop[55] from Indochina. Puncture of the gallbladder and transhepatic cholangiography were the technical precursors of interventional radiology of the biliary tract.

Direct cholangiography is performed today by endoscopic means if no postoperative access to the bile ducts is available. Endoscopic cannulation of the ampulla of Vater was first described in the United States in 1968 by McCune and associates.[56] The clinical applications of retrograde endoscopic cholangiopancreatography were perfected in Japan and Europe. In 1965 Rabinov and Simon, two radiologists in Boston, successfully guided a catheter into the ampulla of Vater for direct cholangiography and pancreatography.[57] Endoscopic retrograde cannulation was technically easier and became the method of choice.

Indirect cholangiography by intravenous means was first reported in 1953 using sodium iodipamide (Biligrafin).[58] It permitted preoperative and postoperative examination of the bile ducts but required added tomography because of low opacification of the bile ducts. Intravenous cholangiography has been replaced today by other imaging techniques after several reports of severe complications. It is still used today in European countries for preoperative investigation for common duct stones if laparoscopic cholecystectomy is scheduled.

Scintigraphy

Biliary scintigraphy was accomplished for many years with rose bengal, providing imaging of the hepatic parenchyma. Bile duct visualization, however, was limited until derivatives of iminodiacetic acid (IDA) were introduced. Harvey et al.[59] demonstrated in 1975 that technetium 99m–HIDA would lead to rapid visualization of liver, bile ducts, gallbladder, and intestine using a serial gamma camera. HIDA and other IDA molecules have none of the undesirable side effects of intravenous cholangiography media, and

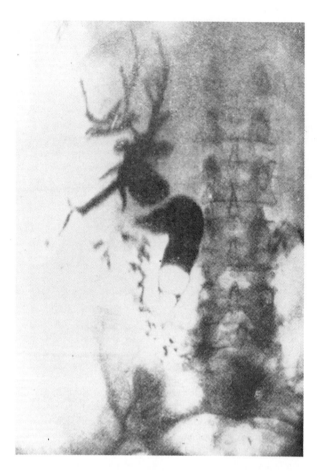

Fig. 1-24 Cholangiogram. Gaston Cotte, a French surgeon, became a biliary specialist early in his career and is credited as the first to suggest the use of intraoperative cholangiography. This radiograph demonstrates two calculi in the distal common bile duct. Contrast material had been injected into a biliary fistula.

radionuclide imaging is today one acceptable method to investigate acute cholecystitis.[60]

LIVER, SPLEEN, AND PANCREAS

Plain film radiography permitted estimation of liver and spleen size, but visualization of the pancreas had to await modern transverse imaging techniques. Early after the turn of the century, Williams and others introduced air into the gut, or performed a pneumoperitoneum, in an attempt to visualize the nonhollow appendages of the alimentary tract.[10,61] Weber[62] in 1913 used oxygen for peritoneography.

One of the substances used in the 1920s for the visualization of solid organs in the abdominal cavity was thorium dioxide. Oki in Japan noticed spleen opacification with this agent in 1929 (Fig. 1-25). Radt[63] in Berlin reported independently in the same year spleen and liver opacification with Thorotrast. Sarcoma of the liver following thorium use was reported in 1947,[64] and subsequent reports of tumors in spleen and bone marrow appeared, leading to the discontinuation of Thorotrast. The image of the pancreas re-

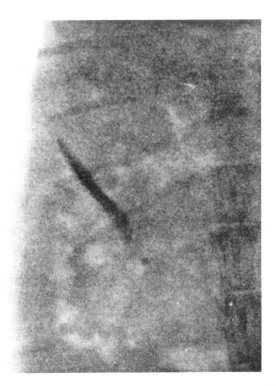

Fig. 1-25 Thorotrast in the spleen. In 1929 Oka of Japan described the accidental imaging of a rabbit's spleen after intravenous injection of thorium dioxide. Subsequently Radt in Germany found that the same agent permitted visualization of the liver as well. The use of this agent to demonstrate these organs continued until the first human neoplasm secondary to thorium was observed in 1947.
From Bruwer AJ: *Classic descriptions in diagnostic roentgenology,* Springfield, Ill, 1964, Charles C Thomas.

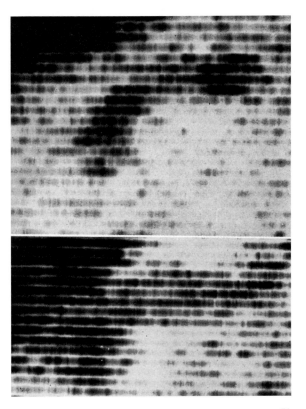

Fig. 1-26 Early pancreas scans by Blau and Bender using ^{75}Se-selenomethionine. The normal organ below the liver is readily recognized in these two patients.
From Blau M, Bender MA: *Radiology* 78:974, 1962.

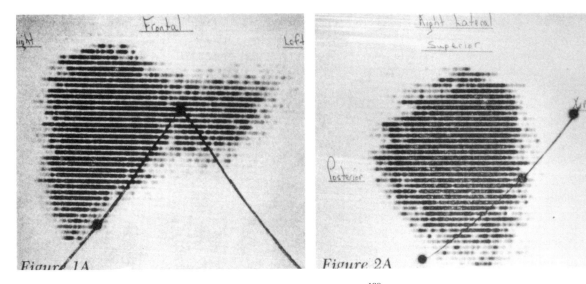

Fig. 1-27 Normal liver scan. This study was performed with ^{198}gold, a commonly used isotope in the 1960s. Better resolution has been achieved with different isotopes and newer imaging cameras.
From Siber FJ: *Radiol Clin North Am* 4:586, 1966.

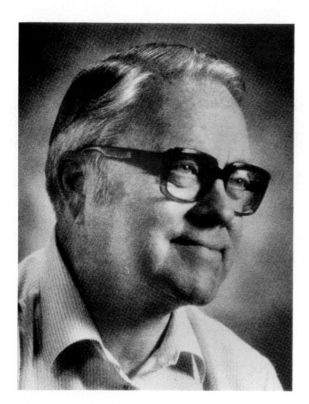

mained elusive until recently (Fig. 1-26). Acute hemorrhagic pancreatitis and chronic pancreatitis with calcification could be diagnosed on plain films, but progress was not made until selective arteriography and radionuclide pancreatography were developed in 1970s. Soon, however, retrograde endoscopic pancreatography became available.

Iodine-labeled rose bengal and radioactive gold permitted radioisotope imaging of the liver (Fig. 1-27).

Seldinger's[65] (Fig. 1-28) ingenious yet simple method for percutaneous catheter insertion in Sweden in 1953 rapidly led to the radiologic subspecialty of selective angiography (Fig. 1-29). The liver, stomach, spleen, and pancreas became accessible. Odman[66] published his monograph on percutaneous selective angiography of the celiac artery in 1958 and Boijsen[67] on selective pancreatic angiography. Many indications for angiography of the solid abdominal organs and the gut developed, and radiologists from many countries travelled to Sweden to acquire expertise in this new subspecialty. Bringing these advances back to their own institutions, radiologists became the specialists to assume the practice of angiography.

Fig. 1-28 Sven-Ivar Seldinger (1921-). Seldinger's initial paper on percutaneous needle placement for arteriography (published in 1953) soon became internationally known.
From *AJR* 142:4, 1984.

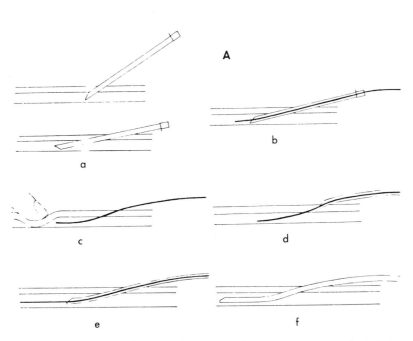

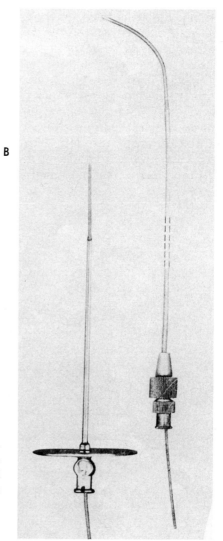

Fig. 1-29 A, Original catheter replacement principle as diagrammed by Seldinger. *a,* Artery is punctured and needle is pushed upward. *b,* Leader is inserted. *c,* Needle is withdrawn and artery is compressed. *d,* Catheter is threaded onto leader. *e,* Catheter is inserted into artery. *f,* Leader is withdrawn. **B,** Original equipment. Stylet is removed and leader is inserted through needle *(left)* and catheter *(right).*
From Seldinger SI: *Acta Radiol* 39:365, 1953.

CROSS-SECTIONAL IMAGING
Ultrasound

Medical ultrasonography owes its origins to sonar—the use of water-transmitted sound waves for the detection of submarines. The effort to develop sonar started during World War I but was not brought to practicality until the mid-1920s and was perfected during World War II.[68]

Ultrasonography was used for diagnostic purposes in industry to detect flaws in materials between the two world wars. The "Reflectoscope," developed by Firestone in 1944 at the University of Michigan, had the same transducer pick up the echoes reflected between the generated pulses and was also used for industrial purposes to detect flaws in metal.[69] As many physicians and engineers were exposed to sonar in the Navy during World War II, the interest to apply this method to medical diagnosis was burgeoning in many countries and, with the improved means of communications, many workers in the field complemented each other's achievements.[68]

Japanese investigators were among the pioneers in the development of ultrasound. At the Nihon Musen Research Laboratories (now Aloka), physicist Rokuro Uchida built Japan's first A-mode ultrasound equipment in 1949. Kikuchi, at the Institute of Radar Science, Tohoku University at Sendai, developed the medical ultrasound scanner for Tanaka and his assistant Wagai of Juntendo University in Tokyo in 1951. Wagai used this instrument to detect cholelithiasis in 1951 and continued to apply ultrasound to various parts of the body. Oka, of Osaka University, started with B-mode scanning in 1954, and a team of investigators led by Satomura and Nimura at the same university pioneered the introduction of Doppler ultrasound to study the cardiovascular system.[70]

Wild, an Englishman who joined the University of Minnesota, discovered the ability of ultrasound to distinguish between cancer and surrounding normal tissue.[71] With engineer Reid, Wild developed the first hand-held contact B-mode scanner, enabling them to make extensive clinical use of this new technique in real time. Howry, working with spare parts in his basement and with the help of physicists and engineers, produced a pulse echo scanner and in 1950 recorded images with a 35-mm camera. His scanner used a large water bath into which the patients had to be immersed.[72] For a very short time, however, inspired by the success of the contact scanners of Wild and Reid and of Donald, two engineers from the Denver team of Howry, Wright, and Meyer, created their own contact scanner and formed a company that manufactured the first commercially available articulated arm hand-held scanner (Fig. 1-30).

A team headed by Donald, at the University of Glasgow, introduced ultrasound into gynecology and obstetrics.[73] This team, displaying a model cooperation between physicians, physicists, and commercial engineers, created the first compound contact scanner in 1957 and continued improving it.[74]

Ultrasonography was applied to abdominal disease from its very clinical beginnings. Ludvig, a young physician in the U.S. Naval Medical Research Institute, investigated the

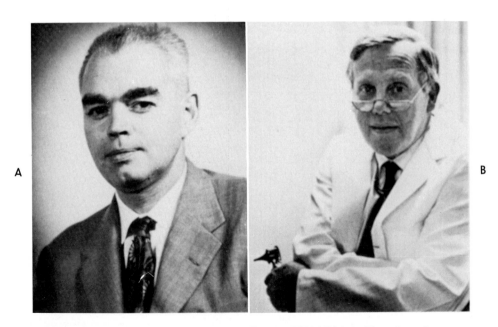

Fig. 1-30 A, Douglass Howry (1920-1969) and, **B,** John Wild (1924-). These investigators were among the earliest ultrasound pioneers. In 1951 Howry developed the technique of compound or sector scanning. Wild used his "echoscope" to conduct experiments demonstrating that ultrasound could distinguish between normal and abnormal tissue.
From King D: *Diagnostic ultrasound,* St Louis, 1974, Mosby–Year Book.

capacity of ultrasound to detect gallstones embedded in tissues in 1949.[71] Transrectal probes, flexible and rigid, were designed and used by Wild in the early 1950s. Howry and his team demonstrated gallstones in an excised gallbladder in 1951.[72,75] In the late 1950s the Denver team led by Holmes produced abdominal ultrasonograms in patients. Although much of the interest of the pioneering teams working in the abdomen was in obstetrics, Donald showed images of liver disease, including cirrhosis.[76] In 1974 Pedersen of the Gentofte Laboratory in Copenhagen, founded by Holm, developed a technique for liver biopsy guided by ultrasound.[77] In the United States several teams advanced ultrasonography—Goldberg at Jefferson,[78] Leopold, first at the University of Pittsburgh and then at the University of California, San Diego,[79] and Asher and Freimanis[80] developed scanning techniques for abdominal organs. Filly and Freimanis[81] reported in 1970 for the first time on the echographic diagnosis of the pancreas (Fig. 1-31).

Doppler ultrasound, first introduced in Japan in the early 1950s by Satomura and Nimura,[82] was further advanced at the University of Washington by Rushmer and Reid. Strandness, a vascular surgeon at the same university, studied waveforms in various vascular conditions.[83] Wells[84] at Bristol developed range-gated Doppler equipment producing pulsed Doppler beams that could be used clinically to separate several moving targets. Color Doppler popularized this approach further and made it clinically very useful particularly in the evaluation of patency of major abdominal vessels and following transplantation of the liver and kidneys.[85-89] Endosonography of the rectum, while a routine procedure in the evaluation of the prostate and the guiding of biopsy, has also been used in the study and staging of cancer of the rectum.

Computed tomography

Cross-sectional tomography was an idea that for many years many laboratories tried to achieve. Takahashi[90] was the first to produce and design a clinically successful axial tomographic machine. The images, however, were blurred. In 1963 and 1964 Cormack,[91,92] a physicist at the Groote Shuur Hospital at Cape Town, South Africa, developed mathematic approaches to compute the radiation dose absorbed by various organs in the radiotherapy field. This led him to the conclusion that multiple x-ray projections of structures had to be obtained at many angles. The mathematic formulas were then tested by Cormack on aluminum and with disks and irregularly shaped phantoms. This was published in the *Journal of Applied Physics* and went virtually unnoticed until unearthed by the Nobel Prize Committee. Many other investigators tried to develop image reconstruction formulas for cross-sectional imaging; Oldendorf[93] developed the formula for radiographic cross-sectional depiction of the brain and published his preliminary results in 1961. Kuhl and Edwards[94] tried to reconstruct cross-sectional images from radionuclide scans. Their techniques, published in 1963, constituted the basic approach on which PET positron-emission tomography (PET) was to be developed.

Modern computed tomography (CT), however, was developed by Hounsfield working for Electronic and Musical Industries Ltd. (EMI) in England. Hounsfield was intrigued by the possibility that "a computer might be able to reconstruct the picture from sets of very accurate measurements taken through the body at a multitude of different angles."[95,96] His original work, with a gamma ray source and using Perspex, produced images; however, it took over 9 days to complete the acquisition of data. Substituting the

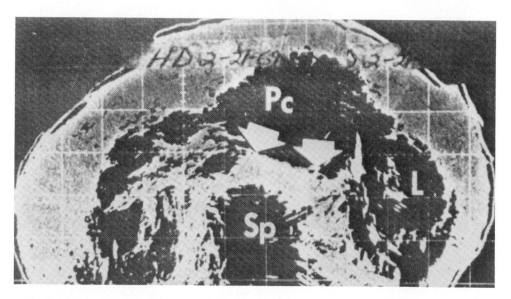

Fig. 1-31 Pancreatic pseudocyst *(Pc)* demonstrated by B-mode scanning. *L,* Liver; *Sp,* cross section of vertebra.
From Filly RA, Freimanis AK: *Radiology* 96:575, 1970.

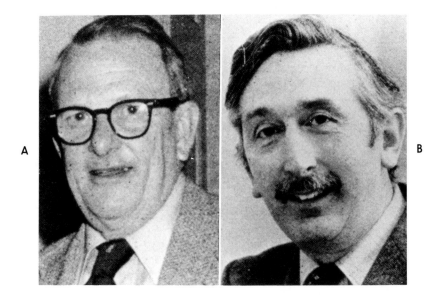

Fig. 1-32 A, Allan MacLeod Cormack (1924-) and, **B,** Godfrey Newbold Hounsfield (1919-). Independent investigations led Cormack and Hounsfield to use computed tomography. Cormack's analyses were published in 1963 and 1964, whereas Hounsfield put CT scanning into practical application in 1972. They shared the 1979 Nobel Prize for medicine for their discoveries. From Montgomery BJ: *JAMA* 242:2380, 1979.

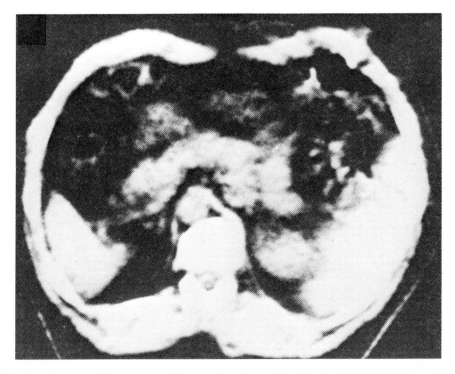

Fig. 1-33 CT scan of the pancreas, demonstrating the quality of early abdominal CT scans. The liver, spleen, and pancreas are fairly well depicted in this 1975 image.

gamma ray source with an x-ray tube, the scan time was reduced to 9 hours and produced better images. Hounsfield then started working on preserved human brain and fresh bull brains and obtained images that had some detail. A prototype scanner was developed in 1969 and 1970, and a clinically applicable machine was installed at the Atkinson-Morely Hospital in the suburbs of London. The first scan, on a woman with a suspected brain tumor, showed a large, cystic lesion in the left frontal lobe. As more patients were scanned by Ambrose, it became obvious that a new revolutionary imaging approach had been born.[97] The first clinical results were presented by Ambrose and Hounsfield in 1972 at the Congress of the British Institute of Radiology. The further obvious success of the approach was due, however, to the rapid advances in small computers, making it possible to develop clinical CT scanners. Since interest for cross-sectional imaging was very intense throughout the United States, Europe, and Japan, it became apparent that such scanners had to be acquired by clinical centers and their uses further developed.[98] The early recognition of the value of this approach was shown by the award of the Lasker Foundation in 1975 to Hounsfield, Kuhl, and Oldendorf. The Nobel Prize in Physiology and Medicine for 1979 was awarded to Cormack and Hounsfield for their discovery of computed tomography (Fig. 1-32).

The instruments for computed tomography, from the very beginning, were in such demand that salesmen for EMI were not taking the time to leave the airport in the cities where institutions that they selected for installation were located, and hospital representatives had to come with cash in hand to conclude the purchase of a scanner to be delivered much later. The original EMI head scanner required long scanning times, but upgrades on newer machines were rapidly introduced, such as the elimination of the water bag to surround the head. In 1974 Ledley,[99] working at Georgetown University in Washington, D.C., constructed and tested a whole body CT scanner. This was soon followed by a total body scanner introduced by Technicare and also EMI. The latter scanner was capable of producing scans in less than 20 seconds and made clinical scanning of the abdomen and chest a reality[100-104] (Fig. 1-33).

Further advances dealt with improvement in spatial resolution by the development of the fan beam and xenon detectors.[105] The original rotate translate machines introduced by Hounsfield were replaced by the rotate machine in which the x-ray tube and the detectors moved rapidly in a circle around the patient.[106] Under a grant by the National Institutes of Health, an instrument with a ring of stationary detectors was developed with only the x-ray tube rotating. Improvement in the units and faster computers allowed scanning to be reduced to 5 and 6 seconds or less, leading to ultrafast scanners in which only electrons shoot out of an electron gun, are focused by magnetic fields, and move and create x rays by scanning rings of tungsten[107] (Fig. 1-34).

The introduction of intravenously administered iodine-

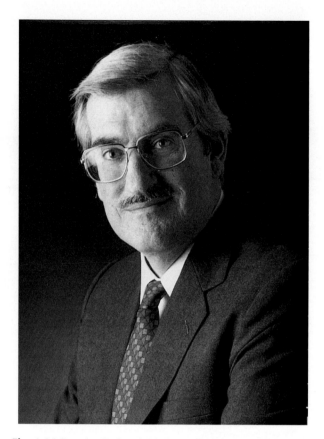

Fig. 1-34 Douglas P. Boyd, Ph.D., co-inventor of the fan beam and xenon detectors for computed tomography. Boyd was also designer and inventor of the ultrafast CT scanner using no rotating parts with scanning performed by electrons.

containing contrast media, ionic, and, later, nonionic and orally administered contrast media, with rapidly improving spatial resolution,[108] have made abdominal computed tomography one of the preferred clinical imaging approaches.

Magnetic resonance

Nuclear magnetic resonance was described almost simultaneously in 1946 by Bloch, then at Stanford University, and Purcell at Harvard University.[109,110] They demonstrated that it is possible to obtain chemical information about the arrangements of atoms in molecules by exposing compounds in static, external magnetic fields to radiofrequency pulses specifically related to the strength of the magnetic field (Fig. 1-35).

Bloch and Purcell received the Nobel Prize for Physics in 1952; Ernst, a professor at the University of Zürich, received the Nobel Prize for Chemistry in 1991 for advancing the field of NMR further and making it the sophisticated, analytic method of today. Until 1973 nuclear magnetic resonance was predominantly used as a sophisticated in vitro chemical test. Biologic applications were first developed by Damadian,[111] who found significant differences in relaxation times, T1 and T2, between normal rat tissue

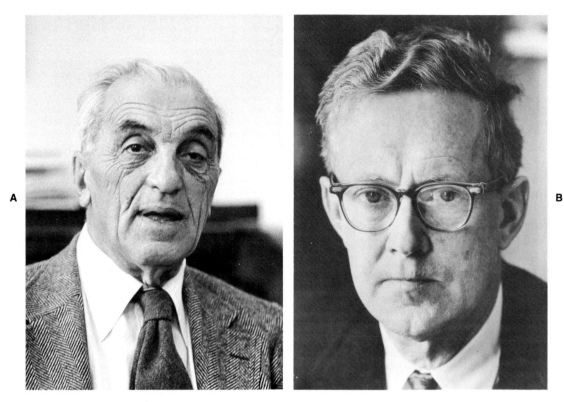

Fig. 1-35 A, Felix Bloch (1905-1983) and, **B,** Edward Purcell (1912-). These two investigators independently discovered nuclear magnetic resonance principles in 1946. They shared the Nobel Prize for physics in 1952.
A courtesy Stanford News Services; **B** courtesy Dr. Purcell.

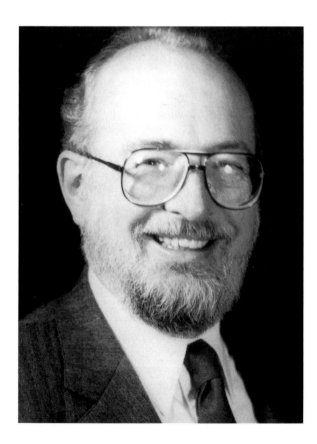

Fig. 1-36 Dr. Paul C. Lautebur. He is considered to be the father of MRI by introducing gradients into the magnetic field, thus permitting localization of emitted frequency signals.

and sarcoma tumors in rats. He published his results in 1971. Nuclear magnetic resonance imaging, however, was developed by Lauterbur,[112] who recognized that the frequency of signals emitted by protons in a static magnetic field depends on the strength of the field, and if magnetic gradients were to be introduced, this could lead to spatial determination of the signals from the known location of the gradients. He published his results with the first magnetic resonance image in 1973 (Fig. 1-36).

In 1977 Damadian performed the first whole body magnetic resonance imaging (MRI) scan.[113] Like a burst of activity following Roentgen's discovery of x rays in 1895, multiple laboratories started working and perfecting MRI. Lauterbur's laboratory at New York State University at Stony Brook and laboratories in Nottingham, Oxford, Aberdeen, London, University of California at San Francisco, the Cleveland Clinic, and Massachusetts General Hospital stood out in this early era. Publications (Fig. 1-37) with images of live animals,[114] human wrist,[115] finger,[116] and later head and body were following each other at a dizzying pace. Rapid advances in reconstructive algorithms, the introduction of spin echo T1- and T2-weighted sequences[117] (Fig. 1-38), cardiac and respiratory gating, gradient recalled echo imaging, and echo planar imaging[118] all advanced the field and made MRI the most versatile and sophisticated imaging approach.

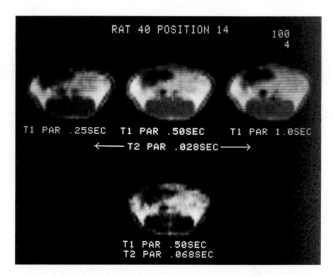

Fig. 1-37 Four images through the abdomen of a live rat obtained in late 1979. Before the nomenclature of TR and TE, T1 par, which was used at that time in the Radiology Imaging Laboratory, is now TR, and T2 par is now TE. The images shown, in effect, were among the early spin echo T1 and T2 images obtained.

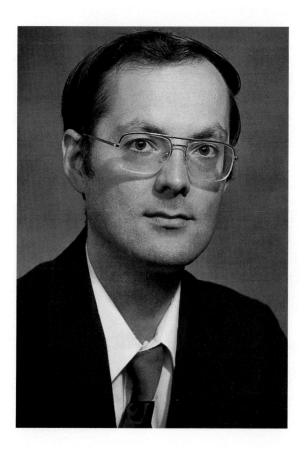

Fig. 1-38 Lawrence E. Crooks, Ph.D., applied the Hahn spin echo sequence to MRI, thus introducing T1 and T2 sequences. He also designed simultaneous acquisition of multiple slices, which made MRI a clinical reality.

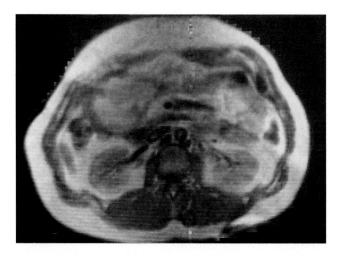

Fig. 1-39 Early spin echo T1 abdominal image obtained in October 1981.

MRI has advantages over other imaging modalities of outstanding soft tissue contrast resolution, direct scanning in any plane (since it depends on multiple physical parameters, and an unlimited number of approaches and sequences that give both morphologic and functional detail. The absence of ionizing radiation made this method rapidly accepted. Abdominal MRI has been relatively slow in coming except for imaging of the liver[119-121] (Figs. 1-39 and 1-40), rectum,[122-124] and esophagus.[125] The absence of a universally accepted oral contrast medium has somewhat delayed the imaging of the esophagus, stomach, duodenum, and rectum. However, although the development of contrast media for the liver has been slow, it shows great promise. MRI, along with CT and ultrasonography, and with the great improvements in endoluminal gut contrast studies and endoscopic advances, have provided great precision and sophistication in imaging of the digestive system.

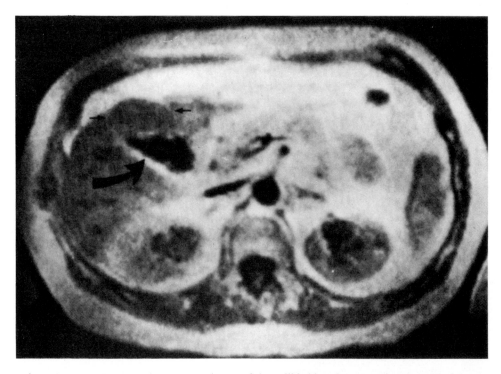

Fig. 1-40 An early magnetic resonance image of the gallbladder, demonstrating the potential use of this modality for imaging intraabdominal structures. Advances have already resulted in improved spatial resolution. MR spectroscopy also holds promise for the diagnosis of intraabdominal disease. *Small arrows,* Bile; *large arrows,* gallstones.
From Hricak H et al: *Radiology* 147:481, 1983.

INTERVENTION

The subspecialty of interventional radiology represents the most active clinical involvement of our specialty. The radiologist participates in patient treatment. Therapeutic extension of diagnostic procedures has occurred in many areas of radiology but started in gastrointestinal radiology when the barium enema diagnosis of intussusception in children was followed by hydrostatic reduction treatment in the 1920s.[126] The term *interventional radiology* was coined by Margulis in 1967.[127] More sophisticated interventional procedures were developed as fluoroscopy and image amplification equipment improved. Interventional radiologic procedures represent an alternative to operative measures but often carry a lower risk and complication rate and can usually be performed without hospital admission. Diagnostic fine needle aspiration biopsy with ultrasound or CT guidance has become a widely practiced technique today and can be followed by an interventional radiologic procedure with percutaneous placement of an abscess drainage catheter without the need for a major surgical procedure.

The introduction of interventional procedures in the intestinal tract includes rapid intestinal intubation in 1968,[128] catheter retrieval of foreign bodies from the gastrointestinal tract in 1971,[129] drainage of enterocutaneous fistulae, placement of percutaneous gastrostomy in 1983,[130] and dilatation of strictures with the use of balloon catheters.[131,132] Even narrow and long strictures that cannot be negotiated by endoscopic means will usually accept a guidewire un-

der fluoroscopic control followed by a dilatation catheter. The same technique is employed for gastroenterostomy or ileostomy strictures.

Intervention of the biliary tract by radiologists started with extraction of retained common duct stones by Burhenne in 1972[133] (Fig. 1-41). He used a steerable catheter for easier instrumentation of the T-tube tract under fluoroscopic control, whereas Bean and Mahorner[134] preferred the use of arterial catheters for basket insertion. Benign strictures of the bile ducts were first dilated with balloon catheters in 1974.[135] Burhenne reported on seven patients with strictures in the intrahepatic and extrahepatic bile ducts and at the hepatojejunostomy anastomosis.[136] This was before the introduction of the balloon-tipped angiographic catheter by Grüntzig and Hopff.[137] Molnar and Stockum[138] first dilated choledochoenterostomy strictures by the transhepatic route in 1978. Ring and colleagues[139] also reported on therapeutic applications of catheter cholangiography in 1978. Transhepatic catheter manipulation through benign and malignant strictures was shown to establish internal drainage into the gastrointestinal tract.[140,141] This was an extension of Molnar and Stockum's[142] report in 1974 on relief of obstructive jaundice through percutaneous transhepatic catheter insertion. The transhepatic percutaneous route, therefore, evolved from cholangiography to external bile drainage[143] in 1956 and since 1974 to internal biliary drainage in obstructive jaundice.[142] The next step was to place permanent stents or biliary prostheses in the same

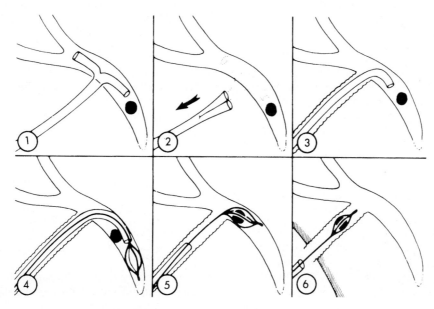

Fig. 1-41 Burhenne technique for nonsurgical removal of common duct stones. *1*, Identification of retained stone; *2*, extraction of T-tube 5 weeks after surgery; *3*, use of T-tube sinus tract for insertion of steerable catheter; *4*, opening of wire basket distally to retained stone; *5*, engagement of stone; *6*, retrieval through sinus tract.
From Burhenne HJ: *AJR* 134:888, 1980.

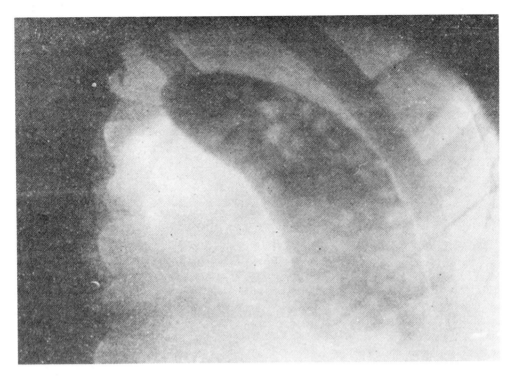

Fig. 1-42 Percutaneous transhepatic cholecystogram. Percutaneous injection of contrast into the gallbladder had its origin in the works of Burckhardt and Mueller. This 1921 radiograph is a result of direct injection of contrast medium into the gallbladder of a cadaver.

fashion[144] or via a retrograde endoscopic approach. Transhepatic catheter placement in bile duct cancer is used for successful palliation with internal irradiation by 192 iridium.[145]

Percutaneous transhepatic gallbladder puncture (Fig. 1-42), first described by Burckhardt and Muller in 1921,[52] was modified in 1976 using ultrasonic guidance for direct injection, first in animals and then in humans.[146-148] This approach is used now for drainage of acute cholecystitis, removal of gallbladder stones, and instillation of methyl *tert*-butyl ether for gallstone dissolution.[149]

Electrohydraulic shockwave fragmentation was first described as a radiologic interventional technique in vitro and in vivo for the treatment of gallstones with intracorporeal probes in 1975,[150] followed by ultrasonic fragmentation of large residual biliary tract stones by passing a flexible ultrasonic drill through the T-tube tract.[151] The most promising noninvasive technique for gallstone fragmentation is the extracorporeal shockwave application, first introduced by Sauerbruch and his group in 1986.[152] Other procedures were recently reviewed in Burhenne's article "The History of Interventional Radiology of the Biliary Tract."[153]

Many interventional radiologic techniques are a modification of the basic Seldinger technique.[65] This is certainly true for the interventional therapeutic extensions of diagnostic angiography in the alimentary tract. Nusbaum and associates[154] introduced the concept of transcatheter injec-

tion of vasoconstrictors in the superior mesenteric artery to reduce portal hypertension. This was extended to mesenteric arterial infusion of vasopressin to control gastrointestinal hemorrhage in 1971.[155] In 1972 Rösch, Dotter, and Brown[156] described a new method for control of acute gastrointestinal bleeding by embolization of the gastroepiploic artery. They used autologous clots. Subsequent embolic agents were bucrylate, Gelfoam, Ivalon, and stainless steel spring coils devised by Gianturco and colleagues in 1975.[157]

Therapeutic interventional procedures in the alimentary tract such as nonoperative stricture dilatation, stone extraction, control of bleeding, and selective instillation of chemotherapeutic anticancer agents have greatly enhanced the medical contributions by radiologists and the reputation of the specialty. Interventional radiology is a rapidly expanding subspecialty with new procedures being described as this publication goes to print.

Endoscopy

Endoscopy started before Roentgen's discovery but was much slower than radiology in becoming an integral part of medical practice. In a lecture published in 1868, Kussmaul described his observations of a tolerant patient, a sword swallower, the interior of whose stomach he demonstrated to the Freiburg society of naturalists by means of a straight, direct-vision gastroscope.[158] Rigid gastroscopes were not without hazard, and the semiflexible gastroscope introduced by Schindler[159] was a major step forward. Japanese workers developed the flexible gastrocamera in the late 1950s, but the clinical breakthrough had to await the development of coherent fiberoptic glass bundles, which was achieved independently by Hopkins[160] in the United Kingdom and by Curtiss[161] in the United States, culminating in the demonstration of a fully flexible gastroscope by Curtiss and Basil Hirschowitz[162] at the University of Alabama in 1957.

Since then, developments have been rapid. Diagnostic and therapeutic instuments for the upper and lower gastrointestinal tract and for the biliary and pancreatic ducts were available by 1970. The replacement of the coherent bundle by the photocell chip led to video endoscopes and to the technology of laparoscopic surgery. Endoscopy has taken its place alongside radiology as a key technology in the imaging and management of gastrointestinal disease.

REFERENCES

1. Phillips CES: *Bibliography of x-ray literature and research* (1896-1897), London, 1897, "The Electrician" Printing and Publishing.
2. Hickey PM: The first decade of roentgenology, *AJR* 20:249, 1928.
3. Becher W: The use of Roentgen procedures in medicine, *Dtsch Med Wochenschr* 22:202, 1896.
4. Rigler LG, Weiner M: History. In Margulis AR, Burhenne HJ, eds: *Alimentary tract radiology,* ed 3, St Louis, 1983, Mosby–Year Book.
5. Thompson EP: *Röntgen rays and phenomena of the anode and cathode,* New York, 1896, D. van Nostrand.
6. Brown P: *American martyrs to science through the roentgen rays,* Springfield, Ill, 1936, Charles C. Thomas.
7. Haenisch F: The value of the roentgen ray in the early diagnosis of carcinoma of the bowel, *Am Q Roentgenol* 3:175, 1911.
8. Brecher R, Brecher E: *The rays: a history of radiology in the United States and Canada,* Baltimore, 1969, Williams & Wilkins.
9. Rumpel T: The clinical diagnosis of fusiform dilatation of the esophagus, *Muenchen Med Wochenschr* 44:420, 1897.
10. Williams FH: *The roentgen rays in medicine and surgery,* New York, 1903, MacMillan.
11. Rieder H: Radiologic examination of the stomach and intestines in the living man, *Muenchen Med Wochenschr* 51:1548, 1904.
12. Rieder H: Beitrage zur Topographie des Magendarm Kanales beim lebenden Menschen nebst Untersuchungen über den zeitlichen Ablauf der Verdauung, *Fortschr Rontgenstr* 8:141, 1905.
13. Hulst H: President's address, *Am Q Roentgen* 1:1, 1907.
14. Beclere A: A physiologic study of vision in fluoroscopic examinations, *Arch Electr Med* 7:469, 1899.
15. Trendelenburg W: Adaptation glasses as an aid for fluoroscopy, *Muenchen Med Wochenschr* 63:245, 1916.
16. Chamberlain WE: Fluoroscopes and fluoroscopy, *Radiology* 38:383, 1942.
17. Morgan RH: Screen intensification: a review of past and present research with an analysis of future development, *AJR* 75:69, 1956.
18. Clairmont P, Haudek M: *Die Bedeutung der Magenradiologie für die Chirurgie,* Jena, Germany, 1911, Fischer.
19. Carman R, Miller A: *Roentgen diagnosis of diseases of the alimentary canal,* Philadelphia, 1917, WB Saunders.
20. Cole LG et al: *The radiologic exploration of the mucosa of the gastrointestinal tract,* Minneapolis, 1934, Bruce Publishing.
21. Hampton AO: A safe method for the roentgen demonstration of bleeding duodenal ulcers, *AJR* 38:565, 1937.
22. Shirakabe H: *Double contrast studies of the stomach,* Stuttgart, 1972, Thieme-Verlag.
23. Miller R, Chernish SM, Skucas J et al: Hypotonic roentgenography with glucagon, *AJR* 121:264, 1974.
24. Simpkins KC: Radiology now: the colon pacified, *Br J Radiol* 49:303, 1976.
25. Carman RD: *The roentgen diagnosis of diseases of the alimentary canal,* ed 2, Philadelphia, 1921, WB Saunders.
26. Cannon WB: *The mechanical factors of digestion,* New York, 1911, Longmans, Green.
27. Béclère A, Mériel C: L'exploration radiologique dans les affections chirurgicales de l'estomac et de l'intestin. 25 Congres Francais de Chirurgerie, 1912.
28. Morse RW, Cole LG: The anatomy of the normal small intestine as observed roentgenographically, *Radiology* 8:149, 1927.
29. Pendergrass EP et al: Studies of the small intestine: effects of foods and various pathological states of gastric emptying and the small bowel pattern, *Radiology* 26:651, 1936.
30. Schwarz G: The roentgenologic detection of deeper stenoses of the small intestine, *Wien Klin Wochenschr* 40:1386, 1911.
31. Pesquera GS: A method for the direct visualization of lesions in the small intestine, *AJR* 22:254, 1929.
32. Gershon-Cohen J, Shay H: Barium enteroclysis: a method for the direct immediate examination of the small intestine by single- and double-contrast techniques, *AJR* 42:456, 1939.
33. Schatzki R: Small intestinal enema, *AJR* 50:743, 1943.
34. Trickey SE, Halls J, Hobson CJ: A further development of the small bowel enema, *Proc R Soc Med* 56:1070, 1963.
35. Golden R: The small intestine and diarrhea, *AJR* 36:892, 1936.
36. Canada WJ: Use of Urokon in roentgen study of the gastrointestinal tract, *Radiology* 64:867, 1955.
37. Schüle A: Über die Sondierung und Radiograhie des Dickdarms, *Arch Verdauungskr* 10:111, 1904.
38. Haenisch GF: The roentgen examination of the large intestine, *Arch Roentgen Ray* 17:208, 1912.
39. Holzknecht G: Die normale peristaltik des colon, *Muenchen Med Wochenschr* 2:2401, 1911.
40. Schwarz G: *Klinische roentgendiagnostik des Dickdarms,* Berlin, 1914, Springer.
41. Fischer AW: A new roentgenologic method for examination of the large intestine: a combination of the contrast material enema and insufflation with air, *Klin Wochenschr* 2:1595, 1923.
42. Welin S: Results of the Malmo technique of colon examination, *JAMA* 199:369, 1967.
43. Burhenne HJ: Intestinal evacuation study: a new roentgenologic technique, *Radiologic Clinica* 33:79, 1964.
44. Brown B St-J: Defecography or anorectal studies in children including cinefluorographic observations, *Can Assoc Radiol J* 16:66, 1965.
45. Mahieu PHG: Defecography. In Margulis AR, Burhenne HJ, eds: *Alimentary tract radiology,* ed 4, St Louis, 1989, Mosby–Year Book.
46. Wakely TH: The new photographic discovery, *Lancet* 1:310, 1896.
47. Churchman JW: Acute cholecystitis with large amounts of calcium soap in the gallbladder, *Bull Johns Hopkins Hosp* 22:223, 1911. In Buckstein J: *Clinical roentgenology of the alimentary tract,* Philadelphia, 1940, WB Saunders.
48. Cole WH: The story of cholecystography, *Am J Surg* 99:206, 1960.
49. Graham EA, Cole WH: Roentgenologic examination of gallbladder: new method utilizing intravenous injection of tetrabromthenolphthalein, *JAMA* 82:613, 1924.
50. Graham EA, Cole WH, Copher GH: Visualizing the gallbladder by the sodium salt of tetrabromthenolphthalein, *JAMA* 82:1777, 1924.
51. Goodman PC: History. In Margulis AR, Burhenne HJ, eds: *Alimentary tract radiology,* ed 4, St Louis, 1989, Mosby–Year Book.
52. Burckhardt H, Muller W: Versuche über die Punktion der Gallenblase und ihre Roentgendarstellung, *Dtsch Z Chir* 162:163, 1921.
53. Cotte G: Sur l'exploration des voices biliaires au lipiodol en cas de fistule, *Medicine* 7:42, 1925. In: Buckstein J: *Clinical roentgenology of the alimentary tract,* Philadelphia, 1940, WB Saunders.

54. Mirizzi PL, Losada CQ: Exploration of the principal biliary pathways during the course of operation, Congreso Argention de Cirurgia Session of October 17, 1931. In Bruwer A: *Classic descriptions in diagnostic roentgenology,* Springfield, Ill, 1964, Charles C Thomas.

55. Huard P, Do-Xuan-Hop: La ponction transhepatique des canaux biliaires, *Bull Soc Med Chir Indochine* 15:1090, 1937.

56. McCune WS, Shorb PE, Moscovitz, H: Endoscopic cannulation of the ampulla of Vater: a preliminary report, *Am Surg* 167:762, 1968.

57. Rabinov KR, Simon M: Peroral cannulation of the ampulla of Vater for direct cholangiography and pancreatography, *Radiology* 85:693, 1965.

58. Frommhold W: Ein neuartiges Kontrastmittel für die intravenöse Cholezystographie, *Fortschr Rontgenstr* 79:283, 1953.

59. Harvey J, Loberg M, Cooper M: Tc 99m-HIDA: a new radiopharmaceutical for hepatobiliary imaging, *J Nucl Med* 16:533, 1975 (abstract).

60. Marton KI, Doubilet P: Diagnosis and treatment: how to image the gallbladder in suspected cholecystitis, *Ann Intern Med* 109:722, 1988.

61. Lorey A: Ueber eine Methode die Organe der Bauchhöhle im Röntgenbilde darzustellen, *Muenchen Med Wochenschr* 61:274, 1914. In Buckstein J: *Clinical roentgenology of the alimentary tract,* Philadelphia, 1940, WB Saunders.

62. Weber E: Uber die Bedeutung die Einführung von Sauterstoff respective. Luft in die Bauchhöhle für die experimentelle und diagnostische Röntgenologie. *Fortschr Geb Rontgenstr* 20:453, 1913. In Buckstein J: *Clinical roentgenology of the alimentary tract,* Philadelphia, 1940, WB Saunders.

63. Radt P: Eine Methode zur röntgenologischen kontrast Darstellung von Milz und Leber, *Klin Wochenschr* 8:2128, 1929.

64. MacMahon HE, Murphy AS, Bates MI: Sarcoma of the liver, *Rev Gastroenterol* 14:155, 1947.

65. Seldinger SI: Catheter replacement of the needle in percutaneous arteriography, *Acta Radiol* 39:365, 1953.

66. Odman P: Percutaneous selective angiography of the celiac artery, *Acta Radiol Suppl (Stockh)* 1:159, 1958.

67. Boijsen E: Selective pancreatic angiography, *Br J Radiol* 39:481, 1955.

68. Goldberg BB, Kimmelman BA: *Medical diagnostic ultrasound: a retrospective on its 40th anniversary,* Rochester, NY, 1988, Eastman Kodak.

69. Firestone FA: The supersonic reflectoscope for interior inspection, *Metal Progress* 48:505, 1945.

70. Satomura S: A study on examining the heart with ultrasonics. I. Principle. II. Instrument, *Jpn Circ J* 20:227, 1956.

71. Wild J: The use of ultrasonic pulses for the measurement of biologic tissues and the detection of tissue density changes, *Surgery* 27:183, 1950.

72. Howry DH, Bliss NR: Ultrasonic visualization of soft tissue structures of the body, *J Lab Clin Med* 40:579, 1952.

73. MacVicar J, Donald I: Sonar in detection of early pregnancy and its complications *J Obstet Gynaecol Br Commwlth* 70:387, 1963.

74. Donald I, MacVicar J, Brown TG: Investigation of abdominal masses by pulsed ultrasound, *Lancet* 1:1188, 1958.

75. Holmes J, Howry D, Posakony G, Cushman CR: The ultrasonic visualization of soft tissue structures in the human body, *Trans Am Clin Climatol Assoc* 66:208, 1955.

76. Donald I: Use of ultrasonics in diagnosis of abdominal swellings, *Br Med J* Nov:154, 1963.

77. Pedersen F: Percutaneous puncture guided by ultrasonic multitransducer scanning, *J Clin Ultrasound* 5:175, 1977.

78. Goldberg BB, Isard HJ, Gershon-Cohen J, Ostrum BJ: Ultrasonic fetal cephalometry, *Radiology* 87:328, 1966.

79. Leopold G, Asher M: Fundamentals of abdominal and pelvic ultrasonography, Philadelphia, 1975, WB Saunders.

80. Asher MW, Freimanis A: Echographic diagnosis of retroperitoneal lymph node enlargement, *Am J Roent Radium Ther Nucl Med* 105:438, 1969.

81. Filly RA, Freimanis AK: Echographic diagnosis of pancreatic lesions, *Radiology* 96:575, 1970.

82. Satomura S: Ultrasonic doppler method for the inspection of cardiac functions, *J Acoust Soc Am* 29:1181, 1957.

83. Strandness DE, Schultz RD, Sumner DS, Rushmer RF: Ultrasonic flow detection: a useful technic in the evaluation of peripheral vascular disease, *Am J Surg* 113:311, 1967.

84. Wells NT: A range-gated ultrasonic doppler system, *Med Biol Eng Comput* 7:641, 1969.

85. Taylor KJW, Burns PN, Woodcock JP et al: Blood flow in deep abdominal and pelvic vessels: ultrasonic pulsed doppler analysis. *Radiology* 154:487, 1985.

86. Ralls PW: Color doppler sonography of the hepatic artery and portal venous system, *AJR* 155:517, 1990.

87. Reuther G, Wanjura D, Bauer H: Acute renal vein thrombosis in renal allografts: detection with duplex doppler US, *Radiology* 170:557, 1989.

88. Namekawa K, Dasai C, Tsukamoto M et al: Imaging of blood flow using autocorrelation, *Ultrasound Med Biol* 8:138, 1982.

89. Hildebrant V, Fifel G, Dhorn G: The evaluation of the rectum by transrectal ultrasonography, *Ultrasound Quarterly* 6:167, 1988.

90. Takahashi S: Rotational radiography, Tokyo, 1957. Society for the promotion of science. In Moss A, Gamsu G, Genant H: *Computed tomography of the body,* Philadelphia, 1983, WB Saunders.

91. Cormack AM: Representation of function by its line integrals with some radiological applications. Part I. *J Appl Phys* 35:2722, 1964.

92. Cormack AM: Representation of function by its line integrals with some radiological applications. Part II. *J Appl Phys* 35:2908, 1964.

93. Oldendorf WH: Isolated flying spot detection of radiodensity discontinuities: displaying the internal structure of a complex object, *IRE Trans Biomed Electronics* 8:68, 1961.

94. Kuhl DE, Edwards RQ: Image separation isotope scanning, *Radiology* 80:653, 1963.

95. Hounsfield GN: Computerized transverse axial scanning (tomography). Part 1. Description of system, *Br J Radiol* 46:1016, 1973.

96. Hounsfield GN: Computed medical imaging, *Science* 210:22, 1980.

97. Ambrose J: Computerized transverse axial scanning (tomography). Part II. Clinical application, *Br J Radiol* 46:1023, 1973.

98. DeChiro G: Of CAT and other beasts, *AJR* 122:659, 1974.

99. Ledley RS et al: Computerized transaxial x-ray tomography of the human body, *Science* 186:207, 1974.

100. Alfidi RJ et al: Computed tomography of the thorax and abdomen: a preliminary report, *Radiology* 117:257, 1975.

101. Korobkin M, Kressel HY, Moss AA, Koehler RE: Computed tomographic angiography of the body, *Radiology* 126:807, 1978.

102. Schellinger D et al: Early experience with the Acta scanner, *Radiology* 114:257, 1975.

103. Segal SS, Stanley RJ, Evens RG: Early experience with motionless whole body computerized tomography, *Radiology* 117:321, 1976.

104. Sheedy PF II et al: Computed tomography of the body: initial clinical trial with the EMI prototype, *AJR* 127:23, 1976.

105. Dreike R, Boyd DP: Convolution reconstruction of fan beam projections, *Comput Graphics Image Processing* 5:459, 1976.

106. Chen ACM et al: Five-second fan beam CT scanner, *SPIE Appl Optical Instr Med* 96:294, 1976.

107. Boyd D et al: A proposed dynamic cardiac 3-D densitometer for early detection and evaluation of heart disease, *IEEE Trans Nucl Sci NS* 26:2724, 1979.

108. Boyd DP, Couch JL, Napel SA, Peschmann KR, Rand RE: Ultrafast cine CT: Where have we been? What lies ahead? *Am J Cardiac Imaging* 1:175, 1987.

109. Bloch F, Hansen WW, Packard M: Nuclear induction, *Physiol Rev* 69:127, 1947.

110. Purcell EM, Torrey HC, Pound RV: Resonance absorption by nuclear magnetic moments in a solid, *Physiol Res* 69:37, 1946.

111. Damadian R: Tumor detection by nuclear magnetic resonance, *Science* 171:1151, 1971.

112. Lauterbur PC: Image formation by induced local interactions: examples employing nuclear magnetic resonance, *Nature* 242:190, 1973.

113. Damadian R, Goldsmith M, Minkoff L: NMR in cancer. XVI. FONAR image of the live human body, *Physiol Chem Phys Med NMR* 9:97, 1977.

114. Lauterbur P: Magnetic resonance zeugmatography, *Pure Appl Chem* 40:149, 1974.

115. Hinshaw WB, Bottomley PA, Holland GN: Radiographic thin section image of the human wrist by nuclear magnetic resonance, *Nature* 270:722, 1977.

116. Mansfield P, Maudsley AA: Medical imaging by NMR, *Br J Radiol* 50:188, 1977.

117. Crooks LE: Overview of NMR imaging techniques. In Kaurman L, Crooks LE, Margulis AR, eds: *Nuclear magnetic resonance imaging in medicine,* New York, 1981, Igaku-Shoin.

118. Mansfield P: Real-time echo-planar imaging by NMR, *Br Med Bull* 40:187, 1984.

119. Hamm B, Karl-Jurgen W, Felix R: Conventional and rapid MRI of the liver and Gd-DTPA, *Radiology* 164:313, 1987.

120. Moss AA et al: Hepatic tumors: magnetic resonance and CT appearance, *Radiology* 150:141, 1984.

121. Stark DD et al: Magnetic resonance imaging of cavernous hemangioma of the liver: tissue-specific characterization, *AJR* 145:213, 1985.

122. Butch RF, Stark DD, Wittenberg J, Tepper JE, Saini S et al: Staging rectal cancer by MR and CT, *AJR* 146:1155, 1986.

123. de Lange EE, Fechner RE, Edge SB, Spaulding CA: Preoperative staging of rectal carcinoma with MR imaging: surgical and histopathological correlation, *Radiology* 176:623, 1988.

124. Gomberg JS, Friedman AC, Radecki PD, Grumbach K, Caroline DF: MRI differentiation of recurrent colorectal carcinoma from postoperative fibrosis, *Gastrointest Radiol* 11:361, 1986.

125. Quint LE, Glazer GM, Orringer MB: Esophageal imaging by MR and CT: study of normal anatomy and neoplasms, *Radiology* 156:717, 1985.

126. Nordentoft JM, Hansen H: Treatment of intussusception in children: brief survey based on 1830 Danish cases (I. 1042 cases 1928-1935. II. 796 cases 1944-1949), *Surgery* 38:311, 1955.

127. Margulis AR: Interventional diagnostic radiology–a new subspecialty, *AJR* 99:761, 1967.

128. Edlich RF: New long intestinal tube for rapid nonoperative intubation, *Arch Surg* 95:443, 1968.

129. Bilbao MK, Krippaehne WW, Dotter CT: Catheter retrieval of a foreign body from the gastrointestinal tract, *AJR* 111:473, 1971.

130. Ho CS: Percutaneous gastrostomy for jejunal feeding, *Radiology* 149:595, 1983.

131. Ball SW, Siegel RS, Goldthorn JC, Kosloske AM: Colonic strictures in infants following intestinal ischemia: treatment by balloon catheter dilatation, *Radiology* 149:469, 1983.

132. London RL, Trotman BW, Di Marino AJ Jr, Oleaga JA, Freiman DB et al: Dilatation of severe esophageal strictures by an inflatable balloon catheter, *Gastroenterology* 80:173, 1981.

133. Burhenne HJ: Extraktion von Residualsteinen der Gallenwege ohne Reoperation, *Fortschr Rontgenstr* 117:425, 1972.

134. Bean WJ, Mahorner H: Removal of residual stones through the T-tube tract, *South Med J* 65:377, 1972.

135. Burhenne HJ: Nonoperative roentgenologic instrumentation technics of the postoperative biliary tract: treatment of biliary stricture and retained stones, *Am J Surg* 128:111, 1974.

136. Burhenne HJ: Dilatation of biliary tract strictures: a new roentgenologic technique, *Radiological Clinica* 44:153, 1975.

137. Grüntzig A, Hopff H: Perkutane Rekanalisation chronischer arterieller Verschlüsse mit einem neuen Dilatations-Katheter, *Dtsch Med Wochenschr* 99:2502, 1974.

138. Molnar W, Stockum AE: Transhepatic dilatation of choledochoenterostomy strictures, *Radiology* 129:59, 1978.

139. Ring EJ, Oleaga JA, Freiman DB, Husted JW, Lunderquist A: Therapeutic applications of catheter cholangiography, *Radiology* 128:333, 1978.

140. Mori K, Misumi A, Sugiyama M et al: Percutaneous transhepatic bile drainage, *Ann Surg* 185:111, 1977.

141. Hoevels J, Lunderquist A, Ihse I: Percutaneous transhepatic intubation of bile ducts for combined internal-external drainage in preoperative and palliative treatment of obstructive jaundice, *Gastrointest Radiol* 3:23, 1978.

142. Molnar W, Stockum AE: Relief of obstructive jaundice through percutaneous transhepatic catheter—a new therapeutic method, *AJR* 122:356, 1974.

143. Remolar J, Katz S, Rybak B, et al: Percutaneous transhepatic cholangiography, *Gastroenterology* 31:39, 1956.

144. Pereiras RV Jr, Owen JR, Hutson D et al: Relief of malignant obstructive jaundice by percutaneous insertion of a permanent prosthesis in the biliary tree, *Ann Intern Med* 89:589, 1978.

145. Herskovic A, Heaston D, Engler MJ et al: Irradiation of biliary carcinoma, *Radiology* 139:219, 1981.

146. Hogan MT, Watne A, Mossburg W et al: Direct injection into the gallbladder in dogs, using ultrasonic guidance, *Arch Surg* 111:564, 1976.

147. Bean WJ, Calonje MA, Aprill CN et al: Percutaneous catheterization of the gallbladder with ultrasonic guidance, *South Med J* 72:612, 1979.

148. Elyaderani M, Gabriele OF: Percutaneous cholecystostomy and cholangiography in patients with obstructive jaundice, *Radiology* 130:601, 1979.

149. Allen MJ, Borody TJ, Bugliosi TF et al: Cholelitholysis using methyl tert-butyl ether, *Gastroenterology* 88:122, 1985.

150. Burhenne HJ: Electrohydrolytic fragmentation of retained common duct stones, *Radiology* 117:721, 1975.

151. Bean WJ, Davies H, Barnes F: Ultrasonic fragmentation of large residual biliary tract stone, *J Clin Ultrasound* 5:188, 1977.

152. Sauerbruch T, Delius M, Paumgartner G et al: Fragmentation of gallstones by extracorporeal shock waves, *N Engl J Med* 314:818, 1986.

153. Burhenne HJ: The history of interventional radiology of the biliary tract. *Radiol Clin North Am* 28:1139, 1990.

154. Nusbaum M, Baum S, Sakiyalak P et al: Pharmacologic control of portal hypertension, *Surgery* 62:299, 1967.

155. Baum S, Nusbaum M: The control of gastrointestinal hemorrhage by selective mesenteric arterial infusion of vasopressin, *Radiology* 98:497, 1971.

156. Rösch J, Dotter CT, Brown MJ: Selective arterial embolization: a new method for control of acute gastrointestinal bleeding, *Radiology* 102:303, 1972.

157. Gianturco C, Anderson JH, Wallace S: Mechanical devices for arterial occlusion, *AJR* 124:428, 1975.

158. Hill W: On gastroscopy and oesophago-gastroscopy, London, 1912, John Bale and Sons Danielsson.

159. Schuman BM: Presentation of the 1985 Rudolf Schindler award to William S. Haibrich, *Gastrointest Endosc* 31:302, 1985.

160. Hopkins HH, Kapany NS: Transparent fibrescopes for the transmission of optical images, *Optica Acta* 1:164, 1955.

161. Curtiss LE, Hirshowitz B, Peters CW: A Long fiberscope of internal medical examinations, *J Opt Soc Am* 47:117, 1957.

162. Hirschowitz B, Curtiss LE, Peters CW, Polland NM: Demonstration of a new gastroscope, the fiberscope, *Gastroenterology* 35:50, 1958.

PART II

ANATOMY AND PHYSIOLOGY

 # 2 *Anatomy*

ELIAS KAZAM
WILLIAM A. RUBENSTEIN
JOHN A. MARKISZ
JOSEPH P. WHALEN
KENNETH ZIRINSKY

The interpretation of any imaging procedure depends on a thorough knowledge of anatomy. Before the advent of the newer imaging procedures, sectional anatomy was considered a valuable tool for the interpretation of conventional radiographs.[1] Over the last decade ultrasound, computed tomography (CT), and magnetic resonance imaging (MRI) have revolutionized abdominal imaging.[2] With these developments sectional anatomy has become simply indispensable.

In this chapter the normal sectional anatomy of the abdomen is illustrated with sagittal, transverse, and coronal cadaver sections. For each anatomic section the corresponding in vivo anatomy is illustrated with ultrasound, CT, and/or MRI scans. Odd figure numbers designate anatomic sections. The corresponding ultrasound, CT, and/or MRI images have been given even numbers, except for the anatomic section in Fig. 2-24 *A*. All transverse and coronal images are displayed with the subject's right side oriented to the reader's left side. All sagittal sections are displayed with the subject's head oriented to the reader's left.

Emphasis has been placed on the use of normal anatomic relationships for recognizing and understanding pathologic anatomy. The anatomic basis for obtaining certain oblique and coronal ultrasound views are discussed. Normal variants, which may mimic pathologic abnormalities, are also illustrated.

Table 2-1 provides an alphabetized list of anatomic abbreviations of abdominal structures and organs and their appearance in pertinent figures. This chapter also gives a brief description of the major structures and organs.

□ **TABLE 2-1**
Alphabetized list of anatomic abbreviations of abdominal structures and organs with pertinent figures

Abbreviation*	Structure/organ	Figure
ac	Ascending colon	2-1, 25, 27
ae	Abdominal esophagus	2-7, 13, 14 *C,D,* 29
ao	Aorta	2-4 *A,B,* 7, 8 *A-C,* 9, 10 *B,C,* 13, 14 *B,C,* 15, 16*A,B,* 17, 18 *C-E,* 19, 21, 22 *A,* 24 *A-D,* 25, 26 *A,B,* 28 *A,B,* 29, 30 *B*
arf	Anterior renal fascia	2-9, 11, 21, 23, 24 *A,* 25, 27, 28 *A*
arv	Arcuate vessel	2-1, 11
as	Accessory spleen	2-15, 16 *D,* 20*B*
ba	Bare area of liver	2-1, 3, 5, 15, 17, 19
bd	Bile ducts	2-1, 5, 7, 18 *A-C*
cd	Common duct	2-3, 4 *A,* 5, 6 *A,C,* 15, 17, 18 *A,C,* 19, 20 *C,D,* 21, 22 *A,C-E,* 23, 24 *A*
ce	Celiac axis	2-7, 8 *A,C,* 10 *B,* 15, 16 *A,* 17, 18 *D,* 20 *D,E,* 29, 30 *A*
ceg	Celiac ganglion	2-20 *D*
cf	Lateroconal fascia	2-21, 23, 24 *A,* 27, 28 *B*
cha	Common hepatic artery	2-5, 6 *B,C,* 8*B,* 15, 16 *A,* 18 *B,D,* 19, 20 *C-E*

*Abbreviations may be capital letters in figures.

□ **TABLE 2-1**

Alphabetized list of anatomic abbreviations of abdominal structures and organs with pertinent figures—cont'd

Abbreviation*	Structure/organ	Figure
chv	Caudate hepatic veins	2-5, 6 *A-C*
cia	Common iliac artery	2-10 *B*
civ	Common iliac vein	2-10 *B*
cl	Caudate lobe of liver	2-4 *C*, 5, 6*A,C*, 10 *B*, 13, 16*F*, 18*A*, 29, 30 *A*
cn	Celiac lymph nodes	2-7, 19
cp	Caudate process of liver	2-3, 4 *C*, 5, 6 *B*, 15, 17, 18 *B,D*, 19, 20 *C,E*, 29
cr	Crural margin of esophageal hiatus	2-7, 14 *D*, 16 *B*
cx	Renal cortex	2-2*A*, 12 *A*, 22 *E*, 24 *A*, 26 *A,B*
cxa	Renal cortical arches	2-1, 2 *C*, 11, 17, 19, 21, 27
cxc	Renal cortical columns	2-1, 2 *C*, 17, 19, 21, 27
cyd	Cystic duct	2-3, 15, 20 *C-E*
d	Diaphragm	2-1, 2 *A,C*, 3, 6 *A,C*, 7, 10 *C*, 11, 12 *A*, 13, 14*A,C-F*, 15, 16 *C*, 17, 27
d1	Duodenal bulb	2-3, 4 *A*, 20 *F*, 21, 22*B-E*, 24*A*, 29
d2	Descending duodenum	2-3, 21, 22 *C-E*, 23, 24 *A,C*, 25, 27, 28 *A*
d3	Transverse duodenum	2-6 *C*, 7, 25, 26*A,B*, 28 *A*
d4	Ascending duodenum	2-7, 24 *A*
dc	Descending colon	2-21, 23, 24 *A*, 30*A,B*
dj	Duodenojejunal flexure	2-9, 21, 24 *A*
dr	Renal "dromedary hump"	2-19
drpv	Dorsal right portal vein	2-1, 2*C*, 4*B*, 21, 17, 18 *A-C*
ef	Epiploic foramen	2-5, 6 *B*, 15, 19
eh	Esophageal hiatus	2-9, 13
epf	Extrapleural fat	2-13, 14 *C,D*
f	Falciform ligament	2-5, 7, 17, 19, 21, 23, 24*A*
fgb	Fissure for gallbladder	2-2 *B*, 22*C,D*
flt	Fissure for ligamentum teres hepatis	2-3, 4*A*, 17, 18 *A-C*, 20 *C*, 22*C,D*
flv	Fissure for ligamentum venosum	2-5, 6 *A*, *B* 13
gan	Gastric antrum	2-4 *C*, 19, 20 *D,E*, 22 *B*, 24 *A*
gb	Gallbladder	2-1, 2 *B,C*, 4 *A*, 19, 20 *D-F*, 21, 22 *C-E*, 24*A*, 30 *A*
gbn	Gallbladder neck	2-20 *D*
gda	Gastroduodenal artery	2-20 *B,E*, 22*A,C-E*
gh	Gastrohepatic space	2-5, 7, 13, 15, 17
go	Greater omentum	2-5, 7, 9, 11, 13, 14 *C*, 15, 17, 19, 21, 23, 24 *A*
gpl	Gastrophrenic ligament	2-11
gs	Gastrosplenic space	2-13
gsl	Gastrosplenic ligament	2-11, 15, 17, 19
ha	Hepatic arterial branch	2-1
hfc	Hepatic flexure of colon	2-2 *C*, 22*E*, 30 *A*
hr	Hepatorenal space	2-19
hrn	Hiatal hernia	2-7, 9, 16 *B*
hzv	Hemiazygos vein	2-14 *C*, 17, 21, 24*A*
icl	Inferior coronary ligament	2-1, 3, 5, 13, 15, 17, 19
icv	Ileocolic vein	2-30 *A*
ilm	Iliacus muscle	2-10 *B*
ilv	Interlobar vessel	2-1, 11, 21
ima	Inferior mesenteric artery	2-25
imv	Inferior mesenteric vein	2-8 *A*, 9, 21, 22 *C,D*, 24 *A*, 25, 30 *A*
ipa	Inferior phrenic artery	2-16 *A*, 18*D*, 19
j	Jejunum	2-11, 16 *D*, 23, 24 *A*, 25, 28 *B*
L1	First lumbar vertebra	2-19
L2	Second lumbar vertebra	2-23, 27
L3	Third lumbar vertebra	2-25
lac	Left adrenal cortex	2-9, 17, 18 *D,E*

Continued.

☐ **TABLE 2-1**
Alphabetized list of anatomic abbreviations of abdominal structures and organs with pertinent figures—cont'd

Abbreviation*	Structure/organ	Figure
lad	Left adrenal gland	2-9, 10 *A,C*, 15, 17, 18 *D,E*
lam	Left adrenal medulla	2-9, 17
larf	Left anterior renal fascia	2-28 *B*
lav	Left adrenal vein	2-16 *A*, 18 *D,E*, 30 *B*
lc	Left diaphragmatic crus	2-9, 10 *C*, 13, 14 *C*, 16 *C,D*, 17, 19, 21, 25
lcia	Left common iliac artery	2-22 *F*
lcl	Left coronary ligament	2-7
lcv	Left colic vein	2-24 *A*, 25
lga	Left gastric artery	2-7, 8 *A*, 8*C*, 15, 30 *A*
lgov	Left gonadal vein	2-10 *A*, 29
lgv	Left gastric (coronary) vein	2-7, 19, 21, 24*A*, 25, 28 *B*
lh	Left renal hilus	2-9, 10 *A*
lhv	Left hepatic vein	2-13, 14 *A-C*
lk	Left kidney	2-9, 10 *A,C*, 11, 12*A,B*, 15, 16 *D*, 17, 18
ll	Left lobe of liver (lateral segment)	2-5, 6*A*, 7, 8 *A-D*, 13, 14 *A-D*, 15, 16 *E*, 17, 18 *A-C*, 19, 20*C*, 22*B*
lma	Lumbar artery	2-25
lmv	Lumbar vein	2-6 *C*, 12 *B*, 25
lo	Lesser omentum	2-5, 13, 15, 17
lp	Left renal pelvis	2-21
lpv	Left portal vein	2-4 *C*, 17
lra	Left renal artery	2-20 *B*, 21, 22*F*, 24 *A,B*
lrl	Lienorenal (phrenicosplenic) ligament	2-11, 15, 19
lrv	Left renal vein	2-7, 8 *A,C*, 10*B*, 20 *B,C*, 21, 22 *A*, 24*A-D*, 29, 30 *A*
ls	Lesser sac	2-5, 7, 9, 11, 13, 15, 17, 19, 24*A*
lu	Lung	2-1, 3, 5, 7, 9, 10 *A*, 11
lv	Left ventricle	2-9, 11, 13, 14 *C*
mc	Transverse mesocolon	2-3, 7, 9, 11, 23, 25
me	Mediastinal esophagus	2-14 *B*
mhv	Middle hepatic vein	2-1, 5, 6 *C*, 13, 14 *A-C*
msm	Muscularis mucosae	2-8 *D*, 22*B*
muc	Mucosa	2-7, 8 *D*
mus	Muscularis	2-7, 8 *D*, 22 *B*
mvs	Mesenteric vessels	2-11
otl	Omental tuberosity of left lobe of liver	2-13, 15, 17
otp	Omental tuberosity of pancreatic body	2-17
pb	Pancreatic body	2-8 *A,C*, 9, 10*B*, 15, 16 *A,D*, 17, 18 *B,E*, 20 *A,B,E*, 22 *A,C-E*
pc	Pericardium	2-11, 13
pcf	Pericardial fat	2-13
pd	Pancreatic duct	2-7, 8 *A*, 9, 11, 22*A,C,D*
pdv	Pancreaticoduodenal vessels	2-5, 22 *C,D*, 24 *A*
pef	Perirenal fat	2-1, 2 *C*, 3, 11, 12*B*, 15, 17, 18 *D*, 21, 23, 24 *A*, 27, 28 *B*
ph	Pancreatic head	2-4 *A,C*, 5, 6*A,C*, 21, 22 *A,C-E*, 23, 24 *A-D*, 26 *A,B*, 27, 28 *A*, 30*A*
pha	Phrenic ampulla of esophagus	2-13
pn	Pancreatic neck	2-21, 22 *A,C,D*
pp	Papillary process of caudate lobe of liver	2-5, 6*B*, 17, 18 *B-E*, 29
ppf	Posterior pararenal fat	2-21, 24 *A*, 25
ppv	Peripancreatic vessel	2-24 *B*
pr	Peritoneum	2-21, 27
prf	Posterior renal fascia	2-11, 21, 23, 24 *A*, 25, 27, 28 *B*
ps	Psoas muscle	2-1, 2 *C*, 3, 4 *C*, 9, 10 *A,B*, 11, 21, 23, 24 *A*, 25, 27, 28 *B*, 30 *B*
pspdv	Posterosuperior pancreaticoduodenal vessel	2-4*A*, 6 *A,B*, 22 *A*
pt	Pancreatic tail	2-10 *B*, 11, 12*A*, 15, 16 *A*, 17, 19, 20 *A,B*, 29, 30 *A*
pv	Portal vein	2-3, 4 *A,C*, 5, 6 *A,B*, 15, 16 *A,F*, 18 *A-C, E*, 19, 20 *C-F*, 29, 30*A*
pvl	Intrapancreatic vessel	2-17, 24 *B*

☐   **TABLE 2-1**

Alphabetized list of anatomic abbreviations of abdominal structures and organs with pertinent figures—cont'd

Abbreviation*	Structure/organ	Figure
py	Renal medullary pyramid	2-1, 2 *A*, 11, 12 *A*, 17, 19, 21, 22 *E*, 24 *A*, 26 *A,B*, 27
pyl	Pylorus	2-3, 22 *B*
pylc	Pyloric canal	2-22 *B*
q	Quadratus lumborum muscle	2-21, 24 *A*, 27
ql	Quadrate lobe of liver	2-1, 2 *C*, 3, 15, 17, 18 *A-C*, 19, 21, 22 *C-E*, 23, 25
r	Rib	2-1, 3, 11, 13, 15, 23, 27
ra	Right atrium	2-5
rac	Right adrenal cortex	2-3, 17, 18 *D,E*
rad	Right adrenal gland	2-3, 4 *B,C*, 10*C*, 15, 17, 18 *D,E*
ram	Right adrenal medulla	2-17
rarf	Right anterior renal fascia	2-28 *B*
rav	Right adrenal vein	2-3, 16 *A*, 18*D,E*, 30 *B*
rc	Right diaphragmatic crus	2-4 *B*, 5, 7, 8*C*, 9, 10 *C*, 12 *B*, 13, 14 *C*, 15, 16 *C,D*, 17, 19, 21, 24*A*, 27
rcia	Right common iliac artery	2-22 *F*
rgepv	Right gastroepiploic vein	2-5, 8 *B*
rgov	Right gonadal vein	2-30 *A*
rh	Right renal hilus	2-3
rha	Right hepatic artery	2-4 *A*, 15, 16*A*, 17, 20 *C*
rhv	Right hepatic vein	2-1, 2*C*, 3, 4*B,C*, 10*C*, 13, 14*A-C*, 21, 30*B*
rihv	Right inferior accessory hepatic vein	2-30*B*
rk	Right kidney	2-1, 3, 4 *C*, 10 *C*, 12 *B*, 21, 24 *A*, 25, 27, 28*B*, 30 *B*
rl	Right lobe of liver	2-1, 2 *B,C*, 3, 4*B*, 10 *C*, 12 *B*, 13, 14*A-D*, 15, 17, 18 *A-C*, 19, 21, 24*A*, 27
rlrv	Retroaortic left renal vein	2-24 *C*
rm	Rectus abdominis muscle	2-17, 25
rp	Renal pelvis	2-27
rplp	Red pulp (spleen)	2-13
rpr	Retropancreatic recess	2-19
rpv	Right portal vein	2-2 *B*, 10 *B*, 17, 18 *A*, 29, 30 *A*
rra	Right renal artery	2-4 *B*, 5, 6*A*, 10 *B*, 21, 22 *A,F*, 23, 24 *A,B*
rrv	Right renal vein	2-4 *B,C*, 5, 23, 24*A,B*
rsf	Renal sinus fat	2-1, 9, 11, 21
rv	Right ventricle	2-5, 7, 11
sa	Splenic artery	2-7, 8 *A,C*, 10*A,B*, 11, 16 *A-C*, 17, 18 *D*, 20 *D*, 29
sbm	Submucosa	2-7, 8 *D*, 22 *B*
scl	Superior coronary ligament	2-1, 3, 5, 13
sdf	Subdiaphragmatic fat	2-13, 14 *D,F*
ser	Serosa	2-7, 8 *D*
sfc	Splenic flexure of colon	2-29
sls	Superior recess of lesser sac	2-13, 17
sma	Superior mesenteric artery	2-7, 8 *A,C*, 10 *B*, 19, 20 *B*, 21, 23, 24*A,B*, 25, 26 *A,B*, 29, 30 *A*
smv	Superior mesenteric vein	2-7, 8 *B,C*, 20 *B*, 21, 22 *C,D*, 23, 24*A-C*, 25, 26 *A,B*
sp	Spleen	2-10 *A-C*, 12 *A,B*, 13, 14 *B-E*, 15, 16 *A-E*, 17, 18*C*, 19, 20 *A,B*, 21
sr	Splenorenal space	2-19
st	Stomach	2-5, 6 *C*, 7, 8 *B,C*, 9, 10 *A,B*, 11, 13, 14 *B-F*, 17, 18 *C,E*, 20 *A*, 21, 23, 24 *A*, 29, 30 *A*
sv	Splenic vein	2-7, 8 *A,B*, 9, 10*A,B*, 11, 15, 16 *A*, 17, 18 *D,E*, 19, 20 *D*, 22 *C-E*, 24 *B*, 29
svl	Splenic vessels	2-12 *A*, 14*C*
T11	Eleventh thoracic vertebra	2-13
T12	Twelfth thoracic vertebra	2-15
t	Ligamentum teres hepatis	2-15, 17, 19, 22 *C,D*

Continued.

☐ **TABLE 2-1**

Alphabetized list of anatomic abbreviations of abdominal structures and organs with pertinent figures—cont'd

Abbreviation*	Structure/organ	Figure
tc	Transverse colon	2-1, 3, 9, 11, 15, 17, 19, 21, 23, 24 A, 25, 27
tf	Transversalis fascia	2-27
tlfm	Thoracolumbar fascia	2-27
tm	Transversus abdominis muscle	2-27
td	Thoracic duct	2-17
tp	Transverse process vertebra	2-13, 15, 19
tpvl	Transverse pancreatic vessel	2-20 B
tz	Treitz' ligament	2-7, 8 C, 16 C, 21
u	Uncinate process	2-8 B, 23, 24 A,D
ulpv	Umbilical portion of left portal vein	2-3, 4A, 16 F, 18 A-C
ur	Ureter	2-23, 25
vb	Vertebral body	2-5, 7
vc	Inferior vena cava	2-4 C, 5, 6A-C, 8 B, 10 B, 13, 14A,C, 15, 16 A,F, 17, 18 A-E, 19, 20 C-F, 22 A,E,F, 23, 24A-D, 26 A,B, 27, 28 A,B, 29, 30 B
vlp	Ventral left portal venous branch	2-17
vrpv	Ventral branch of right portal vein	2-1, 2C, 4 B, 14 A, 17, 18A-C
wplp	White pulp (spleen)	2-13
zv	Azygos vein	2-10 C, 13, 14 C, 17

DIAPHRAGM

The diaphragm is thinnest superomedially in its central tendinous portion and thickest peripherally near the origins of its costal and crural fibers [3-5] (Figs. 2-1, 3, 7, 11, 13).* The costal fibers cannot be delineated on most abdominal sonograms because they lie either too near or too far from the transducer and are obscured by ribs. The echogenic line that marks the location of the diaphragm on upper abdominal sonograms reflects the strength of its acoustic interface with lung rather than its true thickness (Fig. 2-2A,B).

On CT and MRI the costal diaphragmatic fibers are visible at their interfaces with subdiaphragmatic or extrapleural fat (Figs. 2-2 C, 12, 14 C-F). Infoldings of these fibers may indent the liver, stomach, colon, or spleen, forming accessory fissures or pseudotumors, particularly on deep inspiratory scans in elderly individuals[5,6] (Fig. 2-14 D-F).

The *crural fibers* of the diaphragm, especially the thicker right crus, can be seen with all three imaging methods and should not be mistaken for enlarged lymph nodes on transverse sections (Figs. 2-5, 6 A, 9, 10 C). Typically the crura become progressively thinner on consecutive scans from the twelfth thoracic to the third lumbar levels. Superiorly the crura may have nodular contours on deep inspiratory scans, analogous to those formed by the costal fibers of the diaphragm.[5] The margins of the esophageal hiatus are formed predominantly by right crural fibers [4,7] (Figs. 2-9, 13, 14 D, 16B-D), which may appear hypertrophied or nodular in

the presence of hiatal hernia (Figs. 2-9, 16 B,C). The suspensory muscle of the duodenum, or Treitz' ligament, contains right crural fibers in its upper half (Fig. 2-7) and may mimic blood vessels on sonography and MRI (Fig. 2-8 C) or lymph nodes on CT (Fig. 2-16C).

LIVER

The liver is divided topographically into four lobes by three major fissures.[4,6] The *oblique fissure*, or fissure for the gallbladder (Figs. 2-2 B, 22 C,D), separates the right and left lobes. The *sagittal fissure*, or fissure for ligamentum teres hepatis (round ligament of the liver), divides the left lobe into lateral and medial segments (Figs. 2-3, 4 A, 17, 18A-C, 20 C, 22 C,D). The inferior portion of the left medial segment is known as the quadrate lobe (Figs. 2-1, 2 B,C, 3, 15, 17, 18A-C, 19, 21, 22 C-E, 23, 25). The *coronal fissure*, or the fissure for ligamentum venosum (venous ligament), separates the caudate lobe from the more anterior medial and lateral segments of the left lobe (Figs. 2-5, 6 A,B, 13).

The major fissures are important landmarks for locating liver lesions when segmental resection is planned. In addition, the oblique fissure is valuable for locating the gallbladder with ultrasound, CT, or MRI. True accessory hepatic fissures are rare, in contradistinction to the pseudofissures caused by diaphragmatic invaginations, as discussed in the previous section[6,7] (Figs. 2-21, 24 A).

The *right lobe* of the liver is attached posterosuperiorly to the diaphragm by the right superior and inferior coronary ligaments, demarcating a bare area of posteromedial liver that is devoid of peritoneum[8] (Figs. 2-1, 3, 5, 15, 17,

---

*In this chapter, because of the extensive references to figure numbers and parts, "Fig. 2-" will be given only once at the start of a list, followed by appropriate numbers and letters.

19). In contrast, the left lobe is attached to the diaphragm by a single coronary ligament (Fig. 2-7). The right lobe may have a long posteroinferior extension, or Reidel's lobe, which should not be mistaken for hepatomegaly. At its interface with the right kidney, the right lobe has a posterior concavity of variable depth (Figs. 2-1, 3, 21, 23, 25). Loss of this concavity may occur with right lobe enlargement or with absence or ptosis of the right kidney (Figs. 2-22 *C,D,* 24 *B*).

The *lateral segment of the left lobe,* referred to as the "left lobe" in the illustrations, is the most variable portion of the liver. In asthenic individuals this segment appears elongated in transverse dimension, with only a mild posterior convexity, and may curve around the anterior tip of the spleen (Figs. 2-13, 16 *E*). In endomorphic individuals the lateral segment is usually shortened transversely with a prominent posterior omental tuberosity (Fig. 2-17 versus Figs. 2-13, 15). This segment may also be hypoplastic or absent (Fig. 2-16 *F*). In such cases the caudate lobe may be either prominent or rudimentary.[9] Rarely the sagittal and oblique fissures may be congruent, and as a result the left lobe may not be segmented.

The *caudate lobe* lies at the posterosuperior aspect of the liver. At the porta hepatis (portal fissure) the caudate lobe is connected to the right lobe by a caudate process, which extends laterally between the portal vein and inferior vena cava. The most medial portion of the caudate lobe, or the papillary process, protrudes to the left—and at times anteriorly—to invaginate the superior recess of the lesser sac[9] (Figs. 2-5, 6 *B,* 17, 18 *B-E,* 29). The papillary process may also extend inferiorly below the caudate process. The caudate and papillary processes may be separated by a groove of variable depth, which usually is oriented in a sagittal or parasagittal plane but occasionally is in a semicoronal plane (Figs. 2-5, 6 *B,* 29). As a result, the papillary process may appear separate from the liver on transverse sections at and below the porta hepatis, mimicking an extrahepatic structure[9] (Figs. 2-18 *B,D,E*).

HEPATIC VEINS

The systemic hepatic veins form three main trunks near the junction with the inferior vena cava,[10] which are easily seen with sonography, MRI, and contrast-enhanced CT (Figs. 2-1, 2 *C,* 3, 4 *B,C,* 5, 6 *C,* 10 *C,* 13, 14 *A-C,* 21, 30*B*). The *right hepatic vein* drains the posterior and anterosuperior right lobe and courses between the ventral and dorsal branches of the right portal vein, within the plane separating the anterior from the posterior segments of the right lobe of the liver (Figs. 2-1, 2 *C,* 3, 4 *B,C,* 10 *C,* 13, 14 *A-C,* 21, 30 *B*). The *middle hepatic vein* drains the anteroinferior right lobe and the quadrate lobe and is an important internal landmark for separating the right from the left lobes above the oblique fissure. The *left hepatic vein* drains the left lateral segment and the superior portion of the medial segment.

The left and middle hepatic veins usually form a common trunk before emptying into the vena cava. Smaller hepatic veins also drain directly into the cava; these include the relatively constant caudate hepatic veins (Figs. 2-5, 6 *A-C*) and the variable right inferior accessory hepatic veins (Fig. 2-30 *B*), which drain into the vena cava in proximity to the adrenal veins.[10,11]

PORTAL VEINS

The portal veins enter the liver at the porta hepatis with their corresponding bile ducts and hepatic arteries. As is the case with the systemic hepatic veins, the portal veins are easier to see with sonography than with CT. The *right portal vein* extends almost as a direct continuity of the main portal vein into the right lobe of the liver and quickly divides into right ventral and dorsal branches (Figs. 2-2 *B,* 10*B,* 17, 18 *A,* 29, 30 *A*). The right portal vein supplies the right lobe and the lateral aspect of the caudate lobe. The *left portal vein* (Figs. 2-4*C,* 17) courses transversely to the left, where it sends branches to the medial caudate lobe, then courses anteriorly into the fissure of the ligamentum teres, where the umbilical portion of the left portal vein sends branches to the medial and lateral segments of the left lobe[10] (Figs. 2-3, 4 *A,* 16 *F,* 18 *A-C*).

COMMON DUCT

The common duct lies at the right anterolateral aspect of the portal vein in the porta hepatis (Figs. 2-3, 5, 6 *A,C,* 15, 17, 18 *A,C,* 19). This constant relationship forms the basis for accurate imaging of the common hepatic duct with right anterior oblique sonography[12] (Fig. 2-4 *A*). After exiting the porta hepatis, the common duct courses behind the duodenum, then along the posterolateral aspect of the pancreatic head (Figs. 2-3, 4*A,* 5, 6 *A,* 20 *C,D,* 21, 22*A,C-E,* 23, 24 *A*). This portion of the bile duct is often obscured by gas or fat on sonography and can be more reliably imaged with CT. Because the level of the junction between the common hepatic and cystic ducts is variable and difficult to localize accurately with sectional imaging, all portions of the common bile duct have been jointly referred to as the "common duct" in the illustrations.

The *right and left bile ducts* also maintain constant relationships with their corresponding portal veins (Figs. 2-1, 5, 7, 18 *A-C*). The ventral and dorsal right bile ducts parallel their corresponding portal venous branches before joining anterior to the right portal vein to form the right hepatic duct. The left bile duct usually courses along the right lateral aspect of the umbilical portion of the left portal vein, then travels anteriorly to the transverse portion of this vessel. On CT mildly dilated bile ducts may be mimicked by the periportal fat, which invaginates the liver along the portal veins[13] (Fig. 2-18 *B*). This same fat appears echogenic on sonography, whereas dilated bile ducts appear poorly echogenic. Thus ultrasound is more specific than CT for detection of mildly dilated ducts near the porta hepatis. On the other hand, mildly dilated ducts in the periphery of the liver, especially in the portions of the right lobe surrounded by ribs, are easier to detect with contrast-enhanced CT than with ultrasound.

PORTACAVAL SPACE

The portacaval space is a small compartment between the portal vein and the vena cava. This space contains the epiploic (Winslow's) foramen to the lesser sac (Figs. 2-5, 6 B, 15, 19), the caudate and papillary processes of the caudate lobe (Figs. 2-3, 4 C, 5, 6 B, 15, 17, 18 B,D, 19, 20 C,E, 29), and several important vessels and lymph nodes that lie within the superior hepatoduodenal ligament.[14] Retroportal lymph nodes may have oval or rectangular contours on transverse sections (Fig. 2-20 E,F) and therefore may be mistaken for portions of the caudate lobe or pancreatic head. Careful analysis of the contours of the caudate lobe on consecutive sections, as well as comparison of the texture of these structures with the adjacent pancreas, helps to avoid such errors.

Portacaval nodes may be involved by a variety of primary and secondary neoplastic and inflammatory processes. Since both intraperitoneal and retroperitoneal pathologic processes can spread to these lymph nodes, they are often valuable indicators of the extent of disease.[14]

The cystic duct may course inferiorly within the hepatoduodenal ligament, along the posterolateral aspect of the portacaval space, before joining the common duct (Fig. 2-20 D). Portacaval vessels include accessory or replaced right hepatic arteries, which arise from the celiac axis or superior mesenteric artery, and posterior pancreaticoduodenal vessels (Figs. 2-4A, 6 A,B, 22 A, 24B), which accompany the distal common bile duct as it courses inferiorly toward the duodenal papilla. The epiploic foramen communicates with the posterior subhepatic compartment of the greater peritoneal cavity (Morison's pouch), just lateral to the portacaval space.

GALLBLADDER

The gallbladder lies within its oblique fissure at the posterolateral, inferior aspect of the quadrate lobe[4,13] (Figs. 2-1, 2 B,C, 4 A, 19, 20 D-F, 21, 22 C-E, 24A, 30 A). These anatomic landmarks are valuable for localizing the gallbladder when its lumen is not clearly visualized on sagittal or transverse images.[13] Occasionally the oblique fissure may extend peripherally to the anterolateral surface of the liver and may be high in position.[6] In such cases the gallbladder may be anteriorly interposed between the liver and diaphragm.[6] The gallbladder fundus is constantly related to the hepatic flexure of the colon[4] (Figs. 2-1, 22 E, 24 A), even in the presence of anterior colonic hepatodiaphragmatic interposition. Omental fat, which often surrounds the gallbladder (Figs. 2-1, 22C-E, 24 A), may appear as a thick echogenic rind on sonography, mimicking gallbladder wall thickening. This potential source of error does not occur with CT or MRI.

The cystic duct is tortuous and difficult to demonstrate with sectional images. As it extends transversely to join the common duct, the cystic duct may lie anterolateral or posterolateral to the portal vein. This duct may also course inferiorly with the common duct before joining it behind the pancreatic head. Since the cystic duct is often obscured by overlying bowel gas or fat (Fig. 2-20 D), it is the only portion of the gallbladder that may be seen better with CT than sonography.

SPLEEN

The spleen lies in the superolateral left upper quadrant, just below the diaphragm (Figs. 2-10 A-C, 12, 13, 14B-E, 15, 16 A-E, 17, 18 C, 19, 20 A,B, 21). The spleen is often lobulated, especially superiorly (Figs. 2-14 E, 16F), and may be invaginated by infoldings of the diaphragm, analogous to but shallower than those that invaginate the liver. Although intraperitoneal, the spleen extends posterior to the left kidney (Figs. 2-11, 12 A). The spleen's medial portion therefore may be mistaken for a suprarenal or renal mass, particularly if it is separated from the rest of the spleen by an inferior groove (Fig. 2-16 B,C). The spleen is attached to the stomach and kidney by peritoneal folds known as the *gastrosplenic* and *splenorenal ligaments*, respectively. Accessory spleens may be found within these ligaments[4] (Figs. 2-15, 16 D, 20 B).

The *splenic artery* divides into several branches before entering the spleen.[15] Blood flows from these arteries into arterioles and subsequently into sinusoids (*red pulp*). These sinusoids drain into five or more veins, which form the splenic vein in the lienorenal (phrenicosplenic) ligament. Periarteriolar sheaths of lymphoid tissue (*white pulp*) may be visible as whitish dots (malpighian bodies) on the cut surface of the spleen.[15] The white pulp appears to be concentrated within branching islands in the splenic parenchyma and is surrounded by red pulp (Figs. 2-13, 15, 19).

The spleen normally shows transient patchy opacification in the first few seconds of the arterial phase after intravenous contrast injection (Fig. 2-16 A). This probably reflects initial opacification of the white pulp, where the splenic arterioles are concentrated, analogous to early opacification of the renal cortex. Alternatively this opacification may be caused by closure of some of the presinusoidal arteriolar sphincters, leading to a transient radiolucency of the sinusoids these sphincters supply. Whatever the cause of this phenomenon, the hypovascular areas become isodense, together with the remainder of the spleen in a few more seconds, unlike true parenchymal lesions. Prolonged opacifications of the white pulp on dynamic CT scans, accompanied by relative radiolucency of the red pulp, may occur with portal hypertension.

STOMACH

The stomach is globular to the left (*gastric fundus*) and tubular to the right (*gastric body*) (Figs. 2-5, 6 C, 7, 8 B,C, 9, 10 A,B, 11, 13, 14 B-F, 17, 18 C,E, 20A, 21, 23, 24

A, 29, 30 *A*). The gastric cardia marks the junction of the stomach with the cone-shaped abdominal esophagus[16] (Figs. 2-7, 13, 14*C,D,* 29). The abdominal esophagus is often unopacified with oral contrast media and should not be mistaken for a mass. The midportion of this cone-shaped segment is normally oriented horizontally, unlike the posthiatal segment of stomach in the presence of hiatal hernia.[16]

The antrum is the distal portion of the gastric body (Figs. 2-4*C*, 19, 20 *D,E*, 22 *B,* 24*A*). The pyloric sphincter is marked by a focal thickening of the antral wall at its junction with the duodenum (Figs. 2-3, 22 *B*, 24 *A*). The pyloric sphincter should not be mistaken on CT for the prepyloric fold, which is seen more proximally within the antrum, near the angular incisura.

The gastric wall has a multilayered appearance with high-resolution ultrasound[17] (Figs. 2-8 *D*, 22 *D*). The gastric submucosa and the interfaces between gastric mucosa and lumen—or gastric serosa and peritoneum—appear echogenic. On the other hand, the muscularis mucosae and muscularis (propria) layers are poorly echogenic. The normal thickening of the muscularis layer at the pylorus, forming the pyloric sphincter, can also be visualized sonographically (Fig. 2-22 *D*). These findings make sonography a potentially valuable tool for detecting gastric wall abnormalities and assessing the extent of gastric wall involvement.

DUODENUM

The duodenum surrounds the pancreatic head and is separated from it by periduodenal fat and vessels (Figs. 2-3, 4 *A*, 6 *C*, 7, 20 *F*, 21, 22 *B-E*, 23, 24 *A,C*, 25, 26 *A,B*, 27, 28 *A*, 29). The duodenal bulb is usually easy to recognize with sectional images because of its characteristic cone-shaped configuration (Figs. 2-3, 4 *A*, 20 *F*, 21, 22 *B-E*, 24 *A*, 29).

The transverse duodenum extends horizontally across the midline between the aorta and superior mesenteric artery and is a good marker for the inferior pancreas (Figs. 2-6 *C*, 7, 25, 26 *A,B*, 28 *A*). The ascending duodenum and duodenojejunal junction lie just to the left of the midline, below the pancreatic body (Figs. 2-7, 9, 21, 24*A*).

COLON

The ascending and descending colon and the rectum are extraperitoneal structures, whereas the cecum, transverse colon, and sigmoid colon are intraperitoneal[4] (Figs. 2-1, 3, 9, 11, 15, 17, 19, 21, 23, 24 *A*, 25, 27, 30*A,B*). The ascending and descending colon may have a complete mesocolon in 26% and 36% of cases, respectively.[15] In such cases intraperitoneal fluid may appose these portions of the colon along nearly their entire contour. The hepatic flexure of the colon is a constant companion of the gallbladder. This flexure normally lies posterior to the liver—inferior, directly behind, or to the left of the quadrate lobe (Figs. 2-1, 24 *A*). Occasionally the hepatic flexure may be anteriorly interposed between the liver and diaphragm, causing a cold defect on radionuclide liver scans.[4]

Rarely the colon may be posteriorly interposed between the liver and diaphragm, extending up to the tenth or eleventh thoracic vertebral levels.[18] In this high position the colon may mimic posterior liver masses or diaphragmatic defects on sonography. The transverse colon usually lies below the stomach but may be found occasionally anterior and superior to the stomach, especially if the left lobe is hypoplastic. The distal transverse colon, or radiologic splenic flexure, usually lies lateral to the stomach and anterior to the spleen (Figs. 2-16*F*, 17, 18 *C*, 24 *A*, 29). Occasionally the distal transverse colon may be found between the spleen and left kidney, within the splenorenal space.

INTRAPERITONEAL COMPARTMENTS

The peritoneal cavity may be divided into several spaces where fluid is likely to collect.[2,15] The configuration of these compartments is determined by peritoneal folds or ligaments and adjacent organs. Thus the right subphrenic space is separated from the posterior subhepatic space by the right coronary ligaments and bare area of liver[8] (Figs. 2-1, 3, 5, 13, 15, 17, 19). The left subphrenic space is separated from the lesser sac, medially by the left coronary ligament and laterally by the gastrosplenic fold[8] (Figs. 2-7, 11, 17). The superior recess of the lesser sac surrounds the anterior, medial, and posterior borders of the caudate lobe, whereas the epiploic (Winslow's) foramen lies inferior to the caudate process between the main portal vein and vena cava[8] (Figs. 2-5, 6*B*, 15, 19). The lesser omentum separates the lesser sac posteriorly from the gastrohepatic space anteriorly, although these two compartments can communicate along the lateral free edge of the lesser omentum or directly through holes within this cobweblike peritoneal layer (Figs. 2-11, 17).

Intraperitoneal fluid and pancreatic inflammatory effusions may extend from the superior recess of the lesser sac, around the free edge of the lesser omentum, and into the hilum of the liver (Fig. 2-17). Occasionally these fluid collections may also extend into the right and left lobes of liver along the right and left portal veins. The inferior recess of the lesser sac is bounded laterally by the gastrosplenic ligament and inferiorly by the transverse mesocolon and lesser omentum (Figs. 2-5, 7, 9, 11, 13, 15, 17, 19, 24 *A*).

The *posterior peritoneal compartments* may extend behind well-known retroperitoneal structures such as the kidneys and ascending and descending colon.[4,19] Thus the posterior subhepatic (hepatorenal) and splenorenal spaces may extend behind the upper borders of the renal upper poles (Fig. 2-19). The splenorenal space is continuous with the peritoneal compartment behind the pancreatic tail[19] (Fig. 2-19). The paracolic gutters may extend behind the ascending and descending colon, if the peritoneum covering these structures forms a posterior mesocolon. Fluid within these posterior compartments may be mistaken for retroperitoneal collections or for thickened renal fascia.

Text continued on p. 47.

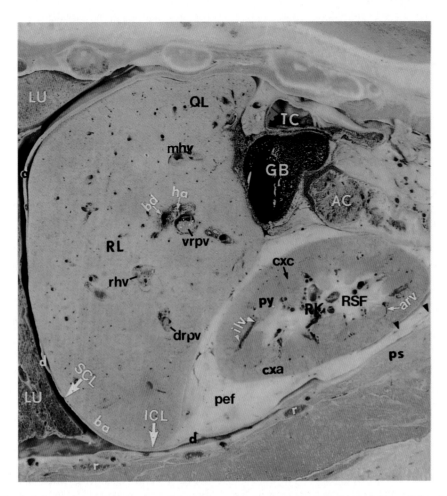

Fig. 2-1 Sagittal anatomic section of the right upper quadrant through the midplane of the right kidney *(RK)*. The right lobe of the liver *(RL)* is attached posteriorly to the diaphragm *(d)* by the superior *(SCL)* and inferior *(ICL)* coronary ligaments. These peritoneal reflections separate the right subphrenic space (anterosuperior to *SCL)* from the posterior subhepatic space (posteroinferior to *ICL)*. Fluid within either of these two spaces cannot extend over the bare area of the liver *(ba)*, which is devoid of peritoneal covering. Ventral *(vrpv)* and dorsal *(drpv)* branches of the right portal vein lie posterior to their respective bile ducts *(bd)* and hepatic arteries *(ha)*. Fibrofatty tissue, continuous with Glisson's capsule, envelops the portal vessels and accounts for the echogenic rind that surrounds them on sonography (see Fig. 2-2). In contrast, the middle *(mhv)* and right *(rhv)* hepatic veins have little, if any, fibrous tissue around them. The middle hepatic vein separates the medial segment of the left lobe—or (inferiorly) the quadrate lobe *(QL)*—from the right lobe, whereas the right hepatic vein courses between anterior and posterior segments of the right lobe of the liver. The fundus of the gallbladder *(GB)* is intimately related to the hepatic flexure of the colon *(AC,* Ascending colon; *TC,* transverse colon). Note the peritoneal (omental) fat around the gallbladder. This may produce an echogenic rind on sonography in obese patients, which should not be mistaken for gallbladder wall thickening. The right lobe of the liver, although intraperitoneal in location, extends posterior to the renal upper pole; if enlarged, it can easily displace the right kidney inferiorly. The renal cortex *(cxa, cxc)* is paler and coarser in texture than the medullary pyramids *(py)*. Columns of the renal cortex *(cxc)* and interlobar vessels *(ilv)* can be seen between medullary pyramids. Arcuate vessels *(arv)* course between the peripheral cortex and medulla. *RSF,* Renal sinus fat; *pef,* perirenal fat; *black arrowheads,* posterior renal fascia; *PS,* psoas muscle. The diaphragm *(d)* is thinner centrally in its tendinous portion but thicker in its peripheral muscular portions. *LU,* Lung; *r,* rib.
Modified from Whalen JP, Bierny JP: *Radiology* 92:1427, 1969.

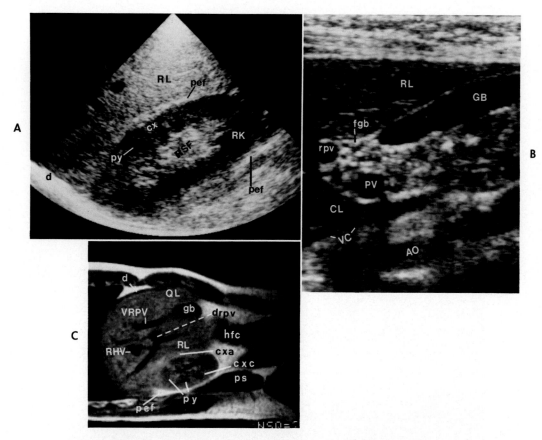

Fig. 2-2 A, Sagittal sonogram at approximate level of Fig. 2-1. Renal sinus fat *(rsf)* and perinephric fat *(pef)* are extremely echogenic. The renal cortex *(cx)* is moderately echogenic, whereas the medullary pyramids *(py)* are poorly echogenic. The echogenic diaphragmatic interface *(d)* is an exaggeration of the true thickness of the diaphragm at this level. **B,** Sagittal oblique sonogram of gallbladder *(gb)*. The fissure for the gallbladder *(fgb)* extends between the gallbladder neck and the right protal vein *(rpv)*. *RL,* Right lobe of liver; *CL,* caudate lobe of liver; *vc,* vena cava; *ao,* aorta. **C,** Sagittal MRI (SE 750/33) corresponding to Fig. 2-1. The gallbladder *(gb)* lies within its fissure between the quadrate *(QL)* and right *(RL)* lobes of the liver. The right hepatic vein *(rhv)* courses between the ventral *(vrpv)* and dorsal *(drpv)* branches of the right portal vein. The anterior muscular portion of diaphragm *(d)* is clearly delineated. The right renal cortex *(cxa, cxc)* is brighter than the medullary pyramids *(py)* on this relatively T1 image. *pef,* Perinephric fat; *hfc,* hepatic flexure of the colon; *ps,* psoas muscle.

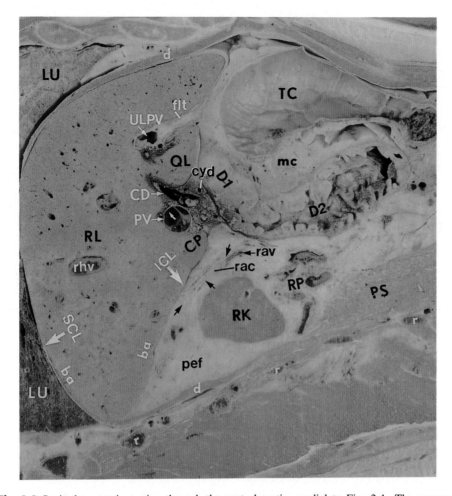

Fig. 2-3 Sagittal anatomic section through the porta hepatis, medial to Fig. 2-1. The common hepatic duct *(CD)* lies anterior to the right edge of the portal vein *(PV)*. Below the porta hepatis, the common duct courses behind the pylorus *(pyl)* and duodenal bulb *(Dl)*. As a result, the proximal common hepatic duct is almost always visible with ultrasound, where the liver serves as a sonic window (see Fig. 2-4 *A*). In contrast, the distal common duct is often obscured by overlying gas and fat. *cyd,* Cystic duct. The left portal vein can be seen on end *(curved white arrow)* at its origin from the main portal vein, then more anteriorly, where its umbilical portion *(ULPV)* lies at superior margin of the fissure for the ligamentum teres hepatis *(flt)*. *QL,* Quadrate lobe; *CP,* caudate process; *RL,* right lobe of liver; *rhv,* right hepatic vein. The superior *(SCL)* and inferior *(ICL)* coronary ligamentous attachments are farther apart than on Fig. 2-1, demarcating a wider bare area *(ba)*. Note that the inferior coronary ligament is contiguous to the perirenal fat *(pef)* rather than to the diaphragm *(d)* at this level, thus forming the *hepatorenal ligament*. The perirenal fat extends superiorly to the diaphragm, along the bare areas of the liver. The right adrenal gland *(black arrows)* lies anterior and superior to the medial upper pole of the right kidney *(RK)*. The cholesterol-laden right adrenal cortex *(rac)* has a very similar texture to the surrounding perinephric fat *(pef)*. *rav,* Right adrenal vein; *RP,* renal pelvis and vessels at the right renal hilus.
Modified from Whalen JP, Bierny JP: *Radiology* 92:1427, 1969.

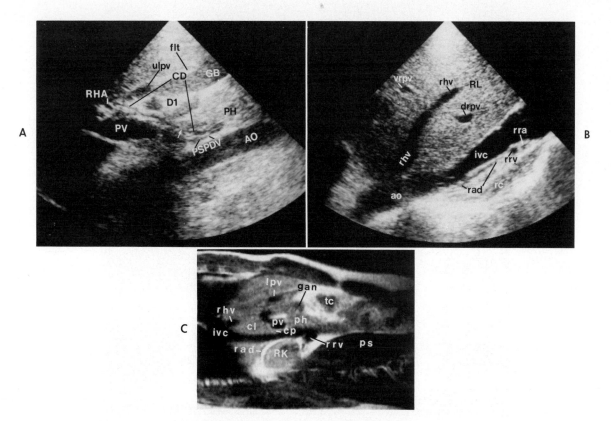

Fig. 2-4 A, Right anterior oblique sonogram of the porta hepatis. The common duct *(cd)* lies anterolateral to the portal vein *(pv)* and courses inferiorly behind the proximal duodenum *(Dl)* to run along the posterior aspect of the pancreatic head *(ph)*. A portion of the common duct *(small arrow)* is obscured by overlying duodenal air *(Dl)*. The right hepatic artery *(rha)* lies behind the proximal common duct, whereas the posterosuperior pancreaticoduodenal vein *(pspdv)* courses behind the distal common bile duct. *ulpv,* Umbilical portion of the left portal vein; *flt,* fissure for ligamentum teres; *gb,* gallbladder wall; *ao,* aorta. **B,** Anterior oblique sonogram just lateral to Fig. 2-4 *A.* The medial portion of the right adrenal gland *(rad)* is visible behind the inferior vena cava. *rrv,* Right renal vein; *rra,* right renal artery; *rc,* right diaphragmatic crus. The right hepatic vein *(rhv)* lies between the ventral *(vrpv)* and dorsal *(drpv)* branches of the right portal vein, within the plane that divides the right lobe of the liver *(RL)* into anterior and posterior segments. *ao,* Upper abdominal aorta. **C,** Sagittal MRI (SE 750/33) at approximate level of Fig. 2-3. The common hepatic duct is not clearly delineated because of the relatively lower spatial resolution of MRI. *Pv,* Main portal vein; *lpv,* left portal vein. The right hepatic vein *(rhv)* is seen near its junction with the inferior vena cava *(vc). cl,* Caudate lobe; *CP,* caudate process; *ph,* pancreatic head; *gan,* gastric antrum; *tc,* transverse colon; *rad,* right adrenal gland; *RK,* medial upper pole right kidney; *rrv,* right renal vein; *ps,* psoas muscle.

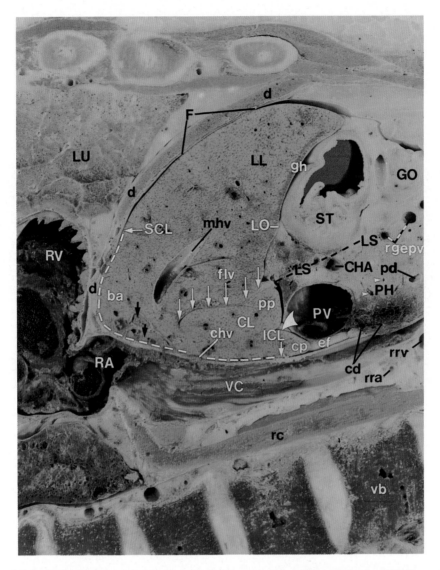

Fig. 2-5 Sagittal anatomic section through the inferior vena cava. The portal vein *(PV)* lies anterior to the vena cava *(VC)*, between the pancreatic head *(PH)* inferiorly and the caudate lobe *(CL)* superiorly. *pd,* Pancreatic duct; *small arrowheads,* pancreaticoduodenal vascular arcade. The distal common bile duct *(cd)* courses along the posterior aspect of the pancreatic head. A small groove *(large arrowhead)* on the inferior surface of the caudate lobe separates the caudate process *(cp)* posteriorly from the papillary process *(pp)* anteriorly. The lesser sac *(LS)* lies anterior to the pancreas and behind the stomach *(ST)* and extends superiorly into the fissure for the ligamentum venosum *(flv, upper white arrows),* anterior to the caudate lobe toward the diaphragm *(d),* forming the superior recess of the lesser sac. Inferiorly, the lesser sac extends behind the stomach *(ST)* and anterior to the pancreas. The gastrohepatic space *(gh)* is separated from the inferior recess of the lesser sac behind it by the lesser omentum *(LO)*. *GO,* Greater omentum; *rgepv,* right gastroepiploic vessels. The caudate process *(cp)* forms the roof of the epiploic foramen *(ef)*. *CHA,* Common hepatic artery. The vena cava follows a gentle anterosuperior course to the diaphragm and is not completely surrounded by the liver along its posterior aspect. The superior *(SCL)* and inferior *(ICL)* coronary ligaments are even further separated than on Fig. 2-3, demarcating the widest bare area *(ba)* of the liver. The small caudate hepatic vein *(chv)* drains the caudate lobe directly into the vena cava. Other small hepatic veins *(black arrows)* drain into the vena cava, independently of the main hepatic veins. *mhv,* Middle hepatic vein; *LL,* left lobe of liver; *F,* falciform ligament; *rc,* right diaphragmatic crus; *rra,* right renal artery; *rrv,* right renal vein. Muscular portions of the diaphragm are clearly demarcated from the thin central tendinous portion, which lies directly beneath the right ventricle *(RV)*. *RA,* right atrium; *LU,* lung; *vb,* vertebral body.
Modified from Whalen JP, Bierny JP: *Radiology* 92:1427, 1969.

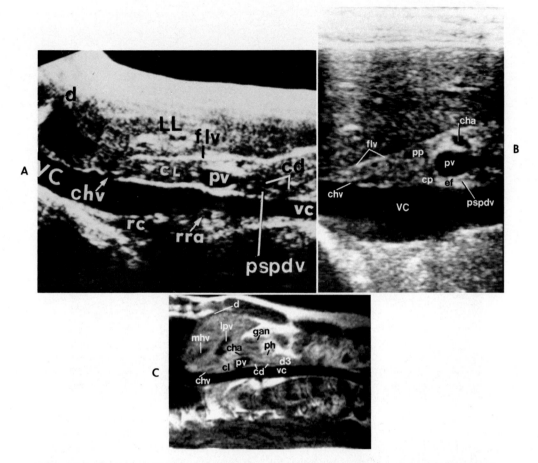

Fig. 2-6 A, Sagittal sonogram corresponding to Fig. 2-5 shows the pancreatic head *(ph)* inferior to the portal vein *(pv)* and anterior to the inferior vena cava *(vc)*. The common bile duct *(cd)* courses through the posterior aspect of the pancreatic head. *pspdv,* Posterior superior pancreaticoduodenal vein; *cl,* caudate lobe; *chv,* caudate vein; *flv,* right superior recess of lesser sac, or fissure for ligamentum venosum; *LL,* left lobe of liver; *rc,* right crus; *rra,* right renal artery; *d,* diaphragm. **B,** Sagittal sonogram through the upper vena cava *(vc)*. The caudate hepatic vein *(chv)* drains directly into the vena cava, whereas the posterior pancreaticoduodenal vein *(pspdv)* courses behind the portal vein *(pv)* at the epiploic foramen *(ef)*. *cha,* Common hepatic artery; *cp,* caudate; *pp,* papillary processes of caudate lobe; *flv,* fissure for ligamentum venosum. **C,** Sagittal MRI (SE 750/33) corresponding to Fig. 2-5. The pancreatic head *(ph)* lies anterior to the vena cava *(vc)* and inferior to the portal vein *(pv)*. *cd,* Distal retropancreatic common duct; *cha,* common hepatic artery; *lpv,* left portal vein; *cl,* caudate lobe; *chv,* caudate hepatic vein, *mhv,* middle hepatic vein; *gan,* gastric antrum; *d3,* third portion of duodenum; *d,* diaphragm; *lmv,* lumbar veins.

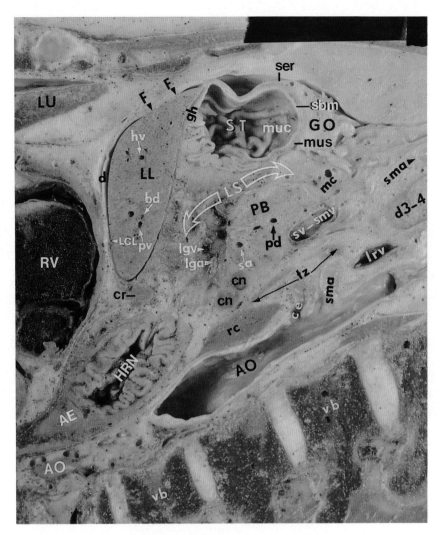

Fig. 2-7 Sagittal anatomic section through the aorta. The abdominal aorta *(AO)* maintains posterior position as it extends superiorly through the aortic hiatus, in contrast to the anterosuperior course followed by the upper vena cava (Fig. 2-5). The proximal celiac axis *(ce)* and superior mesenteric artery *(sma)* are clearly delineated. *lrv*, Left renal vein. The pancreatic body *(pb)* lies anterior to the junction of the splenic *(sv)* and superior mesenteric *(smv)* veins. *sa*, Splenic artery. In contrast, the celiac nodes *(cn)* lie behind the splenic and superior mesenteric vessels. The eccentric location of the pancreatic duct *(pd)* in the posterior aspect of the pancreatic body is a normal variant. The right crus *(rc)* is normally thickened at this level. Extending inferiorly from the right crus are striated muscle fibers that form the superior aspect of the suspensory muscle of the duodenum, or Treitz' ligament *(tz)*. The lower part of this ligament, which is attached to the posterior wall of the duodenojejunal flexure *(d3-d4)*, contains smooth muscle and fibrous tissue only and is therefore not clearly delineated on this anatomic section. The transverse mesocolon *(mc)* is attached posteriorly to the inferior margin of the pancreatic body. As it extends caudally and anteriorly to the transverse colon, which lies just below this section, the transverse mesocolon blends with the greater omentum *(GO)* and forms the inferior wall of the lesser sac *(LS)*. *gh*, Gastrohepatic space; *lga*, left gastric artery; *lgv*, left gastric (coronary) vein. Two portions of the stomach *(ST)* are visible. The body of the stomach lies anteriorly below the left lobe of the liver *(LL)*, whereas the cardia is herniated *(hrn)*, along with the abdominal esophagus *(AE)* between the thickened crural margins *(cr)* of the esophageal hiatus. The gastric mucosa *(muc)*, submucosa *(sbm)*, muscularis *(mus)*, and serosa *(ser)* can be delineated in the inferior aspect of the body of the stomach. A single left coronary ligament *(LCL)* attaches the left lobe of the liver to the left diaphragm *(d)* and separates the anterior subphrenic space just below the diaphragm from the superior portion of the gastrohepatic space. As a result, there is no bare area of the left lobe of the liver. *F*, Falciform ligament; *RV*, right ventricle; *vb*, vertebral body.
Modified from Whalen JP, Bierny JP: *Radiology* 92:1427, 1969.

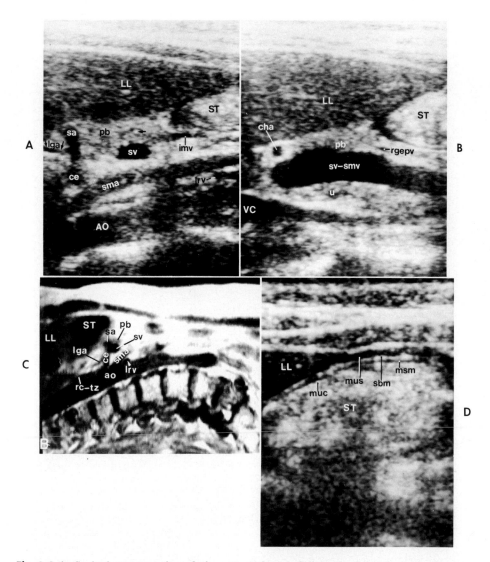

Fig. 2-8 A, Sagittal sonogram through the aorta *(AO)*. *ce,* Celiac axis; *lga,* left gastric artery; *sa,* splenic artery. The pancreatic body *(pb)* lies anterior to the splenic vein *(sv)*. *Arrow,* pancreatic duct. A portion of the inferior mesenteric vein *(imv)* is visible at the caudal aspect of the pancreatic body, posterior to the body of the stomach *(ST)*. *LL,* Left lobe of liver; *sma,* superior mesenteric artery; *lrv,* left renal vein. **B,** Sagittal sonogram just to the right of **A.** The pancreatic body *(pb)* lies anterior to the junction of the splenic and superior mesenteric veins *(sv-smv),* whereas the uncinate process of the pancreatic head *(u)* lies behind *smv. cha,* Common hepatic artery; *LL,* left lobe of liver; *st,* stomach; *rgepv,* right gastroepiploic vessel; *vc,* inferior vena cava. **C,** Sagittal MRI through the abdominal aorta *(ao)*. Major vessels are well shown but appear nearly as black as the right crus *(rc)* and air within the stomach *(ST)*. **D,** High-resolution sonogram of gastric wall. Submucosa *(sbm)* is echogenic, as are mucosal *(muc)* and serosal *(ser)* interfaces. Muscularis mucosae *(msm)* and muscularis *(mus)* layers are echo poor. Air within gastric lumen obscures the far wall of the stomach. *LL,* Left lobe of liver.
C from Kazam E et al: Cross-sectional anatomy of the abdomen. In Taveras JM, Ferrucci JT, eds: *Radiology,* Philadelphia, 1986, JB Lippincott.

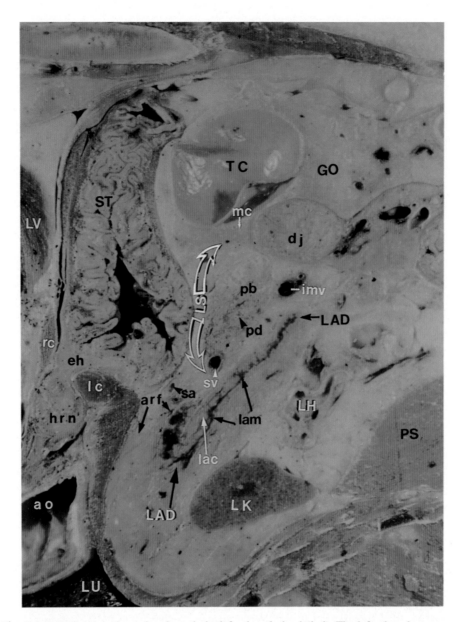

Fig. 2-9 Sagittal anatomic section through the left adrenal gland *(lad)*. The left adrenal appears as a ribbon folded on itself superiorly and extends from just above the medial upper pole of the left kidney *(LK)* to the left renal hilus *(LH)*. The left adrenal cortex *(lac)* has a golden-yellow pigment, whereas the left adrenal medulla *(lam)* has a brownish red pigmentation because of central and medullary veins. The anterior renal fascia *(arf)* separates the left adrenal gland from the splenic vessels *(sa, sv)*. *pb,* Pancreatic body; *pd,* pancreatic duct; *imv,* inferior mesenteric vein; *dj,* duo-denojejunal flexure; *Tc,* transverse colon; *ls,* lesser sac; *ST,* stomach; *eh,* left lateral margin of esophageal hiatus; *hrn,* left lateral margin of sliding hernia; *rc,* right crus; *lc,* left crus; *ao,* de-scending thoracic aorta; *LU,* lung; *LV,* left ventricle; *PS,* psoas muscle.
Modified from Whalen JP, Evans JA, Shanser J: *Am J Roentgenol* 113:104, 1971.

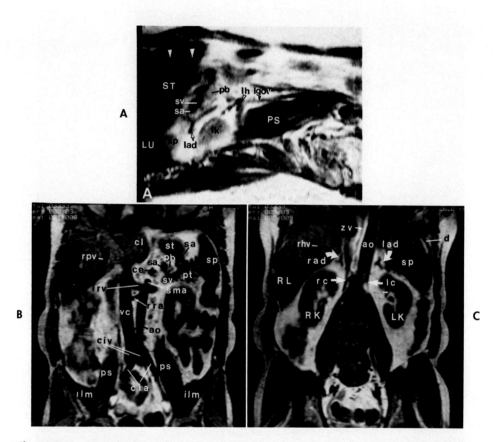

Fig. 2-10 A, Sagittal MRI at approximately the same level as Fig. 2-9. The left adrenal gland *(lad)* has a Y-shaped appearance and extends inferiorly toward the vessels in the left renal hilus *(lh)*. *Igov,* Left gonadal vein; *lk,* medial upper pole of left kidney; *sa,* splenic artery; *sv,* splenic vein; *pb,* pancreatic body; *ST,* stomach with air-fluid level *(arrowheads); sp,* medial spleen; *PS,* psoas muscle; *LU,* lung. **B,** Coronal MRI through aorta *(ao)* and vena cava *(vc)*. The left renal vein *(lrv)* lies anterior to the aorta, directly below the superior mesenteric artery *(sma). rra,* Right renal artery; *ce,* celiac axis. Portions of tortuous splenic artery *(sa)* can be seen cephalad to the pancreatic body *(pb)* and tail *(pt). sv,* Splenic vein; *sp,* spleen; *st,* posterior gastric fundus; *cl,* caudate lobe of liver; *rpv,* right portal vein; *civ,* common iliac veins; *cia,* common iliac arteries; *ps,* psoas muscle; *ilm,* iliacus muscle. **C,** Coronal MRI 2.5 cm posterior to **B.** Left *(lad)* and right *(rad)* adrenal glands are visible at the superomedial aspect of the left *(LK)* and right *(RK)* kidneys. *rc,* Right, and *lc,* left diaphragmatic crura; *zv,* azygos vein; *ao,* aorta; *RL,* right lobe of liver; *rhv,* right hepatic vein; *sp,* spleen; *d,* diaphragm.
A from Kazam E et al: Cross-sectional anatomy of the abdomen. In Taveras JM, Ferrucci JT, eds: *Radiology,* Philadelphia, 1986, JB Lippincott.

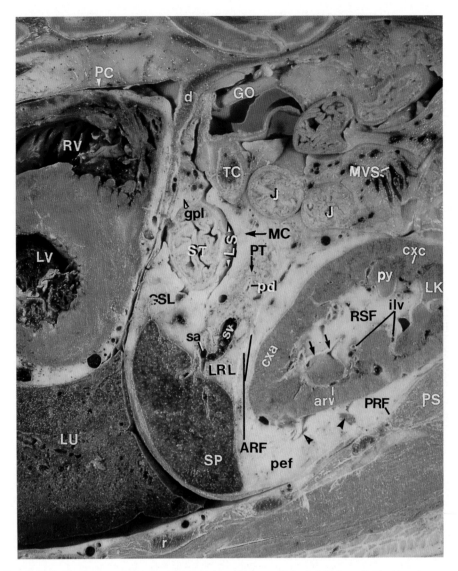

Fig. 2-11 Sagittal anatomic section through the midplane of the left kidney *(LK)*. Abundant renal sinus fat *(rsf)* extends along interlobar *(ilv)* and arcuate *(arv)* vessels. Cortical arches *(cxa)* and columns *(cxc)* have coarser texture than the medullary pyramids *(py)*. Renal calyx *(arrows); pef*, perirenal fat with fibrovascular septa *(arrowheads); ARF*, anterior, and *PRF*, posterior renal fascia. The posteromedial spleen *(sp)* extends posterior to the renal upper pole and, if enlarged, can displace the left kidney inferiorly. The pancreatic tail *(pt)* lies anteroinferior to the splenic artery *(sa)* and vein *(sv)*, surrounded by fat in the lienorenal ligament *(LRL). pd*, Pancreatic duct. The inferior recess of the lesser sac *(LS)* separates the lienorenal ligament from the gastrosplenic ligament *(gsl)*, which extends anteriorly to the stomach *(ST)* and superiorly to the diaphragm *(d)* as the gastrophrenic ligament *(gpl)*. The transverse mesocolon *(mc)*, coursing anteriorly from the caudal aspect of the pancreatic tail to the transverse colon *(TC)*, forms part of the inferior boundary of the lesser sac, which extends anteriorly and superiorly to the greater omentum *(GO)*. From this section, as well as from Figs. 2-7 and 9, the lesser sac and its peritoneal boundaries clearly form an extensive barrier that impedes access of lower intraperitoneal fluid collections to the left diaphragm. One also can easily see that overlying gas and fat obscure the pancreatic tail on sonography, making CT the procedure of choice for noninvasive visualization of this structure. *j*, Jejunum; *mvs*, mesenteric vessels; *PS*, psoas muscle; *LU*, lung; *LV*, left ventricle; *RV*, right ventricle; *PC*, pericardium; *r*, rib.

Modified from Whalen JP, Evans JA, Shanser J: *Am J Roentgenol* 133:104, 1971.

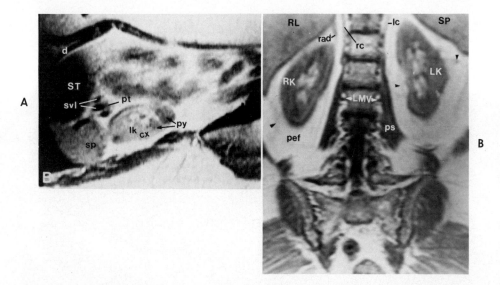

Fig. 2-12 A, Sagittal MRI at approximate level of Fig. 2-11. The spleen *(sp)*, an intraperitoneal organ, extends posterior to the left kidney *(lk)*. The pancreatic tail *(pt)* lies at the anteroinferior aspect of the splenic vessels *(svl)*. *cx,* Renal cortex; *py,* medullary pyramid; *ST,* stomach; *d,* diaphragm. **B,** Coronal MRI through midkidneys *(LK, RK)*. Perirenal fat *(pef)*, with multiple fibrovascular septa *(arrowheads)*, surrounds the kidneys and outlines the lateral contours of the psoas muscles *(ps)*. *rad,* Right adrenal gland; *rc,* right, and *lc,* left diaphragmatic crura. The posteromedial spleen *(sp)* and the right lobe of the liver *(RL)*, both intraperitoneal structures, are well positioned to displace the kidneys inferiorly, if enlarged. *Lmv,* Lumbar veins.
A from Kazam E et al: Cross-sectional anatomy of the abdomen. In Taveras JM, Ferrucci JT, eds: *Radiology*, Philadelphia, 1986, JB Lippincott.

PANCREAS

The pancreas extends obliquely across the abdomen from the hilum of the spleen to the medial border of the duodenal sweep.[15,20]

The *pancreatic tail* is the most proximal portion of the gland and typically has the highest location (Figs. 2-10*B*, 11, 12, 15, 16 *A*, 17, 19, 20*A,B*, 29, 30 *A*). The tail lies anterior and usually caudal to the splenic vessels, within the splenorenal fold of peritoneum, and is therefore an intraperitoneal structure. The pancreatic tail may be thin and tapered (Figs. 2-17, 20 *B*) or thick and bulbous (Figs. 2-19, 20*A*).

The *pancreatic body* extends across the midline, behind the peritoneum and anterior to the splenic and superior mesenteric vessels (Figs. 2-8 *A-C*, 9, 10 *B*, 15, 16 *A,D*, 17, 18 *B,E*, 20*A,B,E*, 22 *A,C-E*). At this point the left renal vein crosses the midline between the aorta and superior mesenteric vessels. Occasionally the pancreatic body is the most superior portion of the gland (Fig. 2-20*D*). This body may have a prominent anterior convexity or omental tuberosity (Fig. 2-17), which may be mistaken for a mass.

The *pancreatic neck* is a thin connection between the pancreatic body and head (Figs. 2-21, 22 *A,C-D*). The neck is contiguous to the right anterolateral margin of the superior mesenteric vein at its junction with the splenic vein.

The *pancreatic head* lies anterior to the vena cava, caudal to the portal vein, and superior to the transverse duodenum (Figs. 2-4 *A,C,* 5, 6 *A,C,* 21, 22 *A,C-E,* 23, 24 *A-D,* 26*A,B,* 27, 28 *A,* 30 *A*). The *uncinate process* is the only portion of the pancreas that lies posterior to the superior mesenteric vessels (Figs. 2-8 *B,E,* 23, 24 *A,D*). The gastroduodenal artery (Figs. 2-20 *B,E,* 22 *A,C-E*) is a good marker for the anterior, but not the lateral, border of the pancreatic head.

The distal common bile duct lies within 5 mm of the posterior border of the pancreatic head but usually does not reliably demarcate its lateral border (Figs. 2-22 *A,C-E,* 24*A*). Thus the pancreatic head can protrude posterolateral to the gastroduodenal artery and common bile duct to invaginate the descending duodenum[18] (Fig. 2-23). This normal variant should not be mistaken for a pancreatic mass. Occasionally the common bile duct courses lateral to the pancreatic head, within the peripancreatic fat medial to the duodenum. Also occasionally, the pancreatic head lies to the left of the midline, anterolateral to the aorta. In such cases the common duct follows a transverse oblique course toward Vater's ampulla.

Text continued on p. 61.

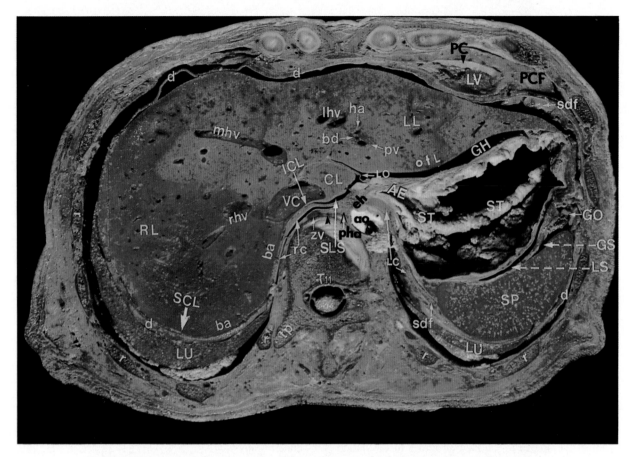

Fig. 2-13 Transverse anatomic section through the upper liver. The middle hepatic vein *(mhv)* divides the liver into right *(RL)* and left *(LL)* lobes of approximately equal volume. *rhv, lhv,* Right, and left hepatic veins. The inferior vena cava *(vc)* is retrohepatic rather than intrahepatic as it runs in a groove on the posterior surface of the liver. Attachments of superior *(SCL)* and inferior *(ICL)* coronary ligaments demarcate the bare area *(ba)* of the liver, which is devoid of peritoneum. Subphrenic fluid cannot extend medial to the *SCL* attachment at this level. The caudate lobe *(CL)* projects into the superior recess of the lesser sac *(sls)*. The lesser omentum *(LO)* extends from the stomach *(ST)* into the anterior part of this superior recess or into the fissure for the ligamentum venosum *(flv)*. The left lobe has mild posterior convexity, or omental tuberosity *(otl)*, toward the lesser omentum. *GH,* Gastrohepatic space; *Go,* greater omentum; *LS,* lesser sac, inferior recess; *GS,* gastrosplenic space. The spleen *(SP)* contains islands of white follicles *(arrows)* representing periarteriolar lymphatic tissue, or *white pulp. Red pulp (arrowheads)* contains splenic cords and sinusoids. *AE,* Abdominal esophagus; *rc, lc,* Right and left crus. The esophageal hiatus *(eh)* lies directly behind the anteromedial aspect of the right crus and contains phrenic ampulla *(pha)* of the esophagus. *ao,* Aorta within aortic hiatus; *zv,* azygos vein; *LV,* left ventricle; *PC,* pericardium; *PCF,* pericardial fat; *sdf,* subdiaphragmatic fat. The eleventh thoracic vertebra *(T11)* has posteriorly angled transverse processes *(tp)*, in contrast to the horizontal transverse processes of the lumbar vertebrae. *r,* Rib.

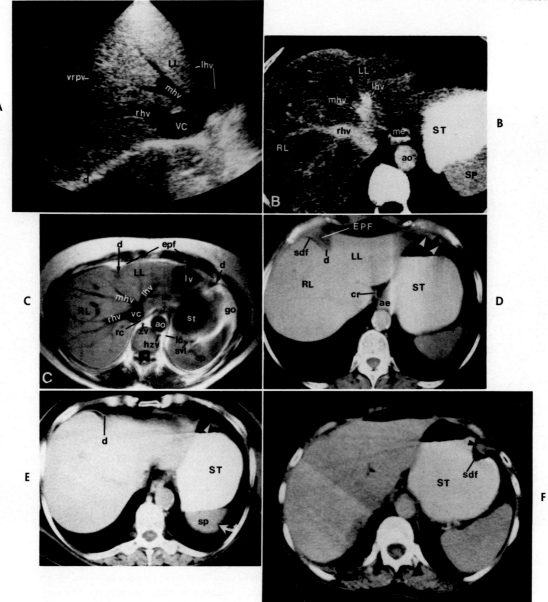

Fig. 2-14 A, Transverse sonogram corresponding to Fig. 2-13. Middle *(mhv)* and left *(lhv)* hepatic veins form a short common trunk just before they join the inferior vena cava *(vc)*. The right hepatic vein *(rhv)* separates right *(RL)* and left *(LL)* lobes of the liver. *vrpv,* Ventral branch right portal vein; *d,* diaphragmatic interface. **B,** Transverse CT at approximate level of Fig. 2-13. The hepatic veins are clearly delineated with intravenous contrast media against a background of fatty liver parenchyma. Middle *(mhv)* and left *(lhv)* hepatic veins form a common trunk before joining the vena cava (see also **A**). *rhv,* Right hepatic vein; *RL, LL,* right and left lobes of liver; *me,* mediastinal esophagus; *ao,* aorta; *ST,* stomach; *SP,* spleen. **C,** Transverse MRI of the upper liver. Right, middle, and left hepatic veins *(rhv, mhv, lhv)* are clearly delineated as black (no signal) tubular structures near their junction with the vena cava *(vc)*. *RL, LL,* Right and left lobes of liver; *ae,* abdominal esophagus; *st,* stomach; *sp,* spleen; *svl,* splenic vessels. Invaginations of the diaphragm *(d)* indent the liver and stomach. *epf,* Extrapleural fat; *go,* greater omental fat; *rc, lc,* right and left diaphragmatic crura; *ao,* aorta; *zv, hzv,* azygos, hemiazygos veins; *lv,* left ventricle. **D-F,** Diaphragmatic pseudofissures and pseudotumors. **D,** CT in deep inspiration shows invagination of the liver by the diaphragm *(d)*, forming an accessory hepatic fissure, at approximate level of junction of the right and left lobes *(RL, LL)*. *EPF,* Extrapleural (extradiaphragmatic) fat; *sdf,* subdiaphragmatic fat. Diaphragmatic infoldings also form pseudotumors or nodules *(arrowheads)* anterior to the stomach *(ST)*. *ae,* Abdominal esophagus; *cr,* crural margin of esophageal hiatus (compare with **C**). **E,** Expiratory CT of approximately same portion of the liver as in **D**. The diaphragm *(d)* appears much thinner than in **D** and does not extend as deeply into the accessory fissure, which appears narrower than in **D**. Diaphragmatic pseudonodule *(arrowhead)* anterior to the stomach *(ST)* is also less prominent than in **D**. Postero-superior spleen is lobulated *(curved arrow)* but not visibly invaginated by the diaphragm at this point. **F,** Infolded diaphragm *(arrowhead)* forms a pseudotumor that indents the stomach *(ST)* but is separated from it by subdiaphragmatic fat *(sdf)*.

B to F from Kazam E et al: Cross-sectional anatomy of the abdomen. In Taveras JM, Ferrucci JT, eds: *Radiology,* Philadelphia, 1986, JB Lippincott.

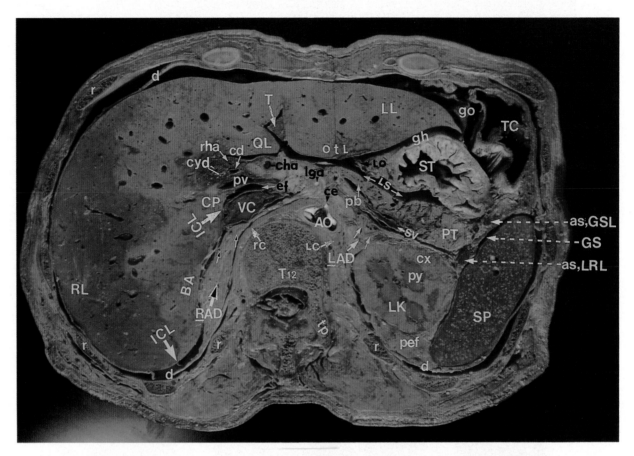

Fig. 2-15 Transverse anatomic section through the upper portion of the pancreatic tail. The pancreatic tail *(pt)* lies behind the stomach *(ST)* within the lienorenal ligament *(LRL)*—a peritoneal fold that extends from the left kidney *(LK)* to the spleen *(SP)*. In essence, the pancreatic tail is an intraperitoneal structure. Fibrofatty interlobular septa traverse the pancreatic parenchyma. The pancreatic body *(pb)* extends to the left, anterior to the celiac axis *(ce)* and aorta *(ao)*. *lga,* Left gastric artery; *sv,* splenic vein. The inferior recess of the lesser sac *(LS)* lies anterior to the pancreas. Its lateral border is formed by the gastrosplenic ligament *(GSL)*, and the inferior recess is separated from the gastrohepatic space *(gh)* by the lesser omentum *(LO)*. Small accessory spleens *(as)* are seen within both the lienorenal and gastrosplenic ligaments. The epiploic foramen *(ef)* to the lesser sac lies between the portal vein *(pv)* and the vena cava *(vc)*. The common duct *(cd)* lies anterior and to the right of the portal vein, whereas the common hepatic artery *(cha)* lies anteriorly and to the left. Portions of undulating cystic duct *(cyd)* are visible lateral to the common duct. *cp,* Caudate process; *RL,* right lobe of liver. The inferior coronary ligament *(ICL)* is attached posteriorly to the diaphragm *(d)* and anteromedially to the right renal fascia to form the hepatorenal ligament. Subphrenic fluid cannot extend medially over the bare area of the liver *(ba)* between attachments of the inferior coronary ligament. Ligamentum teres *(T)*, or obliterated left umbilical vein, can be seen within its fissure, separating the lateral segment of the left lobe of the liver *(LL)* from the medial segment, or quadrate lobe *(QL)*. The right adrenal gland *(RAD)*, surrounded by perirenal fat, has a Y-shaped configuration, with central, medial, and lateral rami *(black-on-white arrows)*. The left adrenal gland *(LAD)* has an inverted-T configuration, also with three major rami *(white arrows)*. Each adrenal gland lies just lateral to its respective diaphragmatic crus *(rc, lc)*.

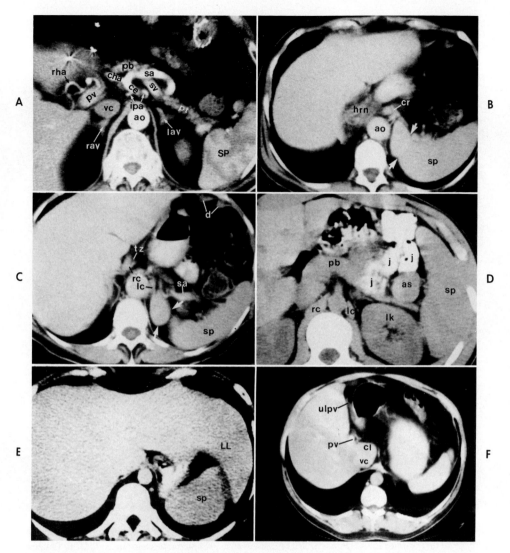

Fig. 2-16 A, CT section through the pancreatic tail *(pt)* shows cobblestone pattern for the pancreatic parenchyma because of fat within the interlobular septa (compare with Fig. 2-15). *pb,* Pancreatic body. The celiac axis *(ce)* is opacified on this contrast-enhanced dynamic scan, along with its common hepatic *(cha),* splenic *(sa),* and inferior phrenic *(ipa)* branches. *ao,* Aorta; *rha,* right hepatic artery. The splenic and portal veins *(sv, pv)* and to a lesser extent the vena cava and adrenal veins *(vc, rav, lav)* are also opacified. The patchy opacification of the spleen *(sp)* is normal and reflects initial enhancement of the periarteriolar white pulp, just before the bolus of contrast reaches the splenic sinusoids. **B-D,** Variations in splenic sectional anatomy. **B,** The spleen *(sp)* has a lobulated medial component *(arrows)* that is nearly contiguous to the aorta *(ao).* *hrn,* Sliding hiatal hernia; *cr,* hypertrophied crural margin of esophageal hiatus. **C,** CT 12 mm below **B.** The spleen *(sp)* now appears totally separated from its medial component *(arrows),* which may mimic a renal or adrenal mass. *sa,* The right and left crura *(rc, lc)* appear hypertrophied. *tz,* Treitz' ligament; *d,* invaginations of the diaphragm. **D,** The accessory spleen *(as)* lies medial to the spleen *(sp)* within the lienorenal ligament. *lk,* Left kidney; *pb,* pancreatic body; *j,* jejunum. **E and F,** Variations in left hepatic lobe anatomy. **E,** The lateral segment of the left lobe *(LL)* is elongated a transversely and curves around the anterior tip of the spleen *(sp).* This configuration is most common in asthenic individuals, especially women. In contrast, endomorphic individuals tend to have a transversely short lateral segment with prominent omental tuberosity (compare with Figs. 2-15 and 17). **F,** The lateral segment of the left lobe is congenitally absent. Umbilical portion of the left portal vein *(ulpv)* is extrahepatic. *pv,* Portal vein; *cl,* caudate lobe; *vc,* vena cava.
From Kazam E et al: Cross-sectional anatomy of the abdomen. In Taveras JM, Ferrucci JT, eds: *Radiology,* Philadelphia, 1986, JB Lippincott.

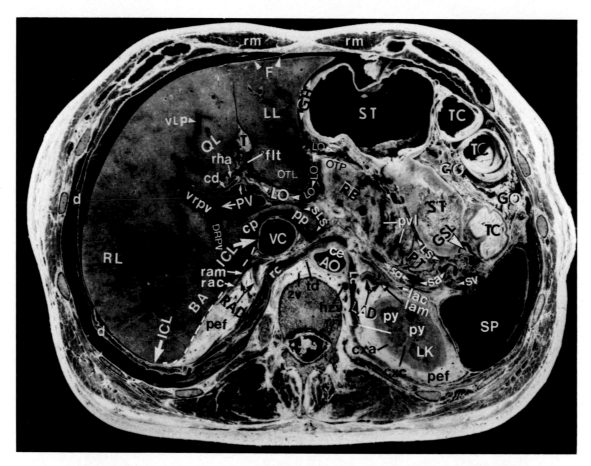

Fig. 2-17 Transverse anatomic section through the pancreatic tail *(PT)*. The pancreatic tail and body *(PB)* lie posterior to the stomach *(ST)* and anterior to the splenic vessels *(sa, sv)*. *OTP,* Omental tuberosity of pancreatic body. Intrapancreatic vessels *(pvl)* traverse the pancreas within the interlobular septa between lobules of glandular tissue. *sp,* Spleen; *LS,* lesser sac; *GSL,* gastrosplenic ligament; *GO, LO,* greater, lesser omentum; *TC,* distal transverse colon. The lateral segment of the left lobe *(LL)* is short in transverse diameter, with prominent omental tuberosity *(OTL),* unlike its appearance in Fig. 2-15. The fissure for the ligamentum teres *(flt)* separates the lateral segment of the left lobe from the medial segment of (inferiorly) the quadrate lobe *(QL). T,* Ligamentum teres; *F,* falciform ligament. The main portal vein *(PV)* divides into a large right branch *(straight arrow)* and a smaller left branch *(curved arrow). vrpv, drpv,* Ventral, dorsal branches of right portal vein; *vlp,* ventral branch of left portal vein to quadrate lobe; *cd,* common duct; *rha,* right hepatic artery. Caudate process of the liver *(cp)* extends between the portal vein and vena cava *(VC)* to connect the right lobe *(RL)* with the caudate lobe. The papillary process of the caudate lobe *(pp)* protrudes into the superior recess of the lesser sac *(sls).* Attachments of the inferior coronary ligament *(ICL)* mark the inferior aspect of the bare area of the liver *(BA).* The right adrenal gland *(RAD)* lies behind the vena cava, lateral to the right crus *(rc),* whereas the left adrenal *(LAD)* lies behind the splenic vessels, lateral to the left crus *(lc).* Cholesterol-laden adrenal cortices *(rac, lac)* have a yellowish pigment, whereas the adrenal medullas *(ram, lam)* have a brownish color mainly because of central veins. *pef,* Perinephric fat; *LK,* left kidney; *cxa, cxc,* renal cortices; *py,* medullary pyramids.

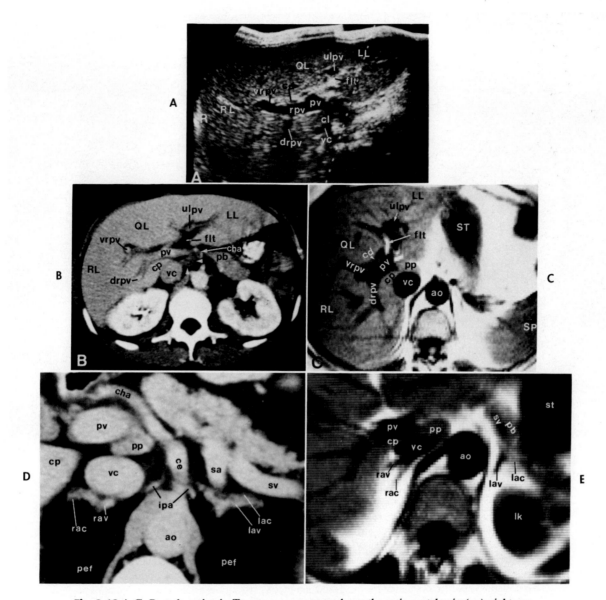

Fig. 2-18 A-C, Porta hepatis. **A,** Transverse sonogram shows the main portal vein *(pv)*, right portal vein *(rpv)*, and its ventral *(vrpv)* and dorsal *(drpv)* branches. *ulpv,* Umbilical portion left portal vein; *flt,* fissure for ligamentum teres; *cd,* common duct; left lobe—lateral segment *(LL)*, quadrate *(QL)*, right *(RL)*, and caudate *(cl)* lobes of liver; *vc,* vena cava. **B,** Transverse CT at approximate level of Fig. 2-17. The portal vein *(pv)* and its branches are isodense with the liver but clearly outlined with periportal fat. Caudate *(cp)* and papillary *(arrowheads)* processes are separated by a groove on the inferior surface of the caudate lobe. **C,** Transverse MRI at approximately the same level as Fig. 2-17. Vascular structures are clearly delineated from the liver by virtue of a signal void associated with flowing blood. **D** and **E,** Adrenal glands. **D,** Contrast-enhanced CT shows clear delineation between the adrenal cortex peripherally *(rac, lac)* and the adrenal medulla and veins centrally *(rav, lav)*. *pef,* Perinephric fat; *ao,* aorta; *ce,* celiac axis; *ipa,* inferior phrenic arteries; *cha,* common hepatic artery; *vc,* vena cava; *sa,* splenic artery; *sv,* splenic vein; *cp,* caudate, and *pp,* papillary processes. **E,** MRI obtained with inversion recovery technique. Good differentiation exists between adrenal veins *(rav, lav)*, which appear black, and the surrounding gray adrenal cortex *(rac, lac)*.

From Kazam E et al: Cross-sectional anatomy of the abdomen. In Taveras JM, Ferrucci JT, eds: *Radiology,* Philadelphia, 1986, JB Lippincott.

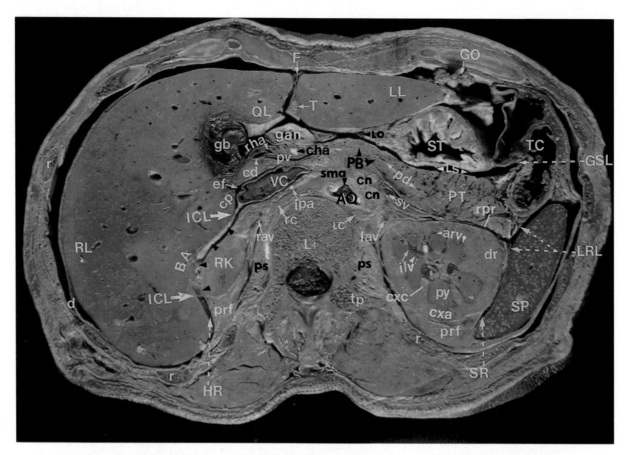

Fig. 2-19 Transverse anatomic section through the pancreatic tail. Lobulated, bulbous contour of the pancreatic tail *(PT)* is a normal variant (compare with Fig. 2-17). Gastrosplenic *(GSL)* and lienorenal *(LRL)* ligaments are continuous medially along the lateral border of the lesser sac *(LS)*. Celiac lymph nodes *(cn)* lie posterior to the splenic vein *(sv)* and posterior to the pancreatic body *(pb)*. Enlargement of these nodes can obscure contours of the adjacent left adrenal gland, which is difficult to see on this section but can be localized by means of the left adrenal vein *(lav)*. *ao,* Aorta; *sma,* superior mesenteric artery. The fissure for the falciform ligament *(F)* is continuous posteriorly with the fissure for the ligamentum teres *(T)*, between lateral *(LL)* and medial segments of the left lobe of the liver. The fetal (left) umbilical vein courses within the falciform ligament to the posterior aspect of the fissure for the ligamentum teres, where it ascends to join the umbilical portion of the left portal vein. The gallbladder *(gb)* lies within its fissure, posterolateral to the medial segment of the left lobe or, at this level, the quadrate lobe *(QL)*. In contrast, the gastric antrum *(gan)* lies posterior and medial to the quadrate lobe. The right anterolateral relationship of the common duct *(cd)* to the portal vein *(pv)* is maintained. *cha,* Common hepatic artery. The right hepatic artery *(rha)* lies anterior to the common duct in this subject but more often courses posterior to the common duct (see Fig. 2-4A). The caudate process *(cp)* protrudes into the lateral aspect of the epiploic foramen *(ef)*, anterior to the vena cava *(VC)*. Attachments of the inferior coronary ligament *(ICL)* demarcate a much narrower bare area of the liver *(ba)* when compared with higher anatomic sections (see Figs. 2-13, 15, 17). Attachment of the inferior coronary ligament to the right renal fascia to form the hepatorenal ligament is indicated by black arrowheads. Posterior subhepatic or hepatorenal space *(HR)*, also known as Morison's pouch, lies behind the upper pole of the right kidney *(RK)* and is marginated anteriorly by the inferior coronary ligament and the right hepatic lobe *(RL)*. Analogous to Morison's pouch is the splenorenal recess *(SR)*, which lies posterolateral to the left kidney and medial to the spleen *(SP)*. The splenorenal recess is continuous anteromedially with the intraperitoneal retropancreatic recess *(rpr)*. The left renal cortical arches *(cxa)* and columns *(cxc)* are clearly delineated from the medullary pyramids *(py)*. The dromedary hump *(dr)* of the left kidney is composed entirely of renal cortex in this subject.

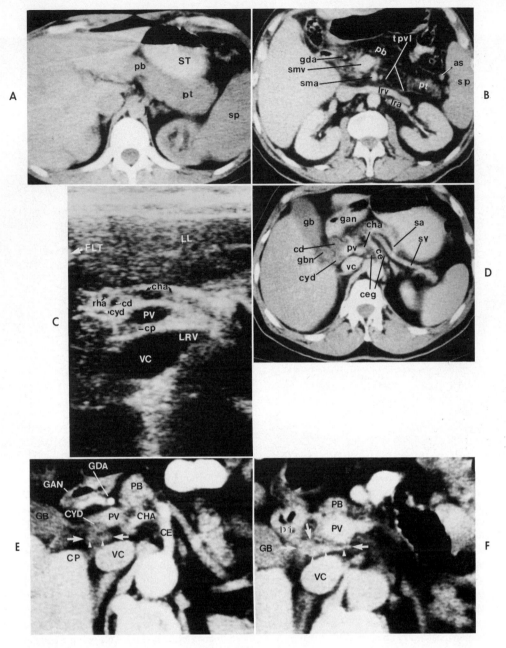

Fig. 2-20 A and **B,** Variations in pancreatic tail morphology. **A,** CT in a young individual shows a thick pancreatic tail *(pt)* with smoothly outlined contours. Interlobular septa seen in Figs. 2-15, 17, and 19 are not visible here. **B,** Fatty atrophy of the pancreas *(pt, pb)* is present in this elderly man. *tpvl,* Transverse pancreatic vessel; *sp,* spleen; *as,* accessory spleen; *sma,* superior mesenteric artery; *smv,* superior mesenteric vein; *gda,* gastroduodenal artery; *lra,* left renal artery; *lrv,* left renal vein. **C,** Transverse portacaval sonogram. The common duct *(cd)* lies at the right anterolateral aspect of the portal vein *(pv)* to the right of the common hepatic artery *(cha). rha,* Right hepatic artery; *cyd,* cystic duct; *cp,* caudate process; *vc,* vena cava; *lrv,* distal left renal vein; *flt,* fissure for ligamentum teres; *LL,* lateral segment of left lobe of liver. **D,** Transverse portacaval CT. Dilated cystic duct *(cyd)* courses along the posterolateral aspect of the portal vein *(pv). cd,* Common duct; *gan,* gastric antrum; *vc,* vena cava; *gb,* gallbladder; *gbn,* gallbladder neck; *cha,* common hepatic artery; *ce,* celiac axis; *ceg,* celiac ganglion, or nodes; *sa, sv,* splenic artery, vein. **E** and **F,** Portacaval (epiploic foramen) lymph nodes. **E,** Dynamic contrast-enhanced CT scan shows a rectangular structure formed by relatively lucent retroportal nodes *(arrows)* and contrast-enhanced pancreaticoduodenal vessels *(arrowheads).* These structures are located within the superior hepatoduodenal ligament at the epiploic foramen. The cystic duct *(CYD)* lies within the same ligament posterior to the portal vein *(PV). VC,* Vena cava. **F,** The CT scan 12 mm below **E** shows a conglomerate of slightly denser retroportal lymph nodes *(arrows)* and vessels *(arrowheads)* within the superior hepatoduodenal ligament, between the portal vein *(PV)* and vena cava *(VC). GB,* gallbladder; *Dl,* duodenal bulb.

A, B, and **D** from Kazam E et al: Cross-sectional anatomy of the abdomen. In Taveras JM, Ferrucci JT, eds: *Radiology,* Philadelphia, 1986, JB Lippincott; **E** and **F** from Zirinsky K et al: *Radiology* 156:453, 1985.

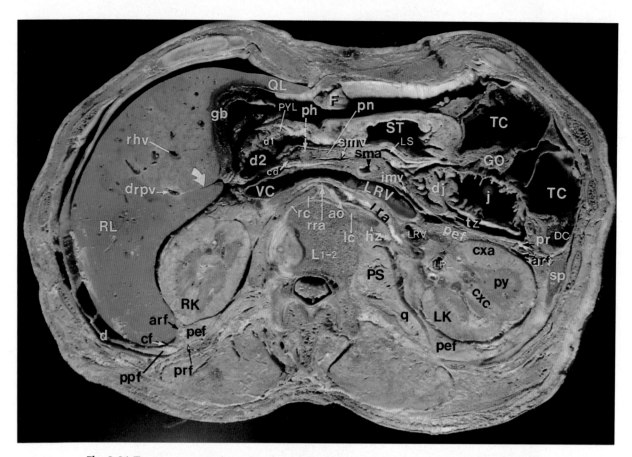

Fig. 2-21 Transverse anatomic section through the upper portion of the pancreatic head. The pancreatic head *(ph)* lies anterior to the vena cava *(VC)* behind the pylorus *(pyl)* and duodenal bulb *(dl)*. The common bile duct *(cd)* is visible at the posterior aspect of the pancreatic head. The pancreatic neck *(pn)* connects the pancreatic head and body and is contiguous to the superior mesenteric vein *(smv)*. The left renal vein *(LRV)* traverses the midline, between the superior mesenteric artery *(sma)* and aorta *(ao)*, to join the vena cava. Thus *LRV* is a good anatomic marker for the upper pancreatic head and neck. *d2,* Descending duodenum; *ST,* lower body of stomach; *LS,* lesser sac. The inferior mesenteric vein *(imv)* courses anteriorly from left to right in front of *LRV* and behind the duodenojejunal flexure *(dj)* to join the splenic or superior mesenteric veins at a higher level. The proximal right renal artery *(rra)* is displaced anteriorly by a rather large right diaphragmatic crus *(rc)* as it courses laterally to the right kidney *(RK)*. The proximal left renal artery *(lra)* is more posteriorly oriented as it courses over the much thinner left crus *(LC)*. This oblique-coronal orientation of origins of the renal arteries from the aorta makes it possible to demonstrate these vessels with oblique-coronal sonography through the right lobe of the liver *(RL)* (see Fig. 2-22 *F*). Right subphrenic and subhepatic spaces are continuous at this level, which is below the attachments of the right coronary ligaments. The gallbladder *(gb)* is again seen within its fossa, posterolateral to the quadrate lobe *(QL)*. A small accessory hepatic fissure *(curved arrow)* extends lateral to the gallbladder fossa toward the dorsal portal venous branch *(drpv)*. *rhv,* Right hepatic venous tributary; *F,* falciform ligament. The greater omentum *(GO)* extends between the stomach and the distal transverse colon *(TC)*, whereas Treitz' ligament *(tz)* can be seen behind the duodenojejunal flexure. The posterior parietal peritoneum *(pr)* is closely approximated to the anterior renal fascia *(arf)* in front of the left kidney *(LK)*, leaving only a thin fat plane between these two layers for the anterior pararenal space. *pef,* Perirenal fat; *rsf,* renal sinus fat. The anterior relationship of the left renal vein to the left renal artery is maintained at the left renal hilum. *LP,* Left renal pelvis. The psoas muscle *(PS)* is contiguous laterally to the perirenal fat. *q,* Quadratus lumborum muscle. On the right, a small amount of posterior pararenal fat *(ppf)* is noted posterolateral to the posterior renal fascia *(prf)* and lateroconal *(cf)* fascia. On the left, the inferior tip of the spleen *(sp)* is visible, but the phrenicocolic ligament, which should course at this level between the junction of the transverse descending colon *(DC)* and the left diaphragm, posteroinferior to the splenic tip, is not clearly delineated.

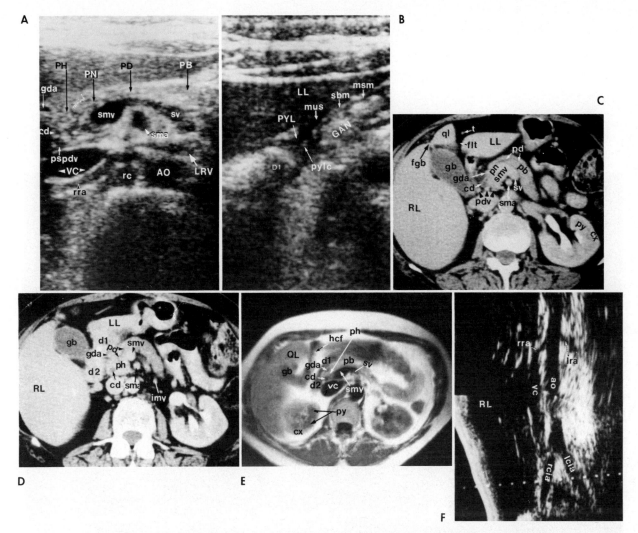

Fig. 2-22 A, Transverse sonogram through the upper pancreatic head *(ph)*. The pancreatic neck *(pn)* extends anterior and to the right of the superior mesenteric vein *(smv)* between the pancreatic head and body *(pb)*. *pd,* Pancreatic duct. The gastroduodenal artery *(gda)* courses anterior to the pancreatic head, whereas the common duct *(cd)* is visible posteriorly. *pspdv,* Posterior superior pancreaticoduodenal veins; *vc,* vena cava; *LRV,* left renal vein; *rra,* right renal artery; *rc,* right crus; *ao,* aorta. **B,** Transverse high-resolution sonogram of the pylorus. Muscularis layer *(mus)* of the gastric antrum *(gan)* shows considerable thickening at the level of the pyloric sphincter *(pyl)*. *pylc,* Pyloric canal; *Dl,* duodenal bulb. Echo-poor gastric muscularis mucosae *(msm)* and echogenic submucosa *(sbm)* are clearly delineated. *LL,* Lateral segment of the left lobe of liver. **C** and **D,** CT scans through the upper pancreatic head and neck. The pancreatic duct *(pd)* is clearly visible as a lucent tubular structure in the pancreatic body and neck *(pb, pn)*, with a characteristic posterior dip into the pancreatic head *(ph)*. *cd,* Common duct; *sv, smv, imv,* splenic, superior, and inferior mesenteric veins; *gda,* gastroduodenal artery; *arrowheads,* pancreaticoduodenal vessels; *d1, d2,* duodenum; *QL,* quadrate lobe; *gb,* gallbladder; *fgb,* fissure for gallbladder; *flt,* fissure for ligamentum teres *(t)*. **E,** Transverse MRI through the upper pancreatic head. The pancreatic body *(pb)* and head *(ph)* lie anterior to the splenic *(sv)* and vena cava *(vc)*, respectively. *gda,* Gastroduodenal artery; *cd,* common duct; *d1, d2,* duodenum; *gb,* gallbladder; *QL,* quadrate lobe; *hfc,* hepatic flexure of colon; *cx,* renal cortex; *py,* medullary pyramid. **F,** Oblique coronal sonogram obtained through the right lobe of the liver *(RL)* with the patient in the left posterior oblique position. Aorta *(ao)*, proximal renal arteries *(rra, lra)*, and proximal common iliac arteries *(rcia, lcia)* are displayed just as they may be seen with aortography. A portion of the vena cava *(vc)* is also visible.

C to **F** from Kazam E et al: Cross-sectional anatomy of the abdomen. In Taveras JM, Ferrucci JT, eds: *Radiology,* Philadelphia, 1986, JB Lippincott.

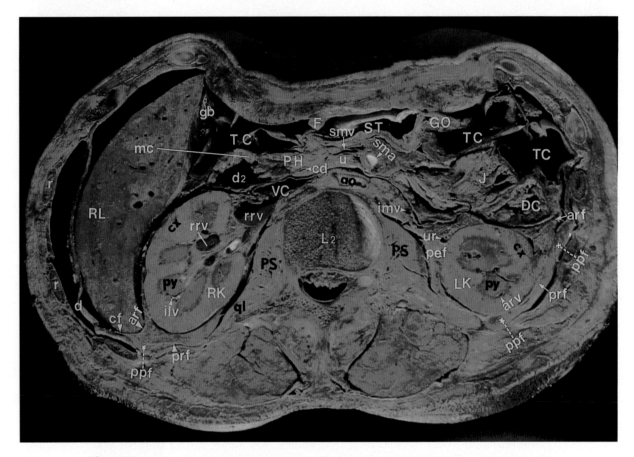

Fig. 2-23 Transverse anatomic section through the lower pancreatic head. The pancreatic head *(PH)* lies anterior to the vena cava *(VC)* and behind the hepatic flexure of the transverse colon *(TC)*. Tonguelike extension of the pancreatic parenchyma between the common bile duct *(cd)* and descending duodenum *(D2)* is a normal variant. Thus the common duct is good marker for the posterior border, but not for the lateral margin, of the pancreatic head. Uncinate process *(u)* is the only portion of the pancreas that lies behind the superior mesenteric vessels *(sma, smv). mc,* Transverse mesocolon; *ST,* inferior part of gastric body; *GO,* greater omentum; *j,* jejunum; *DC,* descending colon.

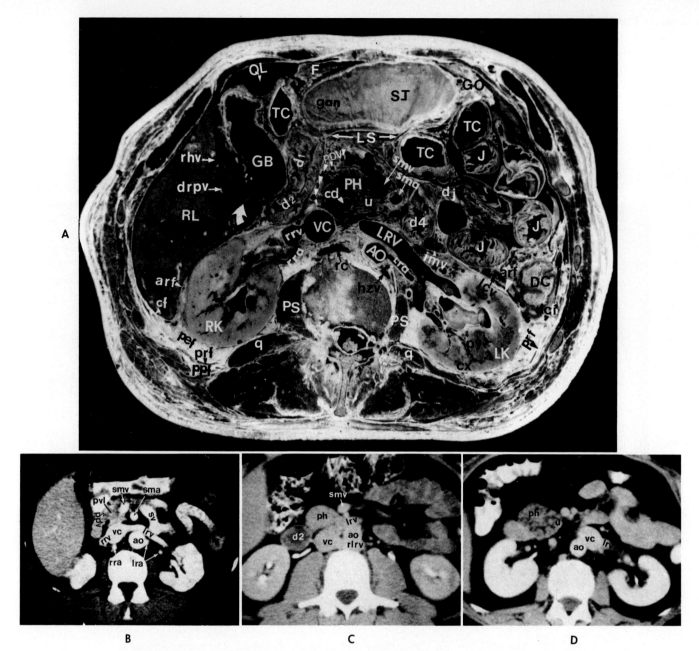

Fig. 2-24 A, Transverse anatomic section through the lower pancreatic head *(PH).* The pancreatic head is thicker in this endomorphic subject than in mesomorphic individual of Fig. 2-23. *u,* Uncinate process; *sma, smv,* superior mesenteric vessels. The distal common bile duct *(cd)* courses through the posterior aspect of the pancreatic head. An arcade of pancreaticoduodenal vessels *(PDV)* lies between the pancreatic head and duodenum *(d1, d2).* The left renal vein *(lrv)* is a good marker for the pancreatic head. *VC,* Vena cava; *rrv,* right renal vein; *ao,* Aorta; *lra, rra,* left, right renal arteries. The gallbladder *(GB)* lies posterolateral to the quadrate lobe *(QL),* whereas the transverse colon *(TC)* and gastric antrum *(gan)* lie posterior or posteromedial to the quadrate lobe. *RL,* Right lobe of liver; *curved arrow,* accessory right hepatic fissure; *drpv,* dorsal-branch right portal vein; *rhv,* right hepatic venous tributary; *RK, LK,* right, left kidneys; *arf, prf,* anterior, posterior renal fascia; *cf,* lateroconal fascia; *pef, ppf,* perinephric, posterior pararenal fat. **B,** Dynamic CT scan through the pancreatic head. There is excellent opacification of the splenic *(sv),* superior mesenteric *(smv),* peripancreatic *(ppv),* and intrapancreatic *(pvl)* veins. The aorta *(ao),* superior mesenteric artery and vein *(sma, smv),* vena cava *(vc),* and both renal veins *(rrv, lrv)* are also opacified. *lra, rra,* Left, right renal arteries. **C,** Transverse CT through the lower pancreatic head *(ph)* shows a relatively thin anteroposterior dimension in this mesomorphic individual (compare with Fig. 2-23). The aorta *(ao)* is surrounded by a circumaortic left renal vein, with anteaortic *(lrv)* and retroaortic *(rlrv)* components. *vc,* Vena cava; *smv,* superior mesenteric vein; *d2,* descending duodenum. **D,** Transverse CT through the lower pancreatic head *(ph)* shows a relatively thick anteroposterior dimension in this endomorphic individual. Interlobular septa are clearly delineated by fat (compare with **A**). The vena cava *(vc)* has crossed to the left of the aorta *(ao)* at this level but was normal in position on higher sections, not shown here. *lrv,* Left renal vein.

B to **D** from Kazam E et al: Cross-sectional anatomy of the abdomen. In Taveras JM, Ferrucci JT, eds: *Radiology,* Philadelphia, 1986, JB Lippincott.

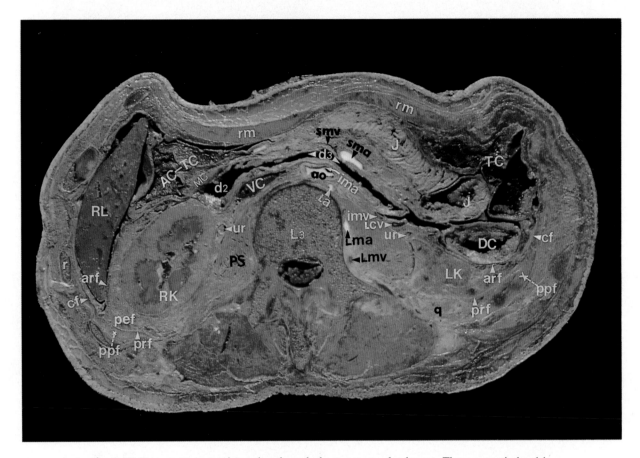

Fig. 2-25 Transverse anatomic section through the transverse duodenum. The pancreatic head is no longer visible. The transverse duodenum *(d3)* crosses the midline anterior to the aorta *(ao)* and posterior to the superior mesenteric artery *(sma)* and vein *(smv)*. The inferior mesenteric artery *(ima)* arises from the aorta just behind the transverse duodenum at the third lumbar vertebral level *(L3)*. The distal descending duodenum *(d2)* rests on the anteromedial surface of the right kidney *(RK)*. The transverse mesocolon *(mc)* extends between the descending duodenum and the hepatic flexure of the colon *(AC-TC)*. The inferior mesenteric *(imv)* and left colic *(lcv)* veins are antero-medial to the left ureter *(ur)*. *LK,* Lower pole of left kidney; *arf, prf,* anterior, posterior renal fascia. Posterior pararenal fat *(ppf)* extends anterolateral to the lateroconal fascia *(CF)* to form a flank stripe. *Lma,* Lumbar artery; *Lmv,* lumbar vein.

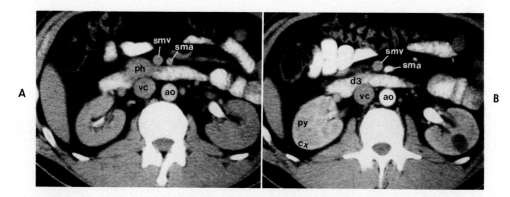

Fig. 2-26 A and **B,** CT scans through the inferior pancreatic head and transverse duodenum. The transverse duodenum *(d3)* marks the inferior boundary of the pancreatic head *(ph)*. The aorta *(ao)* and superior mesenteric artery *(sma)* are opacified in **B,** which was obtained in the arterial phase of dynamic CT scanning. *smv,* Superior mesenteric vein; *vc,* vena cava; *cx,* renal cortex; *py,* medullary pyramid.
From Kazam E et al: Cross-sectional anatomy of the abdomen. In Taveras JM, Ferrucci JT, eds: *Radiology,* Philadelphia, 1986, JB Lippincott.

The *pancreatic duct* has a variable undulating course that may take it close to the anterior and posterior surfaces of adjacent portions of the same pancreas.[15,20] On ultrasound the duct appears as a tubular structure with echogenic walls (Fig. 2-22 *A*). On CT the duct appears as a tubular lucency (Fig. 2-22 *C,D*). The pancreatic duct has a characteristic posterior dip into the pancreatic head (Fig. 2-22 *C,D*). Occasionally the duct runs within a groove on the posterior surface of the pancreas (Figs. 2-5, 7, 9, 11). In such cases it may be difficult to differentiate on CT from the thin fat plane between the splenic vein and pancreatic body or tail.

The *pancreatic parenchyma* is divided into acinar lobules by multiple fibrous septa (Figs. 2-17, 19). These interlobular septa are visible with sectional images when they contain sufficient fat. In such cases the pancreas has a cobblestone texture (Figs. 2-16 *A,* 20 *B,* 24 *D*), which contrasts with its smooth appearance in individuals with minimal septal fat (Figs. 2-18*B,* 20*A,* 24*C,* 26*A*). Parenchymal arteries and veins course along these septa (Fig. 20 *A,* 24 *C,* 26*A*). Parenchymal arteries and veins course along these septa (Fig. 2-17) and may be visible with MRI or contrast-enhanced CT (Fig. 2-24 *B*). Marked parenchymal fatty atrophy may be seen in obese elderly individuals (Fig. 2-20*B*) and should not be mistaken for the fatty atrophy of chronic pancreatitis.

ADRENAL GLANDS

The adrenal glands lie within the perinephric fat at the anterosuperior and medial aspects of the kidneys[15,21] (Figs. 2-3, 4 *B,C,* 9, 10 *A,C,* 15, 17, 18 *D,E,*). The *right adrenal gland* lies posterolateral to the inferior vena cava and is smaller and higher in position than the *left adrenal gland,* which lies behind the splenic vessels and gastric fundus.

Both glands extend inferiorly toward the renal hila (Figs. 2-3, 9, 10*A*). The inferior tip of the longer left adrenal gland lies just above the left renal vein.

In sagittal section the adrenals have the appearance of a ribbon that is folded on itself (Figs. 2-3, 4 *B,C,* 9, 10*A*). In transverse section they may have a Y - or T-shaped configuration with lateral and medial rami on either side of a central ramus (Figs. 2-15, 17, 18 *D,E*). The right lateral ramus is contiguous to the bare area of liver, whereas the right medial ramus extends behind the vena cava toward the right diaphragmatic crus (Figs. 2-15, 17, 18 *D,E*). The left lateral ramus often points posterolaterally behind the splenic vessels, whereas the left medial ramus extends posteriorly or transversely toward the left crus (Figs. 2-15, 17, 18 *D,E*).

The *adrenal cortex* is rich in cholesterol and has a golden-yellow color because of lipochrome pigmentation (Figs. 2-15, 17). The *adrenal medulla* has a reddish brown color, at least partly because of the medullary venous sinusoids and *central vein.* The *right central vein* generally drains anteriorly into the vena cava (Figs. 2-3, 18 *E,* 30 *B*), whereas the *left central vein* drains inferiorly into the left renal vein. The inner vascular portion of the adrenal gland, which includes the central veins and medulla, can be differentiated from the surrounding cortex with ultrasound, contrast-enhanced CT (Fig. 2-18 *D*), and MRI (Figs. 2-10 *A,* 18*E*).

KIDNEYS

The kidneys lie within the perinephric space and are surrounded by the renal fascia. The *renal cortex* forms a continuous arch around each kidney and extends between the *medullary pyramids* to form cortical columns (Figs. 2-1, 2 *A,C,* 11, 12, 17, 19, 21, 22 *E,* 24 *A,* 26 *A,B,* 27). The

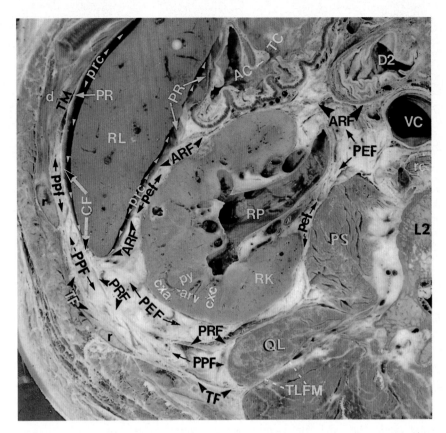

Fig. 2-27 Transverse anatomic section showing extraperitoneal perirenal compartments. The anterior renal fascia *(ARF)* fuses with the posterior renal fascia *(PRF)* behind the posterolateral portion of the right lobe of the liver *(RL)* to form the lateroconal fascia *(CF)*, which in turn continues anterolaterally to fuse with the parietal peritoneum *(PR)*. The anterior pararenal space lies anterior to the anterior renal fascia and posterior to the parietal peritoneum. On the right side, this space contains the ascending colon *(AC)*, descending duodenum *(d2)*, and pancreatic head *(PH)* but is reduced to only a thin potential compartment in the absence of these structures. Similarly, the left anterior pararenal space, which contains the distal duodenum, pancreatic body, and colon, is very narrow in the anteroposterior dimension below the duodenal sweep (see Fig. 2-19). The perirenal space lies between the anterior and posterior renal fascia and contains the kidney *(RK)*, renal pelvis *(RP)* ureter, adrenal, and perirenal fat *(PEF)*. Perirenal fat outlines most of the lateral border of the psoas muscle *(PS)* and blends with fat around the vena cava *(VC)* and aorta. Multiple fibrous septa, some of which contain blood vessels, traverse the perirenal fat. Perirenal fluid collections often extend into the posteromedial perirenal fat, where they obscure the lateral border of the psoas muscle. Note the medial extension of the anterior renal fascia *(ARF)* anterior to the vena cava. There is CT evidence for continuity of perirenal spaces across the midline, behind the anterior renal fascia, and in front of the lower vena cava and aorta. Thus, in effect, the lower aorta and vena cava are located within the midline continuity of perirenal spaces. The posterior pararenal space lies behind the posterior renal fascia *(PRF)* and in front of the transversalis fascia *(TF)* and contains posterior pararenal fat *(PPF)*, which extends anterolaterally to form a flank stripe. Blood in the posterior pararenal space can extend into the flank (Turner's sign) or can continue anteromedially between the transversalis fascia and peritoneum to discolor the umbilicus (Cullen's sign). Medial posterior pararenal fat outlines the lateral contour of the quadratus lumborum muscle *(Q)*. Note the middle layer of the thoracolumbar fascia *(TLFM)*, which fuses with the transversalis fascia behind this muscle. Three extraperitoneal pararenal compartments become continuous below the kidneys.

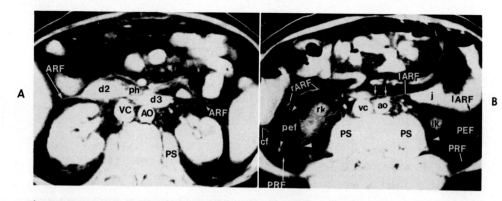

Fig. 2-28 A and **B,** In vivo CT appearance of the renal fascia. **A,** CT scan through midkidneys. The anterior renal fascia *(ARF)* is inseparable from the posterior parietal peritoneum. *ARF* is not visible in the midline, although its projected medial extension would lie anterior to the aorta *(ao)* and vena cava *(vc)*. **B,** CT scan through lower renal poles *(rk, lk)*. The right anterior renal fascia *(rARF)* appears continuous medially with the fascia *(arrows)* in front of the vena cava *(vc)* and aorta *(ao)*. The left anterior renal fascia *(lARF)* is not visualized directly behind the opacified jejunal loop *(j)* but may be seen more medially and laterally. Also seen are the posterior renal fascia *(prf)*, lateroconal fascia *(cf)*, perirenal fat *(pef)* with fibrous septa *(arrowheads),* and psoas muscles *(ps)*.
From Kneeland JB et al: *Radiology* 164:657, 1987.

medullary pyramids are more homogenous in texture than the cortex, probably because of the multiple acoustic interfaces created by the cortical renal corpuscles. There are 1 to 2 million such corpuscles in each kidney,[15] with each unit consisting of a glomerulus and a membranous capsule that forms the beginning of a renal tubule. The papillary tips of the medullary pyramids project into the renal sinus. *Renal sinus fat* surrounds the collecting system and blood vessels at the renal hilum.

The renal cortex and medulla can be differentiated with sonography (Fig. 2-2 *A*), MRI (Figs. 2-2 *C, 12 A, 22 E*), and contrast-enhanced CT, particularly with dynamic scanning (Figs. 2-16*B,* 26 *B*). The renal sinus fat generally appears echogenic on ultrasound (Fig. 2-2 *A*), although it may occasionally contain multiple echo-poor areas mimicking dilated calyces or parapelvic cysts. Fat extending along the interlobar and arcuate vessels accounts for their echogenicity on sonography. On CT and MRI renal sinus fat has a characteristic appearance, resembling perinephric and mesenteric fat.

A *hypertrophied cortical column* is a normal variant that may mimic a mass on intravenous pyelography. This column can be most confidently diagnosed with dynamic CT, which can document its early opacification and isodensity with the renal cortex.

The *dromedary hump* of the left kidney is a normal localized thickening of renal cortex at the medial border of the spleen (Fig. 2-19). Again, this hump can be most confidently diagnosed with dynamic CT scanning.

RETROPERITONEAL COMPARTMENTS

The extraperitoneal space at the level of the kidneys is divided by the renal fascia into three retrospective compartments (Figs. 2-9, 11, 21, 23, 24 *A,* 25, 27, 28 *A,B*). The *anterior pararenal space* lies between the posterior parietal peritoneum and the anterior renal fascia. This space contains the duodenum, pancreatic head and body, and ascending and descending colon. The *perirenal space* lies between the anterior and posterior layers of the renal fascia and contains kidneys, adrenals, and surrounding fat. The perirenal fat outlining the psoas muscle is a valuable landmark for localizing large posterior abdominal masses with CT.[22] The *posterior pararenal space* lies between the posterior renal fascia and transversalis fascia. This space extends into the flank as the properitoneal fat, lateral to the lateroconal fascia, which is formed by the fusion of anterior and posterior renal fascia. Within this posterior compartment retroperitoneal effusions can extend into the flank toward the anterior abdominal wall and umbilicus.

Perirenal fat extends superiorly to outline the medial diaphragms and crura. The two perirenal compartments may communicate with each other anterior to the aorta and vena cava, at and below the third lumbar vertebral level. Thus the aorta and vena cava lie either within the perinephric space or within a compartment of their own, separated from the perirenal space by fibrofatty septa. Multiple fibrovascular septa also traverse the perirenal fat (Figs. 2-12 *B,* 27). Below the kidneys the perinephric, anterior pararenal, and posterior pararenal spaces become continuous.[23]

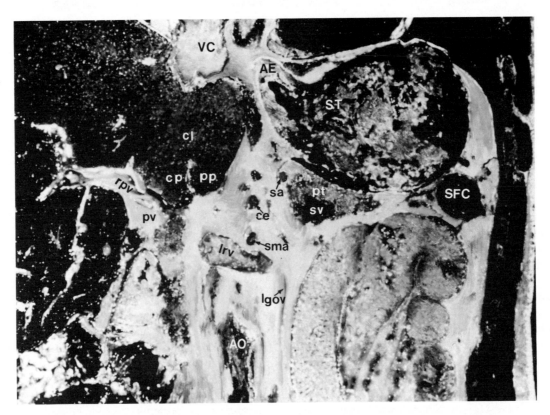

Fig. 2-29 Coronal anatomic section through the porta hepatis. The main portal vein *(pv)* enters the porta hepatis at the inferolateral aspect of the caudate process *(cp)* of the caudate lobe *(cl)*. *rpv,* Right portal vein; *pp,* papillary process. The left renal vein *(lrv)* courses horizontally below the superior mesenteric artery *(sma)* to join the inferior vena cava *(vc)*. *ce,* Celiac axis; *sa, sv,* splenic artery, vein; *pt,* pancreatic tail; *ao,* aorta; *lgov,* left gonadal vein; *ST,* stomach; *AE,* abdominal esophagus; *sfc,* splenic flexure of colon.
Courtesy Dr. Manuel Viamonte, Miami Beach, Fla.

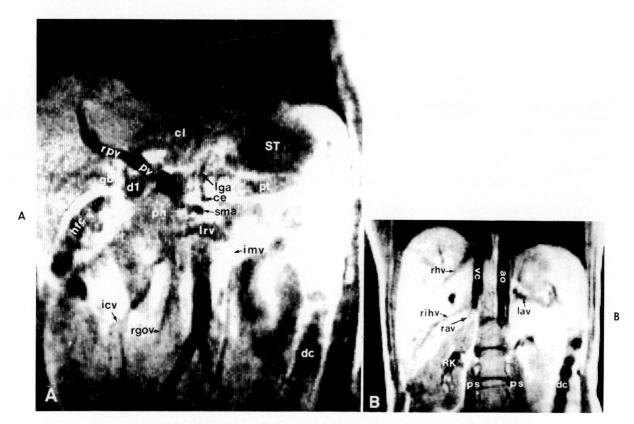

Fig. 2-30 A, Coronal MRI at approximate level of Fig. 2-29 shows the same anatomic relation-ships. Also visible are the pancreatic head *(ph)* and tail *(pt)*, duodenal bulb *(dl)*, celiac *(ce)* and superior mesenteric *(sma)* arteries, left gastric artery *(lga)*, hepatic flexure of colon *(hfc)*, left renal *(lrv)* and right gonadal veins *(rgov)*, ileocolic vein *(icv)*, and inferior mesenteric vein *(imv)*. **B,** Coronal MRI posterior to **A.** The upper aorta *(ao)* and vena cava *(vc)* are visible. *rhv,* Right he-patic vein. The proximity of the junction of the right adrenal vein *(rav)* and right inferior acces-sory hepatic vein *(rihv)* with the vena cava (vc) explains the difficulty usually encountered with selective right adrenal vein catheterization. *RK,* Right kidney; *lav,* left adrenal vein; *dc,* descend-ing colon; *ps,* psoas muscle.
From Kazam E et al: Cross-sectional anatomy of the abdomen. In Taveras JM, Ferrucci JT, eds: *Radiology,* Philadelphia, 1986, JB Lippincott.

ABDOMINAL GREAT VESSELS

The abdominal great vessels and their major branches can be visualized with all three imaging methods (Figs. 2-4 *A-C,* 5, 6 *A-C,* 7, 8 *A-C,* 9, 10*B,C,* 13, 14 *A-C,* 15, 16 *A,B,F,* 17, 18 *A-E,* 19, 20 *C-F,* 21, 22*A,E,F,* 23, 24 *A-D,* 25, 26 *A,B,* 27, 28 *A,B,* 29, 30 *B*). This makes it possible to diagnose major morphologic abnormalities without re-sorting to angiography. On the coronal sections, which are readily available with MRI, the great vessels are displayed just as they appear on angiography (Figs. 2-10 *B,C,* 30 *A,B*). Similar results may be obtained with the versatile and more widely available sonogram, using a coronal oblique view, usually from the right flank[24] (Fig. 2-22 *F*). As al-ready indicated, the abdominal vessels are valuable land-marks for localizing important organs and structures with sectional images. These vessels may also be mistaken for enlarged lymph nodes, especially if they are not opacified on CT.

REFERENCES

1. Whalen JP: *Radiology of the abdomen: an anatomic approach,* Phil-adelphia, 1976, Lea & Febiger.
2. Whalen JP: Caldwell Lecture. Radiology of the abdomen: impact of new imaging methods, *AJR* 133:585, 1979.
3. Kazam E et al: *NMR: anatomic correlations in the body,* New York, 1983, RR Donnelley & Sons.
4. Kazam E et al: Cross-sectional anatomy of the abdomen. In Taveras JM, Ferrucci JT, eds: *Radiology,* vol 4, Philadelphia, 1986, JB Lip-pincott.
5. Rosen A et al: CT appearance of diaphragmatic pseudotumors, *J Com-put Assist Tomogr* 7:995, 1983.
6. Auh YH et al: Accessory fissures of the liver: CT and sonographic appearance, *AJR* 143:565, 1984.
7. Lim JH, et al: The inferior accessory hepatic fissure: sonographic ap-pearance, *AJR* 149:495, 1987.
8. Rubenstein WA et al: The perihepatic spaces: computed tomographic and ultrasound imaging, *Radiology* 149:231, 1983.
9. Auh YH et al: CT of the papillary process of the caudate lobe of the liver, *AJR* 142:535, 1984.
10. Healey JE Jr: Clinical anatomic aspects of radical hepatic surgery, *J Int Coll Surg* 22:542, 1954.

11. Mitty HA, Yeh HC: *Radiology of the adrenals with sonography and CT,* Philadelphia, 1982, WB Saunders.

12. Behan M, Kazam E: Sonography of the common bile duct: value of the right anterior oblique view, *AJR* 130:701, 1978.

13. Kazam E. Schneider M, Rubenstein WA: The role of ultrasound and CT in imaging the gallbladder and biliary tract. In Arger P, Alavi A, eds: *Diagnostic studies in abdominal disease,* New York, 1980, Grune & Stratton.

14. Zirinsky K et al: The portacaval space: CT with MR correlation, *Radiology* 156:453, 1985.

15. Williams PL, Warwick R, eds: *Gray's anatomy,* ed 36, Philadelphia, 1980, WB Saunders.

16. Govoni AF, Whalen JP, Kazam E: Hiatal hernia: a relook, *Radio-Graphics* 3:612, 1983.

17. Machi J et al: Normal stomach wall and gastric cancer: evaluation with high resolution operative ultrasound, *Radiology* 159:85, 1986.

18. Auh YH et al: Posterior hepatodiaphragmatic interposition of the colon: ultrasonographic and computed tomographic appearance, *J Ultrasound Med* 4:113, 1985.

19. Rubenstein WA et al: Posterior peritoneal recesses: assessment using CT, *Radiology* 156:461, 1985.

20. Kazam E et al: Computed tomography of the pancreas. In Wang Y, ed: *CT of the abdomen,* vol 1, Boca Raton, Fla, 1986, CRC Press.

21. Kazam E et al: Sectional imaging of the adrenal glands—CT and ultrasound, with a preview of MRI imaging. In Vaughan ED Jr, ed: *The adrenal glands,* New York, 1988, Thieme.

22. Engal IA et al: Large posterior abdominal masses: computed tomographic localization, *Radiology* 149:203, 1983.

23. Kneeland JB et al: Perinephric spaces: CT evidence for communication across the midline, *Radiology* 164:657, 1987.

24. Pardes JG et al: The oblique coronal view in sonography of the retroperitoneum, *AJR* 144:1242, 1985.

3 Gastrointestinal Physiology

F.P. MCGRATH
GILES W. STEVENSON

ENTERIC NEUROPEPTIDES AND ENTERIC HORMONES

In 1905 Edkins established that the antral mucosa contained a hormone (gastrin) that stimulated the stomach to release acid. Masson was the first to recognize the presence of specialized gut cells in 1914, when he discovered their silver-reducing power. Some 15 distinct endocrine-like cells have since been identified, and the system has been called the *diffuse endocrine system* or the *amine precursor uptake and decarboxylation (APUD) system*.

Major advances in peptide chemistry during the middle of this century allowed elucidation of the structure of many of the gastrointestinal (GI) hormones that had been identified previously based on biologic activity. Gastrin was the first hormone to be purified sufficiently so that its amino acid sequence could be determined[1]; cholecystokinin (CCK)[2] and secretin[3] soon followed. Subsequently, purification and analysis of the amino acid composition of pancreozymin and CCK revealed that they were the same hormone.[2] These structural studies established GI hormones as peptides (i.e., compounds of relatively low molecular weight that, on hydrolysis, yielded two or more amino acids). The recent application of recombinant DNA technology to the field of GI endocrinology has allowed determination of the structure of the DNA that encodes many of these peptides.

Anatomy of the gut-endocrine system

Several substances discovered in recent years function both as neurotransmitters and hormones. Many are found in the brain as well as in the gut and pancreas. In the abdomen they may be produced both by endocrine cells and enteric nerves. They regulate the GI tract in at least four distinct ways—as endocrine, paracrine, neurocrine, and autocrine substances[4] (Fig. 3-1, Table 3-1). Autocrine peptides are released by the same cell upon which they exert their biologic effect. This mode of action has been reported with some small cell carcinomas of the lung that have been shown to synthesize and release gastrin-releasing polypeptide (GRP), but no intrinsic autocrine GI peptides have been reported.[5] Paracrine, neurocrine, and autocrine mechanisms of action ensure that peptides are released in high concentrations locally without being diluted in the bloodstream. This is efficient for conservation of the polypeptide and is also a means by which very high concentrations of potent transmitter substances can be achieved locally without producing systemic effects.

Most functioning endocrine tumors produce one well-defined syndrome, but it is not uncommon for more than one hormone to be produced. However, it is rare for two syndromes to occur simultaneously. Nevertheless, patients with Zollinger-Ellison syndrome who also have hyperinsulinism, adrenocorticotropic hormone (ACTH), melanocyte-stimulating hormone (MSH), or 5-hydroxyindoleacetic acid (5-HIAA) syndromes have been described, which reinforces the concept of the APUD system. The APUD cells share a common neural crest origin and, before differentiation, are pluripotential. When they become malignant, the dominant cell is at a primitive level and secretes any one or a variety of hormones and peptides. Given this concept, it is not surprising that most of the islet cell tumors that secrete multiple peptides have been malignant.

Gastrin

Gastrin is found in G cells in the gastric antrum and duodenum and is released rapidly after ingestion of a meal. This hormone is responsible for the acid secretion that occurs in response to the presence of food. Gastrin also regulates the growth of the acid-producing part of the gastric mucosa. Excessive gastrin from tumor, hyperplasia, or retained antrum produces acid hypersecretion and hyperplasia of acid-secreting mucosa and consequently peptic ulcer and diarrhea.

Interestingly, coffee is a potent stimulator of gastrin release, an effect that persists even after coffee is decaffeinated.[6] Wine also has this effect, but pure alcohol does not,[7] suggesting the presence of unidentified small stimulant peptides in these substances.

Some hormones and neurotransmitters, such as GRP, stimulate the release of gastrin,[8,9] whereas others, such as somatostatin, inhibit release.[10] GRP is the mammalian equivalent of the amphibian peptide bombesin and is the most potent stimulator of gastrin release identified in humans.[9] One recent model proposed by Soll and Berglindh[11] suggests that gastrin interacts with other secretagogues such as histamine and acetylcholine so that the interruption of one step considerably reduces the overall effectiveness of the remaining substances for acid secretion (Fig. 3-2). The effect of H_2 blockers therefore is to limit histamine release

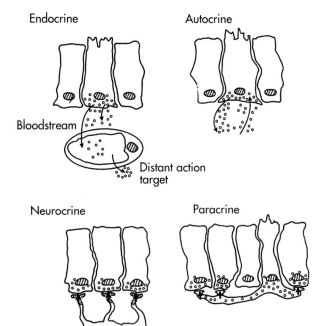

Endocrine   Autocrine

Bloodstream

Distant action
target

Neurocrine   Paracrine

Fig. 3-1 GI tract regulatory peptides—methods of action. The GI regulatory peptides function in at least four distinct ways. *1*, An endocrine substance acts like a classic hormone (i.e., a substance released into the blood to a distant organ to exert its effects). *2*, Autocrine peptides are released by the same cell upon which they exert their biologic effect. *3*, A neurocrine substance is released from nerve endings and acts in the manner of a classic neurotransmitter. *4*, A paracrine substance is released locally to exert its effect on cells in the immediate vicinity of the peptide's cell of origin. Paracrine, neurocrine, and autocrine mechanisms of action ensure that peptides are released in high concentrations locally without being diluted in the bloodstream (see Table 3-1 for a list of the likely roles of many regulatory peptides).

☐ **TABLE 3-1**

Gastrointestinal peptides—likely mechanism of action

Endocrine	Neurocrine	Paracrine
Somatostatin	Somatostatin	Somatostatin
Cholecystokinin (CCK)	Cholecystokinin (CCK)	Peptide YY (PYY)
Gastrin	Gastrin-releasing peptide (GRP)	
Secretin	Opioids	
Insulin	Substance P	
Glucagon	Vasoactive intestinal polypeptide	
Enteroglucagon		
	Neuropeptide Y (NPY)	
Pancreatic polypeptide	Neurotensin	
Neurotensin	Peptide HM (PHM and PHI)	
Motilin	Pancreastatin	
Glucose-dependent insulinotropic peptide (GIP)		
Peptide YY (PYY)		
Urogastrone/epidermal growth factor		

Fig. 3-2 Receptors and pathways regulating parietal cell function. This is a simplified version of the model proposed by Soll and Berglindh[11] for fundic mucosal regulatory pathways based on canine studies. Gastrin, histamine, and acetylcholine *(ACH)*, by acting on their own specific parietal cell receptors, stimulate acid secretion. Somatostatin is the inhibitory pathway through which gastrin, delivered by the capillaries, stimulates a negative feedback control by increasing somatostatin production. Histamine is delivered to the parietal cell by the mast cells located in the lamina propria. Adrenergic cells *(ADR)* appear to have an acid-reducing regulatory role by decreasing mast cell stimulation and enhancing somatostatin production. Conversely ACH, released by postganglionic nerves, produces a positive acid secretory response by reducing somatostatin production and directly enhancing parietal cell acid secretion.

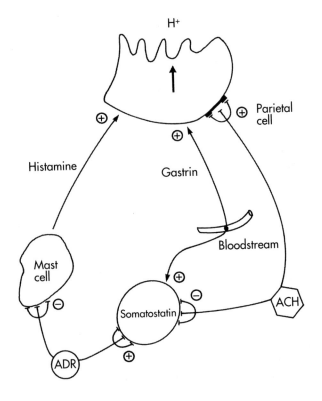

which, based on this model, has a knock-on effect on the other secretagogues.

Cholecystokinin

CCK is secreted by I cells, which are located predominantly in the mucosa of the duodenum and the upper jejunum.[12] Amino acids are a greater stimulant than intact protein for the release of CCK.[8] CCK release is stimulated by a trypsin-sensitive peptide (CCK-releasing peptide [CRP]) that is released into the duodenum.[13] As CCK stimulates pancreatic enzyme secretion, trypsin is released and destroys CRP, thus acting as a feedback control. The physiologic functions of CCK are to stimulate contraction of the gallbladder and the release of pancreatic enzymes into the duodenum.

Secretin

Secretin is produced by the S cells in the duodenal mucosa and is the stimulus for secretion of bicarbonate-rich pancreatic juice. Its release is stimulated by the presence of unbuffered H^+ ions in the duodenum following a meal.

Insulin

A meal is followed by release of enteric hormones that stimulate initial insulin release. This is augmented by the direct effect of rising blood glucose in causing further release of insulin and inhibition of glucagon secretion. The insulin lowers blood glucose by trapping it in the liver for conversion to glycogen and in the muscle and adipose tissue, where more is stored than burned.

Glucagon

Glucagon is best known for its antagonistic action to insulin, raising the blood sugar. Pharmacologically it has an astonishing range of effects and has been very useful to radiologists.[14] It produces an increase in bile flow from the liver and relaxes the gallbladder and Oddi's sphincter. It was advocated as an aid to cholangiography, both scintigraphic and radiologic, and is now used endoscopically to facilitate cannulation of the bile duct. It produces a decrease in gastric and pancreatic secretion, which may improve barium coating. It causes a release of catecholamines from the adrenal medulla, which inhibits the activity of intestinal smooth muscles, producing paralysis. This permits hypotonic barium examination of the stomach and duodenum. The release of catecholamines and the triggering of insulin release, however, provide two contraindications to the pharmacologic use of glucagon, namely in patients with pheochromocytoma or insulinoma, since a crisis can be caused when a pharmacologic dose of glucagon leads to a sudden release of insulin or catecholamine.

The paralytic effect on the lower esophageal sphincter has been used as the therapeutic basis for use of gas granules by mouth, combined with intravenous glucagon, to relieve esophageal bolus impaction. It relaxes the ileocecal valve, increasing the incidence of coloileal barium reflux from 45% to 75%,[15] and also relieves painful colonic spasm and improves the quality of barium enema examinations.

Vasoactive intestinal polypeptide

Vasoactive intestinal polypeptide (VIP) is not found in any endocrine cells but is present in a wide range of neurons in the gut and elsewhere. It probably has a neurotransmitter function in the control of GI relaxation, gut blood flow, and fluid and electrolyte secretion in the pancreas and intestine.

Somatostatin

Somatostatin is the ultimate inhibitory hormone, exciting nothing and inhibiting virtually all exocrine and endocrine functions. It inhibits the release of gastrin, insulin, glucagon, secretin, CCK in the gut and growth hormone from the brain. It is thus a regulatory hormone with no stimulatory effects. It is produced by the D cells of the pancreatic islets.

Distal intestinal peptides

Peptides found within the distal small intestine and colon, such as enteroglucagon, neurotensin, and peptide YY, may function as modulators of the efficiency with which the upper gut handles nutrients. These peptides are released in response to nutrients reaching the distal small bowel and act as an "ileal brake"[16] (Fig. 3-3).

Clinical implications of gut peptides

Virtually every function of the gut appears to be interlinked by a variety of peptide hormones. It is hardly surprising that an alteration in the action or in concentrations of these hormones may be implicated in the pathogenesis of some GI disorders. However, this provides the opportunity to utilize these agents in diagnostic or therapeutic roles.

The *Zollinger-Ellison syndrome* is the most frequently encountered endocrine neoplasm. It is caused by the ectopic secretion of gastrin, which acts as a potent acid secretagogue with the development of recalcitrant peptic ulcers, reflux esophagitis, and diarrhea.[17]

Most islet cell tumors are *insulinomas* (70% to 80%)[18] and produce their clinical effect by hypoglycemia, causing mental confusion, seizures, sweating, tachycardia, and weakness occurring at irregular intervals and relieved by sugar intake (Fig. 3-4). Less than 10% of these B cell tumors will be malignant, and almost all are localized to the pancreas. They are usually single lesions from 1 to 5 cm in size, and their occurrence is evenly distributed throughout the pancreas.[18]

The *Verner-Morrison syndrome* is characterized by profuse watery diarrhea, hypokalemia, achlorhydria, and flushing in 15% of patients and is caused by the ectopic secretion of VIP. VIPomas are located outside the pancreas, especially in the retroperitoneal sympathetic chain and the ad-

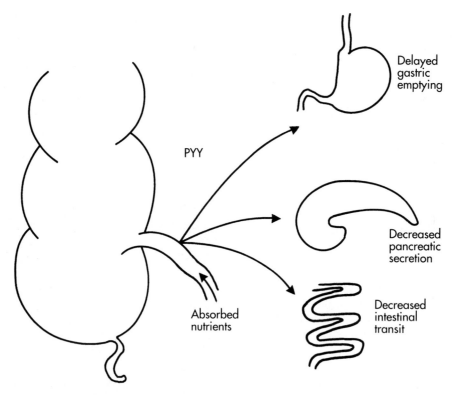

Fig. 3-3 The "ileal brake" concept describes a number of events that promote increased absorption of nutrients bathing the ileum by delaying gastric emptying, decreasing pancreatic secretions, and reducing intestinal motility.[16] Peptide YY *(PYY)* is found in the highest concentrations in the ileum and colon and is thought to play a role in regulating the ileal brake.

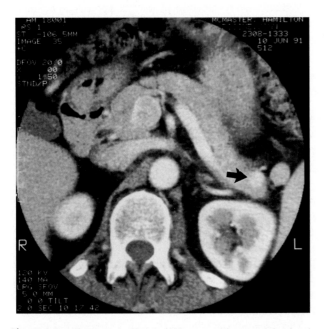

Fig. 3-4 Insulinoma. A 48-year-old man with unexplained episodes of hypoglycemia. CT shows a 1-cm enhancing mass in the pancreatic tail *(arrow)*. Histopathologic assessment found the lesion to be compatible with an insulinoma. The patient's symptoms resolved after a distal pancreatectomy.

renal medulla.[19] Most of these are benign (43%) or malignant (37%) islet cell tumors or islet cell hyperplasia (20%), but 10% are associated with extrapancreatic ganglioneuromas, adrenal tumors, or bronchogenic carcinomas. However, VIP may not always be the sole peptide involved. For example, human pancreatic polypeptide (HPP) is the only peptide known to relax the gallbladder and increase tone in Oddi's sphincter, and gallbladder dilation is a frequent unexplained finding in Verner-Morrison syndrome. Radiologically the principal functional feature is an extremely wet intestine with masses of fluid throughout the GI tract caused by excess secretion and gut relaxation, with the dilated gallbladder serving as a useful clinical clue to the diagnosis.

Other rarer endocrine peptide–secreting tumors include glucagonomas and somatostatinomas. *Glucagonoma* is characterized by an islet cell tumor with hypersecretion of glucagon. Other features include classical skin rash (migrating necrolytic erythema), diabetes mellitus, weight loss, and anemia. The tumor is usually located in the pancreatic body and tail and only rarely in the pancreatic head.[20] Most of these tumors are larger than 3 cm and are relatively easily visualized with the aid of ultrasound, computed tomography (CT), and arteriography. Approximately 70% of these tumors are malignant and metastasize to the liver.[20]

Somatostatinoma is the rarest of the pancreatic endocrine tumors. Patients with this tumor exhibit diabetes mellitus, cholelithiasis, diarrhea, steatorrhea, and gastric achlorhydria. The tumor has a high malignancy potential (50%). Of approximately 20 described in the surgical literature most were located in the pancreatic head.[21,22]

Many of these tumors arise as part of the *multiple endocrine neoplasia syndromes* (MEN), which are predominantly inherited proliferative disorders[23] (Fig. 3-5). Two main types are distinguished. MEN type I is characterized by the combined occurrence of tumors of the pituitary gland, pancreatic islets, and parathyroid. Islet tumors may include gastrinomas, insulinomas, and, rarely, glucagonomas, vipomas, and others. Also a propensity has been noted for carcinoid tumors. MEN type 2A is characterized by pheochromocytoma, medullary thyroid carcinoma, and hyperparathyroidism. MEN type 2B is similar to type 2A but without involvement of the parathyroid glands. It is associated with the development of ganglioneuromas throughout the GI tract and a marfanoid habitus.

Peptide hormones have been used as diagnostic tools for several years.[24] Other peptide hormones are used as adjuncts in a variety of other diagnostic evaluations. In addition to the value of glucagon in radiologic and endoscopic examinations and of CCK as a stimulus to gallbladder contraction, secretin may be used to enhance pancreatic blood flow and aid in the arteriographic demonstration of small pancreatic vessels.

Antagonists to some peptide hormones also have been developed. A long-acting somatostatin analogue (Sandostatin) has proven very useful in alleviating the diarrhea and flushing episodes associated with the malignant carcinoid syndrome, in which there is a hypersecretion of 5 hydroxytryptamine, and has also proven useful in reversing carcinoid crisis[25,26] (Fig. 3-6). The profuse diarrhea associated with Verner-Morrison syndrome (VIPoma) responds well to this agent.[27] Although the only approved uses for Sandostatin are for carcinoid and Verner-Morrison syndromes, there is a long list of possible uses. Those that have raised the most interest are the treatment of enterocutane-

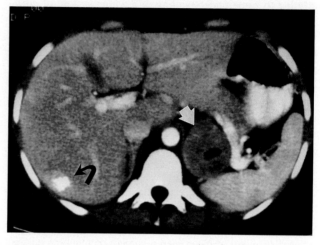

Fig. 3-5 Multiple endocrine neoplasia *(MEN)* type 2A in a 37-year-old woman. CT shows a large adrenal mass *(arrow)*. Fine needle biopsy confirmed the lesion to represent a pheochromocytoma. The dense mass in the right lobe of the liver *(curved arrow)* is a calcified metastasis from a previous medullary carcinoma of the thyroid gland. This tumor also is a component of the MEN type 2A syndrome.

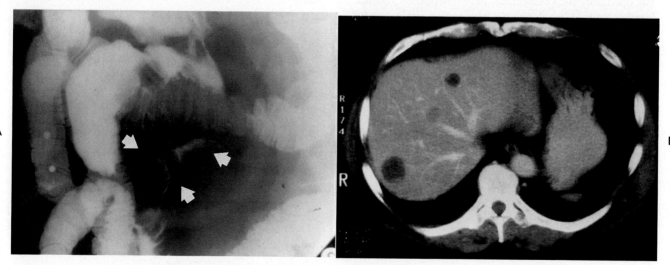

Fig. 3-6 A, Radiograph from a small bowel enema examination in a 46-year-old man with episodes of flushing and diarrhea shows the typical immobile small bowel loop with distorted, thickened, mucosal folds secondary to the local desmoplastic response found with a carcinoid tumor *(arrows)*. **B,** An enhanced CT in the same patient shows metastases in the liver. These were proven at biopsy to be carcinoid deposits and confirmed the clinical suspicion of carcinoid syndrome.

ous fistula[28,29] and of diarrhea in short bowel syndrome.[30] The use of somatostatin to prevent pancreatitis after endoscopic retrograde cholangiopancreatography (ERCP) has not been supported by a recent controlled study,[31] but it may have value in reducing the rate of complications in established acute pancreatitis.[32]

Prostaglandins and the gut

The discovery that human semen has the ability to cause contraction or relaxation of strips of uterine muscle gradually led to some understanding of a whole system of compounds that modify inflammation and whose synthesis is blocked by many of the most widely used antiinflammatory agents, such as aspirin[33] (see Fig. 3-11, A). The prostaglandins are a family of compounds derived from arachidonic acid, a 20-carbon fatty acid that is present in cell membranes and is itself derived from phospholipids. Cyclooxygenase metabolizes free arachidonic acid to cyclic endoperoxidases, which are subsequently altered to various prostaglandin subtypes by tissue-specific processing enzymes. These include prostacyclin (PGI_2), thromboxane, and leukotrienes.

The primary prostaglandins synthesized in the GI mucosa are PGE_2 and $PGF_{2\alpha}$ in a ratio of about 2 to 1.[34] Prostaglandins produced specifically by the gastric mucosal response to acid stimulation have been a subject of much recent interest. Prostaglandins, given orally or intravenously, inhibit both basal and pentagastrin-stimulated gastric acid output, and they also cause an increase in gastric mucosal blood flow, reduction in mucosal H^+ ion back-diffusion, stimulation of mucosal cell turnover, and may be responsible for the increase in blood flow known to occur with acid secretion. In short, they mediate mucosal defense mechanisms.

A deficiency of prostaglandin may predispose to gastric mucosal injury. High doses of adrenocorticosteroids inhibit prostaglandin synthesis by inhibiting the action of phospholipase A_2. Cyclooxygenase inhibitors such as the nonsteroidal antiinflammatory drugs (NSAIDs) and aspirin produce a spectrum of mucosal injury that often leads to ulceration. Indomethacin inhibits prostaglandin synthesis. Pretreatment with prostaglandin protects gastric mucosa against the damage produced by aspirin or indomethacin, an effect called *cytoprotection,* and promotes ulcer healing.[35] Despite much evidence of cytoprotection by prostaglandins, it is still not clear whether it is because of the effect prostaglandins have on reducing gastric acid secretion or the result of a specific cytoprotective effect. However, it is clear that in experimental animals nonalimentary administration of indomethacin, aspirin, or naproxen significantly potentiates gastric mucosal damage by local irritants[36] and that prostaglandins protect small bowel mucosa against NSAID damage. Thus the antral gastric ulcers, usually associated with antiinflammatory drugs, are caused by the drug interfering with the normal protective action of prostaglandin (Fig. 3-7). Currently it appears likely that

prostaglandin analogues (e.g., enprostil) expedite their healing effect by more than one action. Although effective, they lack the potency of the H_2-receptor antagonists. Moreover, diarrhea is reported in 10% to 30% of patients receiving prostaglandin analogues. This is dose related[37] and has limited the widespread use of prostaglandins for duodenal ulceration.

Prostaglandins and irritable bowel

One theory proposed for the etiology of the irritable bowel syndrome is a hypersensitivity reaction to some foods.[38,39] This theory has been supported by the finding of increased levels of PGE_2 content in the stool and jejunal fluid of these patients.[38,40] The increased levels of PGE_2 would be an expected finding in patients who had a gut hypersensitivity reaction to a specific antigen.

Proton pump inhibitors

A new class of antisecretory drugs have recently been developed of which omeprazole is the first to achieve widespread use. This drug acts as an inhibitor of the hydrogen ion pump by limiting the action of H^+/K^+ -ATPase in the gastric parietal cell (see Fig. 3-11, A). It inhibits 90% to

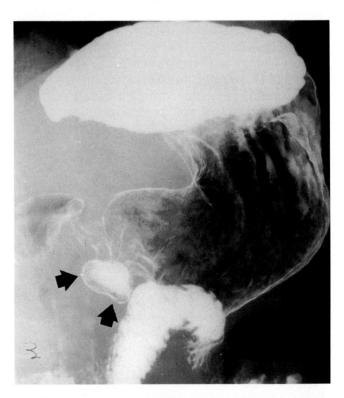

Fig. 3-7 A 78-year-old woman on long-standing indomethacin therapy for rheumatoid arthritis. The barium meal shows a large ulcer crater on the greater curvature of the stomach in the antral region *(arrows).* This is the typical dependent location for ulceration resulting from long-term ingestion of nonsteroidal antiinflammatory medications.

99% of gastric acid secretion in 24 hours as compared with 40% to 68% with conventional doses of H_2 antagonists.[41] It has proved efficacious for acute duodenal ulcers.[42-45] Omeprazole has been shown to yield 4-week healing rates of between 82% to 100%, versus 74% to 80% and 63% to 96%, respectively, for the H_2-receptor antagonists cimetidine and ranitidine.[46] It also appears to have a more rapid ulcer pain relief at 1 to 2 weeks than the H_2-receptor antagonists. Omeprazole has proven very beneficial for the management of gastric acid hypersecretion in patients with Zollinger-Ellison syndrome.[47,48] It is currently the best agent to prevent relapse of treated peptic reflux esophagitis.

OROPHARYNX AND SWALLOWING

The digestive functions of the mouth and pharynx are the mastication of food, mixing it with saliva, and transporting it safely in manageable boluses past the entrance to the airway and into the esophagus. The saliva performs several important functions in the oral cavity. It lubricates the food and the oral and digestive tissues and maintains mucous membrane integrity. Salivary antibiotic activity causes lysis of oral bacteria and has antifungal and antiviral activity, and the neutral pH of saliva also aids in dental protection.[49] Saliva contains a digestive enzyme, amylase, which initiates hydrolysis of starch molecules that reduces food bulk and viscosity and promotes digestion. This enzyme remains active in a bolus of food until it reaches the gastric antrum, where the acid medium has a pH less than 4.

Ninety percent of the volume of saliva comes from the major salivary glands, but 70% of the mucus is secreted by numerous minor salivary glands that are polystomatic (have numerous minor ductules rather than a single duct) and are found in the labial, palatine, buccal, lingual, and sublingual mucosae.

The deficiency of salivary juices produces *xerostomia,* or dry mouth. The cause of this condition is most often iatrogenic and is a result of prescription medications (e.g., antidepressants, antihypertensives, and psychotropic agents). Local causes such as ductal obstruction adenitis may have the same effect. Xerostomia results in increased dental caries, altered taste sensation, poor lubrication of the food bolus, and predisposition to oral infections.

Typically, most individuals swallow from 600 to 1000 times per day, varying from 70 times per hour during waking hours to almost complete absence during deep sleep.[50] The act of swallowing is complex, involving the perfect coordination of some 26 muscles through six cranial nerves and is complete in 1.5 seconds; during this time the radiologist must differentiate normality from abnormality and functional from structural abnormalities.[51] It is clear that motion recording and replay facilities must be an essential requirement for radiologic examination.

Swallowing occurs in two distinct phases. The first is voluntary and involves transfer of the bolus to the oropharynx; the second, involuntary, act sees the bolus swallowed and moved into the esophagus. This is described more fully in Chapters 4-6.

The cricopharyngeal sphincter has intrinsic tone over a length of 2 to 4 cm. The 1-cm band of highest pressure (the upper esophageal sphincter [UES]) represents the loop of cricopharyngeus attached anteriorly on each side to the cricoid cartilage, passing around the pharyngoesophageal junction and compressing the junction against the back of the cricoid. The transverse slit of the closed sphincter thus has higher pressures recorded if the side hole of the recording catheter is anterior or posterior than when it faces laterally. A triangular area of fewer muscle fibers termed *Killian's triangle,* existing posterolaterally between oblique and horizontal components of the cricopharyngeus, is believed to represent the site of Zenker's diverticulum[52] (Fig. 3-8).

Relaxation of the UES is both passive, as forward movement of the larynx changes the laterally oriented slit into a circular space, and active, as electric activity ceases and the muscle actively relaxes. The actual opening of the closed sphincter, however, is passive as the bolus is pushed through by descending peristalsis. Once the peristaltic wave has passed, the larynx falls back and the cricopharyngeus regains its tone.

In one retrospective study of 618 unselected patients who received upper GI barium swallow examinations, evidence of cricopharyngeal abnormalities were seen in 77 patients (10.8%).[53] Dysphagia was found in less than 15% of patients with the cricopharyngeal bar (Fig. 3-9). Most visible cricopharyngeal abnormalities were in fact transient and inconsistent in appearance from swallow to swallow. UES tone is high, up to 142 mm Hg posteriorly,[54] and when acid is instilled into the esophagus, it rises even higher and may cause delayed opening and premature closure of the sphincter. These abnormalities of timing, as well as the transient posterior bulging of the mucosa just above the sphincter, can commonly be observed radiologically. They are usually not associated with dysphagia, may be associated with globus symptoms, and are particularly frequent in reflux disease.[55] Major abnormalities of UES relaxation are uncommon, rarely isolated, and generally occur with lesions affecting the medullary swallowing center (e.g., stroke victims, cerebral trauma).

Esophagus, transit, and acid neutralization

Esophageal and lower esophageal sphincter physiology are discussed in detail in Chapter 11. Although considerable overlap often occurs at the junction between striated and smooth muscle, the control of peristalsis in each of them is quite different.

Contraction of the striated muscle portion is entirely dependent on neural input arising from neurons located in the nucleus ambiguus and is centrally activated by sequential discharge of motor units controlling progressively distal segments in the body of the esophagus. Bilateral vagotomy

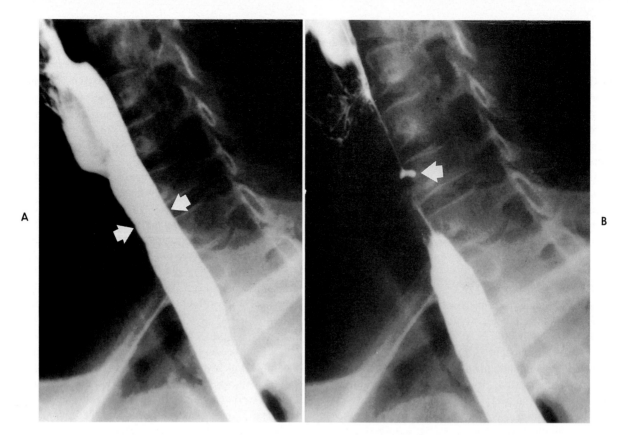

Fig. 3-8 Transient mini-Zenkers diverticulum. **A,** A single spot radiograph from an upper GI swallow examination shows normal distension of the upper esophageal sphincter *(UES)* at the level of the cricopharyngeus *(arrows)*. **B,** As the peristaltic wave sweeps through the UES, a transient weakness at Killian's dehiscence is demonstrated by posterior herniation of the mucosa, lasting less than a second *(arrow)*.

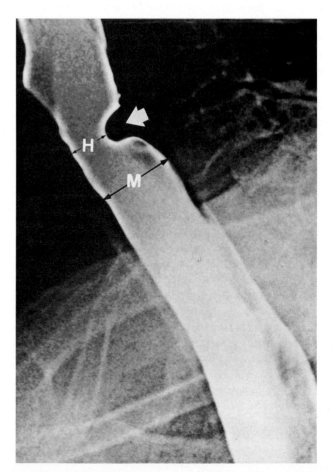

Fig. 3-9 Cricopharyngeal bar. Upper GI swallow examination. The prominent extrinsic defect on the posterior aspect of the cervical esophagus *(arrow)* is caused by hypertrophy and incomplete relaxation of the cricopharyngeus muscle. The degree of hypertrophy *(H)* is calculated as a percentage reduction of the maximal luminal diameter *(M)*, (H/M × 100) in the lateral plane. In this case, 1.5 cm/2.8 cm × 100 is consistent with a 53.6% reduction in maximal luminal diameter.[55]

performed above the origin of the pharyngoesophageal fibers abolishes peristalsis in the striated muscle, whereas peristalsis in the smooth muscle portion can still be stimulated by local distension.[56] The strength and frequency of the peristalsis from striated muscle are affected by both the bolus volume and temperature (i.e., the larger and warmer the bolus the greater the force and duration of the peristaltic wave.[57-59]

In the smooth muscle portion a single inhibitory impulse in nonadrenergic noncholinergic fibers is responsible for the entire esophageal peristaltic wave and the relaxation of the lower sphincter. The progressive nature of the contraction is not caused by central programming but by some property of the muscle itself. If strips of muscle from different points of the esophagus are stimulated, an immediate, brief, unforceful twitch occurs (the "on" response), followed after a latent period by a vigorous response (the "off" response). Muscle from the distal esophagus has a longer latent period than muscle from the mid esophagus.[60] Thus a single inhibitory nerve impulse can produce contractions that occur early in the mid esophagus and later in the distal esophagus. Gradients in potassium concentration appear to be associated with this phenomenon.[61] The same neural impulse inhibits the tonic contraction of the lower esophageal sphincter so that when the bolus arrives the sphincter is relaxed.

Although the lower esophageal sphincter (LES) is tonically contracted, it undergoes periodic collapses of pressure to zero in all normal individuals. When the individual is supine or has a full stomach, gastroesophageal reflux will occur. This happens several times each night and occasionally during the day and is a normal event. When the subject next swallows, the refluxed material is cleared into the stomach by efficient peristalsis. Clearance fails if peristalsis is defective or the individual goes rapidly back into deep sleep, when swallowing does not occur. Peristalsis clears the esophagus of almost the entire volume of fluid, but some hydrogen ions become fixed in the "unstirred" layer of esophageal mucus, so the pH stays low. This acidified mucus layer has to be neutralized by the bicarbonate in saliva, and several dry swallows are required before enough saliva has been swallowed to restore the neutral esophageal pH. This process of dealing with acidified mucus following normal, everyday physiologic reflux is probably one of the most important functions of the salivary glands.

PHYSIOLOGY OF THE STOMACH

There is no gastric absorption of note, apart from alcohol and some drugs. Gastric secretion and motility are the two aspects of interest. Prostaglandin action has given some validity to an old custom involving alcohol. A drink before leaving home "to get in the mood and protect the stomach" once seemed without foundation. However, the administration of a mild gastric irritant has been shown to stimulate prostaglandin release and provide mucosal protection against a later application of the irritant.

Gastric secretion

The stomach secretes five types of substance: acid, pepsin, mucus, intrinsic factor, and a variety of hormones, principally gastrins. Parietal cells secrete acid and intrinsic factor. Chief cells produce pepsinogens that are converted to pepsin by acid, and gastrins are secreted by the G cells of the gastric antrum. Both superficial and neck mucous cells produce mucus. Prostaglandins are secreted by parietal cells and possibly others also.

Acid

Parietal cells or oxyntic cells are generally found in the neck or isthmus of the oxyntic gastric gland and are responsible for gastric acid production and secretion (Fig. 3-10). Food-stimulated acid secretion has traditionally been described in three distinct phases, namely, cephalic, gastric, and intestinal. These phases refer to the site of the stimulus and do not relate to mechanisms of acid secretion.

The three primary stimulants of acid secretion are acetylcholine, gastrin, and histamine (see Fig. 3-2). Acetylcholine is the vagal neurotransmitter and is responsible for most of the cephalic phase of acid secretion. Gastrin is released from antral and duodenal G cells in response to gastric distention and transported to the parietal cell in the bloodstream during the gastric phase. Wine and beer are potent stimuli to acid secretion and serum gastrin. These effects are probably due to amines or amino acids and not

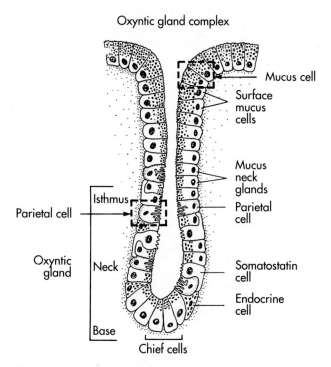

Fig. 3-10 Oxyntic gland complex. The parietal, or oxyntic, cell is found in the isthmus of the oxyntic gland complex, which is located primarily in the gastric antrum and pylorus.
From Ito S: Functional gastric morphology. In Johnson LR, ed: *Physiology of the gastrointestinal tract*, ed 2, New York, 1987, Raven Press.

to a direct alcohol effect.[62] Histamine is a paracrine agent released from mastlike cells of the lamina propria into the intramucosal extracellular fluid, in which it diffuses to the adjacent parietal cell. Balancing inhibitors and stimulators regulate acid secretion. Acid bathing of the gastric antrum powerfully inhibits gastrin production. In the intestine, acid, fat, and hyperosmolar solutions all inhibit gastric acid secretion, although the mechanisms are unclear.

The regulation of acid secretion can be summarized as follows. The parietal cell has three receptors specific for histamine, gastrin, and acetylcholine, with potentiating interactions. The somatostatin cell has receptors for gastrin (excitatory) and acetylcholine (inhibitory), as well as an excitatory receptor from adrenergic nerve fibers (see Fig. 3-2). Thus at the cephalic phase of gastric stimulation, acetylcholine turns on acid production and inhibits somatostatin. Once gastrin and histamine start to respond massively to a meal, the gastrin turns on the regulatory function of somatostatin. The histamine mast cell has several receptors, including one for prostaglandin F2 and an inhibitory receptor for the adrenergic fibers that turn on somatostatin. In the parietal cell the structure changes on stimulation as the tubulovesicles disappear. The collapsed secretory intracellular canaliculus expands from a collapsed, shrivelled state to a swollen sac with long slender microvilli and absorbs the tubulovesicles. In the secretory canaliculus, weak base accumulates, and an H^+, K^+, ATPase high-energy proton pump relocates itself from the tubulovesicles onto the surface of the canaliculus. The pump exchanges potassium for hydrogen ions. When secretion stops the canaliculus collapses, and the intracellular tubulovesicles that store the H^+, K^+, ATPase reappear. Omeprazole, which acts as a proton pump inhibitor and totally prevents release of hy-

drogen ions from the gastric parietal cells, is becoming established as a very effective medical treatment for acid peptic disease and may also provide an effective medical treatment for the extreme acid hypersecretion of Zollinger-Ellison syndrome (Fig. 3-11, *A*).

Pepsin

Proenzyme pepsinogens are secreted by the gastric mucosa in response to food. Concomitant stimulation of the parietal cells provides the acid medium for rapid conversion to the active form, pepsin. Although parietal and chief cells commingle, the density of parietal cells is greater in the upper and midportions of the glands, whereas chief cells are more numerous in the deeper regions of the gland. Only 1% of pepsins are absorbed into the bloodstream—a fundic serum pepsinogen called type I, which is excreted into the urine and might become useful as a tubeless test of gastric secretory capacity. Ninety-nine percent of pepsinogen stays in the stomach and initiates protein digestion. The peptides thus released initiate the release of various hormones, including gastrin and CCK. In this way pepsinogen contributes to the overall regulation of digestion.

Mucus

Mucus secretion is of interest to radiologists, but ways of controlling it for our purposes are not developed.[63] Ninety percent of mucus is water with a glycoprotein matrix, and mucus is a partial barrier to acid and pepsin penetration. Polymerization of the mucus subunits by disulfide bonds is essential for the formation of the hydrated gel.[63] Bicarbonate is secreted by the surface mucosal cells into an unstirred mucus layer, where it is trapped and forms a thin but high concentration barrier to the movement of H^+

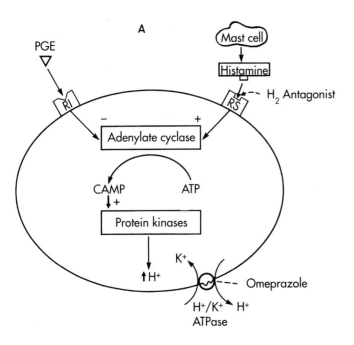

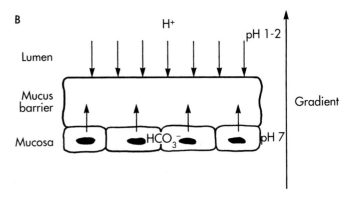

Fig. 3-11 A, Schematic diagram illustrating the sites and mechanisms of action of the more commonly prescribed antiulcer medications (H_2 antagonists, omeprazole, and prostaglandins) within the parietal cell. *PGE,* Prostaglandin E; *RI,* inhibitory receptor; *RS,* stimulatory receptor. **B,** The pH gradient of the gastric mucosa is maintained by a thick mucus barrier. When the barrier becomes destroyed or thinned, the mucosa is subject to the irritating effects of the acid medium.

ions.[64] A large pH gradient is maintained by this barrier between the lumen (pH 1 to 2) and the epithelial cell surface (pH 7)[65] (Fig. 3-11, *B*). It has been suggested that some patients with both gastric and duodenal ulcer have a mucous gel covering that is structurally weaker than in normal subjects.[66] Electron micrographs suggest that the layer of mucus is often thin and patchy, but that it can thicken rapidly in response to stress. This is in keeping with some radiologic observations. Coating of the stomach by barium is variable, and areae gastricae are not routinely detectable because of the covering mucus layer. In one study coating was inferior in individuals who had smoked before their barium meal, perhaps because of a mucus response to smoking.[67]

A solvent such as dilute acetic acid (vinegar) would dissolve mucus but might well excite a vigorous outpouring of fresh mucus, which would defeat the object of obtaining good barium coating. An agent that would temporarily paralyze mucus production while the patient is vigorously turned and shaken to enable the barium to wash off much of the existing mucus layer might provide a more reliable demonstration of the gastric mucosa.

Apical expulsion, exocytosis, and cell exfoliation are the three methods of gastric mucus release in dogs, with exocytosis being slow, apical release a sudden maximal response, and exfoliation a rare method.[68] In humans the mechanism of stimulation for release of mucus from the cell is not well understood. Acetylcholine, which stimulates acid secretion, does stimulate mucous gel production in the dog, but the relevance of this experiment to humans is unclear. Prostaglandins E and F, either systemically or topically, definitely increase the effective thickness of human gastric mucous gel by stimulating bicarbonate secretion and causing release of mucin from the mucosa.[69,70] Indomethacin, as discussed previously, inhibits prostaglandins and is associated with gastric mucosal damage (see Fig. 3-7). A short-lived prostaglandin antagonist might also improve gastric mucosal visualization during barium studies by blocking mucus production.

Intrinsic factor

Intrinsic factor is a glycoprotein present in gastric secretions that is essential for the absorption of cobalamin (vitamin B_{12}) in the terminal ileum. It is synthesized and secreted by the parietal cells.[71] Secretion is stimulated by the same agents as acid secretion, yet the secretory response is not linked to acid secretion.[72] In the complete absence of intrinsic factor, as in pernicious anemia or following total gastrectomy, vitamin B_{12} deficiency ensues. Patients with pernicious anemia have a high incidence of antibodies directed against intrinsic factor (70%). This also results in atrophy of the oxyntic mucosa and achlorhydria. Simple atrophic gastritis may involve low serum B_{12} levels but a normal intrinsic factor—diminished acid and pepsin fail to liberate cobalamin that is bound to food.[73]

Gastric motility
After feeding

Gastric motility comprises accommodation, peristalsis, and emptying. The fundus and upper body dilate by two distinct processes. When the throat or esophagus is mechanically distended, the fundal pressure is reduced and the fundus relaxes, an effect called *receptive relaxation,* which is abolished by vagotomy. Thus the moment a subject swallows a mouthful of barium, the fundus is already starting to relax, and a contracted fundus is seldom visualized. Second, when material is introduced into the fundus, the intragastric pressure hardly rises at all, and relaxation occurs, an effect called *gastric accommodation.* Both effects are probably mediated by the neurotransmitter VIP, and together they give the proximal stomach a reservoir function.

Another fascinating postulated function of the fundus is as a regulator of belching and reflux. A large network of sensory nerve fibers of unknown function spreads over the fundus from the cardia. Some evidence suggests that this supplies a sampling function similar to that of the upper anal canal (discussed later). These nerve endings can then detect whether gas, solid, or liquid is lying against the mucosa adjacent to the cardia, and sphincter relaxation is permitted only if gas is present. According to this model, gastroesophageal reflux disease is a disorder of belching control.

The stomach plays two important roles in digestion: (1) it stores food and controls gastric emptying so that food enters the intestine at rates that can be easily assimilated; and (2) it breaks up food into tiny particles with large surface areas to facilitate digestion. Most of the body and antrum undergo peristalsis after feeding, and this peristalsis mixes and grinds the food into small particles. Only liquid and fine particles are normally allowed to pass the pylorus. There is constant tone at the pylorus; emptying does not occur by peristalsis across the pylorus but by transient abolition of the pyloric tone as an antral peristalsis sweeps toward it. The pylorus relaxes as the antral wave approaches to allow liquid and fine particles to flow through but closes again before the peristaltic wave reaches the pylorus. This produces peristalsis against an obstructed outlet, and the antral solid contents have to escape retrogradely against the oncoming peristaltic squeeze, which contributes to the grinding up of larger particles. The retrograde escape of distal antral contents back into the body of the stomach against peristalsis is regularly observed during barium meal examinations.

Administration of fat into the duodenum produces high-pressure static contractions of the pylorus that effectively close it and prevent any further pyloric emptying. A CCK response occurs at the same time, but it is not known whether CCK is responsible for this pyloric closure, although the pyloric mucosa is particularly well endowed with CCK receptors. Regardless of the mechanism, a cup of coffee with a little milk just before a barium meal may

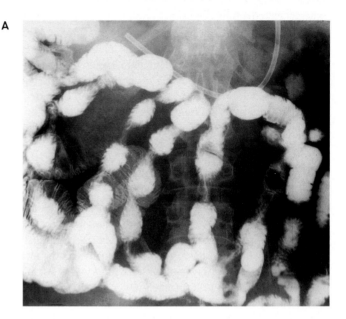

A

Fig. 3-12 The migrating motor complex (MMC) periodically sweeps the small bowel of secretions every 90 to 120 minutes and lasts for about 10 minutes. **A,** This radiograph, taken early in a small bowel enema examination, shows the 1- to 2-cm contractions, separated by 3 to 4 cm long barium-filled intestine typical of the MMC. **B,** A manometric tracing of the MMC in a normal adult. The top two tracings are from the gastric antrum, and the remainder are from the duodenum and proximal jejunum. The motility is traced from left to right in each channel; phase II, III, and I are illustrated sequentially.
From Stevenson GW et al: *Gastrointest Radiol* 13:215, 1988.

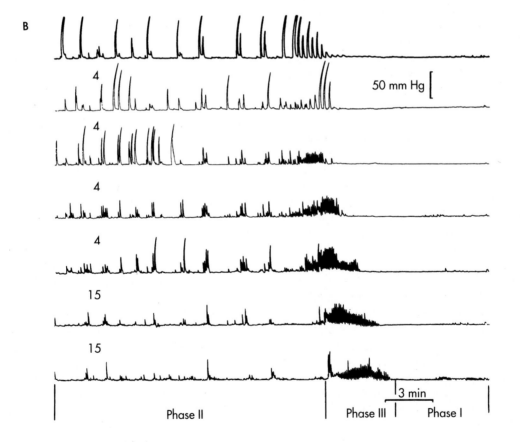

B

Phase II   Phase III   Phase I

effectively close the pylorus for the duration of the examination.

Impaired fundal relaxation or reduced gastric distensibility from any cause accelerates gastric emptying, especially of liquids, during the first few minutes after eating; impairment of gastric peristalsis leads to delayed gastric emptying, especially of solids. Following vagotomy, or with linitis plastica carcinoma, these two abnormalities may coexist.

The effects of fundal tone and antral peristalsis ensure that liquids and solids empty at different rates. This can be confirmed by double isotope tests, in which different isotopes are given in the liquid and solid phases of a meal. Canine studies with indigestible solids (spheres) of 1 to 5 mm in diameter have shown that the rate of passage of spheres through the pylorus is affected by sphere diameter, sphere density, and the presence of liquids to assist passage.[74,75] These fundamentals apply to human gastric physiology as well. Enteric-coated tablets larger than 10 mm do not pass when food is present in the stomach. This is illustrated by the increased blood levels of enteric-coated medications such as salicylates and erythromycin when they are taken with food rather than under fasting conditions.[76]

During fasting

During fasting the migrating myoelectric complex (MMC) occurs every 90 to 120 minutes. This begins with pacemaker potentials arising in the greater curve of the stomach at the junction of the proximal third and distal two thirds of the body. The longest part of the cycle, phase I, sees these pacemaker potentials sweeping down the stomach but not producing muscular contractions and is thus a phase of quiescence. During phase II contractions begin to appear and reach a crescendo in phase III, when for 5 or 10 minutes almost every potential is accompanied by a forceful contraction that sweeps down the stomach, through the antrum, and down the small intestine. These 5-minute bursts of crescendo, phase III activity that sweep along the small bowel are commonly termed the *migrating motor complex* (Fig. 3-12, *A* and *B*). It is interesting that in phase III the pylorus does not close as the peristalsis approaches the antrum (there is usually no fat in the gastric contents at this time) so that larger fragments of undigested food remaining in the stomach may be passed into the duodenum during phase III. Phase IV is a period of diminishing contractility.

DUODENUM AND SMALL INTESTINE
Digestion and absorption

Carbohydrate digestion starts in the mouth with salivary amylase, continues on the inside of food masses in the stomach, and is completed down to the level of disaccharides by pancreatic amylase in the duodenum and jejunum. Since the small intestine is not capable of transporting carbohydrates more complex than monosaccharides, dietary disaccharides and polysaccharides must be cleaved to the monomeric forms. Splitting of disaccharides to monosaccharides for absorption is carried out by enzymes from the brush border of the mature enterocyte present in the upper small intestine. These include lactases, sucrases, and maltases. Deficiency of intestinal lactase is the most common mucosal enzyme deficiency state. Lactase deficiency may be congenital, primary with delayed onset, or secondary. In the congenital form the enzyme is absent from birth. The much more common form, primary with delayed onset, is thought to be a genetic predetermined reduction in enzyme activity during childhood to 5% to 10% of the normal levels. The secondary form of lactase deficiency is caused by an intestinal insult, such as gastroenteritis or celiac disease, that results in insufficient absorptive surface area, reduced contact time between the mucosa and the disaccharide, and decreased mucosal surface area of the intestine. The diagnosis of lactase deficiency should be suggested whenever a patient has discomfort, cramps, and watery diarrhea within 30 minutes to several hours after ingesting milk or milk products. Although conventional small bowel examination findings are normal in patients with lactase deficiency, the addition of 25 g to 50 g of lactose to the barium mixture results in marked dilation of the small bowel with dilution of the barium, rapid transit, and reproduction of symptoms[77] (Fig. 3-13, *A* and *B*). These symptoms develop because of the hyperosmolar effect of the undigested lactose within the intestine. Any of the specific enzyme deficiencies can be tested for in this way by using the disaccharide that is the substrate for the missing enzyme.

Protein digestion is started by pepsins in the stomach. Entrance of food into the duodenum causes release of secretin, which stimulates bicarbonate production by the pancreatic centroacinar cells, and of CCK, which makes the acinar cells release the enzyme precursor granules. The enzyme precursors are inactive at low pH, so bicarbonate is also essential to raise the pH and halt pepsin activity. Enterokinase from the brush border of the duodenal mucosa converts trypsinogen to trypsin, and the trypsin itself converts the other protease precursors, such as chymotrypsinogen, to their active forms. Although much of the protein is absorbed after complete hydrolysis as single amino acids, dipeptides and tripeptides are also absorbed and enhance the amino acid absorption. Dietary protein is the only source of the nine essential amino acids that are required for protein synthesis (valine, leucine, isoleucine, tryptophane, threonine, methionine, phenylalanine, lysine, and histidine). In addition to dietary protein, large amounts of endogenous proteins are digested by the intestine from biliary, gastric, pancreatic, and intestinal secretions, as well as approximately 30 g/day of proteins from intestinal desquamation.[78,79] Congenital abnormalities of transport of specific amino acids across cell membranes are responsible for several rare disorders. However, pancreatic disease, loss

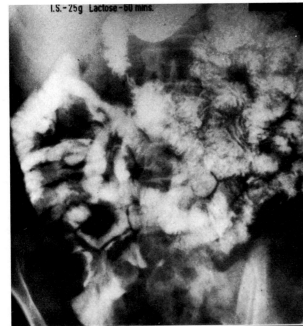

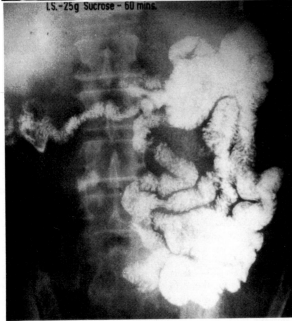

Fig. 3-13 Hypolactasia. **A,** A small bowel meal radiograph taken 60 minutes after a lactose and barium mixture shows a large amount of dilute barium in the small bowel and ascending colon. **B,** A further study taken 60 minutes after a sucrose and barium mixture shows the normal appearance of concentrated barium in the small bowel.

Courtesy J.W. Laws: Disaccharidase deficiency. In Lodge T, Steiner RE: *Recent advances in radiology*, ed 5, London, 1975, Churchill Livingstone.

of intestinal mucosa, such as in celiac disease, and loss of absorptive surface in patients with fistulas or resections are more common causes of nondietary protein deficiency.

Fat, ingested as triglyceride and phospholipid, is emulsified by mechanical action in the stomach. Several pancreatic lipases and colipases are secreted in active form into the duodenum. Together they hydrolyze triglycerides and phospholipids into free fatty acids and monoglyceride, which combine with bile acids to form micelles, which render the lipolytic products water soluble. Micelles diffuse passively across cell membranes, and in the intestinal enterocyte the fatty acids and monoglycerides have to be resynthesized into triglycerides and packaged into chylomicrons so that they can be excreted into the extracellular space for uptake by the lymphatic system.

The formation of bile acids into micelles is crucial to the dispersion of fatty acids in the aqueous phase of intestinal contents. This increases the diffusion across the unstirred layer of mucus to the intestinal mucosal cell by a factor of 100 to 200 times. Ninety-five percent of bile acids (but not bilirubin) are reabsorbed from the lower small bowel so that an enterohepatic circulation of bile acids is set up that facilitates the solubilization and transport of fat from the intestinal lumen to the hepatocyte.

Bile acid deficiency and consequent fat malabsorption may result from impaired hepatic synthesis, as in cirrhosis; from loss of functioning ileum, most frequently in Crohn's disease; or from stasis with bacterial overgrowth—as the bacteria dehydroxylate the bile acids, rendering them insoluble.[80] However, infants with total biliary atresia absorb 50% of their dietary fat, and adults with extensive loss of small bowel usually absorb 75% of ingested fat,[81] so some fat absorption does still occur in the absence of bile acids, although not enough to prevent the development of deficiencies.

Malabsorption

In addition to foods, numerous other essential substances are absorbed from the small intestine: iron, calcium, magnesium, folate, vitamin B_{12}, and other fat- and water-soluble vitamins. Many are affected by malabsorption states, particularly the fat-soluble vitamins D and K, whose deficiencies cause osteomalacia and impaired coagulation. With the exception of cobalamin (B_{12}), the proximal small intestine is more important than the ileum in the absorption of the water-soluble vitamins. For instance, the jejunum is the exclusive site for carrier-mediated folate absorption. The absorption of fat-soluble vitamins, calcium, zinc, and iron also occurs preferentially, but not exclusively, in the proximal small bowel. The stomach is responsible for the absorption of cobalamin.

Other substances that should not be absorbed may be taken up when small intestinal function is deranged. An example is hyperoxaluria, which occurs in many small bowel disorders, especially celiac disease, Crohn's disease, and

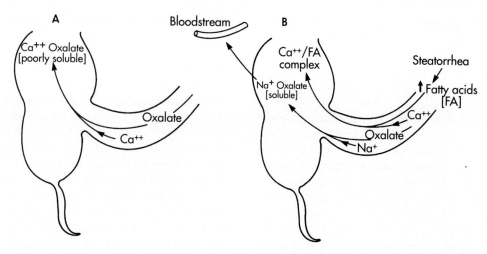

Fig. 3-14 Hyperoxalemia. **A,** Normally, oxalates reaching the distal ileum and cecum link with calcium ions forming a poorly soluble complex. **B,** In malabsorption states there is an increase in the volume of fatty acids *(FA)* reaching the distal small bowel. The *FA* preferentially link with the calcium ions, leaving the oxalates to form a complex with sodium ions. Sodium oxalate is soluble and is reabsorbed. Hyperoxalemia subsequently leads to hyperoxaluria and the development of oxalate urinary tract stones.

any cause of intestinal stasis; it leads to the formation of oxalate urinary stones (Fig. 3-14).

Motility

In addition to the forward propulsion and mixing of intraluminal contents with secretions, small intestinal motor activity is responsible for other functions. For example, after digestion is complete, it keeps the small intestine clear of food residue and desquamated cells. Occasionally it will rapidly move contents in an orad or caudad direction when vomiting or a mass action occurs. The small intestine transports about 9 L of fluid and electrolytes, of which only 1.5 L is from the diet. The rest is from saliva, stomach, pancreas, liver, and the small intestine itself. The small intestine absorbs 7.5 L but can absorb up to 15 to 20 L of isotonic saline daily. Two different patterns of motor activity occur to move this river of fluid along, together with food and the debris from exfoliated cells and mucus.

Fasting state[82]

The initiation of the MMC in the stomach has already been described. Most propulsion occurs in phase III, when regular peristaltic waves sweep slowly down the entire length of the small intestine at 7 cm/min in the upper small bowel. Code and Marlett[83] have observed the MMC fluoroscopically in the dog. The MMC also has been observed fluoroscopically at the start of a small bowel enema. The regularity of the process is striking, with numerous small and identically shaped boluses of barium about 5 cm long separated by about 1 to 2 cm of contraction all moving slowly down the jejunum at identical speed[84] (see Fig. 3-12). The MMC has been called the intestinal house-keeper, with a function of sweeping the intestine clear of debris every hour and a half during fasting. It has been shown experimentally to propel solid boluses rapidly along the small bowel, especially in phase III and to a lesser extent in phase II, the crescendo phase when contractions are beginning to build up to the organized intense activity of phase III.

Giant migrating contractions (GMCs) may perform a similar housekeeping function in the distal small intestine, as well as returning any refluxed fecal material back to the colon. However, the major role of GMCs may be in pathologic states, associated with abdominal cramping and diarrhea. The GMC is responsible for mass movement and will move approximately half the intestinal contents retrogradely into the stomach in preparation for vomiting. In general, GMCs are two to three times greater in amplitude and four to five times longer in duration than individual phasic contractions in the small intestine.[85]

Experience with Golytely indicates that a great deal of mucus and debris appear in the colon overnight. Colonoscopy performed on the same day of Golytely administration reveals a shining clean, if wet, mucosa. If Golytely is given the night before, the colon contains no stool but a moderate amount of mucus and debris, especially in the proximal half.

Fed state

MMCs are replaced by a more or less continual low level of contractile activity in the fed state, suggesting the role of a neurohumoral mechanism rather than a local effect.[86] In humans this myoelectrical pattern is largely disorganized in time and space. These contractions may cause mixing and agitation of intraluminal contents with slow distal propulsion. Occasionally an individual contraction of large amplitude and longer duration migrates over several centimeters and may rapidly propel the contents over this distance. There is a decreasing gradient of contractile activity from the duodenum to the distal ileum, and the postprandial propagation velocity is greater in the small intestine. Antegrade and retrograde movements occur, but antegrade movement predominates. The duration of the fed pattern depends on both the caloric content and qualitative aspects of the ingested meal. For instance, in humans the ingestion of a meal of 345 to 395 kcal can disrupt MMC cycling for more than 90 minutes.[87] In another study on intestinal clearance after feeding, 60% of the meal cleared the intestine in the hour and a half before the return of MMCs, but after the first MMC, clearance had jumped to more than 90%.[88]

In addition to feeding, emotion can interrupt MMCs, and opiates can potentiate them. The combination of gastric distention and apprehension may explain why this normal phenomenon is not seen more often by radiologists during a barium meal.

Immunology

The gut immune system is the largest in the body, serving to protect the 200 to 300 M^2 surface area of the GI tract. The T and B cell system of the gut has unique properties designed to disseminate an immune response over a large surface area. B cells are activated by an antigen and differentiate into plasma cells, which secrete antibodies to bind specifically to the antigen and initiate a variety of elimination responses. T cells operate a cellular defense that is especially effective against fungi, parasites, intracellular viruses, and cancer. There is close dialogue between the two systems. In addition to these two systems, macrophages and mast cells are important for defense.

The GI immune system can be divided into three zones: (1) the organized lymphoid tissue of the tonsils, Peyer's patches, appendix, and colonic lymphoid follicles; (2) the cells of the lamina propria; and (3) the lymphocytes within the gut epithelium itself. An astonishing 25% of gut mucosa is composed of lymphoid cells.[89]

Peyer's patches are covered with thin M cells that lack villi and rapidly transport antigens (whether intact macromolecules or viral particles) across to the interstitial space, where they are processed by the circulating uncommitted B lymphocytes. These lymphocytes then pass through the mesenteric nodes to the thoracic duct and eventually reappear in the lamina propria of the gut, "homing" to the area where the antigen was first encountered. A few also become dispersed in peripheral lymph nodes. The mechanism of the homing phenomenon is unknown. Peyer's patches are thus the source of the B cells that populate the lamina propria and produce an immunoglobulin, IgA.

In response to further antigenic challenge, the activated B cells and plasma cells liberate secretory IgA, which binds antigen and prevents its adherence to the epithelial cell. As adherence is the first stage of colonization, its prevention also inhibits infection. This is typically shown in diseases such as cholera.[90,91] It is purely protective in that it does not initiate any processes that are locally destructive.

If penetration of the epithelium does occur, activation of systemic antibody response and interaction with mast cells occur. IgG is also produced in bowel, but in binding to antigen it sets in motion a cascade of events that may damage the bowel. An imbalance may be harmful; IgG is elevated in patients with inflammatory bowel disease. Mast cells, which are concerned with immediate hypersensitivity, are unique cells involved in antigen recognition and bind IgE. They also release numerous active agents, such as histamine and 5-hydroxytryptamine.

In some circumstances an antigenic challenge leads to acceptance or tolerance, so further exposure to antigen provokes no response.

The lymphoid follicles are crucial in the defense mechanisms of the GI tract. They are larger in children than in adults, which occasionally causes confusion. Radiologists may find them enlarged in the colon after acute infection or in chronic ulcerative colitis. The early lesions of Crohn's disease always start on top of lymphoid follicles. In some hypoimmune states, such as common variable hypogammaglobulinemia, which probably has a variety of causes, the intestinal lymphoid follicles tend to be enlarged. Unusual infections, such as by *Giardia lamblia,* are common.

Intestinal permeability

The intestinal epithelium and its overlying mucus provide a barrier to absorption, particularly to macromolecules. Small amounts do cross the barrier, by intracellular or intercellular routes and through the very thin cell layer at the lymphoid follicle and Peyer's patches. This limited absorption of macromolecules probably normally represents a sampling mechanism by which the immune system monitors the environment. However, passive diffusion of smaller hydrophilic (water-soluble) molecules does occur and can be measured by giving a substance orally that is neither immunogenic nor toxic, is not metabolized nor is a dietary constituent, and is rapidly and completely cleared by the kidneys so that it can be measured in the urine. Such compounds have been called *probes of intestinal permeability* and may be given orally or rectally. There are several molecular probes, such as mannitol. Larger probes include lactulose, polyethylene glycol 400 (PEG-400), and chromium 51-ED7A.[92] In the presence of intestinal inflammation, intestinal permeability and therefore urinary excretion of the larger molecules are increased, whereas the smaller ones show either no change or a decrease in permeability. The tests are inexpensive, noninvasive, and well tolerated.

Their clinical value is unclear,[93] but they may become useful for monitoring activity of diseases such as Crohn's disease[94] and celiac disease. There is a report of increased permeability to PEG-400 in patients with Crohn's disease and their first-degree relatives.[95] A nonspecific activation of the GI immune system resulting from increased intestinal permeability to luminal antigens is one interesting theory for the cause of inflammatory bowel disease.[96] Colonic permeability also increases when bile salts or fatty acids are present in the colon.[97]

Other ways of assessing a leaky bowel are to look for a leak in the opposite direction, to examine loss of white cells or red cells, and to use isotopes.[98] The indium III white cell excretion test shows accumulation in the bowel and can be used to image the bowel in the presence of inflammation, since in normal individuals not enough white cells leak into the intestine to permit imaging. Thus the outlining of the gut may have some value in indicating the degree of disease activity and in localizing inflammation. Isotopes also can be used to quantitate loss of red and white cells in the stool in inflammatory bowel disease.

BILIARY SYSTEM AND LIVER
Anatomy and function

The liver has several functions, including synthesis of proteins, bile lipids, and urea and the secretion of proteins and bile.[99] It has metabolic functions in the control of carbohydrate, fat, and protein metabolism. It normally consists of about 20% to 30% blood by weight but can contract its vascular compartment to expel up to 40% of its blood in response to vasoconstrictors and can vasodilate until it is 50% blood by weight. It plays a role in mediating immunologic responses by means of Kupffer's cells, and it has an astonishing capacity for regeneration, recovering its function and size in a few months after resection of up to 90% of its mass.[100]

To perform such a wide range of tasks the structure of the liver has a number of characteristic features. These include a dual blood supply (portal vein and hepatic artery) and a highly organized hepatic parenchyma and microvasculature that allows efficient exchange between blood and the hepatocytes (Fig. 3-15). The center of a liver acinus consists of a terminal hepatic arteriole, portal venule, bile ductule, lymph vessels, and nerves (portal triad). At the periphery of the acinus are the hepatic venules, each draining part of several acini. The plates of hepatocytes are arranged more or less parallel to each other radiating toward the central hepatic venules. An alternative way to conceptualize the functional acinar unit is to consider the axis between portal triads as the most oxygenated and active zone (Fig. 3-15, *C*) containing interconnecting small portal veins and hepatic arterioles, with a decreasing gradient of metabolic activity toward the central veins. The hepatocytes nearest this axis are the metabolically most active (and most oxygenated), whereas glycogen storage and fat formation occur more peripherally near the central veins. The hepatocytes are arranged in single cell–thick plates so that the two opposite flat surfaces are exposed to the blood of the sinusoids. Around each cell on all the other surfaces is an investing network of bile canaliculi (Fig. 3-16). Each cell can

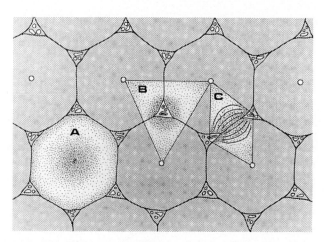

Fig. 3-15 Three representations of liver lobular architecture. *A*, The lobule centered on the hepatic venule. *B*, The lobule of the portal triad. *C*, The functional unit with a gradient of decreasing oxygen tension from the axis between the portal triads toward the central veins.
Courtesy R. Putz, Munich; Rapoport AM, Sasse D: Leberacinus: Die Strukturelle und funktionelle Lebereinheit. In Kühn HH, Wernze TA, eds: *Klinische Hepatologie*, Stuttgart, 1979, Thieme.

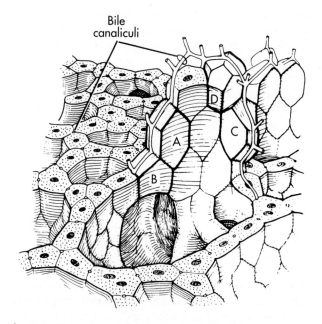

Fig. 3-16 Illustration of the way in which the bile canaliculi invest the hepatocytes on all sides except the two opposite flat surfaces that abut the sinusoids. Cells A, B, C, and D represent the four major shapes that hepatocytes largely conform to: octahedron, pentahedron, decahedron and dodecahedron. These basic shapes vary and depend largely on the regional blood flow.
From Kessel RG, Kardon RH: *Tissues and organs: a text atlas of scanning electron microscopy,* New York, 1979, WH Freeman.

thereby excrete its products into both blood and bile (Fig. 3-17).

The sinusoids are lined by endothelial cells with wide spaces between them and no basement membrane. Between the sinusoidal endothelial cells and the chains of hepatocytes beside them is an extracellular gap called Disse's space (Fig. 3-18), which communicates with the liver lymphatic system. The sinusoids arise from portal venules and empty into hepatic venules, but terminal hepatic arterioles also enter the sinusoids (Fig. 3-17), so sinusoidal blood is a mixture of portal and hepatic arterioles, providing both intestinal nutrient and oxygen to the hepatocytes.

Metabolites in the sinusoids pass freely through the large spaces between the sinusoidal endothelial cells into Disse's space. This space is thus an extracellular space bathed in nutrients and plasma, highly oxygenated, and in direct contact with hepatocyte microvilli (Fig. 3-18). The space is drained by the lymphatic system, so if the pressure on the portal veins is high and albumin is low, the lymphatic system is readily overloaded and ascites will form.

From Disse's space metabolites pass into the hepatocytes by a variety of means, some passively and others actively.[99] Iminodiacetic acid derivatives are taken up by the hepatocyte, and some, such as diisopropyl, are taken up by active transport and excreted even at serum bilirubin levels of 20 mg/100 ml. Since iminodiacetic acid derivatives chelate readily, they can be bound to technetium 99m, which provides excellent scintigraphic imaging of the liver and bile ducts and a functional way of assessing duodenogastric reflux, bile esophagitis, and afferent loop obstruction.

In summary, the flow of metabolic activity starts with the mixing of oxygen and nutrients in the sinusoid. Substances pass from the sinusoid through Disse's space to the hepatocyte. After modification, metabolites leave by one of three routes. They may be transported across the walls between hepatocytes and into the bile canaliculus. Alternatively, they may leave through the other two walls, through which they entered the cell, back into the extracellular Disse's space. From here they may either be drained by the lymphatic system or pass back into the sinusoid to travel out of the liver in the hepatic veins.

Synthesis

Continuous bile acid synthesis from cholesterol is required to maintain the bile acid pool in the enterohepatic circulation. The maximal rate of synthesis is of the order of 4 to 6 g/day.[101] Numerous crucial proteins are also synthesized in the liver, including several concerned with coagulation—fibrinogen, prothrombin, and factors V, VII, IX, and X. All except fibrinogen depend on the fat-soluble vitamin K for synthesis. They are depressed, and coagulation is impaired in many patients with obstructive jaundice because of intestinal malabsorption of fat. The liver is the sole source of plasma fibrinogen, with a steady-state production of 1.7 to 5.0 g/day and with the potential to increase production 20-fold should the need arise. In addition, the liver contributes to coagulation and its control by removing activated clotting factors from the circulation.[102]

Coagulation must be checked and restored before endoscopic sphincterotomy or percutaneous transhepatic procedures. This is not always possible in cases of severe liver disease, a problem that has led to the development of the transjugular liver biopsy, after which bleeding occurs safely into the hepatic veins. The infusion of fresh frozen plasma or platelets should be considered before performance of interventional procedures in patients with marked thrombocytopenia and prolonged coagulation parameters.

Bile acids are derived exclusively from the liver, and cholesterol and phospholipids mainly so.

Almost all urea is synthesized in the liver. Liver failure is followed by diminution in serum urea levels and corresponding elevation in ammonia and amino acid levels. The precise chemical responsible for hepatic encephalopathy has not been identified, but reduction of protein intake and prevention of bacterial ammonia formation in the gut by the use of antibiotics often relieves symptoms of encephalopathy.

Secretion

The hepatocytes secrete proteins in one direction into the sinusoidal blood and lipids from the other wall into the bile canaliculi (see Fig. 3-16). It is not known whether one hepatocyte can produce more than one protein simultaneously. No secretory granules contain multiple substances, as is found in the exocrine pancreatic acinar cells. Production of albumin is quantitatively predominant, with 36% of hepatocytes containing albumin, 8 to 14 g being produced daily. Albumin plays a major role in the prevention of ascites and maintenance of colloid osmotic pressure (discussed later).

The mechanism of secretion of bile acids, lecithins (phospholipids), and cholesterol from hepatocyte to bile duct is unknown, but once they are in the canaliculus an osmotic gradient is set up that draws in water and stimulates flow along the canaliculus. The rate of bile flow correlates directly with the concentration of bile acid in the circulation perfusing the hepatocytes. As delivery of bile acid increases, bile secretion increases. Thus bile flow is partly bile acid dependent. CCK produces a rapid increase in flow of bile into the duodenum and (in dogs) a nonbile salt-dependent increase in bile flow, as well as causing gallbladder contraction.

The ability of CCK or a fat meal to produce a dramatic increase in bile flow is now used as the basis of the fat provocation test for distinguishing obstructed from unobstructed extrahepatic bile ducts on ultrasound examination.[103] An increase in diameter of 2 mm of the extrahepatic duct 45 minutes after stimulation provides good evidence of obstruction, and the test works as well in patients who have had a cholecystectomy as in those who have not. The normal physiologic response is for the extrahepatic duct diameter

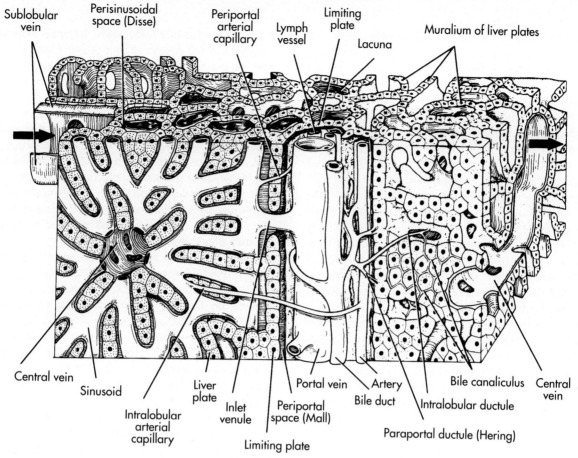

Sublobular vein

Perisinusoidal space (Disse)

Periportal arterial capillary

Lymph vessel

Limiting plate

Lacuna

Muralium of liver plates

Central vein

Sinusoid

Liver plate

Intralobular arterial capillary

Inlet venule

Periportal space (Mall)

Limiting plate

Portal vein

Bile duct

Artery

Intralobular ductule

Bile canaliculus

Paraportal ductule (Hering)

Central vein

Fig. 3-17 Diagram showing the interrelationships of hepatocytes, sinusoids, bile canaliculi, and blood vessels.
From Kessel RG, Kardon RH: *Tissues and organs: a text atlas of scanning electron microscopy,* New York, 1979, WH Freeman.

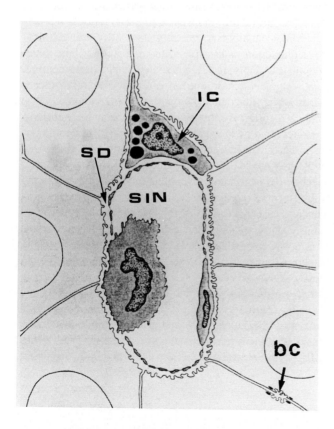

IC

SD

SIN

bc

Fig. 3-18 Sinusoid and Disse's space *(sd).* The sinusoid is shown end on. Note that its endothelial lining has large gaps. Between this endothelium and the villous surface of the hepatocyte is Disse's space, which communicates with the lymphatic drainage of the liver. *sin,* Sinusoid; *bc,* bile canaliculus; *ic,* Ito cell.
Courtesy R. Putz, Munich.

to decrease, because CCK relaxes Oddi's sphincter as bile flow increases, although in some normal subjects there is no change in caliber as flow increases.

A variation on this test is the use of secretin, which produces a rapid increase in flow of pancreatic secretions. One study showed that 8% of normal individuals may have a slight increase in pancreatic duct caliber, but 73% of patients with papillary stenosis have a marked increase in pancreatic duct caliber following secretin administration.[104] Scintigraphy can be used similarly but, despite apparently good results, has not found widespread acceptance.[105] The various iminodiacetic acid derivatives have liver excretion half-times ranging from 18 to 108 minutes. The quicker agents are ideal for intrahepatic and extrahepatic duct visualization but are not necessarily good for the gallbladder.[106] If small bowel imaging is required, CCK administration ensures visualization in normal individuals and improves visualization in patients.

Ninety percent of bile acids are absorbed from the terminal ileum, so very little of the bile acids in the ducts are freshly synthesized. Bilirubin, on the other hand, is not significantly reabsorbed. It is produced from heme by the reticuloendothelial cells, including Kupffer's cells, is conjugated with glucuronide, and is actively transported across the canalicular membrane.

Bile flow

Approximately 600 ml of bile is secreted each day, a little faster during the day than at night, at a pressure of 15 to 25 cm of water, ceasing when the pressure in the common bile duct reaches 35 cm of water. The gallbladder probably undergoes receptive relaxation to a certain volume that varies from one individual to another but is around 60 ml and rarely more than 100 ml. Morphine and, interestingly, secretin cause sphincter contraction. Secretin thus antagonizes CCK, which causes gallbladder contraction and sphincter relaxation, but the secretin response is overwhelmed by the strength of the physiologic response to CCK.

The normal sequence of daily change in biliary flow has been studied by using ultrasound to measure gallbladder volumes. When an individual starts to fast after a meal, the gallbladder is at first almost empty, then slowly begins to fill. After about 100 minutes, phase III of the interdigestive MMC begins to sweep down from the stomach and into the small intestine (probably initiated by the hormone motilin). Coinciding with the onset of phase III, a partial contraction of the gallbladder occurs, producing 20% to 25% emptying.[107] The gallbladder then continues to fill, only to undergo another partial contraction after another hour and a half. Complete filling of the gallbladder thus occurs in a stepwise manner; it takes 6 to 8 hours before it is completely full. Filling is generally thought to be a passive event that occurs as a consequence of the diversion of bile into a relaxed gallbladder.[108]

Once a meal is taken, the MMC pattern is abolished for a while, and the release of endogenous CCK, that occurs when fat reaches the duodenum, produces Oddi's sphincter relaxation, gallbladder contraction, and almost complete gallbladder emptying (down to a volume of 10 to 20 ml). In normal pregnancy, obesity, prolonged parenteral nutrition, and animals given progesterone, both fasting and residual gallbladder volumes are increased. Incomplete emptying may be responsible for the sludge formation so commonly seen on ultrasound examination and the increased incidence of cholelithiasis. The mechanism of partial gallbladder contraction with the MMC is unknown; there is no rise in CCK levels. A weak response to the motilin rise may trigger phase III of the MMC.

Manometric examination of the sphincter of Oddi shows a 4 to 6 mm long segment of increased tone about 5 to 10 mm Hg higher than ductal or duodenal pressures. Superimposed on this are phasic contraction waves three to seven times per minute sweeping along the sphincter,[109] mainly in a downward or antegrade direction, although 14% may normally be retrograde.[110] The proportion of retrograde contractions is increased in patients with stones in the bile duct; however, it is unknown whether this is a contributing factor to stone formation or a consequence of the obstruction. Phasic contractions in the sphincter of Oddi appear to empty or sweep clean only the lumen of the sphincter itself and to impede bile duct emptying,[109] although it also has been suggested that the phasic contractions are responsible for bile duct emptying.[110] Fluoroscopic observation during ERCP after catheter removal reveals quite clearly that sphincter contraction is associated with no flow and that small bursts of transient flow from the distended bile duct follow immediately on sphincter relaxation. Perhaps both observations are correct. Major emptying is probably associated with gallbladder contraction and sphincter relaxation, but small amounts of emptying are associated with phasic contractions, although they appear on observation to occur immediately after rather than with the contraction.

Abnormalities of motility of the sphincter of Oddi have been identified by manometric studies.[111,112] The commonest motor dysfunction of the sphincter of Oddi is increased basal pressure.[113] Increased tone can occur as a consequence of either anatomic (papillary stenosis) or functional (sphincter of Oddi dyskinesia) changes in sphincter performance. The latter can be distinguished by a normal relaxation response of the sphincter to smooth muscle relaxants such as CCK or glucagon. The release of CCK normally results in a decrease in the phasic and tonic contractile activity of the sphincter of Oddi. Occasionally, patients with sphincter of Oddi dysfunction have a paradoxic contractile sphincter response to CCK. This results in duct distention and pain.[114] In humans, the sphincter of Oddi is extremely sensitive to morphine sulphate, which in very small doses (0.05 µg/kg) stimulates phasic wave contractions.[109]

Physiology of ascites

Ascitic fluid may contain blood cells, colloids, and protein molecules, or crystalloids (such as glucose) and water. These are removed from the peritoneum in different ways. Cells are removed almost exclusively from the peritoneal surface of the diaphragm, and the lymph from the diaphragm goes via the right lymphatic duct and not the thoracic duct. Protein from blood diffuses continually into the peritoneum and is removed by the lymphatic system. Crystalloids and water diffuse preferentially into capillaries, not the lymphatic system, and radioactive crystalloids placed in the peritoneal cavity appear more quickly in the urine than in the thoracic duct.[115] A dynamic equilibrium exists between ascites and plasma, and about half the ascites enters and leaves the peritoneum every hour, with rapid transit in both directions.[116]

The factors affecting the development of ascites are principally intravascular osmotic pressure versus hydrostatic portal pressure. Experimental portal hypertension alone, however, will not produce ascites unless the animal is also made hypoproteinemic. Thus colloid osmotic pressure is the major factor. The commonest cause of ascites is cirrhosis of the liver. Hepatic sinusoidal (portal) hypertension causes formation of large amounts of hepatic lymph. This fluid has a relatively high concentration of protein. It is diluted by the outward movement of water from the capillaries of the nonhepatic splanchnic viscera. This outward movement of water into the protein-rich ascitic lymph continues, dropping the osmotic pressure of the ascites, until the gradient of osmotic pressure between plasma and ascites widens sufficiently to balance the hydrostatic pressure gradient of portal hypertension.

One of the most dramatic causes of ascites is the Budd-Chiari syndrome, in which the main hepatic veins are thrombosed, thus increasing the pressure in the hepatic venules distal to the hepatic sinusoids. With the resulting increase in portal and sinusoidal pressure, fluid cannot escape from the liver and seeps through the serosa of the intestine and surface of the liver.

The caudate lobe often drains directly into the inferior vena cava and is therefore frequently spared in Budd-Chiari syndrome, becoming relatively enlarged and being the only part of the liver to opacify normally on sulfur colloid scan.

PANCREAS

The pancreas is 84% exocrine cells, 10% extracellular matrix, 4% ductules and blood vessels, and 2% endocrine cells. The organ has little connective tissue, from which it derives its name (Greek *pan* = all, and *kreas* = flesh). The secretions of the exocrine pancreas—digestive enzymes and bicarbonate—affect the digestion of nutrients. The role of the endocrine pancreas is to produce hormones that regulate metabolism and the breakdown of food within the body.

Endocrine pancreas

The islets of Langerhans contain the cells of the endocrine pancreas. These are distributed throughout the gland but are concentrated mostly in the pancreatic tail. There are three types of cells: an outermost layer of A, or alpha, cells (10% to 20%) that produce glucagon; an intermediate layer of D, or delta, cells (5%) that produce somatostatin, gastrin, and pancreatic polypeptide; and an inner layer of B, or beta, cells (75% to 80%) that produce insulin. Other peptide-secreting cells that may be associated with the islet cells include EC cells containing 5-hydroxytryptamine and PP cells that contain pancreatic polypeptide.

Imaging of the lesions produced by tumors of the different cell types based on their physiology is not yet available. To date this has been done only with the use of ^{131}I-metaiodobenzylguanidine (MIBG), which localizes pheochromocytomas and neuroblastomas. The substance is a norepinephrine analog and is taken up by the adrenal medullary tumor cell by a sodium-dependent process and accumulated in the intracellular storage granules. Scintigraphy with this agent has high sensitivity and specificity, although some false-positive and false-negative results have been obtained, and it is also being used therapeutically for primary tumor and metastases. Generally the best method of localization for gut endocrine tumors has been angiography based on hypervascularity (80% to 90%),[117,118] but this is being superseded by ultrasound (sensitivity 10% to 20%),[118-120] CT (20% to 40%),[118,120] and MRI (10% to 20%)[121] for moderate and large lesions and by endoscopic and intraoperative ultrasound (90%)[122,123] for small lesions.

Exocrine pancreas

The majority of the pancreas is composed of acinar cells. Smaller centroacinar cells are found in the terminal subdivisions of the pancreatic ducts and are responsible for fluid and electrolyte secretion. The acinar cells contain numerous secretory granules, each of which contains the full complement of secretory proteins produced by the pancreas, of which trypsinogen and carboxypeptidase form the highest proportion, with amylase and lipase forming only 5.3% and 0.7%, respectively, by mass. These enzymes are synthesized within the acinar cells and packaged into zymogen granules.[124] Final dissolution of the granule in the lumen of the pancreatic duct probably depends on the presence of bicarbonate from the centroacinar cells.

Secretin is the most potent stimulant of pancreatic fluid and bicarbonate secretion. It is regulated by duodenal pH. CCK is released in response to luminal fatty acids and is a regulator of the postprandial secretion of pancreatic juices.

Alcohol ingestion increases pancreatic secretion and protein concentration and lowers bicarbonate. At least one of these proteins has a high affinity for calcium; the secretions contain more protein precipitates than normal, especially immediately after a period of alcohol abuse. Thus there may be stable calcium-protein precipitates formed in the smaller ducts after alcohol consumption.

Finally, pancreatic duct emptying is assisted by Oddi's sphincter relaxation, which accompanies bile flow after a meal. In the 3% of individuals who have pancreas divisum and have to empty most of the pancreatic secretions through a Santorini's papilla that has a small orifice and no sphincter to relax, alcohol may have an even greater damaging effect. At ERCP it is common to find that in patients with pancreas divisum and chronic pancreatitis, the head, body, and tail draining through Santorini's papilla are severely dilated and contain stones, whereas the portion of the head drained by Wirsung's duct appears normal. Thus it appears that there is a fine balance of factors that maintains pancreatic secretions in solution and ensures adequate drainage of the ducts, and that alcohol and pancreas divisum do not go well together.

Pancreatic cell function tests

Since the pancreas has a vast reserve secretory capacity, changes in secretory function are not found unless disease is far advanced. Thus negative results are not useful in excluding even severe pancreatic loss of function. It is also known that pancreatic secretion may be normal in a large number of patients with radiologic evidence of chronic pancreatitis.[125]

Pancreatic digestion tests

Many indirect tests of pancreatic function exist, but in general the ready availability of ERCP and the rapid improvements in radiologic imaging have rendered pancreatic function tests all but obsolete.

COLON

The functions of the colon are to transport and eliminate stool and absorb water and sodium. Intraluminal contents are also actively biotransformed by colonic bacteria, which adds significantly to the fecal bulk.

Transit

Three types of colonic contractions occur in three functionally distinct but overlapping parts of the colon. The characteristic aspect of motility of the right colon is the rarity of any propagated activity. Most contractions are segmental ring contractions of the circular muscle layer that produce stasis or retrograde movement from the hepatic flexure to the cecum. This pattern was first described by the father of GI radiology, Walter B. Cannon, who used bismuth subnitrate to observe colonic motility in the cat in 1902.[126] The retrograde contractions hold stool in the right colon, produce mixing, and allow time for most of the absorption of water and electrolyte to occur. The retrograde motion is not constant however, and occasionally gives way to tonic segmental contractions that result in forward movement of luminal contents.

Second is the appearance of short static contractions or segmentation mainly in the midcolon, serving to delay passage of stool while some further water and electrolyte absorption occurs.

The third type is the mass action that moves the contents distally over long segments of the colon. Mass actions are purely propulsive contractions that occur two or three times a day and transport stool distally. They often involve only the left colon but may start at the hepatic flexure and move stool to the sigmoid or rectum. The haustral markings disappear abruptly while a bowel motion is moved caudad, following which the haustral markings return. The mass movement may be seen during barium enema, mainly in the very elderly, when they may be repetitive and prevent completion of a barium enema because the barium is evacuated as soon as the head of the column reaches the transverse colon.

Finally, spasm of long segments may be observed radiologically. This is usually nonperistaltic, is often accompanied by pain in patients with irritable bowel, and is even more common in bowel adjacent to acute inflammatory processes, when it may prevent further passage of barium.

Diverticular disease

Diverticula are seen transiently in normal individuals, associated with "spasm" during barium enema (Fig. 3-19). Diverticular disease is associated with increased segmentation contractions with impaired transit and decreased stool weight. Myochosis is a process of thickening of the elastin fibers related to the teniae. It is most often seen with sigmoid diverticulosis in areas of high prevalence.[127] Diverticula usually occur at points of weakness in the colonic wall, where the intramural vasa recta penetrate to the submucosal layers.

The motor activity of the colon increases for up to 1 hour after the ingestion of food. This is commonly known as the *gastrocolic reflex* but is in fact a misnomer, since the source of the stimulus seems to be the small bowel and not the stomach. Furthermore, the response may not be under neural control as was first thought, but hormonally mediated, possibly from CCK or gastrin release.[128,129]

Assessment of colonic function

Wide variability exists in the measures used to define normal colonic function in healthy individuals, making it difficult to establish a definitive diagnosis of colonic motor abnormalities.[130,131] Three methods commonly used are stool frequency, weight and volume, and colonic transit time. In practice the stool frequency, weight, and volume are rarely assessed because the inaccuracies from interpersonal variation in bowel habit. Colonic transit time is a more objective measurement that can reliably be compared from patient to patient and one time to another. Initial attempts at measuring colonic transit time consisted of giving the subject radiopaque markers to swallow, then collecting and ra-

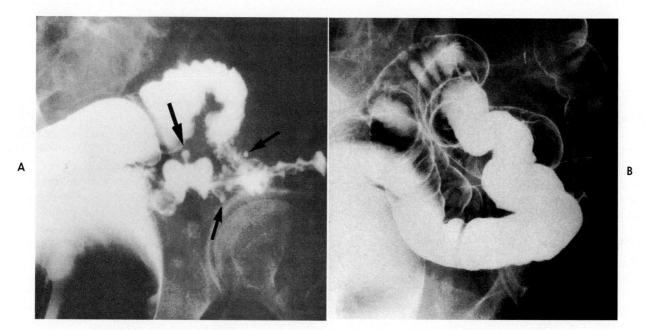

Fig. 3-19 Transient diverticula of the colon. Barium enema. **A,** The single contrast infusion of barium through the sigmoid was obstructed by spasm in a 60-year-old man with altered bowel habit. Diverticula are apparent *(arrows).* **B,** After 20 mg of intravenous buscopan, both the spasm and diverticula disappear.
Courtesy J. Rawlinson and F.J. Brunton.

diographing the stools. Currently, colonic transit is studied by radioactive isotope in a swallowed capsule (radiotelemetry) or, more practically, by following the passage of swallowed radiopaque markers. The radioactive capsule studies have demonstrated slow progress up the ascending colon, with occasional mass actions that transmit stool rapidly to the sigmoid. However, study of abdominal radiographs has revealed immense variation depending on dietary habit.

The simplest and most inexpensive way of studying transit is to give two capsules containing 20 markers each every day for 5 days to set up a steady state while the patient continues to eat a controlled normal diet. A single film on the morning of the sixth day provides a snapshot of bowel function. The typical individual will have less than 48 markers, mainly in the distal colon. A patient with a colonic transit disorder may have numerous markers scattered throughout the colon, whereas a patient with an evacuation problem will have markers held up in the rectum and sigmoid. More frequent films may not be necessary routinely but will demonstrate some interesting events, such as delay and mixing in the right colon, resulting in late markers advancing past earlier ones in the ascending colon. In addition, extra films may be helpful if the patient has an unusual segmental problem.

In one study total colonic transit time was 30.7 hours in men and 38.8 in women, with a ninety-fifth percentile value of 68 hours. Men had a slightly shorter transit time than women, which was most apparent in the right colon. The normal range was so great that only major deviations should be accepted as clinically significant.[132] More information is needed on the normal variation with aging.

Absorption

The colon normally receives about 1500 ml of fluid per day and absorbs 1350 ml of water, as well as sodium, chloride, and bicarbonate. The maximal absorptive capacity is about 3 L, and most water absorption occurs in the ascending colon, in keeping with the radiologic finding that discrete solid food is often visible radiologically at and distal to the hepatic flexure but only proximal to this in very constipated individuals. Only about 100 ml of water will be excreted in the stool. The importance of the right colon in water and salt absorption is relevant for patients with Crohn's disease who require right hemicolectomy. The colon has a large secretory capacity that can be stimulated by luminal toxins or endogenous hormones. The colon also can absorb short-chain fatty acids that are produced by bacterial catabolism of unabsorbed carbohydrates. These fatty acids may often account for an astonishing 10% of ingested calories.[133,134]

Diarrhea
Abnormal absorption (osmotic diarrhea)

Although the maximal absorptive capacity of the small intestine remains undefined, it has been shown that the normal adult capacity is 4 to 5 L per 24 hours. If the absorptive capacity of the small intestine is decreased by 50%, either by disease or pharmacologic agents, the volume of fluid presented to the colon will exceed its absorptive capacity (approximately 4 L). In the colon a decrease in the ability to absorb even the normal 1500 ml of water per day may result in increased fluid content in the stool. This alteration may come about from a failure of absorption of Na^+ and H_2O because of either a deranged epithelial transport mechanism or to the presence of nonabsorbable solutes in the intestinal lumen. The retention of high osmotic pressure substances in the intestine increases small bowel water and produces an osmotic diarrhea, as in lactase deficiency and celiac disease. However, in Crohn's disease, as mentioned previously, there is increased permeability to large molecules and decreased permeability to small ones.

Abnormal secretion (secretory diarrhea)

The discovery of the role of cyclic intracellular nucleotides in initiating intestinal Cl and H_2O secretion led to a completely new concept of diarrhea in 1968.[135] This was subsequently substantiated by the discoveries that neurotransmitters, hormones, bacterial endotoxins, and cathartics all stimulate intestinal Cl and H_2O secretion by way of alteration in the intracellular cyclic adenosine monophosphate (AMP), cyclic glucose monophosphate (GMP), and ionized Ca^{++}. Secretory diarrhea, as in cholera, releases a toxin that increases jejunal secretion by activating cyclic AMP, which triggers enterocytes. These cells then secrete for 2 or 3 days, probably for the rest of their life cycle, until they are shed at the tips of the villi. Absorption, however, is not affected, so oral rehydration therapy is effective. Other secretory agents that in excess cause diarrhea have already been mentioned such as gastrin and VIP. *Escherichia coli* toxins, *Yersinia* toxins, and *Clostridium difficile* toxins all stimulate secretory diarrhea, but not through cyclic AMP; the mechanism is unknown, although calcium is known to be involved.[136]

Contrary to what might be expected, diarrhea is not generally associated with increased colonic contractions but with diminished segmental contractions. Increased segmental contractions impede transit and produce constipation. Increased frequency of mass actions, however, almost certainly does occur in some types of diarrhea.

Physiology of bowel preparation

The exact way in which many laxatives produce diarrhea has been unclear, partly because of what Brunton has called a *certain costiveness* in this area.[137] Laxatives act by one of the four following general mechanisms:

1. They may act directly on colonic mucosa to reduce water absorption (purgatives).
2. By their osmotic properties, they may cause fluid retention (osmotic purges).
3. They may increase motility in the small intestine to decrease transit time.
4. If unabsorbable and isotonic, they may purge simply by a high volume rapid fluid load (balanced electrolyte solutions).

Purgatives are still the most commonly used form of bowel preparation. Stimulant laxatives cause accumulation of water and electrolytes in the intestinal lumen by increasing mucosal permeability, possibly by making tight cell junctions leaky. Recently it was reported that bisacodyl, ricinoleic acid, phenolphthalein, and senna anthraquinones increase colonic mucosal release of prostaglandin E and that pretreatment with indomethacin (an inhibitor of prostaglandin synthesis) inhibited the effect of these laxatives on both fluid movement and prostaglandin E release.[138,139] These agents do, however, tend to cause severe abdominal cramping, often fail to clear the cecum, and may leave fecal residue more distally. A cleansing enema is therefore normally required to supplement the purgative, which is both time consuming for the nursing staff and unpleasant for the patient.

Osmotic purgatives such as the magnesium salts (citrate or sulphate) and nonabsorbed carbohydrate (lactulose, sorbitol, mannitol) have been used extensively as alternatives to cleansing enemas. These are usually added to, or supplement the oral contact purgative. Mannitol is widely used. Its sweet taste can be reduced by cooling, and the nausea may be decreased by premedication with an antiemetic agent such as metoclopramide, 30 minutes beforehand. A risk of explosion exists if electrocautery is performed when the nonabsorbable carbohydrates are used as purgatives for colonoscopy. This is because of the increased hydrogen gas levels from fermentation of intestinal bacteria.[140] The use of CO_2 as the insufflating agent or the aspiration of gas before reinsufflating air will prevent this complication. Magnesium salts are strong purgatives with a rather unpleasant taste, so the more palatable citrus flavor is usually preferred. Lactulose should be more widely used as an agent to prevent solidification of barium after upper GI tract examination in elderly patients. A strong case could also be made for routinely prescribing it after barium examination in institutionalized geriatric patients to avoid barium impaction.

Balanced electrolyte solutions are given orally in 4 to 6 L volumes and give excellent results. Early attempts to use a jejunal flush of balanced electrolytes led to considerable fluid absorption, but large molecules, such as PEG-4000, have proved to be very successful methods of rapid and effective bowel preparation[141] that have at last removed the need for bowel washouts before barium enema examination.[142] They have also made urgent colonoscopy for acute rectal bleeding more rewarding, so that has, to some extent, replaced angiography for this purpose. About 5% of patients are unable to complete the preparation orally because of the taste and the large volumes required. Administration of the PEG agent by nasogastric tube may be necessary to overcome this problem.[143,144]

Certain medications such as oral iron medication and constipating agents should be discontinued before bowel preparation. Oral iron forms organic iron tannites in combination with vegetable residue making the colon contents sticky and difficult to clear. A more optimal cleansing is obtained no matter what regimen is used if a liquid diet is instituted 24 to 48 hours before the examination.

The ideal agent for bowel preparation would achieve optimal bowel cleansing with relatively small volumes, be palatable by most patients, and cause a minimal amount of discomfort. It does not yet exist. The instructions to the patient should be easy to read and comprehend, and the preparation should be simply packaged.

Defecation

The physiology of defecation and the role of imaging in pelvic floor dysfunction are both discussed in Chapters 42-44.

REFERENCES

1. Gregory RA, Tracy HJ: The constitution and properties of two gastrins extracted from hog antral mucosa: Part 1. The isolation of two gastrins from hog antral mucosa, *Gut* 5:103, 1964.
2. Mutt V, Jorpes JE: Structure of porcine cholecystokinin-pancreozymin: 1. Cleavage with thrombin and with trypsin, *Eur J Biochem* 6:156, 1968.
3. Mutt V, Jorpes JE, Magnusson S: Structure of porcine secretin: the amino acid sequence, *Eur J Biochem* 15:513, 1970.
4. Feyrter F: Uber die These von den peripheren Endokrinen (Parakrinen), *Drusen Acta Neurareg* 4:409, 1952.
5. Cuttitta F et al: Bombesin-like peptides can function as autocrine growth factors in human small-cell lung cancer, *Nature* 316:823, 1985.
6. Feldman EJ, Isenberg JI, Grossman MI: Gastric acid and gastrin response to decaffeinated coffee and a peptone meal, *JAMA* 246:248, 1981.
7. Lenz HJ, Ferrari-Taylor J, Isenberg J: Wine and five percent ethanol are potent stimulants of gastric acid secretion in humans, *Gastroenterology* 85:1082, 1983.
8. Walsh JH: Gastrointestinal hormones. In Johnson LR, ed: *Physiology of the gastrointestinal tract,* ed 2, vol 1, New York, 1987, Raven Press.
9. Walsh J, Maxwell V, Ferrari J et al: Bombesin stimulates human gastric function by gastrin-dependent and independent mechanisms, *Peptides* 2:193, 1981.
10. Creutzfeldt W, Arnold R: Somatostatin and the stomach: exocrine and endocrine aspects, *Metabolism* 27:1309, 1978.
11. Soll AH, Berglindh T: Physiology of isolated gastric glands and parietal cells: receptors and effectors regulating function. In Johnson LR, ed: *Physiology of the gastrointestinal tract,* ed 2, vol 1, New York, 1987, Raven Press.
12. Solcia E et al: Endocrine cells of the digestive system. In Johnson LR, ed: *Physiology of the gastrointestinal tract,* ed 2, vol 1, New York, 1987, Raven Press.
13. Lu L, Louie D, Owyang C: A cholecystokinin-releasing peptide mediates feedback regulation of pancreatic secretion, *Am J Physiol* 256:430, 1989.
14. Maglinte DD et al: The minimum effective dose of glucagon in upper gastrointestinal radiography: gastrointestinal radiography with glucagon, *Gastrointest Radiol* 4:1, 1979.
15. Monsein LH et al: Retrograde ileography: value of glucagon, *Radiology* 161:558, 1986.
16. Read NW et al: Effect of infusion of nutrient solutions into the ileum and gastrointestinal transit and plasma levels of neurotensin and enteroglucagon, *Gastroenterology* 86:274, 1983.
17. Wolfe MM, Jensen RT: Zollinger-Ellison syndrome: current concepts in diagnosis and management, *N Engl J Med* 317:1200, 1987.
18. Stefanini P, Carboni M, Patrassi N: Surgical treatment and prognosis of insulinoma, *Clin Gastroenterol* 3:697, 1974.
19. Long RG et al: Clinicopathologic study of pancreatic and ganglioneuroblastoma tumors secreting vasoactive intestinal polypeptide (vipomas), *Br Med J* 282:1767, 1981.
20. Prinz RA et al: Glucagonoma. In Howard JM, Jordan GL, Reber HA, eds: *Surgical diseases of the pancreas,* Philadelphia, 1987, Lea & Febiger.
21. Schusdziarra V et al: Somatostatinoma syndrome: clinical, morphological, and metabolic features and therapeutic aspects, *Klin Wochenschr* 61:681, 1983.
22. Reber HA: Rare islet cell tumors of the pancreas. In Howard JM, Jordan GL, Reber HA, eds: *Surgical diseases of the pancreas,* Philadelphia, 1987, Lea & Febiger.
23. Lips CJ, Vasen HF, Lamers CB: Multiple endocrine neoplasia syndromes, *Crit Rev Oncol Hematol* 2:117, 1984.
24. Isenberg JI et al: Unusual effect of secretin on serum gastrin, serum calcium, and gastric acid secretion in a patient with suspected Zollinger-Ellison syndrome, *Gastroenterology* 62:626, 1972.
25. Bloom SR, Greenwood C: Proceedings of Somatostatin '85, *Scand J Gastroenterol Suppl* 119:1, 1985.
26. Kvols LK et al: Rapid reversal of carcinoid crisis with a somatostatin analogue, *N Engl J Med* 313:1229, 1985.
27. O'Dorisio TM et al: Somatostatin and analogues in the treatment of VIPoma, *Ann NY Acad Sci* 527:528, 1988.
28. Borison DI, Bloom AD, Pritchard TJ: Treatment of enterocutaneous and colocutaneous fistulas with early surgery or somatostatin analog, *Dis Colon Rectum* 35:635, 1992.
29. Nubiola-Calonge P et al: Blind evaluation of the effect of octreotide (SMS 201-995), a somatostatin analogue, on small bowel fistula output, *Lancet* 2:672, 1987.
30. Ladefoged K et al: Effect of a long-acting somatostatin analogue SMS 201-995 on jejunostomy effluents in patients with severe short bowel syndrome, *Gut* 30:943, 1989.
31. Sternlieb JM et al: A multicenter, randomized, controlled trial to evaluate the effect of prophylactic octreotide on ERCP-induced pancreatitis, *Am J Gastroenterol* 98:1561, 1992.
32. Choi TK et al: Somatostatin in the treatment of acute pancreatitis: a prospective randomized controlled trial, *Gut* 30:223, 1989.
33. Moncada S, Flower RJ, Vane JR: Prostaglandins, prostacyclin, thromboxane A2, and leukotrienes. In Gilman AG et al, eds: *Goodman and Gilman's The pharmacological basis of therapeutics,* ed 7, New York, 1985, Macmillan.
34. Johansson C, Bergström S: Prostaglandins and protection of the gastroduodenal mucosa, *Scand J Gastroenterol Suppl* 77:21, 1982.
35. Vantrappen G et al: Effect of 15(R)-15 methyl prostaglandin E2 (arbaprostil) on the healing of duodenal ulcer: a double-blind multicenter study, *Gastroenterology* 83:357, 1982.
36. Whittle BJ, Vane JR: Prostanoids as regulators of gastrointestinal function. In Johnson LR, ed: *Physiology of the gastrointestinal tract,* ed 2, vol 1, New York, 1987, Raven Press.
37. Misoprostol, *Med Lett* 31:21, 1989.
38. Alun Jones V et al: Food intolerance: a major factor in the pathogenesis of irritable bowel syndrome, *Lancet* 2:1115, 1982.
39. Nanda R et al: Food intolerance and the irritable bowel syndrome, *Gut* 30:1099, 1989.
40. Bentley SJ, Pearson DJ, Rix KJB: Food hypersensitivity in irritable bowel syndrome, *Lancet* 2:295, 1983.
41. Jones DB et al: Acid suppression in duodenal ulcer: a metaanalysis to define optimal dosing with antisecretory drugs, *Gut* 28:1120, 1987.
42. De Gara CJ, Gledhill T, Hunt RH: Nocturnal gastric acid secretion: its importance in the pathophysiology and rational therapy of duodenal ulcer, *Scand J Gastroenterol Suppl* 121:17, 1986.
43. Gustavsson S et al: Rapid healing of duodenal ulcers with omeprazole: double-blind dose-comparative trial, *Lancet* 2:124, 1983.

44. Prichard PJ et al: Double-blind comparative study of omeprazole 10 mg and 30 mg daily for healing duodenal ulcers, *Br Med J* 290:601, 1985.

45. Belgian Multicentre Group: Rate of duodenal ulcer healing during treatment with omeprazole: a double-blind comparison of a daily dose of 30 mg versus 60 mg, *Scand J Gastroenterol Suppl* 118:175, 1986.

46. Bianchi Porro G, Parente F: Omeprazole in the treatment of duodenal ulcer, *Scand J Gastroenterol Suppl* 166:48, 1989.

47. Lamers CBHW et al: Omeprazole in Zollinger-Ellison syndrome, *N Engl J Med* 310:758, 1984.

48. McArthur KE et al: Omeprazole: effective, convenient therapy for Zollinger-Ellison syndrome, *Gastroenterology* 88:939, 1985.

49. Mandel ID: The role of saliva in maintaining oral homeostasis, *J Am Dent Assoc* 119:298, 1989.

50. Nelson JB, Richter JE: Upper esophageal motility disorders, *Gastroenterol Clin North Am* 18:195, 1989.

51. Jones G: The radiological investigation of oropharyngeal dysphagia, *Clin Radiol* 45:295, 1992.

52. Van Oberbeck JJM: *The hypopharynx diverticulum: endoscopic treatment and manometry,* Amsterdam, 1977, Van Corcum.

53. Curtis DJ, Cruess DF, Berg T: The cricopharyngeal muscle: a videorecording review, *AJR* 142:497, 1984.

54. Gerhardt DC et al: Esophageal dysfunction in esophagopharyngeal regurgitation, *Gastroenterology* 78:893, 1980.

55. Low V, Somers S, Stevenson GW, Panju A: Cricopharyngeal muscular hypertrophy: relationship to gastroesophageal reflux (in press).

56. Goyal RK, Patterson WG: Esophageal motility. In Woods JD, ed: *Handbook of physiology—the gastrointestinal system,* vol 1, Bethesda, Md, 1989, American Physiological Society.

57. Dodds WJ et al: A comparison between primary esophageal peristalsis following wet and dry swallows, *J Appl Physiol* 35:851, 1973.

58. Winship DH, Viegas de Andrade SR, Zboralske FF: Influence of bolus temperature on human esophageal motor function, *J Clin Invest* 49:243, 1970.

59. Jordan PH, Longhi EH: Relationship between size of bolus and the act of swallowing on esophageal peristalsis in dogs, *Proc Soc Exp Biol Med* 137:868, 1971.

60. Weisbrodt NW, Christensen J: Gradients of contractions in the opossum esophagus, *Gastroenterology* 62:1159, 1972.

61. Decktor DL, Ryan JP: Transmembrane voltage of opossum esophageal smooth muscle and its response to electrical stimulation of intrinsic nerves, *Gastroenterology* 82:301, 1982.

62. Singer MV et al: Action of ethanol and some alcoholic beverages on gastric acid secretion and release of gastrin in humans, *Gastroenterology* 93:1247, 1987.

63. Neutra MR, Forstner JF: Gastrointestinal mucus: synthesis, secretion, and function. In Johnson LR, ed: *Physiology of the gastrointestinal tract,* ed 2, vol 2, New York, 1987, Raven Press.

64. Snary D, Allen A, Pain RH: Structural studies on gastric mucoproteins: lowering of molecular weight after reduction with 2-mercaptoethanol, *Biochem Biophys Res Commun* 40:844, 1970.

65. Allen A, Garner A: Mucus and bicarbonate secretion in the stomach and their possible role in mucosal protection, *Gut* 21:249, 1980.

66. Roberts SH, Heffernan C, Douglas AP: The sialic acid and carbohydrate content and the synthesis of glycoprotein from radioactive precursors by tissues of the normal and diseased upper intestinal tract, *Clin Chim Acta* 63:121, 1975.

67. Rose CJ et al: Cigarette smoking and duodenal coating with barium, *J Can Assoc Radiol* 33:77, 1982.

68. Zalewsky CA, Moody FG: Mechanisms of mucus release in exposed canine gastric mucosa, *Gastroenterology* 77:719, 1979.

69. Kauffman GL, Reeve JJ, Grossman MI: Gastric bicarbonate secretion: effect of topical and intravenous 16, 16-dimethyl prostaglandin E2, *Am J Physiol* 239:44, 1980.

70. Lamont JT et al: Cysteamine and prostaglandin $F_2\beta$ stimulate rat gastric mucin release, *Gastroenterology* 84:306, 1983.

71. Levine JS, Nakane PK, Allen RH: Immunocytochemical localization of human intrinsic factor: the nonstimulated stomach, *Gastroenterology* 79:493, 1980.

72. Donaldson RM: Intrinsic factor and the transport of cobalamin. In Johnson LR, ed: *Physiology of the gastrointestinal tract,* ed 2, vol 2, New York, 1987, Raven Press.

73. King CE, Leibach J, Toskes PP: Clinically significant vitamin B_{12} deficiency secondary to malabsorption of protein-bound vitamin B_{12}, *Dig Dis Sci* 24:397, 1979.

74. Meyer JH et al: Effects of viscosity and fluid outflow on postcibal gastric emptying of solids, *Am J Physiol* 250:161, 1986.

75. Meyer JH et al: Effect of size and density on gastric emptying of indigestible solids, *Gastroenterology* 89:805, 1985.

76. Bogentoft C et al: Influence of food on the absorption of acetylsalicylic acid from enteric-coated dosage forms, *Eur J Clin Pharmacol* 14:351, 1978.

77. Laws JW, Spencer J, Neale G: Radiology in the diagnosis of disaccharidase deficiency, *Br J Radiol* 40:594, 1967.

78. Gardner MLG: Amino acid and peptide absorption from partial digests of proteins in isolated rat small intestine, *J Physiol* 284:83, 1978.

79. Freeman HJ, Sleisenger MH, Kim YS: Human protein digestion and absorption: normal mechanisms and protein-energy malnutrition, *Clin Gastroenterol* 12:357, 1983.

80. McMichael HB: Digestion and malabsorption of fat. In Bouchier IAD et al, eds: *Textbook of gastroenterology,* London, 1984, Bailliere Tindall.

81. Hofmann AF, Poley JR: Role of bile acid malabsorption in pathogenesis of diarrhea and steatorrhea in patients with ileal resection, *Gastroenterology* 62:918, 1972.

82. Wingate DL: Backwards and forwards with the migrating motor complex, *Dig Dis Sci* 26:641, 1981.

83. Code CF, Marlett JA: The interdigestive myoelectric complex of the stomach and small bowel of dogs, *J Physiol* 246:289, 1975.

84. Stevenson GW, Collins SM, Somers S: Radiological appearance of migrating motor complex of the small intestine, *Gastrointest Radiol* 13:215, 1988.

85. Kruis W, Azpiroz F, Phillips SF: Contractile patterns and transit of fluid in canine terminal ileum, *Am J Physiol* 249:264, 1985.

86. McCoy EJ, Baker RD: Effect of feeding on electrical activity of dog's small intestine, *Am J Physiol* 214:1291, 1968.

87. Kellow JE et al: Human interdigestive motility: variations in patterns from esophagus to colon, *Gastroenterology* 91:386, 1986.

88. Kerlin P, Zinsmeister P, Phillips S: Relationship of motility to flow of contents in the human small intestine, *Gastroenterology* 82:701, 1982.

89. Kagnoff MF: Immunology of the digestive system. In Johnson LR, ed: *Physiology of the gastrointestinal tract,* ed 2, vol 2, New York, 1987, Raven Press.

90. Holmgren J, Svennerholm AM: Cholera and the immune response, *Prog Allergy* 33:106, 1983.

91. Clemens JD et al: Field trial of oral cholera vaccines in Bangladesh: results from three-year follow-up, *Lancet* 335:270, 1990.

92. Jenkins RT et al: Small bowel and colonic permeability to ^{51}Cr-EDTA in patients with active inflammatory bowel disease, *Clin Invest Med* 11:151, 1988.

93. Cooper BT: Small intestinal permeability in clinical practice, *J Clin Gastroenterol* 6:499, 1984.

94. Sanderson IR et al: Improvement of abnormal lactulose/rhamnose permeability in active Crohn's disease of the small bowel by an elemental diet, *Gut* 28:1073, 1987.

95. Hollander D et al: Increased intestinal permeability in patients with Crohn's disease and their relatives: a possible etiologic factor, *Ann Intern Med* 105:883, 1986.

96. Stenson WF, MacDermott RP: Inflammatory bowel disease. In Yamada T et al, eds, *Textbook of gastroenterology,* Philadelphia, 1991, JB Lippincott.

97. Freel RW et al: Role of tight-junctional pathways in bile salt–induced increases in colonic permeability, *Am J Physiol* 245:816, 1983.

98. Datz FL, Taylor AT: Cell labeling: techniques and clinical utility. In Freeman LM, Johnson PM, eds: *Freeman and Johnson's clinical radionuclide imaging,* ed 3, vol 3, Orlando, Fla, 1984, Grune & Stratton.

99. Brooks FP: The physiology of the liver. In Herlinger H, Lunderquist A, Wallace S, eds: *Clinical radiology of the liver,* vol 1, New York, 1982, Marcel Dekker.

100. Monaco AP, Hallgrimsson J, McDermott WV: Multiple adenoma (hamartoma) of the liver treated by subtotal (90%) resection, *Ann Surg* 159:513, 1964.

101. Dowling RH, Mack E, Small DM: Effects of controlled interruption of the enterohepatic circulation of bile salts by biliary diversion and by ileal resection on bile salt secretion, synthesis, and pool size in the rhesus monkey, *J Clin Invest* 49:232-242, 1970.

102. Mannucci PM, Forman SP: Hemostasis and liver disease. In Colman RW et al, eds: *Hemostasis and thrombosis: basic principles and clinical practice,* Philadelphia, 1982, JB Lippincott.

103. Darweesh RMA et al: Efficacy of quantitative hepatobiliary scintigraphy and fatty meal sonography for evaluating patients with suspected partial common duct obstruction, *Gastroenterology* 94:779, 1988.

104. Warshaw AL et al: Objective evaluation of ampullary stenosis with ultrasonography and pancreatic stimulation, *Am J Surg* 149:65, 1985.

105. Zeman RK et al: Postcholecystectomy syndrome: evaluation using biliary scintigraphy and endoscopic retrograde cholangiopancreatography, *Radiology* 156:787, 1985.

106. Williams W et al: Scintigraphic variations of normal biliary physiology, *J Nucl Med* 25:160, 1984.

107. Scott RB, Eidt PB, Shaffer EA: Regulation of fasting canine duodenal bile acid delivery by sphincter of Oddi and gallbladder, *Am J Physiol* 249:622, 1985.

108. Ryan JP: Motility of the gallbladder and biliary tree. In Johnson LR, ed: *Physiology of the gastrointestinal tract,* ed 2, vol 1, New York, 1987, Raven Press.

109. Geenen JE et al: Intraluminal pressure recording from the human sphincter of Oddi, *Gastroenterology* 78:317, 1980.

110. Toouli J et al: Action of cholecystokinin-octapeptide on sphincter of Oddi basal pressure and phasic wave activity in humans, *Surgery* 92:497, 1982.

111. Coelho JCU, Moody FG: Certain aspects of normal and abnormal motility of sphincter of Oddi, *Dig Dis Sci* 32:86, 1987.

112. Steinberg WM: Sphincter of Oddi dysfunction: a clinical controversy, *Gastroenterology* 95:1409, 1988.

113. Dodds WJ, Hogan WJ, Geenen JE: Perspectives about function of the sphincter of Oddi, *Viewpoints Dig Dis* 20:2, 1988.

114. Toouli J et al: Manometric disorders in patients with suspected sphincter of Oddi dysfunction, *Gastroenterology* 88:1243, 1985.

115. Kreel L: Ascites and peritoneal fluid. In Herlinger H, Lunderquist A, Wallace S, eds: *Clinical radiology of the liver,* vol 2, New York, 1982, Marcel Dekker.

116. Birkenfield LW et al: Total exchangeable sodium, total exchangeable potassium, and total body water in edematous patients with cirrhosis of the liver and congestive heart failure, *J Clin Invest* 37:687, 1958.

117. Hemmingsson A et al: Diagnosis of endocrine gastrointestinal tumors, *Acta Radiol* 22:657, 1981.

118. Dunnick NR et al: Localizing insulinomas with combined radiographic methods, *AJR* 135:747, 1980.

119. Shawker TH et al: Ultrasound investigation of pancreatic islet cell tumors, *J Ultrasound Med* 1:193, 1982.

120. Hancke S: Localization of hormone-producing gastrointestinal tumors by ultrasonic scanning, *Scand J Gastroenterol Suppl* 53:115, 1979.

121. Frucht H et al: Gastrinomas: comparison of MR imaging with CT, angiography, and US, *Radiology* 171:713, 1989.

122. Charboneau WJ et al: Intraoperative realtime ultrasonographic localization of pancreatic insulinoma: initial experience, *J Ultrasound Med* 2:251, 1983.

123. Norton JA et al: Intraoperative ultrasonographic localization of islet cell tumors: a prospective comparison to palpation, *Ann Surg* 207:160, 1988.

124. Gorelick FS, Jamieson JD: Structure-function relationship of the pancreas. In Johnson LR, ed: *Physiology of the gastrointestinal tract,* ed 2, vol 1, New York, 1987, Raven Press.

125. Malfertheiner P, Büchler M: Correlation of imaging and function in chronic pancreatitis, *Radiol Clin North Am* 27:51, 1989.

126. Cannon WB: The movements of the intestines studies by means of the Röntgen rays, *Am J Physiol* 6:251, 1902.

127. Parks TG: Natural history of diverticular disease of the colon: a review of 521 cases, *Br Med J* 4:639, 1969.

128. Connell AM, Logan CJH: The role of gastrin in gastroileocolic responses, *Am J Dig Dis* 12:277, 1967.

129. Snape WJ et al: The gastrocolic response: evidence for a neural mechanism, *Gastroenterology* 77:1235, 1979.

130. Martelli H et al: Some parameters of large bowel motility in normal man, *Gastroenterology* 75:612, 1978.

131. Drossman DA et al: Bowel patterns among subjects not seeking health care: use of a questionnaire to identify a population with bowel dysfunction, *Gastroenterology* 83:529, 1982.

132. Metcalf AM et al: Simplified assessment of segmental colonic transit, *Gastroenterology* 92:40, 1987.

133. Bond JH et al: Colonic conservation of malabsorbed carbohydrate, *Gastroenterology* 78:444, 1980.

134. Saunders DR, Wiggins HS: Conservation of mannitol, lactulose, and raffinose by the human colon, *Am J Physiol* 241:397, 402, 1981.

135. Field M, Rao MC, Chang EB: Intestinal electrolyte transport and diarrheal disease, *N Engl J Med* 321:800, 1989.

136. Turnberg LA: Pathophysiology of diarrhea. In Misiewicz JJ, Pounder RE, Venables CW, eds: *Diseases of the gut and pancreas,* Oxford, 1987, Blackwell Scientific Publications.

137. Brunton LL: Laxatives. In Gilman AG et al, eds: *Goodman and Gilman's The pharmacological basis of therapeutics,* ed 7, New York, 1985, Macmillan.

138. Beubler E, Juan H: Effect of ricinoleic acid and other laxatives on net water flux and prostaglandin E release by the rat colon, *J Pharm Pharmacol* 31:681, 1979.

139. Beubler E, Kollar G: Stimulation of PGE_2 synthesis and water and electrolyte secretion by senna anthraquinones is inhibited by indomethacin, *J Pharm Pharmacol* 37:248, 1985.

140. Bond JH, Levitt MD: Colonic gas explosion: is a fire extinguisher necessary? *Gastroenterology* 77:1349, 1979.

141. Girard CM et al: Comparison of Golytely lavage with standard diet/cathartic preparation for double-contrast barium enema, *AJR* 142:1147, 1984.

142. Fitzsimons P et al: A comparison of Golytely and standard preparation for barium enema, *J Can Assoc Radiol* 38:109, 1987.

143. Davis GR et al: Development of a lavage solution associated with minimal water and electrolyte absorption or secretion, *Gastroenterology* 78:991, 1980.

144. Reichelderfer M: Colonoscopy preparation: is it better from above or below? *Gastrointest Endosc* 33:301, 1986.

PART III

PHARYNX

4 Normal Anatomy and Techniques of Examination of the Pharynx

EMMETT T. CUNNINGHAM, JR.
BRONWYN JONES
MARTIN W. DONNER

GENERAL INDICATIONS

The pharynx participates in complex and vital bodily functions, including swallowing, respiration, and speech. It is no wonder, therefore, that diseases affecting the pharynx result in considerable clinical disability. Patients with pharyngeal disease typically present with dysphagia, usually described as a sticking sensation in their throat or behind the sternum on swallowing. More subtle manifestations of pharyngeal dysfunction, such as recurrent pneumonias or chronic sore throats and hoarseness, are also common.[1-4] Patients with primary pharyngeal disorders may consult any of a number of clinical subspecialists, including gastroenterologists, pulmonologists, otolaryngologists, and neurologists. In each case, however, radiographic studies that assess the structure and function of the upper aerodigestive tract are indispensable (see Chapter 8). In fact, without modern imaging techniques, the adequate evaluation and management of patients with pharyngeal disease would be virtually impossible.

This chapter reviews the relative advantages and disadvantages of, as well as the indications for performing, the more routine pharyngeal imaging techniques of plain radiography, cinefluorography and videofluorography, computed tomography (CT), magnetic resonance imaging (MRI), and ultrasonography. Examples of some of the more commonly encountered lesions that produce pharyngeal dysfunction are furnished to illustrate the use of the various modalities. Further examples can be found in other chapters throughout this book. Nuclear medicine procedures (scintigraphy) and the more investigative imaging techniques, such as ultrafast CT, are not covered.

PHARYNGEAL ANATOMY

The pharynx constitutes a musculomembranous tube, which, in the adult human, is approximately 12 cm long. It is bordered anteriorly by the nasal cavity, the oral cavity, and the laryngotracheal complex; superiorly by the skull

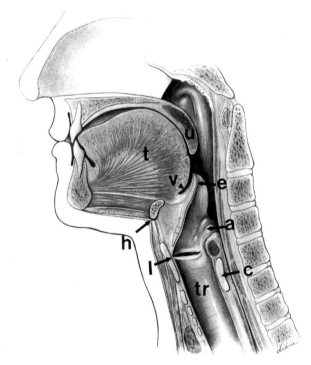

Fig. 4-1 The anatomy of the pharynx. A sagittal view of the principal anatomic landmarks of the mouth, pharynx, upper esophagus, and upper airway. *t*, Tongue; *u*, uvula; *h*, hyoid; *e*, epiglottis; *a*, arytenoid; *l*, larynx; *c*, cricoid cartilage; *tr*, trachea; *v*, vallecula.
From Donner MW, Bosma JF, Robertson DL: *Gastrointest Radiol* 10:196, 1985.

base; and posteriorly by the cervical spine (Fig. 4-1). The pharynx is connected to the oral cavity by the pharyngeal inlet, which is open in the resting state, and to the esophagus by the upper esophageal sphincter, which is closed in the resting state. The healthy pharynx acts as an effective conduit for both the passage of air from the nasal cavity to the larynx and trachea and the transport of food and liquid from the oral cavity to the esophagus.[5-8]

☐ **TABLE 4-1**

Muscles contributing to the pharyngeal stage of swallowing

Muscle	Origin	Insertion	Innervation		Primary action during deglutition
			Nerve	Nucleus	
Mylohyoid	Mandible	Hyoid	Mylohyoid n.	Vm	Elevate and anteriorly displace hyoid and larynx; propel bolus
Anterior digastric	Mandible	Hyoid	Mylohyoid n.	Vm	"
Tensor veli palatini	Scaphoid fossa, auditory tube, mandible	Palatal aponeurosis	Pharyngeal plexus	Pharyngeal plexus	"
Geniohyoid	Mandible	Hyoid	Hypoglossal n.	XII	"
Hypoglossus	Hyoid	Tongue muscles	Hypoglossal n.	XII	"
Styloglossus	Styloid process	Tongue muscles	Hypoglossal n.	XII	Seal pharyngeal inlet
Pterygopharyngeus	Pterygoid plate, mandible	Pharyngeal raphe	Pharyngeal plexus	NA	"
Palatoglossus	Soft palate	Tongue muscles	Pharyngeal plexus	NA	"
Palatopharyngeus	Soft palate	Thyroid cartilage, pharyngeal muscles	Pharyngeal plexus	NA	"
Stylopharyngeus	Styloid process	Thyroid cartilage, pharyngeal muscles	Pharyngeal plexus	NA	"
Salpingopharyngeus	Auditory tube	Pharyngeal muscles	Pharyngeal plexus	NA	"
Levator veli palatini	Temporal bone, auditory tube	Palatal aponeurosis	Pharyngeal plexus	NA	"
Musculus uvulae	Palatal bone aponeurosis	Uvula	Pharyngeal plexus	NA	"
Stylohyoid	Styloid process	Hyoid	Facial n.	VII	"
Posterior digastric	Temporal bone, mastoid notch	Hyoid	Facial n.	VII	"
Superior constrictor	Pterygoid hamulus plate, mandible, tongue muscles	Pharyngeal raphe	Pharyngeal plexus	NA	"
Thyrohyoid	Thyroid cartilage	Hyoid	Hypoglossal n.	C1	Depress and posteriorly displace hyoid and larynx
Sternohyoid	Sternoclavicular joint	Hyoid	Ansa cervicalis	C1-3	"
Sternothyroid	Manubrium	Thyroid cartilage	Ansa cervicalis	C1-3	"
Omohyoid	Superior scapula	Hyoid	Ansa cervicalis	C1-3	"
Hypopharyngeus	Hyoid, stylohyoid ligament	Pharyngeal raphe	Pharyngeal plexus	NA	Clear bolus
Thyropharyngeus	Thyroid cartilage	Pharyngeal raphe	Pharyngeal plexus	NA	"
Cricopharyngeus	Cricoid cartilage	Pharyngeal raphe	Pharyngeal plexus	NA	"
Aryepiglottic	Arytenoid cartilage	Epiglottis	Inferior laryngeal n.	NA	Adduct vocal cords to seal larynx
Lateral cricoarytenoid	Cricoid cartilage	Arytenoid cartilage	Inferior laryngeal n.	NA	"
Transverse arytenoid	Arytenoid cartilage	Arytenoid cartilage	Inferior laryngeal n.	NA	"
Oblique arytenoid	Arytenoid cartilage	Arytenoid cartilage	Inferior laryngeal n.	NA	"
Thyroarytenoid	Cricothyroid ligament	Arytenoid cartilage	Inferior laryngeal n.	NA	"
Cricothyroid	Cricoid cartilage	Thyroid cartilage	Superior laryngeal n.	NA	"

Modified after Cunningham ET Jr, Donner MW, Jones B, Point SM: Anatomical and physiological overview. In Jones B, Donner MW, eds: *Normal and abnormal swallowing: imaging in diagnosis and therapy,* New York, 1990, Springer-Verlag.

n., Nerve; *Vm,* ventromedial; *NA,* nucleus ambiguus.

The pharynx is composed of nearly two dozen individual muscles (Table 4-1),[6,9] which classically have been grouped according to anatomic zones, or segments (Fig. 4-2). The most cephalad segment is the nasopharynx, or epipharynx, and is that portion of the pharynx at and above the level of the soft palate. The most caudal segment is the laryngopharynx, or hypopharynx, and represents that portion that extends from the level of the hyoid bone or pharyngoepiglottic folds down to the cricopharyngeus muscle, or the upper esophageal sphincter. Interposed between these two segments is the oropharynx, or mesopharynx, a structure of bewildering complexity composed of no less than 10 slinglike muscles that suspend the tongue base, the hyoid, and the laryngotracheal complex from the skull base and upper portion of the vertebral column (Figs. 4-2 and 4-3).

Functionally, the events that take place during the pharyngeal phase are deemed either early or late, depending on the position and motion of the hyoid bone and associated aspects of the larynx relative to the bolus[5,9,10] (Figs. 4-3 to 4-5). The early part of the pharyngeal phase is primarily propulsive and consists of:

1. Sealing of the nasopharynx by contraction of the tensor veli palatini, the levator veli palatini, and the musculus uvulae
2. Bolus propulsion and superior and anterior elevation of the hyoid bone and associated larynx by contraction of the mylohyoid, the anterior digastric, the hyoglossus, and the geniohyoid muscles
3. Closure of the pharyngeal inlet by constriction of the styloglossus, the palatoglossus, the pterygopharyngeus, the salpingopharyngeus, the stylohyoid, the stylopharyngeus, the posterior digastric, and the superior constrictor

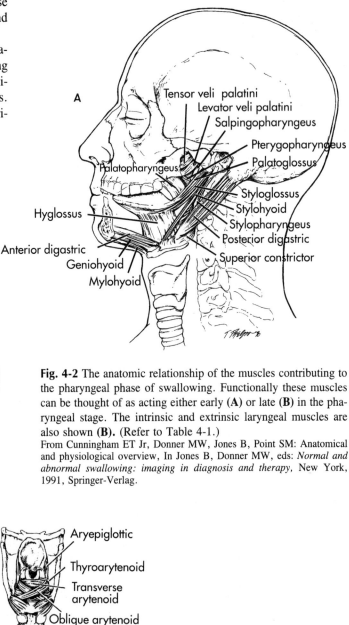

Fig. 4-2 The anatomic relationship of the muscles contributing to the pharyngeal phase of swallowing. Functionally these muscles can be thought of as acting either early (**A**) or late (**B**) in the pharyngeal stage. The intrinsic and extrinsic laryngeal muscles are also shown (**B**). (Refer to Table 4-1.)
From Cunningham ET Jr, Donner MW, Jones B, Point SM: Anatomical and physiological overview, In Jones B, Donner MW, eds: *Normal and abnormal swallowing: imaging in diagnosis and therapy*, New York, 1991, Springer-Verlag.

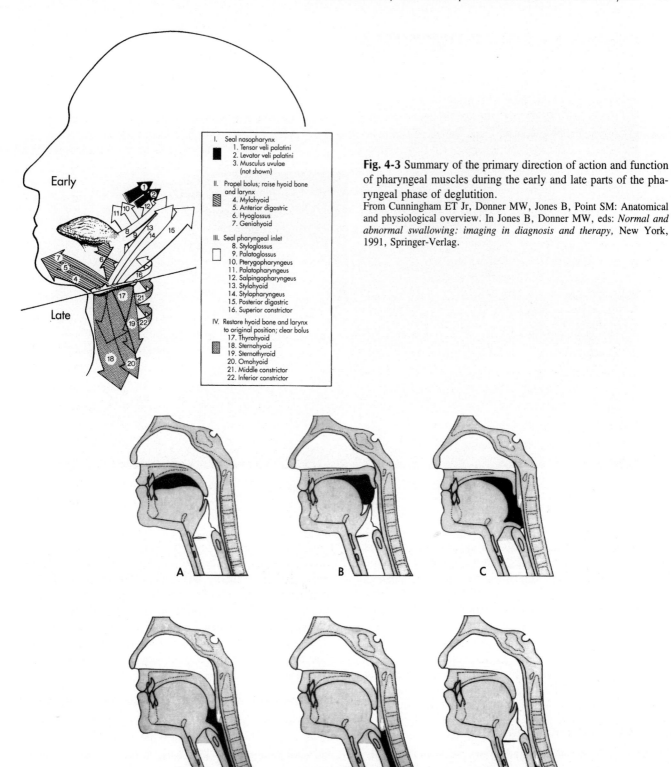

I. Seal nasopharynx
    1. Tensor veli palatini
    2. Levator veli palatini
    3. Musculus uvulae
       (not shown)

II. Propel bolus; raise hyoid bone
    and larynx
    4. Mylohyoid
    5. Anterior digastric
    6. Hyoglossus
    7. Geniohyoid

III. Seal pharyngeal inlet
    8. Styloglossus
    9. Palatoglossus
    10. Pterygopharyngeus
    11. Palatopharyngeus
    12. Salpingopharyngeus
    13. Stylohyoid
    14. Stylopharyngeus
    15. Posterior digastric
    16. Superior constrictor

IV. Restore hyoid bone and larynx
    to original position; clear bolus
    17. Thyrohyoid
    18. Sternohyoid
    19. Sternothyroid
    20. Omohyoid
    21. Middle constrictor
    22. Inferior constrictor

Fig. 4-3 Summary of the primary direction of action and function of pharyngeal muscles during the early and late parts of the pharyngeal phase of deglutition.
From Cunningham ET Jr, Donner MW, Jones B, Point SM: Anatomical and physiological overview. In Jones B, Donner MW, eds: *Normal and abnormal swallowing: imaging in diagnosis and therapy,* New York, 1991, Springer-Verlag.

Fig. 4-4 Lateral view of cinefluorographic frames from a normal swallow sequence. The bolus, in this case barium, is initially held in the oral cavity with the pharyngeal and laryngeal structures at rest **(A).** As the swallow begins, the nasopharynx is sealed and the hyoid and larynx begin to elevate **(B).** The bolus is propelled through the pharynx by an initial tongue thrust **(C)** and a subsequent cephalad-to-caudad pharyngeal stripping wave **(C-E).** The upper esophageal sphincter opens when the hyoid and larynx reach their maximal elevation **(D).** Pharyngeal and laryngeal structures return to their resting position once the bolus has entered the esophagus **(F).**
From Donner MW, Bosma JF, Robertson DL: *Gastrointest Radiol* 10:196, 1985.

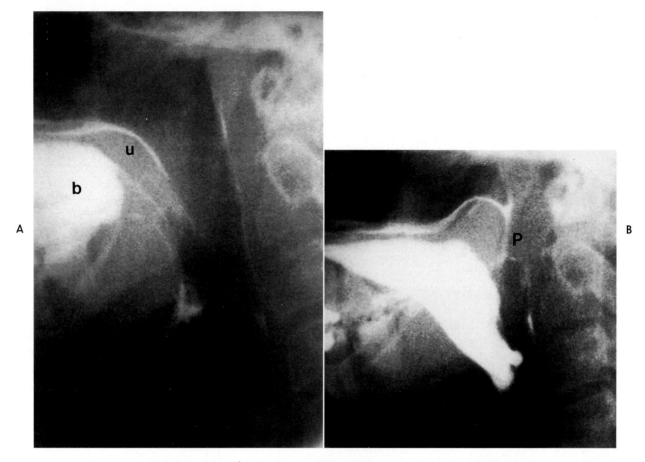

Fig. 4-5 For legend see opposite page.

In contrast, the late part of the pharyngeal phase consists primarily of clearing the bolus, and this involves:

1. Relaxation of the tonically active upper esophageal sphincter
2. Clearance of the bolus by contraction of the middle and inferior constrictor
3. Restoration of the hyoid and associated larynx to their original resting position by the combined forces of gravity and the elastic recoil of the tracheobronchial tree and strap muscles, including the thyrohyoid, the sternohyoid, the sternothyroid, and the omohyoid

NORMAL PHARYNGEAL SWALLOW

The normal pharyngeal swallow represents an artificially isolated component of a larger oral-pharyngeal-esophageal cascade (Figs. 4-1, 4-4, and 4-5). In brief, the normal swallow begins with the oral, or preparatory, phase, which is almost entirely voluntary and involves both ingestion and bolus formation. This is followed immediately by the pharyngeal phase, a largely reflex-mediated sequence in which approximately two dozen muscles that connect the skull base to the tongue and upper airway are activated. Together these muscles form a propulsive conduit that transports the

bolus from the oral cavity to the esophagus, while working in conjunction with the intrinsic laryngeal musculature to protect the upper airway. The details of this remarkable feat of functional anatomy are considered in the next section. The third and final component of a normal swallow is the esophageal phase, which consists of the peristaltic transport of the bolus from the pharynx to the stomach. This last step must be temporally linked to the sequential inhibition of the upper and lower esophageal sphincters.[9,11-14]

NEURAL CONTROL OF THE PHARYNGEAL PHASE

The muscles of the pharynx are controlled in a largely reflex manner by a number of cranial nerve motor nuclei and peripheral nerves (Fig. 4-6). In brief, sensory stimuli sufficient to elicit a swallow are conveyed from the posterior tongue, the soft palate, the tonsillar pillars, and the posterior oropharynx via the superior laryngeal nerve. This nerve terminates centrally in a discrete region of the dorsomedial medulla termed the *nucleus tractus solitarii*. From there, interneurons project directly to those specific subdivisions of the nuclei of cranial nerves, V, VII, IX, X, XI, and XII that are involved in activating the pharyngeal muscles required for swallowing. Reflex control of the phar-

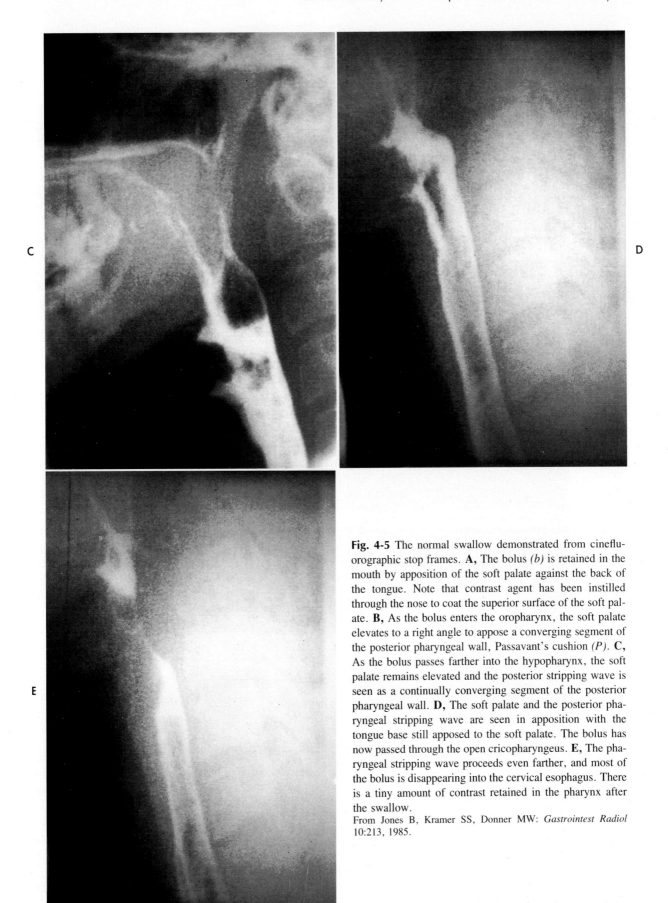

C

D

E

Fig. 4-5 The normal swallow demonstrated from cinefluorographic stop frames. **A,** The bolus *(b)* is retained in the mouth by apposition of the soft palate against the back of the tongue. Note that contrast agent has been instilled through the nose to coat the superior surface of the soft palate. **B,** As the bolus enters the oropharynx, the soft palate elevates to a right angle to appose a converging segment of the posterior pharyngeal wall, Passavant's cushion *(P)*. **C,** As the bolus passes farther into the hypopharynx, the soft palate remains elevated and the posterior stripping wave is seen as a continually converging segment of the posterior pharyngeal wall. **D,** The soft palate and the posterior pharyngeal stripping wave are seen in apposition with the tongue base still apposed to the soft palate. The bolus has now passed through the open cricopharyngeus. **E,** The pharyngeal stripping wave proceeds even farther, and most of the bolus is disappearing into the cervical esophagus. There is a tiny amount of contrast retained in the pharynx after the swallow.
From Jones B, Kramer SS, Donner MW: *Gastrointest Radiol* 10:213, 1985.

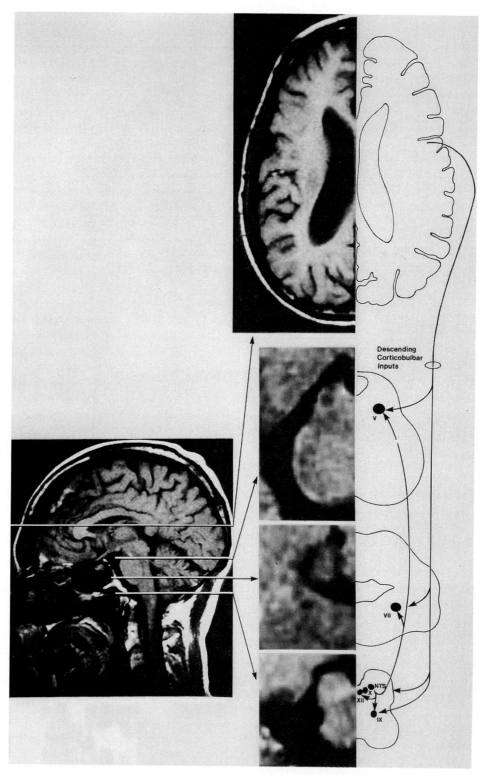

Fig. 4-6 A combined magnetic resonance image and illustration of the central neural levels and pathways involved in the control of the pharyngeal phase of swallowing. Sensory information from the oropharynx is conveyed via the nucleus of the solitary tract (NST) in the dorsal medial medulla. Discrete regions of the NST then project to the fifth, seventh, ninth, and twelfth cranial nerve nuclei to coordinate the sequential activation of pharyngeal and laryngeal musculature. These reflexes may, to some extent, be modified by descending pyramidal (shown here as corticobulbar inputs) and extrapyramidal (not shown) inputs. Projections from the region of the NST to motor neurons of the eleventh cranial nerve that innervate the strap muscles are not shown.

From Cunningham ET Jr, Donner MW, Jones B, Point SM: Anatomical and physiological overview, In Jones B, Donner MW, eds: *Normal and abnormal swallowing: imaging in diagnosis and therapy,* New York, 1991, Springer-Verlag.

ynx may, to some extent, be modified by descending inputs from the midbrain and forebrain, thus involving virtually all levels of the neuraxis. Most of the early, or propulsive, aspect of the pharyngeal phase is under the control of the fifth, seventh, and twelfth cranial nerve nuclei, whereas most of the late, or clearing, aspect of the pharyngeal phase, including relaxation of the upper esophageal sphincter, is under the control of the ninth and tenth cranial nerve nuclei. The eleventh cranial nerve, which arises from spinal levels C1 through C3, controls the strap muscles, which were noted earlier to function in a largely passive fashion during deglutition[11,15-18] (Fig. 4-4).

TECHNIQUES OF EXAMINATION
Choice of studies

A number of imaging techniques are now available for examining the pharynx.[19,20] Each has its own relative merits and shortcomings, so the choice of studies depends primarily on the patient's status, clinical history, and suspected underlying disease. The more commonly used techniques include plain radiography, barium studies such as double-contrast and dynamic pharyngography, CT, MRI, and ultrasonography. The emphasis in this chapter is placed on the relative advantages and disadvantages of these techniques in the evaluation of patients with pharyngeal disease, most typically manifested as dysphagia.

Plain radiography

Plain radiography is the least expensive, least time-consuming, and most common technique for the initial imaging of the pharynx. It is especially useful in the evaluation of trauma, foreign body impaction, and bony disorders of the cervical spine. In addition, it accurately depicts the position of the hyoid bone, the size of the tongue and pharyngeal cavity, and, in the lateral view, the thickness of the muscular layer in front of the cervical vertebral bodies.

Both frontal and lateral views should be obtained in every case, although the frontal view typically yields less information about the pharynx per se because the pharyngeal cavity is radiographically superimposed on the cervical portion of the vertebral column. Exposures of the air-filled pharynx in the lateral view should be timed so that the patient phonates the vowel "eee"; this brings forward the tongue base, hyoid bone, and larynx. In the frontal view the pharyngeal cavity may be enlarged by having the patient forcibly exhale against pursed lips; this is the so-called Jonsson or modified Valsalva maneuver. Soft tissue exposures are often useful because they can also depict bony structures with sufficient clarity for most situations. The prevertebral soft tissues and potential prevertebral space are best visualized at end-inspiration, as the posterior pharyngeal wall thickens at peak expiration and this may mimic the appearance of an abscess or tumor. Cervical spine views obtained at rest as well as in neck flexion and extension may be particularly useful when pharyngeal functions are disrupted as the result of skull base or vertebral abnormal-

ities, for example, the cervical osteophytes seen in osteoarthritis and Forestier's disease (Fig. 4-7)[21,22] or the subluxation typical of rheumatoid arthritis.[19]

Barium studies

Barium studies are best suited for the detailed and dynamic imaging of the pharynx because they provide high-resolution, real-time images. Moreover, only dynamic radiography can furnish "functional" images of the upper aerodigestive tract, whether obtained during swallowing, speech, or respiration.[13,20,23-27] Thus the radiologist may evaluate pharyngeal structure and mobility in response to a provocative challenge or while the patient is trying to reproduce his or her symptoms. However, a complete barium study of the pharynx must also include a thorough evaluation of the oral cavity and esophagus,[23,28] both because oral and, more often, esophageal lesions can give rise to referred pharyngeal symptoms[29-32] and because of the relatively high incidence of synchronous lesions involving the upper aerodigestive tract, a frequency reported to exceed 50% in some patient populations.[33]

The tailored examination

It may seem obvious, and in fact trite, to state that each patient is different. However, this is an extremely important point to keep in mind when performing a barium study of the upper aerodigestive tract, both because of the potential danger of laryngeal penetration or aspiration of large amounts of barium in a severely compromised patient, and because a lesion or defect may be missed in the patient who can compensate for his or her pharyngeal dysfunction under all but the most challenging of circumstances.[34,35] The history and clinical status of each patient must therefore be thoroughly assessed before the examination is initiated.[1,36]

In general, the more ill the patient, the more care must be taken by the radiologist. In the high-risk patient, it is advisable to have the suction apparatus set up and a nurse experienced in videofluorography on hand at the examination to assist with suctioning if necessary. Such precautions are especially important in the poststroke or recently operated patient, particularly when a tracheostomy is in place. Moreover, if there is a history of cough-choke episodes or recurrent pneumonia, and therefore aspiration poses a threat, it is advisable to start the examination with the tube centered over the larynx in the lateral position and to use only 2 to 5 ml of liquid barium. Small volumes should also be used in suspected obstruction because retention above an unexpected high-grade obstructing lesion can provoke overflow aspiration. Localization of an obstruction is usually best accomplished with the patient in the left posterior oblique position, and following the bolus from the pharyngeal inlet to the gastroesophageal junction. The frontal view is particularly helpful if there is pharyngeal asymmetry or displacement, as might occur postoperatively or in the presence of tumors or thyroid disease.

In addition to the standard erect views described later, it

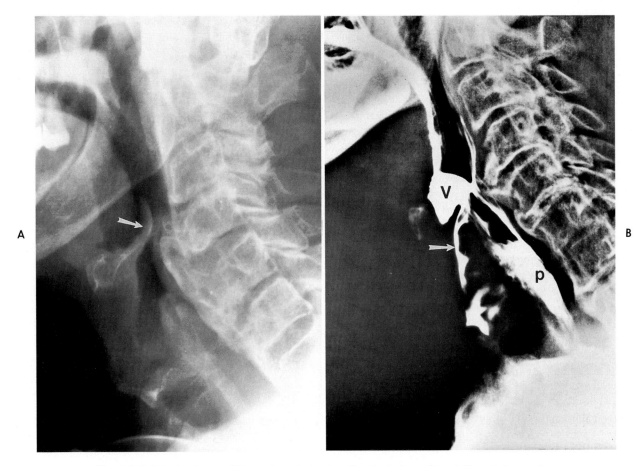

Fig. 4-7 Epiglottic abnormalities and cervical spine disorders. **A,** A lateral film of the cervical spine that also depicts well the soft tissues. There is evidence of Forestier's arthritis, with flowing osteophytes and a large bony ledge extending down the anterior cervical spine from C3 to C7. The epiglottis *(arrow)* is unable to tilt. **B,** A contrast study from another patient shows a similar finding, although the disease in this patient is more focal with large osteophytes at several levels. The epiglottis is unable to invert, remaining at an oblique or semiupright position, and there is marked laryngeal penetration *(arrow)*. Note also the retention in the valleculae *(V)* and piriform sinuses *(P)*.
From Jones B, Donner MW: Interpreting the study. In Jones B, Donner MW, eds: *Normal and abnormal swallowing: imaging in diagnosis and therapy,* New York, 1991, Springer-Verlag.

is essential to examine the capable patient in various horizontal positions, including the supine, semisupine, or prone-oblique.[24,36] Most of the reasons for examining the patient in the horizontal position pertain to the delineation of esophageal pathology. For example, some lesions, such as a significant Schatzki's ring, may be seen only in the prone-oblique position with the patient drinking continuously so that the region of the gastroesophageal junction is maximally distended. In addition, the horizontal position eliminates the propulsive effects of gravity, thus accentuating esophageal peristalsis and facilitating the examination of motility. Similarly, pharyngeal dysfunction is often highlighted in the horizontal position. For example, the supine view places stress on the patient's ability actively to seal the oral and nasal cavities. Consequently, nasal or oral re-

gurgitation, or both, in this position implies weakness of the involved pharyngeal muscles.

The semisupine view, during which the patient rests his or her head against the machine, elicits the maximal contribution of the oral and pharyngeal musculature to the elevation of the hyoid bone and laryngotracheal complex. This maneuver often allows a more detailed evaluation of the moderately compromised patient by minimizing the need for these muscles to maintain an erect head position. The prone-oblique view stresses those pharyngeal and tongue base muscles that elevate and protect the airway during a swallow by adding the weight of the tongue, the hyoid bone, and the laryngotracheal complex, and may thus disclose subtle tongue or pharyngeal weakness, or both. Subtle swallowing abnormalities may also be detected with the patient's head extended or by the fatigue provoked by repetitive swallows.[37]

As already mentioned, it is usually advisable to begin the study with small quantities of thin barium. If no laryngeal penetration or aspiration is observed, larger volumes of thick barium may then be used. When appropriate, barium paste, barium mixed with mechanical soft foods such as rice or applesauce, barium-soaked solids such as graham crackers, or barium-impregnated tablets or marshmallows may also be used. In general, a more solid bolus slows but has no impact on areas of subtle stricture or spasm. Solids are usually indicated, therefore, in the evaluation of those patients who complain of a solid-food sticking sensation but have no obvious luminal narrowing or spasm with liquid barium.

Barium may also be acidified with 37% hydrochloric acid (0.5 ml HCl/100 ml of barium) to try and reproduce symptoms that are thought to stem from gastroesophageal reflux.[38] Similarly, we have occasionally found barium chilled to 4° C useful for reproducing symptoms associated with spasm or distention.[39]

Dynamic recording

In the absence of a history or a clinical presentation suggestive of laryngeal aspiration, evaluation of pharyngeal structure and motility should commence with thick, or high-density, barium (such as E-2-HD). Both an erect lateral and an upright frontal view should be recorded. The radiographic evaluation of pharyngeal structure and function should be done systematically and include analysis of the tongue, soft palate, epiglottis, the valleculae, the piriform sinuses, the aryepiglottic folds, the larynx (including the vocal cords), the lateral and posterior pharyngeal surfaces, and the cricopharyngeus muscle. The following maneuvers should be performed with each patient.[23]

Lateral view
1. A small amount of barium can be instilled intranasally via a catheter to delineate the nasal surface of the soft palate. The movement of the soft palate is recorded while the patient repeats a word that produces maximal soft palate movement, such as "candy."
2. A swallow is recorded high in the pharynx for the evaluation of the tongue, soft palate, and proximal pharyngeal muscles.
3. A second swallow is recorded centered at a slightly lower level for the evaluation of the larynx, the middle and inferior pharyngeal constrictors, and the pharyngoesophageal sphincter. An oblique view may sometimes furnish a better view of the sphincter in large or obese individuals whose shoulders tend to obscure this region.

Frontal view
1. The patient is instructed to enunciate a short "e" with the recorder centered over the vocal cords to examine the symmetry of movement.

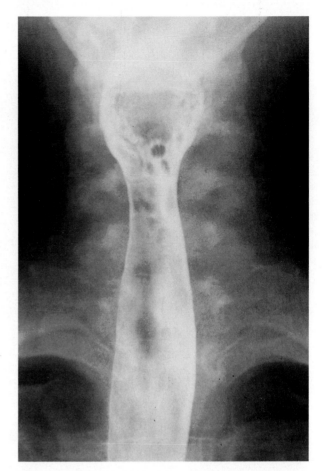

Fig. 4-8 A contrast study showing a normal frontal view during swallowing with symmetric distention of the piriform sinuses and the replacement of piriform sinuses and valleculae by a spherical appearance. The lumen at the cricopharyngeal level is widely patent as the cervical esophagus merges with the thoracic esophagus.
From Jones B, Donner MW: The pharynx. In Taveras J, Ferrucci J, eds: *Radiology diagnosis-imaging-intervention*, Philadelphia, 1990, JB Lippincott.

2. A swallow is recorded centered high in the pharynx, as described for the lateral view.
3. A second swallow is recorded centered at a lower level, as described for the lateral view (Fig. 4-8).

A normal swallow is depicted in Figs. 4-4 and 4-5.

Double-contrast pharyngography

Spot films of the pharynx coated with high-density barium, or double-contrast pharyngography, should be taken for the examination of mucosal detail.[19,25,26,40-44] As in the previous method, both lateral and frontal views should be taken, usually following the respective dynamic recordings. In both views, films at rest and during insufflation should be obtained. In the lateral position, this is accomplished by having the patient enunciate a prolonged "eee," which elevates the soft palate and moves the tongue base anteriorly, thereby revealing the mucosa of the tonsillar pillars, the val-

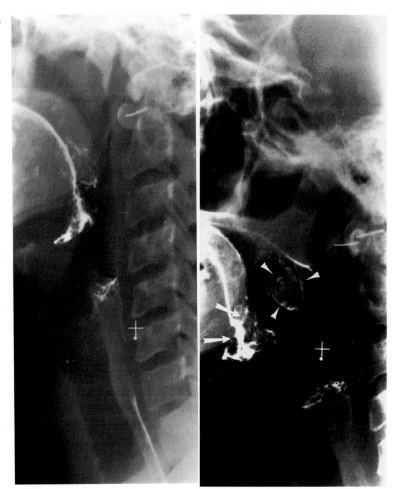

Fig. 4-9 The value of "eee." **A,** A film obtained
at rest shows the barium-coated lateral pharynx,
but the valleculae and piriform sinuses are not
clearly defined. **B,** During the sustained enunciation of "eee," the soft palate elevates to a right
angle, revealing the tonsil *(arrowheads)*. Note
also the nodular filling defects of the tongue base
(arrows) due to the presence of lymphoid tissue.

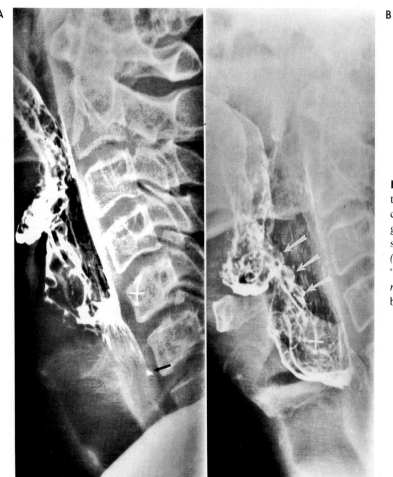

Fig. 4-10 The value of "eee." **A,** A lateral film obtained at rest shows a narrow pharynx and lack of
clear definition of the tongue base area/vallecula/epi-
glottis; the area of the aryepiglottic fold is also not
seen. There is a very tiny Zenker's diverticulum
(arrow). **B,** A film obtained during enunciation of
"eee" shows nodules on the aryepiglottic folds *(arrows)*. Note also how the valleculae have widened
because the tongue base has moved forward.

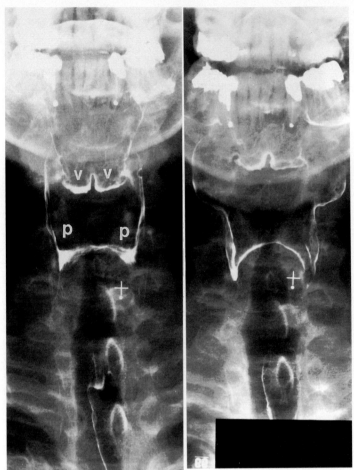

Fig. 4-11 Frontal view at rest and with insufflation. **A,** A film obtained at rest shows the paired valleculae *(V)* and paired piriform sinuses *(P)* coated with high-density barium. The outline of the epiglottis cannot be clearly defined, as its edge is not tangential to the x-ray beam. **B,** On insufflation, the pharynx bulges symmetrically. The bulging is greater above the level of the thyroid cartilage, which prevents the lower piriform sinuses from distending. From Jones B, Donner MW: *Radiology* 167:319, 1988.

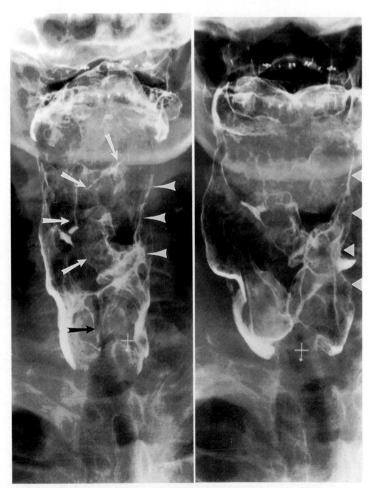

Fig. 4-12 The value of insufflation. **A,** A film obtained at rest discloses severe distortion of the mucosal pattern, with a very large mass extending across the midline *(white arrows)*. There is very subtle infiltration of the lateral wall of the pharynx *(arrowheads)*. The patient has aspirated and there is some contrast agent between the cords *(black arrow)*. **B,** On insufflation, the right side of the pharynx bulges out in a normal fashion, whereas there is no evidence of any change on the left side due to tumoral infiltration. This maneuver therefore accentuates the difference between the normal side and the infiltrated side.

leculae, and the aryepiglottic folds (Figs. 4-9 and 4-10). In the frontal view, pharyngeal distention is best achieved by having the patient blow against pursed lips, puff out his or her cheeks, blow up a balloon, or enunciate a sustained "ooo" (Figs. 4-11 and 4-12). As previously mentioned, the complete study should also involve dynamic and contrast imaging of the oral cavity and esophagus.

Adaptation, compensation, and decompensation

The adjustment of pharyngeal function in response to normal physiologic demands is termed *adaptation,* and that in response to abnormal pathologic demands is termed *compensation.* If pharyngeal structures cannot compensate for underlying pathologic changes, this results in nutritive or respiratory compromise, termed *decompensation.* The signs of adaptation, compensation, and decompensation can be easily recognized on videofluorography. For example, in the supine position, a normal swallow must be assisted by the increased contraction of the palatal and pharyngeal constrictor muscles in order to generate the added propulsion gravity normally provides in the upright position. This is a normal adjustment, or adaptation. In the patient with tongue base weakness or disease, identical changes may be observed in the upright position stemming from an abnormal adjustment to a primary pathologic change, or compensation. Compensation typically takes weeks to months to develop. Further weakening of the tongue base muscles causes either loss of control of the barium bolus with premature leakage into the pharynx prior to initiating the swallow or retention of the barium in the valleculae and piriform sinuses following the swallow. These changes all represent decompensation.[34,35] However, a patient may exhibit signs of both compensation and decompensation. The more commonly encountered radiographic signs of compensation and decompensation are illustrated in Figs. 4-13 to 4-17 and summarized in Table 4-2.

Axial studies

Axial techniques such as CT, MRI, and ultrasonography have revolutionized all aspects of modern radiography, including the examination of the pharynx. Although generally the mucosal detail of the pharynx is studied best with barium contrast, the extraluminal anatomy is demonstrated in unparalleled detail by CT, MRI, and sonography. Axial techniques are therefore most useful as an adjunct to barium studies, particularly for the purposes of tumor staging and the delineation of central and peripheral nervous system lesions producing pharyngeal dysfunction.[45]

The neuroanatomic substrate for pharyngeal control was described earlier, and lesions at any of these levels can present with symptoms of dysphagia, dysarthria, or airway compromise. The anatomy of the peripharyngeal soft tissues has been covered in considerable detail in recent reviews on axial techniques and is not repeated here.[45-54] It should be noted, however, that lesions involving the peripharyngeal tissues are best characterized by their position with regard to one of the four spaces surrounding the pharyngeal cavity: the parapharyngeal space, the masticator space, the retropharyngeal space, and the prevertebral space (Fig. 4-18). The parapharyngeal space can be further divided into the prestyloid and poststyloid compartments. Once the lesion is localized and the normal contents of that

□   **TABLE 4-2**

The more common swallowing abnormalities and their associated radiographic signs of compensation and decompensation

Abnormality	Radiographic sign of compensation	Radiographic sign of decompensation
Tongue base weakness	Palatal prominence or kink to seal the pharyngeal inlet; prominent Passavant's cushion	Inability to initiate a swallow or propel the bolus; repetitive tongue movements; leakage of bolus into pharynx before initiating a swallow; failure of hyoid and laryngeal elevation; failure of epiglottic tilt; oral regurgitation; laryngeal penetration
Palatal weakness	Elevation of the tongue base to seal the pharyngeal inlet; prominent Passavant's cushion	Leakage of bolus into pharynx before initiating a swallow: nasal regurgitation; oral regurgitation
Pharyngeal constrictor weakness	Posterior displacement of tongue base, hyoid, and larynx	Absent or decreased stripping wave; retention of fluid in the valleculae and piriform sinuses; repetitive swallows; laryngeal penetration
Intrinsic laryngeal weakness	Head flexion	Failure of vocal cords to close; laryngeal penetration
Failure of upper esophageal sphincter relaxation	Head flexion	Retention with or without laryngeal penetration; cricopharyngeal prominence or bar; cricopharyngeal tethering with decreased elevation

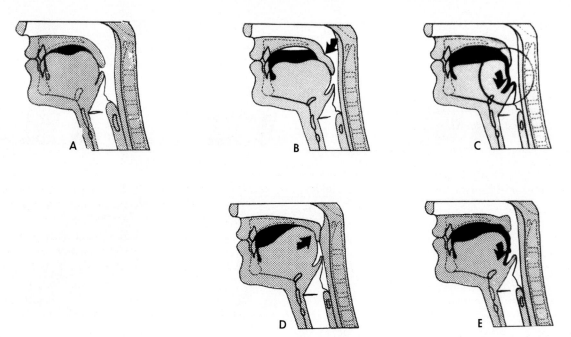

Fig. 4-13 A series of cineradiographic stop frames that illustrate the type of pharyngeal compensation and decompensation observed in the presence of tongue and palatal weakness. Under normal circumstances, the tongue base and palate act together to prevent bolus leakage into the pharynx before a swallow is initiated (**A**). Tongue base weakness, which might result from central neural lesions, tongue base tumors, or surgery, results in a compensatory downward displacement, or kink, in the soft palate that seals the pharyngeal inlet (**B**). Conversely, palatal weakness produces an upward displacement of the tongue base (**D**). When advanced, both palatal (**C**) and tongue base (**E**) weakness may lead to decompensation, with leakage of oral contents into the pharynx and, when severe, laryngeal aspiration.
From Buchholz DW, Bosma, JF, Donner MW: *Gastrointest Radiol* 10:235, 1985.

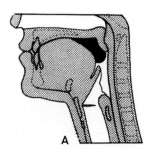
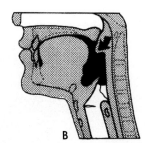
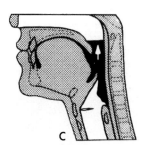

Fig. 4-14 A series of cineradiographic stop frames that illustrate the type of increased prominence of Passavant's cushion that may compensate for palatal weakness to assist in sealing the pharyngeal inlet during swallowing. Compare the normal apposition of the soft palate to Passavant's cushion (**A**) with the compensatory thickening of Passavant's cushion found in the presence of weakness of the soft palate (**B**). Severe weakness results in decompensation, with regurgitation through the nasopharyngeal isthmus (**C**).
From Buchholz DW, Bosma JF, Donner MW: *Gastrointest Radiol* 10:235, 1985.

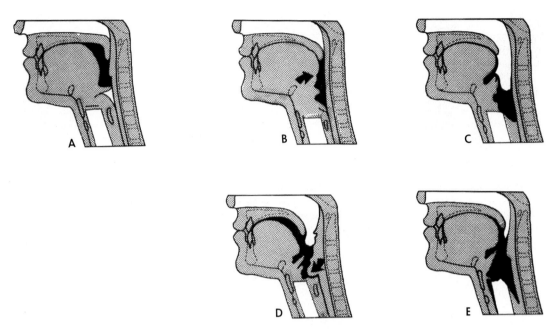

Fig. 4-15 A series of cineradiographic stop frames that illustrate the type of compensatory and decompensatory changes that may accompany weakness of the pharyngeal constrictors. Compare the normal pharyngeal stripping wave **(A)** with the compensatory posterior and superior displacement of the tongue base in response to pharyngeal weakness **(B)** and a prominent stripping wave in response to tongue base weakness **(D).** Severe weakness results in decompensation with retention **(C)** and the possibility of laryngeal penetration **(E).**
From Buchholz DW, Bosma JF, Donner MW: *Gastrointest Radiol* 10:235, 1985.

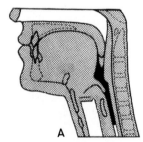
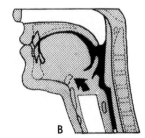
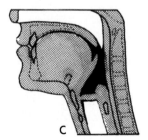

Fig. 4-16 A series of cineradiographic stop frames that illustrate the type of compensatory and decompensatory changes that may accompany weakness of the intrinsic laryngeal muscles. Compare the normal epiglottic tilt and laryngeal elevation and closure **(A)** with the exaggerated laryngeal displacement that may compensate for failed laryngeal closure **(B).** When compensation fails, this results in laryngeal penetration **(C).**
From Buchholz DW, Bosma JF, Donner MW: *Gastrointest Radiol* 10:235, 1985.

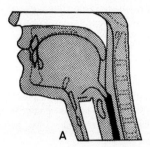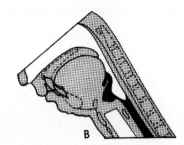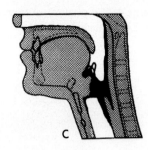

Fig. 4-17 A series of cineradiographic stop frames that illustrate the type of compensatory and decompensatory changes that may accompany failure of the pharyngoesophageal segment to open. Compare the normal opening of the sphincter **(A)** with compensatory head flexion **(B).** Failure of compensation results in retention with the possibility for laryngeal penetration **(C).**
From Buchholz DW, Bosma JF, Donner MW: *Gastrointest Radiol* 10:235, 1985.

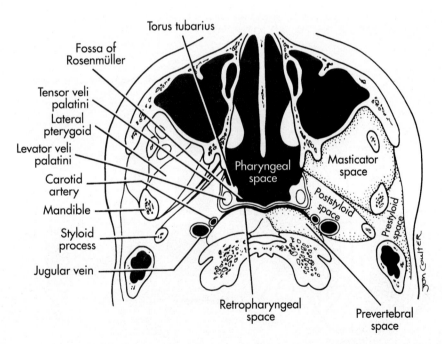

Fig. 4-18 Illustration of the axial section at the level of the oropharynx to show the position and contents of the parapharyngeal spaces, including the masticator space, the pharyngeal space, the parapharyngeal space (composed of the prestyloid and poststyloid compartments), the prevertebral space, and the retropharyngeal space.
From Point SW, Bryan RN, Zinreich ST, Cunningham ET Jr: Integrated approach to cross-sectional imaging and dysphagia. In Jones B, Donner MW, eds: *Normal and abnormal swallowing: imaging in diagnosis and therapy,* New York, 1991, Springer-Verlag.

□ **TABLE 4-3**

The contents of the pharynx and various parapharyngeal spaces and the most common pharyngeal diseases affecting these areas

Space	Contents	Pathologic changes
Pharyngeal space	Tonsils, adenoids, mucosa, muscles	Squamous carcinoma, non-Hodgkin's lymphoma, adenoid cystic and lymphoepithelial carcinoma, adenoma from minor salivary gland, plasmacytoma, melanoma, Tornwaldt's cyst, peritonsillar abscess
Parapharyngeal space		
Prestyloid	Salivary glands, fat, external carotid artery and its branches, fifth cranial nerve, and its branches	Rhabdomyosarcoma (pediatric), parotid tumors, minor salivary gland tumors, lipoma, second branchial cleft cyst, schwannomas, cellulitis, lymphangioma/hemangioma
Poststyloid	Carotid artery, jugular vein, cranial nerves IX to XII, sympathetic chain	Neurogenic tumors, paragangliomas, adenopathy, lymphoma, abscess, extracranial meningiomas
Masticator space	Mandible, muscles of mastication, V3 branch of trigeminal nerve, branches of the external carotid artery	Abscess and cellulitis (odontogenic), minor salivary gland tumor, mandibular metastasis, mandibular or muscular sarcoma, direct spread of squamous-cell carcinoma, lymphoma, hemangioma, neurogenic tumor
Retropharyngeal space	Fat, lymph nodes	Metastatic adenopathy, direct spread of squamous-cell carcinoma, lymphoma, abscess or cellulitis
Prevertebral space	Notochord elements, prevertebral muscles	Chordomas, metastatic disease to spine, osteomyelitis with abscess and/or cellulitis, schwannomas, vertebral body osteophytes
Skull base	Bone, dura mater, muscle, fat, nerve, sphenoid sinus	Local metastatic extension, chordoma, primary bone sarcoma, meningioma, blastocytoma, metastases, glomus tumor, mucocele

Modified from Point SW, Bryan RN, Zinreich SJ, Cunningham ET Jr: Integrated approach to cross-sectional imaging and dysphagia. In Jones B, Donner MW, eds: *Normal and abnormal swallowing: imaging in diagnosis and therapy,* New York, 1990, Springer-Verlag.

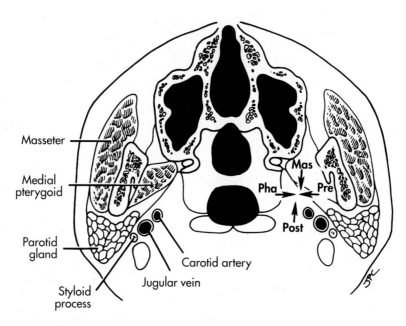

Fig. 4-19 Illustration of an axial section at the level of the oropharynx to show the displacement *(arrows)* of parapharyngeal fat by lesions located in the pharyngeal *(Pha),* masticator *(Mas),* prestyloid *(Pre),* and poststyloid *(Post)* spaces.
From Point SW, Bryan RN, Zinreich ST, Cunningham ET Jr: Integrated approach to cross-sectional imaging and dysphagia. In Jones B, Donner MW, eds: *Normal and abnormal swallowing: imaging in diagnosis and therapy,* New York, Springer-Verlag.

space or compartment thus defined, the list of the more probable pathologic offenders is usually rather limited (Table 4-3).

It is also important to identify the position of the parapharyngeal fat in axial studies, particularly MRI, because displacement of this fat by parapharyngeal lesions follows predictable patterns. Specifically, lesions in the pharyngeal space tend to displace the parapharyngeal fat laterally; lesions in the masticator space tend to displace the parapharyngeal fat posteriorly; lesions in the prestyloid compartment tend to displace the parapharyngeal fat medially; and lesions in the poststyloid compartment tend to displace the parapharyngeal fat anteriorly (Fig. 4-19).

Computed tomography

The axial images produced with CT are based on differential density to a series of radially placed x-rays, and thus the signal interpretation is similar in many ways to that of plain films, with skeletal densities yielding the sharpest image. Similarly, CT is very sensitive for portraying extraskeletal calcification. It also permits reasonable differentiation of fatty from nonfatty soft tissue, and both of these from air and bone. CT is poor, however, at discriminating closely apposed soft tissues of similar density, and is therefore relatively insensitive for distinguishing many of the muscles intrinsic to the tongue base, larynx, and pharynx.[45-47]

Magnetic resonance imaging

MRI contrast is based on the differential content, biophysical state, and movement of protons in various tissues and body fluids. Because the proportion of water, or protons, in most soft tissue is high, MRI affords excellent differential resolution of these structures, including muscles, fat, and intracranial contents. It is for this reason that MRI has become the modality of choice for the detailed imaging of peripharyngeal and central nervous system lesions. Additional advantages include unrestricted slice orientation, a lack of ionizing radiation, and diminished artifact produced by metallic dental amalgams and bone. However, MRI is slightly more expensive to perform, is relatively poor at imaging bony structures, and is contraindicated in patients with pacemakers and internal ferromagnetic materials such as aneurysm clips. In addition, MRI requires longer acquisition times, which makes it more susceptible to motion artifact, a particular problem when studying the upper aerodigestive tract in the very young, the very old, and the very sick.[45,48-54]

Ultrasonography

Sonographic contrast is based on the differential reflectivity of internal tissues to sound waves. Because tissues must be penetrated to be imaged, particularly dense structures such as bone interfere with the imaging of nearby, especially subjacent, echolucent structures. However, for

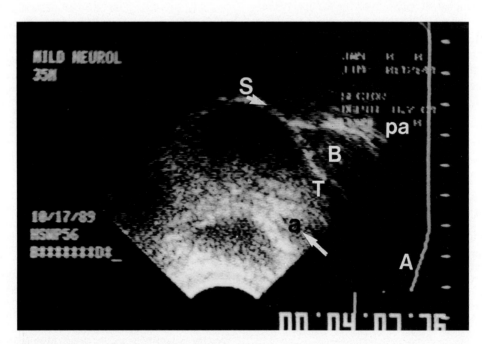

Fig. 4-20 Sagittal sonogram of the oropharynx of a bolus *(B)* immediately before a swallow. Note that the surface *(S)* of the tongue *(T)*, the tongue-bolus interface, air *(a; large arrow)* on the underside of the tongue, and the palate *(pa)* are clearly visible. Anterior is to the right *(A)*.
From Sonies B: Ultrasound imaging and swallowing. In Jones B, Donner MW, eds: *Normal and abnormal swallowing: imaging in diagnosis and therapy*, New York, 1991, Springer-Verlag.

the visualization of superficial soft tissues, such as those in the mouth and pharynx (Fig. 4-20), sonography offers many of the advantages of MRI, including unlimited slice orientation and a lack of ionizing radiation. In addition, sonography has a short acquisition time and can capture dynamic images. Sonography has therefore received considerable attention recently as an excellent tool for imaging the soft tissues of the upper aerodigestive tract, including the pharynx.

Sonographic images of the pharynx are best obtained with the transducer positioned submentally so that neither the mandible nor the hyoid bone hinders imaging. In general, this permits adequate imaging of only the oral cavity, and the nasopharynx and oropharynx, although the entire pharynx may be visible in women and small children. Depending on the area to be imaged and the suspected underlying disease, sagittal, coronal, or transverse views can be taken. The sagittal view is used most typically to image the tongue base and pharyngeal inlet, whereas the coronal and transverse views are superior for imaging the pharyngeal cavity itself. However, ultimately the relative sensitivity and specificity of sonography as an imaging technique in the evaluation of pharyngeal disorders depends in large part on the experience of the sonographer.[55-58]

FUTURE DIRECTIONS IN IMAGING

The recent development of combined cinemanofluorographic techniques for the simultaneous recording of movements and pressures has contributed considerably to the investigation of functional disorders involving the upper aerodigestive tract.[10,14] In addition, shorter acquisition times for both CT and MRI will soon permit dynamic, real-time, cross-sectional studies of this region to be obtained, so-called cine-CT and cine-MRI. To date, however, neither of these techniques has achieved widespread use in the evaluation and management of pharyngeal disorders.

REFERENCES

1. Castell DO, Donner MW: Evaluation of dysphagia: a careful history is crucial, *Dysphagia* 2:65, 1987.
2. Merlo A, Cohen S: Swallowing disorders, *Annu Rev Med* 39:17, 1988.
3. Marshall JB: Dysphagia: diagnostic pitfalls and how to avoid them, *Postgrad Med* 85:243, 1989.
4. Cook IJS: Normal and disordered swallowing: new insights, *Bailliere's Clin Gastroenterol* 5:245, 1991.
5. Bosma JF, Donner MW: Physiology of the pharynx. In *Otolaryngology*, Philadelphia, 1980, WB Saunders.
6. Donner MW, Bosma JF, Robertson DL: Anatomy and physiology of the pharynx, *Gastrointest Radiol* 10:196, 1985.
7. Bosma JF, Donner MW, Tanaka E, Robertson D: Anatomy of the pharynx, pertinent to swallowing, *Dysphagia* 1:23, 1986.
8. Curtis DJ: Radiographic anatomy of the pharynx, *Dysphagia* 1:51, 1986.
9. Cunningham ET Jr, Donner MW, Jones B, Point SM: Anatomical and physiological overview. In Jones B, Donner MW, eds: *Normal and abnormal swallowing: imaging in diagnosis and therapy*, New York, 1990, Springer-Verlag.
10. Cook IJS, Dodds WJ, Dantas RO et al: Timing of videofluoroscopic, manometric events and bolus transit during the oral and pharyngeal phases of swallowing, *Dysphagia* 4:8, 1989.
11. Miller AJ: Deglutition, *Physiol Rev* 63:129, 1982.
12. Dodds WJ: The physiology of swallowing, *Dysphagia* 3:171, 1989.
13. Dodds WJ, Stewart ET, Logemann JA: Physiology and radiology of the normal oral and pharyngeal phases of swallowing, *AJR* 154:953, 1989.
14. Sokol EM, Heitmann P, Wolf BS, Cohen BR: Simultaneous cineradiographic and manometric study of the pharynx, hypopharynx and cervical esophagus, *Gastroenterology* 51:960, 1966.
15. Miller AJ: Neurophysiological basis of swallowing, *Dysphagia* 1:91, 1986.
16. Miller AJ: Swallowing: neurophysiologic control of the esophageal phase, *Dysphagia* 2:72, 1987.
17. Sessle BJ, Henry JL: Neural mechanisms of swallowing: neurophysiological and neurochemical studies on brain stem neurons in the solitary tract region, *Dysphagia* 4:61, 1989.
18. Cunningham ET Jr, Sawchenko PE: Central neural control of esophageal motility: a review, *Dysphagia* 5:35, 1990.
19. Donner MW, Seaman WB, Gayler BW: Radiology. In Burhenne HJ, Margulis AR, eds: *Alimentary tract radiology*, ed 4, St Louis, 1989, Mosby–Year Book.
20. Dodds WJ, Logemann JA, Stewart ET: Radiological assessment of abnormal oral and pharyngeal phases of swallowing, *AJR* 154:965, 1989.
21. Zerhouni EA, Bosma JF, Donner MW: Relationship of cervical spine disorders to dysphagia, *Dysphagia* 1:129, 1987.
22. Davies RP, Sage MR, Brophy BP: Cervical osteophyte induced dysphagia, *Aust Radiol* 33:223, 1990.
23. Jones B, Kramer SS, Donner MW: Dynamic imaging of the pharynx, *Gastrointest Radiol* 10:213, 1985.
24. Jones B, Donner MW: Examination of the patient with dysphagia, *Radiology* 167:319, 1988.
25. Jones B, Donner MW: Interpreting the study. In Jones B, Donner MW, eds: *Normal and abnormal swallowing: imaging in diagnosis and therapy*, New York, 1990, Springer-Verlag.
26. Jones B, Donner MW: Common structural lesions. In Jones B, Donner MW, eds: *Normal and abnormal swallowing: imaging in diagnosis and therapy*, New York, 1990, Springer-Verlag.
27. Gayler BW, Donner MW, Beck TJ: Dynamic radiography of the pharynx and esophagus. In Margulis AR, Burhenne HJ, eds: *Alimentary tract radiology*, ed 4, St Louis, 1989, Mosby–Year Book.
28. Jones B, Donner MW: Pharyngoesophageal interrelationships. In Jones B, Donner MW, eds: *Normal and abnormal swallowing: imaging in diagnosis and therapy*, New York, 1990, Springer-Verlag.
29. Edwards DAW: History and symptoms of esophageal disease. In Vantrappen G, Hellemans J, eds: *Diseases of the esophagus*, New York, 1974, Springer-Verlag.
30. Cherry J, Siegel CI, Margulies SI, Donner MW: Pharyngeal localization of symptoms of gastroesophageal reflux, *Ann Otolaryngol* 79:912, 1970.
31. Jones B, Ravich WJ, Donner MW et al: Pharyngoesophageal interrelationships: observations and working concepts, *Gastrointest Radiol* 10:225, 1985.
32. Jones B, Donner MW, Rubesin SE et al: Pharyngeal finding in 21 patients with achalasia of the esophagus, *Dysphagia* 2:87, 1987.
33. Price JC, Jansen CJ, Johns ME: Esophageal reflux and secondary malignant neoplasia at laryngoesophagectomy, *Arch Otolaryngol Head Neck Surg* 116:163, 1990.
34. Buchholz DW, Bosma JF, Donner MW: Adaptation, compensation, and decompensation of the pharyngeal swallow, *Gastrointest Radiol* 10:235, 1985.
35. Jones B, Donner MW: Adaptation, compensation, and decompensation. In Jones B, Donner MW, eds: *Normal and abnormal swallowing: imaging in diagnosis and therapy*, New York, 1990, Springer-Verlag.

36. Jones B, Donner MW: The tailored examination. In Jones B, Donner MW, eds: *Normal and abnormal swallowing: imaging in diagnosis and therapy,* New York, 1990, Springer-Verlag.

37. Taylor AJ, Dodds WJ, Stewart ET: Pharynx: value of oblique projections for radiographic examination, *Radiology* 178:59, 1991.

38. Donner MW, Silbiger ML, Hookman R, Hendrix TR: Acid-barium swallows in the radiographic evaluation of clinical esophagitis, *Radiology* 87:220, 1966.

39. Ott DJ, Gelfand DW, Munitz HA, Chen YM: Cold barium suspensions in the clinical evaluation of the esophagus, *Gastrointest Radiol* 9:193, 1984.

40. Ekberg O, Nylander G: Double-contrast examination of the pharynx, *Gastrointest Radiol* 10:263, 1985.

41. Semenkovich JW, Balfe DM, Weyman PJ et al: Barium pharyngography: comparison of single and double contrast, *AJR* 144:715, 1985.

42. Balfe DM, Heiken JP: Contrast evaluation of structural lesions of the pharynx, *Curr Probl Diagn Radiol* 15:73, 1986.

43. Rubesin SE, Jessurum J, Robertson D, Jones B, Bosma JF et al: Lines of the pharynx, *Radiographics* 7:217, 1987.

44. Rubesin SE, Jones B, Donner MW: Contrast pharyngography: the importance of phonation, *AJR* 148:269, 1987.

45. Point SW, Bryan RN, Zinreich SJ, Cunningham ET Jr: Integrated approach to cross-sectional imaging and dysphagia. In Jones B, Donner MW, eds: *Normal and abnormal swallowing: imaging in diagnosis and therapy,* New York, 1990, Springer-Verlag.

46. Latchaw RE: Computed tomography of the head and spine. In Bryan RN, McCluggage CE, Horowitz BL, eds: *The normal and abnormal neck,* Chicago, 1985, Mosby–Year Book.

47. Curtin HD: Nasopharynx and paranasopharyngeal space. In Latchaw RE, ed: *Computed tomography of the head and spine,* Chicago, 1985, Mosby–Year Book.

48. Kim W, Buchholz D, Kumar A et al: Magnetic resonance imaging for evaluating neurogenic dysphagia, *Dysphagia* 2:40, 1987.

49. Christianson R, Lufkin RB, Vinuela F et al: Normal magnetic resonance imaging anatomy of the tongue, oropharynx, hypopharynx, and larynx, *Dysphagia* 1:119, 1987.

50. Cross R, Shapiro M, Som P: MRI of the parapharyngeal space, *Radiol Clin North Am* 27:353, 1987.

51. Teresi LM, Lufkin RB, Vinuela F et al: MR imaging of the nasopharynx and floor of the middle fossa: Part I. Normal anatomy, *Radiology* 164:811, 1987.

52. Lufkin RB, Hanafee WN: Magnetic resonance imaging of the head and neck, *Invest Radiol* 23:162, 1988.

53. Kassel E, Keller A, Kuchorczyk W: MRI of the floor of the mouth, tongue and orohypopharynx, *Radiol Clin North Am* 27:331, 1989.

54. Scheillas KP: MR imaging of the muscles of mastication, *AJNR* 10:829, 1989.

55. Shawker TH, Sonies BC, Hall TE, Baum BF: Ultrasound analysis of tongue, hyoid and larynx activity during swallowing, *Invest Radiol* 19:82, 1984.

56. Stone M, Shawker T: An ultrasound examination of tongue movement during swallowing, *Dysphagia* 1:78, 1986.

57. Gritzman N, Gruhwald F: Sonographic anatomy of tongue and floor of the mouth, *Dysphagia* 3:196, 1988.

58. Sonies BC: Ultrasound imaging and swallowing. In Jones B, Donner MW, eds: *Normal and abnormal swallowing: imaging in diagnosis and therapy,* New York, 1990, Springer-Verlag.

5 Benign Structural Diseases of the Pharynx

OLLE EKBERG

Pharyngeal symptoms are much more frequently due to functional abnormalities than to benign structural diseases. Many of the entities described in this chapter are of extrapharyngeal origin. They affect the pharynx because of their anatomic proximity to either the pharyngeal walls themselves, or to nerves and muscles that are adjacent to the pharynx or that control pharyngeal function. The surface mucosa of the pharynx is usually quite irregular, partly because of the richness of lymphoid tissue underneath, and therefore subtle mucosal abnormalities easily escape detection on reasonably adequate double-contrast pharyngograms. This emphasizes both the need for the radiologist to take great care with these examinations and the importance of the clinical examination, both direct and indirect using a mirror. Computed tomography (CT) and ultrasound are both becoming more valuable in the radiologic examination of the pharynx.

BENIGN NEOPLASMS

Benign neoplasms may develop in all types of tissue in the pharyngeal area, including the mucosa, pharyngeal wall, and parapharyngeal spaces.[1] Most benign tumors in the oropharynx (e.g., papilloma, adenoma, fibroma, and lipoma) can be inspected through the mouth, but these entities are actually rare.

Small (less than 1 cm) retention cysts in the valleculae are common. When small, they may resemble aberrant lymphoid tissue, but, even when large, they are not usually symptomatic (Fig. 5-1). However, if a vallecular cyst becomes infected, it usually causes pain during swallowing (Fig. 5-2).

Hemangiomas in the pharyngeal area are uncommon. They may be small innocuous phenomena but occasionally become quite large. They share characteristics with other hemangiomas in the gastrointestinal tract. When large they may impinge on the airways and obstruct both breathing and swallowing. Phleboliths are a diagnostic sign if present.

MUCOSAL ABNORMALITIES

The diagnosis of mucosal abnormalities can be difficult because of the irregularity of the normal pharyngeal mucosal surface. Mucosal lesions caused by candidiasis are seen as plaquelike protrusions. These patients usually have pain on swallowing and often have *Candida* infection in the oral cavity, which can be easily inspected, as well as in the esophagus.

FOREIGN BODIES

Foreign bodies in the pharynx may be located in the vallecula, piriform sinus, or, more commonly, above the cricopharyngeus muscle (Fig. 5-3). A mucosal tear may cause considerable pain even after the foreign body has dislodged, but such tears are notoriously difficult to demonstrate.

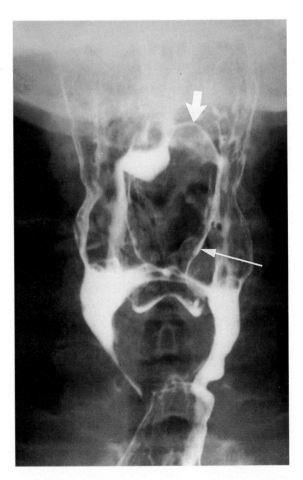

Fig. 5-1 Vallecular cyst. There is a 2-cm retention cyst *(thick arrow)* in the left vallecula. Contrast medium has also entered the laryngeal vestibule *(thin arrow)*.

TRAUMA

Trauma to the neck may cause perforation of the pharynx. Clinically, pain is followed by fever, and crepitus may be found on examination. The first radiologic sign is air in the soft tissue of the neck, usually in the prevertebral area (Fig. 5-4). Initially this may consist only of a small sliver of air, but sometimes massive and widespread air in the soft tissues of the neck and face can develop.

A water-soluble contrast swallow can often reveal the site of the perforation (Figs. 5-5 and 5-6). Trauma may also cause fractures of the thyroid cartilage and the hyoid bone, which may cause severe bleeding, although bleeding may also occur without fractures. The bleeding may then cause considerable swelling and create a mass effect in the neck that obstructs both breathing and swallowing.

Perforation may occur during endoscopy. This characteristically happens above the cricopharyngeus muscle and is more common in patients whose muscle is prominent. In patients with a Zenker's diverticulum, the endoscope may inadvertently be passed into the diverticulum and cause perforation. With the advent of smaller endoscopes and intubation performed under direct vision, such complications are becoming less common.

After a hemithyroidectomy and other surgical procedures in the neck, bleeding may take place in the immediate postoperative period. When large or infected, such a hematoma may cause dysphagia (Fig. 5-7).

LATERAL PHARYNGEAL OUTPOUCHINGS

Outpouchings of the lateral pharyngeal wall are usually mild and caused by defective tonicity of pharyngeal constrictors. When large, they are often called *hypopharyngeal ears* (Fig. 5-8, *A*). Such defects may be unilateral or bilateral. They appear as large, smooth-margined barium- and air-filled bulges. Lateral pouches through the thyrohyoid membrane are located between the hyoid bone and the thyroid cartilage.[1] They protrude through the membrane at a point of weakness where the superior laryngeal vessels penetrate. They are usually encountered in elderly patients and, although not definitely linked to symptoms, may indicate lack of tonicity of the constrictor musculature.[2] In younger

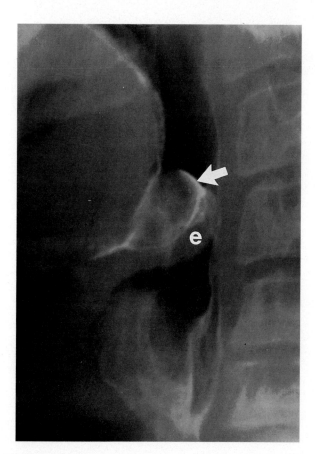

Fig. 5-2 A 3-cm infected cyst *(arrow)* in the vallecular area. The epiglottis *(e)* was dislocated inferiorly and did not move properly during swallowing.

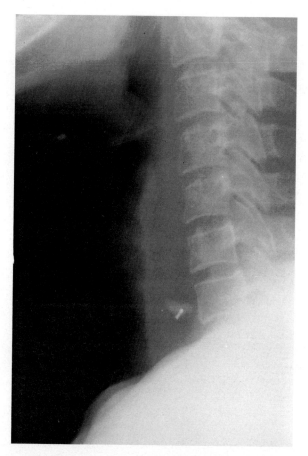

Fig. 5-3 A broken tooth has lodged in the pharyngeoesophageal segment. This patient had severe discomfort and was unable to swallow.

Fig. 5-4 Trauma to the neck with the subtle presence of air in the prevertebral soft tissue *(arrow)*.

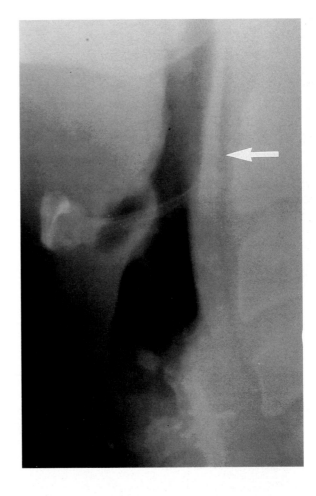

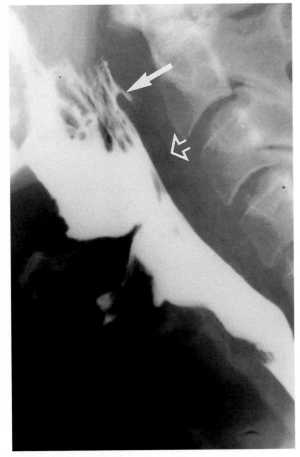

Fig. 5-5 Perforation of the posterior wall of the pharynx. The patient was inadvertently given barium, and some of this can be seen in a small pocket *(solid arrow)* outside the posterior pharyngeal wall in the prevertebral soft tissue. There is also air in the prevertebral soft tissue *(open arrow)*.

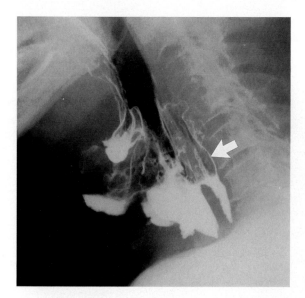

Fig. 5-6 Perforation of the posterior pharyngeal wall made by a retractor used during a Caldwell operation on the cervical spine. There is a major leak of barium into the neck *(arrow)*.

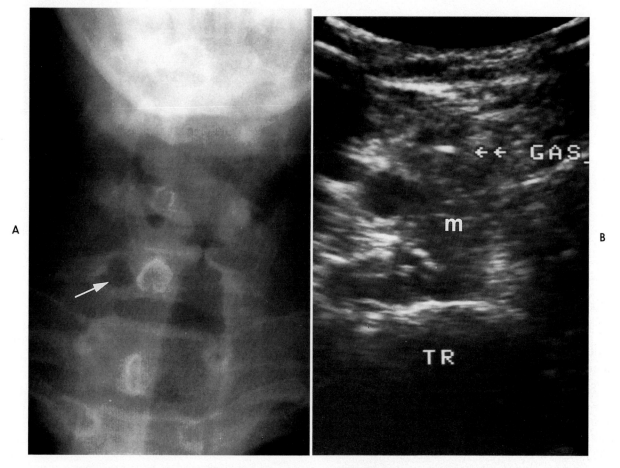

Fig. 5-7 Postoperative hematoma that formed after a right hemithyroidectomy. **A,** Anteroposterior view of the neck shows deviation of the pharynx and the trachea to the left. There is a 1-cm collection of air *(arrow)* to the right of the midline. **B,** Ultrasound image obtained in a transverse projection shows a mass *(m)* with decreased echogenicity due to edema and bleeding as well as the 1-cm air collection *(small arrows)*.

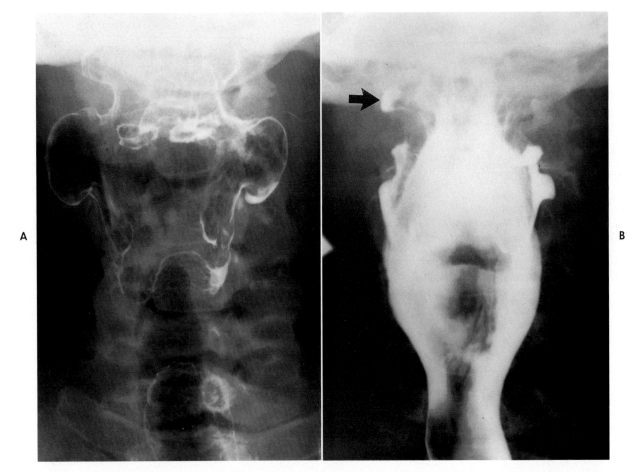

Fig. 5-8 A, Bilateral hypopharyngeal "ears" protruding through a weak thyrohyoid membrane. **B,** A small transient diverticulum *(arrow)* on the right side above the hyoid bone through the tonsillar fossa.

people, they are probably more commonly found in individuals who play wind instruments or in glassblowers. True diverticula in this area are very rare.

Outpouching in the tonsillar fossa, above the hyoid bone, may also occur and is particularly common after tonsillectomy (Fig. 5-8, *B*). Curtis et al.[3] have noted such hypopharyngeal outpouchings to be particularly symptomatic if they appear and disappear early during swallowing.[3]

THE PHARYNGOESOPHAGEAL SEGMENT
Zenker's diverticulum

Zenker's diverticula are located in the midline and usually first appear at a mean age of between 60 and 70. They protrude through Killian's dehiscence between the cricopharyngeus muscle and the inferior constrictor and are usually between 2 and 6 cm in size[4] (Fig. 5-9). When large, they retain food, and affected patients may experience a characteristic regurgitation of food when they lie down even several hours after a meal. However, these patients present with dysphagia or aspiration pneumonia.[5] The opening of the diverticulum is usually rather narrow and has a pro-

nounced neck. Diverticula are found in about 2% of those patients with a nonspecific dysphagia referred for a radiologic evaluation. When large, they protrude to the left of the midline. A Zenker's diverticulum should be distinguished from retention above an incoordinated cricopharyngeus muscle.

Killian-Jamieson's diverticulum

Killian-Jamieson's diverticula are located inferior to the cricopharyngeus muscle and protrude laterally (Fig. 5-10). They are often smaller than Zenker's diverticula. Their neck may be narrow or broad,[2] and they may be bilateral. In addition, they seldom retain swallowed material, and are rare entities.

Webs

Cervical esophageal webs are a common cause of dysphagia and are more common in women.[6] They are typically located at the level of the cricopharyngeus muscle, which is often dysfunctional. They are about 1 mm thick and often localized anteriorly, but may even be circum-

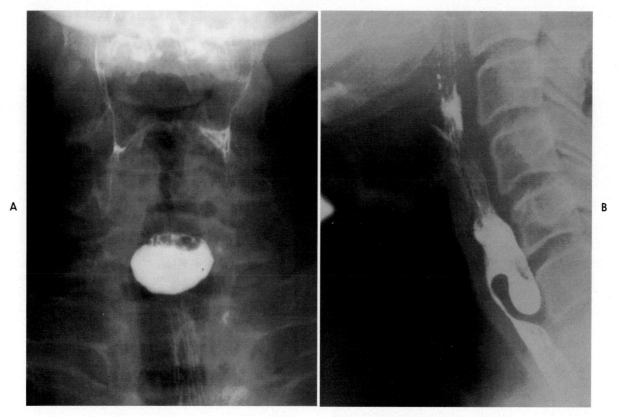

Fig. 5-9 Zenker's diverticulum. **A,** Anteroposterior projection. **B,** Lateral projection.

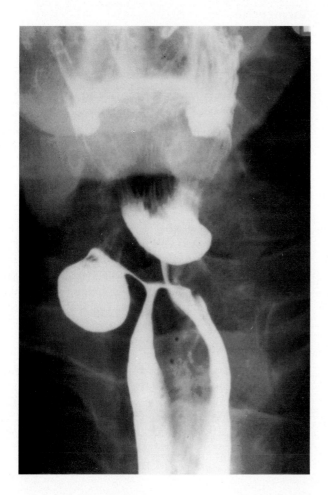

Fig. 5-10 An unusual case in which the patient had both a Zenker's and a right-sided lateral pharyngeal diverticulum.

ferential (Fig. 5-11). They have been associated with anemia and are one of the features of the increasingly rare Plummer-Vinson syndrome.[7] Most webs seem to be asymptomatic,[8] but they may cause dysphagia for solids. Cervical esophageal webs have been regarded as premalignant, but this is a controversial matter.[9,10] Endoscopic dilatation brings about a significant or total elimination of the web and symptoms.

Cricopharyngeal webs are often visible only transiently during a barium swallow and are thus readily overlooked. Cine or video recording can be helpful for disclosing their presence.

Weblike structures can be seen in the floor of the piriform sinuses and, as such, are a normal phenomenon. They are created by a mucosal fold over the inferior laryngeal nerve. Another weblike structure, which may be seen in either of the valleculae, is due to a mucosal fold that covers an aberrant artery or vein, or both.[11]

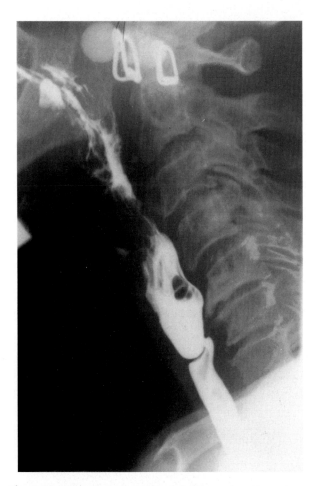

Fig. 5-11 Cervical esophageal web leaving only a 2-mm lumen posteriorly. The patient had severe dysphagia.

BRANCHIAL CLEFT ANOMALIES

Congenital lateral pharyngeal diverticula arising from branchial cleft cysts and tracts are rare.[12,13] If they are derived from the second cleft, their internal opening is located in the area of the valleculae. If they are derived from the third or fourth cleft, the opening is in the area of the thyrohyoid membrane and piriform sinus (Fig. 5-12).

ENLARGED TONSILS

When enlarged, the tonsils are seen as a unilateral or bilateral irregular protruding mass (Fig. 5-13). Rarely a large tonsillar abscess develops after tonsillitis.

PARAPHARYNGEAL ABNORMALITIES
Thyroid gland

An enlarged thyroid gland must reach a considerable size before it can encroach on the cervical esophagus, which is located posteriorly in the neck. However, when enlarged, the posterior lobes of the gland may extend backward and even grow between the trachea and the esophagus. Patients with thyrotoxicosis or inflammatory disease of the thyroid may have pain on swallowing, but the size of the thyroid itself does not usually affect the cervical esophagus in these patients. Rarely the whole thyroid gland, or a part, is ectopically localized in the base of the tongue, and the resulting mass effect may cause swallowing difficulties (Fig. 5-14).

Laryngoceles

A laryngocele seldom extends into the pharyngeal area and does not cause dysphagia. However, when large, the external portion of a laryngocele may encroach on the piriform sinus (Fig. 5-15).

Cervical spine osteophytes, spurs, and kyphosis

Cervical spine spurs may be quite large and impinge on the pharynx (Fig. 5-16). They may also affect the prevertebral space and hinder the smooth upward and downward movement of the pharynx during swallowing.

Parapharyngeal abscesses

Infections in the tonsillar area may perforate into the parapharyngeal space. If this results in the formation of an abscess, it may cause the lateral pharyngeal wall to deviate medially. Cross-section imaging is the modality of choice to assess the spread of infection. Rupture into the prevertebral space allows the abscess to spread into the mediastinum.

Tortuous vessels

The carotid arteries may become elongated and tortuous in elderly or hypertensive individuals and can present as a pulsatile mass in the pharynx. Tinnitus may be another symptom in these patients (Fig. 5-17).

Text continued on p. 126.

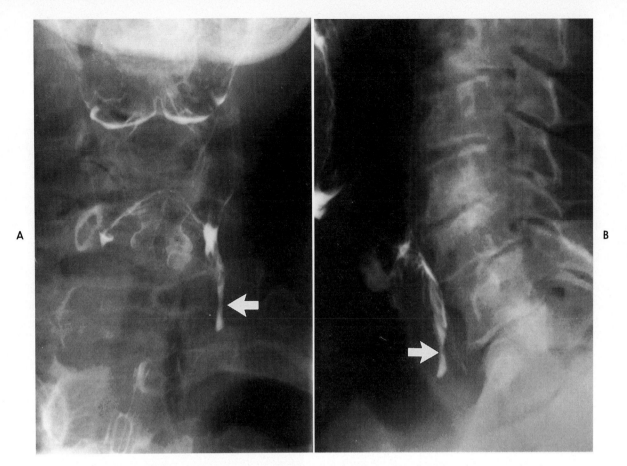

Fig. 5-12 Remnant from the fourth branchial pouch *(arrow)* extending inferiorly from the left piri-form sinus. **A,** Anteroposterior view. **B,** Lateral view.

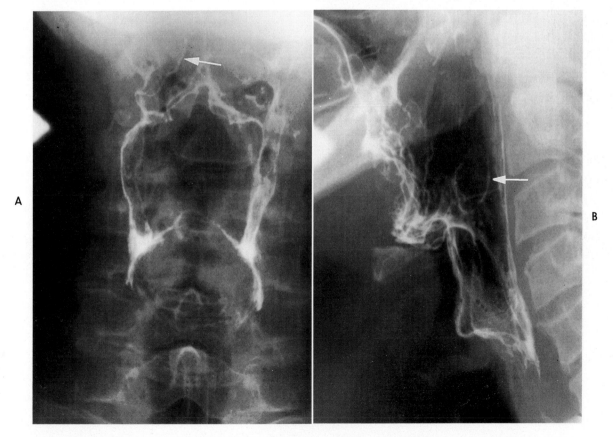

Fig. 5-13 Large tonsil *(arrows)* on the right side. **A,** Anteroposterior projection. **B,** Lateral projection.

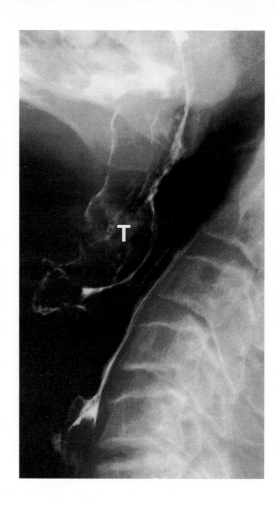

Fig. 5-14 An aberrant thyroid gland located in the base of the tongue *(T)*. A nuclear medicine study showed uptake in this location but none in the normal position.

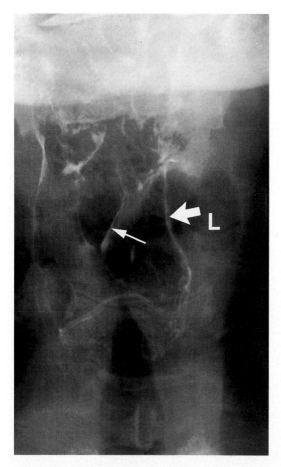

Fig. 5-15 Large external and internal laryngocele that dislocates the left lateral wall of the laryngeal vestibule medially *(thin arrow)*. The external portion *(L)* dislocates the left lateral pharyngeal wall medially *(thick arrow)*.

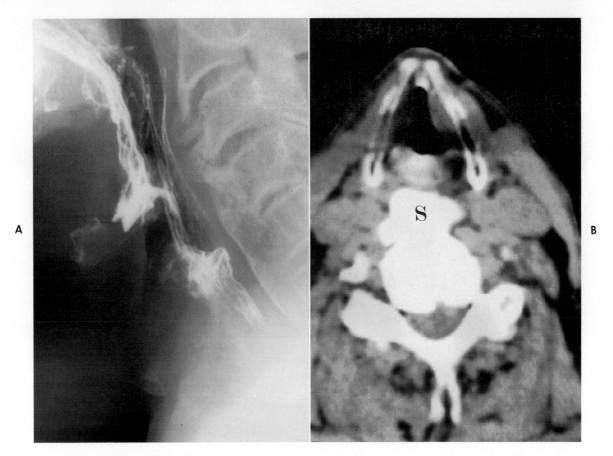

Fig. 5-16 A, Lateral radiogram of the neck shows ossification of the anterior longitudinal ligament and spondylarthrosis that impinge on the posterior wall of the pharynx. **B,** CT scan at the level of the spondylarthrosis *(s)*.

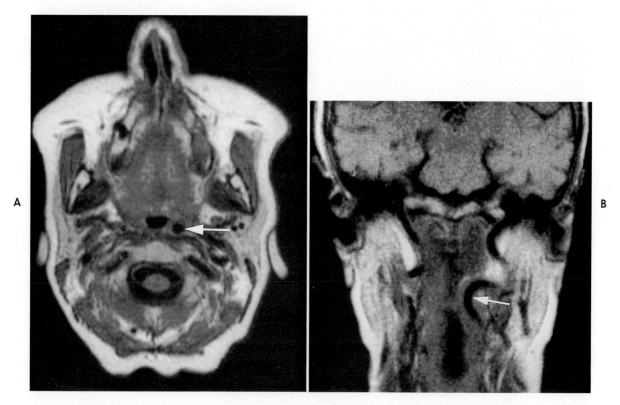

Fig. 5-17 A patient with a pulsative tinnitus in the left ear. **A,** A T1 MRI image showing the internal carotid artery deviating medially *(arrow)*. **B,** A T1 MRI image in the coronal projection showing medial deviation of the internal carotid artery *(arrow)*.

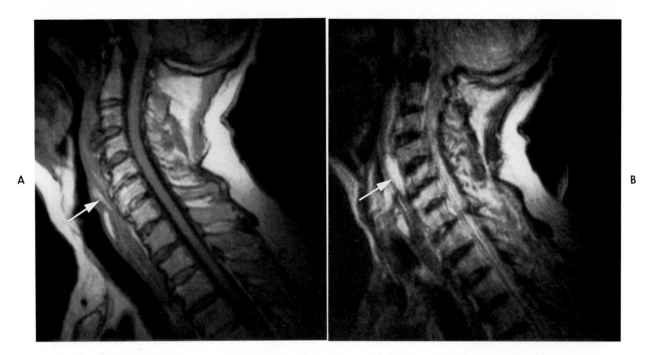

Fig. 5-18 An elderly man with sudden onset of neck pain and dysphagia caused by retropharyngeal tendinitis. **A,** On T1 MRI images, the prevertebral soft tissue is thick. There is spondyloarthrosis and areas that emit medium high-intensity signals *(arrow)*. **B,** On T2 images, this area also gives off a high-intensity signal *(arrow)*, which suggests the presence of an inflammatory process.

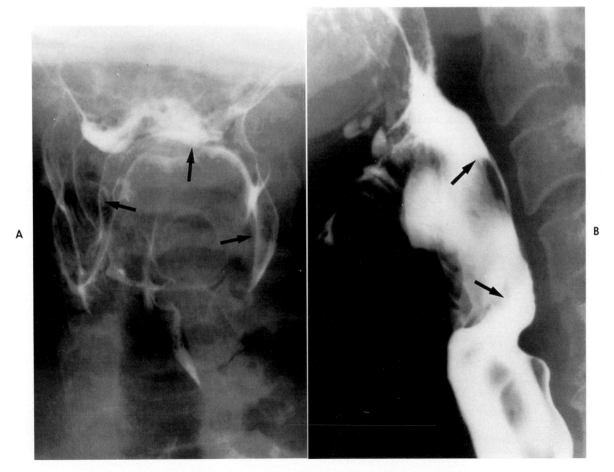

Fig. 5-19 Benign rhabdomyoma. This patient had dysphagia for 8 weeks. A pharyngogram shows a 4-cm mass *(arrows)* arising from the left arytenoid area. **A,** Anteroposterior projection. **B,** Lateral projection.

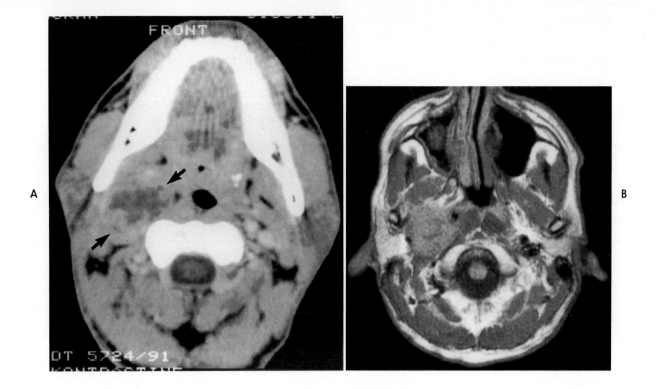

Fig. 5-20 Schwannoma arising from the cervical sympathetic chain in the right side of the neck. **A,** CT scan of the neck shows a 4-cm mass in the right parapharyngeal area *(arrows)*. The periphery of the tumor shows contrast enhancement, and the central part shows necrosis. The lumen of the pharynx deviates somewhat to the left. **B,** A transverse projection of T1 MRI images shows the tumor located between the internal and external carotid artery. **C,** T2 image in the coronal projection shows the tumor to possess a high signal intensity. **D,** Angiogram in the anteroposterior projection shows lateral dislocation of the external carotid artery. The mass exhibited some scattered, small puddles of contrast medium in the midarterial, capillary, and venous phases.

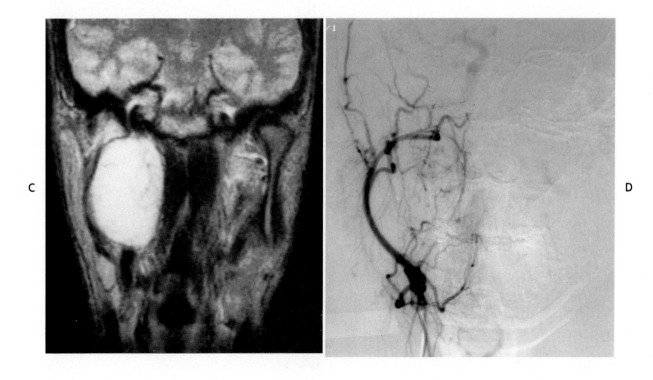

Retropharyngeal tendinitis

Patients with retropharyngeal tendinitis experience the sudden onset of neck pain, which is exacerbated by swallowing and neck movement. They also have a slight fever and leukocytosis. There is usually widening of the prevertebral soft tissue and at times indistinct calcifications. MRI is the most helpful form of imaging for revealing this abnormality (Fig. 5-18).

Thyroglossal cysts

Thyroglossal cysts may present as a midline neck swelling and are located between the foramen cecum in the tongue and the thyroid gland, often posterior to the hyoid bone. Rarely they may be located in a suprahyoid position. They are best visualized with CT and ultrasound, which may show their cystic nature. They extend from the laryngeal ventricle and may protrude laterally and superiorly.

Calcified lymph nodes

One of the most common findings on radiographs of the neck are calcified lymph nodes. They are asymptomatic.

Parapharyngeal neoplasms

Any tumor involving the anatomic structures that surround the pharynx may, if large, encroach on the pharynx. Benign tumors typically cause a soft indentation or deviation of the pharynx (Figs. 5-19 and 5-20); malignant lesions, such as laryngeal carcinoma, may invade the pharyngeal mucosa.

REFERENCES

1. Som PM, Bergeron RT: *Head and neck imaging,* ed 2, St Louis, 1991, Mosby–Year Book.
2. Ekberg O, Nylander G: Lateral diverticula from the pharyngoesophageal junction area, *Radiology* 146:117, 1983.
3. Curtis DJ, Cruess DF, Crain M, Sivit C, Winters C Jr et al: Lateral pharyngeal outpouchings: a comparison of dysphagic and asymptomatic patients, *Dysphagia* 2:156, 1988.
4. Brombart M: *Clinical radiology of the esophagus,* Bristol, 1961, John Wright & Son.
5. Jamieson GG, Curanceau AC, Payne WS: Pharyngo-esophageal diverticulum. In Jamieson GG, ed: *Surgery of the oesophagus,* London, 1988, Churchill Livingstone.
6. Ekberg O, Malmquist J, Lindgren S: Pharyngo-esophageal webs in dysphagial patients, *Fortschr Roentgenstr* 145:75, 1986.
7. Kelly AB: Spasm at the entrance of the oesophagus, *J Laryngol Rhinol Otol* 24:285, 1919.
8. Nosher JL, Campbell WL, Seaman WB: The clinical significance of cervical esophageal and hypopharyngeal webs, *Radiology* 117:45, 1975.
9. Chisholm M: The association between webs, iron and postcricoid carcinoma, *Postgrad Med J* 50:215, 1974.
10. Wynder EL, Hultberg S, Jacobsson F, Bross IJ: Environmental factors in cancer of the upper alimentary tract: a Swedish study with special reference to the Plummer-Vinson syndrome, *Cancer* 10:470, 1957.
11. Ekberg O, Birch-Iensen M, Lindstrom C: Mucosal folds in the vallecula, *Dysphagia* 1:68, 1986.
12. Bachman AL, Seaman WB, Maclean KL: Lateral pharyngeal diverticula, *Radiology* 91:774, 1968.
13. Moore KL: The branchial apparatus and the head and neck. In Moore KL, ed: *The developing human,* ed 4, Philadelphia, 1988, WB Saunders.

6 *Functional Abnormalities of the Pharynx*

OLLE EKBERG

Swallowing in the broad sense takes place at four different anatomic levels. At each of these levels, the abnormalities that cause dysphagia are characteristically different. Motility disorders are almost entirely responsible for abnormalities in the oral stage. In the pharynx, dysmotility is the most frequent abnormality, although structural abnormalities, both intrinsic and extrinsic to the pharynx, do also occur. Structural abnormalities and incoordination may coexist in the pharyngoesophageal (PE) segment. In the esophagus, structural abnormalities are a more common source of dysphagia than is dysmotility.

There are two necessary and fundamentally different aspects to the radiologic evaluation when examining pharyngeal function and dysfunction. One is to observe how the barium bolus is conveyed within the oral cavity and pharynx, especially the nature of the retention and penetration of the barium. The other is to focus on the anatomic structures involved. In this context, defective closure of the laryngeal vestibule is an important finding even if the barium does not enter the laryngeal vestibule during that particular swallow (Fig. 6-1). In the same way, gauging the amount of movement of the constrictor wall is as important as observing the nature of the retention of the barium. Although both observations are important, it is ultimately the movement of anatomic structures that more often enables the radiologist to distinguish between oral, pharyngeal, and PE segment dysfunction.

ORAL STAGE

Abnormalities in the oral stage include those that affect ingestion, containment, processing, and the voluntary initiation of the pharyngeal swallow. An inability to restrict the amount of ingested material may cause severe problems in the processing and initiation of the pharyngeal swallow (Fig. 6-2). Normal individuals can contain the liquid barium bolus within the oral cavity with no, or only minor, movements of the tongue. Incoordinated, jerky movements of the tongue and jaw or chewing gestures are both abnormal signs. Such patients commonly cannot correctly position a bolus on the tongue, and, as a result, the tongue cannot convey the bolus posteriorly. Transfer of the bolus within the oral cavity into a ready-to-swallow position is delayed in this instance.

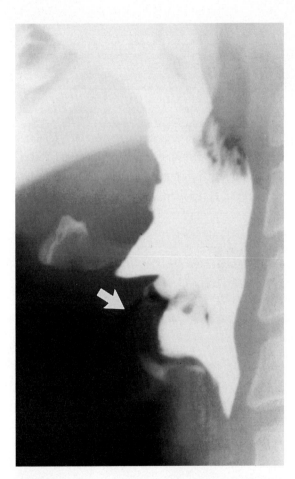

Fig. 6-1 The laryngeal vestibule is open *(arrow)* at a stage when the barium bolus has reached the pharyngoesophageal segment. However, no barium has penetrated into the vestibule.

Defective containment is characterized by the leakage of barium, either anteriorly through the lips, laterally into the buccal pouches, or posteriorly into the pharynx (see Fig. 6-2). The agent may reach the airway if the laryngeal vestibule is not closed, and this is most likely to be the case if there is "dissociation" of the oral stage from the pharyngeal stage by delay in the initiation of the pharyngeal swallow. If the liquid barium bolus leaks or is transported down into the pharynx 1 second or more before initiation of the

127

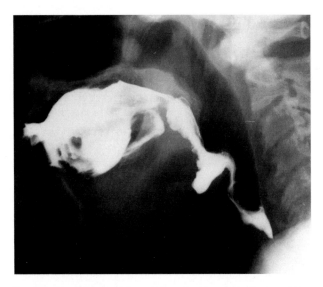

Fig. 6-2 Too large a bolus. Although this patient had problems with ingestion and oral processing, he attempted to swallow too large a bolus. He was then unable to control the barium bolus, which leaked into the pharynx and later into the airway.

pharyngeal swallow (VIP) part of the bolus may enter the vestibule and eventually the trachea. The longer the initiation of the pharyngeal swallow is delayed, the greater the chance for aspiration.

Impaired tongue thrust is characterized by slow and weak posterior movement of the tongue base (Fig. 6-3), but this can be difficult to appreciate radiologically. Retention of the barium in the vallecula is seen as a lack of effacement of the vallecula in the anteroposterior view. If swallowing is abnormal in the oral phase (including impaired lingual movement), this generally leads to a delay in the transfer and clearance of the bolus with a consequent retention of barium in the mouth.

There is a strong correlation between abnormal anterior movement of the hyoid bone and abnormal oral and pharyngeal function as well as defective opening of the PE segment. The crucial oral stage triggers the pharyngeal and PE segment phases of swallowing, in that normal oral transfer is crucial to initiating reflex-mediated pharyngeal and PE segment function and the autonomically controlled esophageal function. An abnormal delay in the initiation of the

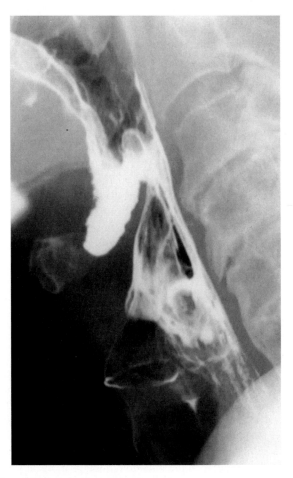

Fig. 6-3 Weak tongue thrust. Retention of barium in the valleculae leading to overflow into the airway.

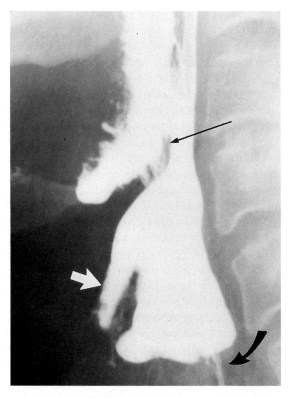

Fig. 6-4 Dissociation between the oral and pharyngeal stages of swallowing. The bolus has been transported down into the pharynx before the pharyngeal swallow has been initiated. The hyoid bone is not elevated, and the epiglottis is not tilted down *(straight black arrow)*. Therefore the vestibule is open and the penetration of barium is massive *(white arrow)*. The pharyngoesophageal segment is not yet open *(curved black arrow)*.

pharyngeal stage of swallowing is easily appreciated because the bolus is conveyed into the pharynx without the pharynx being elevated and without initiation of constrictor activity (Fig. 6-4). Dissociation corresponds by and large to an "open swallow," a term coined by Curtis and Cruess.[1] They reported that 72% of a group of unselected volunteers swallowed by propelling the oral bolus back into an air-filled pharynx so that it fell into the open esophagus, thus the term *open swallow*. In these patients, it was only after the leading edge of the bolus entered the esophagus that the peristaltic wave of the pharyngeal constrictors was initiated in the nasopharynx. In the other 28% of the volunteers, the oropharynx was cleared of air before the arrival of the bolus in the hypopharynx, and the bolus was transported from the oral cavity to the esophagus by peristalsis through an air-tight tube—the closed swallow.

Although the open swallow clearly indicates dissociation between the oral and pharyngeal stages of swallowing, such that elevation of the larynx and pharynx is delayed, it is not a pathologic finding. It may, however, represent a more risky type of swallowing, as the bolus is essentially falling

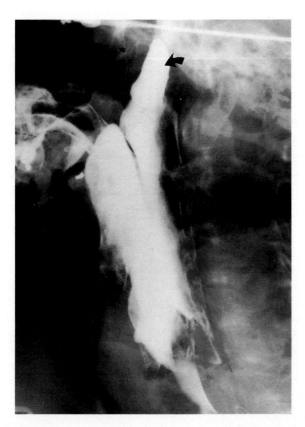

Fig. 6-5 Severe polymyositis. Barium has passed into the epipharynx *(arrow)* because of paresis of the soft palate and the superior constrictor. There is also paresis in the rest of the constrictors with major retention that led to severe aspiration. The patient required a gastrostomy for feeding.

past an open airway with a vertically positioned epiglottis, and this more readily precipitates decompensation in the event of disease. It is, however, associated with an increased incidence of swallowing dysfunction.[2] It may be difficult to appreciate dissociation radiologically when the oral and pharyngeal stages are otherwise normal. A delay in the forward movement of the hyoid in relation to when the bolus appears in the pharynx is the key finding.

Defective closure of the velopharynx allows barium to penetrate superiorly into the nasopharynx. This may be caused by either soft palate dysfunction or by defective functioning of the superior pharyngeal constrictor, or both[3] (Fig. 6-5). During phonation there may be an open nasal quality to the pitch resulting from the defective closure of the nasopharynx, even though, during swallowing, which is controlled by a different brainstem center, closure is normal. Medial movements of the lateral walls are more pronounced in this instance and are easier to appreciate than the anterior movement of the posterior constrictor wall. In addition, movements of anatomic structures are often more pronounced during swallowing than during speech. The compensation developed for impaired muscular function may take the form of an exaggerated Passavant's ridge (see Chapter 5), a protrusion similar to that seen as a compensatory speech maneuver in people with a cleft palate.

PHARYNGEAL STAGE
Hyoid bone

The passive movement of the hyoid bone can be regarded as a phenomenon of both the oral and pharyngeal stage. During chewing and other oral cavity activities, the hyoid bone, which is suspended in muscles attached to the base of the skull, the mandible, and infrahyoid structures such as the larynx, moves superiorly and inferiorly, often in a jerky manner. This is normal, and there are also some anterior and posterior movements of the hyoid. There are several ways of defining when the pharyngeal stage of swallowing commences, that is, when laryngeal elevation starts, when closure of the vocal folds starts, or when the laryngeal ventricles are obliterated. A reliable and conspicuous movement, however, which is easy to recognize radiologically, marks the beginning of the anterior movement of the hyoid.

Closure of the airways takes place at three anatomic levels, namely, the epiglottis, the laryngeal vestibule, and the vocal folds,[4] and abnormalities may arise at all three levels.

Epiglottis

Abnormal movements of the epiglottis always indicate pharyngeal dysfunction.[5-8] A defective second movement of the epiglottis from the horizontal to an inverted position is common (Fig. 6-6), and, on barium swallows, the epiglottis remains in the horizontal position in this instance.[3,5] However, there are a variety of abnormalities in which the

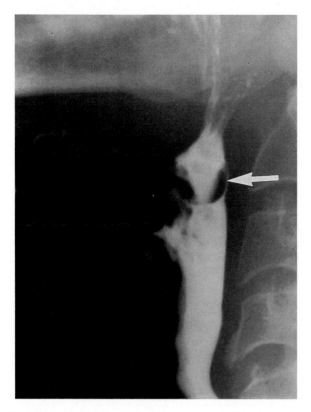

Fig. 6-6 Defective second movement of the epiglottis *(arrow),* which is remaining in a horizontal position.

epiglottis tilts incompletely. This indicates that there is either a variable degree of incoordination of muscle function or a varying degree of paresis. When the first movement from the vertical to the horizontal position is absent, this indicates immobility of the epiglottis usually caused by failure of laryngeal elevation (Fig. 6-4). However, there are always movements transmitted from the back of the tongue, and therefore the epiglottis is rarely completely immobile.

Laryngeal vestibule

Defective closure of the vestibule may either involve the upper part (the subepiglottic portion) or the lower part (the supraglottic portion). Defective closure of the subepiglottic region is usually due to a timing delay, in that the subepiglottic portion closes completely at a later stage. In these patients, the bolus is simply propelled into the pharynx and past the entrance to the vestibule before it has had time to close. This is essentially the same dissociation as that described earlier for an open swallow. Extensive studies that have measured timing in order to define normal and abnormal swallow have been carried out,[9] but the results are unimportant from a clinical perspective.

Defective closure of the supraglottic portion of the laryngeal vestibule may be due to delay. In patients with delayed closure, barium passes into the vestibule and is then expelled either superiorly into the pharynx or inferiorly into the trachea when closure occurs[10-13] (Fig. 6-7). Complete absence of closure of the supraglottic portion of the laryngeal vestibule is rare and is seen only in patients with defective thyrohyoid apposition.

Penetration of barium into the vestibule and trachea can be appreciated in both posteroanterior and lateral views (Fig. 6-8). Abnormal vocal fold apposition is seen in patients with paresis of the recurrent nerve, and this is best assessed in the anteroposterior view.[14]

If barium passes into the larynx or the trachea, or both, this should not necessarily prompt cancellation of the study. There are patients who have massive aspiration into the trachea, but a limited study in these patients is sufficient to indicate whether oral feeding is possible. It is important to evaluate the underlying pathophysiology in these patients. Therefore, when patients can feed themselves orally, a few swallows of a small volume of contrast should be obtained in the lateral projection, even if the patient aspirates the agent during the first swallow.[13] However, in the patient with an obvious swallowing impairment, it is advisable to use a nonionic iodine contrast medium.[4] Suction equipment should also be available with adequately trained staff. Physiotherapy should be instituted if significant aspiration occurs. Overall, sensible clinical judgment should be used in deciding whether the patient can withstand the procedure. The goals of the study should be clear in advance, bearing in mind that the more impaired the patient, the easier the radiologic examination, as only a few relevant clinical questions can then be addressed.

Pharyngeal constrictors

Pharyngeal constrictors play a crucial role in swallowing.[15,16] If they are paretic, the pharyngeal tube will be flaccid, and this will allow abnormal expansion to take place during the compression phase of swallowing because of the piston effect of the tongue. Such a lack of compliance results in the imperfect transit of barium from the oral cavity into the esophagus, even if the tongue functions normally.[17,18] This can be seen as a dilated and wide flaccid pharynx and causes the retention of barium in the pharynx (Fig. 6-9). This abnormality is sometimes best evaluated in the frontal projection (Fig. 6-10). Because the middle pharyngeal constrictor is the most commonly involved, retention typically occurs at the level of the superior laryngeal inlet and may be responsible for causing aspiration after swallowing. Unilateral constrictor paresis is rarely demonstrated during radiologic examination. Because the barium is asymmetrically transported (in the anteroposterior view), it may mimic a pharyngeal tumor on the normal side[17] (Fig. 6-11).

The timing of the pharyngeal events during swallowing has generally not been important from a clinical point of view,[9] but knowing the speed with which constrictor peristalsis progresses inferiorly is potentially valuable. In non-

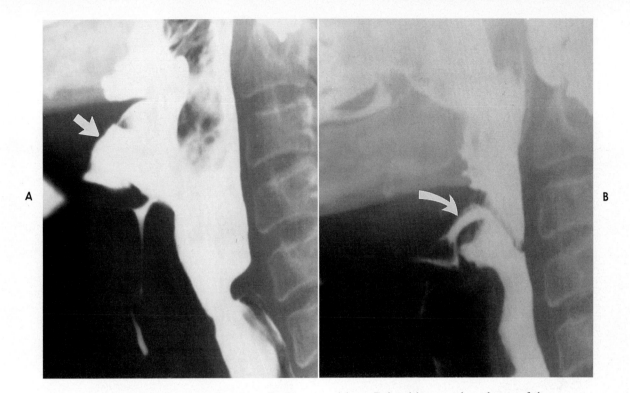

Fig. 6-7 A, Early stage of swallow. **B,** One second later. Delayed but complete closure of the supraglottic segment of the laryngeal vestibule *(arrow)*. When closure occurred, the penetrating bolus was expelled into the pharynx. There is incomplete closure of the subepiglottic segment of the vestibule *(curved arrow)*.

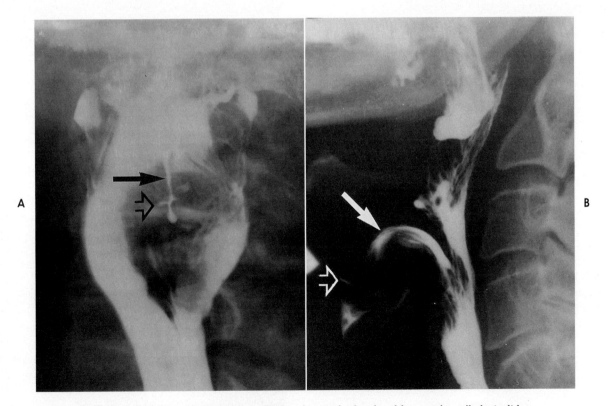

Fig. 6-8 A, Posteroanterior projection. Barium is seen in the closed laryngeal vestibule *(solid arrow)* and laryngeal ventricle *(open arrow),* giving the appearance of a tapered glass. **B,** Lateral projection from the same patient. Barium is seen in the laryngeal vestibule *(solid arrow)* and ventricle *(open arrow)*.

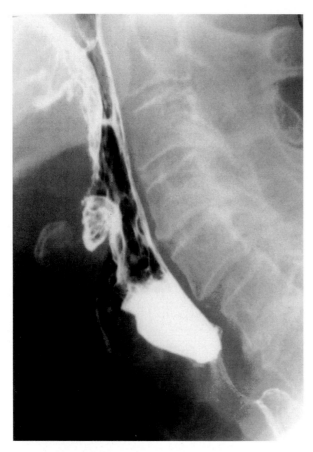

Fig. 6-9 Retention of barium in the piriform sinuses as a result of constrictor paresis.

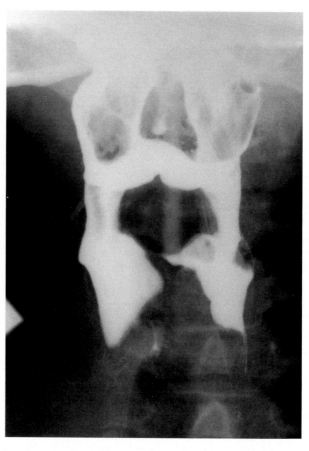

Fig. 6-10 Retention of barium in the valleculae and piriform sinuses caused by paresis of the pharyngeal constrictors.

Fig. 6-11 Postpolio syndrome. There is paresis of the middle and inferior pharyngeal constrictors predominantly on the right side, which bulges. This may mimic a tumor on the left side.

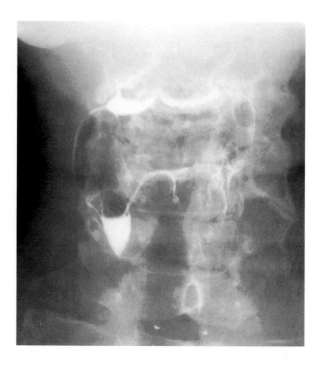

dysphagic normal patients, the speed of peristalsis in a specific individual is always constant and is close to 10 cm per second. In the individual patient with pharyngeal dysfunction, the speed of peristalsis often varies. In some swallows the speed is high, up to 20 cm per second, and in others it may be as low as 3 cm per second. This might become a useful criterion for detecting early dysfunction in patients who otherwise appear normal.

PE SEGMENT DYSFUNCTION

Failure of the PE segment to open may be seen in the context of neurologic disease but is generally not accompanied by abnormal transport of the pharyngeal bolus.[18,19] Failure of the PE segment to open may be because of several factors: (1) defective relaxation, (2) defective distensibility, (3) hypertrophy or hyperplasia, or (4) fibrosis. The differentiation between these four entities is not reliable from either radiologic or manometric studies. The posterior bar intruding into the barium in the PE segment is caused by the cricopharyngeus muscle (Fig. 6-12). It is commonly associated with abnormal motor function in either the preceding segment (i.e., the inferior pharyngeal constrictor) or the following segment (i.e., the cervical esophagus). A cricopharyngeal indentation is the most conspicuous finding but is not the only motor dysfunction that occurs in the PE segment.[19] Major retention of the barium is only rarely observed above such a cricopharyngeal indentation and results from paresis in the inferior constrictor (Fig. 6-13). It is important not to perform a cricopharyngeal myotomy in such patients, as this will only compound an existing severe dysfunction (i.e., constrictor paresis) with a new dysfunction (i.e., cricopharyngeal myotomy).

CAUSE OF DYSFUNCTION

Upper and lower motor neuron diseases as well as left- and right-sided cortical strokes may all cause oropharyngeal swallowing dysfunction. Tumors and tumor surgery in the head and neck area often impair function,[20,21] and a variety of neurologic diseases can be the source of swallowing dysfunction.[22-25] If only two or three swallows are observed in a specific patient, this may disclose only a single abnormality. However, if six or more swallows are observed, a variety of dysfunctions can be identified in the majority of patients.

Upper motor neuron lesions such as cortical and subcortical cerebrovascular accidents interfere chiefly with the oral stage of swallowing,[26] and this is especially true of patients with cognitive deficiencies such as Alzheimer's disease.[27] These patients have a pseudobulbar palsy with intact or exaggerated reflexes and a spastic behavior of the pharynx. Strokes,[26,28,29] Parkinson's disease,[30,31] Wilson's disease, multiple sclerosis, amyotrophic lateral sclerosis,[32] tabes dorsalis, brainstem tumors, and a variety of congenital and degenerative central nervous system disorders all produce this pattern of swallowing dysfunction.

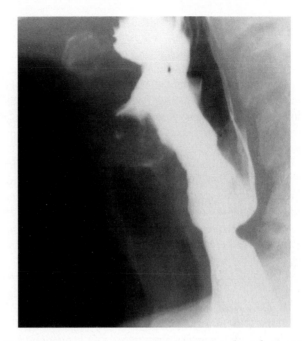

Fig. 6-12 Defective opening of the pharyngoesophageal segment. The cricopharyngeus muscle is seen as a posterior bar.

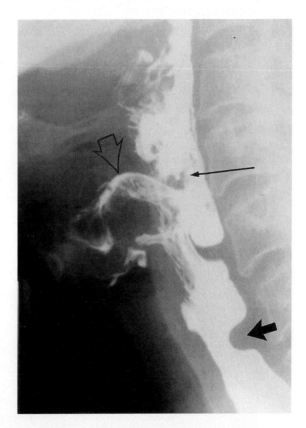

Fig. 6-13 Defective opening of the pharyngoesophageal segment. The cricopharyngeus muscle is seen as a posterior bar *(thick arrow)*. Retention of barium in the pharynx is caused by paresis of the constrictor musculature. There is also penetration of barium into the vestibule *(open arrow)* and defective tilting down of the epiglottis *(thin arrow)*.

Some brainstem lesions, bulbar poliomyelitis,[33] and peripheral neuropathies, such as those resulting from diphtheria, botulism, rabies, and diabetes mellitus, produce a flaccid paralysis that tends to be characterized by pharyngeal constrictor paresis and defective elevation of the larynx and pharynx as well as defective opening of the PE segment. Patients with these lesions are often cognitively intact and are therefore more amenable to recommendations for indirect manipulation, such as positioning, as treatment.

The motor end-plate dysfunction seen in myasthenia gravis[34] and the muscle disorders seen in the muscular dystrophies, dystrophia myotonica,[35,36] primary myositis, metabolic myopathies, amyloidosis, and systemic lupus may all be associated with pharyngeal dysfunction. Patients with Sjögren's syndrome may have difficulties with oral transit because of the lack of saliva.

Not many functional abnormalities in the mouth and pharynx are actually caused by structural lesions (Fig. 6-14). Only when large does a tumor interfere with epiglottic tilting, closure of the laryngeal vestibule, or wall displacement. This may be one reason why a tumor in this region often becomes quite large before the patient seeks medical care. Malignant lesions may be asymptomatic until they infiltrate the parapharyngeal area, and thereby interfere with the innervation that controls swallowing.

There is a strong correlation between epiglottic and vestibular dysfunction. Only in patients with slightly defective closure of the vestibule does the epiglottis move normally. In 80% of those patients with defective closure of the vestibule there is abnormal epiglottic motility.[37,38] There is also a strong correlation between epiglottic and vestibular dysfunction and the presence of pharyngeal constrictor paresis. [37,38] Because a normal epiglottic and vestibular function may sometimes be seen in patients with pharyngeal constrictor paresis, this suggests that the innervation controlling these three functions is separate. As long as elevation of the pharynx and larynx during a swallow is preserved, the thyroepiglottic and the aryepiglottic muscles are able to tilt the epiglottis down and close the vestibule.[37] This is an important ability, since pharyngeal constrictor paresis is usually associated with retention of swallowed material in the pharynx, which may lead to aspiration if airway closure is impaired. However, this is less of a hazard if the sensation is preserved, since such a patient can feel that bolus material is retained and thus will not start breathing but try to compensate for retention. This compensation can take the form of repeated swallowings.

There is also a clear relationship between esophageal and pharyngeal function.[38,39] When patients with high dysphagia are examined, the pharynx may either be normal or the

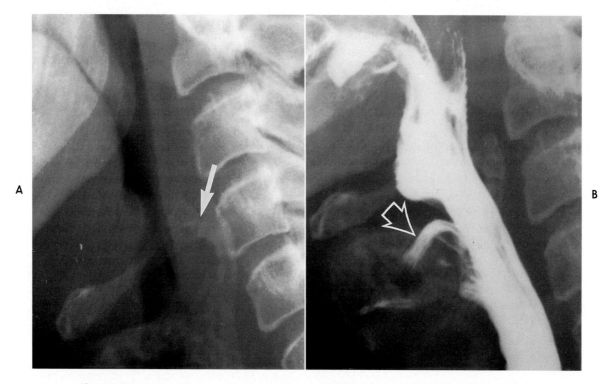

Fig. 6-14 An abnormal connection *(arrow)* between the greater horn of the hyoid bone and the hyoid process of the thyroid cartilage **(A)**, with very limited movement between the two. The complex of hyoid bone and thyroid cartilage did move superiorly and anteriorly during swallowing. However, the important apposition between the hyoid bone and thyroid cartilage was restricted, allowing penetration of liquid into the airway **(B)** *(open arrow)*.

cricopharyngeus muscle may be somewhat prominent, with impaired relaxation giving the appearance of a bar. Gastroesophageal reflux is most commonly associated with such a finding, and the majority of patients with a prominent cricopharyngeus muscle or impaired relaxation are found to have reflux, hiatus hernia, Schatzki's ring, esophageal spasm or other dysmotility, or acid-sensitive esophagus, either singly or in combination. This is not altogether surprising, as it is well known that instilling acid into the esophagus produces a reflex increase in the upper esophageal sphincter pressure, and, therefore, the more proximal the acid instillation, the higher the pressure.[40] However, in addition, such patients frequently have other pharyngeal abnormalities, such as lateral pouches, webs, a Zenker's diverticulum, or asymmetric movement of the epiglottis. Less often, a pharyngeal structural abnormality may be associated with other esophageal disease such as carcinoma.

For this reason, a radiologist should be cautious about interpreting an abnormal pharyngeal study based solely on pharyngolaryngeal findings such as penetration or constrictor paresis. The entire upper gastrointestinal tract should be examined during the assessment, if not at the same examination (Figs. 6-15 and 6-16).

ADAPTATION, COMPENSATION, AND DECOMPENSATION

In terms of swallowing, *adaptation* refers to the ability to adapt to the consistency, viscosity, elasticity, volume, mass, and temperature of the food bolus.[41,42] Patients can also adapt to a mild pharyngeal dysfunction, and this pro-

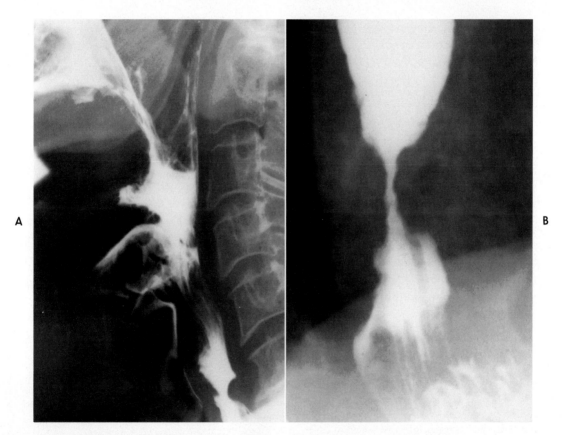

Fig. 6-15 A 65-year-old man with a 2-year history of multiple cerebrovascular accidents that had left him with a left-sided hemiparesis. He also complained of difficulty swallowing. **A,** Functional evaluation of his oropharynx revealed dissociation between the oral and pharyngeal stages of swallowing, leading to penetration of barium into the laryngeal vestibule. However, there was also weakness of the pharyngeal constrictors and delayed opening of the pharyngoesophageal segment. **B,** During the esophageal stage of the examination, a short stricture with tapering edges was also revealed in the distal esophagus, and there were small ulcerations proximal to the stricture. This was due to reflux esophagitis. Further analysis of his dysphagia revealed that he had no problem swallowing liquid, which is usually the main complaint in oropharyngeal dysfunction. The patient was actually found to have dysphagia for solids, specifically for meat, rice, and bread, which is more typical of a structural lesion. After balloon dilatation of the stricture, the patient became asymptomatic, although he still had oropharyngeal dysfunction.

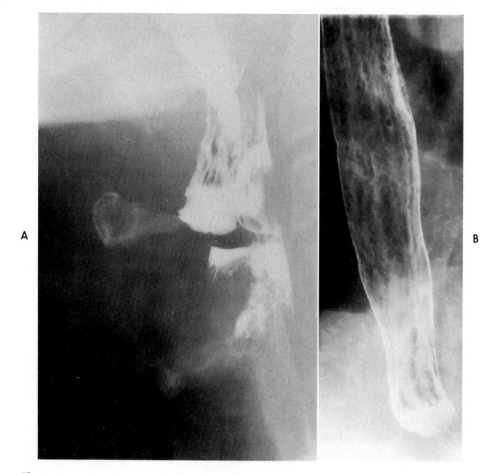

Fig. 6-16 A 72-year-old woman with diabetes who complained of discomfort during swallowing, with a feeling that food stuck in her throat. There was also some pain on swallowing. **A,** Functional evaluation of the oropharynx revealed mild pharyngeal constrictor paresis with some retention of barium, defective tilting down of the epiglottis, and penetration of barium into the subepiglottic segment of the laryngeal vestibule. **B,** Because the patient was able to cooperate, a double-contrast examination of the esophagus was also performed, which revealed multiple millimeter-sized protrusions from the mucosa. These were caused by *Candida* infection. A single-contrast study would probably not have revealed the colonies. After treatment for the candidiasis, she became asymptomatic.

Fig. 6-17 A 75-year-old man who had suffered diphtheria at the age of 7. At that time, he had transient dysphagia. Since then, he had been asymptomatic, until recently, when he started to cough during eating. Oropharyngeal function was found to be severely impaired, with dissociation between the oral and pharyngeal stages of swallowing. The epiglottis did not tilt down during swallow, and the laryngeal vestibule did not close, allowing major penetration of the barium. There was paresis of the constrictor musculature. This patient may well have suffered from pharyngeal dysfunction due to the neurotoxic effect of the diphtheria, but was able to compensate for it over the years. Now, the effects of normal aging have impaired the number of available nerve and muscle fibers, and this additional burden, on top of his prior dysfunction, has led to decompensation with the consequent development of symptoms.

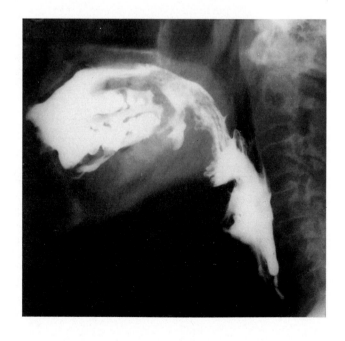

cess, either voluntary or subconscious, is called *compensated swallowing*. When compensation fails, *decompensation* occurs (Fig. 6-17).

Most forms of pharyngeal compensation are obviously involuntary and involve the internal musculature of the pharynx and/or the neck and paraspinal muscles. The voluntary compensation of pharyngeal impairment can be accomplished by a variety of means: food can be specially prepared, patients can chew their food well or mechanically blend it, or they can select food of the right consistency. Patients can also assume a certain posture of the neck when swallowing, such as tilting the head and neck to one side. Many individuals seem to be able to cope well with impairment of one pharyngeal function.[43] Examples of such solitary pharyngeal dysfunction are defective closure of the subepiglottic portion of the vestibule, defective tilting down of the epiglottis from the transverse position, and delayed but complete relaxation of the cricopharyngeus muscle.

The coordination of pharyngeal function deteriorates with aging because the velocity of neuronal impulses is slowed and the elasticity and power of muscles is gradually lost.[44] However, most elderly patients can compensate well for this minor deterioration.

It may be difficult to detect minor compensated pharyngeal dysfunction during a radiologic examination using standard procedures; therefore, an apparently normal study does not exclude dysfunction. Provocative maneuvers may be used to try to demonstrate abnormalities, that is, to provoke decompensation. In some patients, this can be accomplished by extending their neck, giving them a large bolus, or by having them rapidly ingest and then swallow the bolus.[41]

TREATMENT PLANNING

It is helpful to distinguish between an examination intended to diagnose pharyngeal dysfunction and one to plan treatment, and to conduct them at separate times. A diagnostic study is tailored to reveal why the patient has symptoms and to demonstrate the full extent of pharyngeal dysfunction. The treatment planning study, however, is designed to reveal the best possible pharyngeal function that can be achieved. It is often possible to plan treatment and to assess the success of treatment by having patients alter their position and manipulate the bolus to achieve maximal safe swallowing.[21,45-48]

In patients with a posterior leak from the oral cavity, anterior flexion of the head widens the valleculae so that more bolus can be accommodated in the valleculae before spillage occurs into the dangerous area of the superior laryngeal inlet. This prolonged contact optimizes sensory stimulation that may prompt initiation of a pharyngeal swallow with laryngeal closure. Anterior head flexion also facilitates closure of the laryngeal vestibule but may exacerbate dribbling in patients with substantial oral dysfunction.

The treatment planning and assessment studies are best performed with the therapist, often a speech and language pathologist, present, and there are advantages to having the recordings assessed jointly and a joint report issued. These examinations are time consuming but have important clinical implications, since they may determine whether a patient can continue to feed orally, or requires a gastrostomy or the installation of a nasogastric tube.

REFERENCES

1. Curtis DJ, Cruess DF: Videofluoroscopic identification of two types of swallowing, *Radiology* 152:305, 1984.
2. Birch-Iensen M, Borgström PS, Ekberg O: Cineradiography in closed and open pharyngeal swallow, *Acta Radiol* 29:407, 1988.
3. Curtis DJ: Radiologic evaluation of oropharyngeal swallowing. In Gelfand DW, Richter JE, eds: *Dysphagia: diagnosis and treatment*, New York, 1989, Igaku-Shoin.
4. Gray C, Sivaloganathan S, Simpkins KC: Aspiration of high-density barium causing acute pulmonary inflammation: report of two fatal cases in elderly women with disordered swallowing, *Clin Radiol* 40:397, 1989.
5. Ekberg O: Epiglottic dysfunction during deglutition in patients with dysphagia, *Arch Otolaryngol* 109:376, 1983.
6. Curtis DJ, Sepulveda GV: Epiglottic motion: video recording of muscular dysfunction, *Radiology* 148:473, 1983.
7. Ardran GM, Kemp FH: The mechanism of the larynx: II. The epiglottis and closure of the larynx, *Br J Radiol* 40:372, 1967.
8. Curtis DJ, Sepulveda GU: Epiglottic motion: video recording of muscular dysfunction, *Radiology* 148:473, 1983.
9. Curtis DJ, Cruess DF, Dachman AH, Maso E: Timing normal pharyngeal swallow: prospective selection and evaluation of 16 normal asymptomatic patients, *Invest Radiol* 19:523, 1984.
10. Ekberg O: Defective closure of the laryngeal vestibule during deglutition, *Acta Otolaryngol* 93:309, 1982.
11. Ardran GM, Kemp FH: Closure and opening of the larynx during swallowing, *Br J Radiol* 29:205, 1956.
12. Curtis DJ, Hudson T: Laryngotracheal aspiration: analysis of specific neuromuscular factors, *Radiology* 149:517, 1983.
13. Ekberg O, Hilderfors H: Defective closure of the laryngeal vestibule: frequency of pulmonary complications, *AJR* 145:1159, 1985.
14. Ekberg O, Schultze T, Lindgren S: Pharyngeal swallowing in patients with paresis of the recurrent nerve, *Acta Radiol Diagn* 27:697, 1986.
15. Ekberg O, Nylander G: Pharyngeal constrictor paresis in patients with dysphagia: a cineradiographic study, *Clin Radiol* 33:253, 1981.
16. Ardran GM, Kemp FM: Radiologic investigation of pharyngeal and laryngeal palsy, *Acta Radiol Diagn* 46:446, 1956.
17. Thulin A, Welin S: Radiographic findings in unilateral hypopharyngeal paralysis, *Acta Otolaryngol* [Suppl] 116:288, 1954.
18. Curtis DJ, Cruess DF, Berg T: The cricopharyngeal muscle: a video-recording, *AJR* 146:497, 1984.
19. Ekberg O: The cricopharyngeus revisited, *Br J Radiol* 59:875, 1986.
20. Levine FM: Swallowing disorders after skull base surgery, *Otolaryngol Clin North Am* 21:751, 1988.
21. McConnel FMS, Cerenko D, Mendelsohn M: Dysphagia after total laryngectomy, *Otolaryngol Clin North Am* 21:721, 1988.
22. Brin MF, Younger D: Neurologic disorders and aspiration, *Otolaryngol Clin North Am* 21:691, 1988.
23. Donner MW, Siegel L: The evaluation of neuromuscular disorders by cinefluorography. *AJR* 94:299, 1965.
24. Donner MW, Silbiger ML: Cineradiofluorographic analysis of pharyngeal swallowing in neuromuscular disorders, *Am J Med Sci* 251:600, 1966.

25. Silbiger M, Pikielney R, Donner MW: Neuromuscular disorders affecting the pharynx, *Invest Radiol* 2:442, 1967.
26. Veis SL, Logemann JA: Swallowing disorders in persons with cerebrovascular accident, *Arch Phys Med Rehabil* 66:272, 1985.
27. Siebens H, Trupe E, Siebens A et al: Correlates and consequences of eating dependency in institutionalized elderly, *J Am Geriatr Soc* 34:192, 1986.
28. Horner J, Massey EW, Riski JE, Lathrop DL, Chase KN: Aspiration following stroke: clinical correlates and outcome, *Neurology* 38:1359, 1988.
29. Robbins J, Levine RL: Swallowing after unilateral stroke of the cerebral cortex: preliminary experience, *Dysphagia* 3:11, 1988.
30. Calne DB, Shaw DG, Spiers AS, Stern GM: Swallowing in parkinsonism, *Br J Radiol* 43:456, 1970.
31. Robbins JA, Logemann JA, Kirshner HS: Swallowing and speech production in Parkinson's disease, *Ann Neurol* 19:283, 1986.
32. Bosma JF, Brodie DR: Disabilities of the pharynx in amyotrophic lateral sclerosis as demonstrated by cineradiography, *Radiology* 92:97, 1969.
33. Ardran GM, Kemp FM, Wegelius C: Swallowing defects after poliomyelitis, *Br J Radiol* 30:169, 1957.
34. Murray JF: Deglutition in myasthenia gravis, *Br J Radiol* 35:43, 1962.
35. Bosma JF, Brodie DR: Cineradiographic demonstration of pharyngeal area myotonia in myotonic dystrophy patients, *Radiology* 92:104, 1969.
36. Garrett JM, Dubose TE, Jackson JE, Norman JR: Esophageal and pulmonary disturbances in myotonia dystrophica, *Arch Intern Med* 123:26, 1969.
37. Ekberg O, Sigurjónsson SV: Movement of the epiglottis during deglutition: a cineradiographic study, *Gastrointest Radiol* 7:101, 1982.
38. Jones B, Ravich WJ, Donner MW, Kramer SS, Hendrix: Pharyngoesophageal interrelationships: observations and working concepts, *Gastrointest Radiol* 10:225, 1985.
39. Ekberg O, Lindgren S: Gastroesophageal reflux and pharyngeal function, *Acta Radiol Diagn* 27:421, 1986.
40. Gerhardt DC, Schuck TJ, Bordeaux RA, Winship DH: Human upper oesophageal sphincter: response to volume, osmotic, and acid stimuli, *Gastroenterology* 75:268, 1978.
41. Buchholz D, Bosma JF, Donner MW: Adaptation, compensation, and decompensation of pharyngeal swallow, *Gastrointest Radiol* 10:235, 1985.
42. Ekberg O, Nylander G: Cineradiography of the pharyngeal stage of deglutition in 150 individuals without dysphagia, *Br J Radiol* 55:253, 1982.
43. Jones B, Donner MW: *Normal and abnormal swallowing: imaging in diagnosis and treatment,* New York, 1990, Springer-Verlag.
44. Ekberg O, Feinberg MJ: Altered swallowing function in elderly patients: radiologic findings in 56 patients, *AJR* 156:1181, 1991.
45. Linden P, Siebens AA: Dysphagia: predicting laryngeal penetration, *Arch Phys Med Rehabil* 64:281, 1983.
46. Splaingard ML, Hutchins B, Sulton LD, Chaudhuri G: Aspiration in rehabilitation patients: videofluoroscopy vs. bedside clinical assessment. *Arch Phys Med Rehabil* 69:637, 1988.
47. Ekberg O: Posture of the head and pharyngeal swallow, *Acta Radiol Diagn* 27:691, 1986.
48. Siebens AA, Linden P: Dynamic imaging for swallowing reeducation, *Gastrointest Radiol* 10:251, 1985.

7 Malignant Diseases of the Pharynx

HUGH D. CURTIN
THOMAS A. KIM

Almost all malignancies involving the oral cavity and pharynx arise from the mucosa.[1,2] Modern endoscopic equipment, available in many otolaryngologists' offices, allows inspection of virtually the entire mucosa of the pharynx. However, sophisticated equipment is not needed for the detection of most lesions as they are obvious on direct visualization or mirror examination. The purpose of imaging is not usually so much concerned with tumor detection as with determining the extent of a lesion. The diagnosis has actually already been made by the time imaging is performed. Both the radiologist and otolaryngologist must also realize that imaging is not as sensitive as direct visualization and should not be used to exclude the existence of carcinoma of the pharynx.

The clinician can estimate the limits of mucosal disease fairly closely, and imaging is used to assess the tumor's deeper extension, away from the mucosa. The radiologist defines the relationship of the tumor to certain landmarks that are important in planning a surgical resection. Other factors are important to the radiotherapist in planning treatment.

PATHOLOGY

The histologic nature of malignancy of the oral cavity and pharynx reflects the cell populations normally found in the region.[1]

Squamous cell carcinoma

Most of the pharynx and oral cavity is lined with stratified squamous epithelium from which arises the most common malignancy, squamous cell carcinoma, accounting for approximately 90% of the malignancies in the pharynx. These neoplasms arise from the epithelial layer, and carcinogens are strongly implicated as etiologic agents. Tobacco use, including the smokeless varieties, is one of these causes due to its direct irritation of the tissue. Alcohol consumption is also thought to be a contributing cause due to both its local toxic effect and its less clearly defined systemic effects. Substantial alcohol consumption is also associated with significant nutritional deficiencies, and this

may actually have an effect on the immune system. The use of both alcohol and tobacco therefore compounds the problem, and the combined effect may be greater than just simply additive, in that one may potentiate the effect of the other.

Minor salivary gland tumors

The minor salivary glands are small clusters of glands distributed throughout the mucosa, and the tumors that arise in them have the same histopathologic makeup as do tumors that arise in the major salivary glands: the parotid, submandibular, and sublingual glands. However, tumors that arise in the minor salivary glands are more likely to be malignant than those arising within the major glands. Adenoid cystic carcinoma and mucoepidermoid carcinoma are two of the more common histologic types of the minor salivary gland tumors.

Lymphoma

Waldeyer's tonsillar ring includes the lymphoid tissue of the lingual and palatine tonsils as well as the nasopharyngeal adenoids. Lymphoma can involve any part of the pharynx but has a predilection for these areas.

Other

Other much less common malignancies also occur in this region. Various sarcomas can arise from the support structures of the tongue, mouth, and pharynx.

STAGING

Staging of a head and neck tumor takes into consideration the size and location of the primary tumor as well as the extent, if any, of lymph node involvement and distant metastatic spread. A uniform classification system is therefore very important if results are to be compared. Most clinicians use one of two systems, and radiologists should be familiar with these staging systems, even though they do not emphasize the imaging evaluation.

The American Joint Committee on Cancer (AJCC) has published the *Manual for Staging of Cancer,*[3] which is the staging system used in our institution and in most centers in the United States (see the box below). The Union Internationale Contre le Cancer has formulated a separate classification system. Both systems use a TNM classification based on the primary tumor (T), nodes (N), and the presence or absence of distant metastasis (M). As the systems have been further updated and modified, they have become more and more alike.

Imaging

Tumors of the oral cavity and pharynx are usually evaluated by computed tomography (CT) or magnetic resonance imaging (MRI).[4-11] Barium studies may be carried out to evaluate some hypopharyngeal lesions, but many radiolo-gists consider that most information about the lesion is obtained more easily using CT or MRI. Barium studies are effective in evaluating the lower esophagus for the presence of second primaries (see later discussion) but are less sensitive than endoscopy for the detection of early esophageal cancer.

On CT, squamous cell carcinoma is usually isodense with muscle but often enhances slightly when intravenous contrast is instilled. The tumor is denser than fat. On MRI, the tumor is usually dark on T1 images and is isointense with muscle. Often the lesion is brighter (of greater intensity) on a T2 image and also enhances with gadolinium DTPA[12] (Fig. 7-1).

The long image acquisition times required by MRI do

□ DEFINITION OF TNM □

PRIMARY TUMOR (T)

TX   Primary tumor cannot be assessed
TO   No evidence of primary tumor
Tis   Carcinoma in situ
T1   Tumor 2 cm or less in greatest dimension
T2   Tumor more than 2 cm but not more than 4 cm in greatest dimension
T3   Tumor more than 4 cm in greatest dimension
T4   Lip: tumor invades adjacent structures (e.g., through cortical bone, tongue, and skin of neck)
T4   Oral cavity: tumor invades adjacent structures (e.g., through cortical bone, into deep [extrinsic] muscle of tongue, maxillary sinus, and skin)

REGIONAL LYMPH NODES (N)

NX   Regional lymph nodes cannot be assessed
NO   No regional lymph node metastases
N1   Metastasis in a single ipsilateral lymph node 3 cm or less in greatest dimension
N2   Metastasis in a single ipsilateral lymph node, more than 3 cm but not more than 6 cm in greatest dimension; or in multiple ipsilateral lymph nodes, none more than 6 cm in greatest dimension; or in bilateral or contralateral lymph nodes, none more than 6 cm in greatest dimension
   N2a   Metastasis in single ipsilateral lymph node more than 3 cm but not more than 6 cm in greatest dimension
   N2b   Metastasis in multiple ipsilateral lymph nodes, none more than 6 cm in greatest dimension
   N2c   Metastasis in bilateral or contralateral lymph nodes, none more than 6 cm in greatest dimension
N3   Metastasis in a lymph node more than 6 cm in greatest dimension

DISTANT METASTASIS (M)

MX   Presence of distant metastasis cannot be assessed
MO   No distant metastasis
M1   Distant metastasis

OROPHARYNX

T1   Tumor 2 cm or less in greatest dimension
T2   Tumor more than 2 cm but not more than 4 cm in greatest dimension
T3   Tumor more than 4 cm in greatest dimension
T4   Tumor invades adjacent structures (e.g., through cortical bone, soft tissues of neck, and deep [extrinsic] muscle of tongue)

NASOPHARYNX

T1   Tumor limited to one subsite of the nasopharynx
T2   Tumor invades more than one subsite of the nasopharynx
T3   Tumor invades nasal cavity and/or the oropharynx
T4   Tumor invades skull and/or cranial nerve(s)

HYPOPHARYNX

T1   Tumor limited to one subsite of the hypopharynx
T2   Tumor invades more than one subsite of the hypopharynx or an adjacent site, without fixation of the hemilarynx
T3   Tumor invades more than one subsite of the hypopharynx or an adjacent site, with fixation of the hemilarynx
T4   Tumor invades adjacent structures (e.g., cartilage of the soft tissues of the neck)

From Beahrs OH, Henson DE, Hutter RVP, Kennedy BJ, eds: *American Joint Committee on Cancer manual for staging of cancer*, ed 4, Philadelphia, 1988, JB Lippincott.

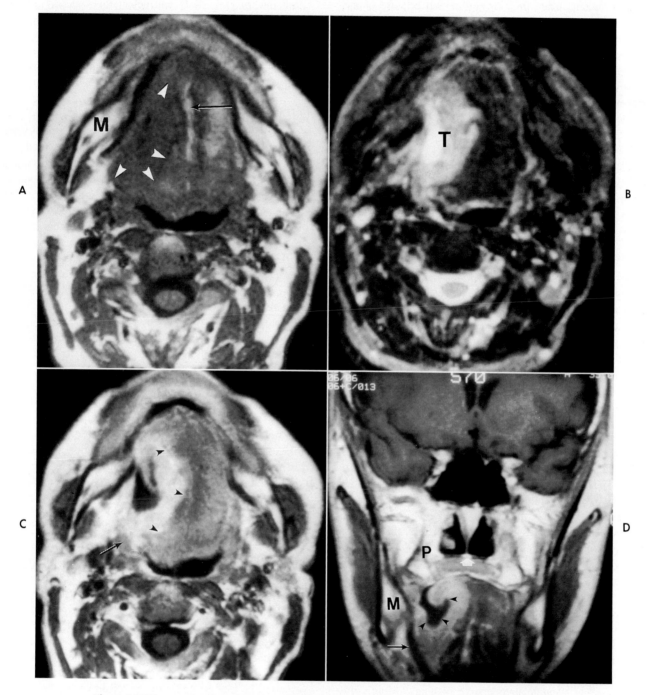

Fig. 7-1 MRI scans showing squamous cell carcinoma of the lateral tongue with submucosal spread across the floor of the mouth. **A,** Axial T1 image. The tumor is seen infiltrating the lateral tongue. The fatty midline *(arrow)* has not been infiltrated by tumor. *M,* mandible; *arrowheads,* margins of the tumor. **B,** T2 image. The bright signal of the tumor relative to the muscle increases its visibility. *T,* Tumor. **C,** Axial T1 view following gadolinium administration. Enhancement of the tumor again causes the lesion to be contrasted against the normal muscle. *Arrowheads,* Margins of the tumor; *arrow,* region of the anterior tonsillar pillar. **D,** Coronal T1 image showing that the tumor involves the undersurface of the lateral free margin of the tongue. The tumor infiltrates inferiorly along the genioglossus muscle and then across the floor of the mouth *(arrowheads)* but does not infiltrate the mylohyoid muscle *(arrow)*. This image shows the relationship of the tumor to the mandible *(M)*. *P,* Pterygoid plate; *white arrow,* hard palate.

cause problems when imaging this region because of the significant artifacts created by breathing and swallowing. Newer imaging techniques, such as fast spin echo and fat suppression, show promise in limiting these artifacts and giving good tissue contrast.

MRI can usually define gross bone involvement by a tumor with invasion of the medullary cavity, but CT is better for detecting subtle erosions of the cortex of a bone or thin bony structures.

Tumor spread

Head and neck malignancies can spread to both contiguous and distant sites. Several modes of tumor spread can be expected in the head and neck, and the radiologist should know when and where to search for each.

Direct encroachment

As the tumor mass increases, it spreads directly into the contiguous structures. The various muscles and fascial layers can initially direct the spread of this growth, or an infiltrating tumor can penetrate aggressively through whatever it comes in contact with. Tumors of the mucosa may be exophytic or infiltrative. An exophytic tumor may be fairly superficial and seem to fungate into the lumen of either the oral cavity or the pharynx. Infiltrative malignancies can invade deeply into the tissues with only a small apparent mucosal component.

Direct encroachment is the most obvious type of tumor spread, and the radiologist is most concerned with identifying the margin of the tumor distant from the mucosal surface. The soft tissues involved should be accurately described and the overall dimensions of the lesion estimated. Determining whether there is bone involvement, and to what extent, is also very important to surgical planning.

Any point where the tumor forms an interface with bone should be identified. The radiologist should indicate whether the tumor merely touches the bone, leaving the cortex apparently intact, whether the cortex is eroded minimally, or whether there is gross destruction of the cortex and replacement of the medullary region of the bone. Although the accuracy of imaging minimal bone involvement is somewhat limited, combining the clinical examination with the imaging findings usually yields enough information to allow accurate preoperative planning. More complete descriptions of certain key methods for assessing osseous structure are provided in appropriate sections dealing with specific anatomic regions.

Although many aggressive tumors seem to destroy whatever tissues they encounter, some types of soft tissue spread can be more subtle. Some tumors are initially limited by the more resistant myofascial structures located throughout the head and neck region. Of special note, however, is submucosal spread,[13,14] in which tumors tunnel beneath the mucosa away from the site of the initial lesion. This phenomenon conveys the tumor away from the obvious mucosal ulceration, and significant clinical understaging results.

Often the imaging study can detect this type of growth, which, though close to the mucosal surface, is not visible to the examining clinician. Submucosal spread usually takes place between the mucosal surface and the constrictor muscles and is extremely common in the oropharynx and hypopharynx.

Perineural spread

Malignancy can follow nerves away from the immediate vicinity of a primary tumor. This perineural spread can carry tumor beyond the limits of the planned resection, and this becomes a prime consideration in the imaging evaluation of any case of head and neck malignancy.[15-17] The course of any major nerve branch that passes near a tumor should be carefully inspected to determine whether there is evidence of this insidious type of tumor spread (see Fig. 7-13).

Perineural spread can occur in the context of many different types of tumor but is particularly typical of adenoid cystic carcinoma arising in the minor salivary glands. Lymphoma can also use the nerve as a conduit to pass from one region to another. The phenomenon is not as characteristic of squamous cell carcinoma but is occasionally seen.

Lymphatic spread

The extensive lymphatic network of the head and neck serves as an important route of spread for malignancy. This type of metastasis is very common in cases of squamous cell carcinoma and is a major consideration in planning treatment for any patient with this disease.[18-21] The location of nodal involvement depends partly on the site of the primary tumor. However, most of the lymphatic pathways of the head and neck converge on certain nodal chains of the neck.

There are many anatomic classifications of the neck nodes, but the deep cervical chains are the most important to the radiologist, as they represent the final common pathway of lymphatic drainage for most of the head and neck. The deep nodes are also the most difficult to palpate, so it is here that the physical examination is least reliable and the radiologic evaluation assumes greater importance.

The internal jugular chain of nodes parallels the carotid artery and jugular vein, passing anterior and lateral to the vessels. The highest nodes of this chain are in the jugulodigastric region at the angle of the mandible, just posterior to the submandibular gland. Many superficial groups of nodes drain into this jugulodigastric area, as do the lymphatics that primarily drain most of the pharynx. The jugulodigastric nodes are therefore very important to assess in the cancer staging process (Fig. 7-2); (see Fig. 7-19).

An important superficial system that drains into this area, and is pertinent to the present discussion, is the lymphatic complex inferior to the mylohyoid. This complex includes the submental (midline) and the submandibular nodes that are often involved in cases of carcinoma of the anterior tongue and floor of the mouth (Fig. 7-3).

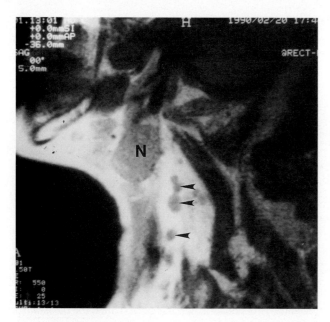

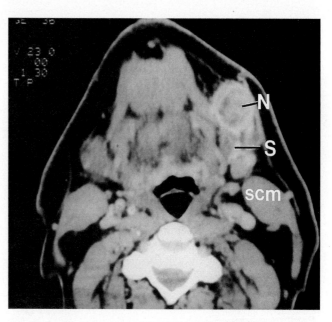

Fig. 7-2 Sagittal T1 image showing metastatic lymphadenopathy. A large metastatic lymph node *(N)* is seen in the jugulodigastric area. The sagittal view also shows multiple nodes, which are normal in size, *(arrowheads)* along the jugular chain.

Fig. 7-3 Metastatic deposit in a submandibular node of a patient with carcinoma of the anterior floor of the mouth. A metastatic node *(N)* is seen anterior to the submandibular gland *(S)*. The node has a low-density center with an enhancing rim. *SCM,* Sternocleidomastoid muscle.

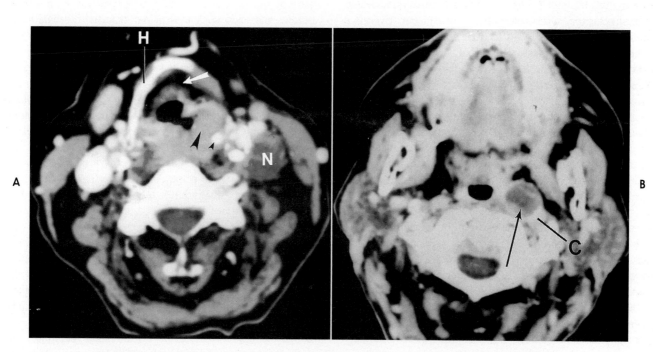

Fig. 7-4 A, Tumor of the hypopharyngeal wall with a metastatic node of Rouviere. Note the tumor extending around the posterior wall and onto the lateral wall of the pharynx *(large arrowhead)*. The preepiglottic fat *(arrow)* is normal. The density just lateral to the tumor represents the upper horn of the thyroid cartilage *(small arrowhead)* and should not be mistaken for the carotid artery. *H,* Hyoid bone; *N,* metastatic node. **B,** A higher slice showing a metastatic node of Rouviere *(arrow)* in a characteristic position just medial to the carotid artery. *(C).*

The spinal accessory chain of nodes follows, at least initially, the spinal accessory nerve (see Fig. 7-24). This chain is posterior to the jugular vein and is sometimes referred to as the *posterior triangle chain*. The spinal accessory nodes extend from the jugulodigastric region down to the lower neck and are located deep to the sternocleidomastoid muscle. They can often be palpated in the posterior triangle just posterior to the sternocleidomastoid muscle. This chain of nodes can receive metastatic deposits from the oropharynx and nasopharynx. Frequently, a posterior triangle node is the first indication of a nasopharynx primary tumor.

The retropharyngeal nodes are situated in the deep soft tissues just medial to the carotid artery close to the prevertebral muscles. These nodes are sometimes called the *nodes of Rouviere* and cannot be detected clinically. Metastatic deposits in these nodes usually originate from tumors in the nasopharynx or oropharynx but occasionally can also come from lesions as low as the hypopharynx (Fig. 7-4).

Positive nodes

Imaging is more accurate than palpation. However, the criteria for judging positive nodal involvement are not absolute. Because imaging cannot detect microscopic deposits, there are false-negative findings in a certain percentage of cases.

A node can be considered positively involved by tumor either based on its size or internal morphology. The upper limit of normal size in the submandibular and jugulodigastric regions is about 1.5 cm.[21] Elsewhere in the jugular and spinal accessory chain, the upper limit is 1 cm. Even if a node is normal in size, an internal abnormality can indicate tumor involvement. This usually consists of a focal low-density defect on a CT scan (see Fig. 7-3 and 7-4). Recently, focal defects have been identified on MRI scans as well.

An irregular margin of an involved node and obliteration of the fat planes contiguous to the node indicate penetration of the node capsule. This so-called extracapsular spread is an important finding because it signifies a substantially worse prognosis (see Fig. 7-22).

Unknown primaries

An enlarging lymph node is often the first indication of the presence of an oral or pharyngeal primary carcinoma. In most cases, the primary tumor can be found by direct inspection, but occasionally the tumor is not obvious and an imaging study may be needed for examining any suspicious areas. In a small percentage of cases, no primary is found even after imaging and thorough endoscopy. A tumor may become obvious at a later time, but occasionally the primary tumor is never found.

Hematogenous metastasis

Although the extent of the primary tumor and the status of the lymph nodes are the principal considerations in the evaluation of malignancies of the pharynx and oral cavity, distant hematogenous metastases do occur.[1] These are unusual at the time of initial presentation but do occasionally develop in the lung, liver, or bone. Metastases may develop later, even if the primary is controlled. Most recurrences are in the area of the primary tumor or in the neck, however.

Second primaries

A patient with primary squamous cell carcinoma of the oral cavity, pharynx, or larynx faces a definite increased risk for having, either concurrently or later, a second separate primary of one of the other regions of the upper aerodigestive system.[1] These second primaries are not part of the same tumor, however, because they do not have either a direct connection to the original tumor or a reasonable potential pathway from it. Rather they are thought to result from exposure of the entire mucosal surface to the same irritants. This phenomenon has been named the *condemned mucosa theory*. Second primaries that occur at the same time as the initially diagnosed neoplasm are referred to as *synchronous,* and those that are separated temporally are called *metachronous*. Such second lesions arise in the oral cavity, oropharynx or hypopharynx, larynx, tracheobronchial tree, esophagus, and even stomach. The nasopharynx appears to be exempt from this increased incidence of second primaries.

This increased incidence of second primaries is a major part of the rationale for evaluating patients with barium studies and endoscopy at the time of initial presentation.

SPECIFIC ANATOMIC LOCATIONS

Imaging of lesions in all locations of the head and neck share certain principles: the local soft tissue involvement should be determined and the overall size of the tumor estimated. The radiologist must always consider the possibility of submucosal spread, bone involvement, perineural extension, and lymph node metastasis.

This chapter considers the oral cavity, oral pharynx, and hypopharynx. Because the nasopharynx is not part of the alimentary tract but is intimately related to the oral pharynx, it is discussed briefly.

Oral cavity
Anatomy

The oral cavity is bound anteriorly by the line of lip closure[13] (Figs. 7-5 and 7-6). The anterior tonsillar pillars and the junction line of hard and soft palates represent the posterior boundary of the oral cavity. A line crossing the tongue at approximately the circumvallate papillae separates the anterior oral tongue from the posterior oropharyngeal segment or base of the tongue.

The oral cavity segment of the tongue has a dorsum and lateral margin as well as a small undersurface just below the lateral free margin. The mucosa of the undersurface of

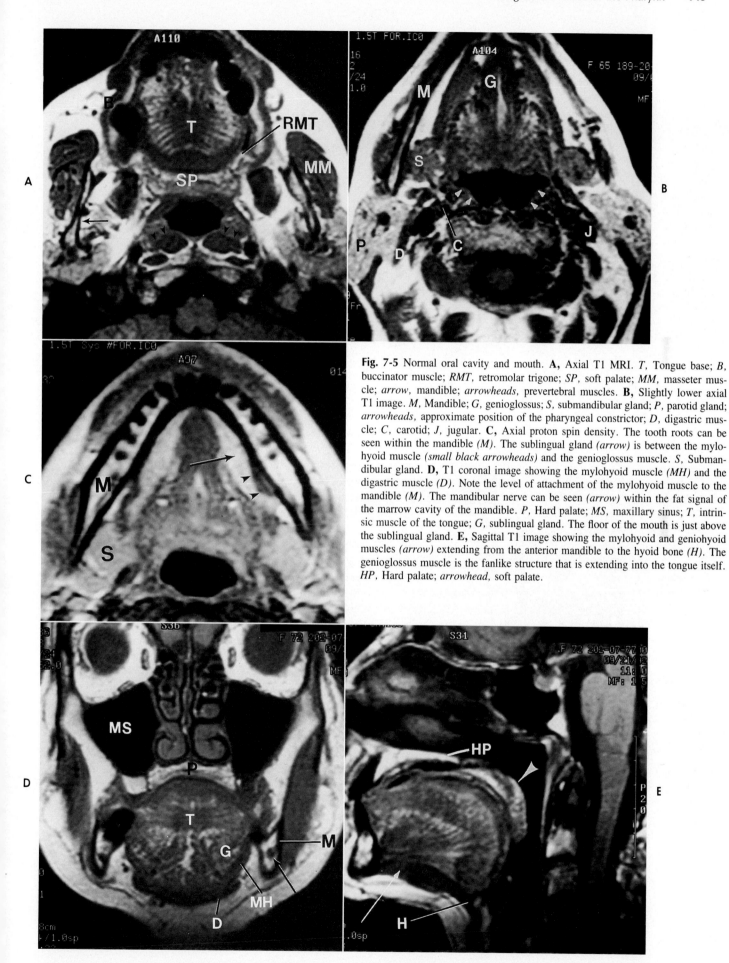

Fig. 7-5 Normal oral cavity and mouth. **A,** Axial T1 MRI. *T*, Tongue base; *B*, buccinator muscle; *RMT*, retromolar trigone; *SP*, soft palate; *MM*, masseter muscle; *arrow*, mandible; *arrowheads*, prevertebral muscles. **B,** Slightly lower axial T1 image. *M*, Mandible; *G*, genioglossus; *S*, submandibular gland; *P*, parotid gland; *arrowheads*, approximate position of the pharyngeal constrictor; *D*, digastric muscle; *C*, carotid; *J*, jugular. **C,** Axial proton spin density. The tooth roots can be seen within the mandible *(M)*. The sublingual gland *(arrow)* is between the mylohyoid muscle *(small black arrowheads)* and the genioglossus muscle. *S*, Submandibular gland. **D,** T1 coronal image showing the mylohyoid muscle *(MH)* and the digastric muscle *(D)*. Note the level of attachment of the mylohyoid muscle to the mandible *(M)*. The mandibular nerve can be seen *(arrow)* within the fat signal of the marrow cavity of the mandible *(M)*. *P*, Hard palate; *MS*, maxillary sinus; *T*, intrinsic muscle of the tongue; *G*, sublingual gland. The floor of the mouth is just above the sublingual gland. **E,** Sagittal T1 image showing the mylohyoid and geniohyoid muscles *(arrow)* extending from the anterior mandible to the hyoid bone *(H)*. The genioglossus muscle is the fanlike structure that is extending into the tongue itself. *HP*, Hard palate; *arrowhead*, soft palate.

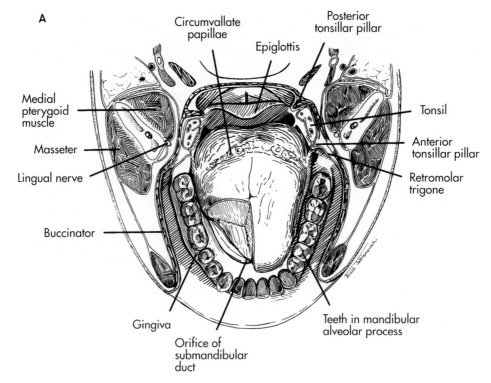

A

Circumvallate
papillae

Epiglottis

Posterior
tonsillar pillar

Medial
pterygoid
muscle

Masseter

Lingual nerve

Buccinator

Tonsil

Anterior
tonsillar pillar

Retromolar
trigone

Gingiva

Orifice of
submandibular
duct

Teeth in mandibular
alveolar process

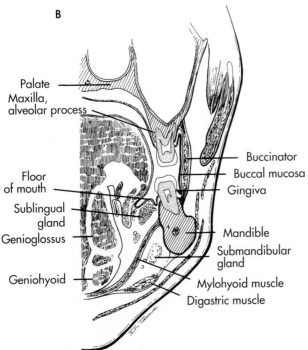

B

Palate
Maxilla,
alveolar process

Floor
of mouth

Sublingual
gland

Genioglossus

Geniohyoid

Buccinator

Buccal mucosa

Gingiva

Mandible

Submandibular
gland

Mylohyoid muscle

Digastric muscle

Fig. 7-6 A, Axial cross section through the mouth with a cut section of the anterior tongue. *RMT,* Retromolar trigone. **B,** Coronal section through the mouth. *FOM,* Floor of mouth.

the tongue is continuous with the mucosa of the floor of the mouth, which covers the sublingual region and glands. After crossing the floor of the mouth, the mucosa becomes the gingiva, which extends over the alveolar ridge of the mandible.

The gingiva is defined as the mucosa that is closely adherent to the alveolar processes of the mandible and maxillae. Laterally and anteriorly, the gingival mucosa is continuous with the buccal mucosa, which represents the outer limit of the oral cavity. The buccal surface sweeps upward from the mandible to meet the gingiva covering the alveolar process of the maxilla. The gingiva of the maxillary alveolus is then continuous with the mucosa covering the hard palate.

The final area of the oral cavity to be considered here is the retromolar trigone (RMT) (see Figs. 7-5 and 7-6). This area of the mucosa covers the anterior edge of the ramus of the mandible and adjacent muscles. It faces roughly anteromedially and is posterior to the maxillary and mandibular molar teeth. Anterolaterally, the RMT merges with the buccal surface, and its posterior medial margin is the anterior tonsillar pillar, which marks the junction of the oral cavity with the oropharynx. Although anatomically the RMT is part of the oral cavity, tumors in this area are often dealt with at the same time as those of the anterior tonsillar pillar because many tumors involve both regions and the clinical concerns and routes of spread are the same.

General considerations

A malignancy in the oral cavity can present as a small sore that does not heal. Larger tumors may be exophytic or ulcerating and invasive. Some tumors, especially adenoid cystic carcinoma, may be almost totally submucosal. As a rule, anterior tumors are smaller when found because they are more obvious to the patient and so discovered earlier.

Tumors of the oral cavity are assigned to one of eight regions of the anatomy based on the site of apparent origin or maximal involvement. These are the lip, buccal region, maxillary gingiva, mandibular gingiva, hard palate, tongue, floor of the mouth, and RMT.[13] The general considerations are the same for the various regions, but the specific anatomic landmarks vary.

Direct extension (soft tissue and bone)

The direct extension of tumors in the oral cavity can introduce the tumor into the contiguous soft tissues or bring it into contact with the bone. Muscle layers such as the buccinator or the mylohyoid muscle can initially contain growth but can be breached by an infiltrating tumor. Any evidence of tumor infiltrating or extending through these muscles should be noted. Tumors arising in the lip can already be outside the boundary musculature and can infiltrate circumferentially outward into the superficial tissues of the face anterior to the lower maxilla and along the anterior surface of the mandible. Tumors of the RMT often extend directly into the soft tissues of the masticator space, where involvement of the pterygoid and temporalis muscles can limit mouth opening.

Within the tongue proper, the radiologist must assess extension toward or across the midline (see Fig. 7-1). Usually there is enough fat in the midline raphe that this landmark can be identified on either T1 MRI or CT scans. Its position can be documented even if a bulky tumor causes displacement. Extension posteriorly brings the tumor into the pharyngeal tongue (base of tongue).

Submucosal spread represents an important type of direct extension, especially in the floor of the mouth and the inferior aspect of the free margin of the oral tongue. Tumor can extend from the inferior free margin of the tongue laterally across the floor of the mouth and reach the mandible (see Fig. 7-1). If the tumor is slightly more posterior, the lateral submucosal extension can introduce the tumor to the lower margin of the anterior tonsillar pillar, which is an important potential submucosal pathway in the oropharynx (see later discussion). These potential submucosal pathways should be carefully examined by the radiologist, since they are difficult to assess clinically. Extension can be in either direction, depending on the location of the primary tumor.

In the area of the gingiva and hard palate, soft tissue extension is of less concern, because, although important in a pathologic sense, it can usually be assessed clinically. Here submucosal extension away from the primary tumor is a consideration as well, with bone involvement the chief concern.

If tumor involves the gingiva, either as a primary lesion or as one spreading from the floor of the mouth, evaluation of the mandible becomes the focus of attention (Figs. 7-7 and 7-8). The radiologist should try to determine whether the cortex is intact, slightly eroded, or completely destroyed. The bony cortex is best evaluated using a bone algorithm on a high-resolution CT scan. Involvement of the medullary cavity may be appreciated as a change from the normal high-intensity signal of the fatty marrow on a T1 MRI scan.

The management of the mandible is one of the key considerations in surgical planning for tumors in the lower oral cavity. The mandible is important cosmetically as well as in mastication and nutrition.

At our institution, the decision about treatment of the mandible is based on the physical examination and the CT scan.[22] If the lesion is not fixed or adherent to the mandible, the bone is left intact.[23] The periosteum may be removed to serve as a margin. If the tumor is fixed to the bone but a bone algorithm CT scan shows little or no irregularity, a marginal mandibulectomy is done. This removes the cortex of the bone along the attachment of the tumor but leaves enough of the opposite cortex so that the basic structure of the bone is maintained. Usually the inferior cortex of the mandible is preserved so that the complete arch from one temporomandibular joint (TMJ) to the other remains.

If there is gross destruction of the mandible and the marrow cavity is involved, the surgeon does a segmental mandibular resection. A complete section is removed, leaving a gap between the TMJ and the opposite side of the mandible. The arch is then incomplete, and a decision must then be made whether to leave it as is or to try to reconstruct it using either a bone graft or metal plate.

If a tumor involves the palate and the alveolar process of the maxilla, bone involvement is again a definite concern (Fig. 7-9). The presence and extent of any bone erosion must be demonstrated. Its proximity to the posterior palate and pterygoid plates is also important. Other questions the radiologist tries to answer are: does the tumor extend through the bone into the maxillary sinus or the nasal cavity?; how much of the palate is eroded?; and does the bone involvement cross the midline? Many of these factors are important to the planning of reconstruction. The defect is usually reconstructed with a prosthesis, and therefore a preoperative estimation of the defect is very helpful. The tumor determines the minimal amount of bone resected, but the surgeon may take slightly more so that the prosthesis is easier to insert and in a more stable position.

When local extension from an RMT malignancy enters the region of the masticator space, the ramus of the mandible can be involved along with the muscles (Fig. 7-10). The anterior edge of the ramus of the mandible is especially at risk, and the same considerations apply here as in the

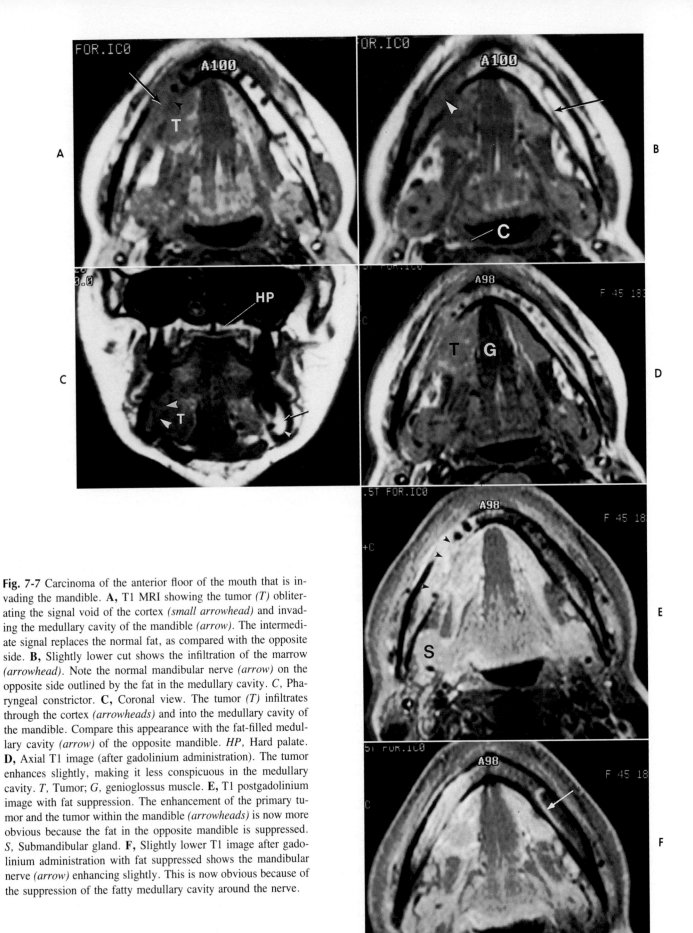

Fig. 7-7 Carcinoma of the anterior floor of the mouth that is invading the mandible. **A,** T1 MRI showing the tumor *(T)* obliterating the signal void of the cortex *(small arrowhead)* and invading the medullary cavity of the mandible *(arrow).* The intermediate signal replaces the normal fat, as compared with the opposite side. **B,** Slightly lower cut shows the infiltration of the marrow *(arrowhead).* Note the normal mandibular nerve *(arrow)* on the opposite side outlined by the fat in the medullary cavity. *C,* Pharyngeal constrictor. **C,** Coronal view. The tumor *(T)* infiltrates through the cortex *(arrowheads)* and into the medullary cavity of the mandible. Compare this appearance with the fat-filled medullary cavity *(arrow)* of the opposite mandible. *HP,* Hard palate. **D,** Axial T1 image (after gadolinium administration). The tumor enhances slightly, making it less conspicuous in the medullary cavity. *T,* Tumor; *G,* genioglossus muscle. **E,** T1 postgadolinium image with fat suppression. The enhancement of the primary tumor and the tumor within the mandible *(arrowheads)* is now more obvious because the fat in the opposite mandible is suppressed. *S,* Submandibular gland. **F,** Slightly lower T1 image after gadolinium administration with fat suppressed shows the mandibular nerve *(arrow)* enhancing slightly. This is now obvious because of the suppression of the fatty medullary cavity around the nerve.

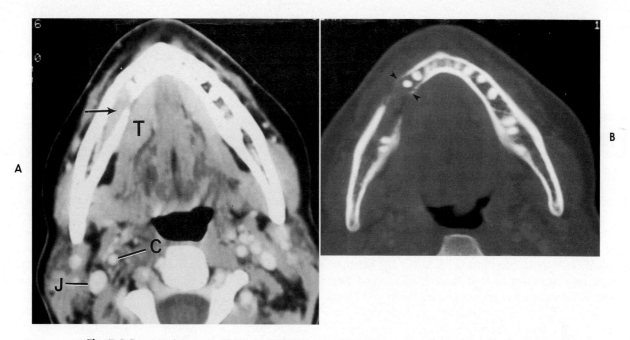

Fig. 7-8 Same patient as in Fig. 7-7. A CT scan obtained using a soft tissue algorithm shows the tumor *(T)* penetrating the cortex and invading the medullary cavity *(arrow)*, where it obliterates the normal fatty density. *C*, Carotid; *J*, jugular. **B,** Use of a bone algorithm reveals the cortical irregularities *(arrowheads)* caused by tumor erosion.

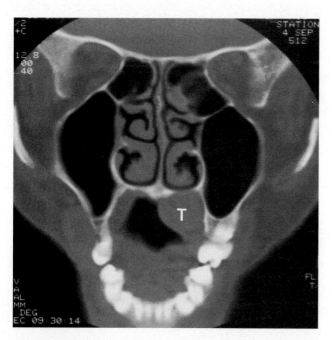

Fig. 7-9 Adenoid cystic carcinoma of the palate. Coronal view shows the tumor *(T)*. The bone is remodeled but not obviously eroded, and there is no tumor in the nasal cavity.

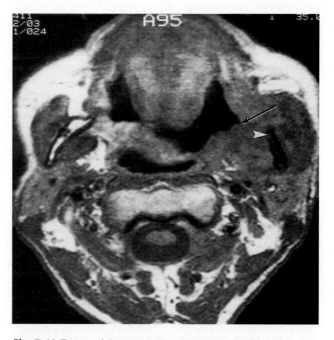

Fig. 7-10 Tumor of the retromolar trigone and tonsillar pillar. The retromolar trigone *(arrow)* is completely infiltrated by tumor, which extends posteriorly into the masticator space. As it invades the mandible, the tumor erodes the cortex *(arrowhead)* and obliterates the fat in the medullary cavity. Compare this appearance with that on the opposite side.

rest of mandible. The radiologist should determine if the tumor touches, erodes, or grossly destroys the bone. Marginal resections or partial (segmental) mandibulectomies with reconstruction can also be carried out in this part of the mandible.

Perineural extension

Perineural extension can follow several nerves in the region of the oral cavity. Almost all are branches of the trigeminal nerve.

The posterior third of the hard palate is of particular concern because it is rich in minor salivary glands, so adenoid cystic carcinoma, with its propensity for perineural spread, is a very common type of cancer in this site. Perineural spread follows the branches of the second division of the trigeminal nerve to the pterygopalatine fossa. The palatine foramina may be infiltrated, and these small passages can be either subtly enlarged or grossly eroded[24] (Figs. 7-11 and 7-12). This finding is best appreciated on high-resolution CT scans. If the tumor reaches the pterygopalatine fossa, the fat is obliterated, a change easily appreciated on either CT or MRI scanning (see Figs. 7-11 and 7-13). If tumor is found in the pterygopalatine fossa, the foramen rotundum should also be carefully examined, as tumor can use this as a conduit to reach Meckel's cave and the cavernous sinus in the middle cranial fossa.

In the lower oral cavity, the third division of the trigeminal nerve is of concern. If there is invasion of the mandible, then the mandibular (inferior alveolar) nerve may act as the conduit conveying the tumor through the body and ramus into the upper masticator space and eventually to the foramen ovale (Fig. 7-14). The radiologist should look for obliteration of the fat near the lingula of the upper mandible where the nerve first enters the bone.

The lingual nerve is the second branch of the third division of the trigeminal nerve and, as such, can carry tumor to the foramen ovale without involving the mandible. This nerve passes along the anterior lateral edge of the medial pterygoid muscle, between the muscle and the mandible, before reaching the upper masticator space beneath the foramen ovale. Again, the radiologist searches for any obliteration of the fat as the tumor grows along the nerve.

Infrequently, tumors from the lip and anterior mouth can infiltrate superiorly and reach the infraorbital foramen and thus can follow the infraorbital nerve to the pterygopalatine fossa. The fat just anterior to the entrance of the canal should be inspected for any obliteration, which indicates the presence of tumor. Tumor passing along the canal can expand the conduit or destroy the surrounding bone. The facial nerve passes along the outer surface of the buccinator muscle and so can be involved, although this is distinctly unusual in carcinoma of the oral cavity.

The hypoglossal and glossopharyngeal nerves also enter the tongue and are discussed in the section on the oropharyngeal part of the tongue.

Nodal metastasis

Nodal metastasis is common in the patient with carcinoma of the oral tongue and floor of mouth, but is less of a problem in lesions of the hard palate.

Lesions of the tongue and floor of the mouth may spread initially to the nodes in the submandibular and submental areas below the mylohyoid muscle. These nodes, in turn, drain to the jugulodigastric nodes and eventually to the jugular chain. The malignancy may skip the more anterior submental and submandibular nodes and go directly to the jugulodigastric nodes. Bilateral involvement is not uncommon, especially in larger tumors and those that cross the midline.

Oropharynx

The oropharynx includes the inferior surface of the soft palate, the tonsillar region, the base of the tongue, and the posterior pharyngeal wall.[13,25] Anteriorly, the boundaries consist of the junction of the soft and hard palates, the anterior margin of the anterior tonsillar pillar, and the circumvallate papillae. Tumors of the RMT readily spread to the anterior tonsillar pillar and tonsillar region and so are often included in descriptions of lateral oropharyngeal wall lesions.

Inferiorly the oropharynx is continuous with the hypopharynx. The line of separation is at the level of the hyoid bone, which is roughly at the level of the valleculae. Superiorly, the oropharynx is continuous with the nasopharynx, with the upper limit of the oropharynx at the level of the soft palate.

Tumors of the base of the tongue and the oropharyngeal wall may be infiltrative or exophytic and characteristically exhibit submucosal spread. The exophytic component can be directly visualized, but the deeper growth is hard to see and palpate.

A tumor infiltrating the wall of the oropharynx may initially be confined by the constrictor muscles that surround the oropharynx (Fig. 7-15). If the tumor does extend through the muscular layer, it gains access to the parapharyngeal spaces laterally or the retropharyngeal region posteriorly. The most significant structures in these regions are the carotid arteries, which can be involved by posterolateral growth. As the tumor approaches or surrounds the carotid artery, the fat planes around the vessel are obliterated.

Direct posterior extension (Fig. 7-16) can involve the prevertebral muscles and eventually the cervical spine. Lateral extension can cross the parapharyngeal space and reach the pterygoid muscles and the mandible. Anterior involvement where the anterior tonsillar pillar borders the RMT of the oral cavity is particularly worrisome. Here the fat planes just anterior and medial to the lower ramus of the mandible can be obliterated, indicating tumor infiltration. When tumors involve the lateral oropharyngeal wall, the radiologist should always try to determine the proximity of the lesion to the ramus of the mandible and more superiorly to

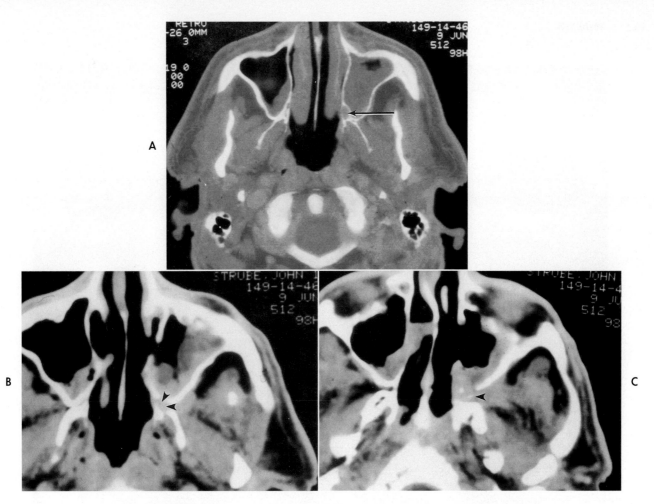

Fig. 7-11 Adenoid cystic carcinoma of the hard palate. A relatively small lesion (not shown) was present on the hard palate close to the junction with the soft palate. **A,** A CT slice through the lower maxillary sinus shows an enlarged pterygopalatine canal *(arrow)* just above the greater palatine foramen. **B,** The tumor *(arrowheads)* reaches the lower pterygopalatine fossa. **C,** Slightly higher, the fat is more obviously obliterated as compared with the opposite side *(arrowheads).*

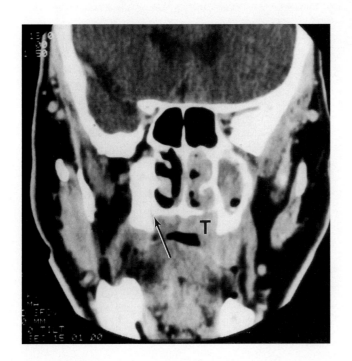

Fig. 7-12 Coronal CT shows tumor *(T)* eroding the bone close to the greater palatine foramen. Note the normal greater palatine foramen on the opposite side *(arrow).*

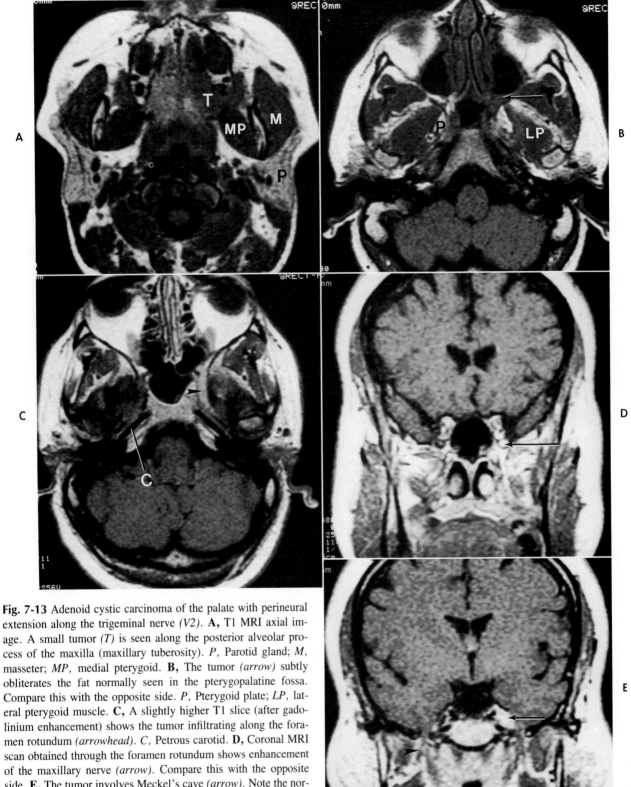

Fig. 7-13 Adenoid cystic carcinoma of the palate with perineural extension along the trigeminal nerve *(V2)*. **A,** T1 MRI axial image. A small tumor *(T)* is seen along the posterior alveolar process of the maxilla (maxillary tuberosity). *P,* Parotid gland; *M,* masseter; *MP,* medial pterygoid. **B,** The tumor *(arrow)* subtly obliterates the fat normally seen in the pterygopalatine fossa. Compare this with the opposite side. *P,* Pterygoid plate; *LP,* lateral pterygoid muscle. **C,** A slightly higher T1 slice (after gadolinium enhancement) shows the tumor infiltrating along the foramen rotundum *(arrowhead)*. *C,* Petrous carotid. **D,** Coronal MRI scan obtained through the foramen rotundum shows enhancement of the maxillary nerve *(arrow)*. Compare this with the opposite side. **E,** The tumor involves Meckel's cave *(arrow)*. Note the normal mandibular nerve *(arrowhead)* extending into the fat beneath the foramen ovale.

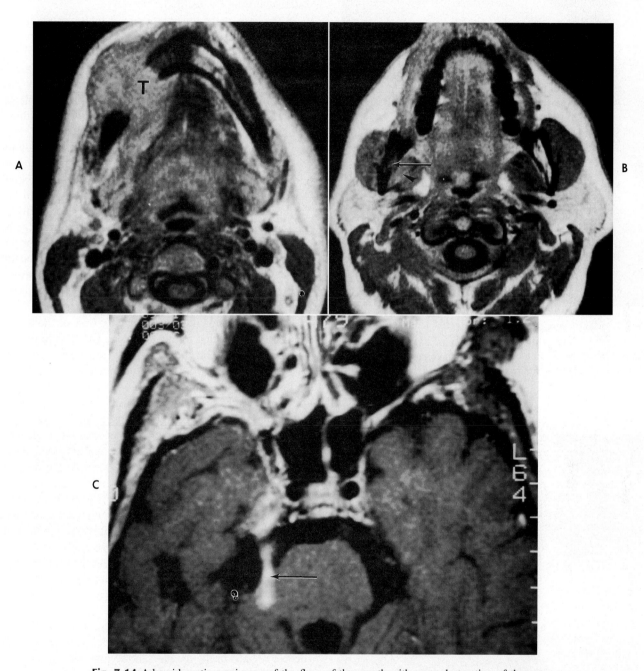

Fig. 7-14 Adenoid cystic carcinoma of the floor of the mouth with gross destruction of the mandible and perineural extension along the mandibular nerve. **A,** T1 MRI showing the tumor *(T)* extending completely through the mandible. **B,** Slightly higher slice. The tumor has followed the mandibular nerve along the mandibular canal to its entry point in the mandibular ramus *(arrow).* The tumor is seen infiltrating the medial pterygoid muscle *(arrowhead).* Compare this with the opposite side. **C,** The tumor followed the trigeminal nerve through the foramen ovale and along the preganglionic segment to the brainstem *(arrow).*
From Kolin ES, Castro D, Jobour RB, Hanafee WN: *Ann Otol Rhinol Laryngol* 100:1032, 1991; and Dr. Robert Lufkin.

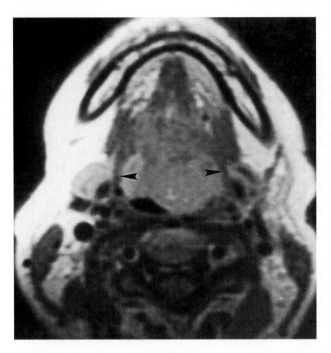

Fig. 7-15 MRI spin-density axial image of a lymphoma of the tongue base. The mass involved the region of the tongue base and lingual tonsil. Note that the margin appears to push the soft tissue *(arrowheads)* rather than to infiltrate deeply.

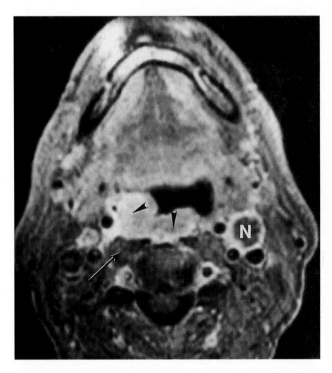

Fig. 7-16 MRI axial fat-suppressed T1 image showing tumor of the oropharyngeal wall. The tumor *(arrowheads)* involves the lateral and posterior pharyngeal walls. The prevertebral muscles *(arrow)* appear to have a normal signal, indicating that they are not infiltrated by tumor. The jugulodigastric node *(N)* shows rim enhancement and a low-intensity center.

the lower pterygoid plates. All of these extensions can be estimated using CT or MRI.

In the base of the tongue the tumor infiltrates the intrinsic musculature. On CT the tumor can assume an appearance very similar to that of the tongue muscle, and therefore its margin may be difficult to ascertain. Some practitioners prefer to use MRI for this purpose, as tumor and musculature can usually be differentiated using multiple sequences. Rapid CT scanning with bolus contrast administration may reduce this advantage.

When tumors affect the base of the tongue, the radiologist should estimate both the size of the lesion and how close the margin is to midline. If the tumor crosses the midline, the opposite lingual artery is threatened. If both lingual arteries are involved, this rules out the possibility of performing a partial glossectomy. The lingual artery can be seen sometimes as a flow void on MRI or may be opacified on CT scans obtained with bolus contrast administration. Even if the artery is not seen, the amount of extension across the midline can serve as a sufficient approximation.

Inferior extension along the posterior base of the tongue brings the tumor first to the valleculae and then to the larynx (Fig. 7-17). The epiglottis forms the posterior surface of the valleculae and actually protrudes up into the lumen of the oropharynx. Tumor can spread superficially onto the surface of the epiglottis or can invade more deeply and infiltrate the fat in the preepiglottic space. Such involvement often means that a laryngectomy is necessary if surgical resection of the primary is done. If a total glossectomy or extensive partial glossectomy is performed, the surgeon must consider doing a laryngectomy as well, even if the larynx is not involved. Most of these patients have significant pulmonary problems, and problems with aspiration, which are unavoidable while the patient is learning to swallow again after glossectomy, may prove fatal.

The tongue attaches laterally to the wall of the oropharynx, and part of the superior constrictor muscle group actually arises from the tongue. Tumor can pass around the limiting barrier of the constrictor muscles in the posterolateral area of attachment. Actually, there is a gap between the constrictor muscles where several nerves enter the deeper regions of the tongue. The styloglossus muscle also passes into and fuses with the tongue musculature. The fat planes abutting the posterolateral margin of the tongue should be examined carefully for signs of tumor infiltration (Fig. 7-18). Again, in this region, carotid artery involvement is a major concern.

Tumors of the oropharynx tend to spread or tunnel beneath the mucosa, so the tumor is actually more extensive than is apparent on direct visual examination.[14] This can happen in any area of the pharynx, but one pathway deserves particular attention. Tumors can follow the tonsillar fossa and especially the anterior tonsillar pillar from one

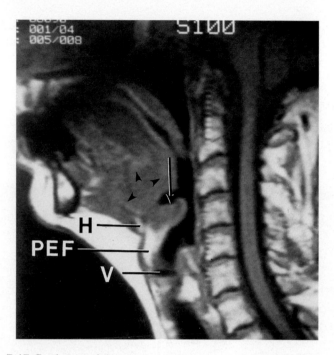

Fig. 7-17 Carcinoma of the tongue base extending posteroinferiorly to reach the larynx. The tumor *(arrowheads)* infiltrates the base of the tongue and extends to the region of the valleculae and on to the vallecular surface of the epiglottis *(arrow)*. Note that the preepiglottic fat *(PEF)* is not infiltrated. *H,* Hyoid bone; *V,* ventricle of the larynx.

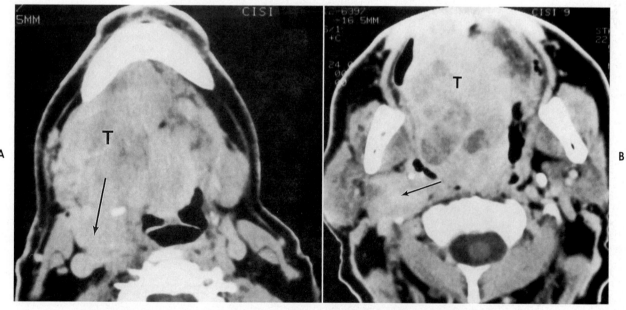

Fig. 7-18 CT scan of an adenoid cystic carcinoma with perineural extension along the hypoglossal nerve. **A,** Large tumor *(T)* infiltrating the tongue and floor of the mouth. Note the posterolateral extension *(arrow)*. **B,** A slightly higher slice shows the tumor *(T)* within the tongue proper. Note the soft tissue mass *(arrow)* in the region of the carotid and jugular. This represented tumor that had followed along the hypoglossal nerve.

area of the oropharynx to another (Figs. 7-19 and 7-20). The palatoglossus muscle forms the anterior tonsillar pillar and extends from the soft palate down into the tongue. This muscle is contained within the constrictor muscles of the pharynx, so tumor appears to follow the muscle or pillar as the line of least resistance rather than invade through the constrictor muscle. This pathway can carry tongue tumors up into the tonsil and eventually the soft palate or even the nasopharynx. Similarly, tonsillar tumors can extend down into the tongue. This type of submucosal spread can be visualized using MRI or rapid bolus contrast-enhanced CT scans.

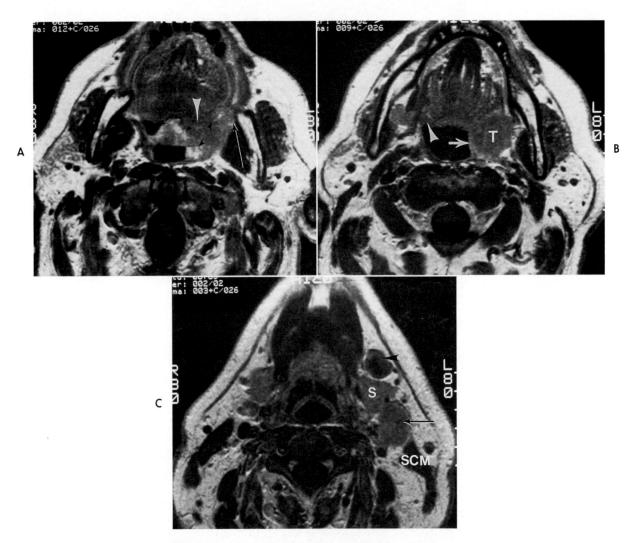

Fig. 7-19 Squamous cell carcinoma of the soft palate and tonsillar pillar with a metastatic node. **A,** Axial T1 MRI showing the infiltrating tumor as an intermediate signal that is approaching the midline and extending toward the ramus of the mandible. Note that the lesion touches *(arrow)* but does not invade the ramus. The margins of the tumor are indicated by black arrowheads. Although the tongue cannot be distinguished from the palate in these images, in fact it is only resting against the palate. If the tongue were to move, the oral airway would intervene between the tumor and the tongue approximately where the white arrowhead is. **B,** A lower slice shows the submucosal tunneling of the tumor *(T)* along the tonsillar pillar. Note the palatoglossus muscle *(arrowhead)* representing the tonsillar pillar on the opposite side. The intrinsic musculature of the tongue is normal at this level. In this case, there was no extension into the tongue itself. An intact mucosa *(arrow)* covers the tumor. **C,** A more inferior slice shows metastatic lymphadenopathy in the jugulodigastric node *(arrow)* and the submandibular nodes *(arrowhead)*. *S,* Submandibular gland; *SCM,* sternocleidomastoid muscle.

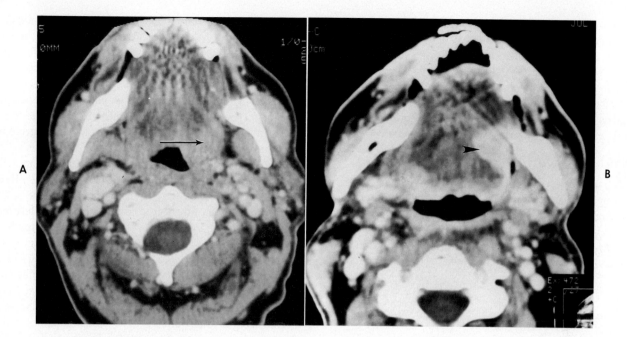

Fig. 7-20 A patient with a large nasopharyngeal tumor (not shown) that infiltrated into the left tonsillar pillar. **A,** An axial scan shows thickening of the tonsillar pillar *(arrow),* but there is no infiltration into the tongue at this time. **B,** One year later, a recurrence is seen in the tongue approximately where the palatoglossus muscle enters. This tumor is thought to have followed the anterior tonsillar pillar into the tongue *(arrowhead).*

Perineural spread

Tumors involving the tongue base have access to the glossopharyngeal nerve and the hypoglossal nerve. Both pass posterolaterally toward the carotid region (see Fig. 7-18). This is the same general area where it is necessary to inspect for direct tumor extension passing inferior to the superior constrictor muscle. The hypoglossal nerve actually passes lateral to the hyoglossus muscle and thus remains outside the constrictors as the nerve passes into the more anterior musculature of the tongue. If tumor is actually using a nerve as the conduit, the lesion obliterates the fat posterior to the carotid, in the sulcus between the artery and the jugular vein.

Tumors involving the lateral oropharyngeal wall or the tongue in the region of the anterior tonsillar pillar can also involve the lingual branch of the second division of the trigeminal nerve. Even though this is unusual, the region along the anterolateral margin of medial pterygoid muscle and the fat planes inferior to the skull base should be inspected for this phenomenon.

Nodes

There is a very high incidence of nodal metastases in patients with oropharyngeal squamous cell carcinoma. The jugulodigastric node and the jugular chain of nodes are the most frequently involved. Tumors of the base of the tongue and pharyngeal wall will also spread to the spinal accessory nodes in the region of the posterior triangle and to the nodes of Rouviere. These latter nodes are particularly important to the radiologist because their location makes them undetectable clinically, and they are not routinely removed at neck dissection.

Hypopharynx

The hypopharynx extends from the level of the hyoid to the lower edge of the cricopharyngeus muscle. Like the oropharynx, the upper posterior wall of the hypopharynx is flat and smooth. The anterior wall and the entire inferior region of the hypopharynx are intimately related to the larynx, and therefore evaluation of tumors arising here entails evaluation of this organ as well as the pharynx itself.

The anterior wall of the hypopharynx includes the mucosa covering the posterior wall of the larynx. The relationship of a tumor to the larynx is one of the most important considerations in deciding whether a patient is a candidate for surgical resection. The aryepiglottic folds curve from the lateral margins of the epiglottis to the interarytenoid notch. Lateral to these folds lie the piriform sinuses, which protrude into the larynx. The mucosa of the piriform sinuses is actually the posterior wall of the paraglottic space of the larynx. (This space is the region between the inner laryngeal mucosa and the outer cartilaginous skeleton of the larynx.)

More inferiorly, the area of the pharynx at the level of the cricoid cartilage is referred to as the *postcricoid region*. The lower limit of this region is the lower edge of the cricopharyngeus muscle. This important landmark is identifiable on CT or MRI scans. The cricopharyngeus muscle stretches from one side of the cricoid to the other and is seen as a linear band at the level of the inferior edge of the cartilage. The esophagus is more circular in appearance.

Direct extension

If hypopharyngeal tumors penetrate through the constrictor ring, the carotid artery and the prevertebral muscles are the most likely structures to be involved, and this can be appreciated on imaging. Fixation of the tumor to the prevertebral musculature and fascia can also be evaluated on a barium swallow (Fig. 7-21). Normally the mucosa slides

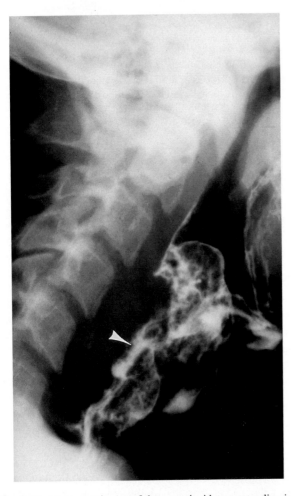

Fig. 7-21 A large carcinoma of the postcricoid area extending into the esophagus. A barium swallow shows a large irregular mass (*arrowhead*) at the level of the larynx. There is definite thickening of the posterior wall. However, on a barium swallow, the entire mass could be seen moving superiorly and inferiorly relative to the spine, indicating that it was not fixed to the prevertebral muscles. The tumor did involve the larynx.

up and down relative to the vertebral bodies, but if a lesion causes fixation, it does not move significantly as the patient swallows. This is often visible on lateral fluoroscopy.

The larynx forms the anterior boundary of the hypopharynx. The relationship of the tumor to the larynx is one of the most important considerations in planning a surgical resection for hypopharyngeal malignancies. Indeed, such a resection often requires a partial or even total laryngectomy to achieve an appropriate margin.

Direct extension anteriorly from the piriform sinus involves the paraglottic space of the larynx (Fig. 7-22). Deep infiltration obliterates the fat that normally exists in the paraglottic region of the upper larynx. Most of the piriform sinus is at the supraglottic level, but the apex extends to the level of the true cord. The lower level of the tumor relative to the true vocal cord should be estimated.[25] The gap between the thyroid cartilage and the arytenoid cartilage becomes an important landmark in this evaluation (see Fig. 7-22). Tumor invading the larynx at the level of the apex of the piriform sinus obliterates the subtle fat planes in this thyroarytenoid gap just above the level of the true cord. Tumor may also widen this gap.

A patient with a lesion high in the hypopharynx and sparing the apex of the piriform sinus may be considered a candidate for a supraglottic partial laryngectomy done in conjunction with resection of the segment of the pharynx.

The postcricoid area is the most inferior part of the hypopharynx. It includes the entire circumference of the hypopharynx, even though only the anterior wall actually abuts the cricoid cartilage. If a lesion in this area is treated surgically, the larynx is almost always removed to obtain a margin.

Determining the inferior extent of the lesion is a key issue in planning a reconstruction of the food passageway. Significant extension below the level of the cricopharyngeus muscle into the esophagus requires a complicated reconstruction using such procedures as a jejunal interposition or a gastric pull-up.

The inferior extent relative to the cricopharyngeus muscle is assessed radiologically, either by imaging or barium swallow (Fig. 7-23).

Perineural and lymphatic spread

Perineural tumor spread is not usually a source of major concern in hypopharyngeal tumors. Although it certainly occurs, it usually has not taken place by the time of diagnosis.

Lymphatic spread is a major consideration in patients with hypopharyngeal tumors, however. There is a very high incidence of metastasis to the jugular nodes from these primaries. Tumor spread can also extend superiorly and reach the nodes of Rouviere at the level of the oropharynx (see Fig. 7-4). Paratracheal nodes are unusual, but this area should nonetheless be examined during CT evaluation.

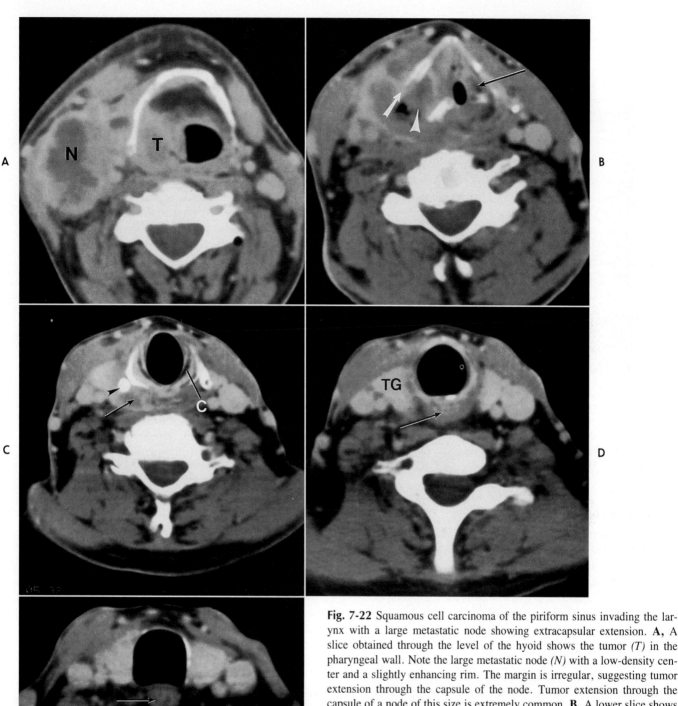

Fig. 7-22 Squamous cell carcinoma of the piriform sinus invading the larynx with a large metastatic node showing extracapsular extension. **A,** A slice obtained through the level of the hyoid shows the tumor *(T)* in the pharyngeal wall. Note the large metastatic node *(N)* with a low-density center and a slightly enhancing rim. The margin is irregular, suggesting tumor extension through the capsule of the node. Tumor extension through the capsule of a node of this size is extremely common. **B,** A lower slice shows the tumor eroding the posterior margin of the thyroid cartilage *(white arrow)* and extending between the thyroid cartilage and arytenoid through the thyroarytenoid gap *(arrowhead)* into the paraglottic fat of the larynx. Normal fat in the paraglottic space on the normal side is shown by the black arrow. **C,** A more inferior slice shows the tumor *(arrow)* following the pharynx to the postcricoid area. Note the level of the cricoid cartilage *(C)* and the lower horn of the thyroid cartilage *(arrowhead)*. **D,** An even more inferior slice shows the curvilinear image of the lower pharynx at the level of the cricopharyngeus muscle *(arrow)*. *TG,* Thyroid gland. **E,** A slightly lower image shows the rounded configuration of the esophagus *(arrow)*.

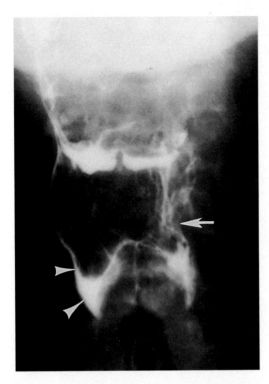

Fig. 7-23 Barium swallow obtained to demonstrate a small lesion of the lateral piriform sinus *(arrow)*. The patient's cheeks are puffed out to show a normal piriform sinus on the right side *(arrowheads)*. A slight irregularity on the opposite side represents a small carcinoma. These areas are fairly easily investigated by endoscopy.

Nasopharynx

The nasopharynx is not part of the alimentary tract and so is only briefly covered in this book. Although the constrictor muscles do not extend to the top of the nasopharynx and the nasopharynx is not required to contract or close to propel the food bolus, it does share many common characteristics with the remainder of the pharynx and so deserves some mention.

The nasopharynx has a roof, posterior wall, and lateral walls. It is open both inferiorly, where it continues into the oropharynx, and anteriorly, where it is continuous with the nasal cavity. The lateral walls are the most complex aspect of the nasopharynx and include the torus tubarius and the orifice of the eustachian tube. The fossa of Rosenmüller is a crevice arching along the upper and posterior margins of the torus tubarius.

Tumors in this area are not quite the same disease process as those found in the remaining pharynx. Most are derived from the squamous epithelium. The World Health Organization (WHO) classification recognizes three types of carcinomas arising from the squamous epithelium: keratinizing, nonkeratinizing, and undifferentiated. The link to tobacco and alcohol use is not as strong as it is to the usual squamous cell carcinoma of the lower pharynx and oral cavity. Adenoid cystic carcinoma can occur in the nasopharynx as well but is not included in the WHO classification, since it does not arise from the squamous epithelium but rather from the minor salivary glands.

Carcinomas of the nasopharynx may present with symptoms relating to obstruction of the eustachian tube, or the first sign of this disease may be an enlarging metastatic node in the posterior triangle of the neck (Fig. 7-24).

Direct extension can carry the tumor into the skull base or laterally into the parapharyngeal soft tissues. Skull base erosion to occurs more laterally than centrally. The key area to inspect on CT or MRI is the foramen lacerum and the petrooccipital fissure. Lateral extension pushes or obliterates the fat planes in the parapharyngeal region. The carotid artery lies immediately outside the posterolateral pharyngeal wall deep to the fossa of Rosenmüller.

Perineural extension has been reported but usually takes place only after significant direct extension. The foramen ovale, pterygopalatine fossa, and jugular foramen should all be carefully examined at the time of imaging.

Nodal metastasis is common. The involvement of posterior triangle nodes is very common and is often the initial indication of disease. The nodes of Rouviere are also frequently involved. In the event of a large tumor, it may be extremely difficult to differentiate between the primary and involved nodes of Rouviere. Finally, the jugular chain must be considered as a potential target of tumor invasion.

RECONSTRUCTION AND POSTOPERATIVE EVALUATION

Once a tumor has been removed, the integrity of the airway and the food passage must be reestablished. The airway is more crucial but usually less of a problem. To accomplish this a tracheostomy is done in the lower neck if the larynx is removed. A partial laryngectomy, which is done with some smaller tumors, maintains a patent airway.

Reconstruction of the food passageway is a more complicated matter, and there are several options available for achieving this.

If the defect is small enough, the surgeon may perform a primary closure by pulling the edges of the remaining tissue together. A skin graft may be used in some areas when significant segments of mucosa are removed.

If the defect is too large to permit primary closure, several options remain. Various flaps, including fat, muscle, and often skin, may be used to provide both bulk and an intact wall for the alimentary tract. These myocutaneous flaps may come from the pectoralis or deltoid region, among others (Fig. 7-25). These flaps retain their original blood supply and are swung up into the surgical field. A flap using the temporalis muscle is often used to provide bulk after resections of the maxilla or upper pharynx (Fig. 7-26).

More recently, advances in the microsurgical reanastomosis of blood vessels have led to the use of free flaps.

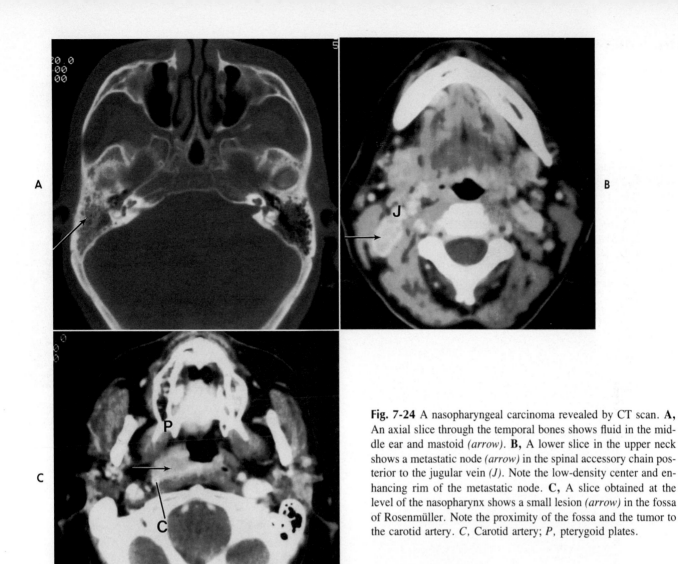

Fig. 7-24 A nasopharyngeal carcinoma revealed by CT scan. A, An axial slice through the temporal bones shows fluid in the middle ear and mastoid *(arrow)*. B, A lower slice in the upper neck shows a metastatic node *(arrow)* in the spinal accessory chain posterior to the jugular vein *(J)*. Note the low-density center and enhancing rim of the metastatic node. C, A slice obtained at the level of the nasopharynx shows a small lesion *(arrow)* in the fossa of Rosenmüller. Note the proximity of the fossa and the tumor to the carotid artery. *C,* Carotid artery; *P,* pterygoid plates.

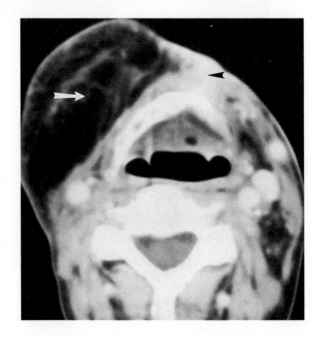

Fig. 7-25 Postoperative CT scan from a patient with a flap reconstruction. The patient had undergone resection of a carcinoma of the tongue that involved the mandible. Most of the flap *(arrow)* has a typical fatty density. However, the soft tissue density *(arrowhead)* just anterior to the hyoid could represent either a tumor or a scar. In this case, there was no tumor.

Fig. 7-26 A flap reconstruction that was done to fill a defect after resection of a nasopharyngeal tumor. The large flap extends across the midline. The linear densities *(small arrowheads)* are characteristic of muscular remnants from the temporalis muscle. The coronoid process *(arrow)* is broken and bent medially to allow positioning of the muscle. The soft tissue density *(large arrowhead)* at the posterior aspect of the flap is a suspicious finding. This most likely represents a portion of the flap, but tumor recurrence could not be excluded because it appears at the edge of the flap.

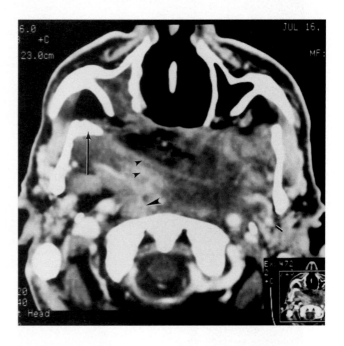

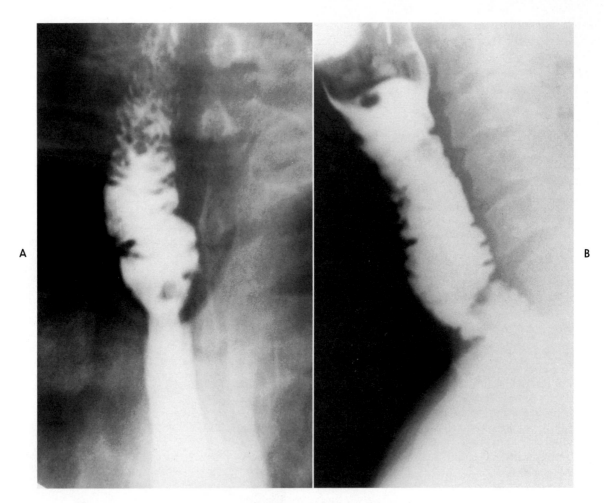

Fig. 7-27 Barium swallow. **A,** Frontal projection. **B,** Lateral projection. The patient had had a laryngopharyngectomy with jejunal interposition. The findings here are normal. The strictures most likely represent the upper and lower anastomoses.

These flaps are removed from the donor area, and their vessels are then reattached to vessels in the neck. This allows surgeons to obtain the most appropriate tissues and removes concern about how far the vascular pedicle can be stretched before the flap loses its viability. Such free flaps can provide both the requisite bulk of muscle and fascia as well as bone for reconstruction purposes, if necessary. Such free flaps include, among others, rectus abdominis flaps and radial forearm flaps, which are often used to reconstruct the oral cavity.

Of special interest in a discussion of the surgical treatment for pharyngeal tumors is jejunal interposition (Fig. 7-27). After the tubular jejunum is harvested from the abdomen, the blood vessels supplying it are reattached to vessels in the neck. The jejunum provides a connection between the remaining pharynx and the esophagus and can be used to reach as high as the soft palate, in which case the jejunum may be opened and spread out to create a wide enough passageway. If there is significant extension of tumor below the cricopharyngeus into the cervical esophagus, then a gastric pull-up must be considered. In this procedure, the stomach is rotated up into the chest, but its original vascular connections are maintained.

Radiologic evaluation after surgery is complicated by the inherent variability of reconstructions. The remaining normal landmarks are often displaced, and the appearance of flaps is inconsistent. Fatty replacement of portions of the flaps often occurs as muscular components atrophy. Usually there are regions of the flap that mimic tumor on either MRI or CT scans. These areas are frequently at the margin of the flap, which unfortunately is also where tumor is likely to recur. At this time, there is no reliable method for distinguishing recurrent or residual tumor from portions of the flap or scar. Familiarity with the type of flap and knowledge of the original position and extent of tumor can both help clarify this matter. The most reliable strategy is to perform an imaging study after about 6 weeks or 2 months, and then to use these examination findings as a baseline for comparison with the findings from future studies. Any increase in soft tissue is regarded as very suspicious.

In the neck, the jejunal interposition can impart a very confusing image because the relocated segment of small bowel can mimic recurrence and may have a very irregular appearance. However, the interposition can be followed superiorly and inferiorly and, if necessary, opacified with contrast to permit differentiation from tumor.

Imaging is the mainstay in the postoperative search for tumor recurrence. Fluoroscopic studies with positive contrast enhancement are less helpful, since scarring and tumor can both cause fixation of the lumen of the food passageway. A Gastrografin (meglumine diatrizoate) swallow is used in the early postoperative period to search for leaks at the site of surgical closure or anastomosis.

SUMMARY

Imaging is targeted at detecting deeper extensions that cannot be found by direct visualization using modern endoscopy. The diagnosis is almost always known before radiologic examination is performed. The radiologist must know the regional anatomy and the potential pathways of tumor spread so that imaging can be put to best use in helping plan therapy. The radiologist must particularly look for direct encroachment (including submucosal spread), bone involvement, perineural extension, and nodal metastasis.

REFERENCES

1. Barnes L, ed: *Surgical pathology of the head and neck,* vols 1 and 2, New York, 1985, Marcel Dekker.
2. Myers EN, Suen JY, ed: *Cancer of the head and neck,* ed 2, New York, 1989, Churchill Livingstone.
3. Beahrs OH, Henson DE, Hutter RVP, Kennedy BJ, eds: *American Joint Committee on Cancer: manual for staging of cancer,* ed 4, Philadelphia, 1988, JB Lippincott.
4. Mancuso AA, Hanafee WN: Larynx and hypopharynx. In Mancuso AA, Hanafee WN, eds: *Computed tomography and magnetic resonance imaging of the head and neck,* ed 2, Baltimore, 1985, Williams & Wilkins.
5. Dillon WP: The pharynx and oral cavity. In Som PM, Bergeron RT, eds: *Head and neck imaging,* ed 2, St Louis, 1991, Mosby–Year Book.
6. Lufkin RB, Wortham DG, Dietrich RB et al: Tongue and oropharynx: findings on MR imaging, *Radiology* 161:69, 1986.
7. Kassel EE, Keller MA, Kucharczyk W: MRI of the floor of mouth, tongue and orohypopharynx, *Radiol Clini North Am* 27:331, 1989.
8. Hoover LA, Wortham DG, Lufkin RB, Hanafee WN: Magnetic resonance imaging of the larynx and tongue base: clinical applications, *Otolaryngol Head Neck Surg* 97:245, 1987.
9. Larsson SG: Computed tomography and magnetic resonance imaging of the base of the tongue and the floor of the mouth, *Acta Radiol Suppl (Stockh)* 372:109, 1988.
10. Parker GD, Harnsberger HR, Jacobs JM: The pharyngeal mucosal space, *Semin Ultrasound CT MR* 11:460, 1990.
11. Silver AJ, Mawad ME, Hilal SK, Sane P, Ganti SR: Computed tomography of the nasopharynx and related spaces, *Radiology* 147:733, 1983.
12. Vogl T, Bruning R, Grevers G, Mees K, Bauer M et al: MR imaging of the oropharynx and tongue: comparison of plain and Gd-DTPA studies, *J Comput Assist Tomogr* 12:427, 1988.
13. Barnes L, Johnson JT: Pathologic and clinical considerations in the evaluation of major head and neck specimens resected for cancer. In Sommers SC, Rosen PP, Fechner RE, eds: *Pathology annual,* part 1/vol 21, Norwalk, CT, 1986, Appleton-Lange.
14. Mancuso AA, Hanafee WN: Elusive head and neck cancer beneath intact mucosa, *Laryngoscope* 93:133, 1983.
15. Laine FJ, Braun IF, Jensen ME, Nadel L, Som PM: Perineural tumor extension through the foramen ovale: evaluation with MR imaging, *Radiology* 174:65, 1990.
16. Curtin HD, Williams R, Johnson JT: CT of perineural tumor extension: pterygopalatine fossa, *AJNR* 5:731, 1984.
17. Kolin ES, Castro D, Jabour BA, Lufkin RB, Hanafee WN: Perineural extension of squamous cell carcinoma, *Ann Otol Rhinol Laryngol* 100:1032, 1991 (imaging case study of the month).
18. van den Brekel MWM, Stel HV, Castelijns JA et al: Cervical lymph node metastasis: assessment of radiologic criteria, *Radiology* 177:379, 1990.

19. Mancuso AA et al: Computed tomography of cervical and retropharyngeal lymph nodes: normal anatomy, variants of normal, and applications in staging head and neck cancer: I. Normal anatomy, *Radiology* 148:709, 1983.

20. Mancuso AA et al: Computed tomography of cervical and retropharyngeal lymph nodes: normal anatomy, variants of normal, and applications in staging head and neck cancer: II. Pathology, *Radiology* 148:714, 1983.

21. Som PM: Lymph nodes of the neck, *Radiology* 165:596, 1987.

22. Close LG, Merkel M, Burns DK, Schaefer SD: Computed tomography in the assessment of mandibular invasion by intraoral carcinoma, *Ann Otol Rhinol Laryngol* 95:383, 1986.

23. Bahadur S: Mandibular involvement in oral cancer, *J Laryngol Otol* 104:968, 1990.

24. Curtin HD: Imaging of the larynx: current concepts, *Radiology* 173:1, 1989.

25. Aspestrand F, Kolbenstvedt A, Boysen M: Staging of carcinoma of the palatine tonsils by computed tomography, *J Comput Assist Tomogr* 12:434, 1988.

8 A Multidisciplinary Approach to the Patient with Swallowing Impairment

BRONWYN JONES
MARTIN W. DONNER

Dysphagia is a symptom, not a disease, and may result from many causes. The true number of dysphagic patients in the general population is unknown, but it seems to be a very common complaint. At our institution, over 1000 swallowing cineradiographic (videofluoroscopic) studies are performed annually, and the numbers increase each year. The incidence of dysphagia in the hospital population ranges from 12% to 15% in general hospitals to greater than 50% in nursing homes.[1] Dysphagia is a common symptom in the elderly, and, as the percentage of the elderly in the population grows, it is bound to increase in incidence. Resuscitation, tracheotomy, and head and neck surgery for the treatment of cancer or benign disease are also contributory causes of dysphagia. Choking is the fourth most common cause of death in the home; in one estimate, 8000 to 10,000 choking deaths occur annually in the United States.

Eating and drinking involve the transport of food or liquid from the mouth (most often evaluated by the dentist or oral surgeon), through the pharynx (the territory of the otolaryngologist or head and neck surgeon and with the advent of more accurate diagnostic modalities, the gastroenterologist), through the esophagus (the gastroenterologist), and into the stomach. Each of these specialists, to name just a few, concentrates their close attention on a specific area of the "swallowing chain." Thus the input of several specialists may be needed before a diagnosis can be reached in a dysphagic patient. It has been estimated that an average of three consultants are needed in the evaluation of the dysphagic patient.[2]

Each of the organs, from the mouth to the stomach, may be involved by a wide spectrum of disorders that affect either motility or structure. The resulting symptoms, however, are frequently nonspecific, and the information given by the patient about the site of the sensation may be misleading. Indeed, because the swallowing process can compensate for deficiencies to a certain extent, the patient may not even be symptomatic, although early signs of decompensation will be visible on videofluorographic studies. Symptoms may be referred or unusual, such as drooling, a nasal voice, cough, or hoarseness, rather than a true dysphagia or a problem with "food sticking," so it may be unclear that a swallowing impairment is the source of the problem.

Both the patient and the physician are therefore often unable to determine which medical specialty is the appropriate one for dealing with the patient's complaints. As a result, the patient may first be seen by a specialist whose expertise turns out to be inappropriate for the clinical question, thus delaying diagnosis and therapy.

In some cases, symptoms of dysphagia may go unexplained, and the patient may be referred to a psychiatrist with a diagnosis of "globus hystericus" or "psychogenic dysphagia," especially if there is a strong psychologic overlay or intense anxiety as a consequence of choking spells or the need for Heimlich maneuvers. Many patients with swallowing problems can become obsessed with their symptoms and many overreact, and, as a result, the psychologic aspects of their problem may dominate the clinical picture.

The structures related to swallowing are thus located at the intersection of various medical and surgical disciplines. To try to address this situation, a multidisciplinary Swallowing Center has been formed at The Johns Hopkins Medical Institution and represents a collaborative approach to the evaluation of the dysphagic patient and the diseases that can cause this symptom.[3] Central specialties include radiology, gastroenterology, neurology, otolaryngology, rehabilitation medicine, speech pathology, psychiatry, and thoracic surgery. Other specialists, such as those in pulmonary medicine, dentistry, rheumatology, and hematology, are available as needed (Fig. 8-1).

The prime objective of the physicians at the center is to evaluate patients together from the outset, to employ the appropriate diagnostic procedures, and to jointly decide the appropriate management after consultation. Emphasis is placed on close communication between the physicians from the different specialties and between the physicians and other allied health professionals. This is a "center without walls" in a conceptual but not a physical sense.

Central to the efficient functioning of this multidisciplinary group is the Swallowing Center coordinator, a lay person who has some medical knowledge. When a referring physician or patient contacts this coordinator, all previously accumulated documents are requested. This information forms the basis for the triage that is performed and the means by which the primary physician is chosen (Fig.

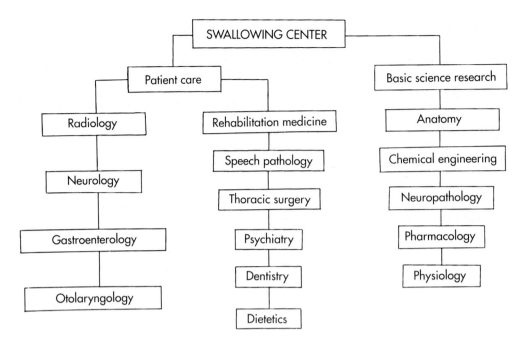

Fig. 8-1 Interdisciplinary organization of the Swallowing Center.
From Ravich WJ, Donner MW, Kashima H et al: *Gastrointest Radiol* 10:255, 1985.

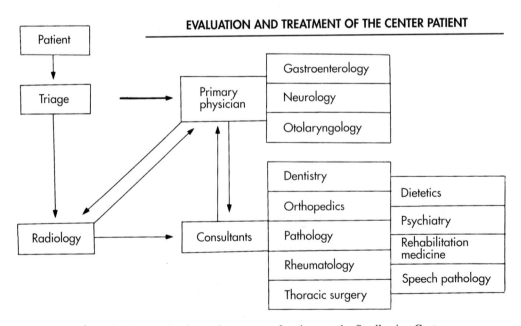

Fig. 8-2 Triage evaluation and treatment of patients at the Swallowing Center.
From Ravich WJ, Donner MW, Kashima H et al: *Gastrointest Radiol* 10:255, 1985.

8-2). The information is reviewed by the clinical director (currently a gastroenterologist) and the coordinator, and triage performed, depending on the diagnosis suggested by the available information. Ultimately the primary physician originally selected may turn out to be inappropriate and the patient may be transferred to a different primary physician as more information becomes available from the clinical or radiologic examination.

Following an initial extensive interview and examination by the primary physician, the patient is sent for an imaging study, usually cinefluorography or videofluorography, to assess motility, and double-contrast films to evaluate mucosal detail. This study and the pertinent clinical data are reviewed at the next weekly joint clinical conference attended by the members of the group. At this meeting, further consultation is arranged as soon as possible, usually within 48 hours. The results of this consultation are then reviewed at the next weekly clinical conference.

The weekly case review conference is the most important forum for communication in the group; at this meeting the clinicians discuss the pertinent clinical, radiologic, and laboratory data for each patient. The imaging studies, which are performed and interpreted by a Swallowing Center radiologist, are reviewed again by the entire group, and these new findings are then correlated with the previous clinical information. On the basis of the conclusions of this review, additional consultations or diagnostic procedures are recommended. If indicated, an additional videofluorographic examination may be performed to assess the effect of other factors on swallowing, such as variations in food consistency, bolus size, or head and neck position. Finally, therapeutic options are discussed. The additional diagnostic or therapeutic procedures are then scheduled by the coordinator, preferably within the same week. The patient's case is then reviewed again at the next weekly meeting. The aim is to complete the diagnostic workup and implement ther-apy expeditiously, ideally within 1 week, especially for patients from outside the immediate metropolitan area.

The emphasis of the program is on close communication and on pooling the expertise of several specialties, rather than having the patient interact independently with several different clinicians. Even among those specialists familiar with the swallowing mechanism, awareness of the diagnostic and therapeutic techniques available in other subspecialties may be quite limited. In the Swallowing Center approach, the specialists learn from each other. A physician dealing with swallowing abnormalities should be knowledgeable about the possibilities and limitations of the "adjacent" specialties.

In conclusion, because a separate subspecialty dedicated to swallowing disorders alone does not yet exist, the multidisciplinary Swallowing Center is an attempt to merge the skills and expertise of many clinical and basic science subspecialties in the diagnosis and management of the patient with swallowing difficulties. This approach has also pinpointed a number of areas that require research, such as the effects of drugs and medications on oral, pharyngeal, and esophageal function, and the need to characterize the rheologic characteristics of foods and liquids. Such work may ultimately find a practical application in the management of patients with swallowing problems. It is our hope that more multidisciplinary centers with an interest in dysphagia will be created, as the resulting exchange of clinical and basic research information will only help to expand the collective knowledge concerning swallowing and swallowing impairment.

REFERENCES

1. Groher ME, Bukatman R: The prevalence of swallowing disorders in two teaching hospitals, *Dysphagia* 1:3, 1986.
2. Donner MW: Personal communication.
3. Ravich WJ, Donner MW, Kashima H et al: The Swallowing Center: concepts and procedures, *Gastrointest Radiol* 10:255, 1985.

PART IV

ESOPHAGUS

9 Normal Anatomy and Techniques of Examination of the Esophagus: Fluoroscopy, CT, MRI, and Scintigraphy

OLLE EKBERG

NORMAL ANATOMY
General radiographic anatomy of the esophagus

The esophagus lies mainly in the posterior mediastinum and is 18 to 22 cm long in adults. Its upper end is at the level of C5-6 where the upper esophageal sphincter forms a 2.5-cm-long high-pressure zone that separates the pharynx from the esophagus. The cricopharyngeus muscle forms a sling, which is attached to the laminae of the cricoid cartilage that loops around the posterior border of the cricopharyngeal junction. In the resting state the sphincter is tonically contracted and closed.

The body of the esophagus enters the thorax behind the trachea, passes a little to the right behind the carina, and then back to the midline as it passes behind the left atrium and ventricle. Finally, it curves to the left and anteriorly to slip between the aorta and left ventricle and pass through the crus of the right diaphragm into the abdomen, with the vagal nerves closely applied to its anterior and posterior walls. On the left side, the aorta is related to the aortic arch, subclavian artery, thoracic duct, and left recurrent laryngeal nerve. Inferiorly on the left the esophagus is enveloped by two layers of pleura, the anterior and posterior left mediastinal pleura, that meet on its lateral border and pass laterally as the inferior pulmonary ligament, which has a free lower margin. This anatomy is important from a clinical perspective in that esophageal rupture usually occurs to the left and escaping air and fluid pass directly into the inferior pulmonary ligament between the leaves of the pleura as a contained air collection. This may be visible early on chest radiographs. Later, further spread usually takes place through rupture into the pleura or infiltration up into the mediastinum, or both.

Inferiorly the esophagus passes anteriorly and to the left for 1 to 2 cm as it passes between the diaphragmatic crura

into the abdomen and enters the stomach at an acute angle. The gastroesophageal junction shows considerable physiologic movement, moving into the hiatus on swallowing and inspiration, and may move above the diaphragm on deep inspiration in normal individuals. The lowest 2 to 3 cm of the esophagus functions as another sphincter, the lower esophageal sphincter, which is a second esophageal high-pressure zone that extends up from the gastroesophageal junction just into the thorax. It corresponds to the slightly more distensible portion of the lower esophagus called the *vestibule* or *phrenic ampulla*. Muscle spasm occasionally occurs at the upper end of the sphincter and is called an *A ring,* to distinguish it from the B ring, or Schatzki ring, which is sometimes seen at the lower end of the sphincter at the gastroesophageal junction. The gastroesophageal junction is also marked by the oblique muscle fibers of the stomach, which hook over the junction and pass down the anterior and posterior walls of the gastric body. These muscles are probably responsible for the acute angle that forms between the stomach and esophagus in patients without a hiatus hernia (Fig. 9-1). The mucosal junction between the stomach and esophagus is very close to the gastroesophageal junction, although mucosa can slide over deeper tissues to a small extent. The Z line of the mucosal junction can be seen only fluoroscopically in the rare patient in whom barium coating of the esophageal mucosa is enhanced by esophagitis. However, its position can often be inferred from the point where the gastric rugal folds cease (Fig. 9-2).

The lower aspect of the closed sphincter can be seen en face through the gas-filled stomach on double-contrast radiographs when the patient is turned on the right side. Herlinger et al.[1] have described four different normal appearances that reflect the degree of tightness or laxness of the sphincter (Fig. 9-3).

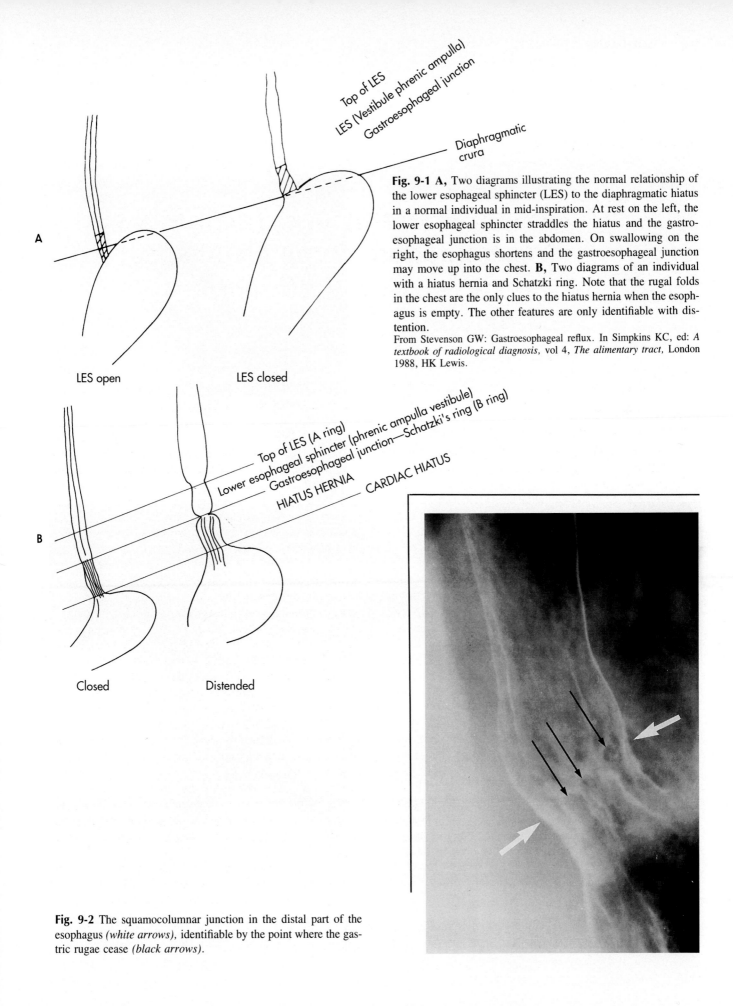

Top of LES
LES (Vestibule phrenic ampulla)
Gastroesophageal junction

Diaphragmatic crura

A

LES open   LES closed

Fig. 9-1 A, Two diagrams illustrating the normal relationship of the lower esophageal sphincter (LES) to the diaphragmatic hiatus in a normal individual in mid-inspiration. At rest on the left, the lower esophageal sphincter straddles the hiatus and the gastroesophageal junction is in the abdomen. On swallowing on the right, the esophagus shortens and the gastroesophageal junction may move up into the chest. **B,** Two diagrams of an individual with a hiatus hernia and Schatzki ring. Note that the rugal folds in the chest are the only clues to the hiatus hernia when the esophagus is empty. The other features are only identifiable with distention.
From Stevenson GW: Gastroesophageal reflux. In Simpkins KC, ed: *A textbook of radiological diagnosis,* vol 4, *The alimentary tract,* London 1988, HK Lewis.

Top of LES (A ring)
Lower esophageal sphincter (phrenic ampulla vestibule)
Gastroesophageal junction—Schatzki's ring (B ring)
HIATUS HERNIA   CARDIAC HIATUS

B

Closed   Distended

Fig. 9-2 The squamocolumnar junction in the distal part of the esophagus *(white arrows),* identifiable by the point where the gastric rugae cease *(black arrows).*

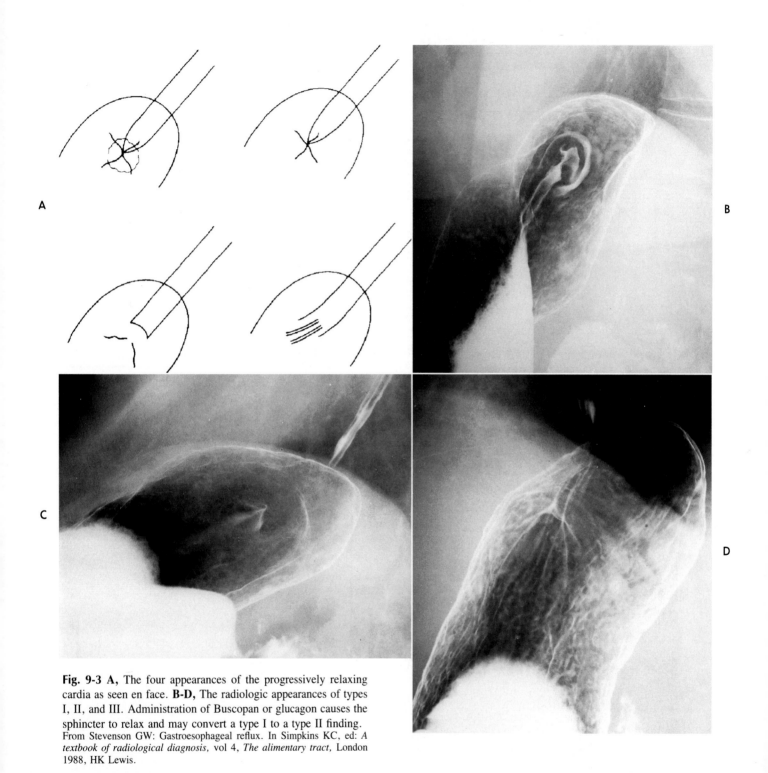

Fig. 9-3 A, The four appearances of the progressively relaxing cardia as seen en face. **B-D,** The radiologic appearances of types I, II, and III. Administration of Buscopan or glucagon causes the sphincter to relax and may convert a type I to a type II finding.
From Stevenson GW: Gastroesophageal reflux. In Simpkins KC, ed: *A textbook of radiological diagnosis,* vol 4, *The alimentary tract,* London 1988, HK Lewis.

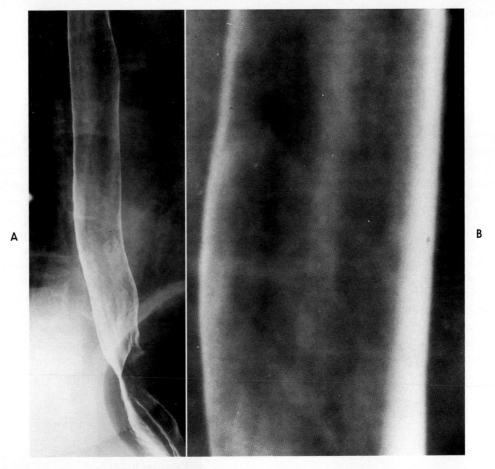

Fig. 9-4 A, Double-contrast study of the esophagus. **B,** Detail from **A** showing the smooth featureless surface.

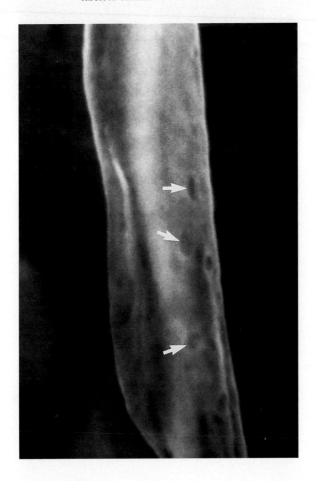

Fig. 9-5 Glycogenic acanthosis of the esophagus, seen as localized millimeter-sized plaquelike nodules *(arrows)*.

The squamous mucosa of the esophagus is smooth and featureless on double-contrast radiographs (Fig. 9-4), and, when distended, the esophageal lumen usually measures between 2 and 3 cm in diameter on radiographs. In the elderly, localized nodules may be seen that represent an accumulation of glycogen in squamous epithelial cells. This is a normal finding and is called *glycogenic acanthosis* [2] (Fig. 9-5). Endoscopically these nodules appear as pale grayish plaques and are common. They are less often seen radiographically, but can occasionally be dramatic and profuse. They may be confused with monilial colonies.

On films taken with the esophagus distended in the right anterior oblique projection, there may be indentations visible on the esophagus. There are usually three of them, and they are due to the aortic arch, left mainstem bronchus (Fig. 9-6), and left ventricle, which is indistinguishable from the left atrium. Patients with heart disease or atheroma frequently exhibit indentations that are due to the left atrium or a dilated descending aorta (Fig. 9-7).

When the esophagus is collapsed so that mucosal relief films can be obtained, the mucosal folds of the esophagus are thin (often between 1 and 2 mm in width) and run parallel to the long axis of the esophagus (Fig. 9-8). Sometimes, transient contractions of the muscularis mucosa can be seen as thin regular folds that run perpendicular to the long axis of the esophagus (Fig. 9-9), and this has been termed the *feline esophagus* [3] because the mucosa of the cat esophagus normally has such transverse striations.

Below the muscularis mucosa are two muscular layers, an inner circular and an outer longitudinal layer. The transition zone from the striated muscle in the upper esophagus and the smooth muscle of the lower esophagus is variable, with the upper 5% exclusively striated and the lower 60% exclusively smooth. There is great individual variation, but that portion of the transition zone that contains mixed elements constitutes an average of 30% of the total length. [4] The esophagus has no serosa but only an outer layer of thin connective tissue separating it from the mediastinal fat and other mediastinal structures.

Venous drainage of the esophagus from the cervical, midthoracic, and abdominal esophagus flows into the inferior thyroid, azygos, and left gastric veins, respectively.

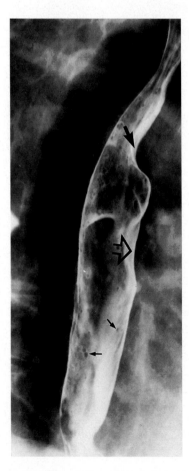

Fig. 9-6 Impression made on the esophagus from the left created by the aortic arch *(arrow)* and the left mainstem bronchus *(open arrow)*. There are also multiple small air bubbles *(small arrows)* caused by the slow release of gas from the effervescent agent.

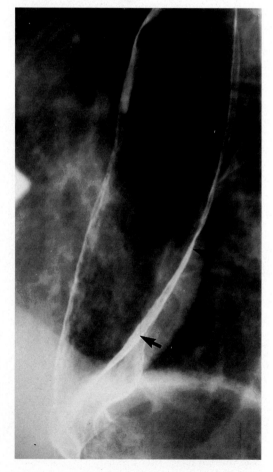

Fig. 9-7 Impression *(arrows)* on the distal part of the esophagus due to a dilated thoracic aorta.

There is also a double system of longitudinal esophageal veins, the submucosal and the paraesophageal, which communicate every 2 to 3 cm by means of perforating veins. These perforators can be identified on endoscopic Doppler ultrasound in patients with portal hypertension by the appearance of blood flowing to the submucosal veins on expiration and out into the paraesophageal veins on inspiration. This double system and its perforators form an anastomosis between the systemic (azygos) and the portal (left gastric) system.

The lymphatic drainage of the esophagus is also a three-way phenomenon. The upper esophagus drains to the cervical supraclavicular nodes, the middle third to the tracheobronchial nodes, and the lower third to the celiac plexus and nearby gastric lymph nodes.

Aspects of cross-sectional anatomy

The thickness of the esophageal wall should be 5 mm or less, and is delineated by the presence of air or contrast agent in the lumen, and, externally, by the presence of periesophageal fat and the airways. However, there is often no fat plane between the posterior wall of the trachea and the esophagus.[5] In the neck the esophagus lies somewhat to the left of the midline and anterior to the spine (Figs. 9-10, *A* and 9-11, *A-C*) and posterior to the trachea. In the right posterior mediastinum the right lung and the esophagus are in direct contact, and this forms an intrusion, called the *azygoesophageal recess,* that extends all the way from the azygos arch to the diaphragm.[6] The edge of this recess is either curved and convex to the left or occasionally straight, but it is never convex to the right.[7] On the left side the esophagus is adjacent to the descending aorta.

At the level of the carina, the esophagus is immediately posterior, often with no visible intervening fat plane, and the thoracic duct, the azygos vein, and the hemiazygos veins and right intercostal arteries are located between the midesophagus and the spine (see Fig. 9-10, *D*). The esophagus is also adjacent to the left atrium (see Fig. 9-10, *E*). The cranial extent of the fissure of the gastrohepatic ligament serves as a landmark for the level of the gastroesophageal junction,[8] but the anatomy of this area is difficult to discern with patients supine because there is frequently an apparent

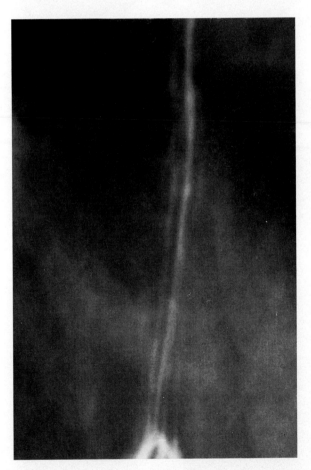

Fig. 9-8 Mucosal relief pattern of the collapsed esophagus. The mucosa is coated with barium sulfate, and thin longitudinal mucosal folds are visualized.

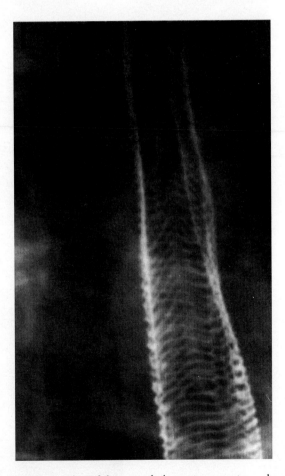

Fig. 9-9 Contraction of the muscularis mucosae creates a characteristic pattern in the esophagus with transverse folds.

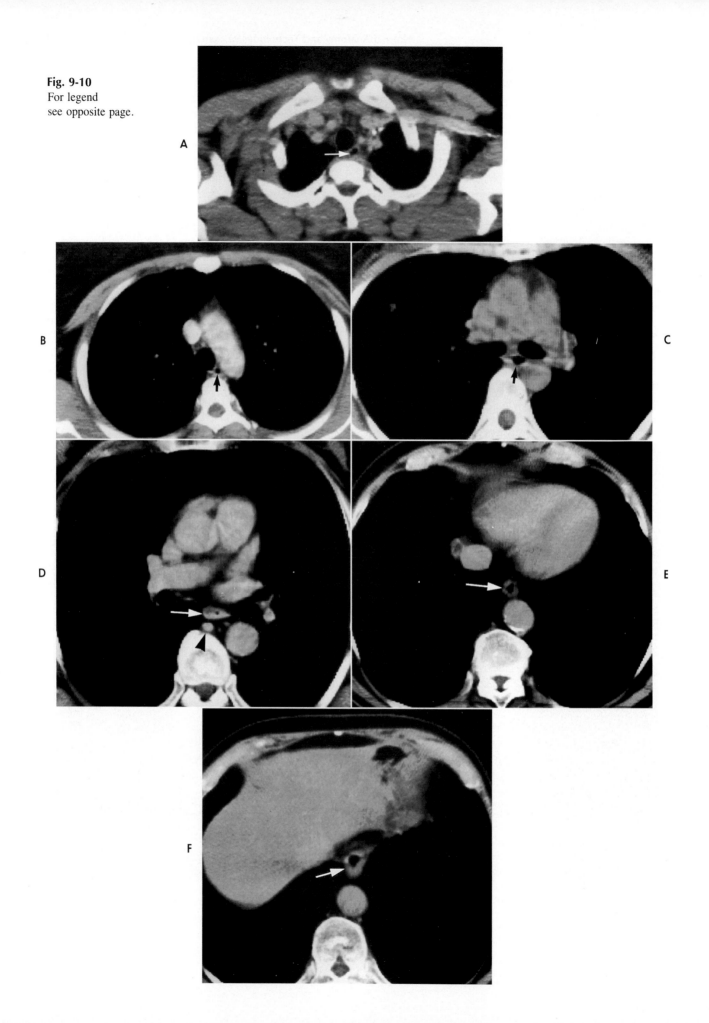

Fig. 9-10
For legend
see opposite page.

Fig. 9-10 A, CT scan of the mediastinum showing the air-filled esophagus *(arrow)* in the neck anterior to the spine. **B** and **C,** The relationship between the esophagus *(arrow)*, aortic arch, trachea, and mainstem bronchi is seen. **D,** The esophagus's *(arrow)* relationship to the azygos vein *(arrowhead)* is seen. **E,** The esophagus *(arrow)* is posterior to the left atrium. **F,** In the gastroesophageal junction, the esophagus is seen to have a thickened wall.

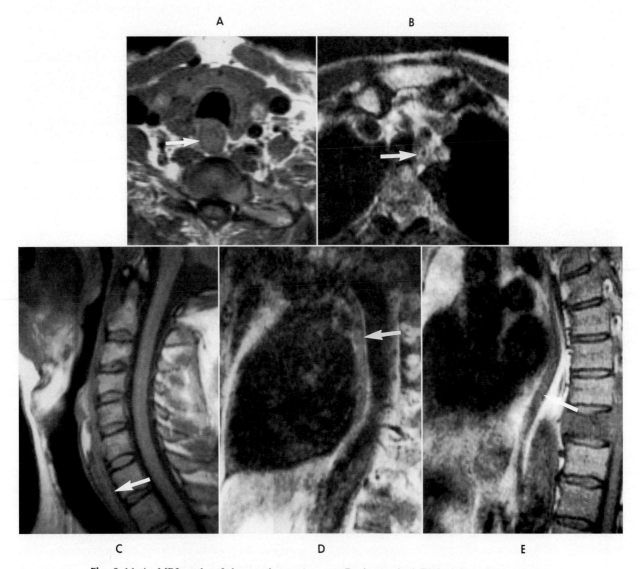

Fig. 9-11 A, MRI study of the esophagus *(arrow)*. During sagittal T1 imaging, the esophagus *(arrow)* can be visualized with a medium signal intensity anterior to the spine. **B,** On T2 images the high signal intensity of the mucosa and submucosa is often seen. **C,** T1 sagittal imaging shows the cervical and upper thoracic part of the esophagus *(arrow)* exhibiting a medium signal intensity. **D,** The upper and mid parts of the esophagus *(arrow)* are visualized with a medium signal intensity on T1 images. **E,** The mid and distal parts of the esophagus *(arrow)*, as well as the gastroesophageal junction, are visualized in T1 images.

thickening or a pseudotumor effect stemming from a combination of incomplete fundal distention and the oblique course of the gastroesophageal junction in relation to the transverse plane of the CT sections (see Fig. 9-10, *F*). Ultrasound is helpful for evaluating the gastroesophageal junction, as the thickness of the wall can be seen more readily.

On MRI scans the normal esophagus exhibits a signal intensity similar to that of the muscle in the chest wall on both T1 and T2 images. In most areas the periesophageal fat is hyperintense, but, as with CT, no fat plane is visible between the esophagus and trachea, and in most patients there is at least partial effacement of the hyperintense fat plane between the esophagus and the aorta.[9] The ability to acquire and display sagittal sections is potentially a very helpful feature for esophageal assessment (see Fig. 9-11, *D* and *E*).

TECHNIQUE OF EXAMINATION
Fluoroscopy
Indications for examination

The indications for an esophageal examination include heartburn, dysphagia, odynophagia (pain on swallowing), chest pain, globus (a feeling of a lump in the throat, related or unrelated to swallowing), pretreatment studies, follow-up studies after therapy. It may also be an incidental investigation as part of an overall evaluation of the upper gastrointestinal tract focused on some other problem. The examination may disclose abnormalities that may be either structural or functional, but are frequently both.

With such a variety of considerations, it is clear that different techniques are required, and some of the techniques that may be helpful under various circumstances are outlined here.

It is becoming routine for gastroenterologists to use endoscopy as the initial procedure in patients with a clinically suspected structural abnormality of the esophagus. However, it is not possible to assess esophageal function endoscopically. In addition, a preliminary radiologic examination permits any subsequent endoscopy to be focused and planned; for example, a pediatric endoscope or dilatation may be needed. For investigating the common symptom of heartburn, either endoscopy or barium radiology is a reasonable initial examination. There is no evidence indicating that either method is superior for the management of most patients with heartburn, although endoscopy is required for dilatation, for biopsy in immunocompromised patients, and for confirmation of the diagnosis and histologic sampling of Barrett's esophagus. For patients with globus, chest pain, or dysphagia, however, barium radiology remains a more useful initial examination. More complex problems may require 24-hour pH monitoring, manometry, or cross-sectional imaging. For most patients with heartburn, the less expensive radiologic study can provide all the information needed for patient management.

Plain film

A plain film is not useful for examining the esophagus, but serendipitously may show fluid levels in the esophagus in a patient with achalasia. In major esophageal dilatation, the esophagus expands to the right, producing a mediastinal edge that runs from the neck to the diaphragm with a single indentation produced by the azygos vein, a finding that can only represent the esophagus. The lateral film can also reveal the thin posterior tracheal stripe, which is a useful finding because thickening of the stripe is occasionally a diagnostic clue to the presence of carcinoma.[10] However, this is neither a sensitive nor specific sign, in that it is also seen in some normal patients when the esophagus is collapsed and in some patients with bronchogenic carcinoma.

The routine multiphasic examination

It remains something of an art to produce a high-quality examination of the esophagus. Each radiologist develops a personal sequence of maneuvers to produce a final hardcopy record. However, the routine examination should include a brief observation of ingestion, swallowing, and esophageal peristalsis, and this should yield films of the whole esophagus in mucosal relief, using both single- and double-contrast modes, as well as films of the gastroesophageal junction. Specific symptoms require additional attention to some particular aspects. Most radiologists start with a brief fluoroscopic examination of the chest.

The double-contrast films are taken at either the beginning or end of the examination with the patient erect. The examination is explained to the patient, who is told to try to avoid burping. The patient is then placed in the left posterior oblique position. A high-density, low-viscosity barium (240% weight per volume [w/v]) is used, and a cup with approximately 70 to 100 ml of barium is given to the patient to hold in the left hand. If the patient has dysphagia, a small first swallow of barium should be observed to confirm that the esophagus can empty. Otherwise, the patient is given the effervescent granules in a cup in the right hand. These may be swallowed dry and then washed down with barium or a little water, or they may be added to 10 ml of water containing antifoam and then swallowed immediately as they start to fizz. The patient then gulps down the barium as fast as possible. This rapid swallowing opens up the lower esophageal sphincter, especially in patients who already have decreased tone, and promotes the reflux of gas up from the stomach to further distend the esophagus. Films are taken rapidly during this swallow, concentrating on timing that yields optimal images rather than lingering to diagnose fluoroscopically. This method usually produces adequate double-contrast images.

Alternatively, after swallowing the effervescent granules, the patient can swallow a single large mouthful of barium and the radiologist then tries to time the exposure for optimal distention. One way to facilitate this is by counting.

The radiologist tells the patient to swallow and then counts. The time delay is noted and the film is exposed on the appropriate count on the next swallow.[11] Rapid-sequence filming is the most certain method, but with a higher radiation dose, and should be used only for settling a specific point rather than as a routine.

For the hard-copy record, three-on-one films with a 17 × 14 inch (42.5 × 35 cm) format are ideal, but many radiologists have only smaller formats. There should be at least one film of each of the three thirds of the esophagus. A 12 × 10 inch (30 × 25 cm) two-on-one format can yield reasonable images, but it is difficult to produce a good hard copy of the whole esophagus using a 9 × 9 inch (22.5 × 22.5 cm) format. In this situation the radiologist may do better to observe the first swallow very carefully and then obtain a hard copy on a second swallow, concentrating on any area of suspicion.

After the double-contrast films have been obtained, the examining table is brought horizontal while the patient continues swallowing (dry swallows if necessary) to prevent eructation. This continuing esophageal peristalsis keeps the carbon dioxide mainly in the stomach.

The patient is given another cup of barium and a straw and is told to make single swallows while esophageal peristalsis is observed. Single-contrast films are obtained. Routinely at least three such swallows should be observed. It is important for the patient to swallow only once for each bolus, as a second swallow will abolish the ongoing esophageal peristalsis and convey a false impression of dysmotility. Having patients open their mouth immediately after a swallow may help in those who habitually double swallow. For the evaluation of peristalsis, it is important to observe the tail of the barium column. This can often provide a high enough view that a second, unwanted, swallow can be detected.

This functional part of the study may be done with the patient either supine-oblique or prone-oblique. In the prone-oblique position, gastric emptying occurs, and this causes duodenal and jejunal contrast to spoil the subsequent gastric films; but, in the supine-oblique position, the views of the gastroesophageal junction are suboptimal. If the supine position is chosen, it may be prudent to check the gastroesophageal junction later with the patient in the prone-oblique position. Most authors recommend use of the prone-oblique position, as it displays the gastroesophageal junction to much better advantage than the supine position (Fig. 9-12). The best view of the distended gastroesophageal junction later is obtained by having the patient take and sustain a deep inspiration as a large bolus of liquid starts to pass through the lower esophagus. After peristalsis has been assessed, the patient is encouraged to rapidly drink dilute barium (40% w/v) so that full-column single-contrast films can be obtained with the esophagus maximally distended (Fig. 9-13). If a gastric examination is to be performed, these full-column films obtained with dilute barium should be deferred until after the double-contrast gastric films have been taken. The compression views of the gastric antrum are more satisfactory after the dilute barium has been swallowed, that is, at the end of the examination.

Finally, at least one film should be obtained with the esophagus collapsed. This can show the fine mucosal relief pattern of the thin longitudinal folds (see Fig. 9-8), especially in the lower esophagus, as this is a very sensitive film for detecting both esophagitis and varices.

Artifacts

A number of artifacts can appear during a fluoroscopic examination of the esophagus.[12] Mucus strands are often coated with barium (Fig. 9-14, *A*). In patients with severe dilatation, disintegration and flaking of barium is sometimes seen, although this is less frequent with the modern barium preparations. Asymmetric flow with poor coating on one side is common (Fig. 9-14, *B*), mainly at the beginning of the study. Any barium spilled onto the patient's gown may project over the esophagus and simulate pathology. Gas bubbles are a frequent artifact, and some effervescent granules can adhere to the mucosa and dissolve slowly, thereby producing a localized 1- to 2-mm filling defect that is usually not as smoothly circular as gas bubbles (see Fig. 9-6). When partly collapsed, a rather coarse mucosal pattern may be seen (Fig. 9-14, *E* and *F*).

Additional techniques
SOLID BOLUS

The results of an examination using liquid barium may be normal in a patient with dysphagia, but not reliably exclude significant strictures, especially if good esophageal distention is not achieved. Whenever a routine swallow is negative in patients with dysphagia, a solid bolus should be administered as well. A barium tablet (Wolf tablet, diameter, 13 mm) is ideal and can be swallowed with water.[13] Alternatively, a non-radiopaque tablet can be swallowed with barium. If tablets stick to the wall of the esophagus, the patient should make several swallows of liquid to differentiate between adherence and obstruction.

Besides revealing strictures overlooked with the liquid swallow, the tablet can provoke bolus-specific symptoms. This method also allows assessment of the size of a stricture and occasionally precipitates bolus-specific dysmotility.

Other practitioners have recommended the use of a marshmallow, whole or cut into three equal parts[14-16] (see Fig. 9-12). These are either swallowed with the barium or can be impregnated with the barium.[17] Bread has also been recommended for this purpose,[18,19] but it does not dissolve as rapidly as a marshmallow.

ADDITIONAL GAS

Some patients have difficulty gulping barium, and a double-contrast examination may thus not be possible. The

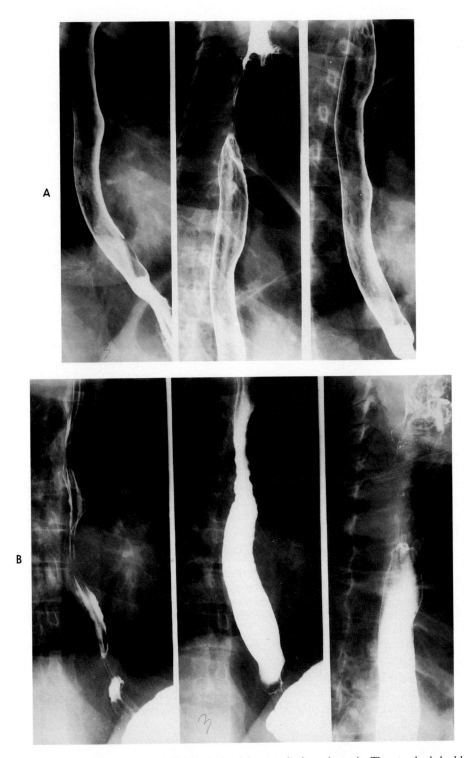

Fig. 9-12 Four views of the esophagus obtained from a single patient. **A,** The standard double-contrast views using a 14 × 14–inch (35 × 35 cm) film format. **B,** There is one mucosal relief film showing a small hiatus hernia and two supine-oblique single-contrast views. Note the suboptimal view of the gastroesophageal junction in the supine projection. **C,** Because the patient had dysphagia, a prone view on full inspiration was obtained and better reveals the hernia, as well as a Schatzki ring. **D,** A marshmallow bolus is shown arrested by the ring.

From Stevenson GW: Gastroesophageal reflux. In Simpkins KC, ed: *A textbook of radiological diagnosis*, vol 4, *The alimentary tract*, London, 1988, HK Lewis.

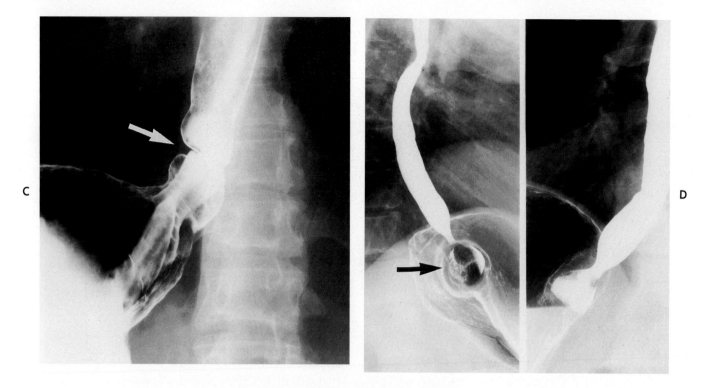

Fig. 9-12, cont'd For legend see opposite page.

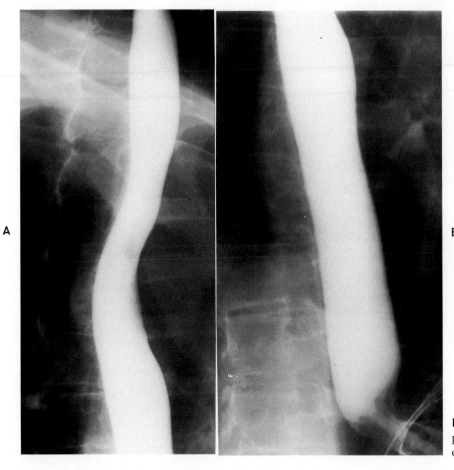

Fig. 9-13 Full-column films showing the proximal half (**A**) and distal half (**B**) of the esophagus.

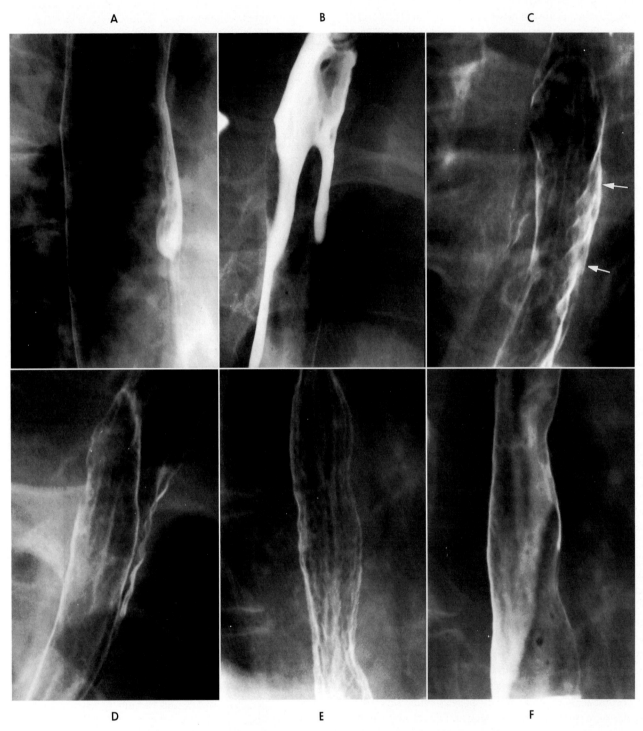

Fig. 9-14 Artifacts observed during a barium examination of the esophagus. **A,** A mucus plug. **B,** uneven coating. **C,** Contrast medium in the trachea simulating a carpet lesion *(arrows).* **D,** The same patient as in Fig. 9-9, *C,* in a more oblique projection. The contrast medium is now clearly outside the esophagus. **E,** When only partly distended the esophageal mucosa may appear coarse. **F,** Same patient as in **E.** When well distended the mucosa is smooth.

patient can drink the barium through a straw with side holes, which allows air to be sucked in. Chilled barium causes the esophagus to relax and enhances the double-contrast effect.[20] However, the most certain method is to perform a tube esophagram using an 8 Fr catheter passed into the esophagus via the nose. Air is then injected through the tube while the patient drinks barium. If the patient is totally unable to drink, the barium is injected through the tube until the esophagus is well coated and then air is injected. This technique is clearly cumbersome, but can produce reasonably good double-contrast images. Elevating the head of the table is a helpful maneuver toward the end of this procedure.

DRUG ENHANCEMENT

Buscopan and glucagon. If there is a high suspicion of esophageal structural disease, or the distention on double-contrast films is unsatisfactory, either glucagon or Buscopan (N-butylscopolammonium bromide) can be injected. Glucagon (0.5 mg) has an effect on the lower esophageal sphincter and may increase gas reflux. It may also promote gastroesophageal reflux, although probably not very much.[21] In addition, it has a transient effect on primary peristalsis that is maximal at 2 minutes; this is usually transient but can persist in some subjects for over 20 minutes.[22] Glucagon has also been shown to reduce the esophageal transit of gelatin capsules,[23] although this is controversial and not all authors have noted an effect on peristalsis.[24] Buscopan (20 mg) has a direct spasmolytic effect on the lower esophageal sphincter and the esophagus, and, for this reason, usually yields an excellent double-contrast effect. Glucagon has not been shown to enhance double-contrast radiography of the esophagus.[25] Neither drug should be used before esophageal motility, reflux, and clearance have been assessed,[22] although the effect of glucagon is much less than that of Buscopan.

Mecholyl and amyl nitrite. The methacholine test at one time was used to reveal denervation in patients with suspected achalasia. When the test result was a positive, however, numerous nonpropulsive contractions occurred, and these were often very painful. It is now only of historical interest and has no place today as a radiologic study.

Of more current interest is the amyl nitrite test, which is a simple test for distinguishing primary from secondary achalasia.[26] In a study that assessed its use, four inhalations of amyl nitrite produced at least a 3-mm increase in the diameter of the lower esophageal sphincter (mean, 4.6 mm) in all of nine patients with idiopathic achalasia; this was accompanied by improved esophageal emptying. Three patients with pseudoachalasia showed no change in the maximal diameter of the lower esophageal sphincter. Dodds et al.,[26] working in a hospital that is a referral center for patients with esophageal disease, encountered one patient with pseudoachalasia for every 35 patients with primary achalasia. However, tachycardia and dizziness were not uncommon in patients who underwent the test, and therefore these patients should be supported at the knees and watched closely for signs of fainting.

Edrophonium chloride. Of those patients with chest pain of suspected esophageal origin, most have reflux disease. However, some have spasm of the esophagus, which may be intermittent. The provocative drugs once used to assess this condition (bethanecol and ergonovine) have potential side effects, especially in patients with cardiac disease, that made their use for radiologic studies imprudent. However, Tensilon (edrophonium chloride) appears to be suitable for this purpose. To quote from Benjamin and Castell,[27] "Although edrophonium did not produce abnormalities in a high percentage of the patients tested, it was the drug most likely to precipitate a motility defect combined with the patients' pain pattern. We suggest therefore that edrophonium be considered the single best provocative agent to be utilized in patients with suspected abnormalities of esophageal function producing a chest pain syndrome." Its relative safety means that it is probably the only drug that radiologists might consider using in a comprehensive esophageal assessment of a patient with chest pain.

In the normal individual, or a patient with gastroesophageal reflux, Tensilon injected in a dose of 80 μg/kg of body weight transiently improves the efficiency of esophageal peristalsis without accompanying symptoms. The experience of one of the editors, however, in 100 consecutive patients admitted to a coronary care unit with noncardiac chest pain was disappointing, with only two patients experiencing minimal chest pain after Tensilon administration. The value of Tensilon as a routine provocative agent thus remains somewhat controversial, but patients with a nutcracker esophagus do exhibit a vigorous response, dramatic nonperistaltic contractions, and chest pain.

Acid barium for pain provocation. For those patients with chest pain due to gastroesophageal reflux, a provocative test using acid barium can be used. This is the "sour barium" test described by Donner and is similar in principle to the Bernstein test, which has largely replaced it. To make acid barium with a pH of 1.7, 100 ml of barium sulfate suspension is combined with 0.5 ml of concentrated hydrochloric acid.[28] The patient is examined recumbent, and the esophageal response to acid barium is compared with that to standard barium. Esophageal peristalsis in normal individuals does not change in the presence of acid barium, but, in some patients with reflux symptoms, segmental nonperistaltic contractions replace peristalsis. Others have the chest pain that originally led them to seek medical help. The patient should take at least five or six swallows of the barium to ensure that the mucosa is adequately exposed to the low pH.

Reflux inducement. Whether it is useful to provoke reflux is discussed in Chapter 11. In some patients, barium refluxes spontaneously; in others, turning on the table, a Valsalva maneuver (by bearing down or by performing a straight leg lift while supine), or dry swallowing may all provoke reflux. Abdominal compression has been quanti-

A

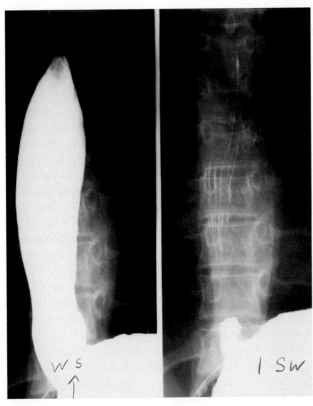

B

fied for isotopic use,[29-31] and an abdominal compression device that exerts 50 mm Hg of pressure has been advocated for radiologic use, but still has a 50% false-negative rate compared with 24-hour pH monitoring.[32]

For fluoroscopic purposes the water siphon test is the most sensitive. It produces a little reflux in normal individuals and tends to flood the esophagus in those with gastroesophageal reflux disease. It may be performed with the patient erect or recumbent; with the patient recumbent, it permits the efficiency of esophageal clearance of refluxed acid to be assessed.

In the erect water siphon test, the patient drinks a large volume of barium and water and then bends forward, thus increasing the intraabdominal pressure. Fluoroscopy is performed in the lateral projection and reflux can be observed. The test is easier to control with the patient recumbent. The stomach should contain a good volume of both barium and gas, such that it is well distended by a large fundal volume of barium. The supine patient is turned briefly to the left to deposit all the gastric barium in the fundus, and then slowly turned to the right to the point where the gastroesophageal junction disappears under the barium puddle, but not so far that the barium runs down into the antrum. Then, holding this oblique position, the patient drinks a glass of water through a straw. Under such provocation, a puff or two of barium refluxes into the lower esophagus in normal individuals but this clears rapidly with peristalsis. In almost all patients with reflux disease, the esophagus becomes flooded, often to the pharynx. A proportion of these patients can clear the acid refluxate within a minute with one or two dry swallows. Others exhibit impaired clearance, even though often fairly normal peristalsis has been observed during the initial assessment of motility with neutral barium (Fig. 9-15). The clinical significance of a positive water siphon test in terms of correlation with symptoms, and the correlation between impaired radiographic clearance and the response to treatment or relapse rate, has never been established. In other words, the water siphon test permits assessment of clearance, but the significance of this is largely intuitive rather than proved.

Gastroesophageal junction

Films of the gastroesophageal junction should be taken in different projections. The best view of the closed junction is obtained as described previously, with the table head elevated 45 degrees and patients on their right side (see Fig. 9-3). The best view of the open sphincter is obtained with the patient prone or prone-oblique and drinking (see Fig.

Fig. 9-15 The positive findings from supine water siphon tests performed on two patients. Both have major reflux on this provocation, **A,** The refluxate has been totally cleared with one swallow. **B,** There is still residual acid and barium after 2 minutes.
From Stevenson GW: Gastroesophageal reflux. In Simpkins KC, ed: *A textbook of radiological diagnosis*, vol 4, *The alimentary tract*, London, 1988, HK Lewis.

9-14). The best view for showing reflux is with the patient supine and the left side elevated and good gastric distention so that the gastroesophageal junction is below the level of the barium-gas interface.

Emergency examination (leak and foreign body)

Emergency examinations may be requested to investigate for a suspected leak or foreign body, or for severe acute odynophagia. In patients with suspected esophageal perforation, a water-soluble contrast medium should probably be used,[33] although some authors believe dilute barium provides superior visualization.[34] This subject has been well reviewed.[35] If initial swallows of small volumes of water-soluble contrast agent reveal no leak, larger mouthfuls should be taken. If still no leak is observed and the esophagus is emptying, the examination should be concluded by having the patient swallow generous volumes of barium sulfate,[35] since any leak not seen at this point must be small. If cost is no object, then low-osmolar water-soluble contrast should be used, but normally such expensive agents should be reserved for those patients who likely have a fistula or who face a definite risk of aspiration to the lungs. It is also recommended for those who have little resistance to a minor insult, such as sick neonates. Hexabrix (ioxaglic acid) is a compromise agent; its cost is moderate and it is safer than Gastrografin if aspirated.

Positioning of the patient is an important part of the examination for perforation of the esophagus. Turning the patient a little to the right and to the left will help, but horizontal-beam radiographs taken with the patient swallowing in right and left decubitus positions improves the diagnostic sensitivity.[36]

In patients with suspected foreign body impaction, often with total dysphagia, the choice of contrast agent depends on what is planned next. If endoscopy is to be performed shortly, barium should not be used, since it ruins the endoscopic view and clogs the endoscope. In addition, if there is associated acute chest pain or any possibility of perforation, a water-soluble contrast agent should be used. Finally, if there is total dysphagia and no swallowing of saliva is possible, a small amount (1 to 2 ml) of nonionic water-soluble contrast agent should be used for the initial assessment because of the risk of aspiration. The pharynx should be assessed carefully, as an acute brainstem lesion may produce pharyngeal dysfunction that mimics esophageal obstruction. Patients should be examined erect and horizontal in two projections at right angles, usually the right and left anterior oblique. If the initial swallows with water-soluble contrast yield negative findings, the examination should always be completed with barium, as the improved visualisation provides a much greater degree of diagnostic confidence.

Many foreign bodies in the esophagus may dislodge if either intravenous relaxants (Buscopan or glucagon) or effervescent granules are given. The latter is especially help- ful in children with coins wedged in the esophagus. In these patients, effervescent granules and some marshmallow to chew often succeed in dislodging the object.

In patients with acute odynophagia, endoscopy is often the first esophageal examination performed, as herpes and other infections are common, and biopsies and fluid aspiration may be successful. If a contrast study is required, it should be performed with the patient erect. Time should be taken to carefully explain the procedure to the patient. Initially, they should take a very small swallow of barium and mucosal relief films obtained. Distention of the esophagus may be painful, so the double-contrast views should be left until the end, even though they may be the most helpful in the diagnosis of herpes or cytomegalovirus infection.

The tailored examination

From what has been described, it is clear that a complete examination cannot, and should not, be performed in every patient. Instead, a barium examination should be tailored to the specific clinical problem at hand. It is poor medical practice for a patient to be referred and examined without a clear understanding of the clinical problem and exactly what questions the barium examination is supposed to answer. The radiologist needs to spend a few moments confirming the given history with the patient and asking specific questions to plan possible modifications of the examination. For example, it is good to clarify in advance whether the dysphagia consists of a problem in initiating a swallow or whether the trouble comes after a swallow has been successfully concluded. If both duodenal ulcer and reflux esophagitis are suspected, the radiologist must decide which to concentrate on, since the examination cannot be optimally tailored for both entities. If the patient has globus as well as heartburn, the examination of the pharynx must be performed in more than the usual detail.

Radiologic equipment

Up until the past year or two, there had been little change in the radiologic equipment used for esophageal examinations since the introduction of the image intensifier. Digital equipment is a significant advance[37] that has at last been refined enough so that it can be used for routine clinical applications. The delay for exposure is less, so getting films with optimal distention is now easier. Although the spatial resolution is slightly less than that yielded by film-screen combinations, the contrast resolution is higher. The ability to stack images efficiently on a work station screen for printing to a laser camera greatly reduces film costs and may force radiologists to carry out more gastrointestinal diagnosis on screen. The immediate availability of images increases room through-put, and the ability to print to a laser camera decreases film costs. It seems likely that digital fluoroscopy will gradually replace conventional units. Computerized radiography with stimulatable phosphor technology also has some advantages, both in terms of reduced cost and radiation dose, as a replacement for spot films in those units that can accommodate a large enough film.

For the functional evaluation, a high-quality video recorder is an essential piece of equipment. Cine recording is now obsolete, other than for some very rapid movements such as in some cardiologic investigations and in research settings where very high frame rates are desired. No doubt the current super VHS and ¾ -inch (2 cm) pneumatic videotape systems will shortly be replaced by videodisk technology, which possesses the huge advantage of permitting the instant selection of desired frame sequences without having to run through a tape.

Cross-sectional techniques
CT examination: indications and technique

The usual indication for obtaining CT scans of the esophagus is to stage an esophageal malignancy or to assess the extent of invasion of a bronchogenic carcinoma that is producing esophageal symptoms. The examination provides considerable information on the intramural and extramural extent of esophageal disease and is also now an indispensable part of the planning for radiation therapy. In the usual technique, no intravenous contrast is used initially and contiguous 8- to 10-mm-thick sections are obtained from the thoracic inlet to the midabdomen, and to the neck if there is a high tumor. In this portion of the examination, the patients are supine and asked to hold their breath. The stomach should be distended with oral contrast medium to ensure a better examination of the cardia. Asking the patient to swallow air may improve delineation of the esophagus, and turning the patient prone and administering effervescent granules as well as preliminary oral contrast greatly improves visualization of the gastroesophageal junction in selected cases.

An alternative method for examining the cardia is to place the patient in the right lateral position, with a nasogastric tube in place for the introduction of air. In the reverse technique the patient drinks a liter of water and is placed in the left lateral position so that the fundus is distended. The water-mucosa interface is the source of fewer artifacts than the air-mucosa interface. If cachexia interferes with delineation of this relationship between the esophagus and the mediastinal structures, or if there are shadows that might be vessels or lymph nodes, then intravenous contrast may be employed to eliminate these problems.[6] Some authors prefer to use routine incremental dynamic scanning starting at the hila during and after the intravenous administration of a bolus of contrast.[38] Thin sections may be obtained for the reexamination of any area of particular concern.

MRI examination—indications and technique

There are no essential indications at present for MRI of the esophagus, and its clinical superiority over CT has not yet been demonstrated. Its potential advantage over CT lies in the variety of projections and superior contrast resolution it offers. The technology, especially sagittal section display, does depict well the relationship of the esophagus to the trachea, the pericardium, the atrium, and the aorta, as well as the gastroesophageal junction. The protocol should include axial, sagittal, and coronal T1 as well as axial T2 scans.[39]

Other techniques
Scintigraphy

The advantages of scintigraphic techniques for the examination of esophageal function are that they are noninvasive, use liquids and solids of a physiologic nature, and produce quantitative data that can be reduced to numeric indices.[40]

Transit tests assess esophageal clearance,[41] but there are some problems with their interpretation.[42] Tests of gastroesophageal reflux include a scintigraphic abdominal binder test,[29] but its results correlate rather poorly with other clinical parameters of reflux disease, and the physiologic reflux test,[30] which has already been described. However, this latter test has a sensitivity of 70% and a specificity of 87%,[43] which are not good enough to make it useful as a screening test for reflux disease. At present, esophageal scintigraphy is probably best suited as a screening test for esophageal dysmotility,[44] and for assessing the results of therapy in some diseases.

REFERENCES

1. Herlinger H, Grossman RG, Laufer I et al: Gastric cardia in double contrast study: its dynamic image, *AJR* 135:21, 1980.
2. Glick SN, Teplick SK, Goldstein et al: Glycogenic acanthosis, *AJR* 139:683, 1982.
3. Gohel VK, Edell SL, Laufer I, Rhodes WM: Transverse folds in the human esophagus, *Radiology* 128:303, 1978.
4. Myer GW, Castell DO: Anatomy and physiology of the esophageal body. In Castell DO, Johnson LF, eds: *Esophageal function in health and disease,* New York, 1983, Elsevier.
5. Moss AA, Schnyder P, Thoeni RF, Margulis AR: Esophageal carcinoma: pretherapy staging by computed tomography, *AJR* 136:1051, 1981.
6. Becker CD, Fuchs WA: Carcinoma of the esophagus and gastroesophageal junction. In Myers MA, ed: *Computed tomography of the gastrointestinal tract,* New York, 1986, Springer-Verlag.
7. Lund G, Lien HH: Computed tomography of the azygo-esophageal recess: normal appearances, *Acta Radiol Diagn* 23:225, 1982.
8. Marks WM, Callen PW, Moss AA: Gastroesophageal region: source of confusion on CT, *AJR* 136:359, 1981.
9. Quint LE, Glazer GM, Orringer MB: Esophageal imaging by MR and CT: study of normal anatomy and neoplasms, *Radiology* 156:727, 1985.
10. Putman CE, Curtis AM, Westfried M et al: Thickening of the posterior tracheal stripe: a sign of squamous carcinoma of the esophagus, *Radiology* 121:533, 1976.
11. Gelfand DW: Techniques for examining the hypopharynx and esophagus. In *Gastrointestinal radiology,* New York, 1984, Churchill Livingstone.
12. Kressel HY, Laufer I: Principles of double contrast diagnosis In Laufer I, ed: *Double contrast gastrointestinal radiology,* Philadelphia, 1979, WB Saunders.

13. Wolf BS: Use of half-inch barium tablet to detect minimal esophageal strictures, *J Mt Sinai Hosp* 28:80, 1961.
14. Kelly JE: The marshmallow as an aid to radiologic examination of the esophagus, *N Engl J Med* 265:1306, 1961.
15. Somers S, Stevenson GW, Thompson G: Comparison of endoscopy and barium swallow with marshmallow in dysphagia, *J Can Assoc Radiol* 37:73, 1986.
16. Ott DJ: Radiologic evaluation of esophageal dysphagia, *Curr Probl Diagn Radiol* 17:1, 1988.
17. McNally EF, Del Gaudio W: The radiopaque esophageal marshmallow bolus, *AJR* 101:485, 1967.
18. Davies HA, Evans KT, Butler F et al: Diagnostic value of bread swallow in patients with esophageal symptoms, *Dig Dis Sci* 28:1094, 1983.
19. Curtis DJ, Cruess DF, Wilgress ER: Abnormal solid bolus swallowing, *Dysphagia* 2:46, 1987.
20. Ott DJ, Gelfand DW, Munitz HA et al: Cold barium suspension in the clinical evaluation of the esophagus, *Gastrointest Radiol* 9:193, 1984.
21. Drane WE, Haggar AM, Engel MA: Glucagon and gastroesophageal reflux, *AJR* 142:709, 1984.
22. Anvari M, Richards D, Dent J et al: Effect of glucagon on esophageal peristalsis and clearance, *Gastrointest Radiol* 14:100, 1989.
23. Channer KS, Bolton R, Al-Hilli S et al: The effect of glucagon on the swallowing of capsules, *Br J Clin Pharmacol* 16:456, 1983.
24. Hogan WJ, Dodds WJ, Hoke SE et al: Effect of glucagon on esophageal motor function, *Gastroenterology* 69:160, 1975.
25. Ott DJ, Chen MY, Gelfand D: Effects of hiatal hernia, reflux esophagitis and glucagon on the quality of the double contrast esophogram, *Gastrointest Radiol* 14:97, 1989.
26. Dodds WJ, Stewart ET, Kishk SM et al: Radiologic amyl nitrite for distinguishing pseudo achalasia from idiopathic achalasia, *AJR* 146:21, 1986.
27. Benjamin SJ, Castell DO: Esophageal causes of chest pain. In Castell DO, Johnson LF, eds: *Esophageal function in health and disease,* New York, 1983, Elsevier.
28. Donner MW, Silbiger ML, Hookman P, Hendrix TR: Acid-barium swallows in the radiographic evaluation of clinical esophagitis, *Radiology* 87:220, 1966.
29. Malmud LS, Fisher RS: Gastroesophageal scintigraphy, *Gastrointest Radiol* 5:195, 1980.
30. Heyman S, Kirkpatrick JA, Winter HS, Treves S: An improved radionuclide method for the diagnosis of gastroesophageal reflux and aspiration in children (milk scan), *Radiology* 131:479, 1979.
31. Velasco N, Pope CE, Gannon RM et al: Measurement of esophageal reflux by scintigraphy, *Dig Dis Sci* 29:977, 1984.
32. Fransson S-G, Sökjer H, Johansson K-G, Tibling L: Radiologic diagnosis of gastroesophageal reflux by means of graded abdominal compression, *Acta Radiol* 29:45, 1988.
33. Nealon TF, Templeton JY, Cuddy KD, Gibbon JH: Instrumental perforation of the oesophagus, *J Thorac Cardiovasc Surg* 41:75, 1961.
34. Foley MJ, Ghahremani GG, Roger LF: Reappraisal of contrast media used to detect upper gastrointestinal perforations, *Radiology* 144:231, 1982.
35. Dodds WJ, Stewart ET, Vlymen WJ et al: Appropriate contrast media for examination of esophageal disruption, *Radiology* 144:439, 1982.
36. Parkin GJS: The radiology of perforate oesophagus, *Clin Radiol* 24:324, 1973.
37. Fowler RC, Bonsor G, Lintott DJ: Description and appraisal of a prototype digital fluorographic system, *Clin Radiol* 40:508, 1989.
38. Quint LE, Glazer GM, Orringer MB, Gross BH: Esophageal carcinoma: CT findings, *Radiology* 155:171, 1985.
39. Herold CJ, Zerhouni EA: The mediastinum and lungs. In Higgins CB, Hricak H, Helms CA, eds: *Magnetic resonance imaging of the body,* ed 2, New York, 1992, Raven Press.
40. Robinson PJ: Scintigraphy in motility disorders of the esophagus. In Simpkins KC, ed: *A textbook of radiological diagnosis,* vol 4, *The alimentary tract,* London, 1988, HK Lewis.
41. Russell COH, Hill LD, Holmes ER et al: Radionuclide transit: a sensitive screening test for esophageal dysfunction, *Gastroenterology* 80:887, 1981.
42. Bartlett RJV: Scintigraphy of the esophagus. In Robinson PJ, ed: *Radionuclide imaging in gastroenterology,* Edinburgh, 1986, Churchill Livingstone.
43. Styles CB, Holt S, Bowes KL et al: Gastroesophageal reflux and transit scintigraphy: a comparison with esophageal biopsy in patients with heartburn, *J Can Assoc Radiol* 35:124, 1984.
44. Åkesson A, Gustafson T, Wollheim F, Brisma J: Esophageal dysfunction and radionuclide transit in progressive systemic sclerosis, *Scand J Rheumatol* 16:291, 1987.

10 *Normal Anatomy and Techniques of Examination of the Esophagus: Endosonography*

JOSE F. BOTET
CHARLES J. LIGHTDALE

FUNDAMENTALS OF INTRALUMINAL SONOGRAPHY

An historical review of the published literature has shown that Wild and Reid[1] in 1957 appear to have been the first to report on the intraluminal use of ultrasound. This event was followed by a lengthy hiatus until 1976, when Lutz and Rosch[2] reported their use of a probe to evaluate the upper gastrointestinal tract.

The technique of endoscopic ultrasonography as it is known today has been in use in Europe and Japan since 1981. The first published series regarding the in vivo experience in humans appeared in 1982.[3,4] In 1986, the *Scandinavian Journal of Gastroenterology* published a series of articles contained in a special supplement in which both Japanese and European physicians reported on their experiences with the technique.[5-11] This specialized equipment became available to a limited number of centers in the United States late in 1986, and, by 1990, it was being sold commercially in this country.

Endoscopic ultrasound essentially represents the successful marriage of a gastrointestinal endoscope and an ultrasound transducer. In the most common arrangement, an endoscope has an ultrasound transducer attached to its tip. The components of the system consist of a transmitter, a transducer in the endoscope, a receiver, and a combination display and recording unit.

How does it work in the gastrointestinal tract? Air is the most resistant medium to the transmission of sound waves at the frequencies (1 to 25 MHz) used in ultrasonography. However, the gastrointestinal tract can be rendered ultrasound friendly either by filling the segment under study with water, which is an excellent medium for the propagation of sound waves, or a latex balloon, which is placed over the transducer tip and may be filled with water through a dedicated channel. This technique facilitates acoustic contact between the gastrointestinal wall and the transducer and permits the evaluation of the gastrointestinal tract from within. In addition, because the area of interest is then so close to the transducer, relatively high-frequency transducers (5 to 12 MHz) can be used. This translates into increased tissue contrast and resolution. The acoustic window pro-

vided by the water also allows the transducer to *see* through the wall and evaluate deep organs such as the pancreas or structures such as the mediastinum, which are not easily evaluated using conventional ultrasound.

Endoscopic ultrasound provides information that other modalities such as conventional ultrasound, computed tomography, and magnetic resonance imaging do not. Because of its high resolution and increased tissue contact, it allows the evaluation of individual layers of the gastrointestinal wall and hence can detect the existence of masses or tumors not seen by these other modalities. Major current applications of this modality include the staging of tumor invasion in the esophagus[12,13] and stomach.[14,15] It also has been very helpful in the detection of postoperative anastomotic recurrences[16] as well as in the evaluation of submucosal tumors and large gastric folds.[17,18] The facility with which it can visualize the pancreas has been of great help in the detection of small neuroendocrine tumors of the pancreas.[19,20]

EVALUATION OF THE GASTROINTESTINAL WALL

The appearance of the gastrointestinal wall depicted by endoscopic ultrasound is the result of multiple interrelated factors. Although a full discussion of these factors is beyond the scope of this book, some of the major ones that have a bearing on the examination are discussed here.

Ultrasound

The term *ultrasound* refers to sound waves in the frequency range of 1 to 25 MHz. In this range, the sound waves propagate ideally in water and may be absorbed by solids such as bone, but propagate very poorly through compressible mediums such as air or gases.

Tissues

Homogeneous tissues exhibit a characteristic acoustic impedance that is comparable to the different tissue densities depicted by x-ray studies. One characteristic of ultrasound is that when a sound wave propagating through an homogeneous tissue reaches a boundary with another tissue having a different acoustic impedance, the sound wave is reflected in part and gives a sharp signal. As more and more interfaces are encountered, the intesity of the sound wave penetrating successive tissues decreases.

Absorption and scatter

Absorption and scatter represent two phenomena by which the sound wave's energy is converted into heat and deviates from its pathway because of boundary layer interactions. They constitute important factors that decrease the intensity of the transmitted sound wave.

Frequency and penetration

Lower-frequency sound waves can travel farther before their energy is dissipated. Conversely, the higher the frequency the greater the resolution.

Focal zone

The focal zone is that distance from the transducer within which images obtained are in focus.

Axial resolution

Axial resolution represents the minimal distance at which two objects placed along the axis of the sound wave may be resolved.

As the preceding discussion makes apparent, it is not normally possible to change the speed of sound in tissues, nor the behavior of absorption or scatter. However, a working frequency appropriate to the procedure can be selected.

THE GASTROINTESTINAL WALL

Histologically the gastrointestinal tract is uniform from the oropharynx to the rectum. It is composed of five layers that are arranged from the inside out in the following order: the mucosa, deep mucosa (lamina propria), submucosa, muscularis propria, and serosa/adventitia. Examination of a normal gastrointestinal wall with an ultrasound transducer in the range of 5 to 20 MHz reveals a five-layered structure similar to that seen in histologic sections (Fig. 10-1). The innermost echogenic band represents the mucosal interface and, it is echogenic because of the significant change in the speed of sound waves that occurs when they travel from water to tissue. This band corresponds histologically, as proved by Tio,[21] to the superficial mucosa, and alterations in this layer, as seen on endosonography, do reflect mucosal abnormalities seen in histopathologic sections. The second layer represents the deep mucosa known as the *lamina propria* and appears endosonographically as a hypoechoic region. The third layer is hyperechoic and corresponds to the submucosa. This layer has a relatively high fat content and this increases its echogenicity. The fourth layer corresponds to the muscularis propria and is hypoechoic, in keeping with its being muscle tissue. This is one of the most variable regions in that it is relatively thin in the esophagus, duodenum, and jejunum; slightly thicker in the normal gastric wall, espe-

cially in the prepyloric and pyloric area as well as in the colon; and thickest in the rectum in the sphincter region. The fifth layer, the serosa/adventitia, appears as a thin echogenic layer and is not a completely reproducible entity. In the esophagus, where no true serosa exists, this fifth layer is commonly seen. As in the case of the mucosa, it may actually represent a strong echo when the speed of propagation changes as it goes from the muscle to the surrounding areolar tissue. However, organs that have a serosa also show a similar echogenic pattern.

THE ESOPHAGUS
Normal anatomy

The esophagus lies between the oropharynx and the cardia. It is approximately 30 cm long, give or take 5 cm. Endoscopically the cardia lies approximately 40 cm from the incisors. This is the most commonly used reference point in the endosonographic examination of the upper gastrointestinal tract. At its origin the esophagus is fixed by the cricopharyngeus muscle, which forms its superior sphincter. Distally the esophagus ends in the cardia. Between these two points the esophagus is a relatively movable structure that can be easily displaced. The esophagus is normally collapsed in its anteroposterior dimension and measures approximately 30 by 20 mm in cross section. When it is normal, it is easily distensible, and, under pathologic conditions such as achalasia, it can distend to 6 or 7 cm in diameter. From an endosonographic point of view, the esophagus is regarded as a 30-cm-long tube that allows the

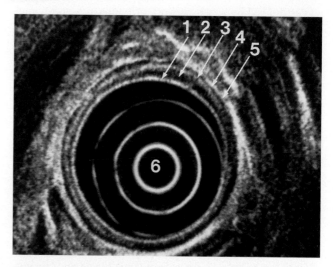

Fig. 10-1 Normal esophageal wall showing five layers. The innermost, hyperechoic area *(1)* corresponds to the mucosa; the second, hypoechoic area *(2)*, to the lamina propria; the third, hyperechoic level *(3)*, to the submucosa; the fourth, hypoechoic area *(4)*, to the muscularis propria; and the fifth and outermost layer *(5)*, which is hyperechoic, to the adventitial interface. *6,* The transducer in the lumen with the water-filled balloon.

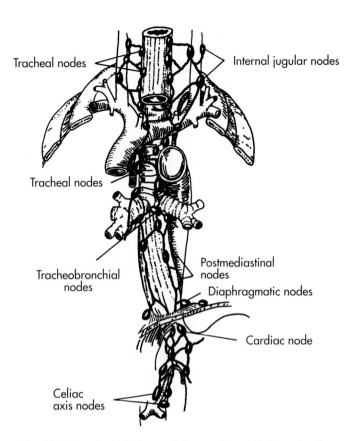

Tracheal nodes

Internal jugular nodes

Tracheal nodes

Tracheobronchial nodes

Postmediastinal nodes

Diaphragmatic nodes

Cardiac node

Celiac axis nodes

Fig. 10-2 Lymphatic drainage of the esophagus. Endoscopic ultrasound can image all the nodes depicted.

placement of an endoscope close to its wall. The esophagus is drained by a rich network of lymphatics and lymph nodes (Fig. 10-2).

The esophagus can be divided arbitrarily into three segments: (1) the upper esophagus, which comprises the area between the oropharynx and the superior aspect of the aortic arch; (2) the middle esophagus, which extends from the aortic arch to the subcarinal region; and (3) the lower esophagus, which constitutes the area between the subcarinal region and the cardia.

Upper esophagus

The upper esophagus originates just below the cricopharyngeus muscle very near the lower cervical and upper thoracic spine. This is an area where bony spurs resulting from degenerative changes of the spine are common, making it difficult to introduce the instrument. It is also a difficult region to image because the patient tends to gag and become restless when the transducer is positioned there. The most proximal portion of the esophagus that can be examined reliably by endosonography is located approximately 3 cm above the aortic arch. This allows the origin and proximal aspects of the first-order branches arising from the aortic arch to be evaluated, namely the left subclavian artery, left

common carotid, and brachiocephalic trunk. This is an important area because of its relationships and lymphatic drainage. At this level the upper thoracic vertebral bodies lie posteriorly and slightly to the right in most patients; the trachea, which lies anteriorly, can be easily and reproducibly differentiated from the surrounding air-filled lung. Anatomically the trachea is formed of cartilaginous rings that cover its anterior and lateral aspect, but its posterior aspect consists of a relatively thin membrane that allows the transmission of sound waves into the tracheal air column, creating a very sharp, echogenic boundary. This is extremely useful when evaluating invasion of the trachea by esophageal tumor or, vice versa, the invasion of the esophagus by tracheobronchial tumors.

The vessels and structures of the mediastinum are surrounded by a lacy type of connective tissue that allows the sharp definition of their margins (Fig. 10-3). Surrounding the vessels, esophagus, and tracheobronchial tree are rich lymphatic node chains. Their drainage pattern has been elucidated in detail and is quite specific. Enlargement or abnormal patterns within specific nodes may provide clues to the origin of malignancy.

Occasionally, when a higher-frequency transducer is used, it may be possible to see the thoracic duct as a single or double duct situated anteriorly and to the left of the upper thoracic vertebral bodies on its way to its termination point in the left jugular vein, venous angle, left subclavian, or innominate vein. In 50% of cases the distal duct forms a localized dilatation just before entering the draining vein.

Middle esophagus

The middle esophagus extends from a point just below the aortic arch, superiorly, to the infracarinal space, inferiorly. In the superior aspect of this region, the esophagus is bound anteriorly by the trachea. Slightly to the right, it may be possible to identify the superior vena cava. This is most commonly identified at its junction with the azygos vein passing anteriorly to join the superior vena cava. At this level the ascending aorta, main pulmonary artery, and both the right and left pulmonary arteries are obscured by the air in the more posterior trachea and main right and left bronchi. The descending aorta posteriorly as well as the aorticopulmonary window are readily visible.

The trachea and carina demonstrate the same sonographic signature as that in the upper esophagus. The membranous portion of the trachea allows a sharp definition of the air column. The carina is well recognized in real-time as the air in the trachea bifurcates. Once the bronchi leave the mediastinum, they cannot be identified, as they are rendered indistinct by the surrounding air in the lungs (Figs. 10-4 and 10-5).

The lymphatic drainage of this area is rich and consists of two main groups of vessels, namely the peritracheal, pericarinal, subcarinal, and peribronchial node group and the periesophageal and subdiaphragmatic group surround-

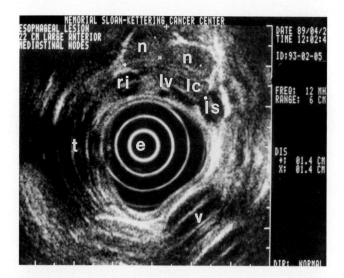

Fig. 10-3 The thoracic inlet. Clockwise beginning at 12 o'clock: *ri*, right innominate (brachiocephalic) artery; *1v*, (variant) low origin of the left vertebral artery; *1c*, left carotid artery (compressed by nodes); *1s*, left subclavian artery; *v*, vertebral body; *t*, trachea; *e*, esophagus. Enlarged lymph nodes surrounding the major vessels of the arch are noted by *n*.

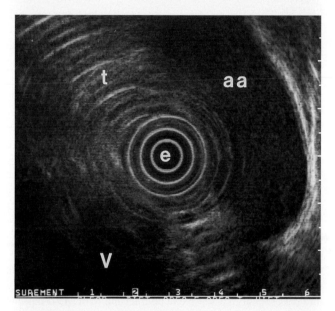

Fig. 10-4 Aortic arch *(aa)*. Notice the layers of the aortic wall as seen at 7.5 MHz and the total absorption of the ultrasound beam by bone. Notice also the parallel lines, which are a signature of the air in the trachea as seen through the posterior membranous portion. *v*, Vertebral body; *t*, trachea; *e*, esophagus.

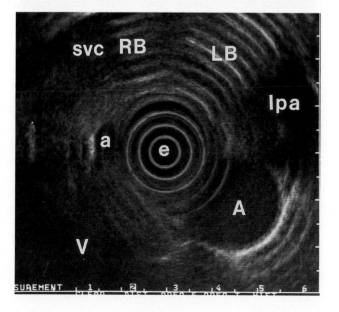

Fig. 10-5 In the carina, notice the widening of the air signature. *RB*, Right main bronchus; *LB*, left main bronchus; *1pa*, left pulmonary artery; *A*, aorta; *V*, vertebral body; *a*, azygos vein moving anteriorly to join the superior vena cava *(svc)*.

ing the azygos and hemiazygos veins. The anterior mediastinal nodes in front of the ligamentum arteriosum are not well visualized. The subcarinal nodes are considered by some to be inferior mediastinal nodes.

The thoracic duct is seen in approximately 75% of patients as a vessel-like structure immediately anterior to the azygos vein. Its course in a cephalad direction should allow its differentiation from a node.

Distal esophagus

The distal esophagus extends from the infracarinal space to the cardia. Anteriorly it is bound by the left atrium. The two layers of the pericardium can be identified easily and reproducibly not only posteriorly but also anteriorly. In 60% to 70% of normal cases it is possible to see them separate from each other during a heart cycle on a real-time examination. Frequently it is possible to identify the coronary sinus traversing almost horizontally anterior to the esophagus. Posteriorly the descending aorta and vertebral bodies are the most important landmarks within the diaphragmatic crux, which also contains the azygos and hemiazygos veins (Fig. 10-6).

The lymphatic drainage in this area is dominated by the periesophageal, cardiophrenic, and crural nodes. Less commonly identified are the pulmonary ligament nodes. As in the middle esophagus, the thoracic duct is seen as a vessel-like structure situated close to the azygos vein.

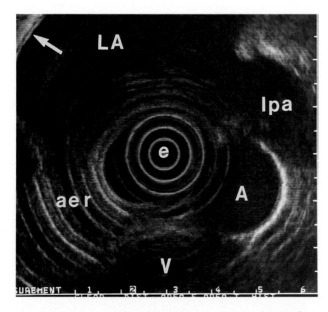

Fig. 10-6 Lower esophagus. Notice the two layers of the pericardium *(white arrow)* and the air signature in the azygos esophageal recess *(aer)*. *LA,* Left atrium; *lpa,* Left inferior pulmonary artery; *A,* aorta; *V,* vertebral body.

Examination technique
Preliminary preparation

Patients are instructed not to eat or drink after midnight. Most procedures are performed on an outpatient basis. Upon arrival, a short history is taken and a physical examination performed by appropriately trained nurses. The procedure and possible risks are explained. These risks consist of those inherent to the endoscopy itself, such as bleeding and perforation of the esophagus, and those associated with intravenous sedation, such as allergic reactions, respiratory depression, and changes in blood pressure or heart rate. Patients' vital signs, such as blood pressure, heart rate, ECG, and oxygen saturation, are monitored. Intravenous sedation is given, usually a combination of Demerol (meperidine hydrochloride) and a short-acting benzodiazepine. The dosage is titrated on an individual basis.

Procedure

There are usually three parts to the procedure: (1) preliminary conventional endoscopy, (2) endoscopic ultrasonography, and (3) if required, endoscopically or sonographically guided biopsies.

Once the patient is sedated, a preliminary endoscopic evaluation of the esophagus and gastric fundus is performed using a conventional endoscope. Suspected abnormalities to be evaluated by endosonography are noted, as well as their distance from the incisors. The most commonly used ultrasound endoscopes have a slightly larger diameter than conventional ones, and this makes their introduction more difficult, especially for the older models which have a straight 5-cm section at the tip. There are several common difficulties that can arise at introduction. If the patient is not well sedated, has degenerative changes of the cervical spine that make it difficult to bend the patient's neck, or has cervical spine spurs that impede the introduction of the instrument into the oropharynx, these can all interfere with smooth performance of the examination. Once the instrument is in the esophagus, it is advanced into the gastric fundus. (Because examination of the fundus is covered in a following section, it is not discussed here.) The balloon at the tip of the endoscope is then filled with water, and the endoscope is slowly withdrawn into the cardia. The examination is actually performed in retrograde fashion, and observations are made using ultrasound imaging as guidance. With real-time images, the exact location of the tip of the probe is known.

It is important to move the endoscope slowly. Respiratory motions may jostle the tip of the transducer as much as 1 cm, but this is far more noticeable in the stomach. These fine respiratory movements are usually all that is necessary for investigating small abnormalities. With the currently available equipment, it is very important to keep the instrument centered within the lumen with the balloon inflated to a 1.0- to 2.0-cm diameter, depending on the distensibility of the esophageal wall and its natural diameter. Three common errors are made in inflating the balloon: (1)

air bubbles within the balloon, which cause streak artifacts that tend to rotate at a lower rate than the transducer; (2) underinflation, which causes poor contact between the esophageal wall and the balloon and allows air to accumulate between them; this artifact tends to stay in a fixed position unless the transducer is moved; and (3) overinflation, which compresses the layers of the esophagus and makes it difficult to differentiate between them. This last problem is a common cause of the so-called three-layered esophageal wall.

REFERENCES

1. Wild JJ, Reid JM: Intraluminal sonogram in the rectum, *Br J Phys Med* 19:248, 1956.
2. Lutz H, Rosch W: Transgastroscopic ultrasonography, *Endoscopy* 8:203, 1976.
3. Di Magno EP, Regan PT, Clain JE et al: Human endoscopic ultrasonography, *Gastroenterology* 83:824, 1982.
4. Tio TL, Tytgat GNJ: Endoscopic ultrasonography in the assessment of intra and transmural infiltration of tumors in the esophagus and papilla of Vater and in the detection of extraesophageal lesions, *Endoscopy* 16:203, 1984.
5. Tio TL, Tytgat GNJ: Endoscopic ultrasonography of normal and pathologic gastrointestinal wall structure: comparison of studies in vivo and in vitro with histology, *Scand J Gastroenterol* 21(suppl 123):27, 1986.
6. Tio TL, Tytgat GNJ: Endoscopic ultrasound in analysing periintestinal lymph node abnormality, *Scand J Gastroenterol* 21(suppl 123):158, 1986.
7. Tio TL, den Hartog Jager FCA, Tytgat GNJ: Endoscopic ultrasonography of non-Hodgkin lymphoma of the stomach, *Gastroenterology* 91:401, 1986.
8. Tio TL, den Hartog Jager FCA, Tytgat GNJ: The role of endoscopic ultrasonography in assessing level of resectability of esophagogastric malignancies: accuracy, pitfalls, and predictability, *Scand J Gastroenterol* 21(suppl):78, 1986.
9. Galetti GC, Bolondi L, Barbara L: Instrumentation and scanning techniques. In Kawai K, ed: *Endoscopic ultrasonography in gastroenterology,* Tokyo, 1988, Igaku-Shoin.
10. Caletti GC, Bolondi L, Zani L et al: Technique of endoscopic ultrasonography investigation: esophagus, stomach and duodenum, *Scand J Gastroenterol* 21(suppl 123):1, 1986.
11. Bolondi L, Caletti GC, Casanova P et al: Problems and variations in the interpretation of the ultrasound feature of the normal upper and lower GI tract wall, *Scand J Gastroenterol* 21(suppl 123):16, 1986.
12. Yasuda K, Nakajimja M, Kawai K: Endoscopic ultrasonography in the diagnosis of submucosal tumors of the upper digestive tract, *Scand J Gastroenterol* 21(suppl):59, 1986.
13. Yasuda K, Nakajima M, Kawai K: Technical aspects of endoscopic ultrasonography of the biliary system, *Scand J Gastroenterol* 21(suppl):143, 1986.
14. Takemoto T, Aibe T, Fuji T et al: Endoscopic ultrasonography, *Clin Gastroenterol* 15:305, 1986.
15. Aibe T, Ito T, Yoshida T et al: Endoscopic ultrasonography of lymph nodes surrounding the upper GI tract, *Scand J Gastroenterol* 21(suppl):164, 1986.
16. Botet JF, Lightdale C: Endoscopic ultrasonography of the upper gastrointestinal tract, *AJR* 156:63, 1991.
17. Yiengpruksawan A, Lightdale CJ, Gerdes H, Botet JF: Mucolytic-antifoam solution for reduction of artifacts during endoscopic ultrasonography: a randomized controlled trial, *Gastrointest Endosc* 37:543, 1991.
18. Tessler FN, Kimme-Smith C, Perella RR, et al: Focal zone placement and artifacts: clinical implications for endoscopic sonography, *Radiology* 173:219, 1989 (abstract).
19. Lux G, Heyder N, Lutz H et al: Endoscopic ultrasonography—technique, orientation, and diagnostic possibilities, *Endoscopy* 14:220, 1982.
20. Heyder N: Endoscopic ultrasonography of tumors of the esophagus and stomach, *Surg Endosc* 1:17, 1987.
21. Boyce GA, Sivak MV, Rosch T et al: Evaluation of submucosal upper gastrointestinal tract lesions by endoscopic ultrasound, *Gastrointest Endosc* 37:449, 1991.

11 *Radiology of the Esophagus*

EDWARD T. STEWART
WYLIE J. DODDS

Three major diagnostic tests are used currently for clinical evaluation of the esophagus: esophagography, endoscopy, and esophageal manometry. Endoscopy is effective for examining esophageal morphology and manometry for esophageal motor function; only radiographic examination is effective for evaluating both morphology and motor function. Generally, esophagography is the preferred initial examination. The findings of a well-done radiologic examination, combined with a salient clinical history, often provide the information needed for diagnosis and treatment without recourse to additional tests.

TYPES OF EXAMINATION

Esophagography brackets multiple methods that differ in materials, performance, and emphasis. Variations include (1) fluoroscopy and spot films with barium; (2) examination with water-soluble contrast medium; (3) spot films for mucosal detail; (4) overhead films of the barium-filled esophagus; (5) double-contrast examination; and (6) studies to record motor function, such as cine, rapid filming, or videotape. Although some overlap in technique and detail exists among the different varieties of examination, these methods differ in emphasis and objective. Knowledge of the salient clinical history is essential for selecting the appropriate examination. Frequently the different methods are combined.

Fluoroscopy with accompanying spot films is the best multipurpose examination for evaluating the esophagus (Fig. 11-1). The contrast medium is generally liquid barium, about 40% weight to volume (w/v). Water-soluble contrast medium is indicated for suspected perforation. Nonionic water-soluble agents are preferable when an esophagotracheal fistula is suspected. The single-contrast examination for mucosal detail is indicated primarily for suspected esophageal varices. For this examination the esophageal folds are coated with thick liquid barium (for example, 250% w/v) or a barium paste preparation, and the esophagus is filmed when collapsed (Fig. 11-1, *B*). Films of the entire esophagus, termed *overhead esophagrams,* are obtained by exposure from an overhead x-ray tube when the esophagus is distended with a full column of barium. For optimal esophageal distention the patient should drink barium rapidly during filming (Fig. 11-1, *A*). Overhead esophagrams are best suited for evaluating esophageal displacement caused by adjacent masses or cardiomegaly,

whereas examination of intrinsic esophageal abnormality is better performed by other methods. Double-contrast examination of the esophagus (Fig. 11-1, *C*) requires thick liquid barium and gas, the latter generally supplied by CO_2 released from ingested granules. The double contrast may also be provided by air injected through an esophageal tube and by swallowed water or methylcellulose solution. Spot films are taken during optimal imaging. The major utility of double-contrast esophagography is to identify small esophageal tumors or subtle mucosal irregularities associated with esophagitis. Satisfactory double-contrast films, however, are not obtained uniformly in all subjects, particularly of the proximal esophagus. Fluoroscopy is adequate to evaluate esophageal motor function, but rapid filming with cine, video, or a 105-mm camera is needed to enable leisurely viewing or to provide a permanent record. Pharyngeal motor function tends to be "quicker than the eye." Consequently, rapid filming is essential for satisfactory evaluation of pharyngeal motor activity. Videoradiography is the optimal method.

The different esophageal examinations often require the use of specific techniques or supplementary maneuvers to achieve a successful examination. Such techniques and maneuvers include wide-bore plastic straws for rapid delivery of barium, perforated straws for delivery of air, esophageal intubation for controlled delivery of contrast, Valsalva's or Müller's maneuvers to enhance varices, abdominal compression by a bolster to retard esophageal emptying, alterations in subject position to promote gastroesophageal reflux, cold barium to suppress esophageal contractions, and pharmacologic agents to suppress or stimulate esophageal motor activity.

PERFORMANCE OF EXAMINATION

A survey of the esophagus and pharynx should be a standard part of any upper gastrointestinal (GI) series. Negligible additional time is required to observe how the barium reaches the stomach. Ambulatory patients are initially fluoroscoped standing. One or two barium swallows are followed from the mouth to the stomach to identify any significant esophageal deviation or obstruction and to evaluate opening of the esophageal sphincters. Double-contrast images are generally obtained while the patient is upright. Subsequently the subject is placed in the right-side-down oblique position, which projects the esophagus free of the

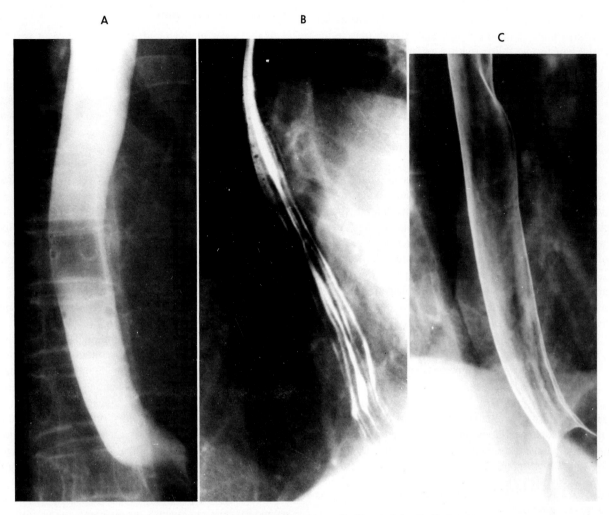

Fig. 11-1 Spot films of esophagus. **A,** Full column. **B,** Mucosal detail. **C,** Double contrast.

spine. Delivery of additional barium to the stomach is observed for several individual swallows of barium, thereby delineating esophageal motor function. The patient is then instructed to drink barium rapidly while several spot films are made of the distended esophagus. Good esophageal distention is essential and often requires use of Valsalva's maneuver or an abdominal bolster to impede esophageal emptying. In cases of dysphagia we routinely ask the patient to swallow a solid bolus, such as a marshmallow at least 1 cm in size. The survey examination of the esophagus and pharynx takes only a few minutes to perform. It can be modified or augmented as indicated. After a double-contrast examination of the esophagus and stomach using thick barium, regular barium should be used to evaluate esophageal motor function and to search for esophageal strictures or rings.

NORMAL ESOPHAGEAL ANATOMY

The esophagus is a straight muscular tube, 20 to 24 cm long, lined mainly with stratified squamous epithelium that has negligible capacity for secretion or absorption. The esophagus joins the hypopharynx just above the sternal notch at the level of the fifth or sixth cervical vertebra and attaches to the stomach behind the xiphoid process. The junctional zone between the hypopharynx and esophagus is demarcated by the cricopharyngeus muscle, which is about 1 cm wide and attaches like a sling to the lamina of the cricoid cartilage. This muscle is the major element of the upper esophageal sphincter (UES). A functional lower esophageal sphincter (LES),[1] 2 to 4 cm long, with minimal muscle thickening exists in the terminal esophagus. The LES segment normally straddles the diaphragmatic hiatus and under resting conditions is partially intraabdominal, partially intrahiatal, and in some instances partially intrathoracic. The esophageal body lies between the two sphincter segments and for descriptive purposes is divided into proximal, middle, and distal thirds. The junction of the proximal and middle third is near the aortic arch level. The proximal 3 to 4 cm of the esophagus lies in the lower part of the neck, whereas the remainder is intrathoracic.

The outer half of the esophageal wall consists of a prominent muscularis arranged into an outer longitudinal and inner circular muscle layer. Striated muscle predominates in the proximal third of the esophagus and smooth muscle in the distal half to two thirds, with a variable zone of overlap. On conventional radiographic or manometric examination it is not generally possible to determine where striated muscle ends and smooth muscle begins. However, certain myogenic or neural disturbances may selectively involve the striated or smooth muscle segments, and some drugs specifically antagonize striated or smooth muscle esophageal function.[2,3]

Extrinsic nerve fibers to the esophagus originate from paired motor nuclei in the brainstem.[4] Motor nerves to the striated muscle of the muscle of the pharynx and the upper esophagus originate in the nuclei ambiguus and pass through the vagal and glossopharyngeal nerves. Cell bodies of motor nerves to esophageal smooth muscle reside in the dorsal motor nuclei, and their axons pass through the vagal nerves. Motor fibers to esophageal striated muscle terminate at motor end-plates without intervening ganglia,[5] whereas motor nerves to esophageal smooth muscle synapse in intramural ganglia and are located mainly in Auerbach's plexus. Both vagal cholinergic excitatory nerves and vagal nonadrenergic inhibitory nerves appear to innervate the esophageal smooth muscle.[6,7] The neural transmitter of the nonadrenergic inhibitory nerves remains unknown.[8,9] These important nerves mediate LES relaxation and relaxation of the esophageal body and participate in peristalsis. Sympathetic adrenergic nerves have a minimal role in regulating esophageal motor function.

NORMAL ESOPHAGEAL PHYSIOLOGY
Resting conditions

The esophageal body, bound by the UES and LES, is normally collapsed during resting conditions. The physiologic sphincters maintain a tonic squeeze recorded manometrically as high-pressure zones that serve to prevent retrograde flow of gastric or esophageal contents (Fig. 11-2).

The main function of the esophagus is to convey ingested material from the pharynx to the stomach. Although gravity assists in bolus transport when the subject is upright, the major mechanism for bolus transport is esophageal peristalsis. Normal peristalsis is capable of moving a bolus against gravity. Swallowing initiates a primary peristaltic sequence that traverses the pharynx and esophagus. For convenience the peristaltic sequence may be envisioned as a rapid wave of inhibition followed by slower wave of contraction.[10] These neuromotor events are integrated and controlled by the medullary swallowing centers and mediated by efferent fibers in the glossopharyngeal and vagal nerves. With deglutition UES tonus falls abruptly within 0.2 to 0.3 second and remains relaxed for about 0.5 second.[10,11] The LES then undergoes receptive relaxation in anticipation of an oncoming bolus (see Fig. 11-2), but does not open unless a bolus is present.[13] LES relaxation persists for about 6 to 8 seconds.[14]

Peristaltic contractions

In the wake of the rapid inhibitory wave, a peristaltic contraction wave traverses the pharynx and esophagus (see Fig. 11-2). This contraction wave sweeps through the pharynx at the rapid rate of 10 to 25 cm/sec and slows in the esophagus to a velocity of 2 to 4 cm/sec. As the peristaltic contractile wave reaches the UES, about 1.5 seconds after swallowing, UES relaxation is completed, and the contraction wave passes across the UES into the esophagus. The peristaltic contraction wave propagates through the esophageal body in 6 to 8 seconds. LES relaxation terminates when the peristaltic contraction reaches the sphincter. Peristalsis in the striated muscle of the pharynx and esophagus is controlled by a descending sequence of neural stimulation programmed in the medulla.[4] Primary peristalsis in esophageal smooth muscle is triggered by stimulation from central nerves at an appropriate instant in the peristaltic sequence,[2] but its propagation through the smooth muscle segment is thought to be controlled primarily by intramural neural circuitry,[6] and perhaps by myogenic spread.[15]

Both the circular and the longitudinal esophageal muscles contract during a peristaltic sequence and also during esophageal distention.[16] However, longitudinal esophageal muscle shortening goes undetected unless metal or anatomic markers, such as esophageal rings or diverticula, are present. Physiologic esophageal shortening during esophageal peristalsis or distention causes intrinsic esophageal structures to make longitudinal excursions, and consequently the esophagogastric junction (Fig. 11-3) is pulled slightly into the chest.[16,17]

Whereas primary peristalsis is initiated by swallowing, secondary peristalsis occurs in response to local esophageal stimulation.[11] The most common stimulus initiating secondary peristalsis is esophageal distention—by gastroesophageal reflux or material left in the esophagus after primary peristalsis. The mechanism is a sensory-motor reflex with either local or central neural connections. Secondary peristalsis acts as a protective mechanism preventing material from collecting in the esophagus that could cause esophagitis or lead to regurgitation and aspiration. Once initiated, secondary and primary esophageal peristalsis have similar features[18] and propagate aborally, irrespective of whether a bolus is present.

Although swallowing or esophageal distention usually elicits peristalsis, the response varies in incidence, force of contraction, and extent of propagation. The incidence of primary peristalsis is defined as the percentage of swallows that initiates a contraction wave that propagates the whole length of the esophagus. Primary peristalsis is incomplete when the peristaltic contraction wave does not traverse the entire esophagus. Aperistalsis, regional or complete, is defined as the absence of peristalsis. In normal adults between 70% and 90% of "dry" swallows and 95% or more of "wet" swallows elicit a complete peristaltic sequence.[14] Emotional disturbances,[19] noise,[20] and aging[21] may cause an in-

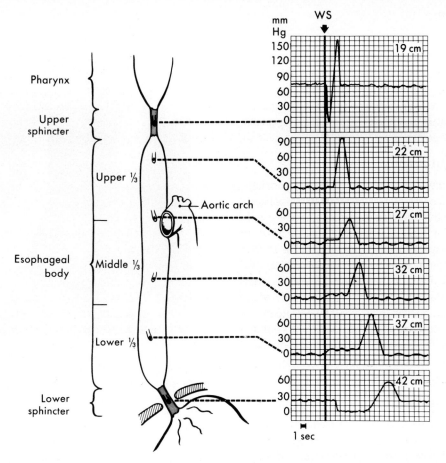

Fig. 11-2 Manometric representation of normal esophageal pressures at rest and following deglutition of barium bolus (8 ml). Tracings are drawn from values obtained in 10 young adults using a high-fidelity recording system.[12] Distance in centimeters of recording tips from nares is indicated on tracings. Pressures are recorded as mm Hg above atmospheric pressure, and the distance between vertical lines in each panel represents a 1-second interval. The heavy vertical line indicates onset of wet shallow (WS). Proximal and distal manometric tips are in the upper and lower esophageal sphincter, respectively, and record resting pressure higher than that in the esophageal body. After swallowing, a wave of inhibition causes upper sphincter relaxation (pressure drop) within 0.2 to 0.3 seconds and lower sphincter relaxation within 1.5 to 2.5 seconds. A peristaltic contraction wave then traverses the upper sphincter, esophageal body, and lower sphincter in an aborally oriented sequence. The contraction wave slows distally. Passage of contraction wave is followed by a sequential return to resting pressure levels throughout the esophagus.

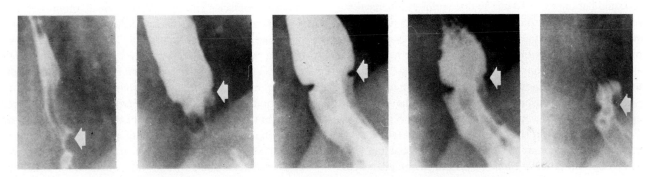

Fig. 11-3 Peristaltic movement of the lower esophageal mucosal ring in an asymptomatic human subject. Cine frames show thin esophageal ring (arrow) representing a transverse mucosal fold at the esophagogastric junction. Note the initial subdiaphragmatic location when the esophagus is collapsed. During peristalsis, the ring makes an oral excursion of 2 to 3 cm and moves slightly above the hiatus. Thus physiologic herniation of a small loculus of stomach into the thorax may occur transiently in association with longitudinal esophageal shortening during peristalsis.

creased incidence of incomplete primary peristaltic sequences. The incidence of secondary peristalsis elicited by esophageal balloon distention ranges from 40% to 65%.[22,23] The LES relaxes in response to nearly 100% of swallows or esophageal distentions in normal young adults. This incidence may decrease with aging.

Nonperistaltic contractions

Any esophageal muscle contraction that is not peristaltic is a nonperistaltic contraction. Nonperistaltic esophageal contractions, generally limited to the smooth muscle esophageal segment, are of variable length and may be feeble or obliterate the esophageal lumen. They may occur spontaneously or after deglutition, are either single or repetitive, and may develop at one or multiple sites. In young adults a nonperistaltic contraction occurs after 10% to 20% of dry swallows. Repetitive, nonperistaltic contractions are rare in young adults but occur after about 5% to 10% of swallows in normal adults in the fourth to sixth decades of life.[24] Spontaneous, repetitive, nonperistaltic contractions are relatively common in the aged.[21]

Radiographic evaluation

Examination of esophageal motor function includes a systematic evaluation of the motor function in the pharynx, both esophageal sphincters, and the esophageal body. Pharyngeal motor function is discussed elsewhere. Both esophageal sphincters are evaluated for abnormal opening or incompetence, whereas the esophageal body is studied for peristaltic and nonperistaltic activity.

Esophageal motor function may be studied satisfactorily fluoroscopically; however, video or cine recording provides a permanent record. Optimally the patient is placed in a right-side-down prone-oblique position. With the patient recumbent, the effects of gravity are evenly distributed along the esophagus and movement of swallowed material is determined predominantly by action of the esophageal musculature. The subject is instructed to take single swallows of liquid barium (5 to 10 ml) so that motor events resulting from a single stimulus can be observed. A second swallow taken before the initial peristaltic sequence is completed may inhibit the initial contractile wave, thereby making it appear abnormal. Rapid, repetitive swallows are used only to distend the esophagus maximally to study morphology.

After deglutition, barium rapidly enters the esophagus coincident with pharyngeal contraction and UES relaxation. The cricopharyngeus is often seen as a notch (about 1 cm high) on the posterior border of the barium column (Fig. 11-4). Barium propelled into the esophagus by pharyngeal contraction generally distributes throughout the esophagus in a continuous column. The head of the column may reach the distal esophagus before LES relaxation occurs (Fig. 11-5). In this circumstance, the barium encounters a momentary delay before entering the stomach, and the proximal margin of the closed LES imparts a V-shaped or bullet-

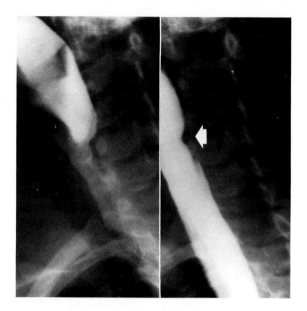

Fig. 11-4 Radiologic appearance of the upper esophageal sphincter (UES) opening during barium swallow. In first frame, subject has just initiated a swallow and, for a fraction of a second, the head of the barium bolus outlines the closed upper margin of the UES, composed mainly of the cricopharyngeus muscle. About 0.1 second later, as seen on right, the relaxed UES is blown open by a propulsive force of pharyngeal peristalsis imparted to the barium bolus. The level of the opened UES is indicated by a shallow posterior indentation *(arrow)* caused by the cricopharyngeus. During swallowing, the cricopharyngeus makes a 1- to 2-cm oral excursion, because it is attached to the lamina of the cricoid cartilage, which makes an oral excursion with swallowing.

shaped configuration to the head of the barium column.[25] Because the relaxed LES is more compliant than the esophageal body, the LES segment, when fully distended, often has a bulbous configuration, termed the *phrenic ampulla,* wherein its diameter exceeds that of the tubular esophageal body. After LES relaxation, the pulsive force of the bolus "blows" the relaxed sphincter open and barium flows freely into the stomach. The upright position is often useful for evaluating esophageal sphincter relaxation and opening.

During primary peristalsis, the lumen-obliterating contraction wave imparts an inverted V-configuration to the proximal end (tail) of the barium column.[26] The peristaltic contraction wave is seen as a progressive stripping movement of the inverted V-shaped tail down the esophageal body (Fig. 11-6, *A*). The point of the tail corresponds precisely to the onset of the peristaltic pressure complex as recorded on manometry.[16] The tail travels fastest in the cervical esophagus and slows distally. Increases in abdominal pressure slow peristalsis in the distal esophagus.[27] In young adults a normal peristaltic wave generally strips all the barium from the esophagus. In some instances, however, some escape of barium (Fig. 11-6, *B*) may occur at the aortic arch level.[13] This phenomenon is a normal variation caused by low peristaltic pressure amplitude in this region.[10,28]

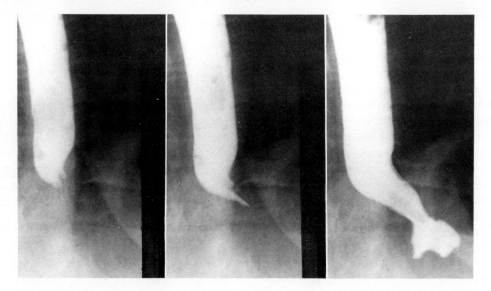

Fig. 11-5 Radiologic appearance of the lower esophageal sphincter (LES) opening after a barium swallow. With the subject upright, three 105-mm films were taken 0.5 second apart beginning 1 second after swallowing. As seen in the first frame, the head of the barium column reaches the LES before its relaxation. The upper margin of the closed sphincter imparts a V- or bullet-shaped configuration to the head of the column. In the middle frame, some barium is seen wedging into the unrelaxed sphincter. As the sphincter relaxes, it is "blown" open by the force of the barium column, and barium flows freely into the stomach.

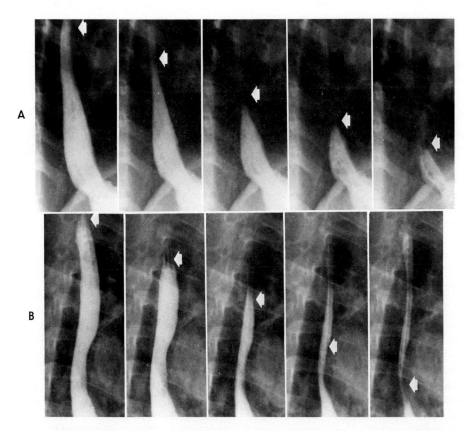

Fig. 11-6 Radiographic appearance of normal primary peristalsis in two recumbent subjects. About 6 to 8 seconds are required for a peristaltic contraction wave to traverse the entire esophagus. **A,** Complete stripping of swallowed bolus. A peristaltic circular contraction wave *(arrows)* imparts an inverted V configuration to the tail of the barium column. The barium tail often develops a flat-top shape in the distal esophagus. **B,** Proximal escape of barium. Circular peristaltic contraction wave *(arrows)* does not quite obliterate the esophageal lumen at the aortic arch level, thereby permitting proximal escape of a modest amount of barium. Below the aortic arch, a peristaltic wave becomes more forceful and obliterates the esophageal lumen, and during its continuation sweeps bulk of swallowed barium into the stomach.

This escape phenomenon becomes more prominent with aging. In the LES segment the peristaltic stripping wave generally develops a rounded or flat-topped configuration. Emptying of barium from the terminal portion of the LES segment often appears as a concentric contraction. In some individuals the stripping wave fades out in the midportion of the LES segment, and barium escapes retrograde into the distal esophageal body. This variation should not be confused with gastroesophageal reflux.

Secondary peristalsis produces the same radiographic appearance as primary peristalsis and is commonly observed after barium from gastroesophageal reflux or a failed primary peristaltic sequence causes sufficient esophageal distention to trigger the stretch reflex. Secondary peristalsis may also be produced by injecting barium into the esophagus through a tube. The tube method is a helpful adjunct in studying esophageal motor function in uncooperative patients or infants.

ESOPHAGEAL MOTILITY DISORDERS

A large number of specific conditions associated with abnormal esophageal motor function are now recognized. Such disorders may be classified as primary or secondary (see box below). In primary motility disorders the esophagus is the major organ involved, whereas in secondary disorders the esophageal motor abnormality results from systemic disease or from physical, chemical, or pharmacologic effects. Many patients with abnormal esophageal motor function do not fit neatly into any one diagnostic category.

Radiographic and manometric features

In esophageal motility disturbances, peristaltic and sphincter function are altered either singly or in combination. Abnormalities of peristalsis include (1) decreased incidence of peristalsis in response to swallowing; (2) incomplete peristaltic sequences; and (3) aperistalsis. Abnormalities of primary peristalsis are readily assessed by radio-

---

□ CLASSIFICATION OF ESOPHAGEAL MOTILITY DISORDERS □

I. Primary
  A. Achalasia
  B. Diffuse esophageal spasm
  C. Intestinal pseudoobstruction
  D. Hypertensive peristalsis
  E. Presbyesophagus
  F. Congenital tracheosophageal fistula
  G. Neonatal chalasia
II. Secondary
  A. Connective tissue
  B. Chemical or physical
    1. Reflux (peptic) esophagitis
    2. Caustic esophagitis
    3. Vagotomy
    4. Radiation
  C. Infection
    1. Fungal: moniliasis
    2. Bacterial: tuberculosis, diphtheria
    3. Parasitic: Chagas' disease
    4. Viral: herpes simplex, cytomegalovirus
  D. Metabolic
    1. Diabetes
    2. Alcoholism
    3. Amyloidosis
    4. Serum pH and electrolyte disturbances (possibly)
  E. Endocrine disease
    1. Myxedema
    2. Thyrotoxicosis
  F. Neurologic disease
    1. Parkinsonism
    2. Huntington's chorea
    3. Wilson's disease
    4. Cerebrovascular disease
    5. Multiple sclerosis
    6. Amyotrophic lateral sclerosis
    7. Central nervous system neoplasm
    8. Bulbar poliomyelitis
    9. Pseudobulbar palsy
    10. Friedreich's hereditary spastic ataxia
    11. Familial dysautonomia (Riley-Day syndrome)
    12. Stiff man's syndrome
    13. Ganglioneuromatosis
  G. Muscular disease
    1. Myotonic dystrophy
    2. Muscular dystrophy
    3. Oculopharyngeal dystrophy
    4. Myasthenia gravis (neuromotor end-plate)
  H. Vascular
    1. Varices (possibly)
    2. Ischemia (possibly)
  I. Neoplasm
    1. Obstruction
    2. Neural invasion
  J. Pharmacologic
    1. Atropine, propantheline, curare, and so on

graphic examination. After swallowing peristalsis may occur normally, or the primary wave may "break" at some level, enabling barium to escape proximally (Fig. 11-7). For the qualitative evaluation of esophageal responses to swallowing, excellent correlation exists between the findings of fluoroscopy and manometry.[29]

The incidence of nonperistaltic contractions increases in many esophageal motility disorders. Because nonperistaltic contractions do not transport barium normally, they are often called *nonpropulsive contractions* when seen radiologically. Nonpropulsive contractions involve esophageal segments of variable length and displace barium both orally and aborally from the contraction site. As the contraction segment relaxes, the contrast material may return to the re-

laxed segment and stimulate a repetition of the sequence. The "to-and-fro" or "yo-yo" motion of barium results from uncoordinated esophageal activity and does not effect orderly esophageal emptying. Feeble repetitive, nonlumen-obliterating, nonperistaltic contractions may impart a scalloped configuration to the barium column, often referred to as *tertiary contractions* (Fig. 11-8). More forceful nonlumen-obliterating contractions may produce a corkscrew appearance, sometimes referred to as *curling* (Fig. 11-9, *A*). Lumen-obliterating, nonperistaltic contractions occurring simultaneously at several sites may cause compartmentalization of the barium column, giving it a rosary bead or shish kebab configuration (Fig. 11-9, *B*).

In selected patients a Mecholyl test may be helpful. An

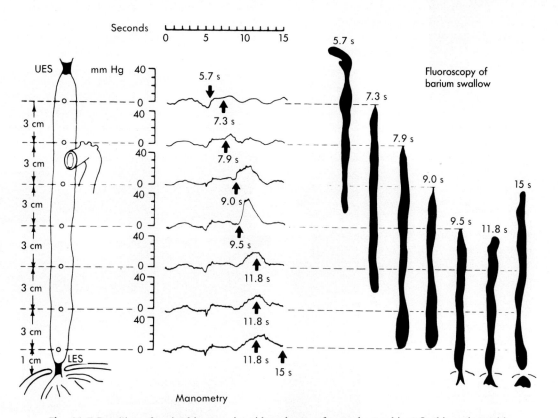

Fig. 11-7 Breaking of peristaltic wave in midesophagus of recumbent subject. In this patient with a nonspecific abnormality of esophageal motor function, 5-ml barium swallow was recorded by concurrent videoradiography and intraluminal esophageal manometry. Seven manometric recording sites, spaced at 3-cm intervals, were distributed along the length of the esophagus. Vertical arrows on each manometric tracing indicate time during swallow sequence that corresponds to video images on right. In the proximal half of the esophagus, normal propagating peristaltic pressure wave strips the swallowed barium bolus toward the stomach. A precise relationship exists between peristaltic pressure wave and video images in that the upstroke onset of peristaltic pressure corresponds to a passage of tail of the barium bolus. In the middle of the esophagus, the peristaltic wave fails, and only a low-amplitude simultaneous pressure wave is seen in the distal esophagus. Because of the failure of the peristaltic contraction wave, the transport of the barium bolus arrests in the distal half of the esophagus (9.5-second image), and then the barium washes back toward the proximal esophagus (15-second image).
From Kahrilas PJ et al: *Gastroenterology* 91:133, 1986.

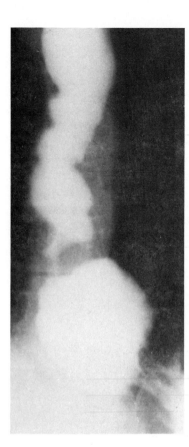

Fig. 11-8 Patient with reflux esophagitis. A sliding hiatus hernia is present. Most peristaltic stripping waves dissipated below the aortic arch level, and tertiary contractions are seen in the distal esophagus.

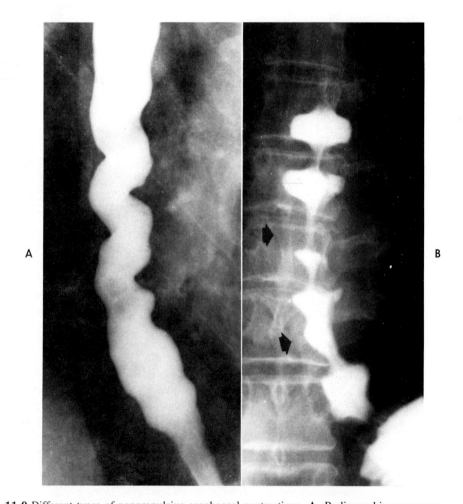

Fig. 11-9 Different types of nonpropulsive esophageal contractions. **A,** Radiographic appearance of "curling" or "corkscrew" esophagus in a patient with presbyesophagus. The helix configuration suggests a possible shortening of the spiral esophageal muscle. **B,** Esophageal segmentation in a patient with a diffuse esophageal spasm. Nonpropulsive, segmental contractions produce multiple areas of pronounced luminal narrowing alternating with areas of sacculation. This pattern causes transient functional obstruction. Esophageal wall *(arrows)* is thickened by muscle hypertrophy.

abnormal response generally indicates a deficiency of esophageal innervation. The cholinergic drug methacholine is injected subcutaneously, starting with a dose of 5 mg. If a positive response does not occur in 10 minutes, the dose is increased by 2.5-mg increments until a dose of 10 mg is reached. When present, an abnormal response occurs about 2 to 5 minutes after injection. On manometry a positive response consists of a sustained contraction of more than 25 mm Hg. For the radiographic examination, the patient is positioned recumbent and the esophagus is filled with barium. A positive response is seen as active, nonperistaltic contractions that culminate in a sustained lumen-obliterating contraction in the distal one half to two thirds of the esophagus (Fig. 11-10). Any significant side effects, such as chest pain, can be rapidly relieved by an intravenous injection of atropine.

Abnormal sphincter function associated with esophageal motility disorders is usually confined to the LES; however, abnormalities of UES function may occur. The UES may demonstrate increased or decreased resting pressure or abnormal relaxation. Abnormal UES relaxation or compliance is reflected as incomplete UES opening and abnormal pharyngeal drainage. Frank UES incompetence is rare and has been observed primarily in a few patients with myotonia congenita. Abnormal UES function is nearly always associated with significant disturbances of pharyngeal motor function.

The LES may show four abnormal patterns on manometry: (1) absent or incomplete relaxation; (2) low resting pressure (hypotensive sphincter); (3) increased resting pressure (hypertensive sphincter); and (4) abnormal peristaltic contractions. Absent or incomplete LES relaxation is seen as an abnormal LES opening on radiographs. In this case barium accumulates above the sphincter until the resting pressure transmitted to the column by an advancing peristaltic wave or hydrostatic forces overcomes the resistance

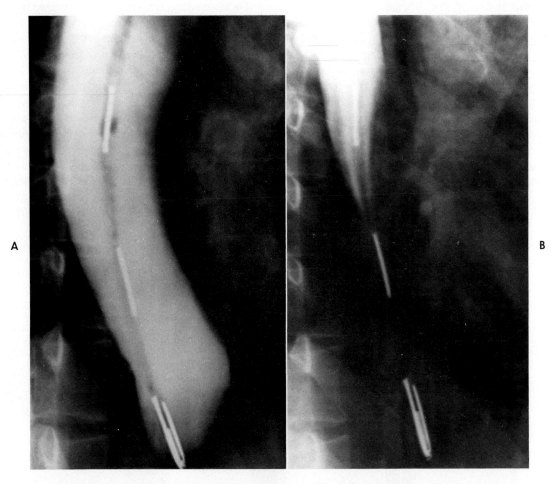

Fig. 11-10 Positive methacholine (Mecholyl) test on radiographic examination. Mercury markers are within monometric tube. Patient is recumbent. **A,** Before methacholine administration, the dilated esophagus is filled with barium. **B,** After administration of methacholine, the distal esophagus undergoes a forceful lumen-obliterating contraction that displaces all of the barium from the distal esophagus.

of the incompletely relaxed sphincter. Barium then wedges the sphincter open slightly and dribbles or squirts into the stomach. In the recumbent patient without normal esophageal body motor activity, swallowed barium often does not traverse the LES, even when the sphincter is relaxed. When the patient is erect, the hydrostatic pressure of the vertical barium column partially overcomes the resistance of an incompletely relaxed sphincter, thereby causing partial opening. It is often difficult, however, to determine whether a narrowed sphincter lumen is caused by incomplete relaxation, failed relaxation, localized stricture, or tumor infiltration. Testing with the smooth muscle relaxant amyl nitrite may distinguish abnormal LES relaxation from mechanical narrowing.[30]

Manometric studies have shown that an excessively low resting LES pressure, such as 5 mm Hg or less, is often associated with gastroesophageal reflux.[31] During the radiographic examination, gastroesophageal reflux of barium may occur in some patients with an incompetent LES. So-called free reflux is unprovoked, whereas stress reflux occurs during maneuvers designed to increase intraabdominal pressure. The radiographic examination, however, is a relatively insensitive method for identifying patients with significant gastroesophageal reflux, and negative results may be misleading.[31,32] Liquid barium is believed to have less tendency to reflux than gastric juice.[33] Also, in some individuals reflux episodes may occur in association with transient LES relaxations that occur intermittently against a background of normal resting LES tone.[34,35] In this circumstance, radiologic detection of gastroesophageal reflux is unlikely during the brief interval of observation.

Primary motility disorders
Achalasia

Clinical symptoms of achalasia are usually insidious in onset and generally develop when the patient is between 30 and 50 years of age. No sex predilection exists. The predominant symptom is dysphagia, which initially is frequently intermittent but later becomes persistent. Symptoms commonly associated with achalasia are foul breath, regurgitation, and aspiration. Chest pain associated with swallowing (odynophagia), a less frequent complaint, may lead to fear of swallowing.

Achalasia is believed to be caused mainly by an impairment or absence of ganglion cells of Auerbach's plexus. This finding, however, is not always present, and electron microscopy has shown degenerative vagal nerve changes and decreased cell bodies in the medullary dorsal motor nucleus.[36] Thus in some patients the primary defect appears to be located in the extraesophageal parasympathetic nerve supply and the esophageal changes are secondary.

On manometry, achalasia is characterized by absent peristalsis in most or all of the esophageal body and by absent or incomplete LES relaxation.[37] Repetitive, nonpropulsive esophageal contractions may be present. Motor function of the pharynx and UES is invariably normal. LES pressure is generally elevated.[37] The response to Mecholyl is nearly always positive,[38] but a positive response may also occur in some patients with diffuse esophageal spasm, Chagas' disease, pseudoobstruction syndrome, and other entities.

On radiographic examination, peristalsis is typically absent in the entire esophageal body, but in some patients peristalsis may progress to the aortic arch level.[39] A strip-

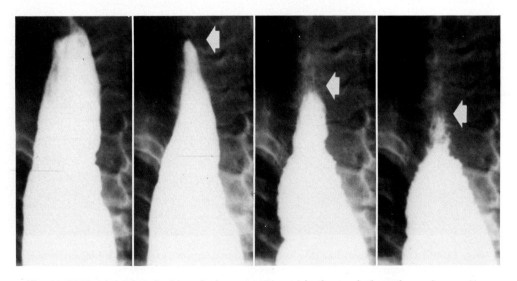

Fig. 11-11 Esophageal peristaltic stripping wave *(arrow)* in the cervical esophagus in a patient with achalasia. (With each swallow, peristalsis "broke" at the level of the thoracic inlet.)

ping wave in the proximal few centimeters of the cervical esophagus (Fig. 11-11) occurs in about one third of patients that otherwise fulfill all criteria for classic achalasia.[40] This finding accompanied by normal function of the striated muscle in the pharynx and UES suggests that achalasia is a disorder of esophageal smooth muscle innervation with secondary decompensation of the striated muscle portion of the esophagus. Nonperistaltic esophageal body contractions occurring spontaneously, after swallows, or both may be a predominant finding, especially when esophageal dilatation is mild to moderate. This variation is sometimes termed *vigorous achalasia*.[22] With severe dilatation, or megaesophagus, the esophagus is usually atonic (Fig. 11-12).

Because the LES does not relax normally, it fails to open normally after a swallow of barium. Barium remains above the closed sphincter until the pressure transmitted through the fluid column by esophageal contractions or hydrostatic pressure overcomes the resistance of the unrelaxed sphincter. The LES is then wedged open, and barium dribbles or squirts into the stomach through the narrow sphincter lumen. The head of the barium column often assumes an elongated V-shaped configuration, likened to a bird's beak (Fig. 11-13). A bird-beak configuration, however, is not specific for achalasia. It may be caused by any disorder associated with failed LES relaxation. For example, some patients with presbyesophagus, diffuse esophageal spasm, or connective tissue disease demonstrate failure of LES relaxation in response to swallows during manometry.[24,41,42] The LES segment may also have a bird-beak configuration in some instances of fibrotic stricture of surrounding hematoma, or when involved with a constricting annular carcinoma ex-

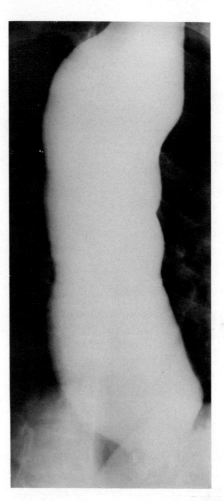

Fig. 11-12 Megaesophagus in a patient with achalasia.

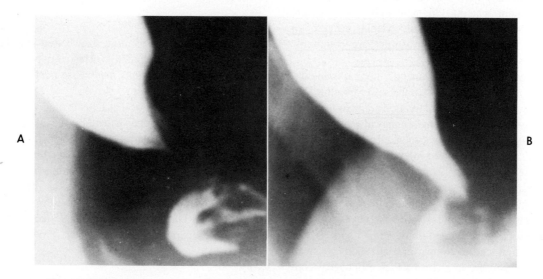

Fig. 11-13 Achalasia. **A,** A failure of the normal lower sphincter opening produces persistent V configuration of the head of the barium column, above the sphincter. **B,** The point of the V elongates (bird-beak appearance) as barium wedges into the sphincter and squirts into the stomach.

tending from the gastric fundus (Fig. 11-14). In this latter circumstance the tumor may cause motor abnormalities in the esophageal body that may be caused by high-grade obstruction or tumor infiltration of the esophageal wall, causing damage to the nerves.[43,44] This condition may simulate achalasia so closely that the true diagnosis is not established until the time of Heller's myotomy. The amyl nitrite test may identify patients with pseudoachalasia.[30] Patients with tumor infiltration of the cardia almost invariably have significant weight loss, and the dysphagia is generally of less than 6 months' duration.[45]

Some patients manifest esophageal motor disturbances, yet unclassified, that approximate achalasia.[46,47] Such patients have clinical complaints similar to those of achalasia, but peristalsis, LES relaxation, or both occur after some swallows.

Diffuse esophageal spasm

Although simultaneous, nonpropulsive esophageal contractions may be associated with a large number of esophageal motility disturbances,[48] Certain individuals manifest a clinical syndrome characterized by (1) symptoms of intermittent dysphagia and chest pain; (2) forceful simultaneous, repetitive contractions on manometry; (3) segmental, lumen-obliterating contractions seen on radiographs; and commonly (4) thickening of the esophageal wall. When this syndrome occurs without obvious cause, it is termed *idiopathic diffuse esophageal spasm* (DES). Occasionally, a DES pattern may result from esophagitis. The patients are usually middle-aged. Dysphagia and pain are characteristically intermittent and frequently elicited by eating, particularly when swallowing a large bolus. Symptoms may also occur spontaneously, even when waking the patient from sleep. The pain may be severe and mimic angina. Occasionally, a patient who has frequent episodes of severe symptoms when eating may lose weight because of odynophagia. Patients with this disorder are commonly classified as psychoneurotics.

On manometry, peristalsis is generally normal in the upper one third of the esophagus.[49] In the lower two thirds of the esophagus, nonperistaltic contractions, single or repetitive, generally follow swallowing but may also occur spontaneously. A normal peristaltic sequence traversing the entire esophagus may be observed intermittently. Generally, the LES relaxes normally.[24,50]

On radiographic examination peristalsis may occur in the upper esophagus in response to some or all swallows. Nonperistaltic contractions are observed in the smooth muscle part of the esophagus. Lumen-obliterating nonperistaltic contractions often cause compartmentalization of swallowed barium, resulting in a shish kebab esophageal configuration (see Fig. 11-9, *B*) and functional obstruction. Barium is displaced both proximally and distally from multiple contraction sites. As the contractions relax, the barium may resume a columnar configuration, only to be disrupted again and again by repetitive contractions. Esopha-

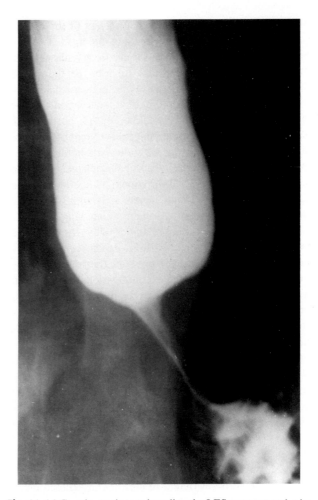

Fig. 11-14 Gastric carcinoma invading the LES segment and mimicking achalasia. Bird-beak appearance of distal esophagus, esophageal dilatation, and aperistalsis were indistinguishable from that of idiopathic achalasia.

geal wall thickening of more than 5 mm may be seen on radiographs of good quality.[49] Muscle hypertrophy or sustained muscle contractions may cause persistent narrowing of the esophageal lumen.

Some workers believe that DES is part of the same spectrum as achalasia. Some patients with DES exhibit a hypersensitive esophageal response to Mecholyl.[51] Transition of a DES pattern into achalasia has been observed,[52,53] and after LES dilatation some patients with achalasia develop a motor pattern simulating DES.[54] On the other hand, electron microscopy of surgical or postmortem specimens from patients with DES and achalasia suggests that the two disorders are separate entities.[55]

Hypertensive peristalsis

A condition of symptomatic hypertensive peristalsis, often termed *the nutcracker esophagus,* is now recognized.[56] Some individuals with this entity experience chest pain or dysphagia associated with excessively forceful peristaltic contractions that register 200 mm Hg or more in the smooth muscle part of the esophagus. At fluoroscopy peristaltic transport of the barium appears entirely normal, and the diagnosis must be made by manometry. Some individuals with hypertensive esophageal peristalsis exhibit intermittent findings of DES.

Idiopathic intestinal pseudoobstruction

Chronic idiopathic intestinal pseudoobstruction (CIIP) is a rare syndrome characterized by symptoms and radiographic findings of intestinal obstruction in the absence of a mechanical obstruction or known underlying cause of paralytic ileus. Accompanying abnormalities of esophageal motor function are commonly present.[57] The underlying abnormality may involve either the neural or myogenic components of intestinal smooth muscle motor function.[58-60] These heterogeneous abnormalities tend to affect most if not all of the alimentary tract. The afflicted patients are of either sex, and the condition is commonly hereditary.[61] Characteristically the patients have recurrent attacks of transient abdominal pain and distention accompanied by vomiting. Commonly, unnecessary abdominal surgery is done for the mistaken diagnosis of mechanical small bowel obstruction. Many patients complain of constipation. Although esophageal symptoms are not common, some patients complain of dysphagia.

On radiographic examination, the small bowel usually exhibits distention and delayed transit, simulating the appearance of small bowel obstruction. The colon is usually redundant, is slightly dilated, and may manifest numerous diverticula. Megacolon may develop. Some patients have gastric distention and delayed emptying. Megaduodenum is a relatively common finding. The esophagus generally exhibits abnormal motor function.[57] Some patients have abnormal peristalsis and feeble nonperistaltic contractions in the smooth muscle part of the esophagus. Others demonstrate abnormal LES opening caused by incomplete LES relaxation and forceful nonperistaltic contractions in the thoracic esophagus. These findings mimic those of achalasia. An atonic megaesophagus simulates classic achalasia, and the Mecholyl test may be positive. With CIIP, esophageal motor dysfunction is unlikely without accompanying abnormalities in intestinal motor function.

Presbyesophagus

Prebyesophagus is an esophageal motor dysfunction associated with aging.[42] Aberrations in esophageal motility occur commonly in elderly persons after age 70 years. About 20% to 50% of elderly individuals manifest some abnormality of esophageal motor function, but generally these individuals are without esophageal symptoms. Occasionally, a patient with presbyesophagus may complain of dysphagia for solids.

The manometric abnormalities of presbyesophagus include (1) a decreased incidence of complete peristaltic sequences; (2) an increased prevalence of nonperistaltic contractions; and (3) an increased incidence of incomplete LES relaxation with swallows.[42,62,63] The proposed underlying cause is a decreased number of esophageal ganglion cells associated with aging.[64] Mecholyl, however, seldom produces an abnormal response. In one study the predominant finding was decreased strength of peristaltic contractions, whereas the incidence of peristalsis and the frequency of nonperistaltic contractions were similar to those of younger subjects.[65] This latter study suggests that the primary defect may be muscle atrophy rather than abnormal innervation. Muscle thickness, however, is reported to be normal in the aged.[64]

On radiographic examination, a spectrum of abnormalities may be observed. Commonly, peristalsis traverses only the upper esophagus, and occasionally no peristaltic activity is identified. Tertiary contractions or other forms of nonperistaltic contractions (see Fig. 11-9, *A*) often involve a long segment of the distal esophagus.[66] The LES segment may demonstrate either normal opening or may consistently fail to relax, imparting a bird-beak configuration to the head of the barium column. Patients with partial or total failure of peristalsis and LES relaxation may have esophageal dilatation that is usually mild to moderate but occasionally may be pronounced. Presbyesophagus may mimic achalasia, diffuse esophageal spasm, connective tissue disorders, or other motility disturbances.[67] The diagnosis is one of exclusion in an elderly patient.

Tracheoesophageal fistula

Children with congenital tracheoesophageal (TE) fistula and esophageal atresia generally have a primary abnormality of esophageal motor function.[68] The motility disturbance is attributed to an embryologic ischemic defect[69] that results in the TE fistula and atresia. In atresia the motility abnormality is not recognized until after operative repair of the TE fistula and esophageal atresia. Despite successful surgery, these children often suffer from aspiration and dysphagia caused by abnormal esophageal motility.[70,71] Radiographic and manometric studies demonstrate a discontinuity of normal peristaltic function in a 6- to 15-cm esophageal segment that extends above and below the surgical anastomosis. In response to swallowing, the abnormal segment either is amotile or exhibits feeble nonperistaltic contraction. Stripping peristaltic contraction waves are often observed proximal and distal to the abnormal segment. The LES may be normal or incompetent.

Children with an H-type TE fistula commonly have esophageal motor dysfunction[72] similar to that described for patients with TE fistula and atresia. The findings of an amotile or hypomotile esophageal segment in a child with recurrent pneumonia should alert the fluoroscopist to the possibility of an underlying H-type TE fistula.

Chalasia

On radiographic examination, some reflux of barium associated with crying or belching is commonly observed in newborn infants. Copious gross reflux in the newborn or

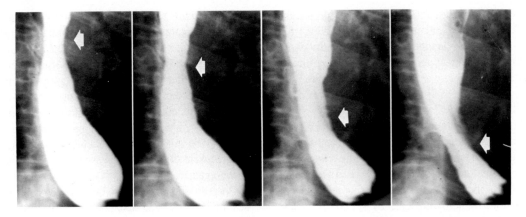

Fig. 11-15 A patient with scleroderma. Feeble, non-lumen-obliterating peristaltic contraction wave *(arrows)* is seen to pass through the distal esophagus. Esophageal peristalsis was normal above the aortic arch level.

moderate reflux after 4 to 6 weeks of age, however, is abnormal.[73] In 1947, a condition in neonates characterized by repetitive episodes of vomiting and cardioesophageal relaxation (chalasia) was described by Neuhauser and Barenberg.[74] The condition was attributed to dysfunction of the LES caused by delayed development of neuromuscular control. Subsequent studies, however, indicated that LES hypotonia is generally not present in infants with undue gastroesophageal reflux.[75] Many of these infants have an associated hiatal hernia.[76] An important mechanism for gastroesophageal reflux in some infants is transient LES relaxation, rather[77] than persistently low basal LES tone.

Secondary motility disorders
Connective tissue disorders

The association of esophageal motor dysfunction and connective tissue disease is documented best for scleroderma (systemic sclerosis). This condition develops insidiously, most often during the third and fourth decades of life, and affects women three times as often as men. Earlier reports suggested that the majority of patients complain of dysphagia.[78-80] but more recent studies establish that the predominant clinical complaint is heartburn.[81] At postmortem examination the esophagus is abnormal in about 75% of the patients.[78] Atrophy of the esophageal smooth muscle is the predominant histologic abnormality.[78,82] A possible explanation is that an intestinal Raynaud's phenomenon causes ischemia that results in smooth muscle atrophy. Neural dysfunction has also been suggested as a cause of impaired esophageal function.[23,82] Fibrosis, when present, appears to replace the atrophic smooth muscle.[78] Findings of reflux esophagitis are common.[78]

Because smooth muscle atrophy is the major abnormality in esophageal scleroderma, the pattern of abnormal function can be readily predicted. Peristalsis is feeble or absent in the distal two thirds of the esophagus, and a hypotonic LES commonly loses its ability to prevent gastroesophageal reflux. On manometry, abnormal peristalsis in the thoracic

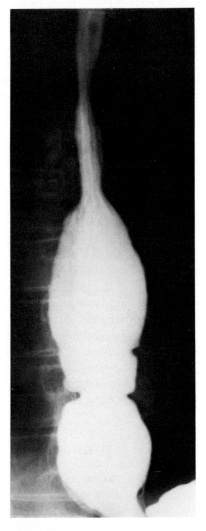

Fig. 11-16 Scleroderma. Distal third of the esophagus is moderately dilated, and a hiatus hernia is present. A feeble peristaltic wave, which allowed the proximal escape of barium, is seen in the midesophagus. During fluoroscopy, no muscular activity was seen in the distal esophagus, and barium refluxed freely from the stomach into the esophagus. Peristalsis was normal in the proximal esophagus.

esophagus is present in 80% to 85% of patients with scleroderma.[79,84] When the motility disturbance is mild, the only abnormality is a reduced incidence of primary peristalsis. With moderate impairment, the amplitude of peristaltic complexes is low and occasionally nonperistaltic contractions occur. Sometimes a DES pattern may be the predominant abnormality early in the course of the disease.[79] With severe impairment, the thoracic esophagus becomes essentially amotile. Nonperistaltic contractions are seldom present. Abnormal peristalsis in the proximal, striated muscle portion of the esophageal segment has been reported[84] but is unusual.[79] LES tone is decreased or absent in about half of the patients.[79,84] Failure of LES relaxation is uncommon but may occur.[41]

On radiographic examination, peristalsis nearly always appears normal above the aortic arch level, but below this level abnormal function is observed in about 70% of patients.[79] Primary peristalsis may be decreased in incidence, and the contractile wave may appear feeble. The latter finding is seen as a nonlumen-obliterating contraction that moves aborally but allows a substantial portion of the barium bolus to escape proximally (Fig. 11-15). Subtle abnormalities in peristalsis may be unmasked by positioning the patient in a 30- to 50-degree headdown position that forces peristalsis to work against gravity. When the motor disor-

der is severe, the amotile distal esophagus may become distended, but esophageal dilatation is generally mild to moderate. With the patient supine, barium pools in the esophagus but readily empties into the stomach when the patient is positioned upright. The LES may be patulous, and free gastroesophageal reflux is often observed. A hiatus hernia (Fig. 11-16) and radiographic features of esophagitis are commonly present.[79]

Abnormal esophageal motility may occur with connective tissue diseases other than scleroderma, such as systemic lupus erythematosus, Raynaud's disease, and dermatomyositis.[80,85] Disturbed esophageal motility accompanying lupus or Raynaud's disease may be similar in pattern to that of scleroderma. In contrast, dermatomyositis often causes abnormal function of the pharynx or proximal striated muscle part of the esophagus.[86] In dermatomyositis, motor dysfunction may also involve the smooth muscle esophageal segment.[41]

Reflux (peptic) esophagitis

Abnormal esophageal motor function is relatively common in patients with reflux esophagitis.[87,88] Functional abnormalities are generally confined to the smooth muscle portion of the esophagus and include abnormal peristalsis, nonperistaltic contractions, and gastroesophageal reflux.

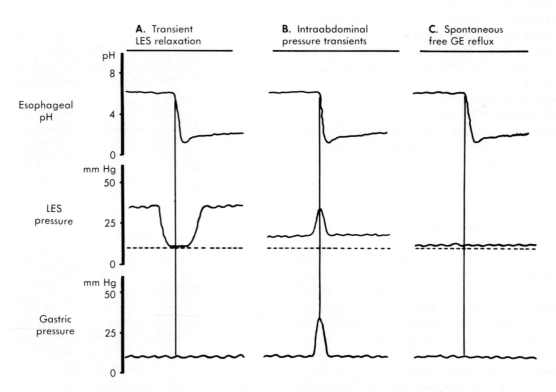

Fig. 11-17 Schematic representation of three general mechanisms responsible for the gastroesophageal reflux. Esophageal pH was recorded from the distal esophagus by a pH electrode. Lower esophageal sphincter (LES) pressure and gastric pressure were recorded concurrently by manometry. Acid gastroesophageal reflux *(vertical line)* may accompany a transient LES relaxation **(A),** develop as stress reflux during transient increase in intraabdominal pressure that overcomes a sphincter with low tone **(B),** or occur as a spontaneous free reflux across the atonic sphincter **(C).** From Dodds WJ et al: *N Engl J Med* 308:1547, 1982.

Earlier studies using low-fidelity manometric recording systems suggested that about two thirds of the patients with mild esophagitis and 85% of patients with moderate or severe esophagitis have esophageal body motor dysfunction.[89,90] A recent study from our manometry laboratory suggests that up to 50% of patients with reflux esophagitis show abnormalities in esophageal body motility and the prevalence of abnormal motor function correlates with esophagitis severity.[88] Resting LES pressure is normal in the majority of patients.[87,91]

On radiographic examination, motor disturbances include (1) a decreased incidence of peristalsis; (2) repetitive breaking of the peristaltic wave in the distal esophagus; (3) nonperistaltic contractions; (4) amotility of the distal esophagus; and (5) gastroesophageal reflux. Motor function of the pharynx, UES, and striated esophageal muscle are almost invariably normal. The most common abnormality is that peristalsis propagates through the proximal esophagus but fails to traverse the entire esophagus, usually the lower one third to one half of the esophagus (Figs. 11-7 and 11-16). Impaired esophageal motor function leads to delayed acid clearance.[92,93] In areas of esophageal narrowing caused by inflammation or stricture, muscle activity is frequently feeble or absent. One report suggests that peptic esophagitis may abolish peristalsis over the entire esophagus,[94] but this variation appears to be rare. Acid barium (pH 1.7) has been proposed as a means of inducing abnormal esophageal motility patterns in patients with esophagitis who demonstrate a normal pattern using standard liquid barium.[95] The test, however, generates false-positive responses and is not widely used at present.

Even with the use of vigorous stress maneuvers, gastroesophageal reflux is demonstrated fluoroscopically in only about 40% of patients who have endoscopic evidence of reflux esophagitis.[31,32] The incidence of gastroesophageal reflux is increased somewhat by employing the water siphon test,[96] but at the expense of obtaining an unacceptably high incidence of positive findings in normal subjects. With this latter test, the LES pressure barrier undergoes physiologic relaxation with swallowing, and the potential for gastroesophageal reflux during this interval is determined by the integrity of esophageal peristalsis and other factors. In the past it was widely believed that LES incompetence in patients with esophagitis was caused by feeble LES tone.[97] The majority of the patients, however, have normal resting LES pressure. What, then, accounts for the paradox that barium reflux cannot be induced in many patients with proved esophagitis? A standard explanation was that barium and gastric juice differ in specific gravity, thereby resulting in different flow dynamics.[33] Recent observations, however, provide an alternative explanation.[34,88] Simultaneous recordings of LES pressure and esophageal pH show that nearly all episodes of gastroesophageal reflux in normal subjects and also the majority of patients with esophagitis are caused mainly by transient LES relaxation lasting 5 to 20 seconds, (Fig. 11-17), rather than by sustained low basal LES pressure. Because these LES relaxations occur intermittently at random, gastroesophageal reflux is unlikely to occur during the short interval of fluoroscopic observation. When LES pressure is more than 10 mm Hg, resistance of the sphincter cannot be overcome by even heroic stress maneuvers that cause substantial increases in intraabdominal pressure. Therefore the radiographic demonstration of reproducible stress or free gastroesophageal reflux, found in 30% to 40% of patients with esophagitis, indicates a feeble LES (Fig. 11-18).

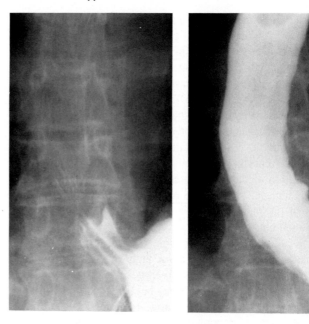

Fig. 11-18 Free gastroesophageal reflux of barium in a recumbent patient with endoscopic evidence of mild esophagitis. **A,** The stomach is filled with barium and a small hiatus hernia is present. **B,** One second later a large amount of barium refluxed spontaneously into the esophagus. On subsequent esophageal manometry, LES pressure measured less than 5 mm Hg.

Postvagotomy syndrome

Postoperative dysphagia is a recognized complication of bilateral vagotomy, particularly transthoracic truncal vagotomy. The dysphagia is severe in about 1% of patients,[98] but mild symptoms may occur in 10% of patients.[99] Swallowing difficulty is first noted 1 to 2 weeks after vagotomy, when a diet of solid foods is started. Postvagotomy dysphagia was attributed initially to interruption of vagal fibers to the LES.[100] Current evidence, however, suggests that the syndrome is usually caused by postoperative edema, hematoma, or fibrosis involving the distal esophagus. Recent animal studies suggest preganglionic fibers to the LES enter the esophagus proximally and then travel intramurally to reach the sphincter.[101] Distal truncal vagotomy would not affect such fibers.

In symptomtic patients radiographic examination generally shows narrowing of the distal esophagus and mild esophageal dilatation, a pattern suggestive of early achalasia. Manometry, esophagography, or a combination of both is usually necessary to determine whether the radiographic abnormalities are caused by postoperative structural changes or vagal denervation. The dysphagia caused by hematoma or vagal denervation usually remits spontaneously in several weeks to several months. Rarely, narrowing caused by fibrosis may persist and require bougienage or surgery.[100]

Metabolic and endocrine disorders

Metabolic disorders such as diabetes[102,103] and chronic alcoholism,[104,105] particularly when associated with peripheral neuropathy, may cause abnormal esophageal motor function. The underlying mechanism is thought to be vagal neuropathy. Despite abnormal esophageal motor function, the clinical symptoms are infrequent. On barium swallows the following abnormalities may be observed in either diabetics or alcoholics: decreased incidence of peristalsis, breaking of the peristaltic waves in the proximal esophagus, delayed esophageal emptying, and nonpropulsive contractions.[103,106]

The GI tract is a site of predilection for amyloidosis, and esophageal involvement may occur. Amyloid deposits in the esophageal musculature may cause loss of peristalsis and megaesophagus.[107]

The effect of systemic acidosis and alkalosis and electrolyte disturbances on esophageal function in humans has not been systematically studied, but abnormal motor function might be anticipated. Hypercalcemia is associated with decreased strength of esophageal smooth muscle.[108]

Abnormalities of esophageal peristalsis have been noted also in patients with myoedema or hyperthyroidism. Myxedema causes a decreased incidence of peristalsis.[109] Thyrotoxicosis may cause a pattern of diffuse esophageal spasm[110] and abnormal relaxation of the UES. In one study the only manometric abnormality demonstrated in thyrotoxicosis was an increased velocity of peristalsis that returned to normal after the patients became euthyroid.[111]

Neuromuscular disease

Swallowing difficulties may accompany a variety of neuromuscular disorders. Esophageal dysfunction in these conditions is often overshadowed by more pronounced pharyngeal abnormalities.[110,112] The pattern of esophageal dysfunction in most of the neuromuscular disorders is generally variable and nonspecific. In practice the diagnosis of neuromuscular disease is usually known, and the examination is done to determine the extent and severity of motor dysfunction rather than as a diagnostic test.

Diseases affecting the central nervous system cause significant disturbances of esophageal function when the supranuclear pathways to the medullary brainstem swallow centers are impaired bilaterally.[112] Diseases of the extrapyramidal nervous system, such as parkinsonism,[113] Huntington's chorea, and Wilson's disease, may also cause abnormal esophageal function. Patients with parkinsonism, for example, may have a decreased incidence of peristalsis, complete loss of peristalsis, or nonperistaltic contractions.[110] Patients with extrapyramidal diseases often exhibit unintentional tremors of the tongue that decrease or disappear during swallowing.[112] Conditions involving the brainstem nuclei, such as vertebrobasilar or posteroinferior cerebral artery insufficiency, amyotrophic lateral sclerosis, multiple sclerosis, neoplasm, or bulbar palsy, may cause feeble or absent peristalsis and nonpropulsive contractions.[114,115] Such conditions may also cause abnormal cricopharyngeal relaxation.[112] Impaired esophageal peristalsis and abnormal cricopharyngeal function also occur in familial dysautonomia[116,117] and hereditary spastic ataxia.[87] In stiff man's syndrome the striated muscle portion of the esophagus may demonstrate spastic contractions.[118] Ganglioneuromatosis associated with multiple endocrine adenomatosis type II syndrome may alter esophageal peristalsis.

Although primary muscle diseases such as myotonia[119,120] and muscular and oculopharyngeal dystrophy[121,122] may cause motor dysfunction limited to the proximal striated muscle esophageal segment, motor dysfunction may also occur in the distal smooth muscle portion of the esophagus. In patients with myotonic dystrophy the UES may be incompetent.[123] The UES segment may occasionally remain open at rest, resulting in an uninterrupted column of barium extending from the pharynx to the esophagus.[123] With myotonia motor function may improve during repetitive swallows.[112] Esophageal dysfunction caused by myasthenia gravis is generally limited to the proximal striated muscle portion of the esophagus (Fig. 11-19). On the initial barium swallow, esophageal peristalsis may appear normal. During repeated swallows, peristalsis in the upper esophagus often becomes feeble or disappears completely.[110] Occasionally, peristalsis may be abnormal in the distal esophagus. Myasthenia is the only disease in which esophageal dysfunction may improve following the administration of a cholinesterase inhibitor, such as edrophonium chloride (Tensilon).[110]

Miscellaneous disorders

Although a variety of different pathogens may cause esophageal motor dysfunction, a characteristic motility disturbance is present only in Chagas' disease. This disease, endemic to areas of South America, is caused by *Trypanosoma cruzi*. Afflicted individuals usually complain of progressive dysphagia. The organism infests the esophageal musculature and damages ganglion cells. Generally, peristalsis is intact initially in esophageal striated muscle and LES pressure values are normal. Initially, multiple uncoordinated contractions occur in esophageal smooth muscle,

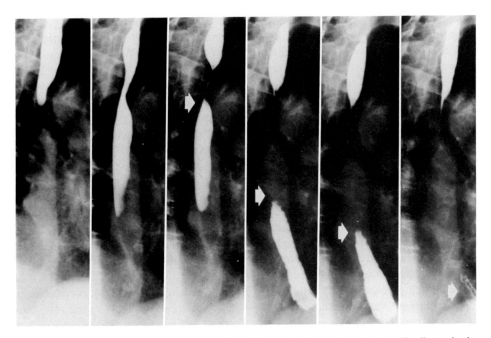

Fig. 11-19 Myasthenia gravis. Patient is supine. After a single swallow, barium distributes in the proximal two thirds of esophagus *(frames 1 and 2)*. No peristalsis occurs in the striated muscle esophageal segment; consequently, barium pools in the upper esophagus. Secondary peristaltic wave *(arrows)*, originating at the level of the aortic arch *(frame 3)*, sweeps barium from the arch level into the stomach.

whereas later the esophagus becomes dilated and amotile.[124] The response to Mecholyl is often positive. On barium examination, Chagas' disease and achalasia are generally indistinguishable.

Monilial esophagitis is commonly accompanied by loss of peristalsis in most or all of the esophagus.[125] Peristaltic function generally returns after successful treatment, unless an underlying motility disorder is present. After caustic ingestion the esophagus often demonstrates shock initially, with loss of peristaltic function. Peristalsis may return after several days, only to be subsequently obliterated if substantial fibrosis occurs.

Malignancy involving the proximal stomach, gastric cardia, or esophagus is occasionally associated with disturbance of esophageal motility and on radiographic and manometric examination may stimulate idiopathic DES[126] or achalasia.[44] In some patients, the motility disturbance may be caused by esophageal obstruction, whereas in others esophageal dysfunction may be caused by invasion of the myenteric plexus by tumor.[43]

Certain pharmacologic agents profoundly affect esophageal motor activity. Most general anesthetics nonselectively depress motor function of the entire esophagus. In contrast, other drugs act selectively on striated muscle or smooth muscle esophageal segments.[3] Striated muscle contraction is diminished by *d*-tubocurare.[127] Anticholinergics, such as atropine, diminish or abolish peristalsis in the distal esophagus and decrease resting LES pressure.[3,128,129] For hypo-

tonic esophagography peristalsis may be abolished by an anticholinergic agent.[130] Glucagon decreases LES pressure but has a negligible effect on motor function of the esophageal body.[131]

Differential diagnosis

Evaluation of esophageal function requires a pertinent clinical history. Important items include not only esophageal symptoms, but also conditions known to cause esophageal dysfunction. The radiographic examination may show different patterns of abnormal esophageal motor function. Consideration of the predominant abnormality may be helpful in approaching the correct diagnosis. Evaluation of the entire GI tract may provide clues about the nature of the esophageal motor abnormality. For example, abnormalities of the small bowel or colon are generally observed in scleroderma, idiopathic intestinal pseudoobstruction, Chagas' disease, amyloidosis, and myotonic dystrophy.

Esophageal dilatation

Severe esophageal dilatation (megaesophagus) is usually caused by idiopathic achalasia (see Fig. 11-12). Other causes of megaesophagus include Chagas' disease, idiopathic intestinal pseudoobstruction, amyloidosis,[107] Ehlers-Danlos syndrome,[132] and presbyesophagus. Tumor infiltration or fibrosis of the cardia must also be considered. Patients with Chagas' disease are nearly always from South America and often have cardiomegaly, megaureters, and megacolon. Amyloidosis of the esophagus is usually accompanied by other intestinal abnormalities. Mild to moderate esophageal dilatation has numerous causes.

Abnormal peristalsis (proximal esophagus)

The finding of feeble or absent peristalsis, primarily in the proximal esophagus, may occur in diseases that affect predominantly striated muscle (myotonic dystrophy, muscular dystrophy, myasthenia gravis [Fig. 11-19], and dermatomyositis), some neurologic disorders involving the brainstem (such as poliomyelitis and amyotrophic lateral sclerosis), and tracheoesophageal fistula. In some instances peristalsis is also abnormal in the distal esophagus. When a neuromuscular disorder causes proximal esophageal dysfunction, abnormalities in pharyngeal motor function are usually present. Myotonia may cause a patulous, incompetent upper esophageal sphincter. Patients with myasthenia often show deterioration of pharyngeal and esophageal striated muscle function during repetitive swallows and improvement of function following administration of edrophonium chloride.

Abnormal peristalsis (distal esophagus)

Feeble or absent peristalsis in the distal two thirds or smooth muscle part of the esophagus occurs characteristically in scleroderma (see Fig. 11-16) but may be found also in other connective tissue disorders and miscellaneous other conditions, including esophagitis, presbyesophagus, alcoholism, diabetes, idiopathic intestinal pseudoobstruction, myxedema, anticholinergic medication, and variants of achalasia. In scleroderma, nonperistaltic contractions are seldom observed. Anticholinergic agents suppress smooth muscle function and may produce a pattern of esophageal dysfunction identical to that of scleroderma. Motor dysfunction of the distal esophageal body caused by esophagitis may be accompanied by gastroesophageal reflux, and generally a hiatal hernia is present. Idiopathic intestinal pseudoobstruction syndrome will invariably have abnormal findings of the intestine. A correct diagnosis of esophageal dysfunction often depends on obtaining the relevant clinical history of alcoholism, diabetes, myxedema, or hyperthyroidism. Esophageal wall thickening suggests DES.

Nonpropulsive contractions

Infrequent nonpropulsive esophageal contractions accompany a large number of esophageal disorders but may also be seen in normal persons. Vigorous, repetitive, nonpropulsive contractions (see Fig. 11-9) are clearly abnormal. They occur most commonly in diffuse esophageal spasm, esophagitis, and presbyesophagus, but also occur in other conditions, including achalasia, scleroderma, metabolic disorders, neuromuscular diseases, and esophageal obstruction. Idiopathic diffuse esophageal spasm and esophagitis are often accompanied by significant thickening of the esophageal wall, hiatus hernia, or both. If free

gastroesophageal reflux is demonstrated (see Fig. 11-18), esophageal dysfunction may be caused by esophagitis.

Abnormal lower esophageal sphincter opening

Abnormal LES opening may be caused by absent or incomplete LES relaxation (see Fig. 11-13), infiltrating neoplasm (see Fig. 11-14), benign stricture, or hematoma. Failure of LES relaxation occurs characteristically in idiopathic achalasia and Chagas' disease. On radiographic examination the unrelaxed sphincter imparts a bird-beak configuration to the head of the barium column, accompanied by some degree of esophageal dilatation and incomplete esophageal emptying. Some patients with DES, presbyesophagus, idiopathic intestinal pseudoobstruction, or other motility disorders may exhibit failure of LES relaxation in response to all swallows during manometry. Esophagoscopy and biopsy may be necessary to exclude organic lesions. Computed tomography (CT) is also useful for demonstrating a malignancy involving the cardia that may present as pseudoachalasia (Fig. 11-20).

Gastroesophageal reflux

Although gastroesophageal reflux of barium is occasionally observed in normal subjects, copious free reflux is rare in healthy individuals. Most individuals who demonstrate free gastroesophageal reflux (see Fig. 11-18) have reflux symptoms and often demonstrate esophagitis on endoscopy and LES hypotension on manometry. An accompanying hiatus hernia is generally present. In addition to garden-variety reflux and peptic esophagitis, other conditions that may be associated with overt gastroesophageal reflux on radiographs include Barrett's esophagus, scleroderma, brain damage, repaired esophageal atresia, and anticholinergic medication.

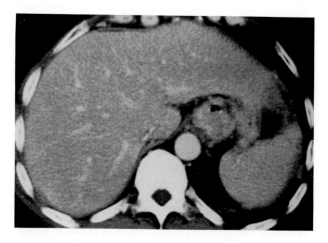

Fig. 11-20 CT of cardia in a patient with pseudoachalasia. A tumor mass is seen involving the distal esophagus and the region of the esophagogastric junction. An eccentric esophagel lumen, identified by a small column of air, is displaced ventrally.

CONGENITAL ANOMALIES

Congenital anomalies of the esophagus are usually apparent clinically in the neonatal period but in some instances may not cause symptoms until later in childhood or during adult life.

Atresia and tracheoesophageal fistula

The incidence of esophageal atresia and TE fistula is about 1 in 2000 live births.[133] There is no sex or familial predilection. Afflicted infants are commonly premature, and about half have other congenital abnormalities.[69] Favored notions of causes include failure of the embryonic esophagus to recanalize and deficiencies in esophageal blood supply. A classification of esophageal atresia and TE fistula is shown in Fig. 11-21.

Esophageal atresia should be suspected in all infants who have unexplained respiratory distress, spit up food, or have a maternal history of polyhydramnios. Infants with esophageal atresia and a TE fistula to the distal esophageal segment often develop gaseous abdominal distention, whereas those with atresia alone or TE fistula to the proximal esophagus have a gasless abdomen. These features as well as findings of pneumonitis or atelectasis are often evident on chest radiographs. In some cases the dilated proximal esophageal pouch may be distended sufficiently with air to compress the trachea. A dilated esophageal pouch needs to be distinguished from cervical gas associated with pharyngeal perforation, commonly caused in infants by false passage of a nasogastric tube.[134]

Definitive diagnosis of esophageal atresia includes the inability to pass a nasogastric tube into the stomach. If necessary, 0.5 to 1 ml of thin barium can be injected into the pouch for visualization and then aspirated. After resection of the atresia and anastomosis of the esophagus, some children demonstrate subsequent narrowing at the anastomotic site. Invariably peristalsis is absent over a long central esophageal segment or occasionally in the whole esophagus.[68] Some children exhibit LES incompetence and may demonstrate reflux esophagitis with stricture. After surgery a TE fistula recurs in 10%.[135]

H-type TE fistulas are frequently not diagnosed until late infancy or early in childhood. The cardinal feature is recurrent unexplained pneumonia. Commonly the initial radiographic examination fails to show the abnormality. A clue to the presence of an H-type fistula, however, is absent peristalsis in the proximal half or middle third of the esophagus.[72] For radiographic diagnosis the esophagus should be intubated with a single-hole catheter and the infant positioned prone or on the side. Most H-type fistulas run cephalad from the esophagus to the trachea and are located in the proximal esophagus (Fig. 11-22). Occasionally, multiple fistulas are present. Dilute barium is injected into the esophagus, beginning just above the LES and progressing proximally. Tracheal filling via an H-type fistula must be distinguished from pharyngeal regurgitation and aspira-

tion. In some instances, only tracheal filling is evident and the tiny H-type fistula may not be visualized directly. Rarely, an H-type fistula is associated with tracheal stenosis caused by ectopic esophageal tissue.[136]

Duplication

Esophageal duplication is rare. About two thirds are found in symptomatic children and the remainder as an incidental finding in adults. In infants the duplication may cause respiratory symptoms by compressing the trachea, rupturing into the esophageal lumen, or bleeding or by perforation when it is lined by functional gastric mucosa.[137] Rarely, the entire esophagus may be involved, giving a double-barrel esophagus when the duplication communicates.[138] Most duplications, however, are segmental and generally located in the lower posterior mediastinum. Esophageal duplications are of two types: (1) intramural cyst, representing true duplications arising from persistent vacuoles that normally reconstitute the esophageal lumen; and (2) neuroenteric cyst, representing foregut anomalies that persist as a remnant of the dorsal part of the notochord.[139] The latter type is often associated with cervical and thoracic spinal abnormalities.

On chest films congenital esophageal duplications often appear as a round or oval posterior mediastinal mass. The mass is closely applied to the esophagus and generally causes deviation or compression. Usually the lesions do not communicate and cannot be easily distinguished from other mediastinal masses. The cystic nature of the lesion is visualized well by CT examination.

Miscellaneous anomalies

Other congenital esophageal malformations include muscle hypertrophy, stenosis, diaphragms, webs, cartilage rings, short esophagus, bronchoesophageal fistula, and laryngotracheal esophageal cleft. All these anomalies are rare. Congenital muscular hypertrophy may involve the whole esophagus[140] or a short segment.[141] The diagnosis of esophageal stenosis is made by identifying esophageal narrowing early in childhood and ruling out other potential causes. Congenital webs, rings, and diaphragms may occur in any portion of the esophagus but are usually proximal. A shortened esophagus, even in infants, is generally caused by esophagitis rather than congenital. Congenital bronchoesophageal fistulas usually originate from lobar or segmental bronchi and may be associated with pulmonary sequestration. A unifying concept suggests that intralobar or extralobar pulmonary sequestrations with or without gastroesophageal communication and esophageal bronchogenic duplications are all bronchopulmonary foregut malformations caused by a supernumerary lung bud.[142] A persistent esophagotracheal lumen known as *laryngotracheal esophageal cleft* causes a variety of pulmonary symptoms and is nearly always evident during the early neonatal period.[143,144]

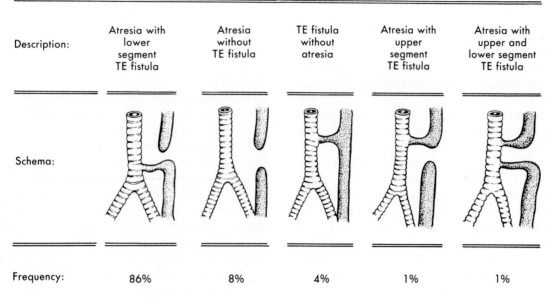

Description:	Atresia with lower segment TE fistula	Atresia without TE fistula	TE fistula without atresia	Atresia with upper segment TE fistula	Atresia with upper and lower segment TE fistula
Schema:					
Frequency:	86%	8%	4%	1%	1%

Fig. 11-21 Types of TE fistula and esophageal atresia.

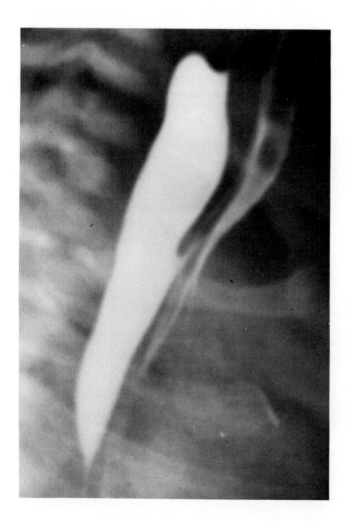

Fig. 11-22 H-type TE fistula in an infant with unexplained pneumonia. H-type fistula is seen between the proximal esophagus and the trachea. A fistula generally takes a diagonal course cephalad to join the trachea.

ESOPHAGEAL DIVERTICULA

Esophageal diverticula are acquired rather than congenital.[145] Diverticula virtually never occur during childhood, seldom develop before age 40 years, and then increase in frequency with age. Small asymptomatic diverticula are commonly observed as a coincidental finding. Like most GI tract diverticula, esophageal diverticula are seldom true diverticula consisting of all wall layers, but are pseudodiverticula with mucosal eventration or herniation through the muscularis.

A tendency exists to classify esophageal diverticula into pulsion Zenker's diverticula, traction diverticula of the midesophagus, and pulsion epiphrenic diverticula of the distal esophagus. Anatomically, Zenker's diverticula originate just proximal to the UES and are properly classified as pharyngeal diverticula. Although diverticula may develop anywhere in the esophagus, they are most common in the middle and distal thirds. Fluoroscopic observations suggest that nearly all esophageal diverticula, regardless of location, are caused by pulsion forces as opposed to traction.[13] Only a few autopsy examples demonstrate traction from mediastinal adhesions. Most esophageal diverticula are oval without any suggestion of traction, are often seen to expand and contract concentrically during peristalsis, and exhibit longitudinal peristaltic excursions without evidence of mediastinal fixation (Fig. 11-23). A small percentage of diverticula in the midesophagus are conical in shape, have no neck, and may be caused by traction.

The causes of pulsion diverticula include esophageal motility disorders, mechanical obstruction, and chronic wear-and-tear forces. The latter category appears to account for most esophageal diverticula. During each normal peristaltic sequence, substantial radial pressure forces exist in the esophagus.[146] Humans swallow about once a minute while awake,[34] which translates into 2 to 3 million swallows per decade. In addition to normal wear-and-tear processes, esophageal diverticula may also be caused by underlying motility disorders, such as achalasia, diffuse esophageal spasm, and hypertensive peristalsis.[146,147]

Most esophageal diverticula are asymptomatic. In some instances, symptoms such as dysphagia may be caused by an underlying motility disorder, diverticulum of large size, or complications from a diverticulum. Complications include erosion with bleeding, inflammation with localized abscess, perforation, fistula formation, retained foreign body, and neoplasm.[148,149]

Some large esophageal diverticula are identifiable on chest films as a soft tissue mass, often containing a gas-fluid level. A retained foreign body or calcified enterolith is occasionally present. On barium swallows, small esophageal diverticula, 0.5 to 2 cm in size, are commonly observed as transient outpouchings that develop only during peristalsis. Large diverticula greater than 4 cm in size commonly empty only by gravity. Those lesions with a narrow neck often retain fluid and gas. Extremely large diverticula may compress the adjacent normal esophagus, and esophageal emptying may occur only by overflow. Epiphrenic diverticula, located just above the LES, generally project to the right, whereas diverticula elsewhere in the esophagus project in any direction except posteriorly. In about 10%

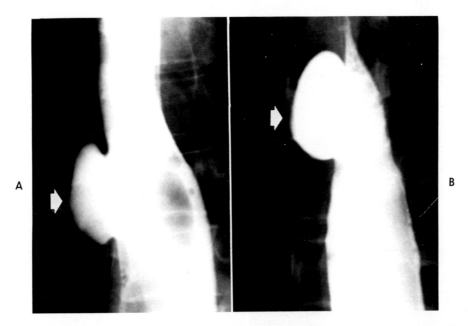

Fig. 11-23 Pulsion diverticulum of the midesophagus. **A,** At onset of swallowing, barium demonstrates a smooth 2 × 3 cm diverticulum *(arrow)* located near the carina. **B,** During esophageal peristalsis, the diverticulum makes a substantial oral excursion without evidence of distortion caused by traction.

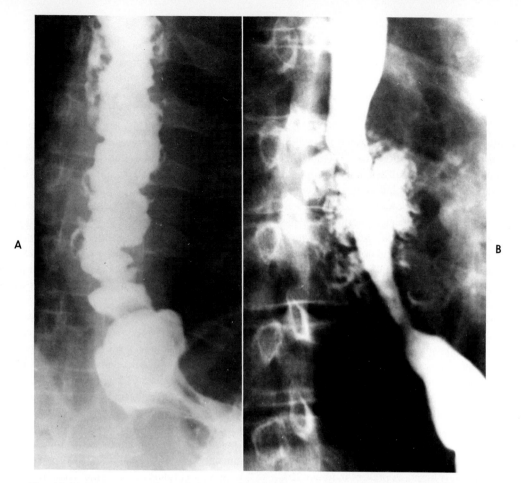

Fig. 11-24 Intramural esophageal pseudodiverticulosis. Numerous sacculations represent dilated esophageal glands. **A,** Diffuse involvement without evidence of stricture. An axial hiatus hernia is present. **B,** Segmental involvement accompanied by an esophageal stricture.

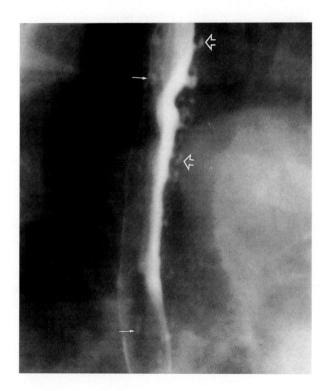

Fig. 11-25 Intramural pseudodiverticulosis of the esophagus. A double-contrast examination of the esophagus demonstrates intramural diverticulosis, both tangentially *(open arrowheads)* and en face *(arrows)*. Most cases of intramural pseudodiverticulosis demonstrate the features seen in this case. Small, flask-like outpouchings from the wall of the esophagus, which represent the dilated, intramural, glandular structures, are unique to this entity. Note that the esophagus is also diffusely narrowed.

to 20% of cases, multiple diverticula are present but seldom number more than three. Evidence of an underlying motility disorder or obstructive lesion may be present.

Intramural pseudodiverticulosis

In 1960 Mendl and co-workers[150] described a condition called *esophageal intramural diverticulosis*.[150] This condition, characterized by numerous small esophageal outpouchings, has been detected in all ages but generally occurs in persons over age 50 years. Later studies showed that the outpouchings were dilated glands located interior to the muscularis, and the condition was renamed *pseudodiverticulosis*.[151,152] The underlying cause is unknown. Nonspecific inflammatory changes of the esophageal mucosa are present in about half the patients.[153] Cultured material often yields monilia. For this reason moniliasis was once suggested as a cause of intramural pseudodiverticulosis, but monilia are simply secondary contaminants in areas of stasis.

Generally, the patients are first seen with dysphagia, often of long duration. On esophagrams multiple cystic or flashlike pouches 1 to 3 mm in size are shown in a short esophageal segment or, in some instance, over the entire length of the esophagus (Figs. 11-24 and 11-25). The pseudosacculations may line up in rows between longitudinal esophageal folds. About two thirds of the patients have one or more esophageal strictures, particularly in the midesophagus.[153] A hiatus hernia is present in about 25%. Most patients exhibit normal esophageal motor function. Therapy for moniliasis does not affect either the patient's symptoms or the radiographic appearance of the pseudodiverticula.

Occasionally, an isolated intramural diverticulum may appear as a solitary lesion in the esophagus.[154] Such a lesion is a sizable pocketlike structure quite distinct from intramural diverticulosis.

TRAUMATIC LESIONS

Esophageal injury may be caused by an ingested foreign body, endoscopy, dilatation procedures, penetrating wounds, blunt trauma, or surgical procedures.

Foreign bodies

Infants, children, and psychiatric patients often swallow different types of foreign bodies. Normal adults may also swallow objects that are held in the mouth, such as tacks and nails. Senile or stuporous patients may swallow dental bridges or dentures. Smooth foreign bodies, such as coins, buttons, dental crowns, and fruit pits, generally pass through the esophagus but may lodge in areas of normal anatomic narrowing at the thoracic inlet, aortic arch, or diaphragmatic hiatus.[155] Sharp objects, such as glass, open safety pins, or needles, may arrest at any esophageal level. The most common foreign body is an unchewed meat bolus that lodges proximal to an area of anatomic or pathologic narrowing.

Young children present clinically with respiratory distress, drooling, or regurgitation.[156] Adults complain acutely of dysphagia, chest pain, or odynophagia. The clinical location of dysphagia frequently does not correspond to the esophageal level of the foreign body. Chronic foreign bodies often cause respiratory symptoms from aspiration. Complications include perforation, bronchoesophageal fistula, aortoesophageal fistula, bleeding, and pericardial injury with tamponade.

Metallic or dense foreign bodies are readily recognized on plain films of the neck or chest. Flat objects, such as coins, are oriented in the coronal plane of the esophagus in contrast to the sagittal plane orientation of flat foreign bodies residing in the trachea. Obstructing foreign bodies may cause a gas-fluid level in the esophagus or tracheal displacement. Signs of perforation may be present. For positive-contrast examination, water-soluble contrast is indicated for the initial swallow to exclude perforation. Barium may be used for subsequent swallows. Cotton balls or marshmallows soaked in barium may be useful to demonstrate a small, hard-to-detect foreign body.

Some blunt esophageal foreign bodies may be removed at fluoroscopy using a straight or balloon catheter. Antecedent relaxation of the esophageal smooth muscle with an anticholinergic agent, such as atropine, or of the LES with glucagon[157] may be helpful. In other patients endoscopy is necessary. Proteolytic enzymes may be digested for an impacted food bolus, but such agents occasionally damage the esophagus and lead to perforation.[65] Some esophageal foreign bodies must be removed surgically.

Esophageal perforation

Nearly all esophageal perforations are caused by trauma.[158] The most common causes are iatrogenic from endoscopy, dilatation procedures (Fig. 11-26, *A*), or thoracotomy. Traumatic perforation also results from penetrating injuries, such as missile or stab wounds, and occasionally from blunt compression when air is trapped in the esophagus. Even so-called spontaneous esophageal rupture is from trauma caused by events such as severe vomiting. Nontraumatic esophageal perforation is generally caused by caustic ingestion or neoplasm. Perforation from peptic esophagitis is rare but may occur occasionally in patients with Zollinger-Ellison syndrome who reflux large amounts of potent gastric juice into the esophagus.[159] Esophageal perforation may also occur when digestive enzymes, such as papain, are used in an attempt to dissolve vegetative esophageal foreign bodies.[160]

In adults about 75% of esophageal perforations occur during endoscopic examinations. The most frequent sites are adjacent to the cricopharyngeus and the distal esophagus. Occasionally, the intraabdominal esophageal segment may perforate into the retroperitoneum or lesser sac.[161] With dilatation procedures, perforation may be immediate or delayed for several days.[162] In infants perforations usu-

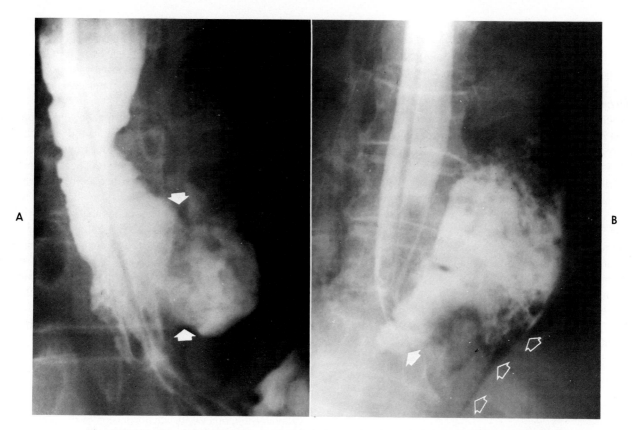

Fig. 11-26 Esophageal perforation. **A,** Achalasia in a patient immediately after pneumatic dilatation of the LES segment. Injection of a water-soluble contrast medium through the esophageal tube shows a perforation, about 4 cm in length *(arrows),* along the left lateral wall of the distal esophagus. **B,** Spontaneous esophageal rupture caused by vomiting (Boerhaave's syndrome). Injection of a water-soluble contrast medium demonstrates a characteristic esophageal tear *(closed arrow),* about 2 cm in length, located along the left lateral margin of the distal esophagus. The contrast medium enters a golf ball-size space within the lower mediastinum. Air has escaped into the mediastinum and dissected beneath the parietal pleura of the left hemidiaphragm *(open arrows).* This later feature contributes to the **V** sign of Nacleiro. ↑ *mediastinal air*

ally occur in the cervical esophagus and hypopharynx. They are generally caused by the passage of tubes.

Spontaneous esophageal rupture, described by Boerhaave in 1724, generally occurs in men and is usually associated with the abrupt onset of chest pain and shock, simulating a heart attack or dissecting aneurysm.[163,164] The classic triad is vomiting, excruciating chest pain, and subcutaneous emphysema. In about 10% to 20% of cases, however, the clinical onset may be insidious and the diagnosis obscure. Neonatal esophageal perforation occurs predominantly in girls.[165] Dyspnea and cyanosis associated with a right tension pneumothorax occur shortly after birth.

The inciting incident for a Boerhaave rupture may be forceful vomiting, straining, childbirth, or a blunt blow to the abdomen or thorax. Gastric contents propelled across the LES cause an abrupt rise in intraesophageal pressure, leading to sudden esophageal distention. Excessive distention initially splits the muscularis, allowing transient mucosal herniation.[166] The abruptly herniated mucosa may

tear, thereby resulting in perforation. The ruptures are vertical tears 1 to 4 cm long. About 90% occur along the left posterolateral wall of the distal esophagus (Fig. 11-26, *B*), where the esophagus is not supported by adjacent mediastinal structures. In infants spontaneous esophageal rupture splits the right side of the distal esophagus and frequently communicates with the right hemithorax.[165]

The radiographic evaluation for suspected esophageal perforation includes a well-exposed chest film and contrast examination of the esophagus.[167] Abnormal findings include pneumomediastinum, mediastinal widening, and cervical emphysema. Fluid and gas in the mediastinal pocket may give a soft tissue density that is easily confused with a hiatal hernia or epiphrenic diverticulum. The finding of a V-shaped radiolucency seen through the heart (Nacleiro sign) represents gas in the left lower mediastinum that dissects under the left diaphragmatic pleura. Although uncommon immediately after esophageal rupture, a left pleural effusion or left hydropneumothorax may develop in 12 to 24 hours. Pulmonary infiltrates are common. Pericardium is rare. In neonatal esophageal rupture, pneumomediastinum is relatively uncommon. A right tension pneumothorax is usually the predominant finding, because the esophagus abuts the right mediastinal pleura in infants. For direct visualization of the esophagus water-soluble contrast should be used initially and augmented by barium if gross perforation is not demonstrated initially. Esophagography should be used liberally in all patients with suspected perforation and in some instances can be used routinely when the risk of perforation is high in patients undergoing dilatation procedures, such as pneumatic dilatation for achalasia.[168]

Miscellaneous lesions

In addition to frank esophageal rupture, abrupt esophageal distention associated with sudden increases in esophageal pressure may cause incomplete tears limited to the esophageal mucosa (Mallory-Weiss syndrome) or involve the submucosa as well. Both these conditions commonly cause gastrointestinal bleeding. When a hiatus hernia is present, Mallory-Weiss tears frequently extend across the

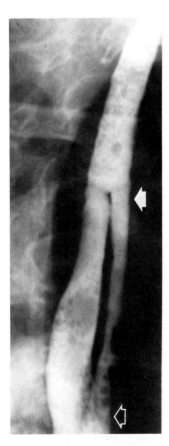

Fig. 11-27 Double-barrel esophagus. False channel *(open arrow)* caused by trauma from endoscopy recommunicates distally *(closed arrow)* to form a double-barrel esophagus.

cardia into the fundus or may be limited to the fundus.[169] Mallory-Weiss tears are rarely demonstrated on an esophagram, but the bleeding site may be shown on selective celiac arteriography. The bleeding usually stops spontaneously, but a vasopressin (Pitressin) infusion is often helpful.

Mucosal tears, caused by overdistention, endoscopy, or foreign bodies, occasionally give rise to a double-channel esophagus (Fig. 11-27). Bleeding from traumatic submucosal injury communicates with the esophageal lumen or remains confined as an intramural hematoma. Esophageal hematomas are generally related to endoscopy, direct trauma, esophageal dilatations, or truncal vagotomy[170,171] but can occur spontaneously in patients on anticoagulants or with bleeding disorders.[172] The hematoma generally causes acute lower chest pain and dysphagia. On radiographic examination, the esophageal lumen is generally compressed by an elongated, eccentric intraluminal mass with smooth, lumpy, or in some instances irregular contours. In some cases, contrast medium fills a false channel.

HIATUS HERNIA

Hiatus hernias are divided into two types: (1) an axial hernia exists when a loculus of stomach and the gastric cardia pass through the hiatus into the thorax; and (2) a paraesophageal hernia exists when a portion of the stomach herniates through the hiatus but the cardia remains normally located. About 99% of hiatus hernias are axial, with only about 1% being paraesophageal. Both types of hernias are usually acquired.

Axial hernias may be fixed in position—for example, by a short esophagus or adhesions—but generally slide in and out of the thorax. Only about half of the axial hernias are associated with a widened hiatus. Occasionally, a widened hiatus is observed without an identifiable accompanying herniation.[173] By strict definition, this latter circumstance simply indicates a patulous hiatus rather than a hiatus hernia. In both circumstances, however, alterations exist in the anatomy of the hiatal region.

A low incidence of axial hiatus hernia exists in infants, whereas hiatus hernias are rare later in childhood. In adults the prevalence of hiatus hernia increases with age. A hiatus hernia as such is seldom accompanied by symptoms unless associated with reflux esophagitis or complicated by bleeding or strangulation.[174]

A sliding hiatus hernia indicates stretching or rupture of the phrenicoesophageal membranes (PEM) that normally tether the distal esophagus at the hiatus.[175] Although the cause of PEM alterations is unknown, considerable evidence suggests that the PEM is forcefully stretched by longitudinal esophageal contraction during esophageal peristalsis.[16,17] In fact, the esophagogastric junction may demonstrate physiologic herniation (see Fig. 11-3) into the thorax during longitudinal esophageal shortening in normal subjects.[13,176,177] Normally the elastic recoil of a healthy PEM restores the cardia to a normal intraabdominal location when peristalsis is complete. This repetitive phenomenon of esophageal peristalsis and PEM stretch occurs about 2 million times per decade of life and may generate wear-and-tear changes of the PEM that lead to stretching or rupture of the membrane and axial herniation.[178]

Radiologic examination is the best method for demonstrating a hiatus hernia. Adequate examination depends on inspection of esophageal function as well as morphology and obtaining maximal esophageal distention during the examination. Distention is enhanced by rapid delivery of barium or impedance of esophageal outflow by Valsalva's maneuver or abdominal bolster. The bolster method is not unphysiologic, because intraabdominal pressure increases only 5 to 10 mm Hg, whereas much higher pressure increases occur during coughing and straining.

Several decades ago, the radiologic anatomy of the distal esophagus and esophagogastric junction (cardia) was poorly understood, resulting in confusing terminology and frequent misdiagnosis. Subsequent studies, however, improved the recognition of the relevant radiologic landmarks, such as the diaphragmatic hiatus, esophagogastric junction, LES segment, and loculus of herniated stomach.[76,173,177,179,180] Because the hiatus is in the mediastinum, its precise level cannot be observed directly but must be estimated by observing its compression on intrahiatal strictures. Sniffing causes a pinch-cock action of the hiatus that identifies its level. The level of the hiatus should not

be judged by the observed level of the left hemidiaphragm. The thin, ringlike structure often seen at the esophagogastric junction (also known as the _B ring_) is a passive ring formed by a transverse mucosal fold, whereas the thicker ring (also known as the _A ring_), which is sometimes present at the upper margin of the sphincter segment, is generated by active muscle contraction.[76,180]

These mucosal and muscle rings (Fig. 11-28) define the margins of the LES and are recognized by their function and morphology.[6] Normally the peristaltic stripping wave passes through the area of the muscle ring but stops at the esophagogastric junction. In the LES segment, the stripping wave generally has a flat-top configuration (see Fig. 11-6, _A_). Some axial hiatus hernias, medium to large in size, exhibit a prominent notch caused by the gastric sling fibers looping around the gastroesophageal junction (Fig. 11-29). This appearance should not be mistaken for a paraesophageal hernia. A herniated gastric pouch may show obvious rugal folds, generally exhibits axial asymmetry, and does not exhibit peristaltic contractions. An increased incidence of axial hiatus hernia may be present in neonates with reflux, children with nonseasonal asthma, after surgical disruption of hiatal structures (for example, during vagotomy), blunt abdominal trauma, scleroderma, diffuse esophageal spasm, and Barrett's esophagus.

The uncommon paraesophageal hernias are generally detected as an incidental finding as a soft tissue density on chest films but may be seen with bleeding or symptoms

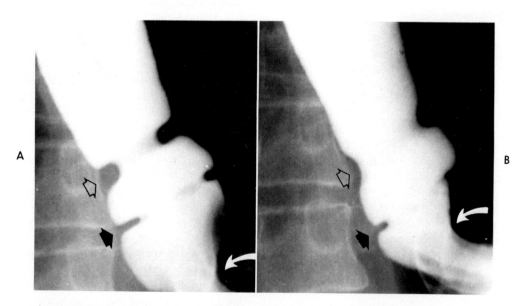

Fig. 11-28 Small axial hiatus hernia. Diaphragmatic hiatus causes a mild constriction (_curved arrow_) of a portion of the stomach within the hiatus. A thin mucosal ring (_closed arrow_) is seen at the esophagogastric junction, whereas a thick muscle ring (_open arrow_) demarcates the upper margin of the lower esophageal sphincter segment from the tubular esophageal body. Muscle ring is contracted in **A,** but relaxes a few seconds later, in **B.** Mucosal fold at the esophagogastric junction shows no change. The herniated portion of the stomach does not contract as part of the esophageal peristaltic sequence.

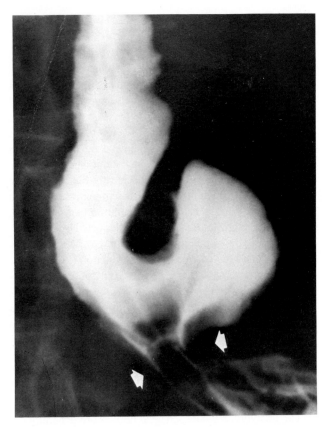

Fig. 11-29 Spurious appearance of a paraesophageal hiatus hernia. A prominent diagonal notch caused by gastric sling fibers causes false appearance of a paraesophageal hiatus hernia. The level of the esophagogastric junction identified by the notch, however, is well above the diaphragmatic hiatus *(arrows)*.

from strangulation. These hernias do not have any association with reflux esophagitis. In some instances, the hernia neck may be sufficiently compressed to delay or even prevent filling of the hernia with barium. Tilting the subject's head down often causes the hernia to fill.

After surgical repair of an axial hiatus hernia, a pseudotumor caused by a fundoplication may exist in the gastric fundus. The defect is more pronounced for the complete wrap of the Nissen procedure than the partial wrap of the Belsey procedure.[181,182] With a split plication, the fundoplication defect may disappear or a complete wrap may slide downward over the stomach (slipped Nissen), thereby giving the stomach an hourglass configuration.

ESOPHAGITIS

Numerous etiologic factors may cause esophagitis. The most common cause is gastroesophageal reflux.

Gastroesophageal reflux disease

Gastroesophageal reflux disease (GERD) is the most common clinical malady of the esophagus. GERD encom-

passes reflux esophagitis and is characterized histologically by inflammatory cells and reflux changes consisting of epithelial hyperplasia without inflammation. The multiple determinant factors in the production of reflux disease include (1) the frequency and volume of gastroesophageal reflux; (2) the volume of gastric contents available to reflux; (3) the potency of the reflux material; (4) the efficacy of esophageal clearance; and (5) the tissue resistance to injury.[31,183]

Heartburn is the most common symptom of gastroesophageal reflux. Other symptoms are regurgitation, chest pain, respiratory complaints, and dysphagia. Dysphagia is usually due to esophageal narrowing. Some patients complain of a lump in the throat (globus). In young children the predominant reflux symptoms are regurgitation, repetitive vomiting, and failure to thrive. Reflux disease may occur occasionally during early childhood but is most common between 30 and 60 years of age.

The radiographic examination for esophagitis consists of fluoroscopy and spot films to evaluate both esophageal function and morphology. With the single-contrast technique, the esophagus should be filmed distended to view esophageal contours and collapsed to evaluate esophageal folds. Full distention is imperative to detect subtle areas of narrowing (Fig. 11-30, *A*). Assessment of gastroesophageal reflux requires 300 to 500 ml of barium in the stomach. Reflux is sought while the patient rolls from the prone to the supine position and during stress maneuvers such as the Trendelenburg, Valsalva, and leg raising done with the patient supine. For the water siphon test, the patient is tilted 15 degrees to the right and takes several swallows of water. The double-contrast examination for subtle morphologic abnormalities may be done before or after the single-contrast study.

Morphologic findings of peptic esophagitis (Figs. 11-30 to 11-34) include irregularity of luminal contour, a granular mucosal pattern, discrete ulcerations, transverse esophageal folds, thickened longitudinal folds, esophageal wall thickening, and segmental narrowing.[184-186] Although not specific, the finding of transverse esophageal ridging or folds (see Fig. 11-33), known as *felinization,* suggests the presence of esophagitis.[187] Morphologic abnormalities are usually absent in mild superficial esophagitis but are generally present in 80% to 90% of patients with proved moderate to severe esophagitis on endoscopy.[188]

Even with the use of vigorous stress maneuvers, reproducible gastroesophageal reflux is demonstrated at fluoroscopy in only about 40% of patients with endoscopic evidence of reflux esophagitis.[31,32] This finding suggests a feeble LES. Esophageal motor function is abnormal in up to 50% of patients with reflux esophagitis. In recumbent patients, abnormal motor function is accompanied by delayed esophageal volume clearance.[189]

A hiatus hernia is present in most patients with reflux esophagitis.[190] At present, however, the relationship between axial hiatus hernia and reflux esophagitis is not clear. Several decades ago an axial hiatus hernia was considered

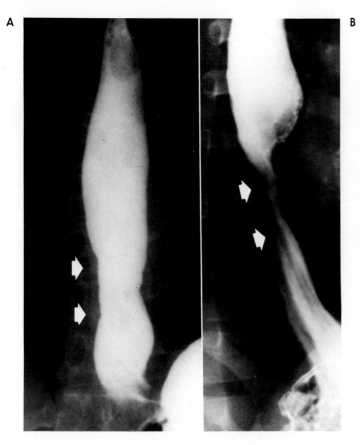

Fig. 11-30 Esophageal strictures caused by reflux esophagitis. **A,** A mild persistent esophageal stricture *(arrows),* 3 to 4 cm in length, was observed only when the esophagus was fully distended by placing the patient over an abdominal bolster. This type of mild stricture is generally missed by endoscopy. **B,** Severe esophageal stricture *(arrows),* approximately 2 to 3 cm in length. A collapsed hiatus hernia is located distal to the stricture.

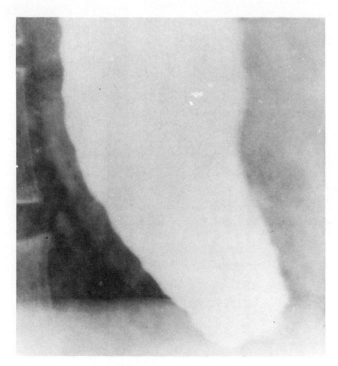

Fig. 11-31 Reflux esophagitis. Luminal contour of the distal esophagus is irregular, and the esophageal wall is thickened.

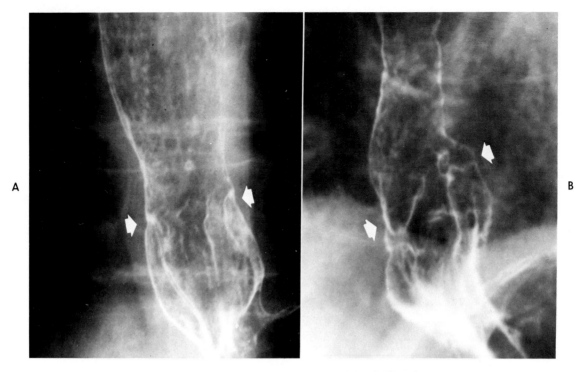

Fig. 11-32 Double contrast esophagrams in two patients with esophagitis. **A,** The level of the esophagogastric junction is indicated by arrows. A small hiatus hernia is present. Esophagitis causes a stippled, granular appearance of the barium. **B,** Arrows indicate the esophagogastric junction. A small hiatus hernia is present. The distal esophagus is narrowed and has an irregular contour.

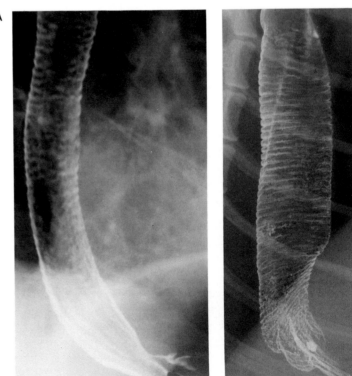

Fig. 11-33 Transverse esophageal folds. **A,** A patient with esophagitis. Well-defined transverse ridges, or folds, are seen in the distal half of the esophagus. This phenomenon has been termed *felinization* of the esophagus. **B,** Cat esophagus demonstrating typical transverse folds present in this species.

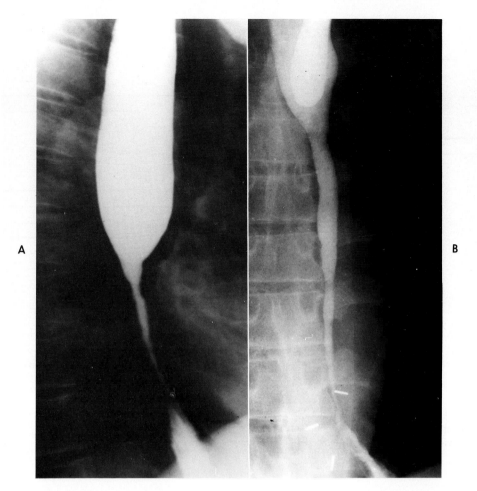

Fig. 11-34 Severe peptic strictures. **A,** A patient with an indwelling nasogastric tube 2 days after abdominal surgery. **B,** A patient with Zollinger-Ellison syndrome. Clips are from a truncal vagotomy.

to be the *sine qua non* of reflux esophagitis, and surgical therapy was directed toward repairing the hernia. Current evidence, however, suggests that most patients with axial hiatus hernia do not have symptomatic esophagitis.[186] Nevertheless, most patients with severe esophagitis do have an accompanying hiatus hernia. In some patients a sliding hiatus hernia may be an incidental finding, while in others it may contribute to gastroesophageal reflux by altering normal hiatal anatomy or perhaps by contributing to a high rate of reflux-associated transient LES relaxations. In a minority of patients with reflux esophagitis, a sliding hiatus hernia may be caused by esophageal shortening.

Recently some workers have proposed that endoscopy should be the primary diagnostic examination for evaluating patients with suspected esophagitis. We believe, however, that the radiographic method remains the optimal initial examination. Although less sensitive than endoscopy for detecting mucosal changes, the radiographic examination provides important information on esophageal motor function and esophageal compliance that is not well examined by endoscopy. The radiographic examination also meets with greater patient acceptance, takes less time, and is less expensive. Subtle esophageal narrowing, observed when the esophagus is well filled with barium, is commonly missed by endoscopy (see Fig. 11-30, *A*). Albeit the radiographic examination fails to detect most patients with mild superficial esophagitis, detectable morphologic abnormalities are exhibited in 50% to 60% of patients with moderate esophagitis and up to 90% of patients with severe esophagitis.[188,191] Such yields may be enhanced by the double-contrast examination (see Fig. 11-32).

In addition to the garden-variety reflux esophagitis commonly observed in adults, severe forms of reflux esophagitis may be observed occasionally in association with repeated vomiting, anesthesia, nasogastric intubation, and the Zollinger-Ellison syndrome (see Fig. 11-34, *A*). Contrary to earlier notions, esophagitis in infants probably is seldom related to LES hypotension from sphincter dysmaturity but is caused by other mechanisms, such as transient LES relaxation.[77]

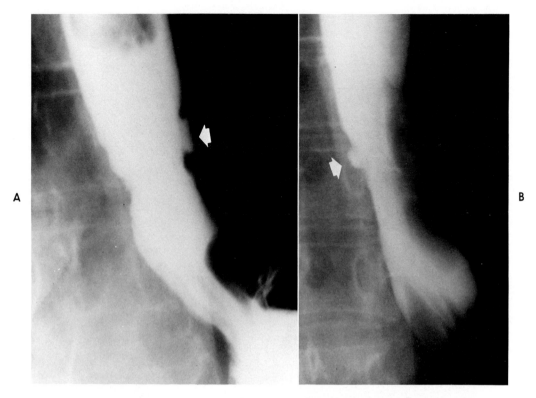

Fig. 11-35 Barrett's columnar-lined esophagus. Two patients with punched-out ulcers *(arrows)* in the distal esophagus. Each patient had a small hiatus hernia that is not well seen, and the columnar epithelium was demonstrated in the distal esophagus by biopsy.

Barrett's esophagus

When the esophagus is partially lined with columnar epithelium, this condition is referred to as *Barrett's esophagus.*[192,193] Although initially considered a congenital abnormality, most workers currently agree that the columnar epithelium reflects an adaptive alteration caused by chronic reflux esophagitis.[109,194,195] Areas of ulcerated squamous epithelium are believed to be replaced by columnar epithelium that extends from the stomach and a variable distance up the esophagus, spreading from islands of columnar cell nests. Chronic reflux esophagitis is due to the effects of acid and pepsin on the esophagus and is presumed to be the most common etiology. Barrett's esophagus has also been observed in patients with total gastrectomy, presumably resulting from bile reflux esophagitis.

There are three types of Barrett's epithelium: (1) specialized columnar epithelium, resembling intestinal mucosa with villiform surface and crypts; (2) junctional-type epithelium, resembling the epithelium of the normal gastric cardia; or (3) gastric fundus–type epithelium, resembling the epithelium of the body and fundus of the stomach. When all three types of epithelium are present, the specialized columnar epithelium is generally seen in the more proximal areas of columnar epithelium. The types of epithelium may be intermingled, even at the same level as the esophagus.

Although Barrett's epithelium is occasionally encountered in children, it is most commonly seen in adults, generally past the age of 40 and as old as age 80. It is more prevalent in whites than in blacks, a feature not clearly explained in epidemiologic terms at this time. Of importance is that patients with a columnar epithelium–lined esophagus are at increased risk for adenocarcinoma.[196] How many such patients ultimately develop adenocarcinoma is not well established, but reports of the coexistence of Barrett's epithelium in patients with adenocarcinoma cite numbers ranging from zero to 45%.

Many cases of adenocarcinoma involving the distal esophagus that were originally thought to be related to tumors originating in the cardia and extending into the esophagus are, in reality, cases of primary adenocarcinoma that developed into Barrett's epithelium. The evolution of adenocarcinoma appears to be related to the presence dysplasia, which forms in Barrett's epithelium and ultimately develops into adenocarcinoma. Because dysplasia frequently arises in Barrett's epithelium, routine follow-up and biopsy are recommended in such patients, and when significant dysplasia appears, the surgical removal of the esophageal

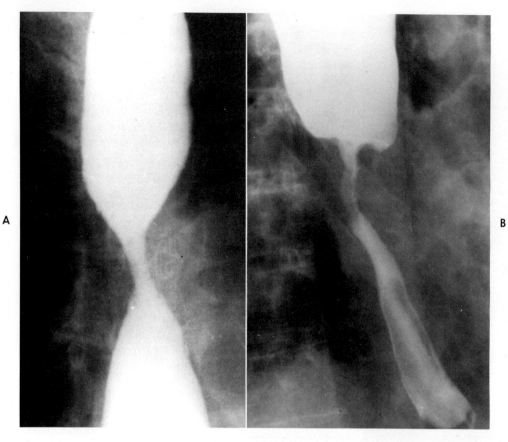

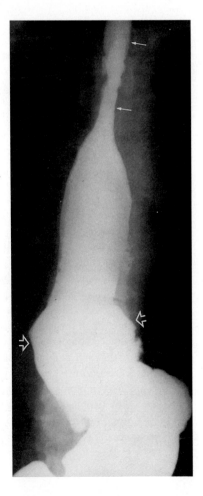

Fig. 11-36 Segmental esophageal narrowing. **A,** Benign stricture at the aortic arch level in a patient with Barrett's columnar-lined esophagus. **B,** Malignant stricture caused by squamous carcinoma of the distal esophagus.

Fig. 11-37 Barrett's esophagus. This single film of the thoracic esophagus demonstrates features of Barrett's esophagus. There is a moderate-size sliding hiatus hernia *(open arrowheads)*. The film was taken during an episode of free gastroesophageal reflux during which the entire thoracic esophagus is filled with barium. There is a stricture *(arrows)* with areas of irregular scarring involving the proximal esophagus. Strictures of the proximal esophagus associated with the features of reflux, as seen in this case, suggest the diagnosis of Barrett's esophagus. In this case the diagnosis was confirmed by endoscopy.

portion containing the columnar epithelium should be seriously considered.

The diagnosis of Barrett's esophagitis is suggested radiologically when a punched-out ulcer or stricture is seen in the mid or proximal esophagus, especially in the presence of a hiatus hernia and gastroesophageal reflux (Figs. 11-35, 11-36, *A,* 11-37, and 11-38). However, its sensitivity in detecting Barrett's epithelium is poor. Although a characteristic "reticular pattern" has been noted in the presence of Barrett's esophagus, the accuracy for detection is quite low.[199] Nevertheless, when patients exhibit symptomatic gastroesophageal reflux at the time of barium examination, a double-contrast examination of the esophageal epithelium may well bring to light this mucosal pattern.[200]

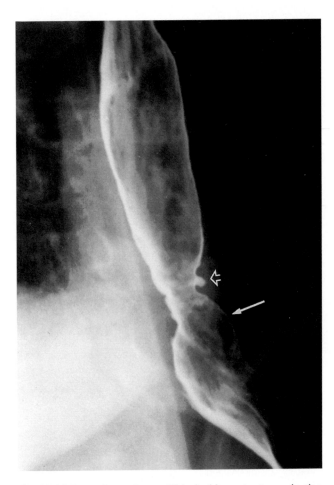

Fig. 11-38 Barrett's esophagus. This double-contrast examination of the esophagus very nicely demonstrates a small, penetrating ulcer involving the distal esophagus *(open arrowhead)*. The ulcer is located above the esophagogastric junction. The ulcer is located in an area of modest stricture as a result of peptic esophagitis. There is a small, sliding hiatus hernia present *(arrow)*. Barrett's esophagus frequently involves the distal esophagus and the presence of a distal esophageal peptic stricture as, in this case, is often encountered in Barrett's esophagus. Although not shown on this image, the gastroesophageal reflux was easily demonstrated in this patient.

Current management of a Barrett's esophagus includes aggressive treatment of the reflux with H$_2$ blockers and antacids, consideration of antireflux procedures, and frequent follow-up with endoscopy and biopsy to detect dysplastic changes. At this time, there is no evidence to suggest that Barrett's epithelium will regress following antacid therapy or antireflux procedures and also none to suggest that aggressive therapy will alter the evolution of adenocarcinoma.[195] Therefore, treatment is instead directed toward relieving the symptoms of esophagitis and healing any active ulceration. Esophageal peristalsis in these patients is usually normal, but some have impaired esophageal motor function and abnormal motor clearance.[201]

Infectious esophagitis

Esophagitis may be caused by a variety of infectious agents. Infectious causes of esophagitis include monilia,[202] herpes simplex,[203] cytomegalic inclusion virus,[204] tuberculosis, lactobacilli,[205] cryptococcoses, blastomycosis, gram-negative bacteria, streptococci,[206] mixed bacterial infections, and diphtheria. In most cases, infectious esophagitis occurs in debilitated individuals; diabetics; immunosuppressed patients; or patients receiving steroids, antibiotics, radiotherapy, or chemotherapy. Infectious esophagitis is seen with increasing frequency in immunosuppressed transplant patients and individuals with impaired T cell function from acquired immunodeficiency syndrome (AIDS). Infectious esophagitis often involves long esophageal segments, particularly with monilia and herpes, but may involve relatively short segments. The typical initial complaint is odynophagia, a symptom rarely encountered with reflux disease. The double-contrast examination has a high sensitivity for detecting infectious esophagitis that compares favorably with that of endoscopy.[207] Additionally, the fine mucosal detail provided by the double-contrast study is essential to detect the discrete ulcerations that may distinguish viral from monilial esophagitis.[208]

Moniliasis

The most common organism infecting the esophagus is *Candida albicans,* a yeast that causes moniliasis. *Candida* organisms are normally present in the mouth, sputum, and feces. Monilial esophagitis occurs almost exclusively in debilitated patients; diabetics; alcoholics; or patients on steroids, immunosuppressants, cytotoxic drugs, or antibiotics. Monilia organisms are a frequent companion of esophageal intramural pseudodiverticulosis. Although monilial esophagitis is usually characterized by the abrupt onset of odynophagia, chest pain, or dysphagia, clinical symptoms are occasionally absent. About half the patients have oral thrush. Monilial esophagitis is currently seen with increasing frequency, especially in immunosuppressed patients or patients with AIDS. The original radiographic description of esophageal moniliasis did not appear until 1956,[209] but numerous cases are now reported.[202,210] The radiographic findings are variable but suggest the correct diagnosis.[211] Esophageal involvement generally occurs over a long segment (Fig. 11-39), and occasionally over the entire esophagus. The luminal contour may show fine speculations, irregularity, a cobblestone pattern,[125] or bizarre thickened folds simulating varices.[212] Ninety-five percent of cases demonstrate a prominent plaquelike formation[207] (Fig. 11-40). Barium may dissect beneath a pseudomembrane, causing a shaggy contour that gives the appearance of ulceration. Esophageal wall thickening is common. The esophagus tends to be atonic. Peristalsis may be feeble or incomplete. Spastic contractions are infrequent but may occur.[212] Because of muscular hypotonia, the esophagus is generally slightly dilated or normal in caliber but may show areas of

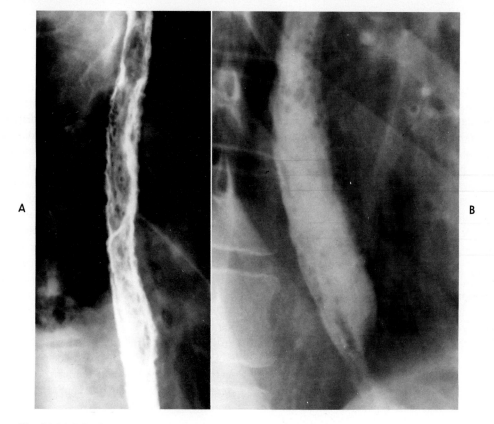

Fig. 11-39 Infectious esophagitis. **A,** Moniliasis. **B,** Herpes simplex. Both patients exhibit diffuse esophagitis of similar radiologic appearance.

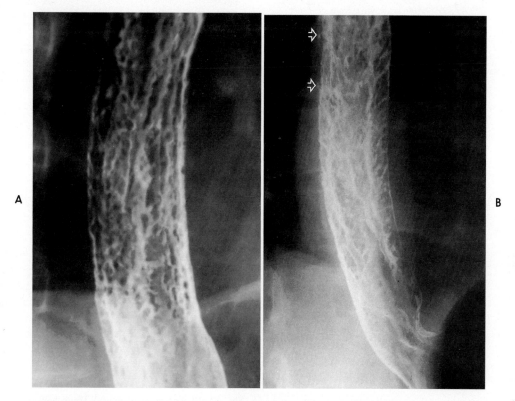

Fig. 11-40 Moniliasis of the esophagus. Two different cases of moniliasis of the esophagus demonstrate the characteristic plaquelike lesions in this entity. **A,** Plaquelike lesions are present, involving the esophageal wall circumferentially. **B,** In another case, similar plaquelike lesions are identified. The proximal esophageal wall is slightly more irregular, indicating that some superficial ulceration also is occurring *(open arrowheads)*.

moderate narrowing. In unusual cases, esophageal moniliasis may appear as a solitary ulcer[213] or develop proximal to an esophageal obstruction.[214] Occasionally, ulcerated nodular lesions are present in the stomach.[210] Endoscopy demonstrates ulceration, friability, and whitish plaques. The diagnosis is confirmed by histologic examination or culture of esophageal scrapings. Treatment with nystatin (Mycostatin) gives prompt relief of symptoms. Esophageal morphology and function generally return to normal in a few weeks,[125] unless a preexisting abnormality was present. Occasionally, moniliasis causes localized masses that simulate carcinoma, segmental strictures, or even narrowing of the entire esophagus.[215,216]

Viral esophagitis

The most common types of viral esophagitis are caused by herpes simplex virus type 1 (HSV-1) and cytomegalovirus (CMV) (Figs. 11-41 and 11-42). Other viral causes, however, include coxsackievirus and retrovirus.[217] These viruses may involve other segments of the GI tract and may affect the esophagus. Diagnosis generally depends on brushings or biopsy material that shows inclusion bodies typical for the virus or that yield a positive culture for the

virus. The diagnosis may be suggested by a rise in virus-specific circulating serum antibodies. It should be remembered that opportunistic infections are often multiple in immunocompromised patients and organisms may coexist in these patients. In the esophagus the differential diagnosis of viral infection is generally limited to either HSV or CMV. Esophageal involvement may occur occasionally in otherwise normal individuals.[218] Although odynophagia is the most common clinical symptom, occasional cases of hemorrhagic esophagitis are manifested by gastrointestinal bleeding.[219] Viral lesions start out as vesicles that quickly rupture to form clear punched-out ulcers with raised margins that are sharply marginated from a normal-appearing mucosa. At this stage, endoscopy reveals the existence of ulcerations typical for a viral infection. Subsequently, these ulcers coalesce, become covered with debris, and may develop a pseudomembrane the presents on appearance similar to that of moniliasis (Fig. 11-39, *B*). The radiographic examination is rarely done while viral esophagitis is in its vesicular stage. The finding of one to several discrete ulcers against a normal mucosal background in immunocompromised patients with odynophagia is nearly pathognomonic for viral esophagitis, generally HSV-1[208,220] or

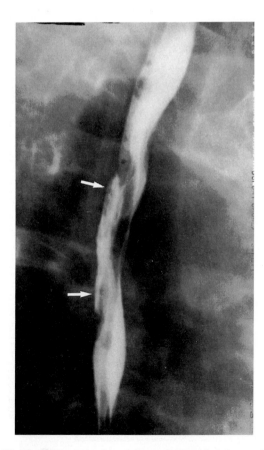

Fig. 11-41 CMV esophagitis. A large shallow ulcer is seen in the midesophagus *(arrows)*. It is surrounded by a rim of edema. This large single ulcer in the midesophagus is caused by CMV esophagitis.

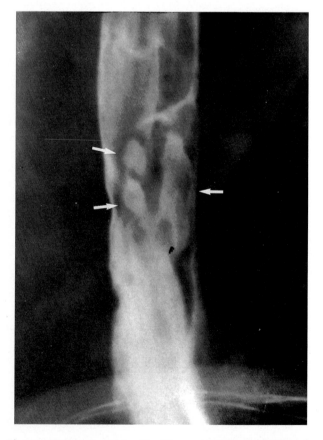

Fig. 11-42 Herpes esophagitis. Three well-defined, shallow ulcers surrounded by a rim of edema and enlarged esophageal folds *(arrows)* are caused by herpes esophagitis.

CMV.[221] Although CMV infection of the alimentary canal can involve virtually the entire GI tract, including the esophagus, stomach, small intestine, colon, bile ducts, and pancreas, the infection is generally manifested as some type of ulceration. In the esophagus, a double-contrast examination appears to be the most sensitive way of detecting CMV esophagitis radiographically. Findings observed in a series of AIDS patients with CMV esophagitis include focal disease, mucosal granularity, erosions, fold thickening, single or multiple deep ulceration in otherwise normal mucosa, and oval or semilunar-shaped ulcerations that project intraluminally. Occasionally, a large plaquelike esophageal ulcer in patients with AIDS is seen in the context of CMV infection.[221,222]

The radiographic findings encountered in herpes esophagitis include widely discrete separated ulcers, plaquelike lesions, a thickening of the esophageal folds, and, when the disease is far advanced, diffuse ulceration with pseudomembrane formation. Because many of these findings are the same as those observed in other types of infectious esophagitis, especially moniliasis, direct visualization and biopsy as well as culture may be necessary to confirm the diagnosis.[221,223,224]

Tuberculosis

Although tuberculous esophagitis is rare, several cases have been diagnosed at our hospital in the past 10 years. Generally, evidence of tuberculosis exists also in the lungs but was absent in two of our patients. Pathways for esophageal infection include extension from adjacent mediastinal nodes, downward extension from the pharynx or larynx, swallowed organisms, or hematogenous seeding.[225] Symptoms include dysphagia and chest pain, but commonly esophageal symptoms are absent. Although the radiographic findings are variable, certain constellations of findings suggest the correct diagnosis. Morphologic abnormalities are often eccentric and may show skip areas. Involvement can occur at any esophageal level, but the middle third of the esophagus is affected most commonly. The luminal contour may show mild irregularity, large or deep ulcers, and sinus tracts. Fistulas are common.[226] The esophageal wall is generally thickened and the lumen often narrowed, sometimes with a masslike appearance that mimics carcinoma.[226] Enlarged mediastinal nodes may displace or compress the esophagus and widen the mediastinum. The finding of a sinus tract accompanied by enlarged mediastinal nodes should suggest the diagnosis (Fig. 11-43); however, these findings may also occur with malignancy and less commonly with actinomycosis or syphilis.

Caustic esophagitis

Caustic ingestion generally occurs accidentally in children and as a suicide attempt in adults. The severity and extent of esophageal injury depend on the type, concentration, and volume of the caustic agent. Injury from caustic agents is similar to that from thermal burns. Alkaline agents can produce deep coagulation necrosis in minutes. Necrosis from acids tends to be more superficial. In addition to esophageal injury, caustic agents may also produce burns of the pharynx and stomach. The initial clinical symptoms are the rapid onset of chest pain and dysphagia. These symptoms tend to resolve in several days. Acute complications include shock, fever, respiratory distress, mediastinitis, and perforation. Late complications are related primarily to fibrosis and stricture, which may cause dysphagia several weeks after the initial injury.[227] Generally, mild injury heals without sequelae, moderate injury leads to stricture, and severe injury causes acute complications.

The radiographic findings vary depending on the severity and extent of esophageal injury. During the first 24 hours, the esophagus often appears normal after a mild insult, but may show blurred margins, contour irregularity, ulceration, or thickened folds when the injury is more severe. Generally, long segments of esophagus are involved. Moderate to severe injury usually abolishes peristalsis. The esophagus is hypotonic and may trap air.[228] In the acute stage the examination should be initiated with water-soluble contrast medium to exclude esophageal or gastric perfora-

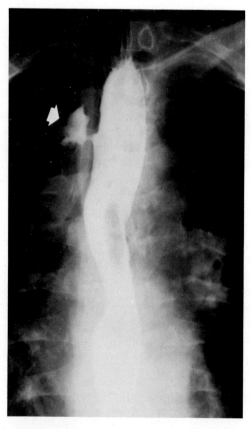

Fig. 11-43 Tuberculosis esophagitis. A sinus tract and small cold abscess *(arrow)* are seen extending from the proximal esophagus. Enlarged carinal nodes indent the right lateral margin of the midesophagus.

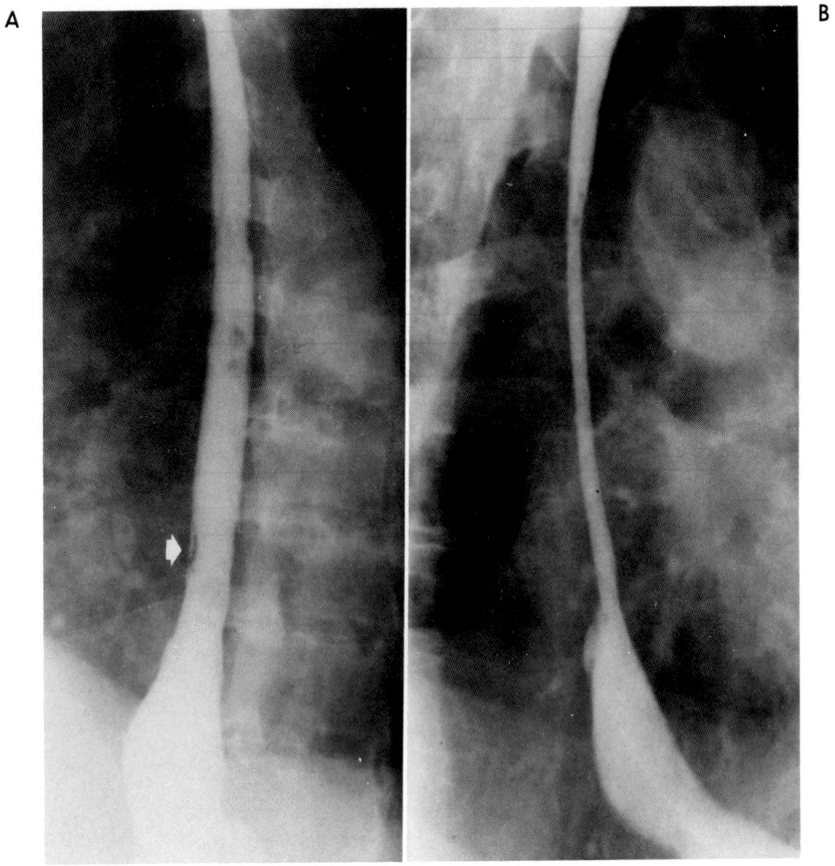

Fig. 11-44 Caustic esophagitis. **A,** Esophagram at 1 week after caustic ingestion shows moderate diffuse esophageal narrowing. In the distal esophagus barium has dissected *(arrow)* beneath the pseudomembrane. **B,** Esophagram 4 weeks after injury shows a severe stricture involving almost the entire esophagus.

tion; then barium may be used.[229] During the first week an acute inflammatory response develops, and areas of significant injury show frank ulceration on esophagrams. A pseudomembrane (Fig. 11-44, *A*) may cause intramural trapping of barium.[228] The esophageal wall is generally thickened, and some luminal narrowing often occurs.[230] By 2 to 6 weeks, healing is well in progress, often accompanied by severe fibrosis (Fig. 11-44, *B*). Commonly, progressive narrowing of the esophageal lumen occurs, heralded by the return or onset of dysphagia. Long stricture segments may involve most or all of the esophagus. The luminal contour may resume a smooth contour after epithelial regeneration, but commonly focal areas of submucosal fibrosis cause nodular defects or scalloping. Coexisting gastric involvement, primarily in the distal part of the stomach, may cause antral ulceration, pyloric stenosis, or frank gastric outlet obstruction.[230]

Drug-induced esophagitis

Drug-induced esophagitis has become generally recognized only during the past decade. Numerous reports indicate that a variety of medications (see box on p. 231) are capable of inducing a focal area of esophagitis by direct action on the esophageal mucosa,[231] analogous to a form of caustic esophagitis. The most common cause is antibiotics, such as tetracycline and doxycycline. Other likely agents are quinidine, antiinflammatory drugs, guanidine, and potassium.[232] When such drugs dissolve in the esophagus, they cause mucosal injury either by creating an acid pH or by a direct irritant effect in the epithelium. Loitering of tablets in the esophagus is favored by swallowing pills while lying down, taking pills without water, abnormal esophageal motility, and cardiomegaly (Fig. 11-45).

Symptoms of drug-induced esophagitis are usually sudden in onset and consist of chest pain, odynophagia, or dysphagia. Bleeding or esophageal perforation may occur. Drug-induced esophagitis usually involves the proximal or middle esophagus but occasionally involves the distal esophagus. A typical location is the aortic arch level, where tablets are delayed because of the aortic indentation on the esophagus and the low contractile force of peristalsis (Fig. 11-46). The radiographic findings consist of luminal irregularity, frank ulceration, and luminal narrowing.[5] Occasionally, the findings may simulate esophageal carcinoma.[233] Generally, the symptoms and radiographic findings resolve rapidly after the offending agent is discontinued. In some instances, however, a permanent stricture may develop (Fig. 11-46, *B*).

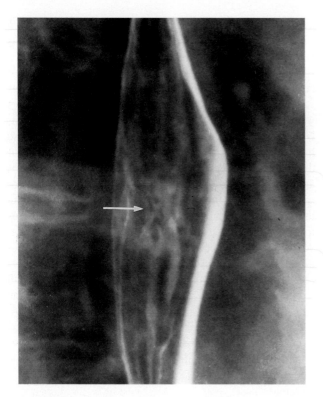

Fig. 11-45 Doxycycline esophagitis. This patient for whom doxycycline had been administered for sinusitis developed odynophagia and dysphagia. This double-contrast examination demonstrates an area of reticular-appearing edema and superficial ulceration in the midesophagus *(arrow)*. This focal area of esophagitis related to doxycycline was confirmed endoscopically.

☐ **DRUGS REPORTED TO CAUSE ESOPHAGITIS** ☐

A. Antibiotics
   1. Tetracycline
   2. Doxycycline
   3. Clindamycin
   4. Lincomycin
B. Antiinflammatory agents
   1. Acetylsalicylic acid
   2. Indomethacin
   3. Phenylbutazone
C. Miscellaneous
   1. Quinidine
   2. Oral potassium
   3. Ferrous sulfate
   4. Ascorbic acid
   5. Fluorouracil
   6. Cimetidine

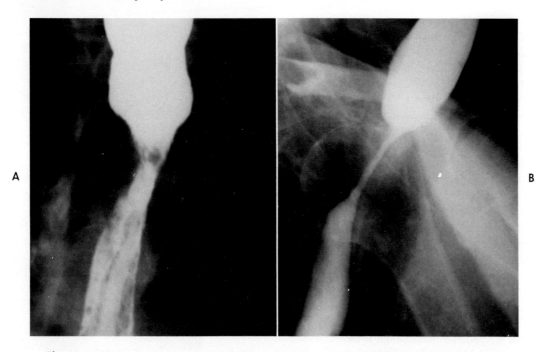

Fig. 11-46 Medication esophagitis in a patient taking quinidine. **A,** At initial presentation the esophageal lumen is narrowed just proximal to the aortic arch, and the mucosal surface is irregular, consistent with ulceration. **B,** Four months later. A tight, benign-appearing stricture is present that required multiple dilatations.

Radiation esophagitis

Symptomatic radiation esophagitis may occur in a small percentage of patients receiving mediastinal radiation. Such patients usually receive 4500 to 6000 rad over a 6- to 8-week period.[234] Symptoms of radiation esophagitis may develop at radiation doses of less than 2000 rad in patients receiving doxorubicin (Adriamycin), an agent that interferes with tissue repair.[235] Clinical symptoms range from mild heartburn to dysphagia.[236] Typically, mild heartburn or dysphagia develops several weeks after the onset of treatment. During this stage, a mild superficial esophagitis is present that heals rapidly. Late symptoms of dysphagia that develop weeks to months after the completion of therapy reflect deep injury to the esophageal muscle or nerves.

The most common radiographic finding in symptomatic subjects is normal esophageal morphology; however, esophageal motor function is generally abnormal.[234] Esophageal peristalsis commonly stops in the proximal esophagus at the upper margin of the radiation field and below this level often degenerates into repetitive, nonperistaltic contractions.[234,237] In some instances the LES may fail to relax. A morphologic abnormality from radiation occasionally consists of diffuse ulceration that may cause pain with swallowing and masquerade as moniliasis. Late findings consist of stricture in the radiation field. Such strictures are generally smooth with tapering margins and rarely show irregularity or ulceration.[234] Occasionally, mucosal bridging may occur.[238]

Miscellaneous causes

Miscellaneous conditions that may be associated with esophagitis include bullous dermatoses, noninfectious granulomatous disease, Behçet's disease, and ulcerative colitis. Bullous dermatoses narrowing squamous mucous membranes may also involve the esophagus. These conditions include pemphigus,[239] pemphigoid,[240,241] epidermolysis bullosa dystrophica,[242,243] toxic epidermal neurolysis,[244] Stevens-Johnson syndrome,[245] and graft-versus-host disease.[246] In these conditions the esophageal lesions consist of vesicles, bullae, desquamation, and ulcers. The lesions often heal without complication, but their repeated formation may lead to significant fibrosis and stenosis. The conditions tend to involve the upper half of the esophagus, but occasionally the whole esophagus may be involved. Whereas pemphigus and pemphigoid are nonhereditary conditions in adults, epidermolysis bullosa dystrophica occurs as an autosomal recessive condition in children. During the acute stage of these conditions, bullae may cause multiple esophageal filling defects on esophagrams, or ruptured bullae may appear as ulcerations. Repetitive insults often lead to strictures that are generally smooth but sometimes have an irregular contour. Epidermolysis commonly produces short stenoses, 1 to 6 cm long, or webs (Fig. 11-47) that may be multiple.[247] Epidermolysis, pemphigoid, and epidermal neurolysis may cause mucosal sloughing as a cast.[241,244,247] Graft-versus-host disease occurs in patients who have undergone bone marrow transplantation.[246]

Although rare, Crohn's esophagitis is probably the most common granulomatous esophagitis without an infectious cause. The most convincing reported cases are in patients with accompanying Crohn's disease of the ileum or colon. Numerous documented cases of esophageal Crohn's disease have been reported.[248,249,250] Clinical symptoms consist of dysphagia and occasionally chest pain. On esophagrams aphthous ulcers may be present,[251] or there may be mucosal irregularity or mild-to-moderate segmental narrowing in the middle or distal esophagus.[248] The morphology tends to resemble Crohn's disease elsewhere in the GI tract. Involvement may be eccentric and simulate a plaquelike neoplasm. Focal nodularity, irregularity, or penetrating ulceration may occur. Fistulas are common[252] and distinguish Crohn's from the rare cases of a sarcoid stricture. Tuberculosis must be excluded. Esophagitis associated with Behçet's disease may cause erosions, focal penetrating ulceration,[253] and spontaneous perforation.[254,255] The few reported cases of esophagitis accompanying ulcerative colitis showed superficial ulceration that may respond to steroid therapy.[256]

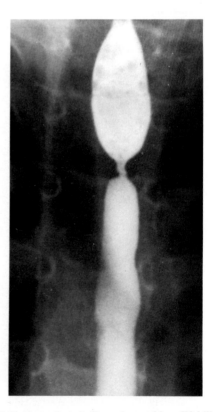

Fig. 11-47 Epidermolysis bullosa dystrophica. Weblike narrowing is seen in the proximal esophagus.

RINGS, WEBS, AND STRICTURES

By common usage the term *web* is generally applied to thick (1 to 2 mm) diaphragm-like membranes that extend partially or completely around the esophageal lumen. The designation *esophageal ring* or *stenosis* is usually reserved for a short annular narrowing, 4 to 10 mm in vertical thickness. Although the morphology of the thin transverse mucosal fold, commonly present at the esophagogastric junction, is similar to an esophageal web, the label *lower esophageal ring* is widely used and will not be tampered with here. Segments of fixed narrowing greater than 1 cm long are generally categorized as strictures.

To accurately diagnose and define esophageal rings, webs, and strictures, it is imperative to achieve adequate esophageal distention during the radiographic examination. Narrow rings at the esophagogastric junction commonly escape detection because the distal esophagus is not distended adequately or the cardia is obscured by an axial hiatus hernia. Esophageal webs, usually located in the proximal esophagus, are inconspicuous and easily overlooked. Incomplete webs tend to be anterior and are commonly seen only on lateral projections. Complete webs occasionally cause a jet effect (Fig. 11-48, *A*) seen at fluoroscopy.[257] The length of esophageal strictures may be overestimated when the normal esophagus distal to the stricture is insufficiently distended. Helpful methods for accomplishing esophageal distention include wide-bored straw for rapid delivery of barium, an abdominal bolster, Trendelenburg position, esophageal intubation, induced gastroesophageal reflux of barium, and hypotonic pharmacologic agents.

Esophageal rings

Excluding the asymptomatic mucosal and muscle rings that commonly demarcate the margins of the LES segment (see Fig. 11-28), the most common esophageal ring seen at radiologic examination is the narrow, symptomatic lower esophageal ring described in 1953 by Schatzki and Gary.[258] Subsequently the term *Schatzki's ring* was applied to the asymptomatic mucosal fold at the esophagogastric junction. The symptomatic Schatzki's ring is an exaggeration of the normal transverse mucosal fold, whereby the fold is thickened to 4 to 5 mm and the luminal aperture is narrowed. The cause of these acquired rings remains unknown but is generally believed to be related to gastroesophageal reflux. On histologic section the rings demonstrate squamous epithelium on their upper surface and columnar epithelium below.[259] The core of the ring consists of lamina propria with-

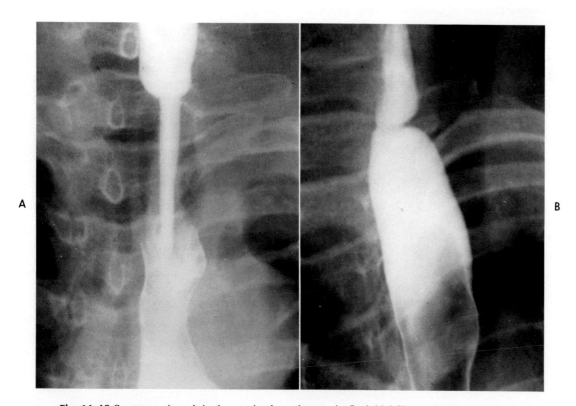

Fig. 11-48 Symptomatic web in the proximal esophagus. **A,** On initial films, a jet effect was seen distal to the web. **B,** Better distention demonstrates a circumferential web at the level of the thoracic inlet. Splitting of the web at endoscopy cured the patient's dysphagia for solid foods.

out inflammation or fibrosis. The muscularis mucosa does not participate in the ring structure.

The symptomatic Schatzki's ring generally produces the characteristic clinical symptoms, called the *steak house syndrome,* of intermittent, episodic dysphagia for solids, often associated with substernal pain. The obstructive symptoms may be relieved by drinking liquid or regurgitation of the ingested material. Occasionally, an impacted bolus must be removed at endoscopy. The typical clinical history should suggest the correct diagnosis before radiographic examination.

On fluoroscopy the symptomatic Schatzki's ring is seen as a thickened, annular narrowing at the esophagogastric junction (Fig. 11-49, *B*). Rings less than 12 mm in luminal diameter are always accompanied by dysphagia. Rings 12 to 20 mm in diameter may or may not cause symptoms, and dysphagia is rare with rings greater than 20 mm in diameter.[260] The symptomatic Schatzki's ring is a passive structure that is easily missed unless sought specifically. Many patients travel from physician to physician seeking relief, carrying reports of negative radiographic examinations. Many are diagnosed as having neurotic dysphagia. The ring is not apparent on radiographs unless the distal esophagus is well distended (Fig. 11-49, *A*). A marshmallow bolus or barium tablet may be useful to demonstrate a narrow ring. A hiatus hernia is generally present.

The radiographic features of an annular peptic structure involving the esophagogastric junction may be identical with those of a Schatzki's ring. Generally, however, patients with an annular peptic stricture have clinical complaints of heartburn in addition to episodic dysphagia, whereas heartburn seldom coexists with a symptomatic Schatzki's ring. Additionally, the annular strictures are often accompanied by morphologic findings, suggesting esophagitis in the distal third of the esophagus.[191]

Careful examination may reveal that an annular inflammatory ring is just above the cardia, rather than precisely at the esophagogastric junction. A ring not precisely at the cardia is not a Schatzki's ring. Distinguishing an annular peptic stricture from a Schatzki's ring is of practical importance, because inflammatory rings are more likely to perforate during dilatation. In many cases, endoscopy may be needed to make the distinction.

The characteristic feature of muscle rings is that they change spontaneously in caliber and configuration (see Fig. 11-28) during fluoroscopy.[28] Occasionally a prominent muscle ring at the proximal margin of the LES segment is of constant configuration, especially when associated with diffuse esophageal spasm. Fixed muscle rings occasionally generate symptoms similar to those caused by a Schatzki's ring.[261] In this circumstance, however, the muscle ring is recognized by its characteristic location and is generally relaxed by administration of amyl nitrite or an anticholinergic agent. Rarely, muscle rings may occur elsewhere in the esophagus, such as the midesophagus or aortic arch level. The same principles apply for their identification as for the

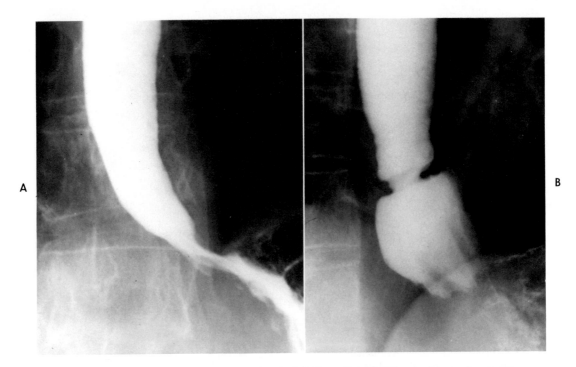

Fig. 11-49 Symptomatic Schatzki's ring. **A,** The initial esophagram did not achieve adequate distention of the distal esophagus and was reported as normal. **B,** Repeat esophagram showing thickened, narrow ring at esophagogastric junction. A fixed passive ring had an aperture diameter of 10 mm.

more common muscle ring at the proximal margin of the LES segment.

Congenital esophageal rings or stenoses may show nonspecific histologic findings or contain remnants of tracheobronchial cartilage and respiratory epithelium. The latter anomaly is thought to result from a failure of respiratory tract tissue to completely separate from the primitive esophagus, as normally occurs during fetal life.[262] Cartilaginous rings are invariably in the distal third of the esophagus, whereas nonspecific congenital rings may occur in the middle third as well. Esophageal dilatation often exists proximal to the ring. Congenital rings are usually found in the neonate or young infant because they cause regurgitation, vomiting, and aspiration.[263] Older children have dysphagia for solids. In infants a congenital ring may be difficult to distinguish from an annular peptic stricture because both are associated with vomiting. With some cartilaginous rings, barium fills linear clefts extending perpendicular to the ring. The clefts represent ducts and cystic spaces lined with respiratory epithelium.[262,263] This finding in a child is virtually specific for a cartilaginous ring, but in adults a similar picture can occur with a localized segment of intramural pseudodiverticulosis or focal tuberculosis with sinus tracts. Intramural congenital esophageal rings also need to be distinguished from vascular rings caused by aberrant blood vessels or a double aortic arch.

Other causes of esophageal rings (Table 11-1) include caustic ingestion, bullous dermatoses, surgical anastomosis, and neoplasm. Caustic ingestion may occasionally result in a short annular web or ring, rather than a long stricture. Annular ring strictures from caustic agents are most likely to occur with the ingestion of Clinitest tablets or irritant drugs, such as doxycycline, quinidine, and ascorbic acid. Bullous skin conditions, such as pemphigus[264] and epidermolysis bullosa, may cause either ringlike stenosis or frank stricture. Short annular esophageal rings may also be caused by carcinoma or a circumferential leiomyoma. These latter lesions, however, are almost invariably more than 1 cm long.

Esophageal webs

Three general types of esophageal webs have been described: (1) nonspecific or idiopathic webs; (2) webs associated with the Plummer-Vinson syndrome,[265] and (3) webs caused by epidermolysis bullosa dystrophica or graft-versus-host disease. Nonspecific esophageal webs are common. They are observed in 5% to 8% of patients referred for barium meals and have an even higher frequency when looked for at autopsy.[266,267] These webs nearly always occur in the cervical esophagus within a few centimeters of the cricopharyngeus (Fig. 11-40, B). They occur predominantly in individuals older than 50 years of age. Histologically the webs are plications of normal squamous mucosa with inflammation. At present the validity of the Plummer-Vinson syndrome, consisting of cervical esophageal webs and iron deficiency anemia, is controversial. This entity is

☐ **TABLE 11-1**

Classification of esophageal rings, webs, and strictures

	Esophagogastric junction	Esophageal body		
		Distal	Middle	Proximal
Esophageal rings				
Transverse mucosal fold	xx			
Symptomatic Schatzki's ring	xx			
Annular peptic stricture	xx	xx		
Muscle ring		xx	x	x
Congenital stenosis				
Cartilaginous		xx		
Nonspecific		xx	xx	
Vascular ring				
Nonpeptic				xx
Caustic agents		x	xx	x
Pemphigus		x	xx	xx
Epidermolysis bullosum		x	xx	xx
Annular tumor				
Carcinoma		xx	xx	x
Circumferential leiomyoma		xx	xx	x
Esophageal webs				
Idiopathic		x	x	x
Plummer-Vinson				xx
Esophageal strictures				
Physical injury				
Peptic esophagitis	x	xx	x	
Caustic esophagitis		xx	xx	x
Radiation		x	xx	x
Sclerotherapy	x	xx		
Infection				
Tuberculosis		xx	xx	xx
Monilial		xx	xx	xx
Congenital				
Cartilaginous		xx		
Nonspecific		xx	xx	
Miscellaneous				
Barrett's esophagus			xx	xx
Pseudodiverticulosis		xx	xx	xx
Epidermolysis bullosa		xx	xx	xx
Graft-versus-host disease		xx	xx	x
Pemphigus		xx	xx	xx
Eosinophilic infiltrate		x	xx	x
Muscular hyperplasia		xx	xx	
Intramural bleed		xx	xx	
Neoplasm				
Carcinoma		xx	xx	x
Invasion		x	xx	x
Metastatic		xx	xx	x
Leiomyoma		xx	xx	
Postoperative				
TE fistula			xx	xx
Nissen repair		xx		
Vagotomy hematoma		xx		

*For a given lesion, **xx,** most common site(s); **x,** less common or unusual site(s).

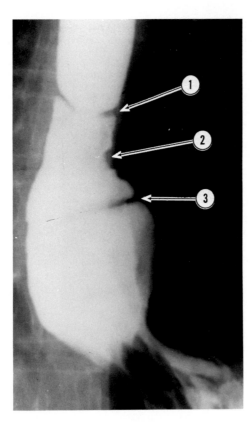

Fig. 11-50 Web in the distal esophagus. A web *(1)* is located 1 cm proximal to the muscle ring *(2)* that identifies the upper margin of the open LES segment. A thin mucosal ring *(3)* at the esophagogastric junction demarcates a hiatus hernia.

allegedly associated with carcinoma of the pharynx or esophagus.[268] In some cases the webs represent patches of heterotopic gastric mucosa.[25] A few patients are observed with multiple esophageal webs[269] or a nonspecific web in the distal esophagus (Fig. 11-50). In some cases webs in the distal esophagus may be associated with esophagitis.[270]

Esophageal strictures

For this discussion an esophageal stricture is considered to represent any persistent intrinsic esophageal narrowing that is longer than 1 cm. The term is nonspecific and does not imply any particular underlying cause. Although the causes of stricture are numerous (see Table 11-1), the most common generic cause is fibrosis from inflammation and neoplasm. The sensitivity of the radiographic method for detecting esophageal stricture equals or exceeds that of endoscopy.[271] It is important to determine whether an esophageal stricture is benign or malignant. Benign strictures characteristically have an hourglass configuration with concentric smooth, tapering margins that gradually merge with the adjacent normal esophageal wall (see Fig. 11-36, *A*). Typically, malignant strictures have an irregular luminal contour, often demonstrating ulceration or tumor nodules.

The narrowing is commonly eccentric, and the margins of the lesion are often shelflike or undercut where they terminate abruptly with adjacent normal esophagus (Fig. 11-36, *B*). However, numerous exceptions occur. A stricture with active inflammation may have an ulcerated, irregular contour and asymmetric margins that simulate malignancy. Fibrosis may cause areas of nodularity. Conversely, malignant strictures with fibrosis may have a benign appearance. Accurate diagnosis may require endoscopy with multiple biopsies.

The most common esophageal strictures are inflammatory strictures caused by reflux peptic esophagitis (see Fig. 11-30). Typically, these strictures are located in the distal third to half of the esophagus, with sparing of the terminal 2 to 3 cm proximal to the cardia. A hiatus hernia is nearly always present.[272] Garden-variety peptic strictures generally vary in length from 2 to 6 cm, and the luminal diameter ranges from a few millimeters to 1 to 2 cm. The esophagus seldom demonstrates substantial dilatation. Occasionally, intramural pneumatosis is adjacent to a stricture.[273] Mild strictures, often unaccompanied by dysphagia, are demonstrated as areas of flattening or reduced compliance only when the esophagus is maximally distended (see Fig. 11-30, *A*). Because of their generous diameter, this latter form of stricture is almost invariably missed by endoscopy. Less common forms of peptic stricture, such as an annular ring or bird-beak tapering of the LES segment, were discussed earlier. Long peptic strictures involving the distal half to two thirds of the esophagus may result from garden-variety reflux esophagitis but more commonly are caused by protracted vomiting, nasogastric intubation (see Fig. 11-34, *A*), the Zollinger-Ellison syndrome (see Fig. 11-34, *B*), or reflux during anesthesia.[159,274] Other causes of long esophageal stricture are caustic ingestion, radiation, and mediastinal fibrosis caused by metastatic breast carcinoma[275] or infection.

Caustic strictures commonly involve a long esophageal segment (see Fig. 11-44, *B*) but may be short or ringlike in appearance. Occasionally, the strictures are multiple. In some instances, the whole esophagus is involved. Luminal narrowing may be uniform or variable. The contour of the lumen may be smooth but usually shows irregularity or nodularity.

Radiation strictures nearly invariably involve the upper half to two thirds of the thoracic esophagus. The luminal contour is generally smooth (Fig. 11-51, *B*). Clues to previous radiation may be provided by geographic paramediastinal lung changes. Other strictures that commonly involve the proximal thoracic esophagus are those associated with columnar-lined Barrett's esophagus (see Fig. 11-36, *A*), medication esophagitis (see Fig. 11-46, *B*), and bullous dermatoses. A benign-appearing stricture in the proximal thoracic esophagus may also be caused by encircling tumor from the adjacent mediastinum (Fig. 11-52).

Stricturelike lesions from a primary esophageal neoplasm

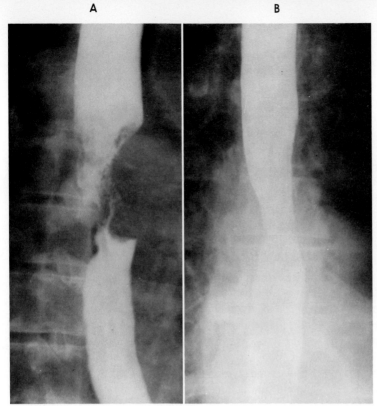

Fig. 11-51 Radiation stricture after radiation therapy for esophageal carcinoma. **A,** Squamous carcinoma of the midesophagus. **B,** One year after radiation therapy, a benign radiation stricture is seen at the location of the previous tumor. Endoscopy and biopsy failed to reveal residual tumor. Radiographic appearance of the stricture remained unchanged on subsequent esophagrams.

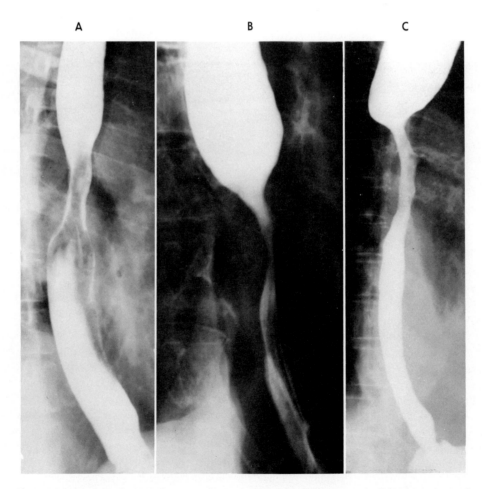

Fig. 11-52 Esophageal narrowing secondary to mediastinal malignancy. **A,** Bronchogenic carcinoma involving the carinal nodes and invading the esophagus. **B** and **C,** Two patients with mediastinal metastases from carcinoma of the breast.

may exist at any esophageal level but occur usually in the distal two thirds of the esophagus. The most common cause is carcinoma. An accompanying hiatus hernia is generally absent.[272] Contour irregularity, ulceration, and nodules are clues to the correct diagnosis. Rarely, coalescing leiomyomas may simulate a stricture.

Miscellaneous esophageal strictures may be caused by congenital abnormalities (Fig. 11-53, *A*), intramural pseudodiverticulosis (Fig. 11-24, *B*), and bullous mucocutaneous disorders, such as pemphigus, epidermyolysis bullosa, and graft-versus-host disease.[240,242,246,276] Tuberculous strictures are often accompanied by a sinus tract or fistula. Rarely, segmental esophageal narrowing may be caused by eosinophilic infiltrate.[277] In rare cases, esophageal stricture may be caused by moniliasis.[278] Muscle hypertrophy may cause persistent narrowing in the smooth muscle portion of the esophagus.[279] Following sclerotherapy for esophageal varices, the esophagus often exhibits mucosal irregularity, wall thickening, luminal narrowing, and even sinus tracts (Fig. 11-54). These changes generally resolve but may lead to a permanent stricture in the distal esophagus.[164,280] Rarely, sclerotherapy of varices may cause an intramural esophageal hematoma with severe dysphagia (Fig. 11-55). Occasionally, stricture of the distal esophagus may be caused by a pseudocyst extending through the diaphragmatic hiatus into the mediastinum. Surgical anastomoses, such as TE fistula repair (Fig. 11-53, *B*), or penetrating injuries may lead to esophageal stricture. The underlying cause of many esophageal strictures is generally evident after a salient medical history is obtained. A Nissen fundoplication for hiatus hernia commonly causes a narrowed esophageal segment in the fundoplication accompanied by a mass defect in the gastric fundus.[281] Other strictures of the distal esophagus may be caused by mediastinal fibrosis[282] or hepatomegaly.[283]

ESOPHAGEAL VARICES

Esophageal varices are dilated, subepithelial veins. Such varices result from increased collateral blood flow via the azygos vein between the intraabdominal portal venous system and the intrathoracic superior vena cava. Generally, the collateral venous flow is "uphill" toward the azygos and superior vena cava. The prevalent cause of esophageal varices is portal hypertension, usually from hepatic cirrhosis, but occasionally the varices are caused by prehepatic portal vein obstruction, posthepatic vein obstruction, or congestive heart failure. In some circumstances, esophageal varices may occur without portal hypertension when portal venous flow is increased because of splenic atrioventricular shunting associated with splenic hemangiomatosis or

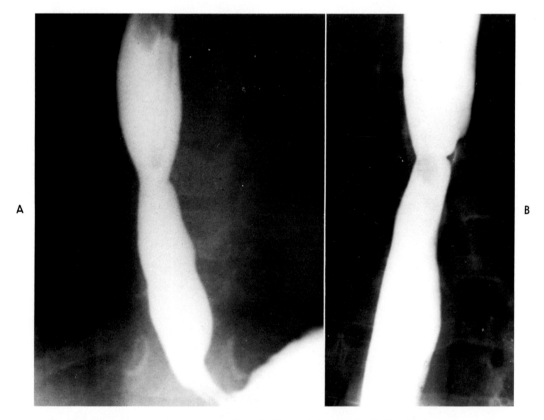

Fig. 11-53 Localized esophageal narrowing. **A,** Congenital stenosis. **B,** Surgical anastomosis for esophageal atresia.

A   B   C

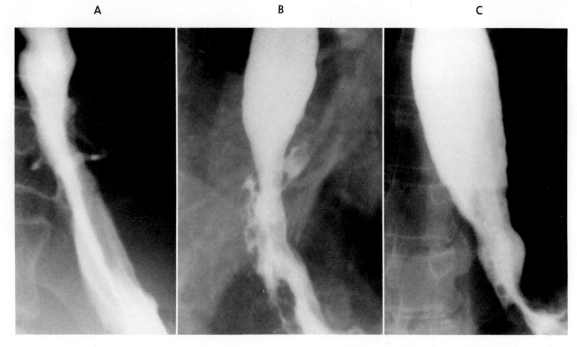

Fig. 11-54 Esophageal changes after sclerotherapy for varices. In each of these three examples, findings of esophageal varices are present. **A,** One week after sclerotherapy, two localized esophageal sinuses developed in the distal esophagus. Sinuses resolved without treatment. **B,** Two weeks after several sclerotherapy treatments. The distal esophagus is narrowed and irregular. Several prominent walled-off sinuses are present. These changes resolved in several months. **C,** A persistent mild esophageal stricture several months after sclerotherapy.

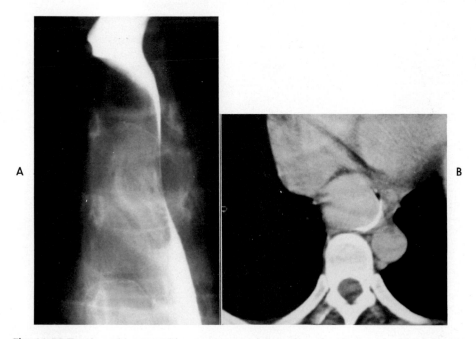

Fig. 11-55 Esophageal intramural hematoma several days after sclerotherapy. **A,** A large intramural hematoma involved the right side of the distal two thirds of the esophagus. The esophageal lumen is compressed and displaced leftward. **B,** CT section through the midesophagus shows an intramural esophageal mass with a crescent of contrast located within the compressed eccentric esophageal lumen. Intramural hematoma resolved completely in several weeks.

Fig. 11-56 CT demonstration of posterior mediastinal varices. Image through the distal esophagus shows substantial esophageal thickening with contrast enhancement from large esophageal varices. Additionally, a large cluster of enhanced varices *(arrow)* shrouds the lateral wall of the descending aorta. These varices were seen as an "ominous" left paraspinous mass on chest radiograph.

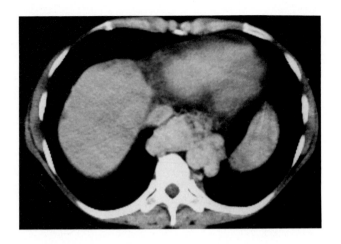

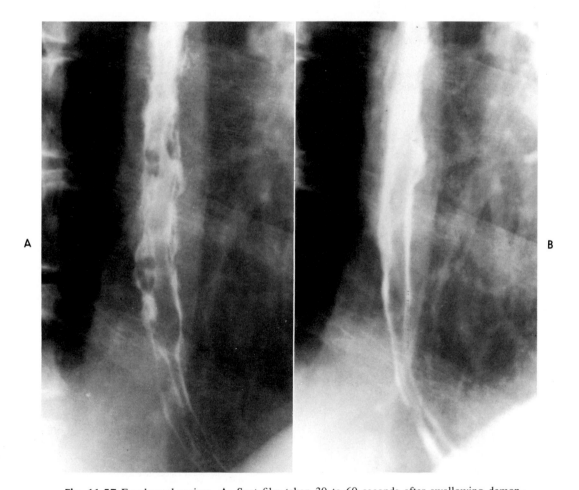

Fig. 11-57 Esophageal varices. **A,** Spot film taken 30 to 60 seconds after swallowing demonstrates multiple esophageal varices. **B,** Spot film in same patient taken immediately after the passage of a peristaltic contraction wave. The peristaltic contraction wave has ironed out the varices so that they are no longer seen. After 30 to 60 seconds, however, the varices refilled and assumed an appearance similar to that in **A.**

marked splenomegaly. Occasionally, "downhill" esophageal varices exist when the superior vena cava is obstructed distal to the entry of the azygos.[284] Usually, downhill varices predominate in the proximal half of the esophagus, whereas the more common uphill varices occur in the distal half of the esophagus. "Hepatofugal" varices are usually associated with portal hypertension, whereas "hepatopetal" varices are present with occlusions of the splenic and/or portal veins. Esophageal varices seldom cause symptoms other than upper gastrointestinal bleeding. Variceal bleeding is generally abrupt in onset and massive. The bleeding site or sites may be associated with venous rupture, mucosal erosion, or ulceration. An earlier report suggested that gastroesophageal reflux could contribute to variceal bleeding,[285] but this proposal was not confirmed by subsequent studies.[286]

Esophageal varices are commonly detected during diagnostic evaluation for upper gastrointestinal bleeding. Small varices are as likely to bleed as large varices. The number or size of the varices do not correlate closely with the magnitude of the portal hypertension. Demonstration of esophageal varices in patients with upper GI bleeding does not necessarily establish the origin of bleeding, because about a third of such patients bleed from other causes, such as a peptic ulcer or Mallory-Weiss tear. In some cases, esophageal varices are detected on barium studies as incidental findings in asymptomatic patients or in patients undergoing evaluation for liver disease. Occasionally, esophageal varices appear initially as posterior mediastinal masses on chest film.[287] The identity of such masses is readily demonstrated by contrast-enhanced thoracic CT (Fig. 11-56).

Optimal radiographic evaluation for esophageal varices depends on adequate mucosal coating with contrast medium, maneuvers designed to enhance variceal filling, and in some instances the use of pharmacologic agents. Although tantalum paste is an optimal contrast medium for demonstrating esophageal varices,[288] this agent is not generally available. For practical purposes barium is the current medium of choice. Standard preparations of liquid barium used for single-contrast esophagrams are often adequate to demonstrate varices. Better esophageal mucosal coating, however, is obtained using high-density liquid barium or paste preparations.

Films of the barium-coated esophagus should be made with the esophagus collapsed, thereby allowing variceal filling and optimal visualization of the esophageal folds. Because peristalsis transiently squeezes and flattens varices,[289] a minimum of 15 to 20 seconds should elapse after esophageal peristalsis to allow variceal refilling before a radiograph is obtained (Fig. 11-57). Overfilling of the esophagus tends to iron out and thereby obscure the varices.

Multiple spot films should be taken of the collapsed esophagus in several different projections. The recumbent position is standard. In some patients, however, the upright position enhances variceal filling, perhaps because the varices fill against the hydrostatic force of the azygos system.

Traditional methods touted to enhance variceal filling are Valsalva's maneuver, Müller's maneuver, and Trendelenburg position. One study suggests the best combination is end-expiratory filming with the patient in the supine left oblique position.[290] No single position or maneuver, however, gives best results uniformly. The highest diagnostic yield is achieved when multiple spot films are obtained in several projections and different provocative maneuvers are used.

On mucosal spot films, esophageal varices seen en face may appear as thickened longitudinal esophageal folds. Fold thickening, however, is a nonspecific finding and is caused most often by esophagitis. Thickened longitudinal esophageal folds are normally exquisitely parallel. Any fusiform separation of the folds suggests the presence of varices. More definite findings are beaded or serpiginous filling defects (Fig. 11-58, A) that characteristically change

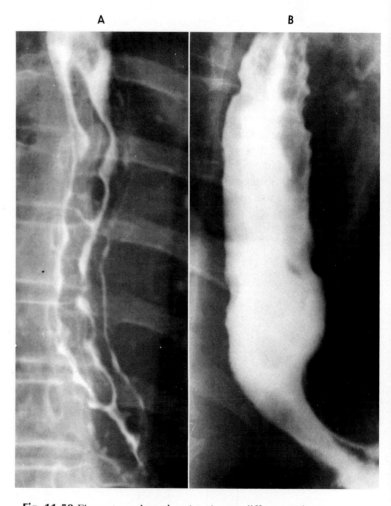

A   B

Fig. 11-58 Flagrant esophageal varices in two different patients. **A,** Mucosal view of a collapsed esophagus demonstrates varices as serpiginous, slightly nodular filling defects when seen en face. **B,** Spot film of a barium-filled esophagus. When seen tangentially, varices cause a scalloped or modular contour to the margin of the barium column.

in size during the examination. Occasionally, a varicoid carcinoma may simulate esophageal varices, but varicoid carcinoma shows areas of rigidity and nodular filling defects that do not change in size or show compression by peristalsis.[291] When seen tangentially varices may appear as nodular filling defects or have a scalloped contour (Fig. 11-58, *B*). Such scalloping may be simulated by tertiary esophageal contractions, but tertiary contractions disappear after esophageal hypotonia is induced with anticholinergic agents.[128] whereas anticholinergic agents tend to enhance the filling of varices.[290,292] Glucagon relaxes the lower esophageal sphincter but does not relax the esophageal body.[131]

Some reports suggest that barium esophagrams detect varices in about one half to two thirds of patients shown to have varices by endoscopy.[290] In some instances, however, the radiographic method demonstrates esophageal varices that go undetected at esophagoscopy. Further, the supplemental use of improved barium preparations and anticholinergic agents that paralyze esophageal smooth muscle enable the radiographic method to compete favorably with endoscopy for detecting esophageal varices.[293] Unlike the radiographic method, however, endoscopy usually establishes whether the varices account for bleeding.

ESOPHAGEAL TUMORS

A number of neoplasms and nonneoplastic conditions cause intramural mass lesions of the esophagus (see box on p. 243). Intrinsic esophageal masses need to be distinguished from an intraluminal foreign body, such as a bolus of meat, or extrinsic conditions that compress the esophagus. On radiographic examination, an intraluminal impaction does not show any point of attachment with the esophageal wall. Rarely, a gastric bezoar regurgitated into the

esophagus may simulate a tumor.[294] Traditional criteria help determine whether an esophageal filling defect is epithelial, submucosal, or extrinsic in origin (Fig. 11-59). Epithelial lesions, such as carcinoma, generally have an irregular contour on tangential views and often have undercut or shelflike margins. In contrast, submucosal tumors generally stretch the esophageal mucosa to form a symmetric, moundlike lesion with exquisitely smooth margins. When seen tangentially, the margins of the lesion taper smoothly to form an obtuse angle with the normal esophageal wall. The estimated center of the mass falls close to or within the projection of the esophageal wall. Axial movement of a lesion during longitudinal esophageal contraction establishes that the lesion is intramural.[13] A filling defect caused by compression from an external mass is generally not as sharply defined as an intramural submucosal lesion. The extrapolated center of the mass falls outside the esophageal wall. Sometimes the radiographic findings are not sufficiently characteristic to enable confident determination of tumor location.

Malignant tumors

In most segments of the GI tract, benign lesions constitute the majority of intraluminal tumors. In the esophagus, however, the majority of intrinsic tumors are primarily carcinomas.

Carcinomas

Carcinoma is the most common tumor of the esophagus and comprises about 4% of all GI tract malignancies. Esophageal carcinoma generally occurs in men older than 50 years of age. High-risk factors are alcohol use; tobacco use; and living in certain geographic areas, such as parts of Iran, China, France, and Japan. Also at risk are patients

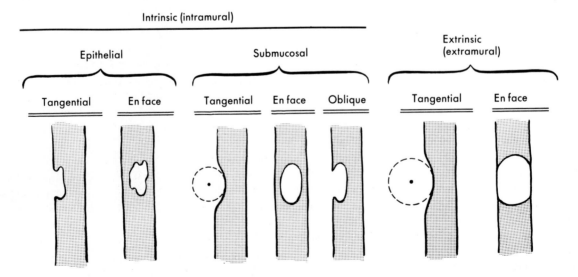

Fig. 11-59 Schematic representation of the three generic categories of polypoid esophageal filling defects.

with Barrett's esophagus, caustic stricture, radiation stricture, achalasia, sprue, Plummer-Vinson syndrome, previous head or neck tumors, and hereditary tylosis.[295-297]

About 90% of esophageal carcinomas are of squamous cell origin. The remainder are adenocarcinomas that arise primarily in the distal esophagus. Rare variants of esophageal carcinoma include verrucous squamous cell carcinoma, oat cell carcinoma, and cylindroma. About 40% of esophageal carcinomas are located in the distal esophagus, 40% in the middle esophagus, and 20% in the proximal esophagus. The predominant clinical complaint is dysphagia, often accompanied by weight loss. Other symptoms include cough, hoarseness, and weakness.

In cases of esophageal carcinoma, chest radiographs generally do not show any abnormalities but may reveal mediastinal widening, a soft tissue mass, an esophageal gas-fluid level, anterior tracheal bowing, or a thickened retrotracheal stripe.[298,299] On esophagrams, esophageal carcinoma presents a variety of morphologic abnormalities (Figs. 11-60 to 11-63). Advanced tumors may appear as an annular apple-core lesion with overhanging margins, irregular narrowed segment, smooth tapering stricture, bulky endophytic mass, large ulceration, varicoid infiltrate, or diffuse nodularity. Moderate-sized lesions, 1.5 to 3 cm in size, generally occur as lobulated sessile lesions that are eccentric and may show evidence of ulceration.[136,300,301] Some lesions are detected as an area of superficial irregularity or a flattened zone of decreased compliance. Small lesions less than 1.5 cm in size may be seen as moundlike sessile polyps, flattened sessile lesions, or a patch of mucosal irregularity (Fig. 11-64). Each of the morphologic patterns of esophageal carcinoma have their own differential diagnosis. For example, areas of irregular narrowing may also be caused by an inflammatory lesion or invasion by an extrinsic malignancy. Varicoid lesions may simulate varices.[291] Small sessile lesions less than 1.5 cm in size may appear as benign lesions.

After radiation therapy, many esophageal carcinomas, even those of substantial size, shrink rapidly and often take on the appearance of a benign esophageal stricture.[302] In some instances, a few small nodules or areas of irregularity remain to suggest the identity of the original lesion. In other instances, all tumor is eradicated and only a benign radiation stricture persists (Fig. 11-51, *B*). Despite the frequent dramatic regression of esophageal carcinoma after radiation, the overall prognosis is poor. Fistulization into the tracheobronchial tree is a frequent complication following radiation treatment for esophageal carcinoma. Fistulization may also occur spontaneously (Fig. 11-65). Fewer than 5% of patients live 5 years—a dismal survival statistic that has shown negligible improvement during the last 30 years. The reason is clear. At initial diagnosis only 25% of patients have a localized, potentially curable lesion. CT examination is often useful for staging (Fig. 11-66) and showing the extent of the lesion.[303-305]

Improvement in patient survival depends on detecting

☐ ESOPHAGEAL TUMORS ☐

I. Malignant neoplasm
  A. Carcinomas
    1. Squamous
    2. Adenocarcinoma
    3. Carcinoid
  B. Sarcoma
    1. Leiomyosarcoma
    2. Fibrosarcoma
    3. Lymphoma
    4. Others
  C. Metastases
II. Benign neoplasm
  A. Mucosal
    1. Papilloma
    2. Adenoma
  B. Submucosal
    1. Leiomyoma
    2. Neurofibroma
    3. Hemangioma
    4. Fibroma
    5. Lipoma
    6. Myeloblastoma
    7. Hemangiopericytoma
III. Nonneoplastic
  A. Fibrovascular polyp
  B. Inflammatory polyp
  C. Cystic lesions
    1. Retention cyst
    2. Enteric cyst
    3. Duplication
  D. Solitary varix
  E. Focal infection
  F. Ectopic tissue
  G. Hamartoma
  H. Hematoma

---

esophageal carcinomas while they are small and asymptomatic. When esophageal carcinoma is confined to the mucosa, 75% are without nodal metastases.[306] For patients with lesions less than 1.5 cm in size, the prognosis is excellent. Patients with lesions 1.5 to 3 cm in diameter have a reasonable chance for survival. Once dysphagia is present, the lesion is generally incurable.

The evaluation of advanced esophageal carcinoma is generally readily accomplished by single-contrast examination. Images of the barium-filled esophagus demonstrate the size and location of lesions sufficiently large to cause dysphagia. Adequate distention is essential to define the lesion's margins. Mucosal views with the esophagus collapsed are often useful for evaluating the fold pattern and surface char-

Text continued on p. 249.

Fig. 11-60, cont'd
For legend see opposite page.

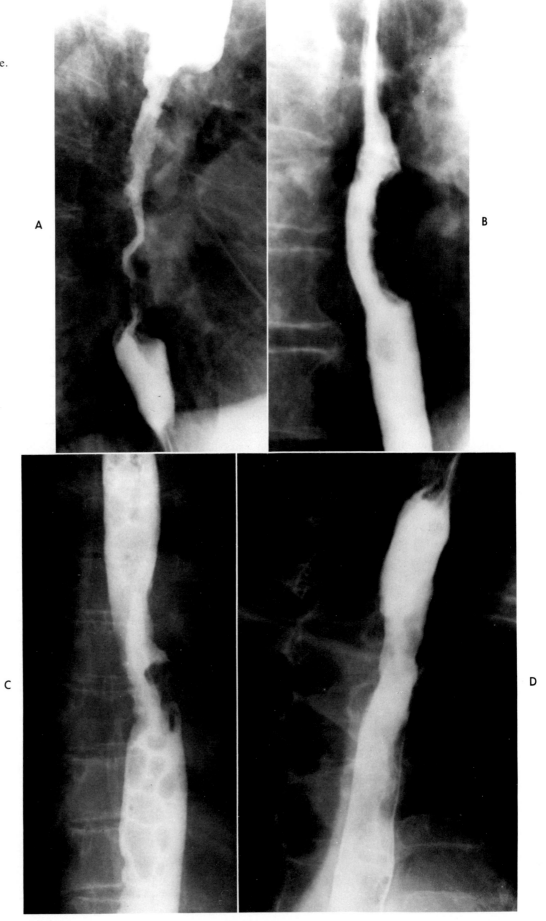

Fig. 11-60 Morphologic varieties of an esophageal carcinoma. **A,** Extensive annular lesion. **B,** Eccentric sessile polypoid lesion 4 cm in length. **C,** Ulcerating flat sessile lesion about 3 to 4 cm in length. **D,** Rigid plaquelike area about 2 to 3 cm in length. Lesion involved 60% of the esophageal circumference.

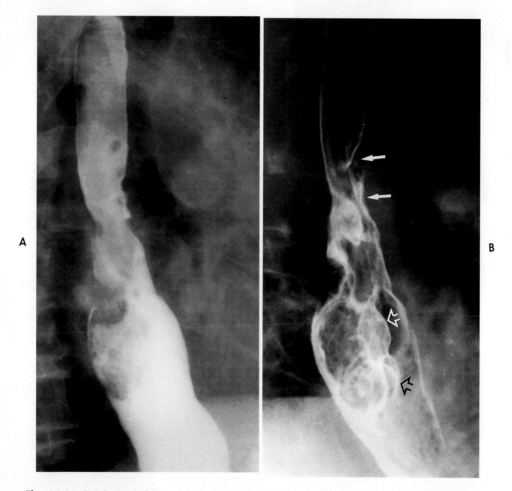

Fig. 11-61 Carcinoma of the esophagus. **A,** A single-contrast examination of a polypoid squamous cell carcinoma of the esophagus demonstrates an extensive mass involving the midportion of the esophagus. Infiltration of the proximal aspect of the tumor into the esophageal wall has resulted in some lack of compliance in this area. The large, irregular intraluminal filling mass is partially outlined in the single-contrast phase of this examination. However, the true polypoid nature is best demonstrated in **B. B,** A double-contrast examination of this same tumor much more accurately depicts the intraluminal polypoid component of the mass *(open arrowheads)*. In this case the squamous cell tumor manifests both intraluminal polypoid mass features as well as evidence of infiltration into the wall of the esophagus proximally *(arrows)*.

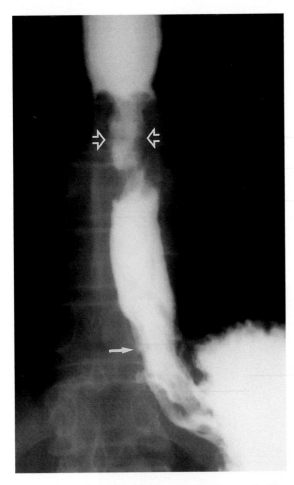

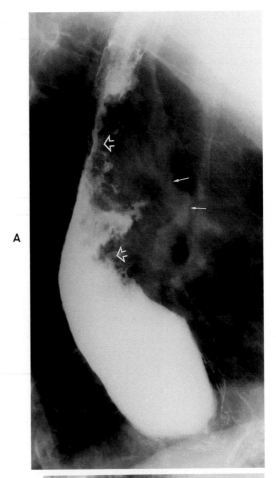

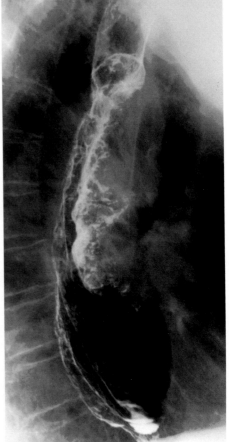

Fig. 11-62 Squamous cell carcinoma of the esophagus. In this case an annular carcinoma is seen in the midportion of the esophagus with circumferential infiltration and overhanging margins *(open arrowheads)*. The tumor has spread submucosally, and a second tumor mass is seen just above the esophagogastric junction *(arrow)*. It is not unusual for tumors originating in the esophagus to spread submucosally in the submucosal lymphatics and reappear at a distant site as in this case.

Fig. 11-63 Squamous cell carcinoma superimposed on long-standing achalasia. **A,** Single-contrast examination of the esophagus demonstrates a very large, irregular, bulky tumor *(open arrowheads)*. The tumor involves the anterior wall of the esophagus, displaces the airway anteriorly, and involves the posterior wall of the distal trachea *(arrows)*. The late onset of symptoms of dysphagia is obviously due to the luminal diameter of the abnormal esophagus involved with achalasia. **B,** A double-contrast examination of the same tumor more accurately depicts the tumor mass and its surface characteristics. The malignant features of this mass are evident on both the single- and double-contrast examinations.

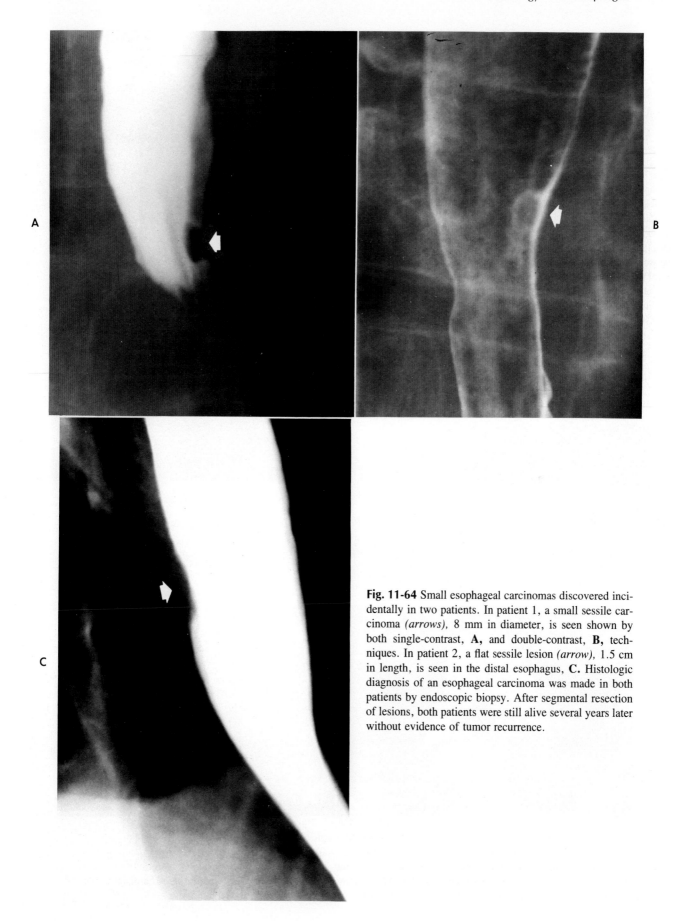

Fig. 11-64 Small esophageal carcinomas discovered incidentally in two patients. In patient 1, a small sessile carcinoma *(arrows),* 8 mm in diameter, is seen shown by both single-contrast, **A,** and double-contrast, **B,** techniques. In patient 2, a flat sessile lesion *(arrow),* 1.5 cm in length, is seen in the distal esophagus, **C.** Histologic diagnosis of an esophageal carcinoma was made in both patients by endoscopic biopsy. After segmental resection of lesions, both patients were still alive several years later without evidence of tumor recurrence.

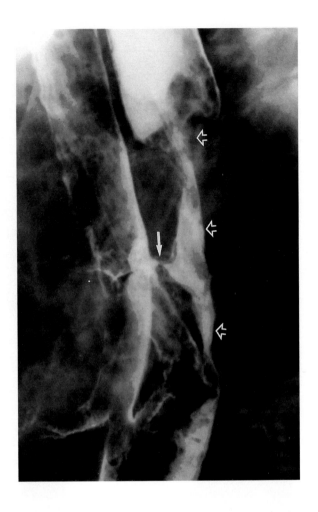

Fig. 11-65 Squamous cell carcinoma of the esophagus with tracheoesophageal fistula. This lateral view of the esophagus was obtained after the development of symptoms of a tracheoesophageal fistula. The patient had been treated with radiotherapy for squamous cell carcinoma of the esophagus. The annular primary esophageal tumor is easily seen *(open arrowheads)*. The fistula between the esophagus and trachea occurs at approximately the level of the carina *(arrow)*. Barium entering the airway through the fistula produces a very nice bronchogram. It is important to document that the appearance of contrast in the airway is caused by fistulization between the esophagus and the airway rather than by aspiration related to obstruction by the esophageal tumor.

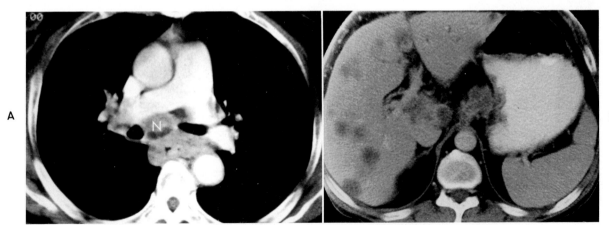

Fig. 11-66 CT examination of two patients with esophageal carcinoma. **A,** Carcinoma involving the middle third of the esophagus. The esophageal wall is substantially thickened by tumor, and a lesion invades the normal fat plane between the esophagus and the descending aorta. Two-centimeter carinal node *(N)* is present. **B,** Carcinoma involving the distal esophagus. The distal esophagus *(arrow)* is seen as an irregular mass. Multiple hepatic metastases are present.

acteristics of the tumor. Small, asymptomatic lesions, however, may be hidden on single-contrast images of the barium-filled esophagus. This fact probably accounts for why more small, asymptomatic carcinomas are not detected fortuitously on upper GI series done for unrelated reasons. Because more than 10 million upper GI series are done annually in the United States, the potential exists to identify several hundred individuals a year with a small, unsuspected esophageal carcinoma. In theory, small lesions, 0.5 to 1.5 cm in size, should be detected with high accuracy, because the esophagus is a clean, straight tube that can be easily projected free of conflicting overlying densities. In some instances, small asymptomatic esophageal tumors may be missed because an adequate screening examination of the esophagus is not included as part of every upper GI series.

The double-contrast esophagram is the best method currently available for identifying small esophageal tumors.[301,306] Adequate double-contrast images, however, are often not obtained for the proximal esophagus, and in about 20% to 30% of studies, satisfactory double-contrast imaging is not obtained for the distal esophagus. Another helpful method for detecting small esophageal tumors is careful observation of the peristaltic stripping wave as it traverses the esophagus. Esophageal peristalsis is intact in the majority of patients with a small esophageal carcinoma and serves as a means of "autopalpation." Small tumors hidden in the barium column are frequently observed during passage of the tail of the barium bolus. The lesions often "pop" into view when squeezed by the aborally directed wave of circular peristaltic contraction. Thus observation of several peristaltic sequences, standard for any upper GI series, offers an opportunity for detecting small esophageal nodules or plaques that are not observed on conventional films of the barium-filled esophagus. Small, sessile esophageal polyps that have a smooth, innocent appearance (see Fig. 11-64) should not be assumed to be benign. For small lesions the morphologic distinction between benign and malignant neoplasm is highly inaccurate, and biopsy is essential.

Sarcoma

Although esophageal sarcomas are rare, one well-described lesion is carcinosarcoma. These lesions have mixed carcinomatous and sarcomatous elements. When metastases occur, they characteristically appear as the sarcomatous element of the primary neoplasm.[307,308] Esophageal carcinosarcomas usually appear as a polypoid, nonulcerated tumor in middle-aged or elderly men. These bulky tumors may pedunculate and give rise to a sausage-shaped mass that fills the esophageal lumen. Partial obstruction may cause proximal esophageal dilatation. Lesions that may have a gross morphology similar to bulky polypoid carcinosarcomas include fibrovascular polyp, adenocarcinoma,

occasional squamous carcinomas, leiomyosarcoma, melanoma, and pseudosarcoma.[309,310] Pseudosarcomas differ from carcinosarcomas in that the carcinomatous and sarcomatous elements are not mixed, and any metastases are squamous carcinoma.[311] These tumors predominate in the midesophagus. The survival prognosis for both pseudosarcoma and carcinosarcoma is better than that for common-variety carcinoma. Other rare esophageal sarcomas include chondrosarcoma, believed to develop from the malignant degeneration of ectopic tracheobronchial elements; fibrosarcoma; liposarcoma; and myosarcoma. Melanoma may be primary[312] as well as metastatic.

Esophageal lymphoma may occur as an isolated lesion or more commonly as part of disseminated lymphoma. Generally, these lesions show contiguous involvement of the distal esophagus and gastric fundus with irregularity and narrowing. Morphologically, the lesions are generally indistinguishable from carcinoma. The radiographic appearances include an ulcerated mass, varicoid filling defects, and multiple submucosal nodules,[313-315] patterns observed with lymphomas elsewhere in the GI tract. A hint as to the identity of such lesions is that the patient often has negligible esophageal symptoms, despite substantial esophageal involvement. The tumors generally regress dramatically following radiotherapy or chemotherapy, and the prognosis for long-term survival is good.[316,317] Rarely, leukemic infiltrates cause multiple intramural filling defects and esophageal narrowing. Similar to lymphoma, leukemic lesions regress dramatically after radiotherapy.[318] Kaposi's sarcoma may involve the esophagus in patients with AIDS.

Metastases

Secondary malignant involvement of the esophagus may be of three general types: (1) direct invasion; (2) involvement from adjacent malignant nodes; and (3) blood-borne metastases.[196] Malignancy of the stomach, lung, thyroid, hypopharynx, and larynx may extend directly into the esophagus. The appearance of these lesions may simulate that of a primary carcinoma. Malignant mediastinal nodes may compress and constrict the esophagus. The common origins are lung and breast carcinoma.[275] Characteristically, metastatic breast carcinoma to the mediastinum elicits an intense fibrotic response that causes smooth, symmetric narrowing of a long esophageal segment,[319] resembling a benign stricture (Fig. 11-52, *B* and *C*). The least common form of secondary esophageal involvement is blood-borne metastases. The primary source may be a melanoma or a malignancy of the pancreas, testes, prostate, liver, or other organs.[320] The radiographic appearance of hematogenous metastases is variable but often simulates primary carcinomas. Metastatic melanoma tends to cause large endophytic lesions that may pedunculate. Similar to lymphoma, secondary metastatic lesions are often considerably larger than the patient's minimal clinical symptoms would suggest.[321]

Benign tumors

Compared with malignant lesions, benign tumors of the esophagus are uncommon. One large autopsy series gives a ratio of six malignant esophageal tumors for every benign tumor.[322]

Leiomyoma

Leiomyoma is by far the most common benign tumor of the esophagus. These tumors occur in patients 20 to 60 years of age and have a predilection for men. The mean age of 35 years is about 20 years younger than that for esophageal carcinoma. Leiomyomas usually occur as solitary masses in the distal third or less commonly in the middle third of the esophagus. About 5% to 10% of leiomyomas arise in the proximal esophagus. The lesions develop primarily from the smooth muscle muscularis externa in the distal two thirds of the esophagus. Occasional lesions appear to arise from the smooth muscle of the muscularis mucosae or blood vessels, accounting for the occasional development of lesions in the proximal esophagus. The lesions generally range from 1 to 6 cm in size, but some are larger and weight as much as 1000 to 5000 g.[323] The lesions are well encapsulated and on cut sections resemble a uterine fibroid. Malignant potential is negligible.

Generally, esophageal symptoms are absent, and the leiomyoma is discovered incidentally during a GI series or occasionally on a chest film. When symptoms are present, dysphagia for solids is the dominant symptom. Occasionally, patients have vague chest pain or respiratory symptoms from aspiration or tracheobronchial compression. Esophageal leiomyomas seldom ulcerate; consequently, bleeding is rare.

On chest films, leiomyomas are occasionally detected as a soft tissue mediastinal density, mediastinal widening, or a calcified mass.[324] Esophagrams usually demonstrate a smooth filling defect[325] with the characteristic features of a submucosal lesion (Fig. 11-67). On tangential views, a semilunar mass with intact mucosa narrows the barium column. Seen face on, the lesion may cause splitting of the barium column, splaying of the longitudinal esophageal folds, and segmental widening of the esophageal diameter. Proximal dilatation seldom occurs. During peristalsis and deep respiration, esophageal leiomyomas usually demonstrate longitudinal movement, thereby demonstrating their intramural origin and lack of fixation. In many cases, a soft tissue companion shadow is observed, caused by the exophytic component of the lesion. Rarely, leiomyomas may grow primarily into the esophageal lumen, causing a lobu-

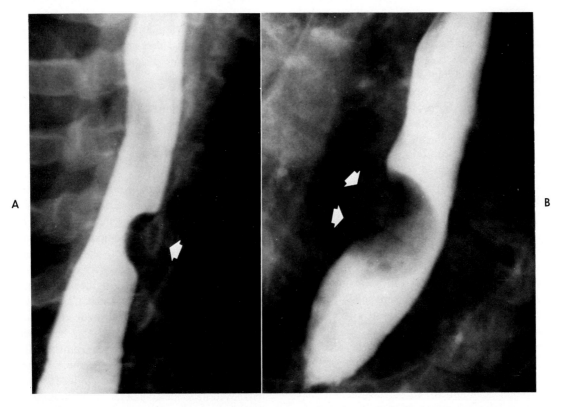

Fig. 11-67 Two patients with esophageal leiomyoma. **A,** Leiomyoma (1.5 cm) *(arrow)* demonstrating a smooth contour with tapering margins. **B,** Leiomyoma (2.5 cm) with sharp margins; the outer margin *(arrows)* of the circular lesion is outlined by the adjacent lung.

lated or pedunculated lesion. Some lesions assume a spiral or annular form and cause significant esophageal narrowing.

Although esophageal leiomyomas occur as solitary lesions, a few develop as multiple lesions, usually no more than two to three in number.[326,327] Rarely, the multiple lesions may be numerous and coalesce. Another rare form is diffuse esophageal leiomatosis.[328] This latter form occurs as a segmental nodular narrowing that involves the distal half of the esophagus and may extend into the stomach. This condition consists of a bizarre form of esophageal smooth muscle hypertrophy often accompanied by fibrosis and hypertrophied nerves.

Other benign submucosal neoplasms include neurofibroma, fibroma, angioma, lipoma, and granular cell tumor. These rare tumors may occur anywhere in the esophagus. Granular cell tumors, formerly termed *myelofibromas*, are believed to have a neural origin and have a predilection for women and blacks.[329,330]

Fibrovascular polyp

Fibrovascular polyps contain varying amounts of fibrous, vascular, and even adipose tissue. At various times they have been called *fibroma, fibrolipoma, myxofibroma,* and *pedunculated lipoma*.[331] The tumor is covered by epidermoid epithelium that may erode and bleed. Some pathologists classify the lesion as a hamartoma. Fibrovascular polyps have a predilection for men and generally develop in the proximal esophagus.[332] Dysphagia is the prevalent clinical symptom. The lesions may appear as small sessile polyps or large bulky lesions that have a sausagelike intraluminal mass. Pedunculation is common (Fig. 11-68). A fibrovascular polyp is the most likely diagnosis for a pedunculated esophageal tumor. Oral regurgitation of the tumor and asphyxiation have been reported. Because the lesions are often highly vascular, they may bleed profusely after biopsy.

Inflammatory polyp

Inflammatory esophageal polyps are sessile lesions consisting of inflamed granulation and fibrous tissue. These polyps have also been called *inflammatory pseudotumors, fibrous polyps,* and *eosinophilic granulomas*. The lesions develop as a response to reflux esophagitis.[333,334] Most patients complain of heartburn. On radiographic examination, inflammatory polyps appear as roundish sessile polyps, usually 0.5 to 2 cm in diameter, that are located near the esophagogastric junction (Fig. 11-69) and often on top of a thickened gastric fold.[150] Often findings of esophagitis are present, such as a reduction in esophageal distensibility and contour irregularity. A hiatus hernia and gastroesophageal reflux are commonly present. The lesions tend to diminish in size and disappear during effective therapy for esophagitis. An inflammatory esophageal polyp needs to be dis-

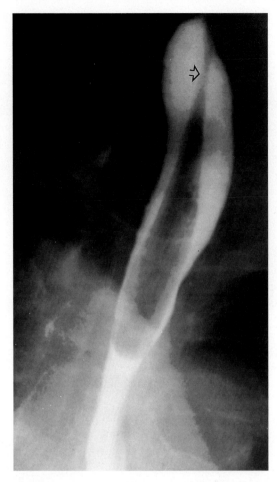

Fig. 11-68 Pedunculated fibrolipoma. This patient's pedunculated fibrolipoma originated in the piriform sinus and extended into the cervical and upper thoracic esophagus. The very long stalk *(open arrowhead)* is identified proximally. The polyp was freely moveable and compressible. The smooth contour is compatible with a benign polypoid lesion.
From Olson DL et al: *Dysphagia* 2:113, 1987.

tinguished from a prolapsed gastric fold, submucosal neoplasm, retention cyst, and small carcinoma.

Papillomas

Papillomas are sessile wartlike excrescences that arise from the esophageal squamous mucosa. Histologically, they demonstrate branching cords of connective tissue stroma covered by normal squamous epithelium. Papillomas are often multiple,[335] ranging from a few in number to numerous nodules.[322,335] They generally occur in the distal third of the esophagus, which suggests that they may be related to irritation caused by gastroesophageal reflux. The lesions are usually seen as small plaques 1 to 4 mm in size. Occasionally, lesions 0.5 to 1.5 cm appear as discrete mucosal tumors. Rare giant papillomas[336] may fill the esoph-

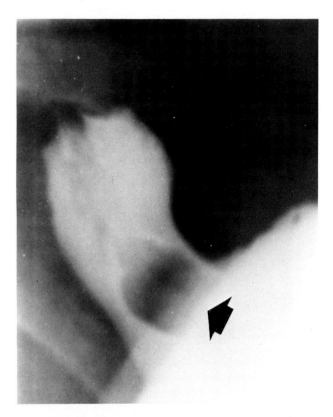

Fig. 11-69 Inflammatory polyp *(arrow)* in the distal esophagus. The patient was examined for heartburn.

ageal lumen and resemble the gross morphology of a villous tumor. Papillomas develop most commonly in elderly men. Generally, the lesions are asymptomatic, and encountered as an incidental finding on esophagrams, endoscopy, or at autopsy. Similarly appearing lesions may be caused by hyperkeratosis, hyperplasia, acanthosis, leukoplakia, and verrucous squamous carcinoma.

Cysts

Esophageal retention cysts are thin-walled, acquired cysts, or mucocele, caused by obstruction of an esophageal mucous gland. They tend to occur in the distal esophagus. They are commonly solitary but may be multiple[337,338] or occur as numerous nodular lesions involving long lengths of the esophagus.[220] The solitary cyst needs to be differentiated from other polypoid lesions in the distal esophagus, such as an inflammatory esophageal polyp, prolapsed gastric fold, leiomyoma, and small carcinoma. Multiple retention cysts have been called *esophagitis cystica,* even though little inflammation is present.[220] The multiple cysts give the esophagus a multinodular or cobblestone appearance. A similar appearance can occur with moniliasis, acanthosis, leukoplakia, squamous papillomata, squamous carcinoma, ganglioneuromatosis, and Cowden's disease.[339,340] Other cystic esophageal lesions, such as enteric cysts and esoph-

ageal duplication, have been discussed earlier under the category of congenital lesions.

Miscellaneous benign tumors

Miscellaneous nonneoplastic esophageal tumors include solitary varix, focal infection, hamartoma, ectopic tissue, and hematoma. A solitary varix may be suspected in patients with cirrhosis or if a lesion changes in size.[341] In such cases, biopsy should be avoided. Small tumorlike masses may be caused also by moniliasis, tuberculosis, or actinomycosis. Esophageal hamartomas may occur as isolated lesions or rarely in patients with Peutz-Jeghers syndrome.

INDENTATIONS AND DISPLACEMENT

The esophagus extends the length of the mediastinum and comes into contact with many vital structures. Consequently it serves as a useful probe for identifying the enlargement of adjacent structures, mediastinal masses, or mediastinal displacement (see box on p. 253). Overhead films of the entire barium-filled esophagus and selected spot films are useful for evaluating the mediastinum and lower part of the neck. Adequate esophageal distention is important to demonstrate compression or indentation of the barium column by adjacent masses.

Indentations

In healthy subjects, several normal structures commonly indent the barium-filled esophagus. Mild indentations are caused commonly by the aortic knob, left mainstem bronchus, and diaphragmatic hiatus.[342] Additionally, the esophagus normally makes a slight arc around the posterior surface of the heart. The impression of the aortic knob becomes more pronounced as the aorta enlarges in elderly subjects. A tortuous innominate or common carotid artery may impinge on the esophagus. Commonly the dilated descending thoracic aorta indents the esophagus just above the diaphragmatic hiatus, where the esophagus passes immediately anterior to the aorta. At fluoroscopy the area of indentation is seen to pulsate. Some reports suggest that ectasia of the descending aorta may rarely cause obstructive symptoms of "dysphagia aortica,"[343,344] especially when accompanied by cardiomegaly (Fig. 11-70). Cervical or thoracic vertebral osteophytes may cause impressions on the proximal esophagus and on rare occasions may also cause dysphagia.[345,346] Symptomatic compression of the proximal esophagus has also been caused by scoliosis.[347] A common cause of esophageal compression as well as displacement is cardiomegaly. Left atrial enlargement causes a localized esophageal impression adjacent to the upper half of the posterior cardiac border. Generalized cardiomegaly causes posterior displacement of the distal half of the thoracic esophagus. These relationships are best shown on lateral views.

Besides a normally positioned aortic arch, other variations of the arch that impress the esophagus are a right-sided

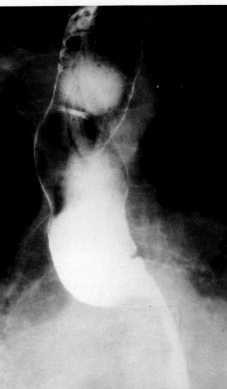

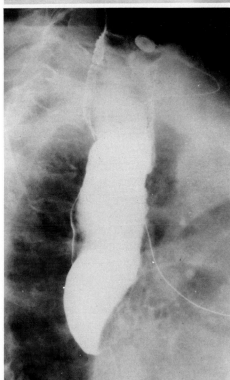

Fig. 11-70 Dysphagia aortica. A patient with cardiomegaly and congestive failure who developed acute onset of dysphagia. **A,** Anteroposterior esophagram demonstrates extrinsic compression on the distal esophagus. **B,** Lateral view demonstrates anterior compression of the esophagus by an enlarged heart pinching the distal esophagus against the dilated aorta. After treatment of congestive failure with a decrease in heart size, dysphagia subsided and extrinsic compression of the distal esophagus was less pronounced.

aortic arch, cervical aortic arch, double aortic arch, and aortic aneurysm. A right aortic arch produces a right-sided indentation slightly higher than the usual indentation of the normal left aortic limb. Two types of right arches occur.[348] In one type, an anterior right arch is a mirror image of the normal left arch. This type is commonly associated with cyanotic congenital heart disease, especially tetralogy of Fallot and truncus arteriosus. In the second type, a posterior right arch is accompanied by an aberrant left subclavian artery that passes behind the esophagus and causes a prominent posterior notch high on the thoracic esophagus. These patients seldom have other congenital abnormalities. With a cervical arch the ascending aorta passes obliquely upward behind the esophagus, causing a prominent posterior indentation, and forms a palpable pulsatile mass on the right side of the neck.[349] Occasionally, the cervical arch is located on the left side of the neck. Double aortic arches exist with variable patterns of brachycephalic vessels; the descending aorta may be on the right or left. Esophagrams usually reveal either bilateral indentations, causing a waist-like narrowing when the arches are at the same level or a kinked appearance when the arches are at different levels. Aortic coarctation usually occurs just distal to the takeoff of the left subclavian artery. Poststenotic aortic dilatation commonly impresses the esophagus just below the normal indentation of the aortic knob. These two indentations on the left side of the esophagus create the reverse-three sign characteristic of aortic coarctation. The diagnosis is generally confirmed by the presence of rib notching.

Esophageal impressions may also be caused by aberrant, anomalous, or enlarged blood vessels. The majority of vascular impressions occur along the upper half of the thoracic esophagus. Vascular impressions rarely cause symptoms unless a complete ring exists around the esophagus and trachea. Symptoms from vascular anomalies in children are almost always respiratory, whereas adults usually have esophageal dysphagia. An aberrant right subclavian artery occurs in about 1 in every 200 people. The aberrant vessel arises distal to the left subclavian and then courses upward and to the right. The aberrant right subclavian almost always passes behind the esophagus, causing an oblique notch or bayonet sign when seen en face. A diverticulum at the takeoff of the aberrant vessel may cause a large oval esophageal indentation.[350] Although an aberrant subclavian may cause "dysphagia lusoria,"[351] obstructive symptoms are rare even when the vascular impression is pronounced on esophagrams. Esophageal indentations may also be caused by other vessels, such as an aberrant left pulmonary artery,[352] anomalous intercostal artery,[141] dilated bronchial artery, left inferior pulmonary vein,[353] dilated hemizygos vein,[354] and an anomalous vein draining below the diaphragm. The aberrant left pulmonary artery arises from the right pulmonary artery and forms a sling behind the trachea as it loops back toward the left lung. The vascular sling generally causes a characteristic notch on the anterior wall

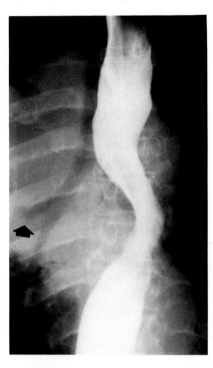

Fig. 11-71 Enlarged carinal nodes indenting and displacing the midesophagus. Bronchogenic carcinoma, metastatic to the carinal nodes, has produced a cut-off sign *(arrow)* of the right upper lobe of the bronchus and consolidation of the obstructed right upper lobe.

of the midesophagus.[355] The vessel may cause sufficient compression of the right main bronchus or trachea to elicit respiratory symptoms.[352] Dilated bronchial arteries, associated with truncus arteriosus, may indent the dorsolateral margins of the midesophagus. A common pulmonary vein draining below the diaphragm may produce an anterior impression along the distal esophagus.

Mediastinal masses that indent the esophagus are caused most commonly by mediastinal adenopathy, particularly enlarged carinal nodes (Figs. 11-43 and 11-71). The indentations are frequently subtle and seen only on oblique views. Mediastinal adenopathy is generally caused by metastases, lymphoma, or infection. Other masses in the middle or posterior mediastinum that may indent the esophagus are mesenchymal neoplasms, cysts, abscess, and hematoma. Parathyroid tumors occasionally cause an impression on the cervical esophagus.

Deviation

Esophageal deviation from the midline may occur as a normal variant or from aortic elongation, mediastinal shifts, or large adjacent masses. In the lower mediastinum, the esophagus is loosely supported by surrounding structures and may move spontaneously to the right or left of the midline. This phenomenon has been referred to as the *wander-*

ing esophagus.[356] In subjects with a narrow sagittal diameter of the thoracic inlet, minimal space may exist for the esophagus between the trachea and cervical spine. Consequently the lower cervical esophagus is often crowded to one side, more commonly to the left,[127] a finding often observed on thoracic CT. With aortic elongation the esophagus often bows to the left to accompany the descending aorta into the left posterior thorax. Mediastinal shifts that displace the esophagus from the midline may be due to pulmonary atelectasis, pulmonary hypoplasia, unilateral emphysema, pneumonectomy, pneumothorax, or hydrothorax.

DIAPHRAGM

The two major functions of the diaphragm are to (1) separate the abdomen into two distinct cavities with different cavitary pressure and (2) serve as the major muscle of respiration. Each hemidiaphragm is innervated by an ipsilateral phrenic nerve consisting of nerve bundles from C3 to C5. Each phrenic nerve originates in the posterior neck and courses through the neck and mediastinum to reach the ipsilateral diaphragm.

Anatomy

The muscle fibers of the diaphragm arise from the xiphoid process, eighth to twelfth ribs, and lumbar spine. They insert into a crescent-shaped central tendon, which corresponds closely to the bare area of the liver, defined by the attachment of the liver suspensory ligaments to the undersurface of the diaphragm. The large right bare area extends substantially posteriorly and caudally, while the smaller left bare area is located near the central part of the left hemidiaphragm. The tough central tendon limits the extension of the hepatic malignancy or other processes either into or through the hemidiaphragm. The most notable exception is a hepatic amoebic abscess, which notoriously may cross the right hemidiaphragm and break into the thorax. The diaphragm has three normal foramina: the esophageal hiatus, the aortic foramen, and the foramen of the vena cava.[357]

Defects

In some individuals, small developmental foramina persist in the diaphragm that allow ascitic or pleural fluid to pass back and forth between the thorax and abdominal cavity. Congenital absence of the diaphragm is a rare congenital anomaly that may be detected in utero by ultrasound.[357] This anomaly is usually left sided. Afflicted infants have a hypoplastic ipsilateral lung and generally exhibit substantial respiratory distress at birth as the herniated gut fills with gas and compresses intrathoracic structures. The appearance on a chest radiograph is characteristic. The abnormality requires immediate surgical correction, but even so, the prognosis is poor.[358]

Well-defined congenital hernias of the diaphragm are of three types: (1) Bochdalek's, (2) Morgagni's, and (3) esoph-

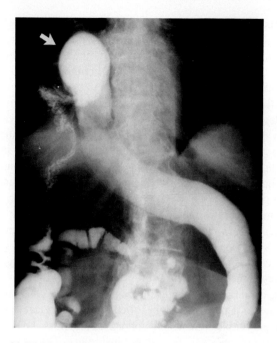

Fig. 11-72 Morgagni's hernia. The hernia is located at the right cardiophrenic angle and contains the proximal transverse colon *(arrow)*.

ageal diaphragmatic hiatus. A posteromedial diaphragmatic hernia may occur through Bochdalek's foramen, a defect that represents incomplete closure of the pleuroperitoneal membrane. When the defect is large, most of the abdominal contents may herniate into the chest, similar to congenital absence of the diaphragm. Generally, the lesion is on the left. When the defect is small, the hernia may be asymptomatic and contain only some retroperitoneal fat or a portion of the spleen or kidney. Such hernias are generally detected incidentally on a chest radiograph. Thoracic CT examinations indicate that small Bochdalek's hernias occur more commonly than thought previously.[359,360]

In Morgagni's hernia the herniation occurs behind the sternum through a persistent diaphragmatic cleft that contains the mammary vessels. Most Morgagni's hernias occur on the right, because the pericardium tends to prevent such herniations on the left. Typically, therefore, Morgagni's hernia presents at the right cardiophrenic angle. Occasionally, Morgagni's hernias occur bilaterally. Usually these hernias are asymptomatic. They generally contain omentum or a portion of transverse colon (Fig. 11-72) but may also contain small bowel or liver. In some cases a Morgagni-type hernia results from blunt abdominal trauma.[361]

Congenital hiatus hernias generally contain only the proximal stomach and appear clinically as excessive reflux and regurgitation. A severe reflux peptic esophagitis occasionally causes an esophageal stricture. Infantile hernias tend to resolve with conservative management but occasionally require surgery.[73]

Acquired diaphragmatic hernias usually are either a sliding hiatus hernia, which is common in the elderly, or occasionally an abrupt diaphragmatic rupture from blunt trauma. A small percentage of hiatal hernias have substantial hiatal enlargement accompanied by herniation of much or all of the stomach into the chest. Typically the stomach undergoes a 180-degree axial rotation, so that the greater curvature is upward. On films of the chest and upper abdomen a large mass with two air-fluid levels is typically seen behind the heart. In many cases the transverse colon enters the hernia because of its connection with the greater curvature of the stomach via the gastrocolic ligament. Such giant hiatal hernias may be encountered incidentally, or the patient may complain of excessive eructation and postprandial symptoms. Occasionally, an obstructed complete gastric volvulus may develop acutely and present as a surgical emergency.

A diaphragmatic rupture, recognized shortly after blunt trauma or penetrating injury, often requires surgical repair. The majority of traumatic diaphragmatic hernias, however, are recognized well after the original injury. They may occur on either side. A traumatic hernia should be expected when a diaphragmatic hernia does not involve the esophageal hiatus or any of the usual locations for congenital hernias. A directed clinical history may uncover a significant episode of blunt trauma, generally a serious automobile accident. About 90% of traumatic hiatal hernias are on the left. Three types of complications may develop, either acutely or after a delay: (1) encroachment of herniated bowel on the lung; (2) obstruction of herniated bowel; and (3) torsion of herniated bowel. The radiographic evaluation of diaphragmatic hernia includes plain films of the chest and abdomen, contrast studies of the upper and lower digestive tract, and, in some cases, CT examination.

Movement and location

The hemidiaphragms generally appear as smooth domes that normally make a synchronous caudal excursion of about 2 to 3 cm during inspiration. Some mesomorphic individuals, however, may breathe mainly by intercostal activity, in which case diaphragm movement may be minimal. Asthenic individuals may show mainly diaphragmatic breathing, with an excursion up to 6 to 8 cm. Bilateral diaphragmatic elevation may occur in association with obesity, ascites, restrictive lung disease, laparotomy, or unconsciousness. The diaphragms are low and flat in patients with pulmonary emphysema.

Unilateral diaphragmatic elevation has numerous causes (see box above). Basically the cause may be related to (1) the ipsilateral lung or thorax; (2) the diaphragm ("eventration") or its innervation; or (3) abnormalities in the abdomen. Additionally, a subpulmonic effusion may simulate an elevated diaphragm. This later condition is readily identified by a decubitus film that demonstrates free pleural fluid. At fluoroscopy an elevated diaphragm may move

---

☐ **CAUSES OF ELEVATED HEMIDIAPHRAGM** ☐

A. Supradiaphragmatic
  1. Pleuritic pain
  2. Fractured ribs
  3. Scoliosis
  4. Atelectasis
  5. Pleural thickening
  6. Partial pneumonectomy
B. Diaphragmatic
  1. Eventration
  2. Muscle dysfunction
  3. Phrenic paralysis
C. Subdiaphragmatic
  1. Abscess
  2. Pseudocyst
  3. Large neoplasm
  4. Organomegaly
  5. Distended gut
D. False appearance
  1. Subpulmonic effusion

---

fairly normally, show feeble movement, not move at all, or show paradoxical movement. Optimally the patient is examined upright. The sniff test is often useful when searching for paradoxical diaphragmatic movement. Paradoxical movement substantiates diaphragmatic paralysis from either a local or central cause. In many cases, however, a paralyzed diaphragm shows no movement. Occasionally, a large pleural effusion may invert the left hemidiaphragm. Such cases show elevation of the pleural fluid during inspiration. Ultrasound and CT are particularly useful for evaluating the process involving or adjacent to the diaphragm. Like fluoroscopy, real-time ultrasound allows direct imaging of diaphragmatic movement.

Neoplasms

Primary neoplasms of the diaphragm are rare. Such neoplasms are generally of mesodermal origin; however, an endothelial mesothelioma may be confined to the diaphragm. About 60% of primary diaphragmatic tumors are benign.[15] Occasionally, metastases may involve the diaphragm by direct extension, seeding, or hematogenous spread. CT is often helpful in evaluating the anatomic location and extent of such lesions.

REFERENCES

1. Liebermann-Meffert D et al: Muscular equivalent of the lower esophageal sphincter, *Gastroenterology* 76:31, 1979.
2. Dodds WJ et al: Pharmacologic investigation of primary peristalsis in the smooth muscle portion of the opossum esophagus, *Am J Physiol* 237: E561, 1979.
3. Kantrowitz, PS et al: Response of the human esophagus to d-turbourare and atropine, *Gut* 11:47, 1970.

4. Doty RW: Neural organization of deglutition. In Code CF, ed: *Handbook of physiology.* VI. *Alimentary canal motility,* vol 4, Washington, DC, 1968, American Physiological Society.

5. Creteur V et al: Drug-induced esophagitis detected by double-contrast radiography, *Radiology* 147: 365, 1983.

6. Diamant, NE, El-Sharkaway TY: Neural control of esophageal peristalsis: a conceptual analysis, *Gastroenterology* 72:546, 1977.

7. Dodds WJ et al: Esophageal contractions induced by vagal stimulation in the opossum, *Am J Physiol* 235: E392, 1978.

8. Goyal RK, Rattan S: Nature of the vagal inhibitory innervation to the lower esophageal sphincter, *J Clin Invest* 55:1119, 1975.

9. Goyal RK, Rattan S: Neurohumoral, hormonal, and drug receptors for the lower esophageal sphincter, *Gastroenterology* 74:598, 1978.

10. Ingelfinger FJ: Esophageal motility, *Physiol Rev* 38: 533, 1958.

11. Fyke FE Jr, Code CF, Schlegel JF: The gastroesophageal sphincter in healthy human beings, *Gastroenterologia* 86:135, 1956.

12. Dodds WJ: Instrumentation and methodology for intraluminal esophageal manometry, *Arch Intern Med* 136:515, 1976.

13. Dodds WJ: Cannon lecture: Current concept of esophageal motor function: clinical implications for radiology, *AJR* 128:549, 1977.

14. Dodds WJ et al: A comparison between primary esophageal peristalsis following wet and dry swallows, *J Appl Physiol* 35:851, 1973.

15. Sarna SK, Daniel EE, Waterfall WE: Myogenic and neural control systems for esophageal motility, *Gastroenterology* 73: 1345, 1977.

16. Dodds WJ et al: Movement of the feline esophagus associated with respiration and peristalsis: an evaluation using tantalum markers, *J Clin Invest* 52:1, 1973.

17. Dodds WJ et al: Effect of esophageal movement on intraluminal esophageal pressure recording, *Gastroenterology* 67:592, 1974.

18. Flesher B et al: The characteristics and similarity of primary and secondary peristalsis in the esophagus, *J Clin Invest* 38:110, 1959.

19. Nagler R, Spiro HM: Serial esophageal motility studies in asymptomatic young subjects, *Gastroenterology* 41:371, 1961.

20. Stacher G, Schmierer G, Landgraf M: Tertiary esophageal contractions evoked by acoustical stimuli, *Gastroenterology* 77:49, 1979.

21. Mandelstam P, Lieber A: Cineradiographic evaluation of the esophagus in normal adults: a study of 146 subjects ranging in age from 21 to 90 years, *Gastroenterology* 58:32, 1970.

22. Bondi JL, Godwin DH, Garrett JM: "Vigorous" achalasia, *Am J Gastroenterol* 58:145, 1972.

23. Winship DH, Zboralske FF: The esophageal propulsive force: esophageal response to acute obstruction, *J Clin Invest* 46:1391, 1967.

24. Creamer B, Donoghue FE, Code CF: Pattern of esophageal motility in diffuse spasm, *Gastroenterology* 34:782, 1958.

25. Williams SM et al: Symptomatic congenital ectopic gastric mucosa in the upper esophagus, *AJR* 148:147, 1987.

26. Zboralske FF, Dodds WJ: Roentgenographic diagnosis of primary disorders of esophageal motility, *Radiol Clin North Am* 7:147, 1969.

27. Dodds WJ et al: Effects of increased intra-abdominal pressure on esophageal peristalsis, *J Appl Physiol* 37:378, 1974.

28. Pope CE II: Effect of infusion on force of closure measurements in the human esophagus, *Gastroenterology* 58:616, 1970.

29. Hogan WJ, Dodds WJ, Stewart ET: Comparison of roentgenology and intraluminal manometry for evaluating esophageal peristalsis (abstract), *Rend Gastroenterol* 5:28, 1973.

30. Dodds WJ et al: Radiological amyl nitrite test for discriminating pseudoachalasia from idiopathic achalasia, *AJR* 1:21, 1986.

31. Dodds WJ, Hogan WJ, Miller WN: A report on reflux esophagitis, *Am J Dig Dis* 21:49, 1976.

32. Kantrowitz PA et al: Measurement of gastroesophageal reflux, *Gastroenterology* 56:666, 1968.

33. Sandmark S: Influence of heavy contrast media on the demonstration of hiatus hernia and gastro-oesophageal reflux, *Acta Radiol* 1:1045, 1963.

34. Dent J et al: Mechanism of gastroesophageal reflux in recumbent asymptomatic human subjects, *J Clin Invest* 65:256, 1980.

35. Dodds WJ et al: Mechanisms of gastroesophageal reflux in patients with reflux esophagitis, *N Engl J Med* 308: 1547, 1982.

36. Cassella RR, Ellis FH Jr, Brown AL Jr: Fine-structure changes in achalasia of the esophagus. I. Vagus nerves, *Am J Pathol* 46:279, 1965.

37. Cohen S, Lipshutz W: Lower esophageal sphincter dysfunction in achalasia, *Gastroenterology* 61:814, 1971.

38. Sheperd JK, Daimant NE: Mecholyl test: comparison of balloon kymography and intraluminal pressure measurement, *Gastroenterology* 63:557, 1972.

39. Ellis FH, Olsen AM: *Achalasia of the esophagus,* Philadelphia, 1969, WB Saunders.

40. Reid DP et al: Achalasia: a reappraisal of manometric and radiographic features (abstract), *Gastroenterology* 62:797, 1972.

41. Creamer B, Andersen HA, Code CF: Esophageal motility in patients with scleroderma and related diseases, *Gastroenterologia* 86:763, 1956.

42. Soergel KH, Zboralske FF, Amberg JR: Prebyesophagus: esophageal motility in nonagenarians, *J Clin Invest* 43: 1472, 1964.

43. Kahrilas PJ et al: A comparison of pseudoachalasia and achalasia, *Am J Med* 82:439, 1987.

44. Lawson TL, Dodds WJ: Infiltrating carcinoma simulating achalasia, *Gastrointest Radiol* 1:245, 1977.

45. Tucker HJ, Snape WJ Jr, Cohen S: Achalasia secondary to carcinoma: manometric and clinical features, *Ann Intern Med* 89:315, 1978.

46. Hogan WJ, Caflisch CR, Winship DH: Unclassified oesophageal motor disorders simulating achalasia, *Gut* 10:234, 1969.

47. Kaye MD: Dysfunction of the lower esophageal sphincter in disorders other than achalasia, *Am J Dig Dis* 18:734, 1973.

48. Bennett JR, Hendrix TR: Diffuse esophageal spasm: a disorder with more than one cause, *Gastroenterology* 59: 273, 1970.

49. Gillies M, Nicks R, Skyring A: Clinical, manometric and pathological studies in diffuse oesophageal spasm, *Br Med J* 2:527, 1967.

50. DiMarino AJ Jr, Cohen S: Characteristics of lower esophageal sphincter function in symptomatic diffuse esophageal spasm, *Gastroenterology* 66:1, 1974.

51. Kramer P et al: Oesophageal sensitivity to Mecholyl in symptomatic diffuse spasm, *Gut* 8:120, 1967.

52. Kramer P, Harris LD, Donaldson RM Jr: Transition from symptomatic diffuse spasm to cardiospasm, *Gut* 8:115, 1967.

53. Millan MS et al: Transition from diffuse esophageal spasm to achalasia, *J Clin Gastroenterol* 1:107, 1979.

54. Vantrappen G et al: Achalasia, diffuse esophageal spasm and related motility disorders, *Gastroenterology* 76:450, 1979.

55. Cassella RR, Ellis FH Jr, Brown AL Jr: Diffuse spasm of the lower part of the esophagus: fine structure of esophageal smooth muscle and nerve, *JAMA* 191:379, 1965.

56. Benjamin SB, Gerhardt DC, Castell DO: High amplitude, peristaltic esophageal contractions associated with chest pain and/or dysphagia, *Gastroenterology* 77:478, 1979.

57. Schuffler MD, Rohrmann CA Jr, Templeton FE: The radiologic manifestations of idiopathic intestinal pseudoobstruction, *AJR* 127:729, 1976.

58. Sarna SK et al: Postoperative gastrointestinal electrical and mechanical activities in a patient with idiopathic intestinal pseudoobstruction, *Gastroenterology* 74:112, 1978.

59. Schuffler MD, Lowe MC, Bill AH: Studies of idiopathic intestinal pseudoobstruction. I. Hereditary hollow visceral myopathy: clinical and pathological studies, *Gastroenterology* 73:327, 1977.

60. Schuffler MD et al: A familial neuronal disease presenting as intestinal pseudoobstruction, *Gastroenterology* 75:889, 1978.

61. Teixidor HD, Heneghan MA: Idiopathic intestinal pseudoobstruction in a family, *Gastrointest Radiol* 3:91, 1978.

62. Hellemans J et al: The presbyesophagus. In *The function of the esophagus,* Odense, Denmark, 1973, Odense University Press.

63. Khan TA et al: Esophageal motility in the elderly, *Am J Dig Dis* 22:1049, 1977.

64. Eckardt VF, LeCompte PM: Esophageal ganglia and smooth muscle in the elderly, *Am J Dig Dis* 23:443, 1978.

65. Holsinger JW Jr, Fuson RL, Sealy WC: Esophageal perforation following meat impaction and papain ingestion, *JAMA* 204:188, 1968.

66. Zboralske FF: The esophagus in the geriatric patient, *Radiol Clin North Am* 3:321, 1965.

67. Zboralske FF, Amberg JR, Soergel KH: Presbyesophagus: cineradiographic manifestations, *Radiology* 82: 463, 1964.

68. Burgess JN, Carlson HC, Ellis FH Jr: Esophageal function after successful repair of esophageal atresia and tracheoesophageal fistula, *J Thorac Cardiovasc Surg* 56:667, 1968.

69. Lister J: The blood supply of the esophagus in relation to oesophageal atresia, *Arch Dis Child* 39:131, 1964.

70. Chrispin AR, Friedland GW, Waterson DJ: Aspiration pneumonia and dysphagia after technically successful repair of oesophageal atresia, *Thorax* 21:104, 1966.

71. Werlin SL et al: Esophageal function in esophageal atresia, *Dig Dis Sci* 26:796, 1981.

72. Thomas PJ, Chrispin AR: Congenital tracheo-oesophageal fistula without oesophageal atresia, *Clin Radiol* 20:371, 1969.

73. Friedland GW et al: The apparent disparity in incidence of hiatal hernia in infants and children in Britain and the United States, *AJR* 120:305, 1974.

74. Neuhauser EB, Berenberg W: Cardio-esophageal relaxation as a cause of vomiting in infants, *Radiology* 48:480, 1947.

75. Moroz SP et al: Lower esophageal sphincter function in children with and without gastroesophageal reflux, *Gastroenterology* 71:236, 1976.

76. Friedland GW et al: Debatable points in the anatomy of the lower oesophagus, *Thorax* 21:487, 1966.

77. Werlin SL et al: Mechanisms of gastroesophageal reflux in children, *J Pediatr* 97: 244, 1980.

78. D'Angelo WA et al: Pathologic observations in systemic sclerosis (scleroderma): a study of fifty-eight matched controls, *Am J Med* 46:428, 1969.

79. Garrett JM et al: Esophageal deterioration in scleroderma, *Mayo Clin Proc* 46:92, 1971.

80. Stevens MB et al: Aperistalsis of the esophagus patients with connective-tissue disorders and Raynaud's phenomenon, *N Engl J Med* 270: 1218, 1964.

81. Miller WN et al: Importance of reflux esophagitis in scleroderma patients with dysphagia (abstract), *Gastroenterology* 68:914, 1975.

82. Treacy WL et al: Scleroderma of the esophagus: a correlation of histologic and physiologic findings, *Ann Intern Med* 59:351, 1963.

83. Cohen S et al: The pathogenesis of esophageal dysfunction in scleroderma and Raynaud's disease, *J Clin Invest* 51: 2663, 1972.

84. Atkinson M, Summerling MD: Oesophageal changes in systemic sclerosis, *Gut* 7:402, 1966.

85. Ramirez-Mata M et al: Esophageal motility in systemic lupus erythematosus, *Am J Dig Dis* 19:132, 1974.

86. O'Hara JM, Szemes G, Lowman RM: The esophageal lesions in dermatomyositis: a correlation of radiologic and pathologic findings, *Radiology* 89: 27, 1967.

87. Dodds WJ et al: Pathogenesis of reflux esophagitis, *Gastroenterology* 81:376, 1981.

88. Kahrilas PJ et al: Esophageal peristaltic dysfunction in peptic esophagus, *Gastroenterology* 91:897, 1986.

89. Alfolter H: Pressure characteristics of reflux esophagitis, *Helv Med Acta* 33:395, 1967.

90. Olsen AM, Schlegel JF: Motility disturbances caused by esophagitis, *J Thorac Cardiovasc Surg* 50:607, 1965.

91. Behar J: Reflux esophagitis: pathogenesis, diagnosis, and management, *Arch Intern Med* 136:560, 1976.

92. Helm JF et al: Determinants of esophageal acid clearance in normal subjects, *Gastroenterology* 85:607, 1983.

93. Helm JF et al: Effect of esophageal emptying and saliva on clearance of acid from the esophagus, *N Engl J Med* 310:284, 1984.

94. Simeone JF et al: Aperistalsis and esophagitis, *Radiology* 123: 9, 1977.

95. Donner MW et al: Acid-barium swallows in the radiographic evaluation of clinical esophagitis, *Radiology* 87:220.

96. Linsman JF: Gastroesophageal reflux elicited while drinking water (water siphonage test): its clinical correlation with pyrosis, *AJR* 94:325, 1965.

97. Cohen S, Harris LD: The lower esophageal sphincter, *Gastroenterology* 63:1066, 1972.

98. Anderson HA, Schlegel JF, Olsen AM: Postvagotomy dysphagia, *Gastrointest Endosc* 13:13, 1966.

99. Dagradi AE et al: Terminal esophageal (vestibular) spasm after vagotomy, *Arch Surg* 85:955, 1962.

100. Guillory JR, Clagett OT: Postvagotomy dysphagia, *Surg Clin North Am* 47:833, 1967.

101. Matarazzo SA et al: Relationship of cervical and abdominal vagal activity to lower esophageal sphincter function, *Gastroenterology* 71:999, 1976.

102. Hollis JB, Castell DO, Braddom RL: Esophageal motor function in diabetes mellitus and its relation to peripheral neuropathy, *Gastroenterology* 73:1098, 1977.

103. Mandelstam P et al: The swallowing disorder in patients with diabetic neuropathy, *Gastroenterology* 56:1, 1969.

104. Hogan WJ, de Andrade SRV, Winship DH: The influence of acute and chronic alcoholism upon oesphageal motor function. In Ottenjann R, Demling L, ed: *International Symposium on Motility of the Gastrointestinal Tract,* Erlangen, July, 1969, New York, 1971, Academic Press.

105. Winship DH et al: Deterioration of esophageal peristalsis in patients with alcoholic neuropathy, *Gastroenterology* 55:173, 1968.

106. Vix V: Esophageal motility in diabetes mellitus, *Radiology* 92:363, 1969.

107. Miller RH: Amyloid disease: an unusual cause of megaloesophagus, *S Afr Med J* 43:1202, 1969.

108. Danielides IC, Mellow AH: Effect of acute hypercalcemia on human esophageal motility, *Gastroenterology* 75:1115, 1978.

109. Christensen J: Esophageal manometry in myxedema (abstract), *Gastroenterology* 52: 1130, 1967.

110. Fischer RA et al: Esophageal motility in neuromuscular disorders, *Ann Intern Med* 63: 229, 1965.

111. Meshkinpour H, Afrasiabi MA, Valenta LJ: Esophageal motor function in Graves' disease, *Dig Dis Sci* 24:159, 1979.

112. Silbiger ML, Pikielney R, Donner MW: Neuromuscular disorders affecting the esophagus, *Invest Radiol* 2:442, 1967.

113. Eadie MJ, Tyrer JH: Radiologic abnormalities of the upper part of the alimentary tract in parkinsonism, *Aust Ann Med* 14:23, 1965.

114. Daly DD, Code CF: Disturbances of swallowing and esophageal motility in patients with multiple sclerosis, *Neurology* 12:250, 1962.

115. Smith AWM, Mulder DW, Code CF: Esophageal motility in amyotrophic lateral sclerosis, *Proc Mayo Clin Staff Meet* 32:438, 1957.

116. Margulies SI et al: Familial dysautonomia: a cineradiographic study of the swallowing mechanism, *Radiology* 90:107, 1968.

117. Sparberg M, Knudsen KB, Frank ST: Dysautonomia and dysphagia, *Neurology* 18:504, 1968.

118. Sulway MJ, Baume PE, Davis E: Stiff-man syndrome presenting with complete esophageal obstruction: report of a case, *Am J Dig Dis* 15:79, 1970.

119. Pierce JW, Creamer B, MacDermot V: Pharynx and oesophagus in dystrophia myotonica, *Gut* 6:392, 1965.

120. Siegel CI, Hendrix TR, Harvey JC: The swallowing disorder in myotonia dystrophica, *Gastroenterology* 50:541, 1966.

121. Duranceau CA et al: Oropharyngeal dysphagia in patients with oculopharyngeal muscular dystrophy, *Can J Surg* 21:326, 1978.

122. Murphy SF, Drachman DB: The oculopharyngeal syndrome, *JAMA* 203:1003, 1968.

123. Seaman WB: Functional disorders of the pharyngo-esophageal junction: achalasia and chalasia, *Radiol Clin North Am* 7:113, 1969.

124. Ferreira SR: Aperistalsis of the esophagus and colon (megaesophagus and megacolon) etiologically related to Chagas' disease, *Am J Dig Dis* 6:700, 1961.

125. Goldberg HI, Dodds WJ: Cobblestone esophagus due to monilial infection, *AJR* 104:608, 1968.

126. Serebro HA et al: Possible pathogenesis of motility changes in diffuse esophageal spasm associated with gastric carcinoma, *Can Med Assoc J* 6: 1257, 1970.

127. Kendall BE, Ashcroft K, Whiteside CG: A physiological variation in the barium-filled gullet, *Br J Radiol* 35:769, 1962.

128. Dodds WJ et al: The effect of atropine on esophageal motor function in man, *Am J Physiol* (in press).

129. Gilbert RJ, Dodds WJ: Effect of selective muscarinic antagonists on peristaltic contractions in esophageal smooth muscle, *Am J Physiol* 13:G572, 1986.

130. Ghahremani GG, Heck LL, Williams JR: A pharmacologic aid in the radiographic diagnosis of obstructive esophageal lesions, *Radiology* 103:289, 1972.

131. Hogan WJ et al: Effect of glucagon on esophageal motor function, *Gastroenterology* 69:160, 1975.

132. Bain NH: Ehler-Danlos syndrome, *AJR* 67:167, 1977.

133. Holden MD, Wooler GH: Tracheo-oesophageal fistula and oesophageal atresia: results of 30 years' experience, *Thorax* 25:406, 1970.

134. Heller RM, Kirchner SG, O'Neill JA: Perforation of the pharynx in the newborn: a near look-alike for esophageal atresia, *AJR* 129:335, 1977.

135. Stringer DA, Ein SH: Recurrent tracheo-esophageal fistula: a protocol for investigation, *Radiology* 151:637, 1984.

136. LaCasse JE, Reilly BJ, Mancer K: Segmental esophageal trachea: a potentially fatal type of tracheal stenosis, *AJR* 134: 829, 1980.

137. Gans SL, Lackey DA, Zucerbraun L: Duplications of the cervical esophagus in infants and children, *Surgery* 63:849, 1968.

138. Ansell G, Edwards FR: Double oesophagus, *J Fac Radiol* 9:154, 1958.

139. Kirwan W, Walbaum B, McCormack R: Cystic intrathoracic derivatives of the foregut and their complications, *Thorax* 28:424, 1973.

140. Blank E, Michael TD: Muscle hypertrophy of the esophagus: report of a case with involvement of the entire esophagus, *Pediatrics* 32:594, 1963.

141. Vargus LL et al: Congenital esophageal stenosis: report of a case of annular muscle hypertrophy at the esophagogastric junction, *N Engl J Med* 255:1224, 1956.

142. Heithoff KB et al: Bronchopulmonary foregut malformations: a unifying etiological concept, *AJR* 126:46, 1976.

143. Blumberg JB et al: Laryngotracheal esophageal cleft: the embryologic implications—review of the literature, *Surgery* 57:559, 1965.

144. Frates RE: Roentgen signs in laryngotracheoesophageal cleft, *Radiology* 88:484, 1967.

145. Bruggeman LL, Seaman WB: Epiphrenic diverticula: an analysis of 80 cases, *AJR* 119:266, 1973.

146. Dodds WJ et al: Radial distribution of esophageal peristaltic pressure in normal subjects and patients with esophageal diverticulum, *Gastroenterology* 69:584, 1975.

147. Kaye MD: Oesophageal motor dysfunction in patients with diverticula of the mid-thoracic oesophagus, *Thorax* 29:666, 1974.

148. Balthazar EJ: Esophagobronchial fistula secondary to ruptured traction diverticulum, *Gastrointest Radiol* 2:119, 1977.

149. Gawande, AS et al: Carcinoma within lower esophageal (epiphrenic) diverticulum, *NY J Med* 72:1749, 1972.

150. Mendl K, McKay JM, Tanner CH: Intramural diverticulosis of the oesophagus and Rokitansky-Aschoff sinuses in the gallbladder, *Br J Radiol* 33:496, 1960.

151. Beauchamp JM et al: Esophageal intramural pseudodiverticulosis, *Radiology* 113:273, 1974.

152. Lupovitch A, Tippins R: Esophageal intramural pseudodiverticulosis: disease of adnexal glands, *Radiology* 113:271, 1974.

153. Fromkes J et al: Esophageal intramural pseudodiverticulosis, *Am J Dig Dis* 22:690, 1977.

154. Schreiber MH, Davis M: Intraluminal diverticulum of the esophagus, *AJR* 129:595, 1977.

155. Bogaars AH: Survey of 100 cases of corpora aliena in the esophagus, *Pract Otorhinolaryngol* (Basel) 24:125, 1962.

156. Smith PC, Swischuk LE, Fagan CJ: An elusive and often unsuspected cause of stridor in pneumonia (the esophageal foreign body), *AJR* 122:80, 1974.

157. Ferruci JT, Long JA: Radiologic treatment of esophageal food and impaction using intravenous glucagon, *Radiology* 125:25, 1977.

158. Phillips LG Jr, Cunningham J: Esophageal perforation, *Radiol Clin North Am* 22:607, 1984.

159. Dodds WJ et al: Severe peptic esophagitis in a patient with Zollinger-Ellison syndrome, *AJR* 113:237, 1971.

160. Davis M, Thomas LC, Guice KS: Esophagitis after papain, *J Clin Gastroenterol* 9:127, 1987.

161. Han SY, Tishler JM: Perforation of the abdominal segment of the esophagus, *AJR* 143:751, 1984.

162. Zegel HG et al: Delayed esophageal perforation after pneumatic dilatation for the treatment of achalasia, *Gastrointest Radiol* 4:219, 1979.

163. O'Connell ND: Spontaneous rupture of the esophagus, *AJR* 99:186, 1967.

164. Tihansky DP et al: The esophagus after injection sclerotherapy of varices: immediate postoperative changes, *Radiology* 153:43, 1984.

165. Harell GS et al: Neonatal Boerhaave's syndrome, *Radiology* 95:665, 1970.

166. Rogers LF et al: Diagnostic considerations in mediastinal emphysema: a pathophysiologic-roentgenologic approach to Boerhaave's syndrome and spontaneous pneumomediastinum, *AJR* 115:495, 1972.

167. Love L, Berkow AE: Trauma to the esophagus, *Gastrointest Radiol* 2:305, 1978.

168. Stewart ET et al: Desirability of roentgen examination immediately after pneumatic dilatation for achalasia, *Radiology* 130:589, 1979.

169. Watts HD: Lesions brought on by vomiting: the effect of hiatus hernia on the site of injury, *Gastroenterology* 71:683, 1976.

170. Bradley JL, Han SY: Intramural hematoma (incomplete perforation) of the esophagus associated with esophageal dilatation, *Radiology* 130:59, 1979.

171. Rabiah FA, Elliott HB: Intramural hematoma of the esophagus: an unusual complication of vagotomy, *Am J Dig Dis* 13:925, 1968.

172. Ashman FC et al: Esophageal hematoma associated with thrombocytopenia, *Gastrointest Radiol* 3:115, 1978.

173. Wolf BS: Sliding hiatal hernia: the need for redefinition, *AJR* 117:231, 1973.

174. Ellis FH Jr: Current concepts: esophageal hiatal hernia, *N Engl J Med* 287:646, 1972.

175. Michelson E, Siegel CI: The role of the phrenico-esophageal ligament in the lower esophageal sphincter, *Surg Gynecol Obstet* 118:1291, 1964.

176. Berridge FR, Friedland GW, Tagart REB: Radiological landmarks at the oesophagogastric junction, *Thorax* 21:499, 1966.

177. Clark MD, Rinald JA Jr, Eyler WR: Correlation of manometric and radiologic data from the esophagogastric area, *Radiology* 94:261, 1970.

178. Dodds WJ et al: Longitudinal esophageal contractions: a possible factor in the genesis of hiatal hernia (abstract), *Invest Radiol* 11:375, 1976.

179. Goyal RK, Bauer JL, Spiro HM: The nature and location of lower esophageal ring, *N Engl J Med* 284:1175, 1971.

180. Goyal RK, Glancy JJ, Spiro HM: Lower esophageal ring, *N Engl J Med* 282:1298, 1970.

181. Feigin DS et al: The radiographic appearance of hiatal hernia repairs, *Radiology* 110: 71, 1974.

182. Skucas J et al: An evaluation of the Nissen fundoplication, *Radiology* 118:539, 1976.

183. Goldberg HI et al: Role of acid and pepsin in acute experimental esophagitis, *Gastroenterology* 56:223, 1969.

184. Dodds WJ et al: Sequential gross, microscopic and roentgenographic features of acute feline esophagitis, *Invest Radiol* 5:209, 1970.

185. Ott DJ, Wu WC, Gelfand DW: Reflux esophagitis revisited: prospective analysis of radiologic accuracy, *Gastrointest Radiol* 6:1, 1981.

186. Ott DJ et al: Current status of radiology in evaluating for gastroesophageal reflux disease, *Clin Gastroenterol* 4:365, 1982.

187. Levine MS et al: Early esophageal cancer, *AJR* 146:507, 1986.

188. Ott DJ, Gelfand DW, Wu WC: Reflux esophagitis: radiographic and endoscopic correlation, *Radiology* 130:583, 1979.

189. Kahrilas PJ, Dodds WJ, Hogan WJ: Effect of peristaltic dysfunction on esophageal volume clearance, *Gastroenterology* 94:73, 1988.

190. Kramer P: Does a sliding hiatus hernia constitute a distinct clinical entity? *Gastroenterology* 57:442, 1969.

191. Ott DJ et al: Esophagogastric region and its rings, *AJR* 142:281, 1984.

192. Allison PR, Johnstone AS: The oesophagus lined with gastric mucous membrane, *Thorax* 8:87, 1953.

193. Barrett NR: Chronic peptic ulcer of the oesophagus and oesophagitis, *Br J Surg* 38:175, 1950.

194. Robbins AH et al: The columnar-lined esophagus: analysis of 26 cases, *Radiology* 123 :1, 1977.

195. Spechler SJ, Goyal RK: Barrett's esophagus. *N Engl J Med* 315:362, 1986.

196. Agha FP: Barrett carcinoma of the esophagus: clinical and radiographic analysis of 34 cases, *AJR* 145:41, 1985.

197. Robbins AH et al: Revised radiologic concepts of the Barrett's esophagus, *Gastrointest Radiol* 3:377, 1978.

198. Anderson, LS, Forrest, JV: Tumors of the diaphragm, *Am J Roengtenol Radiat Ther Nucl Med* 119:259, 1973.

199. Agha FP: Radiologic diagnosis of Barrett's esophagus: critical analysis of 65 cases, *Gastrointest Radiol* 11:123, 1986.

200. Levine MS et al: Barrett's esophagus: reticular pattern of the mucosa, *Radiology* 147: 663, 1983.

201. Holloway RH, Dodds WJ: Esophageal motor function in Barrett's esophagus. In Spechler SJ, Goyal RK, eds: *Barrett's esophagus: pathophysiology, diagnosis, and management*, New York, 1985, Elsevier.

202. Kodsi BE et al: *Candida* esophagitis: a prospective study of 27 cases, *Gastroenterology* 71:715, 1976.

203. Nash G, Ross JS: Herpetic esophagitis: a common cause of esophageal ulceration, *Hum Pathol* 5:339, 1974.

204. Henson D: Cytomegalovirus inclusion bodies in the gastrointestinal tract, *Arch Pathol* 93:477, 1972.

205. McManus JPA, Webb JN: A yeast-like infection of the esophagus caused by *Lactobacillus acidophilus, Gastroenterology* 68:583, 1975.

206. Howlett SA: Acute streptococcal esophagus, *Gastrointest Endosc* 25:150, 1979.

207. Levine MS, Macones AJ Jr, Laufer I: *Candida* esophagitis: accuracy of radiographic diagnosis, *Radiology* 154:581, 1985.

208. Levine MA et al: Herpes esophagitis, *AJR* 136:863, 1981.

209. Andren L, Theander G: Roentgenographic appearance of oesophageal moniliasis, *Acta Radiol* (Stockh) 46:571, 1956.

210. Athey PA, Goldstein HM, Dodd GD: Radiologic spectrum of opportunistic infections of the upper gastrointestinal tract, *AJR* 129:419, 1977.

211. Roberts L Jr et al: Adult esophageal candidiasis: a radiographic spectrum, *Radiographics* 7:289, 1987.

212. Sheft DJ, Shargo G: Esophageal moniliasis: the spectrum of the disease, *JAMA* 213:1859, 1970.

213. Bier SJ et al: Esophageal moniliasis: a new radiographic presentation, *Am J Gastroenterol* 80:734, 1985.

214. Gefter WB et al: Candidiasis in the obstructed esophagus, *Radiology* 138:25, 1981.

215. Ott DJ, Gelfand DW: Esophageal stricture secondary to candidiasis, *Gastrointest Radiol* 2:323, 1978.

216. Rohrmann CA Jr, Kidd R: Chronic mucocutaneous candidiasis: radiologic abnormalities in the esophagus, *AJR* 130:473, 1978.

217. Rabeneck L et al: Unusual esophageal ulcers containing enveloped virus-like particles in homosexual men, *Gastroenterology* 90:1882, 1986.

218. Deshmukh M, Shah R, McCallum RW: Experience with herpes esophagitis in otherwise healthy patients, *Am J Gastroenterol* 79:173, 1984.

219. Fishbein PG et al: Herpes simplex esophagitis: a cause of upper-gastrointestinal bleeding, *Am J Dig Dis* 24:540, 1979.

220. Voirol MW, Welsh RA, Genet ER: Esophagitis cystica, *Am J Gastroenterol* 59:446, 1973.

221. Balthazar EJ et al: Cytomegalovirus esophagitis in AIDS: radiographic features in 16 patients, *AJR* 149:919, 1987.

222. St. Onge G, Bezahler GH: Giant esophageal ulcer associated with cytomegalovirus, *Gastroenterology* 83:127, 1982.

223. Meyers C, Durkin MG, Love L: Radiographic findings in herpetic esophagitis, *Radiology* 119:21, 1976.

224. Teixidor HS et al: Cytomegalovirus infection of the alimentary canal: radiologic findings with pathologic correlation, *Radiology* 163:317, 1987.

225. Williford ME et al: Esophageal tuberculosis: findings on barium swallow and computed tomography, *Gastrointest Radiol* 8:119, 1983.

226. Schneider R: Tuberculous esophagitis, *Gastrointest Radiol* 1:143, 1976.

227. Daly JF: Corrosive esophagitis, *Otolaryngol Clin North Am* p 119, 1968.

228. Martel W: Radiologic features of esophagogastritis secondary to extremely caustic agents, *Radiology* 103:31, 1972.

229. Dodds WJ, Stewart ET, Vlymen WT: Appropriate contrast media for evaluation of esophageal disruption, *Radiology* 144:439, 1982.

230. Franken EA Jr: Caustic damage of the gastrointestinal tract: roentgen features, *AJR* 118:77, 1973.

231. Carlborg B, Densert O: Esophageal lesions caused by orally administered drugs, *Eur Surg Res* 12:270, 1980.

232. Mason SJ, O'Meara TF: Drug-induced esophagitis, *J Clin Gastroenterol* 3:115, 1981.

233. Ravich WJ, Kashima H, Donner MW: Drug-induced esophagitis simulating esophageal carcinoma, *Dysphagia* 1:13, 1986.

234. Goldstein HM et al: Radiological manifestations of radiation-induced injury to the normal upper gastrointestinal tract, *Radiology* 117:135, 1975.

235. Boal DKB, Newburger PE, Teele RL: Esophagitis induced by combined radiation and Adriamycin, *AJR* 132:567, 1979.

236. Seaman WB, Ackerman LV: The effect of radiation on the esophagus: a clinical and histologic study of the effects produced by the betatron, *Radiology* 68:534, 1957.

237. Northway MG et al: The opossum as an animal model for studying radiation esophagitis, *Radiology* 131:731, 1979.

238. Papazian A et al: Mucosal bridges of the upper esophagus after radiotherapy for Hodgkin's disease, *Gastroenterology* 84:1028, 1983.

239. Raque CJ, Stein KM, Samitz MH: Pemphigus vulgaris involving the esophagus, *Arch Dermatol Syph* 102:371, 1970.

240. Agha FP, Raji MR: Esophageal involvement in pemphigoid: clinical and roentgen manifestations, *Gastrointest Radiol* 7:109, 1982.

241. Foroozan P et al: Loss and regeneration of the esophageal mucosa in pemphigoid, *Gastroenterology* 52:548, 1967.

242. Agha FP, Francis IR, Ellis CN: Esophageal involvement in epidermolysis bullosa dystrophica: clinical and roentgenologic manifestations, *Gastrointest Radiol* 8:111, 1983.

243. Orlando RC et al: Epidermolysis bullosa: gastrointestinal manifestations, *Ann Intern Med* 81:203, 1974.

244. Johnson ML: Epidermolysis bullosa acquisita with esophageal casts, *Proc R Soc Med* 60:1272, 1967.

245. Calcaterra TC, Strahan RW: Stevens-Johnson syndrome: oropharyngeal manifestations, *Arch Otolaryngol* 93:37, 1971.

246. McDonald GB, Sullivan KM, Plumley TF: Radiographic features of esophageal involvement in chronic graft-vs-host disease, *AJR* 142:501, 1984.

247. Marsden RA et al: Epidermolysis bullosa of the oesophagus with oesophageal web formation, *Thorax* 29:287, 1974.

248. Ghahremani GG et al: Esophageal manifestations of Crohn's disease, *Gastrointest Radiol* 7:199, 1982.

249. LiVolsi VA, Jaretzki A III: Granulomatous esophagitis: a case of Crohn's disease limited to the esophagus, *Gastroenterology* 64:313, 1973.

250. Miller LJ et al: Crohn's disease involving the esophagus and colon: case report, *Mayo Clin Proc* 52:35, 1977.

251. Degryse HRM, De Schepper MAP: Aphthoid esophageal ulcers in Crohn's disease of ileum and colon, *Gastrointest Radiol* 9:197, 1984.

252. Cynn WS et al: Crohn's disease of the esophagus, *AJR* 125:359, 1975.

253. Brodie TE, Ochsner JL: Behçet's syndrome with ulcerative oesophagitis: report of the first case, *Thorax* 28:637, 1973.

254. Lebwohl O et al: Ulcerative esophagitis and colitis in a pediatric patient with Behçet's syndrome: response to steroid therapy, *Am J Gastroenterol* 68:550, 1977.

255. Mori S et al: Esophageal involvement in Behçet's disease, *Am J Gastroenterol* 78:548, 1983.

256. Knudsen KB, Sparberg M: Ulcerative esophagitis and ulcerative colitis, *JAMA* 201:154, 1967.

257. Shauffer IA, Phillips HE, Sequeira J: The jet phenomenon: a manifestation of esophageal web, *AJR* 129:747, 1977.

258. Schatzki R, Gary JE: Dysphagia due to a diaphragm-like localized narrowing in the lower esophagus ("lower esophageal ring"), *AJR* 70:911, 1953.

259. MacMahon HE, Schatzke R, Gary JE: Pathology of a lower esophageal ring: report of a case, with autopsy, observed for nine years, *N Engl J Med* 259:1, 1958.

260. Schatzki R: The lower esophageal ring: long term follow-up of symptomatic and asymptomatic rings, *AJR* 90:805, 1963.

261. Ingelfinger FJ, Kramer P: Dysphagia produced by a contractile ring in the lower esophagus, *Gastroenterology* 23:419, 1953.

262. Rose JS et al: Congenital oesophageal strictures due to cartilaginous rings, *Br J Radiol* 48:16, 1975.

263. Anderson LS et al: Cartilaginous esophageal ring: a cause of esophageal stenosis in infants and children, *Pediatr Radiol* p 665, 1973.

264. Benedict EB, Lever EF: Stenosis of esophagus in benign mucous membrane pemphigus, *Ann Otol Rhinol Laryngol* 61:1120, 1952.

265. Chisholm M et al: Iron deficiency and autoimmunity in postcricoid webs, *Q J Med* 40:421, 1971.

266. Clements JL Jr et al: Cervical esophageal webs: a roentgen-anatomic correlation, *AJR* 121:221, 1974.

267. Nosher JL, Campbell WL, Seaman WB: The clinical significance of cervical esophageal and hypopharyngeal webs, *Radiology* 117:45, 1975.

268. Howiler W, Goldberg HI: Gastroesophageal involvement in herpes simplex, *Gastroenterology* 70:775, 1976.

269. Longstreth GF, Wolochow DA, Tu RT: Double congenital midesophageal webs in adults, *Am J Dig Dis* 24:162, 1979.

270. Weaver JW, Kaude JC, Hamlin DJ: Webs of the lower esophagus: a complication of gastroesophageal reflux? *AJR* 142:289, 1984.

271. Ott DJ et al: Endoscopic sensitivity in the detection of esophageal strictures, *J Clin Gastroenterol* 7:121, 1985.

272. Ho CS, Rodrigues PRD: Lower esophageal strictures, benign or malignant? *J Can Assoc Radiol* 31:110, 1980.

273. Vanasin B, Wright JR, Schuster MM: *Pneumatosis cystoides esophagi*: case report supporting theory of submucosal spread, *JAMA* 217:76, 1971.

274. Agha FP: Esophageal involvement in Zollinger-Ellison syndrome, *AJR* 144:721, 1985.

275. Anderson MF, Harell GS: Secondary esophageal tumors, *AJR* 135:1243, 1980.

276. Tishler JM, Han SY, Helman CA: Esophageal involvement in epidermolysis bullosa dystrophica, *AJR* 141:1283, 1983.

277. Picus D, Frank PH: Eosinophilic esophagitis, *AJR* 136:1001, 1981.

278. Agha FP: Candidiasis-induced esophageal strictures, *Gastrointest Radiol* 9:283, 1984.

279. Zeller R et al: Idiopathic muscular hypertrophy of the esophagus: a case report, *Gastrointest Radiol* 4:121, 1979.

280. Agha FP: The esophagus after endoscopic injection sclerotherapy: acute and chronic changes, *Radiology* 153:37, 1984.

281. Hatfield M, Shapir J: The radiologic manifestations of failed antireflux operations, *AJR* 144:1209, 1985.

282. Nelson RM et al: Idiopathic retroperitoneal fibrosis producing distal esophageal obstruction, *J Thorac Cardiovasc Surg* 55:216, 1968.

283. Kenneweg DJ, Cimmino CV: Esophageal obstruction and dysphagia caused by hepatomegaly, *Radiology* 91:783, 1968.

284. Mikkelsen J: Varices of the upper esophagus in superior vena cava obstruction, *Radiology* 81:945, 1963.

285. Scobie BA et al: Pressure changes of the esophagus and gastroesophageal function with cirrhosis and varices, *Gastroenterology* 49:67, 1965.

286. Eckardt VF, Grace ND, Kantrowitz PA: Does lower esophageal sphincter incompetency contribute to esophageal variceal bleeding? *Gastroenterology* 71:185, 1976.

287. Jonsson K, Rian RL: Pseudotumoral esophageal varices associated with portal hypertension, *Radiology* 97:593, 1970.

288. Dodds WJ et al: Esophageal roentgenography using tantalum paste, *Radiology* 102:204, 1972.

289. Nelson SW: Roentgenographic diagnosis of esophageal varices, *AJR* 77:599, 1957.

290. Cockerill EM et al: Optimal visualization of esophageal varices, *AJR* 126:512, 1976.

291. Lawson TL, Dodds WJ, Sheft DJ: Carcinoma of the esophagus simulating varices, *AJR* 107:83, 1969.

292. Liu C-I: Enhanced visualization of esophageal varices by buscopan, *AJR* 121:232, 1974.

293. Waldram R et al: Detection and grading of oesophageal varices, *Clin Radiol* 28:137, 1977.

294. Seggie J, Knottenbelt JD: Esophageal obstruction by phytobezoar: rare complication of gastric bezoar, *Dig Dis Sci* 26:90, 1981.

295. Goldstein HM, Zornoza J: Association of squamous cell carcinoma of the head and neck with cancer of the esophagus, *AJR* 131:791, 1978.

296. Harris OD et al: Malignancy in adult coeliac disease and idiopathic steatorrhoea, *Am J Med* 42:899, 1967.

297. Lansing PB, Ferrante WA, Ochsner JL: Carcinoma of the esophagus at the site of lye stricture, *Am J Surg* 118: 108, 1969.

298. Daffner RH, Postlethwait RW, Putman CE: Retrotracheal abnormalities in esophageal carcinoma: prognostic implications, *AJR* 130:719, 1978.

299. Lindell MM Jr, Hill CA, Libshitz HI: Esophageal cancer: radiographic chest findings and their prognostic significance, *AJR* 133:461, 1979.

300. Gloyna RE, Zornoza J, Goldstein HM: Primary ulcerative carcinoma of the esophagus, *AJR* 129:599, 1977.

301. Koehler RE, Moss AA, Margulis AR: Early radiographic manifestations of carcinoma of the esophagus, *Radiology* 119:1, 1976.

302. Levine MS et al: Radiation therapy of esophageal carcinoma: correlation of clinical and radiographic findings, *Gastroenterol Radiol* 12:99, 1987.

303. Daffner RH et al: CT of the esophagus. II. Carcinoma, *AJR* 133:1051, 1979.

304. Picus D et al: Computed tomography in the staging of esophageal carcinoma, *Radiology* 146:433, 1983.

305. Quint LE et al: Esophageal carcinoma: CT findings, *Radiology* 155:171, 1985.

306. Itai Y et al: Superficial esophageal carcinoma: radiological findings in double-contrast studies, *Radiology* 126:597, 1978.

307. Stout AR, Humphreys GH, Rottenberg LA: A case of carcinosarcoma of the esophagus, *AJR* 61:461, 1949.

308. Talbert JL, Cantrell JR: Clinical and pathological characteristics of carcinosarcoma of the esophagus, *J Thorac Cardiovasc Surg* 45:1, 1963.

309. Cho SR et al: Polypoid carcinoma of the esophagus: a distinct radiological and histopathological entity, *Am J Gastroenterol* 78:476, 1983.

310. Olmsted WW, Lichtenstein JE, Hyams VJ: Polypoid epithelial malignancies of the esophagus, *AJR* 140:921, 1983.

311. Nichols T et al: Pseudosarcoma of the esophagus: three new cases and review of the literature, *Am J Gastroenterol* 72:615, 1979.

312. Hendricks GL Jr, Barnes WT, Suter HJ: Primary malignant melanoma of the esophagus: a case report, *Am Surg* 40:468, 1974.

313. Agha FP, Schnitzer B: Esophageal involvement in lymphoma, *Am J Gastroenterol* 80:412, 1985.

314. Levine MS et al: Diffuse nodularity in esophageal lymphoma, *AJR* 145:1218, 1985.

315. Traube M, Waldron JA, McCallum RW: Systemic lymphoma initially presenting as an esophageal mass, *Am J Gastroenterol* 77:835, 1982.

316. Carnovale RL et al: Radiologic manifestations of esophageal lymphoma, *AJR* 128:751, 1977.

317. Nissen S, Bar-Moar JA, Levy E: Lymphosarcoma of the esophagus: a case report, *Cancer* 34:1321, 1974.

318. Al-Rashid RA, Harned RK: Dysphagia due to leukemic involvement of the esophagus, *Am J Dis Child* 121:75, 1971.

319. Chang SF et al: The protean gastrointestinal manifestations of metastatic breast carcinoma, *Radiology* 126:611, 1978.

320. Fisher MS: Metastasis to the esophagus, *Gastrointest Radiol* 1:249, 1976.

321. Wood CB, Wood RAB: Metastatic malignant melanoma of the esophagus, *Am J Dig Dis* 20:786, 1975.

322. Plachta A: Benign tumors of the esophagus: review of literature and report of 99 cases, *Am J Gastroenterol* 38:639, 1962.

323. Tsuzuki T et al: Giant leiomyoma of the esophagus and cardia weighing more than 1,000 grams, *Chest* 60:396, 1971.

324. Gutman E: Posterior mediastinal calcification due to esophageal leiomyoma, *Gastroenterology* 63:665, 1972.

325. Montesi A et al: Small benign tumors of the esophagus: radiological diagnosis with double-contrast examination, *Gastrointest Radiol* 8:207, 1983.

326. Haber K, Winfield AC: Multiple leiomyomas of the esophagus, *Am J Dig Dis* 19:678, 1974.

327. Shaffer HA Jr: Multiple leiomyomas of the esophagus, *Radiology* 118:29, 1976.

328. Kabuto T et al: Diffuse leiomyomatosis of the esophagus, *Dig Dis Sci* 25:388, 1980.

329. Gershwind ME et al: Granular cell tumors of the esophagus, *Gastrointest Radiol* 2:327, 1978.

330. Subramanyam K et al: Granular cell myoblastoma of the esophagus, *J Clin Gastroenterol* 6:113, 1984.

331. Jang GC, Clouse ME, Fleischner FG: Fibrovascular polyp: a benign intraluminal tumor of the esophagus, *Radiology* 92:1196, 1969.

332. Carney JA et al: Alimentary-tract ganglioneuromatosis: a major component of the syndrome of multiple endocrine neoplasia, Type 2b, *N Engl J Med* 295:1287, 1976.

333. Bleshman MH et al: The inflammatory esophagogastric polyp and fold, *Radiology* 128:589, 1978.

334. Staples DC, Knodell RG, Johnson, LF: Inflammatory pseudotumor of the esophagus: a complication of gastroesophageal reflux, *Gastrointest Endosc* 24:175, 1978.

335. Parnell SAC et al: Squamous cell papilloma of the esophagus: report of a case after peptic esophagitis and repeated bougienage with review of the literature, *Gastroenterology* 74:910, 1978.

336. Walker JH: Giant papilloma of the thoracic esophagus, *AJR* 131:519, 1978.

337. Farman J et al: Esophagitis cystica: lower esophageal retention cysts, *AJR* 129:495, 1977.

338. Hover AR et al: Multiple retention cysts of the lower esophagus, *J Clin Gastroenterol* 4:209, 1982.

339. Glick SN et al: Glycogenic acanthosis of the esophagus, *AJR* 139:683, 1982.

340. Hauser H et al: Radiological findings in multiple hamartoma syndrome (Cowden disease), *Radiology* 137:317, 1980.

341. Trenkner SW et al: Idiopathic esophageal varix, *AJR* 141:43, 1983.

342. Chasen MH, Rugh KS, Shelton DK: Mediastinal impressions on the dilated esophagus, *Radiol Clin North Am* 22:591, 1984.

343. Birnholz JC, Ferruci JT Jr, Wyman SM: Roentgen features of dysphagia aortica, *Radiology* 111:93, 1974.

344. Mittal RK et al: Dysphagia aortica: clinical, radiological, and manometric findings, *Dig Dis Sci* 31:379, 1986.

345. Picus D et al: "Discphagia": a case report, *Gastrointest Radiol* 9:5, 1984.

346. Willing S, El Gammal T: Thoracic osteophyte producing dysphagia in a case of diffuse idiopathic skeletal hypertrophy, *Am J Gastroenterol* 78:381, 1983.

347. Mann NS, Brewer H, Sheth B: Upper esophageal dysphagia due to marked cervical lordosis, *J Clin Gastroenterol* 6:57, 1984.

348. Felson B, Palayew MJ: Two types of right aortic arch, *Radiology* 81:745, 1963.

349. Moncada R et al: The cervical aortic arch, *AJR* 125:591, 1975.

350. Salomonowitz E et al: The three types of aortic diverticula, *AJR* 142:673, 1984.

351. Berenzweig H, Baue AE, McCallum RW: Dysphagia lusoria: report of a case and review of the diagnostic and surgical approach, *Dig Dis Sci* 25:630, 1980.

352. Tesler UF, Balsava H, Niguidula FN: Aberrant left pulmonary artery (vascular sling): report of five cases, *Chest* 68:402, 1974.

353. Yeh HC, Wolf BS: A pulmonary venous indentation on the esophagus: a normal variant, *Radiology* 116:299, 1975.

354. Srinivasan MK, Scholz FJ: Hemiazygos vein as a cause of posterior indentation of the esophagus: a case report, *Gastrointest Radiol* 5:13, 1980.

355. Hiller HG, Maclean AD: Pulmonary artery ring, *Acta Radiol* 48:434, 1957.

356. Shahin N: Wandering esophagus, *Isr J Med Sci* 3:462, 1967.

357. Cullen ML, Klein MD, Philippart AI: Congenital diaphragmatic hernia, *Surg Clin North Am* 65:1115, 1985.

358. Benacerraf BR, Greene MF: Congenital diaphragmatic hernia: US diagnosis prior to 22 weeks gestation, *Radiology* 158:809, 1986.

359. Gale ME: Bochdalek hernia: prevalence and CT characteristics, *Radiology* 156:449, 1985.

360. Shin MS et al: Bochdalek hernia of diaphragm in the adult: diagnosis by computed tomography, *Chest* 92:1098, 1987.

361. Ellyson JH, Parks SN: Hernia of Morgagni in a trauma patient, *J Trauma* 26:569, 1986.

Additional Readings

1. Agha FP: Secondary neoplasms of the esophagus, *Gastrointest Radiol* 12:187, 1987.

2. Ahlbom HE: Simple achlorhydric anemia, Plummer-Vinson syndrome and carcinoma of the mouth, pharynx and oesophagus in women, *Br Med J* 2:331, 1936.

3. Balthazar EJ et al: CT evaluation of esophageal varices, *AJR* 148:131, 1987.

4. Benacerraf BR, Adzick NS: Fetal diaphragmatic hernia: ultrasound diagnosis and clinical outcome in 19 cases, *Am J Obstet Gynecol* 156:573, 1987.

5. Binder HJ et al: The effect of cervical vagectomy on esophageal function in the monkey, *Surgery* 64:1075, 1968.

6. Brayko CM et al: Type I herpes simplex esophagitis with concomitant esophageal moniliasis, *J Clin Gastroenterol* 4:351, 1982.

7. Brown WR: Rumination in the adult, *Gastroenterology* 54:933, 1968.

8. Carter MM, Kulkarni MV: Giant fibrovascular polyp of the esophagus, *Gastrointest Radiol* 9:301, 1984.

9. Chen YM et al: Barrett esophagus as an extension of severe esophagitis: analysis of radiologic signs in 29 cases, *AJR* 145:275, 1985.

10. Chen YM et al: Multiphasic examination of the esophagogastric region for strictures, rings, and hiatal hernia: evaluation of the individual techniques, *Gastrointest Radiol* 10:311, 1985.

11. Chisholm M: The association between webs, iron and postcricoid carcinoma, *Postgrad Med J* 50:215, 1974.

12. Code CF et al: *An atlas of esophageal motility in health and disease*, Springfield, Ill, 1958, Charles C Thomas.

13. Craddock DR, Logan A, Walbaum PR: Diffuse esophageal spasm, *Thorax* 21:511, 1966.

14. Cross FS: Esophageal diverticula related neuromuscular problems, *Ann Otol Rhinol Laryngol* 77:914, 1968.

15. Demos RC et al: Spontaneous esophageal hematoma diagnosed by computed tomography, *J Comput Assist Tomogr* 10:133, 1986.

16. Dodds WJ et al: Responses of the feline esophagus to cervical vagal stimulation, *Am J Physiol* 235:E63, 1978.

17. Dodds WJ et al: Gastroesophageal reflux (GER) and esophageal clearance in normal human volunteers and patients with reflux esophagitis. In *Gastrointestinal motility*, New York, 1980, Raven Press.

18. Doman DB, Ginsberg AL: The hazard of drug-induced esophagitis, *Hosp Pract* p 17, 1981.

19. Hollis JP, Castell DO: Esophageal function in elderly men: a new look at "presbyesophagus," *Ann Intern Med* 80:371, 1974.

20. Kahrilas PJ, Dodds WJ, Hogan WJ: dysfunction of the belch reflux: a cause of incapacitating chest pain, *Gastroenterology* 93:818, 1987.

21. Kahrilas PJ et al: Upper esophageal sphincter function during belching, *Gastroenterology* 91:133, 1986.

22. Kapila YV et al: Relationship between swallow rate and salivary flow, *Dig Dis Sci* 29:528, 1984.

23. Kelley ML Jr: Intraluminal manometry in the evaluation of malignant disease of the esophagus, *Cancer* 21:1011, 1968.

24. Kelly AB: Spasm at the entrance of the esophagus, *J Laryngol Rhinol Otol* 34:285, 1919.

25. Koehler RE, Weyman PJ, Oakley HF: Single- and double-contrast techniques in esophagitis, *AJR* 135:15, 1980.

26. Laajam MA: Primary tuberculosis of the esophagus: pseudotumoral presentation, *Am J Gastroenterol* 79:839, 1984.

27. Levine MS, Goldstein HM: Fixed transverse folds in the esophagus: a sign of reflux esophagitis, *AJR* 143:275, 1984.

28. Meeks LW, Renshaw TS: Vertebral osteophytosis and dysphagia: two case reports of the syndrome recently termed ankylosing hyperostosis, *J Bone Joint Surg [Am]* 55:197, 1973.

29. Saladin TA et al: Esophageal motor abnormalities in scleroderma and related diseases, *Am J Dig Dis* 11:522, 1966.

30. Shamm'a MH, Benedict EB: Esophageal webs: a report of 58 cases and an attempt at classification, *N Engl J Med* 259:378, 1958.

31. Shortsleeve MJ et al: Herpetic esophagitis, *Radiology* 141:611, 1981.

32. Skucas J et al: Herpes esophagitis: a case studied by air-contrast esophagography, *AJR* 128:497, 1977.

33. Springer DJ, DaCosta LR, Beck IT: A syndrome of acute self-limiting ulcerative esophagitis in young adults probably due to herpes simplex virus, *Dig Dis Sci* 24:535, 1979.

34. Strawczynski H et al: The behavior of the lower esophageal sphincter in infants and its relationship to gastroesophageal regurgitation, *J Pediatr* 64:7, 1964.

35. Styles RA et al: Esophagogastric polyps: radiographic and endoscopic findings, *Radiology* 154:307, 1985.

36. Sullivan MA et al: Gastrointestinal myoelectrical activity in idiopathic intestinal pseudo-obstruction, *N Engl J Med* 297:233, 1977.

37. Tidman MK, John HT: Spontaneous rupture of the esophagus, *Br J Surg* 54:286, 1967.

38. Vinson PO: Hysterical dysphagia, *Minn Med* 5:107, 1922.

39. Waldenstrom J, Kjellberg SR: Roentgenological diagnosis of sideropenic dysphagia (Plummer-Vinson's syndrome), *Acta Radiol* 20:618, 1939.

40. Walker J, Singer K, Bater P: Disorders of esophageal motility in a family with hereditary spastic ataxia, *Neurology* 19:1212, 1969.

41. Warden HD: Esophageal obstruction due to aberrant intercostal artery: report of a case, *Arch Surg* (Chicago) 83:749, 1961.

12 *Endosonography of the Esophagus*

T. L. TIO

A number of publications describing the technical aspects of the development of fiberoptic endoscopic ultrasound (EUS) have appeared over the last twenty years,[1-12] and the technique has been used by several centers to assess esophageal disease.[13-16] Close contact with the mucosa and a high-frequency ultrasonic beam in the 7- to 20-MHz range have made possible the increased resolution of the esophageal wall and nearby structures and also overcome the problem posed by interference from surrounding lungs and bones that has limited the usefulness of transcutaneous ultrasound for visualizing the mediastinum. Transducers that can mechanically rotate 360 degrees have allowed real-time imaging, and this, in turn, has facilitated anatomic orientation. Color flow Doppler has been developed for transesophageal echocardiography and it is hoped will soon be available for gastrointestinal work. EUS-guided biopsy and cytologic examinations have also recently been described. This chapter describes the usefulness of EUS in the evaluation of esophageal and periesophageal diseases.

INSTRUMENTATION

The quality and ease of use of ultrasound instruments have seen steady progress since 1983. One of the earliest instruments was an echoendoscope (EU-M3), consisting of a small echoprobe attached to the tip of a side-viewing endoscope. The diameter of the echoprobe was almost the same as that of the attached endoscope. In about 25% of the cases of esophageal carcinomas, the stenosis cannot be passed using a standard echoendoscope. Recently, an echoendoscope with a smaller echoprobe and a biopsy channel has become available (Fig. 12-1), and now an immersible Olympus echoduodenoscope with forward-oblique optics is being introduced commercially.

A nonoptic, flexible ultrasonic instrument, consisting of a small echoprobe attached to the tip of a flexible shaft, has also become available mainly for cardiologic assessment. Very small catheter echoprobes have been developed as well. These can be introduced through the biopsy channel of a large-caliber gastroscope or duodenoscope (Fig. 12-2) to accomplish endoscopic-guided ultrasound in patients with a tight luminal stenosis. In addition, other manufacturers are developing interesting new echoendoscopes, including some with a color Doppler probe.

TECHNIQUE

A standard endoscope is routinely used for the initial investigation in patients with esophageal and periesophageal diseases because the side-viewing optics of the EUS instrument do not allow visualization of the esophagus. Then, after the local administration of pharyngeal anesthesia and intravenous administration of diazepam or midazolam for sedation, the echoendoscope is inserted into the pharynx and passed down into the esophagus. The technique is described in more detail in Chapter 10.

Technical features that are specific to the assessment of esophageal carcinoma include the following. The ability of EUS to detect cervical lymph nodes in patients with tumors in the proximal one third is limited because the penetration depth of ultrasound is reduced in this area and because of patient discomfort resulting from tracheal compression produced by the water-filled balloon. The left lobe of the liver should be carefully examined by EUS because small metastatic lesions may be shown better than by transcutaneous ultrasound, although the right lobe of the liver can be more easily and accurately imaged transcutaneously.

In the assessment of tumor infiltration, various sections are necessary to determine the maximal depth of infiltration. This includes cross, oblique, and longitudinal sections whenever possible. The examination should be conducted in a standardized manner so that, for example, cross-sectional images are obtained at the same levels as those obtained by CT. When a patient has a tight stenosis that cannot be passed with an echoendoscope, a small-caliber nonoptic instrument can be used. A catheter echoprobe is the most suitable instrument for passing a filiform stenosis and determining the maximal extent of the carcinoma beyond the stenosis.

The technique for investigating submucosal abnormalities is similar. The instrument should be placed accurately just beyond the target of interest and gradually withdrawn until any extraesophageal abnormalities are clearly imaged. Respiratory excursion produces slight movement, so a stationary position of the probe produces slight movement up and down, clarifying relationships. The relationship between the esophageal wall and mediastinal lesion should be clearly defined so that mucosal abnormalities can be distinguished from extraesophageal lesions. When EUS-guided

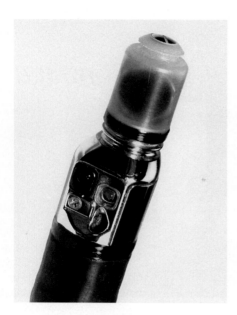

Fig. 12-1 An Olympus echoendoscope with a transducer that is a little narrower than the endoscope, and a biopsy channel.

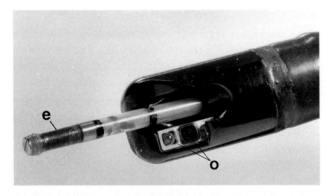

Fig. 12-2 An Olympus catheter echoprobe with a transducer (e) at the tip passing through a side-viewing duodenoscope. O, Illumination and viewing lenses.

aspiration cytology examinations are being performed, the submucosal position of the needle can be imaged by EUS, and appears as an echogenic spot within the mass. The needle tip can be maneuvered under real-time conditions, but this requires an accurate cross-sectional image of the mass and very precise positioning of the needle.

IMAGE INTERPRETATION

The generally accepted interpretation of the five-layered appearance presented by EUS images of the intestinal wall is as follows. The first, which is hyperechoic (echogenic), and second, which is hypoechoic (echo-poor), correspond, respectively, to the mucosa and interface echoes, including the muscularis mucosae. The third pattern, which is hyper-

echoic, corresponds to the submucosa and interface echoes between the mucosa and submucosa and also between the submucosa and muscularis propria. The fourth pattern, which is hypoechoic, corresponds to the muscularis propria minus the interface echoes. The fifth pattern, which is hyperechoic, corresponds to the adventitia (esophagus) or subserosa and serosa (stomach) and interface echoes.[17,18]

The interface echoes created by the ultrasound beam crossing into tissues of varying echogenicity should be taken into consideration, because they appear to be responsible for causing the increased wall thickness shown by EUS, as compared with that seen in histologic specimens. The thickness of the interface echo correlates with the axial resolution of the echoprobe.[18] In other words, the original description of the five layers of alternating echogenicity, corresponding precisely to the histologic mucosa, muscularis mucosae, submucosa, muscularis propria, and serosa, turned out to be too simplistic.[19]

On EUS, a carcinoma is imaged as either a partial or total destruction of one or more of the five layers, depending on the stage of the disease (Fig. 12-3). A tissue diagnosis of carcinoma is the gold standard for confirming the presence of malignancy.

The status of the periintestinal lymph nodes is judged according to the following criteria[20]:

1. Lymph nodes with a hypoechoic pattern and clearly demarcated boundaries imply malignancy.[4]
2. Direct penetration of mural infiltration into adjacent lymph nodes is highly indicative of direct metastatic involvement.

Some authors have suggested that size and shape be used as additional criteria in assessing lymph node involvement to enhance the accuracy, sensitivity, and specificity of the EUS findings.

STAGING OF CANCER

In a prospective study, EUS and CT scanning were performed preoperatively in all 74 participating patients. All these patients had an esophageal carcinoma according to the 1987 UICC TNM classification for EUS and histopathologic staging (see box on p. 266), and this was confirmed in all by endoscopic biopsy.

With regard to tumor staging, the overall accuracy of EUS was 89% compared with 59% for CT (Figs. 12-4 to 12-6). When it came to staging early carcinomas (T1 + T2), the overall accuracy of EUS was 82% and that of CT was 12%, and the difference between the two modalities was significant at $p < 0.0005$. In 26% of the cases the stenosis could not be passed with a regular echoendoscope. The recently available catheter echoprobe, however, can be used even in cases of tight filiform esophageal stenosis (Fig. 12-6). In the staging of regional lymph node metastases, the overall accuracy of EUS was 80% compared with 12% for CT. In this series, it was not possible to pass a stenotic carcinoma in 26% of the cases and thus the EUS accuracy

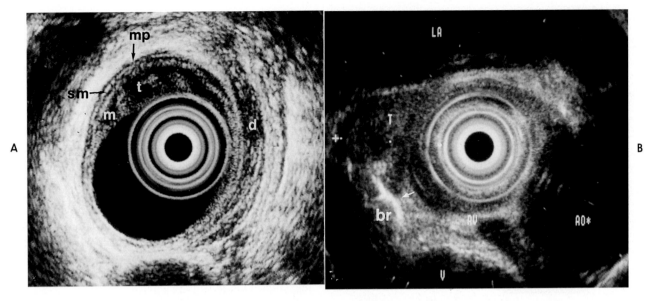

Fig. 12-3 A, Endoscopic ultrasound (EUS) showing a small polypoid carcinoma *(t)* limited to the mucosa adjacent to the esophagogastric junction. Note the left crus diaphragm *(d)* adjacent to the aorta and contralateral to the tumor. *m,* Mucosa; *sm,* submucosa; *mp,* muscularis propria. **B,** EUS reveals a hypoechoic tumor *(t)* that has penetrated into the right bronchus *(br)* contralateral to the aorta *(ao).* Note the anatomic location of the azygos vein *(av)* and the vertebra *(v).*

□ ENDOSCOPIC ULTRASOUND CLASSIFICATION OF TUMOR, REGIONAL LYMPH NODES, AND DISTANT METASTASIS ACCORDING TO THE 1987 TNM SYSTEM □

PRIMARY TUMOR (T)

ES-T1: Hypoechoic tumor localized in the mucosa or submucosa

ES-T2: Hypoechoic T1 tumor with penetration into the muscularis propria

ES-T3: Hypoechoic T3 tumor with penetration into the adventitia

ES-T4: Hypoechoic T3 tumor with penetration into adjacent structures (pericardium, aorta, trachea, diaphragm, or liver)

REGIONAL LYMPH NODE METASTASES AND DISTANT METASTASIS (M)

N0: Hyperechoic, indistinctly demarcated lymph nodes

N1: Hypoechoic, clearly delineated lymph nodes or direct penetration of tumor into the adjacent lymph nodes

M0: No evidence of metastasis in the celiac lymph nodes or liver

M1: Celiac lymph node metastases or liver metastases

STAGE GROUPING

Stage I: T1N0M0

Stage IIA: T2N0M0 or T3N0M0

Stage IIB: T1N1M0 or T2N1M0

Stage III: T3N1M0, T4 any N M0

Stage IV: any T any N M1

for staging celiac lymph nodes was only 68% compared with 82% for CT.

Similar findings were obtained in a prospective study performed at Memorial Sloan-Kettering Cancer Center.[21] In staging the tumor, the accuracy of EUS was 92% compared with 60% for CT, and, for staging regional lymph node involvement, the accuracy of EUS was 88% compared with 74% for CT. In staging distant metastases, the New York group cited a 78% accuracy for EUS, compared to 90% for CT.

In an updated study consisting of 113 patients with esophageal carcinoma, the clinical TNM classification was compared with the pathologic TNM classification based on the observations made on resected specimens.[22] The accuracy of EUS in the evaluation of T1 carcinoma (n = 12) was 83%, T2 carcinoma 85%, T3 carcinoma 92%, and T4 carcinoma 90%. The overall accuracy was 89%. Overstaging and understaging occurred in 6% and 5% of the cases, respectively. In staging lymph node spread (N), the overall accuracy of EUS was 81%, the sensitivity was 95%, and the specificity was 50%. The positive predictive value was 82% and the negative predictive value was 94%. In terms of staging the metastatic spread (M), the accuracy of EUS was 71%, its sensitivity was 60%, and its specificity was 76%. The positive and negative predictive values were 90% and 100%, respectively. If inadequate examinations due to the presence of severe stenosis (25% of cases) were excluded, the overall accuracy was 97%, sensitivity 100%, and specificity 97%.

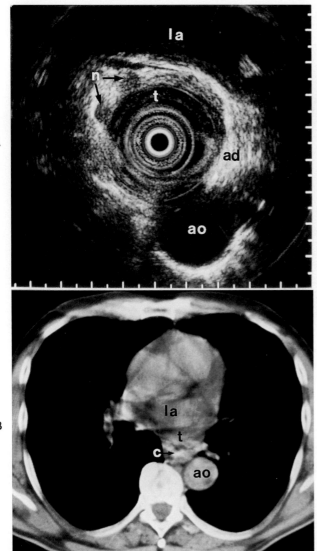

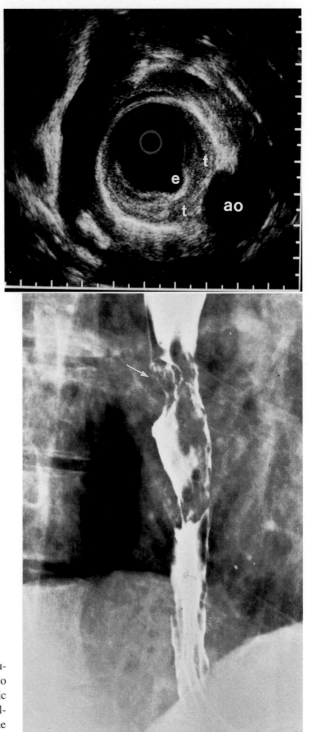

Fig. 12-4 A, Endoscopic ultrasound shows a semicircular transmural hypoechoic tumor *(t)* that has penetrated into the adventitia *(ad)*. Two hypoechoic lymph nodes *(n)* with clearly defined boundaries are adjacent to the left atrium *(la)* (retrocardiac lymph nodes) and are suspicious for metastasis. *ao,* Aorta. **B,** CT scan shows wall thickening *(t)* adjacent to the left atrium *(la)* visualized after the esophageal lumen was filled with contrast *(c)*. *ao,* Aorta.

Fig. 12-5 A, Endoscopic ultrasound shows a semicircular hypoechoic tumor *(t)* that has penetrated into the adventitia *(dots)* directly adjacent to the aorta *(ao)* and is ulcerated *(e)*. The findings are suspicious for aortic invasion compatible with a T4 carcinoma. **B,** Corresponding barium swallow reveals a polypoid tumor *(arrows,* with ulceration, *e)* dorsally in the middle part of the esophagus.

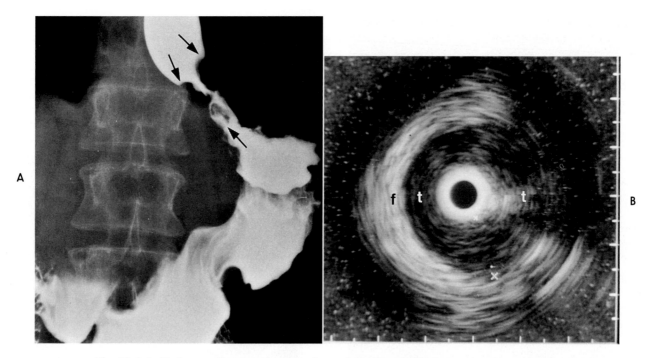

Fig. 12-6 A, Barium swallow reveals a stenotic esophageal carcinoma *(arrows)* at the esophago-gastric junction. **B,** Endoscopic ultrasound image obtained with a catheter echoprobe shows a circular hypoechoic transmural esophageal carcinoma *(t)* with deep penetration *(x)* into the adventitia and periesophageal fat tissue *(f).* The findings are consistent with a T3 carcinoma.

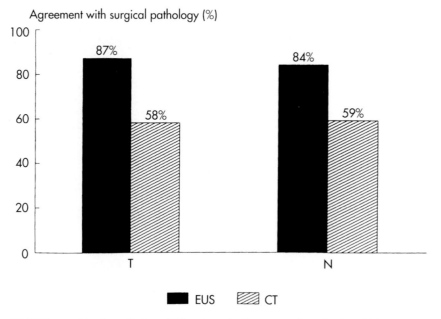

Fig. 12-7 The combined results from 297 patients in five reported studies in which computed tomography and endoscopic ultrasound were used to stage esophageal carcinoma.
From Lightdale CJ, Botet JF: *Gastrointest Endosc* 36(suppl):S11, 1990.

The incidence of lymph node metastasis in T1 carcinomas was 8%; T2 carcinomas, 54%; T3 carcinomas, 75%; and T4 carcinomas, 90%. The EUS findings correctly diagnosed lymph node metastasis in 100% of the T1, 100% of the T2, 92% of the T3, and 96% of the T4 carcinomas.

Fig. 12-7 shows the combined results from five studies that assessed the accuracy of EUS, compared to CT, in staging carcinoma.

ASSESSMENT OF RECURRENCE

Local recurrence of upper gastrointestinal cancer is a common problem, despite aggressive surgery. Lightdale and Botet[21] used EUS to assess 40 patients who had symptoms suggesting tumor recurrence following resection of esophageal or gastric cancer. The results were impressive. EUS results correctly diagnosed recurrent cancer in 23 of 24 patients, based on the finding of a nodular hypoechoic anastomotic thickening. Absence of recurrence was correctly diagnosed in 13 of 16. Thus, its sensitivity for diagnosing recurrence was 95%, the specificity was 80%, the positive predictive accuracy was 88%, and the negative predictive accuracy was 92% in this symptomatic group of patients with a high incidence of recurrence.

In this same report, the results of endoscopy with biopsy and brush cytology were negative in 6 of 23 patients, and CT scans were not useful for detecting anastomotic recurrence, although it was far superior for detecting distant metastases to the lung, liver, and peritoneum. These results suggest that EUS may be the method of choice for detecting anastomotic recurrence of gastrointestinal cancers.

SUBMUCOSAL LESION ASSESSMENT

Tumors of smooth muscle are usually suspected because of a bulge covered with normal mucosa that is found endoscopically or radiographically. However, this may represent only the tip of the underlying disease.[22,23] EUS improves the detection, diagnosis, and staging of submucosal abnormalities because of its ability to image the gastrointestinal wall structures. The most common submucosal abnormalities are leiomyomas, lipomas, leiomyosarcomas, leiomyoblastomas, carcinoid metastases, esophageal or periesophageal varices, and periesophageal metastases arising from breast or gastroesophageal cancers, or lung cancers that have penetrated directly into the submucosa of the esophagus.

Leiomyoma versus leiomyosarcoma, leiomyoblastoma, and other nonepithelial malignancies

The criteria for identifying a leiomyoma are either the local thickening of the muscularis propria or the presence of a hypoechoic homogeneous mass possessing sharply demarcated boundaries (Fig. 12-8). The overlying mucosa is often normal. Occasionally, a central ulcer or blood vessel is found within the mass, particularly when the tumor ex-

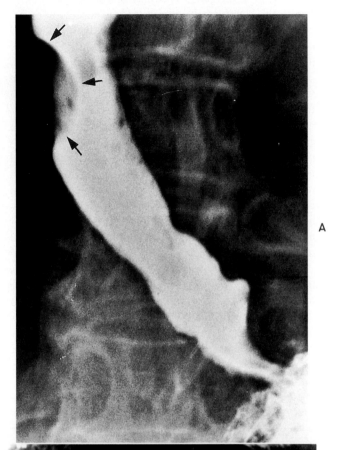

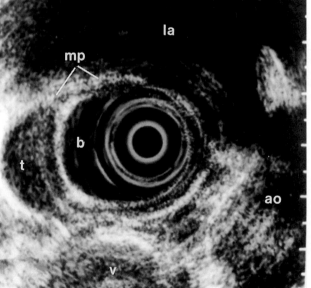

Fig. 12-8 A, Barium swallow reveals a right lateral bulging lesion covered with smooth mucosa in the middle third of the esophagus *(arrows).* **B,** Endoscopic ultrasound reveals a hypoechoic homogeneous tumor with clearly defined boundaries located in the submucosa *(t).* Note the tumor is continuous with the muscularis propria *(mp),* a finding compatible with a local muscular thickening. The findings suggest the existence of a leiomyoma. *b,* Balloon; *la,* left atrium; *ao,* aorta; *v,* vertebra.

ceeds 4 cm in diameter. This may be caused by a reduction in the blood supply, which leads to ulceration or necrosis within the tumor. The mass may exhibit inhomogeneity because of the variety of tissues within it. This may mimic the presence of a malignancy on EUS.

Occasionally, multiple leiomyomas are found, which are similar in appearance to that of uterine myomatosis. A diffuse hypoechoic pattern in the second layer of the esophagus may represent thickening of the muscularis mucosae and is compatible with the presence of myomatosis. A lipoma appears as a hyperechoic (echogenic) circumscribed or large area with an echo pattern similar to that of the periesophageal adventitia, and this area is clearly more echogenic than the muscularis propria. Submucosal carcinoid resembles a leiomyoma in location, size, and echogenicity. EUS-guided cytologic sampling is recommended to rule out or confirm malignancy.

Leiomyosarcomas or leiomyoblastomas are visualized as inhomogeneous masses with either sharply demarcated or irregular margins. The invasion of a hypoechoic tumor into the surrounding structures is highly indicative of malignancy. Occasionally, a fistula penetrates into adjacent structures such as the tracheobronchial tree. Although the tumor size and the occurrence of gross necrosis or fistulization can strongly imply the existence of malignancy, only the biologic behavior of the process actually defines true malignancy in these submucosal tumors. Supplementary findings such as invasion into surrounding structures or the presence of suspicious lymph nodes are helpful for identifying the malignant nature of the disease.[23,24]

An adjacent lung carcinoma may invade the esophageal submucosa and may simulate a leiomyoma in endoscopic studies. EUS-guided cytologic sampling may be helpful in establishing the diagnosis.

EVALUATION OF THE MEDIASTINUM

Transesophageal ultrasound permits clear imaging of the mediastinum and its adjacent structures. The most common lesions are bronchogenic cysts, lymph node enlargement due to sarcoidosis or metastases, aortic aneurysm, and submucosal infiltration by bronchogenic carcinoma. A bronchogenic cyst is imaged as a hypoechoic inhomogeneous or anechoic mass that is adjacent to the hyperechoic bronchus and esophagus. Bronchogenic lesions some distance from the esophagus cannot be imaged because of the limited depth of penetration allowed by the high-frequency ultrasonic beam employed with endoscopic ultrasound. Lymph node conglomerates are imaged as a hypoechoic, clearly demarcated mass next to the esophagus and left atrium. The diameter of lymph nodes can vary between 5 and 40 mm. Paraaortic and paravertebral lymph nodes are often found. Enlarged lymph nodes from inflammatory causes or sarcoidosis may occasionally mimic malignancy. In such cases, EUS-guided cytologic puncture may be helpful in ruling out a malignant disease.

An aortic aneurysm may compress the distal part of the esophagus and simulate the presence of achalasia on a barium swallow.[17] EUS can visualize a dissected aneurysm as an extensive dilated aortic lumen with spontaneous contrast (turbulent bloodstream) and calcification of the aortic wall. The real-time property of EUS allows the clear imaging of blood flow and the distinction between a solid tumor mass and a vascular abnormality or a cystic lesion. In such special cases, duplex sonography is very helpful for imaging the pseudolumen and its abnormal blood flow, and a distinction between achalasia and pseudoachalasia due to a periesophageal tumor mass can be readily made.[11,25,26]

Bronchogenic carcinoma presents the image of a hypoechoic inhomogeneous mass adjacent to the bronchus. The tumor is usually unilateral and compresses or penetrates into the adjacent structures or even the esophagus. Periesophageal lymph node involvement can be clearly imaged with EUS because of its proximity to the target of interest, often more easily than with CT. Moreover, submucosal infiltration of the esophagus can only be detected with EUS because of its ability to image the individual layers of the esophageal wall. To establish the diagnosis, EUS-guided cytologic puncture may occasionally be helpful.

CONCLUSIONS

EUS is now the most reliable imaging technique for the staging of esophageal carcinomas because of its ability to assess the depth of tumor infiltration and lymph node metastases. However, for staging distant metastases, particularly liver metastases, transcutaneous ultrasound or CT, or both methods, are also necessary because the right lobe of the liver cannot be completely examined with EUS. In patients with a severe stenotic carcinoma, CT may also be more helpful. A small-caliber instrument with forward-viewing optics is likely to become popular for the purposes of passing a severe stenosis. A catheter echoprobe will probably become a valuable diagnostic tool that will complement routine endoscopic investigation in the staging of tumor and lymph node metastases. In this manner, endoscopy and EUS can be performed in one session, and, in many cases, will allow the treatment strategy to be planned immediately after the diagnosis is ascertained.

For example, it is important to identify the presence of celiac lymph node metastases so that the surgeon can plan the surgical strategy. If EUS reveals possible lymph node metastasis, abdominal exploration can then be performed before thoracotomy to permit histologic confirmation in advance. There are still limitations to EUS, however. Supraclavicular lymph node metastases due to distal esophageal or cardia carcinoma can be better assessed with CT and transcutaneous ultrasound, and fine-needle aspiration cytology can be performed with transcutaneous guided ultrasound.[27]

With regard to treatment, combined intraluminal irradiation and external radiotherapy may become an alternative treatment for inoperable carcinomas regardless of the presence of T4 cancer.[28] Early stage carcinomas will be treated surgically whenever possible. In high-risk patients, however, endoscopically guided laser-photocoagulation can be performed. Intermediate stage carcinomas will likely still be treated surgically when there are no contraindications. Palliative treatment, consisting of the insertion of an esophageal endoprosthesis, or of endoscopic laser- or thermocoagulation, can be performed when indicated.

Clearly, the management of esophageal cancer is considerably influenced by the stage of the disease, and, for this reason, EUS is likely to become a standard tool in the preoperative, as well as the follow-up, assessment of patients with esophageal malignancy.

REFERENCES

1. Lutz HW, Rosch W: Transgastroscopic ultrasonography, *Endoscopy* 8:203, 1976.
2. Hisanaga K, Hisanaga A: A new real-time sector scanning system of ultra-wide angle and real-time recording to entire cardiac images: transesophagus and transchest methods, *Ultrasound Med* 4:391, 1978.
3. Hisanaga K, Hisanaga A, Hibi N: Highspeed rotating scanner for transesophageal cross-sectional echocardiography, *Am J Cardiol* 41:832, 1980.
4. DiMagno EP, Buxton JL, Regan PT et al: The ultrasonic endoscope, *Lancet* 1:629, 1980.
5. DiMagno EP, Regan PT, Clain JE, James EM, Buxton JL: Human endoscopic ultrasonography, *Gastroenterology* 83:824, 1982.
6. Strohm WD, Phillip F, Hagenmuller F, Classen M: Ultrasonic tomography by means of an ultrasonic fiberendoscope, *Endoscopy* 12:241, 1980.
7. Lux G, Heyder N, Lutz H, Demling L: Endoscopic ultrasonography—technique, orientation, and diagnostic possibilities, *Endoscopy* 14:220, 1982.
8. Tio TL, Tytgat GNJ: Endoscopic ultrasonography in the assessment of intra- and transmural infiltration of tumors in the esophagus, stomach and papilla of Vater and extraesophageal lesions, *Endoscopy* 16:203, 1984.
9. Tio TL, Tytgat GNJ: Endoscopic ultrasonography, *Scand J Gastroenterol* 21(suppl 123):27, 1986.
10. Aibe T, Fuji T, Okita K, Takemoto T: A fundamental study of normal layer structure of the gastrointestinal wall visualized by endoscopic ultrasonography, *Scand J Gastroenterol* 21(suppl 123):6, 1986.
11. Tio TL, Tytgat GNJ: *Atlas of transintestinal ultrasonography*, Aalsmeer, 1986, Mur-Kostverloren.
12. Tio TL: *Endosonography in gastroenterology*, New York, 1988, Springer.
13. Murata Y, Muroi M, Yoshida M, Ide H, Hanyo F: Endoscopic ultrasonography in the diagnosis of esophageal carcinoma, *Surg Endosc* 1:11, 1987.
14. Yasuda K, Kiyota K, Nakayima M, Kawai K: Fundamentals of endoscopic laser therapy for GI tumours: new aspects with endoscopic ultrasonography (EUS), *Endoscopy* 19:2, 1987.
15. Silva SA, Kouzo T, Ogino Y, Sato H: Endoscopic ultrasonography for esophageal tumors and compressions, *J Clin Ultrasound* 16:149, 1988.
16. Tio TL, Cohen P, Coene PPLO, Udding J, den Hartog Jager FCA et al: Endosonography and computed tomography of esophageal carcinoma: preoperative classification compared to the new (1987) TNM system, *Gastroenterology* 96:1478, 1989.
17. Tio TL, Tytgat GNJ: Endoscopic ultrasonography in the assessment of intra- and transmural infiltration of tumours in the oesophagus and papilla of Vater and in the detection of extra-oesophageal lesions, *Endoscopy* 16:203, 1984.
18. Tio TL, Tytgat GNJ: Endoscopic ultrasonography of normal and pathologic gastrointestinal wall structure: comparison of studies in vivo and in vitro with histology, *Scand J Gastroenterol* 21(suppl 123):27, 1986.
19. Kimmey MB, Martin RW, Haggitt RC, Wang KY, Franklin DW et al: Histologic correlates of gastrointestinal ultrasound images, *Gastroenterology* 96:433, 1989.
20. Tio TL, Tytgat GNJ: Endoscopic ultrasonography in analyzing periintestinal lymph node abnormality, *Scand J Gastroenterol* 21(suppl 123):158, 1986.
21. Lightdale CJ, Botet JF: Esophageal carcinoma: preoperative staging and evaluation of anastomotic recurrence, *Gastrointest Endosc* 36(suppl. 2):S11, 1990.
22. Tio TL, Coene PPLO, den Hartog Jager FCA, Tytgat GNJ: Preoperative TNM classification of esophageal carcinoma with endosonography, *Hepatogastroenterol* 27:376, 1990.
23. Tio TL, Tytgat GNJ, den Hartog Jager FCA: Endoscopic ultrasonography for the evaluation of smooth muscle tumors in the upper gastrointestinal tract: an experience with 42 cases, *Gastrointest Endosc* 36:342, 1990.
24. Yasuda K, Cho E, Nakayama M, Kawai K: Diagnosis of submucosal tumors of the upper gastrointestinal tract by endoscopic ultrasonography, *Gastrointest Endosc* 36:S17, 1990.
25. DeViere J, Dunham F, Rickaert F, Bourgeois N, Cremer M: Endoscopic ultrasonography in achalasia, *Gastroenterology* 96:1210, 1989.
26. Ziegler K, Sanft C, Friedrich M, Gregor M, Rieten O: Endosonographic appearance of the esophagus in achalasia, *Endoscopy* 22:1, 1990.
27. van Overhagen H, Lameris JS, Berger MY, van der Voorde F, Tilanus HW et al: Supraclavicular lymph node metastases in carcinoma of the esophagus and gastroesophageal junction: assessment with CT, US, and US-guided fine-needle aspiration biopsy, *Radiology* 179:155, 1991.
28. Tio LT, Blank LECM, Weijers OB, den Hartog Jager FCA, van Dyk JDP et al: Staging and prognosis using endosonography in patients with inoperable esophageal carcinoma treated with combined intraluminal and external irradiation, *Cancer* (submitted for publication).

13 CT and MR Staging of Tumors of the Esophagus and Gastroesophageal Junction and Detection of Postoperative Recurrence

LESLIE E. QUINT
ISAAC R. FRANCIS
GARY M. GLAZER
MARK B. ORRINGER

The esophagram is the radiologic method of choice for evaluating the esophageal mucosal surface and esophageal motility. However, because of their ability to directly image the esophageal wall and surrounding soft tissues, the tomographic imaging modalities, including computed tomography (CT) and magnetic resonance imaging (MRI), can provide complementary information.

COMPUTED TOMOGRAPHY

CT is often performed in patients with esophageal masses and is useful for defining the relationships between esophageal lesions and adjacent mediastinal structures. Usually the esophagus is well visualized by routine thoracoabdominal CT scans in which the heart and mediastinal vessels have been opacified through the bolus injection of intravenous contrast material. Occasionally, it is useful to administer an oral contrast agent such as dilute water-soluble contrast or barium, as this helps distend the esophagus and proximal stomach so that normal collapsed wall can be distinguished from thickening due to tumor. In addition, the contrast agent helps delineate the proximal border of an obstructing esophageal mass. An orally administered dilute barium paste adheres to the esophageal walls and demonstrates the location of the esophageal lumen.[1,2] This is sometimes helpful for delineating esophageal wall thickness and for determining whether a mediastinal mass is esophageal in origin.

The most common esophageal masses are carcinomatous, so most CT studies are focused on evaluating these tumors. However, CT is not the examination of choice when screening for esophageal cancer because endoscopy and barium studies are much more sensitive for detecting small esophageal tumors. In addition, conventional esophagography is more accurate for delineating both gastric tumor extension and the craniocaudal length of a tumor. In some cases, a

hiatus hernia may mimic a distal esophageal cancer on CT scans (Fig. 13-1); this distinction is usually obvious with barium esophagography. Despite these limitations, however, CT is potentially useful in evaluating known primary esophageal tumors.

Normal esophagus

The normal esophageal wall thickness is no more than about 3 mm, depending primarily on the degree of esophageal distention.[3,4] The esophagus is generally surrounded by mediastinal fat, except in extremely thin patients. However, this fat plane may be lost focally at several sites in normal patients, including regions where the esophagus contacts the left atrium, trachea, left mainstem bronchus, or aorta, particularly at the level of the gastroesophageal junction.

Esophageal carcinoma

The only CT finding with small esophageal carcinomas may be a focal or circumferential wall thickening, or the esophagus may appear normal. Tumor invasion through the muscle layer into the mediastinum may manifest as an abnormal soft tissue density in the mediastinal fat (Fig. 13-2). However, mediastinal tumor invasion is often microscopic in nature, and thus is not detected by CT. Loss of the fat plane between the aorta and the esophageal tumor has been used to predict aortic invasion. Picus et al.[5] reported that aortic invasion could be diagnosed with the help of CT if it showed that more than 90 degrees of the aortic circumference of this fat plane was obliterated. If less than 45 degrees was obliterating, this was presumed to indicate no aortic invasion; 45 to 90 degrees of involvement was considered an indeterminate finding (Figs. 13-3 and 13-4). Takashima et al.[6] have suggested that obliteration of the triangular fat space between the esophagus, aorta, and spine

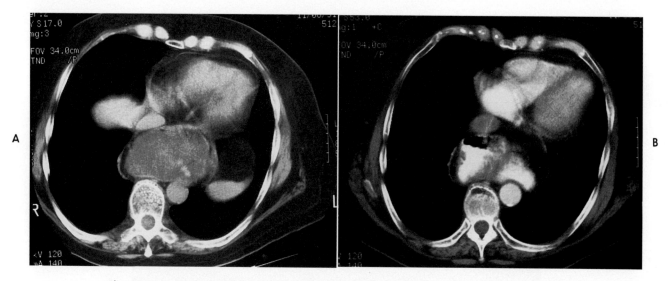

Fig. 13-1 A, Hiatus hernia simulating distal esophageal carcinoma. Presence of fat around the viscus suggests the correct diagnosis, confirmed by the administration of additional oral contrast material **(B).**

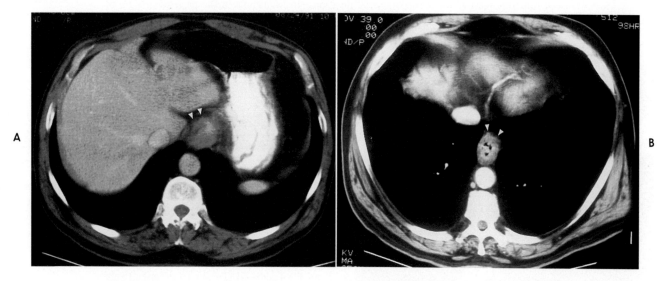

Fig. 13-2 Two cases of esophageal cancer showing circumferential wall thickening and extramural soft tissue stranding, suggestive of mediastinal fat invasion *(arrowheads)* (CT stage T3). At pathologic examination, the tumor was found to be limited to the esophageal wall in one case **(A)** but had spread into the extraesophageal fat in the other **(B).**

indicates aortic invasion. Tracheobronchial invasion may present as compression or displacement of the airway by tumor, or as thickening and irregularity of the tracheobronchial wall (Figs. 13-3 to 13-5). More specific signs of invasion include tracheoesophageal fistula[7] or the finding of tumor tissue within the lumen of the airway. Flattening of the posterior membranous portions of the trachea or mainstem bronchi does not necessarily represent tumor invasion because an adjacent mass effect alone can cause this finding (Fig. 13-5). Tumor spread to the pericardium may assume

the appearance of pericardial thickening, nodularity, and effusion. It is usually difficult to detect pleural tumor extension using CT.

CT staging of esophageal carcinoma
Primary tumor

There is controversy regarding the use of CT for staging esophageal cancer, as evidenced by the large number of studies published on the subject.[5,6,8-25] The majority of patients (59% to 90%)[15,18,21,22,24] present at surgery with T3

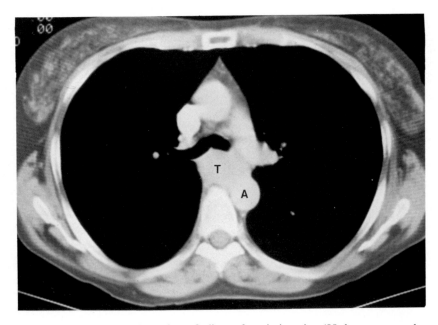

Fig. 13-3 CT scan showing indeterminate findings of aortic invasion (88-degree contact between the tumor *[T]* and the aorta *[A]*). Aortic invasion was found at surgery, confirming that the CT scan was truly positive for tracheobronchial invasion. Note flattening of the posterior margin of the left mainstem bronchus.

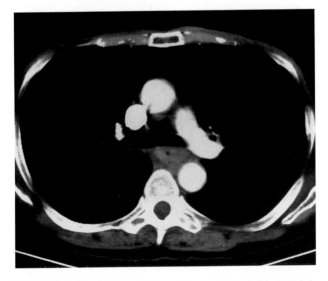

Fig. 13-4 False-positive CT scan for aortic invasion (slightly greater than a 90-degree contact between the tumor and the aorta). The scan was truly positive for invasion of the left mainstem bronchus.

□ **AMERICAN JOINT COMMITTEE TNM STAGING SYSTEM FOR ESOPHAGEAL CANCER** □

PRIMARY TUMOR (T)

TX: Primary tumor cannot be assessed
T0: No evidence of primary tumor
Tis: Carcinoma in situ
T1: Tumor invades lamina propria or submucosa
T2: Tumor invades muscularis propria
T3: Tumor invades adventitia
T4: Tumor invades adjacent structures

REGIONAL LYMPH NODES (N)

NX: Regional lymph nodes cannot be assessed
N0: No regional lymph node metastasis
N1: Regional lymph node metastasis

DISTANT METASTASIS (M)

MX: Presence of distant metastasis cannot be assessed
M0: No distant metastasis
M1: Distant metastasis

From Beahrs OH, Henson DE, Hutter RVP, Myers MH, eds: *Manual for staging of cancer*. American Joint Committee on Cancer, ed 3, Philadelphia, 1988, JB Lippincott.

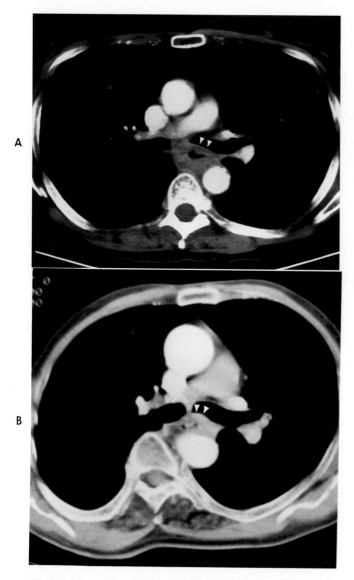

Fig. 13-5 Two different patients show a similar indentation of the left mainstem bronchus by esophageal tumor *(arrowheads),* suggesting tumor invasion. Invasion was surgically confirmed in **A** but absent in **B.** (**A** comes from the same patient as shown in Fig. 13-3.)

or T4 primary tumors (i.e., tumor extension through the wall into the mediastinal fat, with or without invasion into adjacent structures) (see box on p. 274).

The reported accuracy of CT for detecting extraluminal spread ranges from 55% to 100%,[5,8-14,21,22,24] with several of the more recent reports citing accuracies near the lower end of this range.[21,22,24,25] These lower accuracies reflect the difficulty in defining the outer esophageal margin, which is necessary for detecting extraluminal tumor extension (Fig. 13-2). This difficulty is compounded when the patient is cachectic and has little periesophageal fat. The accuracy of CT in detecting invasion of the tracheobronchial tree, although present in only 6% to 20% of proved

cases, has ranged from 74% to 100%.* Aortic invasion is even rarer; in one autopsy series, a 2% prevalence was noted.[26] Depending on the CT criteria used for diagnosing aortic invasion as well as the method of proof, the published CT accuracies range from 55% to 100%.† Using the criteria of Picus et al.[5] (already described), one study showed a CT sensitivity of 100%; however, its specificity was only 52% when indeterminate cases (45 to 90 degrees of involvement) were classified as false positives.[11]

Another source of difficulty in staging the primary tumor arises when patients have already undergone radiation therapy for their esophageal cancer. Radiation therapy often causes blurring of the esophageal-fat interface, in that soft tissue densities found extending into the mediastinal fat on CT scans may simulate tumor spread but actually represent only benign fibrotic tissue. Scans obtained after irradiation or chemotherapy has been carried out may reveal esophageal wall thickening suggesting residual tumor; however, in some cases, pathologic examination of the resected esophagus shows only benign ulceration, fibrosis, and hyperemia, with no residual viable tumor (Fig. 13-6).

Lymph nodes

Esophageal cancers typically spread regionally to paraesophageal and other mediastinal lymph nodes, and this results in nodal enlargement that can be detected by CT. In the cervical esophagus, regional lymph nodes are the cervical nodes, including the supraclavicular lymph nodes. In the thoracic esophagus, regional lymph nodes are mediastinal and perigastric lymph nodes, excluding the celiac nodes. Involvement of more distant nodes is considered distant metastasis. The normal short-axis diameters for the right and left paraesophageal lymph nodes measured on CT scans are reportedly 10 and 7 mm, respectively.[27] However, an esophageal carcinoma can be the source of microscopic metastases to otherwise normal-sized nodes, and, conversely, nodes may be enlarged due to benign causes. Pathologically proved tumor spread to regional lymph nodes has been reported to occur in 10% to 83% of cases.[5,9-13,22,24] The reported accuracy of CT in detecting regional nodal metastases ranges from 55% to 96%.‡ One factor contributing to the low accuracy encountered in some studies was the difficulty in distinguishing esophageal wall thickening from adjacent enlarged lymph nodes. Distant spread to abdominal nodes, occurring in 9% to 89% of reported cases, was diagnosed at CT with an accuracy of 39% to 85%.§ CT's low sensitivity in detecting regional or distant nodal disease, as encountered in several studies, may indicate that microscopic disease commonly occurs within normal-sized nodes.

*References 5,6,11,15,17,18.
†References 5,6,11,14,15,17,18.
‡References 5,9,11,12,17,19,22-24.
§References 5,8,10-15,17,18,22,23.

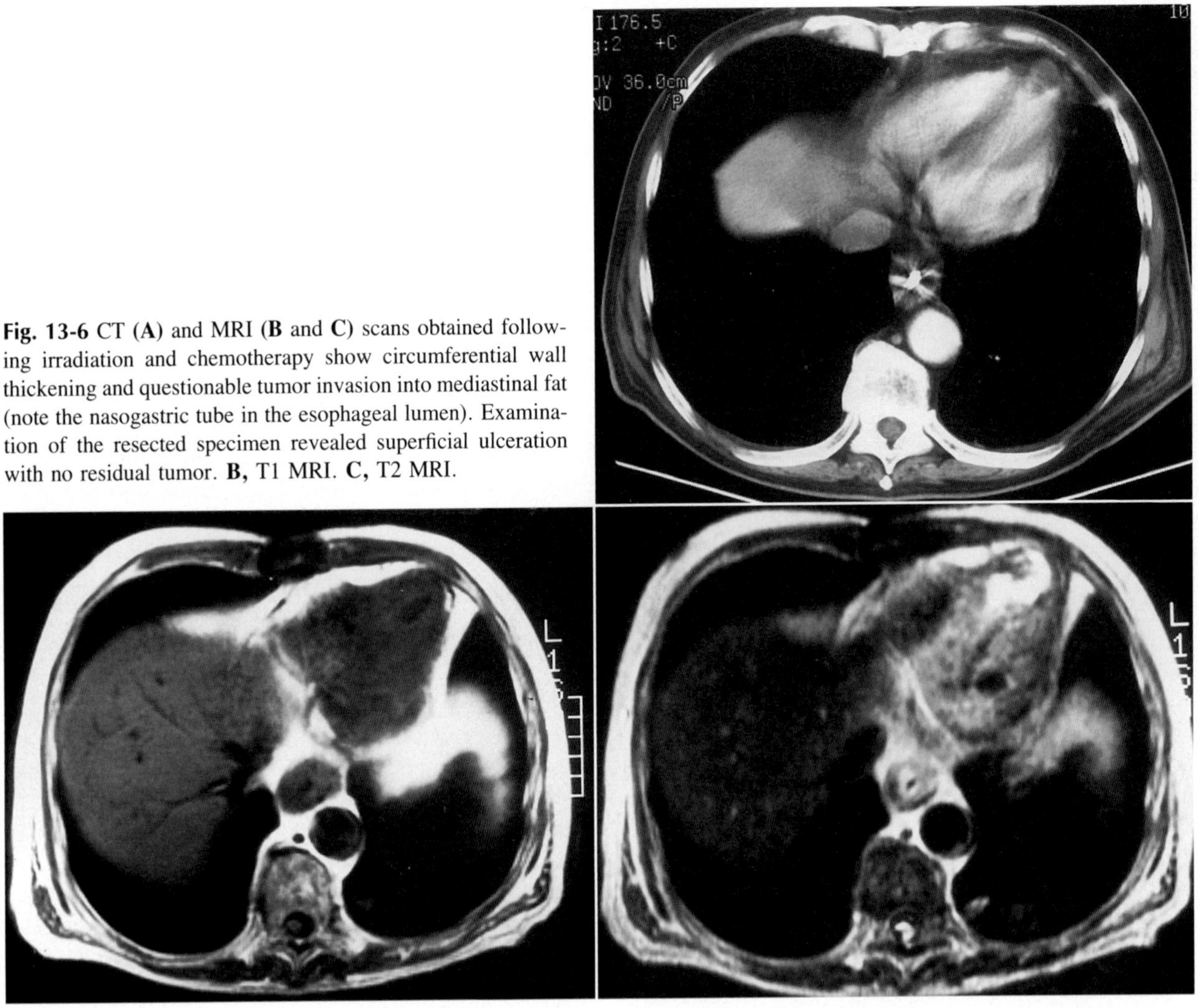

Fig. 13-6 CT (**A**) and MRI (**B** and **C**) scans obtained following irradiation and chemotherapy show circumferential wall thickening and questionable tumor invasion into mediastinal fat (note the nasogastric tube in the esophageal lumen). Examination of the resected specimen revealed superficial ulceration with no residual tumor. **B,** T1 MRI. **C,** T2 MRI.

Metastases

The prevalence of distant metastases at the time of patient presentation is low (range, 0%-12%).[5,8,10,12-14] However, the preoperative diagnosis of distant metastasis is important because its presence generally precludes palliative surgery, as the patient life expectancy is by then so short that major surgery is not really justified. It is generally agreed that CT is highly useful for detecting distant metastases, for example, to the liver, lung, kidneys, adrenals, or occasionally bone.

Overall staging

Not surprisingly, the reported accuracy of CT in the overall staging of esophageal tumors (for example, using the TNM system; Table 13-1) varies greatly, ranging from 39%[11] to 100%.[10] The reasons for these large discrepancies may include differing patient populations and the inclusion of relatively small numbers of patients in each series. Many of the studies lacked precise radiologic, surgical, or pathologic correlation, and thus lacked complete proof of the CT findings. In addition, there were no uni-

form criteria for defining tumor invasion in either CT or surgical terms. Findings were also reported in different fashions and different staging systems were used, thus making it difficult to compare results between the various studies. In several studies, the accuracy of CT in staging the tumor was low because of the difficulty in diagnosing metastases to lymph nodes, particularly in the left gastric and celiac regions.[15,17,18,22] A major factor contributing to the low CT accuracy in other studies was the inability to correctly identify extraluminal spread of tumor into mediastinal fat and adjacent structures.[11,12,18,24] This is an important finding because a large proportion of patients present with it. It has been suggested that CT is significantly more accurate in assessing midesophageal (squamous cell) cancers than in evaluating distal esophageal or gastroesophageal junction adenocarcinomas[14,15]; however, this view is not unanimously held.[18]

Predicting resectability

Most patients with esophageal carcinoma undergo esophagectomy for the palliation of symptoms rather than for cure. However, the exact type of surgical intervention varies among institutions, and thus the surgical criteria for tumor resectability vary. Many surgeons now perform transhiatal esophagectomy without thoracotomy, using a cervical esophagogastric anastomosis. This approach is associated with a much lower morbidity and mortality as compared with conventional esophagectomy via thoracotomy, because it does not make use of a thoracotomy and thus the potential for mediastinitis arising from intrathoracic esophageal anastomotic disruption is eliminated. This procedure entails transhiatal dissection of the esophagus from the mediastinum via cervical and upper abdominal incisions, followed by gastric or colonic interposition.[28] The few contraindications to the performance of blunt esophagectomy primarily consist of aortic or tracheobronchial tumor invasion or dense mediastinal adhesions. Because the prevalence of these features is low, an imaging modality must have a high sensitivity to be efficacious in this setting. Perhaps more importantly, high specificity is needed so that a patient is not denied a palliative and potentially curative operation on false grounds. A University of Michigan study consisting of 33 patients with esophageal carcinoma revealed only a 50% specificity and 55% accuracy in the CT prediction of resectability, yet 91% of the cases proved resectable by transhiatal esophagectomy.[11] At that institution, transhiatal esophagectomy proved possible in 99% of the 395 patients with carcinoma of the intrathoracic esophagus who underwent the procedure.[29] Lehr et al.[18] found that CT was only 63% accurate in diagnosing aortic invasion and 74% accurate in detecting tracheobronchial invasion. The results of these studies therefore suggest that CT is of limited usefulness in the assessment of primary tumor resectability before transhiatal esophagectomy. Takashima et al.[6] cites a higher (84%) CT accuracy in the prediction of resectability, with a 19% prevalence of confirmed aortic or tracheobronchial invasion. Yet, because of multiple false-positive assessments indicating aortic invasion, the specificity was only 80% in this study. A positive CT finding of tracheobronchial invasion can often be confirmed by bronchoscopy before esophagectomy is undertaken, thus avoiding the performance of unnecessary surgery. However, a CT finding of aortic invasion can, in general, only be proved at surgery. It remains to be seen whether newer techniques, such as transesophageal or intravascular transaortic ultrasonography, are more accurate in the preoperative prediction of aortic invasion.

Currently CT is recommended in the preoperative evaluation of all patients with newly diagnosed esophageal cancer so that conditions that would preclude the performance of esophagectomy can be identified. These conditions include tracheobronchial invasion or evidence of metastatic disease to distant lymph nodes or organs. If the biopsy findings are positive under any of these conditions, this would constitute sufficient evidence of inoperability; many of these lesions can be successfully biopsied under CT or ultrasound guidance (Fig. 13-7). However, if the CT find-

□ **TABLE 13-1**

Stage grouping in the TNM system

Stage	Tumor	Node	Metastasis
0	Tis	N0	M0
I	T1	N0	M0
IIA	T2	N0	M0
	T3	N0	M0
IIB	T1	N1	M0
	T2	N1	M0
III	T3	N1	M0
	T4	N1	M0
IV	Any T	Any N	M1

From Beahrs OH, Henson DE, Hutter RVP, Meyers MH, eds: *Manual for staging of cancer. American Joint Committee on Cancer,* ed 3, Philadelphia, 1988, JB Lippincott.

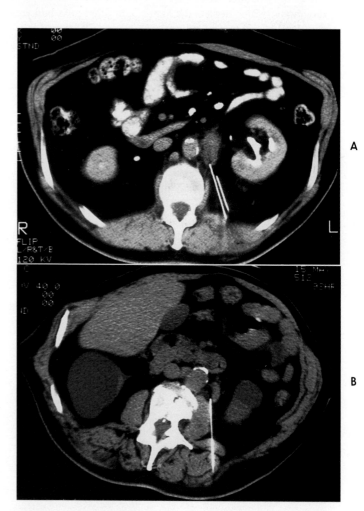

Fig. 13-7 Two patients with newly diagnosed adenocarcinoma of the esophagus and distant abdominal lymphadenopathy that was biopsied under CT guidance (patients prone; images reversed for viewing). The biopsy specimen in **A** showed metastatic adenocarcinoma, precluding esophagectomy. The CT aspiration biopsy in **B** yielded inconclusive findings; subsequent histologic examination of surgically resected thoracic and abdominal nodes showed lymphoma.

ings are positive but the biopsy results are not, this should not be used as a reason to deny the patient surgery.

Recurrent tumor

In contrast to its debatable usefulness in the preoperative assessment of esophageal carcinomas, CT has proved effective in identifying the existence of recurrent tumor after an esophagectomy and gastric pull-through operation[30-33] (Figs. 13-8 to 13-10). In one study, 22 of 35 patients (63%) exhibited evidence of tumor recurrence within 14 months of esophagectomy on routine, follow-up CT studies.[32] Slightly more than half of these patients were clinically asymptomatic at the time. Esophageal cancers tend to recur in the mediastinum outside the area where the intrathoracic stomach has been used for esophageal replacement, although intragastric recurrence or gastric wall invasion by extraluminal tumor is not rare.[33] Conventional barium radiography, which depicts the lumen, can often miss bulky, extraluminal, recurrent tumor[30]; however, CT scans can generally easily detect recurrent disease (Fig. 13-10). The site of the mediastinal recurrence does not necessarily correspond to the location of the primary esophageal lesion[33]; on the contrary, the tumor may recur anywhere throughout the mediastinum (Fig. 13-9), suggesting that the recurrence represents metastatic nodal disease rather than the interim growth of residual, microscopic, extraluminal primary tumor. Concurrent metastatic disease to distant sites is common, including distant lymph nodes (particularly abdominal or cervical), liver, lung, pleura, adrenals, and peritoneum.

Similar to the situation that prevails in the preoperative evaluation of esophageal carcinoma, the specificity of CT in detecting postoperative tumor recurrence is less than desirable.[33] The diagnosis of gastric wall thickening or extraluminal soft tissue mass adjacent to the intrathoracic stomach is often problematic, because incomplete gastric distention may simulate these findings. Patients with recurrent esophageal cancer are generally treated with chemotherapy or radiation therapy for palliative purposes, and tissue proof of CT findings is usually indicated so that unnecessary treatment can be avoided.

MAGNETIC RESONANCE IMAGING

There is little data on the application of magnetic resonance in the imaging of the esophagus.[6,18,34-38] Spin-echo MRI evaluation of the esophagus has been adversely impacted by the prolonged image acquisition times involved, as this results in considerable image blur due to biologic motion. Newer and faster MR image acquisition techniques, used in combination with orally and intravenously administered contrast agents, may considerably improve the effectiveness of MRI in esophageal imaging. In addition, the development of endoluminal surface coils should lead to the improved depiction of esophageal and periesophageal anatomy, including the more accurate assessment of the depth of tumor penetration through the esophageal wall and the better detection of paraesophageal lymph nodes. This endoluminal coil imaging, done in conjunction with phased-array coils, should result in even better signal-to-noise ratios and hence better resolution.

Most of the published studies using MRI have focused on the evaluation of esophageal cancer. In two different studies using spin-echo sequences and a body radiofrequency coil, MRI appeared to show no significant advan-

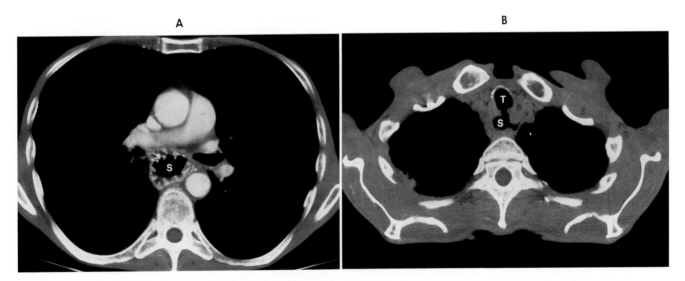

Fig. 13-8 A, Normal postoperative appearance following esophagectomy and a gastric pull-through operation. Note the good visualization of gastric folds in this patient. *S,* Stomach. **B,** Higher section in the same patient shows gastric wall thickening and a malignant fistula between the stomach *(S)* and the trachea *(T).*

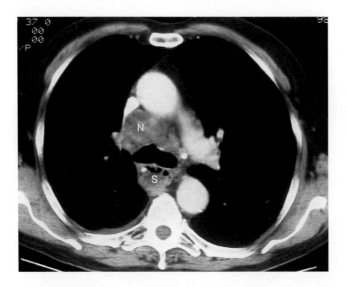

Fig. 13-9 Tumor recurrence in the right and left tracheobronchial lymph nodes *(N)* following esophagectomy and a gastric pull-through operation. The stomach *(S)* is poorly demonstrated because of incomplete distention.

Fig. 13-10 Extensive extraluminal tumor recurrence *(T)* in the upper abdominal lymph nodes following esophagectomy and a gastric pull-through procedure (arrow points to a duodenal gas bubble). Thoracentesis revealed no malignant cells in the large right pleural effusion.

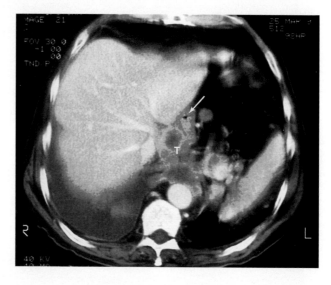

tages over CT in the staging of esophageal cancer.[6,34] Both imaging modalities were similarly weak in defining the anatomic extent of tumor, particularly with respect to invasion through the esophageal wall and into contiguous structures. In one study, MRI correctly detected wall invasion in only 40% of the patients[34] (see Figs. 13-6 and 13-11). An investigation conducted in normal subjects revealed that only 10% with a normal esophagus had a fat plane visible between the aorta and esophagus in all tomographic planes, and only 5% had a definite fat plane visible between the trachea and esophagus.[34] This implies that aortic and tracheobronchial invasion by esophageal cancer may be difficult to evaluate using current MRI technology. The findings from other studies have corroborated these conclusions, in that 13% to 29% of patients with esophageal carcinoma would have been denied surgery on the basis of false-positive MRI findings indicating aortic invasion.[6,18] On the other hand, Petrillo et al.[38] found more encourag-

ing results in their MRI study of 32 patients, all with squamous cell carcinoma of the esophagus. Invasion into the periesophageal fat was diagnosed with an 84% accuracy, and tracheobronchial and aortic invasion were detected with an accuracy of 87% and 91%, respectively.

The in vitro measurement of relaxation times (25 MHz at 25° C) in excised human esophageal tissue has shown significant differences in the T1 times between tumors and adjacent normal esophagus.[36] This suggests that MRI might be useful for accurately depicting tumor extent. However, a more recent in vitro investigation[35] has shown considerable overlap in the T1 times between tumor and adjacent histologically benign segments of esophagus (particularly in dysplastic areas), so it will probably prove unfeasible for MRI to precisely estimate tumor extent. In addition, the considerable variation in the T1 times associated with different esophageal cancers, or regions of a cancer, implies that the measurement of absolute relaxation times will prove

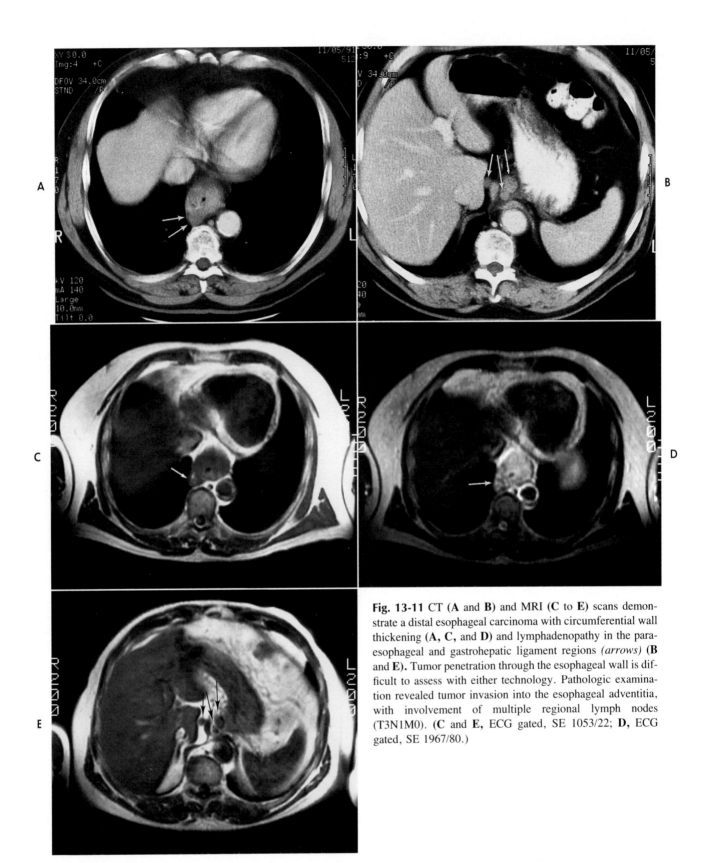

Fig. 13-11 CT (**A** and **B**) and MRI (**C** to **E**) scans demonstrate a distal esophageal carcinoma with circumferential wall thickening (**A, C,** and **D**) and lymphadenopathy in the paraesophageal and gastrohepatic ligament regions *(arrows)* (**B** and **E**). Tumor penetration through the esophageal wall is difficult to assess with either technology. Pathologic examination revealed tumor invasion into the esophageal adventitia, with involvement of multiple regional lymph nodes (T3N1M0). (**C** and **E**, ECG gated, SE 1053/22; **D**, ECG gated, SE 1967/80.)

of little value in the differential diagnosis of esophageal diseases. Instead, the value of MRI will more likely proceed from its ability to provide anatomic information.

As already mentioned, the advent of newer techniques may bring about considerable improvement in MRI's ability to assess the depth of tumor invasion into or through the esophageal wall and to detect regional lymph node involvement. In the event of such developments, MRI would then have a distinct advantage over CT scanning. Nevertheless, because of these weaknesses as well as the time-consuming nature and expense of the examination, MRI is not currently recommended as a routine preoperative imaging study in patients with esophageal cancer. MRI can instead be used for problem solving or as a guide to the planning of radiotherapy.[39] As the technology matures and as newer techniques become available, the role of MRI in esophageal imaging will need to be reassessed.

REFERENCES

1. Cayea PD, Seltzer SE: A new barium paste for computed tomography of the esophagus, *J Comput Assist Tomogr* 9:214, 1985.
2. Conces DJ Jr, Tarver RD, Lappas JC: The value of opacification of the esophagus by low density barium paste in computer tomography of the thorax, *J Comput Assist Tomogr* 12:202, 1988.
3. Reinig JW, Stanley JH, Schabel SI: CT evaluation of thickened esophageal walls, *AJR* 140:931, 1983.
4. Halber MD, Daffner RH, Thompson WM: CT of the esophagus: I. Normal appearance, *AJR* 133:1047, 1979.
5. Picus D et al: Computed tomography in the staging of esophageal carcinoma, *Radiology* 146:433, 1983.
6. Takashima S et al: Carcinoma of the esophagus: CT vs. MR imaging in determining resectability, *AJR* 156:297, 1991.
7. Vaid YN, Shin MS: Computed tomography evaluation of tracheoesophageal fistula, *CT* 10:281, 1986.
8. Daffner RH et al: CT of the esophagus: II. Carcinoma, *AJR* 133:1051, 1979.
9. Freeny PC, Marks WM: Adenocarcinoma of the gastroesophageal junction: barium and CT examination, *AJR* 138:1077, 1982.
10. Moss AA et al: Esophageal carcinoma: pretherapy staging by computed tomography, *AJR* 136:1051, 1981.
11. Quint LE et al: Esophageal carcinoma: CT findings, *Radiology* 155:171, 1985.
12. Samuelsson L et al: CT staging of oesophageal carcinoma, *Acta Radiol Diagn* (Stockh) 25:7, 1984.
13. Terrier F, Schapira CL, Fuchs WA: CT assessment of operability in carcinoma of the oesophagogastric junction, *Eur J Radiol* 4:114, 1984.
14. Thompson WM et al: Computed tomography for staging esophageal and gastroesophageal cancer: reevaluation, *AJR* 141:951, 1983.
15. Becker CD, Barbier P, Porcellini B: CT evaluation of patients undergoing transhiatal esophagectomy for cancer, *J Comput Assist Tomogr* 10:607, 1986.
16. Halvorsen RA Jr et al: Esophageal cancer staging by CT: long-term follow-up study, *Radiology* 161:147, 1986.
17. Lea JW IV, Prager RL, Bender HW Jr: The questionable role of computed tomography in preoperative staging of esophageal cancer, *Ann Thorac Surg* 38:479, 1984.
18. Lehr L, Rupp N, Siewert JR: Assessment of resectability of esophageal cancer by computed tomography and magnetic resonance imaging, *Surgery* 103:344, 1988.
19. Vilgrain V et al: Staging of esophageal carcinoma: comparison of results with endoscopic sonography and CT, *AJR* 155:277, 1990.
20. Rasch L, Brenoe J, Olesen KP: Predictability of esophagus and cardia tumor resectability by preoperative computed tomography, *Eur J Radiol* 11:42, 1990.
21. Lefor AT et al: Computerized tomographic prediction of extraluminal spread and prognostic implications of lesion width in esophageal carcinoma, *Cancer* 62:1287, 1988.
22. Tio TL et al: Endosonography and computed tomography of esophageal carcinoma: preoperative classification compared to the new (1987) TNM system, *Gastroenterology* 96:1478, 1989.
23. Kirk SJ et al: Does preoperative computed tomography scanning aid assessment of oesophageal carcinoma? *Postgrad Med J* 66:191, 1990.
24. Botet JF et al: Preoperative staging of esophageal cancer: comparison of endoscopic US and dynamic CT, *Radiology* 181:419, 1991.
25. Sharma OP, Subnani S: Role of computerized tomography imaging in staging oesophageal carcinoma, *Semin Surg Oncol* 5:355, 1989.
26. Postlethwait R: *Surgery of the esophagus*, ed 2, East Norwalk, Conn, 1985, Appleton-Lange.
27. Glazer GM et al: Normal mediastinal lymph nodes: number and size according to American Thoracic Society mapping, *AJR* 144:261, 1985.
28. Orringer MB: Transhiatal esophagectomy without thoracotomy for carcinoma of the thoracic esophagus, *Ann Surg* 200:282, 1984.
29. Orringer MB, Sterling MC: Transhiatal esophagectomy for benign and malignant disease of the intrathoracic esophagus, *J Thorac Cardiovasc Surg* 105:267, 1993.
30. Gross BH et al: Gastric interposition following transhiatal esophagectomy: CT evaluation, *Radiology* 155:177, 1985.
31. Heiken JP, Balfe DM, Roper CL: CT evaluation after esophagogastrectomy, *AJR* 143:555, 1984.
32. Becker CD et al: Patterns of recurrence of esophageal carcinoma after transhiatal esophagectomy and gastric interposition, *AJR* 148:273, 1987.
33. Carlisle JG et al: CT evaluation of esophageal carcinoma recurrence following transhiatal esophagectomy, Presented at the Annual Meeting of the American Roentgen Ray Society, May 1991, Boston, Massachusetts.
34. Quint LE, Glazer GM, Orringer MB: Esophageal imaging by MR and CT: study of normal anatomy and neoplasms, *Radiology* 156:727, 1985.
35. Ranade SS et al: Significance of histopathology in pulsed NMR studies on cancer, *Magn Reson Med* 2:128, 1985.
36. Shah SS et al: Significance of water proton spin-lattice relaxation times in normal and malignant tissues and their subcellular fractions, *Magn Reson Imaging* 1:91, 1982.
37. Smith FW et al: Oesophageal carcinoma demonstrated by whole body nuclear magnetic resonance imaging, *Br Med J* 282:510, 1981.
38. Petrillo R et al: Esophageal squamous cell carcinoma: MRI evaluation of mediastinum, *Gastrointest Radiol* 15:275, 1990.
39. Poon PY et al: Magnetic resonance imaging of the mediastinum, *J Can Assoc Radiol* 37:173, 1986.

PART V

STOMACH AND DUODENUM

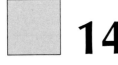

14 *Normal Anatomy and Techniques of Examination of the Stomach and Duodenum*

K. M. HARRIS
G. M. ROBERTS
B. W. LAWRIE

RADIOLOGIC ANATOMY OF THE STOMACH AND DUODENUM

Stomach

The position, shape, and size of the stomach are variable. The stomach is usually a vertically oriented J-shaped structure, particularly in slender individuals. In muscular or obese individuals, it often lies more horizontally.

The radiologic anatomy is similar to that described in standard texts of anatomy. The region of the gastroesophageal junction is termed the *cardia*. The part of the stomach lying above the cardia, which is filled with gas in the erect position, is called the *fundus*. An imaginary line transecting the stomach from the incisura (gastric angulus) on the lesser curve to the greater curve opposite further divides the stomach into the body proximally and the antrum distally. The antrum is then bounded distally by the pylorus, which is continuous with the duodenum.

The stomach lies within the peritoneal cavity; its anterior wall is in contact with the diaphragm above and the anterior abdominal wall below. The fundus lies more posteriorly and is in contact with the dome of the left hemidiaphragm. The lesser (gastrohepatic) omentum attaches the lesser curve of the stomach to the liver. The greater omentum attaches to the convexity of the greater curve of the stomach. The transverse colon is therefore related to the greater curve and may produce a direct impression on the stomach. In a similar fashion, the spleen, which is attached by the gastrosplenic component of the greater omentum, is related to the fundus of the stomach and often produces a characteristic impression. The posterior wall of the stomach forms the anterior wall of the lesser sac (omental bursa) and is therefore intimately related to the pancreas posteriorly.

Knowledge of this three-dimensional anatomy is necessary for the successful performance of a contrast-enhanced examination of the stomach. Correct patient positioning and abdominal compression can then both be used to maximal advantage.

The luminal surface of the stomach has characteristic mucosal folds, or gastric rugae (Fig. 14-1). These are more prominent in the body and fundus, running parallel to the long axis of the stomach and usually measuring between 3 and 5 mm in thickness. In the presence of gastric overdistention, particularly in association with a gastroparetic agent such as glucagon or hyoscine-*N*-butyl bromide (Buscopan; Boehringer Ingelheim), most of these rugae become much less prominent and may even disappear, although those along the greater curve usually persist even with marked distention. Smaller longitudinally oriented folds are seen in the antrum leading up to the thin parallel folds within the pylorus. Multiple fine transverse folds have also been described in the gastric antrum (Fig. 14-2). If present, they persist when the gastric antrum is distended or partially collapsed, and also during peristalsis. They were originally thought to be of no clinical significance,[1] but, more recently, an association between persistent transverse folds and gastritis has been suggested.[2]

The gastric folds in the region of the fundus and cardia have a characteristic pattern. The normal appearance of this region as seen during double-contrast barium examinations has been well described.[3,4] With adequate distention of the stomach, the cardia, when viewed en face, appears as a central fleck of barium with radiating folds, known as the *esophageal rosette*.[3] Several of these folds course for a longer distance along the lesser curvature, and this appearance may mimic ulceration. Normal gastric folds are smooth and regular, and distortion of this pattern should be regarded as a pathologic finding. The normal cardia may appear protuberant and present as a filling defect measuring some 1 to 2 cm in diameter, simulating a tumor.[5] (Fig. 14-3).

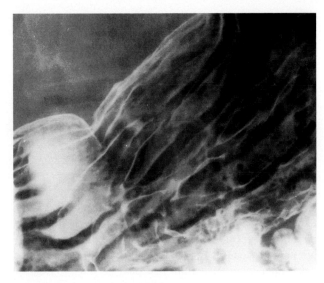

Fig. 14-1 Normal gastric rugae. Note that the folds on the anterior (nondependent) wall appear as "tramlines."

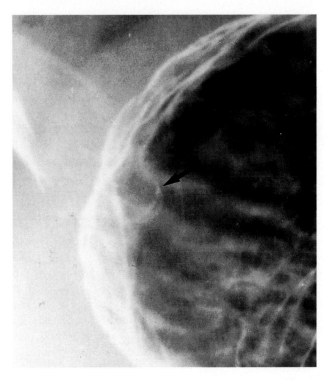

Fig. 14-3 Normal gastroesophageal junction producing the appearance of a pseudotumor *(arrow)*.

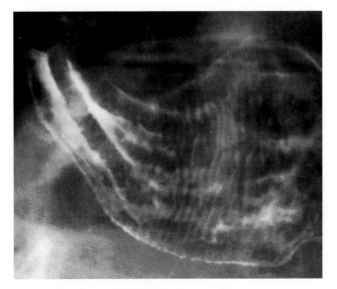

Fig. 14-2 Transverse folds in the gastric antrum.

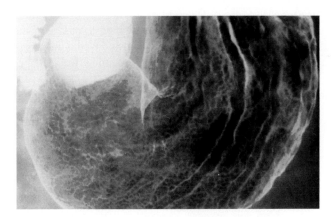

Fig. 14-4 Areae gastricae.

The pylorus, when viewed en face, may also appear as a central collection of barium, and, here again, failure to recognize the normal appearance may lead to the erroneous diagnosis of ulceration.

The micromucosal pattern of the stomach consists of a mosaic of tiny raised nodules with intervening grooves, known as the *areae gastricae* (Fig. 14-4). Their normal histologic appearance is well recognized and correlates well with that seen during double-contrast examination of the stomach.[6] The areae gastricae do not usually exceed 3 mm in diameter and, unlike the gastric rugae, they are visible in both the distended and nondistended states. They are seen most clearly in the antrum but may also extend and be visible throughout the stomach, including the fundus. Their visualization depends on several factors, in particular the density and viscosity of the barium suspension used.

A high-density (250% weight per volume [w/v]) Low-viscosity barium suspension has been shown to demonstrate the areae gastricae or similar fine nodular patterns to best advantage.[7] Another factor shown to affect their demonstration is the thickness of the mucus layer covering the mucosa.[6,8] A thick layer will fill the intervening grooves, and, as the barium suspension is unable to penetrate this layer, a double-contrast meal will fail to show the areae gastricae and the mucosal surface will appear smooth. Gastric mucus is an important factor in the pathogenesis of peptic ulceration, and the correlation between the presence of large areae gastricae and duodenal ulceration can be explained on this basis.[8]

Duodenum

Anatomically the duodenum is the first part of the small intestine but is considered separately by radiologists, as it is usually examined at the same time as the stomach during a barium meal.

The duodenum constitutes the shortest and widest part of the small intestine and, as most of it is retroperitoneal, it is also the most fixed and immobile part.

The duodenum is a C-shaped tube with its concavity facing left. This configuration allows it to be divided into four segments, each having a different orientation. The first part begins at the pylorus and runs superiorly, backward, and to the right. The first 2 cm or so lies invested in the peritoneal folds of the lesser and greater omenta and is therefore relatively mobile. This part is known as the *duodenal cap* or *bulb*. The second, or descending, portion passes downward along the posterior abdominal wall and is covered in front by the peritoneum. It is intimately related posteriorly to the hilum of the right kidney and medially to the head of the pancreas. The third part of the duodenum curves forward from the right paravertebral gutter to pass over the inferior vena cava and aorta and is also covered anteriorly by the peritoneum of the posterior abdominal wall just below the base of the transverse mesocolon. It is crossed near its midpoint by the superior mesenteric vessels. The fourth part passes upward to the left of the aorta and loses its retroperitoneal attachment as it curves forward to the right at the duodenojejunal flexure. Now intraperitoneal, the small intestine continues as the jejunum, attached to the posterior abdominal wall by its mesentery. The duodenojejunal flexure is fixed by firm fibrous tissue known as the *ligament of Treitz*.

The mucosal pattern of the duodenum changes throughout its length.[9] The pear-shaped duodenal bulb has a variable mucosal surface pattern[10,11] (Fig. 14-5). Longitudinal parallel or spiral folds are often present. However, distention of the bulb during a double-contrast examination usually effaces these folds, and they are replaced by a smooth, featureless mucosal surface. Less commonly, a fine reticular mosaic appearance or a more stippled pattern is seen in normal individuals. This appearance has been attributed to small collections of barium that pool between normal but widely spaced villi and resembles the appearance of duodenal erosion.[11] In 6% to 10% of patients the polygonal filling defects of heterotopic gastric mucosa may be observed in the duodenal bulb and probably represent a normal finding. As in the stomach, demonstration of mucosal detail depends in part on the barium suspension used and also on the mucus surface layer of the duodenal mucosa.

In the second and third parts of the duodenum, there are well-developed transverse mucosal folds forming valvulae conniventes, which remain clearly visible even in the presence of distention. The second part of the duodenum is further characterized by the presence of mucosal folds in relation to the papilla of Vater. These landmarks have been described in detail by Ferrucci et al.[12] The papilla of Vater (major duodenal papilla) projects into the lumen on the medial wall of the second part of the duodenum (Fig. 14-6).

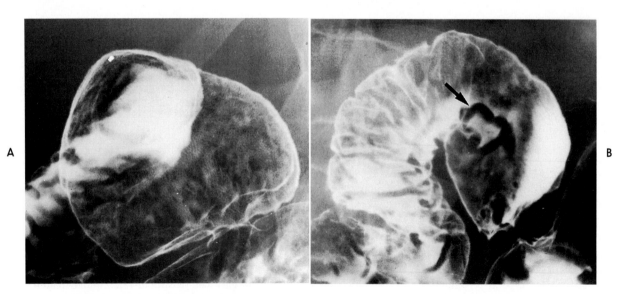

A

B

Fig. 14-5 A, Normal mucosa of the duodenal cap. **B,** Normal folds producing a flexural pseudolesion *(arrow)* in the duodenal cap.
Courtesy of Dr. K. C. Simpkins.

The exact site may vary, and rarely it is seen projecting into the third part.[13] It usually measures less than 1.5 cm in diameter, although normal papillae up to 3 cm in diameter have been described.[12] Through this, the common bile duct and major pancreatic duct (of Wirsung) open into the duodenum.

Three further landmarks have been identified in relation to the papilla—the promontory, the straight segment, and the longitudinal fold. The promontory is a shoulderlike projection of the medial duodenal wall with the major papilla normally situated on or just below it. The appearance of this promontory varies from a gradual slope to an abrupt step. For a few centimeters below this, the duodenal wall is normally rather flat and is termed the *straight segment*. This contrasts with the regular circular mucosal folds that project into the lumen along the lateral wall of the duodenum at the same level. The third landmark, the longitudinal fold, is a raised ridge of mucosa and submucosa that divides superiorly to enclose the major papilla and extends below this for a few centimeters. It runs parallel to the straight segment before dividing into smaller, less obvious ridges. It is uncommon to visualize all of these features in a single examination, but, when present, the major papilla and its associated folds, seen en face, resemble a tadpole.

The accessory papilla of Santorini (or minor papilla) is sometimes seen. It usually lies between 1 and 2 cm proximal and slightly anterior to the major papilla. Because of this relationship the two papillae are seldom seen together en face in the same projection. Its duct (of Santorini) is not usually patent. Although often smaller, its size can vary considerably, and it may even be as large as the major papilla.

NORMAL ANATOMIC VARIANTS AND INDENTATIONS THAT MAY SIMULATE DISEASE
Stomach

Normal anatomic variants of the stomach are uncommon. One such anomaly is the so-called cup-and-spill or cascade stomach. Here the fundus lies behind and below the more proximal part of the body of the stomach. In the normal stomach there is no clear demarcation between the body and fundus, but a distinct ridge is formed between the two in the cascade stomach. Its appearance varies with position and the degree of gastric distention. It is best demonstrated in the erect lateral position and disappears when the subject returns to the supine position. Gaseous distention of the distal transverse colon and splenic flexure is also thought to predispose to this deformity.[14] It should not be mistaken for the pathologic deformity caused by ulceration or tumor involvement of the proximal stomach. Similarly, an extragastric mass, such as a pancreatic pseudocyst or left adrenal mass, can produce such an appearance, but here the distortion persists even when the patient is supine.

When distended and hypotonic during the course of a double-contrast barium meal, the stomach may exhibit characteristic impressions imposed by neighboring structures and organs. The normal left lobe of the liver and the spleen may both produce impressions on the gastric fundus. Various deformities of the fundus have also been described in patients who have undergone splenectomy.[15] An impression either anteriorly on the wall of the body of the stomach or on the greater curve is sometimes seen and is due to prominent anterior left lower ribs, particularly in thin individuals. The normal transverse colon and splenic flexure may produce similar indentations on the greater curve of the stomach. The normal posterior retroperitoneal structures create a characteristic impression on the posterior wall of the stomach, again most noticeable in thin patients.

Duodenum

The anatomic relationships of the duodenum have been described. The normal gallbladder may cause a smooth indentation on the duodenal cap superiorly or even extending to the lateral wall of the descending duodenum. The second, or descending, part, being retroperitoneal, is closely related to the right kidney, which normally produces an impression on its lateral wall. The anatomic relationships between the duodenum and the transverse mesocolon are well described.[16] Fecal loading or even gaseous distention can rarely cause an indentation on the second part of the duodenum anterolaterally.[17] Although widening of the normal

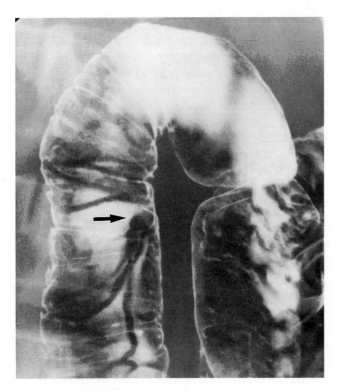

Fig. 14-6 Double-contrast view of duodenum showing arrangement of mucosal folds and major papillae *(arrow)*.
Courtesy of Dr. K. C. Simpkins.

duodenal loop has often been considered an indicator of an abnormal pancreatic mass, such widening may occasionally be seen in obese but otherwise normal individuals.[18] The superior mesenteric vessels cross the third part of the duodenum, and an indentation here is frequently seen. This feature has been confused with the appearances observed in the so-called superior mesenteric artery syndrome.[19]

Armed with prior knowledge and an understanding of the anatomic relationships of the stomach and duodenum, most of these indentations can, based on their characteristic sites and appearances, be reliably considered normal without recourse to further investigations.

BARIUM MEAL TECHNIQUE
Historical perspective

It was not long after the discovery of x rays by Roentgen in 1895 that the first attempts at radiographic examination of the gastrointestinal tract were made. Early experiments were performed on animals using a variety of radiopaque substances. However, many of these contrast agents proved to be toxic. Human studies were conducted shortly afterward, and, during the early 1900s, several contrast agents were tried. Of these, barium sulfate proved to be the safest and most palatable and has been in widespread use ever since.

The potential benefit of a double-contrast technique over these single-contrast studies was soon realized.[20] Ruzicka and Rigler[21] reported on a method of performing a double-contrast barium meal (DCBM) using nasogastric intubation. With the increasing use of endoscopy, it was discovered that small gastric lesions were often missed on conventional single-contrast studies. The higher incidence of gastric cancer in Japan fostered the more widespread use of the double-contrast technique, and, by the 1960s, this type of examination had become standard practice. The Western world, which was faced with a much lower incidence of gastric cancer, was a little slower to adopt these new methods. However, it soon became apparent that the technique was also applicable in the diagnosis of numerous other conditions, and, during the 1970s, the DCBM became an established routine procedure in the practice of medicine in the Western hemisphere.

Numerous modifications to the basic technique followed[22-27] hand-in-hand with improvements in the quality of the barium suspensions and effervescent agents, as well as the selective use of gastroparetic drugs.

Indications

Indications for a barium meal examination are many and varied. One of the most common symptoms prompting such an evaluation is epigastric pain suggestive of peptic ulceration. Others include anorexia, weight loss, vomiting, anemia, heartburn, and dysphagia.

With the advent of alternative imaging modalities, the advisability of performing a barium meal examination under certain circumstances has become questionable. Residual barium in the gastrointestinal tract can create considerable image artifacts on computed tomographic (CT) scans and, at worst, can render such an investigation meaningless. Similarly, as barium can also interfere with both upper gastrointestinal endoscopy and angiography, endoscopy should be the initial investigation in cases of upper gastrointestinal bleeding. This is particularly so because endoscopy is more accurate in localizing the source of bleeding.[28,29]

The referring clinician's request should indicate the suspected abnormality and detail any relevant history, in particular, where previous gastric surgery has been performed. A simple line drawing of the gastroenteric reconstruction is most helpful, as considerable time can be wasted attempting to identify anastomoses and loops that do not exist!

Contraindications

The harmful effects of barium within the peritoneal cavity are well recognized.[30-33] Examination of the upper gastrointestinal tract with barium in cases of suspected gastroduodenal perforation should therefore be avoided. Care should also be taken when there is a history or suspicion of aspiration, and use of an alternative contrast medium should be considered. Suitable alternatives for use in such circumstances are discussed later in the section on contrast media.

Patient preparation

The patient should not eat or drink for at least 6 hours before the examination. Patients who are undergoing a routine study during a morning session are usually told to fast overnight. There is some evidence that cigarette smoking may interfere with optimal barium coating of the mucosa, and patients should therefore probably refrain from smoking.[34,35] The radiologist should be informed at the initial request if the patient is diabetic, and an early morning appointment arranged to avoid prolonged starvation. There does not appear to be any difference in the gastric mucosal coating between DCBMs performed in the morning and those performed in the afternoon.[36] For an examination commencing at 2 PM, patients should fast starting at 8 AM following a light breakfast.

In patients with a clinically suspected gastric outlet obstruction, a preliminary plain abdominal radiograph may demonstrate a large gastric residue. In severe cases a prolonged fast or the intravenous administration of metoclopramide may be ineffective, making nasogastric intubation and aspiration of the contents necessary.

Attempts at improving the quality of the examination by the preliminary administration of metoclopramide, in the belief that it would reduce the volume of residual gastric juice and hence improve mucosal coating, have not proved successful.[37] Similarly, the use of cimetidine to reduce gastric secretion has proved to be of no benefit.[38,39] It would

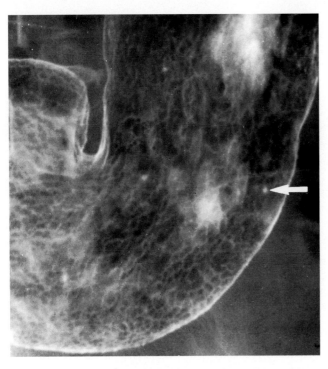

Fig. 14-7 Artifacts caused by barium particle aggregation *(arrow)*.

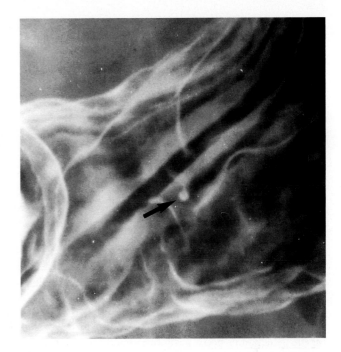

Fig. 14-8 Droplet of barium hanging from the anterior wall of the stomach, seen en face *(arrow)*—the stalactite phenomenon.

appear that mucosal coating depends more on the covering layer of mucus. The deleterious effects of mucus on various barium sulfate suspensions have been described.[40]

Contrast media

A wide range of readily available barium preparations exists for use in examinations of the upper gastrointestinal tract. Numerous studies have investigated the relative importance of the various physical properties of these barium suspensions and how they contribute to mucosal coating and hence the clarity of the mucosal detail.[7,41-43] In particular, the density, viscosity, and particle size have been assessed. The successful demonstration of the areae gastricae has often been deemed a suitable determinant of adequate mucosal coating. However, the areae gastricae vary considerably in their shape, size, and distribution from person to person, even in normal individuals. In vitro methods have been used to assess more objectively the factors that influence mucosal coating.[44] However, it appears that the behavior of barium suspensions often varies considerably between in vitro and in vivo conditions, particularly in terms of double-contrast examinations of the stomach and duodenum.[45]

It is now generally accepted that, for the performance of double-contrast radiography, a high-density (approximately 250 w/v), low-viscosity barium suspension produces the best mucosal coating and hence detail.[7] High-density barium suspensions contain a greater proportion of larger particles than do low-density preparations, but the heterogeneity of particle size is also important for improving muco-

sal coating.[41] Powder preparations need to be mixed with water. The viscosity of the resultant suspension is critically dependent on the volume of water added, as even small changes in the volume can adversely affect mucosal coating.[43] Local variations in the ion content of tap water can be similarly detrimental and result in the formation of small-particle aggregates (Fig. 14-7) or excessive foaming when soft water is used. The use of distilled or deionized water can overcome these problems. These phenomena should not be confused with droplets of barium hanging from the non-dependent wall (stalactite phenomenon), seen en face (Fig. 14-8).

Between 100 and 150 ml of suspension is usually necessary to achieve adequate double-contrast studies of the stomach and duodenum. For single-contrast examinations, a smaller volume (50 ml) of a lower-density suspension (100% w/v, or less) is used, thus allowing some radiographic transparency of the contrast during abdominal compression. This is followed by a larger volume to show distensibility.

Adverse reactions to barium preparations are rare and are usually due to additive agents.[46] Barium embolization to the lungs has been reported following an upper gastrointestinal examination in a patient with active gastroduodenal bleeding.[47] In view of the very large numbers of barium examinations performed, however, these isolated case reports merely emphasize the overall safety of the DCBM examination. Complications associated with alimentary tract radiology have been reviewed by Ansell.[48]

Water-soluble contrast media are indicated when a gastroduodenal perforation is suspected. Meglumine diatrizoate (Gastrografin; Schering) is relatively inexpensive and suitable in most instances. Although such iodinated water-soluble agents are relatively safe and rapidly resorbed after extraluminal leakage, some problems have been reported in connection with their use. Systemic disturbances such as electrolyte imbalance and hypovolemia, which are related to the agents' osmotic effect, have been encountered[49] but are uncommon and appear to be restricted to young infants and elderly debilitated patients. Complications may also arise in connection with aspiration of these agents. When aspirated, hypertonic water-soluble contrast media can produce severe, and occasionally fatal, pulmonary edema.[50,51] A small volume of aspirated barium is relatively innocuous and is rapidly cleared from the healthy lung. However, problems may arise when it is aspirated in larger volumes or in the presence of poor respiratory function.

For these various reasons, selective use of the newer nonionic water-soluble contrast media has been advocated for the detection of upper gastrointestinal perforation when there is a risk of aspiration.[52] This study found that iopamidol (Niopam; E. Merck Limited) was safe, reliable, and free from adverse side effects in the mediastinum, peritoneal cavity, and lungs. At the present time, the main argument against the routine use of such agents is their cost. Some saving can be achieved by using nonsterile unused contrast agent left over from recent vascular investigations.[52]

Paralysis of peristalsis

The abolition of peristalsis during the double-contrast examination of the stomach and duodenum is beneficial,[53] and the effects of various pharmacologic agents on the gastrointestinal tract have been well documented.[54] At present, glucagon and Buscopan (hyoscine-*N*-butyl bromide) are the most suitable and widely used of these drugs.

Glucagon

Glucagon given intravenously produces temporary paralysis of peristalsis with minimal, if any, side effects. It was used initially in relatively large doses of up to 2 mg given intramuscularly or intravenously.[53] Studies were subsequently undertaken to determine the optimum and smallest effective doses.[55] Doses as small as 0.1 mg, given intravenously, have been shown to produce adequate hypotonicity of the stomach and duodenum within 1 minute of administration.[56] If the dose is increased, both the duration and intensity of the response increase. Glucagon slightly prolongs the small bowel transit time, although with small doses (0.1 mg) this delay is not significant. Its use is contraindicated when there is a possibility of a pheochromocytoma or insulinoma, as, when given to a patient with a pheochromocytoma, it may provoke a precipitous rise in blood pressure. Indeed, glucagon has been used in the past as a prov-

ocation test for detecting such tumors.[57] In a patient with an insulinoma, it causes an initial rise in the blood glucose level, followed by profound hypoglycemia. However, the actual risk of such problems when minute doses of glucagon (e.g., 0.1 mg) are used is not known.

Buscopan

The effects of Buscopan, a smooth muscle relaxant with anticholinergic activity, have been known for some time.[54] It inhibits motility in the stomach and colon and slows transit through the small bowel. Buscopan can cause transient pylorospasm, whereas the normal pylorus remains open when glucagon is given. It reduces the lower esophageal sphincter pressure but does not appear to induce gastroesophageal reflux or interfere with the detection of a hiatus hernia in most patients.[58] Its anticholinergic activity is responsible for the transient loss of accommodation experienced by a few patients. Although safe to use on an outpatient basis, this potential side effect should be explained to patients beforehand. Patients are often told not to drive for an hour or so afterward, although there is some evidence that these precautions are unnecessary.[59] Anticholinergic drugs are known to cause an acute rise in intraocular pressure in patients with narrow-angle (shallow anterior) glaucoma. This is an uncommon condition, and routine questioning is unlikely to disclose its existence.[59] Similarly, acute urinary retention may theoretically be precipitated in men with a history of prostatism, but, with the small doses usually given, this is not a problem in practice.

The recommended intravenous dosage is 20 mg, and its effect lasts between 15 and 20 minutes.

Gas-producing agents

Double-contrast examination of the upper gastrointestinal tract is dependent on distention of the stomach with an adequate volume of gas. There should be enough gas to produce distention and straighten the normally convoluted rugae. However, overdistention with too much gas may completely efface most of the rugal folds, with the consequent loss of important radiologic information. Conversely, prominent folds in an underdistended stomach may obscure small mucosal lesions. Underdistention is also responsible for causing the "kissing" artifact, which is due to apposition of the anterior and posterior gastric walls, particularly where the stomach crosses the spine (Fig. 14-9).

In early double-contrast examinations, intubation of the stomach was used as the means to introduce controlled volumes of gas to produce optimal distention. This technique remained popular in Japan but elsewhere was generally considered unacceptable for routine use.[60] Various gas (carbon dioxide)–producing tablets and powders were therefore developed so that the need for intubation could be avoided. The prerequisites for such an agent are the production of an adequate volume of gas (200-400 ml), rapid disintegration leaving no residue, palatability, and low cost.[61] In ad-

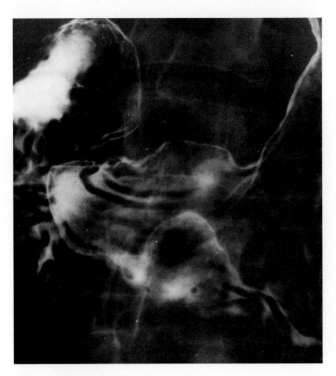

Fig. 14-9 Underdistention of the stomach producing a "kissing" artifact (i.e., contact between dependent and nondependent surfaces) where the stomach crosses the spine.

dition, the normal mucosal coating by the barium suspension should not be adversely affected. Several readily available products now exist that fulfill these criteria, and most also contain an antifoaming agent. Antifoaming agents such as simethicone both enhance the mucosal coating and reduce artifacts,[22] although their addition in excess should be avoided.[62] Alternative methods for introducing gas have been advanced, but none have gained widespread acceptance. These include using "bubbly barium," which is prepared using a refrigerated barium suspension dispensed from a soda syphon,[63,64] or using two freshly prepared barium suspensions that produce gas when combined.[24]

Techniques

Initial claims regarding the increased sensitivity of the DCBM over the single-contrast meal (SCBM) may have been overoptimistic.[65,66] Further studies showed that interpretations based on a combination of both techniques increased the diagnostic accuracy, suggesting the two examinations could complement each other.[67,68] This is the basis of the biphasic examination (see later discussion).

Before describing the technique of the DCBM in detail, the SCBM will be briefly described, as many of the radiographic projections used form the basis of the DCBM. In elderly or immobile patients, a full DCBM may not be feasible, and thus familiarity with the SCBM technique is essential.

The conventional single-contrast barium meal

Although some swallowed air and the gas already within the stomach contribute to a double-contrast appearance, there is no attempt to produce further gaseous distention. A small volume (approximately 50 ml) of relatively low-density (100% w/v) barium suspension is used. This volume, which is sufficient to coat the gastric mucosa (aided by manual compression and palpation), can yield a mucosal relief study. Radiographs of the stomach are taken in the supine right anterior oblique (RAO) and prone left posterior oblique (LPO) positions. With the patient remaining in the latter position, a larger volume of more dilute barium (25% to 50% w/v) is then given using a large-bore straw or plastic tube. This antigravity swallow allows views of the distended esophagus in single contrast to be obtained. At least 100 ml of this more dilute barium is needed to produce the necessary degree of gastric distention, with some authors recommending up to 500 ml.[69] Further radiographs are then taken of the stomach, which should include prone oblique (LPO), supine, supine oblique (RAO), and erect RAO views. Additional spot views of the duodenum using compression as necessary are also taken. Careful compression fluoroscopy is carried out to examine the accessible parts of the stomach, with spot films of positive findings.

Double-contrast barium meal

It is now generally accepted that DCBM is superior to SCBM in the detection of fine mucosal abnormalities such as erosive gastritis.[24,25,70] The development of the DCBM in Japan was prompted by the need for an investigation that could detect the subtle mucosal changes that occur in early gastric cancer.[71] From this origin, the DCBM has evolved to become the primary radiologic investigation of the upper gastrointestinal tract.

The authors' preference is described first, and then a brief description of the alternative methods and their relative merits and limitations follows.[23,25,26,72]

In the authors' approach, the details on the request form are first confirmed with the patient, and the procedure is explained. This brief initial interview can also be used to obtain further information regarding any pertinent previous surgery and other relevant radiologic examinations. Gas-producing tablets or powder are then given, either with a small volume of water or with their accompanying proprietary solution. The patient is instructed not to belch or regurgitate the gas. An intravenous injection of either 0.1 mg of glucagon or 20 mg of Buscopan is then given to produce paralysis of peristalsis.

The patient next stands on the erect fluoroscopic unit in an approximately 30 to 45 degree RAO projection. The patient then swallows about 100 ml of a high-density (250% w/v) barium suspension from a beaker held in the left hand. The barium is swallowed as quickly as possible, and this procedure produces a double-contrast esophagram (Fig. 14-10, *A* and *B*). Images are recorded on small-format (100-

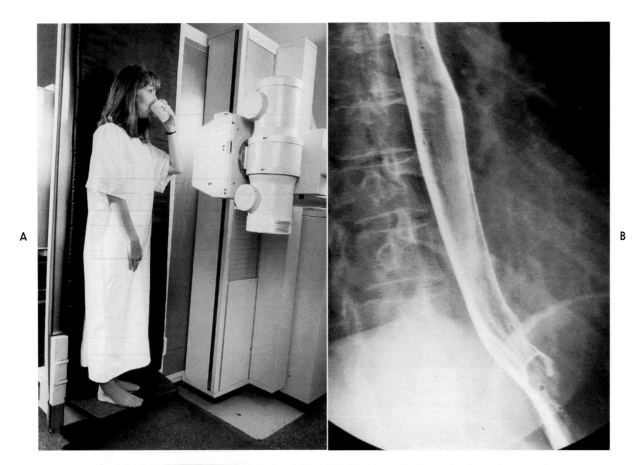

Fig. 14-10 A and **B,** Erect right anterior oblique (RAO) view producing a double-contrast esophagram.   *Continued.*

mm) film with either an undercouch or a remote control overcouch fluoroscopy system. An alternative to these systems is a digital fluoroscopic system, which permits subsequent editing of the images before the production of the hard copy.

The patient is then turned to face the screening table, which is tilted horizontally. This position produces a single-contrast view of the antrum with compression exerted between the spine and the anterior abdominal wall (Fig. 14-10, *C* and *D*). The patient then turns via the left side, to prevent early filling of the duodenum, to lie *supine*. It may be necessary to repeat this maneuver to ensure adequate mucosal coating. A film taken in this position demonstrates the body and gastric antrum in double contrast and the dependent barium-filled fundus in single contrast (Fig. 14-10, *E* and *F*). Both supine oblique projections (RAO and LAO) are obtained, and, after this, the patient lies on the right side. Barium thereby passes under gravity from the fundus into the antrum and enters the duodenum. Double-contrast views of the fundus and barium-filled views of the duodenal cap and loop are obtained (Fig. 14-10, *G* and *H*). Gastroesophageal reflux, if present, may be demonstrated when the patient turns from the supine RAO to LAO positions,

but no further direct attempts to elicit its presence are routinely made.

Further views are taken of the duodenal cap and loop in double contrast. This is best achieved by turning the patient into a steep RAO position (Fig. 14-10, *I* and *J*). Tilting the patient farther into the left lateral position is often helpful for allowing air to enter the duodenum. Another maneuver that is sometimes useful in producing double-contrast views of the cap is to tilt the table 45 degrees head-up (the negative Trendelenburg position) with the patient maintained in the RAO position. An alternative is to tilt the table with the patient supine to allow barium to pass into the second part of the duodenum and then to return the patient to the RAO position.

Another approach to ensuring duodenal distention involves the use of a pad (made from a rolled towel, which is 9 inches [22.5 cm] long and 4 inches [10 cm] in diameter). This is placed so that it compresses the lower body and angulus against the aorta and spine. To do this, once there is sufficient barium in the duodenum, the patient is turned on the left side with the left arm and hand placed behind the body. The pad is placed longitudinally against the epigastrium and the patient is rolled prone onto

Text continued on p. 296.

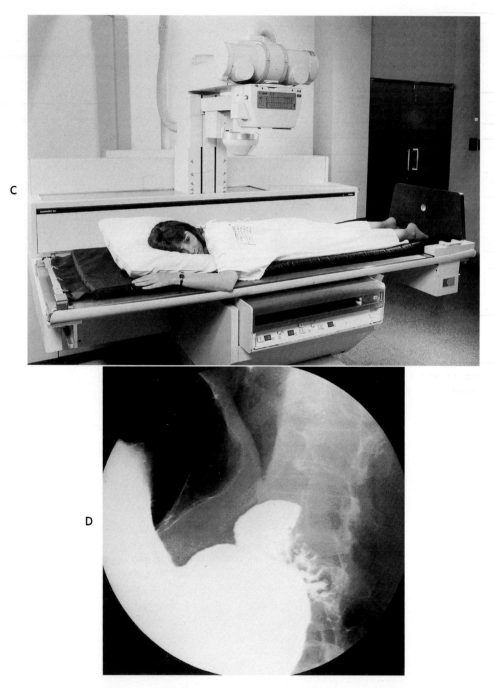

Fig. 14-10, *cont'd* **C** and **D,** Prone position producing a single-contrast study of the body and antrum and a double-contrast study of the fundus.

Continued.

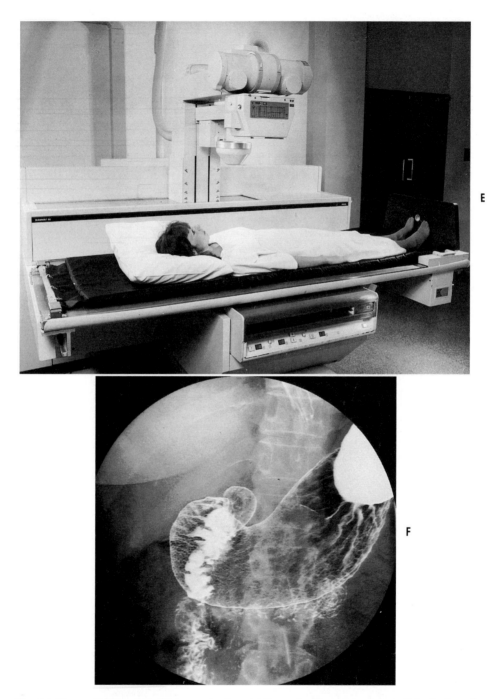

Fig. 14-10, *cont'd* **E** and **F,** Supine projection yielding a double-contrast view of the body and antrum.   *Continued.*

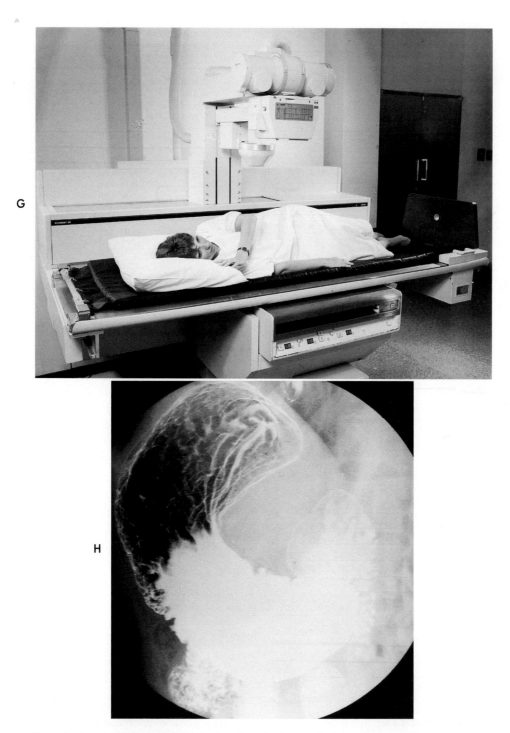

Fig. 14-10, *cont'd* **G** and **H,** Right lateral projection producing a double-contrast view of the fundus and single-contrast view of the duodenum.   *Continued.*

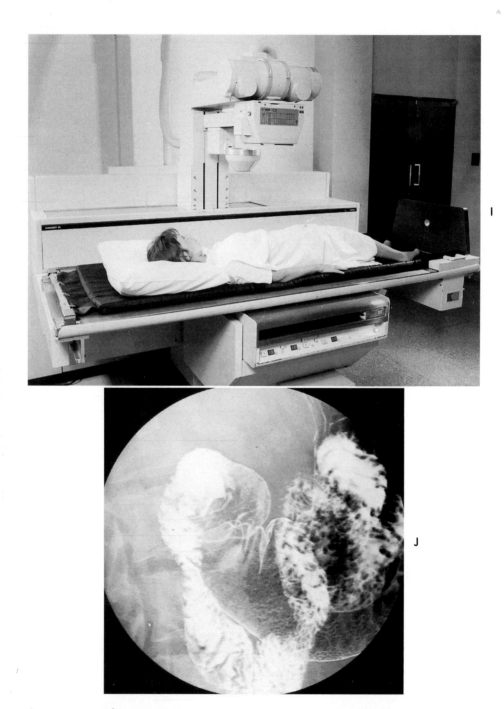

Fig. 14-10, *cont'd* **I** and **J,** Supine RAO position yielding a double-contrast image of the antrum and duodenum. **K** and **L,** Erect view resulting in a double-contrast image of the fundus. **M** and **N,** Prone left posterior oblique view, antigravity swallow.

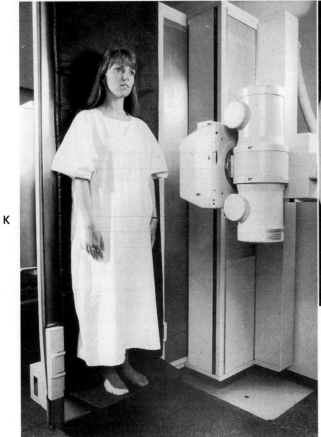

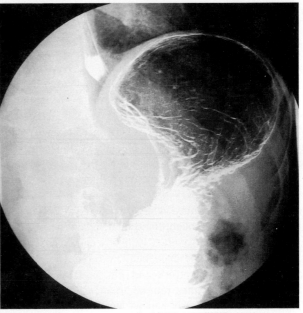

Fig. 14-10, *cont'd*
For legend see opposite page.

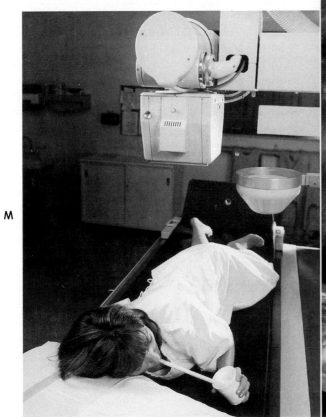

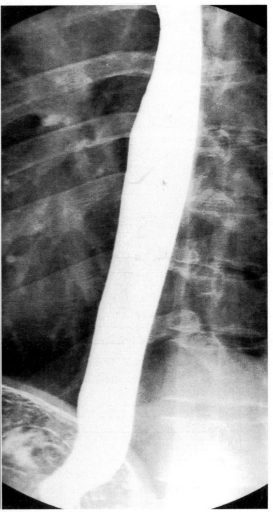

the pad. The pressure from the pad then traps gas in the antrum, which is compressed so that the gas is driven through the pylorus and around the duodenal loop. The patient is then in the proper position for the prone duodenal loop film.

When using a remote-control apparatus with an over-couch tube, tube angulation is available, and this can be used to advantage in certain situations, particularly when the barium-filled third part of the duodenum overlaps the stomach.[73]

Additional gas or barium can be administered at any stage of the examination, although this should seldom be necessary. The patient is finally tilted vertically and erect views of the whole stomach and duodenum are taken using fluoroscopy to guide optimal positioning (Fig. 14-10, *K* and *L*). Care should be taken when returning patients to the erect position, particularly elderly patients who may experience postural hypotension and giddiness. This is potentially more of a problem with a remote-controlled unit, and an assistant should always be on hand to assist the patient if necessary. Alternatively a prone LPO antigravity swallow can be performed at the beginning of the examination (Fig. 14-10, *M* and *N*). In this event, the erect RAO swallow concludes the examination.

Such a routine that includes careful fluoroscopy and the selective use of compression when necessary constitutes a very accurate method of detecting abnormalities of the stomach or duodenum.

Biphasic examination

The biphasic examination combines a single-contrast with a double-contrast examination. Proponents of this type of examination claim its accuracy is better than that of the standard DCBM.[64]

The initial double-contrast series is performed as described in the previous section, although a smaller volume (approximately 75 ml) of high-density barium is used. This is then followed by a primarily single-contrast study in which a larger volume (up to 350 ml) of a much lower-density barium solution (15% to 25% w/v) is used, as already described. By this time the gastroparetic effect of the hypotonic agent is wearing off and any abnormalities of motility can be assessed more accurately.

Techniques for the examination of the duodenum

Demonstration of the duodenum is adequate in the vast majority of DCBMs. Indeed, the study should be considered incomplete if the entire duodenal loop is not visualized. Assessment of the configuration of the duodenal loop and possible mucosal abnormalities, as well as visualization of the papilla and its associated folds, used to play an important role in the investigation of suspected pancreatic disease.[12,74,75] Various techniques therefore evolved for the specific examination of the duodenum.[76-78] For purposes of completeness, a brief description of these methods is given,

even though, with the advent of newer imaging modalities, such techniques are diminishing in importance. Ultrasound, CT, and endoscopic retrograde cholangiopancreatography (ERCP) in particular now play major roles in the investigation of pancreaticobiliary disease.

Hypotonic duodenography
Tubeless studies

Satisfactory double-contrast views of the duodenum are usually obtained during a standard DCBM examination. Paralysis of peristalsis is essential and readily achieved with either glucagon or Buscopan. As previously described in the section on DCBM, the duodenal cap and loop are usually best demonstrated in double contrast using careful fluoroscopy with the patient in the supine RAO position. Tilting the table to a semierect position may also be useful for achieving this.[79] The prone-oblique position has also proved to yield good double-contrast images of the second part of the duodenum; this is achieved by turning the patient prone from the left lateral position.[80]

The gas-filled stomach can sometimes hinder the examination because it causes the duodenum to be rotated more posteriorly.[81] However, various maneuvers can be used to overcome this, including turning the patient a little to the right (LAO) or viewing the duodenum through the gas-filled antrum in the RAO position.

Poor mucosal coating, overlapping of the stomach and duodenum, and inadequate gaseous distention of the duodenum are occasional problems. To overcome some of these problems, a selective tubeless examination has been advocated.[78,82] A small quantity of dilute barium is swallowed while the patient is lying on the right side. This promotes the flow of barium into the duodenum by gravity. A gas-producing agent is then given and, when fluoroscopy reveals the barium in the second part of the duodenum, peristalsis is abolished with Buscopan or glucagon. Turning the patient into the left lateral position allows gas to enter the duodenum, and this achieves the necessary double-contrast effect.

Even using these various techniques, adequate demonstration of the duodenum sometimes proves impossible. Tubeless hypotonic duodenography is not usually effective for the examination of the third and fourth parts of the duodenum. Hypotonic duodenography performed by means of intubation remains an option.

Intubation study

The intubation study was the standard approach to hypotonic duodenography and yielded consistently good results. Any overlap resulting from the presence of contrast within the stomach was avoided and the exact volumes of air and barium could be regulated so that the desired double-contrast effect and degree of distention was achieved. However, patient discomfort resulting from the introduction and manipulation of the duodenal tube, combined with the usually longer duration of the procedure, compared with the tubeless study, made it unpopular for routine use. The technique has been used in combination with fine-needle percutaneous transhepatic cholangiography to evaluate the ampulla and medial wall of the second part of the duodenum in cases of obstructive jaundice.[83]

Several modifications of the Bilbao-Dotter tube are now available. The technique of intubation is described in detail in Chapter 26. In this procedure, once the tip of the tube is satisfactorily placed in the second part of the duodenum, 40 to 50 ml of barium suspension is introduced and peristalsis is abolished. The introduction of air distends the loop and produces a double-contrast appearance. Images are obtained as previously described, but without the problems posed by the overlapping contrast-filled stomach. At the end of the procedure, the tube is simply withdrawn.

MODIFIED BARIUM MEAL TECHNIQUES FOR SPECIFIC CLINICAL SITUATIONS
Suspected gastroduodenal perforation

An chest radiograph with the patient erect or a film of the abdomen with the patient in the left lateral decubitus position may demonstrate the presence of free intraperitoneal gas. In approximately 70% of cases of perforated ulcers, this will disclose the presence of free gas.[84] If a gastroduodenal perforation is suspected and the plain radiographs are unhelpful, a contrast study may be indicated. The choice of contrast media has already been discussed. Provided there is no risk of aspiration, Gastrografin is a suitable agent. To start with, the patient lies on the right side and then either swallows 50 to 100 ml of Gastrografin or it is introduced via a nasogastric tube, if one is in place. Fluoroscopy may reveal a perforation at this stage. If not, an abdominal radiograph should be obtained after 10 to 20 minutes, with the patient continuing to lie on the right side. This may disclose the presence of extraluminal and intraperitoneal collections of contrast, indicating a perforation. Even with careful fluoroscopy, however, the exact site of perforation is often difficult to determine.

If this approach fails to demonstrate leakage, even with adequate duodenal filling, the patient should be placed supine and another film taken after 30 to 40 minutes. Renal excretion of the contrast agent should also be looked for. This confirms the presence of leakage, because it means that the water-soluble contrast has been absorbed from the peritoneal cavity.[85]

Studies performed with water-soluble contrast media are not always successful in demonstrating small perforations or tears, and therefore negative or equivocal findings do not exclude the existence of perforation. It has been suggested that, if the initial examination is negative, immediate reexamination using barium sulfate should be undertaken. This has been shown to be a safe and simple method and to have a higher diagnostic yield in detecting small upper gastrointestinal perforations.[86,87]

Studies of the postoperative stomach and duodenum

Knowledge of the timing and nature of the surgical procedures performed, the site and number of anastomoses, and the specific problem being evaluated is an essential prerequisite to a satisfactory examination.

Early postoperative assessment

The factors influencing the choice of contrast media have already been discussed. Careful fluoroscopy and patient positioning in more than one projection is essential when assessing the integrity of surgical anastomoses, although the discomfort from a recent abdominal operation combined with the often large number of attached tubes and catheters can considerably limit a patient's mobility. Every effort should be made to overcome these problems so that the desired view can be obtained at the patient's first visit. The optimal position to promote drainage of anastomotic loops and pouches can be assessed during the course of the examination, and this information communicated to the staff so that the patient can be cared for accordingly. As with the assessment of patients with a suspected spontaneous gastroduodenal perforation, delayed films may also be helpful.

Late assessment of previous surgery

When confronted with a patient whose surgery took place sometime before, the details of the procedure may not be known. Surgical records, particularly relating to procedures performed in another hospital, are not always available. Although the patient usually knows the nature of the original indication for surgery, the multiplicity of possible procedures makes it difficult to predict the resultant anatomy. The radiologist can assume that the capacity of the stomach has been reduced, however, and modify the DCBM accordingly.

Upper gastrointestinal endoscopy is often the preferred investigation in patients who have undergone gastroduodenal surgery. This allows not only the direct visualization of the gastric remnant, stoma, and anastomotic loops, but also provides the opportunity to perform either random biopsies of the gastric remnant to exclude dysplastic changes or to carry out targeted biopsies of suspicious lesions. When barium studies are performed in these patients, distortion of the anatomy, underdistention of the gastric remnant by either gas, barium, or both, and superimposition of barium-filled small bowel loops are all common problems. However, appropriate modification of the routine DCBM investigation and awareness of these problems can help ensure a satisfactory examination in the majority of cases. Various modifications have been described,[88,89] but paralysis of peristalsis and gaseous distention are essential components of all. A larger dose of glucagon (e.g., 0.5 mg intravenously) has been recommended, as the examination often takes longer than the routine DCBM and paralysis of both efferent and afferent loops can thereby be maintained for several minutes. The patient first swallows the gas-producing agent and then a small volume (40-50 ml) of high-density (250% w/v) barium suspension while lying in the supine RAO position. This prevents overfilling of the gastric remnant. A headdown tilt of 5 to 10 degrees has also been recommended to prevent early filling of small bowel loops.[88] The patient is then turned to ensure adequate mucosal coating, using fluoroscopy to monitor the location of the barium and thereby minimize its loss through the anastomosis. By adjusting the degree of table tilt and the patient's position, satisfactory views of the gastric remnant and stoma can usually be obtained.

When there has been a Polya-type (Billroth II) partial gastrectomy, lying the patient on the right side helps fill the afferent loop. Turning the patient to either a steep posterior oblique or prone position then allows air to fill the loop. If the stoma is patent, filling of the efferent loop is not usually a problem. Compression is sometimes helpful in separating efferent jejunal loops. With a remote-control overcouch tube unit, tube angulation, particularly in a caudad direction, is often useful for overcoming the problem of superimposed bowel.[73] The patient is finally placed in an erect position. This helps in further demonstrating the gastric remnant in double contrast. If required, additional barium can then be given so that the

esophagus can be examined with the patient in the erect RAO position.

Using these modifications, an examination with a useful degree of accuracy is possible in up to 80% of the cases.[89]

Upper gastrointestinal bleeding

Endoscopy should be the initial diagnostic investigation in patients with acute upper gastrointestinal bleeding,[28,29,90] as these patients are often very sick and it is not possible to perform a satisfactory DCBM study. Furthermore, residual barium in the stomach and duodenum may preclude endoscopy and angiography, both of which are of potential therapeutic as well as diagnostic benefit.

Barium studies have been used to demonstrate bleeding ulcers.[91,92] It is also sometimes possible, with a technically satisfactory DCBM study, to identify a possible bleeding site and also to demonstrate features suggestive of recent or active bleeding.[93] These include the presence of adherent blood clot, demonstration of an artery in the ulcer base (Fig. 14-11), or visualization of active bleeding. This last feature may be difficult to detect but sometimes takes the form of an alteration in the mucosal coating produced by blood washing away the barium adjacent to a bleeding lesion (the lava flow effect). A SCBM technique for the localization of a bleeding site that can be performed at the patient's bedside has also been described.[94] If a barium study is to be performed, every attempt should be made to undertake a detailed DCBM in the way described.

THE ROLES OF BARIUM STUDIES AND ENDOSCOPY IN THE INVESTIGATION OF THE STOMACH AND DUODENUM

For many years barium studies were the principal diagnostic procedures for the routine investigation of the upper gastrointestinal tract. Examination using the rigid gastroscope was uncomfortable and incomplete, because the duodenum and large areas of the stomach could not be visualized. This situation changed with the advent of flexible fiberoptic instruments in the late 1960s. By the early 1970s, flexible endoscopes were in widespread use and, for the first time, the diagnostic accuracy of barium examinations was challenged. Since that time, there have been numerous studies comparing the two procedures.[28,95-100] However, the controversy regarding their relative merits continues.

The design of many of these studies was flawed, and consequently they lacked enough statistical power for meaningful conclusions to be drawn. These errors in methodology have been summarized by Dooley et al.[98] When endoscopy is used as the gold standard, radiology is inevitably found to be inferior. Any endoscopic errors then become radiologic errors, further exaggerating the divide. Some studies have also failed to compare equivalent state-of-the-art techniques. Ideally the detailed DCBM study should be compared with the use of modern sophisticated

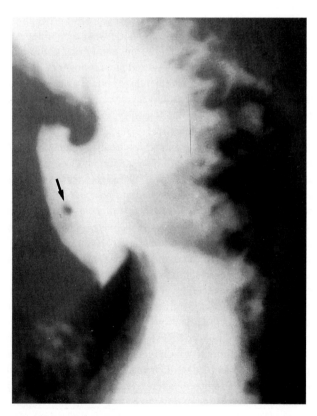

Fig. 14-11 Single-contrast barium meal study demonstrating a large lesser curve gastric ulcer with a vessel in its base *(arrow)*. Active bleeding is producing a "lava flow" appearance.

endoscopes. Similarly, comparing techniques performed by operators with differing experience introduces further errors.[97,99] Randomizing the sequence of examinations, obtaining similar clinical information, and collecting data prospectively are also all essential factors in reaching a valid conclusion. When compared with a third independent diagnostic criterion, such as surgical or postmortem findings, double-contrast radiology and endoscopy appear to possess a similar high degree of diagnostic accuracy. This is particularly so for conditions such as peptic ulceration and carcinoma. More subtle changes in the mucosal pattern, such as those that occur in duodenitis or gastritis, are more reliably detected by endoscopy.[28] Even here, the correlation of radiologic findings with the subsequent endoscopic appearance has led to improvement in the double-contrast techniques and therefore more confident radiologic diagnoses.

For these reasons the diagnostic accuracy rates reported for endoscopy and barium radiology differ widely. In a retrospective study, the accuracy rate of DCBM studies was found to be as high as 96% when compared with endoscopy.[95] The error rate for endoscopy is more difficult to establish, as many studies have used endoscopy as the gold standard and consequently accorded it a 100% accuracy rate. The findings from other studies have suggested the diagnostic accuracy of endoscopy is similar to that of DCBM—96%.[101]

To resolve this issue, a large prospective study in which all patients are examined with both radiology and endoscopy, by experienced technicians using the most sophisticated techniques available, is needed. These results would then need to be compared with a third well-defined standard to determine their relative degrees of accuracy. Clearly such a study would be a considerable undertaking and is unlikely to be mounted because of ethical objections.

It is the authors' belief that endoscopy and barium studies complement each other, and further studies support this view.[96] If symptoms persist once endoscopy reveals normal findings and gastroduodenal pathology is strongly suspected, it seems sensible to perform a DCBM study (or vice versa), rather than to repeat the initial investigation. Barium studies certainly have a role if the endoscopic findings are negative.

The decision to perform either a barium or endoscopic study as the initial primary investigation is determined by several factors.[102]

Clinical diagnosis

Symptoms of peptic ulceration or gastritis are common indications for investigation, although it has been suggested that young patients with a short history of dyspeptic symptoms should be initially managed symptomatically without investigation.[103] The likelihood of serious pathology in these patients is small, and investigation is then reserved for those whose symptoms persist despite adequate treat-

ment. A computer-based preliminary screening program has been devised to attempt to identify, at the outset, those patients at a higher risk of more serious pathology.[104] However, it can be argued that, even in these circumstances, a normal investigation is of benefit,[105] because the expense of a course of antiulcer medication and its potential side effects can be spared.

A technically satisfactory DCBM study performed in a cooperative patient is a highly sensitive examination and will identify most significant pathology.[106,107] The diagnostic accuracy is improved when the films are reviewed by the referring physician and radiologist together. The ability of both endoscopy and the biphasic barium meal to accurately diagnose peptic ulceration and gastric carcinoma is similar.[100] However, endoscopy is more sensitive for detecting small duodenal ulcers and mucosal inflammation. A further study[108] that assessed the two techniques showed that duodenal ulceration was the most common lesion missed radiologically. The significance of not detecting minor mucosal inflammation is debatable, however, because often the results of the investigation do not ultimately change the treatment planned before the tests were requested.[105] The safety aspects of this thinking are discussed later. In the assessment of dyspepsia, Gelfand et al.[109] suggest that the risk from endoscopy alone is greater than that posed by any potentially curable disease that would remain undiagnosed after a DCBM study.

There are certain clinical situations in which endoscopy should be considered as the primary investigation. For instance, endoscopy has a higher diagnostic yield than DCBM in the investigation of acute upper gastrointestinal bleeding.[110] Here again, however, many of the studies comparing the relative merits of endoscopy and DCBM studies are subject to the same methodologic errors. Although one study found endoscopy to have a higher diagnostic accuracy than radiology, there was ultimately no difference in the management approach adopted or the length of survival between the two groups.[111] In those cases in which a third independent criterion could be applied (surgical or postmortem findings), the accuracy rates for endoscopy and DCBM were found to be similar. However, endoscopy does possess several potential advantages. To obtain a DCBM study of the quality needed to achieve an acceptable diagnostic accuracy requires patient cooperation and a degree of mobility that is often lacking in these sick people with their attendant intravenous lines. Such mobility and cooperation are not essential to the success of endoscopy.

A lesion shown by a DCBM study may not be the actual source of bleeding. Although there are radiologic signs that indicate recent or active bleeding,[93] these are often not demonstrated. Cotton et al.[29] showed that approximately one quarter of the patients in their study who had an endoscopically proved duodenal ulcer were in fact bleeding from another site, and approximately 15% of *all* such patients have more than one lesion.[29] Endoscopy can be used to confirm a lesion as the source of blood loss if active bleeding is seen or if the stigmata of recent hemorrhage are present. Besides active bleeding, these features include the presence of blood clot or black slough that is adherent to the lesion and visualization of a vessel that is protruding from the base or margin of the lesion. Such stigmata can be of prognostic value in predicting the likelihood of rebleeding and the need for emergency surgery.[112,113] It has also been suggested that more emphasis be placed on the site of the bleeding lesion rather than on the presence of such stigmata.[114]

Bleeding superficial mucosal lesions may heal very rapidly and, if endoscopy is to be successful in identifying the source of blood loss, it should ideally be performed within 12 hours of the onset of symptoms, but certainly within 24 hours. Foster et al.[113] showed that, when endoscopy was delayed beyond 12 hours after the onset of bleeding, there was a twofold increase in the number of cases without diagnoses. This has been supported by the findings from other studies[115] and has obvious implications regarding the further investigations and management of such patients. However, an accurate diagnosis alone is not necessarily beneficial unless it influences management and improves the patient's prognosis. There is, as yet, no convincing evidence that early endoscopy leads to improved survival.[111,116] This may come with improvements in endoscopic therapy for bleeding gastroduodenal lesions. Fleischer[117] has reviewed these techniques.

Another situation in which endoscopy may yield more rewarding results than barium studies is in the investigation of the postoperative stomach.[102] Disordered anatomy and difficulty in achieving adequate gaseous distention of the gastric remnant can make it difficult to interpret the DCBM findings.

Patient preference

If the accuracy rates of barium studies and endoscopy are similar, then it seems reasonable to take the patients' preference into account. Once they have undergone both investigations, more patients show a preference for upper gastrointestinal endoscopy over a DCBM study.[105,118,119] This is largely due to the amnesic effect of the mild sedation used during endoscopy. Following recovery from sedation, the patient can also often immediately be told the endoscopic findings. This is seldom the case with routine DCBM, and any delay in being told the results increases anxiety.[118]

Other factors are also worthy of consideration. Younger patients, in particular, are often extremely apprehensive about endoscopy, even though with mild sedation they find the procedure is not usually as unpleasant as they expected. The influence of personality traits in the reaction of patients to upper gastrointestinal endoscopy has been studied,[120] and it was found that patients with a high neurosis score are more likely to need premedication with diazepam. Failure to do this jeopardizes future patient willingness to comply.

After a DCBM study, the patient can leave the x-ray department unaided and return to work immediately, whereas after endoscopy with sedation the patient should not drive, must be escorted home, and is off work for up to 24 hours. When sedation is not routinely used, a smaller proportion of patients express a preference for endoscopy. The situation is different in the elderly. Excessive maneuvering is the most common complaint voiced by patients undergoing a DCBM study.[119] Considerable patient positioning is necessary for the performance of a technically satisfactory examination, and this is often difficult, tiring, or distressing for elderly and infirm patients. It would therefore appear sensible to perform endoscopy as the primary investigation in this group. There is also an increased likelihood of malignant disease in these patients, and endoscopy permits biopsy specimens to be obtained for histopathologic confirmation. Endoscopy in elderly patients has been shown to be an efficient, safe, and acceptable procedure.[121]

Safety

Although DCBM studies are considered very safe, endoscopy does carry a mortality rate. In the United Kingdom in 1977 this was 1 in 4400 procedures; however, by 1981 it had improved to less than 1 in 12,000 procedures.[122] With advances in technique and instrumentation, the mortality rate should fall even further. The major complications of diagnostic upper gastrointestinal fiberoptic endoscopy are perforation and cardiorespiratory problems, which are often related to sedation. This topic is discussed in detail elsewhere.[123,124]

Availability and cost

In an ideal world, both investigations would be readily available. However, there is often a delay before the procedure can be carried out, and this length of time varies considerably between centers. The referring gastroenterologists are in control of their own endoscopy schedule, whereas the radiology department controls the availability of barium studies. In addition, some gastroenterologists prefer to "see for themselves" rather than accept a radiologic report. However, it has been suggested that the motives for recommending endoscopy are more complex than this.[125] The fee for an endoscopy performed in the private sector in the United Kingdom is approximately four times that for a DCBM study.[102] With the increasing use of endoscopy, there should be a comparable reduction in the number of barium studies performed, and this has been borne out by data collected by Gelfand et al.[126] from 69 radiologic practices that showed a 24% decrease in the number of upper gastrointestinal barium studies performed between 1975 and 1986. The almost constant decline over this period suggests that it will continue. Although some of this reduction is probably attributable to the increased use of ultrasound and CT, the competition from endoscopy was considered to be the most important factor, and the financial incentives related to the higher cost of endoscopy seem likely to perpetuate this trend.

In the United Kingdom a recent survey conducted in one

health region revealed that the number of barium meal studies was decreasing by 5% per year, in contrast with a predicted 5% rise in the absence of endoscopy. The introduction of an open-access endoscopy service for general practitioners led to a 20% reduction in the number of barium meal studies performed the following year in one hospital,[102] although the benefit to the patient from such a system is questionable. Early reports suggest that this increased emphasis on endoscopy has not in fact translated into either earlier diagnoses of gastric cancer[127] or a reduction in the complication rate from peptic ulceration.[128] A scoring system has been devised that identifies specific risk factors, and this has consequently improved the cost effectiveness of an open-access service.[129] Using such a system, a 32% reduction in the number of endoscopic procedures performed would be achieved while 98% of the cases of serious disease would still be detected. Those patients excluded probably represent young subjects with dyspepsia in whom symptomatic treatment should be the first line of management. Such a system will be of value only if those patients excluded from endoscopy are not subsequently referred for a barium meal investigation.

Gelfand et al.[130] have offered an interesting scenario in this regard:

> One can only imagine the situation if endoscopy had been done alone for several decades, and radiology of the gastrointestinal tract then became available. Suddenly, there is an alternative examination that costs one third of the established method, shows almost as many serious pathologic findings, is associated with negligible mortality and morbidity, and causes little patient discomfort. Radiology would almost certainly be advocated as the more desirable initial examination of the gastrointestinal tract.

UPPER GASTROINTESTINAL ENDOSCOPY

Rigid gastroscopy was an uncomfortable and difficult procedure, and the view it afforded was very limited, in that large areas of the stomach and the entire duodenum could not be examined. The semiflexible lens gastroscopes that became available improved visibility a little, but, with the exception of a few enthusiasts, they remained largely unpopular.

The whole field of endoscopy changed dramatically with the advent of flexible fiberoptic instruments in the late 1960s. By the early 1970s, these endoscopes were being used routinely for upper GI examination.

There is now a large range of instruments available, not only for diagnostic but also for therapeutic purposes. Most recently, with the refinement of the video "chip" endoscope and its associated technology, the facility is available to obtain an accurate permanent color photograph for documentation. This provides a baseline that permits more objective assessment on subsequent follow-up examinations. This system is less tiring to use, and, as the image is displayed on a television monitor, it offers more potential for teaching applications. More complicated therapeutic procedures, such as endoscopic retrograde cholangiopancreatography, can be more informative and interesting for radiographic and nursing personnel.

The forward-viewing gastroscope is the instrument used for the vast majority of routine diagnostic upper gastrointestinal examinations. It allows complete visualization of the esophagus, stomach, and first and second parts of the duodenum. An adequately equipped endoscopy unit should also possess alternative instruments for use in specific circumstances. Side-viewing endoscopes are useful to examine the region of the gastroesophageal junction, the duodenum, and areas around the stoma of a gastroenterostomy that are often hidden from view using a standard forward-viewing instrument. Visualization of a suspicious area en face often makes it easier to obtain biopsy specimens. Smaller pediatric endoscopes are used in young children, and, as they are significantly smaller in diameter, they are less uncomfortable for the patient and can be used more easily without sedation in adult practice. Because of their size, they also cause less respiratory embarrassment, which is of particular importance in the elderly. However, a slightly inferior image quality and a smaller instrument channel limit both the biopsy and therapeutic options.

It is essential to have available the necessary equipment for adequate cleaning and disinfection of the endoscopes and all their nondisposable accessories. Strict adherence to the guidelines for disinfection is mandatory to minimize the risk of cross-infection.

Resuscitation equipment and emergency drugs should be available and all staff should be trained in their use.

Basic technique

There are no absolute contraindications to the performance of upper gastrointestinal endoscopy. Even very sick patients can, if necessary, be examined in the intensive care unit. There is also a definite risk of cross-infection when performing endoscopy in a patient with, for example, HIV infection or hepatitis B. Although these do not represent absolute contraindications, the necessity of the investigation in such patients should be carefully weighed and all the necessary protection, precautions, and disinfection techniques strictly adhered to.

Some endoscopists prefer that any patient presenting with dysphagia has a barium study beforehand. This helps exclude conditions such as a pharyngeal pouch, which can cause problems during endoscopy and increase the likelihood of perforation.

Patient preparation

Many patients, particularly younger ones, are very apprehensive and anxious about endoscopy. Much of this fear can be alleviated by creating a relaxed atmosphere and by the presence of well-trained, caring, and efficient endoscopy staff.

Before a routine investigation, patients should fast for 6 hours. The procedure is also explained to them and informed consent obtained. If sedation is being used, outpatients should have someone available to accompany them home. Any dentures are removed and the patient either changes into a gown, or a plastic bib or apron is used. The pharynx should be anesthetized using a topical local anesthetic agent. This can be given in the form of a spray, which is usually unpalatable, or lozenges. Pharyngeal anesthesia is essential if the examination is being performed without sedation; however, it is less important when using heavy sedation, as is the case during some therapeutic procedures, and may actually be dangerous because of the increased risk of aspiration.

The patient lies in the left lateral position. A mouth guard is inserted, unless the patient is edentulous, although even then it is sometimes useful because it can also act as an airway.

Sedation

The routine use of sedation varies between departments. Overall, patients prefer mild sedation. Some units attempt to perform most routine endoscopic examinations without sedation. This allows the more economical use of staff and resources, as less (if any) patients then need recovery facilities. However, it is the authors' belief that this is an unnecessary and unkind practice, and one that significantly jeopardizes the patient's future willingness to comply. A selective use of sedation is the best policy. Young patients, who are keen to return to work immediately or who have to drive home, should be allowed to have the investigation without sedation, if they wish. Elderly patients and those with reduced pulmonary function may react adversely to sedation, and its use in these groups should sometimes be avoided. Most patients, however, benefit from mild sedation and, because of the amnesic effect, find the procedure is not as unpleasant as they feared. In addition, there is no loss of confidence in the referring physician, and they are happy to undergo a repeat or follow-up examination.

The benzodiazepines, in particular Diazemuls (diazepam emulsion; Dumex Ltd.) or the shorter-acting midazolam (Hypnovel; Roche Products Ltd.) are suitable sedatives for routine use. The dose required is extremely variable, however, and some young patients, particularly those with a history of excessive alcohol intake, require very large amounts. These drugs have a rapid onset of action and, when given by slow intravenous injection, the amount needed can be titrated against the patient's response. Adequate sedation is achieved in most young healthy adults with the intravenous administration of between 5 and 10 mg of Diazemuls. Extreme caution should be exercised in the elderly, because even a fraction of this dose can induce respiratory arrest. Oxygen should be available and given in the appropriate concentration to all elderly patients. There are various types of nasal cannulas and sponges suitable for use and that do not interfere with the procedure. Monitoring using a pulse oximeter should be a standard practice in the elderly and *all* patients receiving sedation.

Flumazenil (Anexate; Roche Products Ltd.), a benzodiazepine antagonist, can reverse some of the central sedative effects of the benzodiazepines and is particularly useful in the elderly. It has been available for some years in Europe, and will hopefully soon be available throughout North America. Some patients become very aggressive under the effects of mild sedation, and risk damaging themselves and the equipment as a result. Merely giving more sedation in these patients is not the answer. It is often more sensible to abandon the procedure, explain the situation to the patient (who usually remembers nothing about it), and try again at a later date, perhaps without sedation.

General anesthesia is very rarely needed for the performance of diagnostic endoscopy. Premedication with other drugs, including narcotic analgesics, is not routinely necessary but may be of benefit in some therapeutic procedures.

Intubation

The methods employed by endoscopists to introduce the instrument vary. A suitable technique, commonly used by the authors, is as follows. The patient lies in the left lateral position, while the operator holds the controls of the endoscope in the left hand and the shaft at the 30- to 35-cm mark in the right hand. The tip of the instrument is introduced blindly into the patient's mouth with the operator controlling the upward and downward flexion of the tip using the thumb of the left hand. Slight downward angulation into the pharynx followed by upward deflection as the endoscope is gently advanced steers a course posteriorly into the esophagus. At this point the patient is encouraged to swallow, which relaxes the cricopharyngeus so that the endoscope passes with a noticeable "give" into the proximal esophagus. The right and left controls should not be needed at this stage, and some practitioners recommend fixing their movement with the brake. When difficulty is encountered during intubation, this is often due to deviation away from the midline. Another method, favored by some, is to introduce the endoscope under direct vision. A third method, which is not recommended, is to use the fingers of the left hand to guide the instrument through the patient's mouth while an assistant holds the controls. Finally, in patients without dysphagia, a soft-tipped cannula may be passed through the upper esophageal sphincter under direct vision for some 15 cm, and this can serve as a guidewire over which the endoscope is gently advanced. Whatever technique is used, *at no time* should insertion of the instrument be forced. It is far better to abandon the procedure at this early stage than to risk serious injury. Nothing is lost by repeating the investigation (or arranging for an alternative study) at a later date.

Once the tip of the instrument is safely in the esopha-

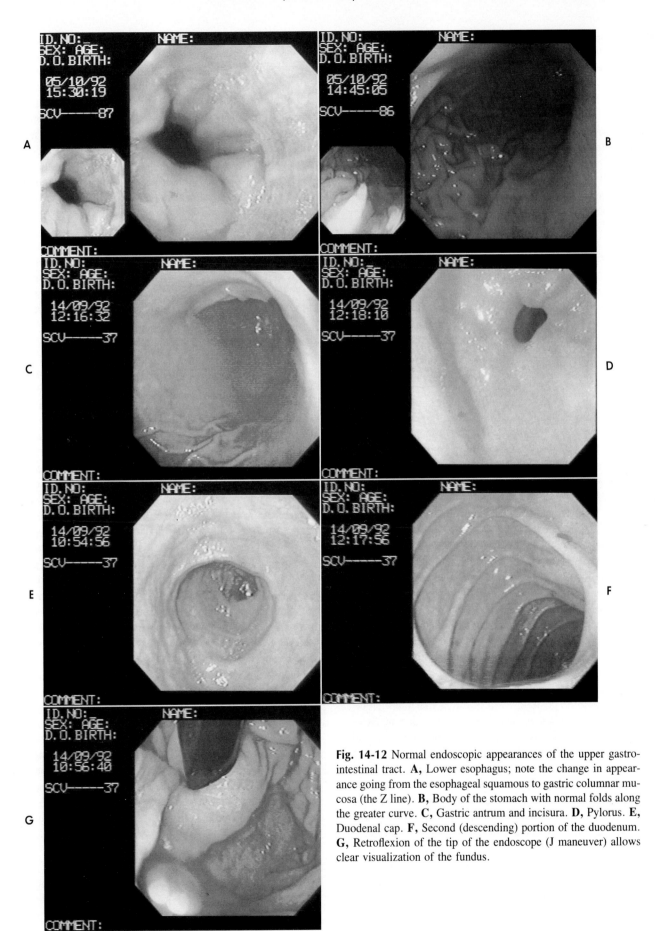

Fig. 14-12 Normal endoscopic appearances of the upper gastrointestinal tract. **A,** Lower esophagus; note the change in appearance going from the esophageal squamous to gastric columnar mucosa (the Z line). **B,** Body of the stomach with normal folds along the greater curve. **C,** Gastric antrum and incisura. **D,** Pylorus. **E,** Duodenal cap. **F,** Second (descending) portion of the duodenum. **G,** Retroflexion of the tip of the endoscope (J maneuver) allows clear visualization of the fundus.

gus, the patient is reassured that the uncomfortable part of the examination is over and is told to breathe normally. If no sedation is used, a running commentary may be welcomed by the patient.

Normal appearances

The normal endoscopic appearance of the upper gastrointestinal tract is illustrated in Fig. 14-12.

Esophagus

The esophagus is seen as a pale pink, relatively featureless tube. Normal indentations (as seen on a DCBM study) produced by the aorta and left main bronchus may be identified. The esophagogastric junction is usually clearly seen where the pale pink esophageal squamous cell mucosa gives way to the orange-red gastric mucosa. This transition is called the Z line. In adults the Z line is normally about 40 cm from the incisor teeth. Indentations from the diaphragm can also be identified and any hiatus hernia assessed. Often the gastric mucosa extends for a centimeter or so above the level of diaphragm.

Stomach

The tip of the endoscope should pass freely into the stomach and usually abuts the proximal lesser curve on entering the stomach, which may temporarily obscure the view. Turning a little to the left and introducing air overcomes this problem. Air is introduced to distend the stomach and the rugal folds then become progressively less prominent, although the longitudinal folds along the greater curve often persist and can act as a landmark and guide down to the antrum. The micromucosal pattern of the areae gastricae are often much less obvious on endoscopy than on DCBM studies. They are sometimes seen when the mucosa is viewed tangentially, but spraying dye such as methylene blue or even simple ink increases their visibility. The instrument is slowly advanced under direct vision at all times. The two main landmarks are the gastric angulus (incisura) and the pylorus. Slight rotation of the whole endoscope in a clockwise direction as the tip passes down through the body into the antrum of the stomach maintains a central position. The lesser curve is seen to the right, the greater curve to the left, and the posterior wall of the stomach at the bottom of the field of view. There is a danger that pools of residual gastric juice may be aspirated, but suction should be used cautiously, as damage to the mucosa can cause a confusing appearance.

A systematic approach is essential to ensure that the entire stomach is visualized. Without this, there may be blind areas that go unrecognized. Individual techniques differ and are described in more detail elsewhere.[131] The lesser curve is one area in particular where a lesion may be missed. With the tip of the endoscope in the antrum, retroflexion of its tip (the so-called J maneuver) affords a good view of the incisura and lesser curve. Gradual withdrawal of the whole instrument with the tip maintained in this position brings into view the proximal lesser curve up toward the cardia. Similarly, 180-degree retroflexion in the opposite direction allows visualization of the greater curve toward the fundus. Withdrawal of the endoscope then enables a detailed examination of the fundus and cardia to be performed. These maneuvers should be performed routinely or areas will be missed. However, they are frequently carried out after the duodenum has been examined "on the way out" to avoid overdistention of the stomach early in the procedure.

Duodenum

As the pylorus is approached, it is seen to open and then close. The tip is gently advanced and maneuvered so that the pylorus fills the field of view. As the pylorus opens, the tip is advanced and easily passes into the duodenum. There is a characteristic change in the color and appearance of the mucosa at this point. The duodenal cap is systematically examined. Because potential blind areas exist just beyond the pylorus, the tip should be gently withdrawn a little. To gain access to the second (descending) part of the duodenum, the tip must be rotated approximately 90 degrees to the right, then angled upward to rotate it around the flexure. The circular folds of the duodenal loop then come into view. By this time, a loop in the endoscope has often formed in the stomach. The endoscope should be gradually withdrawn and, provided its tip is kept rotated to the right, it is possible to advance it farther into the duodenum. The major and minor papillae may be seen tangentially on the medial wall, although a much better view is afforded by the side-viewing duodenoscope.

After making sure that the brakes are not in position, the instrument is now slowly withdrawn and suspicious areas are reexamined. Before leaving the stomach, the air should be sucked out, as gastric distention can be quite uncomfortable. The esophagus should be examined during withdrawal of the endoscope, and a view of the piriform fossae, valleculae, and supraglottic region is obtained immediately before its removal.

Aftercare

If sedation has been used, the patient should remain on the gurney or bed until the effects have worn off. This usually takes about 30 minutes. By this time, pharyngeal sensation should have returned to normal and the patient can be given a drink before leaving the department. A patient who has had sedation should be escorted home and instructed not to drive or operate machinery until the next day. Arrangements for follow-up visits or outpatient appointments can be made before the patient leaves.

Complications

The major complications of endoscopy are perforation and cardiorespiratory problems, which are often related to the sedation or drugs used. These are discussed in detail elsewhere.[123,124]

Who should perform upper gastrointestinal endoscopy?

There is no reason why radiologists, with adequate training, should not perform upper gastrointestinal endoscopy. Who performs the investigation largely depends on the local availability of expertise and the relationship between the referring physician and the radiology department. A gastrointestinal radiologist should be familiar with endoscopy to understand its strengths and weaknesses.[102,132] Ideally, a gastrointestinal radiologist referred a patient with a diagnostic problem should have the expertise and facilities available to investigate the patient as seems most appropriate.[125] This decision would take into account the most likely clinical diagnosis and utilize the imaging modality (endoscopy included) with the highest diagnostic accuracy for that condition, all other factors being equal. Therefore, in certain circumstances, endoscopy would be considered the primary diagnostic investigation, while ultrasonography or barium radiology, for example, would be more appropriate in others.

Practice varies greatly in different countries.[133] In North America, endoscopy was introduced by gastroenterologists, and a major battle was waged in the 1980s before it became an accepted and integral part of surgical training. Currently, the American Society of Gastrointestinal Endoscopy is opposing the efforts of family physicians to start performing upper gastrointestinal endoscopy. There are almost no radiologists practicing endoscopy in North America. In Scandinavia, radiologists have been performing endoscopy for nearly two decades, and, in Sweden, this constitutes an integral part of the service. In the United Kingdom, gastrointestinal radiologists perform endoscopy, and 38% of radiology residents demand to receive endoscopy training, with about half of them getting it. Endoscopy units in that country may be run by gastroenterologists, surgeons, or radiologists, with all specialties participating in the provision of the service. Several units have specially trained family physicians who spend one or two sessions a week helping to provide the service.

Clearly, there are no absolutes operating here. A number of different schemes can work well.[134] In general, when money is not a turf issue, a collaborative interdisciplinary team is easier to establish. In those countries where endoscopy is not a practical possibility for gastrointestinal radiologists, there is more than enough challenge posed by the newer imaging technologies, including interventional. However, it is becoming difficult to adequately train young radiologists in barium techniques, especially when endoscopy is excessively popular.

Concern has been expressed that, if too much of the workload of routine gastrointestinal endoscopy is performed by radiologists, the more traditional facets of radiology would suffer.[135] That too many endoscopies in general are being performed is another matter, and one that has been addressed in some centers by the implementation of a quality assurance program.[136]

Alternative imaging modalities

As indicated previously, both contrast radiology and endoscopy are used routinely as the primary investigations of the upper gastrointestinal tract. Mucosal abnormalities are well demonstrated by both techniques. Information regarding the submucosal and deeper layers of the bowel wall and adjacent structures can, however, only be inferred from indirect signs. CT[137,138] and magnetic resonance imaging (MRI)[139] are both modalities that contribute useful information in such situations.

Computed tomography

CT allows evaluation of the bowel lumen and also the bowel wall and adjacent structures.[140] It may form part of the sequence of investigations in a patient with unexplained weight loss, epigastric or back pain, anorexia, or a palpable abdominal mass. CT may also be used when further information is required about a known abnormality of the stomach or duodenum, such as in the staging of patients with gastric malignancy or in patients who have undergone gastric surgery for removal of a malignancy. CT may also be used to investigate equivocal barium or endoscopic findings, particularly when there is doubt about the extent of the abnormality or if the cause is thought to be extrinsic to the bowel wall.

Technique

As in barium studies of the upper gastrointestinal tract, the patient should ideally fast for 6 hours beforehand. Good distention of the stomach and contrast opacification of the lumen of the bowel are prerequisites to a satisfactory examination. This can be achieved by the administration of 500 ml of 2.5% Gastrografin in two doses, one taken 1 hour and the other 30 minutes before the start of the examination. This is supplemented by an additional 250 ml taken 5 minutes or so before scanning. The agent is made more palatable by the addition of a small quantity of fruit flavoring. Low-density barium suspensions are also commercially available for use in CT examinations and are a suitable alternative.[141]

At the commencement of scanning, 150 ml of 60% iodinated contrast media is rapidly infused intravenously, so that images can be obtained during the arterial phase of enhancement.

The patient lies supine, and, using a scan time of 2 or 3 seconds, contiguous 10-mm images are obtained from the level of the lower esophagus down to below the level of the third (horizontal) part of the duodenum, during arrested respiration. Additional 10-mm sections taken at 15-mm intervals are then obtained through the lower abdomen and

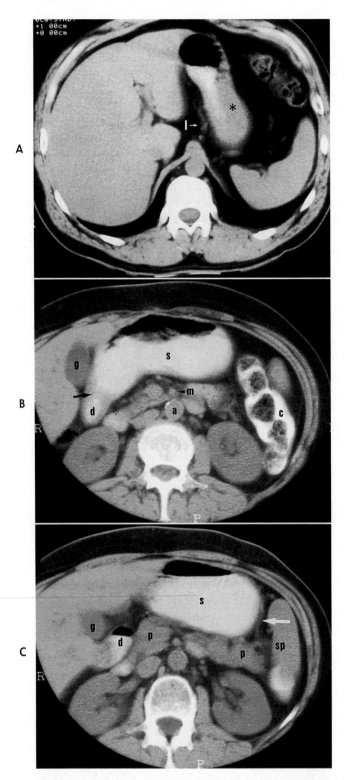

Fig. 14-13 Computed tomographic images of the upper abdomen. **A,** Note the apparent increase in gastric wall thickness (*) due to underdistention and the obliquity of the slice. *l,* Left gastric vessels. **B,** Lower slice showing stomach *(s)* and second part of the duodenum *(d).* Note the retrogastric position of the pancreas *(p)* and the short gastric vessels *(white arrow). sp,* spleen. **C,** Lower slice through the pylorus *(p),* showing the relation of the stomach *(s)* to the gallbladder *(g),* superior mesenteric artery *(m),* and colon *(c). a,* Aorta; *d,* duodenum.
B and **C** courtesy of Dr. S. J. Golding.

pelvis to the level of the symphysis pubis, thus fully evaluating the entire peritoneal cavity for possible occult metastatic disease. These images are then reviewed at appropriate soft tissue window settings (WW400HU and WL+40HU). The liver should also be imaged, but at a narrower window width.

This standard routine should be adequate in most cases. However, various modifications can be made to allow a more detailed "organ-specific" examination. Zerhouni et al.[142] have described a gas-contrast technique for use in the CT examination of the stomach and duodenum. Following an overnight fast, patients are given effervescent granules and an antifoaming agent (as in a DCBM investigation), with a small quantity of water. Scanning then proceeds in the standard manner already described. Specific positioning of the patient may improve visualization of certain parts of the stomach. If the location of the abnormality is known in advance, the patient can be positioned accordingly before scanning. The region of the gastroesophageal junction, posterior gastric wall, and greater curve are best demonstrated with the patient prone. The lesser curve and antrum are seen best in the supine and left lateral decubitus positions. After these images are reviewed, equivocally abnormal areas can be rescanned after further gastric distention is produced with gas or oral contrast or by changing the patient's position according to the site of abnormality.

The duodenum is usually well demonstrated using these techniques. When using the gas-contrast technique, placing the patient in the left lateral decubitus position and administering a hypotonic agent (0.1-0.5 mg of glucagon intravenously) improves duodenal distention. Water[143] and corn oil emulsion[144] have also been used as oral contrast agents, but have not gained widespread acceptance.

Normal CT anatomy

Adequate gastric distention abolishes the mucosal fold pattern. This allows accurate assessment of the gastric wall thickness, which normally is approximately 3 mm but should not exceed 5 mm. Such measurements are subject to errors brought about by gastric underdistention as well as the obliquity of the axial slice through the wall, particularly in the region of the cardia (Fig. 14-13, *A*). An intraluminal bulge at the cardia producing a pseudotumor appearance, similar to what is seen on DCBM studies, is due to a normal gastroesophageal junction.

The lesser (gastrohepatic) omentum and its internal structures are visible on most CT scans (Fig. 14-13, *B*). The normal CT appearance of this region has been well documented.[145] This is a common site of regional lymph node metastases from gastric or lower esophageal tumors. Nonenhancing nodules greater than 8 mm in diameter are likely to represent significant lymphadenopathy.

The anatomic relationships of the duodenum have already been described. Most of the duodenum lies retroperitoneally in the anterior pararenal space. When adequately distended, its wall should not be more than 1 mm thick. Its anatomic location explains why the duodenum may be involved in a variety of disorders arising in adjacent structures, in particular lesions within the pancreatic head, gallbladder, and right kidney. CT is well suited to evaluate such cases.

Magnetic resonance imaging

To date, MRI has failed to make a significant impact on the practice of gastrointestinal radiology, and this is due to several factors, including the limitation of anatomic resolution resulting from cardiovascular, respiratory, and peristaltic motion. Until recently, there was a lack of adequate and readily available oral contrast agents. In addition, images are subject to further degradation because of the need to use a large-diameter receiver coil. Glucagon has been used to abolish intestinal peristalsis, with some improvement in image quality.[146] Fasting for 4 to 6 hours before scanning also results in less image artifact because bowel motion is decreased.

Several imaging sequences have been used in an attempt to reduce the acquisition times and motion artifacts. Gradient motion rephasing[147] and spatial presaturation both improve image quality. An alternative approach is to use ultrafast imaging techniques[148] that "freeze" bowel peristalsis. Images can then be viewed in a cine loop, allowing visualization of the gastrointestinal tract in real time.

A variety of oral contrast agents have been studied.[149] An ideal agent should have all of the following qualities: good contrast effect in all imaging sequences, as well as being nontoxic, palatable, and inexpensive. Substances that produce a brightening of the bowel lumen on both T1 and T2 spin-echo sequences are termed *positive contrast agents*. Conversely, those that cause darkening of the lumen with these sequences are termed *negative contrast agents*. Positive contrast can also be achieved with STIR or T2 imaging, in which water appears hyperintense.

Several positive contrast agents have been described. These include paramagnetic agents such as ferric ammonium citrate and gadolinium (Gd-DTPA). Short T1 contrast agents such as oil emulsions exhibit a high signal intensity on T1 sequences and are suitable for demonstrating the stomach and proximal small bowel, but tend to be absorbed and are consequently inadequate for imaging of the more distal small bowel and colon.

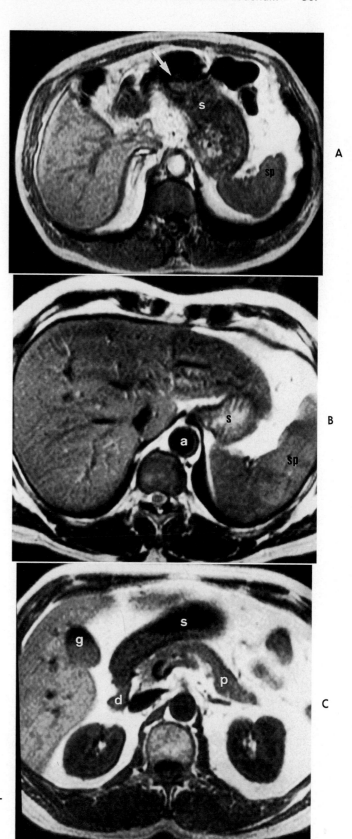

Fig. 14-14 Axial (transverse) magnetic resonance images of the upper abdomen. **A,** Gradient echo sequence obtained during arrested respiration. Note ghost artifact resulting from the aorta *(arrow)*. **B,** T2 fast spin-echo. **C,** T1 fast spin-echo sequence. *a,* Aorta; *d,* duodenum; *g,* gallbladder; *p,* pancreas; *s,* stomach; *sp,* spleen.
Courtesy of Dr. R. Kerslake.

Negative contrast agents include diamagnetic agents such as clay minerals and barium suspensions. Superparamagnetic agents such as superparamagnetic iron oxide also have a negative contrast effect and yield good results. However, their cost, availability, and unproved safety limit their routine use. Good bowel distention is another essential component of successful bowel imaging and is partly achieved with these oral contrast agents. Osmotic agents such as mannitol may further improve distention.[149]

Further clinical work is needed in this area, as it is currently unclear which oral contrast agent is optimal for use in MRI studies of the gastrointestinal tract.

Normal MRI anatomy

As with CT, the stomach is identified between the liver and spleen on transverse (axial) images of the upper abdomen (Fig. 14-14). The gastric wall is seen as a thin region of intermediate signal intensity between the gastric fluid and adjacent surrounding fat. Gas in the stomach produces a signal void on all sequences. As previously discussed, parts of the bowel may not be sharply delineated because of inadequate luminal contrast, poor distention, motion artifacts, and ghost noise arising from non–periodic motion artifacts. With improvements in both contrast agents and imaging sequences, many of these problems should be overcome.

REFERENCES

1. Cho KC, Gold BM, Printz DA: Multiple transverse folds in the gastric antrum, *Radiology* 164:339, 1987.
2. Evans SE, Ferrando JR, Mike N: The significance of transverse folds in the gastric antrum, *Clin Radiol* 42:405, 1990.
3. Freeny PC: Double-contrast gastrography of the fundus and cardia: normal landmarks and their pathological changes, *AJR* 133:481, 1979.
4. Herlinger H et al: The gastric cardia in double-contrast study: its dynamic image, *AJR* 135:21, 1980.
5. Hodges FM, Snead LO, Berger RA: A stellate impression in the cardiac end of the stomach simulating tumor, *AJR* 47:578, 1942.
6. Mackintosh CE, Kreel L: Anatomy and radiology of the areae gastricae, *Gut* 18:855, 1977.
7. Gelfand DW: High density, low viscosity barium for fine mucosal detail on double-contrast upper gastrointestinal examinations, *AJR* 130:831, 1978.
8. Rose C, Stevenson GW: Correlation between visualization and size of the areae gastricae and duodenal ulcer, *Radiology* 139:371, 1981.
9. Kirby JR: Observations on the duodenal mucosa with reference to problems associated with its three dimensional structure, *Clin Radiol* 24:139, 1973.
10. Glick SN, Gohel VK, Laufer I: Mucosal surface patterns of the duodenal bulb, *Radiology* 150:317, 1984.
11. Bova JG et al: The normal mucosal surface pattern of the duodenal bulb: radiologic-histologic correlation, *AJR* 145:735, 1985.
12. Ferrucci JT et al: Radiographic features of the normal hypotonic duodenogram, *Radiology* 96:401, 1970.
13. Lindner HH, Pena VA, Ruggeri RA: A clinical and anatomical study of anomalous terminations of the common bile duct into the duodenum, *Ann Surg* 184:626, 1976.
14. Keller RJ, Khilnani MT, Wolf BS: Cascade stomach, roentgen appearance and significance, *AJR* 123:746, 1975.
15. Ansel HJ, Wasserman NF: Postsplenectomy gastric deformity, *AJR* 139:99, 1982.
16. Meyers MA, Whalen JP: Roentgen significance of the duodenocolic relationships: an anatomic approach, *AJR* 117:263, 1973.
17. Poppel MH: Duodenocolic apposition, *AJR* 83:851, 1960.
18. Op den Orth JO: Duodenum. In Margulis AR, Burhenne HJ, eds: *Alimentary tract radiology,* ed 4, St Louis, 1989, Mosby–Year Book.
19. Anderson JR, Earnshaw PM, Fraser GM: Extrinsic compression of the third part of the duodenum, *Clin Radiol* 33:75, 1982.
20. Hampton AO: A safe method for the roentgen demonstration of bleeding duodenal ulcers, *AJR* 38:565, 1937.
21. Ruzicka FF, Rigler LG: Inflation of the stomach with double contrast, a roentgen study, *JAMA* 145:696, 1951.
22. Obata WG: A double-contrast technique for examination of the stomach using barium sulfate with simethicone, *AJR* 115:275, 1972.
23. Kreel L, Herlinger H, Glanville J: Technique of the double contrast barium meal with examples of correlation with endoscopy, *Clin Radiol* 24:307, 1973.
24. O'Reilly GVA, Bryan G: The double contrast barium meal—a simplification, *Br J Radiol* 47:482, 1974.
25. Laufer I: A simple method for routine double contrast study of the upper gastrointestinal tract, *Radiology* 117:513, 1975.
26. Hunt JH, Anderson IF: Double contrast upper gastrointestinal studies, *Clin Radiol* 27:87, 1976.
27. Young JW, Ginthner TP, Keramati B: The competitive barium meal, *Clin Radiol* 36:43, 1985.
28. Cotton PB: Fibreoptic endoscopy and the barium meal—results and implications, *BMJ* 2:161, 1973.
29. Cotton PB et al: Early endoscopy of oesophagus, stomach and duodenal bulb in patients with haematemesis and melaena, *BMJ* 2:505, 1973.
30. Kay S: Tissue reaction to barium sulfate contrast medium, *Arch Pathol* 57:279, 1954.
31. Almond CH, Cochran DQ, Shucart WA: Comparative study of the effects of various radiographic contrast media on the peritoneal cavity, *Ann Surg* 154(suppl):219, 1961.
32. Cochran DQ, Almond CH, Shucart WA: An experimental study of the effects of barium and intestinal contents on the peritoneal cavity, *AJR* 89:883, 1963.
33. Westfall RH, Nelson RH, Musselman MM: Barium peritonitis, *Am J Surg* 112:760, 1966.
34. Thoeni RF, Goldberg HI: The influence of smoking on coating of the gastric mucosa during double contrast examination of the stomach, *Invest Radiol* 15:388, 1980.
35. Rose C et al: Cigarette smoking and duodenal coating with barium, *J Can Assoc Radiol* 33:77, 1982.
36. Massoud TF, Nolan DJ: Morning or afternoon barium meal? Diurnal variation and the effectiveness of gastric mucosal coating during double contrast studies, *Clin Radiol* 42:407, 1990.
37. Gopichandran TD, Ring NJ, Beckly DE: Metoclopramide in double contrast barium meals, *Clin Radiol* 31:485, 1980.
38. James WB et al: The effect of cimetidine on barium coating of the gastric mucosa, *Br J Radiol* 50:445, 1977.
39. Cohen MD: The value of cimetidine in routine barium meals, *Br J Radiol* 52:408, 1979.
40. Roberts GM et al: Observations on the behaviour of barium sulphate suspension in gastric secretion, *Br J Radiol* 50:468, 1977.
41. Anderson W et al: Barium sulphate preparations for use in double contrast examination of the upper gastrointestinal tract. *Br J Radiol* 53:1150, 1980.
42. Montgomery DP et al: A comparison of barium sulphate preparations used for the double contrast barium meal, *Clin Radiol* 33:265, 1982.
43. Rubesin SE, Herlinger H: The effect of barium suspension viscosity on the delineation of areae gastricae, *AJR* 146:35, 1986.
44. Virkkunen P, Retulainen M: A new method for studying barium sulphate contrast media in vitro. Some factors contributing to the visualisation of areae gastricae, *Br J Radiol* 53:765, 1980.

45. Roberts GM et al: In vivo and in vitro assessment of barium sulphate suspensions, *Br J Radiol* 50:541, 1977.

46. Janower ML: Hypersensitivity reactions after barium studies of the upper and lower gastrointestinal tract, *Radiology* 161:139, 1986.

47. Mahboubi S et al: Barium embolization following upper gastrointestinal examination, *Radiology* 111:301, 1974.

48. Ansell G: Alimentary tract. In Ansell G, Wilkins RA, eds: *Complications in diagnostic imaging,* ed 2, Oxford, 1987, Blackwell Scientific Publications.

49. Harris PD, Neuhauser EBD, Gerth R: The osmotic effect of water soluble contrast media on circulating plasma volume, *AJR* 91:694, 1964.

50. Ansell G: A national survey of radiological complications: interim report, *Clin Radiol* 19:175, 1968.

51. Reich SB: Production of pulmonary oedema by aspiration of water-soluble nonabsorbable contrast media, *Radiology* 92:367, 1969.

52. Bell KE, McKinstry CS, Mills JOM: Iopamidol in the diagnosis of suspected upper gastro-intestinal perforation, *Clin Radiol* 38:165, 1987.

53. Miller RE et al: Hypotonic roentgenography with glucagon, *AJR* 121:264, 1974.

54. Kreel L: Pharmaco-radiology in barium examinations with special reference to glucagon, *Br J Radiol* 48:691, 1975.

55. Miller RE et al: Double-blind radiographic study of dose response to intravenous glucagon for hypotonic duodenography, *Radiology* 127:55, 1978.

56. Miller RE et al: Gastrointestinal response to minute doses of glucagon, *Radiology* 143:317, 1982.

57. Lawrence AM: A new provocation test for pheochromocytoma, *Ann Intern Med* 63:905, 1965 (abstract).

58. Rajah RR: Effects of Buscopan on gastro-oesophageal reflux and hiatus hernia, *Clin Radiol* 41:250, 1990.

59. Sissons GRJ, McQueenie A, Mantle M: The ocular effects of hyoscine–butylbromide (Buscopan) in radiological practice, *Br J Radiol* 64:584, 1991.

60. James WB et al: Double contrast barium meal examination—a comparison of techniques for introducing gas, *Clin Radiol* 27:91, 1976.

61. de Lacey GJ, Wignall BK, Bray C: Effervescent granules for the barium meal, *Br J Radiol* 52:405, 1979.

62. Bagnall RD, Galloway RW, Annis JAD: Double contrast preparations: an in vitro study of some antifoaming agents, *Br J Radiol* 50:546, 1977.

63. Pochaczevsky R: Bubbly barium—a carbonated cocktail for double-contrast examination of the stomach, *Radiology* 107:461, 1973.

64. Op den Orth JO, Ploem S: The standard biphasic-contrast gastric series, *Radiology* 122:530, 1977.

65. Gelfand DW, Ott DJ: Single- vs double-contrast gastrointestinal studies: critical analysis of reported statistics, *AJR* 137:523, 1981.

66. Ott DJ, Gelfand DW, Wallace WC: Detection of gastric ulcer: comparison of single- and double-contrast examination, *AJR* 139:93, 1982.

67. Montagne JP, Moss AA, Margulis AR: Double-blind study of single and double contrast upper gastrointestinal examinations using endoscopy as a control, *AJR* 130:1041, 1978.

68. Gelfand DW, Chen YM, Ott DJ: Multiphasic examinations of the stomach: efficacy of individual techniques and combinations of techniques in detecting 153 lesions, *Radiology* 162:829, 1987.

69. Burhenne HJ, Fache SJ: Technique of radiologic examination. In Margulis AR, Burhenne HJ, eds: *Alimentary tract radiology,* ed 4, St Louis, 1989, Mosby–Year Book.

70. Ott DJ et al: Sensitivity of single- vs. double-contrast radiology in erosive gastritis, *AJR* 138:263, 1982.

71. Gelfand DW, Hachiya J: The double contrast examination of the stomach using gas-producing granules and tablets, *AJR* 93:1381, 1969.

72. Ominsky SH, Margulis AR: Radiographic examination of the upper gastrointestinal tract: a survey of current techniques, *Radiology* 139:11, 1981.

73. Maglinte DDT, Dolan PA, Miller RE: Angled radiography in upper gastrointestinal examinations, *AJR* 137:1082, 1981.

74. Eaton SB et al: Comparison of current radiologic approaches to the diagnosis of pancreatic disease, *N Engl J Med* 279:389, 1968.

75. Kreel L: The pancreas: newer radiological methods of investigation, *Postgrad Med J* 43:14, 1967.

76. Raia S, Kreel L: Gas distension, double-contrast duodenography using the Scott-Harden gastroduodenal tube, *Gut* 7:420, 1966.

77. Bilbao MK et al: Hypotonic duodenography, *Radiology* 89:438, 1967.

78. Goldstein HM, Zboralske FF: Tubeless hypotonic duodenography, *JAMA* 210:2086, 1969.

79. Nolan DJ: The duodenum. In Grainger RG, Allison DJ, eds: *Diagnostic radiology, an Anglo-American textbook of imaging,* Edinburgh, 1986, Churchill Livingstone.

80. Wiljasalo M et al: A comparison of double contrast barium meal and endoscopy. *Diagn Imaging* 49:1, 1980.

81. Stevenson GW, Laufer I: Duodenum. In Laufer I, ed: *Double contrast gastrointestinal radiology,* Philadelphia, 1979, WB Saunders.

82. Sear HS, Friedenberg MJ: Simplified technique for tubeless hypotonic duodenography, *Radiology* 103:210, 1972.

83. Gourtsoyiannis NC, Nolan DJ: Combined fine needle percutaneous transhepatic cholangiography and hypotonic duodenography in obstructive jaundice, *Clin Radiol* 30:507, 1979.

84. Field S: The acute abdomen—the plain radiograph. In Grainger RG, Allison DJ, eds: *Diagnostic radiology, an Anglo-American textbook of imaging,* Edinburgh, 1986, Churchill Livingstone.

85. Jacobson G et al: The examination of patients with suspected perforated ulcer using a water-soluble contrast medium, *AJR* 86:37, 1961.

86. Foley MJ, Rhahremani GG, Rogers LF: Reappraisal of contrast media used to detect upper gastrointestinal perforations, *Radiology* 144:231, 1982.

87. Dodds WJ, Stewart ET, Vlymen WJ: Appropriate contrast media for evaluation of esophageal disruption, *Radiology* 144:439, 1982.

88. Gold RP, Seaman WB: The primary double-contrast examination of the postoperative stomach, *Radiology* 124:297, 1977.

89. Gohel VK, Laufer I: Double-contrast examination of the postoperative stomach, *Radiology* 129:601, 1978.

90. Hoare AM: Comparative study between endoscopy and radiology in acute upper gastrointestinal haemorrhage, *BMJ* 1:27, 1975.

91. Elmer RA, Rousuck AA, Ryan JM: Early roentgenologic evaluation in patients with upper gastrointestinal haemorrhage, *Gastroenterology* 16:552, 1950.

92. Schatzki SC, Blade WR: Emergency X-ray examination in the diagnosis of severe upper gastrointestinal bleeding, *N Engl J Med* 259:910, 1958.

93. Fraser GM: The double contrast barium meal in patients with acute upper gastrointestinal bleeding, *Clin Radiol* 29:625, 1978.

94. Glanville JN: Further experience with the ward acute barium meal, *Clin Radiol* 16:93, 1965.

95. Herlinger H, Glanville JN, Kree L: An evaluation of the double contrast barium meal (DCBM) against endoscopy, *Clin Radiol* 28:307, 1977.

96. Knutson CO et al: Should flexible fibreoptic endoscopy replace barium contrast study of the upper gastro-intestinal tract? *Surgery* 84:609, 1978.

97. Laufer I, Mullens JE, Hamilton J: The diagnostic accuracy of barium studies of the stomach and duodenum—correlation with endoscopy, *Radiology* 115:569, 1975.

98. Dooley CP et al: Double-contrast barium meal and upper gastrointestinal endoscopy, a comparative study, *Ann Intern Med* 101:538, 1984.

99. Moule B et al: A comparative study of the diagnostic value of upper gastrointestinal endoscopy and radiology, *Gut* 16:411, 1975.

100. Chandie Shaw P et al: Peptic ulcer and gastric carcinoma: diagnosis with biphasic radiography compared with fibreoptic endoscopy, *Radiology* 163:39, 1987.

101. Martin TR et al: A comparison of upper gastrointestinal endoscopy and radiography, *J Clin Gastroenterol* 2:21, 1980.

102. Simpkins KC: What use is barium, *Clin Radiol* 39:469, 1988.

103. Mead GM et al: Uses of barium meal examination in dyspeptic patients under 50, *BMJ* 1:1460, 1977.

104. Davenport PM et al: Can preliminary screening of dyspeptic patients allow more effective use of investigational techniques, *BMJ* 290:217, 1985.

105. Stevenson GW et al: Barium meal or endoscopy? A prospective randomized study of patient preference and physician decision making, *Clin Radiol* 44:317, 1991.

106. Salter RH: Upper gastrointestinal endoscopy in perspective, *Lancet* 2:863, 1975.

107. Laufer I: Assessment of the accuracy of double contrast gastroduodenal radiology, *Gastroenterology* 71:874, 1976.

108. Arfeen S, Salter RH, Girdwood TG: A negative double-contrast barium meal—qualified reassurance, *Clin Radiol* 38:49, 1987.

109. Gelfand DW, Ott DJ, Chen YM: Primary panendoscopy: a radiologist's response, *AJR* 149:519, 1987.

110. Stevenson GW, Cox RR, Roberts CJC: Prospective comparison of double-contrast barium meal examination and fibre-optic endoscopy in acute upper gastrointestinal haemorrhage, *BMJ* 2:723, 1976.

111. Dronfield MW et al: A prospective randomised study of endoscopy and radiology in acute upper gastrointestinal tract bleeding, *Lancet* 1168, 1977.

112. Brearley S et al: The influence of stigmata of recent haemorrhage on death from bleeding peptic ulcer disease, *Br J Surg* 71:901, 1984 (abstract).

113. Foster DN, Miloszewski KJA, Losowsky MS: Stigmata of recent haemorrhage in diagnosis and prognosis of upper gastro-intestinal bleeding, *BMJ* 1:1173, 1978.

114. Wara P: Endoscopic prediction of major rebleeding—a prospective study of stigmata of haemorrhage in bleeding ulcer, *Gastroenterology* 88:1209, 1985.

115. Sandlow LJ et al: A prospective randomized study of the management of upper gastrointestinal haemorrhage, *Am J Gastroenterol* 61:282, 1974.

116. Forrest JAH, Logan RFA: Comparative diagnostic accuracy of barium meal and endoscopy, *BMJ* 1:50, 1977.

117. Fleischer D: Endoscopic therapy of upper gastrointestinal bleeding in humans, *Gastroenterology* 90:217, 1986.

118. Walker B, Smith MJ: Upper gastrointestinal endoscopy—a survey of patients' impressions, *Postgrad Med J* 54:253, 1978.

119. Dooley CP, Weiner JM, Larson AW: Endoscopy or radiography?—the patient's choice, *Am J Med* 80:203, 1986.

120. Webberley MJ, Cuschieri A: Response of patients to upper gastrointestinal endoscopy: effect of inherent personality traits and premedication with diazepam, *BMJ* 285:251, 1982.

121. Stanley TV, Cocking JB: Upper gastro-intestinal endoscopy and radiology in the elderly, *Postgrad Med J* 54:257, 1978.

122. Colin-Jones DG: Endoscopy or radiology for upper gastrointestinal symptoms? *Lancet* 1:1022, 1986.

123. Meyers MA, Ghahremani GG: Complications of fiberoptic endoscopy: 1. esophagoscopy and gastroscopy, *Radiology* 115:293, 1975.

124. Lawrie BWE: Endoscopy and endoscopic retrograde cholangiopancreatography. In Ansell G, Wilkins RA, eds: *Complications in diagnostic imaging*, ed 2, Oxford, 1987, Blackwell Scientific Publications.

125. Clark ML: Upper intestinal endoscopy, *Lancet* 1:629, 1985.

126. Gelfand DW, Ott DJ, Chen YM: Decreasing numbers of gastrointestinal studies—report of data from 69 radiologic practices, *AJR* 148:1133, 1987.

127. Holdstock G, Bruce S: Endoscopy and gastric cancer, *Gut* 22:673, 1981.

128. Holdstock G, Colley S: Failure of increased use of endoscopy to influence the complication rate of peptic ulcer disease, *BMJ* 287:393, 1983.

129. Mann J et al: Scoring system to improve cost-effectiveness of open access endoscopy, *BMJ* 287:937, 1983.

130. Gelfand DW et al: Radiology and endoscopy—a radiologic viewpoint, *Ann Intern Med* 101:550, 1984.

131. Cotton PB, Williams CB: *Practical gastrointestinal endoscopy,* ed 3, Oxford, 1990, Blackwell Scientific Publications.

132. Martin DF: Useful collaboration between endoscopy and barium radiology, *Br J Hosp Med* 45:338, 1991.

133. Shorvon P, Stevenson G: Should radiologists perform endoscopy? *AJR* 147:1078, 1986.

134. Rawlinson J, Tate JJ, Shepherd DFC et al: Through the colonoscope: a radiologist's view. *Clin Radiol* 41:253, 1990.

135. Bartram CI: Should radiologists perform gastrointestinal endoscopy, *Clin Radiol* 40:225, 1989.

136. Sapienza PE et al: Impact of a quality assurance program on gastrointestinal endoscopy, *Gastroenterology* 102:387, 1992.

137. Megibow AJ: CT of the stomach. In Megibow AJ, Balthazar EJ, eds: *Computed tomography of the gastrointestinal tract*, St Louis, 1986, Mosby–Year Book.

138. Balthazar EJ: CT of the gastrointestinal tract: principles and interpretation, *AJR* 156:23, 1991.

139. Goldberg HI, Thoeni RF: MRI of the gastrointestinal tract, *Radiol Clin North Am* 27:805, 1989.

140. Scatarige JC, Di Santis DJ: CT of the stomach and duodenum, *Radiol Clin North Am* 27:687, 1989.

141. Hatfield KD, Segal SD, Tait K: Barium sulfate for abdominal computed assisted tomography, *J Comput Assist Tomogr* 4:570, 1980.

142. Zerhouni EA, Fishman EK, Jones B: Principles and techniques. In Fishman EK, Jones B, eds: *Computed tomography of the gastrointestinal tract*, New York, 1988, Churchill Livingstone.

143. Angelelli G, Macarini L, Fratello A: Use of water as an oral contrast agent for CT study of the stomach, *AJR* 149:1084, 1987.

144. Raptopoulos V et al: Fat-density oral contrast agent for abdominal CT, *Radiology* 164:653, 1987.

145. Balfe DM et al: Gastrohepatic ligament: normal and pathologic CT anatomy, *Radiology* 150:485, 1984.

146. Weinreb JC et al: Improved MR imaging of the upper abdomen with glucagon and gas, *J Comput Assist Tomogr* 8:835, 1984.

147. Haake EM, Lenz GW: Improving MR image quality in the presence of motion by using rephasing gradients, *AJR* 148:1251, 1986.

148. Stehling MK et al: Gastrointestinal tract: dynamic MR studies with Echo-Planar imaging, *Radiology* 171:41, 1989.

149. Weissleder R, Stark DD: *MRI atlas of the abdomen,* London, 1989, Martin Dunitz.

15 Endosonography: Normal Anatomy and Techniques of Examination of the Stomach and Duodenum

JOSE F. BOTET
CHARLES J. LIGHTDALE

THE STOMACH
Normal anatomy
The cardia

The cardia constitutes the transitional zone between the esophagus and the stomach. As seen endoscopically, the cardia lies approximately 40 cm from the incisors. It has a five-layered internal structure similar to that of the esophagus and stomach. Anatomically, it is related posteriorly to the aorta and vertebral bodies and laterally to the inferior azygos vein and thoracic duct on the right. Depending on the position of the cardia and the patient's habitus, it is also related to the inferior vena cava and right atrium anteriorly and to the right. On the left is located the hemiazygos vein. The diaphragm also appears to be closely related to the cardia, and this feature may be identified consistently.

The stomach proper lies between two fixed points, the esophageal hiatus and the first portion of the duodenum. Multiple ligaments and other structures tend to fix the stomach's position. Inferiorly, it lies on the transverse mesocolon, to the right it is fixed by the gastrohepatic ligament and on the left by the gastrolienic ligament. Each of these ligaments carries the major vessels that furnish the arterial blood supply and venous drainage along the greater and lesser curve. The major vessels identifiable on endoscopic ultrasonography are the left gastric artery and the arcade of the lesser curve. The gastroepiploic arteries and attending draining veins may also be identified along the greater curve. The short gastric arteries arising from the splenic artery are not commonly seen. The venous drainage may become quite noticeable in patients with portal hypertension. These ligaments are also responsible for conveying a substantial portion of the organ's lymphatic drainage[1,2] (Fig. 15-1).

From an endosonographic point of view, the stomach is a distensible organ that can be filled with water (Fig. 15-2). This permits close evaluation of the gastric wall with a directable endoscope.[3-20] Once the stomach is filled with water, it is possible to see the wall just as clearly as

is the case with regular endoscopy. The stomach can be divided into three arbitrary segments: the fundus, body, and antrum. The boundaries between these segments are not as clearly defined as in the esophagus. There are, however, specific endoscopic relationships characteristic of each segment.

Fundus

The fundal region begins at the cardia and extends inferiorly for an indeterminate length. In its most superior aspect, the anterior relationships of the fundus are variable and depend on the prominence of the left hepatic lobe. In most normal subjects the superior aspect of the left hepatic lobe constitutes the most anterior relationship, but, in patients with small left hepatic lobes, the diaphragm holds this position. In a clockwise direction, the diaphragm is usually seen with the left lower lobe of the lung above it. This usually extends to the 5 o'clock position. At this level the diaphragmatic crura can be seen, with the aorta centrally, the hemiazygos vein to the left, and the azygos vein and thoracic duct on the right. The vertebral body lies posteromedially to the aorta. At the 7 o'clock position is seen the inferior vena cava. Three types of presentation are commonly encountered, and consist of the inferior vena cava and right atrium; the suprahepatic and intrahepatic cavae with the junction of the right, middle, and left hepatic veins. The right hepatic lobe and lateral segment extend from the 7 to 12 o'clock position (Fig. 15-3).

At a slightly lower level, it may be possible to identify the celiac axis (Fig. 15-4). In patients with no variant anatomy, its three branches, the splenic, hepatic, and left gastric arteries, may be followed on real-time evaluation. The left gastric artery and vein can be easily traced along the lesser curve of the stomach, and the gastroepiploic artery and vein may be seen along the greater curve.

The lymphatic drainage of this area is rich and is toward the diaphragm and diaphragmatic hiatus, following the gastrohepatic and gastrosplenic ligaments. Endosonography may visualize nodes as small as 2 mm in these areas.

311

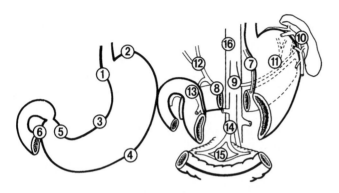

Fig. 15-1 Lymphatic drainage of the stomach. Endoscopic ultrasound can evaluate all the nodes depicted, except for mesenteric and omental nodes 14 and 15.

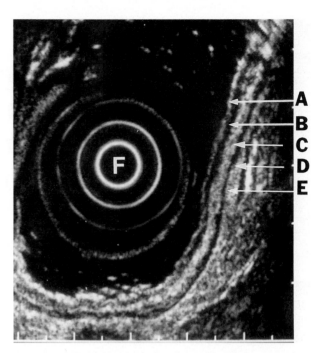

Fig. 15-2 Normal gastric wall showing the five layers. Notice that the balloon is filled with water to maintain the transducer a minimum distance of 1 cm from the wall. *A,* Mucosa (hyperechoic); *B,* lamina propria (hypoechoic); *C,* submucosa (hyperechoic); *D,* muscularis propria (hypoechoic); *E,* serosa (hyperechoic); *F,* transducer in water-filled stomach.

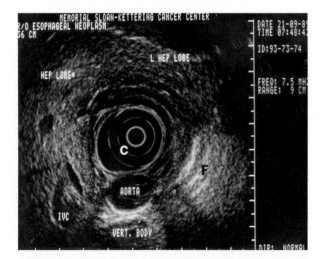

Fig. 15-3 Cardia. Beginning at the 12 o'clock position: *L HEP LOBE,* left hepatic lobe; *F,* air in gastric fundus. The aorta and vertebral body can be seen posteriorly. Notice the elongated shape of the inferior vena cava *(IVC)* in its intrahepatic portion. *C,* Transducer in the cardia.

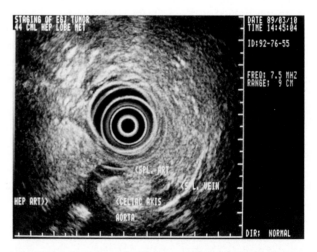

Fig. 15-4 Celiac axis, as seen through the gastric body. Beginning at the 12 o'clock position: *SPL. ART,* Splenic artery; *SPL. VEIN,* splenic vein; *HEP ART,* hepatic artery.

Body

There is a lack of intragastric anatomic landmarks that can be used to define the limits of the three regions. The plane defining the lower end of the fundus and upper end of the body is arbitrary (Fig. 15-5). This also applies to the lower limits of the body, which includes the incisura angularis. This structure surprisingly cannot be identified consistently on endosonography when performed with the stomach fully distended (Fig. 15-6). This area is instead defined by its extragastric relationships, and includes the following landmarks. With regard to the liver, it is possible to identify the most medial aspect of the left portal vein and the spleen is reproducibly seen; this includes the splenic hilum and the splenic artery and vein. These are followed medially to the aorta. Occasionally the left kidney's upper pole may be seen and, in approximately 10% of cases, again depending on the position and shape of the stomach, the left renal vein may be visualized. Posteriorly, the body and tail of the pancreas can be identified consistently.

The major vessels in this area are the celiac axis, splenic vein, and left portal vein (Fig. 15-4).

This area possesses an extremely rich lymphatic drainage. The main lymphatic chains may be followed on real-time imaging by tracing the vessels from the celiac axis to the end-organ and then following the venous drainage back.

Antrum

There is a progressive decrease in the number and prominence of the rugal folds from a maximum at the fundus to a minimum at the antrum. There is a rapid increase in the thickness of the muscularis propria in the immediate prepyloric area (Fig. 15-7). These features allow the sonographer to determine at a glance the position of the scope. As already mentioned, the proximal limits of the antrum are poorly defined. The distal limit is the pylorus. Therefore, this region is also defined by its extragastric relationships.

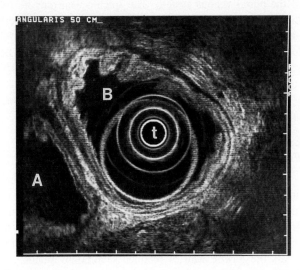

Fig. 15-6 Junction of the body and antrum. Imaging through the lesser curve at the incisura angularis, the antrum *(A)* can be identified. *B,* Body of stomach filled with water; *t,* transducer with water-filled balloon.

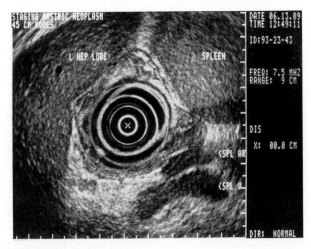

Fig. 15-5 Junction of fundus and body. *L HEP LOBE,* Left hepatic lobe. Posteriorly lie the splenic artery *(SPL AR)* and the splenic vein *(SPL V).*

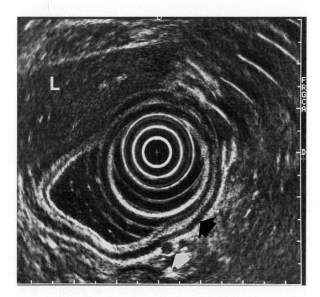

Fig. 15-7 Antrum. Notice the progressive thickening of the muscularis propria *(black arrow).* Also seen are the gastroepiploic artery and vein *(white arrow). L,* Liver.

The inferior aspect of the lateral segment of the left lobe as well as the medial aspect of the right hepatic lobe can be visualized. Important anatomic landmarks are the porta hepatis, usually found at the 10 or 11 o'clock position, and the junction of the splenic and superior mesenteric veins posteriorly (Fig. 15-8). This last relationship defines the uncinate process and the junction of the head and body of the pancreas, which lie posteriorly.

The major vascular relationships at this level are those of the portal venous system. The splenic vein may be followed medially to its junction with the superior mesenteric vein, forming the portal vein. This vessel may then be followed into the porta hepatis, together with the common hepatic artery and the extrahepatic bile duct system. The bifurcation of the portal vein may also be observed.

The lymphatics in this area drain the peripancreatic space and the porta hepatis region.

Examination technique
Preparation

As in the case of the esophageal examination, patients are instructed to neither eat nor drink after midnight the night before the study. A similar preprocedure processing and consent protocol is also used. Patients undergoing the procedure are given an oral preparation, or "cocktail," that clears the gastric wall of retained secretions, mucus, and small clots.[21] The oropharynx is then sprayed with a topical anesthetic. The patient's vital signs are determined at periods varying between 1 and 5 minutes. The patient is then placed in the left lateral decubitus position. An intravenous line is started and the patient receives intravenous sedation, usually a combination of meperidine and a short-acting benzodiazepine.

Procedure

As in the esophageal examination, the usual procedure for examination of the stomach consists of three parts: an initial evaluation with a conventional endoscope, the endosonography proper, and biopsies, if required, performed through a conventional endoscope.

Once the conventional endoscope is removed, the endosonographic scope is introduced and advanced to the first or second portion of the duodenum. Once in the stomach, the scope is advanced through the pylorus. Difficulties may occur here because the most commonly used instrument (Olympus GFM3) is a side-viewing scope and its design makes it difficult to appreciate the position of the pyloric channel. The proximal duodenum is then examined using the water-filled balloon technique as the instrument is slowly withdrawn through the pylorus. Once in the stomach, the organ is distended with 300 to 400 ml of deaerated water. The 2-cm-diameter balloon at the tip of the instrument is kept filled with water so that the tip of the transducer is maintained 1 cm from the gastric wall, providing optimal images in the focal zone.

The examination is performed while the instrument is very slowly withdrawn from the antrum. It is usually advisable to go back in several times to look for specific anatomic landmarks. As mentioned in the section on the esophagus, slow rhythmic respiratory motions move the endoscope back and forth over any area of interest. The greater and lesser curves as well as the posterior and anterior walls of the stomach are usually investigated.

There are several common problems that may be encountered in the evaluation of the stomach.

One of these is residual air in the stomach. In the normal left lateral decubitus position customarily used for the performance of conventional endoscopy, the superior medial aspect of the gastric fundus as well as the distal antrum tend to fill with air. There are two ways in which this problem can be overcome. One is to use the water-filled balloon to obtain acoustic contact between the wall and the transducer, and this strategy usually works in the distal antrum where the lumen narrows. The second approach is to turn the patient supine or in extreme cases into the right lateral decubitus. The latter position usually causes the stomach to empty, which may then require refilling.

Retroflexion of the endoscope may also pose a problem. This can be detected on real time as the image appears to flip 180 degrees, showing a reversal of the normal anatomy.

There may also be problems with residual fluid. Aspirating these through the scope or through a large-bore tube placed in the stomach may eliminate this problem. Usually, however, enough debris is retained to produce significant artifacts (floaters) that can detract from the quality of the images.

THE DUODENUM
Normal anatomy

The duodenum lies between the pylorus and the ligament of Treitz. It is a hollow tube, approximately 30 cm long, that drapes around the head of the pancreas and is located both intra- and retroperitoneally. Masses in the retroperitoneum may affect its usual enlongated C shape. Anatomically, it is divided into four parts.

From an endosonographic perspective, only the first and second portions can be imaged consistently because the scope is not long enough to reach much beyond this point. The third portion can be evaluated in less than 30% of cases.

Once the transducer is passed through the pylorus (Fig. 15-8), it enters the first portion of the duodenum. At this level, the inferior vena cava can be seen as a longitudinal vascular structure. If the common bile duct is dilated, it may also be visualized at this level. As the transducer passes

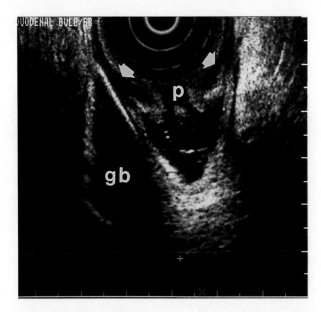

Fig. 15-8 Duodenal bulb. Notice the increased thickening of the muscularis *(arrows)* as the pylorus *(p)* is approached. The bulb is filled with water. Also notice the close relationship to the gallbladder *(gb)*.

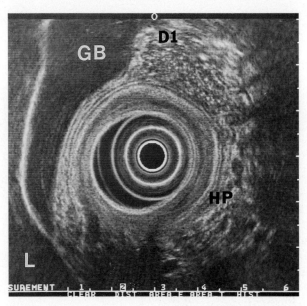

Fig. 15-9 Second portion of the duodenum. Clockwise beginning at the 12 o'clock position, the first portion of the duodenum *(D1)* is filled with water, next is seen the head of the pancreas *(HP)*, the liver *(L)*, and the gallbladder *(GB)*.

the approximate junction of the first and second portion of the duodenum, the gallbladder can be visualized where it is intimately related to the superior anterior wall. The cystic duct may be seen at this level. Medially it is possible to identify the superior aspect of the head of the pancreas.

The second portion of the duodenum is related in its superior and anterior aspect to the gallbladder (Fig. 15-9) and in its medial aspect to the head of the pancreas. The ampulla of Vater can be identified as the site where the pancreatic duct and common bile duct meet.[22] At the junction of the second and third portions of the duodenum, the right renal artery and vein, inferior vena cava (Fig. 15-10), and the superior mesenteric vein, including its junction with the splenic vein to form the portal vein, may be visualized. This area abuts the uncinate portion of the pancreas medially and the upper pole of the right kidney laterally.

The lymphatic drainage in this region is rich, as periduodenal nodes provide drainage for both the duodenum and the pancreas. Nodes are usually found in the immediate periduodenal space. They drain systemically but, of more importance in this context, into the periportal space.[23]

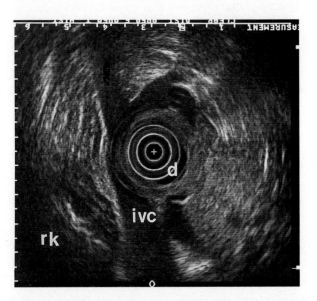

Fig. 15-10 Third portion of the duodenum. The inferior vena cava *(ivc)* appears as a longitudinal structure passing quite close to the duodenum *(d)*. *rk,* Right kidney.

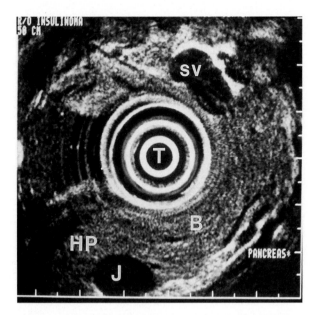

Fig. 15-11 Head and body of the pancreas. Seen in a clockwise direction: *SV,* Splenic vein; *B,* body of pancreas (notice the normal pancreatic duct next to it); *J,* junction of splenic and superior mesenteric vein to form the portal vein; *HP,* head of pancreas. The transducer *(T)* is in the antrum.

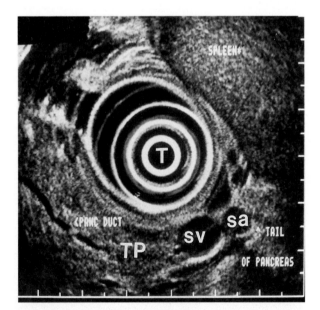

Fig. 15-12 Tail of the pancreas. Seen in a clockwise direction are the spleen and the vessels arising from the splenic hilum; *sa,* Splenic artery; *sv,* splenic vein. Next are seen the tail of the pancreas *(TP)* and the pancreatic duct *(panc duct).* The transducer *(T)* is in the body of the stomach along the greater curve.

The pancreas can be visualized in its entirety through the stomach and duodenum[24-27] (Figs. 15-11 and 15-12).

Examination technique
Preparation

Patients are told to neither eat nor drink after midnight the night before the procedure. The patient goes through a preprocedure interview in which a short clinical history is obtained, vital signs are recorded, and the results of pertinent prior studies and laboratory tests are reviewed. Informed consent is obtained. An intravenous line is started, and the patient drinks a special cocktail to clear secretions from the mucosal wall. The patient's vital signs, including pulse oximetry values, are determined and the patient is placed in the left lateral decubitus position. Oxygen, given via a nasal cannula, is routinely administered at the rate of 2 liters per minute. The oropharynx is sprayed with a topical anesthetic solution and the patient receives intravenous sedation, usually a combination of meperidine and a short-acting benzodiazepine.

Procedure

The procedure is usually divided into three parts. The first is a preliminary endoscopic examination of the upper gastrointestinal tract, in which suspected abnormalities are noted. Next the endosonographic procedure is carried out. The instrument is advanced as far into the duodenum as possible. The duodenal wall and surrounding structures are visualized as the instrument is withdrawn. Acoustic contact can be maintained with the water-filled balloon or, if the duodenum is distended, water can be instilled through the endoscope to fill the duodenal lumen. In such cases, glucagon must be used to halt peristalsis.

There are several common difficulties that may be encountered in this area, one of which is entering the duodenum. Excessive peristalsis poses another common problem. This may require the use of smooth muscle relaxants such as glucagon. Patient intolerance is a third difficulty. To evaluate the distal duodenum, the full length of the scope must be introduced. This is uncomfortable and many patients become restless despite the intravenous sedation. Further sedative doses may thus be required. This makes it essential to have trained personnel to monitor the patient's vital signs.

Duodenal abnormalities are uncommon. However, the water-filled duodenum can act as an acoustic window for the evaluation of surrounding structures such as the pancreas. The examination is tailored to a great extent by the specific suspicious findings that prompted the procedure. It is usually necessary to move the scope only minimally in the evaluation of the pancreas, as respiratory motions move the scope by as much as 1 cm. This has a particular bearing on the examination if identification of the ampulla of Vater is relevant.

REFERENCES

1. Tio TL, Tytgat GNJ: Endoscopic ultrasound in analysing peri-intestinal lymph node abnormality, *Scand J Gastroenterol* 21(suppl 123):158, 1986.
2. Aibe T, Ito T, Yoshida T et al: Endoscopic ultrasonography of lymph nodes surrounding the upper GI tract, *Scand J Gastroenterol* 21(suppl 123):164, 1986.
3. Tio TL, Tytgat GNJ: Endoscopic ultrasonography of normal and pathologic gastrointestinal wall structure. Comparison of studies in vivo and in vitro with histology, *Scand J Gastroenterol* 21(suppl 123):27, 1986.
4. Tio TL, den Hartog Jager FCA, Tytgat GNJ: Endoscopic ultrasonography of non-Hodgkin lymphoma of the stomach, *Gastroenterology* 91:401, 1986.
5. Tio TL, den Hartog Jager FCA, Tytgat GNJ: The role of endoscopic ultrasonography in assessing local resectability of esophagogastric malignancies. Accuracy, pitfalls and predictability, *Scand J Gastroenterol* 21(suppl 123):78, 1986.
6. Caletti GC, Bolondi L, Zani L et al: Technique of endoscopic ultrasonography investigation: esophagus, stomach and duodenum, *Scand J Gastroenterol* 21(suppl 123):1, 1986.
7. Bolondi L, Caletti GC, Casanova P et al: Problems and variations in the interpretation of the ultrasound feature of the normal upper and lower GI tract wall, *Scand J Gastroenterol* 21(suppl 123):16, 1986.
8. Yasuda K, Nakajima M, Kawai K: Endoscopic ultrasonography in the diagnosis of submucosal tumors of the upper digestive tract, *Scand J Gastroenterol* 21(suppl 123):59, 1986.
9. Botet JF, Lightdale C: Endoscopic ultrasonography of the upper gastrointestinal tract, *AJR* 156:63, 1991.
10. Tio TL, Tytgat GNJ: Endoscopic ultrasonography in the assessment of intra and transmural infiltration of tumors in the esophagus and papilla of Vater and in the detection of extraesophageal lesions, *Endoscopy* 16:203, 1984.
11. Lux G, Heyder N, Lutz H et al: Endoscopic ultrasonography—technique, orientation and diagnostic possibilities, *Endoscopy* 14:220, 1982.
12. Heyder N: Endoscopic ultrasonography of tumors of the esophagus and stomach, *Surg Endosc* 1:17, 1987.
13. Boyce GA, Sivak MV, Rosch T et al: Evaluation of submucosal upper gastrointestinal tract lesions by endoscopic ultrasound, *Gastrointest Endosc* 37:449, 1991.
14. Botet JF, Lightdale C, Zauber AG et al: Comparison of endoscopic US and dynamic CT, *Radiology* 181:426, 1991.
15. Tio TL, Coene PPLO, Schouwink MH et al: Esophagogastric carcinoma: preoperative TNM classification with endosonography, *Radiology* 173:411, 1989.
16. Caletti GL, Zani L, Bolondi L et al: Endoscopic ultrasonography in the diagnosis of gastric submucosal tumor, *Gastrointest Endoscop* 35:413, 1989.
17. Yasuda K, Nakajima M, Yoshida T et al: The diagnosis of submucosal tumors of the stomach by endoscopic ultrasonography, *Gastrointest Endoscop* 35:10, 1989.
18. Nakazawa S, Yoshino J, Nakamura T et al: Endoscopic ultrasonography of gastric myogenic tumor. A comparitive study between histology and ultrasonography, *J Ultrasound Med* 8:353, 1989.
19. Lightdale CJ, Botet JF, Kelsen DP et al: Diagnosis of recurrent upper gastrointestinal cancer at the surgical anastomosis by endoscopic ultrasound, *Gastrointest Endoscop* 35:407, 1989.
20. Caletti G, Brocchi E, Baraldini M et al: Assessment of portal hypertension by endoscopic ultrasonography, *Gastrointest Endoscop* 36(suppl):S21, 1990.
21. Yiengpruksawan A, Lightdale CJ, Gerdes H, Botet JF: Mucolytic-antifoam solution for reduction of artifacts during endoscopic ultrasonography: a randomized controlled trial, *Gastrointest Endosc* 37:543, 1991.
22. Yasuda K, Nakajima M, Kawai K: Technical aspects of endoscopic ultrasonography of the biliary system, *Scand J Gastroenterol* 21(suppl 123):143, 1986.
23. Pissa A, Rabischong P: The lymphatic drainage of the pancreas, *Eur J Lymphol* 1:69, 1990.
24. Boyce GA, Sivak MV: Endoscopic ultrasonography in the diagnosis of pancreatic tumors, *Gastrointest Endoscop* 36(suppl):S28, 1990.
25. Lightdale CJ, Botet JF, Woodruff JM et al: Localization of endocrine tumors of the pancreas with endoscopic ultrasonography, *Cancer* 68:1815, 1991.
26. Yasuda K, Hidekazu M, Fujimoto S et al: The diagnosis of pancreatic cancer by endoscopic ultrasonography, *Gastrointest Endoscop* 34:1, 1988.
27. Rosch T, Lightdale CJ, Botet JF et al: Localization of pancreatic endocrine tumors by endoscopic ultrasonography, *N Engl J Med* 326:1721-26, 1992.

16 *Nonneoplastic Diseases of the Stomach*

CHARLES A. ROHRMANN, JR.
SIDNEY W. NELSON

CONGENITAL LESIONS

Congenital lesions of the stomach that are encountered in neonates and children are described in Chapter 98. Those that become symptomatic after childhood or those likely to be discovered incidentally during radiographic examinations in adults are described in this chapter.

Gastric duplication

→non-communicating (common form)
↳communicating (rare)

Gastric duplication, also known as *duplication cyst*, *enterogenous cyst*, *supernumerary stomach*, *gastric cyst*, *embryonal cyst*, *enterocystoma*, and *accessory stomach*, remains a rare phenomenon.[1] The noncommunicating duplication cyst is contiguous with the gastric wall and is lined with alimentary epithelium. In a series of 55 cases collected from the literature, 15 occurred in patients more than 12 years of age, 35 were found along the greater curve, and the size ranged to more than 11 cm.[2] Although gastric duplications do not usually communicate with the stomach lumen, near total duplication has been reported, with barium seen to outline both lumina.[3]

The radiographic appearance of noncommunicating duplications may be indistinguishable from that presented by other intramural masses; in that the margins are smooth, the overlying folds are normal or stretched, and the mucosa is normal. There may be surface ulceration, however (Fig. 16-1).[1] The liquid nature of the cyst contents may permit the configuration to be altered because of the influence of peristalsis or external compression, similar to what happens with alimentary tract lipomas. Computed tomography (CT) and ultrasound can demonstrate the duplication's relationship to the gastric wall and also characterize its content.[1,4]

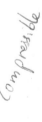
Compressible

Gastric diverticulum

Most gastric diverticula arise from the posteromedial wall of the stomach near the esophagogastric junction, with sizes ranging from 2 to 10 cm.[5] They are easily identified because of their constant location and typical appearance, consisting of a mucosally lined outpouching that varies in size and shape (Fig. 16-2, *A*). They were considered to represent congenital or true diverticula, in which all the layers of the gut are involved, unlike the false, acquired, or pulsion diverticula, which are composed largely of mucosa and submucosa. However, in a series of such diverticula studied after resection, no muscular coat was found in six of seven specimens.[6] This indicates they are false or acquired diverticula, but their constant anatomic location near the esophagogastric junction suggests that an underlying muscle defect may predispose to their development.[7]

Gastric diverticula are rarely symptomatic, but hemorrhage has been reported in up to 10% of them.[8,9] They can simulate an adrenal mass on CT scans (Fig. 16-2, *B*). This has caused some investigators to speculate that the gastric diverticulum herniates through an embryologic retroperitoneal defect near Gerota's fascia.[10,11]

The term *partial diverticulum* has been used to refer to an intramural projection of mucosa without distortion of the serosal layer.[12] These are invariably located along the distal antral greater curve and can be associated with ectopic pancreatic tissue[5] (Fig. 16-3). In rare instances a large diverticulum may occur more proximally on the greater curve of the stomach[13] (Fig. 16-4).

Adenomyosis

The term *adenomyosis* refers to a histologic spectrum of disorders consisting of an excessive proliferation of glandular and other mural tissue in the gastric wall. Included in this category are an ectopic or an aberrant or heterotopic pancreas, Brunner's gland hyperplasia, adenomyoma, myoepithelial hamartoma, and cystic malformation of the stomach.[14-17] Histologically the spectrum ranges from adenomyoma, which consists of poorly differentiated glandular and muscular structures, to well-differentiated lesions containing acini of Brunner's glands or pancreas. It is not possible to differentiate among these submucosal lesions on a radiographic basis unless the characteristic central umbilication of an ectopic pancreas is demonstrated.

Ectopic pancreas

The frequency with which an ectopic pancreas occurs depends on the diligence of the search, and ranges from 1% to 14% in the reports of autopsy series. It is nine times more common in the stomach than is leiomyoma. The lesion is considered to be congenital and is most frequently found incidentally in asymptomatic adults during either an upper gastrointestinal (GI) contrast examination or endoscopy.[17]

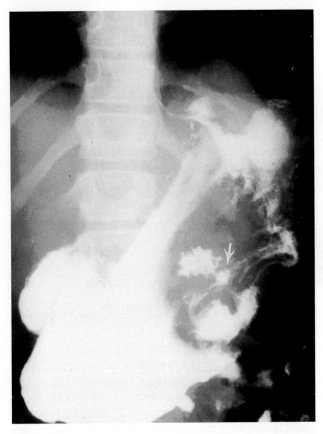

Fig. 16-1 Duplication cyst. A large smooth mass impresses the posterolateral wall of the gastric body, and superimposed small intestine projects over the lesion. The mucosa was normal except for focal ulceration *(arrow)*.

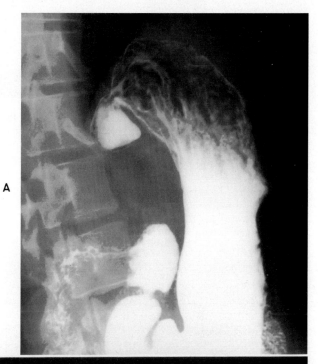

A

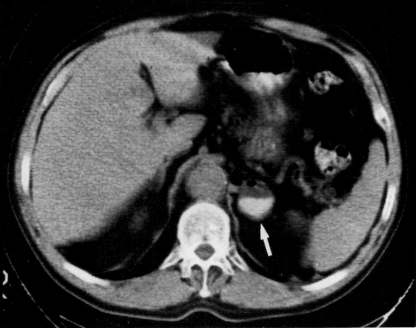

B

Fig. 16-2 Gastric diverticulum. **A,** In the right anterior oblique projection, diverticulum projects posteromedially from the stomach near the esophagogastric junction. Note the normal mucosa extending into the diverticulum. **B,** Computed tomogram shows gastric diverticulum containing contrast material *(arrow)* posterior to the splenic artery.
B Courtesy of Dr. Alan Schwartz.

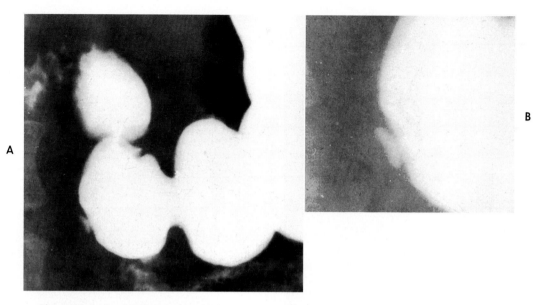

Fig. 16-3 A, Partial diverticulum of the greater curve was associated with ectopic pancreatic tissue. **B,** Detail of the diverticulum.

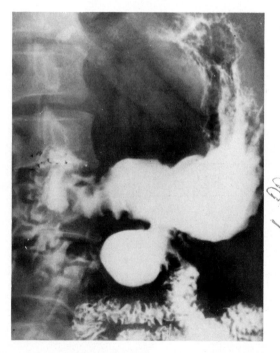

Fig. 16-4 True gastric diverticulum arising from the distal greater curve contained all of the normal layers of the gastric wall. From Dodd GD, Sheft D: *AJR* 107:102, 1969.

Although most foci of ectopic pancreas are asymptomatic and represent incidental findings, obstruction can result if the lesion arises in a strategic location, such as the pyloric channel or periampullary duodenum.[18] All of the pathologic changes that may take place in the pancreas proper have been observed in the ectopic foci, including pancreatitis, carcinoma, and hyperinsulinism.[14]

An ectopic pancreas typically occurs as an umbilicated submucosal nodule on the greater curve of the stomach, which is 1 to 2 cm in diameter and located 3 to 6 cm from the pylorus (Fig. 16-5, *A* and *B*). In a large radiographic series, 40% were found to exceed 2 cm.[19] Some of the larger lesions may consist of most of the pancreatic gland that is embedded in the gastric wall (Fig. 16-6).

The radiographic appearance of these sessile, submucosal masses may be indistinguishable from a leiomyoma unless a ductlike umbilication exists.[20] The characteristic central depression or umbilication is present in 40% to 60% of the cases and represents a rudimentary duct orifice, which variably communicates with functioning pancreatic ducts. The duct orifice may simulate a small ulcer, but the smooth contour of the mass and absence of surrounding inflammatory changes usually permit differentiation. Precise, reliable identification of this condition can be made if ducts are demonstrated by reflux of barium or by endoscopic injection and opacification[21] (see Fig. 16-5, *C*).

Antral diaphragm or web

An antral diaphragm, or web, may vary from a slight crescentic membrane to a nearly complete septum perforated only by a 1-mm opening.[22] Histologically, it consists of normal, noninflamed gastric mucosa located on either side of a membrane of submucosa and hypertrophied mus-

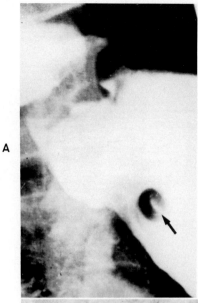

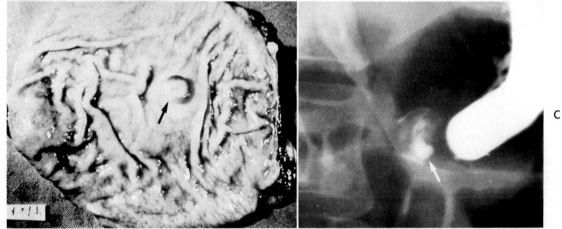

Fig. 16-5 Ectopic pancreas. **A,** Typical antral nodule on the greater curve containing central barium collection *(arrow)*. **B,** Resected gastric antrum showing a 1-cm nodule with central depression *(arrow)*. **C,** In another patient, endoscopic injection of the umbilication shows a rudimentary pancreatic duct system *(arrow)*.

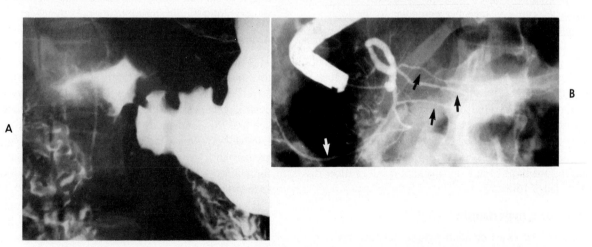

Fig. 16-6 Ectopic pancreas. **A,** Marked fold thickening about the gastric antrum. Contrast reflux into the common bile duct is due to prior sphincteroplasty. **B,** Injection of the pancreatic duct system reveals the presence of an annular duct around the duodenum *(white arrow)* and anomalous ducts in the wall of the gastric antrum *(black arrows)*.
Courtesy of Dr. Martin Green.

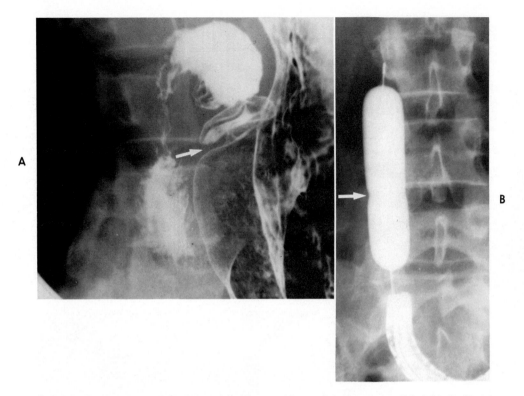

Fig. 16-7 Obstructing antral diaphragm in a 22-year-old woman with postprandial abdominal pain, nausea, and vomiting. **A,** Air contrast view of the antrum shows a constriction 1 cm from the pylorus *(arrow)*. This has produced a "double-bulb" or "double-pylorus" appearance. **B,** At endoscopy, a 3-mm opening was found in a constricting antral web. A transendoscopic wire was placed through the diaphragm and an angioplasty-type balloon catheter was introduced to dilate the web. Note the waist on the balloon *(arrow)* at the web site.

cularis mucosae. It is usually located 1.5 cm away from the pylorus but may be as distant as 7 cm.[23]

In radiographic terms, a constant, symmetric, 2 to 3-mm bandlike deformity is seen perpendicular to the long axis of the antrum. When the stomach distal to this band is distended, this may produce a "double-bulb" effect (Fig. 16-7, *A*). The orifice may be central or eccentric, and peristaltic activity is normal. Associated ulcers are found in 30% to 50% of the cases.[24] Treatment of these lesions consists of the fluoroscopically guided endoscopic placement of a guidewire and balloon dilatation with an angioplasty-type catheter (Fig. 16-7, *B*). Some consider antral diaphragms the sequelae of previous ulcers, because radiographically similar lesions have been a documented result of ulcer disease[25,26] (Fig. 16-8).

Adult pyloric hypertrophy

In a series of cases of adult pyloric obstructions,[27] hypertrophy of the pyloric musculature was found to account for 1%. The pyloric muscle in affected patients is more than 9 mm thick due to both hypertrophy and hyperplasia but without inflammatory changes or fibrosis.[28] The longitudi-

nal muscle is not involved by the hypertrophy and is deficient along the pyloric canal. This causes the pyloric canal to fail to shorten during contraction and explains the classic radiologic finding of elongation of the canal.[29]

Anatomic considerations

Anatomic studies[30] have shown that the circular muscle fibers of the distal stomach are not evenly distributed but form localized thickenings or loops. At the pylorus a muscular loop constitutes the normal division between the stomach and the duodenum, but proximally there is a second, less-well-developed loop. These loops are far apart on the greater curve but intersect on the lesser curve and cross to form a "figure 8," which creates a muscular prominence termed the *torus* (Fig. 16-9).

There are various forms of pyloric hypertrophy,[31] as classified in the box on p. 323. A focal form, limited to the lesser curve where the pyloric muscle loops intersect, is termed *torus hyperplasia*. Diffuse forms of hypertrophy may be associated with benign peptic ulcers, cancer, gastritis, pernicious anemia, and a previous gastroenterostomy.[32-34]

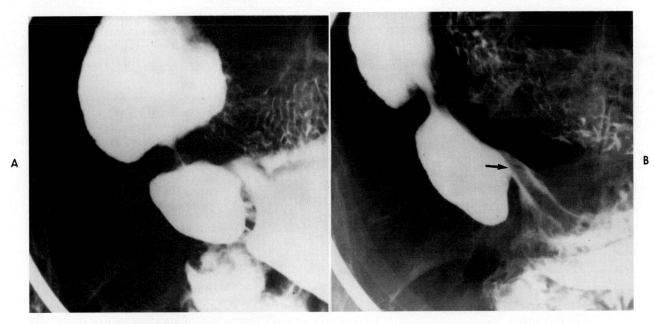

Fig. 16-8 Peptic ulcer scar mimicking an antral diaphragm. **A,** Filled view shows antral septum in a 56-year-old woman with recurrent peptic ulcer disease. **B,** Compression view demonstrates an eccentric lumen *(arrow)*. The "double-pylorus" appearance simulates the antral diaphragm.

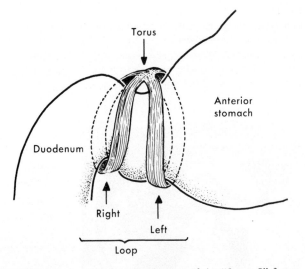

Fig. 16-9 Pyloric musculature. Diagram of the "figure 8" formation of the pyloric muscle fibers based on the description of Torgersen.[30]

☐ **CLASSIFICATION OF PYLORIC HYPERTROPHY** ☐

I. Primary pyloric hypertrophy
   A. Focal form (torus hyperplasia)
   B. Diffuse form without proximal lesion
   C. Diffuse form with proximal lesion
     1. Proximal benign ulcer
     2. Proximal cancer
   D. Diffuse form with associated lesions
     1. Gastritis
     2. Gastroenterostomy
     3. Pernicious anemia
II. Secondary pyloric hypertrophy
   A. Associated with a distal obstructive lesion

Focal pyloric hypertrophy (torus hyperplasia)

In almost all of the 26 reported cases of focal hypertrophy of the pyloric muscle, the hypertrophy seemed to correspond anatomically to the torus.[35] It is not known whether focal hypertrophy represents an early stage of diffuse pyloric hypertrophy or a separate process. Radiographic abnormalities include flattening along the distal portion of the lesser curvature of the antrum and widening of the space between the antrum and the base of the duodenal bulb on the lesser curvature (Fig. 16-10). A rarer manifestation of focal hypertrophy is limited to the proximal muscular loop (Fig. 16-11).

Diffuse pyloric hypertrophy

Although diffuse pyloric hypertrophy can exist in the absence of radiographic abnormalities, certain diagnostic signs are of value in identifying this process in adults.[32,36,37] These abnormalities include elongation and concentric narrowing of the pyloric canal, a cleft or niche at the inferior midportion of the canal (Fig. 16-12), a flexibility or variation in the contour of the narrowed distal an-

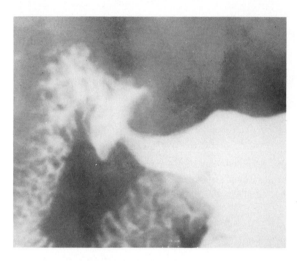

Fig. 16-10 Torus hyperplasia. Flattening of the distal portion of the lesser curve of the antrum due to hyperplasia of the torus portion of the pyloric muscle. A 1-cm nodule of hypertrophied smooth muscle was found at operation.
From Seaman WB: *AJR* 96:388, 1966.

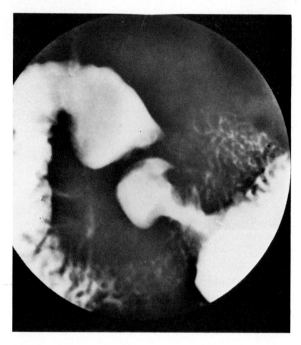

Fig. 16-11 Focal pyloric hypertrophy. The antral narrowing is due to hypertrophy of the proximal or left pyloric muscle loop.
Courtesy of Dr. Gerald Dodd.

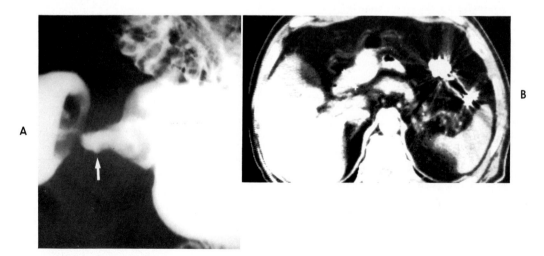

Fig. 16-12 Diffuse pyloric hypertrophy. **A,** Note concentric antral narrowing and the inferiorly directed triangular cleft *(arrow).* This results from mucosa protruding between the two hypertrophied muscular loops. **B,** CT image with cursor measuring a pyloric thickness of 24 mm.

trum, and a proximal benign ulcer, which is an occasional finding.

When relaxed, the normal pyloric canal is 0.5 to 1 cm long. A longer canal is a normal, but transient, phenomenon occurring during the muscular contraction of the distal portion of the stomach. Persistent elongation suggests the presence of pyloric hypertrophy. The elongated canal seen with diffuse pyloric hypertrophy is concentric, straight, or slightly curved, and is occasionally funnel shaped, extending for 3 or 4 cm along the greater curve but only for 2 cm along the lesser curve. Of help in differentiating pyloric hypertrophy from the antral narrowing produced by cancer is that the shape and caliber are seen to vary during a fluoroscopic examination in the benign condition.

The most specific radiographic sign is the triangular cleft or niche in the inferior midportion of the elongated canal (Fig. 16-12, *A*). This cleft probably results from the protrusion of mucosa between the two hypertrophied muscular loops on the greater curve. It may be confused with an ulcer niche, but, unlike the ulcer, the cleft associated with pyloric hypertrophy is transient. Although a specific sign, it is unfortunately found in a minority of cases of pyloric hypertrophy.[32,38] CT and ultrasonography can be used to document the thickening and elongation of the pyloric muscle and to evaluate for secondary signs of neoplasm (Fig. 16-12, *B*).

The combination of a benign gastric ulcer at the lesser curve near the incisura and concentric narrowing of the distal antrum strongly indicates pyloric hypertrophy (Fig. 16-13). Peptic ulceration is common and arises because of obstruction caused by the hypertrophic segment, with consequent stasis, hyperperistalsis, antral distention, and increased gastrin release.[32]

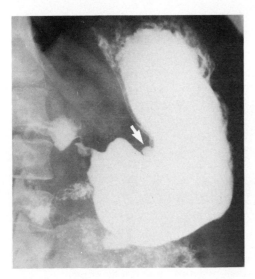

Fig. 16-13 Pyloric hypertrophy and benign gastric ulcer. The combination of an ulcer near the incisura *(arrow)* and a concentric narrowing of the distal antrum strongly suggests pyloric hypertrophy. Irregularity of the narrowed portion is caused by submucosal edema.

INFLAMMATORY DISEASES

Some inflammatory diseases of the stomach are well defined and common (e.g., peptic ulcer disease and specific types of gastritis); some are ill-defined and questionably caused by an inflammatory process (e.g., varioliform gastritis, Crohn's gastritis, eosinophilic gastritis, and eosino-

---

☐ **CLASSIFICATION OF GASTRITIS AND GASTROPATHY** ☐

I. Acute gastritis/ulcer disease
  A. Peptic ulcer disease
  B. Erosive gastritis
  C. Hemorrhagic
    1. Erosive
    2. Stress ulcer
  D. Infectious
    1. Viral
      a. Herpes simplex
      b. Cytomegalovirus
    2. Bacterial
      a. *Helicobacter pylori*
      b. Phlegmonous, emphysematous
    3. Fungal
      a. Histoplasmosis
      b. Candidiasis
      c. Actinomycosis
    4. Parasitic
II. Chronic gastritis
  A. Atrophic fundal gastritis (type A, pernicious anemia)
  B. Antral gastritis (type B, *H. pylori*)
  C. Chronic erosive gastritis (varioliform)
  D. Gastritis following partial gastrectomy, bile reflux
  E. Eosinophilic gastritis
  F. Eosinophilic granuloma
III. Granulomatous gastritis
  A. Crohn's disease
  B. Sarcoidosis
  C. Turberculosis
  D. Fungal disease
  E. Syphilis
IV. Injury gastropathy
  A. Corrosive gastritis
  B. Gastric radiation injury
  C. Medication-induced gastritis
  D. Freezing gastropathy
V. Hypertrophic gastropathy
  A. Menetrier's disease
  B. Zollinger-Ellison syndrome
  C. Pseudolymphoma
  D. Other hypertrophic gastropathies

Modified from Isenberg JI, McQuaid KR, Laine L, Ruben W: Acid peptic disorders. In Yamada T, ed: *Textbook of gastroenterology*, Philadelphia, 1991, JB Lippincott.

philic granuloma); others are more appropriately categorized as "hypertrophic gastropathies" (e.g., Menetrier's disease, Zollinger-Ellison syndrome, and pseudolymphoma). A combined classification, as proposed by experts in gastroenterology,[39] is detailed in the box on p. 325.

Although pathogenetically imprecise,[40] the term *gastritis* has been used traditionally to encompass numerous lesions of the gastric mucosa, of which only some are actu-

ally inflammatory. Of the inflammatory lesions of the stomach, an increasing number are being attributed to specific organisms. The acquired immunodeficiency syndrome (AIDS) epidemic has revealed the potential ability of bacterial, viral, and parasitic processes, previously considered rare, to infect the stomach (see Chapter 40).[41,42] Recent investigations of gastroduodenal inflammation have resulted in identification of *Helicobacter pylori* (formerly *Campylo-*

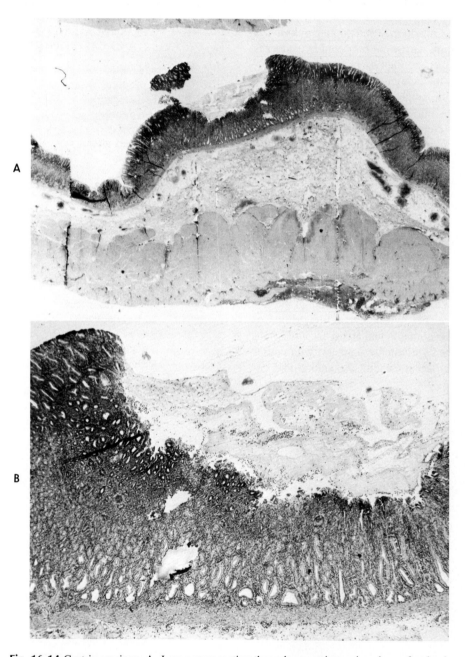

Fig. 16-14 Gastric erosions. **A,** Low-power section through a gastric erosion shows focal submucosal edema, accounting for the halo around the central barium collection. Note that the erosion does not penetrate through the muscularis mucosa. **B,** Higher magnification (×37) through the erosion. Muscularis mucosa in the lower aspect of the image is normal. **C** and **D,** Erosions of the antral greater curvature. Note the small aphthae, one of which protrudes beyond the mucosal surface when viewed in profile *(arrows).*

bacter pylori) as an etiologic agent in some types of gastritis as well as ulcer disease.[43-48] Of the noninfective factors causing gastritis, use of aspirin and other nonsteroidal antiinflammatory agents is the most usual etiology (see box below).

Radiographic signs of gastritis

Patients with histologically defined gastritis may exhibit neither symptoms nor visible endoscopic abnormalities.[49] It is therefore not surprising that even the best radiographic technique using the combined benefits of a single- and double-contrast examination may not detect the disorder.

The most specific radiographic sign of gastritis is the finding of gastric mucosal erosion.[50,51] An erosion is a shallow ulcer that does not penetrate beyond the muscularis mu-

cosa[52] (Fig. 16-14). These are often termed *aphthae (small ulcers)* or *aphthous lesions,* owing to their similarity to the shallow oral ulcer found in infants with thrush. Although frequently found during an endoscopic examination, they are difficult to demonstrate radiographically unless good double-contrast technique is used.[53-55] Erosions have two radiographic appearances. The most common one is the varioliform (smallpox-like) or *complete erosion,* which is situated centrally on a small mound of edema (Fig. 16-15). The term *incomplete erosion* refers to those ulcers that do not possess a halo of edema, and these are particularly difficult to define, even with the best biphasic techniques.[56] Because these may be linear, serpiginous, or irregularly shaped, they can be difficult to differentiate from barium precipitates[55] (Fig. 16-16). Other radiographic signs of gastritis are nonspecific, and include fold thickening and nodularity, which, when seen along the gastric margin, may exhibit a crenulated (undulating) or serrated profile.[51] Ac- ~scalloping?~ centuated transverse antral folds and antral spasm suggest the presence of active antral gastritis.[57] Straightening of the

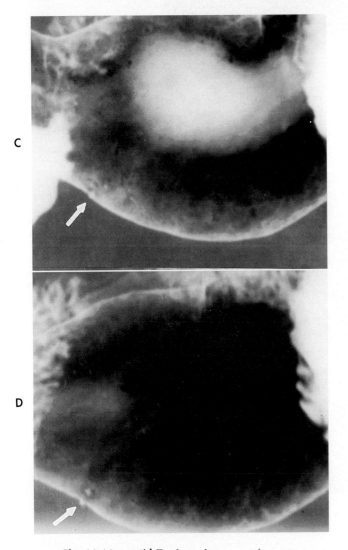

C

D

Fig. 16-14, cont'd For legend see opposite page.

☐ **NONINFECTIVE ETIOLOGIES OF GASTRITIS OR ULCER** ☐

I. Salicylates and other nonsteroidal antiinflammatory agents
II. Other drugs/ingestants
   A. Corticosteroids
   B. Iron
   C. Potassium chloride
   D. Alcohol
   E. Corrosives
   F. Nicotine, smoking
III. Stress
   A. Psychologic
   B. Physical
     1. Trauma, shock
     2. Postoperative
     3. Central nervous system injury (Cushing's syndrome)
     4. Burns (Curling's ulcer)
     5. Sepsis
     6. Organ failure
     7. Nasogastric tubes
   C. Uremia
   D. Ischemia
   E. Radiation
   F. Postoperative bile reflux

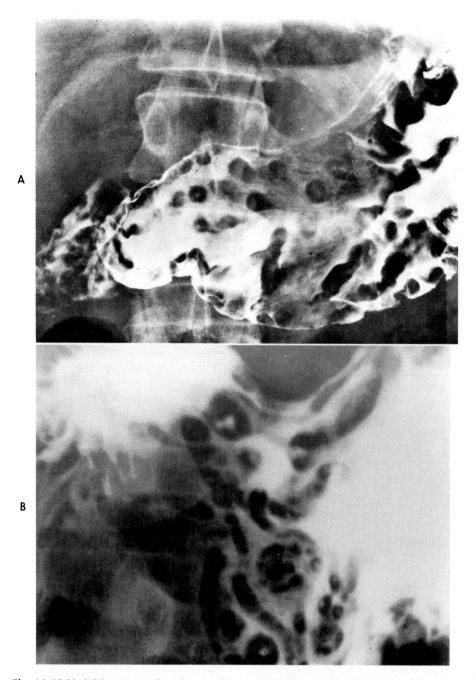

Fig. 16-15 Varioliform type of erosive gastritis. **A,** Note the erosions aligned with the rugae. **B,** Note scalloping of the rugae and the variably sized erosions on mounds of edema.
A courtesy of Dr. Robert Paul.

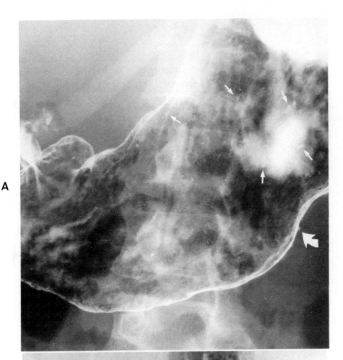

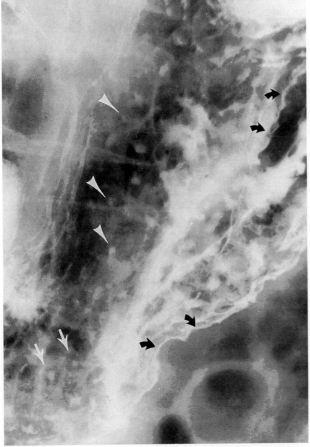

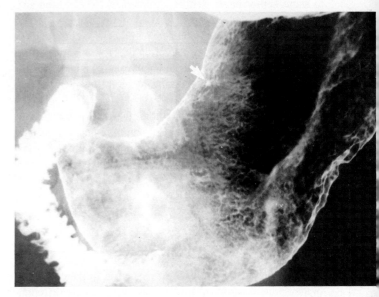

Fig. 16-16 Gastric erosions. **A,** Irregularly shaped, linear, or serpiginous barium collections represent incomplete erosions of the body and antrum of the stomach *(arrows)*. Note that one of these projects beyond the mucosal margin *(curved arrow)*. Unlike the erosions depicted in Fig. 16-15, there is no submucosal edema producing a halo about the erosion. **B,** Diffuse erosion of the stomach with both incomplete *(arrowheads)* and complete *(arrows)* erosions. Note fold thickening with scalloped margins *(curved arrows)*.

Fig. 16-17 Accentuation of the areae gastricae and ulceration. An ulcer in the lesser curvature *(arrow)* in a patient with pronounced areae gastricae.

wall and luminal narrowing are seen in cases of advanced gastritis. Enlargement of the areae gastricae (>4 mm) is an additional sign. When the areae gastricae appear enlarged or prominent, erosions or ulcers should be carefully sought (Fig. 16-17). Except for erosions, these signs are not specific for gastritis and must be evaluated in combination with clinical information to enhance diagnostic accuracy.[51]

Erosive gastritis

Most patients with histologically defined gastritis experience no symptoms, and the clinical diagnosis is suspected only when they exhibit pain, nausea, vomiting, or hemorrhage. The use of corticosteroids or nonsteroidal antiinflammatory drugs (NSAIDs) and alcohol consumption may be causative factors. Gastritis may also develop in patients undergoing operation, experiencing acute stress, receiving radiation therapy, or following a partial gastrectomy. The radiographic demonstration of erosions, as noted previously, aids in the diagnosis, and, if the process is severe and progressive, true ulceration (extension of the process through the muscularis mucosae) may result.

Hemorrhagic gastritis

Although many patients with histologically defined gastritis are silent clinically, profound hemorrhage may be a presenting symptom. It is very likely that hemorrhagic gastritis is not an inflammatory condition but represents a group of diseases with different causes but with the same end result, that is, bleeding mucosa. It has a predilection for the area of stomach that is covered by the fundal epithelium.

Factors and mechanisms similar to those that predispose to the development of acute erosive gastritis can also lead to acute hemorrhagic gastritis. Cortisone, alcohol, and antipyretic drugs are all agents that can reduce mucus secretion, which is the main pathogenetic process leading to mucosal injury. Acute stress ulceration that follows hypovolemic shock and sepsis is probably the result of mucosal ischemia and is due to the shunting of blood away from the mucosa.[58]

Conventional radiographic studies usually yield negative findings. If blood clot does not obscure the mucosa, superficial erosions may be demonstrated using double-contrast techniques, but, in the presence of severe bleeding, neither radiography nor endoscopy can adequately visualize the gastric mucosa.

Chronic gastritis

Chronic gastritis represents a histologic diagnosis that, in general, cannot be correlated with clinical symptoms.[41] For example, the prevalence of dyspepsia in patients with biopsy-proved chronic gastritis is not significantly different from that in those with normal mucosa.[59] It is thought to have no relationship with acute gastritis, which is a reversible condition. Histologically, chronic gastritis is characterized by the replacement of normal epithelial cells with cells that are mainly mucus secreting, a process referred to as *intestinal metaplasia* or *intestinalization*. Although the number of these cells may be increased, producing a thicker mucosa, the end-stage consists of mucosal thinning and atrophy. Chronic gastritis can be defined as either *nonerosive* or *erosive,* but this classification frequently overlaps with other types of gastritis.[40]

Chronic erosive or *varioliform* gastritis is of unknown cause. It is considered to be distinct from peptic ulcer disease,[60] and it has been suggested to have an allergic or viral basis.[61,62] The characteristic radiologic features, which include antral aphthae that are clustered or linearly arranged along gastric folds (see Fig. 16-15), are seen best with a double-contrast technique. Repeat radiographic examination after treatment often shows the lesions persist, even though symptoms may have cleared.

Chronic nonerosive gastritis may be atrophic (type A), as in pernicious anemia, or a type frequently associated with *H. pylori* infections (type B). The latter is much more common, frequently involves the antrum, and may progress to involve the proximal stomach.

H. pylori gastritis

H. pylori is a gram-negative, spiral-shaped bacterium that may inhabit the gastric mucosa in over 50% of asymptomatic individuals.[43,46,47] The organism has, nonetheless, been confirmed as the cause of type B gastritis and may also cause gastric and duodenal ulceration.[47,48] Barium contrast radiography may disclose the nonspecific signs of gastritis, as noted previously. Marked enlargement of the gastric folds, wall thickening, and ulceration may simulate carcinoma, especially on CT scans.[63,65]

Atrophic gastritis

Criteria that establish the radiographic diagnosis of atrophic gastritis that occurs in pernicious anemia include absence of gastric rugae, small or absent areae gastricae, and a narrowed tubular stomach with the greater and lesser curves roughly parallel to each other[66] (Fig. 16-18).

Granulomatous gastritis

Chronic granulomatous inflammation may be precipitated by a variety of agents that elicit a specific cellular reaction of the reticuloendothelial system. The basic lesion—the granuloma—consists of a focus of epithelioid cells, with or without giant cells, surrounded by concentrically arranged reticular fibers. Granulomas are often found under conditions in which foreign material has come into contact with living tissue. Although these conditions are uncommon, the stomach may be involved by a number of infectious and noninfectious granulomatous diseases, including syphilis, tuberculosis, sarcoidosis, histoplasmosis, Crohn's disease, eosinophilic gastritis, and isolated or idiopathic granulomatous gastritis.[67]

The differential diagnosis of granulomatous gastritis in histopathologic terms is difficult. The granulomas found microscopically in the diseases mentioned may not be spe-

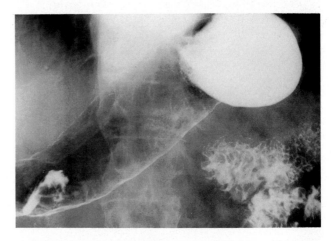

Fig. 16-18 Pernicious anemia. The stomach is devoid of gastric rugae and has a narrowed, tubular configuration with the greater and lesser curves parallel to each other.

cific. In many of the cases of gastritic syphilis and tuberculosis reported in the literature, the specific microorganism in the gastric wall is not identified and the diagnosis was made on the basis of suggestive histology, the response to specific therapy, or the presence of the disease in other parts of the GI tract or in other organs. Gastric abnormalities occurring in patients with disseminated sarcoidosis and regional enteritis elsewhere in the GI tract are usually assumed to be caused by the same disease process.[68] The same is true, although to a lesser extent, in patients with active tuberculosis or syphilis, even though the microorganism is not identified in the gastric tissues.

The radiographic manifestations of such lesions are similar, consisting of nodular accentuation of the rugal pattern or a granular cobblestone mucosa that replaces the normal rugal pattern, together with ulceration, regular or irregular antral narrowing associated with diminished distensibility, and varying degrees of rigidity. Rugal enlargement may be extreme and ulcerations may be large and mimic the appearance of a neoplasm.[69]

Syphilis

Syphilis of the gastrointestinal tract most commonly involves the stomach. Secondary syphilis may cause a diffuse, nonspecific gastritis and duodenitis or an inflammatory mass in the stomach possessing superficial erosions or ulceration.[70,71] The rugae may either be enlarged (Fig. 16-19, *A*) or effaced (Fig. 16-19, *B*). Tertiary syphilis may also involve the stomach, most frequently the antrum, with a granulomatous infiltration. This produces a funnel-shaped narrowing of the antrum with effacement of the mucosal pattern and diminished or absent peristalsis.

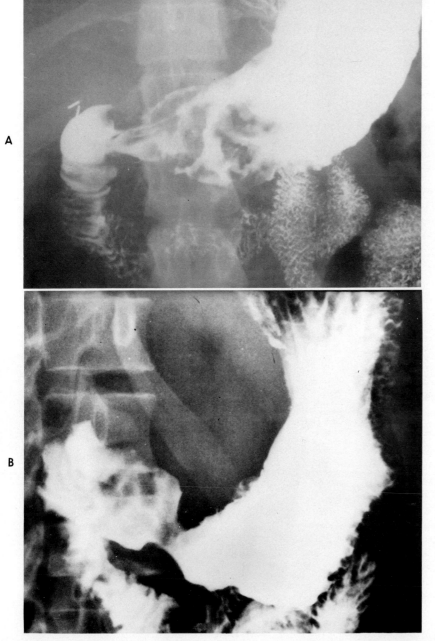

Fig. 16-19 Gastric syphilis. **A,** The antral folds are thickened and erosions and small ulcers are interspersed. **B,** The distal antral contour of another patient is irregular and narrowed and the antral folds are effaced. There are enlarged duodenal folds.
B courtesy of Dr. Leon Love.

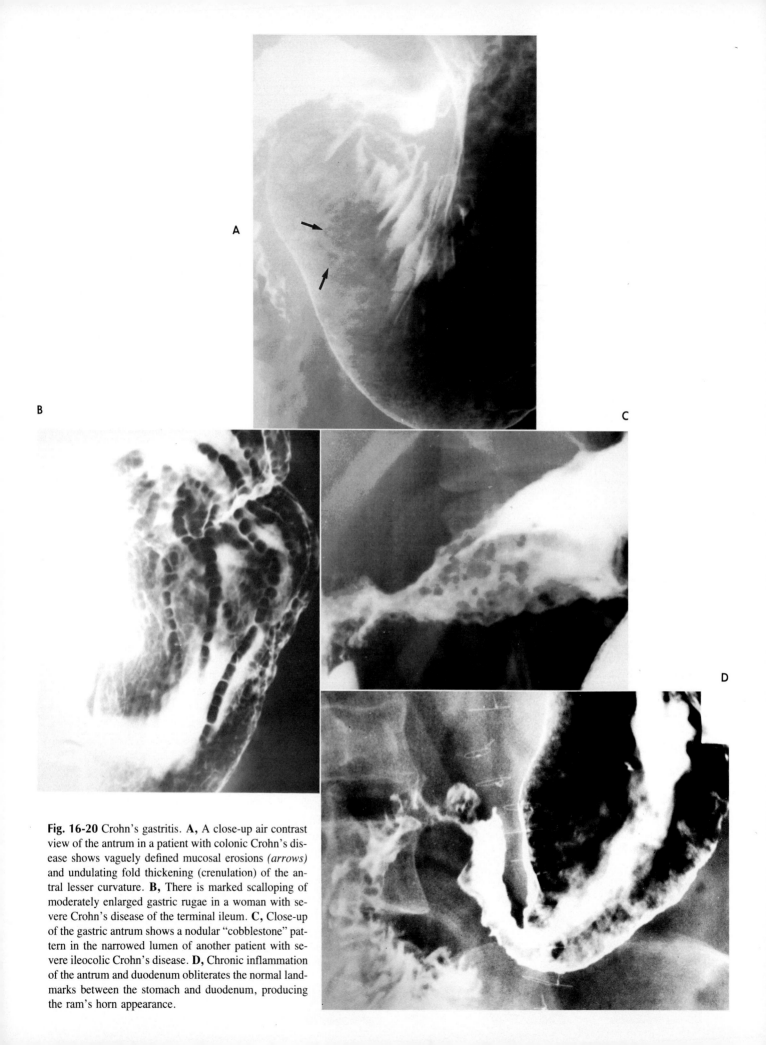

Fig. 16-20 Crohn's gastritis. **A,** A close-up air contrast view of the antrum in a patient with colonic Crohn's disease shows vaguely defined mucosal erosions *(arrows)* and undulating fold thickening (crenulation) of the antral lesser curvature. **B,** There is marked scalloping of moderately enlarged gastric rugae in a woman with severe Crohn's disease of the terminal ileum. **C,** Close-up of the gastric antrum shows a nodular "cobblestone" pattern in the narrowed lumen of another patient with severe ileocolic Crohn's disease. **D,** Chronic inflammation of the antrum and duodenum obliterates the normal landmarks between the stomach and duodenum, producing the ram's horn appearance.

Crohn's disease

The frequency with which the early manifestations of Crohn's disease are identified appears to depend on the techniques of examination. During the acute phases of gastric Crohn's disease, superficial erosions (aphthae) and fold thickening are the usual manifestations (Fig. 16-20, *A*). Using air contrast techniques, aphthae can be demonstrated in as many as 20% to 40% of the cases.[72-76] These lesions represent one of the earliest signs of the disease and are frequently found in asymptomatic patients. They are nonspecific, often associated with fold thickening or scalloping (Fig. 16-20, *B* and *C*), and indistinguishable from erosions of other types of gastritis. The term *ram's horn sign*[77] has been applied to describe the narrowing of the distal stomach that occurs as a late feature of the disease when it involves the antrum (Fig. 16-20, *D*). Frequently, the adjacent duodenum is also involved, and, with obliteration of the normal anatomic landmarks between the duodenal bulb and stomach, a characteristic tubular narrowing, termed the *pseudo-Billroth I sign*,[78,79] can result. Although Crohn's disease preferentially affects the distal stomach, fundal involvement has also been described.[80] Fistula formation is uncommon and is usually associated with a more severely affected distal segment of small bowel or colon.[81]

Gastric sarcoidosis

Involvement of the stomach by sarcoidosis is usually silent clinically and radiologic findings are normal, so its actual prevalence is difficult to assess.[82] In 60 patients with sarcoidosis whose upper GI radiographic findings were normal, biopsy specimens revealed the presence of mucosal granulomas superficial to the level of the muscularis mucosae in 10%.[83] None of these patients exhibited GI symptoms.

Some authors have described the existence of typical benign gastric ulcers that contain sarcoidlike granulomas in the ulcer base and the surrounding tissue.[84] These may be coincidental peptic ulcers and not actually a manifestation of sarcoidosis in the stomach. Other signs include fold thickening and luminal narrowing (Fig. 16-21). There may be similar manifestations in the duodenum.

Infective gastritis

Immune-deficient patients with AIDS, as well as those debilitated by chronic disease, chemotherapy, and immunosuppressive therapy, are susceptible to GI infection caused by a variety of viruses, bacteria, fungi, and parasites. Notable among these are infections due to the herpes simplex virus, cytomegalovirus, tuberculosis, histoplasmosis, and *Crytosporidium*. Many of these infections, which were at one time unfamiliar to the practicing radiologist, will undoubtedly be encountered more frequently in practice. Chapters 25 and 46 consider these processes in some detail. There are two other important gastric infections. One of these, *H. pylori*, has already been considered. The second is phlegmonous gastritis, discussed in the next section.

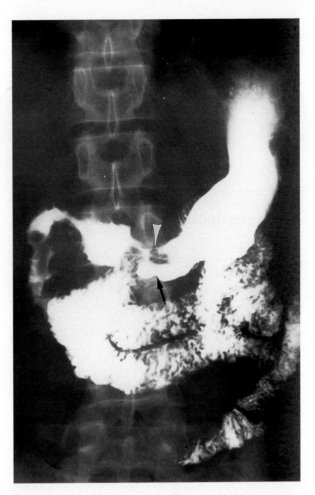

Fig. 16-21 Biopsy-proved gastric sarcoidosis. Fold thickening *(arrowhead)* and luminal narrowing *(arrow)* affect the distal stomach. There is also fold thickening in the second portion of the duodenum.

Phlegmonous gastritis

Phlegmonous gastritis is an acute, fulminant, often fatal, bacterial infection of the stomach characterized by marked polymorphonuclear leukocyte infiltration and necrosis.[85,86] In more than 70% of the cases, alpha-hemolytic streptococci have been identified, but *Staphylococcus aureus*, *Escherichia coli*, *Clostridium welchii*, and *pneumococcus* and *Proteus* organisms have also been found.[87] The clinical picture consists of the acute onset of severe pain, fever, and vomiting. Peritonitis develops in 70% of cases. The mortality is high, but prompt gastrectomy and antibiotic therapy can reduce its threat.

The gastric wall is markedly thickened in the disease and the rugae are swollen, at times to the point of effacement (Fig. 16-22, *A*). Ulcerations are not usually seen, but intramural penetration of the contrast medium may occur, probably through necrotic defects in the mucosa that are often seen on the pathologic specimen. CT or ultrasonography may show wall thickening.[88] If healing occurs, there is marked scarring with shrinkage of the stomach.[87] The condition may be acute, subacute, or chronic in nature. The

Fig. 16-22 Acute phlegmonous gastritis. **A,** The gastric fold pattern is effaced and fluoroscopy showed no peristalsis. **B,** Emphysematous type of phlegmonous gastritis. Note the bubbly appearance of the stomach caused by collections of intramural gas resulting from gas-producing organisms.
A courtesy of Dr. Charles Nice; *B* from Haw SY, Collins LC, Petrany Z: *JAMA* 192:222, 1965.

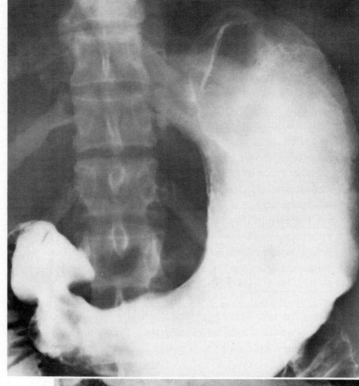

A

☐ **CAUSES OF GASTRIC PNEUMATOSIS** ☐

Phlegmonous gastritis
Necrotizing gastroenteritis
Parasitic infestations
Corrosive gastritis
Infarction
Outlet obstruction
Volvulus
Gastric atony
Gastroscopy or surgery
Vomiting
Pulmonary emphysema
Idiopathic causes

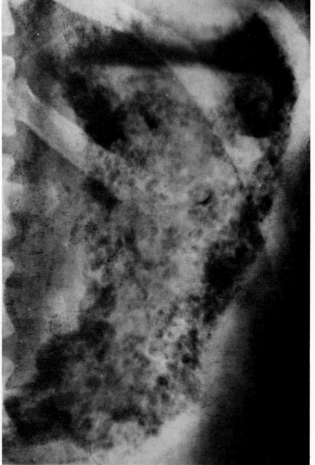

B

chronic form may occasionally be localized to a segment of the stomach.[89]

When the bacterium causing phlegmonous gastritis is a gas-forming organism such as *E. coli* or *C. welchii*, multiple small gas bubbles may be noted radiographically as "intramural pneumatosis"[90,91] (Fig. 16-22, *B*). This condition has also been termed *emphysematous gastritis. Interstitial gastric emphysema* is a more generic term referring to the presence of gas within the gastric wall resulting from a variety of causes, including infection (emphysematous gastritis), increased intraluminal pressure, and, most frequently, the ingestion of corrosive agents.[92-95]

Interstitial gastric emphysema

The terms designating the presence of gas within the wall of the intestinal tract are *intramural pneumatosis* and *pneumatosis intestinalis.* When the process affects the stomach, it may be termed *interstitial gastric emphysema, emphysematous gastritis,* or *gastric pneumatosis*. Gas in the gastric wall does not imply a specific diagnosis or disease, however, but refers to a radiologic or pathologic sign indicating one of several underlying processes that may either allow or cause luminal gas to cross the mucosal barrier (interstitial gastric emphysema) or produce gas in the gastric wall as a result of bacterial action (emphysematous gastritis).[90-99] These processes are listed in the box above.

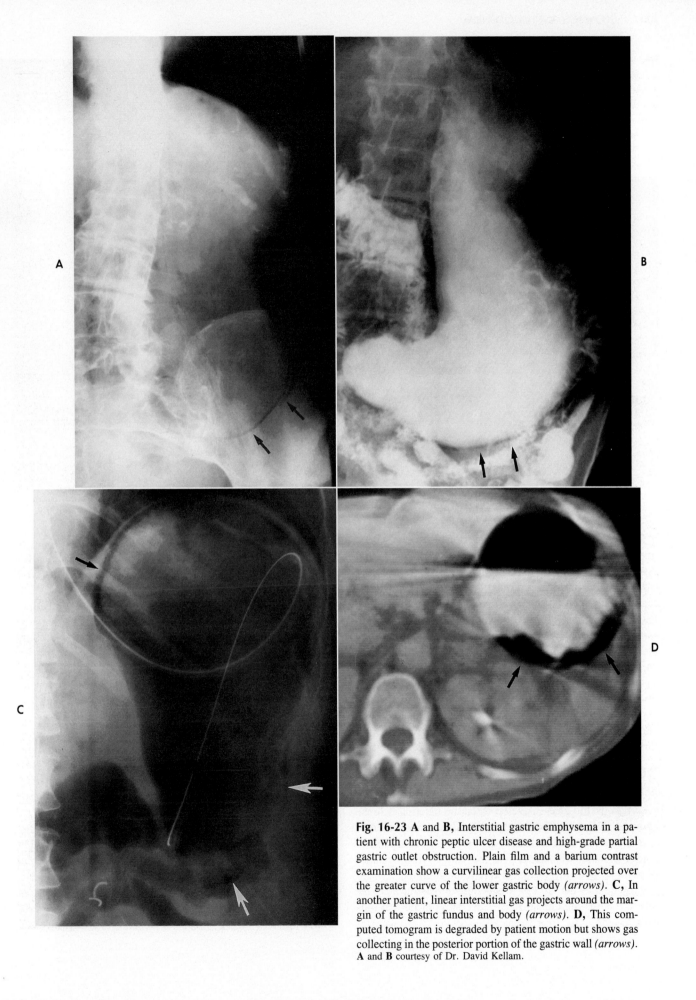

Fig. 16-23 A and **B,** Interstitial gastric emphysema in a patient with chronic peptic ulcer disease and high-grade partial gastric outlet obstruction. Plain film and a barium contrast examination show a curvilinear gas collection projected over the greater curve of the lower gastric body *(arrows).* **C,** In another patient, linear interstitial gas projects around the margin of the gastric fundus and body *(arrows).* **D,** This computed tomogram is degraded by patient motion but shows gas collecting in the posterior portion of the gastric wall *(arrows).* **A** and **B** courtesy of Dr. David Kellam.

Fig. 16-24 Hepatic portal venous gas due to gastric outlet obstruction. **A,** Upright abdominal radiograph shows the branching linear pattern representing gas within the hepatic portal veins. Marked gastric distention is indicated by the location of the air fluid levels in the fundus and antrum *(arrows).* **B,** After nasogastric decompression, contrast material outlines the markedly distended and obstructed stomach. Hepatic portal venous gas has cleared.

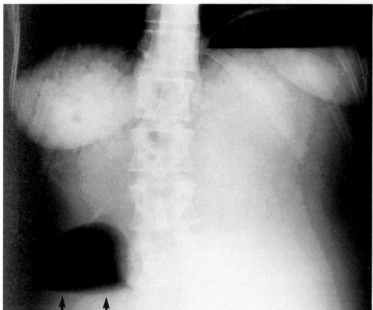

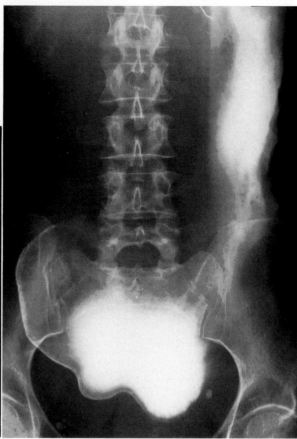

The plain film and CT appearances of interstitial gastric emphysema may vary with the etiology. The transmucosal passage of gas from the lumen into the gastric wall usually produces thin, discrete, and sharply defined streaks in either the submucosa, subserosa, or both[100] (Fig. 16-23). This is in contrast to the formation of gas caused by inflammatory diseases such as emphysematous gastritis, in which the gas tends to be broken up into small bubbles and irregular collections[101] (see Fig. 16-22). These morphologic features, however, do not represent consistently reliable criteria for use in making the differential diagnosis. As is sometimes seen in patients with intestinal pneumatosis, gas from intramural gastric pneumatosis may migrate into the portal venous system of the liver[102] (Fig. 16-24).

PEPTIC ULCER DISEASE
Epidemiology

Benign gastric ulcers develop when the mucosal defense against digestion by acid is reduced or when the normal mucosa is overwhelmed by excess acid production.[103] For example, mucosal defense is reduced by NSAIDs, ethanol use, and *H. pylori* infection, whereas the Zollinger-Ellison syndrome, and the excess production of gastric acid involved, causes inflammation and ulceration of normal mucosa.

Approximately two thirds of benign gastric ulcers can be attributed to specific risk factors such as those listed for gastritis in the box on p. 334.[39] One predominant risk factor is the use of NSAIDs, which is implicated in one third of all ulcer cases. The remainder of ulcer cases are idiopathic, although the possibility that many of these cases are related to type B gastritis of *H. pylori* infection is being actively investigated.[46]

Definitions and location

In contrast to gastric mucosal *erosion*, which does not extend through the muscularis mucosa, gastric *ulcer* involves the submucosa and muscularis propria. If the ulcer extends beyond the serosa, it may *penetrate* into contiguous organs or *perforate* into the lesser sac or greater peritoneal cavity. Although peptic ulcers may arise anywhere in the stomach, most are found along the lesser curve or posterior wall of the body and antrum.[104,105]

The major revolution in the therapy of peptic ulcer disease witnessed in the past 20 years has not only brought about a change in the clinical course of ulcer disease but has altered the diagnostic approach and even the appearance of the ulcers. The "treat first" policy advocated by the American College of Physicians[106] has led to a more efficient and cost-effective medical response to gastric ulcer diagnosis and therapy, and has, at the same time, diminished the role of diagnostic radiology and endoscopy in evaluating patients with peptic ulcer disease. Although most patients respond well to the "treat first" approach and require no further evaluation, persistent symptoms in the patient failing such treatment may necessitate a diagnostic workup. Radiologists are frequently confronted with an ulcer patient who has symptoms of long duration and has failed a variety of treatments. Although some patients may have ulcers in varying stages of healing or with atypical signs, the diagnostic value of the traditional radiographic signs of benign ulcer are of continuing importance.

Plain film evaluation

Benign gastric ulcers and their complications may be visualized on plain films of the abdomen. The ulcer crater, if large enough and optimally placed, may appear as an abnormal gas contour protruding from the body of the gas-

filled stomach (Fig. 16-25, A-D). Complications of gastric ulcer are frequently revealed by plain films, and include gastric outlet obstruction (see Fig. 16-24), perforation with pneumoperitoneum, or abscess formation (Fig. 16-25, E). Complications not usually depicted by plain films are gastroenteric (mainly gastrocolic) fistula, penetration into adjacent organs, and hemorrhage.

Barium contrast examination

Barium contrast radiography for the diagnosis of gastric ulcer is optimally performed using biphasic or multiphasic techniques, which combine the best features of air contrast and mucosal relief methods with palpation and compression spot filming of the coated mucosa in both the en face and profile projections. The examination must be tailored to the ability of the patient to cooperate, and, if possible, should include films made in both the recumbent and erect positions. Using these carefully applied techniques, it is possi-

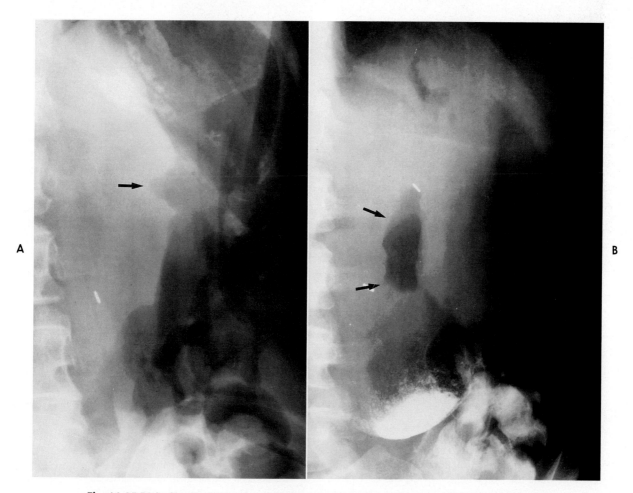

Fig. 16-25 Plain film depiction of a gastric ulcer and its complications. **A,** A gastric ulcer shadow protrudes from the lesser curve of the stomach *(arrow)*. An ulcer mound is suggested at its margins. **B,** Large ulcer of the lesser curve *(arrows)* retains gas adjacent to the collapsed stomach.

Continued.

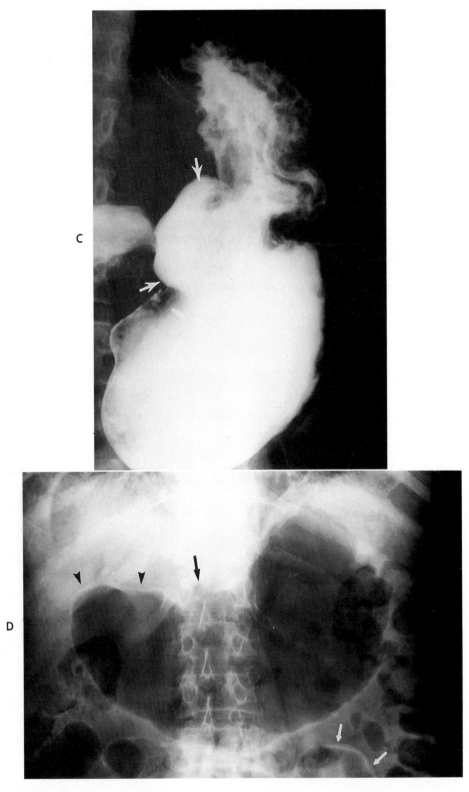

Fig. 16-25, cont'd Plain film depiction of a gastric ulcer and its complications. **C,** Barium contrast examination confirms the presence of a large ulcer in the lesser curve, which penetrates beyond the gastric lumen. **D,** Gastric ulcer perforation. The stomach is distended, and there is the faint shadow of a gastric ulcer along the lesser curve *(arrow)*. There is pneumoperitoneum indicated by the presence of air over the liver and outlining the gastric antrum *(arrowheads)* and bowel wall below the greater curve *(arrows)*.

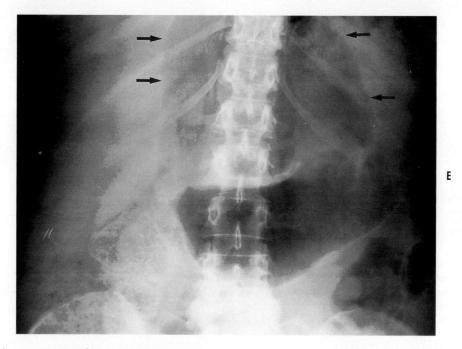

Fig. 16-25, cont'd Plain film depiction of a gastric ulcer and its complications. **E,** Lesser sac abscess due to gastric ulcer perforation. A large gas collection that is superior to the stomach represents gas in the abscess *(arrows)*.

ble to achieve an accuracy approaching that yielded by endoscopy in diagnosing gastric ulcer.[107-112] The details of performing such examinations are described in Chapters 14, 18, and 19.

Radiographic signs of a benign gastric ulcer

The radiologic diagnosis of gastric ulcer depends on the filling or coating of the crater with barium utilizing both the single- and double-contrast components of the multiphasic examination.

To assess the nature of the crater using the air contrast technique, views should be obtained in profile as well as en face.

Most of the profile signs of benign gastric ulcers are best demonstrated with the patient erect. In this position the weight of the barium in the distal stomach produces downward stretching and straightening of the lesser curve, making it easier to recognize penetration of the ulcer beyond the lumen (Fig. 16-26). The more optimal filling out of the contour of the greater curve promoted by the upright position also makes it possible to recognize penetration of ulcers in this location. Conversely, in the prone or prone-oblique positions, the lesser curve is foreshortened, rendering it more difficult or even impossible to assess penetration. It is also easier to profile those lesions against the backdrop of the anterior or posterior wall of the body of the stomach when the patient is erect, because the weight

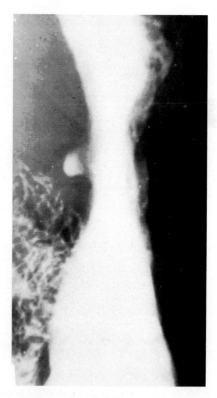

Fig. 16-26 Penetrating benign gastric ulcer. With the patient in the upright position and during compression, the ulcer is seen to clearly penetrate beyond the gastric wall. Also note the prominent ulcer collar.
From Nelson SW: *Radiol Clin North Am* 7:5, 1969.

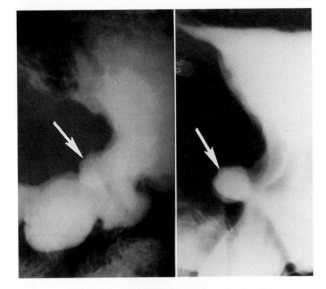

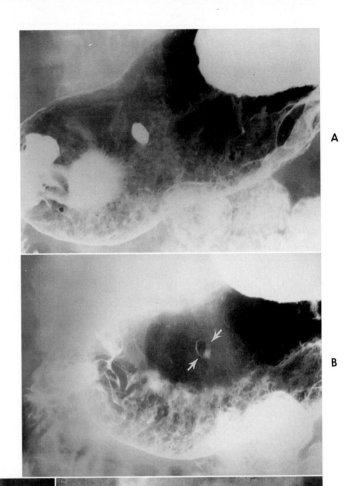

Fig. 16-27 Value of the upright position in demonstrating penetration of a benign gastric ulcer beyond the gastric margin. **A,** Ulcer penetration *(arrow)* is not demonstrated in the prone-oblique position. **B,** With upright positioning the ulcer *(arrow)* clearly projects beyond the lumen. Note the smooth folds radiating to the ulcer.

From Nelson SW: *Radiol Clin North Am* 7:5, 1969.

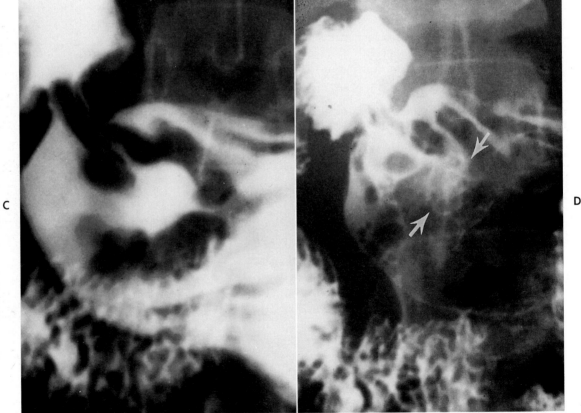

Fig. 16-28 Benign gastric ulcers exhibiting the ring sign. **A,** Posterior wall crater is filled with barium. **B,** Unfilled crater shows ring sign *(arrows)* after barium has drained. The sign is produced by the barium coating the crater walls, which is projected parallel to the x-ray beam. **C,** Filled compression view of the anterior wall crater clearly shows benign ulcer surrounded by an ulcer mound. **D,** Air contrast view shows faint barium coating of the ulcer margin *(arrows)*, producing the ring sign, which could easily be missed.

C and **D** from Nelson SW: *Radiol Clin North Am* 7:5, 1969.

of the barium in the distal stomach pulls the stomach downward so that more of the body of the stomach is below the xiphoid and ribs, making it more accessible for palpation and compression spot filming (Fig. 16-27).

Air contrast techniques can clearly define the shape of a crater and the features of the adjacent mucosa on the dependent wall of the body of the stomach when viewed en face. The well-defined barium-filled ulcer is seen through the overlying air-filled, barium-coated structures (Fig. 16-28, *A*). If the patient's position is changed so that the crater is emptied by gravity, the walls of such a crater when viewed en face can then be defined by an oval-shaped white line (the "ring sign") because the x-ray beam is parallel to the barium-coated walls of the crater (Fig. 16-28, *B*). As the walls of some craters are sloping rather than steep, they may not be clearly seen en face as a ring of barium and may be missed on air contrast studies. However, compression views of the barium-filled lumen can better reveal such craters (Fig. 16-28, *C* and *D*). Air contrast techniques occasionally portray a blood clot as a central "polypoid" defect in the barium-filled crater (Fig. 16-29). This serves as another reliable sign of benign gastric ulcer.

The most important radiographic signs of benign gastric ulcer are illustrated in Fig. 16-30 and consist of:
1. Penetration
2. Radiating fold pattern
3. Blood clot ("polyp") in base of crater
4. Signs of undermining:
   a. "Hampton's line"
   b. "Ulcer collar"
   c. "Collar button" shape
   d. "Crescent" sign
   e. "Straight line" sign
5. "Ulcer mound"

PENETRATION

Penetration of the ulcer beyond the gastric lumen (see Fig. 16-25, *B*, and 16-26) is not a totally reliable sign of benign gastric ulcer because IIc and III early gastric cancers may also show this feature (see Chapter 19). Careful positioning of the patient during the fluoroscopic examination is necessary because penetration can only be demonstrated by imaging the crater in profile, and the erect position is particularly valuable in this regard (see Figs. 16-26 and 16-27).

RADIATING FOLD PATTERN

Uniform, regular, and smooth folds radiating to the edge of or into the crater reliably indicate the benign nature of a

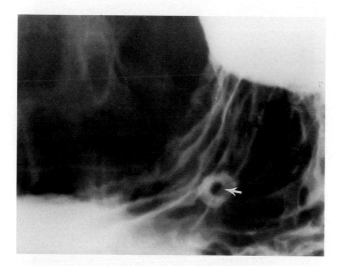

Fig. 16-29 Barium-filled small posterior wall ulcer with clot displacing barium in the base of the crater *(arrow)*. Note that the barium-coated rugae of the nondependent anterior wall project across the ulcer.

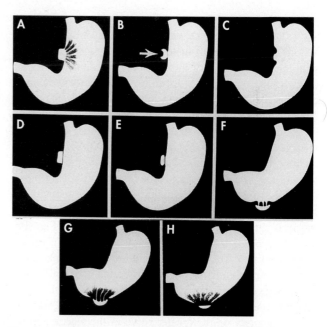

Fig. 16-30 Diagram of the radiographic signs of benign gastric ulcers as viewed in profile. **A,** Folds radiating to the crater edge and penetration. **B,** Penetration assuming a collar button shape in conjunction with a blood clot *(arrow)* in the base of the crater. **C,** Ulcer mound around the crater, which appears to be intraluminal. **D,** Hampton's line and penetration. **E,** Ulcer collar and penetration. **F,** Crescent sign with radiating folds and ulcer mound. **G,** Crescent sign with radiating folds and penetration. **H,** Straight line sign and penetration.

gastric ulcer (see Figs. 16-27, *B,* and 16-31). This sign can be demonstrated on either profile or en face projections. The surrounding edema may be extensive enough to interrupt a few of the folds before they reach the crater margin, but their smooth, nonnodular character is retained.

SIGNS OF UNDERMINING

Hampton's line, ulcer collar, and collar button. The normal gastric mucosa is more resistant than the submucosa to the erosive effects of acid peptic secretions, and this is the situation that fosters the occurrence of undermining. The submucosa is therefore more rapidly destroyed, leaving an overhanging edge or "washer" of mucosa with a relatively normal thickness (1 to 2 mm), known as *Hampton's line* (Fig. 16-32), or a thicker "doughnut" of overhanging edematous mucosa and submucosa, referred to as an *ulcer collar* (Fig. 16-33). Both of these findings are characterized by a linear radiolucent zone that extends across the mouth of the crater. These signs can be seen only when the crater is viewed in profile, because the x-ray beam is then parallel to the interfaces of the barium and the two surfaces of these overhanging margins of mucosa.

The collar button shape of the benign ulcer indicates undermining of the more susceptible deeper layers of submucosa by the erosive process. It may be accentuated by the submucosal and mucosal edema, which forms an ulcer collar.

Straight line sign. In cases of marked submucosal edema and resulting mass effect, undermining may be manifest as a single, straight line, situated at the interface of the ulcer with the undersurface of the overhanging edematous tissue (Fig. 16-34). In the gastric antrum, where associated muscle spasm and fold distortion around the crater may preclude demonstration of a Hampton's line, an ulcer collar, or an ulcer mound, the straight line sign often serves as a reliable indicator of benign ulcer (Fig. 16-34, *D*). Frequently, the sharply defined straight line is slightly concave toward the gastric lumen when the crater is crescent shaped (see Fig. 16-23, *C*). The straight line sign is particularly helpful when intraluminal debris obscures the detail of the mucosal surface of the tissue around the crater (Fig. 16-34, *A* and *B*).

Crescent sign. The crescent sign constitutes a rather spectacular, unusual, and reliable manifestation of extensive undermining, massive edema, and actual prolapse of the overhanging edematous mass of tissue into a large benign ulcer, particularly on the greater curve of the gastric antrum (Fig. 16-35). Before the nature and radiologic significance of this sign were recognized, such lesions were almost always deemed malignant neoplasms because the large lobular mass of markedly edematous tissue overhanging the crater and often projecting into the gastric lumen resembled a tumor. Furthermore, the bizarre, irregular crescent shape of the barium in the crater did not conform to any of the then accepted radiographic configurations of benign peptic ulcers. However, it is now known that this sign is virtually

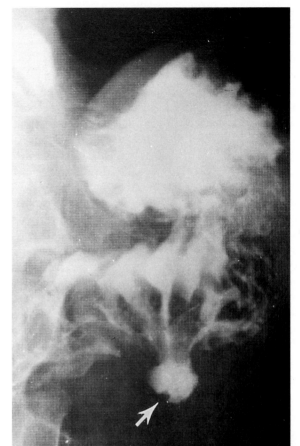

A

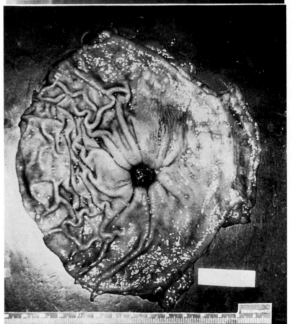

B

Fig. 16-31 Radiating fold pattern typical of a benign gastric ulcer. **A,** Compression view of the ulcer shows folds radiating to the crater, which also has a blood clot *(arrow)* in its base. **B,** Surgical specimen of the ulcer shown in **A** exhibits radiation of the folds to a well-defined ulcer of the greater curve. Note there is no interruption of folds by neoplastic tissue.
From Nelson SW: *Radiol Clin North Am* 7:5, 1969.

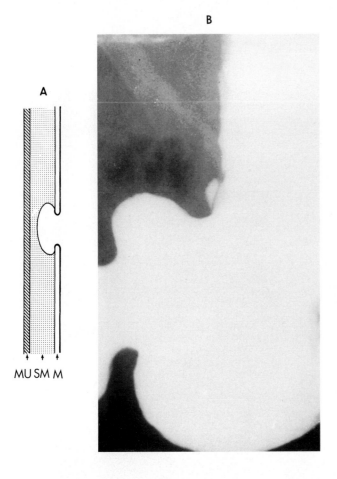

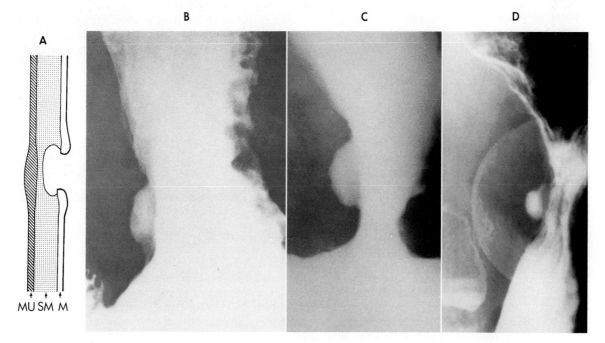

Fig. 16-32 Benign gastric ulcer demonstrating the typical appearance of Hampton's line. **A,** Diagram shows how the overhanging normal mucosa *(M)* contributes to the appearance of Hampton's line. The crater penetrates into the submucosa *(SM)*. The muscularis propria *(MU)* is normal. **B,** Ulcer of the lesser curve in perfect profile elicited by compression. Hampton's line projects as a 1- to 2-mm, sharply defined linear defect across the ulcer neck.

Fig. 16-33 Benign gastric ulcers exhibiting an ulcer collar. **A,** Diagram of the ulcer collar showing it to be composed of swollen mucosa *(M)* and submucosa *(SM)*. The muscularis propria *(MU)* is also swollen but does not contribute to formation of the ulcer collar. The swollen mucosa and submucosa create a thicker, less sharply defined defect than that which causes Hampton's line. **B-D,** Compression spot films of lesser curve ulcers showing the ulcer collar in three patients.

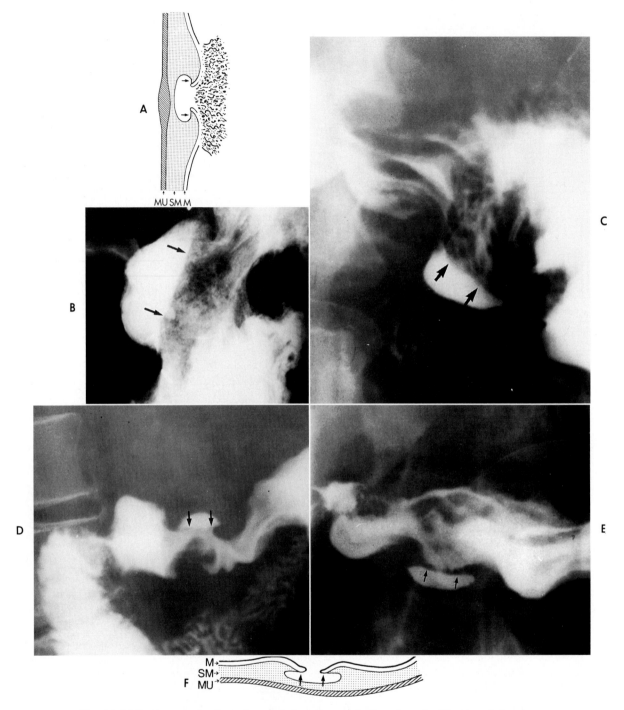

Fig. 16-34 Benign gastric ulcers demonstrating the straight line sign. **A,** Diagram of the ulcer showing the contribution of the overhanging mucosa and submucosa *(arrows)* to the formation of the straight line sign. Extensive edema and debris interfere with visualization of the ulcer signs by contrast-enhanced radiography. **B,** Large ulcer of the lesser curve showing the straight line sign to be a clear indicator of undermining, even though debris obscures the detail of the luminal surface tissue around the crater. **C-E,** Three ulcers exhibiting the straight line sign *(arrows)*. Note the sharp, straight interface of the barium in the crater and the overhanging mucosa and submucosa. **F,** Diagram depicting the contribution of overhanging mucosa *(M)* and submucosa *(SM)* to the formation of the straight line sign *(arrows)* in a patient with an ulcer mound seen in **E.** *MU,* Muscularis propria.

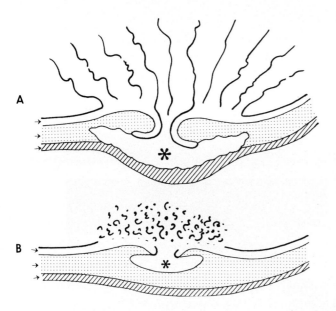

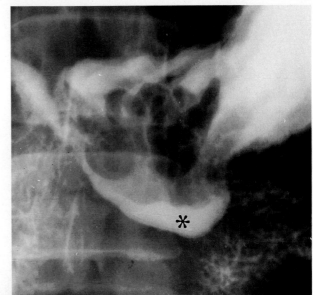

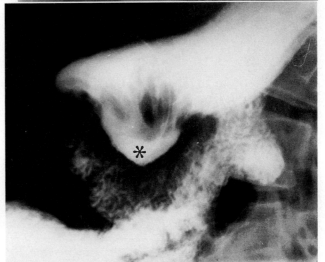

Fig. 16-35 Benign gastric ulcer showing the crescent sign. **A** and **B**, Diagrams showing the marked swelling of the mucosa *(M)* and submucosa *(SM)*, which prolapse into and nearly occlude the ulcer neck. Barium in the crater forms a crescent that projects outside the gastric lumen (*). The muscularis propria may be edematous and eroded **(A)** or normal **(B)**. Debris and edematous folds adjacent to the ulcer neck often limit visualization of the luminal surface **(B)**. **C** and **D**, Typical examples of a benign gastric ulcer in the greater curvature showing how the crescent sign appears in upright anteroposterior **(C)** and lateral **(D)** compression views. The craters (*) frequently retain barium external to the gastric lumen for several days because the orifice is often partially occluded by the large mass of overhanging edematous tissue.

pathognomonic of a benign lesion and is often seen in patients who consume NSAIDs during their waking hours when the erect position favors the contact of these medications with the mucosa of the antrum. The relationship of the sharply defined superior margin of the crescent sign and straight line sign is illustrated in Fig. 16-34, *C*, and Fig. 16-35, in which the undersurface of the overhanging, markedly edematous mound of tissue is shown either as a sharply defined, somewhat concave lobulated line (Fig. 16-35, *C* and *D*) or as a straighter, slightly curved line (see Fig. 16-34, *C*).

Ulcer mound. An ulcer mound results when edema of the mucosa and submucosa is extensive, more so than that which produces an ulcer collar. The ulcer mound, which can be clearly defined in profile (Fig. 16-36, *B* and *C*), is more difficult to evaluate en face, in that filled compres-

sion views often show a mass effect around the crater (Fig. 16-36, *D*) and an indistinct periphery where the mound gradually slopes and blends with the normal mucosa. Conversely, when the ulcer mound is viewed in profile, the interface between the barium in the stomach and the smooth, curvilinear surface of the moundlike mass of tissue is seen as an impression projecting into the lumen (Fig. 16-36, *B* and *C*, and 16-34, *E*). Often when such a large mound of edematous tissue surrounds a benign crater, the presence of intraluminal debris and secretions mixed with the barium precludes optimal tangential visualization of the surface of the large edematous folds. The undermining is still recognizable because of the sharply defined lobulated concave (see Fig. 16-34, *C*) or straight line (see Fig. 16-34, *A* and *B*) seen at the interface between the barium in the crater and the undersurface of the overhanging tissue.

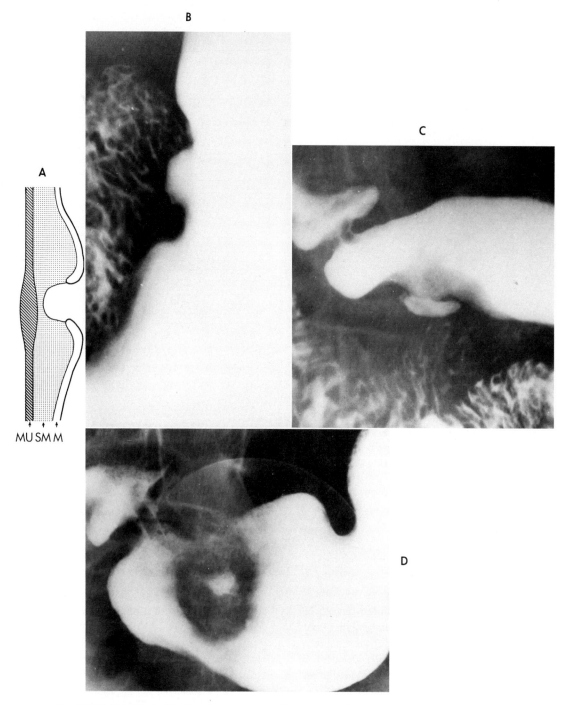

Fig. 16-36 Benign gastric ulcers showing the ulcer mound. **A,** Diagram depicting edema of the mucosa *(M)* and submucosa *(SM)* producing a smooth mass surrounding the ulcer crater. The muscularis propria *(MU)* is often swollen but does not help form the ulcer mound sign. Note the indistinct periphery of the mass as it gradually blends with the normal mucosa. **B** and **C,** Ulcer mounds in two patients viewed in profile are seen as masses that project into the stomach. **D,** In an en face upright compression view, the ulcer mound appears as a smooth mass with indistinct margins as it gradually slopes and blends with normal mucosa.

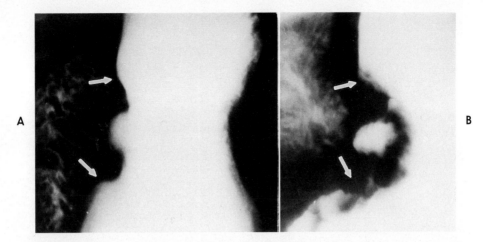

Fig. 16-37 Comparison of an ulcer mound with a neoplastic ulceration. **A,** The benign crater has a smoothly marginated mound of edematous tissue and rounded shoulders, and gradually blends into normal mucosa *(arrows).* **B,** The neoplastic ulcer exhibits abrupt transition between the mound of irregular, nodular neoplastic tissue and normal mucosa *(arrows).*

Differential diagnosis

A benign peptic ulcer can be distinguished from the necrotic area (ulcer) that occurs in a flat sessile neoplasm by the smooth margin of the mound of edematous tissue surrounding its crater and by the gradual transition, or "rounded shoulder" (Fig. 16-37, *A*), at the periphery of this zone of edema where it gradually slopes and blends with the normal mucosa. In contrast, the surface of the malignant lesion is nodular, and the transition between the mound of neoplastic tissue around the crater and the adjacent normal gastric mucosa is abrupt (Fig. 16-37, *B*). These features may be best demonstrated in profile, particularly on filled compression spot films. However, air contrast and en face compression techniques can also clearly depict the surface features of the tissue surrounding the crater and can portray the very subtle nodularity and fold abnormalities associated with shallow, ulcerated neoplasms and depressed superficial carcinomas, as described in Chapters 18 and 19.

If none of the diagnostic signs of benignancy or malignancy is present, the radiologic differentiation between benign and malignant ulceration cannot be made. Such ulcers should be designated as *indeterminate* and endoscopy should be undertaken to allow biopsy of the area. It is very difficult to obtain clear-cut evidence of the benignancy or malignancy of ulcers that are located high on the lesser curvature in the region of the cardia or those in the gastric fundus or greater curve aspect of the upper gastric body. Prominent rugae, sharply curved anatomic contours, and the inaccessibility of these areas to palpation and compression create this diagnostic dilemma. In addition, ulcerating lesions in these locations are statistically more likely to be malignant than those situated along the lesser curvature and posterior wall of the body or those in the region of the angularis, gastric antrum, or pylorus.[105,107,108,110]

Ulcer healing

Ulcer healing (Fig. 16-38) is strong but not absolute proof that a gastric ulcer is benign. The rate of healing is variable, however, and depends on the cause, the size of the ulcer, age of the patient, and the treatment adopted. Benign-appearing gastric ulcers should be followed until complete healing by either endoscopy and biopsy or repeat upper GI series after 8 to 12 weeks. Ulcer scars may be permanent (Fig. 16-39) if the ulcer destroyed portions of the muscularis propria.

Complications

The complications of a gastric ulcer include gastric outlet obstruction (20%), penetration to contiguous organs, perforation (7%), fistula (duodenum, small bowel, and colon), and hemorrhage (20%). Patients who are suspected to have such problems may be evaluated by plain films (see Fig. 16-25), barium-enhanced radiography (Fig. 16-40), or cross-sectional techniques. CT[113,114] and sonography[115] should be considered when penetration into contiguous organs, occult perforation, or abscess is suspected.

HYPERTROPHIC GASTROPATHY

Conditions categorized as hypertrophic gastropathy are characterized by the pathologic and radiographic features of mucosal hypertrophy and enlargement of the gastric folds (hyperrugosity). Diseases in this category include Menetrier's disease, the Zollinger-Ellison syndrome, hypertrophic hypersecretory gastropathy, hypertrophic hypersecretory gastropathy with protein loss, hyperplastic gastropathy, pseudolymphoma, a Menetrier's-like hypertrophic gastropathy that has been identified in AIDS patients and children (which may be reversible and is in some cases probably related to cytomegolvirus infection),[116,117] and a reversible

Fig. 16-38
For legend
see opposite page.

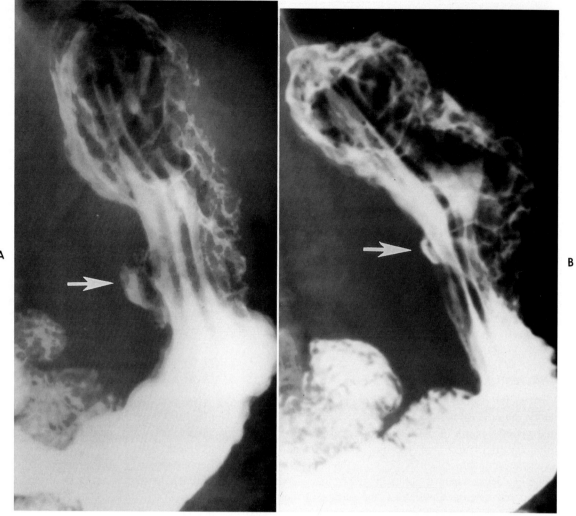

A

B

Fig. 16-39 Ulcer scars revealed by filled compression and air contrast techniques. **A,** A posterior wall gastric ulcer has completely healed, leaving smooth, sharply defined folds radiating toward the scar at the site of the previous ulcer *(arrowhead)*. **B** and **C,** These lesser curve ulcers in two patients have healed, leaving a slight residual deformity to the radiating folds, minimal irregularity of the mucosa, and prominent areae gastricae in the region of the scars *(arrowheads)*.

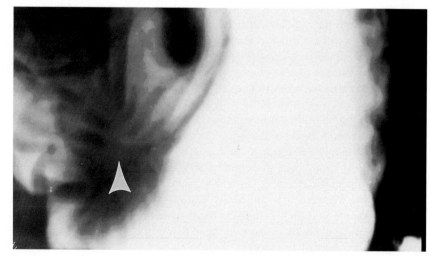

A

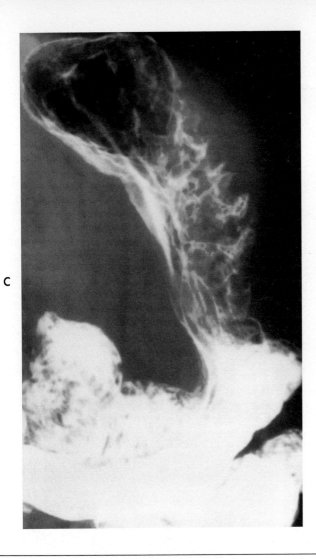

C

Fig. 16-38 Healing of a benign gastric ulcer. **A-C,** Radiographs obtained at 1-month intervals showing complete healing of a benign ulcer located in the lesser curve *(arrows)*.

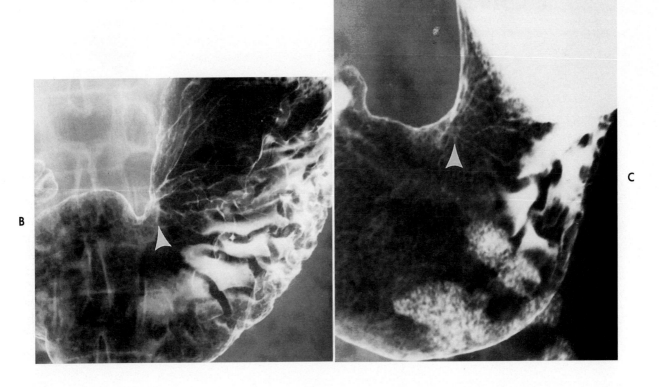

B

C

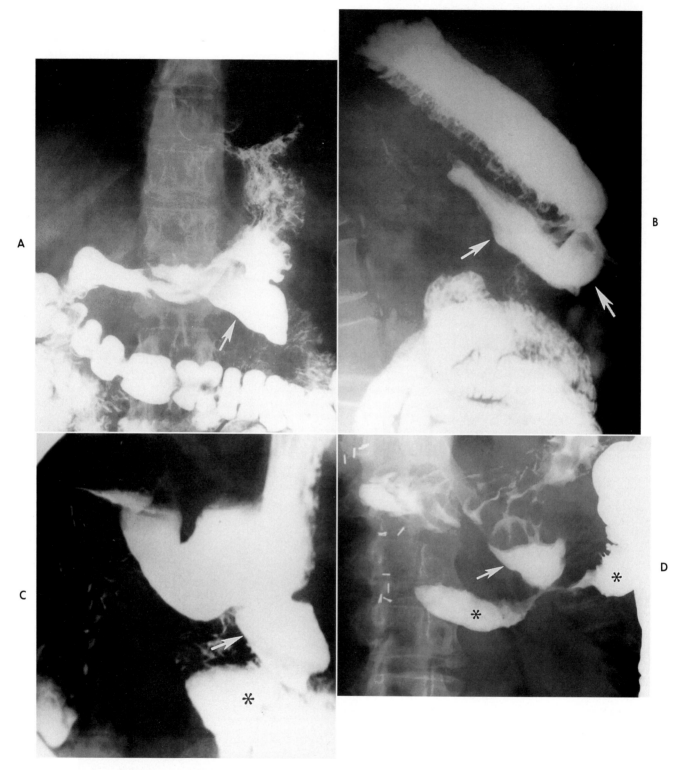

Fig. 16-40 Complications of a benign gastric ulcer defined by barium radiography. **A** and **B,** Perforation into the lesser sac is shown by the presence of contrast material projecting posterior and inferior to the gastric antrum *(arrows)*. **C,** Gastrojejunal fistula through a large ulcer *(arrow)* shows early opacification of the jejunal loops (*). **D,** Gastrocolic fistula through a large ulcer *(arrow)* exhibiting a crescent sign is demonstrated during a barium enema when the agent entered the ulcer from the transverse colon (*).
D courtesy of Dr. Esmond Mapp.

allergic gastropathy that has been identified in adults and may be related to eosinophilic gastritis.[118,119]

Hyperrugosity

Gastric rugae are composed of mucosa, lamina propria, muscularis mucosae, and variable portions of the submucosa. All of these layers may share in fold enlargement, in that edema, infiltration with neoplastic or inflammatory cells, or vascular engorgement can all result in hyperrugosity.

Gastric folds should be considered enlarged when they measure more than 5 cm on radiographs of the distended stomach, especially in the antrum.[120] A more liberal upper limit (1 cm) can be applied to rugae in the setting of a collapsed gastric fundus. Enlarged folds in the gastric fundus and body have been correlated with increased acid secretion, but such is not the case with the enlarged folds in the gastric antrum.[121,122] Normal folds may appear prominent, especially in the gastric antrum of older individuals, owing to loss of elasticity and decreased tone of the muscularis mucosae.

Enlarged and tortuous gastric mucosal folds may be caused by a variety of pathologic conditions, both inflammatory and neoplastic, and may also occur as a normal anatomic variant.[120] The nonneoplastic causes are listed in the box below. The radiologic features that suggest an underlying pathologic reason for fold enlargement include nodularity or focal swelling, asymmetry or segmental distribution, wall rigidity, excess fluid, and erosion or ulceration.[123]

□ BENIGN CAUSES OF HYPERRUGOSITY □

- Gastritis
  - Peptic
  - Infectious
  - Alcoholic
  - Hypertrophic
  - Phlegmonous
  - Parasitic
  - Granulomatous
- Injury gastropathy
  - Alcoholic gastritis
  - Gastric radiation injury
  - Medication-induced gastritis
  - Corrosive gastropathy
- Hypertrophic gastropathy
  - Menetrier's disease
  - Zollinger-Ellison syndrome
  - Pseudolymphoma
- Miscellaneous
  - Amyloidosis
  - Eosinophilic gastritis
  - Pancreatitis
  - Varices
  - Hypoproteinemia
  - Normal variant

Menetrier's disease

Menetrier in 1888 was the first to describe a syndrome in which giant mucosal hypertrophy occurs in conjunction with gastric carcinoma.[124] Although a very rare condition, it has become the standard example of hypertrophic gastropathy. Hypoproteinemia and hypochlorhydria have been accepted as its characteristic features, and it is particularly prevalent in middle-aged men (up to nine times its occurrence in women).[125-130] Variations do occur, in that the characteristic mucosal hypertrophy may be associated with hypoproteinemia and hyperchlorhydria,[127,128] as well as with normal serum protein and gastric acid levels.[126]

The natural history of Menetrier's disease in adults suggests that it is an irreversible process, although there are a few case reports of the spontaneous transformation from a hypertrophic to an atrophic appearance, with associated clearing of the gastric protein loss.[124,129,131] In children the disease usually resolves spontaneously.[123,126,130,132] Its frequent association with eosinophilia in children suggests that it may be a different disease in this age group, possibly a manifestation of eosinophilic gastritis.

Because gastric carcinoma develops in about 10% of the patients with Menetrier's disease,[130,131,133] and because the disease is generally irreversible, gastric resection has been recommended as a reasonable form of therapy.[134]

The histologic findings that typify this form of hypertrophic gastropathy include a grossly thickened mucosa measuring up to 6 mm (the normal thickness ranges from 0.6 to 1 mm). There is also a proliferation of both the mucus-secreting cells of the gastric glands and the surface epithelial cells, but cystic dilatation of the basal portions of the gastric glands is the predominant finding (Fig. 16-41). Chief and parietal cells may be atrophic, thus explaining the decreased acid production seen in the disorder.

The most notable radiographic feature of Menetrier's disease is the marked enlargement of the gastric folds. These large and tortuous gastric rugae are usually present along the greater curve in the fundus and body, but generally spare the antrum. They may, however, exist throughout the stomach (Fig. 16-42, *B*) and occasionally are localized to the fundus, the greater curve, or the antrum[135] (Fig. 16-42, *A*). Erosions and ulcers may also be present. Small intestinal fold enlargement may reflect the presence of edema resulting from the hypoproteinemia.

Zollinger-Ellison syndrome

The Zollinger-Ellison syndrome[136-140] is a hypersecretory type of hypertrophic gastropathy. It is different from Menetrier's disease and its variants in that there is no hypoproteinemia, the serum gastrin levels are elevated, and there are large amounts of gastric secretions. It is caused

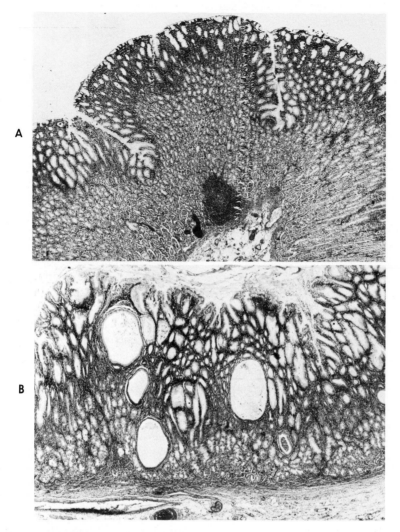

Fig. 16-41 Hypertrophic gastropathy. **A,** Photomicrograph shows some proliferation of the surface epithelial cells, but hyperplasia limited largely to the glandular layer of the mucosa is the dominant finding. **B,** Note the cystic glandular dilatation in an otherwise normal glandular layer.

by a gastrin-secreting tumor, and the clinical picture consists of the following triad of findings[139]:

1. Marked gastric hypersecretion containing an unusually large amount of hydrochloric acid, usually more than 100 mEq every 12 hours.

2. A fulminating peptic ulcer diathesis resistant to medical therapy. The ulcers frequently resemble ordinary peptic ulcer disease of the stomach and duodenal bulb, but they are often situated in the second and third portions of the duodenum and proximal portion of the jejunum. The fulminating peptic ulcer diathesis is characterized by recurrent large marginal ulcers that form after conventional surgical operations for the treatment of peptic ulcer.

3. A gastrin-secreting non-beta islet cell tumor (gastrinoma). About one fourth of the patients with the Zollinger-Ellison syndrome have other endocrine abnormalities associated with multiple endocrine adenomas. Fasting serum gastrin levels are characteristically greater than 1000 pg per milliliter. This high output of gastrin results in the continuous production of hyperacidic gastric secretions.

The striking but nonspecific roentgenographic finding in the stomach is the presence of a large amount of fluid in a fasting patient who otherwise shows no evidence of pyloric obstruction. Films obtained in the erect position usually show this finding (Fig. 16-43). The barium coating of the gastric mucosa is usually poor, due to hypersecretion, and this diminishes the diagnostic quality of double-contrast studies. However, a single- or air-contrast barium examination and CT scans often clearly show the huge gastric folds (Fig. 16-44).

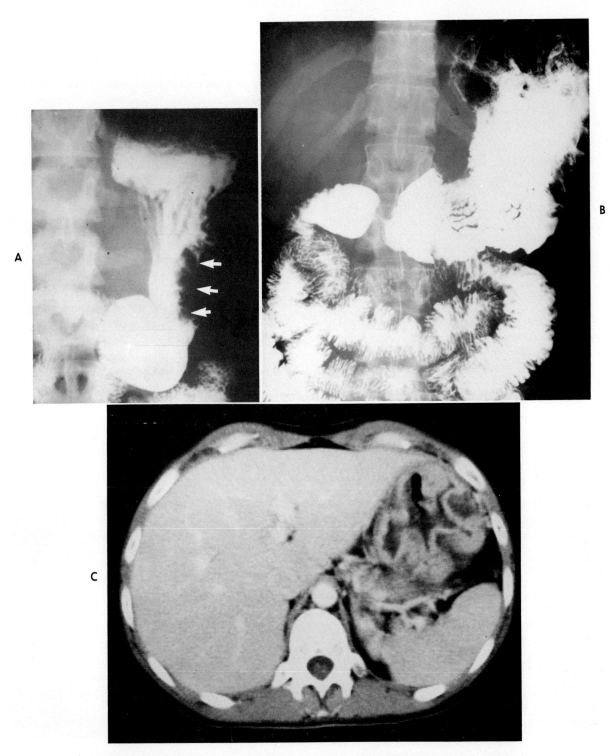

Fig. 16-42 Menetrier's disease. **A,** Focal area of giant rugal hypertrophy along the greater curve of the body of the stomach *(arrowheads).* **B,** An upper GI series in another patient demonstrates diffuse and marked enlargement of the rugal pattern involving the fundus, body, and proximal antrum of the stomach. There is excess fluid in the gastric lumen. **C,** Computed tomogram shows marked enlargement of the gastric folds with redundancy and infolding.
B and **C** courtesy of Drs. Peter Huzyk and Harold Shulman.

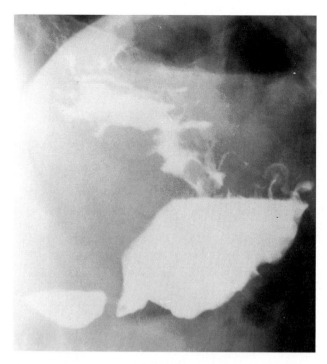

Fig. 16-43 Zollinger-Ellison syndrome. There is marked fluid retention in this fasting patient. Note fluid above the barium and air fluid level near the uppermost portion of the fundus. There is an open pylorus with contrast in the duodenal bulb and no evidence of obstruction.
From Nelson SW, Christoforidis AJ: *Semin Roentgenol* 3:254, 1968.

When a patient has large gastric folds, gastric hypersecretion, and an open pylorus, the presence of *any one* of the following *associated* radiographic abnormalities is highly suggestive, if not diagnostic, of the Zollinger-Ellison syndrome[140]:

1. Multiple ulcers between the duodenal bulb and ligament of Treitz (Fig. 16-45)
2. One or more peptic ulcers in the region of the ligament of Treitz
3. One or more peptic ulcers in the proximal jejunum
4. Perforation of a clinically unsuspected ulcer in the distal duodenum or proximal jejunum
5. Large, rapidly recurrent anastomotic ulcers after operation for peptic ulcer disease.

Pseudolymphoma

Benign lymphoproliferative lesions of the stomach are rare. Although variably designated as *lymphoreticular hyperplasia*, *chronic lymphoid gastritis*, *reactive lymphoid hyperplasia*, and *gastric lymphoid hyperplasia*, recent authors have favored the designation *pseudolymphoma*.[141-144]

Pseudolymphoma of the stomach is an apt name for the lesion, because both its radiologic and gross appearance mimics malignant lymphoma. Both entities exhibit marked gastric fold thickening, may be complicated by ulceration, and may possess a similar color and texture when the specimen is incised.[145] Not until careful microscopic examination of the fixed specimen reveals the characteristic histo-

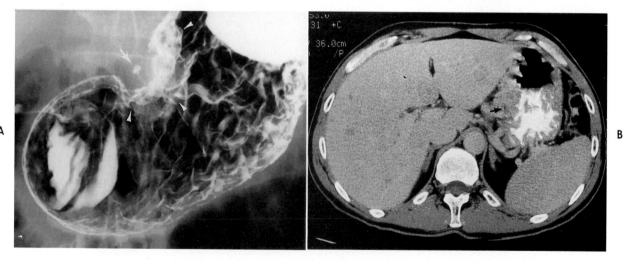

Fig. 16-44 Zollinger-Ellison syndrome. **A,** Double-contrast examination shows hyperrugosity and a deep narrow-necked ulcer in the lesser curve *(arrow)* with a large ulcer mound *(arrowheads)*. **B,** Computed tomogram shows rugal enlargement and a mass (ulcer mound) along the lesser curve. There is a small amount of air in the mass, indicating the presence of an ulcer *(arrow)*.

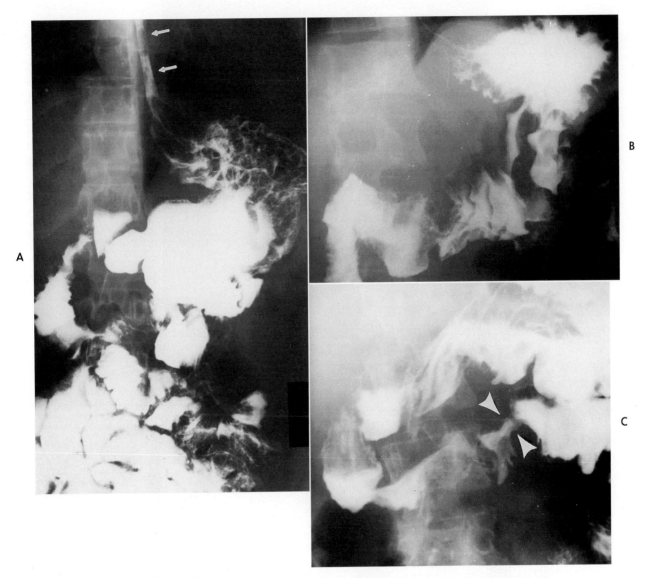

Fig. 16-45 Zollinger-Ellison syndrome. **A,** There are enlarged gastric folds and gastric hypersecretion, together with an open pylorus and enlarged irregular duodenal folds. Esophageal narrowing *(arrows)* is due to severe gastroesophageal reflux disease. **B** and **C,** Another patient with gastric fold enlargement and ulcer in the third portion of the duodenum *(arrowheads)*.
B and **C** from Nelson SW, Christoforidis AJ: *Semin Roentgenol* 3:254, 1968.

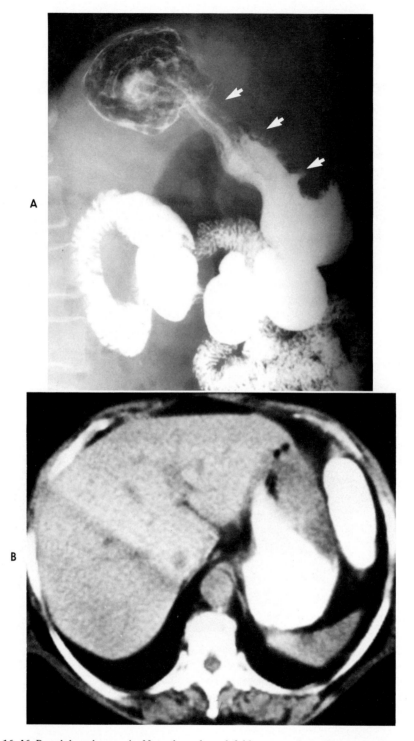

Fig. 16-46 Pseudolymphoma. **A,** Note the enlarged fold pattern along the greater curve of the fundus and body *(arrows)*. The distal stomach is normal. **B,** CT image of the stomach shows focal thickening in the lateral aspect of the gastric wall. There is no hepatosplenomegaly.

logic features is the diagnosis established. These features include a polymorphous cellular infiltrate, lymph follicle hyperplasia with reactive germinal centers, and fibroblastic reaction.[144,146,147] Immunocytochemical processing of deep biopsy tissue may also be necessary to firmly establish the diagnosis.[148]

Until recently, pseudolymphoma was considered most likely to represent an inflammatory response to chronic gastric ulceration, as most cases were associated with ulcer disease.[149,150] Recent authors, however, have proposed that pseudolymphoma is in some way related to true lymphoma.[144,147,148]

Radiographic findings include gastric hyperrugosity, which may be focal (Fig. 16-46, A), intraluminal masses, and multiple ulcerations.[141,149] CT scans show findings similar to those of gastric lymphoma, except that lymphadenopathy and splenic enlargement are not found in the presence of pseudolymphoma (Fig. 16-46, B).

Injury gastropathy

As listed in the box on p. 325, a number of insults can cause gastric inflammation or necrosis. Hemorrhagic gastritis of varying severity may result from alcohol intake or from NSAID and corticosteroid use. More severe lesions have resulted from gastric freezing, which was once used to treat chronic ulcer disease, gastric radiation injury, and the ingestion of corrosive substances.

Corrosive gastropathy

Corrosive agents, which are swallowed either accidentally or with suicidal intent, are usually strong acids or alkalis.[151] The classic teaching was that alkalis chiefly affect the esophagus and spare the stomach.[152] However, the ready availability of strongly alkaline solutions has led to an increased incidence of severe gastric injury. Strong acids tend to severely damage the stomach, and esophageal injury is frequently simultaneous.[153] The coagulation necrosis produced by these agents may affect only the mucosa and submucosa or may involve the entire thickness of the gastric wall.[154]

Radiographic studies obtained soon after ingestion (Fig. 16-47, A, B, and C) show the striking rugal edema, ulcers, atony, dilatation, intramural gas, sloughing of the mucosa, and perforation.[155] Afterward, cicatrization occurs (Fig. 16-47, D and E) in conjunction with varying degrees of gastric outlet obstruction, which may not become apparent for 3 to 10 weeks.[152,154-156] The duodenum may be involved, but an initial intense acute pyloric spasm may limit duodenal exposure. The radiographic appearance of corrosive gastritis may be different if granular corrosives have been ingested in gelatin capsules.[156] The corrosive effect thus spares the esophagus but may produce more focal ulcerative gastritis (Fig. 16-48) and perforation.

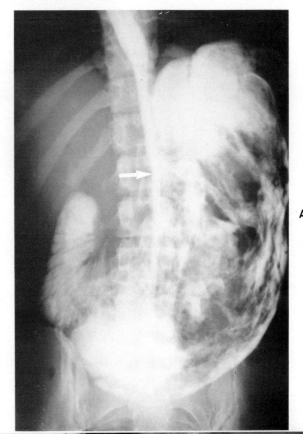

A

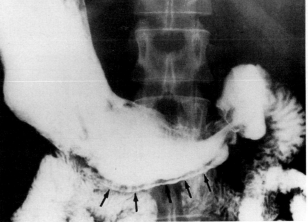

B

Fig. 16-47 Corrosive ingestion. **A,** A 26-year-old woman drank a concentrated solution of drain cleaner. Upper GI series obtained through a nasogastric tube *(arrow)* demonstrates diffuse gastric atony, while necrotic mucosa and other debris fills the enlarged stomach. The duodenum was protected by pyloric spasm. **B,** In another patient who ingested a corrosive substance, there is dissection of barium into the gastric wall beneath the necrotic mucosa *(arrows)*. *Continued.*

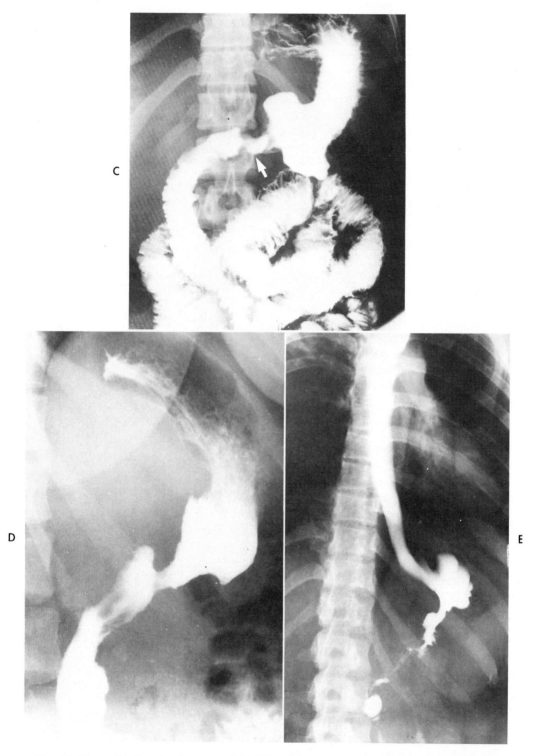

Fig. 16-47, cont'd Corrosive ingestion. **C-E,** This 39-year-old woman accidentally drank cleaning fluid containing hydrochloric acid. **C,** Initial film taken 24 hours after ingestion shows narrowing of the gastric body in the antrum, ulcer in the distal antrum *(arrow),* and enlarged mucosal folds in the duodenum and proximal jejunum. **D,** Two weeks later, after the mucosa had completely sloughed, there is no recognizable mucosal pattern in the stomach or duodenum. **E,** At 5 weeks there is striking stenosis of the stomach and duodenum. Note the relatively normal esophagus.

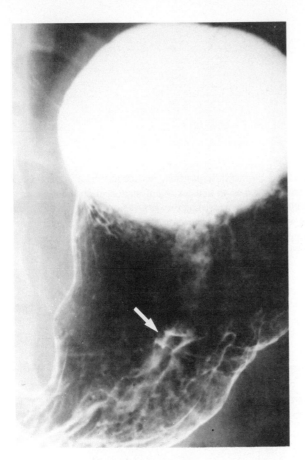

Fig. 16-48 Focal corrosive gastric injury. This 30-year-old man packed granular drain cleaner into gelatin capsules and ingested them in a suicide attempt. Note the focal stellate-shaped ulcer of the stomach *(arrow)*.

Gastric radiation injury

Doses of radiation sufficient to produce radiation gastritis are, on rare occasions, delivered to the stomach during the treatment of upper abdominal malignancies.[157] The radiation effect is ischemia, which stems from endarteritis of the vessels supplying the intestinal wall. The ischemic process results in edema and ulceration in the acute phase, which may progress to become chronic fibrosis with luminal narrowing. These findings are observed when the dose level exceeds 4500 rads administered within 4 to 5 weeks. Radiation ulcer and perforation may occur, typically 4 to 8 weeks after irradiation.[157,158] These ulcers are radiographically indistinguishable from ordinary peptic ulcers. The associated edema and fibrosis may then produce antral rigidity and narrowing with loss of motor activity (Fig. 16-49). These late effects may occur 1 month to 6 years after irradiation, but the median time is 5 months.

MISCELLANEOUS GASTROPATHIES
Eosinophilic gastropathy

Eosinophilic gastropathy embraces such entities as eosinophilic granuloma, inflammatory pseudotumors, and eosinophilic gastroenteritis, all of which are characterized by gastrointestinal infiltration by eosinophils. They probably have an inflammatory etiology, although a history of allergy is found in approximately 50% of the patients.[118,159] The most striking clinical feature of eosinophilic gastroenteritis is the presence of peripheral eosinophilia, which may exist in as many as 60% of the patients. The eosinophilic infil-

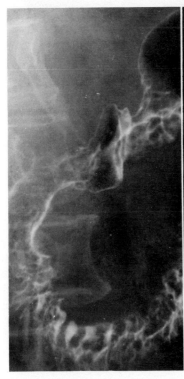

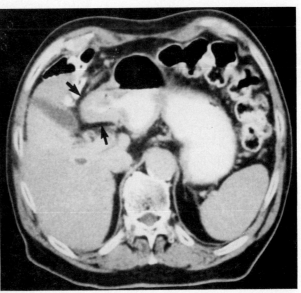

Fig. 16-49 Radiation antritis. Anorexia, nausea, and vomiting developed in this 60-year-old man after he had undergone midline abdominal radiation for the treatment of lymphoma. **A,** Spot film of the antrum and duodenum shows fold thickening. **B,** CT scan demonstrates thickening of the wall of the distal stomach and pylorus *(arrows)*.

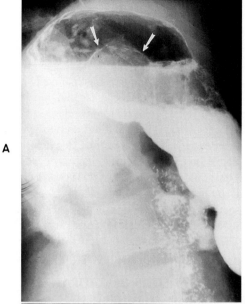

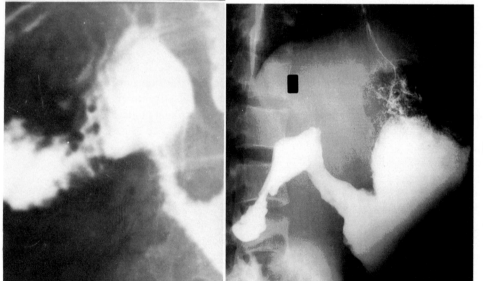

Fig. 16-50 Eosinophilic gastritis. **A,** Lobular mass in the gastric fundus *(arrows)* is an unusual manifestation of eosinophilic gastropathy. **B,** Chronic eosinophilic gastritis involving the distal antrum with a cobblestone appearance to the mucosa. **C,** Antral narrowing and partial gastric obstruction.
A courtesy of Dr. Ronald B. Port; **C** courtesy of Dr. David Christie.

trate, which is considered to be the histologic hallmark of the disease, may involve any or all layers of the gut.[160-162]

The stomach is involved alone in about one half of the cases, with a predilection for the antrum.[161,162] During the acute phase, the radiographic appearance may include enlarged rugae, polypoid lesions (Fig. 16-50, *A*), or signs of gastritis, whereas a contracted antrum simulating scirrhous carcinoma (Fig. 16-50, *B* and *C*) may be seen during the chronic phase.

The term *eosinophilic granuloma* has been given to a circumscribed inflammatory polypoid lesion that arises in the submucosa. It is composed of fibroelastic tissue, numerous blood vessels, and dilated lymphatics, and has a variable degree of eosinophilic infiltration.[163,164] It occurs almost exclusively in the gastric antrum and is not associated with peripheral eosinophilia. A better term is *inflammatory fibroid gastric polyp*.[165] It is not related to eosinophilic granuloma of bone or to eosinophilic gastroenteritis.

Amyloidosis

Gastrointestinal involvement by amyloidosis is common in patients with this disorder and, on occasion, may be confined to the stomach.[166-169] There may be multiple erosions and ulcerations with hemorrhage,[166] or the stomach may exhibit a diffuse infiltration, with generalized thickening of the wall and loss of rugae simulating a scirrhous carcinoma. A localized mass may simulate a polypoid or sessile neoplasm.[168]

Abnormalities of function
Obstruction

Gastric outlet obstruction can be a complication of both malignant and benign diseases of the stomach. The differential diagnosis includes the processes listed in the box on the right, and precise diagnosis can usually be established by the results of barium examination, endoscopy, or both. If gastric obstruction is suspected, but not confirmed by upper gastrointestinal series, the patient should be evaluated for gastric motor dysfunction.

Gastric atony

Gastric retention in the absence of mechanical obstruction can occur in the context of many disease processes and is the result of dysfunction of the gastric neuromuscular system. Many of these processes are listed in the box below. Gastric atony may develop gradually as an insidious process or may occur acutely. The acute type has been given many names that reflect the various etiologic theories proposed to explain the process. These include acute gastric dilatation, cast syndrome, postoperative gastric paralysis, arteriomesenteric ileus, postpartum dilatation of the stomach, acute gastric succorrhea, Wilkie's syndrome, gastric atony or neuropathy, acute duodenal occlusion, and primary ectasia of the stomach.[170-172]

The underlying factors responsible for triggering this neuromuscular dysfunction remain a mystery. The clinical features consist of vomiting, abdominal distention, and vascular collapse. It can develop so rapidly that, within 24 to 48 hours, the stomach fills the entire abdomen and distends to volumes of as much as 7500 ml. The diagnosis is frequently suggested when a large stomach filled with air and fluid is seen on conventional radiographs of the abdomen. The paralysis must be differentiated from gastric outlet obstruction such as that due to ulcer disease, neoplasm, volvulus, or pyloric stenosis. Retention of barium and loss of muscle tone in a dilated stomach without peristaltic activity are radiographic features of diagnostic value. The pylorus is usually patulous, and gastric contents can be manually expressed into the duodenum, which may also be dilated.

Acute gastric dilatation may progress to chronic gastric retention.[173,174] Although the latter implies a milder and more chronic process, in fact the two conditions are not necessarily mutually exclusive. One of the most frequently encountered examples of chronic gastric atony is the decrease in gastric motility with resultant dysfunction or distention, or both, that is encountered in patients with diabetes.[175] The syndrome is now well recognized to be diabetic gastroparesis, which occurs predominantly in diabetics with advanced disease and complications of retinopathy, nephropathy, and peripheral neuropathy.[176-179] These patients may be asymp-

---

□ BENIGN CAUSES OF GASTRIC OBSTRUCTION □

Congenital lesions
  Pyloric hypertrophy
  Antral diaphragm
  Duplication cyst
  Ectopic pancreas
Adjacent lesions
  Pseudocyst, pancreatitis
  Abscess
  Gallstone obstruction
Bezoar and foreign body
Iatrogenic
  Tubes, balloons
  Postoperative stenosis
  Radiation stenosis
Ulcer or gastritis scarring
Crohn's disease
Injury gastropathy
  Corrosive stenosis
Volvulus
Intussusception

□ CAUSES OF GASTRIC ATONY □

ACUTE

Surgical vagotomy, fundoplication
Diabetes
Postoperative effects
Childbirth
Trauma, burns, corrosives
Immobilizing casts
Infection, inflammation
Hypokalemia, hypocalcemia
Medications
Phlegmonous gastritis

CHRONIC

Diabetes
Stroke
Medications
Immobilizing casts
Surgical vagotomy, fundoplication, gastroplasty
Scleroderma, polymyositis
Chronic idiopathic pseudoobstruction
Uremia
Muscular dystrophy
Myxedema
Obesity

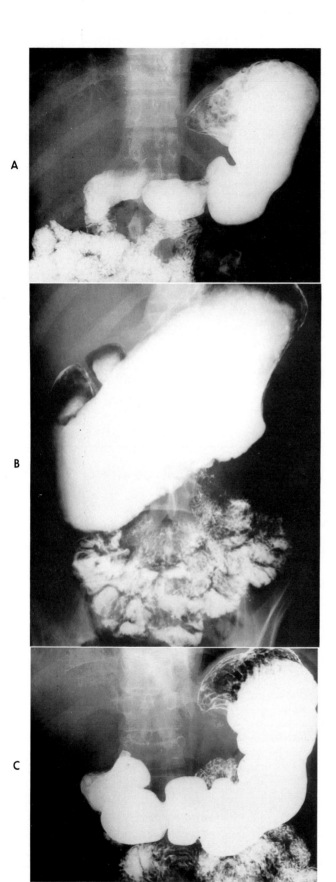

tomatic, have vague abdominal problems, or have vomiting severe enough to suggest pyloric obstruction.

The radiographic manifestations of diabetic gastroparesis (Fig. 16-51) include gastric atony, with (Fig. 16-51, *B*) or without (Fig. 16-51, *A*) dilatation, diminished to absent peristalsis or ineffective hyperperistalsis (Fig. 16-51, *C*) with gastric retention, a patulous or hypertonic pylorus, and a dilated duodenum. Barium may remain in the stomach for 5 or 6 hours in affected patients, even though there is no pyloric obstruction.[172,175] Because barium evaluation is nonquantitative in determining gastric dysfunction, gastric emptying scintigraphy has been utilized instead.[180]

Various acute illnesses, more chronic diseases such as scleroderma,[181] polymyositis, dermatomyositis,[182] myotonic dystrophy,[183] and chronic idiopathic intestinal pseudoobstruction,[184] and the aftermath of vagotomy and gastroplasty may have bezoar formation associated with gastric atony[170,185,186] (Fig. 16-52).

Volvulus

Gastric volvulus is an uncommon condition in which there is an abnormal degree of rotation of the stomach about itself, resulting in gastric obstruction. Although the term *gastric volvulus* has been used to identify abnormalities of gastric position without obstruction, such as the "upside-down stomach," gastric displacement through sliding hiatus hernias, and large paraesophageal hernias, a strong case has been made for using the term *true volvulus* only when there is obstruction.[187] These conditions of torsion, displacement, or chronic volvulus without obstruction should be distinguished from acute volvulus in which there is a strangulating type of obstruction. As much as 180 degrees of twisting may occur without obstruction or strangulation of the blood supply. Twisting beyond 180 degrees usually produces complete obstruction with clinical manifestations of an acute condition in the abdomen[188] and, occasionally, gastric necrosis.[189] The triad of severe epigastric pain, vigorous unproductive attempts to vomit, and inability to pass a tube into the stomach, constitutes the classic clinical presentation of a patient with gastric volvulus.

Fig. 16-51 Diabetic gastropathy. **A,** The stomach is unobstructed with retention of food material. Fluoroscopy revealed diminished peristaltic activity. **B,** In another patient, there is severe gastric distention and retention of contrast material. There was no peristaltic activity, although contrast flowed from the stomach with gravity. **C,** In a 30-year-old diabetic man with gastric enlargement and no obstruction, note the ineffective hyperperistalsis as indicated by the six contraction waves along the greater and lesser curves.

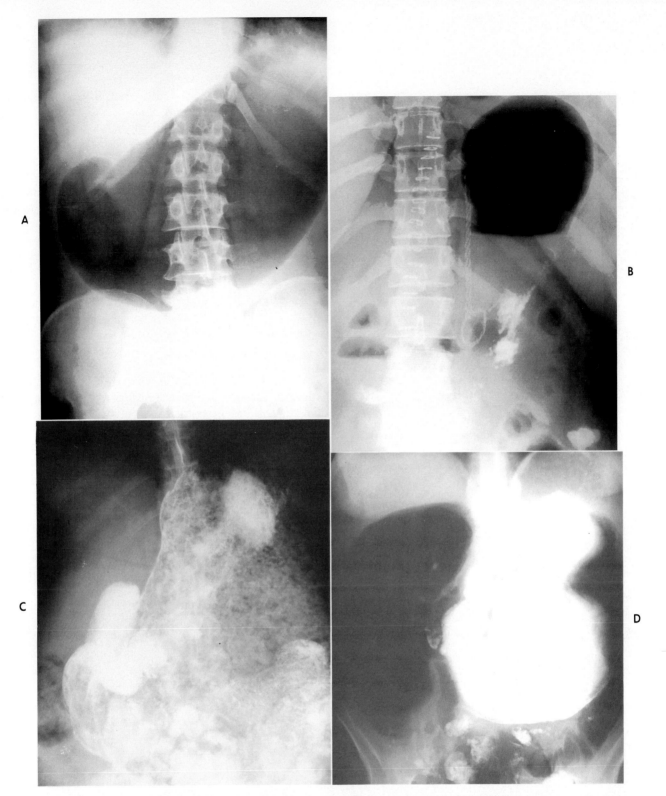

Fig. 16-52 Gastric atony. **A,** Acute gastric dilatation in a patient with acute hepatitis. Note the marked gastric distention and lack of gas in other intestinal segments. **B,** Gastric atony after vertical band gastroplasty was performed. Upright film obtained 3 days after the administration of contrast material shows the retention of contrast within the distal stomach and a large air fluid level. Gastroplasty is frequently performed in conjunction with vagotomy, which can cause gastric atony. **C,** Gastric atony after vagotomy. A 61-year-old woman was examined because of progressive abdominal distention that developed after she underwent vagotomy for the treatment of peptic ulcer disease. The stomach is markedly enlarged and contains much retained solid material. There was no peristaltic activity but barium flowed with gravity into the duodenum. **D,** Chronic idiopathic intestinal pseudoobstruction. A 58-year-old woman was evaluated because of chronic abdominal distention. A 5-hour film shows gastric distention and only minimal contrast in the small intestine. Note the colonic distention.
A courtesy of Dr. Saul A. Rosenblum.

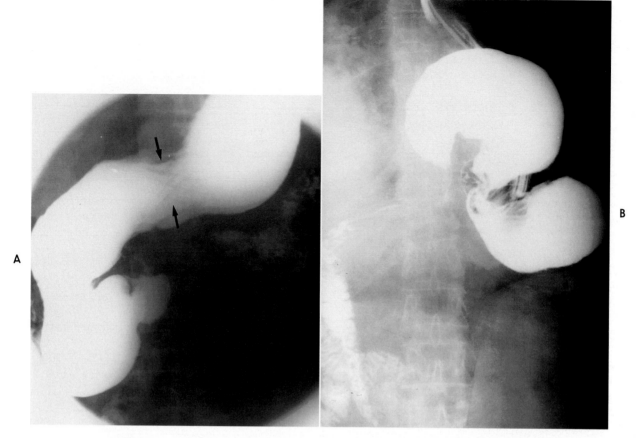

Fig. 16-53 Gastric volvulus. **A,** Partial organoaxial volvulus. This nonobstructing volvulus shows twisting of the fundus and body of the stomach, as indicated by crossing of the mucosal folds *(arrows)*. **B,** Partial mesenteroaxial volvulus exhibits a torsion point between the body of the stomach (marked by a nasogastric tube at the esophagogastric junction) and distal antrum. These examples of partial or nonobstructing gastric torsion illustrate the two types of gastric volvulus. If the volvulus were complete, obstruction at the esophagus or proximal stomach would prevent depiction of the pathologic anatomy seen here.

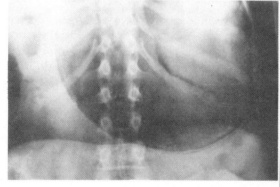

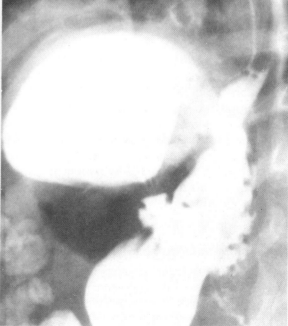

Fig. 16-54 Gastric volvulus with intramural pneumatosis in a 49-year-old woman with a 10-day history of nausea and vomiting. **A,** Large, gas-distended stomach is the result of gastric volvulus. Note the radiolucent lines within the gastric wall on the greater curve caused by submucosal and subserosal gas. **B,** Barium study done several days later reveals the obstruction has disappeared but the gastric torsion persists.

When the rotation occurs about a line extending from the cardia to the pylorus along the longitudinal axis of the stomach, it is classified as an *organoaxial volvulus* (Fig. 16-53, A). If the rotation is about an axis running transversely across the stomach at right angles to the lesser and greater curves, it is designated a *mesenteroaxial volvulus*[190-192] (Fig. 16-53, B). Mixed types are also seen. Laxity or elongation of the four gastric suspensory ligaments (hepatic, splenic, colic, and phrenic) is the underlying cause of volvulus. Most of the reported cases have been associated with diaphragmatic abnormalities, such as enventeration or hernia. About one third of the cases are associated with hiatus hernia, usually of the paraesophageal type.

The large, distended stomach resulting from volvulus can be recognized on abdominal and chest radiographs. Strangulation may lead to mucosal ischemia, with subsequent areas of focal necrosis that permit gas to dissect into the gastric wall, producing intramural emphysema (Fig. 16-54, A). Perforation may result from full-thickness necrosis. A barium study in a patient with acute obstructive volvulus will show failure of the contrast material to enter the stomach and perhaps "beaking" at the point of the twist. Fluoroscopic guidance may help in advancing a nasogastric tube into the obstructed stomach and allow decompression with stabilization of the patient's condition.

The differential diagnosis includes gastric atony, acute gastric dilatation, and other causes of gastric obstruction. In these conditions, however, there is no delay in the passage of barium into the stomach, which has a normal or distended configuration.

Gastric bezoar

In modern medicine the term *bezoar* is used to refer to an intragastric mass composed of accumulated ingested material. A bezoar may be composed of hair (trichobezoar), fruit or vegetable products (phytobezoar),[193] or the concretions, such as resins, asphalt, or other material,[194] listed in the box on right. Phytobezoars are the most common, making up 55% of some series.[195] The classic phytobezoar is caused by the ingestion of unripened persimmons. In modern medical practice, however, the formation of bezoars is more commonly due to altered gastric motility or anatomy that causes ingested food material to be retained in the stomach. These processes include impaired digestion, diminished peristalsis, or partial obstruction.[193] Bezoars of this type (Fig. 16-55) are common following vagotomy and gastroduodenostomy and are less common following gastrojejunostomy.

Trichobezoars (Fig. 16-56) are much less common than phytobezoars and occur almost entirely in long-haired females with trichotillomania. In more than 80% of the reported cases, the patients are under the age of 30 years. Trichobezoars can frequently be palpated as an epigastric mass and may be as large as 6½ pounds (3 kg).[196]

Bezoars cause symptoms that stem from the mechanical presence of either the foreign body or an associated gastric ulcer, which exists in 24% to 70% of the reported cases.[194] The latter finding can be explained by the stasis, antral distention, and increased gastrin secretion provoked by the foreign body. Radiologically, bezoars are not difficult to detect, as they conform to the shape of the gastric lumen and are freely movable. Plain films may show a mottled, mixed-density mass in the area of the stomach (Fig. 16-56, C). This finding can be confirmed by a barium examination in which the agent surrounds and outlines the mass in all projections (Fig. 16-56, B and D). These lesions may fill the entire lumen of a markedly dilated stomach and may extend into the duodenum. They may also be detected by CT or ultrasonography. The latter may show a highly reflective mass with intense shadowing[197] (Fig. 16-56, A).

Varices

Varices are the most common vascular abnormality of the stomach. Although usually located in the fundus and proximal gastric body, they may also be found in the gastric antrum.[198,199] They are dilated peripheral branches of the short gastric and left gastric veins, which represent part of the collateral circulation in patients with portal hyperten-

---

☐ **TYPES OF BEZOARS** ☐

Trichobezoars
  Hair
  Fiber
Concretion bezoars
  Gums
  Resins
  Paraffin
  Shellac
  Tar
  Asphalt
  Antacids
Phytobezoars
  Unripe persimmons
  Orange, grapefruit pith
  Sauerkraut
  Asparagus
  Brussel sprouts
  Coconut
  Pineapple
  Cantaloupes
  Apples
  Figs
  Potato skins
  Artichokes
  Dandelion greens
  Green beans
  Berries

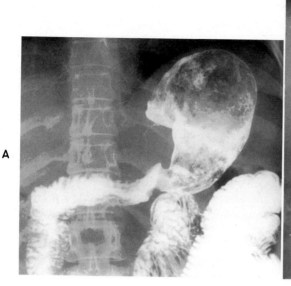
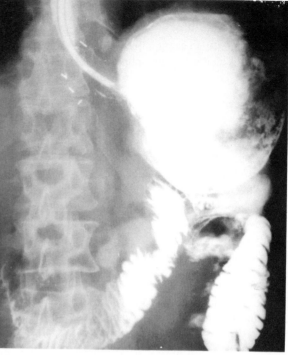

Fig. 16-55 Food bezoars. **A,** Mixed food bezoar that formed as a result of the effects of vagotomy and antrectomy. Note that barium surrounds the entire mass. **B,** Asparagus bezoar after vagotomy and partial gastrectomy were performed to treat radiation antritis. This 60-year-old man was first seen because of anorexia and a firm epigastric mass. There is marked distention of the gastric pouch, which contains a semisolid mass. At endoscopy, the mass was composed mainly of vegetable fiber, which was removed.

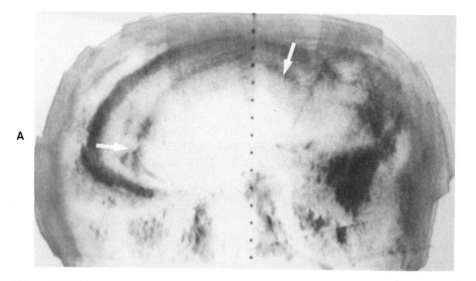

Fig. 16-56 Trichobezoar. **A,** Transverse sonogram shows a large echogenic mass filling the stomach *(arrows)*. **B,** Large trichobezoar extends into the second duodenum. **C,** In another patient, a trichobezoar is seen on a plain radiograph as a mass extending into the gastric fundus. **D,** Barium administered through a nasogastric tube reveals the existence of a large gastric mass that extends into the duodenum. Note that contrast material surrounds the mass. **E,** Mass of hair removed at surgery had formed a cast of the stomach and duodenum.
C to **E** courtesy of Dr. Roscoe E. Miller.

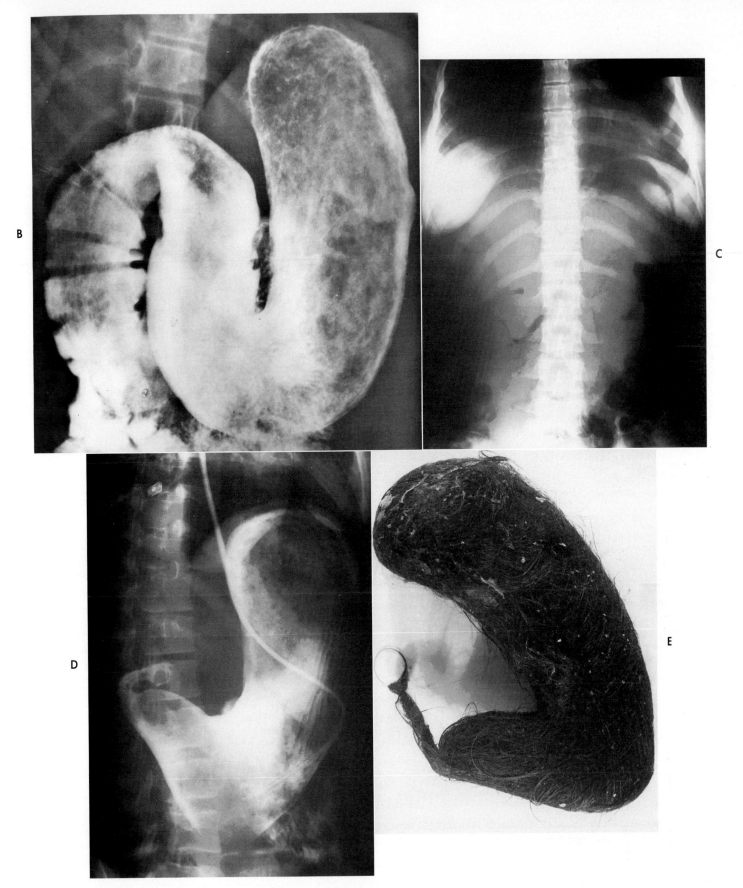

Fig. 16-56, cont'd For legend see opposite page.

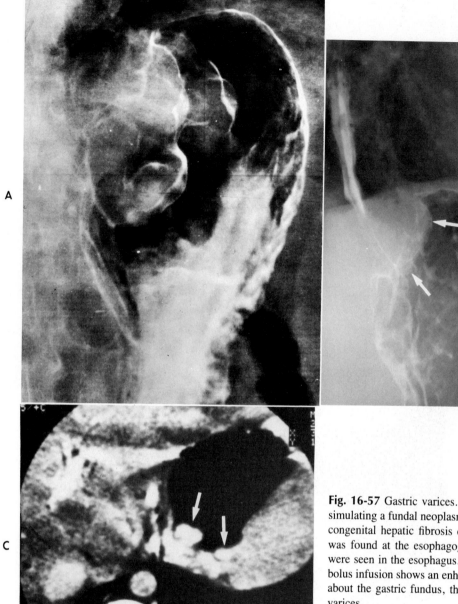

Fig. 16-57 Gastric varices. **A,** A large cluster of gastric varices simulating a fundal neoplasm. **B** and **C,** In a 15-year-old boy with congenital hepatic fibrosis evaluated for anemia, a lobular mass was found at the esophagogastric junction *(arrows)*. No varices were seen in the esophagus. **C,** CT image obtained after contrast bolus infusion shows an enhancing lobular masses *(arrows)* in and about the gastric fundus, thus confirming the presence of gastric varices.

sion or splenic vein obstruction.[200] They are not always associated with esophageal varices.

The radiographic appearance of smooth lobulated filling defects in the fundus or antrum suggests the existence of gastric varices. Gastric varices may also simulate the prominent, irregular rugal fold pattern normally found in the proximal stomach. A history of pancreatitis (splenic vein obstruction) or liver disease, or demonstrable splenomegaly and esophageal varices, can facilitate the diagnosis. The

diagnosis is more difficult when there are no esophageal varices. This can occur in patients without portal vein obstruction when the splenic vein is obstructed by pancreatic cancer, pancreatitis, or pseudocyst, and whose left coronary vein is patent and normotensive.[201] The resultant multilobulated mass in the fundus can be easily mistaken for a neoplasm[202] (Fig. 16-57, *A* and *B*). Varices may also occur when gastric veins are directly anastomosed with retroperitoneal veins. CT done with the bolus injection of contrast material can reveal the existence of well-defined rounded or tubular masses enhancing to the same degree as vascular structures[203] (Fig. 16-57, C).

Gastric varices at sites other than the fundus are less common. Enlargement of the pancreatic, duodenal, right gastroepiploic, and branches of the superior mesenteric vein can cause the formation of varices in the antrum.[200,204] On upper GI examinations, they appear as multiple filling defects in the antrum.

Gastric rupture

An extremely uncommon condition, gastric rupture has devastating consequences.[205] It may be the result of blunt abdominal trauma, including seat belt restraint or performance of the Heimlich maneuver. It may also occur as a complication of gastric obstruction or appear either after a Nissen fundoplication,[206] or after trauma is sustained, such as vigorous emesis, weight lifting, or endoscopy. The site of rupture is usually along the lesser curve when caused by distention and along the greater curve if due to vomiting.[207]

Diagnosis is confirmed by the presence of pneumoperitoneum on plain films, combined with a clinical picture consisting of abdominal distention, shock, subcutaneous emphysema, and peritoneal irritation.

ACKNOWLEDGMENT

The authors wish to acknowledge the significant contributions of William B. Seaman, M.D., an author of prior editions of this chapter, whose original scientific observations and careful review of the work of others have served as the foundation of several sections of this chapter.

REFERENCES

1. Koltun WA: Gastric duplication cyst. Endoscopic presentation as an ulcerated antral mass, *Am Surg* 57:468, 1991.
2. Bartels RJ: Duplication of the stomach: case report and review of the literature, *Am Surg* 33:747, 1967.
3. Agha FP, Gabriele OF, Abdulla FH: Complete gastric duplication, *AJR* 137:406, 1981.
4. Hulnick DH, Balthazar EJ: Gastric duplication cyst: GI series and CT correlation, *Gastrointest Radiol* 12:206, 1987.
5. Palmer E: Gastric diverticula, *Int Abstr Surg* 92:417, 1951.
6. Tillander H, Hesselsjo R: Juxtacardial gastric diverticula and their surgery, *Acta Chir Scand* 134:255, 1968.
7. Lame EL: The gastric cardia and fundus, *Radiology* 75:703, 1960.
8. Brown PW, Priestly JT: Massive and recurrent gastrointestinal hemorrhage from diverticulum of the stomach, *Mayo Clin Proc* 13:270, 1938.
9. Sommer AW, Goodrich WA: Gastric diverticulum, *JAMA* 153:1424, 1953.
10. Schwartz AN, Goiney RC, Graney DO: Gastric diverticulum simulating an adrenal mass: CT appearance and embryogenesis. *AJR* 146:553, 1986.
11. Silverman PM: Gastric diverticulum mimicking adrenal mass: CT demonstration, *J Comput Assist Tomogr* 10:709, 1986.
12. Treichel J, Gerstenberg E, Palme G, Klemm T: Diagnosis of partial gastric diverticula, *Radiology* 119:13, 1976.
13. Dodd GD, Sheft D: Diverticulum of the greater curvature of the stomach, *AJR* 107:102, 1969.
14. Dolan RV, ReMine WH, Dockerty MB: The fate of heterotopic pancreatic tissue, *Arch Surg* 109:762, 1974.
15. Goldberg HI, Margulis AR: Adenomyoma of the stomach, *AJR* 96:382, 1966.
16. Oberman HA, Lodmell JG, Somer ND: Diffuse heterotopic cystic malformation of the stomach, *N Engl J Med* 269:909, 1963.
17. Pang LC: Pancreatic heterotopia: a reappraisal and clinicopathologic analysis of 32 cases, *South Med J* 81:1264, 1988.
18. Feldman M, Weinberg T: Aberrant pancreas: a cause of duodenal syndrome, *JAMA* 148:893, 1952.
19. Kilman WJ, Berk RN: The spectrum of radiographic features of aberrant pancreatic rests involving the stomach, *Radiology* 123:291, 1977.
20. Thoeni RF, Gedgaudas RK: Ectopic pancreas: usual and unusual features, *Gastrointest Radiol* 5:37, 1980.
21. Rohrmann CA Jr, Delaney JH, Protell RL: Heterotopic pancreas diagnosed by cannulation and duct study, *AJR* 128:1044, 1977.
22. Feliciano DV, vanHeerden JA: Pyloric antral mucosal webs, *Mayo Clin Proc* 52:650, 1977.
23. Felson B, Berman Y, Hayumpa AM: Gastric mucosal diaphragm, *Radiology* 92:513, 1969.
24. Ghahremani GG: Non-obstructive mucosal diaphragm or rings of the gastric antrum in adults, *AJR* 121:236, 1974.
25. Huggins MJ, Friedman AC, Lichtenstein JE, Bova JG: Adult acquired antral web, *Dig Dis Sci* 27:80, 1982.
26. Pederson WC, Sirinek KR, Schweoinger WH, Levine BA: Gastric outlet obstruction secondary to antral mucosal diaphragm, *Dig Dis Sci* 29:86, 1984.
27. Quigley RL, Pruitt SK, Pappas TN, Akwari O: Primary hypertrophic pyloric stenosis in the adult, *Arch Surg* 125:1219, 1990.
28. Horwitz A, Alvarez WC, Ascanio H: The normal thickness of the pyloric muscle and the influence on it of ulcer, gastroenterstomy and carcinoma, *Ann Surg* 89:521, 1929.
29. DuPlessis EJ: Primary hypertrophic pyloric stenosis in the adult, *Br J Surg* 53:485, 1966.
30. Torgersen J: The muscular build and movements of the stomach and duodenal bulb, *Acta Radiol Suppl* 45:1, 1942.
31. Skoryna SC, Dolan HS, Gley A: Development of primary pyloric hypertrophy in adults in relation to the structure and function of the pyloric canal, *Surg Gynecol Obstet* 108:83, 1959.
32. Seaman WB: Hypertrophy of the pyloric muscle in adults: analysis of 27 cases, *Radiology* 80:753, 1963.
33. Lumsden K, Truelove SC: Primary hypertrophic pyloric stenosis in the adult, *Br J Radiol* 31:261, 1958.
34. Hajdu N, Hyde I, Riddell V: Antro-pyloric hypertrophy in patients with longstanding gastroenterostomies, *Br J Radiol* 41:49, 1968.
35. Seaman WB: Focal hypertrophy of the pyloric muscle: torus hyperplasia, *AJR* 96:388, 1966.
36. Bateson EM, Talerman A, Walrond ER: Radiological and pathological observations in a series of seventeen cases of hypertrophic pyloric stenosis in adults, *Br J Radiol* 42:1, 1969.
37. Kaynes WM: Simple and complicated hypertrophic pyloric stenosis in the adult, *Gut* 6:240, 1965.
38. Larson LJ, Carson HC, Dockerty MB: Roentgenologic diagnosis of pyloric hypertrophy in adults, *AJR* 101:453, 1967.
39. Isenberg JI, McQuaid KR, Laine L, Ruben W: Acid peptic disorders. In Yamada T, ed: *Textbook of gastroenterology,* Philadelphia, 1991, JB Lippincott.
40. Rubin CE: Histological classification of chronic gastritis: an iconoclastic view, *Gastroenterology* 102:360, 1992.
41. Falcone S, Murphy BJ, Weinfeld A: Gastric manifestations of AIDS: radiographic findings on upper gastrointestinal examination, *Gastrointest Radiol* 16:95, 1991.
42. Megibow AJ, Balthazar EJ, Hulnick DH: Radiology of nonneoplastic gastrointestinal disorders in acquired immune deficiency syndrome, *Semin Roentgenol* 22:31, 1987.

43. Dooley CP, Cohen H, Fitzgibbons PL, Bauer M, Appleman MD et al: Prevalence of *Helicobacter pylori* infection and histologic gastritis in asymptomatic persons, *N Engl J Med* 321:1562, 1989.

44. Iserhard R, Freise J, Wagner S et al: Epidemiology and treatment of gastric *Campylobacter pylori* infection: more questions than answers, *Hepatogastroenterology* 37(suppl 2):38, 1990.

45. Ormand JE, Talley NJ, Shorter RG et al: Further evidence supporting a pathogenic role for *H. pylori* in chronic nonspecific gastritis, *Dig Dis Sci* 36:142, 1991.

46. Clearfield HR: *Helicobacter pylori*: aggressor or innocent bystander? *Med Clin North Am* 75:815, 1991.

47. Graham DY, Molety HM, Evans DG et al: Epidemiology of *Helicobacter pylori* in an asymptomatic population in the United States, *Gastroenterology* 100:1495, 1991.

48. Blaser JM: Hypothesis on the pathogenesis and natural history of *Helicobacter pylori*–induced inflammation, *Gastroenterology* 102:720, 1992.

49. Akdamar K, Ertan A, Angawal NM et al: Upper gastrointestinal endoscopy in normal volunteers, *Gastrointest Endosc* 32:78, 1986.

50. Ott DJ, Gelfand DW, Wu WC, Kerr RM: Sensitivity of single- vs. double-contrast radiology in erosive gastritis, *AJR* 138:263, 1982.

51. Thoeni RF, Goldberg HZ, Omensky S, Cello JP: Detection of gastritis by single- and double-contrast radiography, *Radiology* 148:621, 1983.

52. Tragardt B, Wehlin L, Ohasi K: Radiologic appearance of complete gastric erosions, *Acta Radiol* 19:634, 1976.

53. Laufer I, Hamilton J, Mullens JE: Demonstration of superficial gastric erosions by double contrast radiography, *Gastroenterology* 68:387, 1975.

54. Catalano D, Pagliari U: Gastroduodenal erosions: radiological findings, *Gastrointest Radiol* 7:235, 1982.

55. Levine MS, Verstandig A, Laufer I: Serpiginous gastric erosions caused by aspirin and other nonsteroidal antiinflammatory drugs, *AJR* 146:31, 1986.

56. Shaw PC, van Romunde LK, Griffioen G, Janssens AR, Kreuning J et al: Detection of gastric erosions: comparison of biphasic radiography with fiberoptic endoscopy, *Radiology* 178:63, 1991.

57. Evans SE, Ferrando JR, Mike N: The significance of transverse folds in the gastric antrum, *Clin Radiol* 42:405, 1990.

58. Lucas CE, Sugawa C, Riddle J et al: Natural history and surgical dilemma of "stress" gastric bleeding, *Arch Surg* 102:266, 1971.

59. Roberts DM: Chronic gastritis, alcohol and nonulcer dyspepsia, *Gut* 13:768, 1972.

60. Elta GH, Fawaz KA, Dayal Y et al: Chronic erosive gastritis: a recently recognized disorder, *Dig Dis Sci* 28:7, 1983.

61. O'Brien TK, Saunders DR, Templeton FE: Chronic gastric erosions and oral aphthae, *Am J Dig Dis* 17:447, 1972.

62. Howiler W, Goldberg HI: Gastroesophageal involvement in herpes simplex, *Gastroenterology* 70:775, 1976.

63. Yardley JH: *C. pylori* and large gastric folds, *Radiology* 171:609, 1989.

64. Morrison S, Dahms BB, Hoffenberg E, Czinn SJ: Enlarged gastric folds in association with *Campylobacter pylori* gastritis, *Radiology* 171:819, 1989.

65. Urban BA, Fishman EK, Hruban RH: *Helicobacter pylori* gastritis mimicking gastroenteritis at CT evaluation, *Radiology* 179:689, 1991.

66. Levine MS, Palman CL, Rubesin SE, Laufer I, Herlinger H: Atrophic gastritis in pernicious anemia: diagnosis by double-contrast radiography, *Gastrointest Radiol* 14:215, 1989.

67. Hirsch BZ, Whitington PF, Kirschner BS, Black DD, Bostwick DG, Yousefzadeh DK: Isolated granulomatous gastritis in an adolescent, *Dig Dis Sci* 34:292, 1989.

68. Fahimi HD, Deren JJ, Gottleib LS, Zamcek N: Isolated granulomatous gastritis: its relationship to disseminated sarcoidosis and regional enteritis, *Gastroenterology* 45:161, 1963.

69. Nudelman HL, Rakatonsky H: Gastric histoplasmosis, *JAMA* 195:134, 1966.

70. Reisman TN, Leverett FL, Hudson JR, Kalser MH et al: Syphilitic gastropathy, *Am J Dig Dis* 20:588, 1975.

71. Beckman JW, Schuman BM: Antral gastritis and ulceration in a patient with secondary syphilis, *Gastrointest Endosc* 32:355, 1986.

72. Ariyama J, Wehlin L, Lindstrom CG et al: Gastro-duodenal erosions in Crohn's disease, *Gastrointest Radiol* 5:121, 1980.

73. Gonzalez G, Kennedy T: Crohn's disease of the stomach, *Radiology* 113:27, 1974.

74. Laufer I, Costopoulos L: Early lesions of Crohn's disease, *AJR* 130:307, 1978.

75. Gore RM, Ghahremani GG: Crohn's disease of the upper gastrointestinal tract, *Crit Rev Diagn Imaging* 25:305, 1986.

76. Levine MS: Crohn's disease of the upper gastrointestinal tract, *Radiol Clin North Am* 25:79, 1987.

77. Farman J, Fagenburg D, Dallemond S, Chen C-K: Crohn's disease of the stomach: the "ram's horn" sign, *AJR* 123:242, 1975.

78. Nelson SW: Some interesting and unusual manifestations of Crohn's disease (regional enteritis) of the stomach, duodenum, and small intestine, *AJR* 107:86, 1969.

79. Thompson WM, Cockrill H, Rice RP: Regional enteritis of the duodenum, *AJR* 123:252, 1975.

80. Gray RR, St Louis EL, Grosman H: Crohn's disease involving the proximal stomach, *Gastrointest Radiol* 10:43, 1985.

81. Jacobson IM, Schapiro RH, Warshaw AL: Gastric and duodenal fistulas in Crohn's disease, *Gastroenterology* 89:1347, 1985.

82. Gould SR, Handley AJ, Barnardo DE: Rectal and gastric involvement in a case of sarcoidosis, *Gut* 14:971, 1973.

83. Palmer ED: Note on silent sarcoidosis of the gastric mucosa, *J Lab Clin Med* 52:237, 1958.

84. Ramirez JJ, Ponka JL, Heubrich WS: Massive hemorrhage from sarcoid ulcers in the stomach, *Henry Ford Hospital Med Bull* 12:5, 1964.

85. Crussis-Gonzalez F, Hackett RL: Phlegmonous gastritis, *Arch Surg* 93:990, 1966.

86. Farman J, Dallemand S, Rosen Y: Gastric abscess: a complication of pancreatitis, *Am J Dig Dis* 19:751, 1974.

87. Miller A, Smith B, Rogers AI: Phlegmonous gastritis, *Gastroenterology* 68:231, 1975.

88. Tierney LM, Gooding G, Bottles K et al: Phlegmonous gastritis and *Hemophilus influenzae* peritonitis in a patient with alcoholic liver disease, *Dig Dis Sci* 32:97, 1987.

89. Smith GE: Subacute phlegmonous gastritis, *Gastrointest Endosc* 19:23, 1972.

90. Moosvi AR, Saravolatz LD, Wong DH, Simms SM: Emphysematous gastritis: case report and review, *Rev Infect Dis* 23:848, 1990.

91. Meyers H, Parker J: Emphysematous gastritis, *Radiology* 89:426, 1967.

92. Weens HS: Emphysematous gastritis, *AJR* 55:588, 1946.

93. Gonzalez LL, Schowengerdt C, Skinner HH, Lynch P: Emphysematous gastritis, *Surg Gynecol Obstet* 116:79, 1963.

94. Haw SY, Collins LC, Petrany Z: Emphysematous gastritis, *JAMA* 192:222, 1965.

95. Nelson S: Extraluminal gas collections due to diseases of the gastrointestinal tract, *AJR* 115:225, 1972.

96. Cancelmo JJ: Interstitial gastric emphysema, *Radiology* 63:81, 1954.

97. Berens SV, Moskowitz H, Mellins HZ: Air within the wall of the stomach, *AJR* 103:310, 1968.

98. Kussin SZ, Henry C, Navarro C et al: Gas within the wall of the stomach: report of a case and review of the literature, *Dig Dis Sci* 27:949, 1982.

99. Williford ME, Foster WL, Halvorsen RA, Thompson WM: Emphysematous gastritis secondary to disseminated strongyloidiasis, *Gastrointest Radiol* 7:123, 1982.

100. Seaman WB, Fleming RJ: Intramural gastric emphysema, *AJR* 101:431, 1967.

101. de Lange EE, Slutsky VS, Swanson S, Shaffer HA: Computed tomography of emphysematous gastritis, *J Comput Assist Tomogr* 10:139, 1986.

102. Radin DR, Rosen RS, Halls JM: Acute gastric dilatation: rare cause of portal venous gas, *AJR* 148:279, 1987.

103. Moore SC, Malagelada JR, Shorter RG, Zinsmeister AR: Interrelationships among gastric mucosal morphology, secretion, and motility in peptic ulcer disease, *Dig Dis Sci* 31:673, 1986.

104. Oi M, Sugimura S: Location of gastric ulcer, *Gastroenterology* 36:45, 1959.

105. Gelfand D, Dale WJ, Ott DJ: Location and size of peptic ulcers, *AJR* 143:755, 1984.

106. Health and Public Policy Committee, American College of Physicians: Endoscopy in the evaluation of dyspepsia, *Ann Intern Med* 102:266, 1985.

107. Nelson SW: The discovery of gastric ulcers and the differential diagnosis between benignancy and malignancy, *Radiol Clin North Am* 7:5, 1969.

108. Thompson G, Somers S, Stevenson GW: Benign gastric ulcer: a reliable radiologic diagnosis? *AJR* 141:331, 1983.

109. Thoeni RF, Cello JP: A critical look at the accuracy of endoscopy and double contrast radiography of the UGI tract in patients with substantial UGI hemorrhage, *Radiology* 135:305, 1980.

110. Levine MS, Creteur V, Kressel HY, Laufer I, Herlinger H: Benign gastric ulcers: diagnosis and follow-up with double contrast radiography, *Radiology* 164:9, 1987.

111. Gelfand DW, Ott DJ: Benign gastric ulcers: diagnosis and follow-up with double contrast radiography, *Radiology* 165:878, 1987(letter).

112. Op den Orth JO: Use of barium in evaluation of disorders of the upper gastrointestinal tract: current status, *Radiology* 175:586, 1990.

113. Scatarige JC, DiSantis DJ: CT of the stomach and duodenum, *Radiol Clin North Am* 27:687, 1989.

114. Jacobs JM, Hill MC, Steinberg WM: Peptic ulcer disease: CT evaluation, *Radiology* 178:745, 1991.

115. Joharjy IA, Mustafa MA, Zaidi AJ: Fluid-aided sonography of the stomach and duodenum in the diagnosis of peptic ulcer disease in adult patients, *J Ultrasound Med* 9:77, 1990.

116. Coad NAG, Shah KJ: Menetrier's disease in childhood associated with CMV infection, *Br J Radiol* 59:615, 1986.

117. Marks MP, Lange MV, Kahlstrom EJ et al: Pediatric hypertrophic gastropathy, *AJR* 147:1031, 1986.

118. MacCarty RL, Talley NJ: Barium studies in diffuse eosinophilic gastroenteritis, *Gastrointest Radiol* 15:183, 1990.

119. Lesser PB, Falchuk KR, Singer M, Isselbacher J: Menetrier's disease: report of a case with transient and reversible findings, *Gastroenterology* 68:1598, 1975.

120. Press AJ: Practical significance of gastric rugal folds, *AJR* 125:172, 1975.

121. Burns GP, Laws JW: The radiological assessment of gastric acid secretions, *Lancet* 1:70, 1966.

122. Moghadam M, Gluckman R, Eyler WR: Radiological assessment of gastric acid output, *Radiology* 89:888, 1967.

123. Balthazar EJ, Davidian MM: Hyperrugosity in gastric carcinoma: radiographic, endoscopic, and pathologic features, *AJR* 136:531, 1981.

124. Menetrier P: Des polyadenomas gastriques et de leurs rapports avec le cancer de l'estomac, *Arch Physiol Norm Pathol* 1:322, 1888.

125. Berenson MM, Sannella J, Freston JW: Menetrier's disease: serial morphological secretory and serological observations, *Gastroenterology* 70:256, 1976.

126. Tan DTD, Stempien SJ, Dagradi AE: Clinical spectrum of hypertrophic hypersecretory gastropathy, *Gastrointest Endosc* 18:69, 1971.

127. Freter SS, Richert RR: Hyperplastic gastropathy: analysis of 50 selected cases from 1955-1980, *Am J Gastroenterol* 76:321, 1981.

128. Searcy RM, Malagelada J-R: Menetrier's disease and idiopathic hypertrophic gastropathy, *Ann Intern Med* 100:565, 1984.

129. Scharschmidt BF: The natural history of hypertrophic gastropathy (Menetrier's disease): report of a case with 16 year follow-up and review of 120 cases from the literature, *Am J Med* 63:644, 1977.

130. Baker A, Volberg F, Sumner T, Moran R: Childhood Menetrier's disease: four new cases and discussion of the literature, *Gastrointest Radiol* 11:131, 1986.

131. Frank BW, Kern F Jr: Menetrier's disease: spontaneous metamorphosis of giant hypertrophy of gastric mucosa to atrophic gastritis, *Gastroenterology* 53:953, 1967.

132. Chouragui JP, Roy CC, Brochu P: Menetrier's disease in children: report of a patient and review of sixteen other cases, *Gastroenterology* 80:1042, 1981.

133. Williams SM, Harned RK, Settles RH: Adenocarcinoma of the stomach in association with Menetrier's disease, *Gastrointest Radiol* 3:387, 1978.

134. Scott HW, Skull HJ, Law DH: Surgical management of Menetrier's disease with protein losing gastropathy, *Ann Surg* 181:765, 1975.

135. Olmstead WW, Cooper PH, Madewell JE: Involvement of the gastric antrum in Menetrier's disease, *AJR* 126:521, 1976.

136. Zollinger RM, Ellison EH: Primary peptic ulceration of the jejunum associated with islet cell tumors of the pancreas, *Ann Surg* 142:709, 1955.

137. Zboralske FF, Amberg JR: Detection of the Zollinger-Ellison syndrome: the radiologist's responsibility, *AJR* 104:529, 1968.

138. Deveney CW, Deveney KE: Zollinger Ellison syndrome (gastrinoma). Current diagnosis and treatment, *Surg Clin North Am* 67:411, 1987.

139. Nelson SW, Christoforidis AJ: Roentgenologic features of Zollinger-Ellison syndrome: ulcerogenic tumor of the pancreas, *Semin Roentgenol* 3:254, 1968.

140. Nelson SW, Lichtenstein JE: Zollinger-Ellison syndrome. In Marshak RH, Maklansky D, Lindner AE, eds: *Radiology of the stomach,* Philadelphia, 1983, WB Saunders.

141. Martel W, Abell MR, Allen TNK: Lymphoreticular hyperplasia of the stomach (pseudolymphoma), *AJR* 127:261, 1976.

142. Mattingly SS, Cibull ML, Ram MD et al: Pseudolymphoma of the stomach: a diagnostic and therapeutic dilemma, *Arch Surg* 116:25, 1981.

143. Orr RK, Lininger JR, Lawrence W: Gastric pseudolymphoma: a challenging clinical problem, *Ann Surg* 200:185, 1984.

144. Sigal SH, Saul SH, Auerbach HE et al: Gastric small lymphocytic proliferation with immunoglobulin gene rearrangement in pseudolymphoma versus lymphoma, *Gastroenterology* 97:195, 1989.

145. Sternberg A: Diagnosing gastric pseudolymphoma by gastroscopic biopsy, *Gastrointest Endosc* 33:397, 1987.

146. Smith JL Jr, Helwig EB: Malignant lymphoma of the stomach: its diagnosis, distinction and biologic behavior, *Am J Pathol* 34:553, 1958.

147. Tokunaga O, Watanabe T, Morimatsu M: Pseudolymphoma of the stomach. A clinicopathologic study of 15 cases, *Cancer* 59:1320, 1987.

148. Scoazec JY, Brousse N, Potet F, Jeulain JF: Focal malignant lymphoma in gastric pseudolymphoma. Histologic and immunohistochemical study of a case, *Cancer* 57:1330, 1986.

149. Chiles JT, Platz CE: The radiographic manifestations of pseudolymphoma of the stomach, *Radiology* 116:551, 1975.

150. Graham JR: Gastric pseudolymphoma developing from chronic gastric ulcer: endoscopic diagnosis and the effect of cimetidine, *Dig Dis Sci* 27:1051, 1982(letter).

151. Chong GC, Beahrs OH, Payne WS: Management of corrosive gastritis due to ingested acid, *Mayo Clin Proc* 49:861, 1974.

152. Clearfield HR, Shin YH, Schriebman BK: Emphysematous gastritis secondary to lye ingestion, *Am J Dig Dis* 14:195, 1969.

153. Zargar SA, Kochhar R, Nagi B, Mehta S, Mehta SK: Ingestion of corrosive acids, *Gastroenterology* 97:702, 1989.

154. Ritter FN, Newman MH, Newman DE: A clinical and experimental study of corrosive burns of the stomach, *Ann Otol Rhinol Laryngol* 77:830, 1968.

155. Muhletaler CA, Gerlock AJ, deSoto L, Halter SA: Gastroduodenal lesions of ingested acids: radiographic findings, *AJR* 135:1247, 1980.

156. Johns TT, Thoeni RF: Severe corrosive gastritis related to Drano: an unusual case, *Gastrointest Radiol* 8:1983, 1983.

157. Roswit B: Complications of radiation therapy: the alimentary tract, *Semin Roentgenol* 9:51, 1974.

158. Sell A, Jensen TS: Acute gastric ulcers induced by radiation, *Acta Radiol* [Ther] 4:289, 1962.

159. Cello JP: Eosinophilic gastritis: a complex disease entity, *Am J Med* 67:1099, 1979.

160. Goldberg HI, O'Kieffe, Jenis EH, Boyce HW: Diffuse eosinophilic gastroenteritis, *AJR* 119:342, 1973.

161. Schulman A, Morton PCG, Dietrich BE: Eosinophilic gastroenteritis, *Clin Radiol* 31:101, 1980.

162. Katz AJ, Goldman H, Grand RJ: Gastric mucosal biopsy in eosinophilic (allergic) gastroenteritis, *Gastroenterology* 73:705, 1977.

163. Helwig EB, Ranier A: Inflammatory fibroid polyps of the stomach, *Surg Gynecol Obstet* 96:355, 1953.

164. Ureles AL, Alschibaja T, Lodico D, Stabins SJ: Idiopathic infiltration of the gastrointestinal tract: diffuse and circumscribed, *Am J Med* 20:894, 1961.

165. Johnstone JM, Morson BC: Inflammatory fibroid polyposis of the gastrointestinal tract, *Histopathology* 2:349, 1978.

166. Legge DA, Carlson HC, Wollaeger EE: Radiologic appearance of systemic amyloidosis involving the gastrointestinal tract, *AJR Radium Ther Nucl Med* 110:406, 1970.

167. MacManus O, Okies EJ: Amyloidosis of the stomach: report of an unusual case and review of the literature, *Am Surg* 42:607, 1976.

168. Dastur KJ, Ward JF: Amyloidoma of the stomach, *Gastrointest Radiol* 5:17, 1980.

169. Carlson HC, Breen JF: Amyloidosis and plasma cell dyscrasias: gastrointestinal involvement, *Semin Roentgenol* 21:128, 1986.

170. Dragstedt LR, Dragstedt CA: Acute dilatation of the stomach, *JAMA* 79:612, 1922.

171. Berk RN, Caulson DB: Body cast syndrome, *Radiology* 94:303, 1970.

172. Joffe N: Some unusual roentgenologic findings associated with marked gastric dilatation, *AJR* 119:291, 1973.

173. Malagelada JR: Physiologic basis and clinical significance of gastric emptying disorders, *Dig Dis Sci* 24:657, 1979.

174. Dubois A: Gastric dysrhythmias: pathophysiologic and etiologic factors, *Mayo Clin Proc* 64:246, 1989.

175. Gramm HF, Reuter K, Costello P: The radiologic manifestations of diabetic gastric neuropathy and its differential diagnosis, *Gastrointest Radiol* 3:151, 1978.

176. Kassander P: Asymptomatic gastric retention in diabetics (gastroparesis diabeticorum), *Ann Intern Med* 49:987, 1958.

177. Zitomer BR, Gramm HF, Kozak GP: Gastric neuropathy in diabetes mellitus: clinical and radiologic observations, *Metabolism* 17:199, 1968.

178. Malagelada JR, Rees WDW, Mazzotta LJ, Go VLW: Gastric motor abnormalities in diabetic and post-vagotomy gastroparesis: effect of metoclopramide and bethanechol, *Gastroenterology* 78:286, 1980.

179. Fox S, Behar J: Pathogenesis of diabetic gastroparesis: a pharmacologic study, *Gastroenterology* 78:757, 1980.

180. Horowitz M, Harding PE, Maddox A et al: Gastric and esophageal emptying in insulin-dependent diabetes mellitus, *J Gastroenterol Hepatol* 1:97, 1986.

181. Peachey RDG, Creamer B, Pierce JW: Sclerodermatous involvement of the stomach and the small and large bowel, *Gut* 10:285, 1969.

182. Horowitz M, McNeil JD, Maddern GJ et al: Abnormalities of gastric and esophageal emptying in polymyositis and dermatomyositis, *Gastroenterology* 90:434, 1986.

183. Horowitz M, Maddox A, Maddern GJ et al: Gastric and esophageal emptying in dystrophia myotonica, *Gastroenterology* 92:570, 1987.

184. Rohrmann CA, Ricci MT, Krishnamurthy S, Schuffler MD: Radiologic and histologic differentiation of neuromuscular disorders of the gastrointestinal tract: visceral myopathies, visceral neuropathies, and progressive systemic sclerosis, *AJR* 143:933, 1981.

185. Hom S, Sarr MG, Kelly KA, Hench V: Postoperative gastric atony after vagotomy for obstructing peptic ulcer, *Am J Surg* 157:282, 1989.

186. Christian PE, Datz FL, Moore JG: Gastric emptying studies in the morbidly obese before and after gastroplasty, *J Nucl Med* 27:1686, 1986.

187. Schatzki R, Simeone FA: Gastric volvulus, *Am J Dig Dis* 7:213, 1940.

188. Carter R, Brewer LA, Henshaw DB: *Acute gastric volvulus, Am J Surg* 140:99, 1980.

189. Tanner NC: Chronic and recurrent volvulus of the stomach with late result of colonic displacement, *Am J Surg* 115:505, 1968.

190. Myerson DA, Myerson PJ, Lawson JP: Antral infracolic volvulus of the stomach, *J Can Assoc Radiol* 26:128, 1975.

191. Gerson DE, Lewicki AM: Intrathoracic stomach: when does it obstruct? *Radiology* 119:257, 1976.

192. Figiel LS, Figiel SJ: Acute organo-axial gastric volvulus, *AJR* 90:761, 1963.

193. Emerson AP: Foods high in fiber and phytobezoar formation, *J Am Diet Assoc* 87:1675, 1987.

194. Rogers LF, Davis EK, Harle TS: Formation and food boli following phytobezoar gastric surgery, *AJR* 119:280, 1973.

195. DeBakey M, Ochsner A: Bezoars and concretions: a comprehensive review of the literature with an analysis of 303 collected cases, *Surgery* 4:934, 1938.

196. Hoyt CS, Burke EC, Hallenbeck GA: Trichobezoar, *Mayo Clin Proc* 33:298, 1958.

197. McCracken S, Jorgeward R, Silver TM, Jafri SZH: Gastric trichobezoar: sonographic findings, *Radiology* 161:123, 1986.

198. Marshall JP, Smith PD, Hoyumpa AM: Gastric varices, *Am J Dig Dis* 22:947, 1977.

199. Rice RP, Thompson WM, Kelvin KM et al: Gastric varices without esophageal varices, *JAMA* 237:1976, 1977.

200. Levine MS, Kieu K, Rubesin S, Herlinger H, Laufer I: Isolated gastric varices: splenic vein obstruction or portal hypertension? *Gastrointest Radiol* 15:188, 1990.

201. Itzchak Y, Glickman MG: Splenic vein thrombosis in patients with a normal size spleen, *Invest Radiol* 12:158, 1977.

202. Anderson JF, Dunnick NR: Pseudo tumor caused by gastric varices, *Am J Dig Dis* 22:929, 1977.

203. Balthazar EJ, Megibow A, Naidich D, LeFleur RS: Computed tomographic recognition of gastric varices, *AJR* 142:1121, 1984.

204. Sos T, Meyers MA, Baltaxe HA: Non-fundic gastric varices, *Radiology* 105:579, 1972.

205. Chandrasekhara KL, Iyer SK, Sutton AL, Stanell AE: Spontaneous rupture of the stomach, *Am J Med* 81:1062, 1986.

206. Kurgen A, Hoffmann J, Abramowitz HB: Spontaneous rupture of the stomach: a rare complication of Nissen fundoplication, *Int Surg* 69:357, 1984.

207. Watts HD: Lesions brought on by vomiting: the effect of hiatus hernia on site of injury, *Gastroenterology* 71:683, 1976.

17 *Benign Tumors of the Stomach*

E. MAUREEN WHITE

A wide variety of benign polyps and tumors may originate either from normal histologic constituents within the stomach or from underlying structural anomalies. The exact etiology of these lesions is unknown. Collectively the prevalence of these masses at necropsy has been reported to be as high as 16.6%.[1] The vast majority of lesions are asymptomatic and are discovered incidentally, with approximately 5% producing clinical manifestations.[2] Benign gastric masses are generally classified as epithelial or nonepithelial. Gastric epithelial polyps are identified in less than 1% of autopsies[3] and in 3% to 5% of patients undergoing gastroscopy.[4,5] The incidence of gastric polyps increases in certain disease processes such as pernicious anemia (22% to 37%)[6,7] and chronic atrophic gastritis (6%),[8] as well as in gastric remnants following partial gastrectomy (4% to 20%).[9-11] Polyps are frequently found in patients with gastric carcinoma.[12] Benign nonepithelial tumors of the stomach arise in the submucosal, muscular, or subserosal tissues and include a broad spectrum of pathologic subtypes, the most common of which are myogenic, neurogenic, lipomatous, and vascular neoplasms.

RADIOLOGIC EVALUATION OF BENIGN GASTRIC TUMORS AND POLYPS

Radiologic techniques have an important role in the detection of gastric masses, a large percentage of which represent benign tumors and polyps. Barium examination of the upper gastrointestinal tract provides excellent anatomic detail, particularly of the mucosal surface. Epithelial masses present either as sessile, broad-based polyps or as pedunculated lesions attached to the mucosa by a stalk. These lesions disrupt the normal mucosal pattern and, when sufficiently large, displace adjacent rugal folds. Sessile polyps typically form an acute angle at the interface of the lesion with the surrounding normal mucosa. Intramural tumors tend to form more obtuse angles with adjacent stomach, although exceptions may occur with endogastric extension of large mural masses. Superficial or deep ulcerations within the lesion may be identified on upper GI examination. This finding is diagnostically useful, as certain masses are more likely to ulcerate. These include heterotopic pancreatic rests, leiomyomas, neurofibromas, lipomas, inflammatory fibroid polyps, carcinoid tumors, and plasmacytomas.

Cross-sectional imaging techniques (CT, ultrasound, and MRI) are extremely useful in the detection and delineation of benign gastric masses.[13] Although these modalities do not reliably depict small mucosal polyps, larger lesions are usually well defined. Imaging studies are frequently used to demonstrate the exophytic component of a mass and its relationship with adjacent structures. Furthermore, internal characteristics of the tumor such as necrosis, central ulceration, and dystrophic calcification are generally well shown. CT is most often used to delineate gastric masses because of its excellent spatial resolution and the availability of effective enteric contrast agents. Gastric evaluation is facilitated through oral ingestion of dilute Gastrografin or barium before imaging. When contrast media is not tolerated by the patient, gas-producing agents or water may be helpful to distend the gastric lumen through the use of effervescent granules or by rapid ingestion of up to 800 ml of tap water. In a comparative study of these two techniques, water intake was found to provide more detail of the gastric wall and better delineation of mass lesions.[14] However, in severely ill patients the gas-producing agents were better tolerated. The mean value for normal gastric wall thickness ranges between 2 to 5 mm in the fundus, body, and antrum.[14] The gastroesophageal junction is usually thicker, with a mean wall dimension of 12.5 mm.[14] Ultrasound and MRI may also demonstrate gastric masses, although with more limited overall success than CT. With these techniques, oral agents such as water may also be employed to distend the stomach and define the mass. A prospective investigation of gastric wall thickness using ultrasound revealed an average wall thickness of 5.107 ± 1.100 mm in normal subjects and 15.933 ± 4.471 mm among neoplastic patients.[15]

BENIGN EPITHELIAL POLYPS AND TUMORS

Epithelial polyps account for 5% to 10% of gastric tumors.[16] Certain polyposis syndromes with gastric involvement have a familial mode of transmission, whereas other types of polyps tend to arise in the setting of chronic inflammation. The underlying etiology for development of many gastric polyps is unknown. On pathologic examination, gastric polyps may be nonneoplastic (e.g., hyperplastic polyps) or may represent true neoplasms with a malignant potential (e.g., adenomas. The number of polyps ranges from a solitary mass to innumerable lesions producing the appearance of mucosal "carpeting." Multiple defects are often encountered with hyperplastic and hamartomatous polyps. Furthermore, gastric polyps vary in size from small sessile plaques to large multilobulated masses. Lesions are readily detected on upper GI examination, which provides excellent definition of the gastric mucosa. Polyps typically appear as well-circumscribed filling defects that interrupt the normal mucosal pattern and occasionally displace gastric folds. Superficial ulcerations may be identified and are a potential cause of hematemesis or melena. The major categories of benign gastric polyps are described in the following sections.

Hyperplastic (regenerative) polyps

Hyperplastic polyps account for approximately 75% of gastric polyps.[17] These lesions are more common among the elderly. In the majority of patients the polyps produce no symptoms. Rarely, hemorrhage or prolapse with obstruction may produce clinical manifestations. Hyperplastic polyps are composed of an overgrowth of superficial gastric (foveolar) epithelium, with cystic dilation of elongated mucosal glands. Inflammatory cells may also be present. Hyperplastic polyps are small sessile lesions that appear on upper GI examination as smoothly marginated, circular, or hemispherical filling defects (Fig. 17-1). Occasionally, pedunculated lesions develop. Hyperplastic polyps have an average diameter of 5 to 10 mm, although the size of individual polyps varies from a few millimeters to several centimeters (Fig. 17-2). Superficial erosions often occur at the tip of the polyp.

Lesions are multiple in 20% to 25% of cases. These polyps usually develop in a chronically inflamed gastric mucosa with atrophic changes. Hyperplastic polyps are also found relatively frequently in the peristomal region of gastric remnants.[11] There has been a report of two cases of giant hyperplastic polyps in a gastric remnant simulat-

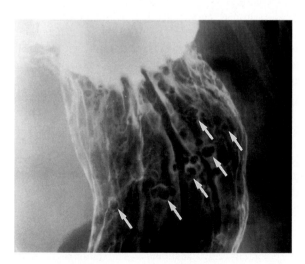

Fig. 17-1 Hyperplastic polyps. Small well-circumscribed sessile polyps *(arrows)* in the proximal half of the stomach.

ing carcinoma on upper GI examination.[18] Hyperplastic polyps rarely if ever degenerate into malignancy,[3,19,20] which tends to develop only in polyps larger than 2 cm in diameter. Whereas it is uncommon for malignancy to arise in hyperplastic polyps, there is a higher incidence of hyperplastic polyps in patients with an independent carcinoma located elsewhere in the stomach.[4] Hyperplastic polyps have been observed to regress spontaneously.[5] In other instances, new lesions may appear on follow-up studies.[21]

Gastric adenomas

Adenomas are the second most common type of benign gastric epithelial mass, following hyperplastic polyps. These lesions account for approximately 8% to 10% of epithelial polyps in the stomach.[22] In contrast to hyperplastic polyps, adenomas represent true neoplasms that are primarily composed of tall, thin columnar cells not usually present in the gastric mucosa. Gastric adenomas are further classified into two histologic subtypes that may coexist. *Tubular adenoma (adenomatous polyp)* consists of branching tubules that surround the lamina propria, whereas *papillary (villous) adenoma* is made up of papillary projections that arise from the lamina propria. When both histologic types are present within a lesion, it is referred to as a *papillotubular adenoma.*

Papillary or papillotubular adenomas are more likely to become malignant than are tubular adenomas, which are usually better differentiated. Carcinoma within a gastric villous adenoma has been detected in 40% to 100% of cases,[23-25] as compared with a 30% incidence of malignancy among colonic villous adenomas.[26] Malignant degeneration occurs most often in larger gastric lesions. An increased incidence of gastric adenoma and a synchronous but separate gastric carcinoma have been reported, particularly with papillotubular and papillary lesions. The greater risk of malignancy in patients with gastric adenomas may relate to its frequent development in patients with severe atrophic gastritis or gastric atrophy.

The incidence of gastric adenoma increases with age, with the average age at detection being 62.6 years.[27] These lesions occur more often (2:1) in males than in females and most commonly develop in the antrum (Fig. 17-3). The majority of adenomas occur as solitary lesions, usually exceeding 2 cm in diameter at the time of diagnosis. On upper GI and cross-sectional imaging examinations, the gastric adenoma usually presents as a sessile polypoid mass that projects into the gastric lumen. Occasionally a pedunculated lesion is found, which is often larger than the sessile mass. Tubular adenoma forms a smooth, rounded mass, whereas papillary or papillotubular tumor frequently presents as a lobulated lesion with an irregular, fissured surface.[28] These topographic features are depicted on upper GI examination as either a smooth or lobulated surface, depending on the underlying tumor type.

Hamartomatous polyps

Hamartomatous polyps of the stomach are <u>rare</u>. These lesions contain various histologic elements that are normally present in the gastric wall, but they assume in a disorganized and proliferative pattern. Hamartomatous polyps usually occur in hereditary polyposis syndromes such as Peutz-Jeghers syndrome and juvenile polyposis. In these disease processes, greater numbers of polyps develop within the intestinal tract than in the stomach. Furthermore, polyps that arise in the stomach may be of different histology compared with those in the intestines. For example, in familial polyposis coli the most common gastric polyp is a distinctive type of hamartoma, whereas the intestinal polyps are typically adenomas. The following sections describe the three primary syndromes associated with hamartomatous gastric polyps—Peutz-Jeghers syndrome, juvenile polyposis, and fundic gland polyp.

Peutz-Jeghers syndrome

Peutz-Jeghers syndrome is an inherited autosomal dominant disorder, with incomplete penetrance and sporadic development through spontaneous genetic mutation. This pathologic process is characterized by gastrointestinal polyps and mucocutaneous pigmentation, with melanin spots developing most often along the lips, buccal mucosa, and digits. These lesions represent hamartomatous polyps, which are found in the small bowel, colon, and stomach, in order of decreasing frequency. The esophagus is spared. Gastric polyps develop in 25% to 50% of patients.[3,29] Polyps are usually multiple and vary in size from a few millimeters to several centimeters. Lesions may arise at any site within the stomach, occurring most frequently in the antrum. These polyps are usually larger than the adenomatous polyps of familial polyposis coli and Gardner's syndrome. The surface is often lobulated, occasionally simulating the gross appearance of a villous tumor.

The majority of patients with Peutz-Jeghers syndrome are relatively asymptomatic. Polyps may become clinically manifest as a consequence of bleeding from ulceration or of abdominal pain from large pedunculated lesions that obstruct or intussuscept the bowel. Occasionally, afflicted individuals have only pigmentation or only polyposis. The potential for malignant degeneration in Peutz-Jeghers syndrome is controversial. In early reports a high incidence of carcinoma was subsequently attributed to misplaced glandular tissue within muscle bundles, misinterpreted as invasion. With exclusion of these cases, the number of individuals with Peutz-Jeghers syndrome and associated gastrointestinal malignancy decreases to 2% to 3%.[30,31] Patients with Peutz-Jeghers syndrome are also believed to be at increased risk for development of extraintestinal malignancies originating most often in the pancreas, breast, and reproductive tract.[32]

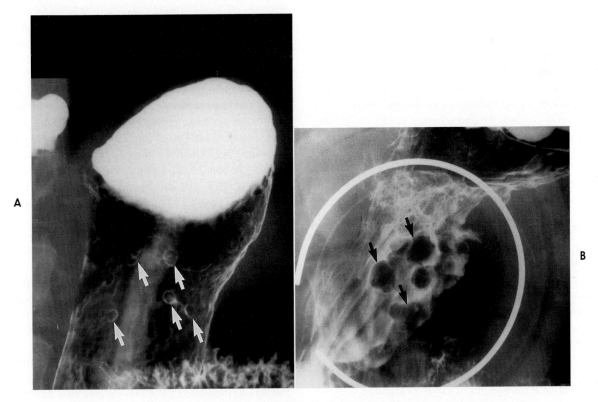

Fig. 17-2 Hyperplastic polyps. **A,** Multiple polyps in the upper gastric body *(arrows),* some with superficial ulceration. **B,** Large hyperplastic polyps *(arrows)* in the body of the stomach.

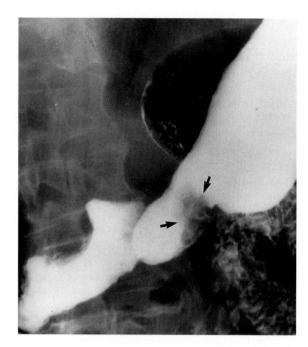

Fig. 17-3 Papillary (villous) adenoma. Lobulated gastric antral mass *(arrows)* with an irregular fissured surface.

Juvenile polyposis syndrome

Juvenile polyposis syndrome occurs primarily in children, although the diagnosis may be established at any age. This syndrome is characterized histologically by numerous dilated glands containing mucus and inflamed stromal tissue. Juvenile polyposis syndrome has four subtypes: solitary juvenile polyp, juvenile polyposis coli, juvenile gastrointestinal polyposis, and familial juvenile polyposis of the stomach. The most frequently encountered is the solitary juvenile polyp, occurring as an isolated rectal or colonic lesion in children without a family history of this disease. Juvenile polyposis coli is associated with numerous colonic polyps and occasionally with polyps in the small intestine. In 40% of these cases, familial transmission is documented. Gastric polyps occur in juvenile gastrointestinal polyposis and in juvenile polyposis limited to the stomach,[33,34] both of which are associated with familial inheritance. The former develops among infants and young children in a recessive genetic pattern and among adults through dominant genetic transmission.[34-38] In both of these polyposis syndromes, the number of lesions varies from a single mucosal mass to numerous polyps. Carcinomas occasionally develop in patients with juvenile polyposis as well as in relatives who do not have polyps. The majority of carcinomas occur in the colon, with occasional gastric carcinomas.

Fundic gland polyp

The fundic gland polyp is composed of normal-appearing fundic glands with increased numbers of parietal and chief cells. The glands are often tortuous and cystically dilated, referred to as *glandular cysts*. There are usually no inflammatory changes. Lesions appear as clusters of small, smooth-surfaced, and primarily sessile masses up to 5 mm in diameter. These polyps are located predominantly in the fundus and body of the stomach and are typically multiple (between 15 to 30). There is a strong female preponderance (3:1) in the incidence of fundic gland polyps. These lesions are usually of no particular significance and may regress spontaneously.[39] In the initial report of 22 patients with fundic gland polyps, six individuals had familial polyposis coli.[40] Patients with this condition may also develop gastric adenomas, occurring more often in the pyloric than the fundic region, as well as carcinomas and carcinoid tumors. Since this report, fundic gland polyps have also been identified in patients with Gardner's syndrome[41,42] as well as in individuals without an underlying polyposis syndrome.[43,44]

Retention polyps (Cronkhite-Canada syndrome)

Retention polyps are rare gastric lesions composed of dilated cystic glands and stromal tissue. These polyps are encountered in middle-aged individuals (average age 60 years) with Cronkhite-Canada syndrome, an entity first described in two patients by Drs. Cronkhite and Canada in 1955.[45] Cronkhite-Canada syndrome is characterized by extensive gastric and intestinal (small bowel and colonic) polyposis, as well as by ectodermal abnormalities including alopecia, cutaneous hypopigmentation, and atrophy of the nails. There is no known etiology or familial tendency associated with this syndrome. Polyps present as sessile or pedunculated lesions that may impart an irregular nodular appearance to the gastric folds, resembling extensive juvenile polyposis. Pathologically the intestinal tract mucosa demonstrates polypoid thickening, with intense edema of the lamina propria and cystic glandular dilation. Rupture of these cysts may lead to inflammatory changes. Frequent symptoms are nausea and diarrhea, related to the severe protein-losing enteropathy and resultant hypoalbuminemia. The clinical course of Cronkhite-Canada syndrome is variable, with remissions occurring between episodic recurrences.[46]

Radiographic manifestations, including the distribution and patterns of involvement, were described in a review of six cases.[47] The stomach was diffusely involved with polyposis in five individuals, and one patient had focal antral lesions. The gastric body and antrum were affected more than the fundus in four cases. Small bowel polyps were present in four patients and colonic polyps in all six. Gastric polyposis presented one of three appearances: (1) innumerable small polyps extending over a portion or all of the gastric mucosa, with or without fold thickening (four patients), (2) scattered polyps of varying size with thick folds (one patient), and (3) minimal involvement with a few small polyps (one patient). The radiographic patterns of gastric and colonic polyposis were in concordance in five of the six patients.

Heterotopic polyps (ectopic pancreas, adenomyoma, Brunner's gland hyperplasia)

Heterotopic tissue from either the adjacent pancreas or duodenum may be found in the stomach, presenting as a polypoid mass. These pathologic entities include aberrant (ectopic) pancreas, adenomyoma, and Brunner's gland hyperplasia.

Heterotopic pancreatic rests

Heterotopic pancreatic rests made up mainly of exocrine glands and ducts with variable numbers of islet cells. This heterotopic tissue may occur in the stomach and in the intestinal tract. Heterotopic pancreas in the stomach accounts for 4% of polypoid lesions, with the greater curve aspect of the prepyloric region being a favored site.[22] On barium examination these lesions appear as a submucosal lesion elevating the overlying mucosal surface and containing a central barium collection.[48] This umbilication may represent the site of an excretory duct (Fig. 17-4). The appearance can be confused with neoplasm or peptic ulceration. The lesions are usually asymptomatic, but gastrointestinal bleeding may occur.

Adenomyomas

Adenomyomas are uncommon gastric lesions made up of ducts epithelialized by columnar cells and arranged in a haphazard pattern. Sometimes, pancreatic tissue is identified. The majority of lesions are less than 2 cm in diameter but may occasionally enlarge to 5 cm. Radiologically and endoscopically, these lesions are indistinguishable from ectopic pancreas, occurring in the same prepyloric area and demonstrating similar features of a smooth, sharply demarcated intramural mass. Clinical symptoms include pain, bleeding, and vomiting.

Brunner's gland hyperplasia

Brunner's gland hyperplasia presents as polypoid lesions composed of tightly organized but normal Brunner's glands. It develops primarily in the duodenum, with rare occurrences in the prepyloric region of the stomach. Lesions located in this area may very rarely produce obstructive symptoms.

Teratoma

The stomach is one of the rarest sites for development of a teratoma. Teratomas have a benign course and usually occur in infants less than 1 year of age. There is a strong male preponderance. The most common gastric location is along the greater curve. Lesions are often large and have both solid and cystic components. Consequently, these tumors often present as a palpable mass. Other clinical features include gastrointestinal bleeding and respiratory com-

promise. Calcifications are present in approximately half of cases. Congenital anomalies coexist in 10% to 15% of patients.

BENIGN NONEPITHELIAL TUMORS

Several histologic varieties of benign nonepithelial gastric tumors have been described. These are often asymptomatic and discovered incidentally on upper GI examination, CT, or endoscopy. The most frequent symptom is gastrointestinal bleeding. Occasionally, these tumors produce symptoms from obstruction or intussusception. Certain tumors, such as smooth muscle and carcinoid neoplasms, are often difficult or impossible to classify as benign or malignant through histologic examination of the primary tumor alone. Rather, the neoplastic behavior and metastatic potential require further elucidation at laparotomy and through clinical follow-up. Similar radiologic features of different masses often preclude a tumor-specific diagnosis. One exception is the gastric lipoma, which, because of homogeneous fat attenuation, has a pathognomonic appearance on CT.

Smooth muscle tumors (spindle cell leiomyoma, epithelioid variant)

By far the largest group of benign nonepithelial gastric neoplasms are smooth muscle tumors, accounting for 34% to 58% of cases.[49,50] Approximately two thirds of all smooth muscle tumors of the gastrointestinal tract arise in the stomach. Most gastric leiomyomas present as a solitary mass, with multiple lesions occurring in 10% of cases. Tumor size varies considerably from small to huge. The common histologic form is spindle cell leiomyoma, composed of uniform spindle cells arranged in whorls. Highly cellular areas alternate with foci of liquefaction and hyalinization. An infrequent anatomic variant is epithelioid leiomyoma, originally termed *leiomyoblastoma*, which is predominantly composed of round or polygonal cells.[51,52] These tumors are considered to have malignant potential somewhere between leiomyoma and leiomyosarcoma. The majority of gastric smooth muscle tumors are benign; however, it is notoriously difficult to predict the malignant behavior of these tumors pathologically. The frequency of mitotic figures is one of the most useful prognostic indicators. When the mitotic count exceeds 5 per 50 high-power microscopic fields, the likelihood of metastasis is high. Tumors with more than 10 mitoses per 10 high-power fields are usually extremely aggressive. Those larger than 6 cm in diameter are also likely to be malignant.

Small leiomyomas tend to be intramural in location. As the lesion enlarges, it usually projects toward the lumen as an endogastric mass (Fig. 17-5) and occasionally from the serosal surface as an exophytic tumor (Fig. 17-6). Dumbbell-shaped lesions have components growing both toward and away from the gastric lumen. Some tumors present as an annular lesion. Larger masses often become

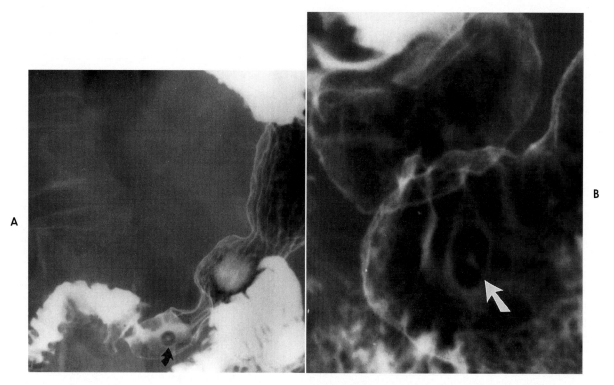

Fig. 17-4 Heterotopic pancreas. **A** and **B,** Typical findings of a gastric antral mass *(arrows)* with central umbilication.

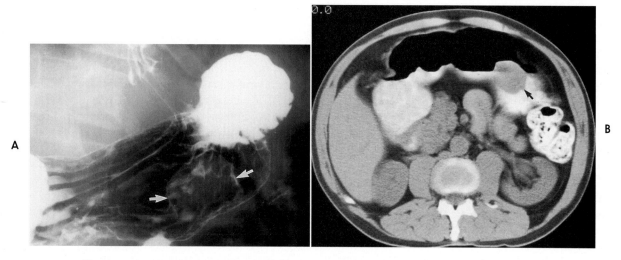

Fig. 17-5 Gastric leiomyoma. **A,** Endogastric mass *(arrows)* arising in the body of the stomach with superficial ulcerations. **B,** CT section through the luminal component of a gastric body mass *(arrow).*

pedunculated and may demonstrate superficial or deep ulcerations as well as central necrosis. Approximately 50% of gastric leiomyomas develop in the body of the stomach, with the remainder distributed equally between the fundus and antrum. This excludes the epithelioid variant, which occurs more often in the distal stomach.

On upper GI examination, smooth muscle tumors usu-ally appear as a smooth, rounded, well-circumscribed filling defect in the stomach. Central ulceration is often identified. Calcifications are occasionally detected within the tumor on conventional radiography or CT, and a rare case of an ossified gastric leiomyoma has been reported.[53] CT provides excellent delineation of the exophytic component of a mass, which is difficult to identify on upper GI examina-

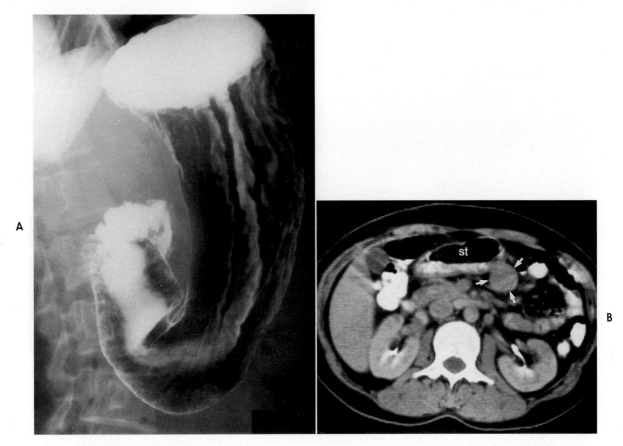

Fig. 17-6 Exophytic leiomyoma. **A,** No luminal abnormalities caused by an exogastric leiomyoma in the distal portion of the stomach. **B,** CT image of a pedunculated mass *(arrows)* projecting from the greater curve of the lower gastric body. *St,* Lumen of stomach.

tion and endoscopy. The majority of leiomyomas are of homogeneous density on CT and have a uniform enhancement pattern.[54] Large myomas occasionally contain necrotic areas. Both transabdominal and endoscopic ultrasound[55] have been used to detect and evaluate these tumors. They typically appear as hypoechoic masses. Irregularly shaped sonolucent foci within the tumor correspond to areas of liquefactive necrosis. Two rare cases of epithelioid stromal tumors of the stomach presenting as multiseptate cystic exogastric masses have been reported.[56]

Smooth muscle tumors are encountered at all ages, with a peak incidence in the fifth to seventh decades. Approximately one third of tumors are found incidentally, and there is no gender predilection. The most common symptom is bleeding, which may be slow or profuse. Other clinical manifestations include abdominal discomfort, nausea, and vomiting. On rare occasion, gastric epithelioid stromal tumors are associated with pulmonary chondromas and functioning extraadrenal paragangliomas, designated as *Carney's triad.*[57] These associated pathologic abnormalities have a marked female predilection and no inheritable tendency. Infrequently, only two of the three elements that de-

fine this entity are manifest, representing an incomplete variant of Carney's triad.[58]

Neurogenic tumors (schwannoma, neurofibroma, paraganglioma, ganglioneuroma)

Neurogenic tumors refer to those neoplasms that arise from nerve sheaths (e.g., schwannomas and neurofibromas), as well as rarer neoplasms containing ganglion cells (e.g., paragangliomas and ganglioneuromas). Together, these tumors constitute about 5% to 10% of all benign gastric tumors,[49] and the majority are asymptomatic. Patients may occasionally present with hemorrhage, pain, or an abdominal mass. These lesions are usually solitary and occur most often along the lesser curve of the stomach, particularly in the antrum. Neurogenic tumors are usually submucosal in location but may develop as a subserosal mass or have elements of both.[59,60] Pedunculation is common. These lesions may be difficult to differentiate microscopically, from smooth muscle tumors. Schwannomas (neurilemomas) arise from the Schwann cells of the nerve sheath rather than from the nerve fiber (Fig. 17-7). These tumors are made up of sheets of spindle cells and have a propen-

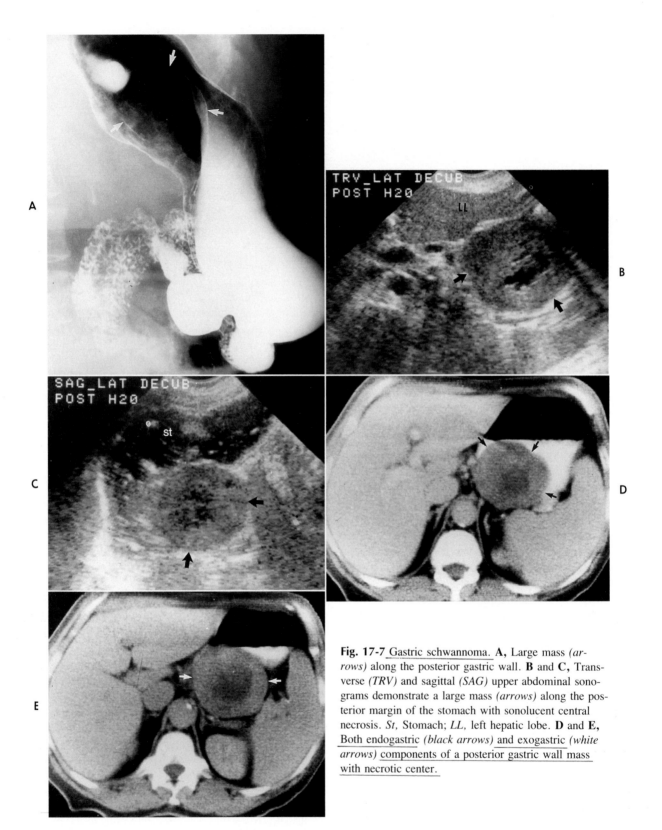

Fig. 17-7 Gastric schwannoma. **A,** Large mass *(arrows)* along the posterior gastric wall. **B** and **C,** Transverse *(TRV)* and sagittal *(SAG)* upper abdominal sonograms demonstrate a large mass *(arrows)* along the posterior margin of the stomach with sonolucent central necrosis. *St,* Stomach; *LL,* left hepatic lobe. **D** and **E,** Both endogastric *(black arrows)* and exogastric *(white arrows)* components of a posterior gastric wall mass with necrotic center.

sity to ulcerate. Neurofibromas also contain spindle cells, which are arranged in a more regular orientation. These tumors originate from the sympathetic fibers of the subserosal myenteric (Auerbach's) plexus and from the submucosal plexus of Meissner. The majority of neurofibromas are small, typically presenting as a well-circumscribed nonencapsulated submucosal mass. Irregular mural thickening is an unusual appearance that results from diffuse involvement along the myenteric plexus. Approximately 15% of patients with gastrointestinal neurofibromas have von Recklinghausen's disease, an autosomal dominant disorder affecting approximately 1 in 3000 persons. Conversely, 25% of patients with von Recklinghausen's disease have neurogenic tumors of the bowel. Sarcomatous degeneration develops in approximately 10% of neurofibromas. Paraganglioma rarely arises in the stomach, usually occurring in the second portion of the duodenum, particularly in the periampullary region.[61] These lesions contain epithelioid polygonal cells and a neural component with large ganglion cells. Ganglioneuroma is also a rare neurogenic gastric tumor. These lesions are composed of proliferations of nerve and Schwann cells, as well as variable numbers of ganglion cells.

Lipoma

The stomach is an uncommon site for development of gastrointestinal lipomas, which occur most often in the colon. Of the benign gastric mural tumors, 3% are lipomas.[62] These lesions present as a submucosal mass in approximately 90% to 95% of cases and as a subserosal lesion in the remaining 5% to 10%.[63] Lipomas are usually solitary and are typically sessile (Fig. 17-8), with occasional pedunculated lesions. On gross inspection the lipoma appears as a yellowish mass that may be either pliable or firm. These tumors are composed of mature adipocytes and are surrounded by a fibrous capsule. The surface is usually smooth, with easy retraction of the mucosa from underly-

ing fat. Seventy percent of gastric lipomas arise in the antrum (Fig. 17-9). Most lesions are small and do not produce symptoms. Surface erosion and central ulceration may develop, resulting in acute or chronic bleeding. Hemorrhage may be severe, producing anemia due to iron deficiency. Large pedunculated tumors often cause pain, particularly with peristalsis. Some lipomas become clinically manifest as a result of obstruction or intussusception. For example, antral lesions may prolapse into the duodenum, producing nausea, vomiting, and gastric distention.

On upper GI examination the lipoma usually presents as a well-circumscribed, intramural mass with a radiolucent appearance.[64] Because of the pliability of the tumor, peristalsis or external compression effects changes in tumor shape. CT examination is extremely useful in confirming the diagnosis, by demonstration of a smoothly marginated homogeneous fatty mass[65] (Fig. 17-10). CT attenuation features are in the range of -80 to -120 Hounsfield units. The lesions are usually hyperechoic on transabdominal or endoscopic ultrasound studies, although fat may sonographically demonstrate variable degrees of increased echogenicity. MRI may be used to characterize the adipose tissue contained within a lipoma. On conventional spin-echo imaging, the lipoma has hyperintense (short) T1 and hypointense (long) T2 signal characteristics. Fat-suppression techniques such as STIR (short tau inversion recovery) imaging may confirm the diagnosis. Malignant transformation is rare, with liposarcomas accounting for less than 0.1% of all gastric tumors.

Inflammatory fibroid polyp

Inflammatory fibroid polyps are uncommon benign gastric tumors. However, within the gastrointestinal tract, the stomach is the most common site for development of these lesions. Gastric inflammatory fibroid polyps occur most often in the antrum near the pyloric sphincter, followed by

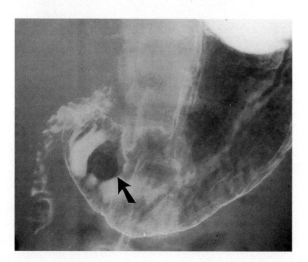

Fig. 17-8 Gastric lipoma. Smoothly marginated radiolucent mass *(arrow)* in the gastric antrum.

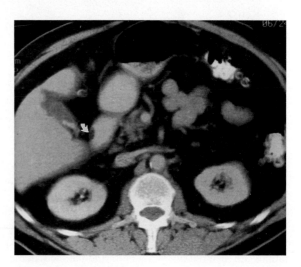

Fig. 17-9 Antral lipoma. Small sessile fatty mass *(arrow)* arising from the gastric antral wall.

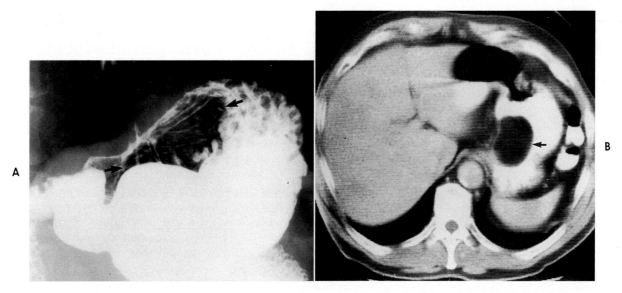

Fig. 17-10 Fundal lipoma. **A,** Radiolucent appearance of a circumscribed gastric fundal mass *(arrows)*. **B,** CT section reveals a typical homogeneous fatty attenuation *(arrow)* characteristic of a lipoma.

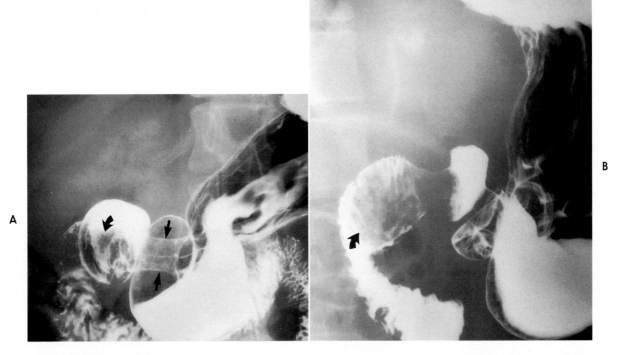

Fig. 17-11 Inflammatory fibroid polyp. **A** and **B,** Large pedunculated mass originating from a stalk in the gastric body *(straight arrows)* and prolapsing into the duodenum *(curved arrows)*.

the body and fundus of the stomach. These polyps typically appear as a solitary, well-circumscribed, smoothly marginated mass with a broad base. Superficial erosions and ulcerations are identified in about half, and the median diameter is approximately 2.5 cm. Large pedunculated intraluminal masses may cause gastric outlet obstruction and intussusception (Fig. 17-11).

Histologically, inflammatory fibroid polyps are nonencapsulated masses composed of fibroblasts and histiocytes within a hypocellular myxoid stroma. Scattered throughout the stroma is a capillary network, as well as inflammatory cells, which usually include numerous eosinophils. These lesions are of unknown etiology and develop in a variable age group, with a mean age at diagnosis of approximately

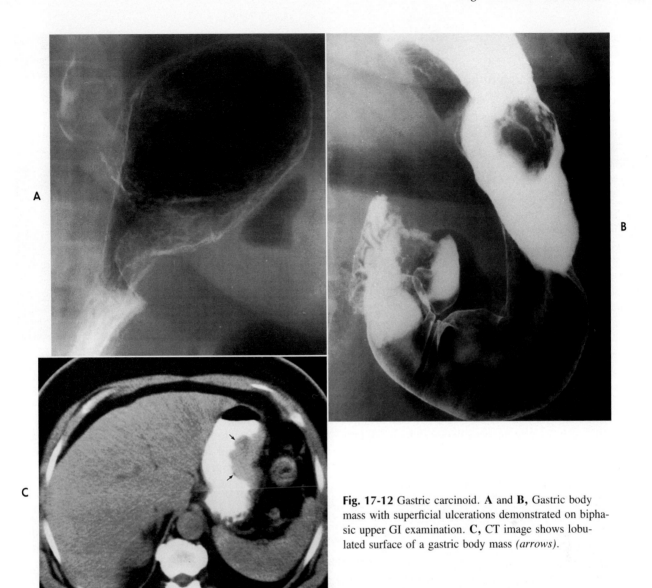

Fig. 17-12 Gastric carcinoid. **A** and **B,** Gastric body mass with superficial ulcerations demonstrated on biphasic upper GI examination. **C,** CT image shows lobulated surface of a gastric body mass *(arrows).*

50 years. There may be a slight gender predilection for males. In a series of 16 patients with gastric inflammatory fibroid polyps, 50% appeared on radiographic studies as a smooth, well-circumscribed intramural mass, and 44% presented as an intraluminal polyp (five pedunculated and two sessile).[66] The remaining case was difficult to characterize because of a poor-quality image.

Glomus tumor

Glomus tumors are rare benign neoplasms that are markedly vascular. The majority of glomus tumors in the alimentary tract occur in the stomach, with the antrum being the most common site. These masses are well circumscribed in contour and intramural in location. Most of these tumors are approximately 2 to 4 cm in diameter but may be larger, with larger lesions being more likely to ulcerate. Histologically, glomus tumors are made up of uniform round cells that are ultrastructurely of smooth muscle origin. These cells are oriented in sheets or clusters that are closely applied to the endothelial walls of capillaries. Vascular spaces form, which vary in size. The mucosal surface of these tumors may necrose and ulcerate. Gastrointestinal hemorrhage is the most common symptom.

Vascular tumors (hemangioma, lymphangioma, hemangiopericytoma, hemangioendothelioma)

Angiomas (hemangioma, lymphangioma, hemangiopericytoma, and hemangioendothelioma) of vascular or lymphatic origin rarely develop in the stomach. Hemangiomas may occur as solitary or multiple lesions. On microscopic examination, these tumors contain either cavernous or small capillary channels. Small calcifications representing phleboliths may be identified and suggest an underlying vascular neoplasm. The malignant counterparts of these neoplasms, such as angiosarcoma, rarely occur in the stomach.

Carcinoid tumor (benign form)

Carcinoid tumors are endocrine neoplasms that may arise anywhere in the alimentary tract. The majority are found in the appendix and small bowel. Approximately 2% to 3% of all carcinoid tumors occur in the stomach.[67] Gastric carcinoid tumors usually present as a well-circumscribed, firm intramural nodule[68] (Fig. 17-12). Multiplicity of these lesions is infrequently encountered. Intact mucosa usually covers carcinoid tumors, although ulceration may occur. The distribution of these lesions in different portions of the stomach is relatively uniform. Carcinoid tumors originate from the Kulchitsky cells of the deep mucosal layer, found in the crypts of Lieberkühn. Diagnosis of carcinoid tumors is established microscopically, with identification of small uniform tumor cells of cuboidal or low columnar type containing cytoplasmic granules. Carcinoid tumors are slow growing and may be benign or malignant. This distinction often requires integration of clinical and microscopic findings. Approximately 20% of these tumors undergo malignant transformation. The size of the neoplasm is a factor in the malignant potential. Lesions smaller than 2 cm are generally associated with a favorable prognosis, whereas most tumors more than 2 cm in diameter demonstrate local invasion and nodal metastases.

Gastric carcinoid tumors usually occur between the ages of 40 and 70 years. A large percentage of afflicted individuals have minimal or no symptomatology. Clinical manifestations are varied and may be secondary to hormone secretion, such as postprandial flushing due to histamine release. Gastric carcinoid tumors differ from midgut neoplasms in primarily secreting 5-hydroxytryptophan rather than 5-hydroxytryptamine (serotonin). Tumors from both sites within the gastrointestinal tract may elevate the urinary levels of the final breakdown product of 5-hydroxyindolacetic acid (5-HIAA). Other secretory products of gastric carcinoids include histamine, gastrin, and rarely ACTH, beta-melanocyte–stimulating hormone (beta-MSH), and epinephrine. Presenting symptoms among tumors lacking endocrine function include nausea, vomiting, pain, and anemia. Bleeding from ulceration of gastric carcinoid tumors is common. Radiographic manifestations of gastric carcinoid tumors are variable and nonspecific. The most frequent appearance is of a solitary, sharply marginated sessile intramural mass. Ulcerations are often demonstrated on upper GI examination. Other manifestations of gastric carcinoid tumors include multiple gastric polyps, a large ulcer, and a polypoid intramural tumor.

Granular cell tumor (myoblastoma)

The granular cell tumor (myoblastoma) is a rare, benign lesion of the stomach. The majority of these tumors within the gastrointestinal tract arise in the esophagus. Granular

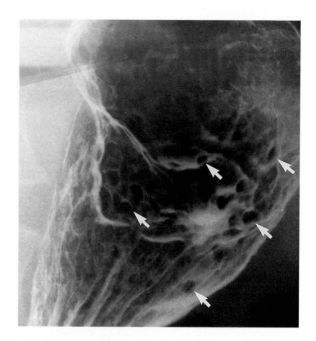

Fig. 17-13 Lymphoid hyperplasia. Multiple small polypoid lesions *(arrows)* in the gastric fundus and body.

cell tumors may occur at any site within the stomach and typically are 1 to 4 cm in diameter. Pathologic examination of the tumor reveals spindle or epithelioid cells that contain coarsely granular eosinophilic cytoplasm.

Lymphoid hyperplasia (Pseudolymphoma)

Lymphoid hyperplasia, also referred to as *pseudolymphoma,* is characterized by focal reactive proliferation of gastric lymphoreticular tissue. This has been identified at various sites within the stomach (Fig. 17-13). The appearance of these lesions varies, often presenting as an umbilicated polypoid lesion[69] or as a submucosal tumor. Other manifestations include an ulcerated or constricting mass that resembles a malignant tumor, a large ulcer crater, an infiltrating lesion, or markedly enlarged rugal folds. Although usually solitary, multiple lesions may occur. Ulceration is present in approximately 70% of cases. Lymphoid hyperplasia is believed to result from chronic inflammation. Histologically, these masses are made up of mature lymphocytes in submucosal follicles, which are increased in number and size. Other cellular elements often identified in these lesions include histiocytes, plasma cells, and fibroblasts. Microscopic findings are distinctive from malignant lymphoma, which does not form follicles and has immature cellular constituents. Radiographic differentiation is difficult, but lymphoma is more rigid, less distensible, and is more likely to contain multiple sites of ulceration.

Plasmacytoma

Primary plasmacytoma of the stomach is rare. Approximately 5% of plasmacytomas are extramedullary; 85% of

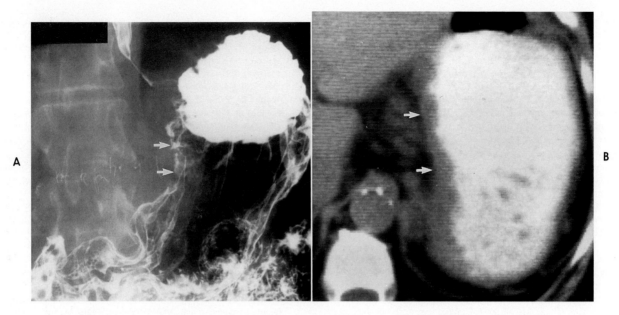

Fig. 17-14 Gastric plasmacytoma. **A,** Ulcerated plaquelike mass *(arrows)* along the upper margin of the lesser curve *(arrows)*. **B,** Irregular mural thickening along the medial aspect of the proximal stomach *(arrows)* due to extramedullary plasmacytoma.

these occur in the upper respiratory tract or conjunctiva.[70] This is followed by the small bowel and stomach in frequency of occurrence. Most tumors present as a solitary submucosal mass[71] (Fig. 17-14) composed of plasma cell infiltration. These lesions usually occur in middle-aged and elderly individuals and are more common in males than females. Gastric plasmacytomas are often associated with symptoms of ulcer disease. Tumors usually present as an ulcerated mass on upper GI examination, but single or multiple polypoid masses are seen occasionally.

REFERENCES

1. Stout AP: Tumors of the stomach. In *Atlas of tumor pathology,* sect 6, Washington, DC, 1953, Armed Forces Institute of Pathology.
2. McNeer G, Pack GT: *Neoplasms of the stomach,* Philadelphia, 1978, JB Lippincott.
3. Ming SC: The classification and significance of gastric polyps. In Yardley JH, Morson BM, eds: *The gastrointestinal tract,* Baltimore, 1977, Williams & Wilkins.
4. Rösch W: Epidemiology, pathogenesis, diagnosis, and treatment of benign gastric tumours, *Front Gastrointest Res* 6:167, 1980.
5. Laxèn F, Sipponen P, Ihamaki T et al: Gastric polyps: their morphological and endoscopical characteristics and relation to gastric carcinoma, *Acta Pathol Microbiol Scand [A]* 90:221, 1982.
6. Elsborg L, Andersen D, Myhere-Jensen O, Bastrup-Madsen P: Gastric mucosal polyps in pernicious anemia, *Scand J Gastroenterol* 12:49, 1977.
7. Stockbrugger RW, Menon GG, Beilby JO et al: Gastroscopic screening in 80 patients with pernicious anaemia, *Gut* 24:1141, 1983.
8. Siurala M: Gastritis, its fate and sequelae, *Ann Clin Res* 13:111, 1981.
9. Janunger K, Domellof L: Gastric polyps and precancerous mucosal changes after partial gastrectomy, *Acta Chir Scand* 144:293, 1978.
10. Ovaska JT, Ekfors TO, Havia TV, Kujari HP: Endoscopic follow-up after resection for gastric or duodenal ulcer, *Acta Chir Scand* 152:289, 1986.
11. Stemmermann GN, Hayashi T: Hyperplastic polyps of the gastric mucosa adjacent to gastroenterostomy stomas, *Am J Clin Pathol* 71:341, 1979.
12. Morson BC: Gastric polyps composed of intestinal epithelium, *Br J Cancer* 9:550, 1955.
13. Yeh HC, Rabinowitz JG: Ultrasonography and computed tomography of gastric wall lesions, *Radiology* 141:147, 1981.
14. Gossios KJ, Epameinondas VT, Demou LL et al: Use of water or air as oral contrast media for computed tomographic study of the gastric wall: comparison of the two techniques, *Gastrointest Radiol* 16:293, 1991.
15. Rapaccini GL, Aliotta A, Pompili M et al: Gastric wall thickness in normal and neoplastic subjects: a prospective study performed by abdominal ultrasound, *Gastrointest Radiol* 13:197, 1988.
16. MacDonald WC: Gastric tumors. In Gitnick G, ed: *Principles and practice of gastroenterology and hepatology,* New York, 1988, Elsevier.
17. Lewin KJ, Riddell RH, Weinstein WM: Inflammatory hyperplastic-type polyps (regenerative polyps, hyperplasiogenous polyps, focal foveolar hyperplasia) and juvenile polyps. In *Gastrointestinal pathology and its clinical implications,* vol I, New York, 1992, Igaku-Shoin.
18. Glick SN, Teplick SK, Amenta PS: Giant hyperplastic polyps of the gastric remnant simulating carcinoma, *Gastrointest Radiol* 15:151, 1990.
19. Remmele W, Kolb EF: Malignant transformation of hyperplasiogenic polyps of the stomach: case report, *Endoscopy* 10:63, 1978.
20. Papp JP, Joseph JI: Adenocarcinoma occurring in a hyperplastic gastric polyp: removal by electrosurgical polypectomy, *Gastrointest Endosc* 23:38, 1976.
21. Joff N, Goldman H, Antonioli DA: Recurring hyperplastic gastric polyps following subtotal gastrectomy, *AJR* 130:301, 1978.
22. Ming SC: Epithelial polyps of the stomach. In Ming SC, Goldman H, eds: *Pathology of the gastrointestinal tract,* Philadelphia, 1992, WB Saunders.
23. Meltzer AD, Ostrum BJ, Isard HJ: Villous tumors of the stomach and duodenum: report of three cases, *Radiology* 87:511, 1966.

24. Miller JH, Gisoold JJ, Weiland LH, Melbrath DC: Upper gastrointestinal tract: villous tumors, *AJR* 134:933, 1980.

25. Robbins SL, Cotran RS, eds: Tumors of the stomach. In *Pathologic basis of disease,* ed 2, Philadelphia, 1979, WB Saunders.

26. Wolf BS: Roentgen diagnosis of villous tumors of the colon, *AJR* 84:1093, 1960.

27. Hirota T, Okada T, Itabashi M, Kitaoka H: Histogenesis of human gastric cancer with special reference to the significance of adenoma as a precancerous lesion. In Ming SC, ed: *Precursors of gastric cancer,* New York, 1984, Praeger.

28. Gaitini D, Kleinhaus U, Munichor M, Duek D: Villous tumors of the stomach, *Gastrointest Radiol* 13:105, 1988.

29. Utsunomiya J, Gocho H, Miyanaga T et al: Peutz-Jeghers syndrome: its natural course and management, *Johns Hopkins Med J* 136:71, 1975.

30. Linos DA, Dozois RR, Dahlin DC, Bartholomew LG: Does Peutz-Jeghers syndrome predispose to gastrointestinal malignancy: a later look, *Arch Surg* 116:1182, 1981.

31. Reid JD: Intestinal carcinoma of the small intestine in father and daughter, *JAMA* 229:833, 1974.

32. Buck JL, Harned RK, Lichtenstein JE, Sobin LH: Peutz-Jeghers syndrome, *Radiographics* 12:365, 1992.

33. Dos Santos JG, de Magalhaes J: Familial gastric polyposis: a new entity, *J Genet Hum* 28:293, 1980.

34. Watanabe A, Nagashima H, Motoi M, Ogawa K: Familial juvenile polyposis of the stomach, *Gastroenterology* 77:148, 1979.

35. Beacham DH, Shields HM, Raffensperger EC, Enterline HT: Juvenile and adenomatous gastrointestinal polyposis, *Am J Dig Dis* 23:1137, 1978.

36. Sachatello CR, Pickren JW, Grace JT Jr: Generalized juvenile gastrointestinal polyposis: a hereditary syndrome, *Gastroenterology* 58:699, 1979.

37. Goodman ZD, Yardley JH, Milligan FD: Pathogenesis of colonic polyps in multiple juvenile polyposis: report of a case associated with gastric polyps and carcinoma of the rectum, *Cancer* 43:1906, 1979.

38. Sachatello CR, Griffin WO Jr: Hereditary polypoid diseases of the gastrointestinal tract: a working classification, *Am J Surg* 129:198, 1975.

39. Iida M, Tsuneyoshi Y, Watanabe H et al: Spontaneous disappearance of fundic gland polyposis: report of three cases, *Gastroenterology* 79:725, 1980.

40. Watanabe H, Enjoji M, Yao T, Ohsato K: Gastric lesions in familial adenomatosis coli: their incidence and histological analysis, *Hum Pathol* 9:269, 1978.

41. Burt RW, Berenson MM, Lee RG et al: Upper gastrointestinal polyps in Gardner's syndrome, *Gastroenterology* 86:295, 1984.

42. Tonelli F, Nardi F, Bechi P et al: Extracolonic polyps in familial polyposis coli and Gardner's syndrome, *Dis Colon Rectum* 28:664, 1985.

43. Grigioni WF, Alampi G, Martinelli G, Piccoluga A: Atypical juvenile polyposis, *Histopathology* 5:361, 1981.

44. Sipponen P, Laxen F, Seppala K: Cystic 'hamartomatous' gastric polyps: a disorder of oxyntic glands, *Histopathology* 7:729, 1983.

45. Cronkhite LW, Canada WJ: Generalized gastrointestinal polyposis: an unusual syndrome of polyposis, pigmentation, alopecia, and onychotrophia, *N Engl J Med* 252:1011, 1955.

46. Daniel ES, Ludwig SL, Lewin KJ et al: The Cronkhite-Canada syndrome: an analysis of clinical and pathologic features and therapy in 55 patients, *Medicine* 61:293, 1982.

47. Dachman AH, Buck JL, Burke AP, Sobin LH: Cronkhite-Canada syndrome: radiologic features, *Gastrointest Radiol* 14:285, 1989.

48. Thoeni RF, Gedgaudas RK: Ectopic pancreas: usual and unusual features, *Gastrointest Radiol* 5:37, 1980.

49. Palmer ED: Benign intramural tumors of the stomach: a review with special reference to gross pathology, *Medicine* 30:81, 1951.

50. Marshall SF: Gastric tumors other than carcinoma: report of unusual cases, *Surg Clin North Am* 35:693, 1955.

51. Martin JF, Bazin P, Feroldi J, Cabanne F: Tumeurs myoides intramurales de l'estomac: considerations microscopiques á propos de 6 cas, *Ann Anat Pathol* (Paris) 5:484, 1960.

52. Stout AP: Bizarre smooth muscle tumors of the stomach, *Cancer* 15:400, 1962.

53. Savit RM, Horrow MM, Agarwal P: Ossified leiomyoma of the stomach: demonstration on computed tomography, *Br J Radiol* 62:79, 1989.

54. Megibow AJ, Balthazar EJ, Hulnick DH et al: CT evaluation of gastrointestinal leiomyomas and leiomyosarcomas, *AJR* 144:727, 1985.

55. Nakazawa S, Yoshino J, Nakemura T et al: Endoscopic ultrasonography of gastric myogenic tumor: a comparative study between histology and ultrasonography, *J Ultrasound Med* 8:353, 1989.

56. Choi BI, Ok ID, Im JG et al: Exogastric cystic gastric leiomyoblastoma with unusual CT appearance, *Gastrointest Radiol* 13:109, 1988.

57. Carney JA, Sheps SD, Go VLV et al: The triad of gastric epithelioid leiomyosarcoma, functioning extraadrenal paraganglioma, and pulmonary chondroma, *N Engl J Med* 296:1517, 1977.

58. Mazas-Artasona L, Romeo M, Felices R et al: Gastro-oesophageal leiomyoblastomas and multiple pulmonary chondromas: an incomplete variant of Carney's triad, *Br J Radiol* 61:1181, 1988.

59. Nussinson E, Vigder L, Kaveh Z et al: Exogastric neurilemmoma presenting as acute abdomen: role of computed tomography in diagnosis, *Gastrointest Radiol* 13:306, 1988.

60. Nielson R, Eiken M: Gastric tumors of neurogenic origin, *Dan Med Bull* 8:121, 1961.

61. Imai S, Kajihara Y, Komaki K et al: Paraganglioma of the duodenum: a case report with radiological findings and literature review, *Br J Radiol* 63:975, 1990.

62. Chu AG, Clifton JA: Gastric lipoma presenting as peptic ulcer: case report and review of the literature, *Am J Gastroenterol* 78:615, 1983.

63. Fernandez MJ, Davis RP, Nova PF: Gastrointestinal lipomas, *Arch Surg* 118:1081, 1983.

64. Taylor AJ, Stewart ET, Dodds WJ: Gastrointestinal lipomas: a radiologic and pathologic review, *AJR* 155:1205, 1990.

65. Heiken JP, Forde KA, Gold RP: Computed tomography as a definitive method for diagnosing gastrointestinal lipomas, *Radiology* 142:409, 1990.

66. Harned RK, Buck JL, Shekitka KM: Inflammatory fibroid polyps of the gastrointestinal tract: radiologic evaluation, *Radiology* 182:863, 1992.

67. Godwin JD: Carcinoid tumors: an analysis of 2837 cases, *Cancer* 36:560, 1975.

68. Marshall JB, Bodnarchuk G: Carcinoid tumors of the gut: our experience over three decades and review of the literature, *J Clin Gastroenterol* 16:123, 1993.

69. Bahk YW, Ahn JS, Choi HJ: Lymphoid hyperplasia of the stomach presenting as umbilicated polypoid lesions, *Radiology* 100:277, 1977.

70. Godard JE, Fox JE, Levinson MJ: Primary gastric plasmacytoma, *Dig Dis* 18:508, 1973.

71. Remigo PA, Klaum A: Extramedullary plasmacytoma of the stomach, *Cancer* 27:562, 1971.

18 *Diagnosis of Gastric Cancer in Europe*

J. ODO OP DEN ORTH

Although its incidence is slowly decreasing, gastric carcinoma is still the second most common cancer in the world.[1] There are important geographic variations in the incidence rates, with the highest in Japan, followed by Europe and then North America.[1] Gastric carcinoma, at least outside Japan, is associated with a poor survival rate. The mortality statistics for Europe demonstrate important regional variations, however. The death rates in Hungary, Poland, Portugal, and Romania are relatively high compared with Denmark, France, and Greece.[2] Gastric carcinoma rarely occurs in children and young adults; most patients are over 50 years old, and it is more prevalent in men than in women.[1,3-8]

A recent British review of more than 31,000 cases[9] revealed an overall age-adjusted survival at 5 years of only 5%. Early gastric carcinoma (EGC) was defined by Japanese practitioners as a carcinoma of the stomach that has invaded only the mucosa and submucosa. Neither the size of the carcinoma nor the presence of metastases influences this definition. Only the depth of tissue infiltration matters. The overall 5-year survival of EGC in a relatively large Japanese series was about 90%.[10] Although there was some skepticism about the prevalence of this form of gastric carcinoma outside Japan, it is now known that the characteristics of EGC in Western countries is similar in clinical, morphologic, and histopathologic respects.[3,8,11-25] Nevertheless, EGC is more frequently diagnosed in Japan than in the Western world. In a Japanese surgical series, 39.6% of the cases were diagnosed in the early stage[26]; in contrast, at the author's institution, EGC was diagnosed in only 19.6% of the resected specimens (9.3% of the entire series).[8] However, in Japan the institution of mass screening programs has led to the discovery of ECG in many more asymptomatic patients, and this has contributed to the better statistics there.

BARIUM EXAMINATION
State-of-the-art technique

Currently, most authors advocate a biphasic examination, combining the advantages of both double- and single-contrast techniques.[27] Drug-induced hypotonia is also widely advocated.[27] Despite an apparent consensus that a biphasic examination is the examination of choice, many radiologists throughout the world still employ pure double-contrast examinations. On a theoretic basis, many lesions of the anterior wall of the distal half of the stomach will be missed if only double-contrast films are obtained. However, in actuality, irregularities of the posterior wall of the stomach can be appreciated to excellent advantage if the examination is performed with the patient supine. As the patient is maneuvered on the table, a layer of barium suspension of varying thickness will flow along the posterior, or dependent, wall of the organ, thereby visualizing in relief virtually every protrusion or excavation of the mucosa of this dependent wall. At the same time, if conditions are optimal, the anterior, or nondependent wall, is coated with a thin, even layer of barium. On the nondependent wall, excavations and protrusions with sloping edges cannot be depicted, but irregularities with abrupt margins may be observed (Fig. 18-1). However, even lesions of the nondependent wall that possess abrupt margins may be missed if the x-ray beam is not parallel with these margins (Fig. 18-1). For most parts of the bowel, radiographs obtained with the patient in the prone dependent position allow optimal visualization of the mucosa of the anterior wall. Prone double-contrast radiographs of the distal half of the stomach are, however, difficult to obtain because the distal stomach is completely filled with barium in this position.[12,27] Single-contrast, graded-compression studies can, however, clearly demonstrate lesions of the anterior wall in the distal half of the stomach (Figs. 18-2 and 18-3). At times, when conditions for compression are optimal, adequate single-contrast, graded-compression studies may be obtained if the patient is given a high-density barium suspension; however, results are often poor because of inadequate x-ray penetration. Medium-density barium suspensions combine the advantages of good mucosal coating in the double-contrast phase with transparency in the single-contrast, graded-compression phase.[12,27-29] Radiologists who prefer to use a high-density barium suspension for double-contrast radiographs can perform a biphasic examination by giving patients a low-density barium suspension after double-contrast radiographs have been obtained.[30-33]

Limitations of barium examination

More than 15 years ago, my colleagues and I tried to define the limitations of the standard biphasic gastric series

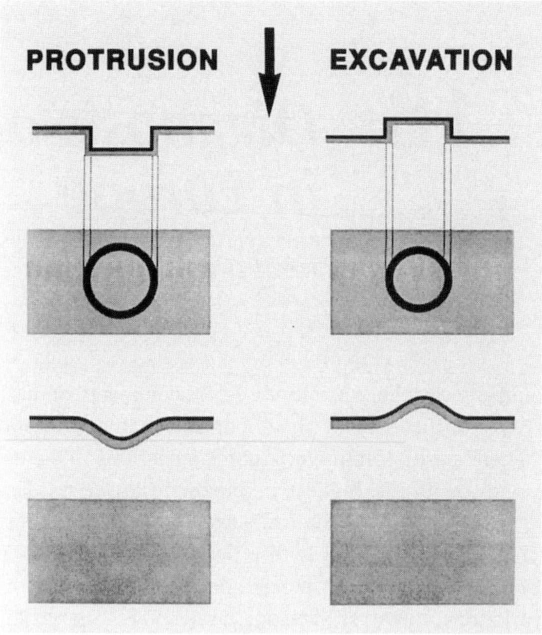

Fig. 18-1 Capabilities and limitations of double-contrast demonstration of lesions of the nondependent wall of the stomach. The upper part of this diagram illustrates how, on the nondependent wall, protrusions and excavations with abrupt margins may be depicted on double-contrast studies if the x-ray beam *(arrow)* is parallel with these margins. The lower part shows how protrusions and excavations with gently sloping edges are missed because there is no significant change in the thickness of barium to be penetrated by the x-ray beam.
From Op den Orth JO: *Radiology* 713:601, 1989.

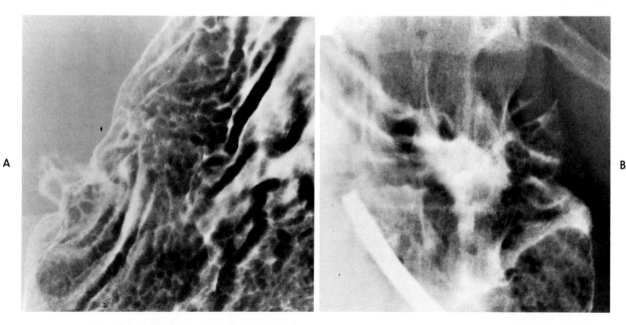

Fig. 18-2 Importance of single-contrast compression studies in diagnosing superficial depressed early gastric carcinoma of the anterior wall of the antrum. **A,** Double-contrast view shows only deformation of the lesser curve in the pyloric region. **B,** The prone single-contrast compression study reveals a nearly flat ulcer in the anterior wall. Biopsy specimens obtained at subsequent endoscopy exhibited adenocarcinoma. Examination of the resected specimen showed the malignant infiltration was restricted to the mucosa and submucosa.
From Op den Orth JO: *Radiology* 713:601, 1989.

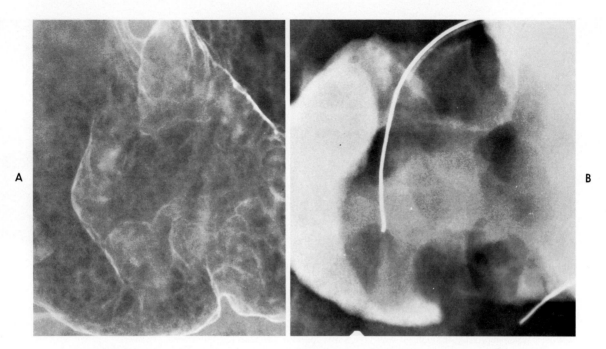

Fig. 18-3 Importance of single-contrast compression studies in depicting ulcerating advanced carcinoma of the anterior wall of the antrum. **A,** Double-contrast view suggests a nearly flat lesion. **B,** Single-contrast graded-compression study demonstrates an ulcerating tumor in the anterior wall of the antrum.

employed at our institution in theoretic terms.[28] Mapping the gastric regions using our standard biphasic examination revealed a high degree of coverage, often with overlapping single- and double-contrast visualization. The anterior wall of the higher body, however, appeared difficult to visualize because the ribs interfere with compression. More recently, the findings from prospective and retrospective studies[8,11,12,24,34-36] have shown that this examination is, in practice, an excellent tool for detecting early and advanced gastric carcinoma in virtually every location. Cross-sectional techniques have been helpful for elucidating the nature of malignant lesions possessing sloping edges and located in the anterior wall of the gastric body (Figs. 18-4 and 18-5).

CROSS-SECTIONAL TECHNIQUES

Barium examinations of the stomach provide detailed information not only on tiny protrusions and excavations of the mucosa, but also on the shape and distensibility of this part of the bowel. Although cross-sectional techniques may supply important additional information on the gastric wall (Figs. 18-4 and 18-5), a barium examination remains the appropriate initial imaging technique for the evaluation of suspected gastric carcinoma. Computed tomography, magnetic resonance imaging, and endosonography are covered in Chapters 14, 21, and 22, but some aspects of transabdominal gastric ultrasound are discussed in the next section.

Transabdominal gastric ultrasound

It is well known that extensive malignant infiltration of the gastric wall can often be detected during routine upper transabdominal ultrasound examinations (Fig. 18-6, *A*). Nevertheless, recently,[37-40] it has been shown that dedicated transabdominal gastric ultrasound performed after the ingestion of water and injection of a hypotonic agent may provide detailed and unique information about both the normal (Fig. 18-7) and abnormal gastric wall (Figs. 18-6, *B, C,* and 18-8). The author's own technique,[40] which consists of the use of a tilt table, the intravenous injection of glucagon, graded-compression, and high-frequency transducers, allows visualization of the five layers of the gastric wall in the distal corpus and the antrum. Although the fundal wall thickness can frequently be measured by this method, the layers of the wall of the gastric fundus can seldom even be visualized (Fig. 18-5, *B* and *C*). Unlike endosonography, there is only limited published information on transabdominal ultrasound. However, transabdominal ultrasound is interpreted in a fashion similar to that used with endosonography. Although specific layer involvement often suggests the underlying pathology and certain ultrasound patterns are highly suggestive of either benignancy or malignancy, this modality does not enable clinicians to make a definitive histologic diagnosis. Especially when ulceration is present, differentiating between carcinomatous infiltration, inflammatory infiltration, and fibrosis is not possible.[41] Nevertheless, a surprisingly high percentage of

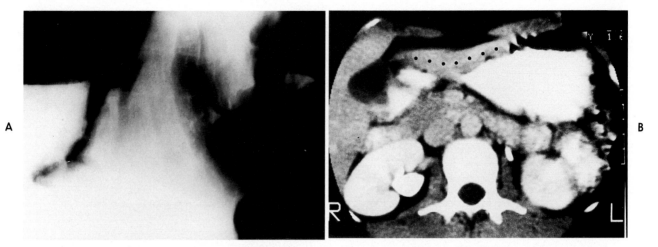

Fig. 18-4 Visualization by barium examination and computed tomography of advanced carcinoma with sloping edges located on the anterior wall of the corpus. **A,** Single-contrast, graded-compression study demonstrates a filling defect in the gastric corpus. Because double-contrast studies were nearly normal, the filling defect suggests an anterior wall mass. **B,** Subsequent CT scan demonstrates well the anterior wall tumor with sloping edges *(dots).* Adenocarcinoma that diffusely infiltrated through all wall layers was found in the resected specimen.

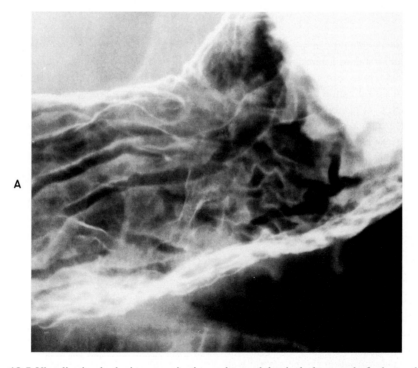

Fig. 18-5 Visualization by barium examination and transabdominal ultrasound of advanced carcinoma of the anterior wall of the corpus. **A,** Double-contrast study shows inadequate distention of the corpus and irregular anterior wall folds. **B,** Transverse transabdominal ultrasound image obtained with a 3.5-MHz transducer after water and glucagon administration shows local thickening of the anterior wall of the corpus *(arrows).* **C,** Ultrasound image obtained with a 7.5-MHz transducer shows the layered structure of a noninvolved part of the anterior wall *(white arrow)* and part of the normal posterior wall at the left side of the film. Autopsy disclosed an adenocarcinoma with a 3-cm diameter that infiltrated all wall layers.

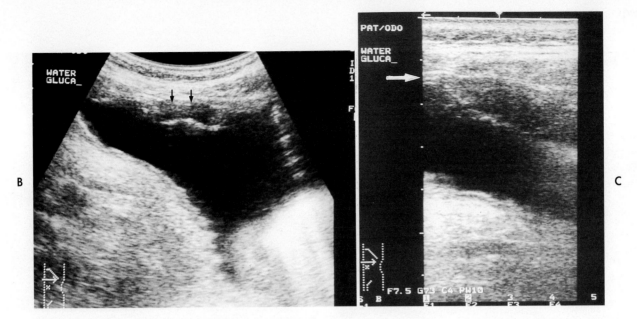

Fig. 18-5, cont'd For legend see opposite page.

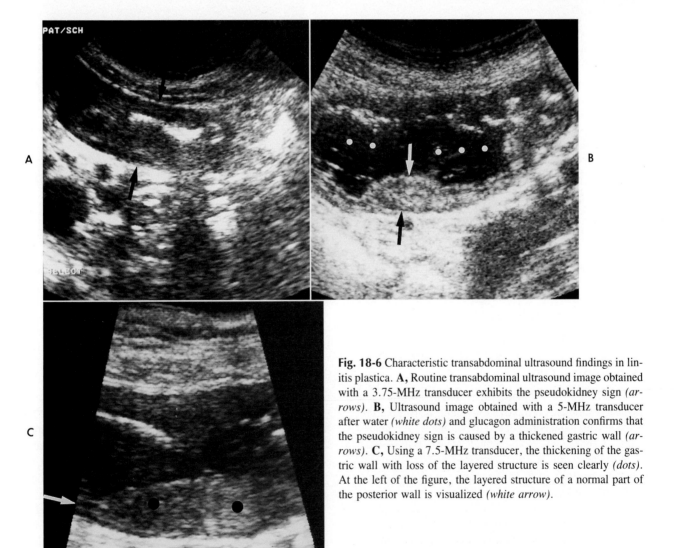

Fig. 18-6 Characteristic transabdominal ultrasound findings in linitis plastica. **A,** Routine transabdominal ultrasound image obtained with a 3.75-MHz transducer exhibits the pseudokidney sign *(arrows)*. **B,** Ultrasound image obtained with a 5-MHz transducer after water *(white dots)* and glucagon administration confirms that the pseudokidney sign is caused by a thickened gastric wall *(arrows)*. **C,** Using a 7.5-MHz transducer, the thickening of the gastric wall with loss of the layered structure is seen clearly *(dots)*. At the left of the figure, the layered structure of a normal part of the posterior wall is visualized *(white arrow)*.

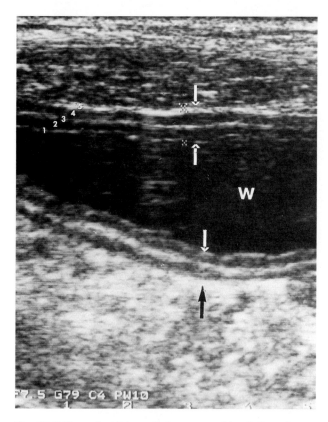

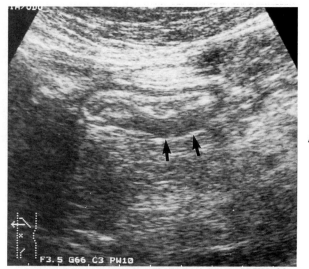

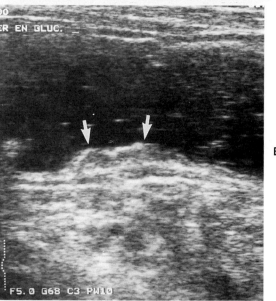

Fig. 18-7 Normal gastric wall demonstrated by dedicated transabdominal gastric ultrasound. A transverse scan of the gastric corpus obtained with a 7.5-MHz transducer after water and glucagon administration. Normal anterior and posterior wall *(arrows)* are shown to good advantage, with thicknesses of 4 and 5 mm, respectively. *1,* Interface between water and mucosa; *2,* mucosa; *3,* submucosa; *4,* muscularis propria; *5,* serosa and subserosal fat; *W,* water.
From Sijbrandij LS, Op den Orth JO: *Eur J Radiol* 13:81, 1991.

Fig. 18-8 Abnormal gastric wall demonstrated by routine and dedicated transabdominal gastric ultrasound. **A,** Transabdominal ultrasound image obtained with a 3.5-MHz transducer suggests thickening of the posterior wall of the antrum *(arrows)*. **B,** Image obtained with a 5-MHz transducer after water and glucagon administration confirms thickening *(white arrows)* involving layers 1, 2, 3, and 4 (see Fig. 18-7). Biopsy specimens demonstrated adenocarcinoma, and resected specimen showed infiltration into the proper muscle layer but none into the serosa.

malignant lesions of the stomach can be visualized on transabdominal ultrasound images if, in elderly patients, the gastric wall (see Figs. 18-5, 18-6, and 18-8) and the gastric contents[42] (Fig. 18-9) are included in the ultrasound examination of the upper abdomen.

DIAGNOSTIC VALUE OF BARIUM EXAMINATION VERSUS ENDOSCOPY

In two prospective, blinded studies, the diagnostic value of biphasic techniques, employing medium-density barium suspension with glucagon-induced hypotonia was compared with that of endoscopy. Both methods appear to have equal merit in the detection of gastric carcinoma.[34-36] The excellent Japanese results in the radiographic diagnosis of gastric carcinoma are generally acknowledged. The sensitivity and specificity values of initial radiographic examinations at the Cancer Institute Hospital in Tokyo have proved to be only slightly lower than the endoscopic values in the diagnosis of gastric cancer, including early and advanced cases.[43,44] However, in these studies the endoscopist often knew what the prior radiographic findings were, and this may have somewhat biased the results. In Japan, radiography has been considered the primary examination for the screening of gastric cancer,[26] with endoscopy reserved for the investigation of suspicious lesions detected at the barium examination. The findings of several studies[8,24,25] have

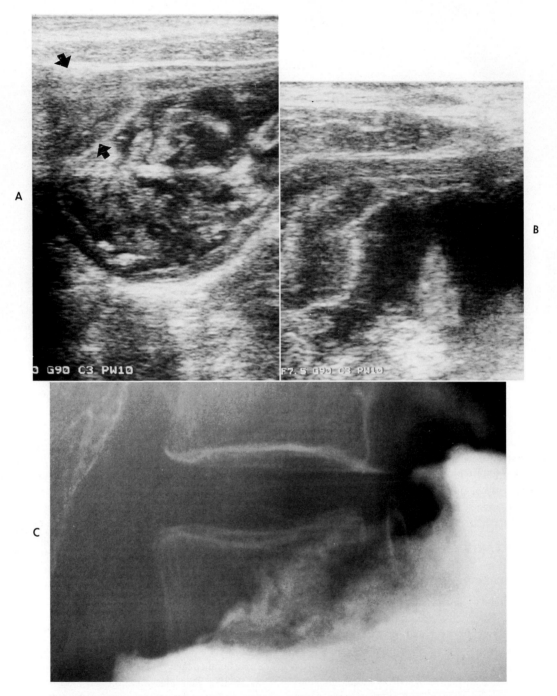

Fig. 18-9 Antral adenocarcinoma with retained material in the stomach demonstrated by transabdominal gastric ultrasound. **A,** Transabdominal ultrasound image obtained with a 5-MHz transducer reveals retained solid material and fluid in the stomach of a patient after an overnight fast. The anterior wall of the prepyloric region is thickened *(arrows)*. **B,** Detailed study of the anterior wall of the antrum obtained with a 7.5-MHz transducer shows that there is still some preservation of a distorted layered structure in the thickened wall. **C,** Barium study confirms the presence of an obstructing antral tumor. Infiltration of the adenocarcinoma through all wall layers was found in the resected specimen.

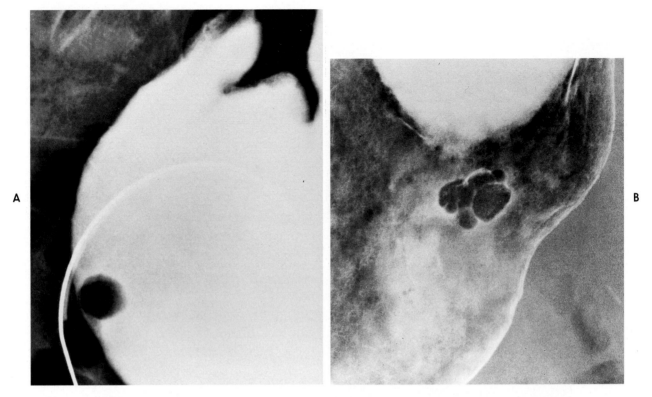

Figs. 18-10 A and **B,** Gastric adenomas in two different patients.
A from Op den Orth JO: *Radiology* 141:289, 1981; **B** from Op den Orth JO: *The standard biphasic-contrast examination of the stomach and duodenum: methods, results and radiological atlas,* The Hague, 1979, Martinus Nijhoff.

demonstrated that, in Europe as well, barium examinations may compare favorably with endoscopy in the detection of EGC. However, only at institutions where the gastric examinations are performed by skilled radiologists can such good results be expected.

DIAGNOSIS OF EARLY AND ADVANCED GASTRIC CARCINOMA
Current role of radiology

The role of radiology in the diagnosis of gastric carcinoma is to detect potentially malignant lesions. Patients with such lesions should undergo endoscopy. The most important role of gastroscopy is to obtain biopsy specimens, of which many should be taken.[45] When biopsy findings are negative despite a suspicion based on radiologic findings, endoscopy should be repeated so that more tissue specimens can be obtained. When there is radiologic evidence of linitis plastica, biopsy findings are often unreliable[46] (see Fig. 18-14). This diagnostic approach, in which endoscopy complements the barium examination, is the safest option. In the early 1980s at the author's institution, endoscopy appeared to be indicated in approximately 12% of the patients who underwent barium examinations; this figure dropped to approximately 8% in the early 1990s. Our results in the diagnosis not only of advanced but also of

early gastric carcinoma[8,12,36] encouraged us to persist in the opinion that a state-of-the-art barium examination is an excellent way to select patients for endoscopy. In a series consisting of 28 patients with EGC, the barium examination findings were negative in only one.[8] This approach permits adenocarcinoma to be diagnosed preoperatively in most instances. However, it is only the pathologist who, when determining the depth of carcinomatous infiltration in the resected specimen, can ultimately classify a carcinoma as EGC.

Macroscopic types of gastric carcinoma

The Japanese classification of EGC includes protruded, superficial (nearly flat), and excavated lesions (Figs. 18-11 to 18-13). This classification can also be applied to carcinomas that penetrate deeper than the submucosa (advanced carcinoma). The diffusely infiltrative type of carcinoma (linitis plastica) (see Fig. 18-14) does not fit comfortably into this classification, however.

Protruded type

If a radiologic examination reveals one or more protruded lesions, the possibility of a malignant or premalignant lesion should be considered. Endoscopic biopsy and endoscopic polypectomy using a diathermy snare are excellent ways to obtain tissue for histologic analysis. Yet, the multiplicity of these polypoid lesions and the fact that they are now frequently found during radiologic examinations in aged and often debilitated people precludes intervention in every case.[47,48] Gastric adenoma, the most common potentially malignant polyp, can reliably be detected radiologically. Gastric adenomas are rare, being seen in approximately 1 in 1000 barium examinations.[47] Adenomas are usually single lesions located in the distal half of the stomach with a diameter of more than 1 cm; in most instances they are sessile or pedunculated, but flat adenomas also occur. Their surface is often irregular, but it is sometimes smooth[47] (Figs. 18-10). The malignant potential appears to correlate with the size of the polyp, such that larger adenomas (particularly with a diameter of 2 cm or more) carry a greater potential for malignant change.[47,48] Fig. 18-12, A, shows a protruded type of EGC caused by malignant degeneration restricted to the mucosa of an adenoma.

Hyperplastic polyps, on the other hand, are not liable to malignant degeneration; they are rather common in elderly people, with an incidence of more than 1%.[47,48] Hyperplastic polyps can arise anywhere in the stomach, are usually multiple, and are smaller than 1 cm. Therefore, a policy of performing endoscopic polypectomy of any polypoid lesion with a diameter of 1 cm or more that does not appear to be a typical submucosal mass seems appropriate.[47,48]

Superficial type

A completely flat lesion will most certainly be missed at a barium examination, but fortunately these lesions are very rare. The flat or, according to the Japanese classification, superficial lesions in practice consist of superficial elevated, superficial depressed, and combined lesions. Barium radiography of the stomach can discern even these slight differences in height (Figs. 18-12, B and C).

Excavated lesions

All gastric ulcers should be regarded as potentially malignant lesions, even if none of the numerous more or less reliable signs of malignancy exists. Therefore, it has become the practice for virtually every patient with a radiologically detected gastric ulcer to undergo endoscopy. However, there is strong evidence that, if the radiographic appearance of a gastric ulcer is unequivocally benign, radiographic monitoring of the lesion until complete healing is achieved,[49,50] may be a good alternative to endoscopic intervention. Fig. 18-13 shows an ulcer in which the radiographic findings suggested malignancy (excavated-type EGC).

Linitis plastica

In linitis plastica, there is extensive infiltration of the tumor along the gastric wall, causing it to thicken and stiffen.

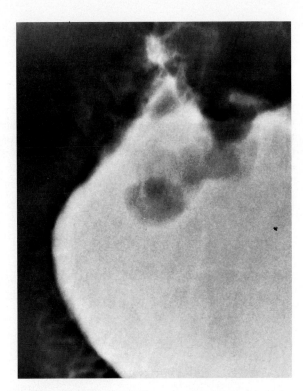

Fig. 18-11 Protruded early gastric carcinoma. Single-contrast, graded-compression study demonstrates a broad-stalked antral polyp. In the resected specimen there was malignant degeneration of a gastric adenoma restricted to the mucosa.
From Op den Orth JO: *Radiology* 141:289, 1981.

The mucosal surface of the stomach may be slightly nodular and necrotic in some areas but macroscopically intact in others. There is infiltration of the muscularis propria. Linitis plastica is usually caused by a primary gastric adenocarcinoma; gastric involvement by metastatic carcinoma of the breast may also be a source.

A barium examination is not the best modality for visualizing the diffuse thickening of the gastric wall that occurs in linitis plastica, although, at times, wall thickening may be suggested by the presence of gas in the surrounding parts of the bowel (Fig. 18-14). The narrowing of the stomach and the stiffening of the gastric wall can, however, be appreciated well. Therefore, if a part of the stomach does not distend under the influence of gravity or when palpated or if fluoroscopic study of peristaltic movements discloses stiffening of the gastric wall, linitis plastica should be suspected. Premedication with a small intravenous dose (e.g., 0.1 mg) of glucagon does not prevent fluoroscopic observation of gastric peristalsis; these movements can be observed as soon as the action of this hypotonic agent has worn off, usually within 10 minutes. Visible peristalsis, however, does not totally exclude the existence of linitis plastica.

Because endoscopic biopsy findings are often negative in

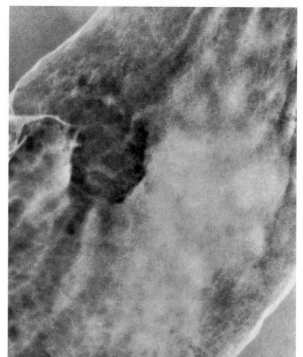

Fig. 18-12 Three cases of superficial early gastric carcinoma. **A,** A superficial elevated lesion; the resected specimen showed malignant degeneration restricted to the mucosa, or a flat adenoma. **B,** A nearly flat combined lesion caused by mucosal carcinoma. **C,** The same superficial depressed lesion as in Fig. 18-2, *B*. The resected specimen demonstrated a malignant ulcer with restriction of malignant infiltration to the mucosa and submucosa.
A from Op den Orth JO: *Radiology* 141:289, 1981; **B** from Op den Orth JO: *Radiology* 713:601, 1989.

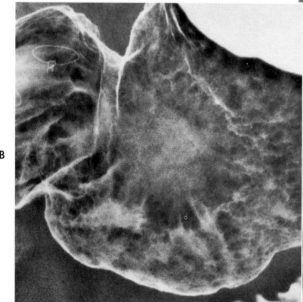

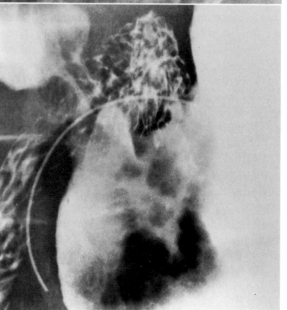

Fig. 18-13 Excavated early gastric carcinoma. The ulcer is in the posterior wall of the gastric antrum, and the gastric folds end *(dots)* fairly far from the center and are deformed. Adenocarcinoma was found in biopsy specimens. In the resected specimen, the carcinoma was shown to involve the muscularis mucosae.

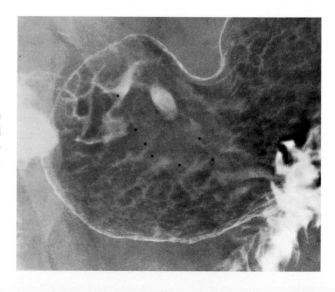

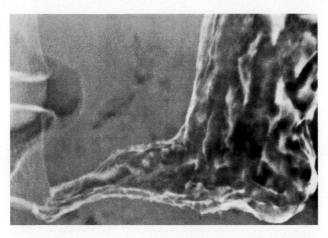

Fig. 18-14 Linitis plastica. There is narrowing of the gastric antrum, and this strongly indicates linitis plastica. No peristaltic waves were noted to pass through the antrum. Two series of endoscopic biopsies (including large-particle biopsies) revealed no signs of malignancy. In the resected specimen the linitis plastica was found to infiltrate the surrounding fatty tissue.
From Op den Orth JO: *The standard biphasic-contrast examination of the stomach and duodenum: methods, results and radiological atlas,* The Hague, 1979, Martinus Nijhoff.

cases of linitis plastica, endoscopy has significant limitations when it comes to confirming the radiologic diagnosis.[12,27,46] Cross-sectional techniques, however, are very useful for visualizing the gastric wall in suspected cases of linitis plastica (see Fig. 18-6), although computed tomography is only able to demonstrate thickening of the gastric wall, which occurs in a great number of conditions besides linitis plastica.

Transabdominal ultrasonography or endosonography not only shows whether the gastric wall is thickened, but also which layers are involved. This helps to limit the otherwise extensive differential diagnosis. If, for example, only the mucosa is thickened, linitis plastica can be excluded. Common causes of mucosal thickening are hypertrophic gastritis and mucosal hyperplasia,[40,51] and peptic ulceration is a common cause of gastric wall thickening involving the deeper wall layers. In practice, however, when a barium examination has excluded the existence of a gastric ulcer, gastric wall thickening involving the deeper layers strongly suggests a malignant cause, either the linitis plastica type of adenocarcinoma or malignant lymphoma.

EXPERIENCE IN A DUTCH GENERAL HOSPITAL

Although its incidence is slowly declining and currently more people die of colonic cancer, gastric carcinoma still represents a formidable problem in the Netherlands. In 1988 more people died of gastric cancer than as the result of road traffic accidents.[7] St. Elisabeth's of Groote Gasthuis is a 450-bed general hospital, where the cooperation between the departments of radiology, internal medicine (which includes a gastroenterology section), and pathology has always been excellent. The results of radiologic examinations

are discussed at daily conferences, and the radiology department is provided with copies of the reports of all endoscopy biopsy and resected specimen findings.

In 1977 we reported on the radiologic, endoscopic, and clinical aspects of 10 cases of EGC.[11] We had found that the symptom pattern was vague and the physical examination findings were usually negative. We therefore concluded that, when persistent vague abdominal complaints were encountered in patients over the age of 40, an optimal radiologic examination should be performed. If this raises even the slightest suspicion of malignancy, gastroscopy and multiple aimed biopsies should then be performed.

In 1979 we confirmed that our technique of barium examination (a biphasic examination with glucagon-induced hypotonia) was a reliable screening method for detecting potentially malignant lesions and for determining which patients should then undergo gastroscopy and biopsy.[12] In the 3650 patients aged 30 years and over who made up our study population, 57 patients were found to have gastric carcinoma. In 12, the resected specimen showed EGC. In all 12, the lesions had been judged to be potentially malignant at the first examination. There was one false-negative radiologic report resulting from an interpretative error; in retrospect, this carcinoma could have been clearly defined.

In 1991 Craanen et al.[8] reported on their 16-year experience at our institution with 302 patients suffering from gastric carcinoma. Twenty-eight patients together had 31 lesions (three had more than one[52]), and the resected specimens were all classified as EGC (9.3% of all patients and 19.4% of the resected specimens). The common symptoms of EGC in these patients were abdominal discomfort, epigastric pain, and pyrosis. A biphasic barium examination with glucagon-induced hypotonia as well as gastroscopy was carried out in 26 patients. Radiologic examination was done before endoscopy in 19 patients; in seven with acute bleeding, endoscopy was the initial examination. Radiologic investigation missed one lesion. In three patients, however, the initial radiologic findings either established a diagnosis of malignancy or were suspicious. On the other hand, endoscopy, performed so that biopsy could be done, needed to be done twice to prove malignancy. The pathology specimens were reexamined. The mean size of the lesions was 19.8 mm (range, 5 to 50 mm), 16 lesions were restricted to the mucosa, and 15 lesions had invaded the submucosa. Lymph node involvement was encountered in only three patients with invasion of the submucosa. The overall 5-year survival rate was 91.3% (100% for mucosal cancer and 85.7% for submucosal cancer). This study[8] once again shows that EGC reported in the Western world is the same as that reported in Japan and that the lesion can be reliably detected radiologically. The problem is that many patients with EGC are asymptomatic, and the implementation of a mass radiologic screening program of asymptomatic people is not considered feasible outside Japan.

REFERENCES

1. Parkin DM, Läärä E, Muir CS: Estimates of the worldwide frequency of sixteen major cancers in 1980, *Int J Cancer* 41:184, 1988.
2. Kurihara M, Aoki K, Tominaga S, eds: *Cancer mortality statistics in the world,* Nagoya, Japan, 1984, The University of Nagoya Press.
3. Barentsz JO et al: Radiologic examination in gastric cancer, *Acta Radiol* 27:547, 1986.
4. Waterhouse JAH: Epidemiology of gastric cancer. In Preece PE, Cuschieri A, Wellwood MA, eds: *Cancer of the stomach,* New York, 1986, Grune & Stratton.
5. Todesursachen, Reihe 4. In *Statistisches Bundesamt* (Fachserie 12), Stuttgart, 1989, Metzler-Poeschel.
6. Adloff M et al: Le cancer superficiel de l'estomac, *Ann Chir* 9:713, 1990.
7. Mortality by some causes of death. In *Vademecum of health statistics of the Netherlands 1991,* The Hague, 1991, CBS.
8. Craanen ME et al: Early gastric cancer: a clinicopathologic study, *J Clin Gastroenterol* 13:274, 1991.
9. Allum WH et al: Gastric cancer: a 25-year review, *Br J Surg* 76:535, 1989.
10. Shirakabe H, Maruyama M: Definition and classification of early gastric cancer. In Shirakabe H et al: *Atlas of x-ray diagnosis of early gastric cancer,* Tokyo, 1982, Igaku-Shoin.
11. Dekker W, Op den Orth JO: Early gastric cancer, *Radiol Clin* 46:115, 1977.
12. Op den Orth JO: *The standard biphasic-contrast examination of the stomach and duodenum,* The Hague, 1979, Martinus Nijhoff.
13. Paulino F, Roselli A: Early gastric cancer: report of twenty-five cases, *Surgery* 85:171, 1979.
14. Rheault MJ et al: Early gastric cancer at the Hôtel-Diue de Montréal: a 30-year review, *Can J Surg* 24:606, 1981.
15. Op den Orth JO: Frühkarzinom des Magens. In Czembirek H, Pokieser H, Wittich G, eds: *Doppelkontrasttechnik in der gastrointestinalen Radiologie,* Vienna, 1982, Fakultas.
16. Montesi A et al: Radiologic diagnosis of early gastric cancer by routine double-contrast examination, *Gastrointest Radiol* 7:205, 1982.
17. Palmer Gold R et al: Early gastric cancer: radiographic experience, *Radiology* 152;283, 1984.
18. Carter KJ, Schaffer A, Ritchie WP: Early gastric cancer, *Ann Surg* 199:604, 1984.
19. White RM et al: Early gastric cancer, *Radiology* 155:25, 1985.
20. Miller G, Gloor F: Das Magenfrühkarzinom, *Schweiz Med Wochenschr* 116:1366, 1986.
21. Biasco et al: Early gastric cancer in Italy, *Dig Dis Sci* 32:113, 1987.
22. Ballantyne KC et al: Accuracy of identification of early gastric cancer, *Br J Surg* 74:618, 1987.
23. Longo WE et al: Detection of early gastric cancer in an aggressive endoscopy unit, *Am Surg* 55:100, 1989.
24. Treichel J: *Doppelkontrastuntersuchung des Magens,* Stuttgart 1990, Georg Thieme.
25. Huguier M et al: Le cancer superficiel de l'estomac. Ne le manquez pas! *Ann Chir* 44:435, 1990.
26. Murata I, Clot JP, Sakabe T: Dépistage précoce du cancer de l'estomac au Japon, *J Chir* (Paris) 124:35, 1987.
27. Op den Orth JO: Use of barium in evaluation of disorders of the upper gastrointestinal tract: current status, *Radiology* 713:601, 1989.
28. Op den Orth JO, Ploem S: The standard biphasic-contrast gastric series, *Radiology* 122:530, 1977.
29. de Lange EE, Schaffer HA: Barium suspension formulation for use with the bubbly barium method, *Radiology* 154:825, 1985.
30. Montagne JP, Moss AA, Margulis AR: Double-blind study of single and double contrast upper gastrointestinal examination using endoscopy as a control, *AJR* 130:1041, 1978.
31. Trenkner SW, Laufer I: Double-contrast examination: I. Esophagus, stomach, and duodenum, *Clin Gastroenterol* 13:41, 1984.
32. Moss AA, Margulis AR: Overview. In Margulis AR, Burhenne HJ, eds: *Alimentary tract radiology,* ed 4, St Louis 1989, Mosby–Year Book.
33. Levine MS et al: Double-contrast upper gastrointestinal examination: technique and interpretation, *Radiology* 168:593, 1988.
34. Chandie Shaw MP et al: Peptic ulceration and gastric carcinoma: diagnosis with biphasic radiography compared with fiberoptic endoscopy, *Radiology* 163:39, 1987.
35. Chandie Shaw MP: Biphasic radiologic examination of the stomach and the duodenum compared with fiberoptic endoscopy, Leiden, 1987, Thesis, University of Leiden.
36. Dekker W, Op den Orth JO: Biphasic radiologic examination and endoscopy of the upper gastrointestinal tract: a comparative study, *J Clin Gastroenterol* 10:461, 1988.
37. Miyamoto Y, Tsujimoto F, Shimpei T: Ultrasonographic diagnosis of submucosal tumors of the stomach: the "bridging layers" sign, *J Clin Ultrasound* 16:251, 1988.
38. Worlicek H, Dunz D, Engelhard K: Ultrasonic examination of the wall of the fluid-filled stomach, *J Clin Ultrasound* 17:514, 1989.
39. Miyamoto Y et al: Ultrasonographic findings in gastric cancer: in vitro and in vivo studies, *J Clin Ultrasound* 17:309, 1989.
40. Sijbrandy LS, Op den Orth JO: Transabdominal ultrasound of the stomach: a pictorial essay, *Eur J Radiol* 13:81, 1991.
41. Ohashi S, Nakazawa S, Yoshino J: Endoscopic ultrasonography in the assessment of invasive gastric cancer, *Scand J Gastroenterol* 24:1039, 1989.
42. Smithuis RHM, Op den Orth JO: Gastric fluid detected by sonography in fasting patients: relation to duodenal ulcer disease and gastric-outlet obstruction, *AJR* 153:731, 1989.
43. Maruyama M: Comparison of radiology and endoscopy in the diagnosis of gastric cancer. In Preece PE, Cuschieri A, Wellwood JM, eds: *Cancer of the stomach,* New York, 1986, Grune & Stratton.
44. Shirakabe H, Maruyama M: Neoplastic diseases of the stomach. In Margulis AR, Burhenne HJ, eds: *Alimentary tract radiology,* ed 4. St Louis, 1989, Mosby–Year Book.
45. Dekker W, Tytgat GN: Diagnostic accuracy of fiberendoscopy in the detection of upper intestinal malignancy, a follow-up analysis, *Gastroenterology* 73:710, 1977.
46. Levine MS et al: Scirrhous carcinoma of the stomach: radiologic and endoscopic diagnosis, *Radiology* 175:151, 1990.
47. Op den Orth JO, Dekker W: Gastric adenomas, *Radiology* 141:289, 1981.
48. Dekker W, Op den Orth JO: Polyps of the stomach and duodenum: significance and management, *Dig Dis* (in print).
49. Thompson G, Stevenson GW, Somers S: Benign gastric ulcer: a reliable radiologic diagnosis? *AJR* 141:331, 1983.
50. Levine MS et al: Benign gastric ulcers: diagnosis and follow-up with double-contrast radiography, *Radiology* 164:9, 1987.
51. Fujishima et al: Scirrhous carcinoma of the stomach versus hypertrophic gastritis: findings at endoscopic US, *Radiology* 181:197, 1991.
52. Brandt D et al: Synchronous early gastric cancer, *Radiology* 173:649, 1989.

19 Diagnosis of Gastric Cancer in Japan

MASAKAZU MARUYAMA
TSUTOMU HAMADA

The mortality rate from gastric cancer has recently begun to decrease in Japan. In 1991, however, Hisamichi et al.[1] reported that gastric cancer was still the leading cause of death in both sexes. In 1988 the mortality rate of stomach cancer was 24.6% in males and 21.6% in females. Consequently, gastric cancer is still an important target for cancer control in Japan. In 1987 Ohta et al.[2] reported that cancer in its early stages accounted for one third of all surgically resected cases during the 33-year period from 1946 to 1978. More recently, however, Nakajima, from the same institution, discovered early cancer constituted nearly half of all the resected cases in the 5-year period from 1985 to 1989 (Fig. 19-1). Liorens et al.[3] encountered 86 cases of early cancer out of 1290 cases of gastric cancer that were diagnosed in the 11 years since 1980. In their series, early cancer accounted for only 6.7% of the total number of cases of gastric cancer.

JAPANESE APPROACH TO THE RADIOGRAPHIC EXAMINATION OF THE STOMACH
Basic approach

In the basic approach to radiographic examination, it is assumed that any lesion that is visible macroscopically can be detected radiographically. The exact reproduction of macroscopic features is therefore the primary goal of the radiographic investigation.[4]

The initial, or routine, radiographic examination consists of a combination of the four examination methods, mucosal relief, a film of the barium-filled stomach, a double-contrast study, and a compression study, although the double-contrast study forms the backbone of the examination. Single-contrast examination by itself is never performed in Japan. Double-contrast radiography is only *one* of the examination methods, however, and overreliance on this method must be avoided. It may be that the successful

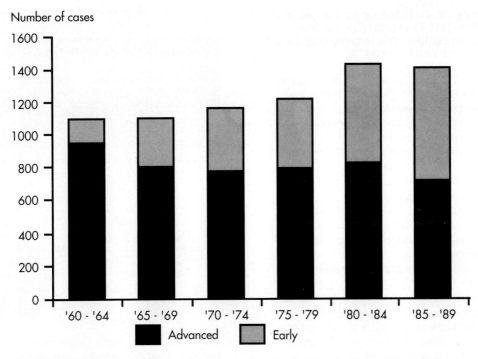

Fig. 19-1 The increase in surgical operations for early gastric cancer from 1960 to 1990 at the Cancer Institute Hospital.
Courtesy of T. Nakajima.

experience with double-contrast studies witnessed in the 1960s and 1970s fostered the myth that double-contrast radiography is omnipotent. However, awareness of its limitations has actually led to further major improvements in the initial radiographic examination. A poor double-contrast examination reveals much less information than do the other examination methods (Fig. 19-2), and all four methods are employed in the initial radiographic examination, with the three other methods playing a vital supplementary role to the double-contrast examination. The initial radiographic examination is started using the sequence of exposures listed in the box below, although there can be some variations in the positioning of the patient and the number of films obtained.

Technical considerations in the initial (routine) study

To perform double-contrast radiography of the stomach, the principal requirements are an adequate volume of barium and gas and frequent repositioning of the patient. At least 200 ml of barium is needed, except in some patients with stomach deformities. Less than 200 ml of barium does not produce a good-quality double-contrast image; a smaller volume cannot wash the entire mucosal surface. Consequently the influence of mucus and gastric juice persists to impair coating.

It used to be generally accepted that the ideal amount of gas was that which made it possible to obtain a double-

contrast image of the middle portion of the body of the stomach in the supine frontal position. This volume of gas may give the impression that the stomach is overdistended. More recently, however, the gaseous distention of the stomach has been obtained in two steps, even for the initial radiographic examination. In the first step the stomach is distended with a small volume of gas using 2 g of effervescent granules. This produces an optimal double-contrast image extending from the gastric antrum to the incisura region (Fig. 19-3, *A*). It is not necessary to use effervescent granules when the volume of gas already in the gastric fornix, including the air swallowed during the intake of barium, allows optimal distention of the gastric antrum and incisura region. This is not infrequently encountered.

Overdistention of this area may obscure a subtle muco-

```
□  SEQUENCE OF RADIOGRAPHIC EXPOSURES
       IN THE INITIAL EXAMINATION OF THE
     STOMACH, INCLUDING THE ESOPHAGUS AND
            THE DUODENUM  □
```

1. Mucosal relief image in the prone position
2. Esophagus in the upright left anterior oblique position (double-contrast view, if possible)
3. Esophagus in the upright right anterior oblique position (double-contrast view, if possible)
4. Barium-filled film in the upright, frontal position (Use 2 g of effervescent granules)
5. Double-contrast image in the supine frontal or left anterior oblique position (Use additional 2 to 3 g of effervescent granules)
6. Double-contrast image in the supine frontal position
7. Double-contrast image in the supine right anterior oblique position
8. Double-contrast image in the supine left anterior oblique position
9. Double-contrast image in the semiupright, right decubitus, or steep left anterior oblique position
10. Barium-filled image in the upright frontal position
11. Double-contrast image in the upright right anterior oblique position (with barium passing through the cardia)
12. Compression images

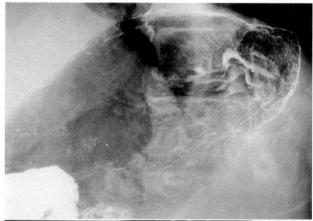

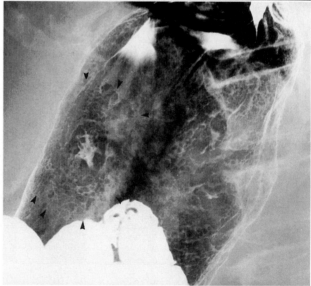

Fig. 19-2 Advanced gastric carcinoma with central ulceration **(B)**, localized superficial elevation, and abnormal mucosa extending for some distance from the ulcer. Note that a film taken earlier in the examination **(A)**, before the mucosa has been well coated, shows no evidence of the tumor.
Courtesy of Dr. Y. Kaku.

sal abnormality, such as a small type IIc lesion (Fig. 19-3, B) and erosions. Even a large advanced cancer may be missed because of the vertical dislocation of the gastric antrum caused by excessive gaseous distention.

In the second step, an additional 2 to 3 g of effervescent granules is given, and double-contrast images of the lower gastric body to the fornix are obtained. Lesions in this area, especially the upper gastric body and cardia, are frequently missed if gaseous distention is inadequate.

The patient's position should be changed frequently to wash the mucosal surface with a rapid flow of barium. By shifting the contrast medium from the fundus to the antrum, adherent mucus is washed away and the gastric juice is mixed with the barium, optimizing barium coating of the mucosal surface.

Difference in image quality of the initial and detailed studies

Western radiologists may question whether there is any real need for a detailed radiographic examination, done after the diagnosis of cancer is already established by endoscopy and biopsy. However, the difference in the image quality between the initial and detailed radiographic examination can be considerable. Frequently, the extent of a depressed-type early cancer is poorly defined in the initial radiographic examination (Fig. 19-4). In particular, the precise distance from its proximal border to the esophagogas-

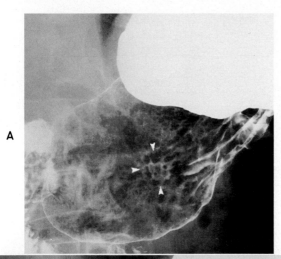

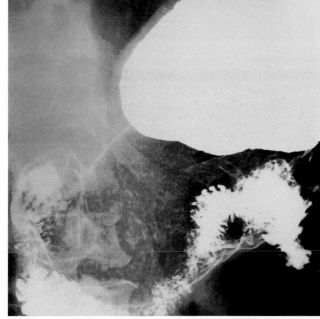

Fig. 19-3 A modest amount of gas produces optimal distention that reveals the features of this type IIc early carcinoma **(A).** More gas, given for proper display of the gastric body, overdistends the antrum and renders the carcinoma almost invisible **(B).**

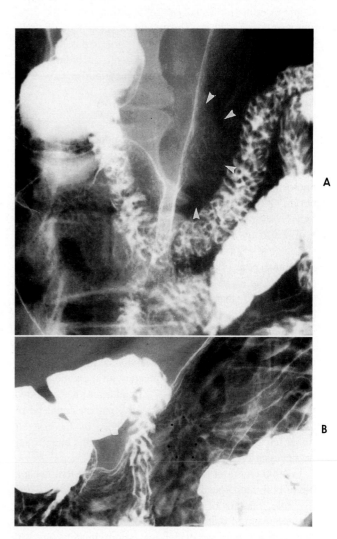

Fig. 19-4 A, Film from an initial radiographic examination in which the lesion is barely perceptible *(arrowheads).* During the detailed examination **(B),** gastric juice has been removed, and efforts have been made to optimize both the degree of distention and the barium coating; thus details of the small superficial tumor with central depression are shown well en face *(dots).*

tric junction should be made clear preoperatively. Moreover, continuing research is now focused on reducing the difference in image quality between the two examinations. It seems that the presence of gastric juice is the decisive factor that interferes with visualization of subtle mucosal abnormalities (see Fig. 19-2, *A*). For this reason, removal of the gastric juice is the minimal requirement of the detailed radiographic examination.

DIAGNOSIS OF GASTRIC CANCER
General considerations

A routine initial diagnostic procedure in Japan may consist of either a radiographic or endoscopic examination, except when a mass is palpable in the abdomen. In this event, computed tomography (CT) ultrasound, or magnetic resonance imaging (MRI) may be the first choice. The combined information from both the radiographic and endoscopic examination usually permits estimation of the depth of invasion of cancer. The recent development of endoscopic ultrasound (EUS) has now made it possible to assess the architecture of the gastric wall, including a cancerous lesion, and its relationship to neighboring structures.

Application of computed radiography to the double-contrast examination

Recent advances in electronic and computer technologies have led to new diagnostic applications. There are two methods of image processing using computers. One uses photostimulable phosphers as the memory material for temporarily storing the radiographic image[5] and is called *computed radiography* (CR). The other method, which directly acquires image data by digitizing video signals from an image intensifier, is called *digital radiography* (DR).[6]

Yamada et al.[7] have reported that a new type of CR demonstrates the areae gastricae pattern with surprising precision, beyond that possible with conventional double-contrast radiography, and that an easy-to-diagnose image could be obtained by processing the digitized image with a computer (see Fig. 19-14, *B*). Furthermore, early gastric cancer in the anterior wall of the stomach was clearly visualized on a double-contrast image with the patient in the supine position (see Fig. 19-14). In addition, it was shown that the x-ray dosage received by the patient could be reduced to less than 10% of that produced by the conventional screen-film system without disturbing the image quality necessary for diagnosis.[7,8]

In 1990 Ogura et al.[9] stated that the DR system is capable of both high-speed image data acquisition and real-time dynamic imaging of the gastrointestinal (GI) tract. They also emphasized that the incident exposure for the DR system with a 9-inch intensifier was approximately one fifth that for the screen-film system which was controlled by the automatic exposure control (AEC).

It was expected that CR and DR would be frequently used in double-contrast radiographic examinations of the gastro-intestinal tract (Fig. 19-5) together with the image-processing system. However, these techniques have not proved as popular as was anticipated due to their cost. In addition, further improvements in the data storage and data archiving and retrieving capabilities are needed before these methods can become an acceptable part of conventional GI radiology.

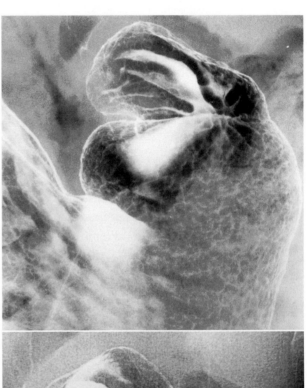

A

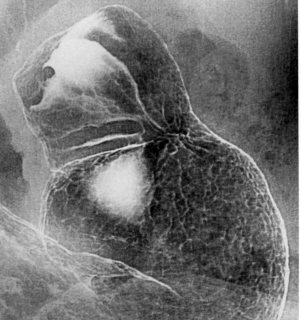

B

Fig. 19-5 Two prone double-contrast films of the gastric antrum obtained by film/screen (**A**) and enhanced digital (**B**) techniques. Note the increased perceptibility of the abnormal areae gastricae in the ill-defined type IIc carcinoma, which extends proximally from an area of scarring.

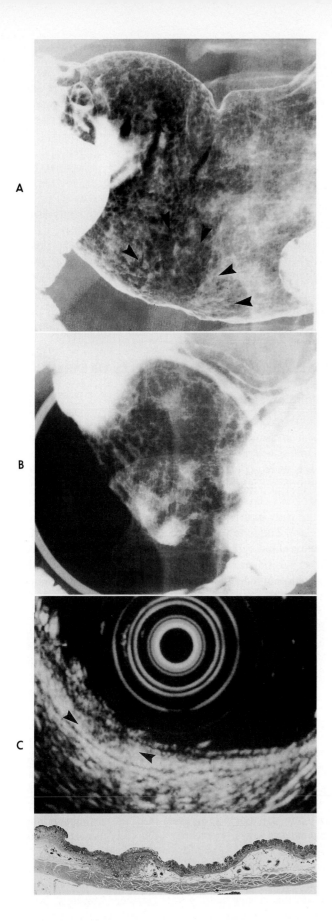

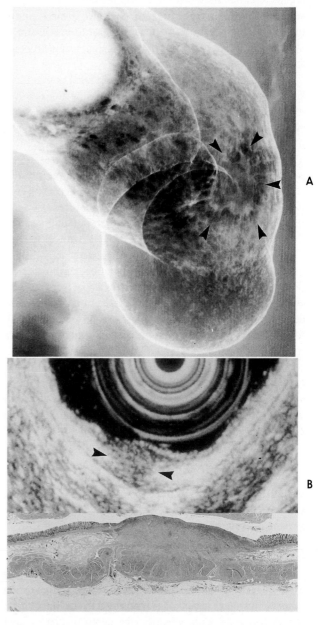

Fig. 19-6 Role of endoscopic ultrasound. The double-contrast film (**A**) shows an abnormal areae gastricae pattern and some stiffness and lack of distensibility of a segment of the greater curve *(arrowheads),* but does not indicate the margins of a lesion. The compression film (**B**) reveals more clearly an area of superficially depressed mucosa (in which barium is trapped), confirming the existence of a lesion. The endoscopic ultrasound film (**C,** with histology below) shows that the cancer has extended from the epithelium perhaps two thirds of the way through the white submucosa but has not reached the black layer of the muscularis propria.
Courtesy of N. Takemoto.

Fig. 19-7 The radiograph (**A**) shows a superficial depressed carcinoma with slightly raised nodular margins (type IIc) *(arrowheads).* **B,** The ultrasound image (and histology) show that the tumor has spread to the margin of, but has not invaded, the muscularis propria.
Courtesy of N. Takemoto.

Role of endoscopic ultrasonography

The advent of EUS has allowed visualization of the internal architecture of gastric lesions as well as the deeper layers of the gastric wall that cannot be seen by radiographic or endoscopic means.

Based on the ultrasonographic study of the normal portions of a resected stomach, the gastric wall has five layers[10] (see Chapter 15).

The recognition of abnormalities in each layer permits the depth of cancer invasion to be estimated, and helps in the differential diagnosis between benign and malignant submucosal tumors. This examination also provides information on the condition of the extragastric space and on the relationship of the stomach to the neighboring structures and organs.

In cases of early cancer without associated peptic ulcer, EUS can be a reliable method for assessing the depth of malignant invasion (Figs. 19-6 and 19-7). However, the results have not been as encouraging in the presence of peptic ulceration.

Peptic ulceration exists in 36.3% of the cases of depressed cancers, including early and advanced ones, which are smaller than 3 cm,[11] and the rate of peptic ulceration complicating cases of depressed cancers rapidly increases as the tumor enlarges. In 1990 Chonan et al.[12] reported that, in the depressed type of early cancer associated with ulceration, EUS correctly assessed the invasive depth in only 50% of the cases with submucosal involvement because of the difficulty in distinguishing cancerous invasion from fibrosis.

A grading system has been devised for assessing the depth of invasion, based on the disruption of the fourth and fifth layers. For a cancer to be deemed intramucosal, the fourth layer must be intact, with only a small wedge-shaped echo in the third layer. When the third layer becomes irregular, submucosal involvement may be suspected.[13]

Chonan et al.[14] reported that the depth of invasion was correctly diagnosed in 55.6% of the tumors involving the propria muscle, in 50% of the those involving the subserosa, in 83.3% of those in which the serosa was exposed, and in 66.7% of those that had invaded neighboring structures. These results were substantiated in a review conducted by a panel of 13 experts.[15] There is no doubt that EUS can assess the depth of cancer invasion, but more experience is required before its clinical utility is known.

Role of computed tomography

On CT examinations, gastric cancer is visualized either as a thickening of the gastric wall or as tumor formation.[16] However, it cannot demonstrate the architecture of the gastric wall. Consequently, the depth of cancer invasion when limited to the gastric wall cannot be ascertained. CT can show whether the serosa is severely involved or whether contiguous structures are involved. Komaki and Toyoshima,[16] however, claim that the diagnostic accuracy of CT in evaluating tumor invasion of adjacent structures is not as high as that reported.

In the general guidelines that are applied in gastric cancer studies that make use of surgical and pathologic findings,[17] serosal invasion based on gross findings is classified into four types:

S0 No serosal invasion
S1 Suspected serosal invasion
S2 Definite serosal invasion
S3 Invasion to contiguous structures

Ohkuma et al.[18] reported that CT could correctly identify the extent of serosal involvement in 80% of the cases of gastric cancer, peritoneal dissemination in only 20%, liver metastasis in 83%, and lymph node metastasis in 59%. On CT images a lymph node exceeding 1 cm in diameter is judged metastatic. However, sometimes a metastatic node measures less than 1 cm,[19] and an enlarged lymph node is not always metastatic, although it may be inflammatory.

DEFINITION AND CLASSIFICATION OF EARLY GASTRIC CANCER
Definition and classification

Early gastric cancer has been defined as "carcinoma in which invasion is limited to the mucosa and submucosa, regardless of lymph nodes and distant metastases."

The macroscopic classification of early gastric cancer was proposed at the time this definition was offered because Bormann's classification of gastric cancer was not applicable to early gastric cancer limited to the mucosa and submucosa. The following classification can be applied in the context of radiographic and endoscopic diagnoses, based on the supposition that exact correspondence between the macroscopic and radiographic findings is possible if an optimal radiographic examination is performed (Fig. 19-8).

I. Polypoid (>0.5 cm in height)
II. Superficial
   A. Elevated (<0.5 cm in height)
   B. Flat—minimal or no alteration in the height of the mucosa
   C. Depressed—superficial erosion, usually not extending beyond the muscularis mucosae
III. Excavated—prominent depression, usually caused by ulceration

An early polypoid cancer is classified as type I (see Fig. 19-12) if it protrudes into the gastric lumen by more than 0.5 cm and as type IIa (see Figs. 19-13, 19-14, *B*, 19-15, and 19-44) if it protrudes by less than 0.5 cm. If the elevation or depression of a lesion from the surrounding normal mucosa is nearly unrecognizable, it is classified as type IIb. This type was added in the anticipation that it might represent a transient phase in the development of gastric cancer, although, at the time the classification was proposed, this change had not been clarified. Currently, however, type IIb is considered in a broader sense than that contained in the original definition. In both the radiographic and endoscopic diagnosis, type IIb now stands for a visible and diagnosable lesion whose appearance of protrusion or

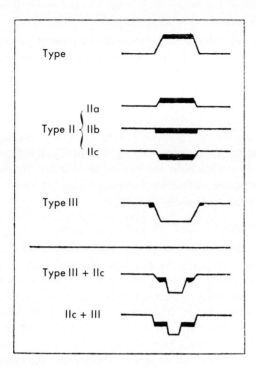

Fig. 19-8 Gross classification of early gastric cancer.
From Japan Gastroenterological Endoscopy Society: *I-to-Cho* 6:1,1971.

depression differs only slightly from that of the adjacent mucosa, and this change is called a *type IIb–like lesion*[20] (see Fig. 19-31). A lesion with a slightly depressed surface is designated as type IIc (see Figs. 19-3, *A*, 19-4, *B*, 19-5, 19-6, 19-22 to 19-24, 19-27 to 19-29, 19-31, 19-45, 19-48, and 19-49). A type III lesion has a prominent excavation that most likely, although not always, indicates an ulcer (see Figs. 19-25, *A*, and 19-26). In the most common presentation, two or more types coexist. The type is rendered such that the predominant pattern precedes the other, for example, type IIc + III (see Fig. 19-25, *B*) or type I + IIa.

In a series of 1000 cases of solitary early gastric cancer, Ohta et al.[2] observed the ratio of the elevated to the depressed type to be one to four.

RADIOGRAPHIC DIAGNOSIS OF EARLY GASTRIC CANCER AND CORRELATION WITH ENDOSCOPY

In Japan the overreliance on endoscopy and biopsy for establishing the final diagnosis has made it difficult to conduct a study that compares the relative merits of the two examinations in the diagnosis of gastric cancer. Recently there has been a trend to conduct an endoscopic investigation using a forward-viewing endoscope as the initial examination for the upper gastrointestinal tract, and to perform a radiographic examination to define further the nature and involvement of tumor so that the surgical removal of a gastric cancer can be planned.

In their early report, Shirakabe et al.[21] noted that the ini-

tial routine radiographic examination detected 86% of all cases of gastric cancer, and the first endoscopic examination, carried out after this, detected another 9%. In the third (1983) edition of this book, the authors reported that the routine radiographic examination missed 10.4% (72/695) of the cases of a single early cancer and 35.1% (39/111) of those of multiple lesions, which were subsequently detected by endoscopic studies or the examination of resected specimens. We found that 17 single lesions in the patients in this study escaped detection in both radiographic and endoscopic investigations.

In 1986 Maruyama[22] reported on the efficiency of radiology and endoscopy in the diagnosis of gastric cancer, based on computer processing of the diagnostic data, and showed that actual malignancy was confirmed in only 36.2% of all the cases deemed early cancer based on the findings from the initial radiographic examination using remote-controlled x-ray television apparatus. Furthermore, the histologic examination after surgery disclosed that only 64.3% of all the cancers considered early based on radiographic findings were actually so. Maruyama also reported that 1.5% of the cases judged normal according to the initial radiographic findings were ultimately confirmed to be cancer based on the subsequent endoscopic findings, using endoscopy as the denominator. In other words, 0.2% (11/5630) of all the cases are misdiagnosed as normal on initial radiographic studies.

In Maruyama's series the sensitivity of the initial radiographic examination was 97.1%, its specificity was 32.3%, and its accuracy was 46.2%. There was only a minor difference in the sensitivity and specificity between radiology and endoscopy in the diagnosis of gastric cancer, including early and advanced forms. This indicates that there are a large number of false positives due to the difference in image quality between the initial and second detailed examination (see Figs. 19-2 and 19-4).

It is not uncommon that the image quality of the initial radiographic examination is inadequate to allow a firm diagnosis of early cancer (see Fig. 19-4, *A*). Controlling the volume of air plays a decisive role in the delineation of subtle mucosal abnormalities, such as those seen in the IIc type of early cancer, not only in the second detailed examination, but also in the initial radiographic examination. In 1988 Hamada et al.[23] reported that only 73.6% of all the cases of early gastric cancer (72.2% of the elevated type and 74.1% of the depressed type) could be detected in the initial radiographic examination, even when cases of vague abnormalities were included.

In 1987 Takasu[24] reported that panendoscopy missed 10.1% of the early cancers and 9.3% of the advanced cancers over an 11-year-period starting in 1976. In 1989 Otsuji et al.,[25] based on their 9-year experience with panendoscopy performed in a fixed asymptomatic group aged 50 years and over, reported that it failed to detect gastric cancer in 7.2%. In a recent report Yao et al.[26] stated that the frequency with which an initial radiographic examination missed a gastric cancer was nearly equivalent to that of endoscopy, when performed for the same purposes. They stressed the importance of achieving a high-quality radiographic examination to optimize the detection rate. In 1990 Nishizawa et al.[27] reported on a study conducted over the course of 10 years and consisting of 306 cases of advanced cancers in which the radiologic examinations were done before the endoscopic studies in the initial evaluation of the patients. They found that seven cases (2%) were missed by radiology and two cases (0.6%) were missed by endoscopy. Based on this experience, they concluded that radiology is apt to overlook advanced cancers in the upper part and anterior wall of the stomach and those simulating type IIc early cancer, and that endoscopy is inclined to overlook advanced cancers of the linitis plastica type. The only endoscopic factor that may improve the rate of diagnosis of early gastric cancer is training endoscopists in improved biopsy techniques.

DIAGNOSIS OF EARLY POLYPOID CANCER
General considerations

The radiographic diagnosis of early polypoid cancer is based on a detailed analysis of the radiographic findings.[28] This analysis starts with identifying the size, form, and surface pattern of the polypoid lesion. These lesions typically range from 1 to 4 cm in their largest diameter. Next, the height of a polypoid lesion on a compression or double-contrast image is estimated, and this can roughly distinguish between type I and IIa lesions when a polypoid lesion is judged malignant. Of most importance to the differentiation between benign and early polypoid cancer versus advanced cancer is the surface pattern of the lesion. The granular or lobular appearance, although irregular and enlarged, is similar to that of the surrounding mucosa (Fig. 19-9). In most cases of early polypoid cancer, which is limited to the submucosal layer, the surface pattern resembles the surrounding areae gastricae. This represents the most reliable radiographic sign for establishing the diagnosis of early cancer in a polypoid lesion.

As the cancerous infiltration extends beyond the submucosal layer, this similarity in the surface pattern is usually replaced by erosion or ulceration. In contrast, even a large early polypoid cancer resembles the surrounding mucosa (see Fig. 19-16).

Gross appearance of polypoid lesions

The gross appearance of the different types of gastric polypoid lesions is basically defined as pedunculated, subpedunculated, or sessile. The sessile lesion is further divided into two subtypes: one with constriction at the base and the other with gradual sloping. The base is constricted in most type IIa cancers, whereas benign epithelial and submucosal lesions show a gradual sloping. The gross classification of gastric polyps suggested by Yamada and Fukutomi[29] (Fig. 19-10) has been widely used because it is simple and approximately defines the form of polypoid lesions in both endoscopic and radiographic terms.

Adenoma

An adenoma should be distinguished both radiographically and clinically from a type IIa carcinoma. Various names have been given to this lesion because of its histologic appearance, which differs from that of hyperplasia in the gastric glands. The names consist of *adenomatous poli*,[30,31] *adenoma*,[32] *IIa-subtype*,[33] *Nakamura's type III*,[34] and *atypical epithelium*.[35] Currently the term *adenoma* is used most frequently in Japan. According to the histologic classification, it is a "tubular adenoma of small intestinal type."[36]

Adenomas occur most often in patients older than 50.[36] The gross appearance of an adenoma is a flat mucosal elevation or polypoid lesion. In most cases it does not exceed 2 cm, and approximately 50% of these lesions measure 1 cm. The gastric antrum is the most common site of an adenoma; it is rarely seen in the upper portion of the stomach.

Long-term follow-up studies have disclosed that the site of an adenoma remains the same for several years, although exceptions are seen.[32,36] Many authors have stated that adenomas develop slowly over a long time. Malignant transformation is estimated to not exceed 0.4%.[37] However, of clinical importance is the fact that a very well-differentiated adenocarcinoma cannot be distinguished histologically from

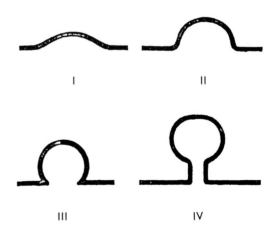

Fig. 19-10 Classification of polypoid lesions of the stomach. From Yamada T: *I-to-Cho* 1:145, 1966.

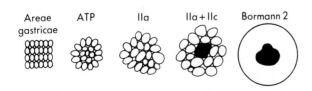

Fig. 19-9 Surface pattern of polypoid lesions of the stomach.

an adenoma.[38] In other words, a certain number of cases of potential carcinoma are included among those cases of lesions that are currently diagnosed as adenoma according to biopsy findings. Endoscopic resection is the preferred method for the diagnosis and treatment of these lesions.

Yamada[39] stated that the radiographic surface pattern of an adenoma is more like that of the surrounding areae gastricae than that of a type IIa cancer (Fig. 19-11).

Types I and IIa

Early polypoid cancer (types I and IIa) is most frequently seen in the elderly population, usually in those 60 to 70 years old, and constitutes approximately 25.4%[40] of all the cases of gastric carcinomas that occur in Japan. Type I is less common than type IIa, and is usually sessile with an irregular surface pattern that simulates the areae gastricae (Fig. 19-12). The type I tumor is larger than 2 cm in most cases and is rarely pedunculated.

Most pedunculated lesions are benign hyperplastic polyps with a surface pattern that is nearly always smooth, unlike the granular surface and lobulation typical of early polypoid cancers, or the areae gastricae pattern characteristic of adenomas. Subpedunculated lesions are primarily benign hyperplastic polyps, although some can be malignant.[28] Currently, endoscopic polypectomy appears to be the treatment of choice for pedunculated lesions.

Type IIa lesions have a flat mucosal elevation not higher than 0.5 cm and are constricted at their base. They usually exceed 2 cm in diameter and the surface pattern exhibits a somewhat irregular granularity (Figs. 19-13 to 19-15), compared with that of an adenoma (see Fig. 19-11). A gradual sloping lesion is usually not malignant but represents an atypical submucosal tumor.

In the radiographic examination of type I and IIa tumors the compression method is best suited for the detection and delineation of the lesion. Double-contrast radiography is indispensable for comparing the lesion's surface pattern to that of the surrounding areae gastricae.

Types IIa + IIc and IIc + IIa

Macroscopically a type IIa + IIc lesion usually possesses a flat mucosal elevation with a recognizable central depression. Its diameter ranges from 1 to 3 cm but is sometimes larger. The central depression is usually irregular (Fig. 19-16). The size and depth of the central depression are closely related to the depth of cancer invasion, in that, the larger and deeper the depression, the deeper the invasion. Accordingly, there is a risk that invasion may actually be deeper than the submucosal layer in a polypoid lesion possessing a substantial central depression, and the likelihood of lymph node and liver metastases in this form is then high. The depression in a polypoid lesion is not always in its center. A diagnosis of type IIc + IIa cancer is made when the type IIc portion predominates (Fig. 19-17, *B*).

On radiographic examinations, type IIa + IIc lesions are best delineated using the compression method, especially the exact form of the central depression (see Figs. 19-16, *C* and 19-17, *B*). The existence of IIa + IIc–type early cancer is suggested when the surface pattern of the raised mucosa is similar to that of the areae gastricae (see Figs. 19-16 and 19-17).

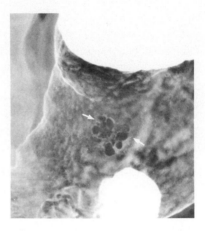

Fig. 19-11 Double-contrast radiograph of an adenoma. Note that, in this case, the areae gastricae–like surface of the lesion shows great variation in size and shape, more typical of a type IIa lesion, although this was an adenoma. However, note that much greater irregularity of the type IIa lesions in Figs. 19-13 to 19-15.

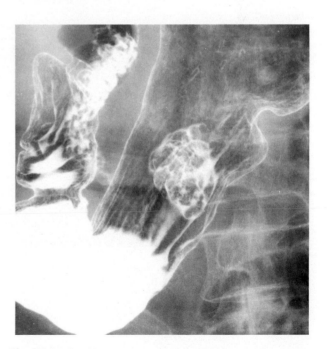

Fig. 19-12 Double-contrast radiograph of type I early cancer, which is limited to the mucosa.

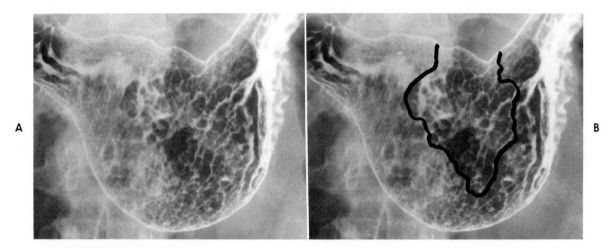

Fig. 19-13 A, Double-contrast radiograph of a type IIa early mucosal cancer. **B,** The extent of the tumor.

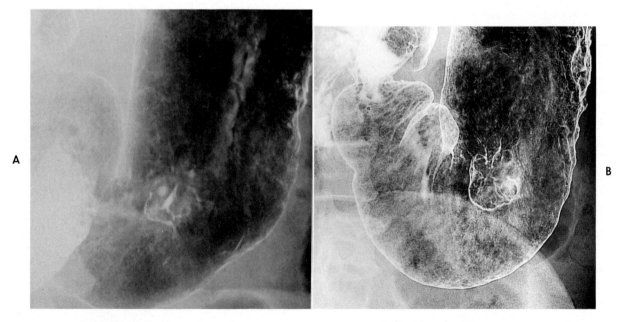

Fig. 19-14 A, Supine double-contrast conventional film showing an anterior wall type IIa submucosal cancer. **B,** The computed radiograph shows the lesion much more clearly.
Courtesy of Dr. T. Yamada.

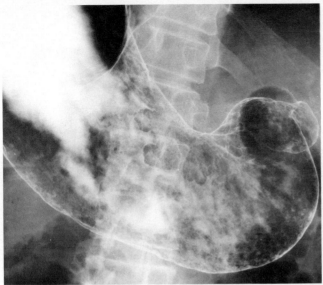

Fig. 19-15 Prone double-contrast radiograph showing superficial spreading carcinoma type IIa of the anterior wall. The full extent of the lesion is readily overlooked, as its margins are some distance from the most obvious nodular lesions nearer the center
Courtesy Dr. T. Hamada.

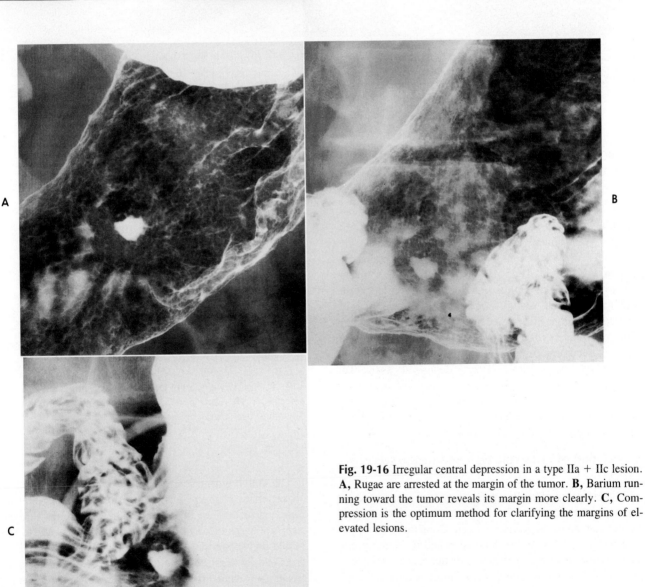

Fig. 19-16 Irregular central depression in a type IIa + IIc lesion. **A,** Rugae are arrested at the margin of the tumor. **B,** Barium running toward the tumor reveals its margin more clearly. **C,** Compression is the optimum method for clarifying the margins of elevated lesions.

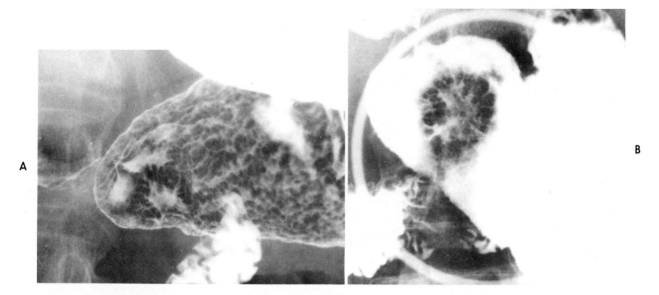

Fig. 19-17 Type IIc + IIa tumor. The margins and central depression are a subtle finding on a double-contrast image **(A)**, but much more distinct on a compression image **(B)**.
From Hamada T et al: In Maruyama M, Kimura K: *Review of clinical research in gastroenterology,* Tokyo, 1988, Igaku Shoin.

RADIOGRAPHIC DIAGNOSIS OF EARLY DEPRESSED CANCER
General considerations

The invasion pattern in the early depressed form of cancer is regarded as two dimensional and in advanced cancer, as three dimensional.[41] The diagnosis of early depressed cancer is based on the nature of the depression and its converging folds (Fig. 19-18). The depression is analyzed in terms of its outline, surface, and depth. It is usually irregular and has a serrated or spiculated margin, whereas a benign ulcer usually has a sharp, straight margin. An irregular margin, however, is sometimes seen in cases of recurrent peptic ulcers, which cannot always be distinguished from that of an early depressed cancer. The margin of an early depressed cancer is usually distinct, but sometimes shifts gradually without an abrupt transition to normal mucosa. The extent of early depressed cancer is therefore frequently difficult to determine.

Correlation of histologic type and depressed early cancer

In most cases of early depressed cancer, the surface of the depression is uneven because of the irregular proliferation of cancerous tissue (Fig. 19-19). Sometimes an island-like nodule remains in the depression and is a more prominent feature than the unevenness of the cancer depression (Fig. 19-20). This nodule is made up of regenerative epithelium, and its presence strongly suggests early cancer. The depth of the depression varies depending on the degree of cancer erosion and associated peptic ulceration.

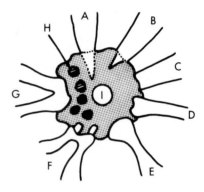

Fig. 19-18 Various appearances of converging fold terminations and central mucosa in early depressed cancer. **A,** Gradual tapering. **B,** Abrupt tapering. **C,** Abrupt termination, **D** and **E,** Clubbing. **F,** Fusion with abrupt tapering. **G,** Fusion (with V-shaped deformity). **H,** Uneven base with nodules or depressions. **I,** Smoother regenerative epithelium.

The converging folds in early depressed cancer exhibit characteristic changes, such as tapering, clubbing, interruption, and fusion (see Fig. 19-18). These abnormal fold patterns are signs of early depressed cancer. It was also suggested by Nakamura and Sugano[42] that these abnormal patterns can be separated into those features that indicate *differentiated* and those that indicate *undifferentiated* carcinomas, and that the difference between these two histologic types is visualized in well-documented radiographic studies.[43]

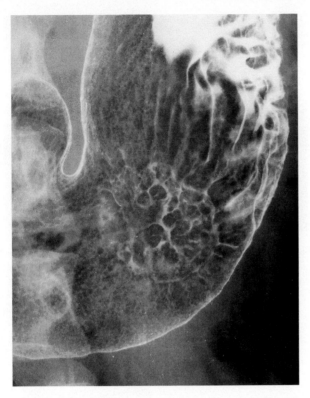

Fig. 19-19 Uneven surface of tumor due to irregular proliferation of nodules of undifferentiated cancer.

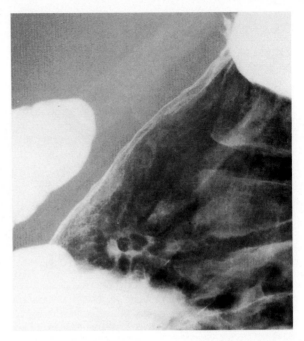

Fig. 19-20 The two nodules are more obvious in this type IIc lesion than is the full extent of the tumor, represented by the white area around it, which is the depressed cancer extending to the margins of the interrupted folds.

The radiographic characteristics of early depressed cancer are better understood when it is classified into the two histologic types just mentioned. This is a major classification of gastric carcinoma, one that corresponds to Lauren's intestinal and diffuse types,[44] and to Ming's expanding and infiltrative types.[45] The concept of poorly differentiated adenocarcinoma proposed by the Japanese Research Society for Gastric Cancer (JRSGC)[17] has not been incorporated in the classification and typing formulated by the WHO.[46] Clinically, this type is regarded as undifferentiated carcinoma.

In 1991, Hirota et al.[47] reported the following distributions by histologic type for all cases of resected cancers of the stomach seen at the National Cancer Centre Hospital: 11.1%, papillary adenocarcinoma; 17.2%, well-differentiated adenocarcinoma; 18.4%, moderately differentiated adenocarcinoma; 25.9%, poorly differentiated adenocarcinoma; 23.6%, signet-ring cell carcinoma; and 3.6%, mucinous adenocarcinoma. These authors used the classification and typing recommended by the JRSGC. Thus, differentiated adenocarcinoma (papillary and well-differentiated, moderately differentiated, and mucinous forms) accounts for 50.5% and undifferentiated adenocarcinoma (poorly differentiated and signet-ring cell carcinoma) accounts for 49.5%. The distribution between differentiated and undifferentiated types of early cancer was nearly the same as that observed for all cancers resected.[47]

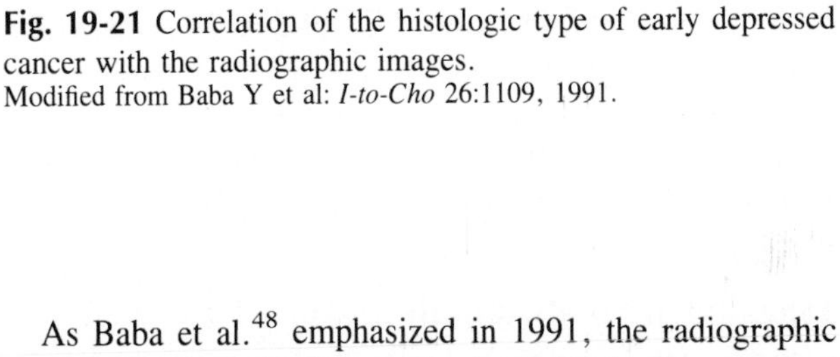

Undifferentiated type	Differentiated type

Fig. 19-21 Correlation of the histologic type of early depressed cancer with the radiographic images.
Modified from Baba Y et al: *I-to-Cho* 26:1109, 1991.

As Baba et al.[48] emphasized in 1991, the radiographic images seen in early depressed cancer are closely correlated with their undifferentiated or differentiated nature (Fig. 19-21). Significant differences in their radiographic images can be recognized, and recognition of the histologic type from the radiographic images assists in estimating the depth of invasion and the extent of horizontal spread of early cancer.

In undifferentiated early cancers, a depression generally consists of an irregular granularity (Fig. 19-22) or nodularity (see Fig. 19-19), and the depression is sharply defined

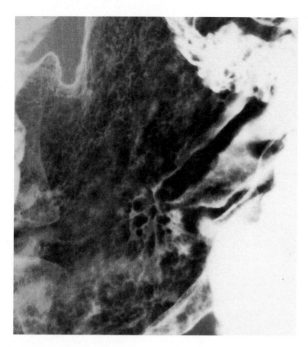

Fig. 19-22 Typical appearance of an undifferentiated type of early IIc cancer, with small nodules superimposed on a well-defined area of depressed malignant mucosa and clearly defined ends of the converging folds.

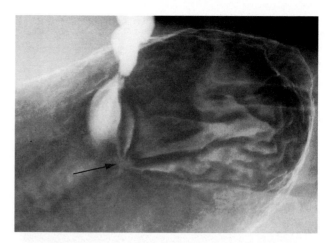

Fig. 19-23 Small area of depression with converging folds, whose ends are not very clearly defined, in a differentiated (intestinal) type IIc carcinoma located close to the cardia.

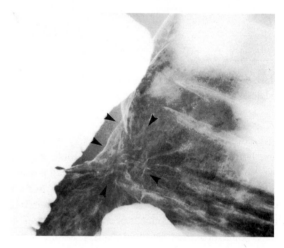

Fig. 19-24 Very poorly defined area of depressed mucosa with radiating folds *(arrowheads)*. Although there is clearly a lesion, it is impossible to accurately determine its margins. This is common with intestinal types of differentiated early gastric cancers.

(see Figs. 19-19, 19-20, and 19-22). Abrupt interruption and tapering of the converging folds (see Figs. 19-19, 19-20, and 19-22) also imparts a well-defined margin to the depression in the undifferentiated type. Intestinal metaplasia of the surrounding mucosa is less prominent in the undifferentiated type (see Figs. 19-27 to 19-29).

On the other hand, a depression that lacks both granularity and nodularity, showing instead a pattern similar to that of the normal surrounding mucosa, is seen in the differentiated type. Usually the depression is outlined by subtle, but irregular, spiculation (Fig. 19-23). The converging folds may be clubbed at the margin of the depression, and gradually tapered in the depression (Figs. 19-23 and 19-24). In the differentiated type, there is moderate to severe intestinal metaplasia in the surrounding mucosa, even when a lesion is small.

Types IIc, IIc + III, and III

Types IIc and III cancers may be distinguished radiographically by the thickness of the contrast medium that has collected in a depression. A relatively thick collection in the depression of a peptic ulcer indicates a type III lesion, (Figs. 19-25, *A*, and 19-26) and a thinner collection indicates a type IIc lesion (see Figs. 19-19, 19-20, and 19-22). Thus, a combination of the two different depths is designated type IIc + III (see Fig. 19-25, *B*), or type III + IIc. Usually the deeper part (type III) is in the center of the depression, surrounded by the shallow aspect. The density of

the contrast medium in the depression of a type IIc lesion is not uniform. The scar left by a healed ulcer may sometimes be seen as a slight depression. The same may be true for an erosion or a healing peptic ulcer.[49] In these instances, however, the depression is more faint than that of a type IIc lesion, and there is a homogenous density to the contrast medium.

On radiographic examinations, a type IIc lesion is best demonstrated with the double-contrast method (see Figs. 19-19, 19-20, and 19-22). For the precise delineation of a type IIc lesion, postural maneuvers must be performed carefully during the examination so that the contrast medium does not flow out of the depression.[4]

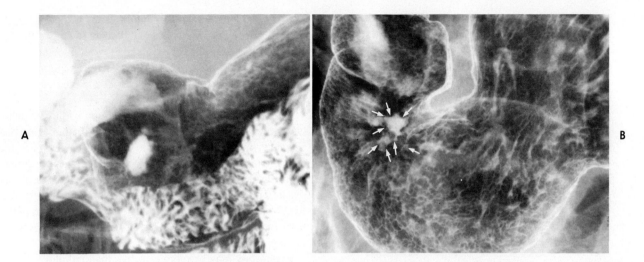

Fig. 19-25 A, Double-contrast radiograph of type III early cancer. Two months later **(B),** the ulcer has healed and has been replaced by a type IIc lesion limited to the mucosa, the extent of which is indicated by arrows.

Type III lesions have depth, whereas type IIc lesions may be scarcely recognizable at the periphery of a deeper ulcer depression. In such cases the presence of cancer is identified radiographically as the slightest change in a type IIc lesion or an irregularity of the niche itself (see Fig. 19-26). This irregularity can surround the niche either totally (see Fig. 19-25, *A*) or partially.[50] Close scrutiny may discern the irregularity of the niche. Sometimes the radiolucent defect surrounding the niche may be prominent in a type III lesion when an acute peptic change has taken place.

Careful attention should be directed to a profile niche that does not appear irregular. In type III + IIc lesions, the profile niche is so prominent that the surrounding type IIc lesion may be missed[4] and a benign peptic ulcer diagnosed instead. Thus the Hampton line alone is not a totally reliable sign of a benign peptic ulcer. A frontal view of the niche and the surrounding mucosa is required to detect a type IIc lesion at the ulcer margin. During follow-up studies the niche in type III lesions may decrease in size as the ulcer heals with treatment, and the surrounding type IIc lesion increases, and may then be recognized more clearly (see Fig. 19-25, *B*). The niche finally disappears and a fairly large type IIc lesion then becomes evident.[4] This phenomenon of healing seen with peptic ulceration in a carcinoma has been called the *malignant cycle*[51] and has been observed by many radiologists and endoscopists.[52,53]

Early cancer smaller than 1 cm

The detection of an early tumor smaller than 1 cm is very difficult in the initial radiographic examination. In 1990 Hamada et al.[54] stated that the limit of initial radiographic detection was 0.6 cm for early polypoid cancer and 0.5 cm for early depressed cancer. They also stated that the detection rate was 52% for early polypoid cancer, 50% for early

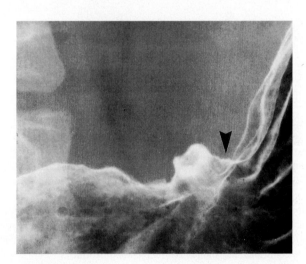

Fig. 19-26 Type III + IIc early cancer. This is a predominantly benign peptic ulceration occurring in a type IIc cancer. The superior margin of the ulcer is slightly irregular. This is not sufficient to allow a confident diagnosis, but is suspicious enough to direct the endoscopist to biopsy in this area. Endoscopy and biopsy should be repeated if they yield negative findings the first time.

depressed cancer less than 0.5 cm, and 56.9% for early depressed cancers ranging from 0.6 to 1.0 cm.

Most depressed carcinomas smaller than 1 cm are not accompanied by ulceration.[11] Consequently, it is extremely difficult to detect such a lesion. Hamada et al.[54] also reported that early cancer not associated with ulceration was detected radiologically in only 30.2% of the cases, whereas that associated with ulceration was detected in 82.4% of the cases. If a lesion is situated in an area where double-contrast radiography provides a good view of the mucosal

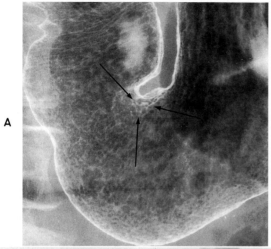

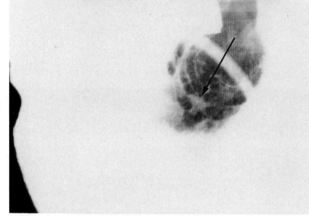

Fig. 19-27 Type IIc lesion. The abnormality on the double-contrast radiograph (**A**) is obvious once attention is drawn to it *(arrows)* but can be readily overlooked. In this case, it would be the routine compression films of the angulus (**B**) that would draw attention to the irregular nodules adjacent to a small depressed area. Once detected by compression fluoroscopy, the lesion can be confirmed and studied on double-contrast films.

details, malignancy can be diagnosed by adhering to the general principles of radiographic diagnosis (Figs. 19-27 to 19-29). A lesion that is associated with ulceration can thereby be easily detected and diagnosed as malignant. The presence of mucosal convergence is a particularly good clue.

When a lesion is smaller than 0.5 cm in its largest diameter (microcarcinoma), the radiographic diagnosis of malignancy is not always possible because the lesion is too small to be eligible for the criteria of malignancy. Sometimes an irregular surrounding translucency, which is unusual in the context of a benign ulcer, strongly suggests malignancy. In such instances, double-contrast radiography is less likely to detect the lesion than the compression method.[19]

Endoscopy may be more effective than radiology for the detection of ulcerated microcarcinoma. The microcarcinomas have now attracted the attention of endoscopists because they can be treated endoscopically. Even a type IIc lesion lacking ulcerative changes can be excised using an endoscopic snare.[11]

Type IIb–like lesion

A type IIb lesion can be considered cancerous in its earliest phase. This was confirmed when purely type IIb lesions were discovered incidentally in the stomach during surgical procedures performed to remove other primary lesions; all were smaller than 0.5 cm.[42] Many clinical cases that were not classified as purely type IIb, however, have mimicked type IIb lesions. Only a subtle difference could be discerned in the elevation or depression from the normal surrounding mucosa, and consequently the border of these lesions was not clearly defined. This appearance has been designated a *type IIb–like* lesion[20] (Fig. 19-30). The two histologic types possess different radiographic appearances. The surface pattern of a differentiated carcinoma may simulate the surrounding normal mucosa (see Fig. 19-

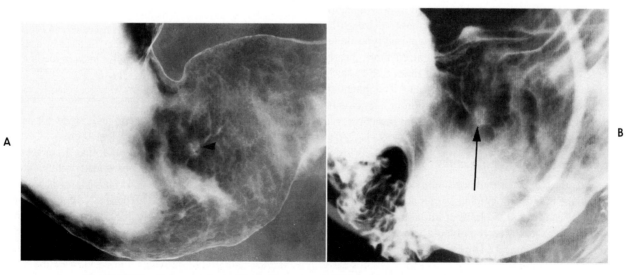

Fig. 19-28 Small depressed type IIc carcinoma on double-contrast (**A**) and compression (**B**) films.

30), whereas that of an undifferentiated carcinoma is nearly homogeneous. The undifferentiated carcinoma showing type IIb–like spread is frequently covered with normal foveolar epithelium containing scattered microerosions.[43]

The proximal limit of the type IIb–like lesion should be defined as precisely as possible so that the line of the surgical excision can be determined. The endoscopic approach, including the dye-spraying method and carbon ink injection, is indispensable for this purpose.[55,56]

Superficial spreading carcinoma

The first mention of superficial spreading carcinomas appears in the report by Stout[57] published in 1924. He collected 15 cases of depressed cancer that spread along the mucosa, which he called "superficial spreading carcinomas." The first case was an intramucosal carcinoma with a horizontal spread that measured 9 × 6 cm. Stout did not strictly define superficial spreading carcinoma based on the extent of its horizontal spread; for example, the horizontal spread of the second case measured only 3.2 × 3 cm, which is not significant enough to be deemed a superficial spreading carcinoma. Rather, it should be classified as a typical type IIc or type IIc + III early carcinoma in light of the Japanese experience to date.

In Japan a strict definition of superficial spreading carcinoma has not yet been established. The term is generally employed, however, to refer to a superficial early carci-

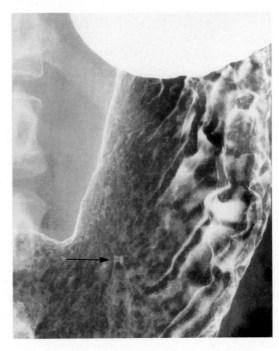

Fig. 19-29 Tiny type IIc carcinoma, well shown because it lies in the middle of the posterior wall of the lower body in the easiest position to find, and the degree of distention is appropriate.

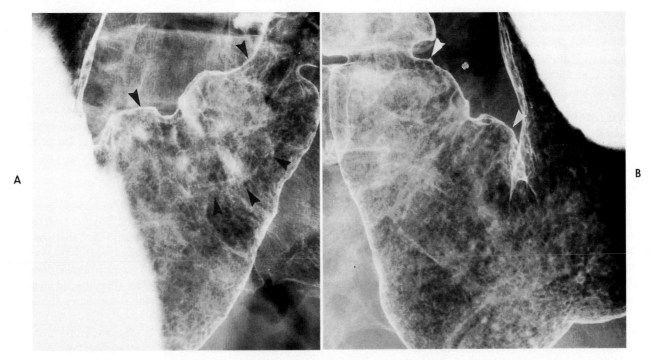

Fig. 19-30 Prone (**A**) and supine (**B**) double-contrast films of a type IIb–like early cancer. The tumor is very hard to detect. All that can be said is that the pattern of the areae gastricae is not normal, in that it is less well defined and the coating is a little thicker in a patchy manner on the prone film, suggesting some patchy depression of the mucosa. Although the margins of a lesion cannot really be defined, the uneven coating raises enough suspicion to recommend biopsy.

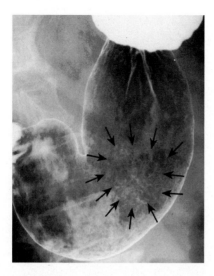

Fig. 19-31 Superficial spreading carcinoma of the IIa type, with margins that can be appreciated with a little difficulty, and shown by arrows. Slightly less distention would facilitate easier margin definition.

noma, that is, a type II early carcinoma. In this type of early carcinoma, the product (S) of its greatest diameter (a) and the diameter perpendicular to the greatest diameter (b), or $(S = a \times b)$, is greater than 5 cm^2.[58]

The diagnosis of superficial spreading carcinoma based on radiographic findings is simple, except for type IIb–like lesions (Fig. 19-30). A typical type IIa (Fig. 19-31) or IIc lesion with surface dimensions of 25 to 36 cm^2 is easily diagnosed by double-contrast radiography. The diagnostic difficulty arises, however, when the surface dimensions exceed 36 cm^2,[59] because the affected mucosa is then so large that it is difficult to recognize the mucosal abnormality in contrast to the small part of normal mucosa remaining.

RADIOGRAPHIC DIAGNOSIS OF ADVANCED CANCER
General considerations

The radiographic diagnosis of advanced gastric cancer may be established when a tumor mass formation is noted on x-ray studies. The tumor may be demonstrated using either the compression or double-contrast method. In a definite case of advanced cancer, one of four types of invasion patterns may be recognized, following the Bormann classification (Fig. 19-32). All views of such an advanced cancer will depict a filling defect, a surrounding raised margin, and shrinkage of the affected portion of the entire thickness of the stomach.

A lesion is sometimes encountered, which slightly or moderately involves the propria muscle, that macroscopically simulates type IIc early cancer. Rarely there is invasion of the entire thickness of the gastric wall or direct invasion of adjacent structures (see Fig. 19-42). This is called an *advanced cancer simulating type IIc,* and is designated a Bormann type 5 according to the JRSGC classification.[17]

Classification

Advanced cancer is defined as a lesion that involves at least the muscularis propria or the deeper layers of the gastric wall (subserosa and serosa). Although the classification of gastric cancer is claimed to be confusing in the Western literature,[60] the Bormann classification (originally proposed in 1926) has been accepted and is used exclusively in Japan[18] (see Fig. 19-32). This classification is based solely on gross appearances. In what is considered an "old" classification,[60] elements partially overlap in each category, thus lessening its meaning because the gross and microscopic criteria are intermingled. In the manual prepared by the JRSGC,[17] two types were added to the Bormann classification: early cancer (type 0) and lesions unclassifiable into the Bormann categories (type 5). A more simplified classification than that of Bormann, the Kajitani classification (see Fig. 19-32), is also often used because it allows easy recognition of the infiltrating pattern of advanced cancer.

Bormann types 1 and 2

A Bormann type 1 lesion is a large polypoid lesion that usually exceeds 3 cm in its greatest diameter and possesses a large irregular lobulation. Sometimes a slight surface depression may exist. A Bormann type 1 lesion is seen to have a large, irregular filling defect in its margin on radiographs of a barium-filled lesion and as an irregular tumor shadow with rough lobulation on double-contrast (Fig. 19-33) and compression radiographs. Occasionally a large pedunculated lesion may be an early carcinoma that also falls into the original classification of Bormann type 1.

The Bormann type 2 lesion is visible as a localized filling defect of the gastric wall on a compression radiograph. These depict an irregular crater with a greatly raised margin that is sharply set off from the normal surrounding mucosa (Figs. 19-34 and Fig. 19-35). It usually exceeds 3 cm in its greatest diameter. The smaller Bormann type 2 lesion is difficult to distinguish from early type IIa + IIc cancer with involvement of the submucosa (Figs. 19-34 and 19-35).

Bormann type 3

Usually the Bormann type 3 lesion is larger than the type 2. Radiographs obtained after barium filling disclose a filling defect and stiffening of the gastric wall (Fig. 19-36). A compression radiograph shows a large, irregular crater and the surrounding radiolucent defect (Fig. 19-36), which is not as well defined as that of the Bormann type 2 lesion. Double-contrast radiographs show best the whole aspect of Bormann type 3 lesions (Fig. 19-37). Stiffening of the gastric wall extends beyond the cancer crater because of the diffuse infiltration of the gastric wall (Fig. 19-37, *B*). Usually the mucosal convergence is interrupted at the margin of the crater (Fig. 19-37, *B*), which is not as prominent as that seen with a Bormann type 2 lesion. Sometimes a component of type IIc may surround the crater; in this event, a

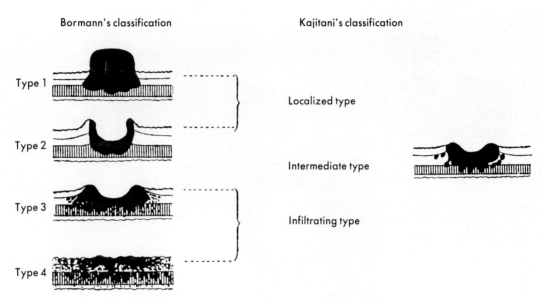

Fig. 19-32 Gross classification of advanced gastric cancer.

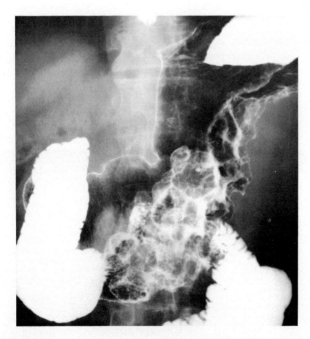

Fig. 19-33 Double-contrast radiograph of a Bormann type 1 lesion, consisting of a huge mass invading neighboring structures.

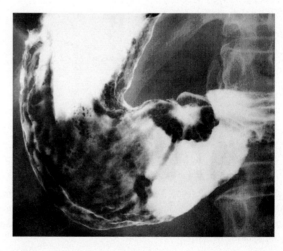

Fig. 19-34 Bormann type 2 carcinoma. This prone compression film shows the well-defined mass with an irregular central ulcer.

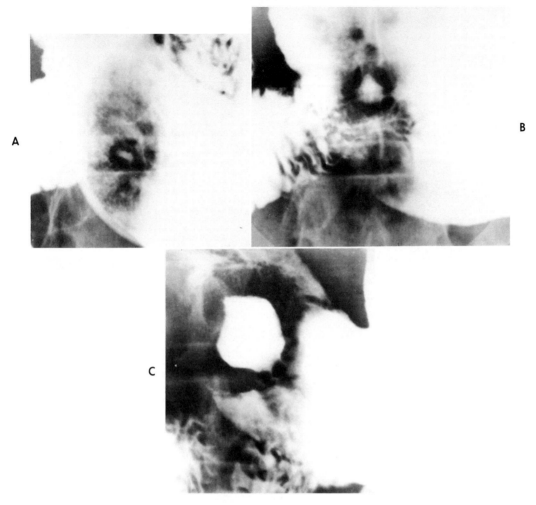

Fig. 19-35 Erect compression radiograph (**A**) shows a small central depression and surrounding elevation characteristic of type IIa + IIc early cancer. The patient declined surgery. **B** and **C** document tumor enlargement as this cancer progresses into a typical Bormann type 2 lesion.

Fig. 19-36 Bormann type 3 advanced cancer. The mass is more prominent than the ulcer and the edges of the tumor are more poorly defined than they are in the Bormann type 2 lesion, as the lesion spreads laterally.

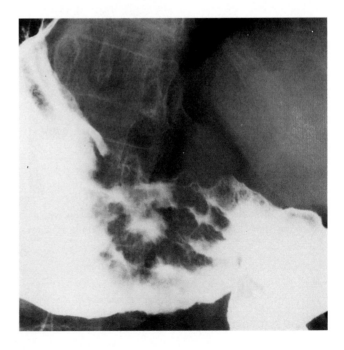

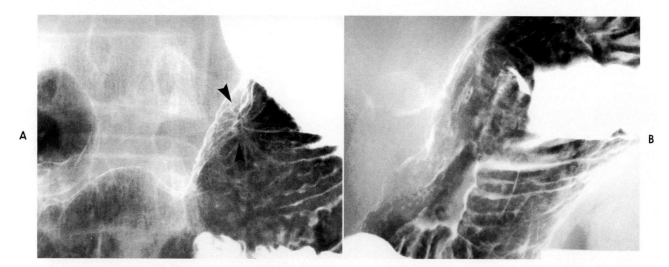

Fig. 19-37 Initial film (**A**) showing a small cancer, but with some wall stiffening. The patient declined treatment, and some months later (**B**) the typical appearances of a Bormann type 3 tumor are present, consisting of an irregular mass and interrupted folds adjacent to the ulcer and an infiltrating lesion without clear margins.

greater or lesser deformity of the stomach, resulting from extensive cancerous infiltration, may be revealed.

Bormann type 4

A Bormann type 4 lesion is referred to as a *diffuse infiltrative carcinoma* in the Western literature. Bormann called it *diffuse carcinoma*. Thickening of the gastric wall caused by diffuse cancerous infiltration and pronounced proliferation of fibrotic tissue are macroscopic characteristics of this type of growth. Linitis plastica is a Bormann type 4 lesion.

The Bormann type 4 lesion is seen on barium radiographs as a deformity of the stomach. The gastric antrum is the typical site of involvement and is greatly narrowed (Fig. 19-38). A double-contrast radiograph demonstrates poor distensibility of the gastric wall and often depicts the primary site as an erosion or ulceration (Fig. 19-39). At a late stage, this primary site is enlarged, imparting a disturbed appearance to the mucosal surface. Ultimately this surface is extensively replaced by a large, irregular erosion. A pattern of malignant folds with enlargement and twisting is not prominent in most Bormann type 4 lesions. No definite tumor forms are present in this type. Sometimes the proximal limit of infiltration may be difficult to define, but double-contrast radiography may be effective for this purpose (Fig. 19-38, *B*).

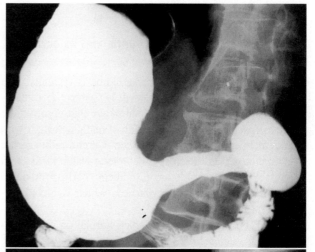

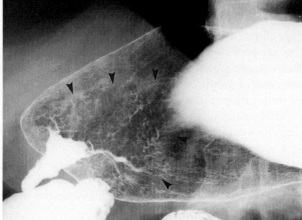

Fig. 19-38 Single-contrast film (**A**) showing an infiltrated rigid and narrowed antrum due to Bormann type 4 linitis plastica carcinoma. The double-contrast film (**B**) shows the proximal extent of the mucosal lesion, but these tumors may spread submucosally far beyond the mucosal edge of the lesion.

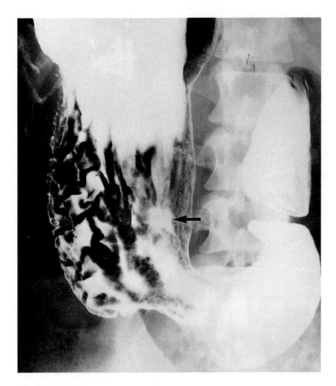

Fig. 19-39 Prone double-contrast films showing the lack of distention due to the presence of an infiltrating Bormann type 4 tumor, as well as the ulcerated lesion that was probably the site of origin of the cancer.

Linitis plastica–type of carcinoma and its early phase

The linitis plastica–type of carcinoma is typically seen in patients younger than 40 years. It is characterized radiographically by a deformity and shrinkage that involves the entire stomach. A pattern consisting of malignant folds with enlargement and twisting is also seen. Careful radiographic examination should disclose a depressed lesion in the area where the mucosal folds are prominent, corresponding to the primary focus of linitis plastica, which is most common in the gastric body.[61]

A stomach that had been deemed normal on routine radiographic studies may transform into a "leather bottle" structure within a few months. On retrospective evaluation of the first radiographic examination, only the slightest abnormality of the gastric wall may be discerned. Much effort has been directed toward detecting the early phase of linitis plastica; it is the only problem that remains in the diagnosis of gastric cancer, even now when the diagnosis of early gastric cancer has been well established.

Nakamura et al.[61] estimated that it may take from 3 to 8 years for a cancer to evolve into linitis plastica, with a mean of 6 years. They theorize that the early detection of linitis plastica is facilitated by the discovery of a type IIc lesion smaller than 2 cm in the mucosa of the fundus.

The radiographic diagnosis of early linitis plastica should

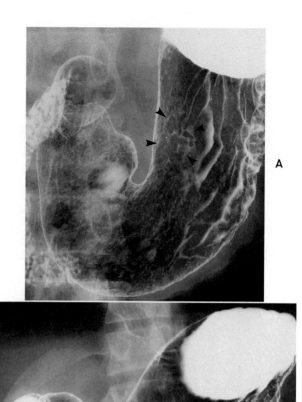

Fig. 19-40 Linitis plastica type of carcinoma (the entire stomach was involved). The rugae adjacent are rather prominent and indicate linitis plastica infiltration (**A**). However, the administration of more gas (**B**) effaces the folds, which are therefore not apparently abnormal and there is thus no evidence of the advanced cancer.

include detection of (1) the pathologic changes characteristic of linitis plastica before shrinkage of the stomach and (2) early undifferentiated cancer in the mucosa of the fundus (Fig. 19-40). Attention should therefore be directed toward discovering a type IIc lesion in the mucosa.[62] Double-contrast radiography using as much gas as is needed to separate the prominent mucosal folds is required for this purpose (Fig. 19-40, *B*). The first condition is indicated when abnormalities such as slight spiculation and stiffening of the mucosal folds are noted. Accumulated experience with cases of linitis plastica in which the stomach does not shrink is necessary for obtaining clinical proof that type IIc lesions develop into linitis plastica.

Advanced cancer simulating type IIc

Macroscopically, advanced cancers that mimic a type IIc lesion are not definite advanced cancers. The submucosal involvement of an early cancer is generally slight and limited to the central aspect. Consequently, radiographic evidence of extensive submucosal involvement suggests an advanced cancer simulating a type IIc cancer. Extensive translucency surrounding a lesion, visible on a compression image, implies involvement that is deeper than the submucosal layer.[41] Such a translucency, however, is not always present in association with lesions.

To estimate the depth of invasion, it may be useful to change the volume of gas. The resulting changing appearance of the depression and the converging folds can provide invaluable information for estimating the pattern of invasion as well as the depth.[63]

A mucosal cancer or a cancer with slight submucosal in-

volvement does not produce a tumor shadow on a double-contrast image, even with a small volume of gas. In a lesion that extensively involves the submucosa and slightly to moderately involves the propria muscle, a tumor shadow, which is visualized on a double-contrast image with a moderate to large amount of gaseous distention, is effaced by excessive gaseous distention.[4] A compression image can consistently reveal a pronounced translucency of the tumor shadow. These radiographic findings establish the existence of advanced cancer.

In addition to the analysis of the radiographic findings already mentioned, EUS and CT (Fig. 19-41) are indispensable for assessing the thickness of the affected gastric wall, although EUS provides the best information on the architecture of the invasive pattern. Sometimes, extensive involvement of abdominal lymph nodes may be observed in an advanced cancer simulating a type IIc cancer (Fig. 19-41).

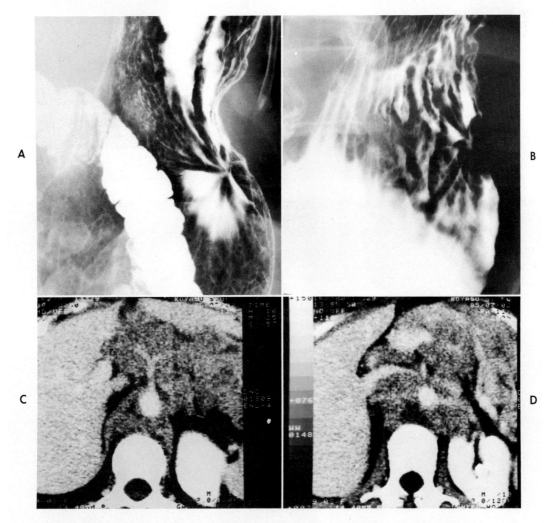

Fig. 19-41 A, Double-contrast radiograph of advanced cancer simulating type IIc. **B,** Compression film reveals that there is a tumor mass. **C** and **D,** CT scan showing a conglomerate mass consisting of metastatic lymph nodes and lesser omentum, and direct invasion of the liver.
B courtesy of Y. Masuda; **C** and **D** courtesy of M. Hori.

ESOPHAGEAL INVASION BY GASTRIC CANCER

The esophagus is frequently involved by a cancer located in the gastric cardia or in the vicinity of the esophagogastric junction. Even an early cancer may involve the lower esophagus. Generally the invasion pattern of the esophagus depends on the histologic type of the gastric cancer. In the differentiated type, an affected portion of the esopha-

gus usually shows obvious filling defects due to tumor formation (Figs. 19-42 and 19-47, *C*), and cancerous invasion replaces the esophageal mucosa. The undifferentiated type, on the other hand, diffusely invades the submucosa and beneath, often not affecting the esophageal mucosal surface. A smooth enlarged fold is not infrequently the only sign of esophageal involvement (Fig. 19-43).

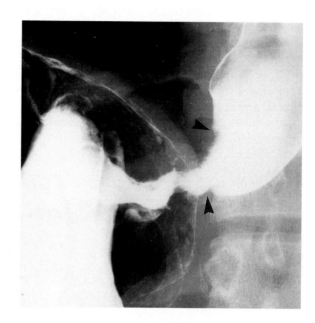

Fig. 19-42 Differentiated (intestinal) cancer invading the esophagus with mucosal ulceration.
Courtesy of Dr. Y. Kaku.

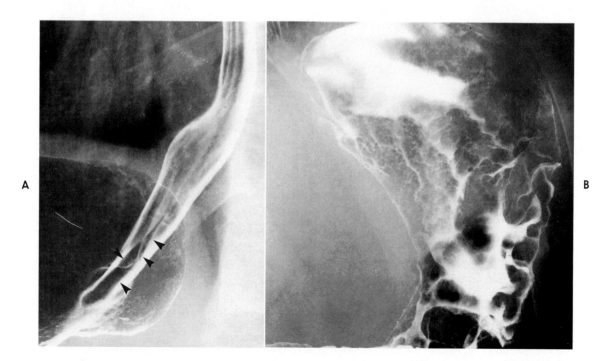

Fig. 19-43 A, A widened fold is present in the lower esophagus, and this is the only abnormality visible here. However, the stomach (**B**) shows the presence of a large fungating tumor, of undifferentiated type, that is invading the esophagus submucosally.
Courtesy of Dr. Y. Kaku.

CARCINOMA OF THE GASTRIC STUMP AFTER GASTRECTOMY
General considerations

Cancer of the gastric stump or gastric remnant is divided grossly into two groups: (1) that arising after an initial gastrectomy for a benign lesion and (2) that arising after an initial gastrectomy for cancer. The first group includes cancer of the cut end, cancer of the stoma (anastomotic site), and cancer of the stump (cancer of the gastric remnant that does not involve the stoma and suture line). The second includes residual, recurrent, and multiple cancers.

For radiographic diagnosis, double-contrast radiography with very considerable gaseous distention is usually necessary. Sometimes, however, a large volume of gas may obscure the abnormalities present along the lesser and greater curves. Double-contrast radiography can detect even an early cancer of the gastric stump. The compression method is best suited for the assessment of the anastomotic site and suture line, if possible, but it cannot be applied in most patients with a gastric remnant because of its anatomic location.

Carcinoma of the gastric stump after gastrectomy for benign lesions

A recent report issued by the National Cancer Centre Hospital[64] in Tokyo cites that, between 1962 and 1988, 52 patients underwent surgery for gastric stump cancer after they had undergone gastrectomy for benign lesions and that 61 patients underwent surgery for gastric cancer after gastrectomy for malignancies. During this time, there was a total of 6169 patients who were operated on for gastric cancer. The first group of patients accounted for 0.8% of all those patients who underwent surgery for gastric cancer, and 9 of 52 patients had early cancers, comprising 17.3%.

The gastric remnant should be well distended for the demonstration of early cancer (Figs. 19-44 and 19-45).

Residual and recurrent cancer of the gastric stump

Residual cancer refers to a stomal cancer when the cut end of the resected stomach proves cancerous. Improvements in surgical technique have minimized the incidence of this problem. From the standpoint of radiographic diagnosis, the risk still exists that a second type IIb–like lesion is the cause of an apparent residual cancer (Fig. 19-46).

Recurrent cancer is a cancer that involves the gastric stump and may result from intragastric metastases. It is rare, and the diagnosis may be difficult to establish histologically. Peritoneal dissemination or direct invasion of the gastric stump from metastatic lymph nodes is common in cases of recurrent cancer of the stomach. In such instances the signs of peritonitis carcinomatosa or of a palpable mass are much more prominent than the abnormality of the gastric stump. Ascites and a recurrent mass in the abdomen, including lymph node metastases, are best appreciated by CT. However, peritoneal dissemination without ascites is difficult for CT to detect.

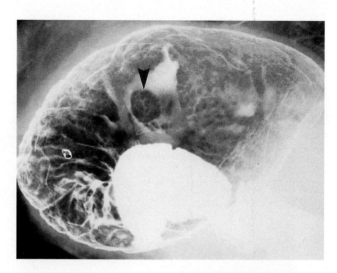

Fig. 19-44 Early cancer in the gastric remnant several years after a Billroth I gastrectomy.

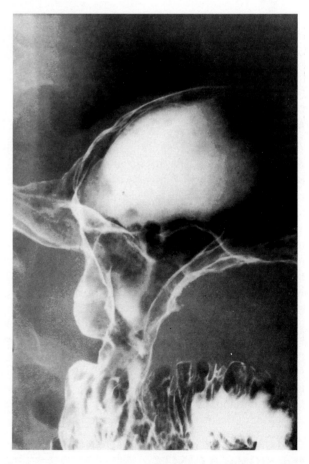

Fig. 19-45 Advanced gastric cancer 27 years after a Billroth II gastrectomy for peptic ulcer. The symptom was early satiety and had lasted for only 3 weeks.

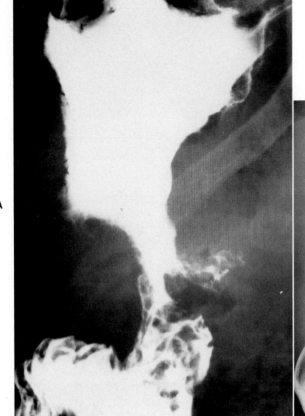

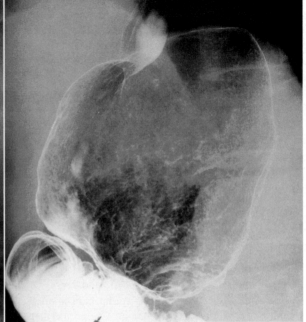

Fig. 19-46 A, Extensive infiltrating advanced cancer several years after a distal gastrectomy. **B,** Review of the previous barium meal shows an irregular areae gastricae pattern that could be gastritis, but is focal (*arrows*) and therefore suspicious for type IIb early carcinoma. Note that good distention is necessary to assess the mucosa in gastric remnants.

Multiple cancers

A late recurrence of a residual cancer of the stump may develop several years after the initial gastrectomy and may be difficult to distinguish from synchronous multiple cancers near the stoma. The oval wedge of the initially resected specimen should undergo careful histologic examination, and the presence of a minute satellite focus of synchronous multiple cancer thereby excluded.[6] Several cases of metachronous early cancer have been reported.[65,66] Special attention should be paid to the possible development of cancer in a stomach that has been reconstructed as part of a procedure for esophageal cancer resection.[67-69]

For radiographic diagnosis, as much compression as possible should be exerted on the stoma and its vicinity.[70] Appropriate double-contrast radiography facilitates the diagnosis not only of advanced cancer (Fig. 19-47, *A* and *B*), but also of early cancer (Figs. 19-44, 19-46, *B,* and 19-48) of the gastric stump. Endoscopy and biopsy, however, are essential for evaluating a radiographic abnormality.

EVALUATION OF A MASS SCREENING PROGRAM FOR STOMACH CANCER
Value of mass screening

In Japan a gastric mass screening program, involving a barium meal study imaged by an indirect x-ray device, was instituted in 1960. Since then it has been gradually implemented nationwide. A total number of 5,157,778 people underwent mass screening in 1987. Gastric cancer was detected in 0.13% (6661) of them and surgery was performed in 97.2%. Early cancer comprised 52.1% of the detected cases and 60.7% of the resected cases.[1] It is well known that the prognosis in cases of gastric cancer diagnosed by screening is much better than that for symptomatic patients,[40] although lead time bias and length bias should be taken into consideration in this comparison.[71] A long-term follow-up study of those patients with cancer detected by mass survey revealed that the likelihood of recurrence decreased rapidly over the immediate 7 years and remained low after that. Yamazaki and colleagues[72] concluded that about two thirds of them were successfully cured of their disease.

In Japan there have been many reports dealing with the value of mass screening for gastric cancer, although it has not been proved in a randomized controlled trial. In 1983, The Health and Medical Services Law for the Aged came into effect, and The Ministry of Health and Welfare set up a policy to achieve 30% of an annual coverage rate for gastric mass screening for people aged 40 and over.

There is an ongoing randomized controlled trial for evaluating this mass screening program, which was started in

1985. However, it was necessary to implement it on an individual-based randomization because the target population had already been screened at the time the trial was started.[1] In fact, the present situation in Japan makes it very difficult to conduct a randomized controlled trial that examines the efficacy of gastric mass screening. Consequently, second-best methods have been adopted to substantiate the validity of gastric mass screening instead of an actual randomized controlled trial. These methods include time trend analysis, retrospective cohort study, correlation of screening rate and change in mortality, and case-control study.

Based on the results of a case-control study, Oshima et al.[73] reported that the mass screening program is effective in reducing the mortality associated with stomach cancer.

Method of mass screening

In recent years, photofluorography using an image intensifier has been used for the mass screening program, and usually seven radiographic images are documented on a 100-mm roll film (the seven-film method) in the following order, although there are some variations in the sequence of radiography and in the number of films obtained: (1) prone mucosal relief image; (2) prone barium-filled image; (3) supine frontal double-contrast image; (4) supine right anterior oblique double-contrast image; (5) semi-upright left anterior oblique double-contrast image; and (6) upright frontal barium-filled image.[74]

Murakami et al.[74] found that the quality of 100-mm photofluorography using an image intensifier is nearly equiva-

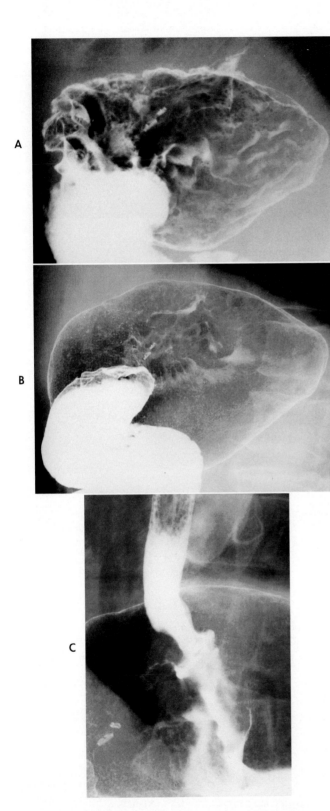

Fig. 19-47 An examination with inadequate distention and poor coating (**A**) reveals no lesion, but, when more gas is given and the mucus is cleared from the mucosa, an advanced carcinoma is revealed (**B**), extending into the esophagus (**C**).

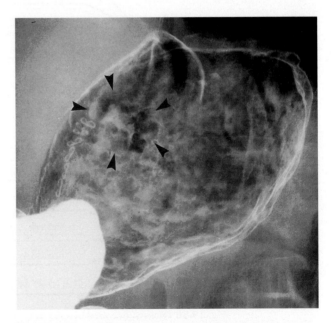

Fig. 19-48 Type IIa + IIc early gastric cancer in the gastric remnant. Excellent distention and washing of all mucus from the stomach with sufficient barium is necessary to achieve good mucosal coating in postoperative patients. A relaxant is essential.

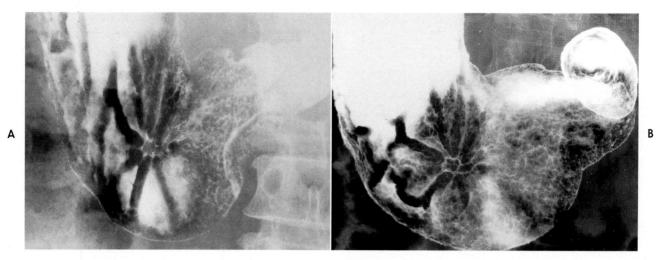

Fig. 19-49 Two prone films. **A,** 100-mm mass screening radiography clearly displays early gastric cancer on the anterior wall. **B,** Detailed study carried out before surgery.

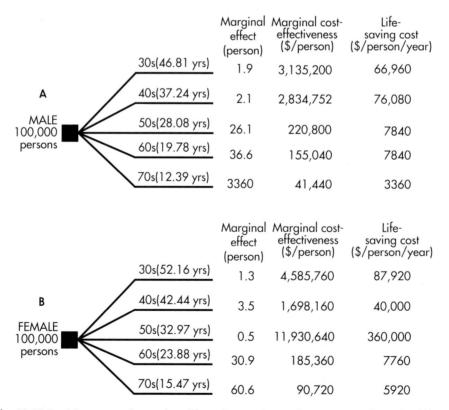

Fig. 19-50 Decision tree used to analyze life-saving cost in gastric mass survey for males **(A)** and females **(B).**
From Hamajima C et al: *Gastroenterol Mass Survey* 89:22, 1990.

lent to that of direct radiography. In fact, it can detect early cancers without difficulty (Figs. 19-49).

Cost-effectiveness analysis

Based on their experience in the Miyagi prefecture, which is located in the northern part of Honshu Island, Hisamichi et al.[1] cited sensitivity of gastric mass screening of 85%, and specificity of 90% in a target population of 100,000 people. In an individual-based mass screening program, Hamajima et al.[75] found that the sensitivity of mass screening was 79% and the specificity was 79%.

The value of mass screening has recently been evaluated in terms of its cost and life-saving effect.[75] The marginal cost-effectiveness (cost of mass screening for 100,000 persons minus the cost for outpatient visits over the same time period divided by marginal effect) was found to be $220,800, which represented the total cost of screening to save one person aged 50 from death due to gastric cancer. The cost in terms of life-saving for a male aged 50 is $7,840 per year of life saved (Fig. 19-50, *A*). The figures for women are quite different (Fig. 19-50, *B*).

Calculation of the life-saving cost is controversial. Fig. 19-50, *A*, shows that, for both sexes, mass screening is most effective in the 70-year-old age group, whereas it is very expensive in those of working age. Nevertheless, the morbidity resulting from treatment for even early gastric cancer is higher in the elderly, and the 40- and 50-year-old group are important as a screening target because they are responsible for their families spiritually as well as economically, and because they bear most of the socioeconomic expense. Nevertheless, the elderly are able and have the right to enjoy productive and meaningful lives.

REFERENCES

1. Hisamichi S et al: Evaluation of mass screening programme for stomach cancer in Japan: In Miller AB, Chamberlain J, Day NE, Hakama M, Prorok PC, eds: *Cancer screening*. Cambridge, 1991, Cambridge University Press.
2. Ohta H et al: Early gastric carcinoma of the stomach with special reference to macroscopic classsification, *Cancer* 60:1099, 1987.
3. Llorens P et al: Diagnostico del cancer gastrico y terapeutica endoscopica de las leiones gastricas incipientes, *Gastroenterol Latinoam* 2:29, 1991.
4. Maruyama M: Early gastric cancer. In Laufer I, ed: *Double contrast gastrointestinal radiology with endoscopic correlation*, Philadelphia, 1979, WB Saunders.
5. Sonoda M et al: Computed radiography utilizing laser stimulated luminescence, *Radiology* 148:833, 1983.
6. Ogura T et al: Technical and clinical evaluations of a 2048 × 2048 matrix digital radiography system for gastrointestinal examinations, *Image Physics*, vol 1443, Proceedings Preprint, The International Society for Optical Engineering, San Jose, Calif, Feb 23–March 1, 1991.
7. Yamada T et al: Clinics of FCR: the gastrointestinal tract, *J Med Imag* 4(suppl 1):34, 1984.
8. Unayama F: Upper gastrointestinal tract. In Tateno Y, Iinuma T, Takano M, eds: *Computed radiography*, Tokyo, 1987, Springer-Verlag.
9. Ogura T et al: Technical and clinical evaluations of a 2048 × 2048-matrix digital radiography system for gastrointestinal examinations: Image Physics 1443, In *Proceedings of The International Society for Optical Engineering*, February 1991.
10. Matsue H: Ultrasonographic examination and diagnosis of stomach diseases. In Maruyama M, Kimura K, eds: *Review of clinical research in gastroenterology*, Tokyo, 1988, Igaku-Shoin.
11. Takekoshi T, Takagi K, Kato Y: Radical endoscopic treatment of early gastric cancer. In Oguro Y, Takagi K, eds: *Endoscopic approaches to cancer diagnosis and treatment* (Gann Monograph on Cancer Research 37:111), Tokyo, London, 1990, Japan Scientific Societies Press.
12. Chonan A et al: Clinical evaluation of endoscopic ultrasonography (EUS) on estimation of the depth of invasion in advanced gastric cancer with depressed lesion, *Gastroenterol Endosc* 32:493, 1990.
13. Kida M et al: Endoscopic ultrasonography in diagnosis of the degree of gastric cancer invasion, *J Med Ultrasonogr* 52:441, 1988.
14. Chonan A et al: Clinical evaluation of endoscopic ultrasonography (EUS) on the diagnosis for depressed type early gastric cancer associated with ulceration, *Gastroenterol Endosc* 32:1081, 1990.
15. Yao T: Advanced cancer simulating early cancer: Introduction, a brief summary on the case conference on the estimation of invasive depth of gastric cancer, *I-to-Cho* 25:1381, 1990.
16. Komaki S, Toyoshima S: CT's capability in detecting gastric cancer, *Gastrointest Radiol* 8:307, 1983.
17. Japanese Research Society for Gastric Cancer: The general rules for the gastric cancer staging in surgery and pathology. Part I. Clinical classification. Part II. Histological classification of gastric cancer, *Jpn J Surg* 11:127, 1981.
18. Ohkuma K, Hisa N, Hiramatsu K: Computed tomography staging of gastric cancer, *I-to-Cho* 19:1313, 1984.
19. Hori M et al: Detection of lymph nodes of the stomach cancer with computed tomography, *Rinsho Geka* 39:543, 1984.
20. Kumakura K, Maruyama M, and Sugiyama N: Radiological diagnosis of type IIb- and IIb-like lesions of the stomach, *I-to-Cho* 7:21, 1972.
21. Shirakabe H et al: Comparison of x-ray and biopsy examination for the diagnosis of early gastric cancer, *Jpn J Clin-Oncol* 2:93, 1972.
22. Maruyama M: Comparison of radiology and endoscopy in the diagnosis of gastric cancer. In Preece PE, Cushieri A, Wellwood JM, eds: *Cancer of the stomach*, San Diego, 1986, Grune & Stratton.
23. Hamada T, Kaji F, Shirakabe H: Detectability of gastric cancer by radiology as compared to endoscopy. In Maruyama M, Kimura K, eds: *Review of clinical research in gastroenterology*, Tokyo, 1988, Igaku-Shoin.
24. Takasu Y: Detection of early cancer by panendoscopy: recent progress in diagnosis of cancer and treatment of digestive diseases, *J Jpn Soc Intern Med* 77:1651, 1988.
25. Otsuji M et al: Assessment of small diameter panendoscopy for diagnosis of gastric cancer: comparative study with follow-up survey data, *I-to-Cho* 24:1291, 1989.
26. Yao T et al: Failure to detect gastric cancer at the initial examination and measures against it, *I-to-Cho* 25:27, 1990.
27. Nishizawa M et al: Methodology to avoid missing advanced gastric cancer, *I-to-Cho* 25:49, 1990.
28. Maruyama M, Yamada T, Matsue H: Theoretical basis for the radiographic diagnosis of polypoid early cancer. In Shirakabe H et al, eds: *Atlas of x-ray diagnosis of early gastric cancer*, Tokyo, 1982, Igaku-Shoin.
29. Yamada T, Fukutomi H: Polypoid lesions of the stomach, *I-to-Cho* 10:1479, 1975.
30. Ming SC, Goldman H: Gastric polyps: a histogenic classification and its relation to carcinoma, *Cancer* 18:721, 1965.
31. Morson BC: Gastric polyps composed of intestinal epithelium, *Br J Cancer* 9:550, 1955.

32. Enjoji M, Watanabe H: Adenoma of the stomach: a borderline lesion, *I-to-Cho* 10:1443, 1975.

33. Fukuchi S, Hiyama M, Mochizuki T: Endoscopic diagnosis of IIa-subtype of polypoid lesions which belong to borderline lesions between benignancy and malignancy. *I-to-Cho* 10:1487, 1975.

34. Nakamura T: The concept of gastric polyp, *I-to-Cho* 1:539, 1967.

35. Takagi K et al: Type IIa and ATP: problems on early gastric cancer, *I-to-Cho* 3:15, 1968.

36. Fukuchi S, Mochizuki T: IIa-subtype (gastric adenoma of small intestinal type): a clinical, endoscopic and histological study. In Maruyama M, Kimura K, eds: *Review of clinical research in gastroenterology,* Tokyo, 1988, Igaku-Shoin.

37. Nakamura K, Takagi K: Some considerations on lesions of atypical epithelium of the stomach, *I-to-Cho* 10:1455, 1975.

38. Fuchigami T, Iwashita A: Clinical course of group III elevated lesions of the stomach, *I-to-Cho* 25:927, 1990.

39. Yamada T: X-ray diagnosis of borderline lesion between malignancy and benignancy, *I-to-Cho* 10:1479, 1975.

40. Kampschoer GHM, Fujii A, Masuda Y: Gastric cancer detected by mass survey, *Scand J Gastroenterol* 24:813, 1989.

41. Maruyama M et al: Radiodiagnostic possibility of gastric carcinoma involving the proper muscle layer, *I-to-Cho* 11:855, 1976.

42. Nakamura K, Sugano H: Carcinoma of the stomach in incipient phase; its histogenesis and histological appearances, *Gann* 59:251, 1968.

43. Baba Y et al: A comparative study between radiologic and macroscopic findings of early gastric carcinoma with IIb-like intramucosal spread: with special reference to radiologic definition of proximal boundary, *I-to-Cho* 12:1087, 1977.

44. Lauren P: The two histological main types of gastric carcinoma: diffuse and so-called intestinal type carcinoma. An attempt at a histo-clinical classification, *Acta Pathol Microbiol Scand* 64:31, 1965.

45. Ming SC: Gastric carcinoma. A pathobiological classification, *Cancer* 39:2475, 1977.

46. Watanabe H, Jass JR, Sobin LH: *Histological typing of esophageal and gastric tumors,* ed 2 (WHO International, Histological classification of tumors), Berlin, 1990, Springer-Verlag.

47. Hirota T et al: Significance of histologic type of gastric carcinoma as a prognostic factor, *I-to-Cho* 26:1149, 1991.

48. Baba Y et al: Histological classification of gastric cancer related to radiological and endoscopic manifestations, *I-to-Cho* 26:1109, 1991.

49. Maruyama M, Kumakura K, Yarita T: Radiographic diagnosis of peptic ulcer. In Shirakabe H, et al: *Atlas of x-ray diagnosis of early gastric cancer,* Tokyo, 1982, Igaku-Shoin.

50. Kumakura K et al: Limitation in radiological diagnosis of malignant ulcer of the stomach, *I-to-Cho* 8:1183, 1973.

51. Murakami T: New concept for an ulcer-cancer of the stomach, *Juntendo Igaku Med J* 13:157, 1967.

52. Okabe H: Analysis of gastric cancer followed up under the diagnosis of benign ulcer, *I-to-Cho* 3:705, 1968.

53. Sakita T et al: Observations on the healing of ulcerations in early gastric cancer: the life cycle of the malignant ulcer, *Gastroenterology* 60:835, 1971.

54. Hamada T et al: Detection of early gastric cancer less than 1 cm in diameter during routine radiological examination, *I-to-Cho* 25:39, 1990.

55. Takekoshi T et al: Significance of endoscopic carbon ink injection method in recognition of boundary of gastric carcinoma, with special reference to defining proximal boundary, *I-to-Cho* 12:1031, 1977.

56. Ujiie T: A study on intramural injection of the stomach under direct vision by mean of fiberscope, *I-to-Cho* 6:211, 1971.

57. Stout AP: Superficial spreading type of carcinoma of the stomach, *Arch Surg* 44:651, 1942.

58. Yasui A et al: Pathology of superficial spreading type of gastric carcinoma, *I-to-Cho* 8:305, 1973.

59. Kumakura K et al: X-ray diagnosis of superficial spreading carcinoma of the stomach, *I-to-Cho* 8:1313, 1973.

60. Palmer WL: Pathology: classification, In Bockus HL, ed: *Gastroenterology,* vol 1, ed 3, Philadelphia, 1974, WB Saunders.

61. Nakamura K, et al: Growing process to carcinoma of linitis plastica type of the stomach from cancer development, *I-to-Cho* 15:225, 1980.

62. Igarashi T et al: Estimation of the depth of invasion in type IIc cancer: from the view of dynamic observations by double contrast study, *I-to-Cho* 12:433, 1977.

63. Nishimata H et al: Diagnostic ability of screening x-ray examination to pick-up type IIc early gastric cancers in the fundic gland area—early detection of linitis plastica type gastric cancers, *I-to-Cho* 22:1027, 1987.

64. Sasako M et al: Surgical treatment of carcinoma of the gastric stump, *Br J Surg* 78:822, 1991.

65. Hoshino H et al: Three cases of recurrent gastric cancer more than ten years after the initial operation, *I-to-Cho* 12:41, 1977.

66. Takagi K et al: Four cases of gastric cancer recurrence with free interval of more than 10 years after gastrectomy, *I-to-Cho* 12:47, 1977.

67. Akiyama H et al: Double cancer of the esophagus and stomach: cancer developing in the reconstructed esophagus, *Geka Chiryo* 28:245, 1973

68. Iizuka T et al: Carcinoma of the stomach tube after radical operation of esophageal carcinoma, *I-to-Cho* 12:433, 1977.

69. Kinoshita I et al: Metachronous double cancers of the esophagus and stomach: cancer developing in the reconstructed esophagus, *Jpn J Cancer Clin* 22:482, 1976.

70. Hamada T et al: Roentgen diagnosis of carcinoma of the postoperative stomach, *Radiat Med* 2:116, 1984

71. Oshima A: Screening for stomach cancer: the Japanese program: In Chamberlain J, Miller AB, eds: *Screening for gastrointestinal cancer:* 65, Bern, Stuttgart, 1988, Hans Huber.

72. Yamazaki et al: A long-term follow-up study of patients with gastric cancer detected by mass screening, *Cancer* 63:613, 1989.

73. Oshima A, et al: Evaluation of a mass screening program for stomach cancer with a case-control study design, *Int J Cancer* 38:829, 1986.

74. Murakami R et al: Estimation of validity of mass screening program for gastric cancer in Osaka, Japan, *Cancer* 65:255, 1990.

75. Hamajima C et al: A study of gastric mass survey by age groups, *Gastroenterol Mass Survey* 89:22, 1990.

20 *Malignant Tumors of the Stomach*

HENRY I. GOLDBERG

In this chapter, malignant tumors of the stomach other than adenocarcinoma are discussed. Such tumors are rare in the stomach, and include lymphoma, leiomyosarcoma, metastasis (melanoma, breast, lung), Kaposi's sarcoma, carcinoid tumors, villous adenomas, and leukemic infiltrate.

LYMPHOMA

The most common of the gastric malignancies other than adenocarcinoma is lymphoma. This tumor represents 1% to 5% of all gastric malignancies.[1] Ten percent of the cases are primary gastric malignancies, and the rest are part of a generalized lymphoma process.[1] Both Hodgkin's and non-Hodgkin's lymphomas occur in the stomach, but Hodgkin's disease is much rarer.[2] In 2% to 3% of patients with generalized non-Hodgkin's lymphoma, the stomach is involved.[3] The stomach is the most common site of extranodal involvement.

Gross and histologic appearance

The early phase of lymphoma has been classified[2] based on the depth of invasion, similar to the classification for early gastric adenocarcinoma. This classification includes superficial depressed lesions, polypoid lesions, ulceropolypoid lesions, and giant rugal enlargement. In this classification, early gastric lymphoma is limited to the submucosa of the stomach.

The more advanced phases are generally polypoid and ulcerating with infiltration of the gastric rugae or nodular tumor formation.[2] The superficial infiltrating type of lymphoma mimics the type 2C early gastric cancer.

Endoscopic superficial biopsies frequently are nondiagnostic in patients with suspected gastric lymphoma.[3] This is particularly true in the infiltrative or giant rugal type. However, the polypoid or ulcerative forms of lymphoma, which involve the gastric muscosa itself, are often diagnosed by endoscopic appearance and concomitant biopsy findings.

Radiographic findings—upper GI barium examination

The features of lymphoma demonstrated on the upper GI series are a manifestation of the depth of involvement of the lymphoma infiltrate and the amount of superficial ulceration present. Early in the disease process, the upper GI series may show evidence of a mass projecting into the lumen of the stomach with or without superficial erosion or ulceration. These masses may simulate gastric carcinoma. Multiple small polypoid lesions may be seen throughout the stomach (Fig. 20-1). If the lymphoma has infiltrated into and through the submucosa, the gastric rugae will be thickened locally. If the infiltration is advanced, the rugal thickening may be more extensive. One of the causes of giant rugal hypertrophy is this type of lymphoma. Usually the folds retain their flexibility with compression and the stomach is distensible. Ulcerations of these enlarged folds are not uncommon. The more advanced lymphomas of the stomach appear as sessile polypoid masses projecting into the lumen of the stomach, and they may reach several centimeters in size. In the most advanced cases, smoother, larger masses may occur, indicating the basic submucosal origin of the tumor. As lymphomas infiltrate submucosally, they are reflected in the presence of large rugal folds. Large ulcers within lymphomatous masses may be difficult to distinguish from benign gastric ulcer and advanced cancer. Fold enlargement may be focal or diffuse, involving most of the stomach (Fig. 20-2). The process may continue across the pylorus to involve the duodenal bulb.[4]

Ultrasound findings

External abdominal ultrasound performed to evaluate gastric lesions may reveal a markedly thick gastric wall. A spectrum of findings may be encountered, from mild thickening of the hypoechoic mucosal layer to circumferential smooth and nodular thickening to marked transmural bulky tumor.[5] The more advanced forms of lymphoma may therefore be detected in the water-filled stomach by virtue of this gastric wall thickening. However, the findings are not specific for lymphoma. Endoscopic transluminal ultrasound, by virtue of its ability to define the layers of the gastric wall, has the potential to detect processes that are submucosal. Therefore, in a patient in whom an endoscopic or barium examination demonstrates what appear to be large folds or submucosal masses, endoscopic luminal ultrasound may help in identifying the tumor as well as in characterizing it as diffusely infiltrating, which is suggestive of one form of lymphoma.

CT findings

The CT features of gastric lymphoma and adenocarcinoma may be similar.[6] Both may exhibit wall thickening, mural mass, ulceration, extension into perigastric fat, regional lymphadenopathy, and spread to peritoneum. How-

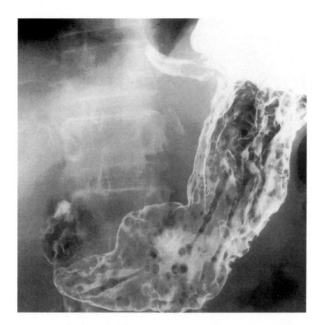

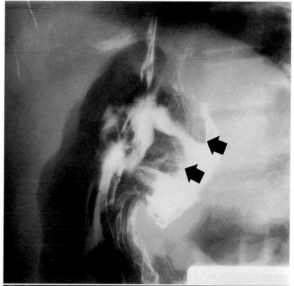

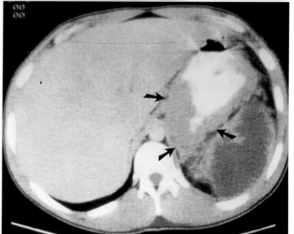

Fig. 20-1 Lymphoma of the stomach. Multiple small nodular lesions are distributed throughout the stomach in this double-contrast study. This appearance is one end of the spectrum that includes larger masses with or without ulceration and large irregular gastric rugae. The differential diagnosis of these multiple small polypoid nodules includes multiple polyps, polyposis syndromes, metastatic lesions from melanoma, or Kaposi's sarcoma.

Fig. 20-2 Lymphoma of the stomach. **A,** A limited single-contrast barium examination of the stomach shows enlarged distorted folds in the fundus *(arrows)*. **B,** A CT scan demonstrates extensive gastric wall thickening, greater than 2 cm in some portions *(arrows)*. The spleen is also involved by lymphoma.

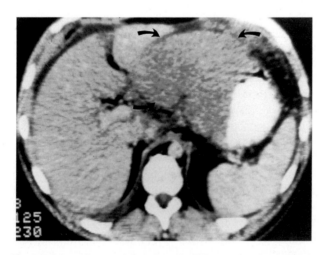

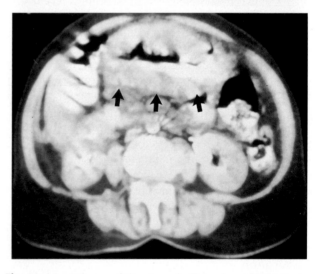

Fig. 20-3 Lymphoma of the stomach. CT scan showing an enormous mass extending from the medial portion of the fundus of the stomach *(arrows)*. Gastric masses of this size, with little intraluminal component, are either lymphomas or leiomyosarcomas.

Fig. 20-4 Lymphoma of the stomach. Extensive wall thickening (2 cm) circumferentially around the antrum of the stomach *(arrows)* is typical of lymphoma infiltrate of the gastric wall. Occasionally, adenocarcinoma of the scirrhous type may produce a similar appearance, although not usually with as much gastric wall thickening.

ever, some CT features are highly suggestive of lymphoma. Thickening of the gastric wall greater than 1 cm (Figs. 20-2 and 20-3), involving most or all of the stomach circumferentially, is most suggestive of lymphoma[1] (Fig. 20-4). The outer wall of the gastric lesion is often lobulated but smooth in contour with preservation of the fat planes between the tumor and adjacent organs.[1] Although this is often the case, in one third of cases a portion of the fat plane is obliterated.[7] Inhomogeneity in the CT appearance of the thickened gastric wall has been reported[4]; it is thought to result from tumor necrosis and hemorrhage. These necrotic tumors may perforate and fistulize into adjacent organs or into the lesser sac, producing a lesser sac or subphrenic fluid collection. Rapidly growing lymphomas or those respond-ing to chemotherapy or radiation therapy are more likely to perforate.[8] When a diffusely thickened gastric wall is detected on CT scan in the stomach distended with contrast material, lymphoma should be strongly considered, even if superficial mucosal biopsies have not been diagnostic, because endoscopic biopsies are not uncommonly negative in patients with lymphoma[9] (Fig. 20-5). In lymphoma, perigastric lymphadenopathy may involve the nodes in the gastrohepatic and gastrosplenic ligaments and in the peripancreatic and portahepatis regions, as well as the periaortocaval retroperitoneal nodes. This usually indicates disseminated disease, but it has been pointed out that reactive hyperplasia of nodes may occur with primary gastric lymphoma.[7]

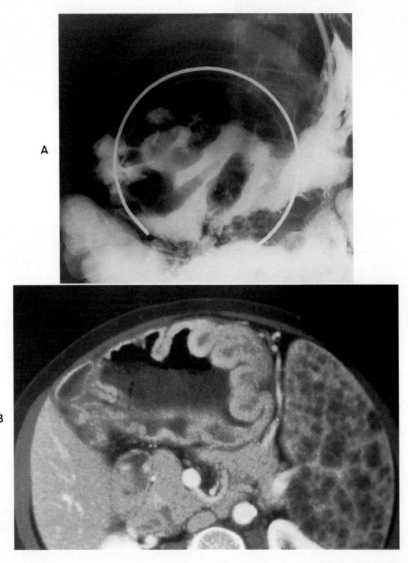

Fig. 20-5 Lymphoma of the stomach and spleen. **A,** Extensive enlargement of gastric folds is present on barium radiograph of the stomach. **B,** Markedly thickened gastric rugae are present in the body of the stomach. In addition, multiple low-density lesions are present in an enlarged spleen. Two superficial endoscopic biopsies revealed only chronic inflammation. However, a third, deeper endoscopic biopsy demonstrated non-Hodgkin's lymphoma.

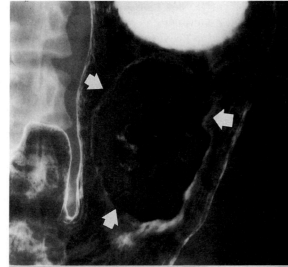

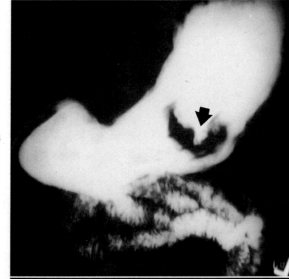

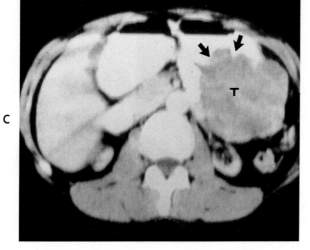

LEIOMYOSARCOMA

Leiomyosarcomas are rare gastric tumors that arise from gastric wall smooth muscle and are estimated to represent 1% to 3% of primary gastric malignancies.[10] Patients harboring gastric leiomyosarcomas may present with abdominal pain, a palpable mass, or gastrointestinal bleeding. Some of these tumors are not discovered until they are over 10 cm in size and have ulcerated, thereby explaining the clinical findings. While leiomyosarcomas grow to a very large size, most of the tumor mass is extramural, projecting into the perigastric space. Usually only a small portion of these mural tumors projects into the gastric lumen. However, ulceration frequently occurs in the intraluminal portion.

The diagnosis of leiomyosarcoma is based on histologic evidence, either from endoscopically obtained biopsy or surgically obtained biopsy of pleomorphism and the presence of myotic figures along with hypercellularity and tumor necrosis.[11] About half of these tumors metastasize, the most common site being the liver. Direct extension into the omentum retroperitoneum and adjacent organs such as the liver and pancreas may occur.

Radiographic features

Typically, leiomyosarcomas appear as smooth, rounded masses projecting into the lumen in the fundus and body of the stomach (Fig. 20-6). They are best seen on double-contrast examinations.[2] A central depression representing ulceration is often present. The ulceration may vary in size, depth, and contour, so it may in some instances occupy a large portion of the tumor mass. If the exogastric portion of the tumor is large, the stomach may be displaced by the mass as may be a part of the transverse colon. The differential diagnosis on barium radiography includes all other types of submucosal tumors (leiomyoblastomas, fibromas, lipomas, neurogenic lesions, carcinoids). Radiographic differentiation of leiomyoma and leiomyosarcoma is based mainly on size, the sarcomas being larger.

Fig. 20-6 Leiomyosarcoma of the body of the stomach. **A,** Double-contrast gastric examination demonstrates a large, smooth, but somewhat lobulated mass, seen en face, on the posterior wall of the stomach *(arrows)*. Irregular barium collections in the center suggest central ulcerations. **B,** An overhead radiographic study obtained after fluoroscopy also suggests the presence of an ulceration *(arrow)* in the mass. **C,** A CT scan illustrates the intraluminal portion of the tumor *(arrows)*. The surface is irregular on the anterior portion, consistent with ulceration. The majority of the tumor *(T)* projects beyond the gastric wall into the perigastric space. These findings are typical of gastric leiomyosarcoma.

Ultrasound features

Endoscopic ultrasonographic features of leiomyosarcomas have been recently described.[12] These leiomyosarcomas may be seen to arise from the outer muscularis propria layers as rounded hypoechoic enlargements of this layer, often greater than 3.5 cm in size, with lobulated borders and a central heterogeneous appearance.

CT features

On CT scans of the upper abdomen, leiomyoscarcomas often appear as bulky soft tissue density masses that have their base in the wall of the stomach but extend outside the stomach into the adjacent perigastric tissue[10] (Figs. 20-6, and 20-7). Most often they have a smooth contour to the surface projecting into the stomach lumen and a lobulated contour on the external surface. The ulceration seen on the gastric lumen surface may be deep enough to be detected by CT scans. Leiomyosarcomas often have areas of central necrosis, which appear on intravenous contrast CT scans as low-density areas against the background of the enhanced vascular portion of the tumor. Calcifications may also been seen in the tumor.[7] Liver metastases from leiomyosarcoma are also vascular and contain areas of central low density representing necrosis (Fig. 20-7). Hematogenous metastases also occur in the lungs and bones. Direct extension of leiomyosarcomas into other organs such as spleen, pancreas, and omentum can be detected best by CT scanning. Metastasis to regional lymph nodes is uncommon.[6] In general the combination of barium and CT scan features permit adequate differentiation of leiomyosarcomas from adenocarcinoma and lymphoma.[6,13]

METASTASES

Hematogenous metastasis to the stomach is a rare occurrence (0.2% to 2.3% of gastric malignancies).[2] The most common primary tumors that metastasize to the stomach are breast, lung, melanoma, ovary, and thyroid (Fig. 20-8). In addition, esophageal squamous carcinomas may occasionally invade the gastric fundus (Fig. 20-9). Direct extension of pancreatic carcinoma and carcinoma of the transverse co-

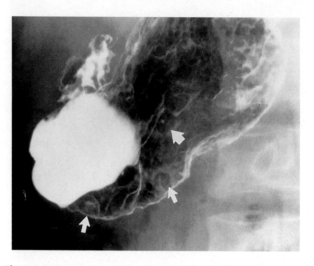

Fig. 20-8 Metastatic gastric melanoma. On double-contrast examination, multiple large mucosal nodules are seen *(smaller arrows)*. These metastatic melanoma masses sometimes contain central ulcerations *(large arrow)*. The differential diagnosis of this appearance includes lymphoma and Kaposi's sarcoma.

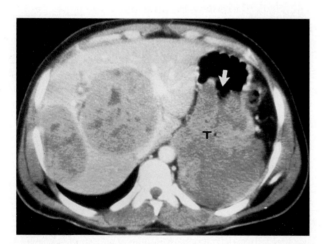

Fig. 20-7 Gastric leiomyosarcoma. Only a small portion of this tumor *(T)* projects into the gastric lumen, and that portion appears to contain a central ulceration *(arrow)*. Most of the tumor is in the perigastric space and has a heterogeneous CT density. Liver metastases are present that have areas of higher CT density suggesting vascular enhancement.

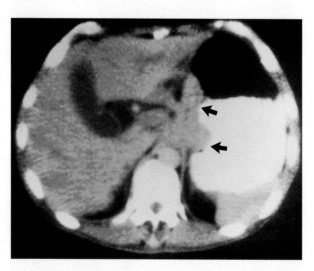

Fig. 20-9 Metastatic esophageal carcinoma to fundus of stomach. Squamous carcinoma of the esophagus may occasionally metastasize to gastric wall and adjacent lymph nodes, illustrated on this CT scan *(arrows)*.

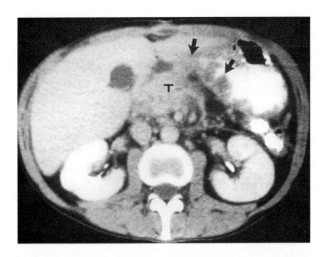

Fig. 20-10 Pancreatic carcinoma directly invading the stomach. A pancreatic tumor *(T)* invades the gastric wall and extends along the gastric wall producing nodular masses *(arrow)*.

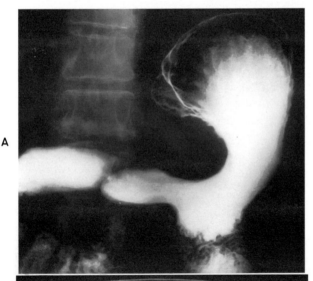

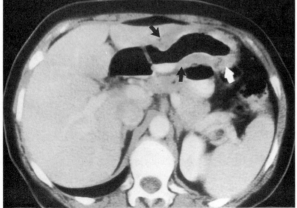

lon into the stomach may occur[6] via gastrocolic splenorenal, and gastrosplenic ligaments (Fig. 20-10). Most metastatic lesions involve the submucosa of the stomach, resulting in a smooth mass with an obtuse to straight angle with the gastric mucosa. These masses are often ulcerated. This is best seen with double-contrast or single-contrast upper GI examinations. Multiple metastases may involve the gastric wall, producing multiple nodular lesions on barium studies. The ulceration seen in the center of metastatic lesions has been called the "bull's eye sign" and is typical of melanomas[14] but has also been seen with lung, pancreas, and colon.[2] On CT scans, these lesions seen in profile appear as intramural masses with gastric wall thickening locally and cavitation in the mass resulting from superficial ulceration. Diffuse gastric wall thickening, suggestive of linitis plastica on both barium studies and CT, may be produced by metastatic breast cancer[6] (Fig. 20-11).

CARCINOID TUMORS

Carcinoid tumors are rare tumors of the stomach that are derived from neuroectodermal cells and originate in the deep layer of the mucosa from Kulchitsky's cells in the crypts of Lieberkühn. The carcinoids of the stomach are capable of endocrine activity, secreting 5-hydroxytryptophan (not serotonin). Thus the carcinoid syndrome is almost never observed with gastric carcinoids.[15]

Although these tumors may secrete other hormones, they usually cause clinical findings by virtue of their mass effect and ulceration. Pain, nausea and vomiting, and gastrointestinal bleeding are common clinical presentations.[16] Carcinoid may be malignant and may metastasize to local lymph nodes and the liver. The prognosis appears to be related to the size of the lesion, with tumors 2 cm or larger more likely to exhibit local invasion.[15] The most common radiographic appearance on single- or double-contrast upper GI barium study is that of a single intramural mass. These are well circumscribed, smooth, and 1 to 3 cm in size. Often an ulcer is seen in the center. Carcinoids have a similar appearance to small leiomyomas or any other intramural tumor. Other forms of gastric carcinoid include polypoid lesions and large ulcerating masses simulating carcinoma.

Fig. 20-11 Breast carcinoma metastatic to antrum of stomach. **A,** On the gastric barium examination, the distal body and antrum are diffusely narrowed. This appearance can be seen with breast metastasis, but also results from scirrhous gastric carcinoma (linitis plastica) after radiation, after caustic ingestion, and from syphilis. **B,** CT scan shows diffuse gastric wall thickening involving the antrum *(arrows)* but sparing the duodenal bulb.

KAPOSI'S SARCOMA

Kaposi's sarcoma is an unusual tumor of the stomach that has been recently reported in patients with AIDS.[12,17-19] Patients with AIDS have a high likelihood of developing GI tract Kaposi's sarcoma.[18] The gastric involvement may be part of multifocal involvement of the GI tract including the esophagus, duodenum, small bowel, and colon. Findings on upper GI series are most typically of polypoid or nodular lesions, plaques, or raised lesions with umbilications, thickened folds, and actual masses. The CT appearance of Kaposi's sarcoma most likely reflects the size of the nodular lesions and the amount of gastric wall thickening associated with this (Fig. 20-12).

VILLOUS ADENOMA

Recently, four cases of villous adenoma of the stomach were reported in the radiologic literature.[20] Two of these were found histologically to contain malignancy. All were discovered on upper GI series as fairly large solitary lobulated lesions 2 to 6 cm in diameter. They occurred in the midbody of the stomach.

GASTRIC INVOLVEMENT BY LEUKEMIA

Leukemic infiltration of the gastric wall has been noted recently.[21] In five patients, diffuse gastrointestinal involvement was present with nausea and vomiting. The gastric findings reflected the infiltrative nature of the leukemic cell, demonstrating a generalized scirrhous appearance with thick folds in the body of the stomach and an abnormal granular mucosal pattern seen on double-contrast studies and endoscopy.

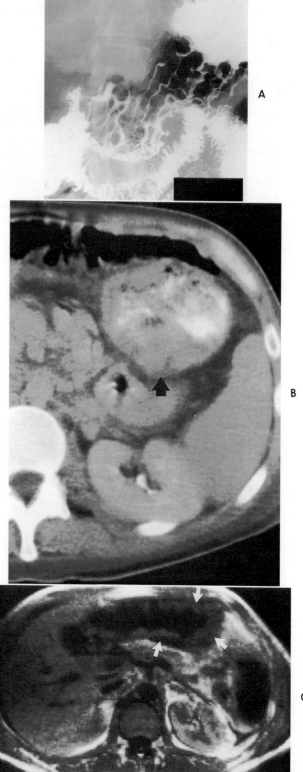

Fig. 20-12 Kaposi's sarcoma of the stomach. **A,** The gastric barium examination shows multiple nodular masses in the stomach associated with thickened gastric rugae. The nodular masses are typical of Kaposi's sarcoma and are seen in patients with AIDS. Metastatic melanoma, lymphoma, or multiple polyps may have a similar appearance. **B,** The CT scan shows that the disease process has also thickened the gastric wall (*arrow*). **C,** A T1 MRI scan demonstrates both nodularity of the lumenal contour and thickening of the gastric wall (*arrows*).

REFERENCES

1. Moss AA: Computed tomography in staging of gastrointestinal carcinoma, *Radiol Clin North Am* 20:771, 1982.
2. Shirakebe H, Mariyama M: Neoplastic diseases of the stomach. In Margulis AR, Burhenne HJ, eds: *Alimentary tract radiology,* ed 4, St Louis, 1989, Mosby–Year Book.
3. Davis GR: Neoplasms of the stomach. In Sleisenger and Fordtran, eds: *Gastrointestinal disease,* ed 3, Philadelphia, 1983, WB Saunders.
4. Maklansky D, Linder A, Kurzban JD: Gastric neoplasms, In Traveras J, Ferrucci JT, eds: *Radiology,* Philadelphia, 1987, JB Lippincott.
5. Goerg C, Schwerk WB, Goerg K: Gastrointestinal lymphoma: sonographic findings in 54 patients, *AJR* 155:795, 1990.
6. Scatarige JC, DiSantis DJ: CT of the stomach and duodenum, *Radiol Clin North Am* 27:687, 1989.
7. Thoeni RF, Moss AA: The gastrointestinal tract. In Moss AA, Gamsu G, Genant HK, eds: *Computed tomography of the body,* ed 2, Philadelphia, 1991, WB Saunders.
8. Megabow AJ: Gastrointestinal lymphoma: the role of CT on diagnosis and management, *Semin Ultrasound CT MR* 7:43, 1986.
9. Fork FT, Haglund U, Hogstrom H, Wehlin L: Primary gastric lymphoma versus gastric cancer: an endoscopic and radiographic study of differential diagnostic possibilities, *Endoscopy* 17:5, 1985.
10. Nauert TC, Zornoza J, Ordonez N: Gastric leiomyosarcomas, *AJR* 139:291, 1982.
11. Spjut H: Stomach and duodenum pathology. In Margulis AR, Burhenne HJ, eds: *Alimentary tract radiology,* ed 4, St Louis, 1989.
12. Nakazawa S, Yoshino J, Nakamura T, et al: Endoscopic ultrasonography of gastric myogenic tumor: a comparative study between histology and ultrasonography, *J Ultrasound Med* 8:353, 1989.
13. Megibow AJ, Bathazar EJ, Hulnick DH: CT evaluation of gastrointestinal leiomyomas and leiomyosarcomas, *AJR* 144:727, 1985.
14. Pomeranz H, Margolin HN: Metastasis to the gastrointestinal tract from malignant melanoma, *AJR* 88:712, 1962.
15. Belthazar EJ: Carcinoid tumors. In Marshak RH, Lindner AE, Maklansky D, eds: *Radiology of the stomach,* Philadelphia, 1983, WB Saunders.
16. Honig LJ, Weingarten G: A gastric carcinoid tumor with massive bleeding, *Am J Gastroenterol* 61:40, 1974.
17. Finger DH, Frager JD, Brandt LJ et al: Gastrointestinal complications of AIDS: radiologic features, *Radiology* 158:597, 1986.
18. Wall SD, Ominsky S, Altman DF et al: Multifocal abnormalities of the gastrointestinal tract in AIDS, *AJR* 146:1, 1986.
19. Jones B, Fishman EK: CT of the gut in the immunocompromised host, *Radiol Clin North Am* 27:763, 1989.
20. Gaitini D, Kleinhaus U, Munichor M, Duck D: Villous tumors of the stomach, *Gastrointest Radiol* 13:105, 1988.
21. Utsunomiya A, Hanada A, Terada A, Kodama M, Uematsu T et al: Adult T cell leukemia with leukemic cell infiltration into the gastrointestinal tract, *Cancer* 61:824, 1988.

21 CT and MR Staging of Gastric Carcinoma

ROBERT A. HALVORSEN

Although the prevalence of gastric carcinoma has steadily declined worldwide since 1930, it remains a significant health risk in the United States. In this country, the death rate from gastric carcinoma has declined from 30/100,000 in 1930, when this disease was the most frequent cause of cancer death, to 4/100,000 in 1990. US rates are now among the lowest in the world. Gastric carcinoma is now ranked fifth to sixth in importance among cancer deaths. However, stomach cancer remains more common in older people as the cause of cancer death in the United States. Approximately 23,200 new cases of gastric carcinoma and 13,700 deaths resulting from the disease were estimated to have occurred in 1990.[1] The unexplained decrease in this highly lethal malignancy is particularly striking when considered in the context of the very high incidence rates of gastric carcinomas in countries such as Japan and Costa Rica. Dietary factors that have been associated with a high incidence of gastric cancer include smoked food, salted food, and aflatoxin.[2]

Although during this century the incidence of all types of gastric carcinoma has fallen sharply in this country, adenocarcinoma of the gastric cardia has become more common.[3] The annual incidence and mortality associated with all types of gastric adenocarcinomas reached a minimum in 1976 when 22,900 new cases were reported. However, the incidence of gastric cancer has been slowly and steadily rising, with 24,400 cases expected in 1992. Despite the low rate of stomach cancer overall, an alarming trend exists: adenocarcinoma of the gastric cardia has increased dramatically, far outpacing increases in other tumors such as melanoma, lung cancer, and non-Hodgkin's lymphoma. The more proximal gastric carcinomas are more aggressive than distal adenocarcinomas and account for almost half of all gastric cancers in white men. Men are four times more likely than women to be diagnosed with proximal lesions, whereas distal lesions are equally common between the sexes.

Gastric cancer is more common among the lower socioeconomic groups and people who emigrated to the United States as compared with native-born Americans.[2] Several conditions appear to predispose patients to malignancy. Patients with pernicious anemia have been reported to have gastric carcinoma 20 times more frequently than the general population.[2] Intestinal metaplasia and atrophic gastritis appear to be precursor lesions of gastric cancer. Intestinal metaplastic change, defined as a replacement of the stomach epithelium by intestinal epithelium containing goblet cells, is more frequent in countries where the incidence of gastric cancer is high. Intestinal metaplasia occurs with known gastric carcinogens but also occurs in patients after gastric resection for benign peptic ulcer disease. Postoperative patients have decreased gastric acid, which may favor the development of intestinal metaplasia of the stomach.

PATHOLOGY

Approximately 95% of malignant neoplasms of the stomach are adenocarcinoma. While other tumors such as adenoacanthoma, squamous cell carcinoma, and carcinoid tumors do occur in the stomach, they are infrequent, representing less than 1% of gastric malignancies. Leiomyosarcomas of the stomach are more frequent, accounting for between 1% and 3% of gastric malignancies. Gastric lymphoma is the most frequent site of primary GI tract lymphoma and is usually a non-Hodgkin's lymphoma. Secondary involvement of the stomach is more frequent than primary gastric lymphoma.

There are four types of gross pathologic features with gastric carcinoma. First, the majority of gastric carcinomas are ulcerative.[4] Second, polypoid lesions account for approximately 10% of gastric carcinomas. The third type of gastric cancer is the scirrhous type, which also represents approximately 10% of gastric adenocarcinomas. In scirrhous lesions there is a desmoplastic reaction within the gastric wall leading to a stiffened stomach giving the appearance of linitis plastica. The appearance of a scirrhous pattern has prognostic significance, since this type of tumor is almost uniformly fatal. The fourth type of gastric carcinoma is the superficial variety, which is uncommon, and is characterized by sheetlike collections of cancer cells replacing the normal mucosa.

Early gastric cancer is defined as tumor confined within the mucosal or submucosal layers without metastasis. Once a tumor extends beyond the submucosa, the lesion is defined as an advanced gastric cancer and the probability of metastases increases substantially.

ANATOMIC CONSIDERATIONS

The patterns of spread of gastric cancer include direct extension, nodal metastases, vascular metastases, and peritoneal metastases. Direct spread includes extension into the stomach, pylorus, and duodenum or the ligamentous attachments of the esophagus such as the lesser omentum and gastrocolic ligament. Lymphatic spread may lead to local or distant lymph node metastases. Vascular metastases gener-

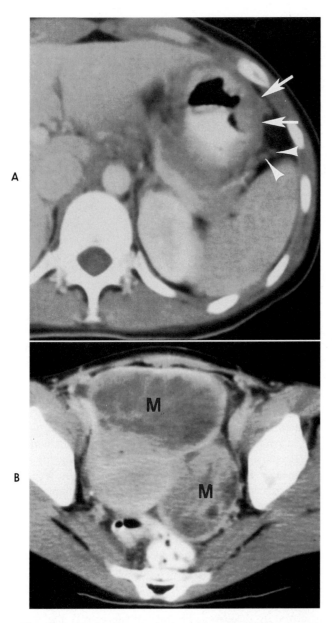

Fig. 21-1 Gastric adenocarcinoma with peritoneal drop metastases. **A,** CT of left upper quadrant demonstrates tumor *(arrows)* along greater curve of stomach with adjacent small lymph nodes *(arrowheads)* and obliteration of fat plane between stomach and pancreas posteriorly. **B,** Pelvic metastases *(M)*. Note large metastasis anterior to uterus and second smaller lesion in left adnexa representing Krukenberg's tumor.

ally involve the liver first because of the venous drainage of the stomach, but pulmonary, bone, or brain metastases are not uncommon. Peritoneal metastases occur when there is spillage of tumor cells from the serosal surface of the stomach or, less probably, from the lumen of the stomach at the time of an operative procedure. Peritoneal metastases can be disseminated through the abdominal cavity or can be found in the pelvis with such lesions as drop metastases to Blumer's rectal shelf, or to the ovary as a Krukenberg's tumor (Fig. 21-1).

Direct spread of gastric cancers can occur into contiguous organs such as esophagus and duodenum. Involvement of the greater and lesser omentum is frequent with gastric carcinoma. Anatomically, the omenta are a continuation of the gastric serosa and are easily involved once the cancer spreads to the serosal surface. While direct extension into the omentum is the most frequent type of omental involvement, lymphatic, hematogenous, or peritoneal spread can also occur to these structures. Direct extension along the gastrocolic ligament may involve the transverse colon (Fig. 21-2). Tumors can extend into the gastrosplenic ligament along the left side of the greater curve of the stomach directly to the spleen. Tumors that involve the lesser curve of the stomach may extend directly to the liver via the gastrohepatic ligament. Posterior lesions may extend into the lesser sac and secondarily into the pancreas or the transverse mesocolon and indirectly into the transverse colon.

The lymphatic drainage of the stomach can be divided into three major systems: the left gastric chain, the splenic chain, and the hepatic chain.[2] The lymphatic pathways are complex and interconnected; the lymphatic channels generally follow the pathways of the major vascular supply to the stomach. When there is early blockage of lymphatic channels, the lymphatic drainage pattern is altered, causing retrograde lymphatic flow. Because of the rich lymphatic supply to the stomach and the possibility of altered flow direction, it is generally difficult to predict which lymph nodes will be involved with a particular tumor location. However, distal gastric lesions are less frequently found to metastasize to the lymphatics in the splenic chain.

STAGING

In 1988 the American Joint Committee on Cancer published new TNM staging criteria for gastric cancer.[5] The new staging criteria represent a simplification of the previous system. In the staging of the primary tumor (T), the depth of invasion through the gastric wall is the only criterion assessed with the new system; the size of the tumor is of no consequence. Involvement of regional lymph nodes (N) has been simplified, with the N categories reduced from five to four. Many abdominal lymph nodes previously considered regional nodes are now considered distant metastases. Therefore the definition of distant metastases (M) has been redefined to include more abdominal lymph node groups.

For the purpose of staging, the stomach is divided into three anatomic regions: the upper, middle, and lower thirds.

Staging systems

Staging is divided into clinical and pathologic staging. Clinical staging is designated as *cTNM* and is based on physical examination, imaging findings, endoscopy, and biopsy. Pathologic staging, designated *pTNM,* is based on data acquired clinically and on results of surgical exploration and examination of the resected specimen or biopsy. In general, if there is doubt concerning the correct T, N, or M assignment, the lower or less advanced category is selected.

Primary site (T)

The new staging criteria for the primary tumor (T) are listed in the box on the right. Note that the size of the tu-

☐ **PRIMARY TUMOR** ☐

TX	Primary tumor cannot be assessed
TO	No evidence of primary tumor
Tis	Carcinoma in situ: intraepithelial tumor without invasion of the lamina propria
T1	Tumor invades lamina propria or submucosa
T2	Tumor invades the muscularis propria or the subserosa
T3	Tumor penetrates the serosa (visceral peritoneum) without invasion of adjacent structures
T4	Tumor invades adjacent structures

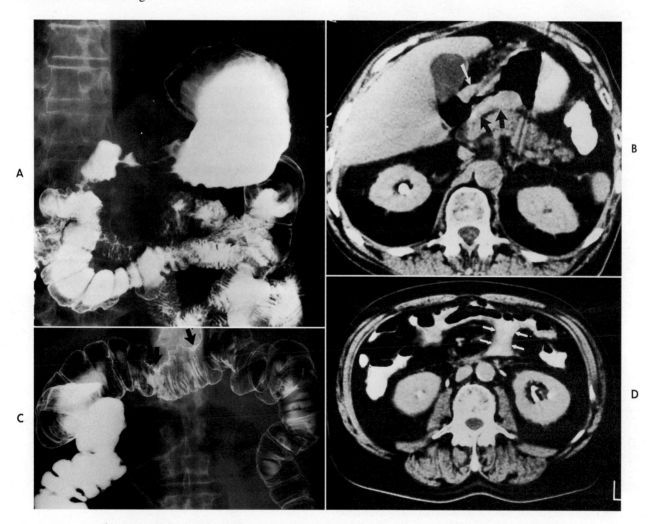

Fig. 21-2 Direct tumor extension along gastrocolic ligament and transverse mesocolon. **A,** Antral carcinoma with circumferential narrowing of distal stomach. **B,** CT demonstrates circumferential antral tumor *(arrows).* **C,** Air contrast barium enema reveals irregular nodular masses *(arrows)* along superior aspect of transverse colon. **D,** CT demonstrates soft tissue mass *(arrows)* extending from transverse colon posteriorly along transverse mesocolon.
From Halvorsen RA Jr, Thompson WM: *Semin Ultrasound CT MR* 10:467, 1989.

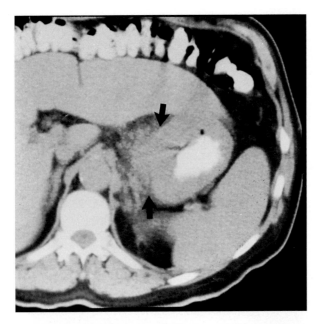

Fig. 21-3 Gastrohepatic ligament extension (T2). Note circumferential tumor with no abnormality in perigastric fat laterally, but ill-defined margin medially *(between arrows)*. Tumor had spread directly into gastrohepatic ligament at surgery.

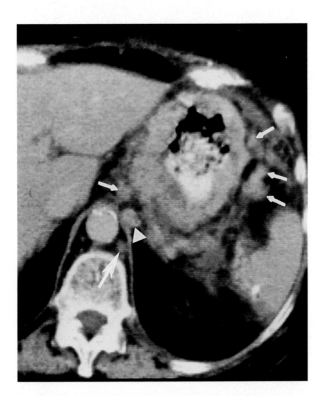

Fig. 21-4 Regional lymph nodes. Circumferential adenocarcinoma in midstomach. Note multiple lymph node metastases *(small arrows)* along greater and lesser curvature. Nodes have ill-defined outer margins. One node is in direct contact with left diaphragmatic crus *(arrowhead)*. Note enlarged lymph node in retrocrural space *(large arrow)*, which represents a distant metastasis—*not a regional lymph node*.

mor is not used to define T, only the depth of invasion. With the new staging system a tumor may penetrate the muscularis propria with extension into the gastrocolic or gastrohepatic ligaments or into the greater or lesser omentum without perforation of the visceral peritoneum covering these structures and still be considered a T2 lesion (Fig. 21-3). Only when there is perforation of the visceral peritoneum covering the gastric ligaments or omenta is the tumor upgraded to a T3.

When there is intramural extension into the duodenum or distal esophagus, the tumor is classified by the depth of the greatest invasion in any of these sites, including the stomach. Esophageal or duodenal extension is not considered invasion of an adjacent structure. For TNM classification the adjacent structures of the stomach are the spleen, transverse colon, liver, diaphragm, pancreas, abdominal wall, adrenal gland, kidney, small intestine, and retroperitoneum.

Regional lymph nodes (N)

The definition of regional lymph nodes varies depending on the location of the tumor in the gastric wall. N1 nodes are defined as metastases in perigastric lymph nodes (S) within 3 cm of the edge of the primary tumor. N2 nodes are defined as metastases in perigastric lymph nodes more than 3 cm from the edge of the primary tumor (Fig. 21-4) or in lymph nodes along the left gastric, common hepatic, splenic, or celiac arteries (Fig. 21-5).

The previous TNM system (the second edition) included an N3 category. Many of the nodes that were previously considered N3 are now considered distant sites and should be recorded as M1. These include the paraaortic, hepatoduodenal, retropancreatic, and mesenteric lymph node groups.

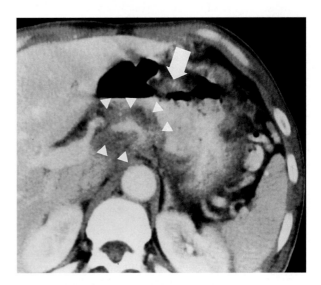

Fig. 21-5 Gastric adenocarcinoma anteriorly *(arrow)* with extensive retrogastric adenopathy enwrapping hepatic artery *(arrowheads)* defined as N2 nodal involvement.

Distant metastases (M)

Metastases are classified as either M0 (no distant metastases) or M1 (distant metastases present). Metastases are most frequently encountered in the liver (Fig. 21-6). The next two most common sites of metastases are the peritoneum and omentum, which are involved only half as often as the liver. The lung and the adrenal glands are the most commonly involved distant organs.

Stage grouping

The stages are listed in Table 21-1. In the new staging system there are seven stage groupings for finer discrimination. Stages I and III have been subdivided into A and B groupings. Any metastasis results in a stage IV classification, but N2 regional nodes more than 3 cm from the primary tumor may result in a IIIA, IIIB, or stage IV classification depending on the associated staging of the primary tumor.

Histopathologic staging

The staging recommendations apply only to carcinomas and not to other tumor types such as lymphomas or sarcomas. Adenocarcinomas are divided into three subtypes: intestinal, diffuse, and mixed. The prognosis is worse for the diffuse type of tumor. Histopathologic grading (G) is rated: *GX*, grade cannot be assessed; *G1*, well differentiated; *G2*, moderately well differentiated; *G3*, poorly differentiated; *G4*, undifferentiated.

COMPUTED TOMOGRAPHIC STAGING OF GASTRIC CARCINOMA

Computed tomography (CT) can detect local invasion, enlarged tumor-containing lymph nodes, and distant metastases in patients with gastric cancer. However, the role of CT in the staging of gastric carcinoma is controversial. The ability of CT to accurately determine the degree of local invasion and the presence of tumor within normal and abnormal size lymph nodes has been questioned.[6] Some argue that a CT procedure is unnecessary for staging because many gastric cancer patients require surgery either for attempted cure or palliation, and staging of the cancers could be done at that time.[7] However, more than 25% of patients who receive surgical exploration have no procedure other than open biopsy because of the advanced stage of disease encountered.[8-10]

Initial reports were enthusiastic. In a series of 40 patients, 28 of whom had gastric adenocarcinoma studied by CT, Moss et al.[11] reported no instances of inaccurate staging of

☐ **TABLE 21-1**
Stage grouping

Stage	Primary tumor	Regional lymph nodes	Distant metastases
Stage 0	Tis	N0	M0
Stage IA	T1	N0	M0
Stage IB	T1M	N1	M0
	T2	N0	
Stage II	T1	N2	M0
	T2	N1	
	T3	N0	
Stage IIIA	T2	N2	M0
	T3	N1	M0
	T4	N0	M0
Stage IIIB	T3	N2	M0
	T4	N1	M0
Stage IV	T4	N2	M0
	Any T	Any N	M1

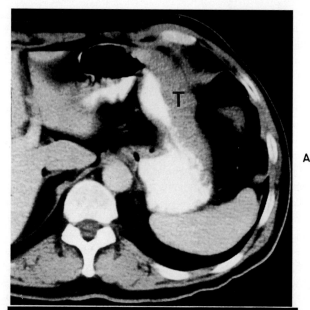

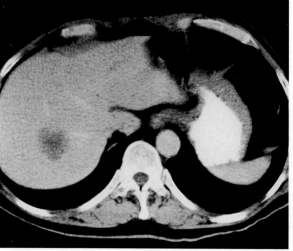

Fig. 21-6 Liver metastases. **A,** Primary tumor *(T)* has smooth inner and outer margins with no evidence of extension into perigastric fat. **B,** Solitary metastasis in posterior segment of right lobe of liver makes tumor M1 and therefore stage IV lesion.

gastric carcinoma by CT. Another early report of eight patients with gastric carcinoma recommended CT as a valuable method for the preoperative workup of patients with malignant gastric neoplasms.[12] However, the authors report that CT did not detect one case of gastrohepatic ligament extension, was unable to detect involvement of perigastric lymph nodes, and missed one case of liver metastases. In a study of 12 patients reported by Balfe et al.,[13] obliteration of the fat plane between the posterior wall of the stomach and the pancreas correctly identified retrogastric spread of tumor in three patients. They concluded that CT could provide valuable information regarding the extent of the tumor or involvement of adjacent organs but was not the primary diagnostic modality in the evaluation of gastric neoplasms. In another study the potential economic impact of preoperative staging of gastric adenocarcinoma using CT was analyzed.[14] Moss et al. suggested in a review of 22 patients with proven gastric adenocarcinoma that CT staging correlated closely with surgical findings and was superior to other diagnostic modalities in the evaluation of local extension, regional adenopathy, and the size of tumor mass. They compared the cost of CT staging with the cost of surgical exploration and concluded that CT not only was accurate but that it was also a cost-effective method of preoperatively staging gastric carcinoma.

In an editorial rebutting Moss et al.'s conclusions, two surgeons, McFee and Aust,[15] stated that Moss et al. had failed to appreciate a fundamental point. They wrote that "abdominal exploration in visceral carcinoma, and especially in gastric cancer, is not done primarily to stage the disease. It is done to remove the disease and effect a cure or as significant a palliation as possible." They also state that where there were laparotomies in patients with gastric carcinoma performed routinely "only to stage the extent of gastric neoplastic spread, a very considerable case could be made for substituting the CAT scan. They [laparotomies] are not." Because the surgical procedure provides the only relief from the disease in question, CT studies should not be used to preclude patients from operative intervention.

In another study evaluating the ability of CT as an alternative to laparotomy for predicting the stage and resectability of gastric carcinoma, Cook et al.[16] evaluated 37 patients with gastric adenocarcinoma who received preoperative CT scanning. The extent of the disease found during the operation and at pathology was compared with the CT findings. In 19 patients (51%), there was more extensive disease than was predicted by CT. Of the six patients predicted by CT to have widespread disease, three (50%) were found at operation to have disease confined to the stomach or regional lymph nodes. They concluded that there is a continued role for laparotomy in managing patients with gastric adenocarcinoma, since a significant percentage of patients whose disease is believed to be unresectable based on CT findings have potentially curable lesions at operation.

In what is the largest series of patients with gastric adenocarcinoma and in whom preoperative CT findings were compared with surgical and pathologic findings, Sussman et al.[17] reported the findings in 75 patients. We concluded that CT does not accurately display the true extent of disease in patients with gastric carcinoma and therefore should not be used for routine staging of patients with gastric carcinoma. CT was found to be incapable of accurately predicting involvement of lymph nodes or direct pancreatic invasion and was inaccurate in predicting TNM staging.

Adenopathy

In our study,[17] CT was insensitive in detecting adenopathy, with a sensitivity of only 67%. Five of the 14 false-negative cases of lymph node involvement not detected with CT were patients who had peritumoral lymph nodes confluent with the primary tumor. The inability of CT to detect lymph nodes adjacent to the primary tumor mass has been described by others[12,16,18] and represents a pitfall of CT's ability to stage gastric cancer (Fig. 21-7). The other missed lymph node metastases occurred in patients with metastases in normal-sized lymph nodes (Fig. 21-8). Lymph nodes were considered abnormally enlarged if they were larger than 8 mm in the gastrohepatic ligament, 6 mm in the retrocrural space, and 15 mm in greatest diameter in other locations in the abdomen.

Enlarged lymph nodes detected by CT but found to be free of malignancy at surgery were noted in 13 patients, resulting in a poor specificity of only 61%. The lymph node enlargement may have resulted from reactive hyperplasia or benign enlargement of these lymph nodes caused by adjacent inflammation or infection. In another study of 33 patients with gastric adenocarcinoma studied with CT, Botet et al.[19] also demonstrated poor results in determining whether nodes contained malignancy. Using larger than 1 cm as the criterion for lymph node enlargement, they reported a concordance of only 48% between the CT study and pathologic findings for lymph node involvement.

Komaki[20] has suggested two concepts that might decrease the number of false-positive CT examinations of lymph nodes.[20] He recommends that adenopathy be characterized as either massive or solitary. In his series, massive adenopathy represented metastatic disease in 96% of cases, whereas solitary adenopathy represented metastatic disease in only 48% of cases. In the study by Sussman et al.,[17] the majority of the false-positive CT studies for adenopathy (62%) demonstrated only solitary adenopathy. Therefore a single enlarged lymph node is less likely to contain a metastasis than is a group of enlarged lymph nodes.

The second point Komaki made is the benefit of using dynamic CT in assessing nodal enhancement. In his series, enhancement was found in 82% of normal lymph nodes, whereas no enhancement was found in lymph nodes replaced by metastatic disease.

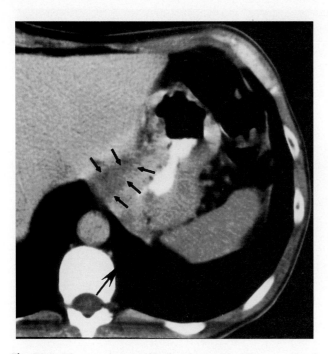

Fig. 21-7 Adenocarcinoma of body of stomach. Note area of soft tissue density medial to stomach of slightly lower density than primary tumor *(small arrows)*, representing matted gastrohepatic ligament lymph nodes inseparable from primary tumor at surgery.

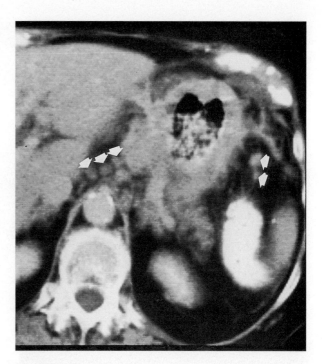

Fig. 21-8 Tumor in normal-sized lymph nodes. Adenocarcinoma with bulky circumferential tumor with multiple lymph nodes *(arrows)* in gastrohepatic ligament and along greater curvature that were normal in size but contained tumor at surgery.

Pancreatic invasion

Pancreatic invasion is typically predicted when CT studies demonstrate the absence of the fat plane between the gastric tumor and an adjacent organ such as the pancreas (Figs. 21-9 to 21-11). In the study by Sussman et al., CT failed to accurately predict pancreatic invasion. In eight patients, CT demonstrated an intact fat plane between the tumor mass and the pancreas, whereas surgery and pathologic examination showed direct invasion to be present, resulting in a sensitivity of only 27% for pancreatic invasion. Other authors have also found that CT is insensitive in detecting pancreatic invasion. Cook et al.[16] reported a sensitivity of only 60% for detection of pancreatic invasion, and Frasier et al.[21] reported CT missing pancreatic invasion in 9 of 11 patients in whom invasion was found at surgery. Absence of the peripancreatic fat plane appears to be an unreliable indicator of direct invasion, perhaps because patients with gastric carcinoma are often cachectic. Another potential cause of obliteration of the peripancreatic fat plane is inflammation due to pancreatitis or other adjacent inflammatory processes. For instance, Dehn et al.[22] described four cases in which both CT and surgical findings suggested direct pancreatic invasion, but pathologic examination showed only an inflammatory response. Because of the large number of false-positive studies combined with the small number of true-positive studies, the positive predic-

tive value for the CT finding of pancreatic invasion was only 38%.[17]

TNM staging

CT did not accurately predict the stage of the tumors, underestimating the stage in 31% and overestimating in 16% (Table 21-2). In a similar fashion, Cook et al.[10] reported understaging 51% and overstaging 18% of their patients with adenocarcinoma. In the study by Sussman et

□ **TABLE 21-2**

CT staging versus surgical staging (n=75)

| | Surgical stage | | | | |
CT stage	I	II	III	IV	Total
1	1	0	0	0	1
2	0	10	8*	3*	21
3	0	4†	8	12*	24
4	0	2†	6†	21	29
TOTAL	1	16	22	36	75

Modified from Sussman SK, Halvorsen RA Jr, Illescas FF, Cohan RH, Saeed M et al: *Radiology* 167:335, 1988.
*CT understaged.
†CT overstaged.

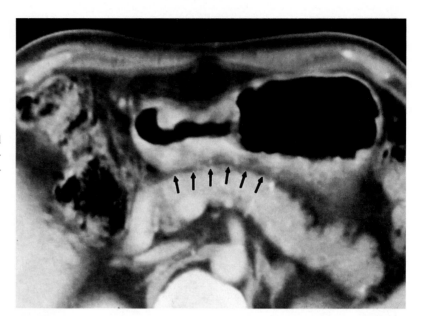

Fig. 21-9 Intact peripancreatic fat plane. Antral carcinoma with distinct fat plane *(arrows)* separating tumor from pancreas. No invasion of pancreas at surgery.

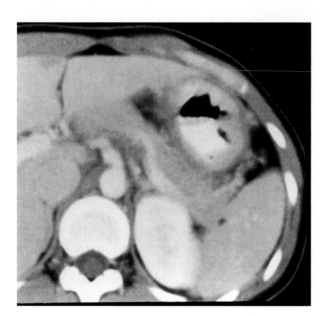

Fig. 21-10 Obliterated peripancreatic fat plane. Circumferential adenocarcinoma with obliteration of peripancreatic fat plane suggesting direct invasion.

Fig. 21-11 Pancreatic invasion. Bulky antral tumor *(T)* directly invades body of pancreas. Note obliteration of fat plane between tumor and pancreas in midline with preserved fat plane laterally *(arrows)*.

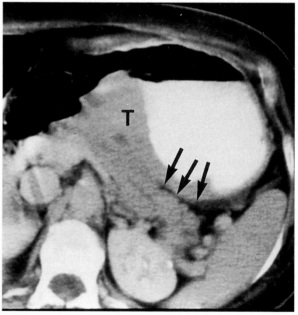

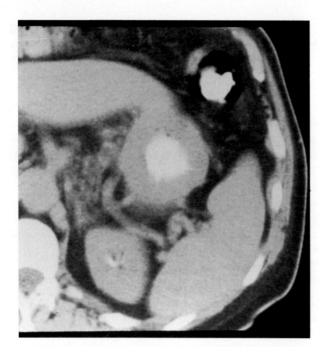

Fig. 21-12 False-negative lymph node involvement. Circumferential adenocarcinoma with extensive infiltration of perigastric fat along gastrohepatic ligament, but no discernibly enlarged lymph nodes. Lymph node metastases found at surgery.

al.,[17] 12 patients were overstaged based on the CT findings. The error was fairly equally divided between overdiagnosing adenopathy and overdiagnosing invasion of contiguous organs. Of the 23 patients understaged, error was equally divided among three areas: direct organ invasion, adenopathy, and peritoneal carcinomatosis.

Another study comparing the ability of CT to accurately stage gastric carcinoma reached slightly more optimistic conclusions. Kleinhaus and Militianu[23] found an overall accuracy for CT staging of 72%. In their comparison of CT and surgical findings in 31 patients, they found that local lymph node involvement and invasion of adjacent organs were unreliable (Fig. 21-12). They concluded that CT staging of gastric carcinoma was of little value. They state that the causes of understaging were microscopic local nodal involvement, small peritoneal metastases, and small liver metastases.

MAGNETIC RESONANCE IMAGING OF THE STOMACH

Despite the availability of magnetic resonance imaging (MRI) equipment for approximately 10 years, little has been written about the use of MRI in the evaluation of the stomach. As occurred with CT, MRI was initially used to evaluate the central nervous system with less emphasis on other organ systems. The role of MRI in the evaluation of the GI tract has been limited primarily to the esophagus and the colon.[6,24-30] Evaluation of the stomach has been limited to a certain extent by motion artifacts noted in upper abdominal spin echo sequences, as well as the lack of a commer-

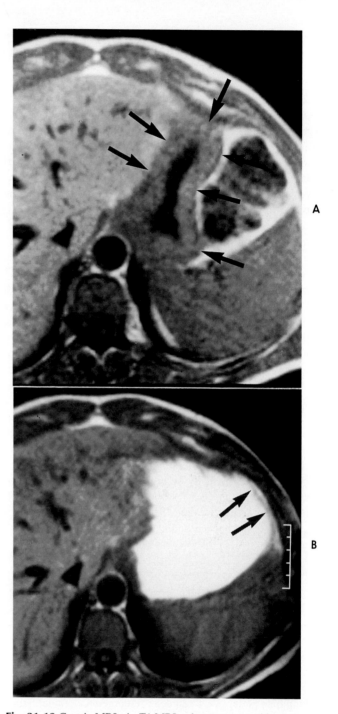

Fig. 21-13 Gastric MRI. **A,** T1 MRI pulse sequence without contrast media demonstrates apparently thickened gastric wall (arrows). **B,** After ingestion of experimental oral contrast media (OMR, Oncomembrane, Seattle, Wash.) note excellent gastric distension. Gastric wall (arrows) now seems to be of normal thickness.

cially available oral contrast agent to opacify the GI tract. A number of contrast media are approaching FDA approval that will allow better evaluation of the stomach (Fig. 21-13). Currently, scans can be obtained either without contrast media, or with water, barium, or a variety of over-the-counter substances, such as Geritol.[31-33]

The potential application of MRI of the stomach is theoretically greater than with CT. With CT it is impossible to differentiate the various layers of the gastric wall. However, with intravenous administration of gadopentetate dimeglumine, MRI allows identification of layers within the gastric wall. There is a hyperintense inner zone and a hypointense outer zone.[34] The enhanced inner zone presumably represents the mucosa and submucosa, and the hypointense unenhanced zone presumably represents the muscular layer of the gastric wall. The ability of MRI to differentiate two components of the normal gastric wall may prove to be of benefit in the staging of gastric tumors. To date, no study has evaluated the ability of MRI to stage gastric carcinoma.

The appearance of diffusely infiltrating gastric carcinoma with MRI has been reported.[35] A patient with infiltrating mucus-producing adenocarcinoma was studied with both CT and MRI. CT demonstrated a concentrically thickened body of the stomach. MRI also demonstrated concentric thickening of the gastric wall; the abnormal gastric wall had low signal intensity on T1 MRI that decreased in signal intensity relative to muscle on the T2 MRI pulse sequence. With infiltrating gastric carcinoma, the most prominent histologic characteristic is deposition of fibrous tissue. The T2 signal characteristic of the gastric wall was suggestive of fibrous tissue, not the higher signal intensity expected with most carcinomas. One other case of linitis plastica has been reported with similar findings. There were areas of decreased signal intensity on both T1 and T2 MRI spin echo sequences in this case.[36] In both these cases with infiltrating adenocarcinoma, the MRI characteristics were those of scar tissue rather than tumor.

CONCLUSION
Role of CT

Because CT is unable to accurately detect lymph node metastases or local invasion, it cannot be used to accurately stage all patients with gastric carcinoma. However, CT has a role in the evaluation of patients with gastric carcinoma because of its ability to detect distant metastases. Identification of multiple hepatic masses, peritoneal studding, or omental caking is diagnostic of metastatic disease and can help plan therapy. CT can detect enlarged abdominal lymph nodes that may not be readily accessible to visual inspection in surgery. For instance, Sussman et al.[11] encountered a number of cases with retrocrural adenopathy that the surgeons stated would have been difficult to identify without scanning guidance. Also, many surgeons feel that preoperative staging can be helpful in predicting patients in whom a palliative procedure should be planned, rather than a curative approach, especially when obvious metastatic disease is present.[37] Therefore patients with adenocarcinoma should receive preoperative CT in the search for enlarged distant lymph nodes and peritoneal, omental, or liver masses. The decision of whether to operate should not be based on CT findings of enlarged local nodes or local invasion because these findings do not necessarily indicate advanced disease.

Role of MRI

Currently, MRI is an effective tool useful in detecting liver metastases in patients with gastric cancer, but it has unproven use in identifying other types of metastases, nodal involvement, and direct spread of tumor. The potential of MRI is great, especially when faster scanning techniques and oral contrast agents become available. However, because CT does allow detection of enlarged nodes and peritoneal metastases, as well as liver lesions, CT should remain the procedure of choice in the preoperative evaluation of patients with gastric adenocarcinoma.

REFERENCES

1. Silverberg E, Boring CC, Squires TS: *Cancer statistics, 1990, CA-Cancer J Clin* 40:9, 1990.
2. MacDonald JS, Cohen I Jr, Gunderson LL: Cancer of the stomach. In DeVita VT Jr, Helman S, Rosenberg SA, eds: *Cancer principles and practice of oncology*, ed 2, Philadelphia, 1985, JB Lippincott.
3. Richmond E, ed: What's new in stomach cancer, *Patient Care* 430:27, 1992.
4. Borchard F: Classification of gastric carcinoma, *Hepatogastroenterology* 37:223, 1990.
5. Beahrs OH, Henson DE, Hutter RVP, Myers MH: *Manual for staging of cancer*, ed 3, Philadelphia, 1988, JB Lippincott.
6. Halvorsen RA Jr, Thompson WM: Primary neoplasms of the hollow organs of the gastrointestinal tract: staging and follow-up, *Cancer* 67:1181, 1991.
7. Halvorsen RA Jr, Thompson WM: CT for staging gastrointestinal malignancies: I. Esophagus and stomach, *Invest Radiol* 22:2, 1987.
8. Cassell P, Robinson JO: Cancer of the stomach: a review of 854 patients, *Br J Surg* 63:603, 1976.
9. Costello CB, Taylor TV, Torrance B: Personal experience in the surgical management of carcinoma of the stomach, *Br J Surg* 64:47, 1977.
10. Lundh G, Burn JI, Kolig G, Richard CA, Thomson JWW et al: A cooperative international study of gastric cancer, *Ann World Coll Surg, Engl* 54:219, 1974.
11. Moss AA, Schnyder P, Candardgis G, Margulis AR: Computed tomography of benign and malignant gastric abnormalities, *J Clin Gastroenterol* 2:401, 1980.
12. Lee KR, Levine E, Moffat RE, Bigongiari LR, Hermreck AS: Computed tomography staging of malignant gastric neoplasms, *Radiology* 133:151, 1979.
13. Balfe DM, Koehler RE, Karstaedt N, Stanley RJ, Sagel SS: Computed tomography of gastric neoplasms, *Radiology* 140:431, 1981.
14. Moss AA, Schnyder P, Marks W, Margulis AR: Gastric adenocarcinoma: a comparison of the accuracy and economics of staging by computed tomography and surgery, *Gastroenterology* 80:45, 1981.
15. McFee AS, Aust IB: Gastric carcinoma and the CAT scan, *Gastroenterology* 80:196, 1981.
16. Cook AO, Levine BA, Sirinek KR, Gaskill HV: Evaluation of gastric adenocarcinoma: abdominal computed tomography does not replace celiotomy, *Arch Surg* 121:603, 1986.
17. Sussman SK, Halvorsen RA Jr, Illescas FF, Cohan RH, Saeed M et al: Gastric adenocarcinoma: CT vs. surgical staging, *Radiology* 167:335, 1988.
18. Megibow AJ: Stomach. In Megibow AJ, Balthazar EJ, eds: *Computed tomography of the gastrointestinal tract*, St Louis, 1986, Mosby–Year Book.

19. Botet JF, Lightdale CJ, Zauber AG, Gerdes H et al: Preoperative staging of gastric cancer: comparison of endoscopic ultrasound and dynamic CT, *Radiology* 181:426, 1991.
20. Komaki S: Gastric carcinoma. In Meyers MA, ed: *Computed tomography of the gastrointestinal tract,* New York, 1986, Springer.
21. Frasier I, Nash R, James DC: Computed tomography in gastric cancer (letter), *Br J Surg* 72:249, 1985.
22. Dehn TCB, Reznek RH, Nockler IB, White FE: The preoperative assessment of advanced gastric cancer by computed tomography and surgery, *Br J Surg* 71:413, 1984.
23. Kleinhaus U, Militianu D: Computed tomography in the preoperative evaluation of gastric carcinoma, *Gastrointest Radiol* 13:97, 1988.
24. Rohde H: Staging of gastric cancer: clinical, surgical, and pathological. In Sugarbaker P, ed: *Management of gastric cancer,* Boston, 1991, Kluwer Academic Publishers.
25. Smith FW, Hutchison JM, Mallard JR et al: Oesophageal carcinoma demonstrated by whole-body nuclear magnetic resonance imaging, *Br Med J* 282:510, 1981.
26. Halvorsen RA Jr, Thompson WM: Gastrointestinal cancer, diagnosis, staging, and the follow-up role of imaging, *Semin Ultrasound CT MR* 10:467, 1989.
27. Ross RJ, Thompson JS, Kim K, Bailey R: Nuclear magnetic resonance evaluation of a leiomyosarcoma, *Magn Reson Imaging* 1:87, 1982.
28. Church J, Bodie B, Jagelman DG, Buonocore E: Primary rectal lymphoma staged by magnetic resonance imaging: case report of an unusual cause of rectal bleeding, *Cleve Clin Q* 51:477, 1984.
29. Quint LE, Glazer GM, Orringer MB: Esophageal imaging by MR and CT: study of normal anatomy and neoplasms, *Radiology* 156:727, 1985.
30. Halvorsen RA, Herfkins RJ, Wolfe WG et al: *Comparison of magnetic resonance to computed tomography for staging esophageal carcinoma,* Miami Beach, 1987, American Roentgen Ray Society Proceedings.
31. Ros PR, Steinman RM, Torres GM, Burton SS et al: The value of barium as a gastrointestinal contrast agent in MR imaging: a comparison study in normal volunteers, *AJR* 157:761, 1991.
32. Mitchell DG, Vinitski S: Principles of protocol optimization for MR of the abdomen and pelvis, *Crit Rev Diagn Imaging* 31:117, 1990.
33. Marti-Bonmati L, Vilar J, Paniagua JC, Talens A: High density barium sulphate as an MRI oral contrast, *Magn Reson Imaging* 9:259, 1991.
34. Hamed MM, Hamm B, Ibrahim ME, Taupitz M, Mahfouz AE: Dynamic MR imaging of the abdomen with gadopentetate dimeglumine: normal enhancement patterns of the liver, spleen, stomach, and pancreas, *AJR* 158:303, 1992.
35. Schmidt HC, Tscholakoff D, Hricak H, Higgins CB: MR image contrast and relaxation times of solid tumors in the chest, abdomen, and pelvis, *J Comput Assist Tomogr* 9:738, 1985.
36. Winkler ML, Hricak H, Higgins CB: MR imaging of diffusely infiltrating gastric carcinoma, *J Comput Assist Tomogr* 11:337, 1987.
37. Bralow SP: Diagnosis and staging of esophageal and gastric cancer, *Cancer* 50:2566, 1982.

22 *Endoscopic Ultrasound of the Stomach*

JOSE F. BOTET

From an historical perspective the radiologic evaluation of the stomach has undergone a series of transformations. It began with abdominal radiographs and progressed through single, double, and multiphasic contrast studies, endoscopy, and biopsy. Since 1970, transcutaneous ultrasound, computed tomography (CT), and, to a lesser extent, magnetic resonance imaging (MRI) have allowed us to view structures adjacent to the stomach. These techniques, however, have not demonstrated in detail the internal structure of the gastric wall, although high-resolution transcutaneous ultrasound can in some circumstances provide limited information.[1,2] Unfortunately the presence of air in the stomach, of intervening organs and air-filled bowel loops between the transducer and the target organ, and of occasional intervening bone structures, as well as the need to image through the skin and subcutaneous tissues, all significantly decrease the resolution provided by the transcutaneous approach.

With the advent of endoscopic ultrasonography (EUS) almost all of the limitations of conventional ultrasound have been overcome. The use of high-frequency transducers has for the first time allowed routine demonstrations of the internal layered structure of the gastric wall. The advantages of these techniques are being put to good use in evaluating benign and malignant processes that involve the gastric wall, although the technology is in use in only a few centers at present, and its role in routine clinical practice is still being assessed.

BENIGN PROCESSES
Inflammatory processes

Hypersecretory states in the stomach are often accompanied by changes in the normal structure of the gastric layers, usually with hypertrophy of specific layers. In mild gastritis there may not be any specific layer thickening, although the hypersecretory state is documented on endoscopy by the presence of increased gastric secretion and a relatively low pH of the aspirated material.[3] In moderate gastritis the mucosa and lamina propria are usually thickened (Fig. 22-1) with sparing of other layers. In severe gastritis the inflammatory process may result in hypertrophy of all layers (Fig. 22-2). An extreme example of this is commonly found in patients with the Zollinger-Ellison syndrome.[4]

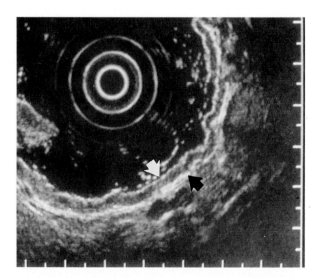

Fig. 22-1 Moderate gastritis. Note the thickening of the mucosa/lamina propria *(white arrowhead)* and submucosa *(black arrowhead)*. The muscularis is normal.

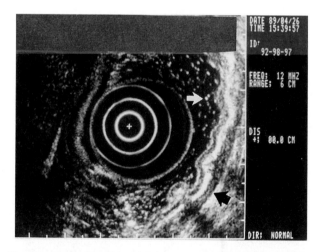

Fig. 22-2 Severe gastritis. All layers are diffusely thickened *(black arrowhead)*. Notice the increased number of "floaters" *(white arrowhead)* despite the use of a special cocktail, indicating significantly increased gastric secretion.

Gastric ulcers may be diagnosed by endoscopy or by barium meal examination,[5,6] but those that fail to heal on adequate medical treatment pose the problem of possible malignancy. In this situation, and when conventional endoscopic biopsy findings are negative or equivocal, endosonography may help differentiate benign and malignant disease (Figs. 22-3 and 22-4). It should be stressed, however, that endoscopic ultrasound tends to overstage ulcerated malignant gastric tumors; it has proved difficult to differentiate the inflammatory component from the tumor.

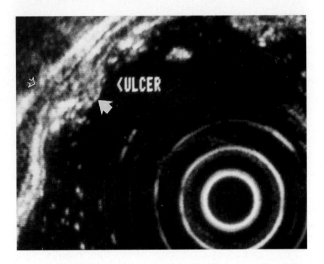

Fig. 22-3 Small ulcer *(white arrowhead)* with surrounding inflammation, the so-called ulcer mound. Notice that the muscularis is intact. The mound mimics a malignant tumor *(open arrowhead)*. Differentiation on the basis of endosonography alone is not possible in some cases.

Two of the major uses of endoscopic ultrasound in benign gastric conditions have been in evaluating large gastric folds and in studying submucosal tumors.

Large gastric folds

We studied 91 patients referred for the evaluation of large gastric folds (Table 22-1) and identified three patterns. All the patients with increased thickening of the gastric wall but with preservation of the internal architecture had benign disease (Figs. 22-1 and 22-2). A second pattern consisted of disruption of some or all layers, and this was seen in patients with lymphoma or linitis plastica (Figs. 22-5 and 22-6). Finally, a third pattern was identified in which hypoechoic disruptions of the submucosa were seen, and this represented varices[7,8] (Fig. 22-7).

Submucosal tumors

Early in our experience we conducted a multiinstitutional study evaluating submucosal tumors of the stomach (Table 22-2). Further cases have confirmed that EUS is an ideal tool for evaluating these tumors (Fig. 22-8) because we can identify the specific layer or layers from which they arise.[9] Others, notably Yasuda[10] and Nakasawa[11] in Japan, have come to the same conclusion.

☐ **TABLE 22-1**
Large gastric folds

Disruption (46)	Hypertrophy (41)	Hypoechoic (4)
Lymphoma (32)	Gastritis (28)	Varices (4)
Linitis plastica (14)	Ulcer(s) (5)	
	Zollinger-Ellison (4)	
	Other (4)	

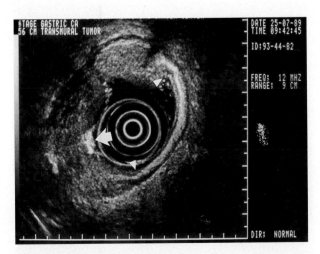

Fig. 22-4 Malignant ulcer *(white arrow)*. The surrounding tumor with its characteristic transition *(small arrowheads)* allows us to make the correct diagnosis.

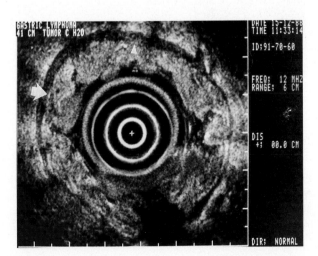

Fig. 22-5 Lymphoma. Notice the loss of definition of layers in the mucosa and submucosa *(white arrow)* as well as the segmental infiltration of the muscularis propria *(small arrowheads)*.

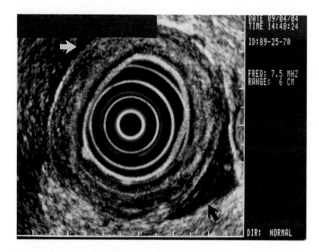

Fig. 22-6 Linitis plastica. Notice the gross involvement with loss of definition of individual layers. The presence of ascites *(black and white arrowheads)* is well demonstrated.

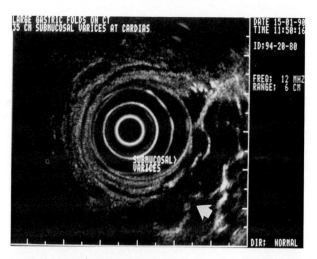

Fig. 22-7 Gastric varices. Notice the presence of large submucosal and extragastric varices *(white arrowhead)* mimicking a large gastric fold. Endoscopic biopsy of such a fold could potentially be disastrous.

☐ **TABLE 22-2**
Submucosal tumors of the stomach

Diagnosis	No. of patients	Findings on EUS	Agreement with pathology
Leiomyoma	9	Within muscularis propria hypoechoic with occasional hyperechoic focus in larger tumors, smooth border	9/9
Leiomyosarcoma	2	Within muscularis propria, hypoechoic or hyperechoic, irregular margin	2/2
Neurolemoma	2	Mixed echogenicity within submucosa and muscularis	2/2
Varix	7	Submucosal and extragastric hypoechoic	7/7
Others	5		4/5

Modified from Boyc GA, Sivak MV, Rosch T et al: *Gastrointest Endosc* 37:449, 1991.

Fig. 22-8 Submucosal tumors. Ectopic pancreas *(white arrow).* Note the small duct *(small white arrowhead)* emptying into the antral lumen.

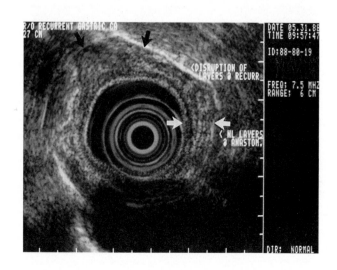

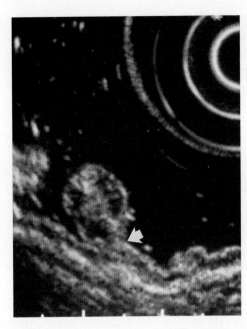

Fig. 22-9 Gastric polyps. Close-up view of a gastric adenomatous polyp. Notice that it arises from the mucosa *(white arrowhead)*. The lamina propria, submucosa, and muscularis are not involved. On malignant transformation there is progressive invasion of these layers.

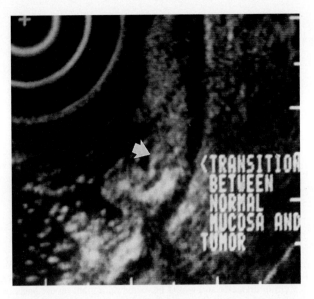

Fig. 22-10 Transition between normal mucosa and tumor in a gastric cancer *(white arrowhead)*. Below the transition the individual layers of the gastric wall can be seen. Above it, we see confluence of the mucosa, lamina propria, and submucosa with increased thickening of the muscularis propria.

Polyps

Barium meal examination and endoscopy also can readily demonstrate gastric polyps.[12] There are limitations, however, in the assessment of invasion, especially in the case of adenomatous polyps with malignant change. Although no peer-reviewed papers have appeared regarding this use of EUS, there are enough anecdotal cases to support the contention that it may prove helpful in evaluating invasion (Fig. 22-9).

MALIGNANT TUMORS

A large variety of malignant tumors both primary and metastatic can involve the stomach. The initial diagnosis may be made by barium meal, endoscopy, or on occasion, ultrasound or CT. Histologic confirmation by endoscopic biopsy may not be sufficient to decide the course of action, and many surgeons require an attempt at staging of primary tumors during the initial workup. Most stagings are based on the TNM system. Other than EUS, the currently available imaging tools provide little information on the depth of invasion of the tumor and for the most part provide limited information on nodal involvement. Two major studies have addressed this issue using the model of the gastric adenocarcinoma.

Gastric cancer

This is the most common primary malignant tumor of the stomach. In the United States approximately 20,000 new

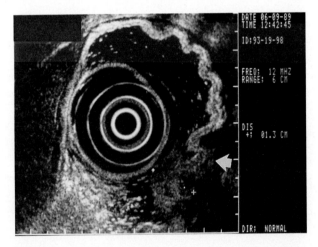

Fig. 22-11 Characteristic hypoechoic appearance of a localized transmural tumor (T3) of the greater curvature *(white arrowhead)*.

cases will be diagnosed in 1993 and approximately 14,000 patients will die of the disease.

Adenocarcinoma of the stomach arises from the mucosa (Figs. 22-10 and 22-11). As it progresses it penetrates other layers and invades surrounding organs and vascular structures. EUS allows excellent visualization of this process. Lymphatic involvement can also be staged using EUS because most of the immediate drainage node groups are within the range of the transducer. A major difference between EUS and CT is that the differentiation of reactive

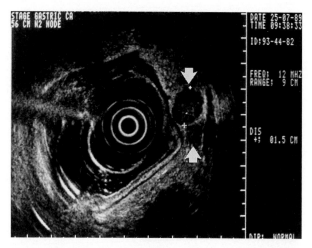

Fig. 22-12 Nodal disease. Notice the presence of two rounded, hypoechoic nodes *(white arrowheads)*. The largest one measures 1.5 cm in diameter and would be called malignant on the basis of CT or MRI. The smaller one is also rounded and hypoechoic but only measures 7 mm in diameter. This would be indeterminate for both CT and MRI, yet following EUS criteria, it would be called malignant with a great degree of confidence.

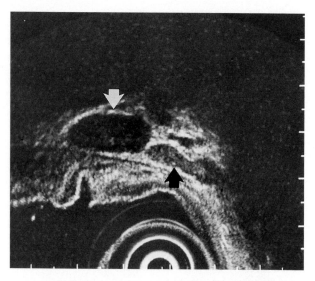

Fig. 22-13 Nodal disease. Two nodes of the same length (15 mm). One is round and hypoechoic *(white arrowhead)*; this was proven malignant. The other is elongated and echogenic *(black arrowhead)*; this was found to be reactive at pathologic examination.

□   **TABLE 22-3**

Tumor stage in gastric cancer: concordance of endoscopic US versus dynamic CT in staging depth of tumor invasion (T) and regional node involvement (N) with pathologic classification

Pathologic classification	Endoscopic US					Dynamic CT				
	T0	T1	T2	T3	T4	T0	T1	T2	T3	T4
T0										
T1		4						1	1	
T2		1	6	1		2	1	2	1	
T3			1	30		1		8	7	3
T4				1	6				3	3

NOTE: Numbers are number of tumors.
p<.00042.

Pathologic classification	Endoscopic US			Dynamic CT		
	N0	N1	N2	N0	N1	N2
N0	10	0	1	3	0	2
N1	7	15		7	7	3
N2	1	2	14	2	3	6

Modified from Botet JF, Lightdale CJ, Zauber AG et al: *Radiology* 181:426, 1991.
NOTE: Numbers are cases of lymph node metastasis.
p < .038.

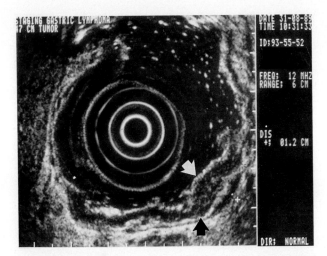

Fig. 22-14 Early gastric lymphoma. Notice the localized thickening of the submucosa *(black arrowhead)* in the presence of an intact mucosa *(white arrowhead)*. This is typical of early lymphoma.

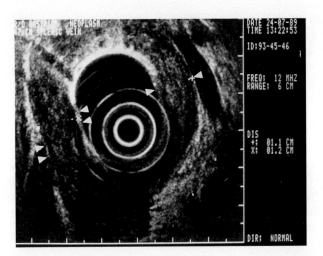

Fig. 22-15 Advanced gastric lymphoma. Notice the involvement of all layers with associated thickening of the gastric wall, which measures 11 mm *(single arrowhead)* and 12 mm *(double arrowhead)* in cross section. Circumferential tumor involvement is noted as well.

nodes and malignant ones is not based on size criteria but actually on the intrinsic characteristics of the node (length-to-width ratio and echogenicity). These parameters reflect better than size the true nature of the nodal involvement (Figs. 22-12 and 12-13). A ratio of length to width greater than 2:1 usually indicates a benign lymph node and less than 2:1 favors malignancy. Currently EUS can detect nodes as small as 2 mm in diameter.

EUS does not, however, reliably detect, or exclude, metastatic spread. This is a result of the limited field of view and the limited depth of field, which do not allow evaluation of regions such as lung and other distal metastatic sites. In studies comparing EUS and dynamic CT, EUS proved significantly more accurate in the staging of T (tumor invasion) and N (nodal involvement)[13,14] (Table 22-3).

Gastric lymphoma

Bolondi et al.[15] reported a study of the endosonographic differentiation of carcinoma and lymphoma of the gastric wall and were able to differentiate the two. In our experience it is difficult to differentiate between primary gastric lymphoma and linitis plastica, because in most cases both diseases tend to involve all gastric layers diffusely. Tio[16] has reported similar findings (Figs. 22-14 and 22-15).

Others

There has been limited and essentially anecdotal reference to gastric involvement by other rare tumors such as leiomyoma, leiomyoblastoma, and leiomyosarcoma.[9,10]

Anastomotic recurrences

The radiologic assessment of anastomotic recurrence after surgery for malignant gastric tumors has been disappointing in the past. Endoscopy is only able to detect in-

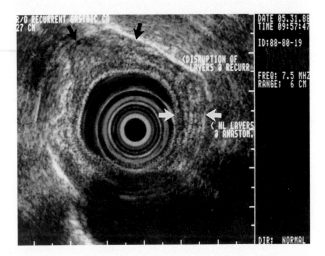

Fig. 22-16 Anastomotic recurrence. The tumor is seen as a disruption *(black arrowheads)* of the normal layered structure in the noninvolved portion of the anastomosis *(white arrowheads)*.

☐ **TABLE 22-4**

Anastomotic recurrences: comparison of endoscopic ultrasound (EUS) and dynamic computed tomography (DCT)

	EUS	DCT
Symptomatic patients	40	40
Recurrences present	23/24* (95%)	8/24*(33%)
Recurrences absent	13/16 (81%)	15/16 (93%)

Modified from Lightdale CJ, Botet JF: *Gastrointest Endosc* 36(suppl):S11, 1990.
*p<.003.

traluminal recurrences. Endosonography allows us to investigate both the wall and the immediate extraluminal tissues. We have performed a study in symptomatic patients comparing EUS with dynamic CT, and the results in favor of EUS were statistically significant[17] (Table 22-4, Fig. 22-16).

SUMMARY

EUS appears to be an effective tool that significantly complements conventional imaging studies of the stomach. The ability to evaluate the individual layers of the gastric wall and to a lesser degree the internal architecture of nodes allows us a glimpse of the gastroenterologic imaging of the twenty-first century.

REFERENCES

1. Fleischer AC, Dowling AD, Weinstein ML et al: Sonographic patterns of distended, fluid-filled bowel, *Radiology* 133:681, 1979.
2. Bluth EI, Merritt CRB, Sullivan MA: Ultrasonic evaluation of the stomach, small bowel, and colon, *Radiology* 133:677, 1979.
3. McGuigan JE, Trudeau WL: Differences in rates of gastrin release in normal persons and patients with duodenal ulcer, *N Engl J Med* 288:64, 1973.
4. Frucht H et al: Secretin and calcium provocative tests in the Zollinger-Ellison syndrome: a prospective study, *Ann Intern Med* 11:713, 1989.
5. Levine MS, Rubesin SE, Herlinger H, Laufer I: Double contrast upper gastrointestinal examination: technique and interpretation, *Radiology* 168:593, 1988.
6. Silverstein FE, Tytgat GNJ: *Atlas of gastrointestinal endoscopy,* Philadelphia, 1987, WB Saunders.
7. Fujishima H, Misawa T, Chijiiwa Y et al: Scirrhous carcinoma of the stomach versus hypertrophic gastritis: findings at endoscopic ultrasound, *Radiology* 181:197, 1991.
8. Botet JF, Lightdale CJ: Endoscopic US in the evaluation of patients with large gastric folds, *Radiology* 177:115, 1990 (abstract).
9. Boyce GA, Sivak MV, Rosch T et al: Evaluation of submucosal upper gastrointestinal tract lesions by endoscopic ultrasound, *Gastrointest Endosc* 37:449, 1991.
10. Yasuda K, Nakajima M, Yoshida T et al: The diagnosis of submucosal tumors of the stomach by endoscopic ultrasonography, *Gastrointest Endosc* 35:10, 1989.
11. Nakasawa S, Yoshino J, Nakamura T et al: Endoscopic ultrasonography of gastric myogenic tumors: a comparative study between histology and ultrasonography, *J Ultrasound Med* 8:533, 1989.
12. Sarre RG, Frost AC, Jagelman DG et al: Gastric and duodenal polyps in familial adenomatous polyposis: a prospective study of the nature and prevalence of upper gastrointestinal polyps, *Radiology* 165:588, 1987 (abstract).
13. Botet JF, Lightdale CJ, Zauber AG et al: Endoscopic ultrasonography in the preoperative staging of gastric cancer: a comparative study with dynamic CT, *Radiology* 181:426, 1991.
14. Tio TL, Coene PPLO, Schouwink MH et al: Esophagogastric carcinoma: preoperative TNM staging with endosonography, *Radiology* 173:411, 1989.
15. Bolondi L, Casanova P, Caletti GC et al: Primary gastric lymphoma versus gastric carcinoma: endoscopic US evaluation, *Radiology* 165:821, 1987.
16. Tio TL, den Hartog Jager FCA, Tytgat GNJ: Endoscopic ultrasonography of non-Hodgkin's lymphoma of the stomach, *Gastroenterology* 91:401, 1986.
17. Lightdale CJ, Botet JF, Woodruff JM et al: Diagnosis of recurrent upper gastrointestinal cancer at the surgical anastomosis by endoscopic ultrasound, *Gastrointest Endosc* 35:407, 1989.

23 Radiology of the Stomach After Gastric Surgery for Obesity

CLAIRE SMITH

The medical complications of obesity have long been recognized as serious health threats.[1,2] Although chronic obesity is a common disease and the clinical characteristics have been well described, the pathogenesis of obesity is poorly understood.[3] As a result, treatment methods have varied. Unfortunately, few morbidly obese patients achieve long-term weight loss after dietary or behavioral therapy or with the use of nonoperative aids such as intragastric balloons.[4] During the past two decades, gastric restrictive surgery has evolved as the cornerstone of surgery for morbid obesity.[5,6] Gastric bypasses and vertical gastroplasties have been found to be effective operations that induce weight loss and decrease associated health hazards in many obese patients, and are currently the standard operations for obesity.[3-6] This chapter reviews the basic principles of gastric restrictive surgery, describes the radiologic methods used to evaluate patients who have had these operations, outlines the normal radiologic appearance of the stomach after surgery for weight control, and discusses the acute and long-term complications that may occur in these patients.

GENERAL OVERVIEW

Gastric surgery to control obesity evolved as an outgrowth of the empiric observation that patients who had partial gastric resections for other diseases lost weight after their gastric surgery. The factors that determined this weight loss were not specifically known, but the rationale for operation was that if the stomach volume could be minified and if the egress of food from the small gastric pouch could be slowed, then satiety should occur quickly and the patient's oral intake would be limited. Ideally, these effects should produce modified eating habits and result in calorie restrictions and sustained weight loss without the unacceptable risks found to be associated with the malabsorption that developed in patients who underwent small bowel shunts for weight control.[5]

Although gastric bypass and gastroplasty procedures were introduced in the late 1960s, their popularity increased in the 1970s when automatic stapling devices facilitated the technical aspects of these procedures.[5,7,8] Over the years, numerous procedural variations appeared, but several basic principles evolved. Based on early observations, great importance has been attached to the attainment of very small,

precisely measured gastric pouches. Pouch volumes of 15 to 30 ml are created. The diameters of the channels or outlets were controlled at 1 cm or less. Operations tended to be successful when these measurements were maintained, when staple lines were reinforced, and when gastroplasty channels were stabilized by supporting materials.[9-11]

GASTRIC BYPASS

In gastric bypass, the small gastric pouch is anastomosed to a loop of small bowel by a loop type or Roux-en-Y anastomosis[7,10,12] (Figs. 23-1 and 23-2). The Roux-en-Y configuration is preferred currently. The caliber of the anastomosis is restricted and gastric transection is optional.

In addition to the effects imposed by these external factors, patients with gastric bypass procedures may experience unpleasant symptoms of the dumping syndrome when large amounts of sweets are ingested. The nausea, vomiting, and lightheadedness associated with the ingestion of carbohydrates theoretically add to the adverse conditioning needed to help patients who are "sweet-eaters" maintain reasonable diets.[3,12,13] With gastric bypass, a mild degree of malabsorption related to the exclusion of the duodenum from the food pathway may also contribute to weight loss.[10,12]

GASTROPLASTY

With the gastroplasty or gastric partition approach, staple lines change the food path without major rearrangement of the upper alimentary tract anatomy. Technically, gastroplasty is less complicated than gastric bypass. Currently the vertical gastroplasty is the approach of choice.[3,11,14] Studies have shown that the horizontal approach and unsupported gastrogastrostomies have a high rate of complications, and they are no longer favored as weight control procedures.[6,15,16]

With the vertical gastroplasty, two double rows of staples placed as close together as possible form a triangular gastric pouch on the lesser curve side of the stomach. There are several ways to create and support the narrowed channel to the distal stomach. An opaque silastic tubing placed directly around the channel as a ring or a nonopaque mesh placed around the channel through a gastric window can be used to reinforce the channel[6,8,11,14] (Figs. 23-3 and 23-

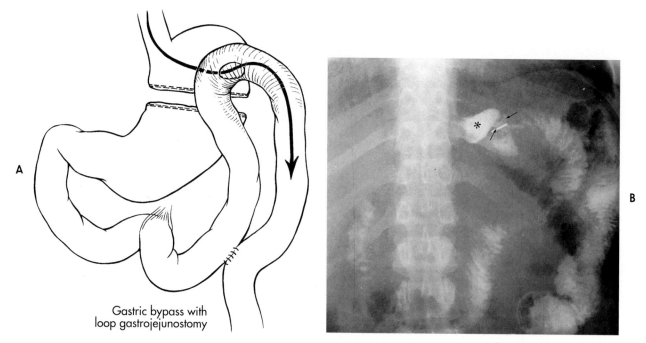

Fig. 23-1 Gastric bypass with loop gastrojejunostomy. Diagram **(A)** and contrast material study **(B).** Water-soluble contrast material has emptied from the proximal pouch *(asterisk)* through the narrowed channel *(arrows)* into the small bowel. Contrast material fills the afferent loop to the duodenum but has not refluxed into the distal stomach. Contrast material is seen in normal caliber efferent small bowel distally.
From Smith C et al: *Radiology* 153:321, 1984.

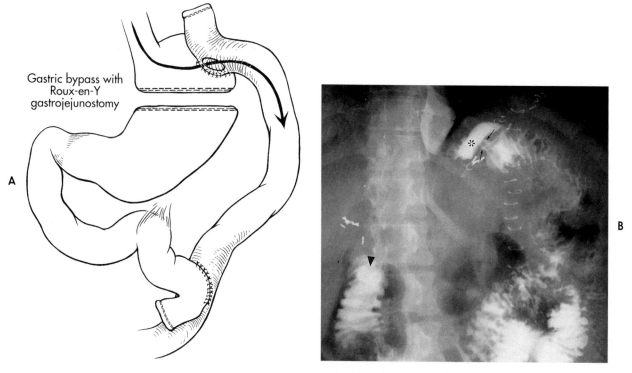

Fig. 23-2 Gastric bypass with Roux-en-Y gastrojejunostomy. Diagram **(A)** and contrast material study **(B).** The proximal pouch *(asterisk)* empties via the narrowed channel *(arrows)* into the small bowel. The exact site of the patient's enteroenterostomy is not visualized, but contrast material is present in the descending duodenum *(arrowhead).*
From Smith C et al: *Radiology* 153:321, 1984.

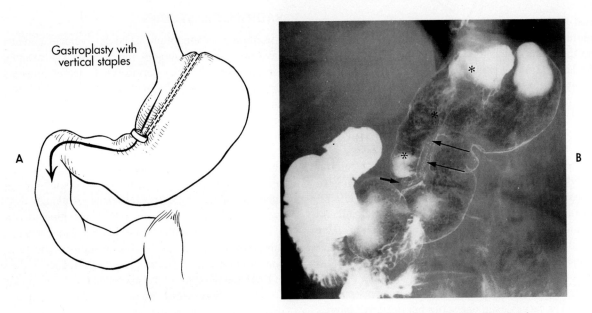

Fig. 23-3 Vertical banded gastroplasty. Diagram **(A)** and biphasic contrast study **(B).** The proximal pouch *(asterisks)* is located along the lesser curvature portion of the stomach. An opaque ring *(short arrow)* supports the narrowed channel. The parallel vertical lines of staples *(long arrows)* are seen near the channel but are obscured by contrast material in the pouch more proximally.
From Smith C et al: *Radiology* 153:321, 1984.

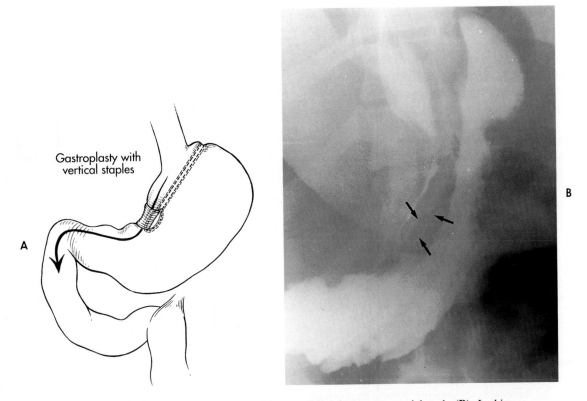

Fig. 23-4 Vertical banded gastroplasty. Diagram **(A)** and contrast material study **(B).** In this vertical banded gastroplasty, a nonopaque mesh supports the channel through a "gastric window." The ring of staples *(arrows)* making the window is barely apparent.
From Smith C et al: *Radiology* 153:321, 1984.

4). Food passes directly from the proximal gastric pouch through the channel into the distal stomach and duodenum without diversion of the food pathway or gastric transection. Malabsorption, dumping, and metabolic effects do not occur with this procedure.

WEIGHT CONTROL

In recent years, clinical studies that evaluate postoperative complications, sustained weight loss, and assessment of risk reductions have become available.[17-26] Unfortunately, side-to-side comparisons of these studies are impossible because of differences in definitions of the criteria for success or failure of the operation.[27] In many patients, although there may be only modest weight reduction, there may be major decreases in obesity-related diseases such as hypertension, diabetes, and left ventricular wall thickness that are not readily appreciated when figures that only reflect weight loss are considered.[23] These patients may be categorized as successes in one series but operative failures in another. In addition, lack of a defined method to list patients lost to follow-up makes it difficult to assess the true postoperative experience.[24,25]

In addition to the clinical follow-up, studies have attempted to elucidate factors that govern weight control and to relate these factors to the anatomic variations caused by gastric restrictive operations.[28-32] For gastroplasty, it has been found that pouch volume and channel diameter do not seem to correlate accurately with weight loss obtained.[29-31]

In studies that measured the rate of pouch emptying for solids, semisolids, and liquids by scintigraphic methods, pouch emptying rate for the gastroplasty approach was not found to be an important determinant of weight loss.[30,31] Gastric emptying after gastric bypass has been shown to be rapid for liquids with some delay in emptying for solid food.[32] The rapid pouch emptying for liquids may in turn be responsible for symptoms of dumping that can occur after the ingestion of high-carbohydrate liquids.[3,13,32] These studies and others suggest that further elusive factors are likely to be important determinants of weight loss.[28,29,31] In many cases, investigators feel that a failure of weight loss may result not from stomal dilatation, staple line dehiscence, or pouch dilatation, but rather from a change in the patient's diet to high caloric liquids or semisolid foods that readily pass through the gastric pouch into the distal stomach or small bowel.[13,28] Gross dietary indiscretion and failure of patients to eat slowly and to stop eating when hunger ceases are equally important causes for inadequate weight loss.[17]

Despite some of the shortcomings in the studies mentioned above, it has been shown that surgical gastric restrictive methods of weight control can yield successful and durable weight reduction in many patients* and can significantly improve the quality of patients' lives with minimal surgical complications.[23]

---

*References 4, 6, 13, 15, 23, 24.

RADIOLOGIC STUDIES

Radiologists are often asked to evaluate patients who have had previous surgery for obesity. The examinations may be needed in the perioperative period or years after the operation was performed. Although examination techniques vary with individual patients, certain underlying principles have been found to result in successful diagnostic studies.[33,34]

Before attempting any examination of patients who have had gastric surgery, the radiologist must be aware of the surgical approach, the specific clinical complaints, and the concerns of the referring physicians. Although this background information search may be frustrating, it is a critical step in the radiologic consultation. Time spent gaining this information before the examination begins saves time and radiation exposure during the performance of the study.

Plain radiography of the abdomen has been shown to be a vital and necessary component of the radiologic examination. Plain films allow detection of unsuspected abnormalities, including abnormal gas collections, distended bowel loops, soft tissue masses, and foreign bodies.[35] In patients who have had gastric restrictive surgery, the pattern of the surgical staples also provides a reliable indicator as to the type of surgery that was performed.[33,34] The staple pattern for a vertical gastroplasty does not vary significantly from patient to patient and is easily recognized. Staple configurations in gastric bypasses are more variable but can be identified accurately.

Once the plain film has been reviewed and the staple pattern has been characterized, contrast material administration can begin. In patients who are in the immediate postoperative period or those who have failed to lose weight, fluoroscopic evaluation is difficult to impossible. It has been found that these patients require prompt filming of the very first contrast swallow without prolonged attempts at fluoroscopic observation.[33,34,36] Also, patients must be turned into the best possible starting position to optimize chances at obtaining a diagnostic study (Table 23-1). Patients who

---

☐ **TABLE 23-1**

Staple-line geometry predicts optimal initial examination position

Staple geometry; initial position	Probable surgery	Optimal
Vertical; posterior oblique	Gastroplasty, lesser curvature channel	Right
Horizontal; posterior oblique	Gastroplasty, greater curvature channel	Left
Mixed or confusing; oblique	Gastric bypass	Left posterior
Oblique	Revision operation: unknown anatomy	Left posterior
Oblique	Vertical gastroplasty	Right posterior

From Smith C et al: *Radiology* 153:321, 1984.

have had vertical gastroplasties should be turned into the right posterior oblique position with relationship to the fluoroscopic table. Patients who have had gastric bypasses and horizontal gastroplasties are best examined when turned to the left.[33]

Positioning of obese patients throughout the examination may be difficult. They cannot move quickly, are not able to lie prone, and may not be able to be positioned laterally, and examination techniques must reflect these limitations.[33,34,36,37] It is not sensible to expect the same degree of agility from these obese patients as from smaller patients, and limitations must be accepted. In general, asking technologists to help turn these patients should be limited to assistance with IV tubing and catheters, or back injuries may occur. At the kilovolts used, scattered radiation is very high, and technologists should stand farther back from the table than is usually necessary—this may be verified by having the technologist wear an audible radiation monitor.

Choice of contrast material depends on the clinical question. When leaks or perforations are suspected, water-soluble contrast material is used.[35,37] Barium sulfate suspension, in either a single-contrast or biphasic study, is used for examinations in the late postoperative period. No matter which contrast agent is chosen, it should be administered slowly to prevent overdistention of the proximal pouch, vomiting, and a nondiagnostic study.

Agents that induce bowel hypotonia are optional. Their use may increase the chance of manipulating contrast material into the distal stomach in patients who have had gastric bypasses. Currently, the use of either percutaneous contrast injection into the distal stomach or retrograde endoscopy around the loop provides a more reliable method to evaluate the distal stomach after gastric bypass.[38-40]

IMMEDIATE COMPLICATIONS
Anastomotic leak and abscess

Leaks or anastomotic breakdowns are serious perioperative complications that may require urgent surgery.[3,6,15] Although any operation on the gastrointestinal tract is associated with a risk of leak and abscess, there is an increased incidence of leak in morbidly obese patients when compared with nonobese patients.[3,41]

When there is frank extravasation of contrast material, identification of the leak is straightforward (Figs. 23-5 and 23-6). If the patient has a gastrostomy tube in place, contrast material must be injected through the tube to ensure that portions of the stomach not outlined by ingested materials are examined adequately. If there is no gastrostomy tube in place, contrast material can be introduced percutaneously into the distal stomach after gastric bypass.[38,39] All portions of the postoperative gastrointestinal tract should be filled with contrast material, since leakage can occur at any operative site.

Ultrasound and CT scanning may be useful adjuncts if an abscess is suspected and if contrast studies fail to demonstrate a leak (Fig. 23-7). Unfortunately, these examina-

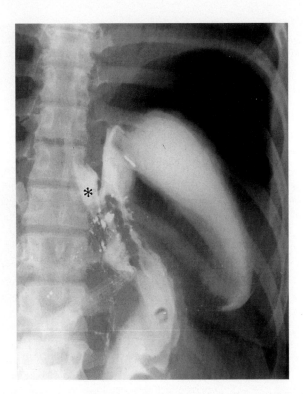

Fig. 23-5 Vertical banded gastroplasty with staple line leak. When the patient ingested contrast material, the proximal pouch was seen to be normal *(asterisk)*. During the later stages of the study, contrast material passed into the distal stomach, refluxed back into the fundus, and extravasated freely from the proximal end of the staple lines into the left upper quadrant.

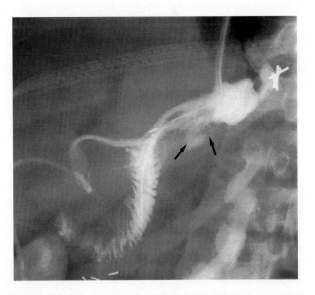

Fig. 23-6 Gastric bypass with anastomotic leak. Contrast study shows faint wisps of contrast material *(arrows)* below the anastomotic site. Adjacent surgical drains are outlined with the extravasated contrast material.

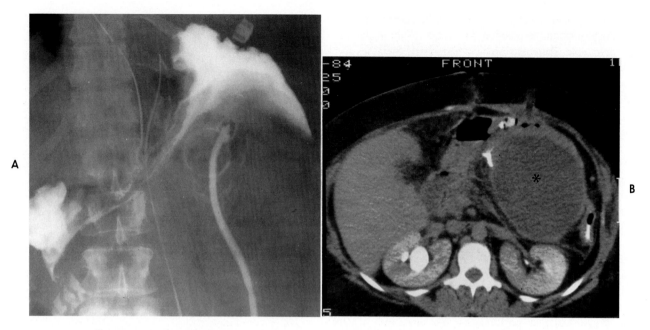

Fig. 23-7 Abscess after vertical banded gastroplasty: contrast study (**A**) and CT scan (**B**). During the initial stages of the examination the proximal pouch was seen to be normal. Injection of contrast material into the gastrostomy tube in the distal stomach shows that there is effacement and mass effect along the lower portion of the stomach without gross extravasation of contrast material. CT scan shows an abnormal fluid collection *(asterisk)* in the left side of the abdomen. This fluid collection did not contain any contrast material and was found to be an abscess at surgery. There was no associated staple line leak.

tions are limited by the patient's body size and physical state. Ultrasonography may be nondiagnostic because of body bulk, bowel gas, or wounds and accompanying surgical dressings, despite the use of state-of-the-art equipment.

The ability to use CT may be limited because the weight and size of these patients may exceed recommended guidelines for equipment. Contrast material should be used liberally during the CT examination to outline all portions of the gastrointestinal tract, since nonopacified fluid-filled portions of the stomach after either gastric bypass or gastroplasty may exactly mimic an abnormal extraluminal fluid collection.

Scintigraphic studies can be used to localize postoperative abscesses in obese patients when other methods fail. Since high-energy isotopes are employed, there is minimal image degradation despite patient body size. The limiting factor for scintigraphy is that the normal tissue changes from surgery demonstrate increased uptake of radionuclides. If gallium 67 citrate is used, a 2-week interval is recommended before scanning the perigastric area. A 1-week delay is needed if indium 111–labeled leukocytes are used. Earlier scanning may result in unreliable conclusions. If there is suspicion of an abscess remote from the site of surgery, nuclear medicine studies can be performed immediately.

If a leak or abscess is identified, percutaneous catheter drainage has become a safe and accepted alternative to immediate reoperation in some patients.[42,43]

Pouch perforation

Perforations of the proximal gastric pouch remote to the staple lines or anastomoses can occur (Figs. 23-8 and 23-9). The etiology is uncertain, although hyperacidity, ischemia, and the use of large nasogastric tubes postoperatively are thought to contribute.[3,34] Currently the prophylactic use of medications that block or neutralize acid production or release and the change from a horizontal staple configuration to a vertical gastroplasty may help to decrease the risk factors for pouch perforation.[3]

Staple line dehiscence

Early staple line dehiscence is thought to result from some type of technical failure intraoperatively. The failure is usually an unrecognized mechanical misfiring of the stapling device.[3] Risk of staple line dehiscence is increased if channel obstruction and vomiting occur in the early postoperative period. Most patients have decompressing nasogastric tubes or gastrostomy tubes to minimize the adverse sequelae caused by overdistention of the proximal pouch.

With disruption of the staple lines, gastric emptying occurs both by the normal channel and through the area of

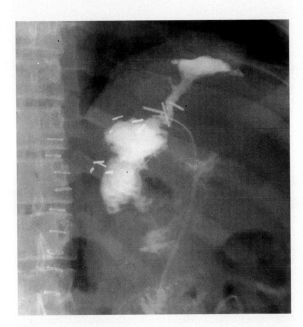

Fig. 23-8 Pouch perforation after gastric bypass. Water-soluble contrast material tracks from the superior surface of the proximal pouch into the left upper quadrant.

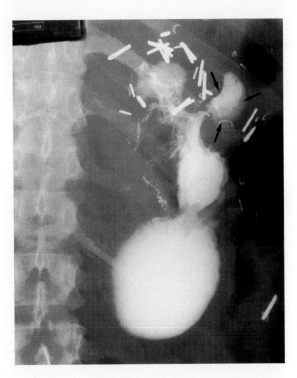

Fig. 23-9 Pouch perforation after horizontal gastroplasty. A small contrast collection *(arrows)* is present in the lateral perigastric tissues. It is near the greater curvature channel in this patient, who had a horizontal approach. Because of the high degree of ischemia along this portion of the stomach with the horizontal approach, it is no longer favored as a weight-control procedure.

dehiscence. If the stomach has not been transected between the staple lines, dehiscence does not result in frank extravasation of gastric contents into the abdomen (Figs. 23-10 to 23-12).

In light of the recent data that suggest a lack of specific correlation between pouch volumes, channel diameters, and pouch emptying, the significance of detecting staple line disruption is uncertain concerning the final outcome of the procedure in terms of weight loss. In theory, a staple line disruption should contribute to some degree of failure of weight loss, but there is no reliable evidence to support this.

Channel obstruction

Perioperative outlet obstruction at the channel or anastomosis is usually caused by edema. Other iatrogenic causes have been seen occasionally (Figs. 23-13 and 23-14). Since patients are on liquid or semisolid diets after surgery, obstruction by food particles is not encountered in the early stages. Prompt decompression of the pouch is indicated so that increased pressure in the obstructed pouch, subsequent ischemia, pouch perforation, and staple line dehiscence are avoided.

Obstruction of the distal stomach after gastroplasty does not occur commonly. Afferent limb obstruction after loop gastric bypass is a problem, but obstruction at the enteroenteric anastomosis in Roux-en-Y procedures is not encountered frequently. In the past, afferent limb obstruction was difficult to detect if a gastrostomy tube was not left in place. Current percutaneous methods of contrast injection into the stomach make it feasible to demonstrate the obstruction directly. Less invasive methods that suggest the diagnosis of

afferent limb obstruction include the identification of fluid-filled portions of the stomach and upper alimentary tract by CT or ultrasound and abnormal accumulation of nuclear medicine hepatobiliary agents in the bypassed bowel.

DELAYED COMPLICATIONS
General principles

Patients who are past the immediate postoperative period may have abdominal pain, emesis, failure of weight loss, or excess weight reduction. Radiographic studies using barium sulphate suspension or endoscopic examinations are ordered frequently. In patients who have experienced significant weight loss, fluoroscopic observation may be improved in comparison with fluoroscopic capabilities when the patient was obese. Despite this favorable factor, prompt filming of the first contrast swallow with the patient in the optimal starting position is recommended. Continued examination should proceed only when the postoperative anatomy is clearly defined.

The size, configuration, and relationship of the gastric pouch to the channel or anastomosis can be delineated with contrast material. Since pouch diameters and volumes change significantly depending on the amount of gastric distension, and since measurements have not been found to be reliable predictors of successful weight loss, attempted quantitation by radiographic measurements with elaborate

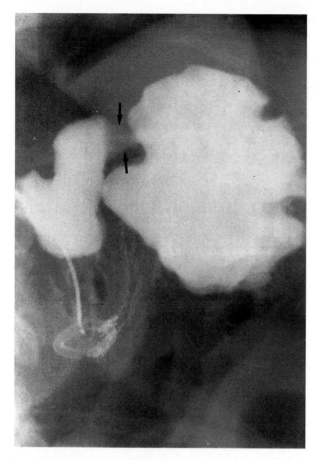

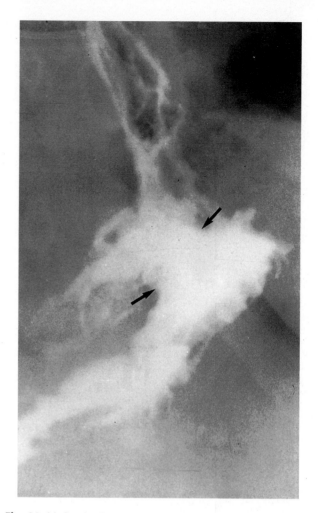

Fig. 23-10 Staple line dehiscence after vertical banded gastroplasty. Water-soluble contrast material does not pass via the normal channel into the distal stomach but egresses abnormally through the upper end of the staple line *(arrows)*. Since the stomach is not transected, staple line dehiscence does not result in spillage of gastric contents into the abdomen.
From Smith C et al: *Radiographics* 5:193, 1985.

Fig. 23-11 Staple line dehiscence after vertical banded gastroplasty. There is a large area of dehiscence *(arrows)* along the superior end of the staple line. Almost all of the contrast material passes quickly into the distal stomach.
From Smith C et al: *Radiographics* 5:193, 1985.

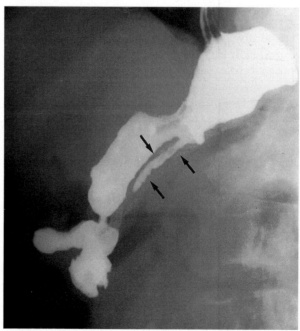

Fig. 23-12 Partial staple line dehiscence after vertical banded gastroplasty. Incomplete dehiscence of the staple lines allows contrast material to insinuate in the combined space between the staple lines *(arrows)*. This situation requires urgent surgical revision, since increased pressure within this small volume space can lead to ischemia of the adjacent stomach.

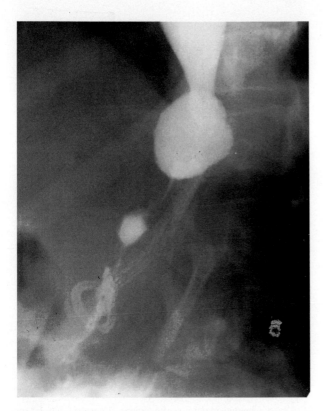

Fig. 23-13 Channel obstruction after vertical banded gastroplasty. There is delayed passage of contrast material from the proximal pouch with two areas of narrowing. The patient had surgery 7 days before this study and the stenoses were thought to be on the basis of edema. A follow-up study 2 weeks later showed complete resolution and a normal proximal pouch.

extrapolation for magnification is no longer recommended. Rather, contrast studies have been found to be important sources of information about the patient that may be unavailable to the surgeon otherwise. For example, the radiologic examination can reveal the degree of pouch distention a patient will tolerate without complaint, estimate the amount of nausea or type and location of abdominal pain that occurs when the pouch and stomach are distended with contrast material, and demonstrate both the amount of gastroesophageal reflux and any symptoms it produces during the study. This type of information may be much more valuable to the surgeon in assessing the success or failure of a gastric restrictive procedure than measurements of the gastric pouch size and volume and of channel diameter.

As a result, upper GI studies should not be used to "predict" the outcome of gastroplasty procedures directly. They should be used in conjunction with meticulous patient follow-up that entails specific, goal-directed patient evaluation by the surgeon.

Pouch dilatation

Studies evaluating the stability of pouch size and volume vary. Most recent studies strongly suggest that pouch size increases over time.[30] Radiographically, a significant change in pouch size from a baseline study can be identified readily (Fig. 23-15). Reoperation can be performed in selected patients to reduce the pouch volume.[44] However, revision surgery based only on the radiographic appearance of the postoperative stomach, and the coincident failure to

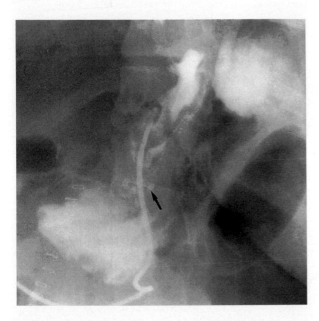

Fig. 23-14 Outlet obstruction after vertical banded gastroplasty. Note that the gastrostomy tube in the distal stomach has migrated in a cephalad direction through the channel and has its tip in the proximal pouch *(arrow)*. Repositioning of the gastrostomy tube with relief of the obstruction was accomplished easily.

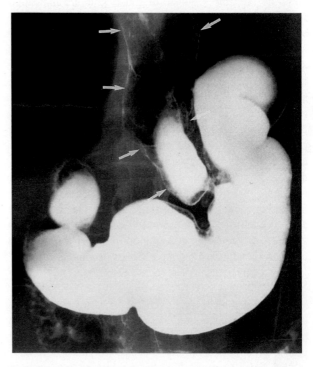

Fig. 23-15 Pouch dilatation after vertical banded gastroplasty. This biphasic study shows a large-volume proximal pouch *(arrows)* in this patient who had surgery 4 years ago. Despite the enlarged pouch volume, she continued to lose weight.

lose weight, may not be considered as promptly as it was in the past. Revision surgery is usually not undertaken until the surgeon is confident that dietary indiscretion, whether it be purposeful or unwitting, is not the basis for unsatisfactory weight loss.

Staple line dehiscence

Causes of staple line disruption in the delayed postoperative period usually relate to gross dietary indiscretion or outlet obstruction with prolonged increased pouch pressure and subsequent tissue damage.[45] Staples may pull apart from the gastric wall and create alternate and additional routes to the normal channel for the gastric pouch to empty.

Channel widening

Channel reinforcement after gastroplasty and the creation of smaller channels have decreased the incidence of channel widening. Delaying the intake of solid food in the 6- to 8-week period after surgery also allows the channel to undergo sufficient fibrosis to prevent dilatation.[46]

Widening of the channel after gastric bypass may increase the vasomotor symptoms related to the dumping syndrome (Fig. 23-6). This situation may in fact contribute to weight loss rather than to weight gain. Currently, as in pouch dilatation, the identification of channel widening alone does not always necessitate surgical revision.

Channel stenosis and obstruction

Channel stenoses with significant symptoms of reflux, vomiting, and the sequelae of esophagitis are indications for prompt therapy. Unfortunately, patients may be reluctant to seek follow-up care because of the dramatic weight loss and may endure painful symptoms (Fig. 23-17). Endoscopic studies are usually the first examinations performed when patients have symptoms suggesting channel stenosis.[47] Foreign bodies may be removed and stenoses may be dilated at the time of the diagnostic procedure (Fig. 23-18). Endoscopic balloon dilatations are effective alternatives to surgical revision and can be successful even in cases when the reinforced channel appears no larger than a pinhole.[48] If severe channel angulation is present, surgical revision is usually required.[47,48] Outlet obstruction caused by food impaction can occur (Fig. 23-18). The usual causes are ingestion of pills, large-sized foods with a tough consistency, or premature consumption of fiber through noncompliance with postoperative dietary recommendations.[47]

Ulceration

Gastritis and ulcers in the proximal gastric pouch and distal stomach are uncommon but increase with medication intake[47,49] (Figs. 23-19 and 23-20). Stomal ulceration after gastric bypass occurs rarely.[3,47] Gastritis and inflammation of the distal stomach after gastric bypass have recently come into focus with the increasing use of endoscopy to study the bypassed stomach.[40] This inflammation is thought to be related to bile reflux, is a definite cause of patient

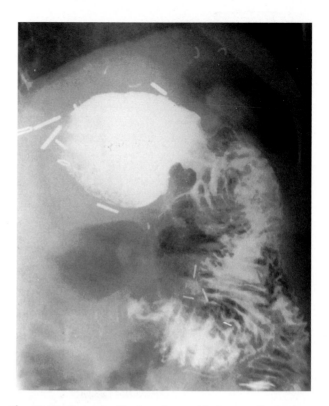

Fig. 23-16 Channel widening after gastric bypass. Contrast material passes freely from the proximal pouch through the widened channel into the small bowel. Despite a large channel, the patient had sustained weight loss.

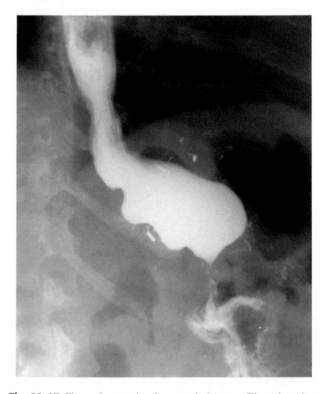

Fig. 23-17 Channel stenosis after gastric bypass. There is only a slow trickle of contrast material from the proximal pouch into the small bowel. Most of the contrast material refluxes into the esophagus, which is ulcerated.

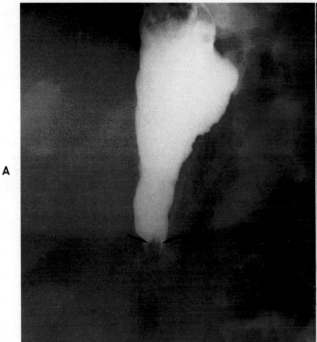

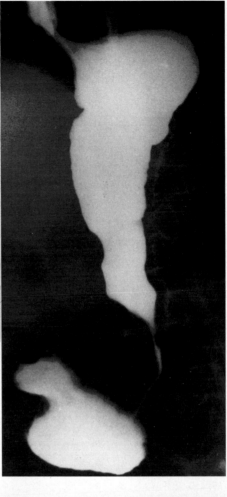

Fig. 23-18 Outlet obstruction caused by food impaction after vertical banded gastroplasty. Contrast material study **(A)** and a follow-up examination **(B)**. Endoscopy showed that the filling defect *(arrows)* at the distal end of the proximal pouch near the channel was a peanut lodged in the channel. Follow-up study shows that the channel is pinpoint in diameter. Multiple endoscopic dilatations were needed for successful channel enlargement.
From Smith C et al: *Radiographics* 5:193, 1985.

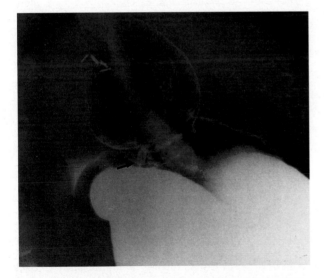

Fig. 23-19 Gastritis after horizontal gastroplasty. There is dilatation of the proximal pouch, widening of the channel *(solid arrows),* and superficial ulcerations in the proximal pouch *(open arrows).* This patient had a history of ulcerogenic medication intake.

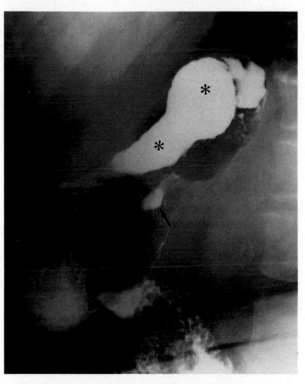

Fig. 23-20 Vertical banded gastroplasty with ulceration. This lateral view obtained during a contrast study shows the proximal pouch *(asterisks)* overlapping the distal stomach. There is an ulcer 15 mm in diameter *(arrow)* in the distal stomach along the posterior wall.

discomfort, and may lead to ulceration, bleeding, or perforation.[47] Metaplasia with the possibility of carcinoma is still an unknown risk and requires further study.[40]

SUMMARY

In summary, many patients have had gastric surgery for obesity over the last several decades. Many had surgical procedures that are no longer the currently favored approaches but are still intact, and some of these patients may need to be examined radiologically. The radiologist performing studies on patients who have had gastric surgery for weight control must be aware of the possible anatomic configurations that can occur, the normal appearance of the stomach postoperatively, and the array of complications that may be seen.

REFERENCES

1. National Institutes of Health Consensus Development Panel: Health implications of obesity: National Institutes of Health Consensus Development Conference statement, *Ann Intern Med* 103:147, 1985.
2. Manson JE et al: Body weight and longevity: a reassessment, *JAMA* 257:353, 1987.
3. Moody FG, McGreevy JM: Complications of gastric surgery. In Greenfield LJ, ed: *Complications in surgery and trauma*, ed 2, Philadelphia, 1990, JB Lippincott.
4. Hall JC et al: Gastric surgery for morbid obesity: the Adelaide study, *Ann Surg* 211:419, 1990.
5. Linner JH: Overview of surgical techniques for the treatment of morbid obesity, *Gastroenterol Clin North Am* 16:253, 1987.
6. Benotti PN et al: Gastric restrictive operations for morbid obesity, *Am J Surg* 157:150, 1989.
7. Mason EE, Ito C: Gastric bypass in obesity, *Surg Clin North Am* 47:1345, 1967.
8. Mason EE: Vertical banded gastroplasty for obesity, *Arch Surg* 117:701, 1982.
9. Eckhout GV, Willbanks OL, Moore JT: Vertical ring gastroplasty for morbid obesity: five-year experience with 1463 patients, *Am J Surg* 152:713, 1986.
10. Flickinger EG, Sinar DR, Swanson M: Gastric bypass, *Gastroenterol Clin North Am* 16:283, 1987.
11. Willbanks OL: Gastric restrictive procedures: gastroplasty, *Gastroenterol Clin North Am* 16:273, 1987.
12. Flickinger EG, et al: The Greenville gastric bypass: progress report at 3 years, *Ann Surg* 199:555, 1984.
13. Sugerman HJ, Starkey JV, Birkenhauer R: A randomized prospective trial of gastric bypass versus vertical banded gastroplasty for morbid obesity and their effects on sweets versus non-sweets eaters, *Ann Surg* 205:613, 1987.
14. Mason EE: Morbid obesity: use of vertical banded gastroplasty, *Surg Clin North Am* 67:521, 1987.
15. Yale CE: Gastric surgery for morbid obesity: complications and long-term weight control, *Arch Surg* 124:941, 1989.
16. Shearman CP, Baddeley RM: Which gastroplasty for the correction of massive obesity? *Ann R Coll Surg Engl* 68:139, 1986.
17. Halverson JD, Koehler RE: Gastric bypass: analysis of weight loss and factors determining success, *Surgery* 90:446, 1981.
18. Linner JH: Comparative effectiveness of gastric bypass and gastroplasty: a clinical study, *Arch Surg* 117:695, 1982.
19. Pories WJ et al: The effectiveness of gastric bypass over gastric partition in morbid obesity: consequence of distal gastric and duodenal exclusion, *Ann Surg* 196:389, 1982.
20. Makarewicz PA et al: Vertical banded gastroplasty: assessment of efficacy, *Surgery* 98:700, 1985.
21. Hocking MP, Kelly KA, Callaway CW: Vertical gastroplasty for morbid obesity: clinical experience, *Mayo Clin Proc* 61:287, 1986.
22. Nightengale ML et al: Prospective evaluation of vertical banded gastroplasty as the primary operation for morbid obesity, *Mayo Clin Proc* 66:773, 1991.
23. Carr ND et al: Vertical banded gastroplasty in the treatment of morbid obesity: results of three-year follow-up, *Gut* 30:1048, 1989.
24. Brolin RE et al: The dilemma of outcome assessment after operations for morbid obesity, *Surgery* 105:337, 1989.
25. MacLean LD, Rhode BM, Forse RA: Late results of vertical banded gastroplasty for morbid and super obesity, *Surgery* 107:20, 1990.
26. Ismail T et al: Vertical silastic ring gastroplasty: a 6-year experience, *Br J Surg* 77:80, 1990.
27. Benotti PN: Vertical banded gastroplasty in the treatment of severe obesity (editorial), *Mayo Clin Proc* 66:862, 1991.
28. Villar HV et al: Mechanisms of satiety and gastric emptying after gastric partitioning and bypass, *Surgery* 90:229, 1981.
29. Salmon PA: Failure of gastroplasty pouch and stoma size to correlate with postoperative weight loss, *Can J Surg* 29:60, 1986.
30. Behrns KE et al: Anatomic, motor, and clinical assessment of vertical banded gastroplasty, *Gastroenterology* 97:91, 1989.
31. Andersen T et al: A randomized comparison of horizontal and vertical banded gastroplasty: what determines weight loss? *Scan J Gastroenterol* 24:186, 1989.
32. Horowitz M et al: Gastric emptying after gastric bypass, *Int J Obesity* 10:117, 1986.
33. Smith C et al: Gastric restrictive surgery for obesity: early radiologic evaluation, *Radiology* 153:321, 1984.
34. Smith C et al: Radiology of gastric restrictive surgery, *Radiographics* 5:193, 1985.
35. Burhenne HJ: The postoperative stomach. In Taveras JM, Ferrucci JT, eds: *Radiology: diagnosis—imaging—intervention*, Philadelphia, 1986, JB Lippincott.
36. Smith C, Gardiner R: The postoperative stomach and recurrent abdominal pain. In Thompson WM, ed: *Common problems in gastrointestinal radiology*, Chicago, 1989, Mosby–Year Book.
37. Baer JW: Radiology of obesity surgery, *Gastroenterol Clin North Am* 16:349, 1987.
38. McNeely GF et al: Percutaneous contrast examination of the stomach after gastric bypass, *AJR* 149:928, 1987.
39. Rankin RN, Grace DM: Examination of the distal stomach after gastric bypass for obesity, *J Can Assoc Radiol* 36:146, 1985.
40. Sinar DR et al: Retrograde endoscopy of the bypassed stomach segment after gastric bypass surgery: unexpected lesions, *South Med J* 78:255, 1985.
41. Alexander-Williams J, Hoare AM: The stomach: Part II. Partial gastric resection, *Clin Gastroenterol* 8:331, 1979.
42. Mishkin JD et al: Interventional radiologic treatment of complications following gastric bypass surgery for morbid obesity, *Gastrointest Radiol* 13:9, 1988.
43. van Sonnenberg E et al: Percutaneous abscess drainage: current concepts, *Radiology* 181:617, 1991.
44. Cates JA et al: Reoperative surgery for the morbidly obese: a university experience, *Arch Surg* 125:1400, 1990.
45. Carey LC, Martin EW Jr: Treatment of morbid obesity by gastric partitioning, *World J Surg* 5:829, 1981.
46. Goodman P, Halpert RD: Radiological evaluation of gastric stapling procedures for morbid obesity, *Crit Rev Diagn Imaging* 32:37, 1991.
47. Freeman JB: The use of endoscopy after gastric partitioning for morbid obesity, *Gastroenterol Clin North Am* 16:339, 1987.
48. Sataloff DM, Lieber CP, Seinige UL: Strictures following gastric stapling for morbid obesity: results of endoscopic dilatation, *Am Surg* 56:167, 1990.
49. Nunes JR et al: Suture line ulceration: a complication of gastric partitioning, *Gastrointest Radiol* 9:315, 1984.

24 *Radiology of Benign and Malignant Diseases of the Duodenum*

JACQUES W.A.J. REEDERS
G. ROSENBUSCH

Endoscopy has had an enormous impact on the diagnosis of duodenal disease, while paraduodenal and extrinsic diseases, which had to be diagnosed 20 years ago mainly by hypotonic duodenography, are now more accurately assessed by ultrasound (US), computed tomography (CT), magnetic resonance imaging (MRI), and endosonography. It remains important, however, for radiologists to recognize the various diseases on barium studies.

Double-contrast examination of the duodenal bulb with hypotonia and distension shows mostly a smooth featureless surface, and in about 5% to 10% of cases, a fine, lacy reticular pattern.[1] There may be very small rounded lucent areas corresponding to the villi.[1,2]

In distension, Kerckring's folds (valvulae conniventes) are transverse, sometimes circular in the descending part. They are 1 to 2 mm thick and 5 to 10 mm apart from each other. At the medial side in the midportion they end at the straight segment and the longitudinal fold produced by the papilla of Vater and the distal common bile duct. When the duodenum is not distended, the mucosal pattern is feathery.

CONGENITAL AND MISCELLANEOUS ABNORMALITIES
Congenital positional anomalies

Congenital position anomalies and mesenteric bands can be important in childhood because they may cause recurrent partial obstruction. Sometimes they are encountered in adults as incidental findings. Because of disturbances in fixation and rotation, the duodenal loop can be absent or incomplete (malrotation, nonrotation) when the duodenal sweep ends before or in the midline. In these cases the small intestine and the large bowel wall show atypical position, too. When angiography is performed in cases with recurrent obstruction, the superior mesenteric artery and the superior mesenteric vein can be twisted around the mesenteric root with dilatation of the draining veins.

As a result of defective attachment, the duodenum can show increased mobility, which can be observed during examination in the upright and supine positions. In the case of an inverted duodenum, the duodenum runs craniad from the bulb.

Congenital diaphragm of the duodenum

A diaphragm or web (membrane) of the duodenum is a congenital anomaly. When the membrane is complete, obstruction is complete, and symptoms are present from birth.[3] When the membrane is perforated or incomplete, symptoms can develop later and depend on the degree of stenosis. The diaphragm may be silent or provoke only slight pain in the midabdomen, or vomiting.[4] The membranes are located near the papilla of Vater. They have mucosa on both sides and muscularis mucosae in between.

On barium study, a weblike lesion can be seen. Usually there is no abnormality of transit, but it can be obstructive, causing proximal duodenal dilatation (megaduodenum). There may be associated anomalies such as duplication of the gallbladder.

Ladd's bands

Ladd's bands result from a rotation anomaly, with obstruction of the third or fourth part of the duodenum.[5] Usually this anomaly manifests immediately after birth or in early childhood. Rarely the symptoms present in adolescents or adults.

Clinically and radiologically an acute and chronic form are distinguished. The radiologic feature of the acute form is high-grade duodenal obstruction, and in the chronic form there is dilatation with increased duodenal peristalsis. The site of obstruction may be anywhere from the crossing of the superior mesenteric artery to the ligament of Treitz.

Annular pancreas

Annular pancreas is a rare anomaly. It results from failure of the embryologic central anlage to rotate and join the dorsal limb.[6] Although it may present during infancy, the condition becomes apparent more frequently in adults during the third to fifth decades.[6,7] Coexisting congenital anomalies (congenital heart disease, duodenal stenosis or atresia, mongolism, tracheoesophageal fistula with or without esophageal atresia, and malrotation of the intestines) may be present in 20% to 70% of cases.[7]

Annular pancreas may be found as the underlying cause of duodenal stenosis or atresia in 40% of cases in infancy. In childhood the characteristic radiographic feature is a "double bubble sign." In a series of 266 patients with symptomatic annular pancreas, 52% were children and 48% adults.[6]

The condition may be entirely asymptomatic unless complications occur, such as peptic ulceration (22%), acute pancreatitis (15% to 50%), and bile duct obstruction.[7,8] Varying degrees of duodenal obstruction occur with secondary symptoms such as colicky upper abdominal pain (86%), nausea, vomiting, and weight loss. The following radiologic signs may be seen in annular pancreas (Fig. 24-1):

1. A small annular filling defect in the upper midportion of the descending duodenum, with massive dilatation of stomach and duodenal bulb
2. Extrinsic compression arising from the lateral wall, proximal to the stenotic area[9,10]
3. At the level of the annulus, retraction of the duodenum toward the head of the pancreas by the encircling tissue
4. A notchlike defect with eccentric luminal narrowing, generally 1 to 2 cm long; the diameter of the duodenal lumen distal to the annulus is normal.

At endoscopy a stenotic area or complete obstruction is present beginning generally within 3 cm of the apex.[10] Just above the stenotic area a nonspecific increase of duodenal folds may be seen.[11] Endoscopic retrograde cholangiopancreatography (ERCP) can show the corresponding duct of the annular pancreas running around the constriction of the duodenum.[9,10] At ultrasonography a narrow echo-dense band around the fluid-filled and hypotonic duodenum can be demonstrated.[12] The fine echo-free line in the center of the echo-dense band may be caused by the pancreatic duct.

In the differential diagnosis, cholecystoduodenocolic bands, postbulbar peptic ulcer stricture, primary neoplasm, and duodenitis need to be considered.

Duodenal diverticulum

Diverticula of the duodenum can be congenital or acquired. They are found in 1% to 6% of all upper radiologic GI series but are found much more often during autopsy.[13] The duodenum is the second most common location of diverticula, after the colon.

Congenital diverticula are herniations of all layers of the duodenal wall through muscular defect, especially where

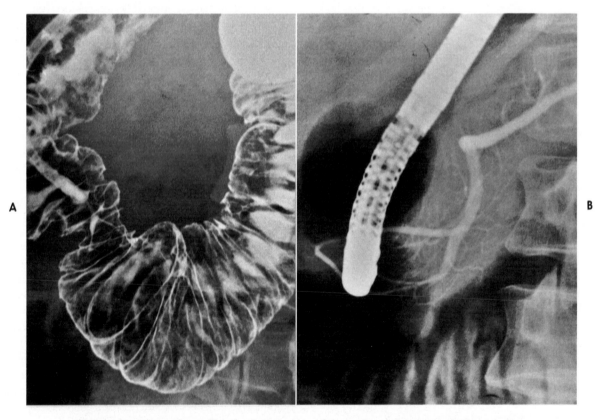

Fig. 24-1 Annular pancreas. The circular extension of the pancreatic head around the second portion of the duodenum causes a circular constriction with intact folds. The anomaly of the ventral anlage of the pancreas can best be demonstrated by endoscopic retrograde cholangiopancreatography (ERCP), which shows the corresponding duct running around the constriction of the duodenum. **A,** Hypotonic duodenography. **B,** ERCP.

arteries enter the wall. They are rare and mostly located on the medial duodenal wall. *Acquired* duodenal diverticula consist only of the mucosal and submucosal layers with some scattered muscle fibers. They are discovered mainly in the fifth and sixth decades. The incidence increases with age and is the same in males and females. Most duodenal diverticula remain asymptomatic. When located near the papilla of Vater they can compress the common bile duct or the pancreatic duct and cause obstruction. When the common bile duct or the pancreatic duct terminates in a juxta-Vaterian diverticulum, there is increased risk for obstructive inflammatory disease of both bile duct and pancreas.[14]

Congenital and acquired diverticula cannot be differentiated radiologically. In more than 10%, the diverticula are multiple. Their main location is on the inner sweep. The most frequent location is adjacent to the papilla of Vater, followed by the third and fourth parts. Postbulbar sites and sites on the outer side of the duodenum are rare.

Most diverticula are between 0.3 and 3 cm in size. The larger ones are mostly found at the duodenojejunal flexure when the mouth and neck are much smaller than the sac. Mucosal folds enter the neck of the diverticula (Fig. 24-2; see Fig. 24-17, *C* and *D*).

Contrast media may remain longer in the diverticulum than in the duodenum itself. Sometimes food particles can be seen in the diverticulum. During examination some change in size and form of the diverticulum can be observed, and lobulation may be seen. Fluid levels may be seen on erect films. On US, fluid-filled diverticula can mimic pancreatic pseudocysts. A change in size during the examination aids in diagnosis, as does the finding of air in the diverticulum.

The diagnosis of diverticulum on CT is facilitated by use of oral iodinated contrast medium. Because the diverticulum can penetrate the parenchyma of the pancreas, filling with contrast medium is important to differentiate it from pancreatic pseudocyst. Gas or food particles may also be seen on CT.[15] A small diverticulum can mimic a gastric ulcer or polyp when projecting over the stomach; conversely, a giant ulcer of the duodenal bulb or postbulbar region may readily be mistaken for a diverticulum. Adhesions or scars can lead to traction with diverticula-like outpouchings.

Complications of diverticula include ulceration, hemorrhage, and perforation. Abscesses or fistulas can complicate such peptic ulcers. Perforation is usually into the retroperitoneal space or in the mesenteric root, rarely into the peritoneal cavity. Fistulas are possible to both the gallbladder and the colon.[16] When such complications are suspected, the examination must be performed with an iodinated contrast medium, not barium. Carcinoma in a diverticulum is a rarity.

The clinical symptoms of duodenal diverticulitis may be those of cholecystitis, pancreatitis, peptic ulcer disease, colitis, and retrocecal appendicitis. Duodenal diverticulitis is rarely diagnosed by upper GI series because the diverticulum may fail to fill. On a plain film sometimes a mottled extraluminal gas pattern can be seen in a paraduodenal location. On US, retroperitoneal gas shows brightly echogenic foci perirenally.[13] On CT studies, extraluminal fluid collections, extraluminal gas, wall thickening, hazy soft tissue density, as well as strands in adjacent fat may be evident.[17]

Intraluminal diverticulum

Intraluminal duodenal diverticulum is rare compared with the common duodenal diverticulum. It is a congenital

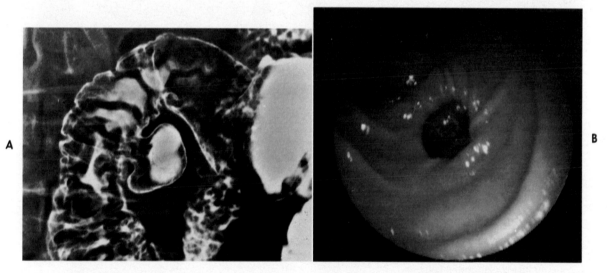

Fig. 24-2 Duodenal diverticulum. Mucosal folds radiating into a large diverticulum arising from the second part of the duodenum. **A,** Upper GI barium study. **B,** Endoscopy.

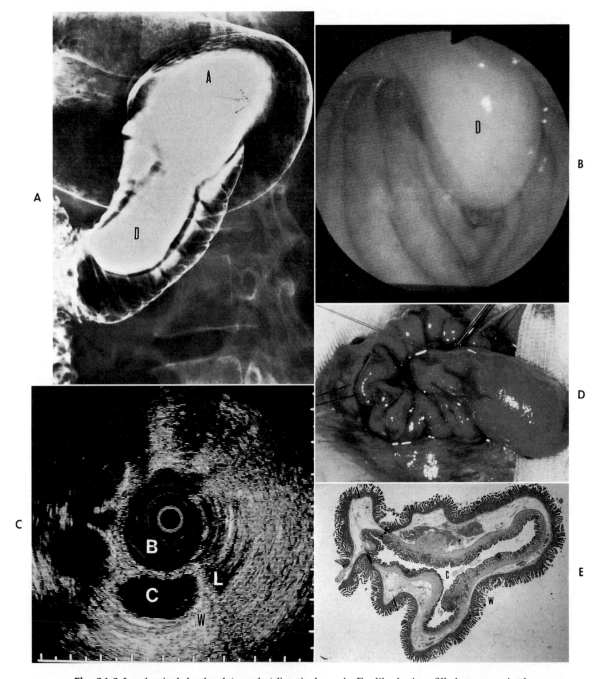

Fig. 24-3 Intraluminal duodenal (pseudo-)diverticulum. **A,** Egglike barium-filled structure in the duodenal lumen. A thin radiolucent line surrounds the diverticulum *(D)* caused by its wall. Although the true lumen of the duodenum is almost empty, the diverticulum is still filled with barium. *A,* Antrum. **B,** Submucosal mass covered by normal mucosa in the second part of the duodenum just distal to the papillary orifice. **C,** EUS demonstrates the "cystic" nature of the lesion. *B,* Water-filled balloon serving as an acoustic window; *L,* intestinal lumen; *W,* wall of cyst; *C,* diverticulum. **D,** Resection specimen shows saclike structure with a normal mucosal epithelium. **E,** On both sides the intraluminal diverticulum has a mucous membrane with a thin layer of muscularis mucosae in between.

anomaly. Essentially it is an incomplete septum or diaphragm in the second and occasionally in the third part of the duodenum. When the stomach contents are expelled into the duodenum, this septum, which results from abnormal canalization of the duodenum, is caudally distended.[18] This intermittent distension, increased by peristalsis of the duodenum for many years, leads to a saclike structure called an *intraluminal diverticulum*. The size is usually 2 to 4 cm, but the length can be up to 12 cm, the width up to 6 cm, and the opening up to 2 or 3 cm.[19] On both sides this diverticulum has epithelium with a thin layer of muscularis mucosae in between.

On barium studies, this fingerlike or egglike diverticulum fills with barium (Fig. 24-3). A thin radiolucent line surrounds the diverticulum, representing its wall. Rarely a small distal opening facilitates emptying of the diverticulum. More often, the diverticulum remains filled with barium after the true lumen of the duodenum has emptied. When such an intraluminal diverticulum is packed with food, no barium can enter it, and a changeable oval filling defect is seen in the second part of the duodenum.

When small, an intraluminal diverticulum is asymptomatic, but when larger it produces pain in the right upper quadrant or signs of postprandial discomfort. This may explain why the diagnosis is often made in the third and fourth decades of life.

Bleeding can occur from laceration. Pancreatitis is possible when the flow of pancreatic juice is impeded by compression. Eventually, symptoms of obstruction may develop.

The intraluminal diverticulum occurs sometimes with other congenital anomalies, such as duplication of the gallbladder and anomalies of the heart. Endoscopic incision or excision of the diverticulum has been described[18]; this form of treatment may render open surgery unnecessary.

Wall cysts of the duodenum

Duodenal wall cysts (also known as enterogenic cysts or duplication cysts) may be congenital or the result of chronic pancreatitis caused by heterotopic pancreatic tissue present in the duodenal wall or from cystadenomas.[20] They occur in the first or second part of the duodenum. Most cysts do not have a communication with the duodenal lumen. They are much more often diagnosed in children than in adults.

Patients can have vague epigastric discomfort associated with nausea and vomiting. A relationship with chronic relapsing pancreatitis is reported, probably because of obstruction of the pancreatic duct by the cystic lesion.[20] Because these lesions are intramural, they are recognized on a barium study as smooth, spherical intramural filling defects on the medial wall of the descending part. They are 2.5 to 8 cm long and can sometimes change their form with compression, since they contain fluid.

With US the intramural lesion is sonolucent or sometimes has a complex echo pattern. The cystic wall is usually thick, regular, and similar to the gut wall. Internal septa can be present.[21] Sometimes the pancreas shows calcifications and a dilated duct and pseudocysts.

On CT the lesion density may vary from solid to water. The contents can be inhomogeneous. Calcifications caused by mobile enteroliths in the cysts have been described.[22] Ductal changes of chronic pancreatitis are sometimes present. Cystic wall lesions of the duodenum have to be differentiated from other intramural lesions such as leiomyomas, choledochoceles, and intraluminal diverticula, as well as from pancreatic pseudocysts.

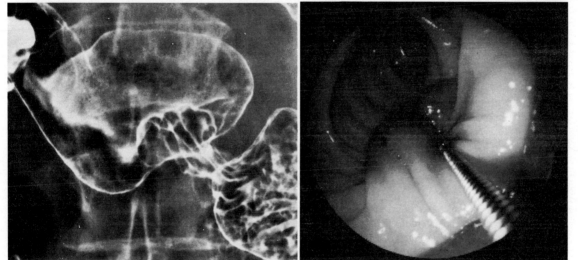

Fig. 24-4 Prolapse of antral mucosa. **A,** Prolapse of antral mucosa into the duodenal bulb. Well-delineated filling defects are seen along the base of the bulb on both sides of the pylorus. The picture changes during examination. **B,** Prolapse of the mucosa into the duodenum, grasped by a forceps.

Antral mucosal prolapse

Redundant mucosa of the gastric antrum can prolapse through the pylorus and produce a changeable mushroom-like filling defect in the base of the duodenal bulb[23,24] (Fig. 24-4). The filling defect may vary in size during the examination depending on the degree of gastric peristalsis. Usually it is of no clinical importance.

Intussusception

Duodenal intussusception is less frequent than intussusception of the small intestines because of the fixed retroperitoneal duodenal position.[25] Intussusception starts more easily from the first duodenal portion because of the greater mobility resulting from its connection with the lesser omentum.[26]

Duodenal tumors—benign or malignant—may act as the lead point for intussusception. However, benign tumors (polyposis, fibroadenoma, lipoma, papilloma, Brunner's gland adenoma, prolapsing gastric tumor) do so more frequently because they are more mobile.[27,28]

The symptoms of duodenal intussusception lack specificity; they include episodes of crampy epigastric pain and occult blood loss. The classic radiologic manifestation is a "coiled spring" appearance caused by the intussusceptum

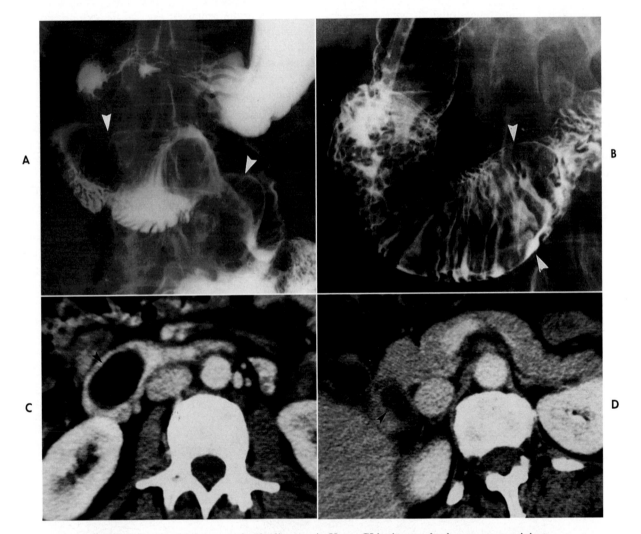

Fig. 24-5 Duodenal intussusception by lipoma. **A,** Upper GI barium study shows a mass originating in the second part of the duodenum, intussuscepted in the jejunum. The jejunum shows a coiled-spring pattern. The intussusceptum goes the shortest way in curves, simulating two separated masses *(arrows)*. **B,** Three days later hypotonic duodenography reveals a polypoid mass in the inferior duodenal flexure *(arrows)*. The intussusception has resolved spontaneously. **C** and **D,** Contrast-enhanced CT scans show the hypodense lipoma *(arrow)* of the inferior duodenal flexure and the intussusception in the form of a double concentric lumen *(arrow)*, the duodenum being opacified with water.
From Van Beers B et al: *Gastrointest Radiol* 13:24, 1988.

invaginating and foreshortening the receiving bowel[25] (Fig. 24-5).

Several entities should be considered in the differential diagnosis of duodenal intussusception, including intraluminal diverticulum, duodenal hematoma, pancreatitis, pancreatic mass, and postbulbar duodenal ulcer.

Paraduodenal hernias

More than 50% of all internal abdominal hernias occur in the paraduodenal region. They are congenital and are located on the left or right side (see Chapter 94).

INFLAMMATION
Nonspecific duodenitis

It is still not clear whether duodenitis is a distinct clinical entity or represents part of the spectrum of peptic ulcer disease.[29-31] Gastric hyperacidity[32] and duodenal ulceration are frequent associated findings. The radiographic criteria of spasm, irritability, thickening of duodenal folds greater than 4 mm, mucosal nodularity (Fig. 24-6), erosions, and bulbar deformity are relatively unreliable for diagnosing duodenitis.[33] Using these criteria the radiologic sensitivity in literature varies from 52% to 80%[33,34]; however, the rate of false-positive findings related to mucosal pits in the duodenum, mimicking erosions on double-contrast studies and false-negative radiologic diagnoses, in the study by Levine et al. was 50%.[2,34] They found swelling of duodenal folds in only 44%, mucosal nodularity and bulbar deformity in less than 12%, and duodenal erosions in less than 8% of their patients.

The diagnosis can best be made by the endoscopic appearance and by the characteristic histopathologic findings on biopsies.[35] Reddening of the bulb with pale areas of intervening mucosa, focal erosions, and confluent or patchy erythema are common findings.

Erosions

Duodenal erosions are uniform and may be numerous; they are superficial, punctate, and focal. They are usually located in the proximal bulb and often surrounded by a faint radiolucent halo caused by edema, but they can present as white dots on nodular folds.[36]

The differential diagnosis should include peptic ulcer disease and aphthoid ulcers in Crohn's disease.

Crohn's duodenitis

Approximately 200 cases of Crohn's duodenitis have been reported in the literature. Over 80% of these patients have had coexistent lesions in the more typical segments such as terminal ileum, right colon, or both.[37-41] The duodenum, most frequently proximally (including the antrum of the stomach), is involved in 2% to 20% of cases of Crohn's duodenitis.[41]

The main symptoms, which may be overshadowed by the severity of those from disease in the small bowel or colon, include persistent or intermittent postprandial upper epigastric pain associated with nausea, vomiting, weakness, and weight loss. The *initial* phase of Crohn's duodenitis is usually characterized radiologically by superficial tiny defects mimicking erosive lesions. These defects are scattered over

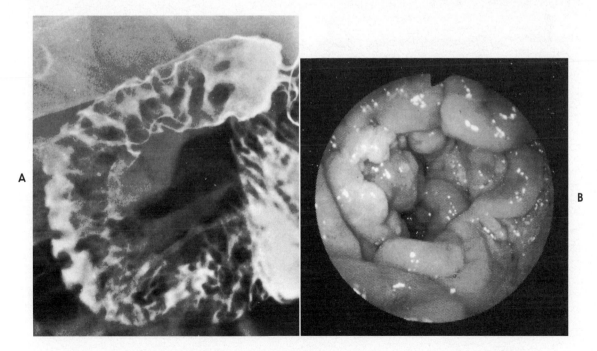

Fig. 24-6 Nonspecific bulbarduodenitis. **A,** Duodenal erosions as punctate collections of barium, surrounded by nodular mounds of edema on thickened duodenal folds. **B,** Endoscopy: thickening of duodenal folds with erosions.

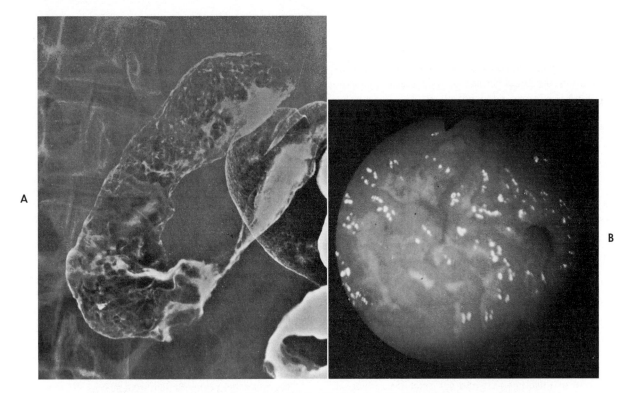

Fig. 24-7 Crohn's duodenitis. **A,** Asymmetric distribution of multiple serpiginous and solitary aphthoid ulcers in D1 and D2. Coarsening of the mucosal pattern with deformity of the descending duodenum. **B,** Endoscopy shows the coarsening of the duodenal mucosa with serpiginous and solitary aphthoid ulcers.

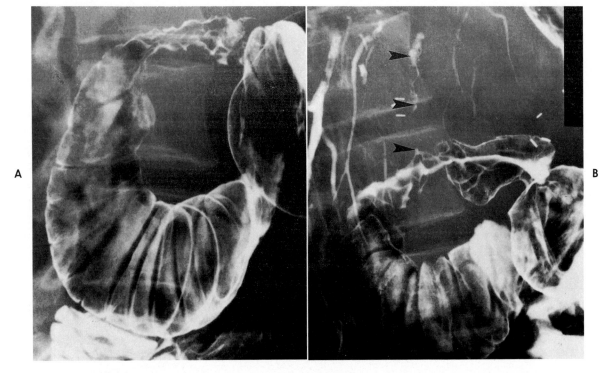

Fig. 24-8 Duodenal stricture in Crohn's disease. Postbulbar irregular but symmetric stricture with longitudinal ulcerations and a fistulous tract from the duodenum into the common bile duct *(arrows)* as complication in long-standing Crohn's duodenitis.

edematous folds, which may appear nodular because of lymphoid or glandular hyperplasia. When erosions are detected endoscopically they are demonstrated by radiography in 50% of patients.[37,41,42] In the *subacute* phase "cobblestone" nodularity of the mucosa may be apparent.[43]

In the *chronic* progressive phase the transmural inflammation causes luminal narrowing of the thickened and rigid duodenal wall. A short segmental stricture or multiple stenotic segments may also develop, most frequently in the first and second parts of the duodenum, separated by pseudodiverticula and dilatation of the intervening "skip" areas.[44] These pseudodiverticula tend to be on the outer side of the duodenal sweep, unlike the diverticula described previously. The third part of the duodenum may be involved, and disease sometimes progresses distally to involve the ligament of Treitz[45] (Fig. 24-7). Ulcerations are rarely seen in this stage. The pyloric channel is distorted and frequently becomes patulous and continuous with the duodenal bulb ("ram's horn"). When stomach and duodenum are both involved it may have a pseudo-Billroth I configuration.

Reflux of barium into the biliary tract and pancreatic duct may be observed during barium examination of the upper gastrointestinal tract.[44,46] Sinus tracts and duodenobiliary fistulas (Fig. 24-8), duodenocolic fistulas (Figs. 24-9 and 24-10), or duodenoenterocutaneous fistulas may complicate Crohn's duodenitis[37,44] in the first and second parts of the duodenum.

Radiographic observation of progressive duodenal narrowing or ulceration (Fig. 24-8) should stimulate careful endoscopic evaluation and biopsy to exclude malignant degeneration of Crohn's duodenitis. Patients with Crohn's disease of the duodenum and small bowel are at risk for developing malignant degeneration of chronically inflamed loops.[37,47,48] This occurs more proximally; the frequency in the duodenum is twice that in the jejunum and four times that in the ileum.[48] It develops more frequently (30%), however, in a bypassed segment. The endoscopic appearance of Crohn's duodenitis includes lack of distensibility, poor contractions, aphthoid ulcers or erosions, deep serpiginous ulcers,[43,49] a diffuse nodular pattern (cobblestones), thickening or stiffening of antral and duodenum folds, and eventually stenosis.[49]

On CT Crohn's duodenitis may demonstrate wall thickening, with enhancement after intravenous contrast administration. Extramucosal complications (such as abscesses and fistulas) can be seen better by CT.[37]

The most important differential diagnoses are sarcoidosis, tuberculosis, non-Hodgkin's lymphoma, peptic ulcer disease, primary duodenal carcinoma, metastases (from breast, lung, colon, and kidney carcinoma), pancreatitis, and eosinophilic gastroenteritis.

Eosinophilic gastroduodenitis

Although an uncommon site, the duodenum may be involved as a continuation of the disease from the prepyloric antrum of the stomach. In a patient with prominent indu-

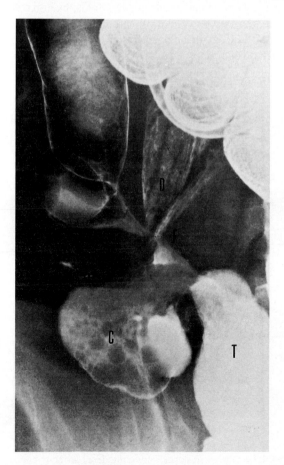

Fig. 24-9 Coloduodenal fistula caused by Crohn's disease. There is a severe Crohn's stricture at the junction of the cecum with the ascending colon. *D,* Duodenum; *C,* cecum; *T,* terminal ileum; *F,* fistula.

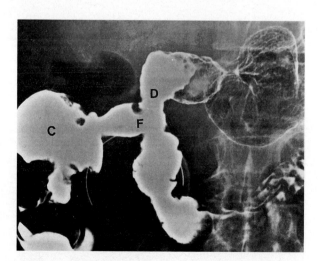

Fig. 24-10 Coloduodenal fistula caused by Crohn's disease. Fistula between hepatic flexure of the colon and the descending portion of the duodenum in long-standing Crohn's colitis and Crohn's duodenitis. *D,* Duodenum; *F,* fistula; *C,* colon.

rated prepyloric antral folds and eosinophilia, the diagnosis of duodenal involvement is considered even if endoscopy shows only nonspecific erythema or nodularity.[50] Radiologic signs are irritability and fold thickening of the duodenum, almost always with jejunal involvement.

Radiation ischemic duodenitis

Although the duodenum is an uncommon site for ischemia, it may occur in patients who receive more than 4000 rads (for metastatic carcinoma of the cervix, testicular carcinoma, or primary right-sided retroperitoneal tumors) to the entire abdominal paraortic lymph node chain or to the right upper retroperitoneal area. Diffuse thickening of mucosal folds caused by submucosal edema, hemorrhage with "scalloping" (thumb printing) of the duodenal margins, wall thickening, ulceration, and stricture formation may be observed radiographically (Fig. 24-11). On endoscopy there is in addition either focal or diffuse nonspecific erythema and coarsening of the mucosal villous pattern.

Chronic radiation ischemia may result in stricturing of varying lengths (Fig. 24-12). These appearances also may be caused by emboli, venous or arterial thrombosis, vascular invasion by tumors, and vasculitis.

Caustic ingestion

Caustic ingestion may lead to duodenitis, always in conjunction with antral lesions (scattered ulceration), eventually leading to stricture formation and, rarely, to jejunal ulceration.

Infective duodenitis
Tuberculosis

The diagnosis of localized duodenal tuberculosis is seldom made preoperatively because it is extremely rare [51] even in patients with pulmonary tuberculosis. The clinical presentation includes epigastric pain, weight loss, fever, nausea, vomiting, and ascites.[52] Sometimes gastric outlet obstruction is found. The possible routes of tuberculous spread are hematogenous, lymphatic, directly from adjacent structures, or via ingestion. Radiologic signs are edematous coarsening of mucosal folds and small superficial ulcerations, giving a spiculated outline of the duodenal wall mimicking Crohn's disease (Fig. 24-13).

Granulating mucosal pseudopolyps with or without ulcers may be seen. The disease may progress or heal with resulting fibrosis and subsequent stricturing of the second portion of the duodenum. Caseation with abscess formation may occur. Submucosal and extrinsic masses (enlarged tuberculous lymph nodes indenting the duodenal wall) may cause obstruction and simulate malignancy of the duodenum.

Sinuses and fistulas are uncommon complications. A chest radiograph in these patients often shows evidence of pulmonary tuberculosis, while a normal chest x ray makes a diagnosis of duodenal tuberculosis unlikely. On endoscopy deep irregular ulcerations are seen, with markedly enlarged and erythematous surrounding folds; masslike deformities are common. The most common conditions considered in the differential diagnosis are Crohn's duodenitis and duodenal neoplasm.

Parasites

Giardia, Strongyloides, Ascaris lumbricoides, and *Ancylostoma duodenale* may all affect the duodenum. They are described in Chapter 46.

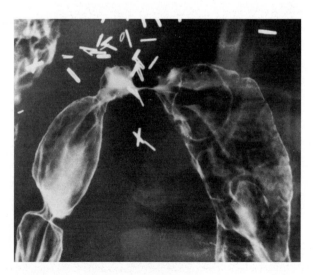

Fig. 24-11 Postbulbar radiation-induced stricture (11 months after radiation of colonic metastatic carcinoma).

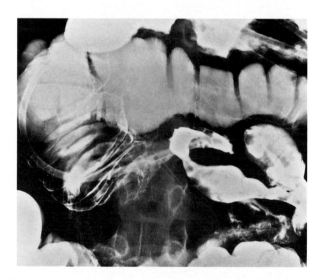

Fig. 24-12 Iatrogenic postischemic duodenal stricture caused by accidental ligation of superior mesenteric artery. Severe destruction of mucosal folds and transmural thickening *(arrowheads)* at the third part of the duodenum are visible; enteroclysis: transverse colon is already filled.

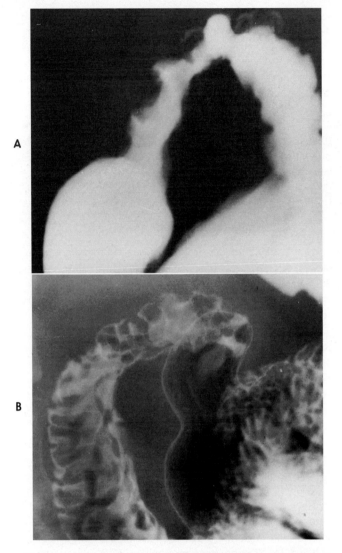

Fig. 24-13 Tuberculous duodenitis. Duodenal bulb deformed by edematous, coarsened and ulcerated mucosal folds. The duodenal bulb and postbulbar region are indented by enlarged tuberculous lymph nodes. **A,** Single-contrast study, left anterior oblique view. **B,** Double-contrast study, right anterior oblique view.

Organisms associated with immunologic deficiency

In patients with immunologic dysfunction (posttransplant, AIDS), a multitude of opportunistic infections of the GI tract may occur. The most common infections involving the duodenum are cytomegalovirus (CMV) and *Cryptosporidium,* with *Candida* and *Histoplasma capsulatum* being less common.

CYTOMEGALOVIRUS

Duodenal and small intestinal disease account for the greatest percentage of GI abnormalities seen radiographically in AIDS patients. Duodenal abnormalities may be found in 82% of AIDS patients with upper GI abnormalities.[53] On barium studies CMV may produce a diffuse du-

odenitis, submucosal nodules (0.25 to 0.75 cm), thickening of folds, discrete erosionlike to deep round or serpiginous scattered ulcerations of various sizes and depths, and narrowing of the lumen.

Duodenal obstruction and perforation may occur. They are attributed to the ischemic necrosis secondary to vasculitis induced by CMV inclusion bodies found in the endothelial cells and the small vessels of the bowel wall.[54] Biopsy specimens from these lesions may reveal typical cells with prominent intranuclear inclusions. On CT the duodenum wall may be thickened.

CRYPTOSPORIDIUM

Cryptosporidiosis has been shown to be an important cause of severe infections of the duodenum and small bowel in patients with disordered immunoregulation in AIDS. The clinical symptoms may vary from moderately severe diarrhea to uncontrollable dehydration and electrolyte disturbances. Barium studies show thickened duodenal folds, fragmentation and flocculation of barium caused by hypersecretion, spasm, and dilatation. Differential diagnosis includes giardiasis, *Strongyloides,* Zollinger-Ellison syndrome, cystic fibrosis, acquired hypogammaglobulinemia, and alpha chain disease.

CANDIDA

Candida overgrowth of the duodenum can occur in a compromised immune state, especially within the base of an ulcer.[55] Duodenal plaquelike pseudomembranes, focal candidal ulceration, or both may be found at endoscopy and radiography.

HISTOPLASMA CAPSULATUM

Although the small bowel is the commonest GI site for dissemination of histoplasmosis in immunocompromised patients, duodenal involvement is uncommon[56] (2%). Diarrhea and malabsorption are common symptoms. No radiologic manifestations are known. The diagnosis can be made only by (blind) endoscopic biopsy.

PEPTIC ULCER
General aspects

Duodenal ulcers are common, four times as frequent as gastric ulcers. The incidence is 3 to 10 times as great in males as in females with a peak age between 30 and 40 years, about 10 years earlier than with gastric ulcers. The major symptoms are epigastric pain, typically but not invariably relieved by food, and waking the patient at night. Uncommonly, duodenal ulcers are found in patients with no pain, especially elderly patients. Symptoms that suggest complications include recurrent duodenal bleeding, hematemesis, weight loss, intractable abdominal or back pain, and vomiting caused by residual or progressive stricture formation. About 30% of duodenal ulcer patients have an associated gastric ulcer. There is an association with smoking.

It has recently become clear that the overwhelming single factor in the etiology of peptic ulceration is infection with the organism now called *Helicobacter pylori*. This organism meets Koch's postulates as the causative agent for chronic type B gastritis and is probably the cause of most non-drug-related gastritis. Antral chronic type B gastritis is found in all patients with duodenal ulcer, most of whom also have gastric metaplasia in the duodenal bulb. *H. pylori* can be found in these metaplastic cells and is thus a constant feature in patients with duodenal ulcer, as it is with gastric ulcer (apart from ulcers caused by antiarthritis medication or aspirin). Now that the sequence of causation of the intestinal type of gastric cancer is known (from gastritis through atrophy and intestinal metaplasia to dysplasia and finally to carcinoma), *H. pylori* may be considered a major cause of gastric cancer of the nondiffuse type.[57]

If *H. pylori* is a pivotal agent in gastritis, gastric ulcer, duodenal ulcer, and gastric cancer, is endoscopy and biopsy required to diagnose its presence in every patient with dyspepsia?[58] Morrissey and Reicheldorfer[59] have suggested that the answer is no, that there is no need to perform endoscopy in a patient who has had a duodenal ulcer diagnosed radiologically, for two reasons.[59] First, the organism will be recovered from over 90% of such patients, so its presence can be assumed. Second, antimicrobial therapy is not very often successful. Development of a successful treatment and demonstration that relapse was uncommon after eradication of the organism might change this as would development of simple serologic tests to permit detection and monitoring of *H. pylori* infection without the need for biopsy.[58] A number of regimens are being evaluated for the elimination of *H. pylori* infection, for example, omeprazole combined with amoxicillin, and these research efforts require multiple endoscopies and biopsies.

Peptic ulcers occur with increased frequency during corticosteroid therapy, in hyperparathyroidism, in liver cirrhosis, in renal transplantation, and with exocrine pancreatic insufficiency. Duodenal ulcer may also be found in association with annular pancreas (43%).

Acute ulcers can heal without significant scarring, whereas in chronic ulcers radiating folds develop. The recurrence rate of duodenal ulcers is very high. There is no malignant degeneration of duodenal ulcers.

The majority of duodenal ulcers are small (less than 1 cm), frequently multiple, and occur preferentially in the first 3 cm of the bulb. About 50% of duodenal ulcers are located on the anterior wall, 25% on the posterior wall, 20% at the cranial side, and 5% at the caudal side. About 5% to 10% are postbulbar. Ulcers beyond the level of the ampulla of Vater are uncommon; if present, Zollinger-Ellison syndrome should be suspected,[60] which is responsible for 0.1% to 1.0% of peptic ulcers.

Radiologic features

The radiologic diagnosis of a duodenal ulcer depends on the demonstration of an ulcer niche.[60,61] Before the introduction of hypotonia, indirect signs were sometimes considered enough for diagnosing an ulcer. For diagnosis, characterization, and localization, such older techniques as barium-filled views, compression, and examination in different positions such as left anterior oblique (LAO), right anterior oblique (RAO), supine, and prone have to be employed, as well as double-contrast (multiphasic) study.

The typical picture of an acute ulcer is a niche with a mound caused by adjacent inflammatory edema. This ulcer mound is smooth, but in chronic disease radiating folds are seen that end at the edge of the ulcer. The niche is round or oval, but can be linear too (see below), with regular or irregular margins (Figs. 24-14 and 24-15, *D-F*). The size varies from some millimeters to some centimeters (see Giant Duodenal Ulcer).

Ulcers should always be demonstrated in two projections or with different techniques. They should be examined with graded compression and in full-column in LAO. In the latter position, differentiation of anterior or posterior wall ulcers is possible.

Posterior wall ulcers can readily be visualized on double-contrast films in the supine position, whereas an anterior ulcer empties in this position and is visible only as a ringlike structure,[62] representing the ulcer margin. In the prone position, however, the anterior wall becomes dependent, and an anterior wall ulcer is well seen, filled with barium.

Ulcers on the superior or inferior surface are best seen in profile, that is, the RAO position, when the bulb is fully distended, and on full-column view and double-contrast films.

When two ulcers touch with the duodenum collapsed, usually when they are directly opposite each other on the anterior and posterior walls, they are called *kissing ulcers* (Fig. 24-16). Double-contrast films in the supine position show the ulcer on the dependent wall filled with barium, whereas the one on the nondependent wall empties and is depicted as a ring. With compression of the barium-filled bulb, both ulcers are seen superimposed, and on the LAO position they can be seen anteriorly and posteriorly.

A shallow ulcer with gently sloping margins localized at the dependent surface may be difficult to see on double-contrast films. Barium may run out of it in the supine position and only a ringlike shadow remain. In such a case, when a second (kissing) ulcer is present on the nondependent wall, two ringlike structures may be visible in double-contrast.

When an ulcer has a collar at the entrance and is located at the nondependent wall, it can show two concentric rings in double-contrast films, caused by the collar and sides of the wider ulcer base.

Fibrotic tissue around a chronic ulcer can lead to shrinkage, resulting in converging folds and pseudodiverticula that resemble a clover leaf (Fig. 24-17, *A*). The pyloric channel can be eccentric and the fornix flattened (Fig. 24-18). *Text continued on p. 484.*

Text continued on p. 484.

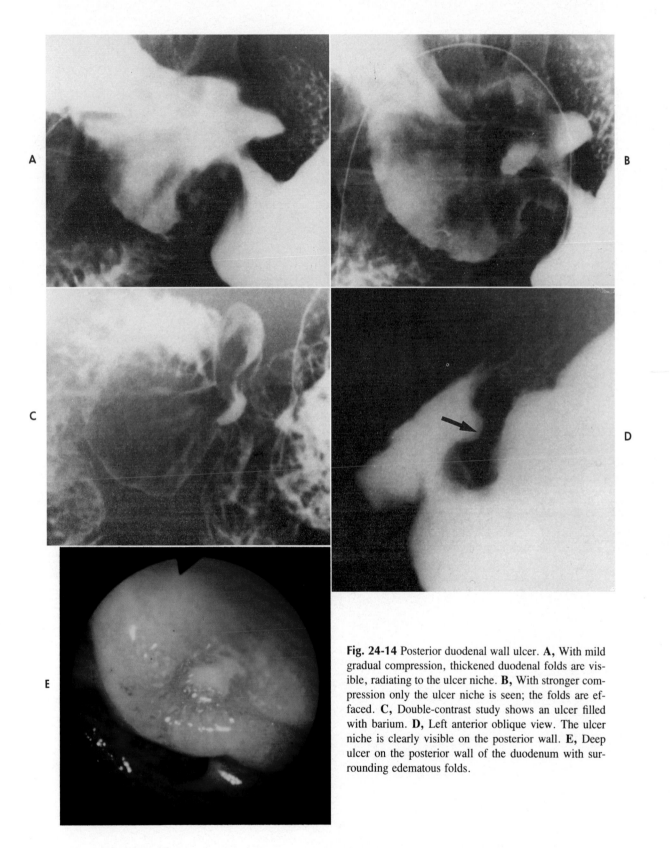

Fig. 24-14 Posterior duodenal wall ulcer. **A,** With mild gradual compression, thickened duodenal folds are visible, radiating to the ulcer niche. **B,** With stronger compression only the ulcer niche is seen; the folds are effaced. **C,** Double-contrast study shows an ulcer filled with barium. **D,** Left anterior oblique view. The ulcer niche is clearly visible on the posterior wall. **E,** Deep ulcer on the posterior wall of the duodenum with surrounding edematous folds.

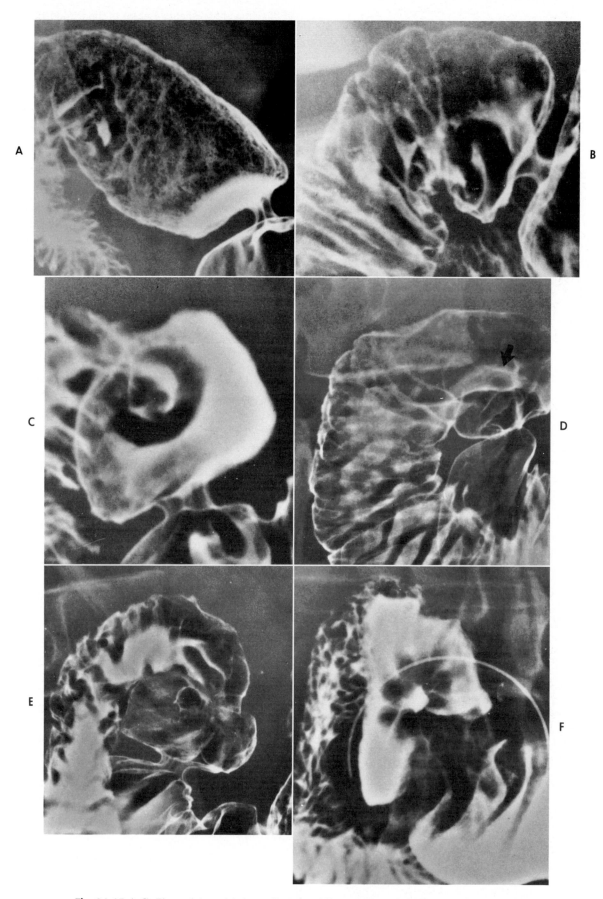

Fig. 24-15 A-C, Flexural (pseudo)ulcers. Round and linear barium collections between redundant mucosa of a relatively mobile bulb, simulating duodenal ulcer. Endoscopy showed solitary fold thickening without evidence for ulcerative disease. **D** and **E,** Ulcer niche of the nondependent anterior wall of the duodenum. The empty ulcer crater appears as a ring. **F,** Posterior duodenal wall ulcer (compression view) with surrounding edematous radiating folds.
A-C from R.E. Kottler.

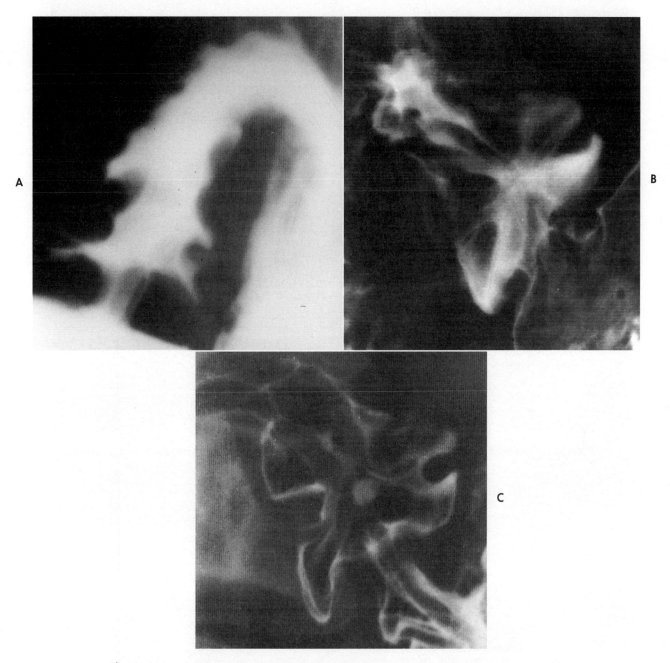

Fig. 24-16 Kissing ulcers. Ulcers of the anterior and posterior walls of the duodenal bulb. **A,** Left anterior oblique view. The duodenal bulb shows two ulcers, one on the anterior wall and one on the posterior wall. **B** and **C,** With slight compression and in double contrast, both ulcers are seen as one niche, because they are projected over each other.

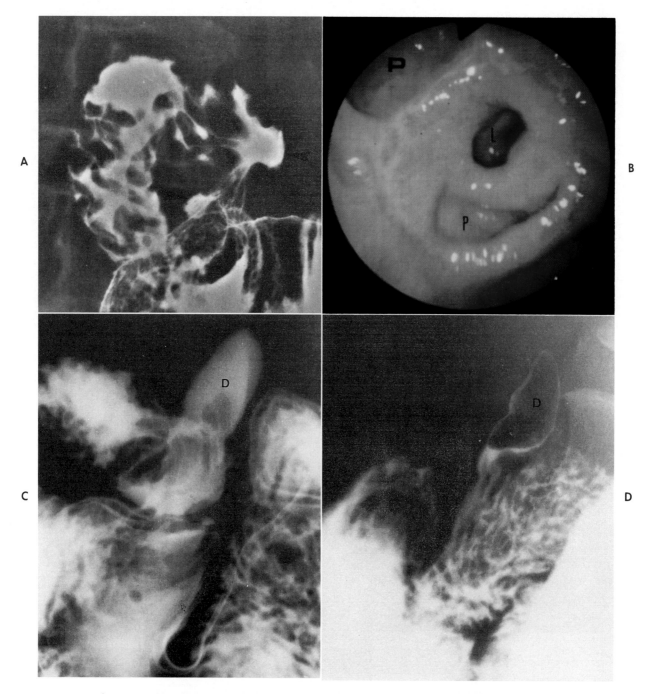

Fig. 24-17 Pseudodiverticula versus diverticula of the duodenum. **A,** Duodenal bulb deformed from previous duodenal ulcer disease showing pseudodiverticula *(arrows)* (cloverleaf deformity). **B,** Endoscopy shows the pseudodiverticula (*L,* Lumen; *P,* pseudodiverticula). **C** and **D,** Diverticulum of the third part of the duodenum. By applying different projections it is possible to differentiate the diverticulum from a giant ulcer. *D,* Diverticulum.

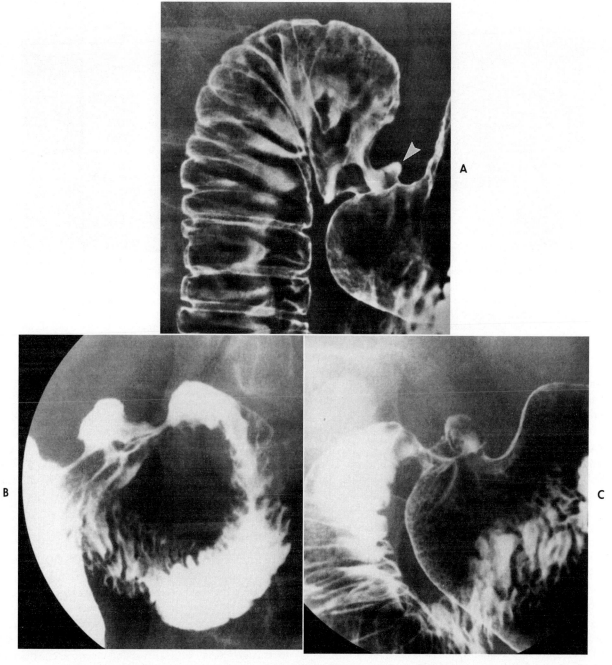

Fig. 24-18 Pyloric ulcer with deformity of the anteroduodenal junction. **A,** Deformity of the base of the duodenal bulb with a deep penetrating ulcer at the pylorus. Ovoid barium collection *(arrow)* on the posterior wall of the pylorus associated with lumen narrowing and wall retraction. Right anterior oblique position in filling state. **B,** Right anterior oblique view in prone position. **C,** RAO in supine position: converging folds with swelling around the niche. *U,* Ulcer.

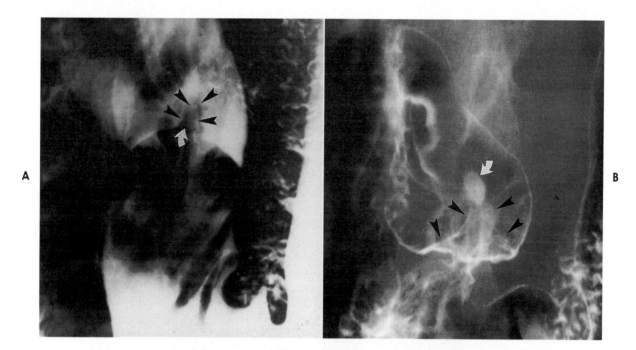

Fig. 24-19 Baseline tenting sign. **A,** Upright compression view of the duodenal bulb shows sharply interrupted baseline *(arrow)* and two perpendicular lines *(arrowheads)* converging at the site of an ulcer. **B,** Supine left posterior view shows baseline tenting sign *(arrowheads)* and a round ulcer crater *(arrow)*. No other bulb deformities are present.
From Lu CC, Murakami J, Barloon T, Ell SR, Franken SA: *Gastrointest Radiol* 12:109, 1987.

In the healing phase, "baseline tenting" occurs in 84% of patients with acute or chronic duodenal ulcer[61] (Fig. 24-19). It is characterized by interruption of the baseline of the bulb with two associated perpendicular lines extending from the base and converging to a point in the duodenal bulb. In the normal duodenal bulb the baseline is either straight or slightly convex toward the apex, extending from the superior to the inferior fornix.[61] A negative baseline tenting sign does not exclude the diagnosis of duodenal ulcer. In an acute ulcer there may be only edema and interruption of the baseline without tenting, particularly if the ulcer is near the base. With a giant ulcer or severely deformed bulb, the baseline is usually distorted, so the baseline tenting sign is not applicable. In the differential diagnosis of baseline tenting, prolapse of antral mucosa has to be considered.

In the scarred bulb a small depression often persists, so radiologically it is difficult to decide whether or not an ulcer is still present. This is important when a patient with known ulcer disease is coming for a new upper GI series. If an examination was performed after treatment, no comparison is possible, and in this case, endoscopy is preferred if further examination is absolutely necessary.[63]

On ultrasound examination of patients with duodenal ulcer an echogenic focus (hyperechoic center) may be seen in various shapes and sizes, localized in the wall of the ulcerated lesion. This echogenic focus corresponds to necro-inflammatory material found on the surface of ulcerated lesions and is visualized because of the interface between this tissue and edema of the adjacent layers of the duodenal wall,[64,65] which are visible as a hypoechoic halo surrounding the echogenic focus. A specific sonographic diagnosis can seldom be made even within the appropriate clinical setting (Fig. 24-20).

Linear ulcer

Linear ulcers are found in 6% to 7% of all duodenal ulcers[66,67] and represent the healing phase of some ulcers. They are transversely oriented. The transverse niche on the deformed bulb can be demonstrated when well distended in double-contrast, and even better with graded compression.[66] The niche may be a fuzzy line with radiating folds to its edge[66] (Fig. 24-21). A round ulcer can coexist with a linear ulcer. Kissing linear ulcers have been described. They occur most often in the clover-leaf bulb but are also seen in nondeformed duodenal bulbs as acute ulcers heal.

Giant duodenal ulcer

Duodenal ulcers exceeding 2 cm in diameter or involving the whole bulb have been termed *giant duodenal ulcers*.[68] Giant duodenal ulcers (2 to 6 cm) may be difficult to recognize on upper GI studies because they are mistaken

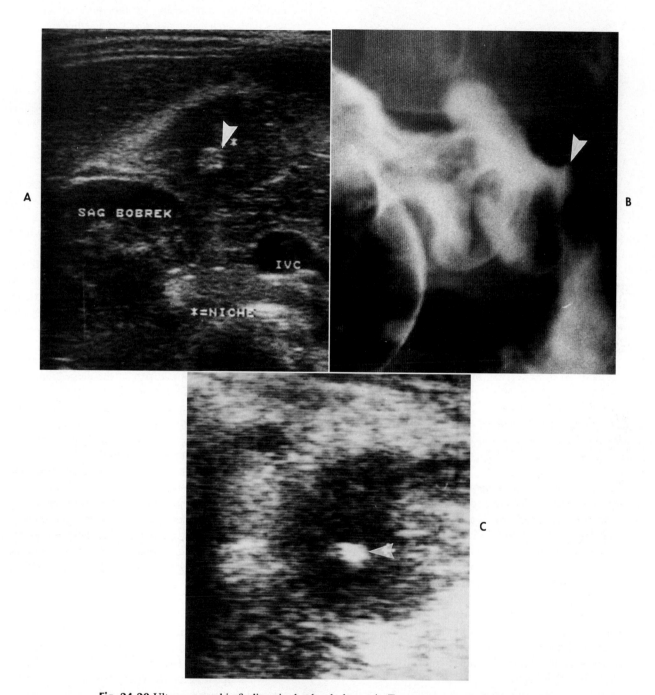

Fig. 24-20 Ultrasonographic findings in duodenal ulcers. **A,** Transverse sonography demonstrates an echogenic core surrounded by a thick hypoechoic halo lateral to the head of the pancreas *(arrow).* **B,** Ulcer with spasm at the apex of the duodenal bulb *(arrow; prone position).* **C,** An echogenic area surrounded by a thick hypoechoic rim *(arrow)* caused by duodenal ulcer.
From Tuncel E: *Gastrointest Radiol* 15:207, 1990.

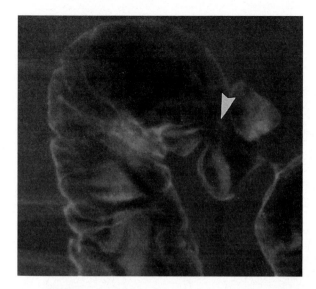

Fig. 24-21 Linear duodenal ulcer. En face view of a fine linear barium collection at the center of radiating folds caused by healing duodenal ulcer.

for a deformed duodenal bulb or diverticulum, especially if the gastroduodenal ulcer has completely destroyed the posterior wall of the bulb and is eroding into the pancreas. In giant duodenal ulcer the risk of hemorrhage and perforation is increased. The accuracy rate of radiologic diagnosis ranges from 45% to 84%.[68-70] When using traditional and new criteria, giant duodenal ulcers can be diagnosed correctly 100% of the time.[68] The main problem is to think of the diagnosis. Criteria for diagnosing a giant duodenal ulcer include the following:

1. Constancy in size and shape of the niche throughout the examination. The crater does not contract like the duodenal bulb, because it is a cavity with rigid walls; barium may be drained by changing the position of the patient. Late films, hours after examination, may show residual barium in the niche.
2. Loss of mucosal pattern; often round or oval, sometimes irregular, sharp crater outline.
3. Ulcer/bulb ratio: greater than 0.8.
4. Air-filled, barium-coated cast of cavity visible.
5. Consistent alterations in the appearance of the pylorus proximally and of the duodenum distally to the gastroduodenal ulcer.
6. Filling defects resulting from the nodularity of the floor of the ulcer crater, simulating carcinoma; constriction of the duodenal lumen distal to the crater.
7. "Ulcer-within-an-ulcer" appearance (31%). This appearance is important because the radiologist may diagnose the smaller ulcer as the only ulcer and fail to recognize that it is superimposed on a giant duodenal ulcer. The crater of a gastroduodenal ulcer may be mistaken for the entire bulb, for a pseudodiverticu-

lum of the bulb, or for a true diverticulum. The appearance of the gastroduodenal ulcer depends on the position of the patient, the projection (en face or in profile), the relationship of the ulcer to anatomic structures such as the pylorus, and whether an inflammatory mass is present.

The constancy of size and shape of the giant duodenal ulcer in contrast to the changeability of the outline of a normal bulb is the major differential criterion. Endoscopically a giant duodenal ulcer can be distinguished from a normal bulb, diverticulum, or pseudodiverticulum by the absence of a normal mucosal pattern.

Postbulbar ulcer

Postbulbar ulcers account only for about 5% of duodenal ulcers, but their demonstration is important because they may lead to pancreatitis, bleeding, and, when fibrosis occurs, to stenosis. It occurs mainly in males in their fifties after several years of ulcer symptoms.[57]

The postbulbar ulcer can be difficult to detect radiologically because the interest of the examiner is concentrated on the bulb. As spasm, edema, and poor coating obscure the ulcer, hypotonic duodenography is very important and helpful for its demonstration; indeed, it is usually essential.

Usually, the ulcers are located at the medial or posteromedial aspect of the proximal part of the descending duodenum (Fig. 24-22). Ulcers distal to the papilla of Vater are very rare. The atypical localization of duodenal ulcers, especially when mucosal folds are thickened, should suggest the Zollinger-Ellison syndrome. The form of the ulcer niche can be either longitudinal or round.

The size can vary from a few millimeters to several centimeters in length and depth. On the opposite side of the ulcer there is spasm in the form of an incisura, an almost constant and diagnostic feature that may be more obvious than the ulcer itself until intravenous relaxants are given. When the ulcer is chronic, the indentation on the opposite side does not disappear with hypotonia because fibrosis is already present.

Complications

The most common complications of peptic ulcer are, in decreasing frequency, stricture,[62,71] obstruction, bleeding, penetration of adjacent organs, and perforation (3% to 13%).[72] In duodenal strictures with obstruction, an upper GI series will show excessive fluid in a dilated stomach with delay in emptying.

Fifty percent of all duodenal ulcers may bleed, which may be diagnosed by endoscopy or angiography.[73] Selective angiography of the celiac trunk can show the bleeding site; when a penetrating ulcer of the posterior wall erodes the gastroduodenal artery, bleeding can be catastrophic.

Free perforation (10% to 35%) is demonstrated on plain films. In 50% of the patients with free perforation, it is the

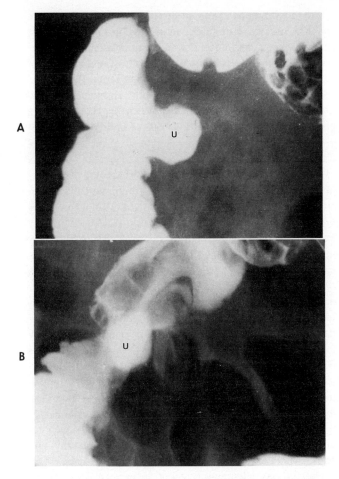

Fig. 24-22 Giant postbulbar ulcer at the medial site. **A,** Tangential view. **B,** En face view.

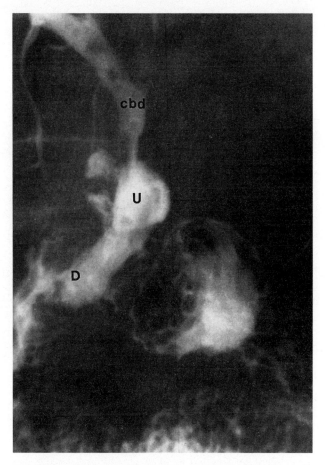

Fig. 24-23 Duodenocholedochal fistula caused by ulcer perforation. Filling of the common bile duct *(CBD)* from a big ulcer *(U)* niche.

first symptom of peptic disease. A water-soluble contrast examination may occasionally be necessary to confirm the diagnosis. Often there is a continued perforation, usually because adhesions have already developed before perforation has occurred. Perforation into adjacent organs, especially the pancreas, and fistula formation (i.e., duodenocolic, duodenocholedochal [Fig. 24-23] and duodenocholecystic) have been described.

Ultrasonography may help diagnose perforation and penetration complicating peptic ulcer because 11% of patients with perforated ulcer show no free intraperitoneal air or gas on radiography. After perforation, the intestinal contents may be visible on ultrasound, initially as an echo-free, and later, an echogenic effusion.

Focal peritonitis caused by a perforated ulcer is usually located in the right upper quadrant, which is accessible to sonographic evaluation. Sometimes the site and extent of penetration may be detected on ultrasonography.[72]

Although CT may occasionally demonstrate large ulcers,

its chief utility lies in assessing patients with suspected complications, such as perforation, lesser sac abscess, or penetration-induced pancreatitis.[72]

Differential diagnosis and pitfalls

A false-positive radiologic diagnosis of peptic ulcer is possible, with confusion arising from a wide variety of normal variants, lesions, and other diseases, including:
- Flexural pseudolesion[74,161] (Fig. 24-15, *A-C*)
- Overprojection of adjacent structures, such as diverticula of the duodenojejunal flexure
- Diverticula; the mucosal folds run up to the neck of the diverticulum; the diverticula are usually smooth and can contain food particles
- Ectopic pancreatic tissue
- Pseudodiverticula in "clover-leaf deformity"
- Adenoma, metastasis of melanoma, or submucosal lesion as leiomyoma, when a slight depression is present, which can be caused by ulceration

- Inflammation of such adjacent organs as the pancreas or gallbladder
- Nonpeptic ulceration
- Tuberculosis
- Aortoduodenal, duodenocolic, or duodenorenal fistula
- Extension of carcinoma of adjacent organs such as the pancreas, gallbladder, right kidney, or right colon

X ray versus endoscopy

When a multiphasic examination is performed (i.e., double-contrast, single-contrast, graded compression) and different projections are used, a 10% to 20% improvement in overall sensitivity can be expected.[75,76] In a prospective blinded study, Chandieshaw et al.[75] found a lower sensitivity and specificity for duodenal ulcers with radiography than with endoscopy, but this difference disappeared if very small erosion-like ulcers were excluded. Because a duodenal ulcer never becomes malignant, duodenoscopy with biopsy is much less important than in gastric ulcer.

In young patients with dyspeptic symptoms, an upper GI series is sufficient for demonstration of peptic ulcer, even if it is slightly less accurate than endoscopy.

TUMORS

Small bowel tumors are rare lesions. Twenty percent to 45% of the benign tumors in the small intestine occur in the duodenum, and 20% to 50% of these are of epithelial origin.[77]

Adenoma

Adenomas, although uncommon, have been encountered with increasing frequency.[77] They are divided into villous, tubular, and tubulovillous adenomas.

Villous adenomas (papillary adenoma, adenomatous papilloma, papillary tumor) with high malignant potential (21% to 47%) should be distinguished from other adenoma-like forms, such as Brunner's gland "adenomas," which never degenerate, and Lieberkühn's "adenomas."[77-81]

Widespread application of upper GI endoscopy and more frequent endoscopic surveillance of patients with polyposis syndromes have resulted in identification of more and younger patients with duodenal adenomas. The average age for patients with villous adenoma is 57 years with a male to female sex ratio of 1:1. For nonvillous adenoma the average age is 53 years, and the sex ratio is 2:1[77] These adenomas generally occur as isolated lesions (Fig. 24-24). Ninety-four percent of nonvillous adenomas occurred in the bulb and first or second parts of the duodenum, whereas 87% of the villous adenomas were found between the first and second parts, especially periampullary (82%).[82] The average size of villous adenoma was 4.6 cm (range, 0.4 to 10 cm).[10-23] Twenty-seven percent of villous adenomas lead to obstruction of the duodenum or obstructive jaundice.[83]

Compression spot films are useful in defining the extent and characteristics of tumor margins. On double-contrast examination, a radiolucent rounded nodular mass may be seen as a filling defect, interspersed in a fine lacework of barium ("cauliflower," "soap bubble" appearance) in villous adenomas. This appearance is caused by entrapment of barium in the intervillous spaces between the fine frondlike projections of the tumor[83] (Figs. 24-25 and 24-26).

Tubular and tubulovillous adenomas are more often pedunculated (Fig. 24-27), and villous adenomas appear as cauliflower-like masses (Fig. 24-26). Endoscopy and barium studies are complementary rather than mutually exclusive techniques. False-negative results are found in 9.5% of barium studies.[77] The sensitivity of upper GI endoscopy exceeds that of double-contrast studies.[81] Endoscopy permits accurate identification and localization of duodenal adenomas and biopsy for histologic classification, which can prove useful for planning the appropriate operative procedures.[81] In some cases endoscopic polypectomy is possible. However, endoscopy is limited with regard to duodenal tumors because of submucosal tumor growth, inability to assess the distal extension of large tumors that cause duodenal obstruction, and occasionally, the patient's intolerance to endoscopy. Although Fork et al.[81] did not find tumor size to be a predictor of invasive carcinoma, other authors place more diagnostic value on size; any lesion larger than 0.5 cm should be suspected of malignant degeneration until proved otherwise.[81] However, the margins and adjacent mucosal deformity may be unreliable signs.[84] Duodenal villous adenomas without invasive cancer can be managed successfully by local transduodenal submucosal excision, but invasive carcinoma requires radical resection (radical pancreaticoduodenectomy).[82]

Adenocarcinoma

Malignant tumors of the duodenum are uncommon, accounting for 0.3% to 0.4% of gastrointestinal neoplasms. Long-term survival is poor. Of malignant neoplasms of the small intestine, 25% to 45% occur in the duodenum.[85] Duodenal adenocarcinomas are located in the periampullary and intraampullary regions, with extremely rare involvement of the duodenal bulb.[86-88] There is an association with Gardner's syndrome, celiac sprue, Crohn's disease, and Peutz-Jeghers syndrome.[85,86,89]

Most patients present in the sixth to eighth decades of life and usually have symptoms 6 to 10 months before the definitive diagnosis is made. The female to male ratio is 1.2:1.0.[85] The early symptoms of duodenal malignancy are nonspecific (abdominal pain, nausea, weight loss, anemia), and the established diagnostic methods (double-contrast upper GI radiograph, upper GI endoscopy, enteroclysis) often fail to include the whole duodenum.[89,90] In addition, the third and fourth parts of the duodenum are often more difficult to evaluate because of overlapping of a stomach or jejunum filled with contrast medium.

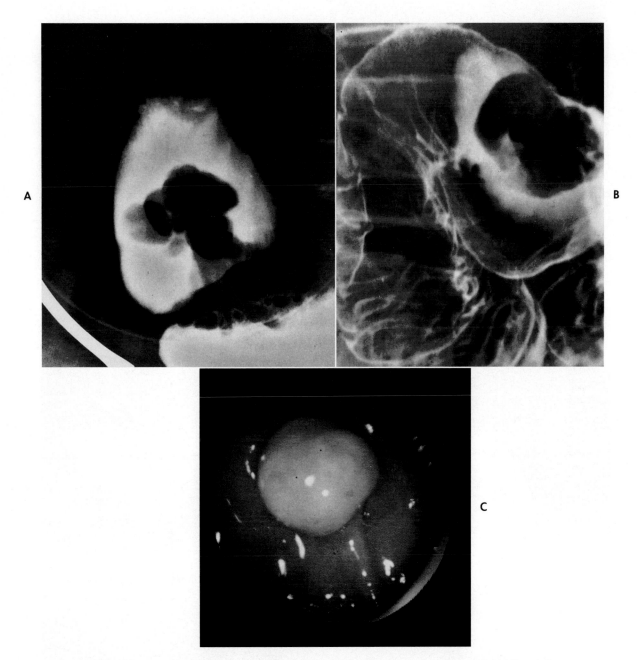

Fig. 24-24 Nodular duodenal protrusions. **A,** Pedunculated polyp in the duodenal bulb. **B** and **C,** Pedunculated polyp in the duodenal bulb shown on radiography (**B**) and endoscopy (**C**).

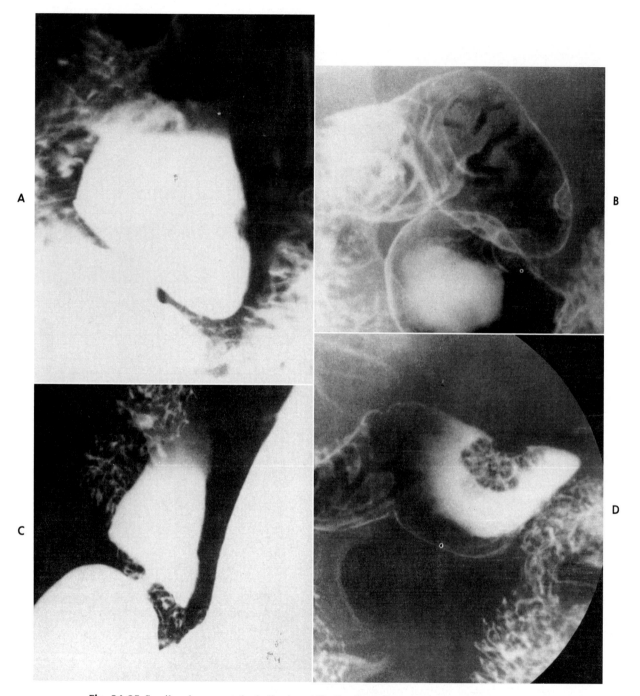

Fig. 24-25 Sessile adenoma at the bulb. **A** and **B,** Small sessile polypoid lesion in the bulb. **C,** The lesion is hidden in the barium pool. **D,** Four years after **A-C.** Growth of the lesion. The surface of the lesion has a netlike structure. (Histology: villous adenoma with dysplasia.)

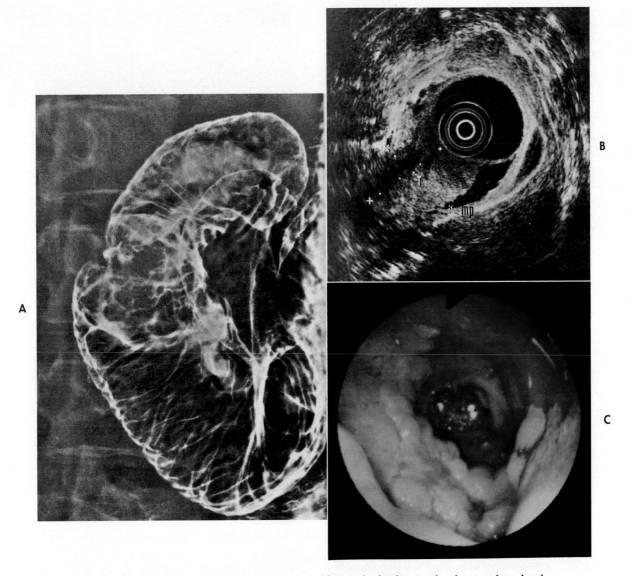

Fig. 24-26 Large duodenal villous adenoma. **A,** Hypotonic duodenography: large pedunculated bulky mass with barium interspersing the intervillous spaces, at the second portion of the duodenum, leading to subtotal obstruction. **B,** EUS shows the bulky mass *(T)* penetrating the muscularis propria *(mp)*. **C,** Endoscopy: cauliflower mass of the villous adenoma.

It may be difficult to maintain good contrast coating and distension of the entire duodenum.[89] On double-contrast radiography a solitary eccentrically (Figs. 24-27 and 24-28) or concentrically growing soft tissue mass may be found, causing lumen narrowing and dilatation of the proximal duodenal segment.

Although ultrasonography of the fluid-filled duodenum in hypotonia[12] may lead to the diagnosis (Figs. 24-28, *C*, and 24-29, *B*), it cannot be considered a satisfactory screening technique because of the inherent problems with gas-filled bowel loops.

On CT an intrinsic mass with wall thickening may be seen, usually without adjacent lymph node enlargement[91] (Fig. 24-28, *B*). Unfortunately, loss of normal fat planes between the mass and adjacent structures has not proved reliable in predicting local invasion.[89,91,92] Despite these major limitations in preoperative staging, thin-section CT obtained with gas or contrast enhancement and hypotonia of the duodenum is particularly helpful in differentiating pancreatic carcinoma, malignant lymphoma, metastatic cancer, and leiomyosarcoma from periampullary duodenal primaries in patients with obstructive jaundice.[26,91] Furthermore, CT is useful for detecting remote and hepatic metastases.

Early diagnosis is essential for successful treatment. Poor prognostic factors include a poorly differentiated tumor and metastatic spread to regional lymph nodes, liver, and lungs. However, 33% to 49% of patients have metastases at the time of diagnosis.[85]

Kaposi's sarcoma

Patients with AIDS and AIDS-related disorders are predisposed to develop Kaposi's sarcoma (KS). KS has been seen in 27% of reported AIDS cases and was present in 29% of patients in our series.[93]

In a clinicopathologic study by Niedt and Schinella[94] 52 of 56 patients dying of AIDS proved to have KS. There are visible cutaneous and oral lesions in 95% of AIDS patients with KS; common sites of involvement include skin (93%), lymph nodes (72%), lungs (52%), liver (34%), and rarely, the brain. The GI tract is involved in 41%.[58,61] The small bowel and the stomach are common sites, with the duodenum and colon rarely affected.

Radiologic studies usually fail to show KS if the lesions are flat (Fig. 24-29, *C*), but elevated lesions may appear as intraluminal filling defects (discrete sharp submucosal nodules 6 mm to 3 cm in size) of variable size and number (Fig. 24-29); central umbilication may be seen. There is normal intervening mucosa without ulceration. Multiple coalescent lesions may produce thickened nodular folds. Diffuse thickening of folds cannot be differentiated radiologically from lymphoma. Differentiation is possible with endoscopy, which shows early superficial lesions in the form of small macular discoloration of the mucosa. Characteris-

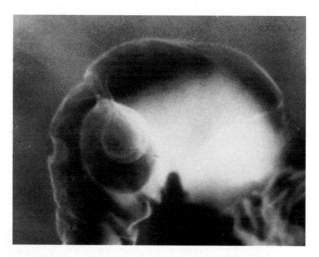

Fig. 24-27 Pedunculated tubular adenoma. Postbulbar, a pedunculated polypoid mass with smooth margins is visible. Slight retraction at the base of the stalk, originating at the lateral surface (histology: benign tubular adenoma). A smaller sessile adenoma distal from the stalk is visible.

tically the lesions are intensely red on endoscopy because of the underlying histopathology, which is that of a capillary hemangiosarcoma with endothelial proliferation.

There is a high incidence of retroperitoneal and mesenteric lymphadenopathy (50%) in this disease. CT or MRI may be helpful in showing the extent of involvement.

Carcinoid

The incidence of carcinoid of the duodenum varies from 0.2% to 5.5% of all GI carcinoids; these tumors form 2% to 3% of all duodenal tumors.[95] Carcinoid produces indefinite symptoms (nausea, vomiting, bleeding, hematemesis, abdominal pain, weight loss) except when the carcinoid syndrome has developed. The incidence of peptic ulcer disease may be increased in those with carcinoid tumor.[95]

Carcinoids of the duodenum are located most frequently in the first portion of the duodenum (57%) and in the ampullary region (23%).

The radiographic appearance can vary from a benign-appearing intramural submucosal mass lesion to a large bulky ulcerating lesion (Fig. 24-30), with deformity of the duodenum and duodenal irregularities. The radiographic findings are nonspecific (Fig. 24-30), but demonstration of a filling defect or multiple defects on upper GI studies should suggest the diagnosis, particularly if the lesions have a sessile appearance. Carcinoid tumors must be considered malignant, although 25% do not metastasize. CT shows a homogeneous ill-defined mesenteric mass with calcification and radiating soft tissue strands of the mesentery (stellate pattern) with displacement of surrounding bowel loops.[26]

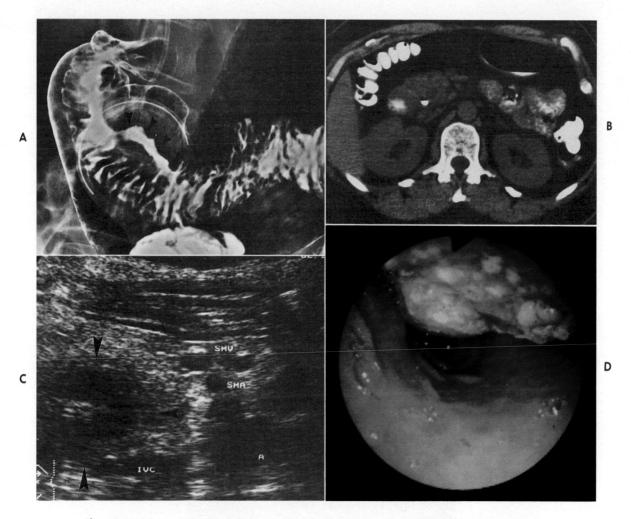

Fig. 24-28 Adenocarcinoma of the duodenum. **A,** Deep penetrating malignant ulcer *(arrowheads)* at the medial border of the duodenal flexure. **B,** CT shows an intrinsic mass lesion at the descending duodenum in front of the inferior caval vein with local invasion into the adjacent pancreatic head. **C,** Ultrasonography shows the intrinsic duodenal mass as a sonolucent structure. The strictured duodenal wall shows hypoechogenicity. **D,** Endoscopy shows the ulcerating tumor mass.

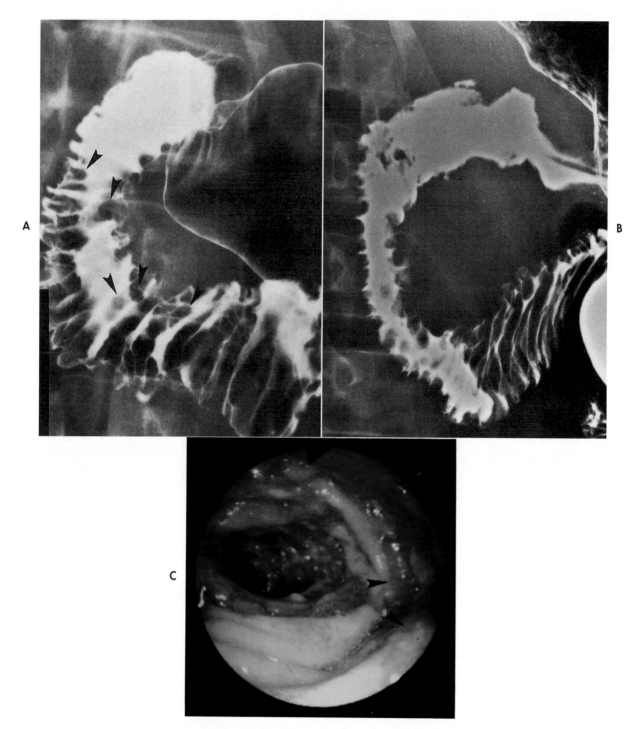

Fig. 24-29 Kaposi's sarcoma. **A** and **B,** Multiple elevated polypoid-like mucosal nodules in D2 and D3 caused by Kaposi's sarcoma. **C,** Superficial flat reddish lesions at the mucosal surface of the duodenum are visible endoscopically but not radiographically.

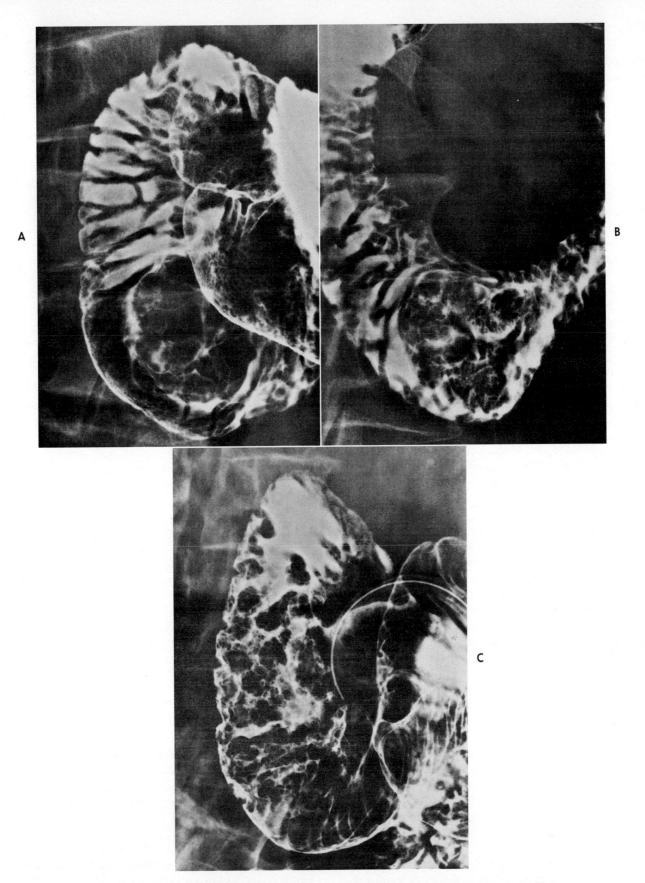

Fig. 24-30 Differential diagnosis of carcinoid. **A,** Carcinoid; large intramural submucosal filling defect at the inferior duodenal flexure. Barium is trapped within the mass, mimicking villous adenoma (histology: carcinoid). **B,** Adenocarcinoma. Large round solitary polypoid mass at the inferior duodenal flexure with ulceration (histology: adenocarcinoma). **C,** Multiple adenomas; multiple round and oval filling defects interspersed with barium (histology: tubular adenomas).

Nonepithelial tumors
Leiomyoma and leiomyosarcoma

Twenty percent to 24% of these lesions are located in the small bowel; they account for 1% of GI tract neoplasms and 10% to 33% of all the malignant duodenal tumors.[96] Over half (52%) of the tumors arise in the second portion of the duodenum, and the rest are found in the third (28%), fourth (12%), and first (8%) portions.[96]

About 70% to 80% of all leiomyosarcomas occur in the fourth to sixth decades. Leiomyosarcomas grow exophytically (63% to 75%), intraluminally (19% to 23%), or both intraluminally and extraluminally (6% to 14%).

Symptoms vary depending on the size, location, and malignant potential of the lesion. The lesions may become very large without clinical (obstructive) symptoms. The most common symptoms are hemorrhage (melena), palpable abdominal mass, anemia, weight loss, and abdominal pain.[96,97]

On double-contrast examination, benign submucosal (60%) tumors produce filling defects characterized by sharp angles with the bowel wall and an intact mucosa with flattening of the rugal folds[97] (Fig. 24-31). The subserosal lesions (35%) can grow larger. "Dumbbell" tumors (5%) show combined features of subserosal and submucosal lesions. Leiomyosarcoma of the duodenum is often mistaken for duodenal ulcer, carcinoma of the pancreatic head, or pancreatic cysts. Their tendency to grow exophytically limits the value of conventional barium studies in documenting the full extent of the mass and its relation to surrounding structures. CT is useful in depicting the origin and extent of these lesions. Leiomyomas are usually eccentric, homogeneous, sharply marginated, and smooth-walled lesions with low attenuation centers.

The CT findings of leiomyosarcoma (Fig. 24-31, C and D) are an irregular bulky eccentric lobulated (larger than 5 cm) low-attenuation tumor, with or without well-defined margins and an irregular central area of water density (liquefactive necrosis), surrounded by variously thickened soft tissue–density walls.[97] Intramural gas-barium levels can frequently be recognized because of cavitation or tumoral ulceration.[96] Calcification is uncommonly seen.

Dynamic CT shows a staining rim surrounding the tumor, similar to the wall of a cystic mass and without central enhancement.[96] Comparison of the CT appearance of leiomyomas and leiomyosarcomas suggests that the malignant lesions are larger, less uniform in shape, and variably attenuating.[97] The ultrasonographic appearance of these masses may be complex: hyperechoic or hypoechoic lesions with echo-free spaces (caused by liquefactive necrosis) may be seen with a hyperechoic rim.[96-99]

In cases where the mass is extremely large, preoperative *selective angiography* is usually necessary to localize the predominant blood supply (Fig. 24-31, B). When a nonlo-calized infiltrative lesion is present, angiography may be useful in differentiating these more highly vascular tumors from less vascular lymphomas.[97] Angiography shows dilated feeding arteries, irregular neovascularization, early venous return, intensive tumor staining, and pooling of contrast at different phases of the study.[98]

Leiomyosarcomas are larger and less vascular than leiomyomas and have indistinct margins.[96] They cannot be distinguished easily from benign leiomyomas by angiography.[96] When angiography shows a tumor larger than 5 cm with an irregular lobulated outline in the capillary phase, it is highly suggestive for leiomyosarcoma rather than leiomyoma.[96]

Tumor spread almost always occurs by local infiltration into adjacent structures, but hematogenous spread occurs to the liver (CT: multiple low-density lesions), peritoneal cavity (CT: discrete rounded masses often with necrotic centers), and omentum. Lymphogenic spread is uncommon. MRI may be useful for preoperative assessment of vessel invasion (Fig. 24-31, E).

Surgical resection of the tumor is the therapy of choice, by either partial duodenectomy or radical pancreaticoduodenectomy. Histologic differentiation of leiomyoma from leiomyosarcoma is almost impossible. The three most helpful indicators of malignancy are metastatic spread, local invasion, and size greater than 5 or 6 cm.

Lipoma

Lipomas are small tumors (2 to 3 cm) specifically located in the descending duodenum at the apex rather than in the bulb itself. They are less common than leiomyomas.[100] Gastrointestinal bleeding or intussusception is an occasional finding.[100] Radiographically, lipoma may present as a sessile polyp with smooth overlying mucosa, usually not umbilicated or ulcerated. Endoscopically they have a slightly yellowish coloration. On CT, lipomas can be differentiated from leiomyomas, Brunner's gland adenoma, and adenomatous polyps by their characteristic fatty density and low attenuation values on CT.[98]

Non-Hodgkin's lymphoma

Primary lymphoma is extremely rare, but as secondary involvement it is the second most common malignancy of the duodenum.[101] CT findings consist primarily of asymmetric thickening of the duodenal wall indistinguishable from the appearance of adenocarcinoma. In addition, there is usually associated retroperitoneal adenopathy.

Mastocytosis

Mastocytosis is a rare disorder characterized by mast cell proliferation in the skin (urticaria pigmentosa), bones, lymph nodes, and parenchymal organs.[102,103] The GI tract is involved in 16% of cases.[102,104,105] Radiologic studies

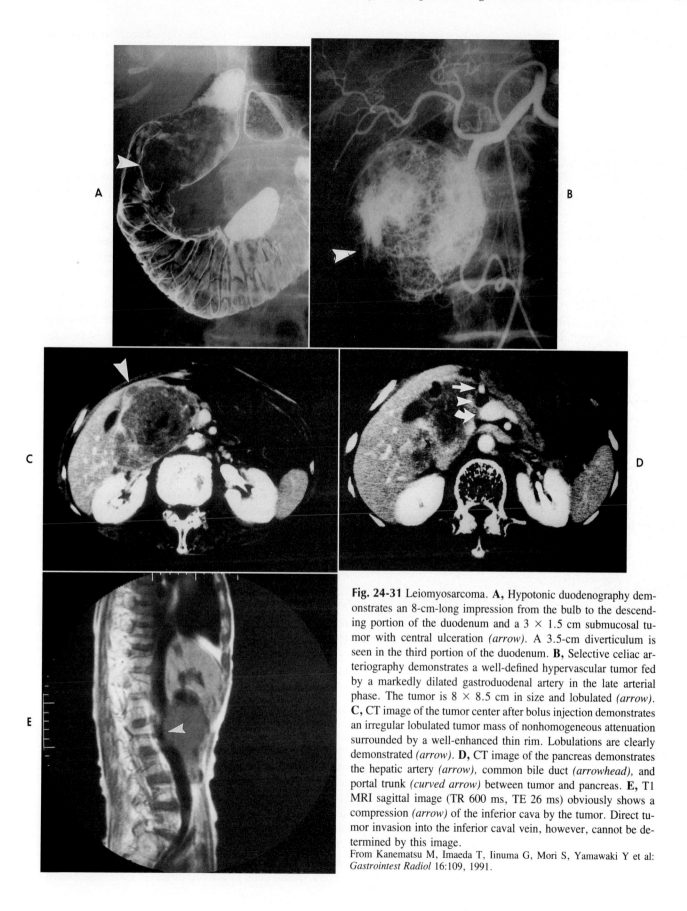

Fig. 24-31 Leiomyosarcoma. **A,** Hypotonic duodenography demonstrates an 8-cm-long impression from the bulb to the descending portion of the duodenum and a 3 × 1.5 cm submucosal tumor with central ulceration *(arrow)*. A 3.5-cm diverticulum is seen in the third portion of the duodenum. **B,** Selective celiac arteriography demonstrates a well-defined hypervascular tumor fed by a markedly dilated gastroduodenal artery in the late arterial phase. The tumor is 8 × 8.5 cm in size and lobulated *(arrow)*. **C,** CT image of the tumor center after bolus injection demonstrates an irregular lobulated tumor mass of nonhomogeneous attenuation surrounded by a well-enhanced thin rim. Lobulations are clearly demonstrated *(arrow)*. **D,** CT image of the pancreas demonstrates the hepatic artery *(arrow),* common bile duct *(arrowhead),* and portal trunk *(curved arrow)* between tumor and pancreas. **E,** T1 MRI sagittal image (TR 600 ms, TE 26 ms) obviously shows a compression *(arrow)* of the inferior cava by the tumor. Direct tumor invasion into the inferior caval vein, however, cannot be determined by this image.

From Kanematsu M, Imaeda T, Iinuma G, Mori S, Yamawaki Y et al: *Gastrointest Radiol* 16:109, 1991.

show thickening of duodenal folds secondary to mast cell proliferation in the lamina propria, mucosal nodularity (2 mm to 5 mm) secondary to (unproven) urticarial changes,[102,105-107] and bull's-eye lesions (see the box below).

There is an increased incidence of peptic ulcer disease and malabsorption.[102,106,107] Males and females are affected with the same frequency. Although it is predominantly a disease of childhood, adults are involved in up to 30%. The late stage of the disease is characterized by fibrosis of the involved organs.[102]

Tumorlike lesions
Aberrant pancreas

Aberrant pancreatic tissue may occur anywhere in the duodenum or proximal small intestine. Usually it is asymptomatic. It is more common in the gastric antrum. Radiologically it is a plaquelike or hemispheric polypoid lesion, 1 to 2 cm in diameter with a central dimple that corresponds with the draining duct. Other polypoid lesions, such as adenomas and aphthoid ulcers, can look similar.

Heterotopic gastric mucosa

Heterotopic gastric mucosa (HGM) is being reported in the literature with increasing frequency[108,109] because of continued technical development and widespread use of upper GI endoscopy. It has been observed in 1% to 12% of all duodenal endoscopies.[108,110-113] Clinical symptoms may be dyspepsia and gastrointestinal bleeding. Very rarely, intussusception may lead to obstruction.[114]

HGM occurs in patients ranging in age from the teens to the eighties. Metaplastic gastric epithelium in the duodenum has been associated with erosions and peptic ulcerations (1%), hyperacidity, and alcoholic and uremic duodenitis.[80,110,112,113,115] It is commonly observed on the anterior wall of the duodenal bulb,[110-113] but it may be found anywhere in the GI tract from the oral cavity to the rectum.[115] It has also occurred in the gallbladder and bile ducts, airways, spinal column, and urinary bladder.[116]

Heterotopic gastric mucosa is classified on the basis of its histopathologic features into congenital and acquired types, both of which can be found in the duodenum. The *congenital* HGM is composed of well-differentiated gastric mucosa of the fundic type with normal glandular elements that excrete an alkaline juice for cytoprotection against the hydrochloric acid. The *acquired* HGM represents patchy replacement of the native mucosa by gastric epithelium after inflammatory or peptic processes. These lesions are categorized as solitary (0% to 30%) or multiple elevations (70%). Radiographically the solitary lesions are hemispheric. Large solitary lesions tend to have a central depression. The multiple lesions are small multifaceted or platelike nodules of 2 mm to 5 mm diameter (Fig. 24-32). They are best visualized in DC, using glucagon-induced hypotonia and with compression.[109]

The endoscopic appearance is distinct: pale salmon red mucosa or patches or clusters of nodules raised above the normally pink mucosa of the duodenum. The application of 1% Congo red solution as a pH-sensitive stain during endoscopy results in black discoloration of the acid-producing HGM.

Endoscopic biopsy and histologic examination are necessary to diagnose HGM and differentiate it from other entities that may cause polypoid or nodular mucosa (hyperplasia of Brunner's glands or lymphoid follicles, adenomas, polyposis syndrome). If the association of duodenal bulb HGM with *H. pylori* infection is proved to be a constant one,[108] then the recognition of the lesion may have clinical utility in showing that the patient is, or has been, infected, and is therefore at risk for peptic ulcer disease.

Hyperplasia of Brunner's glands

Brunner's glands seem to protect the duodenal surface epithelium of the first part of the duodenum by neutralizing gastric acid through the secretion of bicarbonate. They are most numerous in the first portion of the duodenum, just distal to the pylorus and gradually diminish toward the second and third portions of the duodenum. The anatomic distribution therefore reflects their physiologic role.[117,118] They are not found beyond the ligament of Treitz. The actual number of Brunner's glands varies from a thin layer of widely spread cells to a more localized collection beneath

---

☐ **BULL'S-EYE LESIONS IN THE GASTROINTESTINAL TRACT** ☐

SINGLE

Primary neoplasms
    Spindle cell tumor
    Lymphoma
    Carcinoid
    Carcinoma
Kaposi's sarcoma
Aberrant pancreas
Eosinophilic granuloma

MULTIPLE

Metastases
    Melanoma
    Breast
    Lung
    Kidney
    Kaposi's sarcoma
Lymphoma
Mastocytosis

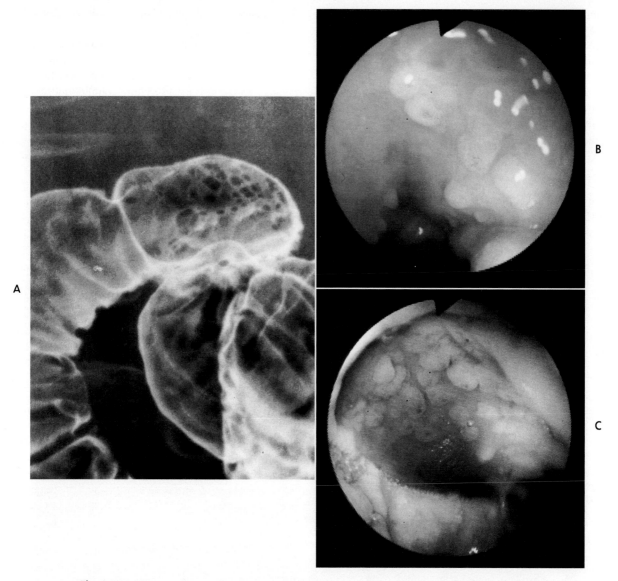

Fig. 24-32 Heterotopic gastric mucosa. **A,** Small ovoid and polygonal faceted nodules of various sizes in the duodenal bulb caused by metaplastic gastric epithelium. **B** and **C,** Endoscopy shows clusters of nodules raised above normal mucosa of the duodenum; the application of methylene blue results in better delineation of these benign lesions.

the muscularis mucosae.

While atrophy of Brunner's glands may occur in the elderly, hyperplasia of Brunner's glands is a common acquired condition, in which the submucosal glands of the duodenum enlarge in response to prolonged stimulation by gastric hyperacidity. It is frequently associated with peptic duodenitis. Duodenal abnormalities are demonstrated in 31% to 55% of patients with chronic renal failure.[119-122] In uremia the incidence and severity in duodenitis increase directly with the increase of Brunner's gland hyperplasia. Peptic ulceration (10%) may be found.[119,121-123]

The mucosal patterns of the duodenum in Brunner's glands hyperplasia can be classified into five categories[124]:

1. *Focal* Brunner's gland hyperplasia: a solitary submucosal nodule or a cluster of several adjacent nodules beneath the mucosa of the duodenal bulb.

2. *Diffuse* Brunner's gland hyperplasia: a myriad of round oval nodules measuring 2 mm to 5 mm, scattered throughout the bulb and duodenal loop. The diffuse form is the most frequent.

The lesions can often be differentiated from lymphoid hyperplasia in that the polygonal mucosal lesions in the latter condition are usually uniform and smaller (1 mm to 3 mm in diameter). Endoscopically, single or multiple submucosal nodules of variable size may be seen, covered by either normal or thickened edematous or hemorrhagic mucosa.

3. *Multifocal* Brunner's glands hyperplasia: multiple well-defined polygonal masses from 5 to 15 mm.

4. Brunner's gland hyperplasia *combined with duodenitis:* prominent nodular mucosa of the bulb and post-bulbar segments. The endoscopist may see erythema, mucosal congestion, and hemorrhage, whereas the ra-

diologist will notice thickened or nodular duodenal folds.[33]

5. *Brunner's gland hyperplasia* masked by severe erosive duodenitis: distorted mucosal pattern.

Giant brunneromas, solitary or multiple sessile or pedunculated masses larger than 15 mm, could be added as a sixth category (Fig. 24-33). At least 12 cases of giant brunneromas have been reported.[125]

Most giant brunneromas are solitary lesions of hamar-

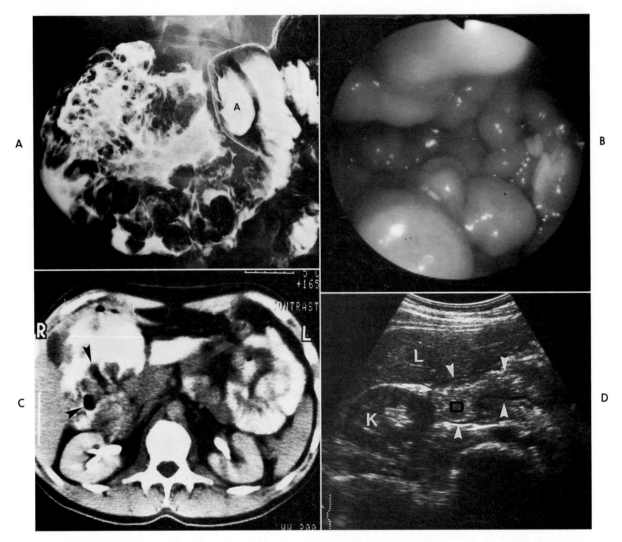

Fig. 24-33 Giant brunneromas. **A,** Multiple large polypoid lesions in a dilated duodenum. **B,** Endoscopy shows multiple smooth polyps in the duodenal bulb. **C,** CT shows fat densities (−50 Hounsfield units [HU]) in some of the polypoid lesions *(arrows).* **D,** Ultrasonography shows a dilated duodenum *(D)* with intact submucosal lining *(arrows)* and intraluminal masses. *K,* Kidney; *L,* liver.
From Van Rooij WJJ, van der Horst JJ, Stuifbergen WNHM, Pijpers PM: *Gastrointest Radiol* 15:285, 1990.

tomatous rather than neoplastic origin because of mature adipose tissue (fat) in these tumors. They arise in the duodenal bulb rather than the second portion of the duodenum.[117,125]

Brunneromas are not considered premalignant.[117] The clinical manifestations, if any, depend on tumor size. There may be vague abdominal pain, nausea, vomiting, and melena. Complications include bleeding from an ulcerated surface and duodenal stenosis.

The radiographic appearance of a solitary brunneroma is of a sessile or pedunculated smooth polypoid filling defect.[117,125]

The differential diagnosis includes mesenchymal tumor (lipoma, leiomyoma, fibroma), villous adenoma, neurogenic tumor, hemangioma, carcinoid, aberrant pancreatic tissue, prolapsed gastric mucosa, and duodenal duplication cyst. Round polypoid filling defects in the duodenal bulb should suggest the diagnosis of Brunner's gland hyperplasia with a possibility of duodenitis, benign lymphoid hyperplasia, or heterotopic gastric mucosa.[33,115,124,126]

Pedunculated brunneromas may be excised endoscopically even if they are large (3 cm to 4 cm).[125] Sessile brunneromas larger than 2 cm may need surgical excision.

Benign lymphoid hyperplasia

Benign lymphoid hyperplasia is characterized by a benign proliferation of lymphoid follicles of the submucosal layer. It may be a part of diffuse lymphoid hyperplasia of the stomach, duodenum, small bowel, colon, and rectum, associated with malabsorption, giardiasis, and hypogammaglobulinaemia (IgA deficiency).[126]

A radiographic cobblestone appearance of the mucosa may be seen, with multiple, small, rounded, polypoid, umbilicated filling defects. The striking endoscopic feature is that of numerous round raised 1 to 2 mm nodules that cover the entire surface of the duodenal bulb.[126]

Metastases into the duodenum

See p. 508.

VASCULAR ABNORMALITIES
Vascular malformation

Approximately 8% to 33% of endoscopically diagnosed upper GI tract angiodysplasia is found in the duodenum. It is usually a single lesion in the duodenal bulb, between 2 and 4 mm. It is not elevated and cannot be detected with a barium study.[11]

Lymphangioma in the duodenum has been described. The cavernous type is smooth, elevated, and pliable and cannot be differentiated from other submucosal lesions.[127]

Duodenal varices

Duodenal varices mainly develop in extrahepatic portal vein and splenic vein obstruction, when the blood from the spleen or the mesenteric veins is drained by the gastroepiploic, pancreaticoduodenal, and coronary veins into the portal vein. Patients often simultaneously have a duodenal ulcer.

Duodenal varices can occur in portal hypertension when esophageal varices are present, rarely in long-standing occlusion of the inferior caval vein, and when collateral vessels have developed via lumbar, azygos, and hemiazygos veins and the portal venous system.[128]

Patients with duodenal varices can present with hematemesis, melena, or both. On a barium study duodenal varices can show as polypoid thickened folds, which run in a somewhat irregular or serpiginous fashion.[129] They may change a little depending on the filling state and the tone of the duodenum. An isolated varix in the bulb or postbulbar region is rare. Antral folds are often thickened. In patients with extrahepatic portal hypertension, splenomegaly is seldom present.

When duodenal varices are present without esophageal varices and the spleen is not enlarged, splenic vein obstruction is very likely. Duplex (color) Doppler examination is necessary for evaluating the portal circulation. More information about the cause and location of the obstruction and the collaterals can be obtained by indirect portography with intraarterial digital subtraction angiography of the superior mesenteric and celiac arteries.

Arterioduodenal fistula

The most common arterioduodenal fistula is aortoduodenal fistula. Mesentericoduodenal and hepatoduodenal fistulas are much rarer.

Aortoduodenal fistula

When an aortoduodenal fistula develops between an aortic aneurysm and the ascending duodenum, it is called *primary*. It is caused by necrosis of the duodenal wall from pressure, as the ascending duodenum is fixed where it runs between the aorta and superior mesenteric artery. When the wall of the duodenum is necrotic, the enteric succus can digest the aortic wall, which often leads to fatal bleeding.[130,131]

When an aortoduodenal fistula develops between the duodenal lumen and the prosthetic graft for aortic aneurysm, it is called *secondary*.[132] It is caused by a pseudoaneurysm that erodes the duodenum. Prosthetic infection can also lead to such a fistula with massive bleeding. The first sign is usually fever, 1 to 2 weeks postoperatively.

On upper GI examination, only a broad impression on the duodenum can be seen with ventral displacement. The diagnosis is most often made by endoscopy. CT, MRI, and angiography are the appropriate imaging methods for diagnosing an aortoduodenal fistula.

On CT, graft infection is characterized by increased perigraft soft tissue, ectopic gas, and bowel wall thickening.[133] Early diagnosis is imperative because the bleeding is often catastrophic.[134]

Mesentericoduodenal fistula

Mesentericoduodenal fistulas develop in the same way as aortoduodenal fistulas. A fistula between a pseudoaneurysm of the common hepatic artery and the duodenum has been reported.[134]

Traumatic changes of duodenum

With blunt trauma of the upper abdomen, especially from traffic accidents, the fixed duodenum is compressed against the spine. In children who have suffered blunt trauma, the possibility of abuse must be considered. Blunt trauma can lead to intramural hemorrhage and to partial or complete laceration of the duodenum.[135] The most frequent location is the second and third parts of duodenum[136] (Fig. 24-34).

Other causes of trauma of the duodenum are sudden increase in intraluminal pressure or direct trauma with sharp objects. Duodenal perforation during intubation for enteroclysis is very rare.[137]

When complete rupture occurs, a gas collection can usually be seen retroperitoneally. If an upper GI series is requested, a water-soluble iodinated contrast medium should be used. Clinical symptoms of duodenal rupture in the retroperitoneum are subtle, and the radiologist should maintain a high index of suspicion.[138] On CT, fluid, gas, or both may be demonstrated in the right anterior pararenal space. If water-soluble iodinated contrast medium has been administered, fluid with high attenuation may be seen in the right anterior pararenal space (Fig. 24-35).

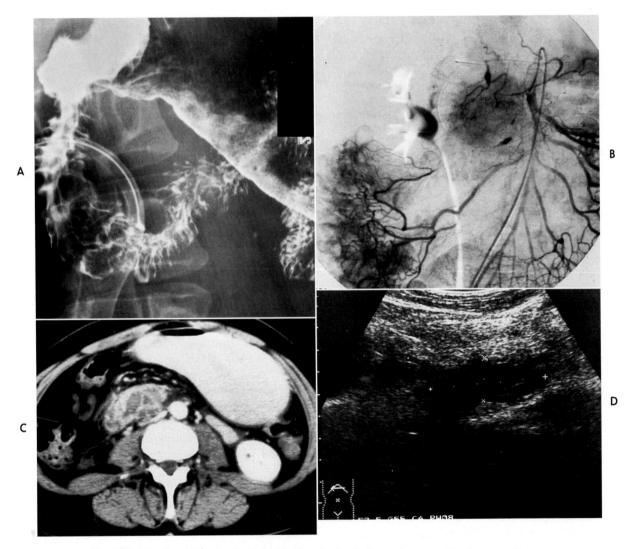

Fig. 24-34 Duodenal hematoma. **A,** Incomplete duodenal obstruction caused by intramural hematoma 5 days after blunt trauma. **B,** Angiography shows the site of hemorrhage at the gastroduodenal arterial junction. **C,** Enhanced CT shows a curvilinear area of high density with a central low attenuation. **D,** Ultrasonography shows a well-delineated sonolucent mass that is difficult to differentiate from a pancreatic pseudocyst.

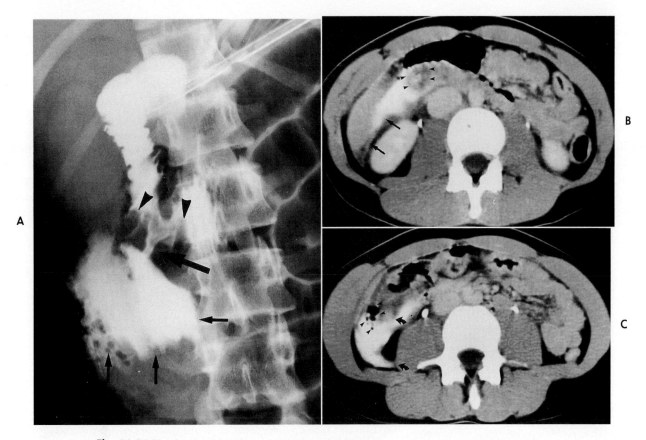

Fig. 24-35 Duodenal perforation. **A,** Gastrografin upper gastrointestinal series demonstrates extraluminal contrast and air *(arrows)* and duodenal fold thickening *(arrowheads)*. Site of perforation *(large arrow)*. **B,** CT scan of the abdomen at the level of the lower third of the right kidney demonstrates extraluminal contrast in the right anterior pararenal space *(arrows)* and a ring of thickened duodenal wall *(arrowheads)*. **C,** CT scan below the level of the kidneys demonstrates extraluminal contrast *(arrows)* and gas *(arrowheads)* in the infrarenal retroperitoneal (extraperitoneal) space.
From Hofer GA, Cohen AJ: *J Comput Assist Tomogr* 13:430, 1989.

Intramural hematoma

Most intramural hematomas are caused by blunt trauma. They can also occur with anticoagulant therapy, in hemophiliacs from postoperative stress ulcers,[139] with rupture of aneurysms, with acute pancreatitis,[140] in panarteritis nodosa, after endoscopic biopsy, with intubation for enteroclysis,[73,141,142] in abused children, and even with duodenal ulcer.

The bleeding often starts in the submucosa, less often in the subserosa. The bleeding may be diffuse or very localized. When the bleeding is diffuse, the mucosal folds get thicker and disorganized, producing a coiled-spring appearance. Spiculation ("picket fence" or "stacked coin" appearance) is described when circular folds have disappeared.[143] With localized massive bleeding in the submucosa the signs are those of an intrinsic lesion, which widens the duodenal sweep and may even obstruct the duodenum. The most frequent site of intramural hematoma is the second or third

part of the duodenum[141] (Figs. 24-34 and 24-36).

On CT, intramural hematomas show inhomogeneous wall thickening, with a submucosal mass that narrows the lumen and has a relatively high attenuation.[135,144] At the site of acute hemorrhage, a curvilinear area of high density may appear ("ring sign").[92,145] With time the attenuation diminishes. Old hematomas can be indistinguishable from other fluid collections, including abscesses and necrotic tumors. A dense rim can result from formation of a pseudocapsule.[143] MRI scans show a mass containing a ring with short T1 and long T2 relaxation times[143,146] (Fig. 24-37). With ultrasound, an intramural hematoma appears as a sonolucent mass anteromedial to the right kidney, and is sometimes difficult to differentiate from a pancreatic pseudocyst, a renal cyst, a necrotic tumor, or a fluid-filled duodenum.

Smaller hematomas are resorbed spontaneously. The filling defect diminishes, and small nodular lesions appear.[147]

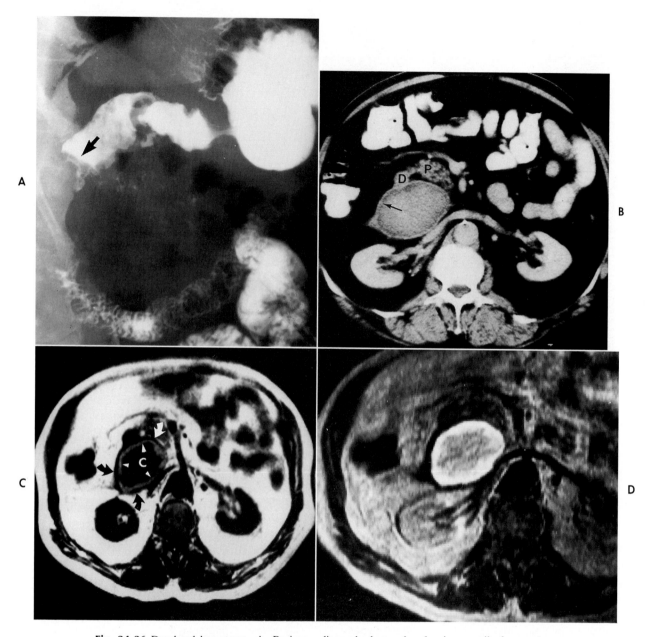

Fig. 24-36 Duodenal hematoma. **A,** Barium radiograph shows sharply circumscribed mass *(arrow)* partially obstructing the descending duodenum. **B,** CT scan with both oral and intravenous contrast media shows a 10-cm mass compressing the duodenum *(D)* and elevating the pancreatic head *(P)*. There is a thin soft tissue rim *(arrow)* surrounding a center of lower signal intensity. **C,** SE 310/20/12 (T1 MRI) transverse image. **D,** SE 2350/60/3 (T2 MRI) image. A concentric ring appearance *(arrowheads* in **C)** is again demonstrated. On the SE 310/20/12 sequence, the middle, high-intensity ring is thin and sharply demarcated from the central core. On the T2 MRI image the middle ring is coarser and is not sharply demarcated from the core.
From Hahn PF, Stark PD, Vici LG, Ferrucci JT: *Radiology* 159:379, 1986.

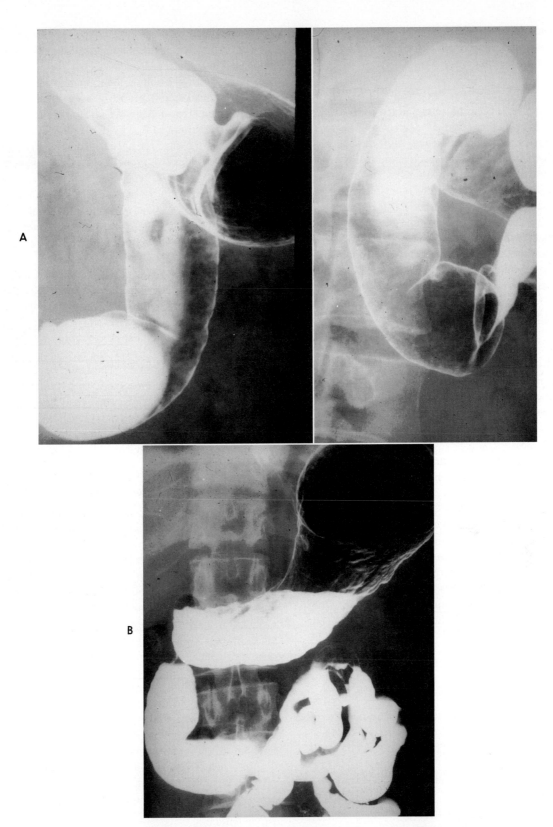

Fig. 24-37 A, Complete loss of valvulae conniventes in a 27-year-old man in whom heartburn was the only presenting symptom of celiac disease. **B,** The erect radiograph shows retained food in the stomach and that the loss of valvulae extends to the jejunum, which looks more like the ileum—a characteristic sign of celiac disease. The ileum showed valvulae of jejunal pattern. The heartburn resolved on a gluten-free diet.

Bigger hematomas have to be evacuated. Fibrotic reaction in the wall can result in narrowing of the duodenum, without destruction of the mucosa.

Superior mesenteric artery compression syndrome

When the angle between the aorta and the superior mesenteric artery gets smaller (from 37 degrees to 8 degrees), the duodenum can be compressed as it passes between them. The main factor leading to such compression is loss of weight with decrease of retroperitoneal fat (nutcracker syndrome). Increased lordosis of the lumbar spine, aortic aneurysm, changes of motility and peristalsis of the duodenum as in scleroderma and dermatomyositis, Chagas' disease, disturbances of innervation, and medical treatment with tranquilizers may all hamper emptying of the duodenum and increase duodenal dilatation. Long bed rest, duodenal ulcer, and loss of tone of the duodenal wall are predisposing factors, too.[148] On upper GI examination there is dilatation of the first and second portions of the duodenum, which ends almost vertically in the midline or just to the right of the vertebra.[149] When the barium finally passes after many to-and-fro peristaltic movements, a small vertical impression on the duodenum can be seen with normal mucosal folds. With hypotonic duodenography, intact mucosa at the point of compression can be demonstrated.[150] Arteriography with lateral exposure is seldom performed today.

If there is stasis in the duodenum with the patient in the left decubitus position, an organic obstruction should be suspected.

This syndrome occurs in children but is more often seen in adults. The symptoms are vomiting, abdominal distension, postprandial epigastric pain, and weight loss. In the prone position, the patient may have relief from symptoms. When the patient has gained weight (and retroperitoneal fat), the angle between the aorta and the superior mesenteric artery increases,[149] and symptoms may resolve. Strict diagnostic criteria should be applied before surgery is considered for this condition.

DUODENAL INVOLVEMENT AS PART OF MORE EXTENSIVE DISEASE
Celiac disease

The clinical symptoms of celiac disease are malabsorption with weight loss, abdominal distension, and diarrhea. The duodenal mucosal surface appears smooth in the presence of subtotal villous atrophy. The duodenal folds may be normal or prominent and erythematous.[43,151] In more advanced disease, atrophy of the valvulae may lead to a smooth duodenum and proximal jejunum (ilealisation). With indigo-carmine or methylene blue dye scattering technique a mosaic pattern or a finely convoluted appearance may be seen. In many patients no abnormality is found radiographically, but multiple small, often hexagonal nodules

in the duodenal bulb give it a bubbly appearance[152] (Fig. 24-38). In these cases the other parts of the duodenum show thickened and coarsened folds.

The most striking radiographic manifestations are duodenal fold thickening, probably as a result of mucosal edema in patients with a low serum albumin level, and fragmentation of barium caused by marked hypersecretion. Endoscopically the mucosa appears superficially normal or pale and atrophic with a pronounced vascular pattern.[153,154]

Whipple's disease

Whipple's disease is an uncommon systemic disease in which many organs are involved (see Chapter 32). It is found in the United States and Northern Europe. Untreated, death by cachexia follows after some years.[155]

The duodenum is involved in about half of the patients, the jejunum almost always. Radiologically the folds of the duodenum and small intestine are slightly broadened (2.5 to 3.5 mm thick) and distorted by tiny nodular lesions. The sometimes foamlike appearance should not be mistaken for small gas bubbles.[156] On CT mesenteric and paraaortal lymph nodes can be enlarged. The bowel wall may show a somewhat low attenuation because of fatty deposits.

In the differential diagnosis intestinal lymphangiectasia must be considered. In intestinal lymphangiectasia the folds are broadened and the bowel wall thickened. There may be dilatation and a nodular mucosa. The duodenal bulb never shows changes.

Progressive systemic sclerosis (scleroderma)

In progressive systemic sclerosis the small intestine, including the duodenum, is involved in up to 50% of patients. The symptoms may include diarrhea, abdominal pain and distension, malabsorption, and weight loss. The disease is characterized by fibrin deposits in the intima of small mesenteric arteries. The smooth muscle cells become atrophic and are replaced by fibrous tissue.

Radiologically the duodenum appears hypotonic and dilated. Sometimes no peristalsis at all is observed in the duodenum or small intestine. Because patients can be thin, emptying of the dilated duodenum may be further hampered by compression by the superior mesenteric artery. Hypotonicity of the esophagus, stomach, and small intestine supports the diagnosis of scleroderma. Sacculation can develop when dilatation of the duodenum is extreme.[156] In the differential diagnosis of hypotonic duodenum, other collagen diseases such as systemic lupus erythematosus and dermatomyositis or amyloidosis should be considered, along with *Strongyloides* infection and drugs.

Cystic fibrosis

In cystic fibrosis there is thickening and coarsening of duodenal folds. Multiple small nodular elevations may be present; these can be seen in the proximal jejunum as well.

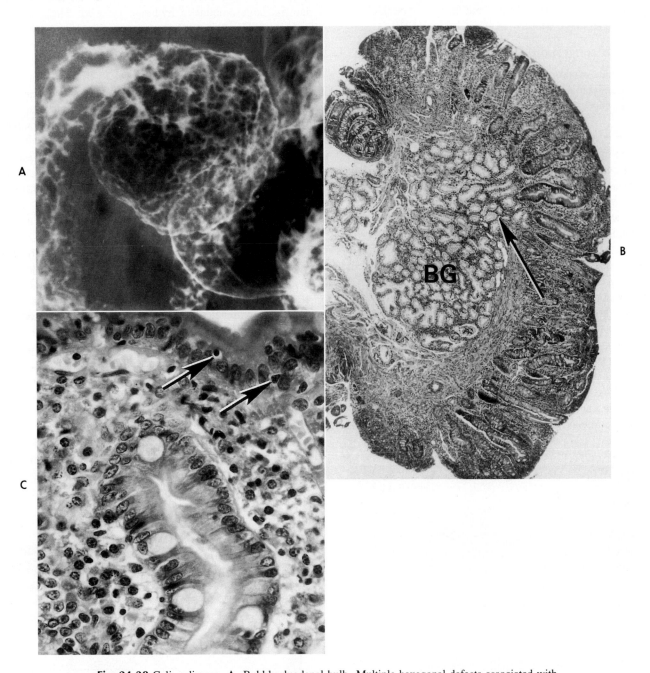

Fig. 24-38 Celiac disease. **A,** Bubbly duodenal bulb. Multiple hexagonal defects associated with nodularity and fold thickening in the descending duodenum. **B,** Biopsy specimen of the descending duodenum (low-power photomicrograph). Flat luminal surface reflects absence of villi owing to celiac disease. Prominent submucosal Brunner's glands *(BG)* extend through muscularis mucosae into mucosa *(arrow)*, representing findings of peptic disease. *H & E,* ×45. **C,** High-power photomicrograph: epithelial features of celiac disease. Surface epithelium is cuboidal with numerous intraepithelial lymphocytes *(arrows)*, whereas crypt epithelium lacks evidence of injury. *H & E,* ×400.
From Jones B, Bayles TM, Hamilton SR, Yardley JH: *AJR* 142:119, 1984.

Amyloidosis

In amyloidosis the duodenum can appear normal even if biopsy specimens are positive, but there may be thickened and coarse folds. Motility is often decreased.[157]

Venous congestion, hypoproteinemia

Venous congestion and hypoproteinemia, especially hypoalbuminemia, can lead to thickening of Kerckring's folds of the duodenum and proximal jejunum.

Zollinger-Ellison syndrome

This syndrome, described in 1955, is characterized by peptic ulcer disease, diarrhea, gastric acid hypersecretion, and gastrin-producing tumors. Initially, most of these tumors were thought to be in the pancreas, but newer studies indicate that most of the tumors are found in the gastrinoma triangle—superiorly the confluence of the cystic and bile ducts, caudally the border of the second and third portions of the duodenum, and medially the junction of the head and body of the pancreas.[158] Extrapancreatically, the duodenum is a common location. Many other localizations of gastrinomas are also reported.

Of patients with peptic ulcer disease, 0.1% to 1% have Zollinger-Ellison syndrome. Most patients are between 30 and 50 years of age, and males dominate by 2:1 to 3:2. About 25% of Zollinger-Ellison patients have the multiple endocrine neoplasia type I (MEN-I) syndrome. Hypergastrinemia caused by the gastrin-producing tumors (gastrinoma) stimulates the parietal cells of the stomach to hyperplasia and acid hypersecretion. The pancreatic bicarbonate output, although often increased, is insufficient to neutralize the large amount of hydrochloric acid. The resulting very low pH in the duodenum and proximal jejunum inactivates digestive enzymes and damages the mucosa. Clinically, malabsorption develops, resulting in diarrhea, steatorrhea, and maldigestion.[159]

The radiologic signs are a relatively hypotonic duodenum with a nodular appearance of the bulb caused by hypertrophy of Brunner's glands (Fig. 24-39); peptic ulcers, sometimes atypically located in the second, third, or rarely fourth portion of duodenum or even in the jejunum; and sometimes coarsening and broadening of the mucosal folds caused by edema and infiltration, increased amount of fluid, and often hyperperistalsis of the jejunum.[160]

Metastasis to the duodenum

Besides the extension of malignant tumors from adjacent organs, the duodenal wall can be involved by transperitoneal spread (Fig. 24-40). Retroperitoneal lymph node metastasis and malignant tumors of the pancreas, colon, right kidney, suprarenal gland, and gallbladder can invade the duodenum. Depending on the degree of the extension, only the outer layers of the duodenum may be involved with identation, or there may be ulceration when the whole wall is penetrated by the tumor. Hematogenous metastasis is described from cancer of the breast and lungs and from melanoma. When only outer layers are involved, the lumen is narrowed but the folds are not destroyed. In melanoma more often the mucosa is ulcerated, leading to bull's-eye lesions. Usually other parts of the GI tract reveal similar lesions.

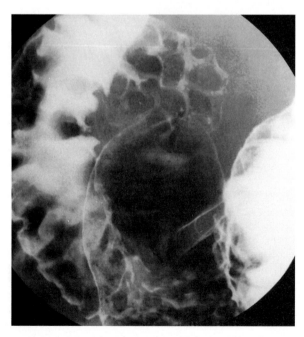

Fig. 24-39 Zollinger-Ellison syndrome. Polypoid lesions in the duodenal bulb corresponding to hypertrophy of Brunner's glands. Thickening of Kerckring's folds in the vertical portion of the duodenum.

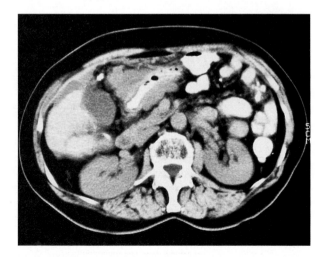

Fig. 24-40 Metastatic spread of ovarian carcinoma into the duodenum. Contrast-enhanced CT shows a large, irregular, lobulated soft tissue mass surrounding the first and second parts of the duodenum with narrowing of the lumen and peritoneal thickening.

ACKNOWLEDGMENT

We gratefully acknowledge Dr. G.N.J. Tytgat, professor in the department of gastroenterology at the Academic Medical Center in Amsterdam, The Netherlands, who supplied the endoscopic pictures.

REFERENCES

1. Glick SN, Gohel VK, Laufer I: Mucosal surface patterns of the duodenal bulb: subject review, *Radiology* 150:317, 1984.
2. Bova JG, Kamath V, Tio FO, Peters JE, Goldstein HM: The normal mucosal surface pattern of the duodenal bulb: radiologic-histologic correlation, *AJR* 145:735, 1985.
3. Pratt AD: Current concepts of the obstructing duodenal diaphragm, *Radiology* 100:637, 1971.
4. Bachmann KD: Die angeborene Duodenalstenose, *Dtsch Med Wochenschr* 105:1428, 1980.
5. Friedland GW, Mason R, Poole GJ: Ladd's bands in older children, adolescents, and adults, *Radiology* 95:363, 1970.
6. Kiernan PD, ReMine SG, Kiernan PC, ReMine WH: Annular pancreas: Mayo Clinic experience from 1957 to 1976 with review of the literature, *Arch Surg* 115:46, 1980.
7. Lloyd-Jones W, Mountain JC, Warren KW: Annular pancreas in the adult, *Ann Surg* 176:163, 1972.
8. Dharmsathophorn K, Burrel M, Dobbins J: Diagnosis of annular pancreas with ERCP, *Gastroenterology* 77:1109, 1979.
9. Glazer GM, Margulis AR: Annular pancreas: etiology and diagnosis using endoscopic retrograde cholangiopancreatography, *Radiology* 133:303, 1979.
10. Clifford KMA: Annular pancreas diagnosed by ERCP, *Br J Radiol* 53:593, 1980.
11. Blackstone MO: Endoscopic interpretation. In *Normal and pathologic appearances of the gastrointestinal tract,* New York, 1984, Raven Press.
12. Brambs HJ, Spamer C, Volk B, Holstege A: Diagnostic value of ultrasound in duodenal stenosis, *Gastrointest Radiol* 11:135, 1986.
13. Pugash RA, O'Brien SE, Stevenson GW: Perforating duodenal diverticulitis, *Gastrointest Radiol* 15:156, 1990.
14. Neill SA, Thompson NW: The complications of duodenal diverticula and their management, *Surg Gynecol Obstet* 120:1251, 1965.
15. Stone EE, Brant WE, Smith GB: Computed tomography of duodenal diverticula, *J Comput Assist Tomogr* 13:61, 1989.
16. Yasui K, Tsukaguchi I, Ohara S, Sato K, Ono N et al: Benign duodenocolic fistula due to duodenal diverticulum: report of two cases, *Radiology* 130:67, 1979.
17. Van Beers B, Trigaux JP, De Ronde T, Melange M: CT findings of perforated duodenal diverticulitis; case report, *J Comput Assist Tomogr* 13:528, 1989.
18. Soreide JA, Seime S, Soreide O: Intraluminal duodenal diverticulum: case report and update of the literature 1975–1986, *Am J Gastroenterol* 83:988, 1988.
19. Economides NG, McBurney RP, Hamilton FH: Intraluminal duodenal diverticulum in the adult, *Ann Surg* 185:147, 1977.
20. Stelling T, van Rooij WJJ, Tio TL, Reeders JWAJ, Bartelsman JJWM et al: Pancreatitis associated with congenital duodenal duplication cyst in an adult, *Endoscopy* 19:171, 1987.
21. Procacci C, Portuese A, Fugazzola C, Pederzoli P, Caudana R et al: Duodenal duplication in the adult: its relationship with pancreatitis, *Gastrointest Radiol* 13:315, 1988.
22. Bar-Ziv J, Katz R, Nobel M, Antebi E: Duodenal duplication cyst with enteroliths: computed tomography and ultrasound diagnosis, *Gastrointest Radiol* 14:220, 1989.
23. Teplick SK, Glick SN, Keller MS: The duodenum. In Putman CE, Racin CE, eds: *Textbook of diagnostic imaging,* Philadelphia, 1988, WB Saunders.
24. Feldman M, Myers P: The roentgen diagnosis of prolapse of gastric mucosa into the duodenum, *Gastroenterology* 20:90, 1952.
25. Van Beers B, Trigaux JP, Pringot J: Duodenojejunal intussusception secondary to duodenal tumors, *Gastrointest Radiol* 13:24, 1988.
26. Laurent F, Raynaud M, Biset JM, Boisserie-Lacroix M, Grelet P et al: Diagnosis and categorization of small bowel neoplasms: role of computed tomography, *Gastrointest Radiol* 16:115, 1991.
27. Kleinhaus U, Weich YL, Maoz S: Gastroduodenal intussusception secondary to prolapsing gastric tumors, *Gastrointest Radiol* 11:229, 1986.
28. Rieth KG, Abbott GF, Gray G: Duodenal intussusception secondary to Brunner's gland hamartoma: a case report, *Gastrointest Radiol* 2:13, 1977.
29. Greenlaw R, Sheehan DG, DeLuca V et al: Gastroduodenitis: a broader concept of peptic ulcer disease, *Dig Dis Sci* 25:660, 1980.
30. Jolfe SN: Relevance of duodenitis to nonulcer dyspepsia and peptic ulceration, *Scand J Gastroenterol* 17(suppl):88, 1982.
31. Gelzayd EA, Gelfand DW, Rinaldo JA: Nonspecific duodenitis: a distinct clinical entity? *Gastrointest Endosc* 19:131, 1973.
32. Myren J: Gastric secretion in duodenitis, *Scand J Gastroenterol* 17(suppl):98, 1982.
33. Gelfand DW, Dale WJ, Ott DJ, Wu WC, Kerr RM et al: Duodenitis: endoscopic-radiologic correlation in 272 patients, *Radiology* 157:577, 1985.
34. Levine MS, Turner D, Ekberg O, Rubesin SE, Katzka DA: Duodenitis: a reliable radiologic diagnosis? *Gastrointest Radiol* 16:99, 1991.
35. Whitehead R: Nonphysiological aspects of duodenitis, *Scand J Gastroenterol* 17:80, 1982.
36. Catalano D, Pafliari U: Gastroduodenal erosions: radiological findings, *Gastrointest Radiol* 7:235, 1982.
37. Meiselman MS, Ghahremani GG, Kaufman MW: Crohn's disease of the duodenum complicated by adenocarcinoma, *Gastrointest Radiol* 12:333, 1987.
38. Gore RM, Ghahremani GG: Crohn's disease of the upper gastrointestinal tract, *Crit Rev Diagn Imaging* 25:305, 1986.
39. Kelvin FM, Gedgaudas RK: Radiologic diagnosis of Crohn's disease (with emphasis on its early manifestations), *Crit Rev Diagn Imaging* 16:43, 1981.
40. Levine MS: Crohn's disease of the upper gastrointestinal tract, *Radiol Clin North Am* 25:79, 1987.
41. Nugent FW, Richmond M, Park SK: Crohn's disease of the duodenum, *Gut* 18:115, 1977.
42. Ariyama J, Wehlin L, Lindstrom CG, Wenkert A, Roberts GM: Gastroduodenal erosions in Crohn's disease, *Gastrointest Radiol* 5:121, 1980.
43. Silverstein FE, Tytgat GNJ: *Atlas of gastrointestinal endoscopy,* New York, 1987, Churchill Livingstone.
44. Flueckiger F, Kullnig P, Melzer G et al: Colobronchial and gastrocolic fistulas: rare complication of Crohn's disease, *Gastrointest Radiol* 15:288, 1990.
45. Marshak RH, Maklansky D, Kurzban JD, Lindner AE: Crohn's disease of the stomach and duodenum, *Am J Gastroenterol* 77:340, 1982.
46. Barthelemy CR: Crohn's disease of the duodenum with spontaneous reflux into the pancreatic duct, *Gastrointest Radiol* 8:319, 1983.
47. Traute J, Simpson S, Riddell RH, Levin B, Kirsner JB: Crohn's disease and adenocarcinoma of the bowel, *Dig Dis Sci* 25:939, 1980.
48. Slezak P, Rubio C, Blomquist L, Nakano H, Befrits R: Duodenal adenocarcinoma in Crohn's disease of the small bowel: a case report, *Gastrointest Radiol* 16:15, 1991.
49. Danzi JT, Farmer RG, Sullivan BH et al: Endoscopic features of gastroduodenal Crohn's disease, *Gastroenterology* 70:9, 1976.
50. Caldwell JH, Mekhjian HS, Hurtubisc PH, Beman FM: Eosinophilic gastroenteritis with obstruction: immunological studies of seven patients, *Gastroenterology* 74:825, 1978.
51. Tishler JMA: Duodenal tuberculosis, *Radiology* 130:593, 1979.
52. Black GA, Carsky EW: Duodenal tuberculosis, *AJR* 131:329, 1978.
53. Wall SD, Ominskey S, Altman DF: Multifocal abnormalities of the gastrointestinal tract in AIDS, *AJR* 146:1, 1986.

54. Meiselman MS, Cello JP, Margareten W: Cytomegalovirus colitis in AIDS, *Gastroenterology* 88:171, 1985.

55. Peters M, Weiner J, Whelan G: Fungal infection associated with gastroduodenal ulceration: endoscopic and pathologic appearances, *Gastroenterology* 78:350, 1980.

56. Orchard JL, Luparello F, Brunskill D: Malabsorption syndrome occurring in the course of disseminated histoplasmosis: case report and review of gastrointestinal histoplasmosis, *Am J Med* 66:331, 1979.

57. Wyle FA: *Helicobacter pylori:* current perspectives, *J Clin Gastroenterol* 13(suppl 1):114, 1991.

58. Vaira D, Holton J, Osborn J et al: Use of endoscopy in patients with dyspepsia, *Br Med J* 299:237, 1989.

59. Morrissey JF, Reicheldorfer M: Gastrointestinal endoscopy, *N Engl J Med* 325:1142, 1991.

60. Rodriguez HP, Aston JK, Richardson CT: Ulcers in the descending duodenum: postbulbar ulcers, *AJR* 119:316, 1973.

61. Lu CC, Murakami J, Barloon T, Ell SR, Franken EA: Base line tenting: a sign of duodenal ulcer disease, *Gastrointest Radiol* 12:109, 1987.

62. Lubert M, Krause GR: The "ring" shadow in the diagnosis of ulcer, *AJR* 90:767, 1963.

63. Kawai K, Ida K, Misaki F, Akasaka Y, Kohli Y: Comparative study of duodenal ulcer by radiology and endoscopy, *Endoscopy* 5:7, 1973.

64. Martinez-Noguera A, Mata J, Matias-Guiu X, Donoso L, Coscojeula P: Echogenic focus in the gastrointestinal wall as a sign of ulceration, *Gastrointest Radiol* 14:295, 1989.

65. Tuncel E: Ultrasonic features of duodenal ulcer, *Gastrointest Radiol* 15:207, 1990.

66. de Roos A, Op den Orth JO: Linear niches in the duodenal bulb, *AJR* 140:941, 1983.

67. Braver JM, Paul RE, Philipps E, Bloom S: Roentgen diagnosis of linear ulcers, *Radiology* 132:29, 1979.

68. Eisenberg RL, Margulis AR, Moss AA: Giant duodenal ulcers, *Gastrointest Radiol* 2:347, 1978.

69. Lumsden K, MacLarnon JC, Dawson J: Giant duodenal ulcer, *Gut* 11:592, 1970.

70. Kirsch IE, Brendel T: The importance of giant duodenal ulcer, *Radiology* 91:14, 1968.

71. Ball RP, Segal AL, Golden R: Postbulbar duodenal ulcer and ring-stricture, *Radiology* 100:27, 1971.

72. Madrazo BL, Hricak H, Sandler MA, Eyler WR: Sonographic findings in complicated peptic ulcer, *Radiology* 140:457, 1981.

73. Radin DR: Intramural and intraperitoneal hemorrhage due to duodenal ulcer, case report, *AJR* 157:45, 1991.

74. Burrell M, Toffler R: Flexural pseudolesions of the duodenum, *Radiology* 120:313, 1976.

75. Chandieshaw P, van Romunde LKJ, Griffioen G, Janssens AR, Kreuning J et al: Peptic ulcer and gastric carcinoma: diagnosis with biphasic radiography compared with fibreoptic endoscopy, *Radiology* 163:39, 1987.

76. Laufer I, Mullens JE, Hamilton J: The diagnostic accuracy of barium studies of the stomach and duodenum: correlation with endoscopy, *Radiology* 115:569, 1975.

77. Delpy JC, Bruneton JN, Drouillard J, Lecomte P: Non-vaterian duodenal adenomas: report of 24 cases and review of the literature, *Gastrointest Radiol* 8:135, 1983.

78. Schulten MF, Oyasu R, Beal JM: Villous adenoma of the duodenum; a case report and review of the literature, *Am J Surg* 132:90, 1976.

79. Spira IA, Wolff WI: Villous tumors of the duodenum, *Am J Gastroenterol* 67:63, 1977.

80. Smithuis RHM, Vos CG: Heterotopic gastric mucosa in the duodenal bulb: relationship to peptic ulcer, *AJR* 152:59, 1989.

81. Fork FT, Haglund U, Hogstrom H, Wehlin L: Primary gastric lymphoma versus gastric cancer: an endoscopic and radiographic study of differential diagnostic possibilities, *Endoscopy* 17:5, 1985.

82. Bjork KJ, Davis CJ, Nagorney DM, Mucha P: Duodenal villous tumors, *Arch Surg* 125:961, 1990.

83. Miller JH, Gisvold JJ, Weiland LH, McIlrath DC: Upper gastrointestinal tract: villous tumors, *AJR* 134:933, 1980.

84. Ring EJ, Ferrucci JT, Eaton SB, Clements JL: Villous adenomas of the duodenum, *Radiology* 104:45, 1972.

85. Alwmark A, Andersson A, Lasson A: Primary carcinoma of the duodenum, *Ann Surg* 191:13, 1980.

86. Barloon TJ, Lu CH, Honda H, Walker WP, Murray J: Primary adenocarcinoma of the duodenal bulb: radiographic and pathologic findings in two cases, *Gastrointest Radiol* 14:223, 1989.

87. Craig O: Duodenal carcinoma, *Br J Surg* 56:39, 1969.

88. Bosse G, Neeley JA: Roentgenologic findings in primary malignant tumors of the duodenum, *AJR* 170:111, 1969.

89. Cwikiel W, Andrén-Sandberg A: Diagnostic difficulties with duodenal malignancies revisited: a new strategy, *Gastrointest Radiol* 16:301, 1991.

90. Maglinte DDT, Lappas JC, Kelvin FM, Rex D, Chernish SM: Small bowel radiography, how, when, and why, *Radiology* 163:297, 1987.

91. Farah MC, Jafri SZH, Schwab RE, Mezwa DG, Francis IR et al: Duodenal neoplasms: role of CT, *Radiology* 162:839, 1987.

92. Scatarige JC, DiSantis DJ: CT of the stomach and duodenum, *Radiol Clin North Am* 27:687, 1989.

93. Reeders JWAJ, ed: *Diagnostic imaging of AIDS,* New York, 1992, Thieme.

94. Niedt GW, Schinella RA: AIDS: clinicopathologic study of 56 autopsies, *Arch Pathol Lab Med* 109:727, 1985.

95. Clements JL, Roche RR: Carcinoid of the duodenum: a report of six cases, *Gastrointest Radiol* 9:17, 1984.

96. Kanematsu M, Imaeda T, Iinuma G, Mori S, Yamawaki Y et al: Leiomyosarcoma of the duodenum, *Gastrointest Radiol* 16:109, 1991.

97. Megibow AJ, Balthazar EJ, Hulnick DH, Naidich DP, Bosniak MA: CT evaluation of gastrointestinal leiomyomas and leiomyosarcomas, *AJR* 144:727, 1985.

98. Subramanyam BR, Balthazar EJ, Raghavendra BN, Madamba MR: Sonography of exophytic gastrointestinal leiomyosarcoma, *Gastrointest Radiol* 7:47, 1982.

99. Kaftori JK, Aharon M, Kleinhaus U: Sonographic features of gastrointestinal leiomyosarcoma, *J Clin Ultrasound* 9:11, 1981.

100. Reddy RR, Schuman B, Priest RJ: Duodenal polyps: diagnosis and management, *J Clin Gastroenterol* 3:139, 1981.

101. Balikian JP, Nassar NT, Shamma'a MH et al: Primary lymphomas of the small intestine including the duodenum, *AJR* 107:131, 1969.

102. Quinn SF, Shaffer HA, Willard MR, Ross S: Bull's eye lesions: a new gastrointestinal presentation of mastocytosis, *Gastrointest Radiol* 9:13, 1984.

103. Ammann RW, Vetter D, Deyhle P, Tschen H, Sulser H et al: Gastrointestinal involvement in systemic mastocytosis, *Gut* 17:107, 1976.

104. Dantzig PI: Tetany, malabsorption, and mastocytosis, *Arch Intern Med* 135:1514, 1975.

105. Janower ML: Mastocytosis of the GI tract: a report of a case, *Acta Radiol* 57:489, 1962.

106. Clemett AR, Fishbone G, Levine RJ, James AE, Janover M: Gastrointestinal lesions in mastocystosis, *AJR* 102:405, 1967.

107. Lucaya J, Perez-Candela V, Aso C, Calvo J: Mastocytosis with skeletal and gastrointestinal involvement in infancy, *Radiology* 131:363, 1979.

108. Yoshimitsu K, Yoshida M, Motooka M, Sakurai T, Kitagawa S et al: Heterotopic gastric mucosa of the duodenum mimicking a duodenal cancer, *Gastrointest Radiol* 14:115, 1989.

109. Langkemper R, Hoek AC, Dekker W, Op den Orth JO: Elevated lesions in the duodenal bulb caused by heterotopic gastric mucosa, *Radiology* 137:621, 1980.

110. Weingart J, Seib HJ, Elster K, Ottenjann R: Magenschleimhaut heterotopien im oberen Gastrointestinaltrakt, *Leber Magen Darm* 14:155, 1984.

111. Uraoka M, Fujitani T, Lida M, Iwashita A: Clinicopathological investigation of heterotopic gastric mucosa of the duodenum, *Gastroenterol Endosc* (abstract in Japanese) 28:3078, 1986.

112. Lessels AM, Martin DF: Heterotopic gastric mucosa in the duodenum, *J Clin Pathol* 35:591, 1982.

113. Spiller RC, Shousha S, Barrison IG: Heterotopic gastric tissue in the duodenum, *Dig Dis Sci* 27:880, 1982.

114. McWey P, Dodds WJ, Slota T, Stewart ET, Hogan WJ: Radiographic features of heterotopic gastric mucosa, *AJR* 139:380, 1982.

115. Agha FP, Ghahremani GG, Tsang TK, Victor TA: Heterotopic gastric mucosa in the duodenum: radiographic findings, *AJR* 150:291, 1988.

116. Cynn WS, Rickert RR: Heterotopic gastric mucosal polyp in the duodenal bulb associated with congenital absence of the gallbladder, *Am J Gastroenterol* 60:171, 1973.

117. van Rooij WJJ, van der Horst JJ, Stuifbergen WNHM, Pijpers PM: Extreme diffuse adenomatous hyperplasia of Brunner's glands: case report, *Gastrointest Radiol* 15:285, 1990.

118. Weinberg PE, Levin B: Hyperplasia of Brunner's glands, *Radiology* 84:259, 1965.

119. Cassar-Pullicino VN, Davies AM, Hubscher S, Burrows F: The nodular duodenum in chronic renal failure, *Clin Radiol* 41:326, 1990.

120. Fraser GM, Pitman RG, Lawrie JH et al: The significance of the radiological finding of coarse mucosal folds in the duodenum, *Lancet* 2:979, 1964.

121. Wiener SN, Vertes V, Shapiro H: The upper gastrointestinal tract in patients undergoing chronic dialysis, *Radiology* 92:110, 1969.

122. Zukerman GR, Mils BA, Koehler RE et al: Nodular duodenitis: pathologic and clinical characteristics in patients with end-stage renal disease, *Dig Dis Sci* 11:1018, 1983.

123. Dodd GD, Fishler JS, Park OK: Hyperplasia of Brunner's glands; report of two cases with review of the literature, *AJR* 60:814, 1953.

124. Merine D, Jones B, Ghahremani GG, Hamilton SR, Bayless TM: Hyperplasia of Brunner glands: the spectrum of its radiographic manifestations, *Gastrointest Radiol* 16:104, 1991.

125. Bastlein C, Decking R, Voeth C, Ottenjann R: Giant brunneroma of the duodenum, *Endoscopy* 20:154, 1988.

126. Govoni AF: Benign lymphoid hyperplasia of the duodenal bulb, *Gastrointest Radiol* 1:267, 1976.

127. Davis M, Fenoglio-Preiser C, Haque AK: Cavernous lymphangioma of the duodenum: case report and review of the literature, *Gastrointest Radiol* 12:10, 1987.

128. Greenspan A, Bryk D: Duodenal varices secondary to inferior vena cava obstruction, *Dig Dis Sci* 18:983, 1973.

129. Itzchak Y, Glickman MG: Duodenal varices in extrahepatic portal obstruction, *Radiology* 124:619, 1977.

130. Wyatt GM, Rauchway MI, Spitz HB: Roentgen findings in aortoenteric fistulae, *AJR* 126:714, 1976.

131. Zeppa MA, Forest JV: Aortoenteric fistula manifested as an intramural duodenal hematoma, *AJR* 157:47, 1991.

132. O'Mara CS, Williams GM, Ernst CB: Secondary aortoenteric fistula, *Am J Surg* 142:203, 1981.

133. Low RN, Wall SD, Jeffrey RB, Sollitto RA, Reilly LM et al: Aortoenteric fistula and perigraft infection: evaluation with CT, *Radiology* 175:157, 1990.

134. Aggarwal S, Berry M: Duodenal fistula: complication of a pseudoaneurysm of the common hepatic artery, *Gastrointest Radiol* 13:230, 1988.

135. Hofer GA, Cohen AJ: CT signs of duodenal perforation secondary to blunt abdominal trauma, *J Comput Assist Tomogr* 13:430, 1989.

136. Cleveland HC, Wadell WR: Retroperitoneal rupture of the duodenum due to nonpenetrating trauma, *Surg Clin North Am* 43:413, 1963.

137. Diner WC: Duodenal perforation during intubation for small bowel enema study, *Radiology* 168:39, 1988.

138. Toxopeus MD, Lucas CE, Krabbenhoft KL: Roentgenographic diagnosis in blunt retroperitoneal duodenal rupture, *AJR* 115:281, 1972.

139. Blakemore WS, Baum S, Nusbaum M: Diagnosis and management of massive hemorrhage from postoperative stress ulcers of the descending duodenum, *Surg Clin North Am* 50:979, 1970.

140. Baum S, Ward S, Nusbaum M: Stress bleeding from the mid-duodenum: an often unrecognized source of gastrointestinal hemorrhage, *Radiology* 95:595, 1970.

141. Felson B, Levin EJ: Intramural hematoma of the duodenum; a diagnostic roentgen sign, *AJR* 63:823, 1954.

142. Sadry F, Hauser H: Fatal pancreatitis secondary to iatrogenic intramural duodenal hematoma: a case report and review of the literature, *Gastrointest Radiol* 15:296, 1990.

143. Hahn PF, Stark PD, Vici LG, Ferrucci JT: Duodenal hematoma: the ring sign in MR imaging, *Radiology* 159:379, 1986.

144. Plojoux O, Hauser H, Wettstein P: CT of intramural haematoma of the small intestine: a report of 3 cases, *Radiology* 144:559, 1982.

145. Yoshino MT: Duodenal hematoma: CT demonstration of the ring sign, *Gastrointest Radiol* 12:330, 1987.

146. Martin B, Mulopulos GP, Butler HE: MR imaging of intramural duodenal hematoma; case report, *J Comput Assist Tomogr* 10:1042, 1986.

147. Mahboubi S, Kaufman HJ: Intramural duodenal hematoma in children; the role of the radiologist in its conservative management, *Gastrointest Radiol* 1:167, 1976.

148. Wallace RG, Howard WB: Acute superior mesenteric artery syndrome in the severely burned patient, *Radiology* 94:307, 1970.

149. Marchant EA, Alvear DT, Fagelman KM: True clinical entity of vascular compression of the duodenum in adolescence, *Surgery* 168:381, 1989.

150. Gondos B: Duodenal compression defect and the "superior mesenteric artery syndrome," *Radiology* 123:575, 1977.

151. Marn CS, Gore RM, Ghahremani GG: Duodenal manifestations of nontropical sprue, *Gastrointest Radiol* 11:30, 1986.

152. Jones B, Bayles TM, Hamilton SR, Yardley JH: "Bubbly" duodenal bulb in celiac disease: radiologic-pathologic correlation, *AJR* 142:119, 1984.

153. Cheli R, Aste H: *Duodenitis,* Stuttgart, 1976, Thieme.

154. Ottenjan R, Classen M: *Gastroenterolgoische Endoskopie; Lehrbuch und Atlas,* Stuttgart, 1991, Enke Verlag.

155. Comer GM, Brandt JL, Abissi CJ: Whipple's disease: a review, *Am J Gastroenterol* 78:107, 1983.

156. Sellink JL, Miller RE: *Radiology of small bowel: modern enteroclysis technique and atlas,* The Hague, 1982, Martinus Nijhoff.

157. Carlson HC, Breen F: Amyloidosis and plasma cell dyscrania: gastrointestinal involvement, *Semin Roentgenol* 21:128, 1986.

158. Stabile BE, Morrow DJ, Passaro E: The gastrinoma triangle: operative implications, *Am J Surg* 127:25, 1984.

159. Deveney CS, Deveney KE: Zollinger-Ellison syndrome (gastrinoma): current diagnosis and treatment, *Surg Clin North Am* 67:411, 1987.

160. Rosenbusch G, Lamers CBH, van Tongeren JHM, Boetes C, Snel P et al: Röntgendiagnostik beim Zollinger-Ellison Syndrom, *Fortschr Röntgenstr* 129:168, 1978.

161. Nelson JA, Sheft DJ, Minagi H, Ferruci JT: Duodenal pseudopolyp—the flexure fallacy, *AJR* 123:262, 1975.

PART VI

SMALL BOWEL

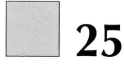 **25** *The Small Bowel: Anatomy and Nontube Examinations*

SAT SOMERS
GILES W. STEVENSON

ANATOMY

The small bowel begins at the pylorus and ends at the ileocecal valve where it joins the colon. Its length, in postmortem studies, is 6 to 7 meters, and its caliber gradually diminishes distally. The length is related to sex and height[1]: in females the average length is 5.92 meters, and in males it is 6.37 meters.[2] In patients undergoing surgery for nonintestinal disorders an average length of 6.5 m[3] has been recorded. Radiologically, it is not as easy to determine the length of the small bowel, but measurements taken during enteroclysis show a much shorter length than the postmortem figures, with an average length of 2.8 m.[4] Measurements made after small bowel resection to determine residual length can be sufficiently accurate to help in management decisions, especially when the remaining bowel is short and it is all visualized on one film.[5]

Most of the small bowel is framed by the colon and lies in the central and lower parts of the abdominal cavity. A portion of it may reach the pelvis and lie in front of the rectum. It is attached to the posterior abdominal wall by a fan-shaped mesentery. The pleated intestinal border of the mesentery measures approximately the length of the small bowel, whereas its root is only 15 cm long. The distance between the root of the mesentery and the small bowel varies; the average distance is about 20 cm. It is longest in the mid small intestine and shortest at the proximal and distal ends of the mesenteric root. The mesenteric border of the small bowel loops can be identified as the concave margin seen when the lumen is distended. The two peritoneal layers of the mesentery contain, in addition to the jejunum and ileum, the jejunal and ileal branches of the superior mesenteric vessels, nerves, lymphatic channels, and lymph nodes, together with a variable amount of fat. This fat makes the small bowel particularly amenable to computed tomographic (CT) study.

There is an arbitrary division of the small bowel beyond the duodenum, into the jejunum, which comprises the proximal two fifths of the small bowel, and the ileum. The je-

junum and ileum, because of their mesentery, have considerable mobility within the abdomen. The jejunum usually occupies the upper left and the periumbilical area, and the ileum the lower right hypogastric and pelvic portions of the abdominal cavity (Fig. 25-1).

The jejunum has a diameter of about 4 cm and a wall that is thicker than the ileum. Its circular mucosal folds are frequent and large (Fig. 25-2, *A*), and the villi are also larger than in the ileum. A few small, discoidal, aggregated lymphatic follicles are present in the distal jejunum. They are almost totally absent from the proximal jejunum.

The ileum has a maximal luminal diameter of about 3.5 cm with a wall that is thinner than the jejunum. There are a few circular folds proximally, but these disappear almost entirely in its distal part (Fig. 25-2, *B*). There are, however, numerous aggregated lymphatic follicles, which are large and obvious in children and young adults, up to 3 to 4 mm in diameter, although more usually 1 to 2 mm.

Although the anatomic calibers of the jejunum and ileum measure 4 cm and 3.5 cm, the luminal diameter should not exceed 3.5 cm in the jejunum and 3 cm in the ileum during a nontube examination of the small bowel.[6] The wall thickness usually measures between 1 mm and 2 mm.[7]

In about 3% of subjects an ileal diverticulum (Meckel's diverticulum) is present on the antimesenteric border of the distal ileum (Fig. 25-3), about 1 meter from the ileocecal valve. Its length averages 5 cm, and the blind end of the diverticulum is either free or connected with the anterior abdominal wall or another part of the intestine by a fibrous band. It represents the persistent proximal part of the vitelline (yolk) duct and is supplied by the vitellointestinal artery, which is sometimes identifiable on angiography. The diverticular mucosa is ileal in type, but small areas occasionally may have a gastric structure with oxyntic cells secreting acid as well as heterotopic areas of pancreatic or other tissues.

The wall of the small intestine contains the usual layers found in bowel. From the serosa to the lumen, they are the

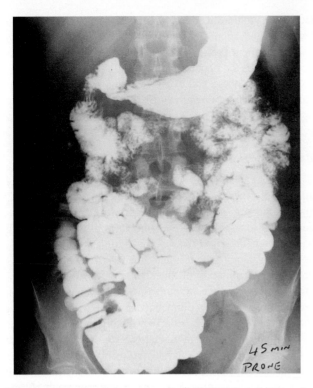

Fig. 25-1 This film from a primary small bowel meal shows the jejunum with its many valvulae in the left upper quadrant and most of the smoother ileum in the lower abdomen. Note that at 45 minutes the right colon is filling, the stomach still contains plenty of barium, and the whole of the small bowel is filled.

serous, muscular, submucosal, and mucosal layers. The serosa is visceral peritoneum with a subserous layer of loose connective tissue. The muscularis is made up of a thin external longitudinal and a thick internal circular layer of nonstriated myocytes. Auerbach's autonomic nerve plexus is located between the two muscular layers and plays a role in peristalsis. The muscularis externa is thicker in the proximal intestine.

The submucosa is loose connective tissue carrying blood vessels, lymphatic channels, and nerves. Meissner's plexus is situated in its deeper part. In the proximal half of the duodenum, the submucosa is filled with Brunner's glands.

The mucosa has three recognizable layers. The outermost layer is the muscularis mucosae. It is a few cells thick and made up of an external longitudinal and an internal circular layer of nonstriated myocytes. It separates the submucosa from the lamina propria, the connective tissue layer of the mucosa. The innermost layer of the mucosa is the epithelium, consisting of absorptive columnar cells and interspersed mucin-producing goblet cells.

The surface area of the small bowel is increased by infoldings of mucosa and submucosa called the *valvulae conniventes.* They begin to appear about 2.5 to 5 cm beyond the pylorus. Proximally they are large and close together; distally they diminish gradually until the midileum and then disappear almost entirely in the distal ileum. The width of the jejunal folds is up to 2 mm and that of the ileum from about 1 to 1.5 mm. The mucosal fold height is about 3.5 to 7 mm in the jejunum and 3.5 mm or less in the ileum.[8] The jejunal folds, unlike those in the stomach, do not dis-

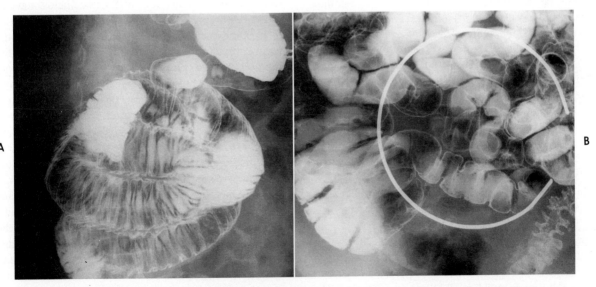

Fig. 25-2 A, An oblique projection film of the jejunum taken after an oral effervescent agent was given shows the jejunal folds to be frequent and large in comparison to the ileum. **B,** Pelvic ileal loops that have been separated with a paddle after carbon dioxide insufflation distended the terminal ileum and distal small bowel. Note that the circular ileal folds are quite thin, infrequent, and often incomplete.

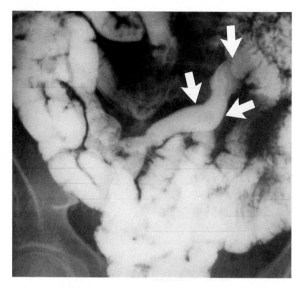

Fig. 25-3 A Meckel's diverticulum *(arrows)* demonstrated on a primary small bowel meal.

appear on distention. The ileal folds, however, become obliterated with even minor distention.

The absorptive surface of the mucosa is further enhanced by the presence of villi. These are highly vascular processes that project from the entire intestinal mucosa. They give the surface a velvety texture. The villi are very small when compared with the mucosal folds and are at or just below the limits of radiologic visualization unless they are pathologically enlarged.[9] When seen en face, they appear like minute soft-tissue projections into the barium. Large lacteals extend into the lamina propria of each villus, and thus any disease process that extends into the lamina propria will readily spread to the mesenteric and paraaortic lymph nodes.

EXAMINATION TECHNIQUES

Enteroclysis is discussed in Chapters 26 and 27. This section describes other ways to examine the small bowel with radiography and fluoroscopy, ultrasound, CT, and magnetic resonance imaging (MRI).

Barium examination

Barium sulphate preparations are ideal for most routine examinations of the small bowel. Water-soluble contrast is used when perforation is suspected, when there may be concern about colonic obstruction (it is advisable in this instance to begin with a colon examination), and in very small infants. A variety of compression devices are an essential requirement for performing small bowel examinations. The F spoon, the Mayo spoon, and an inflatable balloon compression device are all excellent for different situations. A rolled-up and taped towel in a cylinder shape 9 inches long and 3 to 4 inches in diameter is useful. Finally the Malmo

technique includes a rolled and taped firm cloth cylinder 3 feet long and about 3 inches in diameter that can be used with the patient prone. This long cloth is positioned transversely under the upper abdomen and slowly pulled down. Except in the obese and excessively muscular, the individual loops of small bowel can be seen in turn because they are compressed while they slide slowly past the cylinder as it is being pulled down the table.

Barium meal and follow-through

A barium meal and follow-through is the traditional study and is still very widely used.[10-12] The esophagus, stomach, and duodenum are typically examined first with high-density barium, followed by some 450 ml of a more dilute barium preparation. Often, overhead films are taken at half-hour intervals until the terminal ileum is reached, and a fluoroscopic examination of this area is performed with compression views. There are numerous disadvantages with this procedure, and we recommend that it be abandoned as a routine study, although it is occasionally indicated.

The first disadvantage is that the follow-through is ordered, tacked on to an upper GI series, too often with poor indications, "just in case" it might show something. This leads to a large number of normal examinations. Performing large numbers of examinations often leads to cursory study with no fluoroscopy until the cecum is reached, with risk of false-positive examinations (Figs. 25-4 and 25-5). The literature also documents a high false-negative rate for this examination.[11,13] Transit is slow, and there is poor distension of loops, often with overlap. The mixture of dense and less dense barium with effervescent agents is often unsatisfactory. If this study is carried out, the same attention to detail should be given as is described below for the dedicated small bowel meal. When a patient in whom the major suspicion is for small bowel disease arrives in the department, scheduled for upper GI series and follow-through, the best compromise is to perform the barium meal with small bowel barium using single contrast, mucosal relief, and compression techniques, and then to continue as for a dedicated small bowel meal.

Dedicated small bowel meal

If a radiology department announces that the barium meal and follow-through examination will no longer be available as a combined procedure and that patients may be booked for a dedicated small bowel meal or enteroclysis, the number of referrals drops dramatically—not because the patients are being sent elsewhere, but because referring physicians exercise more care in the selection of patients for this "additional" procedure. The decrease in numbers and in percentage of normal examinations enables the radiologist to spend more time with each patient, and this encourages more attention to detail. The dedicated small bowel meal needs a large volume of moderate-density barium to maintain a rapid flow rate. The administration of a prelim-

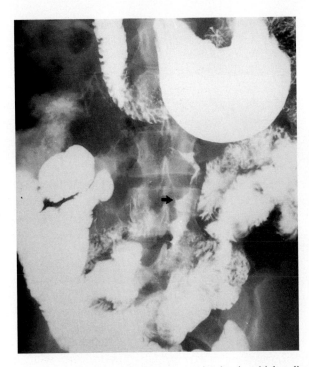

Fig. 25-4 A conventional follow-up examination in which a diagnosis of Crohn's disease was made on the basis of a single abnormal-appearing segment *(arrow)*. This loop was normal on reexamination. Fluorosopic confirmation of suspicious findings is important, especially findings at the leading or trailing edges of the barium column.

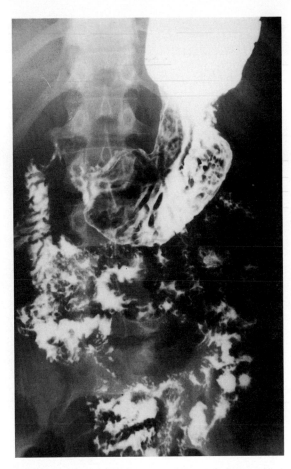

Fig. 25-5 An early follow-up examination done after a barium meal. A malabsorption disease was suggested. A repeat primary small-bowel study was normal. It is not uncommon for unusual appearances to be seen at the front of the barium column, and overinterpretation is a hazard.

inary laxative does not decrease the transit time,[14,15] although it does clear the right colon, which is advantageous if a peroral pneumocolon is planned (see below). The single most important factor in obtaining rapid transit of barium through the small bowel is to keep the stomach well filled with barium[15] (Fig. 25-1). As soon as the stomach empties, forward movement of barium slows, often almost to a halt. Therefore as soon as a film or fluoroscopic examination shows the stomach is no longer well filled, another cup of barium should be given. Once patients appreciate that this shortens the study, there is seldom difficulty in motivation. However, constipation is a concern, and in addition to instructions on drinking plenty of fluids afterward, patients with a tendency to constipation, especially the elderly, should be given a mild laxative or oral lactulose.

Overhead films are taken every 15 minutes. Fluoroscopy is carried out at 30 minutes and again when the cecum is reached. This is usually between 30 and 45 minutes if the stomach is kept filled. A total of 1 liter of barium is commonly required (Fig. 25-6).

Examination of the distal ileum may require the loops to be brought up out of the pelvis. Prone compression with an inflated balloon positioned just above the symphysis pubis often accomplishes this (Fig. 25-7). If this fails and

loops are stuck by adhesions in the pelvis, a lateral view of the pelvis may be helpful.

Small bowel meal with pneumocolon

One problem with both the dedicated small bowel meal and the follow-through is that the terminal ileum, although seen quite well, is seldom distended. It is therefore often difficult to be sure whether apparently thickened folds in the terminal ileum are normal. The peroral pneumocolon often resolves this issue.

The colon has to be relatively clean, which apparently reduces patient discomfort considerably during the insufflation of gas; the gas passes around a clean colon with less distention. It also reduces artifacts caused by stool content being refluxed into the cecum and small bowel. One recommended preparation is a normal breakfast on the day before the examination. At noon the patient takes a bottle of magnesium citrate (Citro-Mag, Rougier) followed by a glass of water. This is followed by a glass of clear fluid

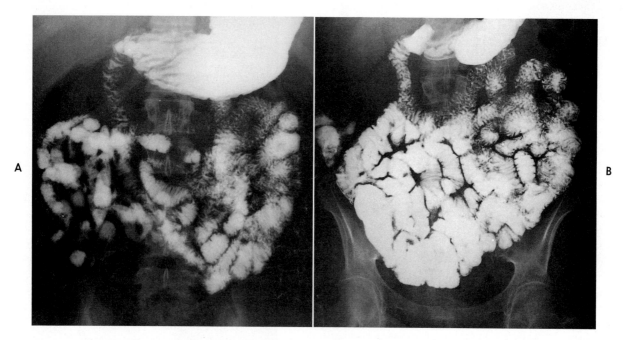

Fig. 25-6 A, 15- and **B,** 25-minute films of a patient having a primary small bowel meal examination. The 25-minute film shows contrast in the proximal ascending colon.

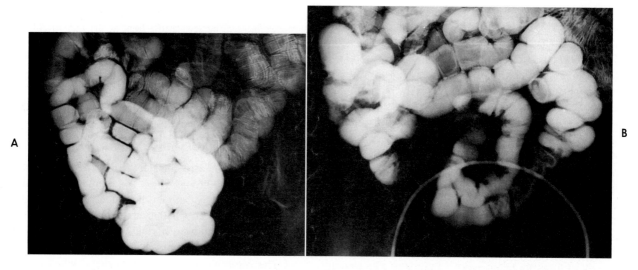

Fig. 25-7 Before compression (**A**) the pelvic loops are overlying and overlapping each other. Prone compression with an inflatable paddle (**B**) brings the normal ileal loops out of the pelvis and separates them.

every hour until bedtime. No solid food is allowed for the rest of the day. At 6 PM the patient takes two biscodyl tablets (Dulcolax, Boehringer Ingelheim). Patients who are insulin-dependent diabetics are asked to take a can of Ensure (Ross) at lunch and supper and half a can as an evening snack. They are told to continue with their normal insulin routine except for the morning of the study, when only half the insulin dose is taken. Patients taking other medications are asked to take them at least 2 hours before the small bowel examination unless they happen to be on iron. All iron medications should be stopped at least 2 days before the examination.

The examination is started with about 400 to 500 ml of barium. A 71% weight/volume suspension made up with 1350 g of Ultra-R barium (E-Z-EM, Inc., Westbury, NY) and 1500 ml of distilled water is satisfactory.

The first film is taken 5 to 10 minutes after the barium has been ingested. The timing of the following films depends on the transit through the small bowel. Typical films are as for the dedicated small bowel meal (Fig. 25-6). During the examination, the overlapping loops should be palpated and separated under fluoroscopic control. An inflatable paddle or an F spoon (Fig. 25-8) is helpful in separating the bowel loops.[16]

Once the terminal ileum and cecum have been opacified, a pneumocolon is performed. This is accomplished by inserting an 18 Fr pediatric enema tip (Fig. 25-8) into the rectum and insufflating air until there is reflux into the terminal ileum.[17-19] If the ileocecal valve does not relax enough to allow reflux of the air, a smooth muscle relaxant such as glucagon (Lilley), up to 0.5 mg, or hyoscine butylbromide (Buscopan, Boehringer Ingelheim), 10 to 20 mg, is given by intravenous injection. If carbon dioxide (CO_2) is readily available,[20] it should be used instead of air, as the postprocedure discomfort is considerably less.[21]

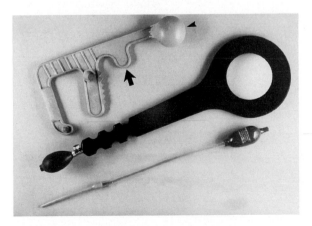

Fig. 25-8 Tools for a small bowel examination. *From top to bottom,* The F spoon *(arrow)* with a compression cone that has two small metallic markers, an inflatable paddle, and a 10 Fr pediatric enema catheter attached to a puffer.

Obtainable from F Spoon Co., Dover, Mass.; Pneumatic Compression Paddle, New Px Imaging, Philadelphia; and E-Z-EM, Westbury, NY, respectively.

The air-insufflated terminal ileum films usually display the mucosal surface very clearly (Fig. 25-9). An added bonus is the clear visualization of the pelvic loops, enhanced not only by the double-contrast view but also by the inflated rectum and sigmoid colon lifting and spreading the pelvic ileal loops (see Fig. 25-2, *B*). A compression paddle assists in further separation of the bowel loops.

The double-contrast views of the terminal ileum help to demonstrate mucosal disease (Fig. 25-10) or to confirm normality (Fig. 25-9). They may show complete normality in patients mistakenly diagnosed on a follow-through film as having inflammatory bowel disease (Fig. 25-11). True disease found on nondistended routine spot films of the terminal ileum as a spastic, narrowed segment with thickened mucosal folds (Fig. 25-12, *A*) are often better displayed with the pneumocolon, which produces a clearer demonstration of the distensibility of the distal ileum and the extent of the disease (Fig. 25-12, *B*). The pneumocolon is particularly useful in patients who have had an ileocolic resection with an anastomosis between large and small bowel. The minor changes of recurrent disease, manifest as aphthoid ulcers in the neoterminal ileum, are easily visualized (Fig. 25-13). When adherent diseased pelvic ileal loops are present, not only does the insufflation make them easier to see by distending the small bowel, but also the distended rectum and sigmoid colon push the normal small bowel out of the way (Fig. 25-14, *A*). A lateral projection is very helpful when there are adherent diseased pelvic loops because the location of the adhesions, the severity of the disease, and any strictures present can be readily determined (Fig. 25-14, *B*). Surprisingly good views of the colon may also be obtained with this examination (Fig. 25-15), but only if bowel preparation has been given.

In advanced disease the diagnosis can sometimes be made without compression, palpation, or insufflation. In such patients the bowel loops may already be separated because the wall is edematous and thick, as in graft-versus-host disease (Fig. 25-16) and milk allergy enterocolitis (Fig. 25-17).

Double-contrast study with oral effervescent agent

A nontube double-contrast study of the small bowel can also be achieved with an orally administered effervescent agent.[22] A small bowel meal is performed. When the column of barium has reached the cecum, enough of an effervescent agent to produce about a liter of gas is given. Any effervescent agent used for a double-contrast upper gastrointestinal series can be used, although delayed-release preparations under development may be superior and easier for patients to tolerate. The patient is then placed in a left posterior oblique or lateral decubitus position. The patient's head is lowered to a slight Trendelenburg's position. This positioning facilitates rapid gas filling of most of the small bowel. Spot films of the entire small bowel are then taken with the patient supine. Compression is used as necessary.

Text continued on p. 524.

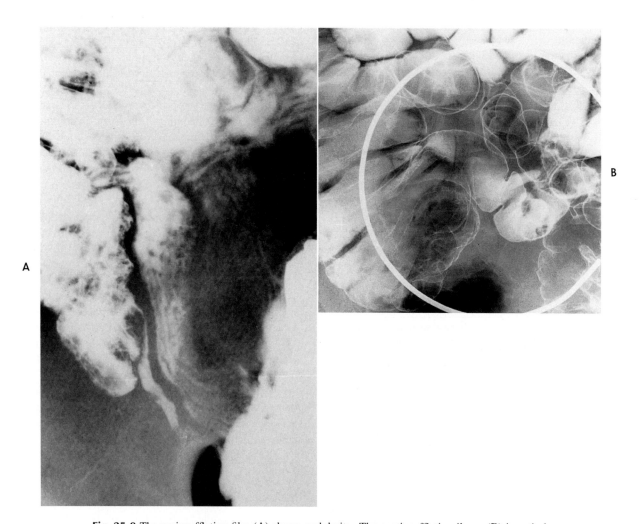

Fig. 25-9 The preinsufflation film (**A**) shows nodularity. The postinsufflation ileum (**B**) is entirely normal, suggesting that the nodules were normal soft lymphoid follicles. The double-contrast film allows a high degree of confidence in a normal report.

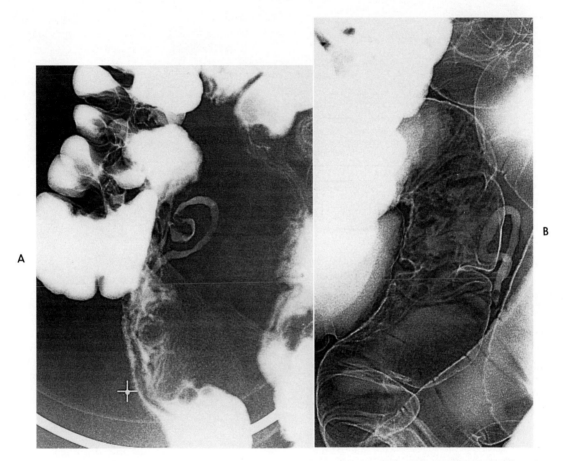

Fig. 25-10 Preinsufflation (**A**) and postinsufflation (**B**) films of the terminal ileum. The postinsufflation film shows mild mucosal changes, which proved on biopsy to be Crohn's disease.

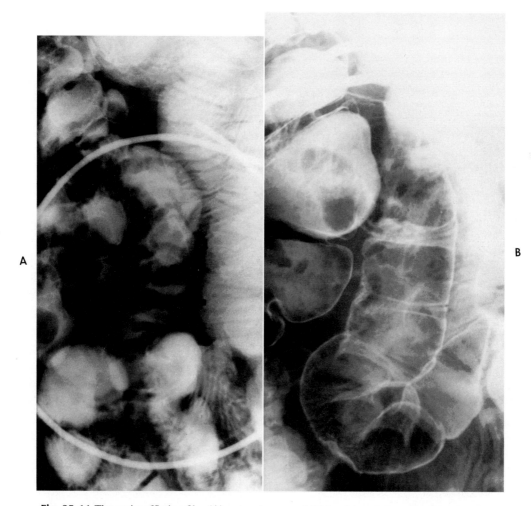

Fig. 25-11 The preinsufflation film (**A**) suggests mucosal thickening, whereas the distended ileum (**B**) is normal.

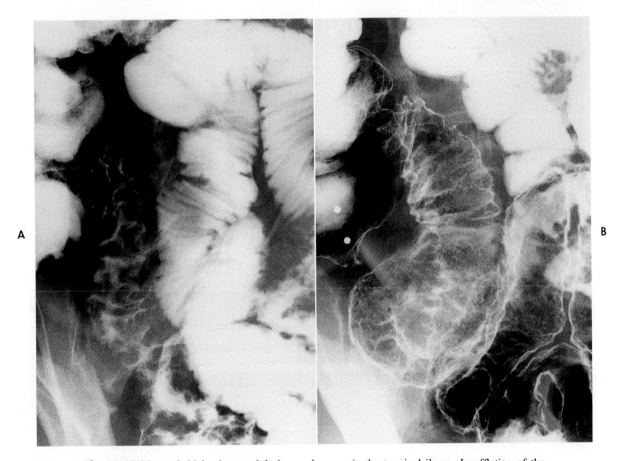

Fig. 25-12 Mucosal thickening, nodularity, and spasm in the terminal ileum. Insufflation of the terminal ileum shows its degree of distensibility and the extent of the Crohn's disease. Both films are useful. The double-contrast film confirms (or sometimes refutes) the validity of the single-contrast images and is better for showing extent of mucosal disease.

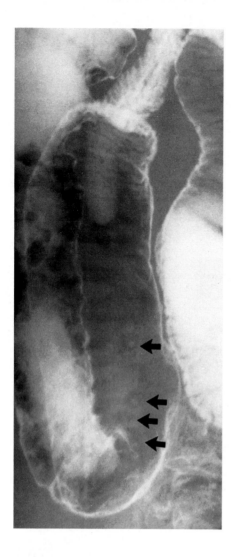

Fig. 25-13 Aphthous ulcers demonstrated in the neoterminal ileum of a patient with an ileocolic resection.

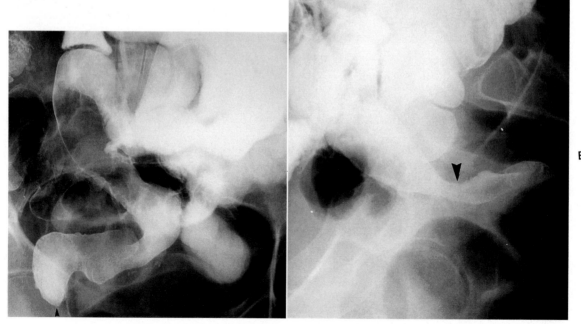

Fig. 25-14 The anterior-posterior view **(A)** demonstrates an adherent *(arrowhead)* diseased distal ileum. The normal bowel has been pushed out of the pelvis by the distended sigmoid colon and rectum. The lateral film **(B)** shows the diseased bowel to have a narrow segment *(arrowhead)* and be adherent to the posterior part of the pelvis.

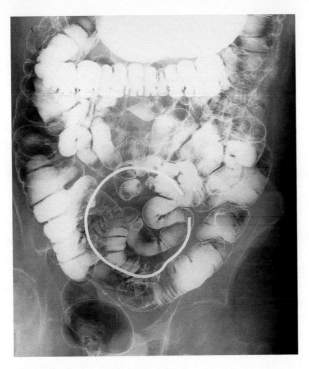

Fig. 25-15 An almost-complete double-contrast examination of the small bowel can be achieved with a pneumocolon in some patients.

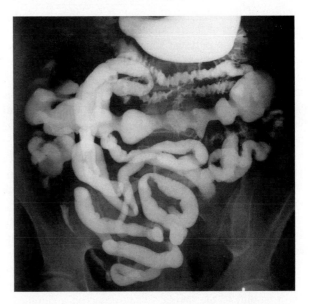

Fig. 25-16 Edematous, thick-walled, separated loops of small bowel demonstrated without the benefit of compression in a patient with graft-versus-host disease.

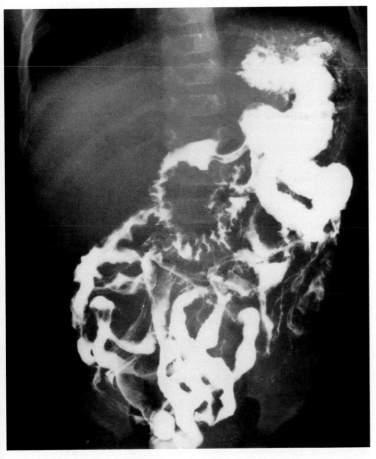

Fig. 25-17 A child with milk allergy enterocolitis in whom compression or double contrast would be superfluous.

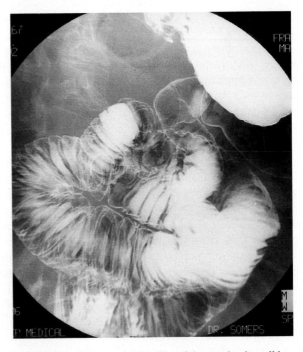

Fig. 25-18 An oblique projection film of the proximal small bowel taken after enough oral effervescent agent was given to produce about a liter of gas. The gas agent was given after the barium had reached the midjejunum. See also Fig. 25-2, *A*.

We have found this method inconsistent for good visualization of the entire small bowel. It is, however, useful for visualization of the proximal small bowel, especially if given early when only the jejunum is opacified. The positioning and filming are as described above, except at this time the examination is limited to the small bowel that is opacified and distended (Fig. 25-18; see Fig. 25-2, *A*). The gas often not only distends the bowel but also accelerates the barium. Therefore it is sometimes possible to visualize most of the small bowel in double contrast. Long loops of proximal jejunum can often be seen concurrently, since rapid distention may promote a transient decrease in peristalsis. In the mid small bowel, peristalsis is usually brisk with oral gas, so only short segments may be seen as distended at a time. The distal small bowel may be examined later with a pneumocolon when the contrast has reached the terminal ileum and cecum.

Fraser and Adam[23] suggested a modification of this type of examination by adding 10 ml of meglumine diatrizoate (Gastrografin) to the barium. They observed a significant decrease in transit time, from 78 to 60 minutes (using a small-volume technique of 300 ml total contrast administered), and postulated that it resulted from release of serotonin from the small bowel mucosa as a result of the meglumine. This finding confirmed the observation by Goldstein et al.[24] that 10 ml of meglumine was sufficient to produce the effect, and 30 ml was no better.

Ileostomy examination

Opinions differ as to the safest method of performing a retrograde small bowel examination. Some GI radiologists advocate never blowing up the balloon of a Foley catheter inside an ileostomy or colostomy because of the risk of perforation. They prefer to use a soft catheter with or without nipple attachments, or to use a Foley catheter with the inflated balloon outside the stoma and pressed against it. Others regard the practice of inflating a balloon inside the stoma as safe if practiced with certain precautions. Both techniques are described in some detail in the section on colostomy enemas (see Chapter 34). The risks are probably greater with an ileostomy than a colostomy because the lumen is smaller, and there is often inflammatory bowel disease adjacent to the stoma. If an intraluminal balloon is used, the balloon should be positioned well inside the ileum away from the stoma; contrast should be injected first to verify the position of the balloon; the balloon should then be inflated under fluoroscopic control by the radiologist; the balloon should not be overinflated relative to the lumen of the ileum and should not be inflated in a diseased segment of ileum; inflation should be stopped if the patient feels any discomfort.

If stomal dysfunction is suspected, single-contrast examination with dilute barium is most helpful. Careful fluoroscopy should be carried out early to look for fistulas. Then plenty of barium should be given to opacify several loops of ileum. If mucosal disease is being assessed, a double-contrast technique is more helpful with a medium-density small bowel barium, usually around 200 ml, followed by CO_2 or air. At the end of the study, the balloon, if used, is deflated and the catheter quickly removed under fluoroscopy. As the gas or contrast rushes out, the distal lumen is assessed. This is important because stomal malfunction caused by fascial scarring may otherwise be missed.[25,26]

Retrograde small bowel examination[12,27]

Retrograde small bowel examination is seldom performed now, although it is quick and easy. The patient must have a bowel preparation, unless the problem is questionable large bowel or distal small bowel obstruction. Without bowel preparation, the procedure is much more distressing for the patient, and vomiting of barium that has come back through an unprepared colon is both disagreeable and dangerous. Indeed, once the cecum and terminal ileum have been shown in an unprepared examination, it is better to allow the patient to evacuate the colon. Then, depending on the condition and age of the patient, a decision can be made either to continue with the retrograde study, to defer it for 24 hours, or to perform an antegrade study.

The single-contrast retrograde study provides good small intestinal distension. It therefore has a role when an enteroclysis is technically difficult (after some types of gastric surgery) and when small bowel distension is required, such as in finding mild strictures. Glucagon or Buscopan are helpful,[27-29] and dilute contrast is run in under fluoroscopic control. The small bowel loops are assessed as the contrast passes up through each loop in turn, and flow is stopped when the ligament of Treitz is reached. The last part of the examination should be performed slowly so that barium does not continue into the stomach once the flow has been turned off.

One occasional use for a retrograde study is to examine the terminal ileum in double contrast after an enteroclysis or follow-through has given unsatisfactory results. This may be performed as a standard or limited double-contrast barium enema, but the small bowel meal and peroral pneumocolon are usually preferable and give comparable results.

Disadvantages include difficulty in seeing ileal loops with sigmoid overlap. This can be partly overcome by switching to water once the distal ileum has filled. Reflux into the ileum does not always occur, but its likelihood can be increased from around 45% to 75% by the use of glucagon intravenously.[29]

Drug assistance in small bowel studies

Drugs may be given to make the small bowel move contents faster or to arrest peristalsis and promote relaxation and distension. Hurry has been induced with neostigmine bromide or methylsulfate (Prostigmin) (in the 1960s), and more recently with metoclopramide, cisapride, and ceruletide.[24,30,31] For enteroclysis, an accelerant helps both

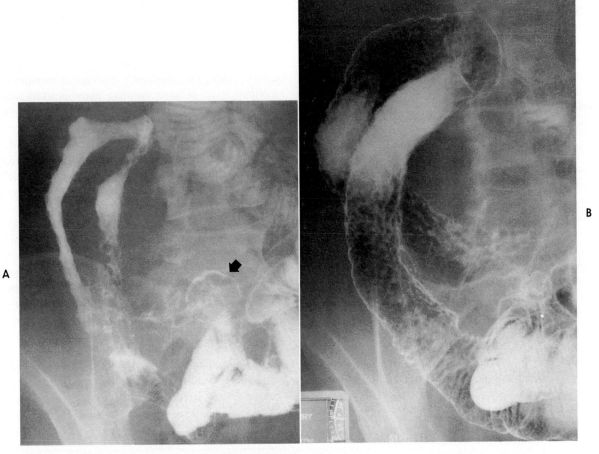

Fig. 25-19 An ileostomy study with a pneumocolon in a patient with recurrent Crohn's disease. **A,** A contracted diseased neoterminal ileum. Barium outlines the ileostomy *(arrow)*. **B,** After insufflation, not only can distensibility be assessed better, but the nature and extent of the mucosal disease are also apparent.

with tube placement and with early onward movement of the small volume of barium, since there is no drive from gastric distention.[32] In general, for nontube examination we believe there is rarely a need for accelerants if the stomach is kept full.[15]

Relaxants are very helpful at the end of the examination to assess the distensibility of various loops and particularly to display optimally the mucosa of the terminal ileum. Buscopan, 10 to 20 mg, is our preferred drug for this purpose,[34] but glucagon works equally well, although at greater expense.[27,29,33,35] The dose of glucagon should not exceed 0.5 mg intravenously, to minimize side effects of nausea and retching, which are more likely to occur when this dose is exceeded.[35]

Summary: nontube barium examinations

To demonstrate both normality and any abnormalities that may be present, examination of the small bowel must be meticulous. Enteroclysis has a major advantage here be-

cause by design it forces the radiologist to spend the maximal amount of time in conducting the examination, at the cost of increased radiation, and it is excellent for detecting minor strictures and adhesions. However, a primary small bowel meal with a pneumocolon can be equal to or almost as good throughout the small bowel in most clinical circumstances, if performed with proper care and dedication. In addition, the dedicated small bowel meal with rectal gas insufflation provides superior images of the terminal ileum and is the examination of choice for this region. Follow-through after a barium meal should be abandoned as a routine study. The dedicated small bowel meal without rectal gas insufflation is a good examination, and the increased attention to the study that goes with it plays a part in avoiding false-positive calls based on a single film (Figs. 25-4 and 25-5). However, the small bowel meal does not provide the same confidence in normality of the terminal ileum as can be obtained with retrograde introduction of gas (Fig. 25-9). Double-contrast films also reduce false-positive calls (Fig. 25-11) from spasm on single-contrast compression views of the terminal ileum. The dedicated small bowel meal with rectal insufflation of CO_2 can be recommended as an excellent examination for the routine study of the small bowel.[17-19,36] All the other methods described have virtues that make them appropriate for certain circumstances. All methods require careful fluoroscopic examination and the use of compression devices.

Ultrasound examination
Anatomy

When there is fluid in the lumen, the small bowel can be visualized as a tubular structure in longitudinal axis and as a target structure on cross section. While valvulae can be identified in fluid-filled jejunum, the ileum appears featureless.[37] The wall of the small intestine is normally less than 4 mm in thickness.[7]

The fetal small bowel can be identified only in about 30% of infants after 34 weeks of gestation, and its diameter should rarely exceed 6 mm near term and never exceed 8 mm.[37-39] Meconium should not normally be seen in the small bowel, although it is routinely identified in the fetal colon.[38] Small bowel peristalsis may normally be seen, and small amounts of sonolucent intraluminal fluid. Herniation of intestine into the umbilical cord may be noted in early (8 to 11 weeks) gestation.[39]

Blood vessels in the mesentery can often be seen, and color-flow Doppler identifies smaller mesenteric vessels. In the presence of ascites, the intestine can often be seen in loops arranged around the periphery of the fan-shaped echogenic mesentery.[37] The mesenteric leaves can be visualized in many normal subjects, with a thickness from 7 mm to 17 mm. The mesenteric vessels can be more readily identified if an oblique scanning plane is used, approximately parallel to the vessels being studied.[40] Given recognition of these normal structures, mesenteric abnormalities and associated vascular changes may be appreciated.

In infants the superior mesenteric vein (SMV) normally lies to the right of the superior mesenteric artery (SMA). When the vein is on the left, midgut rotation may confidently be diagnosed. When the vein is anterior, rotation was present in 28% in one study, and a normal right-sided vein did not exclude malrotation, which was present in 3% of the 91% overall who had a right-sided SMV.[41]

Enlarged mesenteric lymph nodes may be well visualized in children and patients who are not obese.[42] In obese individuals, CT is superior. However, the examination is sufficiently reliable in children that ultrasound should seriously be considered instead of CT, for example, in lymphoma follow-up, to reduce radiation exposure.

Ultrasound findings have been described for a variety of small bowel conditions, from cystic duplications through Crohn's disease to tumors. It is often the first imaging test to lead to suspicion of such problems, and a careful survey

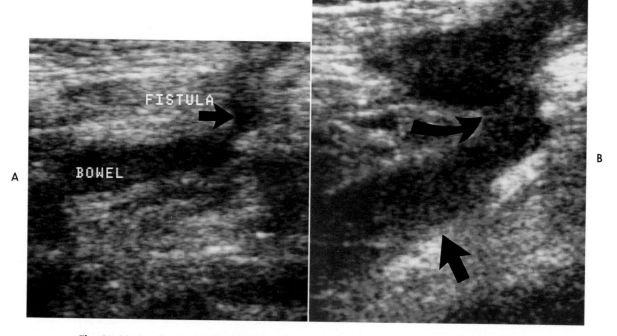

Fig. 25-20 An ultrasound examination can demonstrate not only the thickened loops of bowel associated with Crohn's disease but also may show any fistulous tracts that may be present. **A,** The thickened bowel and the fistula leading from it to the skin surface *(arrow)*. **B,** Another patient with Crohn's disease. The fistula leading to the skin surface *(curved arrow)* is much larger than on the previous patient. The thickened bowel is shown by the straight arrow.

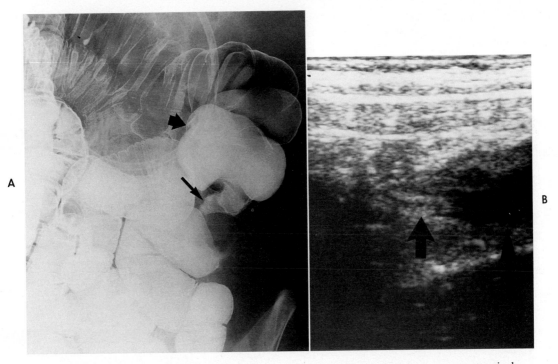

Fig. 25-21 A, The barium study in a patient with Crohn's disease shows a narrow neoterminal ileum *(small, thin arrows)* and a normal-caliber colon *(short, wide arrow)* just distal to the anastomosis. **B,** An ultrasound examination of this area also demonstrates the narrowed, thickened neoterminal ileum *(thick arrow)* and the normal-caliber colon *(long, thin arrow).*

of the intestine, mesentery, and mesenteric root should be part of the routine abdominal examination. Its value in excluding such problems is limited, however, especially in the presence of bowel gas or obesity. It is useful in the assessment of Crohn's disease and its complications, such as fistulas (Fig. 25-20), obstruction (Fig. 25-21), and bowel wall thickening (Fig. 25-22).

CT examination
Anatomy

Although the small bowel has been one of the last of the abdominal organs to be evaluated by CT scanning, the technique has several inherent advantages that make it attractive. In particular, the ability to image the lumen, bowel wall, mesenteric fat, blood vessels, and lymph nodes as well as relevant distant structures provides an overview that neither barium study nor endoscopy can ever hope to rival.

The CT appearances of the normal small bowel mesentery and its vessels have been described.[43] Even with 1983 technology and only half the patients receiving intravenous contrast, the jejunal and ileal branches of the SMA were identified in all patients. Analyses of normal appearances of the small bowel itself are few. One such study in adults[44] reported luminal diameters of 2 to 3 cm in 47 of 50 normals and less than 3.5 cm in 3. Attenuation values of intraluminal contrast were the same in the jejunum and ileum. The

wall was measurable in only half the subjects and was less than 3 mm thick. Jejunal valvulae were seen in all cases and did not exceed 3 mm thickness. No valvulae were seen in the distal ileum, and only a few in the proximal ileum. Attenuation values of mesenteric fat were identical to those of retroperitoneal and subcutaneous fat in the same patient. Branching, serpentine soft tissue attenuation structures of the SMA and SMV were identified in all normal subjects. No mesenteric structure measured more than 4 mm.

Although this report was criticized by reviewers for its retrospective analysis of findings in disease,[45] it provided a very useful starting point for further prospective detailed studies of the role of CT in various disease states, and such studies are beginning to appear for Crohn's disease,[46] tumors[47-49] (Fig. 25-23), obstruction[50,51] (Fig. 25-24), and parastomal hernias,[52] to mention only a few. Normal appearances of the small bowel and its mesentery in children have also been described.[53] The most useful signs for presence of disease were thickening of the bowel wall, increase in attenuation of mesenteric fat, and increase in number of mesenteric vessels.

Technique

All authors agree on the importance of oral and intravenous contrast in assessing the small bowel and the mesentery. Water-soluble contrast has not been replaced by spe-

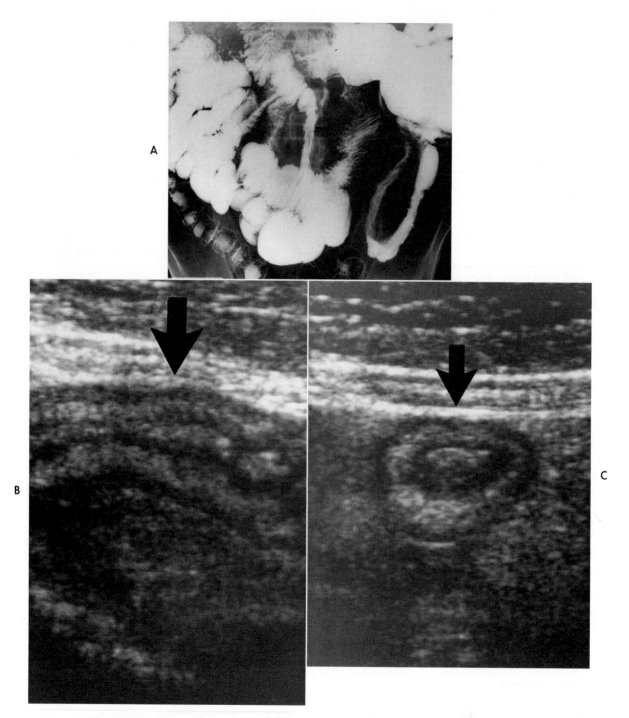

Fig. 25-22 This small bowel barium examination (**A**) shows Crohn's disease manifest by an irregular mucosal pattern with separated loops and skip areas. The ultrasound examination demonstrates the thickening of the bowel wall and the narrowed lumen in both the longitudinal (**B**) and transverse projections (**C**).

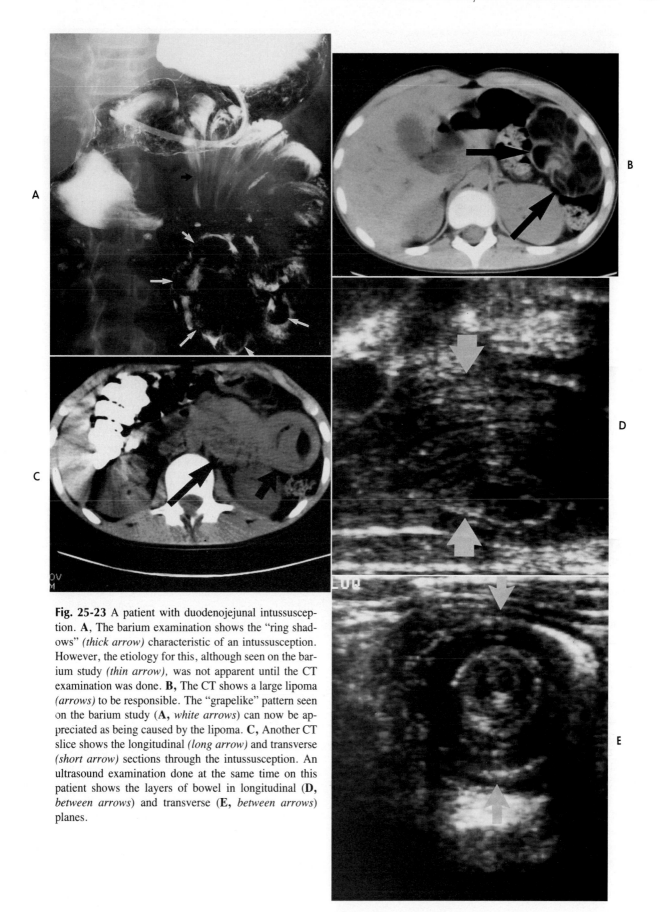

Fig. 25-23 A patient with duodenojejunal intussusception. **A,** The barium examination shows the "ring shadows" *(thick arrow)* characteristic of an intussusception. However, the etiology for this, although seen on the barium study *(thin arrow),* was not apparent until the CT examination was done. **B,** The CT shows a large lipoma *(arrows)* to be responsible. The "grapelike" pattern seen on the barium study (**A,** *white arrows*) can now be appreciated as being caused by the lipoma. **C,** Another CT slice shows the longitudinal *(long arrow)* and transverse *(short arrow)* sections through the intussusception. An ultrasound examination done at the same time on this patient shows the layers of bowel in longitudinal (**D,** *between arrows*) and transverse (**E,** *between arrows*) planes.

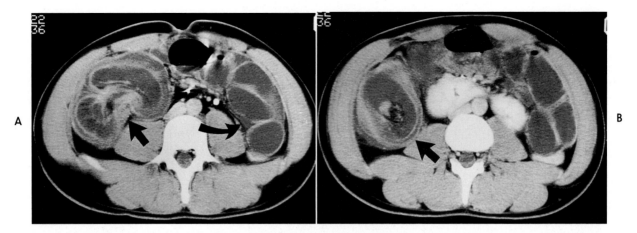

Fig. 25-24 A CT examination can be useful in diagnosing obstruction. It always shows the dilated bowel (**A**—*curved arrow* shows dilated small bowel). In this patient the etiology of the obstruction is also apparent, an ileocolic intussusception *(straight arrow)*. **B,** The intussusception has extended into the proximal ascending colon *(straight arrow)*. This figure also shows the oral contrast to have remained in the proximal small bowel, the distal bowel being full of fluid only. This is not unusual in an obstruction.

cially formulated dilute barium solutions despite possible more even contrast distribution and better taste.[54] Not all patients prefer it,[55] and both barium and water-soluble contrast are still widely used. Telebrix has also been evaluated and was rated better than Gastrografin by patients, with equivalent visualization of the small bowel,[56] and has been preferred by children as well as adults.[57] In one study a 12.5% corn oil emulsion as oral agent led to better delineation of the intestinal wall[58] but was also disliked by about one quarter of the patients.

Oral contrast must be given 30 to 60 minutes before the scan, and further contrast is given 10 minutes before. Total volumes from 250 to 1000 ml of oral contrast are recommended by different authors.[44,49,52,54]

Intravenous contrast is best given by a rapid (1.5 to 2.5ml/sec) 50 ml bolus, followed by a sustained infusion at 0.8 ml/sec for the remainder of the contrast to a total dose of about 45 g of iodine. The spacing of the slices depends on the problem under study. For small bowel obstruction, section thickness of 10 mm with 12 mm spacing over the liver and 15 mm spacing through the remainder of the abdomen has been recommended as an initial scan,[50] with, in selected cases, repeat images over the area of interest with 5 mm collimation and interleaving section indexing. Alternatively, 10 mm contiguous sections through the area of interest may be adequate.[44]

It is clear that CT can be very helpful in assessing diseases of the small bowel and mesentery and can have a considerable impact on clinical management.[59] For example, the cause of small bowel obstruction was correctly determined by CT scan in 73% of patients examined. CT may now be the examination of choice, rather than barium studies, in patients with high-grade obstruction when early surgery is likely, in long-standing obstruction associated with hypoperistalsis, and in suspected bowel infarction.[60]

MRI examination

MRI for the first few years had little to offer in the abdomen, but liver MRI has been clinically useful now for several years. MRI of the pelvis has moved out of the research arena, and MRI of the great vessels of the abdomen is developing rapidly. The intestines are the last of the abdominal organs to yield to improving technology. Now that fast sequences are close to becoming a reality so that respiratory artifact will cease to be an issue, MRI examination of the abdomen for diseases of the alimentary tract will soon be amenable to evaluation against CT and ultrasound to define the particular advantages and roles of each.

It is important to have a contrast agent to distend the lumen of the bowel and permit clear imaging of the wall, and a great deal of work is being done in this area. The desirable characteristics have been described as easy administration, uniform effect throughout the bowel, no stimulation of peristalsis, high patient acceptance, and similar effect with all commonly used pulse sequences.[61] Tart et al.,[61] in comparing five possible agents, found 12% corn emulsion to be the most acceptable to patients and to provide the best images, delineating both small bowel and pancreas well using gradient echo sequences. It is interesting that it has also been rated as the preferred contrast agent for CT examination of the small and large bowel.[58] Others have tried various commercial baby milk preparations and achieved excellent results with lyophilized milk in the stomach and very proximal small bowel, and also of the lower GI tract when given by enema for evaluation of rectal tumors.[62] It is not suitable for most of the small bowel because it is absorbed and inhomogeneously distributed in the lower small bowel. In another study of nine different agents, Similac with Iron provided excellent signal characteristics on several pulse sequences. In vivo, however, although it provided excellent contrast in the upper abdomen, it was less predictable in the distal small bowel because it was not uniformly distributed, so small bowel could not clearly be differentiated from colon. [63] The ability of MRI to demonstrate the great vessels of the abdomen has been well shown, and clinically useful flow measurements are now possible.[64] MRI may well soon have a role in assessing low flow states and ischemic disease of the intestine.[65]

To date there have been few reports of the role of MRI in evaluating small bowel disease. However, the ability to provide coronal and other planes of imaging has been shown to be an advantage in assessing fistulas and sinus tracts in patients with Crohn's disease.[66] T1 MRI provided good delineation of the extension of fistulas in relation to sphincters. T2 MRI showed fluid collections within the fistulas, localized fluid collections in extraintestinal tissues, and inflammatory changes within muscles. The supralevator and infralevator compartments were well defined on coronal images so that the relationship of fistulas to the levator ani could reliably be demonstrated. That these changes can be illustrated by MRI is now clear. Whether there are clinical advantages over CT and ultrasound is not yet clear. The only certainty is that further progress in applying MRI to the management of intestinal disease will be rapid.

REFERENCES

1. Underhill BML: Intestinal length in man, *Br Med J* 4950:1243, 1955.
2. Jit I, Grewel SS: Lengths of the small and large intestine in North Indian subjects, *J Anat (India)* 24:89, 1975.
3. Hackman L, Hallberg D: Small intestinal length: an intraoperative study in obesity, *Acta Chir Scand* 140:57, 1974.
4. Fanucci A, Cerro P, Fraracci L, Letto F: Small bowel length measured by radiography, *Gastrointest Radiol* 9:349, 1984.
5. Nightingale J, Bartram CI, Lennard Jones JE: Length of residual small bowel after partial resection: correlation between radiographic and surgical measurements, *Gastrointest Radiol* 16:305, 1991.
6. Herlinger H: Small bowel. In Laufer I, ed: *Double contrast gastrointestinal radiology with endoscopic correlation*, Philadelphia, 1979, WB Saunders.
7. Fleisher A, Muhletaler C, James AE Jr: Sonographic assessment of the bowel wall, *AJR* 136:887, 1981.
8. Herlinger H, Maglinte D: Anatomy of the small intestine. In Herlingor H, Maglinte D, eds: *Clinical radiology of the small intestine*, Philadelphia, 1989, WB Saunders.
9. Gelfand DW, Ott DJ: Radiographic demonstration of small intestinal villi on routine clinical studies, *Gastrointest Radiol* 6:21, 1981.
10. Chen MY, Ott DJ, Kelley TF, Gelfand DW: Impact of the small bowel study on patient management, *Gastrointest Radiol* 16:189, 1991.
11. Taverne PP, Van der Jagt EJ: Small bowel radiography: a prospective comparison of three techniques in 200 patients, *Fortschr Röntgenstr* 143:293, 1985.
12. Thoeni R: Radiography of the small bowel and enteroclysis: a perspective, *Invest Radiol* 22:930, 1987.
13. Gurian L, Jendrzewski J, Katon R et al: Small bowel enema: an underutilized method of small bowel examination, *Dig Dis Sci* 27:1101, 1982.
14. Garvey CJ, de Lacey G, Wilkins RA: Preliminary colon cleansing for small bowel examinations: results and implications of a prospective survey, *Clin Radiol* 36:503, 1985.
15. Richards DG, Stevenson GW: Laxatives prior to small bowel follow-through: are they necessary for a rapid and good-quality examination? *Gastrointest Radiol* 15:66, 1990.
16. Scholz FJ: Manual compression device for fluoroscopy, *Radiology* 170:564, 1989.
17. Fitzgerald EJ, Thompson GT, Somers S, Franic S: Pneumocolon as an aid to small bowel studies, *Clin Radiol* 36:663, 1985.
18. Kressel HY, Evers KA, Glick SN, Laufer I, Herlinger H: The peroral pneumocolon examination: technique and indications, *Radiology* 144:414, 1982.
19. Kelvin FM, Gedgaudas RK, Thompson WM, Rice RP: The peroral pneumocolon: its role in evaluating the terminal ileum, *AJR* 139:115, 1982.
20. Bernier P, Coblentz C: CO$_2$ delivery system for double-contrast barium enema examinations, *Radiology* 159:264, 1986.
21. Coblentz CL, Frost RA, Molinaro V, Stevenson GW: Pain after barium enema: effect of CO$_2$ and air on double-contrast study, *Radiology* 157:35, 1985.
22. Fraser GM, Preston PG: The small bowel barium follow-through enhanced with an oral effervescent agent, *Clin Radiol* 34:673, 1983.
23. Fraser GM, Adam RD: Modifications to the gas-enhanced small bowel barium follow-through using gastrografin and compression, *Clin Radiol* 39:537, 1988.
24. Goldstein HM, Pole GJ, Rosenquist CJ et al: Comparison of methods for acceleration of small bowel radiographic examination, *Radiology* 98:519, 1971.
25. Fleischner FG, Mandelstam P: Roentgen observations of the ileostomy in patients with idiopathic ulcerative colitis: ileostomy dysfunction, *Radiology* 70:469, 1958.
26. Zagoria RJ, Gelfand DW, Ott DJ: Retrograde examination of the small bowel in patients with an ileostomy, *Gastrointest Radiol* 11:97, 1986.
27. Miller RE: Complete reflux examination of the small bowel, *Radiology* 84:547, 1985.
28. Violon D, Steppe R, Potvliege R: Improved retrograde ileography with glucagon, *AJR* 136:833, 1981.
29. Monsein LH, Halpert RD, Harris ED, Feczko PJ: Retrograde ileography: value of glucagon, *Radiology* 161:558, 1986.
30. Grumbach K, Herlinger H, Laufer I, Levine MS: Metoclopramide-ceruletide assisted small bowel examination, *Fortschr Röntgenstr* 149:47, 1988.
31. Kreel L: The use of metoclopramide in radiology, *Postgrad Med J* (July suppl):42, 1973.
32. Maglinte DDT, Lappas JC, Kelvin FM et al: Small bowel radiography: how, when and why, *Radiology* 163:297, 1987.
33. Simpkins KC: Radiology now. The colon pacified, *Br J Radiol* 49:303, 1976.
34. Kreel L: Pharmacoradiology in barium examinations with special reference to glucagon, *Br J Radiol* 48:691, 1975.
35. Miller RE, Chernish SM, Brunelle RI: Gastrointestinal radiography with glucagon, *Gastrointest Radiol* 4:1, 1979.
36. Wolf KJ, Goldber HI, Wall SD, et al: Feasibility of the peroral pneumocolon in evaluating the ileocecal region, *AJR* 145:10, 1985.
37. Sauerbrei EE, Nguyen KT, Nolan RL: *Abdominal sonography*, New York, 1992, Raven Press.
38. Nyberg DA, Mack LA, Patten RM, et al: Fetal bowel—normal sonographic findings, *J Ultrasound Med* 6:3, 1987.
39. Parulekar SG: Sonography of normal fetal bowel, *J Ultrasound Med* 10:211, 1991.
40. Derchi LE, Solbiati L, Rizzato G, De Pra L: Normal anatomy and pathological changes of the small bowel mesentery: US appearance, *Radiology* 164:649, 1987.

41. Dufour D, Delaet MH, Dassonville M et al: Midgut rotation, the reliability of sonographic diagnosis, *Pediatr Radiol* 22:21, 1992.

42. Levitt RG, Loehler RE, Sagel SS, et al: Metastatic disease of the mesentery and omentum, *Radiol Clin North Am* 20:501, 1982.

43. Silverman PM, Kelvin FM, Korobkin M, Dunnick NR: Computed tomography of the normal mesentery, *AJR* 143:953, 1984.

44. James S, Balfe DM, Lee JKT, Picus D: Small bowel disease: categorisation by CT examination, *AJR* 148:863, 1987.

45. Gerkins SM, Dunnick NR: Reviewers' comments, *Invest Radiol* 23:410, 1988.

46. Kleinhaus U, Weich Y: Computed tomography of Crohn's disease—reevaluation, *Fortschr Röntgenstr* 146:607, 1987.

47. Lorigan JG, Dubrow RA: The computed tomographic appearances and clinical significance of intussusception in adults with malignant neoplasms, *Br J Radiol* 63:257, 1990.

48. Dudiak KM, Johnson CD, Stephens DH: Primary tumours of the small intestine: CT evaluation, *AJR* 152:995, 1989.

49. Laurent F, Raynaud M, Biset JM et al: Diagnosis and categorization of small bowel neoplasms: role of computed tomography, *Gastrointest Radiol* 16:115, 1991.

50. Megibow AJ, Balthazar EJ, Cho KC et al: Bowel obstruction: evaluation with CT, *Radiology* 180:313, 1991.

51. Fukuya T, Hawes DR, Lu CC, Chang PJ et al: CT diagnosis of small bowel obstruction: efficacy in 60 patients, *AJR* 158:765, 1992.

52. Etherington RJ, Williams JG, Hayward MWJ et al: Demonstration of para-ileostomy herniation using computed tomography, *Clin Radiol* 41:333, 1990.

53. Siegal MJ, Evans SJ, Balfe DM: Small bowel disease in children: diagnosis with CT, *Radiology* 169:127, 1988.

54. Carr DH, Banks LM: Comparison of barium and diatrizoate bowel labelling agents in computed tomography, *Br J Radiol* 58:393, 1985.

55. Mitchell DG, Bjorgvinsson E, terMeulen D et al: Comparison of Telebrix Gastro and Gastrograffin in abdominal computed tomography, *Eur J Radiol* 9:179, 1989.

56. Bach DB: Telebrix: a better-tasting oral contrast agent for abdominal computed tomography, *J Can Assoc Radiol* 42:98, 1991.

57. Tannous WN, Azouz EM: Bowel opacification for abdominal computed tomography in children: a clinical trial of oral Telebrix 38, *J Can Assoc Radiol* 42:102, 1991.

58. Raptopoulos V, Davis MA, Davidoff A et al: Fat density oral contrast agent for abdominal CT, *Radiology* 164:653, 1987.

59. Merine D, Fishman EK, Jones B: CT of the small bowel and mesentery, *Radiol Clin North Am* 27:707, 1989.

60. Rubesin SE, Herlinger HH: CT evaluation of bowel obstruction: a landmark article—implications for the future, *Radiology* 180:307, 1991.

61. Tart RP, Li KCP, Storm BL et al: Enteric MRI contrast agents: comparative study of five potential agents in humans, *Magn Reson Imaging* 9:559, 1991.

62. Balzarini L, Aime S, Barbero L et al: Magnetic resonance imaging of the gastrointestinal tract: investigation of baby milk as a low cost contrast agent, *Eur J Radiol* 15:171, 1992.

63. Biset GS: Evaluation of potential practical oral contrast agents for pediatric magnetic resonance imaging: preliminary observations, *Pediatr Radiol* 20:61, 1989.

64. Tamada T, Moriyasu F, Ono S et al: Portal blood flow: measurement with MR imaging, *Radiology* 173:639, 1989.

65. Wilkerson DK, Mesrich R, Drake C et al: Magnetic resonance imaging of acute occlusive intestinal ischaemia, *J Vasc Surg* 11:567, 1990.

66. Koelbel G, Schmiedl V, Majer MC et al: Diagnosis of fistulae and sinus tracts in patients with Crohn disease: value of MR imaging, *AJR* 152:999, 1989.

26 Biphasic Enteroclysis with Methylcellulose

DEAN D.T. MAGLINTE

There are more variations of the enteroclysis examination method than there are of barium contrast examinations of the upper gastrointestinal tract and the colon combined.[1-4] This suggests that there is no enteroclysis technique that everyone agrees is the best. The ease and speed of infusion of low-density mixtures and the ability to modify the technique for a secondary double-contrast examination are reasons given by proponents of single-contrast enteroclysis. In the past, Sellink[4] used water as a flush to augment the single-contrast study, but surface coating of the lumen is less optimal and fleeting. Flocculation occurs rapidly.[2] Luminal surface pattern depiction and the ability to see through overlapping pelvic ileal segments where compression can be difficult are the main reasons given by proponents of primary double-contrast enteroclysis methods using air or methylcellulose. The primary air technique popular in Japan is difficult to reproduce and is uncomfortable to the patient because of its effect on peristalsis. Additionally, air passes through areas of minimal narrowing readily without inciting a flow gradient. The ability of infusion to exaggerate distention proximal to an area of mild narrowing may not be seen. The advantages of enteroclysis in the evaluation of small bowel obstruction is therefore negated by the use of air, which limits the usefulness of this technique in various clinical situations.

Radiologic techniques to examine the small bowel have shown little progress in recent decades. Difficulty in reproducing the various enteroclysis techniques described may be a factor. A survey of members of the Society of Gastrointestinal Radiologists has shown, however, that double-contrast enteroclysis using methylcellulose is the most commonly used method of enteroclysis examination in North America.[5] Two variations of enteroclysis using methylcellulose have been popularized by Maglinte and Herlinger.[1,2] The differences between these two methods have lessened in recent years. Routinely, methylcellulose double contrast is used to augment diagnostic information obtained during the single-contrast phase of the Maglinte biphasic enteroclysis method, and more and more value is placed on compression during the single-contrast phase of the methylcellulose small bowel enema method advocated by Herlinger. Peripheral features of the technique, such as catheters, use of pump, and preparation of the patient, are similar. The remaining difference is the somewhat greater emphasis placed on the quality and value of the single-contrast phase in the biphasic method of Maglinte and the double-contrast phase in the methylcellulose small-bowel enema method of Herlinger.[2,3] In the Maglinte method, 350 to 500 ml of a 50% weight per volume (w/v) mixture is the barium suspension used, the amount varying depending on the length of the small bowel. The Herlinger methylcellulose small bowel enema (SBE) uses 160 to 240 ml of a 95% w/v barium mixture. The methylcellulose suspension (1500 to 2000 ml of a 0.5% methylcellulose suspension) is similar in both techniques. The amount and density of barium mixture used in the biphasic enteroclysis technique allow for a completed single-contrast evaluation of the distal ileum.

A modification of the methylcellulose SBE has been reported by Antes and Lissner[6] and by Wittich et al.[7] The only difference between these techniques and the Herlinger method is the lesser density of the barium mixture used (24% to 48% and 60% w/v, respectively); the difference in the amount of contrast material used was insignificant (300 ml and 200 ml, respectively). The lesser amount of barium with the Herlinger technique allows single-contrast evaluation of the jejunum and proximal ileum; evaluation of the distal ileum relies mainly on the double-contrast effect. With the Maglinte biphasic method, single-contrast evaluation with the amount of barium suspension given is diagnostic for the entire small intestine and consistently provides enough coating of the barium for the distal ileum, which eliminates the need for adjunct techniques to visualize the distal ileum. In patients with pelvic adhesions, the barium mixture can become denser, and the result can be a clumped, featureless overlapping of segments of pelvic ileum after methylcellulose or water infusion.[8] This can happen when 600 ml or more of barium suspension is infused and not enough methylcellulose is given to reach the distal segments. In the Maglinte biphasic method, the maximal amounts of barium and methylcellulose suspension infused prevent this occurrence. The timing of infusion and the sequence of filming allow a double look at every segment. The biphasic method makes full use of the value of fluoroscopy and compression radiography of the entire small bowel during the single-contrast phase, and of the hypotonia and the depiction of the luminal surface pattern by the double-contrast effect of methylcellulose. It is a simple, flexible, and reproducible alternative to the many techniques described and can be used routinely for all indications of enteroclysis.

METHYLCELLULOSE FOR DOUBLE-CONTRAST SMALL BOWEL RADIOGRAPHY

The use of methylcellulose to produce double-contrast radiography of the small intestine was popularized by Herlinger,[9] who described a modified technique for the methylcellulose double-contrast small bowel enema based on a method first introduced by Trickey et al.[10]

Introducing methylcellulose after the injection of barium achieves five purposes:[2] (1) to propel the barium column through the more distal small bowel into the right colon without increasing the density of adherent loops of pelvic small bowel; (2) to dilate the entire small bowel lumen to straighten the plica circularis and render them evaluable; (3) to produce an interface of contrast between the density of the barium coating the mucosa and the water density of the methylcellulose distending the lumen; (4) to permit viewing and study of mucosal surface features in areas where two or even three bowel loops overlap; and (5) to promote evacuation of barium.

Patient preparation

Although the presence of feces in the colon does not preclude a diagnostic-quality enteroclysis, bowel preparation is advisable because the enteroclysis may require more barium suspension and may cause more discomfort to the patient who has not had a laxative.[1] No preparation is necessary in urgent enteroclysis done for obstruction.

A nonresidue diet is given the day before the study—synthetic juices, carbonated drinks, decaffeinated coffee or tea without milk, clear broth, and gelatin dessert. Magnesium citrate is taken during the early afternoon of the day preceding the examination. This is followed by a dose of castor oil in the late afternoon if the magnesium citrate is ineffective. No colonic cleansing enemas are to be used because this refluxes fluid or fecal debris into the distal ileum and results in suboptimal coating.

Nothing is taken by mouth on the day of the procedure. If fluid is present in the stomach, the pylorus does not close firmly and duodenogastric reflux becomes more likely. The reduction of normal fluid and cell outpouring into the small bowel lumen as a result of a diet restriction improves the quality of the examination.[11] If patients are taking medications that inhibit peristalsis, the recommended dosage for metoclopramide is increased.[12] Premedication with a benzodiazepam or midazolam (Versed, Roche) should be routine unless contraindicated. Conscious sedation with diazepam (Valium, Roche) and the selective use of midazolam have made enteroclysis a hassle-free routine procedure in our institution.

Intubation

The procedure is explained to the patient, and the patient is asked to sniff through each nostril with the other one blocked, to see if one has much better air flow than the other. The nostril with the best flow is selected, and, with the patient supine, Xylocaine (viscous) is injected into the nostril in 1 ml aliquots to a total of 3 ml, and the patient again sniffs to draw the Xylocaine into the posterior nasopharynx. The throat may be sprayed with Xylocaine spray.

The enteroclysis tube is checked, and the guidewire is withdrawn some 18 inches from the tip. The patient is then given sedation, usually with 5 mg diazepam, although elderly patients or those with pulmonary disease may require less, and metoclopramide 10 mg is also given intravenously. The tube is then passed *vertically* through the nose, that is, directly posteriorly with the patient supine (avoiding angling superiorly, which will trap the tip under the turbinates and make passage more difficult). Once the tube is in the oropharynx the patient is asked to swallow to enable the tip to enter the esophagus. The patient then turns on the right side, and the tube is advanced to some 60 cm.

Fluoroscopy may then reveal that the tip is in the antrum, in which case the guidewire is advanced to within 5 to 10 cm of the tip, and slow advance usually carries the tube through the pylorus and around the duodenum, assisted by the peristaltic effect of the metoclopramide. As the tube is advanced around the duodenum the tip of the guidewire should be kept near the pylorus. If initial fluoroscopy shows that the tip of the tube is in the fundus and there is a loop in the stomach, advancing the guidewire to the distal stomach and slowly withdrawing the tube takes the tip of the tube distally from the fundus into the antrum and undoes the loop.

Finally, to advance the tip around the duodenojejunal flexure, it is sometimes helpful to turn the patient prone. Once the tip is positioned in the jejunum, the balloon is inflated with 18 to 20 ml of water.

Contrast materials

A 50% w/v barium suspension (Entrobar, Lafayette Pharmacal, Lafayette, Ind.) is preferred. It is free of sorbitol, contains suspending agents that are intended to prolong mucosal coating in the small bowel, and has a shelf life of 2 years. An average of 400 ml is infused followed by the infusion of up to 2 liters of Entrocel (Lafayette Pharmacal, Lafayette, Ind.), a 0.5% solution of hydroxypropyl methylcellulose.

Fluoroscopy and filming sequence

Most lesions are detected during the single-contrast infusion phase. Double contrast, primarily used to ascertain normality in the Maglinte method, is used to demonstrate folds in bowel loops that are beyond the reach of single-contrast compression, such as pelvic segments in the posterior cul-de-sac involved by adhesions. Overreliance on the double-contrast phase should be avoided because occasionally lesions become less conspicuous when the methylcellulose diffuses into the barium. Washing-away of barium by the methylcellulose infusion and the increasing contamination of the methylcellulose with barium through diffusion can result in decreased depiction of lesions. Given a careful and correct technique, a satisfactory single- and double-contrast examination can be obtained with the biphasic method in almost all examinations not involving high-grade partial mechanical obstruction of the small intestine.

The progress of the barium column is observed with intermittent fluoroscopy. The lead portion in the supine patient is intermittently compressed using various obliquities and tube angulations to assess for nonobstructive adhesions. Radiographs are taken whenever a lesion is seen. Our filming sequence in a patient without obstruction, using a remote-control fluoroscopic unit, is detailed in the following sections.

Single-contrast phase

1. A compression radiograph is obtained to show the proximal jejunum after 300 ml of barium have been infused (Fig. 26-1, *A*). After filling of the ileum, a compression radiograph of the pelvic ileum is obtained (Fig. 26-1, *B*). If the distal ileum has been outlined with barium using less than the full amount, the infusion of barium is stopped and that of methylcellulose is commenced.

2. Compression radiographs of the distal ileum, including the terminal ileum, complete the single-contrast examination (Fig. 26-1, *C*). Methylcellulose infusion is continued until all the segments are adequately distended and are shown to be normal or abnormal. Brief intermittent checks for possible reflux into the stomach are made throughout the examination.

Double-contrast phase

3. Radiographs during mild compression are obtained starting from the duodenojejunal segments, progressing distally until all segments have been imaged in double contrast (Figs. 26-1, *D* and *E*). Overcompression results in the dispersal of the barium coating the lumen. Lateral or steeply oblique radiographs are taken of pelvic segments of ileum before contrast fills the descending colon (Fig. 26-1, *F*).

4. A prone radiograph (14 × 17 inches) is obtained when possible at the end of the infusion before tube withdrawal (Fig. 26-1, *G*). Additional compression radiographs are then obtained of suspicious or abnormal segments as desired. Radiographs of the jejunum should be examined before tube removal so that more barium can be infused to examine for questionable abnormalities. Because the proximal jejunum is exposed to methylcellulose longer than the rest of the small intestine, double-contrast coating deteriorates first in this segment (Fig. 26-2). The need to examine the duodenum should be determined before tube removal, especially in patients referred for unexplained gastrointestinal bleeding.

The above sequence of filming allows imaging of proximal jejunum and pelvic segments before barium fills the colon, which can obscure them. Additional radiographs of questionable segments may be obtained after tube withdrawal or after colonic evacuation. Adequate double-contrast coating remains for a few minutes and then deteriorates with the passage of time. With the methylcellulose methods, a bedpan should be readily available for patients with a history of incontinence once contrast is noted in the descending colon to prevent accidental voiding.

Infusion rates

An understanding of the control of flow and distention of the small bowel is important for a fast and reproducible biphasic enteroclysis technique. Lack of understanding of this aspect of enteroclysis results in artificial distention of more proximal segments, inability to appreciate flow gradients at points of low-grade partial obstruction, poor coating of folds of distal small bowel, and a prolonged examination with the possible danger of aspiration caused by gastric overdistention from reflux (Fig. 26-3).

Much of the understanding of the rates of enteroclysis flow derives from the work of Oudkirk.[13] There is no fixed ideal rate of infusion. From experience, it is better to start at lower flow rates. For single-contrast enteroclysis, 65 to 85 ml per minute is the recommended range of infusion. This is slightly lower than our initial recommendation.[1] The motility of the small bowel has a variable response to the different rates of infusion and is also influenced by medications, particularly metoclopramide, sedatives, and antidiarrheal agents. Infusions administered too slowly produce inadequate luminal distention and an irregular fold pattern similar to a follow-through examination. Faster rates of flow distend the lumen and improve the demonstration of the fold pattern but can prolong the examination if they are too fast. Excessively fast rates of infusion cause reflux into the stomach and later vomiting and induce reflux atony, resulting in prolonged transit that requires more barium.

An average of 400 ml of barium suspension is required to reach the cecum in the shortest possible time during single-contrast enteroclysis. For the biphasic technique, it is suggested that the rate be adjusted to give moderate distention of small-bowel loops without totally abolishing peristalsis.[14] In a patient given 10 mg of metoclopramide intravenously and mild sedation, this rate, monitored continuously using an electrically controlled peristaltic tube pump, varies between 65 and 125 ml per minute. A higher rate of infusion is occasionally needed when hyperperistalsis is observed fluoroscopically. The rate should constantly be adjusted as the examination progresses: flow rate is increased if less peristalsis is desired, and flow rate is decreased if more peristalsis is necessary to ensure uniform distention from jejunum to ileum (Fig. 26-4).

A lack of understanding of how the small bowel reacts to varying rates of infusion and luminal distention is usu-

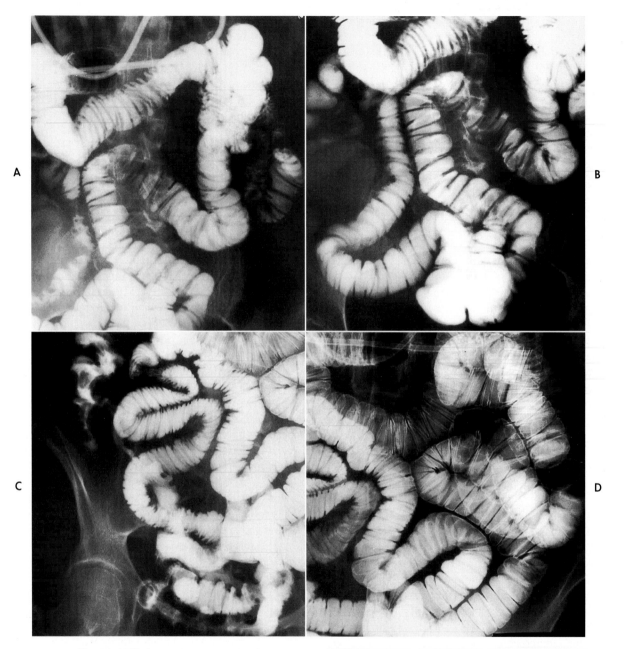

Fig. 26-1 Filming sequence and minimum requirement of radiographs. **A,** A single-contrast radiograph (with or without compression) of jejunum is obtained after infusion of 300 ml of barium. **B,** A single-contrast radiograph of partially filled pelvic segments of ileum (approximately 400 ml) follows. Methylcellulose infusion is started at this point. **C,** The single-contrast phase is completed by a radiograph of the rest of the pelvic segments and distal ileum. The fluoroscopic search for an abnormality is done with compression during this phase. Note demonstration of Crohn's disease of pelvic segments and terminal ileum. Double-contrast effect is now beginning in more proximal segments. **D,** Full double contrast is now present in the jejunum. Supine radiograph with mild compression or a prone radiograph is obtained. The jejunum is imaged before barium fills the transverse colon.

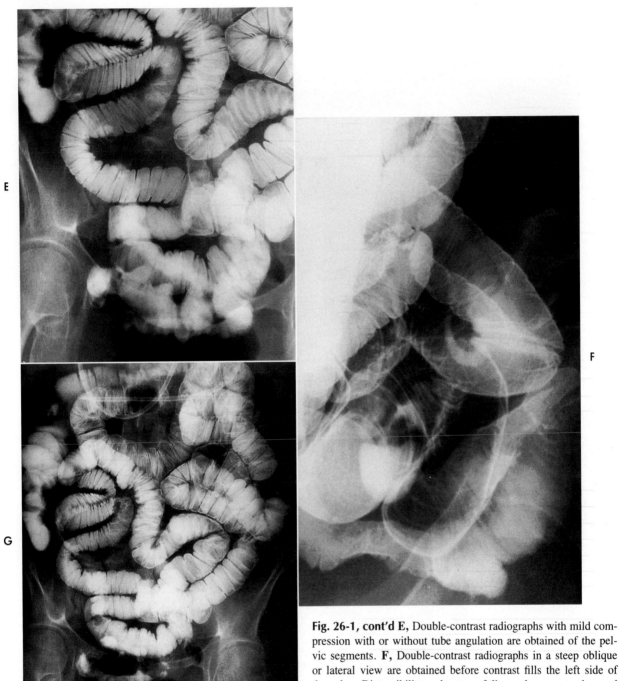

Fig. 26-1, cont'd E, Double-contrast radiographs with mild compression with or without tube angulation are obtained of the pelvic segments. **F,** Double-contrast radiographs in a steep oblique or lateral view are obtained before contrast fills the left side of the colon. Distensibility and extent of diseased segments obscured by overlapping in the frontal projection are sometimes better demonstrated in this view. The anterior abdominal wall is also scanned in this projection for unsuspected ventral hernias. **G,** Overview of entire small bowel in double contrast. The prone position is preferred if possible. Additional radiographs of abnormal or suspicious segments are taken after the minimum number of required radiographs are obtained. If this sequence is followed and the minimum number of required radiographs are taken, all segments of the small intestine are seen in both single and double contrast before overlap by the contrast-filled colon occurs. Note the absence of barium in the left side of the colon.

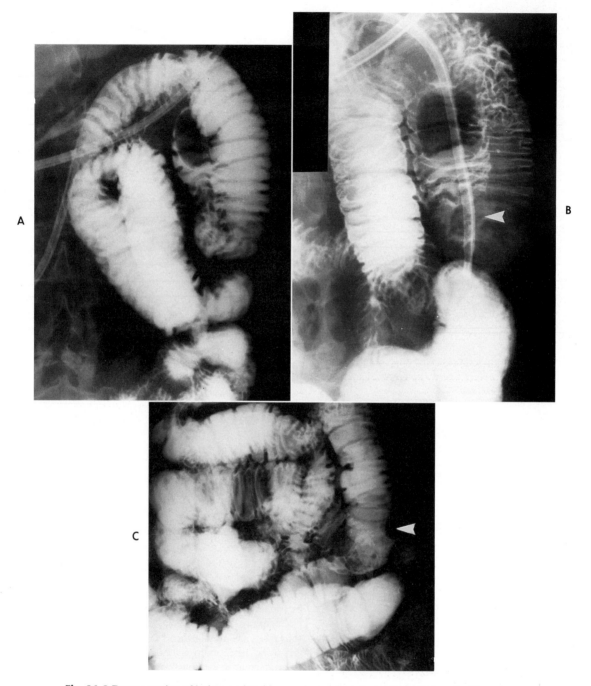

Fig. 26-2 Demonstration of lesion rendered inconspicuous by poor methylcellulose double-contrast coating. **A,** Single-contrast radiograph of proximal jejunum appears unremarkable. Small mural defect from metastatic melanoma was not appreciated at fluoroscopy. **B,** Poorly coated double-contrast radiograph shows area better distended, and a nodule was suspected *(arrowhead)*. **C,** Re-infusion of barium to clarify suspicious defect in **B** was carried out after completion of the minimum number of required radiographs. Nodular defect *(arrowhead)* is apparent. The enteroclysis tube has been withdrawn to the horizontal duodenum, and the balloon is deflated.

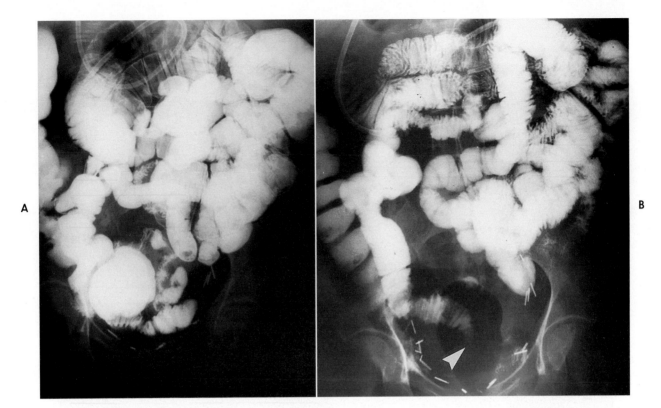

Fig. 26-3 Influence of flow rate in the demonstration of small bowel abnormality. **A,** Emergency enteroclysis done by inexperienced house staff shows extensive pelvic adhesions, but no focal point of obstruction was demonstrated. Note artificial distention of the jejunum caused by a fast infusion rate. Overgrading of degree of obstruction can result because of fast flow rates. **B,** Repeat enteroclysis 3 days later with flow rates appropriately adjusted shows a focal stenosis *(arrowhead)* secondary to a dense adhesive band (confirmed at surgery).

ally manifested by an enteroclysis study showing an overly distended jejunum with excessive reflux into the stomach even with a balloon catheter in place[15] and an incompletely distended distal ileum (Fig. 26-3, *A*). The net result is a prolonged examination, even in a nonobstructed patient. In patients with hyperperistalsis (i.e., in some patients with an exaggerated response to metoclopramide, patients with irritable bowel syndrome, or patients with mild intestinal anoxia [early ischemial]), a very high flow rate may be required (more than 125 ml per minute) to achieve moderate distention and a double-contrast effect. With the use of appropriate flow rates, the passage of too much barium into the colon is deferred until small bowel loops have been shown distended and in double contrast, and this diminishes the chance of inadvertent rectal emptying on the fluoroscopic table. The aim of adjusting the flow rate is to ensure that the degree of distention of the entire small intestine from jejunum to ileum is uniform. Too fast an infusion rate is the most common technical error noted among the inexperienced.

Double contrast with methylcellulose is considered to be established when the terminal ileum at fluoroscopy is adequately distended and transradiant. The examination is terminated at this point. In some patients (i.e., patients with incomplete colonoscopy), delayed radiographs to outline the colon will be of diagnostic value (Fig. 26-5).

It is recommended that outpatients wait for an additional 15 to 20 minutes before leaving the department so that accidental evacuation of contrast does not happen in transit. Because of the use of sedation in our practice, outpatients are required to have a driver for transportation.

Technique-related problems: avoidance and solutions
Prolonged examination

A prolonged examination is usually related to improper flow rates, primarily use of too high infusion rates during the single-contrast phase, as stated above. This can be remedied by decreasing the flow rate and allowing motility to resume. If no response is noted, giving an additional intravenous injection of metoclopramide (10-mg doses) usually restores peristalsis.

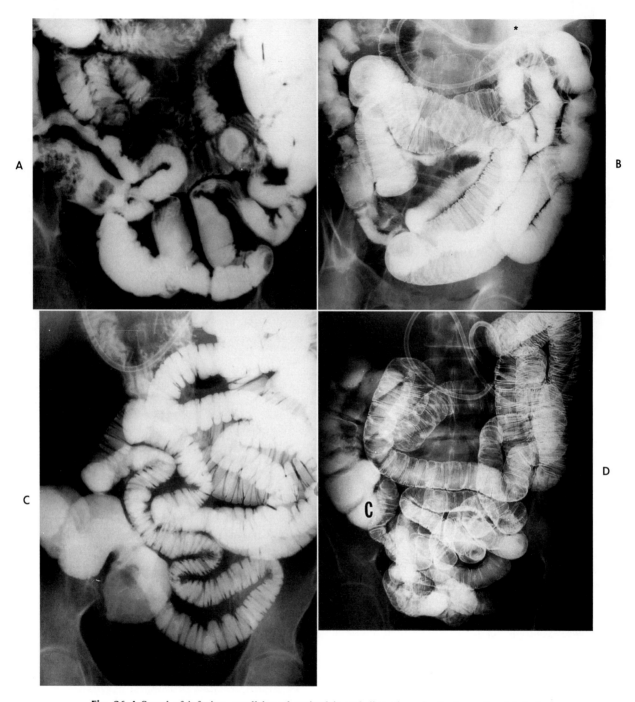

Fig. 26-4 Speed of infusion, small bowel peristalsis and distention. **A,** A slow rate of infusion (<55 ml/min) results in uneven distention and poor visualization of folds. The cecum fills early. **B,** The use of high flow rates (>90 ml/min) induces temporary paralysis of more proximal segments, requiring more contrast to fill the entire small intestine and prolonging the examination. Note reflux into stomach (*). **C,** The use of the optimal rate of infusion during the single-contrast phase (55 to 90 ml/min) results in moderate distention of all folds with mild peristalsis still present. Folds can be assessed. **D,** A slightly higher flow rate during methylcellulose infusion results in uniform distention of the entire small intestine and clear definition of folds from jejunum to terminal ileum without totally abolishing peristalsis of the jejunum. Note the absence of contrast in the left side of the colon, a hallmark of properly adjusted flow rates during infusion. *C*, Cecum.

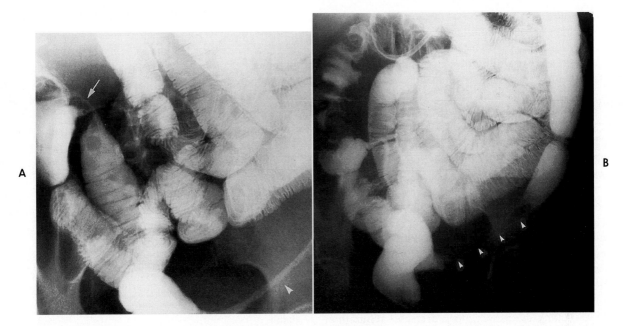

Fig. 26-5 Colon radiography after assessment of small intestine. **A,** Spot film of terminal ileum shows stenosing Crohn's disease with partial obstruction *(arrow)*. Long stenosed sigmoid *(arrowhead)* accounts for inability to pass colonoscope through sigmoid. **B,** Overview of small intestine and colon after assessment of small intestine shows extent of Crohn's stricture of sigmoid *(arrowheads)*.

Incomplete distention of the small bowel

Incomplete distention of small bowel with barium already in the colon in less than 5 minutes is related to slow infusion flow rates or excessive dose or response to metoclopramide. Once recognized, increasing flow until moderate distention and decreased peristalsis are seen salvages the examination. In antegrade examinations, we have not used glucagon to decrease peristalsis since our adoption of the infusion pump to deliver contrast to the small bowel.[14] Glucagon has been utilized to decrease peristalsis in retrograde per ileostomy enteroclysis.

Prolapse of small bowel into the pelvis

It is not uncommon for a few loops of ileum to dip into the pelvis. Angled compression radiography allows lifting of pelvic segments when no adhesions are present. However, in patients with pelvic adhesions from prior pelvic inflammatory disease, hysterectomy, or other pelvic surgical procedures, several loops occupy the entire pelvis, and puddled barium obscures fold assessment in this segment. These are best managed by promoting full double-contrast effect and imaging the pelvis in lateral or steep oblique projections (Fig. 26-1, *F*). The prone angled view also gives additional information. A mobile cecum overhanging the pelvis can also obscure segments of pelvic ileum. However, if the patient is turned prone and the fluoroscopic table tilted head down with balloon compression between the table and the suprapubic area, the cecum usually empties and the terminal ileum becomes visible.

Poorly distended terminal ileum

A poorly distended terminal ileum is related to poor understanding of flow rates. The usual cause is too high an infusion rate and no progression of contrast from jejunum to more distal segments.

Inappropriate amount of barium given

Other than for exceptional patients with a long small bowel, the use of more than 500 ml of barium is discouraged because this prolongs the examination and increases the amount of methylcellulose needed to produce double contrast. A requirement for additional barium is usually related to too high infusion rates. When insufficient barium is given, the problem is usually that infusion rates are too slow. If a patient has had prior small bowel resection surgery, a reduction in the total amount of barium is necessary.

Fecal material in the terminal ileum

An incompetent ileocecal valve allows material from the right side of the colon to enter the terminal ileum. This is not uncommon in unprepared patients, and is also observed in patients who are chronic users of laxatives or are taking long-term mild sedation. Although this may interfere with the single-contrast phase of the examination, diagnostic radiographs are obtainable after infusion of an adequate amount of methylcellulose, which will push the debris into the colon. An additional dose of metoclopramide in these patients serves to speed up the examination.

Reflux into duodenum and stomach

The problem of reflux into the duodenum and stomach is usually related to too fast an infusion rate. The incidence has been decreased by the use of the balloon enteroclysis catheter.[15] Care should be exercised during the entire procedure to ensure that the faintly visible methylcellulose does not overdistend the stomach, which could result in propulsive copious vomiting. Adjusting the flow rates appropriately and positioning the balloon immediately distal to the ligament of Treitz or at least beyond the impression produced by the superior mesenteric artery reduces reflux into the duodenum and stomach. Additional metoclopramide also decreases the amount of reflux if the balloon does not prevent it. Putting the patient prone decreases reflux into the stomach by producing a self-compression effect by the midline barrier (spine, abdominal aorta, and inferior vena cava) on the horizontal duodenum. In patients with small bowel obstruction, preliminary decompression of the stomach and proximal jejunum decreases reflux. The prone position is also safer if vomiting does occur since it reduces the risk of serious aspiration.

Faint opacification of terminal ileum

Faint opacification of the terminal ileum is a common problem when the technique is being learned and gives rise to the criticism that enteroclysis is marvelous for the jejunum but not useful for the distal small bowel. The problem is again caused by difficulties with resultant atony, all the barium being delivered by the time the head of the column has reached mid small bowel. If methylcellulose is then started quickly, once peristalsis eventually returns (because of decreased flow rate or additional metoclopramide), the methylcellulose appears to "overtake" the barium and arrives first in the terminal ileum. If this happens a few times, the radiologist may become discouraged with the technique. Careful attention to flow rates as described above avoids the problem.

The single-contrast technique is easier in this respect, since good terminal ileal distention is more readily achieved by less experienced radiologists. However, the single-contrast technique has less potential for providing mucosal detail.

Modifications of the technique
Ileostomy enteroclysis

A patient with an ileostomy can be safely examined by a retrograde biphasic enteroclysis. The standard balloon cath-

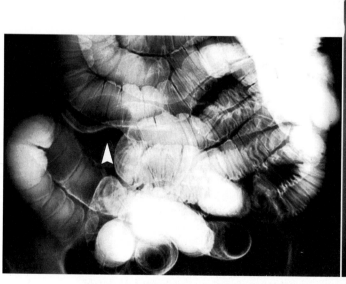
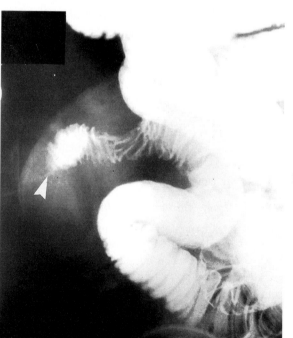

Fig. 26-6 Per ileostomy enteroclysis. **A,** The inflated balloon *(arrowhead)* acts as a seal from within against the narrower, less distensible opening through the abdominal fascia. The balloon should be inflated slowly under fluoroscopic guidance using enough air to produce a resistance to gentle withdrawal of the catheter. This method results in a "clean" examination. **B,** Prestomal segment is evaluated after balloon is deflated. Tangential spot films are taken while some of the instilled contrast overflows through the stoma *(arrowhead)*.

eter can be used for this purpose. The catheter is gently introduced into the ostomy until resistance is felt. The balloon is gradually inflated under fluoroscopy and retracted gently until it is just beyond the peritoneal reflection. The purpose of the inflated balloon is not to occlude the bowel lumen proximal to the stoma, but to act as a seal from within against the usually narrower and nondistensible opening through the abdominal fascia. The balloon should be inflated slowly, using only enough air to produce a resistance to gentle withdrawal of the catheter. Before introducing contrast material, 0.5 mg glucagon intravenously should be given to abolish peristalsis. It is important to evaluate the prestomal portion of the ileostomy because fascial scarring can be a common cause of stomal malfunction. To avoid obscuring the prestomal area, the balloon catheter should be deflated toward the end of the procedure and tangential spot films taken while some of the instilled barium overflows through the stoma. A biphasic technique using less barium (250 ml) followed by methylcellulose allows evaluation of the entire small intestine (Fig. 26-6). In patients with pelvic adhesions, severe discomfort may ensue during infusion, and an analgesic (such as meperidine) may be required. The degree of partial obstruction is more reliably assessed with the antegrade route.

Enteroclysis in patients with high-grade partial small bowel obstruction

Even if fluid is present in the small bowel proximal to the point of obstruction, methylcellulose in lesser amounts is still infused to keep the barium in suspension and to facilitate evacuation of barium. The use of a tube designed to both facilitate decompression of the obstructed small bowel and to perform enteroclysis has made the procedure less complicated and easier for both patient and radiologist. It eliminates the need to replace the nasogastric tube (which cannot be used for enteroclysis) with an enteroclysis catheter and the added discomfort of positioning an enteroclysis catheter alongside the nasogastric tube. The nasogastric-nasoenteric decompression enteroclysis tube (MDEC-1400, Cook Inc., Bloomington, Ind.) is a modification of the the Maglinte balloon enteroclysis catheter.[16] An understanding of the construction of this triple-lumen catheter enables the user to appreciate how the tube works and how to care for it (Fig. 26-7). The catheter can be used similarly to a nasogastric tube if the tip is positioned in the stomach. Because of the smaller size of the catheter (14 Fr compared with the 18 Fr nasogastric tube) it is tolerated better by patients and is easier to maneuver into the duodenum and proximal jejunum. Because of the sump port, efficient decompression is possible (Fig. 26-8).

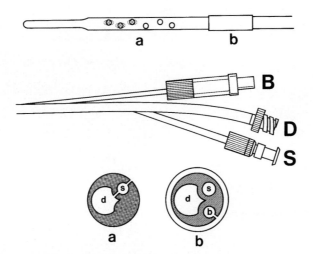

Fig. 26-7 Diagram of internal construction of decompression enteroclysis catheter. The uppermost drawing shows the distal end of the catheter, the middle drawing shows the proximal end, and the bottom diagrams are cross sections at the level of the distal sideports *(a)* and at the level of balloon attachment *(b)*. The distal sideports shown in the uppermost drawing *(a)* connect the intestinal lumen with the sump lumen *(s)*, which in turn communicates with the decompression (suction) lumen *(d)*. The most distal sideports *(a)* are diagrammed to show the longitudinal communication between the sump and decompression (suction) lumens. The sideports communicating with the sump and suction lumens allow flushing from proximal attachment *S* to clear any blockage of the sideports during decompression. The staggered position of the sideports also helps prevent tissue blockage of the ports during suction. The tapered end results in less nasal mucosal irritation during intubation. The sump lumen *(s)* is connected externally at *S* and the suction lumen at *D*. The balloon lumen *(b)*, which is provided with a one-way check valve proximally *(B)*, communicates with the circularly disposed silicone balloon at level *(b)*.

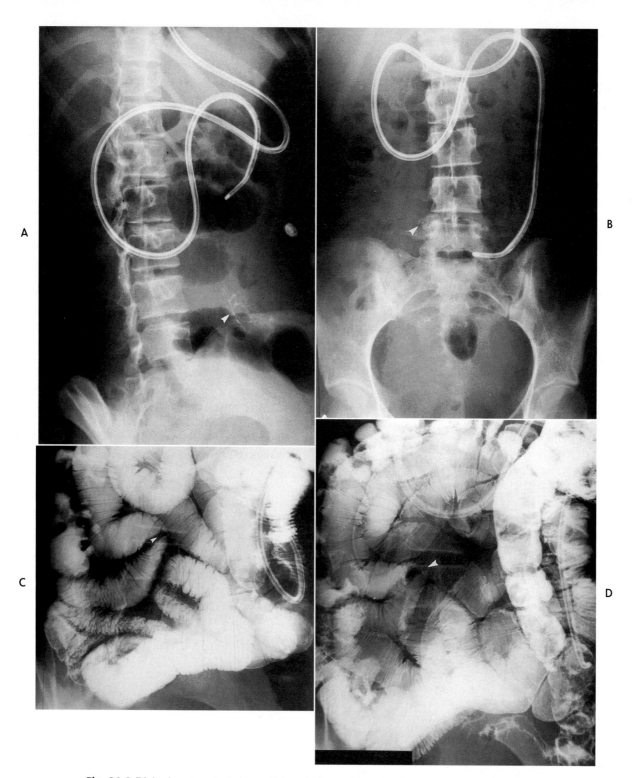

Fig. 26-8 Biphasic enteroclysis in small bowel obstruction: use of a decompression enteroclysis tube. **A,** Decompression enteroclysis tube positioned in proximal jejunum after initial suction of stomach. Low intermittent suction was applied for 24 hours in this patient admitted with intestinal obstruction. Note sutures *(arrowhead)* in abdomen from prior intestinal surgery related to motor vehicle accident. **B,** Follow-up abdominal radiograph the next day shows satisfactory decompression of distended small bowel. **C,** Single-contrast and **D,** double-contrast enteroclysis radiographs identify an adhesive band *(arrowhead)* causing low-grade partial mechanical obstruction. Although the abnormality is better shown in the single-contrast phase, infusion of methylcellulose facilitated passage of all contrast through the point of obstruction and promoted colonic evacuation. The use of this dual-purpose tube simplifies performance of enteroclysis and is better tolerated by patients than the 18 Fr nasogastric tubes currently in use in most hospitals.

A fluid-filled distended stomach should be decompressed before the catheter tip is positioned in the proximal jejunum, the ideal position of the decompression enteroclysis catheter. Because of the smaller lumen of the small intestine as compared with the capacious stomach, the small bowel wall collapses readily around a decompression tube, clogging the suction sideports. The box below gives a set of instructions for nursing or allied health personnel to ensure efficient suction using the decompression enteroclysis catheter.

The technique of enteroclysis is modified depending on the severity of obstruction.[17] The immediate performance of enteroclysis is discouraged if the proximal small intestine is atonic and fluid filled. Computed tomography appears to be more appropriate in this situation.[18] Compared with other long tubes used for decompression (Miller-Abbott tube and others), which rely on peristalsis for propagation, positioning of this tube into the proximal jejunum is readily accomplished.

Combined enteroscopy and enteroclysis

For a proximal enteroscopy performed for malabsorption or for evaluation of unexplained upper gastrointestinal bleeding, a combined enteroscopy-enteroclysis procedure has been described.[19] For this purpose, an exchange wire with a flexible tip is introduced through the endoscope at the end of the examination and is advanced toward the je-

junum.[2] The patient, with the wire left in position, is sent to the radiology department for enteroclysis. An infusion catheter of reduced wall thickness and greater flexibility is threaded over the replacement wire and passes quickly into the jejunum. The patient is still affected by the premedication for endoscopy and is barely aware of the catheter. The biphasic enteroclysis examination then proceeds in standard fashion. For best results, carbon dioxide rather than air is indicated for endoscopic insufflation.

BIPHASIC ENTEROCLYSIS FOR EVALUATION OF UNEXPLAINED GASTROINTESTINAL BLEEDING

Unexplained gastrointestinal bleeding is a frequent indication for enteroclysis. The duodenum should be examined in detail either simultaneously with or after the jejunoileal assessment. When the balloon is deflated, some contrast refluxes into the duodenum. During the period of the in-

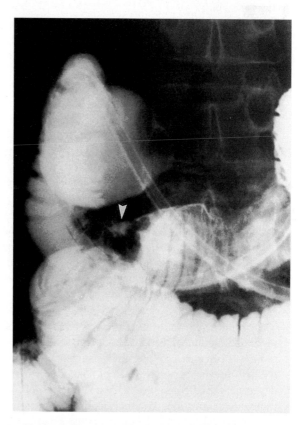

Fig. 26-9 Evaluation of the duodenum before enteroclysis tube removal in patients with unexplained gastrointestinal (GI) bleeding. Initial upper GI endoscopy was unremarkable. An ulcerating mass *(arrowhead)* is demonstrated during infusion of barium after the enteroclysis tube has been retracted to the horizontal segment. Repeat endoscopy and biopsy confirmed presence of a villous adenocarcinoma. This maneuver should be performed routinely in the evaluation of anemia or unexplained GI bleeding because the segment of duodenum distal to the ampulla may not be routinely visualized at esophagogastroduodenoscopy.

□ **INSTRUCTIONS FOR SUCTION WITH THE DECOMPRESSION ENTEROCLYSIS TUBE** □

1. Connect decompression (suction) port (identified by rubber adapter) to *low intermittent* suction; modify as needed.
2. Remove cap from sumping port (labeled "DISTAL AIR") and inject 2 ml of air into the channel as soon as suction is started. Do *not* recap the air channel while suction is being applied. During suction this port allows air to enter and bubble back up the suction channel almost continuously. If "bubbling" is not observed, proceed to step 3. Check that all connections are tight.
3. Irrigate decompression port every 4 hours with 20 ml saline and p.r.n. to prevent clogging of the suction port.
4. Inject the sumping port with 2 ml air every 4 hours and p.r.n. Do not aspirate this port. Steps 3 and 4 can be done at the same time.
5. Any time the decompression port is disconnected, reapply caps to both the suction and the sump ports to prevent fluid leak. Repeat step 2 each time the decompression tube is reconnected for suction.
6. Do not use balloon channel. This port is used only during enteroclysis.

creased flow rate used for methylcellulose infusion, further reflux and distention of the duodenum result. Morphologic assessment of the duodenum is then possible. If this is not possible, the duodenum is evaluated before tube removal. The tube tip is retracted into the proximal horizontal duodenum and infused with barium. Radiographs are then obtained in different projections. If the proximal transverse colon is filled with contrast, the patient is sent to the toilet with the catheter in place, and barium is infused in the duodenum after the colon has emptied. In spite of a report of a negative endoscopic examination, the radiologist should examine the duodenum in detail, especially if the extent of endoscopic assessment is not known (Fig. 26-9). Evaluation of the stomach after an enteroclysis is suboptimal because some methylcellulose usually refluxes into the stomach.

Advantages

The advantages of enteroclysis with methylcellulose include the following:

1. The regulatory action of the pylorus is bypassed, and contrast can be administered at the desired rate. The regulated infusion of barium and methylcellulose reduces flocculation.
2. Enteroclysis challenges the distensibility of the intestinal wall by the accelerated inflow of contrast. Reduced distensibility caused by ulcers, tumors, or low-grade adhesive obstruction stands out against proximal lumen dilatation. Small sinus tracts or fistulas are better shown.
3. The fluid overload temporarily decreases motor activity. This hypotonic state makes possible a better assessment of straightened folds, especially during the double-contrast effect of methylcellulose. Mucosal abnormalities and smaller luminal defects become more clearly visible and normality can be ascertained.
4. The entire small bowel can be demonstrated in a state of distention. All loops can be studied by fluoroscopy spot films and angled views to advantage.
5. The examination can usually be done in one session of 20 to 30 minutes. Continued supervision by the radiologist becomes an essential component of the method. In comparison with the prolonged stay in the department usually required with small bowel follow-through examination, enteroclysis is a logistically more practical method of examining the small bowel in critically ill or elderly patients.
6. The infusion of methylcellulose facilitates evacuation of the barium. This allows abdominal imaging by other methods with less delay.
7. The reliability of a normal enteroclysis is high. This is important in the clinical examination of an organ where the prevalence of disease is low and symptoms of disease are mimicked by disease of adjacent organs.

Complications

Potential complications always exist when foreign objects or fluids are introduced into the body.[20,21] Serious complications can be prevented by understanding the principles of intubation and the response of the small bowel to different rates of infusion. Radiologists who want to start performing enteroclysis should observe the procedure being done in departments performing the study regularly. Patients who are disinclined to be intubated in spite of persuasion and the offer of light sedation must have their wishes accepted, since alternative methods of small bowel examination are available and are informative when done correctly.[22] Perforations or mucosal dissections are possibilities if the guidewire is allowed either to extend beyond the tip of an endhole catheter or to pass through a sideport of sidehole catheters or if the catheter is pushed against resistance. The catheter should never be pushed against any resistance. The injection of a small amount of air into the infusion lumen will sometimes incite peristalsis and direct the tube tip in the appropriate direction. Otherwise, a small amount of barium should be injected to assess the problem. Intubation should be a gentle process with patient comfort in mind.

Minor complications are infrequent. Vomiting caused by substantial reflux into the stomach occurs if excessive flow rates are used, even if a balloon catheter is used. The use of methylcellulose decreases the appreciation of reflux into the stomach. Careful observation is necessary. The danger of aspiration of refluxed contrast into the bronchial tree in cases of aged or very ill patients should be recognized. Should significant reflux be observed, all infusion should be stopped. Methylcellulose and barium refluxed in the stomach should be aspirated before tube removal. Some patients may complain of abdominal fullness or crampy pain during the infusion of methylcellulose. The examination should not be continued if discomfort persists after adjusting the rate of infusion. If enough barium has been infused, the examination can be continued as a fluoroscopic small bowel meal augmented by adjunct procedures to decrease some of the inherent limitations of the follow-through.[12,22]

REFERENCES

1. Maglinte D, Herlinger H: Single-contrast and biphasic enteroclysis. In Herlinger H, Maglinte D, eds: *Clinical radiology of the small intestine,* Philadelphia, 1989, WB Saunders.
2. Herlinger H, Maglinte D: The small bowel enema with methylcellulose. In Herlinger H, Maglinte D, eds: *Clinical radiology of the small intestine,* Philadelphia, 1989, WB Saunders.
3. Shirakabe H, Kobayashi S: Air double-contrast barium study of the small bowel. In Herlinger H, Maglinte D, eds: *Clinical radiology of the small intestine,* Philadelphia, 1989, WB Saunders.
4. Sellink JL: Single contrast enteroclysis. In Margulis AR, Burhenne HJ, eds: *Alimentary tract radiology,* St Louis, 1983, Mosby.
5. Barloon TJ, Lu CC, Franken EA Jr et al: Small bowel enteroclysis survey, *Gastrointest Radiol* 13:203, 1988.

6. Antes G, Lissner J et al: Double-contrast small bowel examination with barium and methylcellulose: results in 300 cases, *Radiology* 148:37, 1983.

7. Wittich G, Salomonowitch E, Szepsi T et al: Small bowel double-contrast enema in stage III ovarian cancer, *AJR* 142:299, 1984.

8. Miller RE, Sellink JL: Enteroclysis: the small bowel enema. How to succeed and how to fail, *Gastrointest Radiol* 4:269, 1979.

9. Herlinger H: A modified technique for the double-contrast small bowel enema, *Gastrointest Radiol* 3:201, 1978.

10. Trickey SE, Halls J, Hodson CJ: A further development of the small bowel enema, *J Roy Soc Med* 56:1070, 1963.

11. Losowsky MS, Walker BE, Kelleher J: *Malabsorption in clinical practice,* Edinburgh, 1974, Churchill Livingston.

12. Maglinte D, Lappas JC, Kelvin FM, Chernish SM: Small bowel radiography: how, when and why, *Radiology* 163:297, 1987.

13. Oudkirk N: Infusion rate in enteroclysis examination. Thesis submitted to Leiden, The Netherlands, 1981, Leiden University.

14. Maglinte D, Miller RE: A comparison of pumps used for enteroclysis, *Radiology* 152:815, 1984.

15. Maglinte D: Balloon enteroclysis catheter, *AJR* 143:761, 1984.

16. Maglinte D, Stevens L, Hall R, Kelvin F, Micon L: Dual-purpose tube for enteroclysis and nasogastric-nasoenteric decompression, *Radiology* 185:281, 1992.

17. Herlinger H, Maglinte D: Small bowel obstruction. In Herlinger H, Maglinte D, eds: *Clinical radiology of the small intestine,* Philadelphia, 1989, WB Saunders.

18. Megibow AJ, Balthazar EJ, Cho KC, Medwid SW, Birnbaum BA et al: Bowel obstruction. Evaluation with CT, *Radiology* 180:313, 1991.

19. McGovern R, Barkin JS: Enteroscopy and enteroclysis: an improved method for combined procedure, *Gastrointest Radiol* 15:327, 1990.

20. Diner W: Duodenal perforation during intubation for small bowel enema study, *Radiology* 168:39, 1988.

21. Ginaldi S: Small bowel perforation during enteroclysis. *Gastrointest Radiol* 16:29, 1991.

22. Herlinger H, Maglinte DDT: Nonintubation barium methods. In Maglinte D, Herlinger H, eds: *Clinical radiology of the small intestine,* Philadelphia, 1989, WB Saunders.

27 Double-Contrast Enteroclysis with Air

TSUNEYOSHI YAO

The air double-contrast study of the small intestine has been used for a long time. Since the earliest description by Gershon-Cohen and Shay in 1938,[1] various modifications have been employed.

In Japan, stimulated by detailed double-contrast study of the stomach and large intestine developed by Shirakabe et al.,[3] double-contrast examination of the small bowel was attempted many years ago. However, most trials were unsuccessful, partly because the examinations took too long, since a 100% weight per volume (w/v) suspension of barium was used. In 1967 Bilbao et al.[3] reported a feasible method of duodenal tube insertion. Sellink[4] studied and reported on suitable concentrations and the specific gravity of several contrast media. These reports showed Japanese investigators that the time required for an examination could be shortened by injecting a 40% to 50% w/v barium suspension and air through a duodenal tube. This prompted the reports of Nakamura, myself, and other colleagues[5] and of Kobayashi et al.[6] on double-contrast studies of the small intestine.

This technique has been widely accepted in Japan since then.[7-9] However, some problems remain that limit the value of the technique as a routine examination.

TECHNIQUE
Patient preparation

Since the transit of barium is influenced by feces, laxatives are given the night before the examination. Nothing is to be taken by mouth after 7:00 PM the night before the examination.

Barium

A 50% to 70% w/v barium sulfate (Barytgen, [Fushimi Pharmaceutical Co., Kagawa, Japan] or Barosperse [Mallinckrodt, St. Louis, Mo.]) mixed with simethicone is used.

At a rate of approximately 60 ml/min, using a 100-ml syringe, 150 to 200 ml of barium suspension is injected slowly. The progress of the barium column is observed by interval fluoroscopy. When peristalsis stops and the barium column arrests, an additional 50 to 100 ml of barium is injected. Generally, a total quantity of 350 to 500 ml is required to make the barium suspension reach the distal ileum. However, for the purpose of fine radiography of the small intestinal loops in double contrast, it is desirable to limit the total amount of barium to 350 ml and to make the barium column progress by changing the patient's position. It is necessary to take compression films when any abnormalities are found under fluoroscopic observation.

Air

Since air cannot propel barium as forcibly as methylcellulose, air should be injected after the head of the barium column has reached the distal ileum.

Initially, 200 ml of air is injected slowly at a rate of approximately 100 ml/min in a right anterior oblique position, using a 100-ml syringe. After observing the progress of the air and barium distally by fluoroscopy, an additional 200 ml of air is injected. Then 100 to 200 ml of air is added several times, preventing barium pooling at any point by making the patient assume various positions—supine, prone, head up, lateral decubitus, and oblique. Optimal double-contrast views of the small intestine in the pelvic cavity are obtained by air injection with the patient in the prone position. Generally, a total amount of 600 to 1000 ml of air is necessary for double-contrast views of the whole small bowel.

When the air reaches the distal ileum in sufficient amount to produce adequate double-contrast views of both the jejunum and the ileum, an antispasmodic agent is injected intravenously or intramuscularly.

Radiography

If the examination is unduly slow, it may be wise to take double-contrast films of the upper small bowel before the injection of an antispasmodic agent. Very prolonged double contrast leads to progressively impaired coating. Generally, however, double-contrast views of the entire small intestine are taken on several films when hypotonicity has been obtained by antispasmodic injection (Fig. 27-1). Light compression using a ball made of cloth may sometimes help to separate superimposed loops. Control of respiration and

548

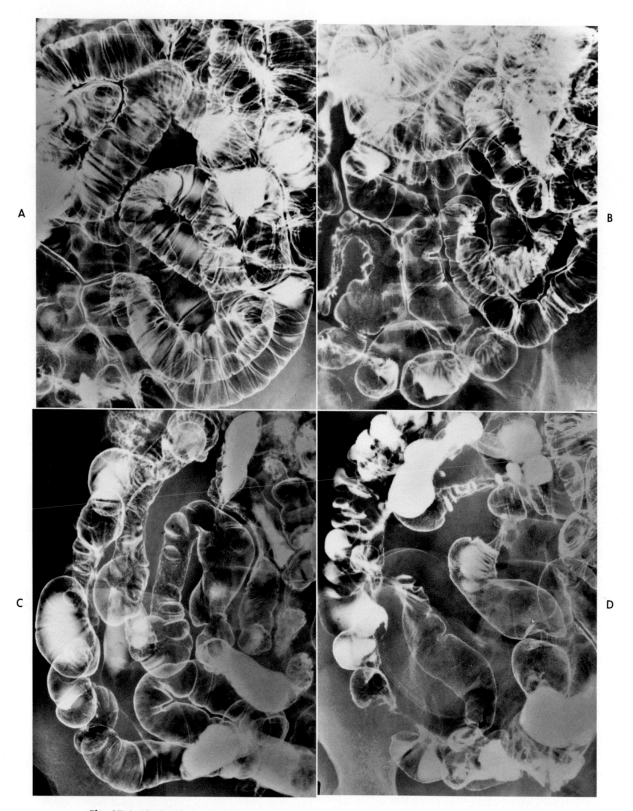

Fig. 27-1 Air double-contrast study in a case of Crohn's disease. Double-contrast views of jejunum (**A**), distal jejunum and proximal ileum (**B**), ileum (**C**), and distal ileum (**D**). Radiography of all loops should be separately taken on several films. Eccentric deformity *(arrowheads)* and bilateral deformity *(arrows)* are seen. Dots show distal ileum. Faint shadow *(short arrows)* indicates a cloth ball used for light compression.

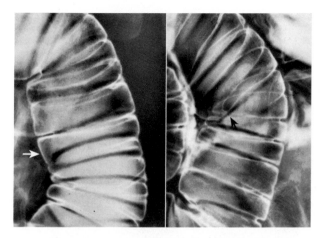

Fig. 27-2 Air double-contrast views showing scarring of jejunum of unknown cause *(arrows)*. These were confirmed by endoscopy.

changes in the patient's position are also required for optimal demonstration of the various loops of small bowel on double contrast.

PROBLEMS

The examination can usually be completed within an hour. In patients with organic lesions such as stenosis, however, transit of barium to the distal ileum may be prolonged for more than an hour, and satisfactory double-contrast views cannot be obtained. In such cases it may be advisable to take double-contrast views of the jejunum only, leaving the ileum for later. To examine only the ileum in such cases, a duodenal tube is passed 2 or 3 hours after oral ingestion of 250 ml of 70% w/v barium, and double-contrast views of the ileum are taken after injection of air.

Because of these problems, the air double-contrast study is not performed in Japan as a routine examination of the small intestine. However, when the examination is successful, it produces exquisite surface detail, such as aphthous lesions and minute scars (Figs. 27-2 and 27-3). Although sometimes these small lesions are not recognized during the fluoroscopic examination, they can be easily seen on the radiographs. When an ulcerative lesion is demonstrated en face, the activity of the disease can be diagnosed, which is helpful in evaluating the treatment (Fig. 27-4, *B*).

The surface detail seen on the air double-contrast study of the small intestine is superior to that of any other examinations, including methylcellulose double-contrast small bowel enema (Fig. 27-4). Despite the intricacy of the technique, air double-contrast studies are employed selectively in Japan to provide a detailed examination of the small bowel.

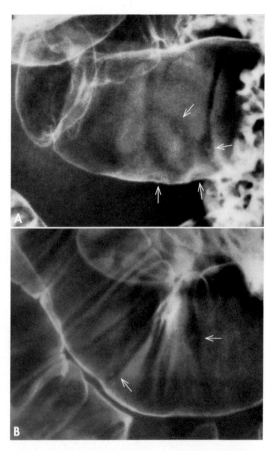

Fig. 27-3 Air double-contrast views. **A,** Multiple aphthoid ulcers in Crohn's disease *(arrows)*. **B,** Aphthous lesions of unknown cause *(arrows)*. Both lesions could not be recognized by fluoroscopic observation and were picked up on radiographs.

REFERENCES

1. Gershon-Cohen J, Shay H: A method for the direct immediate examination of the small intestine by single and double contrast techniques, *AJR* 42:456, 1939.
2. Shirakabe H et al: *Atlas of x-ray diagnosis of early gastric cancer,* Tokyo, 1966, Igakushoin Ltd; Philadelphia, 1966, JB Lippincott.
3. Bilbao MK et al: Hypotonic duodenography, *Radiology* 89:438, 1967.
4. Sellink JL: *Examination of small intestine by means of duodenal intubation,* Leiden, 1971, Steinfert Kroese.
5. Nakamura Y et al: X-ray examination of the small intestine by means of duodenal intubation—double contrast of the small bowel, *Stom Intest* 9:1461, 1974.
6. Kobayashi S et al: Double contrast study of the small bowel (in Japanese), *Jpn J Clin Radiol* 19:619, 1974.
7. Yao T et al: Roentgenographic analysis of tuberculosis of the small intestine, *Stom Intest* 12:1467, 1977.
8. Tanaka K et al: Double contrast study of the minute lesions of Crohn's disease of the small intestine, *Stom Intest* 17:871, 1982.
9. Tsukasa S et al: Roentgenographic diagnosis of Crohn's disease of the small intestine, *Stom Intest* 13:335, 1978.

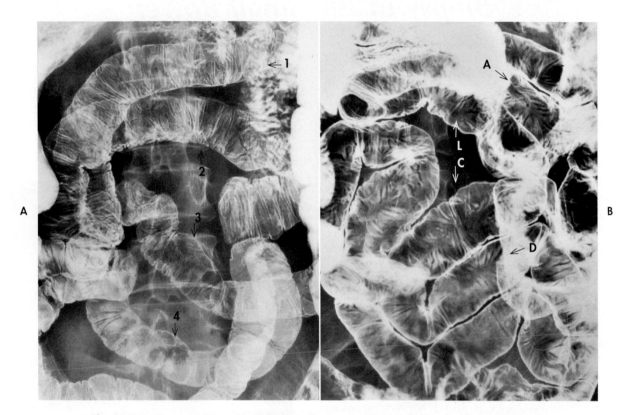

Fig. 27-4 Radiographs in a case of Crohn's disease. **A,** Methylcellulose double-contrast enema; 250 ml of 70% w/v barium (Barytgen Deluxe) and 1200 ml of methylcellulose. Time required for the examination was 30 minutes after injection of barium started. Loops of small intestine are well separated, and more loops are demonstrated in double-contrast views than on the air double-contrast study. However, the loops are not adequately distended. Consequently, although convergence of multiple folds is demonstrated, the arrangement of ulcers is not clearly distinguished. The fine pathologic details on the folds are not very clearly displayed. **B,** Air double-contrast study in the same case as **A;** 300 ml of 70% w/v barium (Barytgen Deluxe) and 600 ml of air. Lesions indicated as *a, l, c,* and *d* in **B** are almost identical to those indicated as *1, 2, 3,* and *4* in **A.** Intestinal loops are not so well separated and are not as extensively demonstrated on double-contrast as compared with those in **A.** However, the loops that are demonstrated on air double-contrast are adequately distended, and it can now be recognized that most lesions with convergence of folds are scars and that they are arranged in a longitudinal fashion or are longitudinal ulcers. This case seems to be a good example showing the advantages and disadvantages of air double contrast. Arrows show an active longitudinal ulcer. The others are evaluated as scars.

28 *Percutaneous Fine-Needle Aspiration Cytology and Peroral Biopsy of the Small Bowel*

SIGMUND DAWISKIBA
ANDERS LUNDERQUIST
ROGER WILLÉN

Neoplasms of the small bowel are rare, despite the fact that the small bowel represents 75% of the length and over 90% of the mucosal surface of the alimentary tract. The small intestine is the site of only 3% to 6% of gastrointestinal (GI) tumors, and only 1% of them are malignant. Symptoms of small bowel lesions are nonspecific, and these lesions are often not diagnosed until lesions of other parts of the GI tract have been excluded.

In patients with malabsorption symptoms clinical findings might suggest celiac disease; small bowel mucosal biopsy gives the final diagnosis. In patients with long-standing celiac disease, malignancy can develop, and the most common is lymphoma.

PERORAL BIOPSY

Biopsy with the Crosby-Kugler capsule has been the most widely used technique for obtaining mucosal specimens for histology. The capsule is attached to the tip of a flexible catheter, which the patient swallows. The capsule contains a spring-loaded blade, which is activated by suction through the catheter. The disadvantage of this technique has been that the capsule cannot be directed to a specific target, and only one specimen can be obtained, after which the catheter has to be removed for the capsule to be emptied. An alternative has been developed with a hydraulic capsule from which the specimen can be flushed to the surface with the capsule still in position. The blade is automatically reset, and multiple specimens can be obtained before the capsule is removed.[1] Complications are rare (0.1% to 4%) and include hemorrhage and bowel perforation.

Mucosal biopsy is an essential investigation in patients suspected of having a diffuse disease of the small bowel. The technique fails in up to 12% of cases; in an additional 8% inadequate biopsy specimens may be obtained.

In celiac disease it is no longer necessary to perform the biopsy in the jejunum. Endoscopic mucosal biopsy has been compared with jejunal capsule biopsy regarding adequacy and ability at arrive at the diagnosis of celiac disease. It

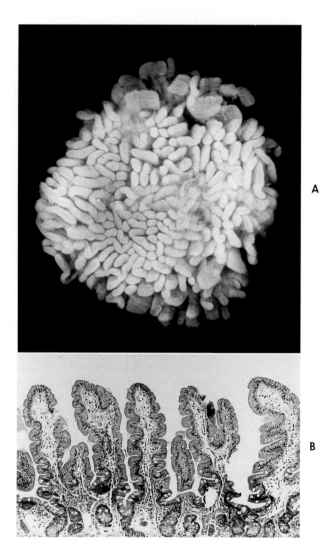

Fig. 28-1 A, Normal small intestine biopsy specimen with fingerlike projections (dissection microscope, ×10). **B,** Light microscopy of normal intestine demonstrating normal slender villi and no inflammatory changes (H&E stain, ×25).

was shown that endoscopic forceps biopsy of the descending duodenum was more reliable than capsule biopsy.[2]

In the department of pathology at the University Hospital of Lund, 1352 biopsies from the small intestine were analyzed for the 5-year period 1986 to 1990. In the age group 0 to 4 years, 126 of 297 (42.4%) were positive for celiac disease. In the age group 5 to 19 years 41 of 110 (37%) were positive, and in the age group 20 years and older, 69 of 945 (7.3%). The biopsy specimens in the first age group were mainly taken with the Crosby capsule, whereas in older persons three or more endoscopic biopsy specimens were taken from the distal duodenum in each patient. The latter technique produced just as good results as the capsule technique.[1-5] This study also demonstrated that older patients with subtle complaints, anemia, or both quite commonly turned out to have celiac disease (see Fig. 28-2, *A*). Examination of the biopsy specimens with a dissecting microscope before histologic sectioning is of considerable diagnostic help. Fig. 28-1, *A*, shows normal small intestine for comparison with the specimen in celiac disease in Fig. 28-2, *B*, which showed gaping crypt openings and rudimentary villi formation. The fingerlike villi of the normal intestine are easily demonstrated in the normal light microscopy slides (Fig. 28-1, *B*), whereas they are lacking in celiac disease (Fig. 28-2, *C*).

Complications in celiac disease, such as lymphoma, collagenous sprue (Fig. 29-3), and broadened villi in the kwashiorkor patient are all easy to demonstrate in 4- to 5-μ slices with light microscopy technique. Kwashiorkor patients often have giardiasis[6] (Fig. 28-4). Granulomas in Crohn's disease are common, and in AIDS patients a variety of superimposed infectious agents are recognized,[7-11] such as cytomegaloviruses (Fig. 28-5), atypical mycobacteria, cryptosporidiosis, coccidiosis, and *Pneumocystis carinii,* among others.

Polyps and polyplike features are often present and when localized in the proximal jejunum or distal ileum may be reached with the endoscope. We have seen adenomas, carcinoids, and carcinomas of polypoid appearance. A newer entity, the inflammatory fibroid polyp[12,13] (Fig. 28-6),

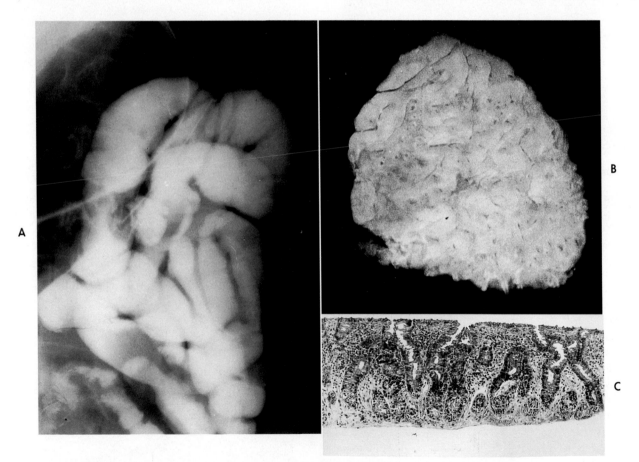

Fig. 28-2 A, Small bowel enteroclysis in a 60-year-old patient with long-standing celiac disease. "Moulage" sign—ilealisation of jejunum with loss of valvulae. **B,** Celiac disease of small intestine with subtotal villous atrophy. Gaping crypt openings and flat mucosa (dissection microscope, ×10). **C,** Light microscopy of celiac disease with total villous atrophy, intense enrichment of lymphoplasmocytic cells in the stroma, and crypt elongation from the surface down to the muscularis mucosa (H&E stain, ×25).

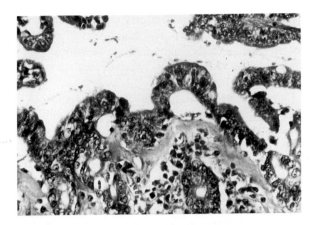

Fig. 28-3 Shortened and broadened villi, collagen proliferation, and intense chronic inflammation in a case of tropical sprue (H&E stain, ×25).

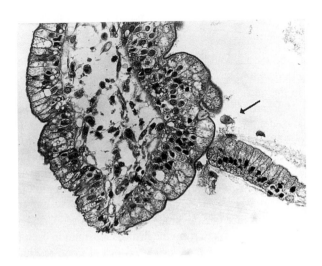

Fig. 28-4 Patient with kwashiorkor with broadened villi with edema and enhancement of lymphoplasmocytic cells. At the surface, note evidence of giardiasis *(arrow)* (H&E stain, ×25).

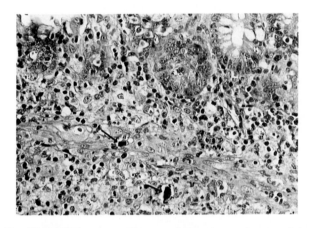

Fig. 28-5 AIDS patient with severe inflammatory changes of the small intestine of aphthous type containing cells with PAS-positive inclusion bodies *(arrows)* as a result of cytomegalovirus infection (PAS stain, ×90).

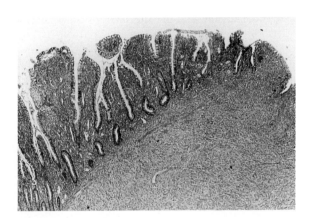

Fig. 28-6 Case of inflammatory fibroid polyp of the small intestine demonstrating granulation tissue, inflammatory cells, and vascular projection with ulcerated surface to the right, broadened and dilated villi to the left.

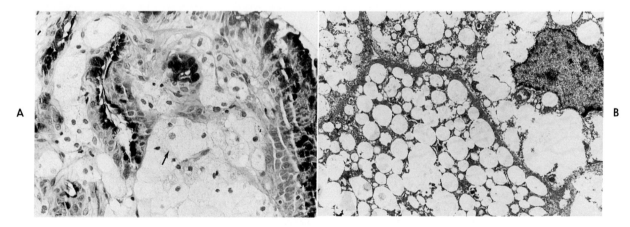

Fig. 28-7 A, Specimen with xanthomatous histiocytes *(arrow)* with granular cytoplasm in the submucosa of the small intestine (H&E, ×90). **B,** Electron micrograph of xanthomatous lesion of the small intestine with fat-laden vacuoles (electron micrograph, ×2.900).

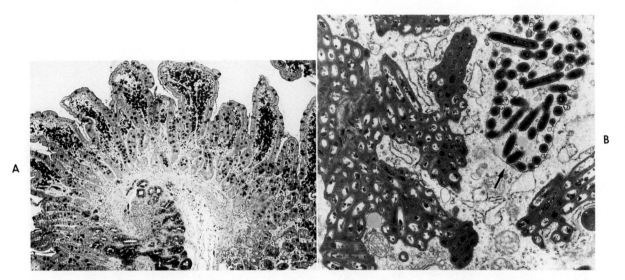

Fig. 28-8 A, Whipple's disease; stromal area contains a rich amount of PAS–positive laden histiocytes (PAS stain, ×25). **B,** Electron micrograph of Whipple's disease demonstrating a large number of bacteria in a honeycombed structure *(arrow)* together with a conglomeration of partly degenerated and compounded bacteria (TEM, ×20,000).

sometimes looks like a malignant lesion but is an inflammatory overgrowth, mainly of granulation tissue of unknown cause. Expansions of the villi by xanthomatous cells[14] (Fig. 28-7, *A*), PAS-positive histiocytes as in Whipple's disease[15-17] (Fig. 28-8, *A*), and malacoplakia[18-21] (Fig. 28-9, *A*) are also found. Here transmission electron microscopy (TEM) is of great help in the subclassification of the lesions. Good results are achieved even with fixation in glutaraldehyde after deparaffination of paraffin-embedded tissue (Figs. 28-7, *B,* 28-8, *B,* and 28-9, *B*).

In a small intestinal biopsy from a 69-year-old woman with light microscopy we demonstrated changes consistent with Waldenström's disease[22] (Fig. 28-10, *A*). Histochemistry and TEM (Fig. 28-10, *B*) further substantiated these changes. Urine and bone marrow investigations verified the diagnosis. Besides carcinoma, benign tumors such as granular cell tumors and leiomyomas[23,24] can be diagnosed. Malignant stromal cell tumors are not infrequently seen[23-27] (Fig. 28-11, *A*). Immunohistopathologic methods[24,26] that can be applied to paraffin-embedded material are very helpful in subtyping these tumors. Antibodies against vimentin, desmin, and S-100 protein facilitate the evaluation of the type of filaments, thus enabling us to evaluate the cellular phenotype. DNA ploidy is sometimes helpful in determining growth potential. Thirty micrometer paraffin slices can easily be used in flow cytometric measurement systems[28] (Fig. 28-11, *B*). X-ray diffraction analysis using a scanning transmission electron microscopic (STEM) mode turned out to be helpful in analysis of intracellular crystal contents, for example, in malakoplakia (Fig. 28-12).

In summary, small intestinal endoscopic biopsy has opened up a fascinating and vast area and has made it possible for us to evaluate subtle changes and diseases with the aid of complementary methods. We can also follow therapeutic results and apply quantitative criteria in the grading of different tissue lesions.

In the localization and diagnosis of circumscribed lesions of the small bowel, radiologic examination after barium administration may be performed either as a barium follow-through examination or as a double-contrast enteroclysis. The findings are often nonspecific, demonstrating a stricture with or without ulceration, a polypoid lesion, or signs of an extraluminal mass. It is surprising that percutaneous fine-needle aspiration cytology (FNAC), now widely used in the diagnosis of lesions in the lungs, liver, pancreas, and lymph nodes and in palpable tumors, has not been used more in the final diagnosis of lesions demonstrated with a barium examination of the small bowel, where endoscopic biopsy cannot be performed.

CYTOLOGIC ASPIRATION TECHNIQUE

A barium examination provides excellent guidance for percutaneous fine-needle aspiration of circumscribed small bowel lesions. Under local anesthesia, a 0.7-mm thin biopsy needle with stylet and clear plastic hub is advanced toward the target under fluoroscopic control. Entering the lesion can easily be recognized by motion of the contrast-filled bowel and the lesion (Fig. 28-13).

Needle thickness is important in cytologic technique. A thin, long needle produces a higher capillary aspiration power and decreases the risk of puncture bleeding or hematoma. It simultaneously increases the chance of obtaining more diagnostic cellular material. We do not recom-

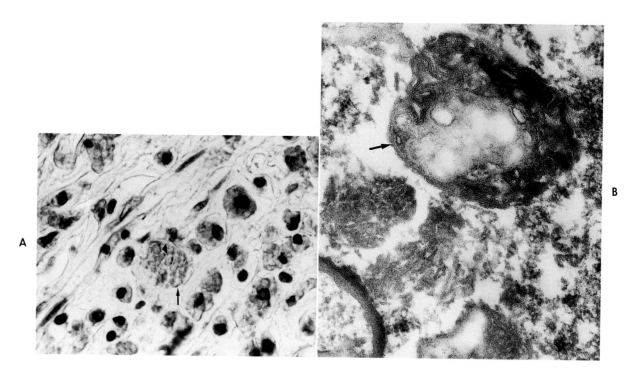

Fig. 28-9 A, Example of malacoplakia demonstrating granular histiocytes *(arrow)* and Michaelis-Gutmann bodies centrally in the cytoplasm *(arrowhead)* (H&E stain, ×800). **B,** Electron micrograph of the same case of malacoplakia demonstrating complex swirled membranes (Michaelis-Gutmann body, *arrow*) (TEM, ×50,000.)

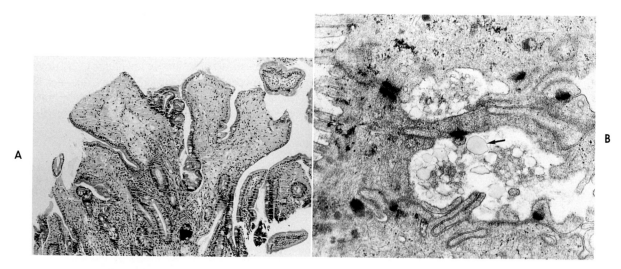

Fig. 28-10 A, Small intestine containing a rich amount of protein-laden histiocytes in the stroma and partly dilated villi in a case of Waldenström's disease (H&E stain, ×25). **B,** Electron micrograph of the same case of Waldenström's disease demonstrating vacuoles with encapsulated proteinaceous material *(arrow)* (TEM, ×20,000).

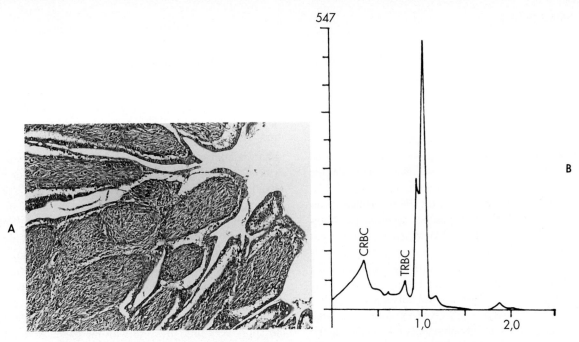

Fig. 28-11 A, Case of leiomyosarcoma of the small intestine with elongated malignant leiomatous cells distending and filling up the submucosal area of the villi (H&E stain, ×25). B, Cytofluorometric DNA pattern of the same case of leiomyosarcoma demonstrating a hypodiploid aneuploid tumor with an s-phase percentage of 3.5. DNA index 0.93, resp. 1.01. CRBC (chicken) and TRBC (trout) internal standard erythrocytes.

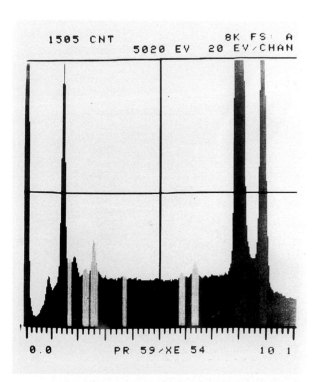

Fig. 28-12 X-ray microanalysis (EDAX). Pattern of Michaelis-Gutmann bodies in small intestinal malacoplakia. The smaller light peaks indicate from *left to right:* silica, sulfur, chloride, calcium, magnesium, and iron. The four larger black peaks indicate copper, presumably from the grids.

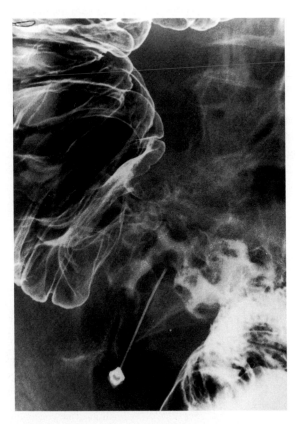

Fig. 28-13 Double-contrast barium examination with reflux of contrast into distal ileum where an irregular tumor is found. Percutaneous biopsy guided by the barium examination. Diagnosis: malignant lymphoma.

mend the use of thicker needles because of the greater risk of an unwanted volume of blood in the aspirate, which interferes with slide making for light microscopy. Spinal needles of Westcott (22 gauge 3.5, Recorder No. 8265 and Yale 22 gauge 3, Ref. No. 05171; Becton Dickinson, Stockholm, Sweden), notched or unnotched, 9 to 15 cm in length with a clear plastic hub, are most suitable for the majority of tumors of the small bowel. Notched needles are more useful in compact, fibrotic tumor tissues (Fig. 28-14). Use of the CAMECO Syringe Pistol (Fibre Medical, Vellinge, Sweden) for 10-ml disposable syringes facilitates one-hand manipulation (Fig. 28-14). When the lesion is entered with the needle, the stylet is removed, the needle is attached to the syringe with the CAMECO handle, and the plunger of the syringe is retracted for negative pressure. The needle is moved back and forth a few times within the tumor mass. When material is observed to come up into the needle's clear plastic hub, the plunger is released while the needle is still within the tumor. Otherwise the aspirated material, with some air, disappears into the barrel of the syringe and cannot be used because it will very quickly become air dried. The needle is withdrawn and detached from the syringe. The syringe is filled with air and reattached to the needle.

The bevel of the needle is directed toward the upper end of a clean glass slide, and its contents are squirted onto the slide with the needle close to the slide. The slides should be marked with patient identification number, puncture site, and fixation technique. The material is expelled on two to four glass slides, spread with another glass slide placed over it, and then the two slides are pulled apart (Fig. 28-15). Half the slides are air dried for May-Grünwald-Giemsa stain and the other half of the slides are ethanol fixed for staining with hematoxylin-erythrosin or Papanicolaou. For quick staining, hematoxylin eosin–Harris staining is used. Wet

fixation in 95% ethanol requires immediate fixation while the samples are still wet. This is necessary to preserve the cellular features needed for microscopic interpretation, because even minimal air drying of the sample alters cellular features. Cells become swollen and lose details important for correct microscopic diagnosis. The time for ethanol fixation is approximately 1 hour, but a shorter fixation time can also be sufficient. Slides that are air dried or ethanol fixed have to be so marked for proper staining.

Benign or normal cells with fixation artifacts can mimic malignant cells on light microscopy (Fig. 28-16). When air-dried areas are observed during the smearing of the material on the slide, it is better to let the slide completely air dry for May-Grünwald-Giemsa stain to prevent ethanol fixation artifacts, which can make microscopic diagnosis impossible.

During the smearing of the sample on the slide one has to apply very little pressure with the hand. Note that cells from malignant tumors are often very vulnerable to pressure. Hard smearing can completely destroy cytologic material (Fig. 28-17, *A*) and make interpretation impossible. Even normal cells, for example, from lymph nodes and bone marrow, are very vulnerable to pressure, whereas other cells from gastrointestinal epithelium, breast, thyroid, pancreas, and prostate are much more resistant. One has to

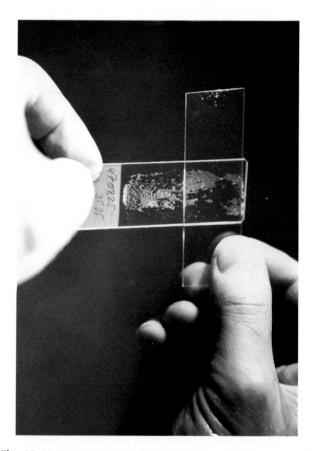

Fig. 28-15 The smearing technique. The second slide is placed over the first, and the two are pulled apart.

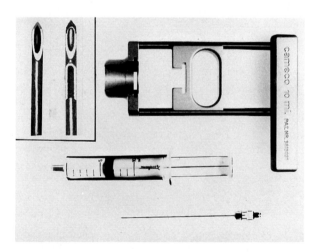

Fig. 28-14 CAMECO syringe pistol for 10-ml disposable syringes. Spinal needle of Westcott with the notched or unnotched needle stylet *(insert)*.

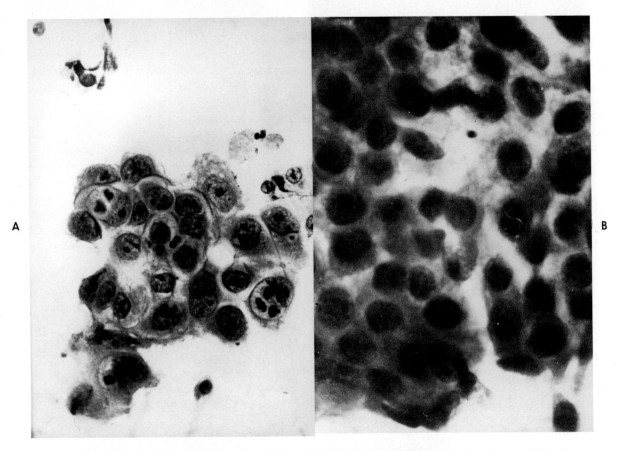

Fig. 28-16 A, An epithelial cancer cell group of well-smeared and well-fixed (ethanol) material. Note the distinct nuclear border, nucleoli, distinct cytoplasm, and inflammatory cell phagocytosis by cancer cells. **B,** Ethanol fixation artifacts. Note the unsharp cell borders and mostly indistinct nuclear morphology. The cells often become swollen and benign or normal cells can mimic malignant cells (H&E, ×80).

strive to attain properly smeared thin cell spreads of monolayer specimens. (Fig. 28-17, *B*). Sometimes different errors can be seen together on the same slide, for example, the combination of hard smearing and late wet fixation in 95% ethanol (Fig. 28-17, *C*). Thus initial macroscopic examination can help to decide if the smears are satisfactory or unsatisfactory.

If the volume of the specimen seems too great for the slide, one can tilt the slide and remove blood that flows to the low side with absorbent tissue. Cystic fluid is collected and enriched with centrifugation or a filter technique. A second aspiration toward the cyst bed—if such is still visible—is sometimes required.

When FNAC is satisfactory and obtained samples are sufficient, the cytologic diagnosis sometimes can be definitive and equivalent to histopathologic diagnosis. Mostly, cytologic examination can differentiate inflammatory conditions from tumors, benign from malignant tumors, and cancer from sarcomas, lymphomas, and carcinoids (Fig. 28-18).

In a small percentage of cases, light microscopic exam-

ination cannot differentiate cancer from lymphomas or sarcomas.

In this situation a further FNAC may be performed, and a cell suspension in HANK's saline solution (Fig. 28-19) is made for preparation of additional cytologic specimens for immunocytologic staining by centrifugation and fixation of glass slides in 96% alcohol. Several immunocytochemical methods have been developed to demonstrate cellular antigens in epithelium, soft and lymphoid tissues, endocrine cells, and other sites. The number of glass slides prepared should be the same as the number of antibodies to be tested. In recent years the use of monoclonal antibodies has increased the sensitivity of the technique.

One can perform additional aspirations for diagnostic electron microscopy. In the case of small round cell malignancies, ultrastructural examination has proved to be of special value, that is, in the distinction of metastatic rhabdomyosarcoma and malignant melanoma, poorly differentiated leiomyosarcoma, neuroblastoma, or sometimes carcinoid tumors versus malignant lymphomas.

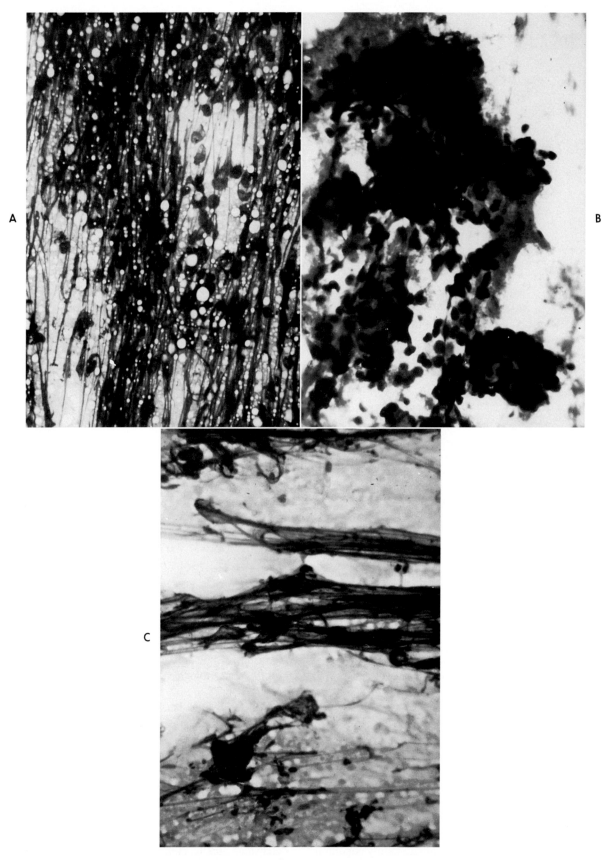

Fig. 28-17 Examples of smearing artifacts, **A,** Hard smearing. The cytologic material is completely destroyed, which makes diagnostic interpretation impossible. May-Grünwald-Giemsa stain, ×80). **B,** Thick smearing. Too much material on one glass slide leads to multilayer cell distribution, which can also make microscopic diagnosis impossible (H&E stain, ×80). **C,** The different errors together on the same glass slide. Here there is combination of hard smearing and late wet fixation in 95% ethanol (H&E stain, ×80).

For electron microscopy the needle containing the aspirate is flushed through with 2% glutaraldehyde in 0.1 mol/L sucrose-cacodylate buffer, pH 7.4, and the aspirated material is immediately ejected into a small glass tube, sealed at one end with a lens paper and unwaxed dental floss, which act as a filter during fixation. This small glass tube is put in a glass vial (Fig. 28-20). The paper filter with aspirates is used for further preparation and embedding for electron microscopy.

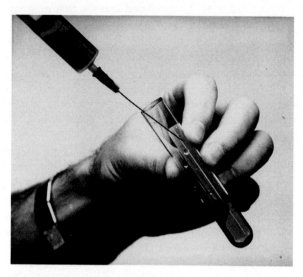

Fig. 28-19 Aspiration technique for immunocytologic staining. Preparation of cell suspension in HANK's saline solution. After the needle content has been injected into the fluid, the needle is repeatedly flushed to remove additional cells.

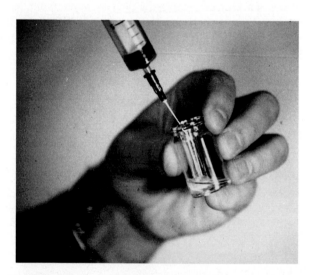

Fig. 28-20 Aspiration technique for diagnostic electron microscopy. Fixation of aspirates in 2% glutaraldehyde and preparation of cell sampling on paper filter. Aspirated material is ejected into a small glass tube and sealed at one end with a lens paper and unwaxed dental floss, which act as a filter during filtration.

A

B

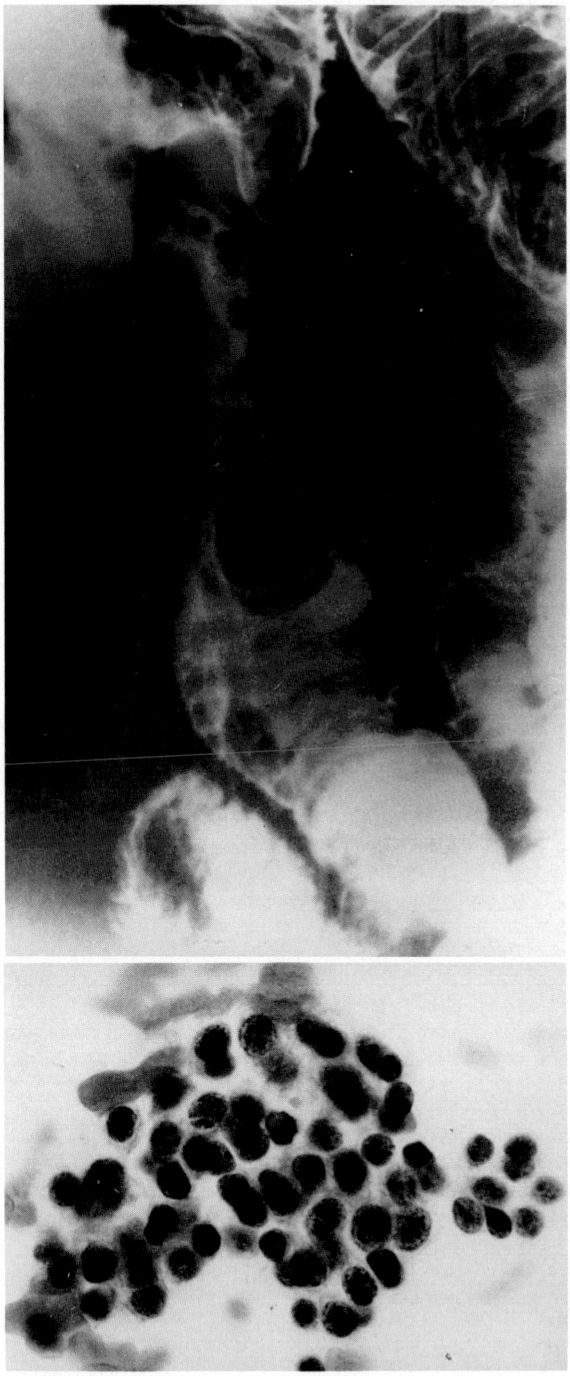

Fig. 28-18 Small-bowel carcinoid. **A,** Small bowel enteroclysis demonstrates polypoid lesion in distal part of ileum. Percutaneous biopsy was performed guided by the barium examination. **B,** Fine-needle aspirate from the same patient. Monolayer of monomorph cells with indistinct cytoplasm and nuclei. "Light-and-dark cell" appearance (H&E stain ×500).

COMPLICATIONS OF FINE-NEEDLE ASPIRATION CYTOLOGY

Fine-needle aspiration of abdominal masses has been found to be a safe and accurate procedure with a very low complication rate.[29] Intraperitoneal hemorrhage or hematoma, bacteremia, peritonitis, and fistulas are extremely rare in patients with normal general immunity. Very close collaboration with cytologists can reduce the risk of complications to a minimum by making a single aspiration pass and then waiting for the cytologist's answer. Ferrucci et al.[30] and Kidd et al.[31] have found that the first pass supplies adequate material in 75% of cases.

Cutaneous needle-tract seeding after percutaneous fine-needle aspiration is an unusual complication. The incidence is unknown, but was estimated at 1 in 21,000 procedures in Smith's study,[32] for an incidence of 0.005%. He found only three cases of needle-tract seeding in more than 63,000 transabdominal fine-needle aspirations. One of these was a patient with pancreatic carcinoma. A few other reported cases were in patients with cecal carcinoma,[33] hepatocellular carcinoma, bronchogenic carcinoma, and renal carcinoma.[34-37] Probably the risk for cutaneous tumor cell seeding increases when the tumors are extremely cellular, undifferentiated, or anaplastic. For highly malignant tumors, it may be wise to remove the needle tract during the subsequent surgical treatment.[38,39] To our knowledge there are no reports published concerning hemorrhage or cutaneous needle-tract seeding after FNAC of small bowel. A fatal outcome has been reported in four cases of abdominal FNAC among 63,108 cases, for an incidence of 0.006% or approximately 1 in 15,000. In three patients, hemorrhage occurred after the FNAC, and one patient developed hemorrhagic pancreatitis after FNAC of a pancreas mass.[32]

Riska and Friman[40] reported a fatal outcome in one patient with liver cirrhosis and hepatoma after FNAC from hemorrhage. Another patient developed necrotizing pancreatitis after FNAC of the pancreas.

To minimize any risk of hemorrhage, the patient's coagulation status should be examined before FNAC.

FNAC is a safe means of obtaining a morphologic tumor diagnosis. Cytologic diagnosis is teamwork and requires close collaboration among radiologists, cytologists, and clinicians.

ACKNOWLEDGMENTS

This work was supported by grants from the University of Lund Research Funds.
We are very grateful to Jenny and Michael Pettersson for designing figures and photographs, and to Birgitta Carlén for help with electron microscopy.

REFERENCES

1. Shiner M: Small bowel biopsy. In Bockus HL, ed: *Gastroenterology*, ed 3, Philadelphia, 1976, WB Saunders.
2. Mee AS, Burke M, Vallon AG et al: Small bowel biopsy for malabsorption: comparison of the diagnostic adequacy of endoscopic forceps and capsule biopsy specimens, *Br Med J* 291:769, 1985.
3. Achkar E, Carey WD, Petras R et al: Comparison of suction capsule and endoscopic biopsy of small bowel mucosa, *Gastrointest Endosc* 32:278, 1986.
4. Maksimak M: A rapid, safe small bowel biopsy technique in children, *Gastrointest Endosc* 37:358, 1991.
5. Saverymutta SH, Sabbat J, Burke M, Maxwell JD: Impact of endoscopic duodenal biopsy on the detection of small intestine villous atrophy, *Postgrad Med J* 67:47, 1991.
6. Vierin Y, Barbet JP, Saglio O et al: Giardia intestinalis et biopsie du grêle pour retard de croissance, *Arch Fr Pediatr* 45:374, 1991.
7. Carter TR, Cooper PH, Petri WA Jr et al: Pneumocystis carinii infection of the small intestine in a patient with acquired immune deficiency syndrome, *Am J Clin Pathol* 89:679, 1988.
8. Rene E, Marche C, Chevalier T et al: Cytomegalovirus colitis in patients with acquired immunodeficiency syndrome, *Dig Dis Sci* 33:741, 1988.
9. Rijpstra AC, Canning EU, van Ketel RJ et al: Use of light microscopy to diagnose small intestinal microsporidiosis in patients with AIDS, *J Infect Dis* 157:827, 1988.
10. Sachs MK, Dickinson GM: Intestinal infections in patients with AIDS, *Postgrad Med* 85:309, 1989.
11. Schofield JB, Lindley RP, Harcourt-Webster JN: Biopsy pathology of HIV-infection: experience at St Stephen's Hospital, London, *Histopathology* 14:277, 1989.
12. Carlén B, Willén R: Inflammatory fibroid polyp of the ileum: case report, *Acta Chir Scand* 154:325, 1988.
13. Johnstone JM, Morson BC: Inflammatory fibroid polyp of the gastrointestinal tract, *Histopathology* 2:349, 1978.
14. Coletta U, Sturgill BC: Isolated xanthomatosis of the small bowel, *Hum Pathol* 16:422, 1985.
15. Arce Salinas CA, Delgado Toledano MA, Larraza Hernandez O et al: Whipple's disease: a case report and review of the literature, *Rev Gastroenterol Mex* 55:231, 1990.
16. Wilson KH, Blitchington R, Frothingham R, Wilson JA: Phylogeny of the Whipple's disease–associated bacterium, *Lancet* 24:338, 474, 1991.
17. Winberg CD, Rose ME, Rappaport H: Whipple's disease of the lung, *Am J Med* 65:873, 1978.
18. Lou T, Teplitz C: Malakoplakia: pathogenesis and ultrastructural morphogenesis: a problem of altered macrophage (phagolysosomal) response, *Hum Pathol* 5:191, 1974.
19. Perez-Atayde A, Lack E, Katz AJ: Intestinal malakoplakia in childhood: case report and review of literature, *Pediatr Pathol* 1:337, 1983.
20. Stanton MJ, Maxted W: Malacoplakia: a study of the literature and current concepts of pathogenesis, diagnosis and treatment, *J Urol* 125:139, 1981.
21. Willén R, Stendahl U, Willén H, Tropé C: Malacoplakia of the cervix and corpus uteri: a light microscopic and x-ray microprobe analysis of a case, *Int J Gynecol Pathol* 2:201, 1983.
22. Brandt LJ, Davidoff A, Bernstein LH et al: Small intestinal involvement in Waldenström's macroglobulinemia. Case report and review of the literature, *Dig Dis Sci* 26:179, 1981.
23. Appelman HD: Smooth muscle tumors of the gastrointestinal tract. What we know now that Stoud didn't know, *Am J Surg Pathol* 10:83, 1986.
24. Miettinen M: Gastrointestinal stromal tumors. An immunohistochemical study of cellular differentiation, *Am J Clin Pathol* 89:601, 1988.
25. Pike AM, Lloyd RV, Appelman HD: Cell markers in gastrointestinal stromal tumors, *Hum Pathol* 19:830, 1988.
26. Saul SH, Rast ML, Brooks JJ: The immunohistochemistry of gastrointestinal stromal tumors, *Am J Surg Pathol* 11:464, 1987.
27. Weiss RA, Mackay B: Malignant smooth muscle tumours of the gastrointestinal tract: an ultrastructural study of 20 cases, *Ultrastruct Path* 2:231, 1981.

28. Fernö M, Baldetorp B, Åkerman M: Flow cytometric DNA ploidy analysis of soft tissue sarcomas. A comparative study of pre-operative fine needle aspirate and post-operative fresh tissue and archival material. *Anal Quant Cytol Histol* 12:251, 1990.

29. Livraghi T, Damascelli B, Lombardi C, Spagnoli I: Risk in fine-needle abdominal biopsy, *J Clin Ultrasound* 11:77, 1983.

30. Ferrucci JT, Wittenberg J, Mueller PR, et al: Diagnosis of abdominal malignancy by radiologic fine-needle aspiration biopsy, *AJR* 134:323, 1980.

31. Kidd F, Freeny PC, Bartha MM: Single pass fine-needle aspiration biopsy, *AJR* 133:333, 1979.

32. Smith EH: The hazards of fine-needle aspiration biopsy, *Ultrasound Med Biol* 10:629, 1984.

33. Persson M: Implantation metastases after fine-needle biopsy from a carcinoma of the caecum, *Ugeskr Laeger* 147:880, 1985.

34. Bush WH Jr, Burnett LL, Gibbons RP: Needle tract seeding of renal cell carcinoma, *AJR* 129:725, 1977.

35. Moloo Z, Finley RJ, Lefcoe MS et al: Possible spread of bronchogenic carcinoma to the chest wall after a transthoracic fine needle aspiration biopsy: a case report, *Acta Cytol* 29:167, 1985.

36. Sakuari M, Seki K, Okamura J, Kuroda C: Needle tract implantation of hepatocellular carcinoma after percutaneous liver biopsy, *Am J Surg Pathol* 7:191, 1983.

37. Shenoy PD, Lakhkar BN, Ghosh MK, Patil UD: Cutaneous seeding of renal carcinoma by Chiba needle aspiration biopsy. Case report, *Acta Radiol* 32:50, 1991.

38. Bergenfeldt M, Genell S, Lindholm K et al: Needle-tract seeding after percutaneous fine-needle biopsy of pancreatic carcinoma, *Acta Chir Scand* 154:77, 1988.

39. Ryd W, Hagmar B, Eriksson O: Local tumour cell seeding by fine-needle aspiration biopsy: a semiquantitative study, *Acta Pathol Microbiol Immunol Scand,* 91:17, 1983.

40. Riska H, Friman C: Fatality after fine-needle aspiration biopsy of liver (letter), *Br Med J* 1:517, 1975.

29 Idiopathic Inflammatory Disease of the Large and Small Bowel

RUEDI F. THOENI

Today the examination of the colon relies on the barium enema, fiberoptic endoscopy, and, more recently, computed tomography (CT). To evaluate the small bowel, barium examination is still the most frequently used method. Recently, however, a small bowel endoscope has been introduced. Its use and indications are not yet sufficiently documented for final conclusions on its place in the armamentarium of tests to be performed for idiopathic inflammatory small bowel disease. While CT is also frequently used to assess complications of Crohn's disease, magnetic resonance imaging (MRI) has not established itself in the evaluation of inflammatory bowel disease for the colon or small bowel because of limited spatial resolution, artifacts resulting from breathing and peristalsis, and lack of a good oral and rectal contrast agent. In the past few years, ultrasound has been used to demonstrate inflammatory changes in the bowel such as wall thickening with or without abscesses, and scintigraphy with indium 111–labeled leukocytes has been used to assess activity of idiopathic inflammatory bowel disease, particularly for follow-up of patients undergoing treatment.

TECHNIQUES AND INDICATIONS FOR FLUOROSCOPIC EXAMINATIONS IN LARGE AND SMALL BOWEL
Plain films of the abdomen
Large bowel

Plain films of the abdomen can provide useful information in patients with inflammatory bowel disease. One study showed that, based on plain films, colitis was diagnosed or strongly suggested in 45% of the patients in the study.[1] A combination of increased thickness of the colonic wall, irregularity of the mucosal surface, and absence of stool in these areas can suggest colitis (Fig. 29-1). Ischemic changes may present in a similar fashion, but the extent of the abnormal bowel segments follows the distribution of a major artery, which is different from inflammatory colitis (e.g., rectal involvement is rare in ischemic disease).

The stool pattern in normal bowel is different from that in patients with colitis: the amount of feces is usually large but varies widely and is seen either throughout the colon or limited to the right side. Rarely, an empty colon is seen in a patient without colonic cleansing. In patients with inflammatory bowel disease, however, feces do not accumulate next to inflamed mucosa, and increased peristalsis moves fecal material to distal segments of the colon. Several studies have shown that the proximal limit of feces can indicate the extent of active inflammatory colonic lesions.[2,3]

In one study of 100 children with inflammatory bowel disease,[4] plain film abnormalities were seen in 73% (76% with Crohn's disease and 72% with ulcerative colitis) and in 20% of 50 matched controls. No correlation between the barium enema and the plain film was obtained because all patients had undergone a colonic preparation. An abnormal stool pattern was found in 47% and an abnormal gas pattern in 38% of these 100 children. In 9% of these children, other findings such as hepatosplenomegaly, bony abnormalities, or renal calculi were found.

Although plain films are not a reliable indicator of the presence or extent of inflammatory bowel disease, careful analysis of abdominal films obtained for screening may pro-

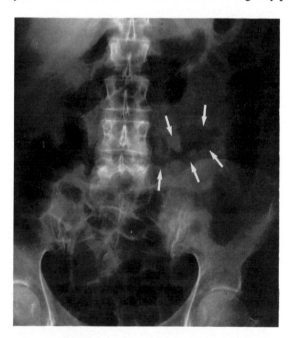

Fig. 29-1 This plain film shows thumbprinting *(arrows)* in the transverse colon due to pseudomembranous colitis. The colon is devoid of stool in the absence of colonic cleansing.

vide useful information. This is particularly important in patients with nonspecific symptoms such as decreased growth rate or vague abdominal pain in children. The use of plain films to detect toxic megacolon is discussed in the section on complications in ulcerative colitis.

Small bowel

Plain films of the abdomen taken before a radiologic examination of the small bowel are useful to determine whether a patient is adequately prepared and to exclude the presence of barium remaining from previous barium examination. Plain films also help to decide the best radiographic method for evaluating patients with suspected small bowel disease (e.g., a patient with distention of only proximal bowel loops would be examined best with enteroclysis, whereas a patient with distention of the entire small bowel could benefit from retrograde examination). An upright film will show whether a large amount of fluid is present in stomach or small bowel loops and should be aspirated before a radiographic small bowel examination. However, fluid content in stomach and small bowel also can be visualized during initial fluoroscopy. Furthermore, free intraperitoneal air, displacement of bowel loops by a mass, and calcifications can be demonstrated.

Barium examinations
Large bowel

Many gastroenterologists hesitate to use barium enema examinations in patients with inflammatory bowel disease because of fear of perforation and toxic megacolon.[5-7] Thus far, however, no investigation has conclusively shown that toxic megacolon was caused by a barium enema examination.[8-10] While there is some suggestion that vigorous bowel preparation or antispasmodic drugs (morphine and similar drugs) may cause toxic dilation,[8,11,12] Welin and Welin[13] recommended the use of atropine during double-contrast barium enema examination without apparent ill effect. Bacteremia has been said to occur in up to 12% of patients with lower intestinal lesions,[14] but another study has questioned this conclusion.[15] Bacteremia also has been found after sigmoidoscopy and colonoscopy. Given these conflicting results, the risk of bacteremia is a contraindication to a double-contrast barium enema examination in patients with inflammatory bowel disease.

Before a barium enema examination is requested for a patient suspected of having inflammatory bowel disease, several factors must be considered: the overall condition of the patient, the severity of the acute inflammatory disease, the information that can be gained from the radiographic procedure, and the relevance of this information to patient care and prognosis. In many instances the barium enema examination is unnecessary because the diagnosis can be made with the help of sigmoidoscopy with biopsy, laboratory tests, and histology of the biopsy specimen. However, in patients who have been treated with steroid enemas or

in whom the rectum and sigmoid colon are spared by the inflammatory process, barium enema examination may establish the presence and extent of disease, which are important prognostic indicators.[16]

No study has reliably compared the single-contrast barium enema examination with the double-contrast technique in patients with inflammatory bowel disease. There is no doubt, however, that whereas both methods detect severe disease, the double-contrast method is superior in detecting superficial mucosal lesions and early changes and can therefore detect the extent of disease more accurately than the single-contrast method.[17-21] Both methods produce similar colonic pressures for given colonic diameters, as shown in the canine model,[22] and the double-contrast method may therefore be used in all patients for whom a barium enema examination is feasible, except in patients with suspected fistulization, which is better demonstrated by a single-contrast technique.

The double-contrast barium enema can be performed by the standard method. However, care must be taken not to overdistend the large bowel and to administer the air slowly to avoid cramping. Patients are subjected to a 24- to 48-hour liquid diet, and water enemas are administered in the evening before the barium enema examination and in the morning before the radiographic procedure. No additives should be used in the water enema. We prefer not to use any laxatives, although some authors have suggested the use of mild laxatives such as mineral oil or bisacodyl.[23] A preliminary film of the abdomen should always be obtained to exclude the presence of a toxic megacolon and to assess the fecal residue. Often the number of overhead films can be limited to three or four (prone, upright, left lateral decubitus, and angled rectal films) to minimize patient discomfort. A postevacuation film is not useful in the double-contrast technique.

Glucagon or Buscopan should be used to relax spasms because patients with inflammatory bowel disease often have difficulty with introduction and retention of the barium and air during the examination.[24] In these patients, we administer 1 mg of glucagon intravenously. Glucagon also should be used for a peroral pneumocolon examination, which may clarify involvement of the terminal ileum in examinations where there is a lack of reflux into the small bowel, or help to further evaluate the right colon. In cases of pancolitis, involvement of the terminal ileum can be used to distinguish ulcerative colitis from granulomatous colitis.[25]

An alternative approach to the standard double-contrast barium enema technique is the instant enema described by Young[26] and Bartram and Walmsley.[27] This method consists of a double-contrast examination without bowel preparation and is based on the fact that fecal residue does not adhere to inflamed mucosa. This technique is useful in ulcerative colitis, which usually starts distally and involves the colon in continuity to its full extent. Fecal material will therefore be limited to the area of the large bowel proximal to the inflammation. This method is indicated to assess the severity and extent of disease in patients with proctitis established by sigmoidoscopy, although the widespread availability of flexible sigmoidoscopy is diminishing the role of the instant barium enema, and to determine the type of disease in patients with acute attacks of colitis in whom a standard double-contrast barium enema is not advisable. The instant enema has been used in patients with acute attacks for over 13 years without complications and can be considered safe.[28] The contraindications to an instant enema in patients with long-standing inflammatory bowel disease are the same as for the standard double-contrast technique, but in addition it should not be used in patients with long-standing inflammatory disease and a high risk of carcinoma or in patients with Crohn's disease, because skip lesions may be obscured.

The single-contrast barium enema demonstrates severe and long-standing disease and permits the presence of edema in the bowel wall to be determined on the basis of the postevacuation film. In the evaluation of idiopathic inflammatory bowel disease, the single-contrast method is best used for patients with suspected bowel obstruction and for patients with suspected fistulas or sinus tracts.

Small bowel

For the radiographic evaluation of the small bowel in patients with suspected idiopathic inflammatory bowel disease, several types of barium studies are available: the conventional small bowel follow-through, the dedicated small bowel follow-through, and enteroclysis. If only the terminal ileum needs to be evaluated, the peroral pneumocolon is the examination of choice. The retrograde small bowel examination, which consists of introducing barium per rectum and refluxing it through the ileocecal valve into the small bowel, has been abandoned today. Enteroclysis can achieve better results and is more comfortable than the retrograde technique. Furthermore, it does not suffer from barium-filled large bowel overlapping small bowel loops. The reader may like to compare the techniques discussed in the following sections with those described in Chapters 25, 26, and 27.

SMALL BOWEL FOLLOW-THROUGH

The small bowel follow-through (SBFT) as practiced in most radiology departments in the United States is usually performed after an upper gastrointestinal series (UGI) in patients who were fasting, starting after a light supper on the day before the examination. In our department and many other institutions, a single-contrast phase (450 ml Barosperse; Mallinckrodt, Inc., St. Louis, Mo.) follows the double-contrast study in the UGI tract. The initial 200 ml of barium given for the small bowel follow-through should be diluted (about 20% to 24% weight per volume [w/v]) to decrease the high-density effect from the double-contrast of

the UGI. The remaining amount of barium is given as a 40% to 45% w/v suspension. Once this is completed, a series of overhead films is obtained at half-hour or 1-hour intervals until the terminal ileum is reached, and at that point compression views of this area are taken. Additional compression views are obtained whenever an overhead film shows an area of abnormality.

DEDICATED SMALL BOWEL FOLLOW-THROUGH

A dedicated SBFT is a barium examination of the small bowel that is completely separate from the UGI. Again, the patient is asked to fast after midnight on the day before the examination. Barium (at UCSF we use approximately 600 to 900 ml Barosperse) is administered orally, and the patient is brought to the fluoroscopy room where compression views are obtained to visualize the proximal jejunal loops. The patient is then placed on the right side to encourage emptying of the stomach, and more spot films are subsequently taken in the area of the mid and distal jejunum. Overhead films are taken at 15 minutes, 30 minutes, 1 hour, 1½ hours, and 2 hours. Delayed films are taken at hourly intervals thereafter until the terminal ileum is reached. Frequent fluoroscopy is performed to assess progression of the barium column, and compression spot films are obtained of the distal small bowel as well. Finally, compression views of the terminal ileum are taken. Careful compression of individual small bowel loops is essential for optimal visualization of the extent of inflammatory changes and to demonstrate fistulas and sinus tracts.

If the transit time of barium through the small bowel is slow, medication such as metoclopramide (Reglan; A.H. Robbins, Richmond, Va) can be given to accelerate the passage.[29] In some instances, a large amount of barium, iced water, or an addition of Gastrografin to the barium is used to achieve a similar goal.[30]

A double-contrast small bowel follow-through can be performed by introducing an effervescent agent that produces approximately 750 to 1000 ml of gas, once the barium has reached the cecum. After administration of the effervescent agent, the patient is placed in the left lateral or left oblique and slight Trendelenburg position so that gas can enter the duodenum and small bowel. In most instances, gas reaches the distal ileum in 5 to 10 minutes. Radiographs with slight compression in the different areas of the small bowel can then be obtained. In one published series, this technique produced good double-contrast images in 43%, with good distension of the small bowel loops in 96% and separation of loops in 85% of all patients.[31]

ENTEROCLYSIS OR SMALL BOWEL ENEMA

Enteroclysis is described in Chapter 26.[32-35]

PERORAL PNEUMOCOLON

The peroral pneumocolon (PPC) technique is used to evaluate the distal ileum. To perform a PPC, the patient is given a colonic preparation similar to the one for a barium enema, and barium is administered orally. When barium has reached the right and proximal transverse colon, air or carbon dioxide is insufflated per rectum and refluxed into the distal small bowel.[36-40] Glucagon or Buscopan can be used for relaxing the ileocecal valve. Multiple spot films are obtained of the terminal ileum and distal ileal loops.

ILEOSTOMY STUDY

For patients with protracted or long-standing ulcerative colitis and occasionally for patients with Crohn's disease, several surgical procedures may be performed: ileorectal anastomosis, permanent ileostomy, continent ileostomy (Koch pouch), or ileoanal pouch.[40] Currently, only the permanent ileostomy or the ileoanal pouch procedure is used. The ileoanal pouch is performed in two steps. The first step consists of a total colectomy and creation of an ileoanal pouch with proximal ileostomy and distal muco-cutaneous fistula (double-loop ileostomy), and the second step is take-down of the ileostomy. Therefore the radiologist is asked to perform an ileostomy enema or a pouchogram (antegrade or retrograde filling of the ileoanal pouch) to assess the condition of the pouch before take-down of the ileostomy or to detect the presence or absence of complications with the pouch such as leakage or abscess formation.

The patient with a permanent ileostomy is best examined with a retrograde study. If a patient is suspected of having an ileostomy dysfunction, the state of the ileostomy stoma and the distal loop should be examined perorally as well as in a retrograde fashion. If the ileostomy functions normally, the distal prestomal ileum does not distend. In patients with ileostomy dysfunction, copious uncontrolled discharge from the ileostomy may be seen. For the retrograde study, a soft catheter should be carefully inserted into the stoma. A cone-shaped device or a catheter with inflatable balloon can be used. If the balloon is inflated inside the stoma, placement and inflation should be performed with great care under fluoroscopic control with contrast to prevent distention of the balloon in an abnormal loop, which could lead to disruption of the stoma or perforation of the distal loop. We initially introduce the catheter into the distal small bowel loop, place the ileostomy bag over the tube, and attach the ileostomy bag to the skin with stoma adhesive. When the procedure is performed in this fashion, the tube can be removed after the procedure is finished and the ileostomy bag clamped without any spillage of bowel content, barium, or hypaque.

To assess the postoperative ileostomy, radiographs of the stoma in profile must be obtained for good detailed views of the distal loop and its passage through the anterior abdominal wall. These views should be taken before and after evacuation. In patients with stoma dysfunction, the diameter of the distal ileum does not reduce significantly after evacuation.[41]

In patients with ileoanal anastomosis, the pouch is best distended with a retrograde study through the ileostomy because hypaque can distend the pouch adequately without loss of contrast agent through the ileostomy. The pouchogram can also be performed per rectum, but distention of the ileoanal loop cannot be controlled completely. The pouchogram permits assessment of the presence or absence of pouchitis, abscess, fistulas, or sinus tracts. The rectal approach may be beneficial in patients with a suspected fistula or sinus tract near the ileoanal anastomosis. In patients with obstructive symptoms after take-down of the ileostomy, an enteroclysis or retrograde study via the anal route often demonstrates a stenosis at the site of reanastomosis of the proximal and distal small bowel loops. This area of narrowing may be caused by postsurgical edema or may represent a true stricture.

Indications for barium examinations
Large bowel

The barium enema examination is indicated in patients with inflammatory bowel disease when it is necessary to establish the presence or extent of colitis, to determine the type of inflammatory disease, or to assess complications resulting from inflammatory bowel disease (e.g., carcinoma, stricture formation, and fistulas). It is contraindicated in patients with toxic megacolon because of the risk of perforation and bacteremia,[42] in patients with a suspected perforation, and immediately after endoscopy with a deep biopsy.[43,44] It is advisable to delay the examination in patients with a fulminant attack, as evidenced by profuse diarrhea, high fever, and constant rectal bleeding, until the disease has reached a less active stage.

Small bowel

Many studies of the small bowel are ordered when there is only a slight suspicion of small bowel disease.[45] A study in 1029 patients showed that the detection rate of small bowel abnormality was much higher if the radiographic examination was obtained for high suspicion of a small bowel pathologic state (14.2%) than for low suspicion (4.9%).[46] Therefore small bowel studies should be obtained only for clear indications.

Enteroclysis should be used as the primary method in most instances, but particularly for intermittent or partial small bowel obstruction and Crohn's disease, if surgery is planned, or if the full extent of disease needs to be assessed. As enteroclysis can demonstrate fine mucosal abnormality with greater ease than any other radiographic small bowel examination, it is particularly helpful in patients with superficial disease. It should be the first investigation in patients with suspected tumors; with occult GI bleeding; when a UGI, barium enema, and an upper and lower endoscopy have been negative; and in any patient with suspected obstructive symptoms after abdominal surgery, particularly in those with pelvic surgery. In any equivocal result with dedicated SBFT, or in any patient with a negative SBFT but strong clinical suspicion for inflammatory disease of the small bowel, enteroclysis is the best method to ascertain normality or pathologic changes.

Because of the ease of performance and the low level of cost and radiation, the dedicated SBFT should be the initial radiographic test in any patient in whom there is a low suspicion for small bowel disease. It should be the method of choice in patients with suspected complete or near-complete bowel obstruction if presurgical delineation of the cause of obstruction is deemed necessary, particularly if the point of obstruction is high in the jejunum. It should be used for patients who may have Crohn's disease[47] unless the diagnosis is already established or surgery is planned, and in patients who refuse placement of a nasogastric tube. Recommendations on ways to improve the oral SBFT have been published[31,48,49] and should help to render the conventional methods more reliable. The double-contrast SBFT using effervescent agents, which achieves adequate distention in 96%,[31] represents a considerable improvement on the conventional SBFT.

PPC or the retrograde small bowel examination should be reserved for evaluation of the terminal ileum and right colon if further clarification of these areas is needed. It can directly follow an SBFT or an enteroclysis.

To achieve such a tailored small bowel examination, clinicians and radiologists need to be educated on the proper use of the different methods based on their accuracies, advantages, disadvantages, costs, and radiation exposures. This is a process that needs some time. At UCSF, the use of enteroclysis has increased from 7% of all small bowel examinations during 1985 to over 50% in 1992. This is a reflection of the increasing enthusiasm of the clinicians for enteroclysis and increasing familiarity with enteroclysis among residents, fellows, and faculty.

PATHOLOGY

Experimental studies in the small bowel of dogs with dysentery toxin can be used as a general model for changes caused by inflammatory disease in the gut.[50] Shock leads to vasoconstriction of arterioles, microaggregation of erythrocytes and platelets, and impaired venous return.[50] Finally, hyaline thrombi form in arterioles and venules, causing necrosis and hemorrhage along with consumption of the coagulation factors and blockage of the reticuloendothelial system.[51] In the wall of the small bowel the toxins lead initially to hyperemia along with thickening of the mucosa and exudation into the submucosa, creating a subepithelial space by lifting up the epithelium. With the formation of hyaline thrombi, more fluid accumulates in the subepithelial space, resulting in necrosis of the tip of the villi in the small bowel. In the subacute stages the necrotic portion is cleared away mechanically or by leukocytes, and ulcers develop that may extend to the muscularis. In the chronic stages, secondary proliferation of the mucosa starts at the edges of the ulcer and leads to pseudopolyposis.

Involvement of the colonic mucosa varies according to the different types of inflammatory bowel disease.[52] Some of them show more fibrin exudate than others. We can distinguish the following four major groups of inflammatory changes:

1. A superficial, uniform reaction involving large portions of the mucosa with deep ulcerations in the subacute stages. Small clusters of inflammatory cells accumulate around the bases of the mucosal crypts and may become crypt abscesses. The ulcer may reach the muscularis, but the disease is largely limited to the mucosa and submucosa. Examples of this type are ulcerative colitis, ischemic bowel disease, shigellosis, salmonellosis, and amebiasis[53,54] (Figs. 29-2 to 29-5).

2. A superficial process with marked mucosal swelling and severe necrosis of the mucosa and submucosa. Fibrinous exudates predominate in the gross and histologic picture. This type is seen in pseudomembranous colitis, uremia, and, occasionally, severe ischemic disease.[55-58]

3. A transmural process with a nonuniform, patchy distribution and deep longitudinal and transverse ulcers and fissures that may lead to fistulas, sinus tracts, or perforation.[59-61] This process typically is seen in patients with Crohn's colitis, tuberculosis, amebiasis, schistosomiasis, or blastomycosis, but severe ischemic disease also may present in a similar fashion (Figs. 29-6 to 29-9).

4. A proliferative phase with an abundance of pseudopolyps, filiform polyps, and mucosal bridging that is associated with total or partial healing in the area surrounding the proliferation.[62-64]

The wide spectrum of inflammatory bowel diseases ranges from mild mucosal edema to severe, deep ulceration. Possible reactions to colonic injury may include superficial ulcers or deep, penetrating ulcers, fistulas, pericolonic abscesses, and sinus tracts, depending on the stage and severity of the disease. While superficial changes usually are caused by ulcerative colitis or infectious diseases related to bacteria or viruses, transmural processes are caused by Crohn's colitis, tuberculosis, or mycotic or amebic infections. Bacterial, amebic, and mycotic inflammations may present as superficial or transmural processes.[65] Even in Crohn's disease and ulcerative colitis, an overlapping spectrum exists in which approximately 15% of cases of ulcerative colitis resemble granulomatous colitis or vice versa.[53,65-67] The number of equivocal cases from double-contrast barium enema is similar to the number found pathologically,[19] but this number is much higher for the single-contrast technique.[53,66] The pathologist's diagnosis depends on the biopsy site or the location from which a colonic specimen is resected. Variability in the severity and depth of the involvement of the colon may result in contradictory pathologic reports, with Crohn's disease diagnosed

Text continued on p. 573.

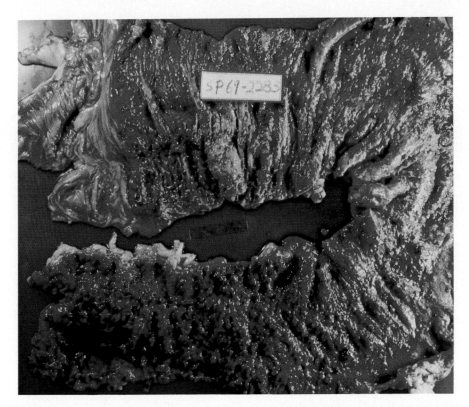

Fig. 29-2 Macroscopic view of a resected colonic segment afflicted by chronic ulcerative colitis shows diffuse granularity of mucosa.
Courtesy of Dr. Caroline Montgomery.

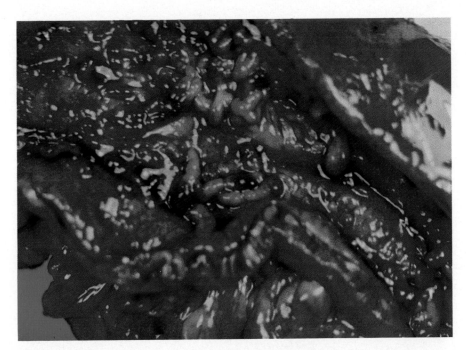

Fig. 29-3 Macroscopic view of severe chronic ulcerative colitis demonstrates deep serpiginous ulcerations and nodular mucosal remnants (pseudopolyps). The mucosa is diffusely erythematous.
Courtesy of Dr. Caroline Montgomery.

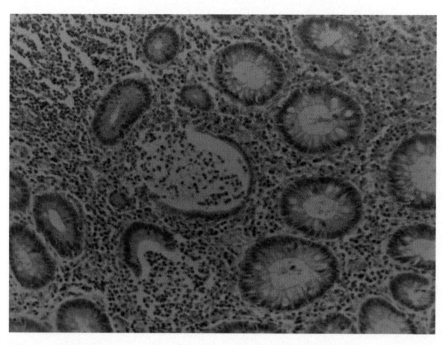

Fig. 29-4 Rectal biopsy from patient with chronic ulcerative colitis demonstrates mucosal atrophy, cellular infiltration, and crypt abscesses.
Courtesy of Dr. Caroline Montgomery.

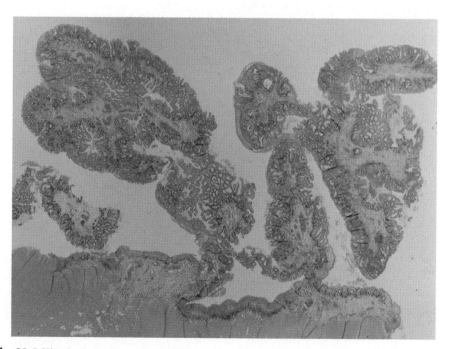

Fig. 29-5 Histologic section through filiform polyp from patient with ulcerative colitis.
Courtesy of Dr. Caroline Montgomery.

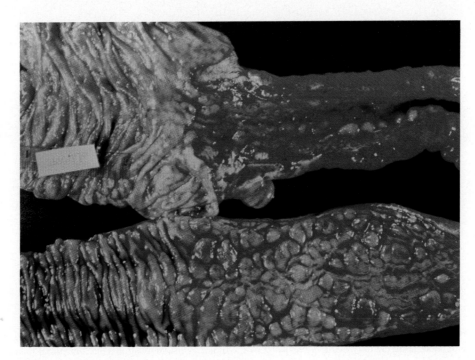

Fig. 29-6 Resected specimen of colon from a patient with Crohn's colitis shows cobblestoning resulting from protuberant mucosa between linear transverse and longitudinal ulcers. Normal colon is seen on the left side.
Courtesy of Dr. Caroline Montgomery.

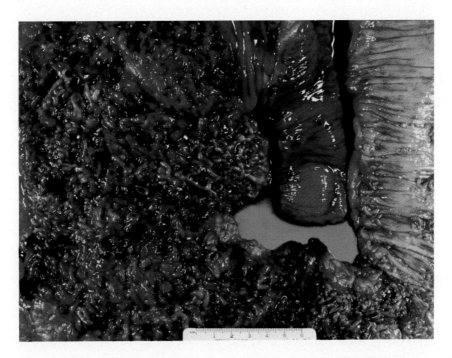

Fig. 29-7 En face view of resected segment of colon from a patient with granulomatous colitis demonstrates filiform polyposis on the left side and normal colon on the right side.
Courtesy of Dr. Caroline Montgomery.

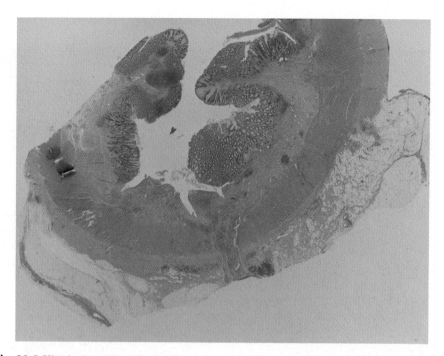

Fig. 29-8 Histologic section of colon from a patient with granulomatous colitis shows a deep fissure penetrating the muscularis in the center of the figure. This demonstrates the transmural nature of this disease.
Courtesy of Dr. Caroline Montgomery.

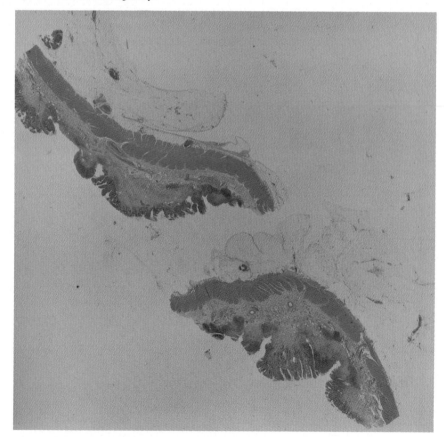

Fig. 29-9 Linear ulcers are seen on this histologic section of colon from a patient with Crohn's disease.
Courtesy of Dr. Caroline Montgomery.

in an area of deep involvement and ulcerative colitis diagnosed in an area of more superficial disease.

The clinical picture and the presence or absence of fistulas and sinus tracts help to distinguish ulcerative from granulomatous colitis. Histologic features are very useful in distinguishing between the two idiopathic inflammatory diseases of the colon: transmural disease is present in 98% of cases of Crohn's disease but only 28% of cases of ulcerative colitis; serositis is present in 96% of cases of Crohn's disease but only 27% of cases of ulcerative colitis; lymphedema is present in 80% of cases of Crohn's disease but only 7% of cases of ulcerative colitis; and crypt abscesses are present in only 56% of Crohn's disease but in 95% of cases of ulcerative colitis.[52] Granulomas, if present, are diagnostic of Crohn's disease but are found in only a small percentage of patients.[68]

ULCERATIVE COLITIS
Pathologic and clinical features

The cause of ulcerative colitis is not known, and most of the histologic features may be seen in other inflammatory diseases. Among the etiologic hypotheses, infectious agents, endotoxins, destructive enzymes, psychogenic mechanisms, metabolic defects, genetic disorders, and immunologic mechanisms have been mentioned.[69] The diagnosis of chronic ulcerative colitis is therefore based on a combination of clinical and histologic criteria.

Cryptitis or crypt abscesses of the crypts of Lieberkühn, considered the primary lesions (see Fig. 29-3), are not initially visible to the naked eye but, through lateral extension and coalescence, may form ulcerations that reach the lamina propria and undermine the mucosa on three sides, resulting in excrescences or so-called pseudopolyps[54] (see Fig. 29-3). At this intermediate stage, the ulcers have a collar-button or flask-shaped configuration. With lateral extension, this configuration is lost, and large areas of bowel wall muscle may be almost completely denuded. The ulcerations and pseudopolyps are visible during endoscopy. Almost immediately, a reparative phase starts, with granulation tissue formation and some minimal fibrosis. If the disease lasts over a long period, the muscularis mucosa hypertrophies. Minimal cellular infiltration of the muscularis propria may be seen. While all of these features are nonspecific and can be seen in shigellosis, gonococcal colitis, and amebiasis, a large number of crypt abscesses, profuse development of granulation tissue, and chronicity of the inflammatory process are more typical of ulcerative colitis than of infectious types of colitis. The disease is intermittently acute, and in the quiescent phase the mucosa may heal but appear atrophic with decreased numbers of crypts, distorted mucosal architecture, and thickening of the lamina propria.

All of these histopathologic features are important for understanding the clinical features. Bleeding results from highly vascular and friable granulation tissue, as well as ulcerations and hyperemia, and the diarrhea results from damage that impairs the ability of the mucosa to perform its major function: reabsorption of water and sodium.[70] Because the disease is limited to the mucosa and submucosa, perforation, fistulization, peritoneal signs, and sharply localized pains are usually absent. Even though foreshortening and apparent stricture formation are seen on radiographs, they may be reversible, because often these findings result from muscular hypertrophy of the bowel wall and spasm.[71,72] If the disease is more severe, it may extend beyond the mucosa and submucosa into the muscularis or to the serosa. In instances where the disease reaches the serosa, the colon may perforate or, if the disease arrests before perforation, severe fibrosis may ensue. The apparent deep involvement of all areas of the bowel wall when the muscularis is affected explains the dilation of the colon, by loss of motor tone, in cases of toxic megacolon. Because the disease may vary in the depth of involvement of the bowel wall, be limited to the rectosigmoid, or even be segmental, besides showing diffuse uniform colonic inflammation, the clinical picture varies greatly, sometimes with dramatic segmented dilatation.

The greatest incidence of chronic ulcerative colitis is in the second, third, and fourth decades of life. The condition is more common in white women.[73] The disease may vary greatly in its severity, course, and prognosis. The onset may be insidious or abrupt, and minor bleeding is often thought to be related to hemorrhoids rather than to colitis. Most patients (60% to 70%) afflicted with this inflammatory process have intermittent disease, with complete remission between attacks.[74] A few patients have one acute episode and then remain symptom free for years, and a few have a protracted course without remission.

Severe disease has a higher mortality and is more prone to treatment failure.[74] One study[75] correlated mortality from ulcerative colitis and Crohn's disease with various occupations of men and women in England and Wales. It found no significant correlation in women. For men, high mortality from idiopathic inflammatory bowel disease tended to be associated with physically less demanding work, sedentary occupations, and type of work that is done indoors, whereas a relatively low mortality was found in men who did physical work, farmed, or had lower social status. The best parameters for assessing the severity of the disease are clinical signs and symptoms. Large volumes of diarrhea indicate severe disease. Also, large amounts of blood in the stool, a low hematocrit value, hypoalbuminemia, sustained high fever, and a markedly elevated erythrocyte sedimentation rate all indicate severe disease.

Radiographic assessment of the extent of the disease by itself is not a reliable indicator of the severity of the disease. Diffuse colitis may be seen in up to 20% of patients with mild colitis; however, diffuse disease with deep ulcerations points to a severe form of inflammatory bowel disease. Foreshortening and narrowing of the colon are indicators of chronicity rather than of severity of disease. Arbitrarily, three degrees of severity are distinguished: mild, moderate, and severe or fulminant. The mild form is characterized by less than four bowel movements a day and the absence of systemic signs.[76] This disease is most commonly seen in segmental distribution but may involve the entire colon.[77] Diarrhea may or may not be present. Most patients (about 60%)[78] afflicted with ulcerative colitis fall into this category. Anorectal complications and extracolonic manifestations such as arthritis or erythema nodosum may occur. Moderate disease is seen in about 25% of ulcerative colitis patients.[78] Symptoms are usually more intense, and diarrhea is a major manifestation. Severe or fulminant ulcerative colitis occurs in about 15% of all patients.[78] The symptoms are usually sudden in onset, with profuse diarrhea and constant rectal bleeding. Weakness, fever, and weight loss are usually profound. Hypoalbuminemia is characteristic in this group.

Endoscopic findings

Initially, loss of the vascular pattern, mild hyperemia, fine granularity, petechiae, and minor bleeding after wiping with a cotton swab are seen. These changes may progress to increased friability, edema, mucopurulent exudate, pseudopolyps, and ulcers with spontaneous bleeding.

In later stages, polyps (inflammatory polyps and hyperplastic or filiform polyps), strictures, and in long-standing disease, mucosal abnormalities suggesting malignancy may be identified. After treatment in mild to moderately severe cases, complete healing with grossly normal-appearing mucosal surface may be present. However, in many instances, granularity remains because of a healing process with granulation tissue covering the muscularis propria. Detailed descriptions of the endoscopic appearance of the mucosa are found in the next section, which compares endoscopic and radiographic findings.

Extraintestinal manifestations

In addition to toxic megacolon,[11,12,79-82] stricture formation,[83] carcinoma,[83-86] uveitis, arthritis, pyoderma gangrenosum, erythema nodosum, and stomatitis may be seen in patients with ulcerative colitis.[87-89] Other pathologic changes related to ulcerative colitis are hematologic abnormalities, hepatobiliary disease, thromboembolic disease, renal disease, and amyloidosis.[90-95] Also, musculoskeletal abnormalities consisting of sacroiliitis and spondylitis (incidence 1% to 26%) and peripheral arthritis (incidence 10% to 12%) are encountered.[96,97]

Liver disease

Approximately 7% of patients with ulcerative colitis have some type of liver abnormality. Some of the abnormalities found in the livers of these patients include fatty liver (40%), postnecrotic liver cirrhosis, pericholangitis (35% to 50%)[98] sclerosing cholangitis (50% of all cases have chronic ulcerative colitis[99]) cholangiocarcinoma (1% to 4%),[99-103] and chronic active hepatitis (1% to 13%).[102] The cause of these changes remains unknown. It is possible that genetic factors predispose patients to both ulcerative colitis and liver pathology. There may be an association of pericholangitis and sclerosing cholangitis because many patients who had biopsies before full-blown sclerosing cholangitis developed had evidence of pericholangitis. The frequency of sclerosing cholangitis in patients with ulcerative colitis has been recognized very readily since the introduction of endoscopic retrograde cholangiopancreatography (ERCP). Patients with sclerosing cholangitis frequently present with recurrent attacks of jaundice, right upper quadrant pain, fever, leukocytosis, and evidence of cholostasis. Unfortunately, many of these patients with primary sclerosing cholangitis develop secondary biliary cirrhosis.

Carcinoma of the biliary ducts is found more frequently in patients with ulcerative colitis than in the general population and almost exclusively in patients with sclerosing cholangitis or pericholangitis. These lesions are often multicentric, and radiographically it is sometimes quite difficult to differentiate cholangiocarcinoma from sclerosing cholangitis or pericholangitis in this patient population.

Fatty infiltration may be caused by malnutrition and protein depletion resulting from chronic illness; it is reversible. Hepatomegaly may be the only finding on physical examination. The cause of chronic active hepatitis in patients with ulcerative colitis is unclear. It may be non-A, non-B hepatitis related to blood transfusions, an autoimmune hepatitis, or extension of disease from the pericholangitis. These patients may present with hepatic failure or portal hypertension. In general, medical therapy of ulcerative colitis does not modify the outcome of the associated hepatobiliary disease.

Hematologic disease

Among the hematologic abnormalities of patients with ulcerative colitis, chronic iron deficiency anemia caused by chronic colonic blood loss is most common. Some patients have a hemolytic anemia, which may be drug related. Leukocytosis and thrombocytosis, usually without associated coagulation defects, are also encountered. Deficiencies in coagulation factors may complicate ulcerative colitis and lead to colonic blood loss through increased prothrombin time. This hypothrombinemia probably results from advanced liver disease, malnutrition, and prolonged antibiotic use. A serious complication from ulcerative colitis is thromboembolic disease, which can be fatal. This complication usually occurs in patients with severe acute ulcerative colitis or after colectomy. In one study[104] deep venous thrombosis or pulmonary embolism occurred in 60% of patients with ulcerative colitis.

Musculoskeletal disease

Arthritic changes may be found in 10% to 24% of adults or children with ulcerative colitis.[105] The serologic tests for rheumatoid factor are negative. Symptoms from arthritis usually occur at the same time as ulcerative colitis, but occasionally they predate the bowel disease. Arthritis associated with ulcerative colitis tends to be migratory, monoarticular, or pauciarticular. Large joints are more often involved than small joints. Arthritis in ulcerative colitis is gradually progressive but independent of the bowel disease activity. Ankylosing spondylitis is seen in ulcerative colitis with a frequency 10 to 20 times that of the general population. It usually precedes the onset of bowel disease. It does not regress and often progresses even after remission of the colitis or colectomy. The incidence of sacroiliitis is even higher than that for ankylosing spondylitis. Osteoporosis probably caused by long-standing steroid therapy, may also be seen.[106]

Ocular disease

Ocular lesions may be present in 3% to 10% of patients with ulcerative colitis.[107] The pathogenesis is not clearly understood, but a systemic immune process may be the underlying cause. It often is associated with peripheral arthritis, erythema nodosum, and aphthous ulcers of the oral cavity. Iritis and uveitis are the most common pathologic changes, and in 50% of the cases the disease is bilateral. Other ocular changes include episcleritis, interstitial keratitis, retinitis, and retrobulbar neuritis.

Dermatologic disease

In 2% to 4% of patients with ulcerative colitis, dermatologic changes are seen, mainly erythema nodosum.[108] This disorder is more common in women. Erythema nodosum should always lead to consideration of inflammatory bowel disease. Erythema nodosum typically occurs as a single episode but may recur in up to 20% of patients. Pyoderma gangrenosum is seen in 2% to 5%. These lesions usually appear during an active bout of colitis. Persistent severe pyoderma gangrenosum is a reason for total colectomy. Aphthous ulcers are seen in about 4% and are most frequent during severe acute attacks. They may be complicated by candidiasis. Occasionally, patients with ulcerative colitis develop drug reactions (maculopapular eruptions, urticaria, or erythema multiforme).

Renal disease

Renal disease is seen in the form of pyelonephritis and nephrolithiasis or urolithiasis. The cause of pyelonephritis is unclear. Dehydration may be a cause. Stone formation may be caused by dehydration, immobility (calcium mobilization), and changes in the composition of the urine pre-

disposing to stone formation. In rare instances, glomerulonephritis may develop.

Radiographic features

Ulcerative colitis predominantly involves the large bowel. Therefore we will discuss the radiographic findings in the colon first. A separate paragraph is dedicated to the radiographic findings of ulcerative colitis in the small bowel, which are distinctly different from those found in Crohn's disease.

Large bowel
GRANULARITY

The early findings of ulcerative colitis that may be detected by radiography are changes in the mucosa related to edema and granulation tissue. With sigmoidoscopy, submucosal inflammation and edema are evidenced by impaired visibility of the ramifying submucosal vessels and irregularity of the mucosa caused by subepithelial infiltration, edema, and crypt abscesses. These changes give the mucosa a granular appearance[17,23,109-111] (Fig. 29-10; see Fig. 29-2).

The mucosa loses its even texture and reveals an amorphous or finely stippled appearance through the barium coating of the mucosa—so-called granularity[21] (Fig. 29-11). Occasionally, these superficial changes cannot be seen, and the only sign of inflammation in the rectosigmoid colon is the blunting of the normally acute angles of the rectal valves (seen in 43% of cases of ulcerative colitis).[112] When the disease progresses, superficial erosions develop that give the mucosa a stippled appearance (Figs. 29-12 and 29-13). In the chronic stages of ulcerative colitis, granula-

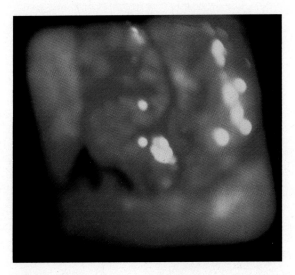

Fig. 29-10 Endoscopic view of acute ulcerative colitis in the transverse colon shows granularity and friability with several bleeding ulcerations.
Courtesy of Dr. John P. Cello.

tion tissue develops that creates a coarse granular mucosal appearance (Figs. 29-14 and 29-15).

The single-contrast barium enema examination is unable to demonstrate the early mucosal changes of ulcerative colitis but may demonstrate inflammatory disease by the failure of the colonic walls to collapse and by abnormal fold patterns on the postevacuation film. These signs are not very reliable.[112] Normal innominate lines demonstrated by the single-contrast method may be confused with irregularities caused by inflammatory disease.

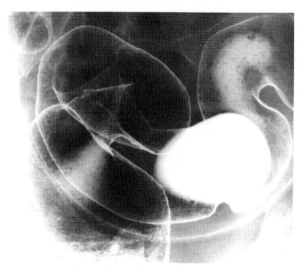

Fig. 29-11 Granularity caused by edema and hypervascularity in a patient with early ulcerative colitis.

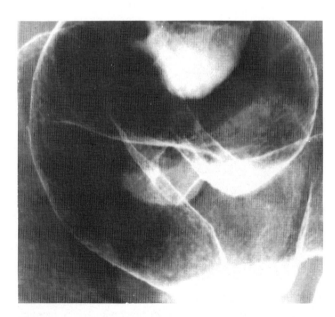

Fig. 29-12 Diffuse granularity of mucosa along with slight stippling related to superficial erosions.

ULCERATION

If an acute attack is superimposed on chronic disease, the mucosa shows multiple ill-defined collections of barium on a background of coarse granularity (Fig. 29-16). These collections represent mucosal ulcerations. Ulcers are often seen best in profile because they are linear in relation to the tenial attachment and undermine the mucosa.[27] They usually have a T-shaped, flask-shaped, or "collar-button" appearance. The term *collar-button ulcer* most frequently is used to describe an acute exacerbation of a chronic stage of ulcerative colitis.[113] These collections are not diagnostic of this idiopathic inflammatory bowel disease, however, because they can be seen in cases of tuberculous colitis, shigellosis, amebiasis, and ischemic colitis.[114] Occasionally, double tracking can be seen, which is caused by the submucosal extension of ulcers. The demonstration of ulcerations by radiographic means is important because these changes indicate clinically and pathologically severe disease.

In the chronic stages, collar-button ulcers may also be demonstrated by the single-contrast method because they are best demonstrated in profile.

POLYPOID CHANGES

Polypoid changes may be seen at any stage of ulcerative colitis. They may occur in the acute stage from ulcerations

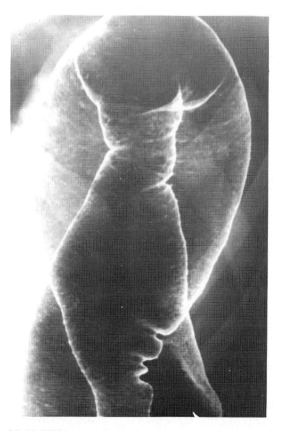

Fig. 29-13 Diffuse granularity is present along with several linear ulcers.

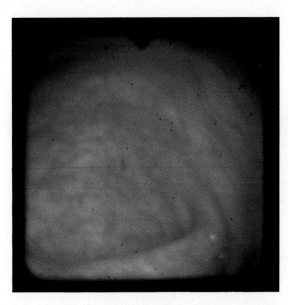

Fig. 29-14 Endoscopic picture of chronic ulcerative colitis reveals coarsely granular and erythematous mucosa. Lumen is straight and narrow.
Courtesy of Dr. John P. Cello.

or in the healed and quiescent stage from mucosal tags.[27,115]

Pseudopolyps. In the acute severe attack, islands of inflamed edematous mucosa are seen between denuded and ulcerated areas. These islands are called *pseudopolyps* because they represent the actual mucosa and not polypoid protuberances. Occasionally, granulation tissue covering the denuded muscularis propria in patients with ulcerative colitis becomes coarse and mimics pseudopolyps. In Crohn's disease the pseudopolyps are larger and more irregular than in ulcerative colitis and are usually referred to as "cobblestoning." If the mucosal ulcerations of Crohn's disease are extensive, small rounded pseudopolyps similar to the ones in ulcerative colitis are evident.

Inflammatory polyps. Inflammatory polyps are areas of inflamed mucosa resulting in polypoid elevations on a background of granular mucosa in patients with low-grade activity of inflammatory bowel disease (Fig. 29-17). These inflammatory polyps may be sessile, or they may have a stalk.

Postinflammatory polyps. Postinflammatory polyps are seen in the quiescent phase of ulcerative colitis. They are seen in 10% to 20% of patients with ulcerative colitis.[83]

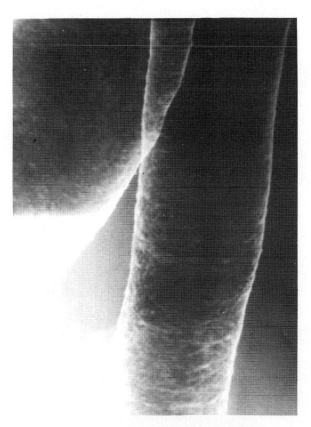

Fig. 29-15 Coarse granularity of colonic mucosa with multiple erosions in a patient with chronic ulcerative colitis.

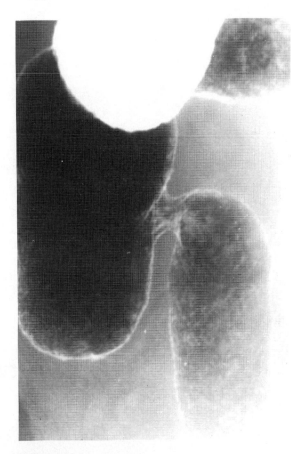

Fig. 29-16 Blotchy collections of barium represent ulcers superimposed on diffuse granularity. The terminal ileum shows similar changes ("backwash ileitis").

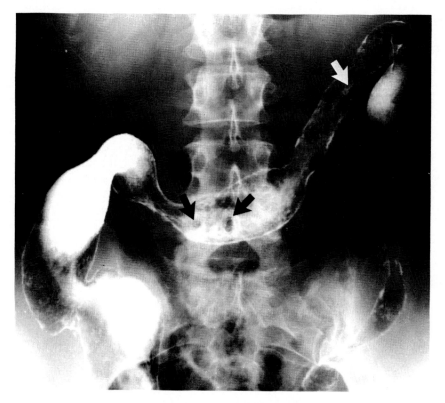

Fig. 29-17 Tubular foreshortened colon in a patient with chronic ulcerative colitis. Several inflammatory polyps *(arrows)* are shown. The underlying mucosa is coarse and granular.

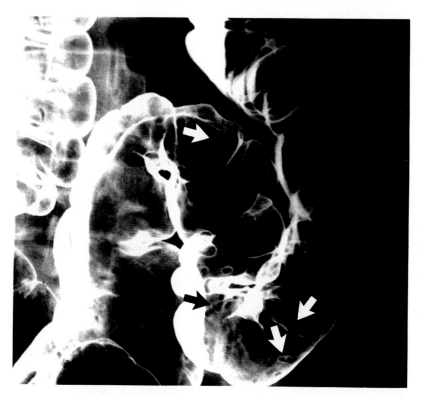

Fig. 29-18 Multiple filiform polyps *(arrows)*. This patient is in quiescent phase of chronic ulcerative colitis.

They may be composed of normal or inflamed mucosa and are thought to have originated from elevations of the mucosa during severe undermining by deep ulcers. Epithelization prevents these mucosal lesions from fusing in a reparative phase, thus creating a multitude of polypoid changes such as sessile nodules, long fingerlike outgrowths called *filiform polyps,* or mucosal bridges created by the fusion of two islands over an area of reepithelization[62-64] (Fig. 29-18; see Fig. 29-5).

The exact significance of these lesions is not yet known. Filiform polyps have been found particularly in patients with long-standing treatment with sulfasalazine. These polyps may represent excessive repair. All of these different polyps are usually easily recognized as being related to the inflammatory bowel disease if other changes indicate ulcerative colitis. Occasionally, however, these polyps are present in a normal-appearing colon[116] and are the only indicators of previous inflammatory disease. Inflammatory polyps on a background of normal mucosa may easily be confused with adenomas or even small carcinomas, and only endoscopy with biopsy can give the correct diagnosis. Adenomas have stalks more often than do inflammatory polyps and occur only rarely in patients with ulcerative colitis. Occasionally, postinflammatory polyps assume a bushlike appearance that mimics a villous adenoma.

In some cases, giant inflammatory polyps may develop that produce symptoms independent of inflammatory disease such as abdominal pain because of their large size, acute bleeding, or chronic blood loss.[117] These giant polyps are more frequent in Crohn's disease than ulcerative colitis, occur usually in the transverse colon, and may mimic a colonic neoplasm. Occasionally, giant inflammatory polyps lead to obstruction that necessitates surgical intervention.[118]

SECONDARY CHANGES

Secondary changes can be easily seen on single- and double-contrast barium enema examinations. The main signs of chronic disease are foreshortening of the colon, lack of haustration, and tubular narrowing of the colon that gives the large bowel the appearance of a garden hose or stovepipe (Fig. 29-19). The narrowing of the colon is often related to spasms and smooth muscle hypertrophy, which explains the fact that a colon that was severely affected by ulcerative colitis may revert to normal. Occasionally, fibrosis and stricture formation develop (Fig. 29-20), and the changes seen in such chronic cases generally are not reversible.

Another secondary sign is increased presacral space (Fig. 29-21). This sign is often used as an indicator of inflammatory disease that involves the rectum. A presacral space measuring 1 cm or less is considered normal.[119] The width of the presacral space usually is inversely related to the width of the rectum. A correlation has been demonstrated between the duration of inflammatory disease and increased

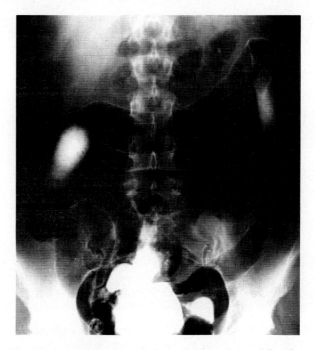

Fig. 29-19 Tubular colon with lack of haustration and foreshortening in a patient with chronic ulcerative colitis. The terminal ileum is very dilated because of backwash ileitis.

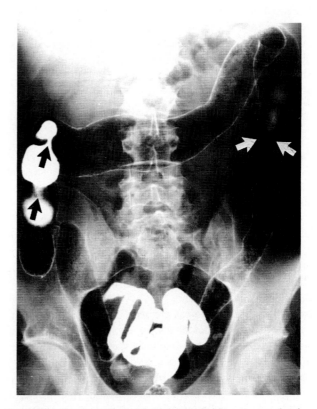

Fig. 29-20 Tubular colon with backwash ileitis and several strictures *(arrows)* as manifestations of the chronic form of ulcerative colitis.

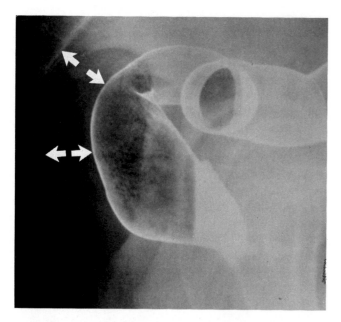

Fig. 29-21 Increased presacral space *(arrows)* in patient with chronic ulcerative colitis and granular pattern in rectum. Note also the limited distention of rectum and rectosigmoid colon.

widths of the presacral space, but no correlation has been found between the severity of the disease in the rectum and increased width of the presacral space.[120,121] Generally, reversal to a normal presacral space is rare. Many other conditions, such as retroperitoneal fibrosis, pelvic lipomatosis, obesity, lymphogranuloma venereum, radiation colitis, and abscesses, may enlarge the presacral space.

Small bowel

TERMINAL ILEUM

In the large majority of patients with ulcerative colitis the terminal ileum is normal.[19] In up to 39% the terminal ileum shows atonia, a widely gaping ileocecal valve, and occasional granularity of the mucosa, which represents the so-called backwash ileitis.[66,122-124] The terminal ileum of patients with long-standing ulcerative colitis may be so dilated that it is interpreted as part of the ascending colon with a stricture. In these cases, careful analysis of the radiographs usually reveals the presence of an ileocecal valve. Ulcers in the terminal ileum are not features of backwash ileitis (see Figs. 29-16 and 29-19). Whenever ulcers, thickened folds, and skip areas are seen in the terminal ileum, Crohn's disease, tuberculosis, or *Yersinia* should be considered. The differential diagnosis should also include cathartic colon. If multiple strictures are present, ulcerative colitis may be difficult to differentiate from a cathartic colon with abnormal contractions simulating the strictures found in chronic colitis (see Strictures, under Complications of Ulcerative Colitis).

The terminal ileum usually is abnormal in a patient with long-standing subacute disease. The most exact radiologic method of determining the presence or absence of inflammatory disease of the terminal ileum is by a peroral pneumocolon examination. In patients in whom ulcerative colitis is the diagnosis, enteroclysis is not indicated because the small bowel is never involved beyond the terminal ileum. Enteroclysis should be reserved for patients with an "overlapping spectrum" of findings that does not permit a definitive diagnosis. The single-contrast method often demonstrates a falsely abnormal terminal ileum based on slight irregularities of the ileal margins.

Accuracy of radiographic examination

With respect to ulcerative colitis, the accuracy of the radiographic examination refers to its ability to show the extent and severity of mucosal disease. Because of the ability of the double-contrast examination to show mucosal surface changes, this method is more accurate in detecting early and mild disease. Because the early manifestations of ulcerative colitis are related to vascular changes along with capillary dilatation and edema that can be detected by endoscopy as changes in the light reflex and vascular pattern, it is not surprising that radiography underestimates the extent of the inflammatory disease. The mucosal surface has to be sufficiently altered to be detected by radiography. This is the major reason why radiography does not detect early disease as accurately as endoscopy. One series shows that in two thirds of the patients examined, inflammatory lesions were found to be more widespread by colonoscopy than by double-contrast radiography.[125]

Endoscopy also underestimates the extent of inflammatory disease if compared with histology. This has been well demonstrated by means of multiple biopsies.[126] The true significance of "histologic colitis" is not known.[110]

Because of these shortcomings of double-contrast enema examinations, it is advisable to talk about "extensive colitis" when radiography detects disease probably extending to the hepatic flexure. This terminology suggests that total colitis is present and consists of radiographically detectable colitis and additional histologic colitis. The radiographic assessment of the true extent of disease is important because long-standing and total colitis are criteria for an increased risk of carcinoma in patients with ulcerative colitis.[86]

Ulcerative colitis can be differentiated from granulomatous colitis in the acute stage because the radiographic features of each disease are most distinct in this phase. Table 29-1 provides useful criteria for the distinction between these two idiopathic inflammatory bowel diseases.

After multiple attacks, remissions, and chronic disease, the typical mucosal patterns are distorted, and distinctions become more difficult. In the acute stages, ulcerative colitis can be distinguished from granulomatous colitis in at

☐ **TABLE 29-1**

Radiographic features of ulcerative, granulomatous, and infectious colitis

Radiographic features	Ulcerative colitis	Granulomatous colitis	Infectious
Granular mucosa	+	−	
Ulcerations			
Small, shallow	−	+	*Yersinia*, Behçet's syndrome, ischemia, tuberculosis, amebiasis, salmonellosis
Confluent, shallow	+	(+)	Amebiasis
Confluent, deep	−	+	Ischemia, amebiasis, tuberculosis, strongyloidiasis
Rectum			
Diffusely involved	+	−	Amebiasis, shigellosis
Patchy distribution	−	+	
Continuity			
Continuous	+	(+)	Shigellosis
Discontinuous	(+)	+	Lymphogranuloma venereum
Stricture			
Symmetric	+	−	Lymphogranuloma venereum (tuberculosis)
Asymmetric	−	+	Ischemia, tuberculosis
Fistulas	−	+	Lymphogranuloma venereum (tuberculosis, ischemia, Behçet's)
Terminal ileum	(+)	+	*Yersinia*, pseudomembranous colitis, tuberculosis
Inflammatory polyp	+	+	Schistosomiasis, colitis cystica profunda (ischemia), strongyloidiasis
Toxic megacolon	+	(+)	Ischemia, amebiasis, (salmonellosis, pseudomembranous colitis)

(), Occurs rarely in that disease.

least 95% of all cases.[23] However, an overlapping spectrum remains, which is estimated to amount to approximately 10% to 15% of cases[17,53,65-67] (Fig. 29-22). This condition is called *indeterminate* or *cross-over* colitis. Confusion is most likely to occur in patients with toxic megacolon or fulminant disease. Some patients diagnosed with ulcerative colitis may be confirmed as having Crohn's disease if they are followed-up for 1 year or longer. Occasionally, diverticular disease in patients with ulcerative colitis can render the radiographic diagnosis difficult.[127]

It was also found in one study that histologically the diagnosis can be made more accurately if the biopsy specimen is obtained during a quiescent phase rather than during acute disease with its nonspecific picture of acute inflammation.[125] The extent of disease is less accurately detected by the single-contrast barium enema examination than by the double-contrast method because of its inability to show minor mucosal surface changes.

For a long time it was believed that the rectum is always and most severely involved in ulcerative colitis.[128,129] Only a few reports mention the occasional lack of rectal involvement as evidenced in radiographs as well as by proctoscopy.[19,27,109] One of the reasons for a low activity of disease in the rectum in patients afflicted with ulcerative colitis is the fact that many of these patients receive steroid enemas before examination.

Complications
Toxic megacolon

One of the most important complications that radiography can detect is the presence of toxic megacolon. Its detection relies on the plain film. Because of the high risk of perforation during a barium enema examination in a patient with toxic megacolon, a preliminary film of the abdomen is mandatory before the examination is begun.

In a review of 200 patients with toxic megacolon, a medical and surgical mortality of 21.5% was found.[6] Suggested precipitating factors include a barium enema examination, endoscopy, the use of opiates and anticholinergic drugs, and progressive metabolic alkalosis.[82,130] However, it has never been conclusively shown that a barium enema examination precipitated or caused toxic megacolon.[8]

Toxic megacolon is best defined as toxic dilatation associated with fulminant colitis. It is based on the clinical status of the patient and radiographic evidence of severe mucosal disease and marked dilatation of the colon. If toxic megacolon is present, the disease has become transmural with neuromuscular degeneration. The most prominent features include smooth muscle destruction and serosal inflammation. The radiographic diagnosis of toxic megacolon is based on colonic dilatation and, more importantly, abnormality of the colonic wall. In general, a diameter of 5.5 to 6.5 cm is considered the upper limit of normal (Fig. 29-

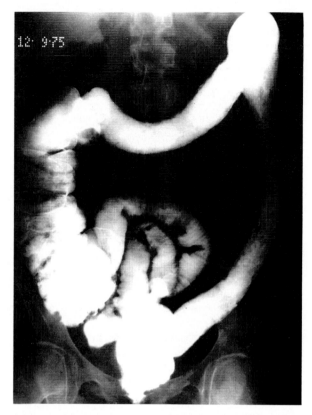

Fig. 29-22 A patient with histologic diagnosis of Crohn's disease shows symmetric narrowing of the colon and multiple pseudopolyps. The right side of the colon appears radiographically to be less severely involved, and the splenic flexure is of a larger caliber than the transverse and descending colons. The rectum is also involved, and the terminal ileum is normal. Based on radiographic appearance, ulcerative colitis is more likely, but a questionable skip area in the splenic flexure favors the diagnosis of Crohn's disease. This case is an example of the overlapping spectrum of idiopathic inflammatory bowel disease.

☐ ETIOLOGY OF TOXIC MEGACOLON ☐

- Ulcerative colitis
- Crohn's disease
- Ischemia
- Pseudomembranous colitis
- *Campylobacter* colitis
- Amebiasis
- Strongyloidiasis
- Bacillary dysentery
- Behçet's syndrome
- Typhoid fever
- Cholera

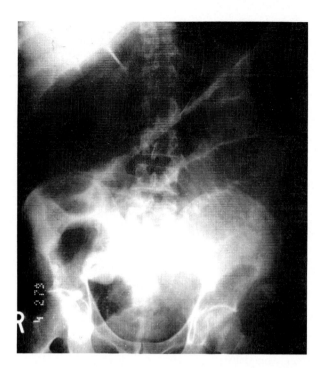

Fig. 29-23 Marked distention of the transverse colon with a diameter larger than 8 cm. The mucosa appears to be normal, indicating that megacolon may be imminent.

23). Often, destruction of mucosa can be inferred on plain films from thinned bowel walls, interrupted by thickened bowel wall caused by subserosal edema and congested mucosa, and mucosal islands that often resemble polyps[131] (Fig. 29-24). Some thumbprint-like impressions on the air column in the early stages of toxic megacolon suggest neuromuscular disorder as well as edema in the bowel wall. While toxic megacolon is most frequently associated with ulcerative colitis, it can be seen in other pathologic conditions (see the box at left).

Perforation

Spontaneous perforation does not occur frequently in ulcerative colitis[132-133] unless toxic megacolon develops. Perforation in toxic megacolon is common and is associated with extremely high morbidity and mortality (44%).[134] It usually is seen in the sigmoid colon during an initial attack.[83] Occasionally, air is seen in the bowel walls, suggesting imminent perforation. In less severe ulcerative colitis perforation is more frequently caused by intervention such as colonoscopy or inflation of a rectal balloon during a barium enema examination in a patient with a severely narrowed rectal pouch.[135]

Strictures

Strictures are seen more frequently in cases of ulcerative colitis than was thought previously (7% to 11% of patients with ulcerative colitis).[83,136] They may be benign or ma-

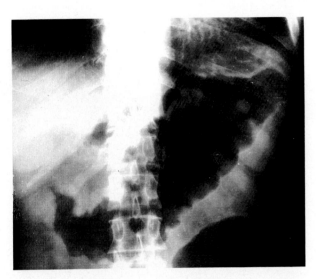

Fig. 29-24 Toxic megacolon in a patient with chronic ulcerative colitis shows thickened edematous bowel wall and several polypoid masses.

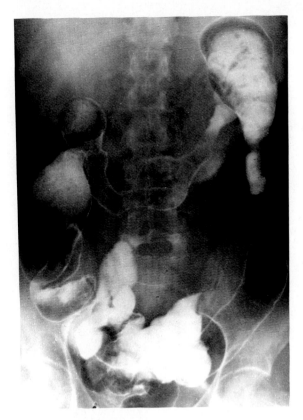

Fig. 29-25 Colon is tubular and shows several areas of narrowing in a patient with chronic laxative abuse. Distinction from ulcerative colitis is difficult without clinical history.

lignant, but the majority are benign.[137] Many strictures are caused by muscular hypertrophy and are potentially reversible. Benign strictures occur only in long-standing and severe cases of ulcerative colitis, and they may be multiple. Occasionally, mucosal dysplasia is found in a stricture. Because of the risk of malignancy in ulcerative colitis, all strictures should be viewed with suspicion, and colonoscopy is indicated in these cases. Benign strictures are smoothly tapering areas of narrowing with a central lumen, whereas malignant strictures may sometimes show irregular narrowing, abrupt edges, overhanging shoulders, and an eccentric lumen.[138] Often the mucosa is markedly irregular.

If multiple strictures are present, ulcerative colitis may be difficult to differentiate from a cathartic colon, with abnormal contractions simulating the strictures found in chronic colitis. A cathartic colon is seen in patients with chronic laxative abuse.[139] Chronic irritation of the mucosa is caused by drugs such as senna, castor oil, bisacodyl, and podophyllum. The radiographic changes found in patients with chronic laxative abuse mimic those of ulcerative colitis, and the mucosa is atrophic, with scattered shallow ulcers, submucosal chronic inflammation, and thickening of the muscularis mucosae. Radiographically, a narrowed colon with a complete lack of haustration is present (Fig. 29-25). The cecum and ascending colon are usually and primarily involved (Fig. 29-26), which is helpful in differentiation from ulcerative colitis, but occasionally diffuse colonic involvement may occur, and the terminal ileum may show superficial ileitis.[140] Often, multiple bizarre contractions are apparent, whereas true strictures are rare but may be seen because of fibrosis and atrophy of the bowel wall. The correct diagnosis can be made only on the basis of the

clinical history, and from endoscopy and biopsy, which may show melanosis.

Malignancy

Epithelial dysplasia is considered a precancerous lesion that occurs in long-standing cases of ulcerative colitis. It may be diagnosed radiographically on the basis of nodularity and irregularity of the mucosa with sharply angular edges. Its detection is an absolute indication for colonoscopy with a biopsy.[141]

As previously mentioned, patients with long-standing disease and total or universal colitis have an increased risk of developing colonic cancer.[86,142-145] However, in one series the observed-to-expected ratio of colorectal cancer was 8 in left-sided ulcerative colitis as compared with 26 in pancolitis.[146] It is therefore important to recognize that while patients with total colitis run a high risk of developing a cancerous lesion, cancer may also be seen in patients with left-sided ulcerative colitis but usually after a greater duration of disease than in pancolitis. In patients with ulcerative colitis confined to the rectum, the risk of developing cancer is the same or minimally increased if compared with the normal population.[147] Colorectal cancer in patients with ulcerative colitis appears to be more often multiple (23%

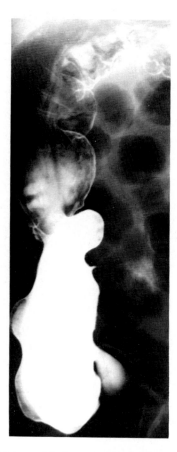

Fig. 29-26 Strictures, tubular narrowing, and pseudosacculations related to asymmetric fibrosis in a patient with a history of chronic senna abuse.

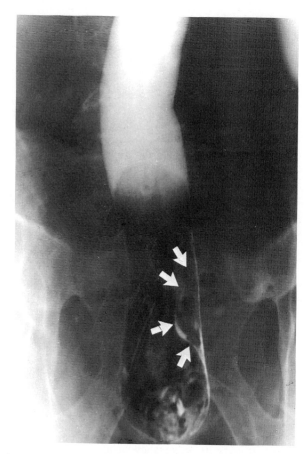

Fig. 29-27 Large plaquelike lesion *(arrows)* in the left lateral rectal wall. The rectum and rectosigmoid colon appear to be narrowed. This patient had had chronic ulcerative colitis for 20 years and now had cancer of the rectum.

to 40%)[84,148,149] and more proximal in location than in the noncolitis population,[150] although a more recent study showed even distribution of cancer in patients with ulcerative colitis, similar to the distribution seen in the general population.[151] The long-term mortality from colitis associated with cancer does not appear to be worse than that for colorectal cancer in the general population,[148] and the risk of developing cancer begins approximately 10 years after the onset of the disease but may be earlier.[84] Thereafter, the risk of cancer increases 10% for every 10 years of the disease.[83,84] In one recent study from England[152] the cumulative probability of developing cancer and severe dysplasia was 4% at 15 years, 7% at 20 years, and 13% at 25 years after onset of ulcerative colitis. These numbers were based on 401 patients who were observed over a period of 22 years. Whether the risk of cancer is higher if the onset of the disease occurs in childhood is debated.[86,146,153] However, regardless of reasons, an early onset of disease is a poor prognostic sign.

The radiographic signs of carcinoma in ulcerative colitis include recognition of mucosal dysplasia based on small plaquelike or nodular, faceted filling defects. Irregularities or nodularity of the mucosa[154] are changes typical of carcinoma of the colon in the general population. The carcinoma in ulcerative colitis is often flat, infiltrating, and difficult to detect because of its plaquelike appearance. Scirrhous carcinoma and annular carcinoma are seen frequently, but polypoid lesions are unusual (Fig. 29-27). Carcinoma associated with a stricture has been seen in 23% to 27% of cases of ulcerative colitis.[86,146,147] Carcinomas that develop in ulcerative colitis tend to be the colloid or mucinous type of neoplasm and usually of high grade. This may be a result of the younger age of the patients rather than the colitis per se. The incidence of lymphomas and leukemia is increased in patients with ulcerative colitis.[155,156] The cause is unclear but is probably multifactorial and involves the immunologic deficiencies present in inflammatory bowel disease, as well as the immunosuppressive treatment used in these patients.

Surgical procedures

For a long time, total colectomy with ileostomy has been the procedure of choice for patients with severe, long-

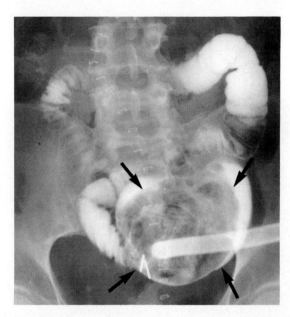

Fig. 29-28 Koch ileostomy. Barium is infused through an irrigation tube or other device, and the ileal pouch with valve for continence is evaluated. In this patient, pouch contained blood clot *(arrows)*.

standing ulcerative colitis. However, because an ileostomy was not a viable or acceptable surgical option for many young patients with active life-styles, other surgical procedures were introduced.

Initially, a total colectomy was performed and an ileorectal anastomosis created. However, this approach has the obvious disadvantage that recurrent or persistent proctitis may occur and, additionally, the patient has to be under constant surveillance for development of cancer in the rectum. These problems led to the development of a continent ileostomy (Koch pouch) after total colectomy. This procedure was successful in some cases, but it is rarely performed today.[157,158] The radiographic appearance of the continent ileostomy has been well described[156] (Fig. 29-28).

More recently, an ileal pouch and ileoanal anastomosis have been used. This procedure consists of mucosal proctectomy and total colectomy with ileoanal anastomosis and ileal pouch immediately above the anastomosis to maintain reservoir function. The reservoir is created from 15 to 20 cm of ileum and may have a side-to-side configuration, a J-shape, or an S-shape[159] (Fig. 29-29). Because of the higher complication rate with S-pouches, most surgeons now favor the J-pouch.

The construction of an ileoanal pouch is a two-step procedure: initially, patients undergo a total colectomy, and an ileal pouch with mucutaneous fistula and a temporary ileostomy are created. The ileal loop is fashioned into a pouch with a stapled blind end, the elbow of the loop is incised, and the opening so created is stapled to the anal verge. The second step consists of take-down of the ileos-

tomy. Before definitive hook-up, most patients are examined radiographically either for a routine checkup or for suspected complications. In these patients, a catheter with an inflatable balloon can be introduced into the ileum (antegrade study) or into the pouch through the anus (retrograde study), a small amount of barium is administered, and the balloon is carefully inflated (Fig. 29-30) (for the technique of this examination, see Ileostomy Study). If the procedure is cautiously performed, no danger of perforation or disruption of the ileostomy exists, and leakage of barium from the stoma is not a problem.

Complications with the J-pouch procedure include pouchitis, leakage, fistula, sinus tract, abscess (Fig. 29-31), and obstruction. Pouchitis is thought to be related to stasis before permanent hook-up and usually resolves spontaneously after ileostomy take-down. Complications with ileostomies include obstruction, ileitis, ileostomy dysfunction, leakage, fistula, sinus tract, or herniation.

CROHN'S DISEASE
Clinical features

The cause of Crohn's disease is unknown but etiologies similar to those in ulcerative colitis have been suggested.[69,160] Crohn's disease is increasing in frequency, and this increase is larger for Crohn's colitis or ileocolitis than for ileitis.[161] The worldwide increase is almost entirely in the young. A study from Scotland showed that in the 1970s, Crohn's disease tripled in frequency.[162] Some of this increase may be a result of increased awareness, but multiple studies appear to indicate that this change is genuine.

Crohn's disease usually occurs in the second to fourth decade of the patient's life, but it may be present at any age.[163] Cases have been reported that demonstrate onset of granulomatous ileocolitis in very early life or extreme old age. Extensive jejunoileitis tends to be more common in younger patients, whereas older patients have more localized regional enteritis. Patients with anorectal disease are affected later in life (mean age, approximately 40 years) and have a shorter duration of symptoms.

Crohn's disease is more common among patients of European origin, particularly among the Jewish population (three to eight times more common in Jews than in non-Jews), and it is consistently more common in whites than in other races. The disease in nonwhite races usually begins at an earlier age and runs a more severe course.[164] A family aggregation has been observed, but the family history often includes relatives with ulcerative colitis as well as Crohn's disease. There are only a few reports of Crohn's disease in husband and wife.[165]

The clinical picture of Crohn's disease may be markedly different from that of ulcerative colitis.[166] Often, patients with granulomatous colitis first seek the help of a physician because of complications related to Crohn's disease such as an anorectal fistula, perirectal sinuses and ab-

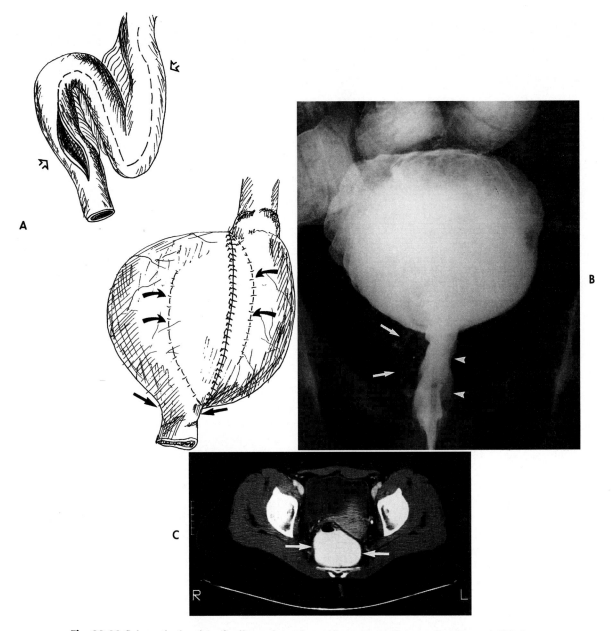

Fig. 29-29 Schematic drawings for ileoanal pouches with corresponding pouchogram and CT. **A,** Schematic drawing of an S-pouch created from an S-shaped loop of ileum resulting in separation of the distal ileal portion from the pouch. **B,** Pouchogram: S-pouch. Note the distal portion of the ileum *(arrowheads),* which is separate from the actual pouch. Complications are more common with this type of procedure. A fistula *(arrows)* is seen in this patient. **C,** CT of S-pouch demonstrating large main pouch *(arrows).*

scesses, intestinal obstruction, or symptoms of abdominal fistulas or abscesses. Often these patients have insidious symptoms (low-grade fever, mild or moderated diarrhea without blood, or mild weight loss and moderate anemia).

In contrast to ulcerative colitis, rectal bleeding is rare in the early stages of Crohn's disease. Bleeding usually occurs in a patient with involvement of the rectum or the rectosigmoid colon. Cramping pain is experienced in the right lower quadrant.[59,166] Often a gradual weight loss is

related to the impaired absorption of bile salts, and anemia may result from the impaired absorption of vitamin B_{12}.[167] In children with Crohn's disease, growth may be markedly stunted for several months before the diagnosis is made. A reduced concentration of conjugated bile salts and increased amounts of unabsorbed irritating bile salts cause steatorrhea and increased diarrhea.

About 10% of patients with Crohn's disease have anal fissures, sinuses, or perirectal abscesses, and 20% to 30%

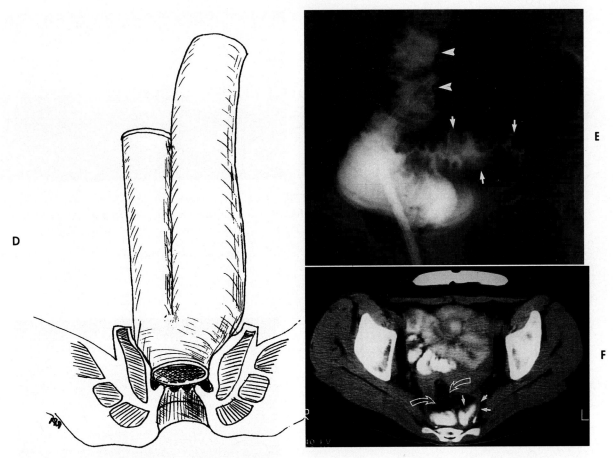

Fig. 29-29, cont'd D, Schematic drawing of J-pouch created from U- or J-shaped ileal loop, which is stapled directly into the anal verge. **E,** Pouchogram: J-pouch. Note the blind-ending stump *(arrows)* and the ileum *(arrowheads)* leading to the remainder of the small bowel. **F,** CT of J-pouch clearly identifies the raphe between the two limbs of the J-pouch. Note the blind-ending stump *(arrows).* The mesentery *(open arrows)* is visible in front of the pouch.
From Thoeni RF et al: *AJR* 154:73, 1990.

have a palpable abdominal mass. Patients often have symptoms of diarrhea for years without being examined for it. Arthritis and skin involvement (erythema nodosum or pyoderma gangrenosum) may be found in another 10%, and these extracolonic manifestations may be the presenting features. Physical examination may reveal a fatigued, pale patient with vague abdominal pain or extreme tenderness in the right lower quadrant. Extremely ill patients appear dehydrated, hypotensive, wasted, and feverish.

Endoscopic findings

Sigmoidoscopy may show a normal rectum in 50% of patients with Crohn's colitis. The transmural process may cause protrusion of islands of mucosa into the lumen or sloughing of mucosa with deep linear and punched-out ulcers. "Skipping" (leaving areas of normal mucosa between severely diseased segments of bowel) and an asymmetric, patchy distribution of the disease are typical. In marked

contrast to ulcerative colitis, the ulcers are deep and form long tracks or clefts between protruding inflamed and edematous mucosal islands ("cobblestoning") (see Figs. 29-6, 29-8, and 29-9). Biopsies may reveal changes similar to those of ulcerative colitis, or lymphoid hyperplasia and noncaseating granulomas, which are nonspecific and can be seen in a large variety of colonic diseases, such as tuberculosis, amebiasis, or fungal infections.

Early changes seen on colonoscopy are hyperemia and edema or sharply edged aphthoid ulcers, which can also be detected by a double-contrast barium enema examination or enteroclysis.[168] The advanced disease shows cobblestoning (Fig. 29-32).

Behçet's syndrome involves the clinical triad of relapsing iritis and painful ulcers of the mouth and genitalia. The skin lesions tend to remit spontaneously and then recur. Other features such as arthralgia and thrombophlebitis have been described in this syndrome, and in some of these pa-

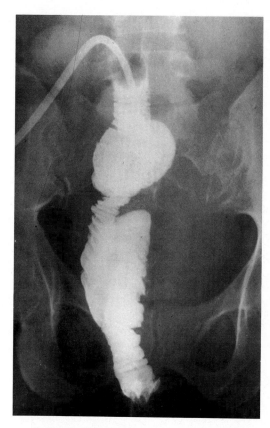

Fig. 29-30 Antegrade pouch study. Total colectomy was performed in this patient with ulcerative colitis, and an ileoanal S-pouch created for continence. This study, which was normal, was performed to evaluate the pouch before definitive hook-up to the remainder of the small bowel. The pouch is not rounded and enlarged before definitive hook-up. Special caution is advised when using an inflated balloon within ileostomy.

tients colitis similar to that found in Crohn's disease is seen.[169-171] Behçet's syndrome therefore is not discussed separately in this chapter.

Extraintestinal manifestations

Patients with Crohn's colitis develop manifestations outside the gastrointestinal tube as frequently as patients with ulcerative colitis. In one series, 25% had more than one extraintestinal feature, and systemic features appeared to be somewhat more common in patients with perianal disease.[172]

Musculoskeletal disease

The reported incidence of musculoskeletal abnormalities in Crohn's disease is higher in recent publications (15% to 22%)[173,174] than previously reported (2% to 4%).[175,176] This may be because the more recent investigations were performed by bone specialists. The most common extraintestinal involvement is arthritis, which may present as a migratory arthritis involving the large joints, as sacroiliitis, or

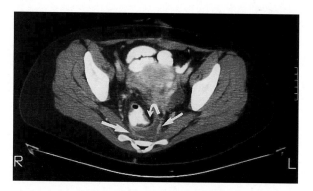

Fig. 29-31 CT of pouch with abscess. CT scan shows a low-density mass with an enhancing rim *(straight arrows)* posterior to the pouch, corresponding to an abscess and slightly thickened pouch wall *(curved arrow).*
From Thoeni RF et al: *AJR* 154:73, 1990.

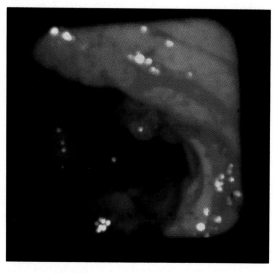

Fig. 29-32 Colonoscopic view of descending colon afflicted by Crohn's disease demonstrates edematous and hyperemic mucosa with deep linear ulcers. Lumen is narrowed, and cobblestoning is evident in inferolateral side of colon.
Courtesy of Dr. John P. Cello.

as ankylosing spondylitis. Spondylitis and sacroiliitis often are present for years before intestinal symptoms of Crohn's disease appear. There is no relationship between the course of the arthritis and the course of Crohn's disease. Peripheral joint disease is more common in Crohn's disease than in ulcerative colitis. Migratory monoarthritis that involves large joints can be seen in both ulcerative colitis and Crohn's disease, but the course of the joint disease follows exacerbations of the bowel disease more closely in ulcerative colitis than in Crohn's disease. Generally, the arthritis associated with Crohn's disease is less severe.

Liver disease

An uncommon extraintestinal manifestation of Crohn's disease is liver disease. Changes include mild abnormalities of liver function and pericholangitis (60% of patients)[101,177]; rarely, sclerosing cholangitis, possibly associated with cholangiocarcinoma; cirrhosis,[101,177] and granulomatous hepatitis. Cholelithiasis (seen in 30%)[93,178] appears to be unrelated to ileal resection. Fatty liver, often seen in autopsy of these patients, is probably more a reflection of severe illness and malnutrition than a specific form of liver abnormality.

Amyloidosis

Amyloidosis is a rare but serious complication of Crohn's disease and is more frequent in Crohn's disease than in ulcerative colitis.[177,179] The diagnosis often can be made with a biopsy of liver or rectum, but occasionally a renal biopsy is needed. The development of nephrotic syndrome or hepatosplenomegaly should alert the physician to the possibility of secondary amyloidosis in a patient with Crohn's disease. Resection of diseased bowel segments has been followed by arrest or reversal of amyloidosis.

Genitourinary disease

Genitourinary complications have been reported in 4% to 23% of patients. They include urinary tract infections caused by enterovesical fistulae, urinary tract calculi, and ureteral obstruction caused by contiguous inflammation of bowel loops .[93,112,164,180-183] Oxalate stones and hyperoxaluria have been related to steatorrhea. Fat malabsorption in these patients increases the availability of dietary oxalate for absorption, particularly from the colon. Also, calcium and fluid intake influence development of renal stones.

Ocular and dermatologic disease

Inflammatory manifestations of the eye, skin, and mucous membranes also may develop during the course of Crohn's colitis and enteritis. Iritis and episcleritis are the common ocular manifestations, whereas erythema nodosum and pyoderma gangrenosum are the major skin manifestations in these patients. Aphthous ulcers on the tongue and buccal mucous membranes are particularly incapacitating.

Thromboembolic disease

Thromboembolic complications are seen in about 1% of patients with Crohn's disease.[104] Crohn's disease appears to be more common in users of contraceptives.[184]

Radiographic features

In contrast to ulcerative colitis, Crohn's disease is a transmural process, and in advanced cases it can be distinguished easily from ulcerative colitis. If the entire colon is involved, however, distinctions may be difficult. Some authors estimate that approximately 20% to 25% of all patients with Crohn's disease cannot be differentiated with certainty from those with ulcerative colitis.[53,66,185] Marshak's many publications[81,186,187] have helped greatly in identifying features that can be used to distinguish these two idiopathic types of colitis. Discontinuity and asymmetry of disease are typical for Crohn's disease, which is remarkably different from ulcerative colitis with its symmetric, continuous, and diffuse involvement of the colon. These distinguishing features can be seen in early as well as advanced stages. While the advanced stages can be recognized easily by a single-contrast barium enema examination and the radiographic findings correspond well with those from surgery and pathology, a double-contrast barium enema can detect the more subtle surface changes and thus detect early Crohn's disease with a high degree of accuracy.

Unlike ulcerative colitis, Crohn's disease may involve any part of the small bowel,[60] the stomach,[188] the duodenum,[189-191] and, on rare occasion, the esophagus.[192] The most commonly involved areas are the cecum and the terminal ileum, and it is unusual to find Crohn's disease of the right colon that does not extend into terminal ileum.[193] Based on several series of patients with Crohn's disease,[194,195] the anatomic distribution of disease was found to be as follows: 29% in small bowel only, 50% in small bowel and colon, 19% in colon only, and 2% in anorectal area only.

Large bowel

Overall, involvement of the colon by Crohn's disease is seen with increasing frequency, and the incidence of Crohn's colitis and ileocolitis is higher for adult-onset or late-onset in whites as well as in other races. This is in contrast to young patients who are more prone to have jejunoileitis. Therefore the distinction between ulcerative colitis with or without backwash ileitis and Crohn's colitis with or without involvement of the terminal ileum becomes increasingly important and represents a challenge to the radiologist and pathologist.

EARLY DISEASE

The earliest pathologic finding of Crohn's disease is granulomatous inflammation, which probably originates from the submucosa and mucosa. On radiographs, the earliest findings are tiny elevations or mammillations of 1 to 2 mm in diameter, which probably represent exaggerated lymphoid follicles.[110,196] Many of these lesions develop ulcerations in their centers and then become radiographically visible as "target lesions" or so-called aphthous ulcers[189,197] (Figs. 29-33 and 29-34). Radiographically they are collections of barium with halos around them.[110,198-200] Because they are shallow lesions, they are not seen in profile.[201] They usually are multiple and are found on a background of normal mucosa. Such ulcers have been seen in *Yersinia* enterocolitis, amebic colitis, and other specific inflammations.[169,202,203] Because many of the infectious types of colitis are not as common as Crohn's disease in the United

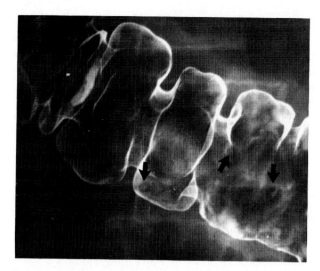

Fig. 29-33 Several aphthous ulcers *(arrows)* are seen on background of normal mucosa in patient with acute Crohn's disease of colon.

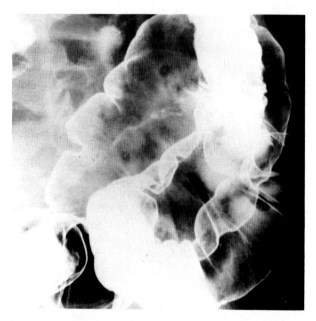

Fig. 29-34 Multiple collections of barium are surrounded by halo in this patient with granulomatous colitis.

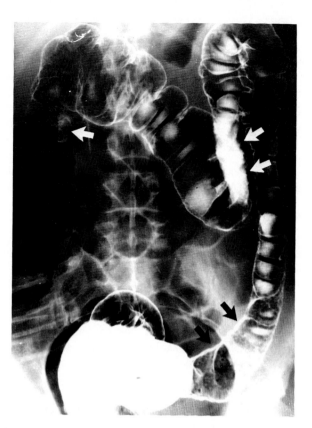

Fig. 29-35 Typical skip lesions *(white arrows)* mimic Crohn's disease in a patient with Behcet's syndrome. Filiform polyposis *(black arrows)* is present in the distal descending colon and in the sigmoid colon.

States, aphthous ulcers still are found most frequently in Crohn's disease. Aphthous ulcers can be demonstrated by a single-contrast barium enema examination but are best seen by the double-contrast technique. They are rapidly changing lesions,[204] and they may regress or develop into the longitudinal and transverse folds commonly seen in advanced disease. Aphthous ulcers may also be seen in other parts of the gastrointestinal tract.

Marshak[187] described the earliest findings of Crohn's disease based on single-contrast barium enema examination as consisting of irregular nodules measuring 5 mm in diameter and often ulcerating. He also found rigidity of the walls and thickening of the haustra to be useful signs for detecting early disease. These findings, however, represent a later stage of the disease than the ones shown by the double-contrast technique.

INTERMEDIATE DISEASE

Asymmetric involvement is another typical feature of Crohn's disease.[199,200] In the intermediate stage, one wall of a bowel segment may be irregular and covered with aphthous ulcers, whereas the opposite wall is completely normal (Figs. 29-35 to 29-37). The mesenteric wall becomes stiff and spiculated, and the antimesenteric side shows scalloping. Ulcers are mostly in the mesenteric area. These features are more readily identified in the small bowel.

ADVANCED DISEASE

The most important features of the advanced stage of Crohn's disease are discontinuity of the disease, asymmetry, strictures, fistulas, and sinuses. Fistulas and sinuses are much more common in the small bowel. Discontinuous dis-

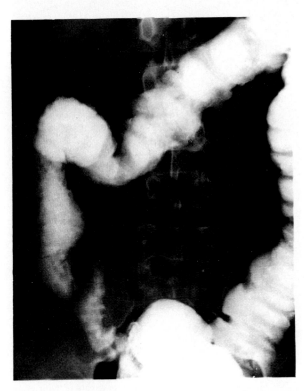

Fig. 29-36 Single-contrast barium enema examination shows asymmetric involvement of the proximal transverse colon. The right side of the colon and terminal ileum are also afflicted by Crohn's disease.

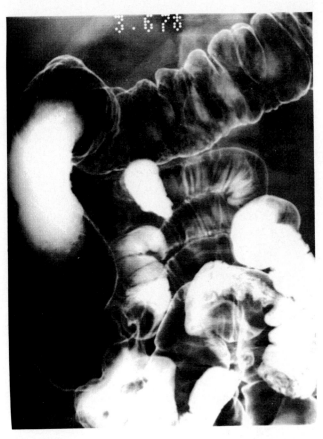

Fig. 29-37 Same patient as in Fig. 29-36. One year later, double-contrast barium enema examination shows asymmetric involvement of the transverse and right side of colon. Several aphthous ulcers are seen in patient with granulomatous colitis.

ease is seen in 90% of all patients with Crohn's disease of the colon[19] (see Fig. 29-33). It is important to remember that ulcerative colitis and Crohn's colitis cannot always be distinguished from one another, but ulcers on a background of granular mucosa are not seen in Crohn's disease, whereas they are typical of ulcerative colitis.

In the advanced stages, fibrosis shrinks the involved bowel wall (mesenteric side) and creates "pseudosacculations" on the opposite normal wall (Fig. 29-38), as can be seen in scleroderma and occasionally in ischemia. Scleroderma, however, does not show mucosal abnormalities. These changes are seen in the intermediate phase but become more pronounced in the advanced phase associated with marked wall thickening. Eventually, the involved segment shrinks to the point that the scalloping can no longer be discerned.

Typical findings in Crohn's disease of the colon and small bowel are marked thickening of the wall and mesentery. Deep longitudinal and transverse ulcers crisscrossing each other and surrounding edematous mucosa create the well-known cobblestone pattern of advanced disease.[19,205,206] (Fig. 29-41). Giant inflammatory polyps occasionally develop, which may produce distinctive signs and symptoms[117,207] (see Inflammatory Polyps).

Strictures are often found in Crohn's disease (Fig. 29-42) but need not be examined for malignancy. Narrowing of the terminal ileum, often referred to as a *string* sign, was originally described as being related to spasms and not to actual stricture formation. Both spasms and stricture may occur in the colon and small intestine of patients with granulomatous colitis. Fistulas and abscesses are uncommon in ulcerative colitis but are seen very frequently in Crohn's disease. Intramural and paracolonic fistula tracts may be seen in patients with Crohn's disease, particularly in the presence of diverticula, but are not reliable indicators for Crohn's disease because they may also be seen in patients with diverticulitis alone.

If the rectum is involved in Crohn's disease (50%),[208] the disease is not uniform but is patchy in distribution and may show deep collar-button ulcers in the rectal ampulla in addition to the characteristic rectal and perirectal sinus tracts. Rectal involvement by Crohn's disease cannot always be demonstrated radiographically because of the patchy distribution. As with ulcerative colitis, all three types of polyploid lesions can be seen (pseudopolyps, inflammatory polyps, and filiform polyps)[209] (Fig. 29-43; see Fig. 29-7). Neoplastic polyps are rare in Crohn's disease.

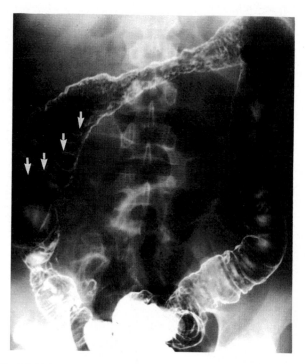

Fig. 29-38 Pseudosacculations *(arrows),* skip lesions, and filiform polyposis are seen in this patient with Crohn's disease of the colon.

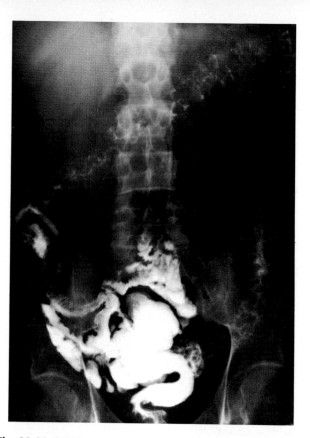

Fig. 29-39 Cobblestoning is well shown in a patient with granulomatous colitis. Note that the rectum appears to be less severely involved.

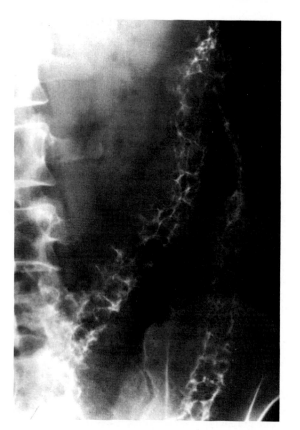

Fig. 29-40 Close-up film of splenic flexure in same patient as seen in Fig. 29-39 demonstrates transverse and longitudinal ulcers of Crohn's disease.

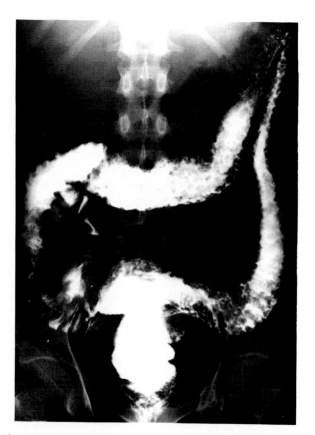

Fig. 29-41 Cobblestoning and pseudopolyposis are easily visible in patient with pancolitis related to granulomatous colitis.

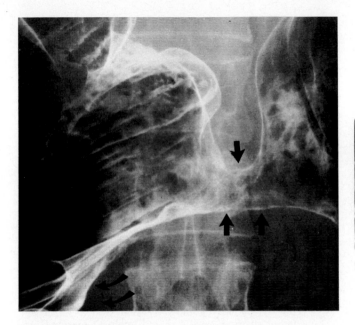

Fig. 29-42 Stricture *(arrows)* in a patient with partial colonic resection and reanastomosis. The terminal ileum is on left side *(curved arrows)*.

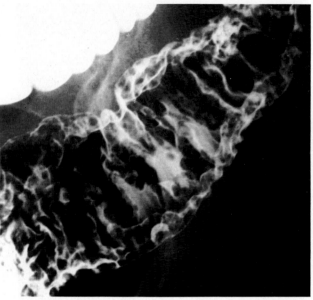

Fig. 29-43 Multiple postinflammatory polyps, some of which are filiform, in a patient with granulomatous colitis.

REVERSIBILITY

Crohn's disease is reversible to a certain degree, more often in the colon than in the small bowel. Aphthous ulcers may fluctuate or regress, but usually the disease progresses to more severe manifestations.[210] Because of the transmural involvement it is rare for the colon to appear completely normal after regression of the acute manifestations of inflammation. Some type of scarring (pseudosacculations, asymmetry, or narrowing) usually remains. Brahme and Fork[204] described regression with remaining scarring in 7% of 86 patients.

RECURRENCE

The high incidence of recurrence of Crohn's disease after partial resection and reanastomosis is still controversial. In a series of 114 patients with a resection for ileocecal Crohn's disease, 28 had recurrence.[211] A significantly higher risk (93%) was found for postoperative recurrence if surgery left behind colonic lesions. Some authors have reported a postoperative spread of disease to a previously normal colon,[204,212-214] which may be explained by preoperative colonic lesions being overlooked during the barium enema examination and surgery.

Submucosal edema that is nonspecific and that may occur in any type of colitis may be seen without evidence of preoperative disease left behind (Fig. 29-44). Recurrence in the new distal ileum in addition to persistent granulomatous colitis occurred in 11 of 12 patients. Disease spread across the ileocecal anastomosis in 92 patients in an oral direction but never in an aboral one[211] (Figs. 29-45 to 29-

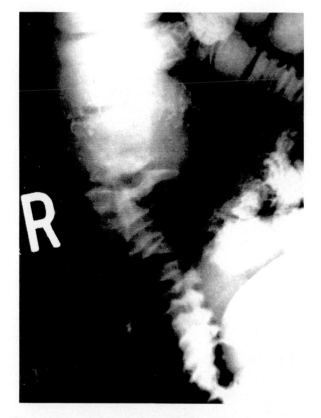

Fig. 29-44 Ileocolic anastomosis in a patient with Crohn's disease is normal. Folds in the terminal ileum are mildly thickened, which may represent nonspecific inflammation if inflammatory changes do not progress to clear manifestations of Crohn's disease.

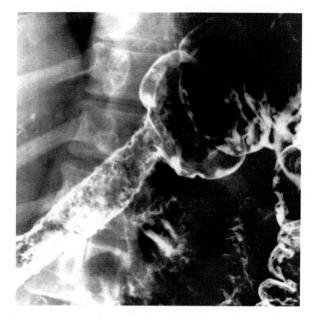

Fig. 29-45 Peroral pneumocolon (PPC) in a patient with resection of the ascending colon and reanastomosis of the transverse colon and ileum for Crohn's disease. Recurrence of disease at anastomosis is seen along with narrowing of the terminal ileum associated with deep ulcers.

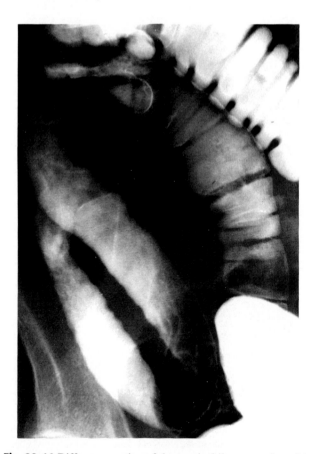

Fig. 29-46 Diffuse narrowing of the terminal ileum together with irregular ileal margins and mucosal nodularity suggest recurrence of disease 1 year after surgery.

47). It appears therefore that recurrence at the anastomotic site is largely related to the exacerbation of disease in the colonic segments that were involved preoperatively and left behind, and not to new recurrent disease. Spread to the distal ileum is facilitated by the anastomosis. Patients who once had pancolitis should always be considered as having diffuse colitis.

Small bowel
CLASSIFICATION OF SEVERITY OF DISEASE

Granularity (edema in intestinal villi), thickening of the folds, nodularity (nodular pattern caused by edema and inflammation in the submucosa, varying in degree from "notching" seen in profile to confluence of nodules), and ulceronodular pattern (progression of disease with deep ulcers between the individual nodules) are features seen in acute Crohn's disease of the small bowel. Aphthous ulcers are considered early lesions and correspond to erosions overlying hyperplastic lymphoid follicles. If erosions become larger, they appear as smooth, convex marginal defects (ulcers), which are oval or stellate, on top of nodular elevations of the mucosa.

To assess severity of disease, Engelholm et al.[201] proposed a radiologic classification system. In this classifica-

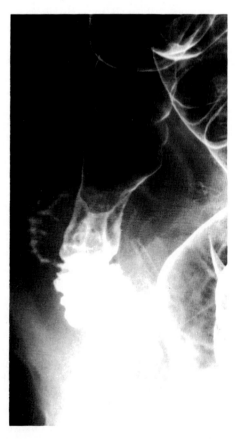

Fig. 29-47 Narrowing and edema in patient with recurrent Crohn's disease at anastomosis.

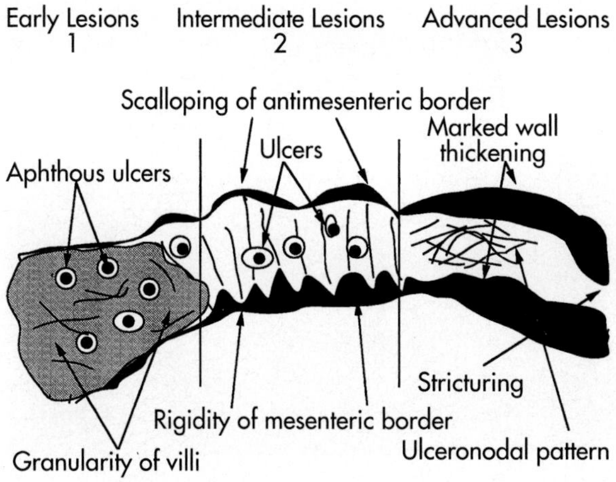

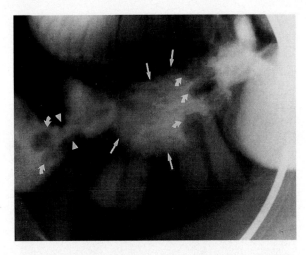

Early Lesions   Intermediate Lesions   Advanced Lesions
1   2   3

Scalloping of antimesenteric border

Marked wall thickening

Aphthous ulcers   Ulcers

Stricturing

Rigidity of mesenteric border

Granularity of villi

Ulceronodal pattern

Fig. 29-48 Schematic drawing for classification of pathologic changes produced by Crohn's disease.
Modified from Engelholm L, de Toeuff C, Herlinger H, Maglinte D: Crohn's disease of the small bowel. In Herlinger H, Maglinte D, eds: *Clinical radiology of the small intestine,* Philadelphia, 1989, WB Saunders.

Fig. 29-49 Granular *(straight arrows)* and nodular *(curved arrows)* pattern in a patient with acute Crohn's disease of the terminal ileum. Note concentric hourglass stricture *(arrowheads).*

tion, three major stages are distinguished: early lesions, intermediate lesions, and advanced lesions (Fig. 29-48).

Early lesions are characterized by aphthous ulcerations or villous abnormality (granularity of the villi) and mild fold thickening. Spasm is noted during fluoroscopy, and the distensibility of the involved intestinal wall is preserved. Also, increased fluid may be present in the area immediately proximal to the involved segment (Figs. 29-49 and 29-50). Intermediate lesions produce a nodular pattern associated with ulcerations (Figs. 29-50 to 29-52), rigidity of the mesenteric border, and scalloping of the contractile antimesenteric border (Fig. 29-53). Ulcerations are present mostly on the mesenteric border. The bowel wall is moderately thickened, and the mesentery may be involved.

Advanced lesions are manifested by an ulceronodular pattern associated with a completely stiff segment (Fig. 29-53). Fistula and sinus tract formation, deeper ulcers, and stricture development indicate advanced disease (Fig. 29-54 to 29-56). Involvement of the mesentery and marked thickening of the intestinal wall also are findings of advanced disease.

TERMINAL ILEUM

The terminal ileum is the most common site of involvement by Crohn's disease, and it can be examined by means of reflux from the cecum during a double-contrast barium enema examination, during enteroclysis, or during a peroral pneumocolon examination that consists of a small bowel follow-through and air insufflation through the rectum to distend the cecum and terminal ileum (see Fig. 30-43). Often, reflux from the cecum into the terminal ileum does not occur during a barium enema examination because of an edematous, spastic ileocecal valve. The examination

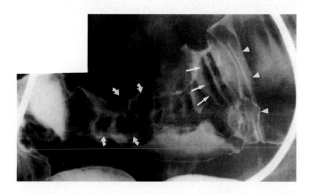

Fig. 29-50 Thickened folds *(straight arrows)* and nodular pattern *(curved arrows)* are seen in a patient with acute exacerbation of Crohn's disease. Note abrupt change from normal mucosa to granulomatous jejunitis *(arrowheads).*

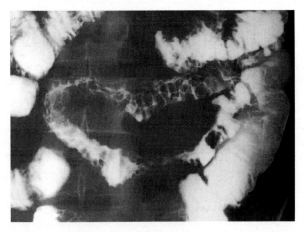

Fig. 29-51 Typical ulceronodular pattern. Note separation of bowel loops.

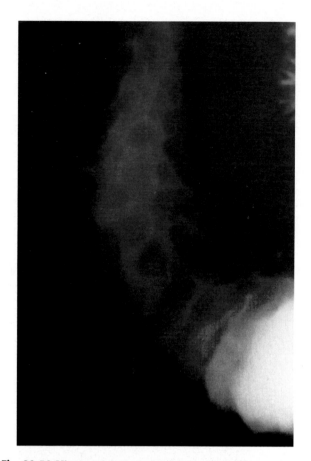

Fig. 29-52 Ulceronodular pattern of the terminal ileum.

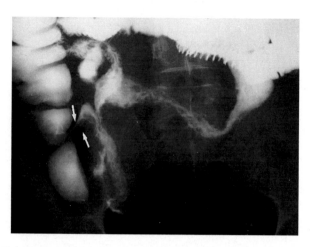

Fig. 29-53 Long tubular narrowing of the ileum with stenosis of segment near the ileocecal valve *(arrows)*.

BASIC PATTERN

Fine granular pattern. A granular appearance of the mucosal surface can be observed over a variable length of small bowel in the transitional zone between normal intestine and the main lesions (see Fig. 29-49). This pattern represents villous hypertrophy and "bridging" caused by edema, vascular congestion in the lamina propria of the small bowel wall, or both. Similar changes can be found in protein-loosing enteropathy, radiation enteritis, backwash ileitis, and small bowel ischemia.

Thickening of folds. Because of the submucosal edema and the "wet" mucosal surface, the folds appear thickened, swollen, somewhat blurred, irregular, and occasionally nodular and straightened (see Fig. 29-50).

Nodular pattern. The profile of the bowel lumen is characterized by large notches related to filling defects as the main radiologic sign. This pattern usually is diffuse, depending on the degree of confluence of these nodules, and the wall is relatively pliable (see Figs. 29-49 to 29-51).

Ulceronodular pattern. With progression of the disease, transverse and longitudinal ulcerations appear in the small bowel with residual islands of inflamed mucosa between them (Fig. 29-57; see Fig. 29-52). These ulcerations produce the cobblestone pattern characteristic of Crohn's disease. At this point, the bowel wall loses its pliability, and the lumen is often reduced by spasm.

String sign. This sign refers to the tubular appearance of the involved small bowel segment (see Fig. 29-53). If the luminal narrowing is caused by fibrous thickening of the small bowel wall, the diameter of the lumen remains constant. When the narrowing is caused by spasm and edema, the degree of stenosis is not constant. In the case of fibrosis, the lining of the lumen is replaced by a fibrinonecrotic membrane in which some islands of mucosa may be interspersed. The contour of the bowel is markedly spiculated, with some of the longer spikes representing deep fissures in a markedly thickened wall.

of the terminal ileum is even easier in patients with ileocecal reanastomosis because of the open communication.

The terminal ileum normally has circular folds that are thin and straight, and the margins of the bowel appear smooth. Occasionally, lymphoid hyperplasia is present in the terminal ileum, which is a normal finding consisting of tiny nodular filling defects. The differentiation of normality from disease may be a particular problem in teenagers who normally have large lymphoid follicles.

During the early stages of Crohn's disease in the terminal ileum, nodularity of the folds, spasms, spiculation of the wall, and aphthous ulcers may be seen. These are all manifestations of mucosal and submucosal disease. In the more advanced stages, marked narrowing, deep ulcerations, cobblestoning, and fistulas are present. Often an impression is noted on the medial cecal wall that is related to small bowel involvement and mesenteric thickening.[215] A similar finding may be seen in cases of appendicitis with abscess formation, but Crohn's disease usually has more severe mucosal disease with deeper ulcerations. An impression may also be present in the sigmoid colon and is related to the inflamed small bowel and contiguous involvement of the sigmoid.

Ulcerations. Aphthous ulcers are early lesions arising from hypertrophic lymphoid follicles in which noncaseating granulomas may be found. En face, they appear as round to oval filling defects with central flecks of barium representing the erosions. Depending on the size of this central fleck of barium, it may appear round, oval, or even stellate. In profile, the aphthous ulcer appears as a smooth nodule with a central collection of barium on the top of its convex surface. The diameter of these nodules varies between 5 mm and 15 mm. Aphthous ulcers may be found alone but are usually seen in combination with deep ulcers and other signs of more severe bowel involvement. They are usually seen at either end of the main lesion in both the initial stages and in recurrent disease. Larger ulcers assume a round, oval, or diamond shape aligned in the longitudinal axis. Convergence of folds may be associated with these ulcers as well as shrinkage of the bowel margin facing the ulcer. These ulcers may be near the main lesion or at some distance from it (skip lesions). Hourglass concentric narrowings may be demonstrated; they are caused by annular ulcers (Fig. 29-58; see Figs. 29-49 and 29-56). Often there is no associated dilatation of the segments proximal to these annular ulcerations despite the apparent narrowing of the lumen. A long, deep ulcer may be present along the mesenteric attachment of the small intestine, which is continuous with the main lesion (see Fig. 29-54). This feature is characteristic of the intermediate stage (see Fig. 29-48).

Filiform polyps. These fingerlike mucosal protrusions are described in the section on Crohn's colitis and are most commonly found in the large bowel. They are rarely seen in the small bowel or stomach and represent repair and scarring from ulcerations.

Fistulas and sinus tracts. These appear in deep longitudinal ulcerations or in intramural fissures. They are seen in the advanced stages of Crohn's disease and occur together with strictures (Fig. 29-59; see Figs. 29-54 to 29-56). They tend to be proximal to strictures.

Thickening and retraction of mesentery. This is a constant feature and involves the mesentery opposite the intestinal lesions. The mesentery is thickened, and the fat spreads over the involved bowel loop until it meets the site where the intestinal lesion is most prominent ("creeping fat"). Regional lymph nodes in this area are always enlarged. The mesenteric thickening and the thickened wall of the involved bowel produce a mass effect that separates intestinal loops or small bowel loops and colon (see Fig. 29-51). The degree of mesenteric thickening contributes to the stiffness of the mesenteric border of the intestine. Occasionally, loops of small bowel assume the shape of the Greek letter omega (Ω), which may also be present in patients with

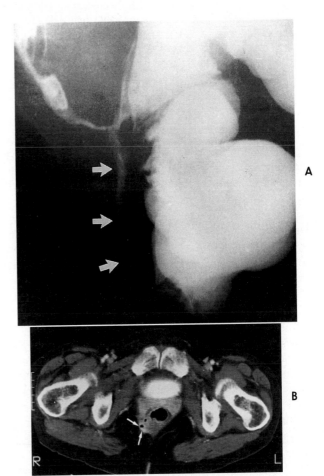

A

B

Fig. 29-55 Perineal fistula in a patient with Crohn's disease. **A,** Fistulous tract *(arrows)* is noted extending from the ileum to perineum associated with rectal inflammation. **B,** CT in the same patient shows air-containing fistula *(arrows)* and thickening of adjacent rectal wall.

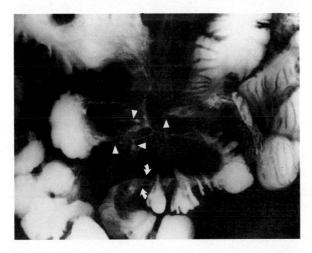

Fig. 29-54 Multiple fistulas *(arrowheads)* are extending between the ileum and jejunum. Note sacculations caused by shrinkage of the mesenteric border and longitudinal ulcer proximal to concentric lesions *(curved arrows)* indicative of intermediary segment.

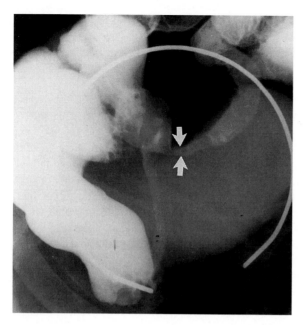

Fig. 29-56 Concentric narrowing of the ileum *(arrows)* with long fistulous tract to the vagina of a patient with Crohn's disease and discharge from vagina.

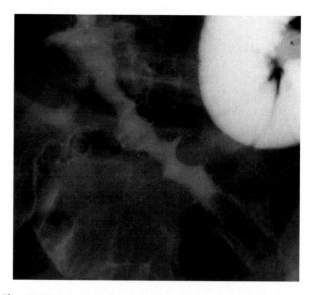

Fig. 29-57 Deep transverse fissures representing ulcers and diffuse narrowing are noted in a patient with advanced Crohn's disease.

peritoneal carcinomatosis, carcinoid tumor, or mesenteric lipomatosis.

SEGMENTAL ARRANGEMENT OF LESIONS

Gradation in the severity of lesions within the involved intestinal loop and mesentery and the tendency for lesions to manifest themselves preferentially on the mesenteric side of the intestine with asymmetry and sacculation are the most typical features of Crohn's disease and are the most important factors for reaching a specific diagnosis. In the characteristic form of Crohn's disease, a transitional zone is observed in which the lesions become progressively less severe in the area between the more pronounced lesions in the ileal loops and the more proximal small bowel.[216] As mentioned above, in the transitional zone between the normal intestine and the main lesions, a fine granular pattern can be seen, which represents edema in the mucosa and submucosa. In segmented forms of the disease, similar transitional zones are observed between more severely involved segments, or if discontinuous disease is present (skip lesions), between severely damaged segments and normal segments of the small bowel (see Fig. 29-50).

The tendency for lesions to preferentially manifest themselves on the mesenteric side of the intestine and the creation of asymmetric involvement and sacculation is another very characteristic sign of Crohn's disease (see Figs. 30-54 and 30-58). Japanese researchers recently published a study in which they called the longitudinal ulcer along the mesenteric attachment of the small intestine "the most characteristic feature of Crohn's disease in Japan."[217]

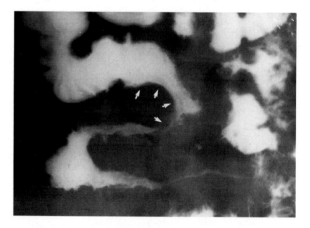

Fig. 29-58 Omega sign associated with concentric narrowing. Note curvilinear and rigid mesenteric border *(arrows)*.

A true intermediary segment meets the following criteria: (1) a curvilinear, rigid mesenteric border (thickened mesentery and thickened bowel wall); (2) a longitudinal ulcer along the mesenteric margins with the folds arrested close to the ulcer; (3) mucosal folds visible on the surface of the loop converging toward certain areas on the mesenteric border (Fig. 29-60); and (4) a scalloped antimesenteric border showing a change in the radiographic pattern on contraction, which indicates that pliability is not completely lost. With increasing shrinkage of the antimesenteric border toward the mesenteric border, asymmetric segments are created. If shrinkage is acute and severe, pseudodiverticula and eccentric stenosis are observed.

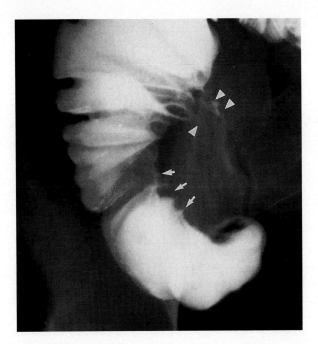

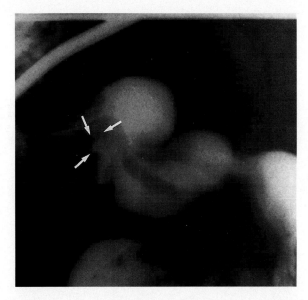

Fig. 29-60 Small ulcer *(arrow)* and converging folds are seen in the ileum of a patient with Crohn's disease.

Fig. 29-59 Spiculation *(arrows)*, fistulas *(arrowheads)*, and large impression on the medial wall of the cecum are present in a patient with terminal ileitis and marked mesenteric thickening caused by Crohn's disease.

CROHN'S DISEASE IN SMALL INTESTINE OTHER THAN TERMINAL ILEUM

While involvement of the terminal ileum is very common, jejunitis or ileitis also can be seen, either as diffuse involvement found in very young patients or as multiple skip areas throughout the small bowel in the adult population.[218] Often, confluence of nodules is evident if the edema is pronounced. However, as with involvement of the terminal ileum, a gradation in severity of lesions is often seen. With increasing progression of disease, asymmetry and discontinuity of disease may be apparent and cobblestoning becomes visible, created by longitudinal and transverse ulcerations. Here also, longitudinal ulcers located on the mesenteric border and shrinkage produce the sacculations of the antimesenteric border. Strictures and fistulas are less common in the jejunum and proximal ileum than in the terminal ileum.

CROHN'S DISEASE IN ESOPHAGUS, STOMACH, AND DUODENUM

Esophagus. Granulomatous changes in the esophagus are the least frequent manifestation of Crohn's disease. Patients with granulomatous esophagitis complain of dysphagia and chest pain. Usually, when granulomatous changes are found in the esophagus, Crohn's disease is also present in the ileum and colon. Diffuse or discrete esophageal ulcerations may be seen. Changes of mild esophagitis can progress to a cobblestone pattern of the mucosa with or without for-

mation of sinus tracts, esophageal stenosis, or esophagobronchial fistulas. Involvement may be eccentric, and focal nodularity, irregularity, and penetrating ulcerations may occur. In patients with documented Crohn's disease elsewhere in the gastrointestinal tract, the presence of ulcerations, especially aphthous ulcers, and intramural fistulous tract(s) should suggest the diagnosis of Crohn's disease. Tuberculous esophagitis can present in a similar fashion and even fistulous tracks are common with this infectious type of esophagitis.

Stomach. As with Crohn's disease in the colon or small intestine, erosions or aphthous ulcers are the earliest finding in the stomach (Fig. 29-61). The erosions are often accompanied by fold thickening or scalloping. The antrum may be narrowed, which is a late manifestation of Crohn's gastritis. The appearance of the stomach in these patients has been referred to as "ram's horn" sign or "pseudo–Billroth II" (Fig. 29-62). Often the duodenum is also involved, and the stomach may assume a tubular narrowing with complete obliteration of the normal anatomic landmarks between duodenum and stomach. In patients who have Crohn's disease elsewhere in the gastrointestinal tract, gastroduodenal involvement is found in 2% to 20%. Fundal involvement, although rare, also has been described.

Duodenum. Only a small percentage of patients with Crohn's disease develop granulomatous changes in the duodenum. The exact incidence of duodenal involvement is difficult to establish, but is estimated to be approximately 10%. The duodenum simply may show thickened folds, but the whole gamut of basic patterns including the ulceronodular form may be seen (Figs. 29-63 to 29-65). As in other areas of the gastrointestinal tract, single or multiple stric-

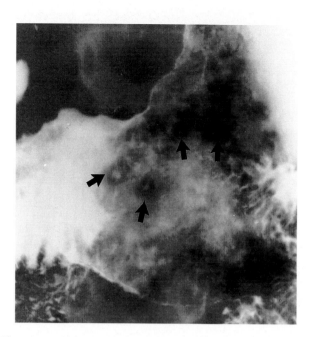

Fig. 29-61 Multiple aphthous ulcers *(arrows)* are present in the body of the stomach of a patient with Crohn's disease first diagnosed in the terminal ileum. The findings in the stomach are nonspecific and could be seen in various types of erosive gastritis.

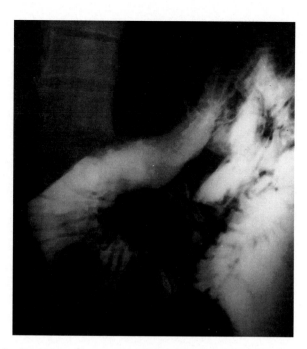

Fig. 29-62 Ram's-horn stomach produced by obliteration of anatomic boundaries between the stomach and duodenum in a patient with biopsy-proven Crohn's disease of the terminal ileum, stomach, and duodenum.

tures may be present. Because patients with Crohn's disease of the duodenum usually have granulomatous changes in the colon, small bowel, or both, the radiographic diagnosis is easier for the duodenum if the granulomatous process is demonstrated in these other areas.

Accuracy of radiographic examination

As with ulcerative colitis, the accuracy of radiographic detection of Crohn's disease of the colon is high, but minor lesions such as aphthous ulcers are demonstrated accurately only if the patient has a clean colon and when the quality of a double-contrast barium enema examination is excellent.[210] The extent of the disease, as mentioned previously, is often underestimated by radiography even if the double-contrast technique is used. Overlooked disease may result in incomplete surgical resection, increasing the risk of recurrence.

Because idiopathic colitis is still the most common type of colitis in the United States and Europe, the differential diagnosis of inflammatory bowel disease usually is narrowed down to ulcerative colitis and Crohn's colitis. Marshak,[187] Marshak and Lindner,[136] and Laufer and Hamilton[19] have facilitated the differential diagnosis of ulcerative and granulomatous colitis. The distinction between these two diseases is important, because the respective prognosis, treatment, recurrence, and risk of cancer are different.

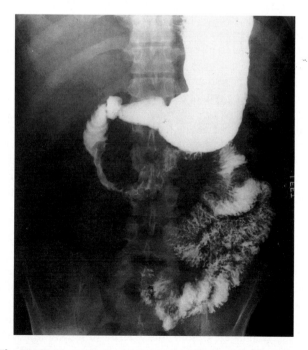

Fig. 29-63 A narrowed second portion of the duodenum and nodular changes in the third part of the duodenum are present with granulomatous disease in the ileum, jejunum, and colon.

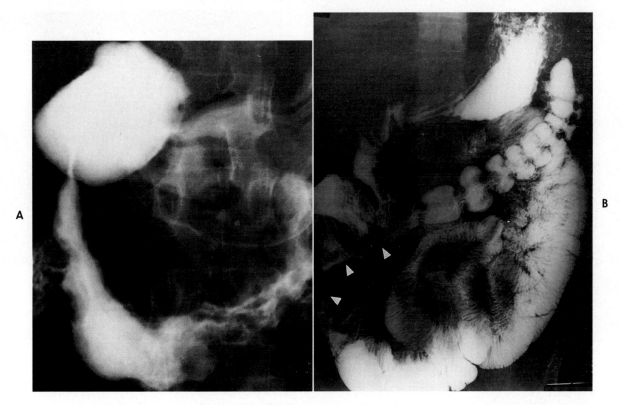

Fig. 29-64 Crohn's disease in the duodenum and jejunum. **A,** Nodular pattern is observed in the duodenum. **B,** Fistulas make impression on the cecum *(arrowheads),* and displacement of bowel loops in the right lower quadrant is noted. CT is needed to rule out abscess.

In most cases of early disease (in 75% to 95% of cases), the distinction between ulcerative and granulomatous colitis is made possible by the findings summarized in Table 29-1. An overlapping spectrum of inflammatory bowel disease remains, however.[53,67-67] Long-standing ulcerative colitis with many remissions and acute attacks, as well as total Crohn's colitis, manifested only by a narrowing of the colon and thickening of the mucosa (walls thicker than 5 mm),[219] make the radiographic determination of the correct diagnosis difficult. The distinction between the two diseases may be impossible in acute, fulminating illness, even with examination of the colectomy specimen.

While small bowel follow-through can diagnose intermediary and advanced Crohn's disease of the small bowel with relative ease, the radiographic features of early Crohn's lesions are difficult to detect by this method. In these early cases, enteroclysis is superior and can show even minor superficial changes of the mucosa and assess the true extent of disease with greater accuracy than any other radiographic technique used for examining the jejunum and ileum.[168] In a recent study on the value of enteroclysis for assessing Crohn's disease, the classification system proposed by Engelholm et al.[201] was used, and an impressive accuracy of 99.3% was found.[168]

Complications
CARCINOMA

There is a slightly higher risk of carcinoma in patients with Crohn's disease than in the general population,[220-222] but the incidence of colonic malignancies is much lower than in ulcerative colitis.[220,221,223] Based on two studies, each consisting of over 500 patients, the incidence of bowel malignancy in patients with Crohn's disease was 3.0% to 3.5%.[224,225] The overall frequency was four times lower than that of colon cancer in patients with ulcerative colitis. The risk of developing a carcinoma in Crohn's disease is similar to that in ulcerative colitis that involves the left side of the colon only.[226]

The mean age of occurrence of carcinoma in patients with Crohn's disease is in the forties. Malignancy may occur in the small bowel or colon, but it is more common in the latter. In the colon, tumors in Crohn's disease have a fairly even distribution.[227,228] In the small bowel, tumors in patients with Crohn's disease, as compared with the normal population, have a preponderance in the ileum.[228,229] There is also a higher incidence of tumors in the area of the anal canal and in fistulas.[228,230]

Carcinomas in Crohn's disease, like those in ulcerative colitis, tend to be colloid or mucinous and frequently infil-

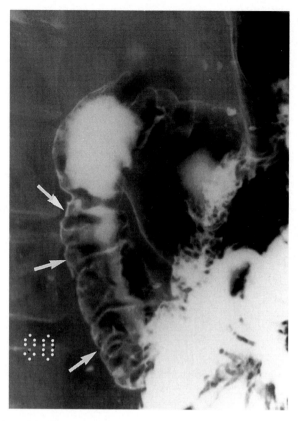

Fig. 29-65 Thickened folds in the duodenum *(arrows)* of a patient with granulomatous colitis. Findings are nonspecific, and peptic disease is more often responsible for this appearance than Crohn's disease.

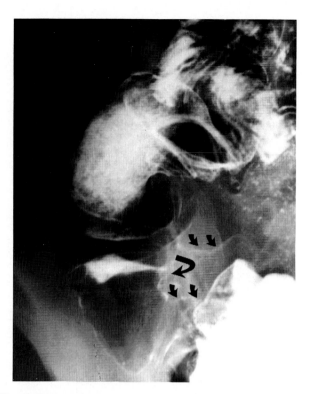

Fig. 29-66 Impressions on medial wall of cecum *(curved arrow)* and thin fistula tracts *(small arrows)* are seen in a patient with acute exacerbation of granulomatous colitis.

trate through and along the bowel wall. Because of this type of spread, the radiographic diagnosis of Crohn's carcinoma is often difficult. Strictures (see Fig. 30-40) and thickening of the bowel wall are features seen in uncomplicated Crohn's disease and cannot be used for diagnosing malignant degeneration. Also, tumors in fistulas are usually not well evaluated by radiographic methods. Any progressive change in the appearance of fistulas or strictures should be viewed with suspicion. CT can help in some of these cases, but biopsy is necessary for confirmation. For both ulcerative colitis and Crohn's disease, an increased incidence of lymphomas and leukemias have been found.[231-233]

FISTULAS

Fistulas occur frequently in Crohn's disease and may extend from the cecum and ascending colon to the terminal ileum or to the sigmoid colon (Figs. 29-66 and 29-67). Also, sinuses from the rectum or sigmoid to the perineum are highly suggestive features of Crohn's disease. As previously mentioned, fistulas are best shown by a single-contrast barium enema examination. Mesenteric thickening may mimic a mass and displace loops of small bowel or

impress on the colon. These features may be difficult to distinguish from an extraluminal abscess. Fistulization and close proximity of an inflammatory mass, abscess, or phlegmon caused by Crohn's disease may lead to nonspecific changes in bowel segments. The radiographic feature of nonspecific involvement consists of focal fold thickening, either in relation to the site of entry of fistulas or, together with mass effect, in response to the extrinsic inflammatory process.[234] This feature can be distinguished from bowel changes caused by actual Crohn's disease. Recognition of this nonspecific involvement is important because it reverts to normal if the area involved by Crohn's disease has been resected. Radiography is helpful in making the correct preoperative diagnosis and preventing unnecessary surgical resection.

PERFORATION

Perforation of the colon related to Crohn's disease is rare[167] but may occur spontaneously. However, perforation with frank diffuse peritonitis does occur and may even be the initial presentation.[235]

DIVERTICULOSIS

Because the incidence of Crohn's disease and ulcerative colitis shows a second peak in the older age group (between 50 and 60 years), diverticulosis is often present in these pa-

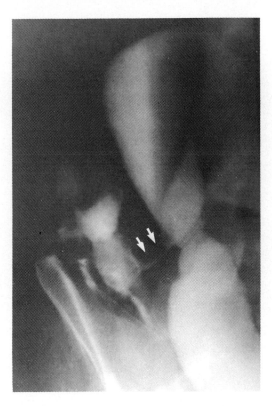

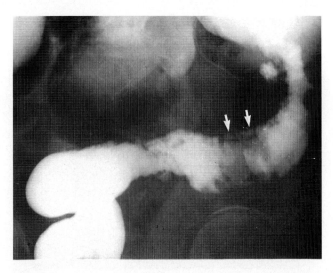

Fig. 29-68 Longitudinal pericolonic tract *(arrows)* in a patient with granulomatous colitis and diverticulitis. Complications of granulomatous colitis are more severe in the presence of diverticulitis. Longitudinal pericolonic tracts may be seen in Crohn's disease as well as in diverticulitis.

Fig. 29-67 Fistula *(arrows)* and large paracolonic abscess are seen in the ascending colon. Patient had had granulomatous colitis for 10 years.

tients and can render the diagnosis of inflammatory bowel disease very difficult.[236] On one hand, if diverticulosis and Crohn's colitis coexist, diverticulitis occurs much more frequently. On the other hand, if diverticulitis is present, complications with Crohn's colitis are more serious.[237] At the site of a diverticulum, only a thin layer of mucosa and submucosa and occasionally some muscle fibers cover the dome of the diverticulum. Because Crohn's disease is a transmural disease, aphthous ulcers may perforate and paracolonic abscesses may develop. Often, paracolonic sinus tracks and mass impressions from the abscess and, occasionally, fissuring in the bowel wall are seen in diverticulosis complicated by granulomatous colitis[238-240] (Fig. 29-68). The fact that granulomatous colitis causes haphazard ulcerations, and in diverticulosis the interdigitating clefts are smooth and more regular, helps differentiate the two conditions.[241]

HEMORRHAGING

Massive bleeding may occur in Crohn's disease but is not very common.[242,243] Microscopic sections of segments of bowel involved by Crohn's disease show hypervascularity and dilation of lymphatics that may lead to massive bleeding if the disease erodes into these dilated vessels. Frank bleeding, either with dark red or bright red blood,

can occur during the course of Crohn's colitis in 25% to 50% of patients with colonic disease. Frank bleeding may be the first symptom of granulomatous colitis. However, insidious bleeding with iron-deficiency anemia in the absence of melena or hematochezia is overall much more common. Frank bleeding also may be seen in ulcerative colitis.[244] Arterial vasopressin infusions have been shown to help stop bleeding in cases of Crohn's disease of the colon and ulcerative colitis.

TOXIC MEGACOLON

Toxic megacolon is most frequently seen with ulcerative colitis,[186] but it has been found in cases of Crohn's disease (incidence 2%), Behçet's disease, ischemic disease, amebiasis, bacillary dysentery, typhoid fever, cholera, *Campylobacter,* pseudomembranous colitis, and salmonellosis.[245-247] The same precautions are indicated as those described for ulcerative colitis.

DIFFERENTIAL DIAGNOSIS OF ULCERATIVE COLITIS AND CROHN'S DISEASE

The features of ulcerative colitis can be found in many infectious types of colitis, whereas Crohn's disease is mimicked by only a few types of colitis.[248-250] The latter group includes tuberculous ileocolitis,[251-255] blastomycosis,[256,257] actinomycosis,[258] pseudomembranous colitis (postantibiotic colitis)[259-263] (Figs. 29-69 to 29-71), ischemia[58,264-272] (Figs. 29-72 to 29-76), and rarely lymphogranuloma venereum[273] (Fig. 29-77). Occasionally, amebiasis presents with skip lesions, which makes distinguishing it from Crohn's disease more difficult.

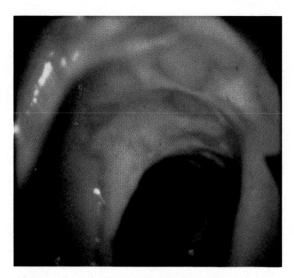

Fig. 29-69 Colonoscopic view of the transverse colon in a patient with hyperemic mucosa related to pseudomembranous colitis shows several slightly elevated lesions (plaques) of variable size. Courtesy of Dr. John P. Cello.

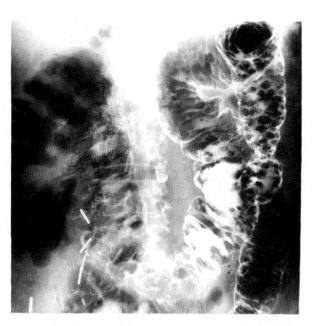

Fig. 29-70 Severe pseudomembranous colitis related to the administration of penicillin. Multiple plaques are well shown, suggesting the correct diagnosis.

Most of the diseases in the differential diagnosis of ulcerative colitis can be excluded by history or laboratory tests. Among the group of specific colitides, bacterial colitis (shigellosis,[126,274-276] salmonellosis,[277-285] colitis caused by staphylococci, *Yersinia*,[202,203,286] *Campylobacter fetus*,[285,287-292] lymphogranuloma venereum,[237,293] [see Fig. 29-77], *Neisseria* [gonorrheal proctitis][294-298] [Fig. 29-78] *Escherichia coli*, clostridium,[299-310] and chlamydia[311,293]) and fungal infections (*Actinomycosis*,[258] *Histoplasmosis*,[312-314] *Mucormycosis, Candidiasis*[312,315]) should be considered.

Among the viral types of colitis, infections with cytomegalovirus, rotavirus, and herpes simplex or zoster come to mind.[267,316-321] Infections by parasitic agents are increasingly seen as a result of AIDS and increased travel to, and newly arrived immigrants from, countries where these infections are endemic. Parasitic infections include *Entamoeba*[322-329] (Fig. 29-79), *Cryptosporidium*,[330,331] and helmintic infections (nematodes: strongyloidiasis[332,333] and *Ascaris;* and trematodes [flukes]: schistosomiasis[334-336]).

Also, the group of pseudomembranous colitis (postantibiotic colitis), uremia, large bowel obstruction with preobstructive distention simulating ulcerative colitis, hypoxia, and postoperative colitis needs to be considered, even though the radiographic picture more frequently suggests Crohn's disease than ulcerative colitis. The changes seen in preobstructive distention of the colon appear to be related to ischemia[337] (see Fig. 29-76).

For differential diagnosis among the group of noninfectious colitis, one needs to consider anaphylactic reaction[338] (Fig. 29-80), cathartic colon[139,140] (see Figs. 29-25 and 29-26), radiation colitis[339] (Fig. 29-81), retractile mesenteritis

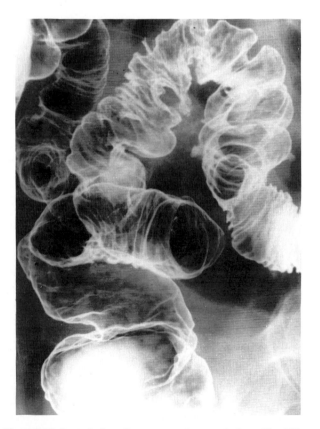

Fig. 29-71 Irregularity of mucosa and several plaquelike filling defects are seen in a patient with pseudomembranous colitis.

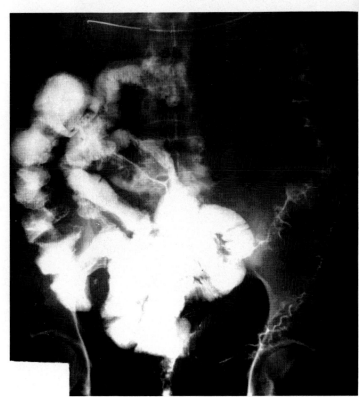
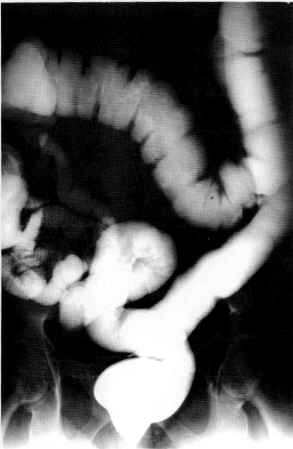

Fig. 29-72 A, Diffuse thumbprinting and edematous mucosa are seen in single-contrast barium enema examination. Patient suffered from acute ischemic colitis. **B,** Same patient as seen in **A.** One week after the initial examination, a repeat single-contrast barium enema examination shows a completely normal colon. Transient ischemia of the bowel is the most common form of ischemic bowel disease.

with direct colonic involvement (Fig. 29-82), nonspecific ulcerative proctitis,[77,113,141] caustic colitis, amyloidosis, diverticulitis, solitary rectal ulcer, diversion colitis, and colitis cystica.[340-342] Among these types of noninfectious colitis, radiation colitis (usually localized to the port of radiation), nonspecific ulcerative colitis, solitary rectal ulcer, and colitis cystica profunda are pathologic changes that are localized to a specific area of the colon, with the remainder of the colon uninvolved in the same process.

All these types of inflammatory changes in large and small bowel with specific etiologies are discussed in Chapters 31, 32, 36, 37, and 46. Some of the more common infections of the colon leading to the radiographic appearance of ulcerative and granulomatous colitis are listed in Table 29-1.

The differential diagnosis of inflammatory changes of the small bowel that may mimic Crohn's disease includes acute terminal ileitis and *Yersinia* ileitis or enterocolitis (both of which are confined to the last 10 to 15 cm of the terminal ileum); lymphoid hyperplasia (normal in children but in adults associated with *Yersinia* ileitis, infections with *Shi-*

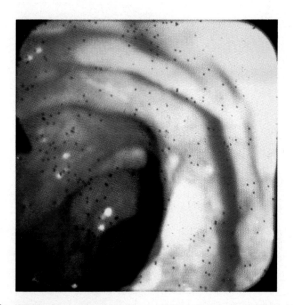

Fig. 29-73 Sigmoidoscopic view of the colon in a patient with ischemic colitis reveals slightly polypoid lesions with blue-black discoloration representing underlying submucosal hemorrhage. Courtesy of Dr. John P. Cello.

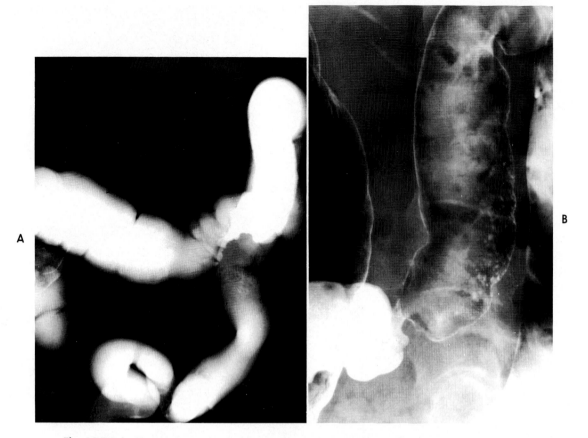

Fig. 29-74 A, Single-contrast barium enema examination shows irregular narrowing of the distal transverse colon. **B,** Double-contrast barium enema examination shows persistence of narrowing even after injection of glucagon. Patient had stricture caused by ischemia from systemic lupus.

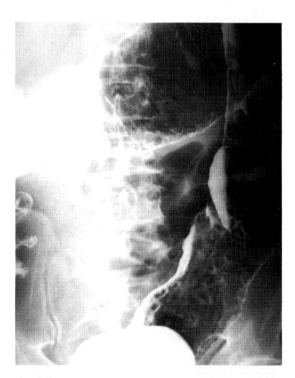

Fig. 29-75 Polypoid filling defects and narrowing of the colon are present in a patient with sequelae of ischemic bowel disease.

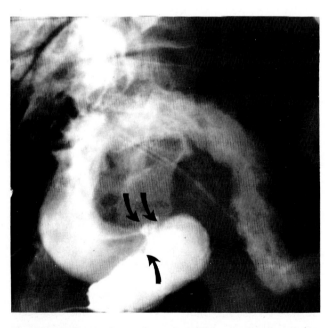

Fig. 29-76 Ulcerated margins and multiple pseudopolyps in the distal descending and sigmoid colons mimic ulcerative colitis in a patient with ischemic changes and bacterial infection proximal to carcinoma of rectosigmoid *(arrows).*

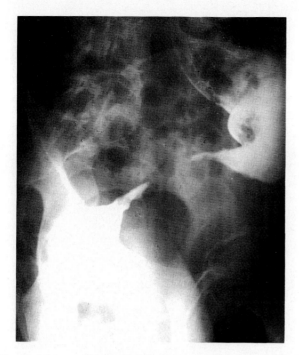

Fig. 29-77 Marked narrowing of the rectosigmoid colon is seen in a patient with lymphogranuloma venereum.

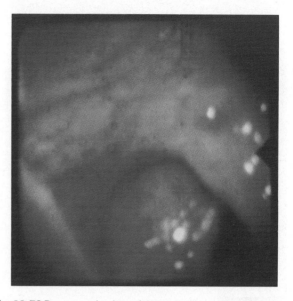

Fig. 29-78 Proctoscopic view of the rectum in a patient with gonococcal proctitis shows diffusely erythematous mucosa. Several tiny punctate ulcers are seen on the background of friable mucosa. Courtesy of Dr. John P. Cello.

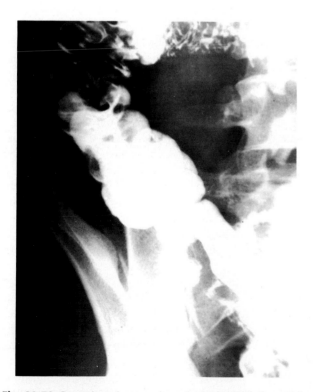

Fig. 29-79 Cone-shaped cecum in patient with chronic amebiasis. The terminal ileum is normal. This type of cecal alteration is not often seen in amebiasis.

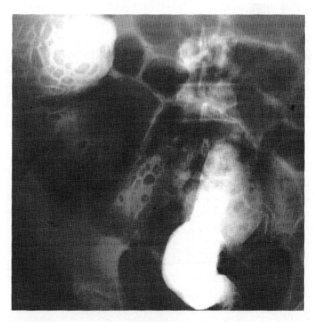

Fig. 29-80 Anaphylactic changes of the colon are shown by means of polygonal angular filling defects. The colon is diffusely dilated.

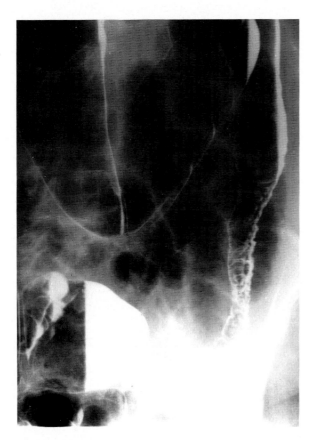

Fig. 29-81 Spiculation, edematous mucosa, and narrowing of lumen are present in a patient with radiation colitis. Distinction from ulcerative colitis is difficult without clinical history.

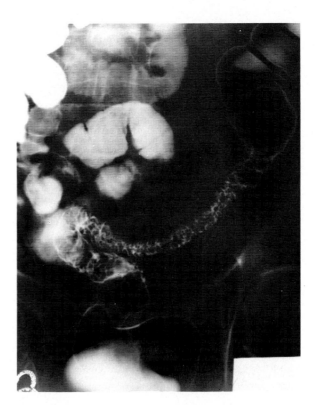

Fig. 29-82 Retractile mesenteritis causes changes similar to ulcerative colitis, ischemia, or radiation colitis. A mesenteric mass usually can be seen on small bowel examination, which helps in reaching correct diagnosis.

gella, or *Salmonella,* adenovirus, immunodeficiency, and malignant lymphoma); primary nonspecific ulcer (idiopathic or benign ulcer); chronic nongranulomatous ulcerative jejunoileitis; acute infectious ileitis (by *Shigella* [usually in distal colon] or *Salmonella* [usually in ascending colon and terminal ileum], *Campylobacter fetus,* and cytomegalovirus); tuberculous enteritis or enterocolitis, and other chronic infectious ileitis or ileocolitis (blastomycosis, actinomycosis, Whipple [usually jejunum], pseudo-Whipple [*Mycobacterium avium intracellulare*]); segmental ischemia; radiation enteritis; eosinophilic gastroenteritis (in any part of the gut from esophagus to colon, but usually only in stomach and proximal small bowel); and very rarely pseudomembranous enteritis or enterocolitis (much more common in colon alone).

ROLE OF COLONOSCOPY

The introduction of fiberoptic endoscopy and endoscopic biopsies has led to an improved understanding of many disease processes. The correlation of radiography, colonoscopy, and pathology helps determine the nature of the disease, its extent, and its clinical course. Colonoscopic-radiographic correlation has been proved to be particularly

helpful in assessing the findings of a double-contrast barium enema examination. Many radiographic findings, such as inflammatory changes, plaques, and polypoid filling defects or masses, can be further investigated by endoscopy to establish a histologic diagnosis for inflammatory bowel disease or to exclude the presence of malignancy. In general, the radiographic examination is only slightly less accurate than colonoscopy in determining the extent of disease, but cases of extensive colitis have been found during colonoscopies after normal results were obtained from a barium enema examination.[27,126,343] If an acute, severe hemorrhage occurs in a patient with colitis, colonoscopy can be used to determine the site of bleeding by direct visualization. Because of the danger of perforation in patients with fulminant colitis, colonoscopy may be dangerous in these patients.

Patients with ulcerative colitis in the high-risk cancer group should be followed-up with endoscopy and radiography. The double-contrast barium enema can show epithelial dysplasia and carcinoma and help determine which patients should undergo close follow-up examinations. However, radiology cannot reliably predict the absence of dysplasia, and therefore the use of radiographic examinations as the primary surveillance technique is not warranted. Colonoscopy combined with multiple biopsies is the primary diagnostic tool in the surveillance of patients with chronic ulcerative colitis.[144,344,345] Radiography should be performed in patients with dysplasia shown on biopsy or with some type of intraluminal lesions detected during a colonoscopy. In patients with ulcerative colitis, double-contrast radiography has the advantages of demonstrating even subtle abnormalities in colonic contour, elevations, or both, and of visualizing strictures. Many of these findings may be imperceptible from the intraluminal perspective of the endoscopist.

Unfortunately, endoscopic and radiographic diagnosis of malignancy in Crohn's disease is much more difficult. Therefore any progressive changes in the appearance of strictures, fistulas, and polyps should be carefully observed and multiple biopsy specimens obtained in the involved areas. Increasing awareness of the malignant potential in patients with long-standing Crohn's disease should lead to an aggressive diagnostic approach, particularly in patients who develop sudden changes in symptomatology such as obstruction, persistent fistulas, or bleeding from fistulas.

The results of colonoscopy and radiography should be carefully analyzed together. Because strictures are usually benign, they are not particularly indicative of cancer. In patients with ulcerative colitis, treatment of consistently positive biopsy specimens for dysplasia, especially for high-grade dysplasia, and treatment of colon cancer consist of total colectomy because of the high risk of multiple lesions.[142,346] In patients with Crohn's disease, treatment consists of local excision of the malignancy.

In patients with fulminant ulcerative colitis and frequent acute attacks, in patients with progressive disease, and in patients with therapy-resistant or chronic disease after 10 years, an aggressive surgical approach is appropriate. This approach has become more acceptable since the development of the ileoanal pouch. However, for Crohn's disease, a surgical approach is only used if absolutely necessary. These patients undergo surgery only for complications of Crohn's disease such as strictures, extensive fistulas, sinus tracts, or abscesses.

ROLE OF RADIOLOGIC FOLLOW-UP EXAMINATIONS IN EVALUATION OF THERAPY

The recent successes with the use of wide-spectrum antibiotic treatment in most types of colitis,[347] except for amebiasis and tuberculosis, have shown that bacteria and their endotoxins are largely responsible for damage to the colonic wall. The pathologic and radiographic findings are similar in a large number of these diseases because of the limited fashion in which the colon can respond to injury. During treatment with antibiotics, radiography shows remission in most patients suffering from inflammatory bowel disease. Radiography shows complete reversal to normal, or at least marked improvement, in many patients with Crohn's disease who undergo antibiotic treatment[348] and in patients with ulcerative colitis who undergo steroid treatment.

The National Cooperative Crohn's Disease Study does not recommend the routine use of radiographic examinations in either the quiescent or the active stage of granulomatous disease of the bowel. It found that the radiographic pattern and the extent of Crohn's disease do not correlate well with the clinical symptoms or response to drug therapy. The conclusion of that cooperative study, however, was based on the single-contrast technique, and the results may not therefore be completely applicable to patients examined by the double-contrast method. Radiographic examinations seem to be recommended only for postsurgical patients with Crohn's disease who develop symptoms of recurrence or for patients with acute severe exacerbation to determine whether strictures with fistula or obstruction are present.[349]

SCINTIGRAPHY FOR INFLAMMATORY BOWEL DISEASE

For assessment of patients with acute inflammatory disease of the bowel with or without abscesses, indium 111–labeled leukocyte scanning has been successfully used.[350-355] However, the accumulation of indium-labeled leukocytes is not specific for idiopathic inflammatory bowel disease and can be seen in ischemic disease, pseudomembranous colitis (Fig. 29-83), cytomegalovirus colitis, and other types of infectious colitis associated with an immunocompromised state such as AIDS,[356] or drug-reactive colitis.[357] So far, positive results have not been seen in irritable bowel syndrome.

Indium 111–labeled leukocyte scintigraphy not only can

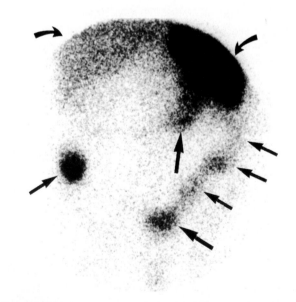

Fig. 29-83 Scintigraphy for inflammatory bowel disease. Uptake in the colon *(arrows)* suggests colitis. Hepatosplenomegaly *(curved arrows)* is also noted in this renal transplant patient with pseudomembranous colitis.
Courtesy of Dr. David Price.

detect abdominal abscesses but also can identify sites of disease activity in inflammatory bowel disease, especially in the colon. It is thought that scintigraphy could be used to monitor response of acute disease to steroid treatment.

COMPUTED TOMOGRAPHY FOR INFLAMMATORY DISEASE OF THE COLON

Barium studies have been and remain the most effective radiographic technique for establishing the diagnosis of inflammatory bowel disease, and computed tomography (CT) is reserved for further study of displacement of bowel loops seen on barium studies, or of complications such as extent of fistulas or abscesses. In suspected malignancy associated with idiopathic inflammatory disease, CT can be used to determine the extent of the neoplasm.

Idiopathic inflammatory bowel disease produces changes in the wall of small and large bowel as well as in the tissue surrounding the involved bowel, and these changes can be demonstrated by CT. For best visualization of these changes, oral and rectal contrast material is essential, and a rapid bolus of intravenously administered contrast agent ensures optimal enhancement of vessels and inflamed tissue. Good opacification of the vasculature helps differentiate adenopathy and vessels and optimizes detection of even small abscesses and areas with granulation tissue. CT can thus detect abnormalities of the colon and small bowel produced by ulcerative (Fig. 29-84) or Crohn's colitis[358-363] (Figs. 29-85 to 29-90) as well as colonic pathology produced by a large variety of infectious types of colitis such as amebiasis or pseudomembranous colitis,[364,365] diverticulitis[366-369] (Figs. 29-91 and 29-92), appendicitis (Fig. 29-93), and drug-induced nonpseudomembranous colitis.[370] Also, ischemic changes of the large and small bowel can be visualized by CT[371,372] (Fig. 29-94), but CT distinction of inflammatory and ischemic changes is possible only when the involvement

of bowel loops follows a typical vascular distribution pattern or if the clinical history is strongly suggestive of a vascular compromise. The detection of wall thickening by CT is nonspecific and a large differential diagnosis is needed, but usually additional features such as clinical history, physical examination, and laboratory tests render the CT diagnosis more specific (see the box below).

In comparison to Crohn's disease, uncomplicated ulcerative colitis shows only minimal wall thickening and few if any changes in the pericolonic fat (see Fig. 29-84). Most infectious types of colitis, with the exception of pseudomembranous colitis, also produce relatively minor wall thickening. This finding is in clear contradistinction to Crohn's disease, pseudomembranous colitis, and ischemia, in which wall thickening is quite prominent. Occasionally, wall thickening in inflammatory bowel disease is caused by submucosal fat deposition rather than inflammation.[207] Such deposition may result from steroid therapy. Bowel wall thickening is nonspecific and may be caused by conditions other than idiopathic and infectious inflammatory bowel disease or ischemia, such as edema resulting from cirrhosis, hypoproteinemia, ascites, amyloidosis, or a local inflammatory process (e.g., pancreatitis, perforation, diverticulitis).

In Crohn's disease, several CT features are highly sug-

☐ **DIFFERENTIAL DIAGNOSIS OF COLONIC WALL THICKENING** ☐

- Crohn's disease
- Infectious colitis
- Pseudomembranous colitis
- Diverticulitis
- Intramural abscess (trauma)
- Perforation with inflammation
- Ischemia/hemorrhage
- Vasculitis
- Ulcerative colitis (minimal)
- Typhlitis (focal)
- Neoplasm
  Adenocarcinoma
  Lymphoma
  Leiomyosarcoma
  Metastases
- Muscular hypertrophy (particularly of sigmoid colon)
- Endometriosis
- Amyloidosis
- Generalized edema (heart failure, uremia, and so on)
- Hemolytic-uremic syndrome
- Angioneurotic edema
- Retractile mesenteritis
- Plication defects after surgery (focal)

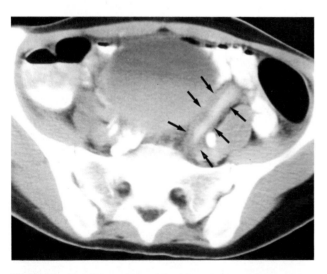

Fig. 29-84 CT of the colon. Thickening of the descending colon *(arrows)* is noted in a patient with ulcerative colitis.

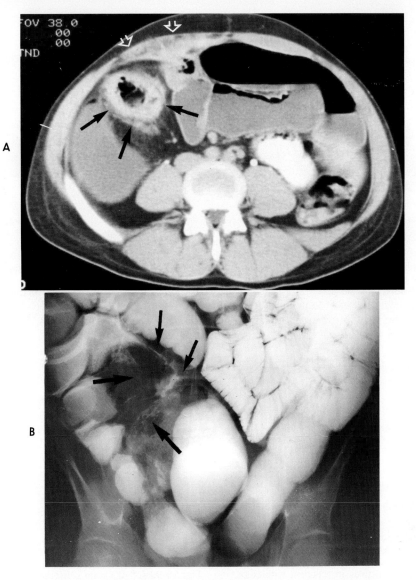

Fig. 29-85 A, CT of the colon in a patient with Crohn's disease. **A,** Note marked thickening of the cecal wall *(arrows)* and pericolonic inflammation. The anterior abdominal wall is also thickened *(open arrows)* in a patient with Crohn's disease. **B,** Multiple ileoileal and ileocolonic fistulas *(arrows)* and abnormal ileal segments are identified during enteroclysis. The mesentery is thickened with displacement of loops of small bowel.

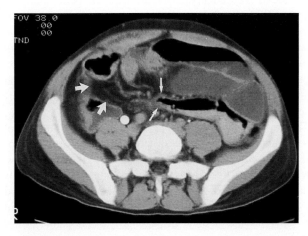

Fig. 29-86 CT of the terminal ileum in a patient with Crohn's disease. Fibrofatty proliferation *(thick arrows)* is shown adjacent to the thickened wall of terminal ileum *(thin arrows)*.

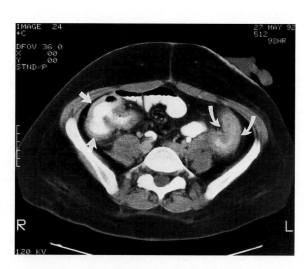

Fig. 29-87 CT of the terminal ileum and cecum in a patient with Crohn's disease. Marked thickening of the wall *(straight arrows)* of the cecum and ileum is noted. The ileal loop on the left *(curved arrows)* representing a skip lesion also is involved.

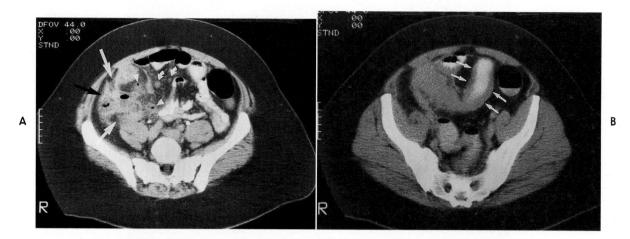

Fig. 29-88 CT of the pelvis in a patient with active Crohn's disease. **A,** Multiple small-bowel loops are matted together in the right lower quadrant *(arrows).* Fistulas are easily seen as small air-filled structures *(arrowheads).* Note nodes *(curved arrows)* near matted loops. **B,** Ileal loop with marked wall thickening *(arrows)* in pelvis of same patient as in **A.**

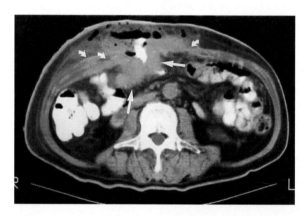

Fig. 29-89 CT of subcutaneous fistulas in a patient with colostomy and recurrent Crohn's disease. Note marked bowel wall thickening *(straight arrows)* and thickening of the abdominal muscle *(curved arrows)* caused by contiguous inflammation.

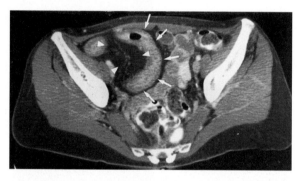

Fig. 29-90 CT of Crohn's disease. Thickening of the terminal ileum *(straight arrows)* and fibrofatty proliferation *(arrowheads)* are seen. CT enables the clinically important differentiation of displacement of bowel loops caused by fibrofatty proliferation from that caused by phlegmon or abscess.

gestive of enteritis, colitis, or both: marked bowel thickening (see Figs. 29-85, 29-87, and 29-88), often associated with stricture formation; increased fat (see Figs. 29-86 and 29-90) in the region surrounding the involved bowel segment (creeping fat or fibrofatty proliferation); adenopathy; increased density in mesentery (phlegmonous reaction); skip lesions (see Fig. 29-87); and perianal sinus tracts and fistulas (see Figs. 29-88 and 29-89). These findings may all be present or only a few of them, but marked bowel wall thickening and fibrofatty proliferation are the most common features encountered on CT scans of patients with Crohn's enterocolitis.[373]

Complications associated with idiopathic inflammatory bowel disease, such as abdominal or pelvic abscesses, fistulas[182,374,375] with or without abscess formation, bowel perforation,[376] and even neoplasm can be detected by CT

and contiguous involvement of adjacent structures assessed. In patients with thickened colonic wall and pericolonic abscess, CT cannot distinguish between diverticulitis with abscess formation, Crohn's disease with abscess, and colon cancer with perforation. The differential diagnosis of wall thickening associated with soft tissue stranding is quite extensive, and additional data such as clinical history and other information are necessary for a definitive diagnosis (see the box on p. 614). In patients with Crohn's disease, CT can determine the degree of thickening of the bowel wall and mesentery; permit differentiation of fibrofatty proliferation, phlegmonous reaction of mesentery, and abscess; detect fistulous tracts between bowel loops and sinus tracts into mesentery and soft tissue near bowel loops and around a stoma; and identify abscesses that cannot be demonstrated by conventional studies. In patients with idiopathic bowel

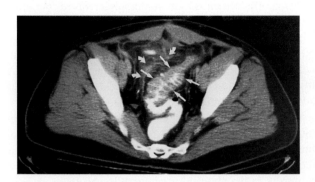

Fig. 29-91 CT of diverticulitis. Note the thickened wall of the sigmoid colon *(straight arrows)*, which is caused by a combination of muscular hypertrophy and inflammation. Pericolonic soft stranding *(curved arrows)* is clearly evident. In comparison to Crohn's disease, the ridges created by edematous muscular hypertrophy and uncomplicated diverticulitis are regular without distortion of anatomy and mass effects, which are signs of Crohn's disease.

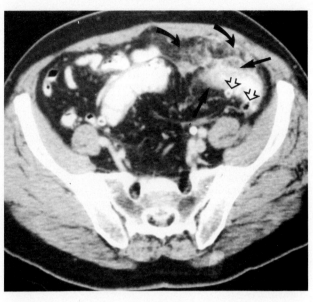

Fig. 29-92 CT of the colon in a patient with diverticulitis. Note thickening of sigmoid wall *(straight arrow)*, pericolonic stranding caused by inflammation *(curved arrows)*, and diverticula *(open arrows)*.

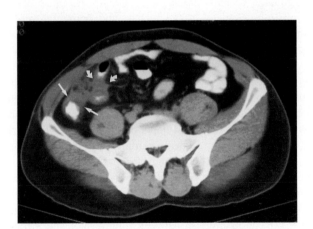

Fig. 29-93 CT of appendicitis. The cecum *(straight arrows)* and terminal ileum *(curved arrows)* have thickened walls, and pericolonic stranding *(arrowheads)* is seen. Based on this CT image, Crohn's disease could not be ruled out.

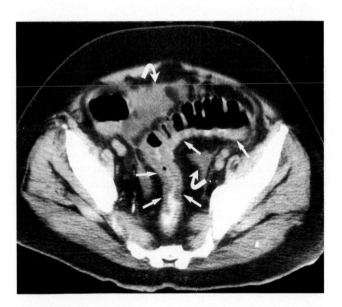

Fig. 29-94 CT of the colon. Thickening of the wall of the rectosigmoid and sigmoid colon *(arrows)*. Some ascites *(curved arrows)* is also noted. Patient suffered from ischemic colitis.

disease and separation of bowel loops seen on enteroclysis or small bowel follow-through, treatment often can be based on findings obtained by CT.

Appendiceal abscesses appear as well-demarcated fluid collections in the right lower quadrant of the abdomen or right pelvis with or without soft tissue strands in the peri-appendiceal fat. Occasionally, thickening of the appendiceal wall alone is seen, which appears as three concentric rings: an outer and inner ring of enhancement separated by a ring of low attenuation, usually associated with peri-appendiceal soft tissue stranding. This type of bowel wall abnormality also can be observed in Crohn's disease and

---

☐ **DIFFERENTIAL DIAGNOSIS OF BOWEL WALL THICKENING WITH STRANDING** ☐

Idiopathic inflammatory bowel disease
Infectious colitis
Ischemia, intramural bleeding
Diverticulitis without abscess
Abscess with
   Diverticulitis
   Pelvic inflammatory disease with contiguous colorectal inflammation
   Rectal perforation
   Prostatitis and contiguous inflammation
Status postpelvic radiation
Invasive neoplasm
Adenocarcinoma
Lymphoma
Cloacogenic carcinoma
Metastases
Giant condyloma accuminata
Endometriosis
Pancreatitis extending to transverse colon or splenic flexure
Transplants of pancreas and kidney with rejection or pancreatitis and contiguous involvement of colon or rectum
Peritonitis with inflammation of bowel

---

ischemia but only when CT scans are obtained during a large and rapidly delivered bolus of contrast material and during rapid dynamic scanning. Solid or ringlike calcifications within a pericecal inflammatory mass indicate an appendicolith and high likelihood of appendicitis.[377] Appendicitis with contiguous inflammation of cecum and terminal ileum may be difficult to distinguish from Crohn's disease (Fig. 29-93).

Pneumatosis coli is diagnosed by demonstrating gas bubbles within the intestinal or colonic wall. These gas bubbles are arranged in a linear fashion and best visualized with the window setting used for demonstrating lung detail such as vessels and bronchi. Pneumatosis coli or intestinalis may be benign in nature (e.g., idiopathic, associated with COPD, steroid treatment, or scleroderma) or associated with ischemia, severe colitis, or bone marrow transplants. A variety of etiologic factors may contribute to pneumatosis intestinalis or coli in patients with bone marrow transplants: graft-versus-host disease, infection, radiation, or chemotherapy. Pneumatosis has even been reported in the stomachs of these patients.[378] When pneumatosis coli is caused by ischemia, gas may also be seen in the portal venous system, and the intestinal wall is thickened. Also, fluid or soft tissue stranding may be seen surrounding the affected ischemic bowel segment.

CT may be helpful in neutropenic colitis, also called *ty-phlitis* or *necrotizing enteropathy*, which is an infectious condition associated with severe neutropenia. It is a complication of acute leukemia, aplastic anemia, or cyclic neutropenia. The cecum is most commonly involved, but other portions of the colon or the terminal ileum may also be affected. In patients with typhlitis, CT shows thickening of the cecal wall with areas of low density caused by edema, hemorrhage, necrosis, or even pneumatosis.[379,380] The thickening of the cecal wall is caused by mucosal ulcerations resulting from ischemia, which may be related to distention of the bowel alone and may be increased by intramural hemorrhage and the effects of steroids, antimetabolites, and folic acid antagonists. The damaged mucosa is then penetrated by bacteria, viruses, and fungi, which grow profusely in the absence of neutrophils. All these changes lead to the wall thickening observed by CT. Frequently, the remaining bowel loops are distended related to a paralytic ileus. Decrease of wall thickening on follow-up examinations indicates recovery from neutropenic colitis. CT is useful in patients with leukemia and nonspecific symptoms of abdominal pain, nausea, and vomiting that could be considered side effects of chemotherapy, because in these instances, recognition on CT of thickened cecal wall can expedite timely and effective medical and possibly surgical management. CT findings similar to those described above for neutropenic typhlitis can be observed in patients with renal, liver, or cardiac transplants and in patients with bone-marrow transplants.

Although Crohn's disease is frequently the cause of inflammatory changes in the rectum and perirectal space, other processes also need to be considered when CT shows rectal wall thickening, perirectal inflammation, or abscesses.[381] Such abscesses can also be seen in patients after corrective surgery for Hirschsprung's disease,[382] after subtotal colectomy and reanastomosis, and in patients with perforated rectal neoplasm such as is seen in advanced adenocarcinoma or in rectal lymphoma. In patients with perirectal inflammation, clinical examination without anesthesia may be quite difficult, and CT provides a noninvasive means to assess the perirectal space reliably and to distinguish patients who need percutaneous drainage or surgery from those who can be managed conservatively. In particular, CT can distinguish between supralevator and infralevator abscess. It is important to differentiate a simple perianal abscess or ischiorectal abscess from one that is a caudal extension of a large supralevator abscess. Failure to recognize such extension of a supralevator abscess leads to inadequate surgical drainage and recurrence of abscess.

CT also can be used in patients with ileoanal pouches before take-down of the ileostomy to detect leakage from the pouch, fistulas, sinus tracts, abscess, or pouchitis.[40,383] CT has been found to be very accurate in the detection of complications with the ileoanal pouch, particularly abscesses.[40] If any of the above-mentioned complications, with the exception of pouchitis, is present, take-down of the ileostomy should be delayed until complications have resolved. Based on CT, decisions can be made on the appropriate treatment for these patients and the success of therapy monitored.

SONOGRAPHY FOR INFLAMMATORY BOWEL DISEASE

In recent years, an increasing number of studies have appeared that explored the use of ultrasonography to assess the intestinal wall and inflammatory bowel disease.[384-387] Inflammatory changes that were examined by ultrasound included *Yersinia* terminal ileitis,[384] acute Meckel's diverticulitis,[388] cecal diverticulitis, appendicitis,[389] and typhoid fever.[390] Ultrasonography has also been used to diagnose pneumatosis of the small bowel,[391] and in vitro studies confirmed its diagnostic use for inflammatory bowel disease.[392] Ultrasonography has also been used in patients with ischemic bowel disease (Fig. 29-95).

Several clinical studies have assessed the value of ultrasound for diagnosing idiopathic inflammatory bowel disease and diverticulitis. The sensitivity of ultrasonography for Crohn's disease (Fig. 29-96) is higher in the colon than in the small bowel and higher in the pediatric patient group than in the adult population.[393]

Gut wall thickening, pericolic and intramural fluid col-lections, and edema of pericolonic fat could be demonstrated by ultrasound.[394-396] The abnormal intestine in Crohn's disease appears as a thickened, sonolucent mantel corresponding to the thickened wall that surrounds a central area of high echogenicity representing the narrowed intestinal lumen. On transverse sections, this ultrasound appearance of abnormal bowel loops has been referred to as a target sign, or "bull's-eye" lesion. A similar observation can be made on CT, which demonstrates this target sign as three concentric rings on transverse sections. On longitudinal sections, ultrasound shows a tubular structure with an echo-poor thickened wall and a narrowed lumen with bright central echoes[393] (see Fig. 29-96).

Sonographic characteristics that may lead to the diagnosis of Crohn's disease include symmetric or circular thickening with a uniform increase in wall thickness, predominantly of the mucosa and submucosa; preservation of integrity of wall layers, and matted bowel loops. Rigid bowel segments without any peristaltic motion and stiff bowel segments with reduced peristalsis may also suggest Crohn's disease. In addition, matting of intestinal loops filled with fluid and, if obstruction is present, prestenotic bowel dilatation with hyperperistalsis are additional helpful features.

Diverticulitis can also be readily diagnosed by ultrasound, based on bowel wall thickening and inflamed

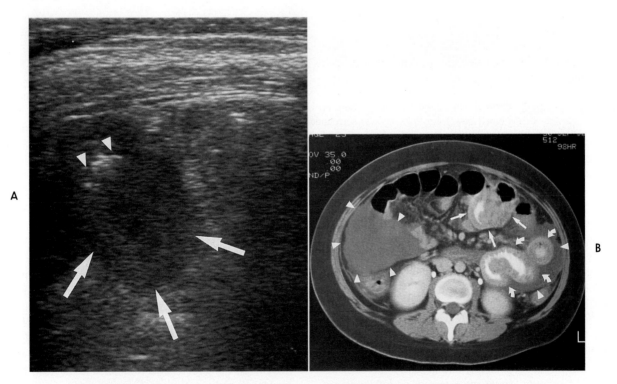

Fig. 29-95 Ischemia of the small bowel. **A,** Ultrasound demonstrates marked thickening of a jejunal loop in the left upper quadrant. Note thickened wall of low echogenicity *(straight arrows)* and high echogenicity of bowel lumen *(arrowheads)*. **B,** CT demonstrates the same bowel loop as shown in **A.** Note ascites *(arrowheads),* nonuniform thickening of the intestinal wall *(small arrows),* and marked thickening of additional jejunal loops *(curved arrows).*

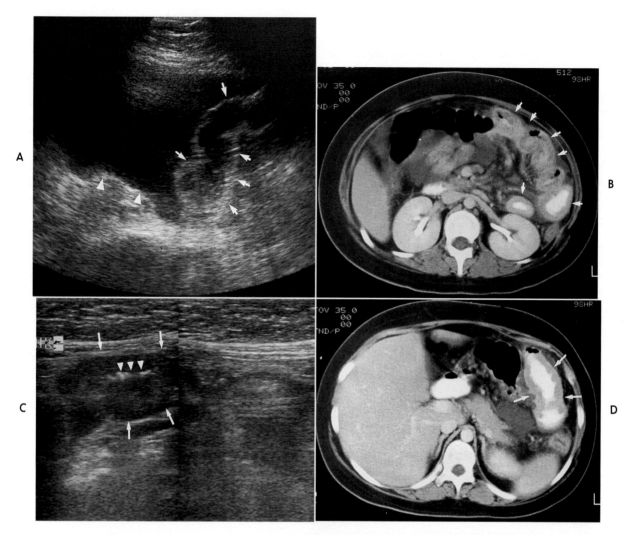

Fig. 29-96 Crohn's disease of the jejunum. **A,** Ultrasound demonstrates markedly thickened loops of the small bowel *(straight arrows)* surrounded by ascites *(arrowheads).* **B,** CT visualizes the same bowel loops. Note extensive wall thickening and minimal ascites. **C,** Ultrasound demonstrates another intestinal loop in the left upper quadrant as a tubular structure *(arrows)* with a markedly thickened wall. Note echogenic lumen *(arrowheads).* **D,** CT shows corresponding area in the small bowel *(arrows)* with a small amount of pericolonic stranding.

diverticula.[397-399] It cannot always be differentiated from Crohn's disease when only colonic involvement is present. However, if clinical suspicion is high for an abscess or if the sonogram is equivocal or poor because of gas, CT should be employed in either case. In Verbanck et al.'s study[397] all cases of diverticulitis with significant pericolic disease were correctly assessed. For acute diverticulitis, ultrasonography appears to be an excellent initial imaging tool because of its ready availability and accuracy. In many instances of Crohn's disease, the extent of an inflammatory process outside the bowel loop, including abscesses, is better defined by CT than by ultrasound, which is often impaired gas present in abscesses or in distended and stiff bowel loops.

MAGNETIC RESONANCE IMAGING FOR INFLAMMATORY BOWEL DISEASE

Currently the use of oral and intravenous paramagnetic and diamagnetic substances for magnetic resonance imaging (MRI) is still in its research phase with several agents undergoing clinical trials.[400-403] Technical problems resulting from slow scanning, inferior spatial resolution, lack of a good oral and rectal contrast agent, and persistently impaired image quality with fast imaging sequences such as fast gradient echo technique or echoplanar imaging are presently limiting MRI for the evaluation of the colon and small bowel. Glucagon injected intramuscularly or subcutaneously to reduce peristaltic motion and administration of air are helpful for better

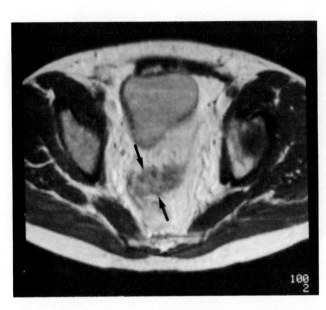

Fig. 29-97 T2 MRI of the colon (TR 2000 msec; MR 60 msec), transverse image. Thickening and increased signal intensity of the sigmoid wall are noted in a patient with diverticulitis *(arrows).* Crohn's disease may appear in a similar fashion.

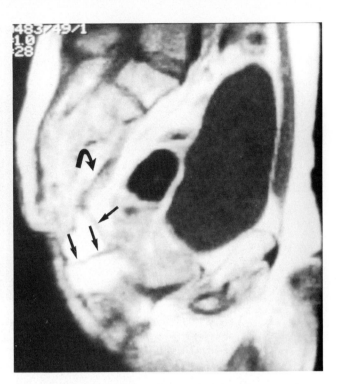

Fig. 29-98 MRI of Crohn's disease. Fistula tracts *(straight arrows)* extend posteriorly to the presacral abscess *(curved arrow).* The rectal wall is thickened and of higher signal intensity.

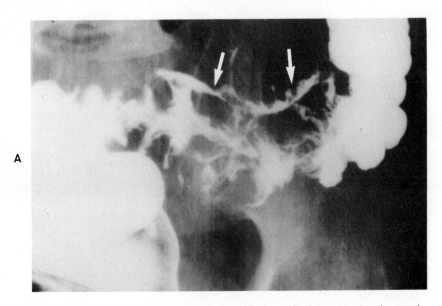

Fig. 29-99 A, An intramural fistula *(arrows)* is well shown by barium enema in a patient with diverticulitis. *Continued.*

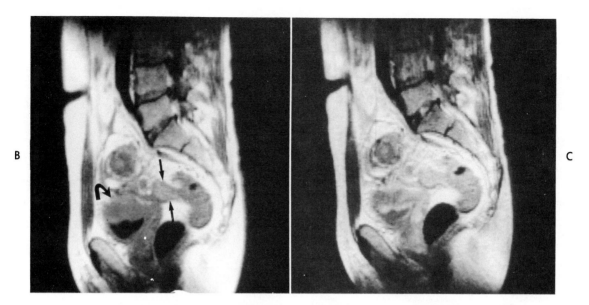

Fig. 29-99, cont'd B, Sagittal T1 MRI (TR 700 msec; TE 15 msec) demonstrates a pericolonic abscess *(arrows),* thickened colonic wall, and thickened bladder wall *(curved arrows).* **C,** Compared to T1 MRI **(B),** T2 MRI sagittal image (TR 2000 msec; TE 60 msec) shows increased signal intensity in the colonic wall, suggesting inflammation.

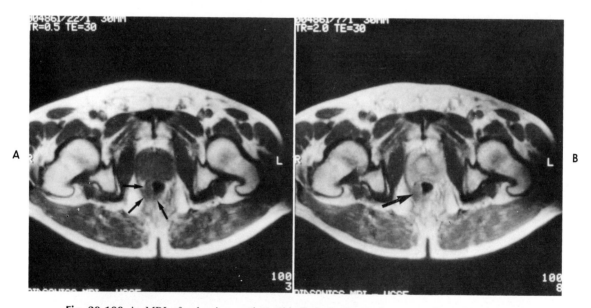

Fig. 29-100 A, MRI of colon in a patient with Crohn's disease in rectum. T1 MRI transverse image (TR 500 msec; TE 30 msec). A thickened rectal wall *(arrows)* and stranding in perirectal fat posterior to the rectum are seen. **B,** T2 transverse image (TR 2000 msec; TE 30 msec). Thickened rectal wall shows increased signal intensity *(arrows).* The signal intensity of some of the soft tissue strands is increased indicating inflammatory changes surrounding the rectum of a patient with Crohn's disease.

assessment of the thickness and surface appearance of the intestinal and colonic wall.

MRI is particularly successful in the rectum because it is a fixed structure in the pelvis. Meticulous cleansing of the colon is needed to avoid confusing feces with thickening of the bowel wall. In the evaluation of the rectum, coronal views are especially helpful because they can distinguish between the supralevator and infralevator compartments. This distinction is important for consideration of treatment. However, to assess complications of idiopathic inflammatory bowel disease such as staging of rectal tumors, MRI only adds additional and useful information to what CT can already provide if rectal coils are employed. These coils permit assessment of the depth of involvement within the rectal wall by invasive tumor. They may also help determine the nature of nodes in the immediate perirectal area of patients with suspected rectal malignancy, but their use is limited to the rectum and possibly rectosigmoid junction. Studies of large series using these rectal coils have yet to be published. For widespread use of rectal coils, conditions such as acceptance by patients and general availability of the device have to be fulfilled.

Very few published data are available on the use of MRI for inflammatory changes in the large bowel (Figs. 29-97 to 29-100). One study[404] found that fistulas could be well visualized on images based on linear structures of low signal intensity on T1 scans and high signal intensity on T2 scans. In 13 of 17 patients in this recent series,[404] the orifice of fistulas or sinus tracts in the bowel was correctly delineated and their connections to muscles, hollow viscera, and skin were shown. However, at present, no definite advantage is apparent for MRI over CT in assessing patients with inflammatory changes of the large and small bowel. Some of the apparent problems with the use of MRI are related to the lack of a commercially available oral and rectal contrast material.

REFERENCES

1. Rice RP: Plain abdominal film roentgenographic diagnosis of ulcerative diseases of the colon, *AJR* 104:544, 1968.
2. Bartram CI: Plain abdominal x-ray in acute colitis, *Proc R Soc Med* 69:617, 1976.
3. Halls J, Young A: Plain abdominal films in colonic disease, *Proc R Soc Med* 57:893, 1964.
4. Taylor GA et al: Plain abdominal radiographs in children with inflammatory bowel disease, *Pediatr Radiol* 16:206, 1986.
5. Jalan KN et al: An experience of ulcerative colitis: I. Toxic dilation in 55 cases, *Gastroenterology* 57:68, 1969.
6. Strauss RJ et al: The surgical management of toxic dilatation of the colon: a report of 28 cases and review of the literature, *Ann Surg* 184:682, 1976.
7. Whorell PJ, Isaacson P: Toxic dilatation of the colon in Crohn's disease, *Lancet* 4:1334, 1981.
8. Goldberg HI: The barium enema and toxic megacolon: cause-effect relationship? *Gastroenterology* 68:617, 1975.
9. Wolf BS, Marshak RH: Toxic segmental dilation of the colon during the course of fulminating ulcerative colitis: roentgen findings, *AJR* 82:985, 1959.
10. Roys G, Kaplan MS, Juler GL: Surgical management of toxic megacolon, *Am J Gastroenterol* 68:161, 1977.
11. Binder S, Patterson JF, Glotzer D: Toxic megacolon in ulcerative colitis, *Gastroenterology* 66:909, 1974.
12. Rosenberg M: Toxic megacolon, *West J Med* 124:122, 1976.
13. Welin S, Welin G: *The double contrast examination of the colon: experiences with the Welin modification*, Stuttgart, 1976, Georg Thieme Verlag.
14. LeFrock T et al: Transient bacteraemia associated with barium enema, *Arch Intern Med* 135:835, 1975.
15. Schimmel DH et al: Bacteraemia and the barium enema, *AJR* 128:207, 1977.
16. Cello JP, Meyer JH: Ulcerative colitis. In Sleisenger MH, Fordtran JS, eds: *Gastrointestinal disease: pathophysiology, diagnosis, management,* vol 2, Philadelphia, 1978, WB Saunders.
17. Laufer I: The radiologic demonstration of early changes in ulcerative colitis by double contrast technique, *J Can Assoc Radiol* 25:116, 1975.
18. Laufer I: The double contrast enema: myths and misconceptions, *Gastrointest Radiol* 1:19, 1976.
19. Laufer I, Hamilton JD: The radiologic differentiation between ulcerative and granulomatous colitis by double contrast radiology, *Am J Gastroenterol* 66:259, 1976.
20. Laufer I: *Double contrast gastrointestinal radiology*, Philadelphia, 1979, WB Saunders.
21. Welin S, Brahme F: The double contrast method in ulcerative colitis, *Acta Radiol* 55:257, 1961.
22. Thoeni RF, Margulis AR: Intracolonic pressures during barium enema studies using the single- and double-contrast techniques. *Invest Radiol* 14:162, 1979.
23. Bartram CI, Laufer I: Inflammatory bowel disease. In Laufer I, ed: *Double contrast gastrointestinal radiology with endoscopic correlation*, Philadelphia, 1979, WB Saunders.
24. Thoeni RF, Vandeman F, Wall S: The effect of glucagon on diagnostic accuracy of double-contrast barium enema examinations, *AJR* 142:111, 1984.
25. Kellett JM, Zboralske FF, Margulis AR: Peroral pneumocolon examination of the ileocecal region, *Gastrointest Radiol* 1:361, 1977.
26. Young AC: The instant barium enema in proctocolitis, *Proc R Soc Med* 56:491, 1963.
27. Bartram CI, Walmsley K: A radiological and pathological correlation of the mucosal changes in ulcerative colitis, *Clin Radiol* 29:323, 1978.
28. Apsimon HT: The single phase double contrast enema, a technique for the average department, *Clin Radiol* 21:188, 1970.
29. Thoeni RF: Pharmacologic enhancement of radiological studies of the gastrointestinal tract. In Margulis AR, Gooding CA, eds: *Diagnostic radiology,* San Francisco, 1983, Extended Programs in Medical Education, San Francisco, University of California.
30. Goldstein HM et al: Comparison of methods for acceleration of small intestinal radiographic examination, *Radiology* 98:519, 1971.
31. Fraser GM, Preston PG: The small-bowel barium follow-through enhanced with an oral effervescent agent, *Clin Radiol* 34:673, 1983.
32. Miller RE, Sellink JL: Enteroclysis: the small-bowel enema: how to succeed and how to fail, *Gastrointest Radiol* 4:269, 1979.
33. Herlinger H: A modified technique for the double-contrast small bowel enema, *Gastrointest Radiol* 3:201, 1978.
34. Lappas JC, Maglinte DT: Enteroclysis edges in on follow-through methods, *Diag Imag* 88, 1987.
35. Thoeni RF: Radiography of the small bowel and enteroclysis: a perspective, *Invest Radiol* 22:930, 1988.
36. Fitzgerald EJ, Thompson GT, Somers SS et al: Pneumocolon as an aid to small-bowel studies, *Clin Radiol* 36:633, 1985.
37. Kelvin FM et al: The peroral pneumocolon: its role in evaluating the terminal ileum, *AJR* 139:115, 1982.

38. Kressel HY et al: The peroral pneumocolon examination: technique and indications, *Radiology* 144:414, 1982.

39. Wolf KJ, Goldberg HI, Wall SD et al: Feasibility of the peroral pneumocolon in evaluating the ileocecal region, *AJR* 145:10, 1985.

40. Thoeni RF et al: Ileoanal pouches: comparison of CT, scintigraphy and contrast enemas for diagnosing postsurgical complications, *AJR* 154:73, 1990.

41. Fleischner FG, Mandelstam P: Roentgen observations of the ileostomy in patients with idiopathic ulcerative colitis: ileostomy dysfunction, *Radiology* 70:469, 1958.

42. Ritchie JK: Results of surgery for inflammatory bowel disease, a further survey of one hospital region, *Br Med J* 1:264, 1974.

43. Harned RK et al: Barium enema examination following biopsy of the rectum or colon, *Radiology* 145:11, 1982.

44. Maglinte DDT et al: Barium enema after colorectal biopsies: experimental data, *AJR* 139:693, 1982.

45. Fried AM, Poulos A, Hatfield DR: The effectiveness of the incidental small-bowel series, *Radiology* 140:45, 1981.

46. Rabe FE et al: Efficacy study of the small-bowel examination, *Radiology* 140:47, 1981.

47. Carlson HC: Perspective: the small-bowel examination in the diagnosis of Crohn's disease, *AJR* 147:63, 1986.

48. Maglinte DT, Burney BT, Miller RE: Lesions missed on small-bowel follow-through: analysis and recommendations, *Radiology* 144:737, 1982.

49. Ott DJ et al: Detailed per-oral small-bowel examination vs enteroclysis. Part I: expenditures and radiation exposure, *Radiology* 155:29, 1985.

50. Kroneberg G, Sandritter W: Kreislaufkollaps und morphologische Veränderungen bei der Vergiftung mit Flexner-Ruhr-Endotoxin, *Medizin* 120:329, 1953.

51. Sandritter W, Lasch HG: Pathologic aspects of shock. In Jasmin G, Cantin M, eds: *Methods and achievements of experimental pathology*, Basel, 1966, S Karger.

52. Farmer RG, Hawk WA, Turnbull RB: Clinical and pathological correlations in inflammatory bowel disease, *Cleve Clin Q* 46:35, 1979.

53. Margulis AR et al: The overlapping spectrum of ulcerative and granulomatous colitis: a roentgenographic-pathologic study, *AJR* 113:325, 1971.

54. Mottet NK: *Histopathologic spectrum of regional enteritis and ulcerative colitis*, Philadelphia, 1971, WB Saunders.

55. Markely JC, Carson RP, Holzer CE: Pseudomembranous enterocolitis, *Arch Surg* 77:452, 1958.

56. Penner A, Bernheim AI: Acute postoperative enterocolitis: a study on the pathologic nature of shock, *Arch Pathol* 17:1966, 1939.

57. Pittmann FE, Pittman JC, Humphrey CD: Colitis following oral lincomycin therapy, *Arch Intern Med* 134:368, 1974.

58. Whitehead R: Ischemic enterocolitis: an expression of the intravascular coagulation syndrome, *Gut* 12:912, 1971.

59. Lewin K, Swales JD: Granulomatous colitis and atypical ulcerative colitis: histological features, behavior and prognosis, *Gastroenterology* 50:211, 1966.

60. Morson B: Histology of Crohn's disease, *Proc R Soc Med* 61:79, 1968.

61. Williams WJ: Histology of Crohn's disease, *Gut* 5:510, 1964.

62. Goldberger LE, Neely HR, Stammer JL: Large mucosal bridges: an unusual roentgenographic manifestation of ulcerative colitis, *Gastrointest Radiol* 3:81, 1978.

63. Hammerman AM, Shatz BA, Sussman N: Radiographic characteristics of colonic "mucosal bridges," sequelae of inflammatory bowel disease, *Radiology* 127:611, 1978.

64. Zegel H, Laufer L: Filiform polyposis, *Radiology* 127:615, 1978.

65. Schachter J: Chlamydial infections (first of three parts), *N Engl J Med* 298:428, 1978.

66. Kirsner JB: Problems in the differentiation of ulcerative colitis and Crohn's disease of the colon: the need for repeated diagnostic evaluations, *Gastroenterology* 68:187, 1975.

67. Price AB: Overlap in the spectrum of nonspecific inflammatory bowel disease—"colitis indeterminate," *J Clin Pathol* 31:567, 1978.

68. Hill RB, Kent TH, Hansen RN: Clinical usefulness of rectal biopsy in Crohn's disease, *Gastroenterology* 77:938, 1979.

69. Kraft SC: Modern clinical aspects of inflammatory tissue diseases, *Radiol Clin North Am* 25:213, 1987.

70. Harris J, Shields R: Absorption and secretion of water and electrolytes by the intact human colon in diffuse untreated proctocolitis, *Gut* 11:27, 1970.

71. Goulston SJM, McGovern VJ: The nature of benign strictures in ulcerative colitis, *N Engl J Med* 281:290, 1969.

72. Morson BC, Dawson IMP: *Gastrointestinal pathology*, Oxford, 1972, Blackwell Scientific Publications.

73. Bonnevie O, Riis P, Anthonsien P: An epidemiological study of ulcerative colitis in Copenhagen County, *Scand J Gastroenterol* 3:432, 1968.

74. Edwards FC, Truelove SC: The course and prognosis of ulcerative colitis: II. Long-term prognosis, *Gut* 4:309, 1963.

75. Sonnenberg A: Occupational mortality of inflammatory bowel disease, *Digestion* 46:10, 1990.

76. Truelove SC, Witts LJ: Cortisone in ulcerative colitis, a preliminary report on a therapeutic trial, *Br Med J* 2:375, 1954.

77. Sparberg M, Fennessy J, Kirsner JB: Ulcerative proctitis and mild ulcerative colitis: a study of 220 patients, *Medicine* 45:391, 1966.

78. Edwards FC, Truelove SC: The course and prognosis of ulcerative colitis: I. Short-term prognosis, *Gut* 4:299, 1963.

79. Carman R, Jannuccilli EA, Thayer WR: Toxic megacolon in inflammatory bowel disease: a new perspective, *RI Med J* 128:935, 1977.

80. Gilat T et al: Ulcerative colitis in the Jewish population of Tel-Aviv Yafo. III. Clinical course, *Gastroenterology* 70:14, 1976.

81. Marshak RH, Lindner AE: Granulomatous colitis and ileocolitis with emphasis on the radiologic features, *Prog Gastroenterol* 1:357, 1968.

82. Norland CC, Kirsner JB: Toxic dilatation of the colon (toxic megacolon): etiology, treatment, and prognosis in 42 patients, *Medicine* 48:229, 1969.

83. deDombal FT et al: Local complications of ulcerative colitis: stricture, pseudopolyps, and carcinoma of the colon and rectum, *Br Med J* 1:1442, 1966.

84. Cook MG, Path MRC, Goligher JC: Carcinoma and epithelial dysplasia complicating ulcerative colitis, *Gastroenterology* 68:1127, 1975.

85. Devroede G, Taylor W: On calculating cancer risk and survival of ulcerative colitis patients with the life table method, *Gastroenterology* 71:505, 1976.

86. Edwards FC, Truelove SC: The course and prognosis of ulcerative colitis: IV. Carcinoma of the colon, *Gut* 5:15, 1964.

87. Johnson ML, Wilson TH: Skin lesions in ulcerative colitis, *Gut* 10:255, 1969.

88. McEwen C, Lingg C, Kirsner JB: Arthritis accompanying ulcerative colitis, *Am J Med* 33:923, 1962.

89. Wright R et al: Abnormalities of the sacroiliac joints and uveitis in ulcerative colitis, *Q J Med* 34:229, 1965.

90. Breuer RJ, Gelzayd EA, Kirsner JK: Urinary crystalloid excretion in patients with inflammatory bowel disease, *Gut* 11:314, 1970.

91. Dobbins J, Binder HJ: Importance of the colon in enteric hyperoxaluria, *N Engl J Med* 296:1977.

92. Enker MD, Block GE: Occult obstructive uropathy complicating Crohn's disease, *Arch Surg* 101:319, 1970.

93. Greenstein AJ, Janowitz HD, Sachar DB: The extra-intestinal complications of Crohn's disease and ulcerative colitis: a study of 700 patients, *Medicine* 55:401, 1976.

94. Lam A et al: Coagulation studies in ulcerative colitis and Crohn's disease, *Gastroenterology* 68:245, 1975.

95. Yassinger S et al: Association of inflammatory bowel disease and large vascular lesions, *Gastroenterology* 71:844, 1976.

96. Dekker-Saeyes BJ et al: Ankylosing spondylitis and inflammatory bowel disease: II. Prevalence of peripheral arthritis, sacroiliitis, and ankylosing spondylitis in patients suffering from inflammatory bowel disease, *Ann Rheum Dis* 37:33, 1978.

97. Jalan KN et al: Arthropathy, ankylosing spondylitis, and clubbing of fingers in ulcerative colitis, *Gut* 11:748, 1970.

98. Wee A, Ludwig J: Pericholangitis in chronic ulcerative colitis: primary sclerosing cholangitis of the small bile ducts? *Ann Intern Med* 102:581, 1985.

99. Roberts-Thompson IC, Strickland RG, Mackey IR: Bile duct carcinoma in chronic ulcerative colitis, *Aust N Z J Med* 2:264, 1973.

100. Cello JP: Cholestasis in ulcerative colitis, *Gastroenterology* 73:357, 1977.

101. Eade MN: Liver disease in ulcerative colitis: I. Analysis of operative liver biopsy in 138 consecutive patients having colectomy, *Ann Intern Med* 72:475, 1970.

102. Mistillis SP: Pericholangitis and ulcerative colitis: I. Pathology, etiology, and pathogenesis, *Ann Intern Med* 63:1, 1965.

103. Perrett AD et al: The liver in ulcerative colitis, *Q J Med* 40:211, 1971.

104. Talbot RW et al: Vascular complications of inflammatory bowel disease, *Mayo Clin Proc* 61:140, 1986.

105. Passo MH, Fitzgerald JF, Brandt KD: Arthritis associated with inflammatory bowel disease in children, *Dig Dis Sci* 31:492, 1986.

106. Compston JE et al: Osteoporosis in patients with inflammatory bowel disease, *Gut* 28:410, 1987.

107. Billison FA et al: Ocular complications of ulcerative colitis, *Gut* 8:102, 1967.

108. Mir-Madjlessi SH, Taylor JS, Farmer RG: Clinical course of erythema nodosum and pyoderma gangrenosum in chronic ulcerative colitis: a study in of 42 patients. *Am J Gastroenterol* 80:615, 1985.

109. Fraser GM, Findlay JN: The double contrast enema in ulcerative and Crohn's colitis, *Clin Radiol* 27:103, 1976.

110. Laufer I: Air contrast studies of the colon in inflammatory bowel disease, *CRC Crit Rev Diagn Imaging* 9:421, 1977.

111. Persigehl M et al: Feinreliefveraenderungen des Kolons in Fruehstadium der Colitis ulcerosa und Colitis granulomatosa, *Fortschr Roentgenstr* 129:177, 1978.

112. Shield DE et al: Urologic complications of inflammatory bowel disease, *J Urol* 115:701, 1976.

113. Beranbaum SL: Roentgenologic diagnosis of idiopathic nonspecific ulcerative colitis with special reference to early manifestations, *Dis Colon Rectum* 7:135, 1964.

114. Lichtenstein JE, Madewell JE, Feigin DS: The collar button ulcer, *Gastrointest Radiol* 4:79, 1979.

115. Buck JL, Dachman AH, Sobin LH: Polypoid and pseudopolypoid manifestations of inflammatory bowel disease, *Radiographics* 11:293, 1991.

116. Lesher DT, Phillips JC, Rabinowitz JG: Pseudopolyposis as the only manifestation of ulcerative colitis, *Am J Gastroenterol* 70:670, 1978.

117. Kelly JK et al: Giant and symptomatic inflammatory polyps of the colon in idiopathic inflammatory bowel disease, *Am J Surg Pathol* 10:420, 1986.

118. Balazs M: Giant inflammatory polyps associated with idiopathic inflammatory bowel disease: an ultrastructural study of five cases, *Dis Colon Rectum* 33:773, 1990.

119. Edling NPG, Eklof O: The retrorectal soft tissue space in ulcerative colitis: a roentgen diagnostic study, *Radiology* 80:949, 1963.

120. Alp MH, Sage MR, Grant AK: The significance of widening of the presacral space at contrast radiography in inflammatory bowel disease, *Aust NZ J Surg* 48:175, 1978.

121. Farthing MJG, Lennard-Jones JE: The rectosacral distance and rectal size in ulcerative colitis, *Br Med J* 2:1266, 1977.

122. Counsell B: Lesions of the ileum associated with ulcerative colitis, *Br J Surg* 185:276, 1956/57.

123. Gardiner GA: "Backwash ileitis" with pseudopolyposis, *AJR* 129:506, 1977.

124. Golligher JC: Primary excisional surgery in the treatment of ulcerative colitis, *Ann R Coll Surg Engl* 15:316, 1965.

125. Gabrielsson N: Extent of inflammatory lesions in ulcerative colitis assessed by radiology, colonoscopy, and endoscopic biopsies, *Gastrointest Radiol* 4:395, 1979.

126. Dilawari JB et al: Colonoscopy in the investigation of ulcerative colitis, *Gut* 14:426, 1973.

127. Berenbaum SL, Yaghmai M, Berenbaum ER: Ulcerative colitis in association with diverticular disease of the colon, *Radiology* 85:880, 1965.

128. Bargen JA: Chronic ulcerative colitis: diagnostic and therapeutic problems: a lifelong study, *AJR* 99:5, 1967.

129. Brahme F: Granulomatous colitis: roentgenologic appearance and course of lesions, *AJR* 99:35, 1967.

130. Vernia P et al: Intestinal gas in ulcerative colitis, *Dis Colon Rectum* 22:346, 1979.

131. Brooke BN, Sampson PA: An indication for surgery in acute ulcerative colitis, *Lancet* 2:1272, 1964.

132. Bucknell NA, Williams GT, Bartram CI: Depth of ulceration in acute colitis, *Gastroenterology* 79:19, 1980.

133. deDombal FT et al: Interperitoneal perforation of the colon in ulcerative colitis, *Proc R Soc Med* 58:713, 1965.

134. Greenstein AJ, Aufses AH: Differences in pathogenesis, incidence, and outcome of perforation in inflammatory bowel disease, *Surg Gynecol Obstet* 160:63, 1985.

135. Nelson JA, Daniels AU, Dodds WJ: Rectal balloons: complications, causes, and recommendations, *Invest Radiol* 14:48, 1979.

136. Marshak RH, Bloch C, Wolf BS: The roentgen findings in strictures of the colon associated with ulcerative and granulomatous colitis, *AJR* 90:709, 1963.

137. Hunt RH et al: Colonoscopy in the management of the colonic strictures, *Br Med J* 3:360, 1975.

138. Simpkins KC, Young AC: The differential diagnosis of large bowel strictures, *Clin Radiol* 22:449, 1971.

139. Urso FP, Urso MI, Lee CM: The cathartic colon: pathological findings and radiological-pathological correlation, *Radiology* 116:557, 1975.

140. Kim SK, Gerle RD, Rozanski R: Cathartic colitis, *AJR* 131:1079, 1978.

141. Folley JH: Ulcerative proctitis, *N Engl J Med* 282:1362, 1970.

142. Butt JH, Lennard-Jones JE, Ritchie JK: A practical approach to the risk of cancer in inflammatory bowel disease: reassure, watch, or act? *Med Clin North Am* 64:1203, 1980.

143. Faintuch J, Levin B, Kirsner JB: Inflammatory bowel diseases and their relationship to malignancy, *CRC Crit Rev Oncol Hematol* 2:323, 1985.

144. Rosenstock E et al: Surveillance for colonic carcinoma in ulcerative colitis, *Gastroenterology* 89:1342, 1985.

145. van Heerden JA, Beart RW: Carcinoma of the colon and rectum complicating chronic ulcerative colitis, *Dis Colon Rectum* 23:155, 1980.

146. Greenstein AJ et al: Cancer in universal and left-sided ulcerative colitis: factors determining risk, *Gastroenterology* 77:290, 1979.

147. Hinton JM: Risk of malignant change in ulcerative colitis, *Gut* 7:427, 1966.

148. Goldgraber MB, Kirsner JB: Carcinoma of the colon in ulcerative colitis, *Cancer* 17:657, 1964.

149. Fennessy JJ, Sparberg MB, Kirsner JB: Radiological findings in carcinoma of the colon complicating chronic ulcerative colitis, *Gut* 9:388, 1968.

150. Dobbins WO: Dysplasia and malignancy in inflammatory bowel disease, *Ann Rev Med* 35:33, 1984.

151. Maglinte DD et al: Colon and rectal carcinoma: spatial distribution and detection, *Radiology* 147:669, 1983.

152. Lennard-Jones JE et al: Precancer and cancer in extensive ulcerative colitis: findings among 401 patients over 22 years, *Gut* 31:800, 1991.

153. Prior P et al: Cancer morbidity in ulcerative colitis, *Gut* 23:490, 1982.
154. Frank PH et al: Radiological detection of colonic dysplasia (precarcinoma) in chronic ulcerative colitis, *Gastrointest Radiol* 3:209, 1978.
155. Bashiti JO, Kraus KT: Histiocytic lymphoma complicating chronic ulcerative colitis, *Cancer* 46:1695, 1980.
156. Fabry TL, Sachar DB, Janowitz HD: Acute myelogenous leukemia in patients with ulcerative colitis, *J Clin Gastroenterol* 2:225, 1980.
157. Montagne JP et al: Radiologic evaluation of the continent (Koch) ileostomy, *Radiology* 127:325, 1978.
158. Schoetz DJ, Coller JA, Veidenheimer MC: Alternatives to conventional ileostomy in chronic ulcerative colitis, *Surg Clin North Am* 65:21, 1985.
159. Hillard AE et al: The ileoanal J pouch: radiographic evaluation, *Radiology* 155:591, 1985.
160. Chiodini RJ et al: Possible role of mycobacteria in inflammatory bowel disease: an unclassified *Mycobacterium* sp. isolated from patients with Crohn's disease, *Dig Dis Sci* 29:1073, 1984.
161. Mayberry J, Rhodes J, Hughes L: Incidence of Crohn's disease in Cardiff between 1934 and 1977, *Gut* 20:602, 1979.
162. Kyle J: An epidemiologic study of Crohn's disease in northeast Scotland, *Gastroenterology* 61:826, 1971.
163. Evans J, Acheson J: An epidemiological study of ulcerative colitis and regional enteritis in the Oxford area, *Gut* 6:311, 1965.
164. Goldman CD et al: Clinical and operative experience with non-Caucasian patients with Crohn's disease, *Dis Colon Rectum* 29:317, 1986.
165. Whorwell PJ et al: Crohn's disease in a husband and wife, *Lancet* 2:186, 1978.
166. Farmer RG, Hawk WA, Turnbull RB: Clinical pattern in Crohn's disease—a statistical study of 615 patients, *Gastroenterology* 68:627, 1975.
167. Cello JP, Meyer JH: Crohn's disease of the colon. In Sleisenger MH, Fordtran JS, eds: *Gastrointestinal disease: pathophysiology, diagnosis, management*, vol 2, Philadelphia, 1978, WB Saunders.
168. Maglinte DD et al: Crohn's disease of the small intestine: accuracy and relevance of enteroclysis, *Radiology* 184:541, 1992.
169. Baba S et al: Intestinal Behçet's disease, report of five cases, *Dis Colon Rectum* 19:428, 1976.
170. O'Connell DJ, Courtney JV, Riddell RH: Colitis of Behçet's syndrome—radiologic and pathologic features, *Gastrointest Radiol* 5:173, 1980.
171. Smith GE, Kime LR, Pitcher JL: The colitis of Behçet's disease: a separate entity? Colonoscopic findings and literature review, *Am J Dig Dis* 18:987, 1973.
172. Rankin GB et al: National Cooperative Crohn's Disease Study: extraintestinal manifestations and perianal complications, *Gastroenterology* 77:914, 1979.
173. Crohn B, Yamis H: *Regional ileitis*, ed 2, New York, 1958, Grune & Stratton.
174. Van Patter WN et al: Regional enteritis, *Gastroenterology* 26:347, 1954.
175. Ansell BM, Wigley RAD: Arthritis manifestations in regional enteritis, *Ann Rheum Dis* 23:64, 1964.
176. Hammer B, Ashurst P, Naish J: Diseases associated with ulcerative colitis and Crohn's disease, *Gut* 9:17, 1968.
177. Eade MN, Thompson H: Liver disease in Crohn's colitis, a study of 21 consecutive patients having colectomy, *Ann Intern Med* 74:518, 1971.
178. Kurchin A et al: Cholelithiasis in ileostomy patients, *Dis Colon Rectum* 27:585, 1984.
179. Shorvon PJ: Amyloidosis and inflammatory bowel disease, *Am J Dig Dis* 22:209, 1977.
180. Amendola MA et al: Detection of occult colovesical fistula by the Bourne test, *AJR* 142:715, 1984.
181. Bagby RJ et al: Genitourinary complications of granulomatous bowel disease, *AJR* 117:297, 1973.
182. Goldman SM et al: CT in the diagnosis of enterovesical fistulae, *AJR* 144:1299, 1985.
183. Stein EJ, Banner MP, Pollack HM: Rectourethrocutaneous fistula in Crohn's disease, *Urol Radiol* 5:103, 1983.
184. Lesko SM et al: Evidence for an increased risk of Crohn's disease in oral contraceptive users, *Gastroenterology* 1046, 1985.
185. Nelson JA et al: Ulcerative and granulomatous colitis: variation in observer interpretation and in roentgenographic appearance as related to time, *AJR* 119:369, 1973.
186. Marshak RH et al: Toxic dilatation of the colon in the course of ulcerative colitis, *Gastroenterology* 38:165, 1960.
187. Marshak RH: Granulomatous disease of the intestinal tract (Crohn's disease), *Radiology* 114:3, 1975.
188. Laufer I, Trueman T, deSa D: Multiple superficial gastric erosions due to Crohn's disease of the stomach: radiologic and endoscopic diagnosis, *Br J Radiol* 49:726, 1976.
189. Laufer I, Costopoulos L: Early lesions of Crohn's disease, *AJR* 130:307, 1978.
190. Thompson WG, Cockrill H Jr, Rice RP: Regional enteritis of the duodenum, *AJR* 123:252, 1975.
191. Wise L et al: Crohn's disease of duodenum, a report and analysis of 11 new cases, *Am J Surg* 121:184, 1971.
192. Cynn WS et al: Crohn's disease of the esophagus, *AJR* 125:359, 1975.
193. Hildell J, Lindstrom C, Wenckert A: Radiographic appearances in Crohn's disease: I. Accuracy of radiographic method, *Acta Radiol [Diagn]* 20:609, 1979.
194. Donaldson RM Jr: Crohn's disease. In Sleiseuger MH, Fordtran JS, eds: *Gastrointestinal disease: pathophysiology, diagnosis, management*, Philadelphia, 1989, WB Saunders.
195. Farmer RG, Whelan G, Fazio VW: Long-term follow-up of patients with Crohn's disease: relationship between the clinical pattern and prognosis, *Gastroenterology* 88:1818, 1985.
196. Laufer I, deSa D: The lymphoid follicular pattern: a normal feature of the pediatric colon, *AJR* 130:51, 1978.
197. Simpkins KC: Aphthoid ulcers in Crohn's colitis, *Clin Radiol* 28:601, 1977.
198. Lockhart-Mummery HE, Morson BC: Crohn's disease (regional enteritis) of the large intestine and its distinction from ulcerative colitis, *Gut* 1:87, 1960.
199. Lockhart-Mummery HE, Morson BC: Crohn's disease (regional enteritis) of the large intestine, *Gut* 5:493, 1964.
200. Pringot J et al: The features of granulomatous colitis in double contrast radiography, *J Belge Radiol* 60:25, 1977.
201. Engelholm L, de Toeuff C, Herlinger H, Maglinte D: Crohn's disease of the small bowel. In Herlinger H, Maglinte D, eds: *Clinical radiology of the small intestine*, Philadelphia, 1989, WB Saunders.
202. Bradford WD, Noce PS, Gutman LT: Pathologic features of enteric infection with *Yersinia enterocolitica*, *Arch Pathol* 98:17, 1974.
203. Vantrappen G et al: Yersinial enteritis and enterocolitis: gastroenterological aspects, *Gastroenterology* 72:220, 1977.
204. Brahme F, Fork FT: Dynamic aspects of colonic Crohn's disease, *Radiologe* 15:463, 1975.
205. Thoeni RF, Margulis AR: Radiology in inflammatory disease of the colon: an area of increased interest for the modern clinician, *Invest Radiol* 15:281, 1980.
206. Welin S, Welin G: A pathognomonic roentgenologic sign of regional ileitis (Crohn's disease), *Dis Colon Rectum* 16:473, 1973.
207. Jones B et al: Submucosal accumulation of fat in inflammatory bowel disease: CT pathologic correlation, *J Comput Assist Tomogr* 10:759, 1986.
208. Korelitz BI, Sommers SC: Differential diagnosis of ulcerative and granulomatous colitis by sigmoidoscopy, rectal biopsy, and cell counts of rectal mucosa, *Am J Gastroenterol* 61:460, 1974.

209. Bernstein JR, Rosenberg JL: Localized giant pseudo-polyposis in granulomatous colitis, *Gastrointest Radiol* 3:431, 1978.
210. Hildell J, Lindstrom C, Wenckert A: Radiographic appearances in Crohn's disease; II. The course as reflected at repeat radiography, *Acta Radiol (Diagn)* 20:933, 1979.
211. Hildell J, Lindstrom C, Wenckert A: Radiographic appearances in Crohn's disease: III. Colonic lesions following surgery, *Acta Radiol (Diagn)* 21(1):71, 1980.
212. Brahme F, Wenckert A: Spread of lesions in Crohn's disease of the colon, *Gut* 11:576, 1970.
213. Marshak RH, Lindner AE, Janowitz HD: Granulomatous ileocolitis, *Gut* 7:258, 1966.
214. Simpkins KG: The barium enema in Crohn's colitis. In Weterman IT, Pena AS, Booth CC, eds: *The management of Crohn's disease*, Amsterdam, 1976, Excerpta Medica.
215. Berridge FR: Two unusual radiological signs of Crohn's disease of the colon, *Clin Radiol* 22:443, 1971.
216. Pringot J: Aspetti radiologici delle lesioni localizzate non tumorali del tenue. In Pistolese G, ed: *La radiologia del tenue et del colon*, Padova, Italy, 1976, Bertoncello.
217. Yamagata S et al: Crohn's disease in Japan. In *Abstracts of papers presented at the 6th World Congress of Gastroenterology*, Madrid, 1978, Editorial Garsi.
218. Mekhjian HS et al: Clinical features and natural history of Crohn's disease, *Gastroenterology* 77:898, 1979.
219. Bartram CI, Herlinger H: Bowel wall thickness as a differentiating feature between ulcerative colitis and Crohn's disease of the colon, *Clin Radiol* 30:15, 1979.
220. Darke SG et al: Adenocarcinoma and Crohn's disease: a report of two cases and analysis of the literature, *Br J Surg* 60:169, 1973.
221. Greenstein AJ, Janowitz HD: Cancer in Crohn's disease: the danger of a bypassed loop, *Am J Gastroenterol* 64:122, 1975.
222. Jones JH: Colonic cancer and Crohn disease, *Gut* 10:651, 1969.
223. Greenstein AJ et al: Cancer in Crohn's disease after diversionary surgery: a report of seven carcinomas occurring in excluded bowel, *Am J Surg* 135:86, 1978.
224. Greenstein AJ et al: Patterns of neoplasia in Crohn's disease and ulcerative colitis, *Cancer* 46:403, 1980.
225. Gyde SN et al: Malignancy in Crohn's disease, *Gut* 21:1024, 1980.
226. Greenstein AJ et al: A comparison of cancer risk in Crohn's disease and ulcerative colitis, *Cancer* 48:2742, 1981.
227. Hamilton SR: Colorectal carcinoma in patients with Crohn's disease, *Gastroenterology* 89:398, 1985.
228. Stahl D, Tyler G, Fischer JE: Inflammatory bowel disease—relationship to carcinoma, *Curr Probl Cancer* 5:1, 1981.
229. Korelitz BI: Carcinoma of the intestinal tract in Crohn's disease: results of a survey conducted by the National Foundation for Ileitis and Colitis, *Am J Gastroenterol* 78:44, 1983.
230. Chaikhouni A, Regueyra FI, Stevens JR: Adenocarcinoma in perineal fistulas of Crohn's disease, *Dis Colon Rectum* 24:639, 1981.
231. Cohn EM, Pearlstine B: Inflammatory bowel disease and leukemia, *J Clin Gastroenterol* 6:33, 1984.
232. Glick SN et al: Development of lymphoma in patients with Crohn's disease, *Radiology* 153:337, 1984.
233. Hanauer SB et al: Acute leukemia following inflammatory bowel disease, *Dig Dis Sci* 27:545, 1982.
234. Herlinger H et al: Nonspecific involvement of bowel adjoining Crohn's disease, *Radiology* 159:47, 1986.
235. Greenstein AJ et al: Free perforation in Crohn's disease: I. A survey of 99 cases, *Am J Gastroenterol* 80:682, 1985.
236. Batest J, Kaminsky V: Diverticulitis and ulcerative colitis, *Br J Surg* 61:293, 1974.
237. Bartram CI: Radiology in the current assessment of ulcerative colitis, *Gastrointest Radiol* 1:383, 1977.
238. Ferrucci JT, Ragsdale BD, Barrett PJ: Double tracking of the sigmoid colon, *Radiology* 120:307, 1976.
239. Marshak RH, Lindner AE, Maklansky D: Paracolic fistulous tracts in diverticulitis and granulomatous colitis, *JAMA* 243:1943, 1980.
240. Meyers MA et al: Pathogenesis of diverticulitis complicating granulomatous colitis, *Gastroenterology* 74:24, 1978.
241. Schmidt GT, Lennard-Jones JE, Morson BC: Crohn's disease of the colon and its distinction from diverticulosis, *Gut* 9:7, 1968.
242. Homan WP, Tang CK, Thorbjarnarson B: Acute massive hemorrhage from intestinal Crohn disease, *Arch Surg* 111:901, 1976.
243. Polodny GA: Crohn's disease presenting with massive lower gastrointestinal hemorrhage, *AJR* 130:368, 1978.
244. Tsuchiya M et al: Angiographic evaluation of vascular changes in ulcerative colitis, *Angiology* 31:147, 1980.
245. Kean BH et al: Fatal amebiasis: a report of 148 fatal cases from the Armed Forces Institute of Pathology, *Ann Intern Med* 44:831, 1956.
246. Miller WT et al: Ischemic colitis with gangrene, *Radiology* 94:291, 1970.
247. Schofield PF, Mandal BK, Ironside AG: Toxic dilatation of the colon in salmonella colitis and inflammatory bowel disease, *Br J Surg* 66:5, 1979.
248. Gardiner R, Stevenson GW: The colitides, *Radiol Clin North Am* 20:797, 1982.
249. Patel AS, DeRidder PH: Amebic colitis masquerading as acute inflammatory bowel disease; the role of serology in its diagnosis, *J Clin Gastroenterol* 11:407, 1989.
250. Yoon JH et al: Atypical clinical manifestations of amebic colitis, *J Korean Med Sci* 6:260, 1991.
251. Carrera GF, Young S, Lewicki AM: Intestinal tuberculosis, *Gastrointest Radiol* 1:147, 1977.
252. Hoshino M et al: A clinical study of tuberculous colitis, *Gastroenterol Jpn* 14:299, 1979.
253. Lewis EA, Kolawole TM: Tuberculosus ileocolitis in Ibadan, a clinical review, *Gut* 13:646, 1972.
254. Thoeni RF, Margulis AR: Gastrointestinal tuberculosis, *Semin Roentgenol* 14:283, 1979.
255. Werbeloff L et al: The radiology of tuberculosis of the gastrointestinal tract, *Br J Radiol* 46:329, 1973.
256. Conant NF: Medical mycology. In Toklik WF, Smith DT, eds: *Microbiology*, New York, 1972, Appleton-Century-Crofts.
257. Wilson JW, Plunkett OA: South American blastomycosis (paracoccidioidomycosis). In *The fungus diseases of man*, Berkeley, 1965, University of California Press.
258. Weese WC, Smith IM: A study of 57 cases of actinomycosis over a 36-year period: a diagnostic "failure" with good prognosis after treatment, *Arch Intern Med* 135:1562, 1975.
259. Beavis JP, Parson R, Salfield J: Colitis and diarrhea: a problem with antibiotic therapy, *Br J Surg* 63:299, 1976.
260. Devroede G et al: Lincomycin-clindamycin colitis is not an entity, *Can J Surg* 20:326, 1977.
261. Stanley RJ, Tedesco FJ: Antibiotic-associated pseudomembranous colitis, *CRC Crit Rev Clin Radiol Nucl Med* 8:255, 1976.
262. Tedesco FJ, Barton RW, Alpers DH: Clindamycin-associated colitis, *Ann Intern Med* 81:429, 1974.
263. Tully TE, Feinberg SB: Those other types of enterocolitis, *AJR* 121:291, 1974.
264. Bartram CI: Obliteration of thumbprinting with double-contrast enemas in acute ischemic colitis, *Gastrointest Radiol* 4:85, 1979.
265. Fagin RR, Kirsner JB: Ischemic diseases of the colon, *Adv Intern Med* 17:343, 1971.
266. Gore RM, Goldberg HI: Computed tomographic evaluation of the gastrointestinal tract in diseases other than primary adenocarcinoma, *Radiol Clin North Am* 20:781, 1982.
267. Greenberg HM, Goldberg HI, Axel L: Colonic "urticaria" pattern due to early ischemia, *Gastrointest Radiol* 6:145, 1981.
268. Iida M et al: Ischemic colitis: serial changes in double-contrast barium enema examination, *Radiology* 159:337, 1986.

269. Kilpatrick ZM et al: Vascular occlusion of the colon and oral contraceptives: possible relation, *N Engl J Med* 278:438, 1968.

270. Marston A et al: Ischemic colitis, *Gut* 7:1, 1966.

271. Tomchik FS, Wittenberg J, Ottinger LW: The roentgenographic spectrum of bowel infarction, *Radiology* 96:249, 1970.

272. Williams LF: Vascular insufficiency of the intestine, *Gastroenterology* 61:757, 1971.

273. Annamunthodo H, Marryatt JP: Barium studies in intestinal lymphogranuloma venereum, *Br J Radiol* 34:53, 1961.

274. deLorimer AA, Moehring HG, Hannan RR: *Clinical roentgenology,* vol 4, Springfield, Ill, 1956, Charles C Thomas.

275. Keusch GT: Shigella infections, *Clin Gastroenterol* 8:645, 1979.

276. Teplick JG, Haskin ME, Schimert AP: *Roentgenologic diagnosis,* vol 1, Philadelphia, 1967, WB Saunders.

277. Cherigie E, Laporte A, Verspyck R: Aspect radiologique du grele chez les typiques, *J Radiol Electrol* 34:522, 1953.

278. Day DW, Mandal BK, Morson BC: The rectal biopsy appearances in *Salmonella* colitis, *Histopathology* 2:117, 1978.

279. Golden R: *Radiologic examination of the small intestine,* ed 2, Springfield, Ill, 1959, Charles C Thomas.

280. McGovern VJ, Slavutin LJ: Pathology of salmonella colitis, *Am J Surg Pathol* 3:483, 1979.

281. Postes JF: Disorders of the small intestine, *CIBA Clin Symposia* 12:107, 1960.

282. Saffouri B, Bartolomeo RS, Fuchs B: Colonic involvement in salmonellosis, *Dig Dis Sci* 24:203, 1979.

283. Schinz HR et al: *Roentgen diagnosis,* vol 5, New York, 1967, Grune & Stratton.

284. Turnbull PCB: Food poisoning with special reference to salmonella—its epidemiology, pathogenesis, and control, *Clin Gastroenterol* 8:663, 1979.

285. Wolfe MS: Diseases of travelers, *Clin Symp* 36:2, 1984.

286. Lachman R, Soong J, Wishon G et al: *Yersinia* colitis, *Gastrointest Radiol* 2:133, 1977.

287. Blaser MJ, Reller LB: *Campylobacter* enteritis, *N Engl J Med* 305:1444, 1981.

288. Blaser MJ et al: *Campylobacter* enteritis: clinical and epidemiologic features, *Ann Intern Med* 91:179, 1979.

289. Blaser MJ, Parsons RB, Wang WL: Acute colitis caused by *Campylobacter fetus* ss *jejuni, Gastroenterology* 78:448, 1980.

290. Kollitz JPM, Davis GB, Berk RN: *Campylobacter* colitis: a common infectious form of acute colitis, *Gastrointest Radiol* 6:227, 1981.

291. Loss RW, Mangia JC, Pereira M: *Campylobacter* colitis presenting as inflammatory bowel disease with segmental colonic ulcerations, *Gastroenterology* 79:138, 1980.

292. Michalak DM et al: *Campylobacter fetus* ss *jejuni:* a cause of massive lower gastrointestinal hemorrhage, *Gastroenterology* 79:742, 1980.

293. Schachter H, Kirsner J: Definitions of inflammatory bowel disease of unknown etiology, *Gastroenterology* 68:591, 1975.

294. Corey L: Sexually transmitted diseases. In Sherris JC, ed: *Medical microbiology: an introduction to infectious diseases,* New York, 1984, Elsevier.

295. Klein EJ et al: Anorectal gonococcal infection, *Ann Intern Med* 86:340, 1977.

296. Owen RL, Hill JL: Rectal and pharyngeal gonorrhea in homosexual men, *JAMA* 220:1315, 1972.

297. Perisher H, Marino AF: Gonorrhea—frequently unrecognized reservoirs, *South Med J* 63:198, 1970.

298. Sider L et al: Radiographic findings of infectious proctitis in homosexual men, *AJR* 139:667, 1982.

299. Birnbaum D, Laufer I, Freund M: Pseudomembranous enterocolitis: a clinicopathological study, *Gastroenterology* 41:345, 1961.

300. Brown RL: The gastrointestinal tract and stool following aureomycin therapy, *Antiobiot Chemother* 2:5, 1952.

301. Gelfand MD, Krone CL: Nonstaphylococcal pseudomembranous colitis, *Am J Dig Dis* 14:278, 1969.

302. Gibson GE, Rowland R, Hecker R: Diarrhoea and colitis associated with antibiotic treatment, *Aust N Z J Med* 5:340, 1975.

303. Goulston SJM, McGovern VJ: Pseudomembranous colitis, *Gut* 6:207, 1965.

304. Groil A et al: Fulminating noninfective pseudomembranous colitis, *Gastroenterology* 58:88, 1970.

305. Newman RJ, McCollum CM: Pseudomembranous colitis due to cephradine, *Br J Clin Pract* 33:32, 1979.

306. Pettet JD et al: Postoperative pseudomembranous enterocolitis, *Surg Gynecol Obstet* 98:546, 1954.

307. Reiner L, Schlesinger MJ, Miller GM: Pseudomembranous colitis following auremycin and chloramphenicol, *Arch Pathol* 54:39, 1952.

308. Stanley RJ, Melson GL, Tedesco FJ: The spectrum of radiographic findings in antibiotic-related pseudomembranous colitis, *Radiology* 111:519, 1974.

309. Swartzberg FE, Marasca RM, Remington JS: Gastrointestinal side effects associated with clindamycin: 1000 consecutive patients, *Arch Intern Med* 136:876, 1976.

310. Tedesco FJ: Pseudomembranous colitis: pathogenesis and therapy, *Med Clin North Am* 66:655, 1982.

311. Schachter J: Chlamydial infections (second of three parts), *N Engl J Med* 298:490, 1978.

312. Chretien JH, Garagusi VF: Current management of fungal enteritis, *Med Clin North Am* 66:675, 1982.

313. Perez CA et al: Some clinical and radiographic features of gastrointestinal histoplasmosis, *Radiology* 86:482, 1966.

314. Sturim HS, Kouchoukos NT, Ahlvin RC: Gastrointestinal manifestations of disseminated histoplasmosis, *Am J Surg* 110:435, 1965.

315. Boyd WP Jr, Bachman BA: Gastrointestinal infections in the compromised host, *Med Clin North Am* 66:743, 1982.

316. Cheatham WJ: Relation of heretofore unreported lesions to pathogenesis of herpes zoster, *Am J Pathol* 29:401, 1953.

317. Henson D: Cytomegalovirus inclusion bodies in the gastrointestinal tract, *Arch Pathol* 93:477, 1972.

318. Khilnani MT, Keller RJ: Roentgen and pathological changes in the gastrointestinal tract in herpes zoster generalisata, *Mt Sinai J Med* 38:303, 1971.

319. Lewis GW: Zoster sine herpete, *Br Med J* 3:418, 1958.

320. Menuck LS et al: Colonic changes of herpes zoster, *AJR* 127:273, 1976.

321. Wyburn-Mason R: Visceral lesions in herpes zoster, *Br Med J* 1:678, 1957.

322. Bablikian JP, Uthman SU, Khouri NF: Intestinal amebiasis: a roentgen analysis of 19 cases including two case reports, *AJR* 122:245, 1974.

323. Cardoso JM et al: Radiology of invasive amebiasis of the colon, *AJR* 128:935, 1977.

324. Hardy R, Scullin D: Thumbprinting in a case of amebiasis, *Radiology* 98:147, 1971.

325. Kolawole TM, Lewis EA: Radiologic observations on intestinal amebiasis, *AJR* 122:257, 1974.

326. Levine SM et al: Ameboma, the forgotten granuloma, *JAMA* 215:1461, 1971.

327. Patterson M, Schoppe LE: The presentation of amoebiasis, *Med Clin North Am* 66:689, 1982.

328. Stauffer JQ, Levine WL: Chronic diarrhea related to *Endolimax nana:* response to treatment with metronidazole, *Am J Dig Dis* 19:59, 1974.

329. Turner JA, Lewis WP, Hayes M: Amebiasis—a symposium, *Calif Med* 114:44, 1971.

330. Berk RN et al: Cryptosporidiosis of the stomach and small intestine in patients with AIDS, *AJR* 143:549, 1984.

331. Bird RG, Smith MD: Cryptosporidiosis in man: parasite life cycle and fine structural pathology, *Pathology* 132:217, 1980.

332. Civantos F, Robinson MI: Fatal strongyloidiasis following corticosteroid therapy, *Am J Dig Dis* 14:643, 1969.

333. deFigueriredo N et al: Hallazgos histopatologicos del intestino delgado en differentes enteroparasitosis, *Bol Chil Parasitol* 28:57, 1968.

334. Chait A: Schistosomiasis mansoni: roentgenologic observations in a nonendemic area, *AJR* 90:688, 1963.

335. Dimmette RM, Sproat HF: Rectosigmoid polyps in schistosomiasis, *Am J Trop Med* 4:1057, 1955.

336. Medina JT et al: The roentgen appearance of schistosomiasis mansoni involving the colon, *Radiology* 85:682, 965.

337. Senturia HR, Wald SM: Ulcerative disease of the intestinal tract proximal to partially obstructing lesions, *AJR* 99:45, 1967.

338. Berk RN, Millman SJ: Urticaria of colon, *Radiology* 99:539, 1971.

339. Mason GR et al: The radiological findings in radiation-induced enteritis and colitis: a review of 30 cases, *Clin Radiol* 21:232, 1970.

340. Bentley E et al: Colitis cystica profunda: presenting with complete intestinal obstruction and recurrence, *Radiology* 160:284, 1986.

341. Epstein SE et al: Colitis cystica profunda, *Am J Clin Pathol* 45:186, 1966.

342. Goldberg HI, Buchignani J, Rulon DB: RPC of the mouth from AFIP, *Radiology* 96:447, 1970.

343. Teague RH, Salmon PR, Read AE: Fiberoptic examination of the colon: a review of 255 cases, *Gut* 14:139, 1973.

344. Blackstone MO et al: Dysplasia-associated lesion or mass (DALM) detected by colonoscopy in long-standing ulcerative colitis: an indication for colectomy, *Gastroenterology* 80:366, 1981.

345. Fuson JA et al: Endoscopic surveillance for cancer in chronic ulcerative colitis, *AJR* 73:120, 1980.

346. Lennard-Jones JE et al: Cancer in colitis: assessment of the individual risk by clinical and histological criteria, *Gastroenterology* 73:1280, 1977.

347. Moss AA, Carbone JV, Kressel HY: Radiologic and clinical assessment of broad spectrum antibiotic therapy in Crohn's disease, *AJR* 131:787, 1978.

348. Pearce C, Dineen P: A study of pseudomembranous enterocolitis, *Am J Surg* 99:292, 1960.

349. Goldberg HI et al: Radiographic findings of the National Cooperative Crohn's Disease Study, *Gastroenterology* 77:925, 1979.

350. Becker W et al: Three-phase white blood cell scan: diagnostic validity in abdominal inflammatory disease, *J Nucl Med* 27:1109, 1986.

351. Froehlich JW: Nuclear medicine imaging of inflammatory bowel disease, *Radiol Clin North Am* 25:133, 1987.

352. Khaw KT, Saverymuttu SH, Joseph AE: Correlation of 111-Indium WBC scintigraphy with ultrasound in the detection and assessment of inflammatory bowel disease, *Clin Radiol* 42:410, 1990.

353. Loréal O et al: Scintigraphic assessment of indium 111–labeled granulocytes splenic pooling: a new approach to inflammatory bowel disease activity, *J Nucl Med* 31:1470, 1990.

354. Rothstein RD: Role of scintigraphy in the management of inflammatory bowel disease, *J Nucl Med* 32:856, 1991.

355. Saverymuttu SH et al: Assessment of disease activity in inflammatory bowel disease: a new approach using In-111 granulocyte scanning, *Br Med J* 287:1751, 1983.

356. Fineman DS et al: Detection of abnormalities in febrile AIDS patients with In 111–labeled leukocyte and GA 67 scintigraphy, *Radiology* 170:677, 1989.

357. Palestro CJ et al: In 111–labeled leukocyte and Ga 67 scintigraphy in cytomegalovirus colitis, *Clin Nucl Med* 15:848, 1990.

358. Goodman P, Raval B, Potter GD: Spontaneous free perforation of the ileum in Crohn disease: CT demonstration, *Comput Med Imag Graph* 13:473, 1989.

359. Gore RM et al: CT findings in ulcerative, granulomatous, and indeterminate colitis, *AJR* 143:279, 1984.

360. Gore RM: CT of inflammatory bowel disease, *Radiol Clin North Am* 27:717, 1989.

361. Gore RM, Calenoff L, Rogers LF: Roentgenographic manifestations of ischemic colitis, *JAMA* 241:1171, 1979.

362. Jabra AA, Fishman EK, Taylor GA: Crohn disease in the pediatric patient: CT evaluation, *Radiology* 179:495, 1991.

363. Merine DS, Fishman EK, Jones B: CT of small bowel and mesentery, *Radiol Clin North Am* 27:707, 1989.

364. Fishman EK et al: Pseudomembranous colitis: CT evaluation of 26 cases, *Radiology* 180:57, 1991.

365. Goodman PC, Federle MP: Pseudomembranous colitis, *J Comput Assist Tomogr* 4:403, 1980.

366. Balthazar EJ et al: Cecal diverticulitis: evaluation with CT, *Radiology* 162:79, 1987.

367. Hulnick DH et al: Computed tomography in the evaluation of diverticulitis, *Radiology* 152:491, 1984.

368. Johnson CD et al: Diagnosis of acute colonic diverticulitis: comparison of barium enema and CT, *AJR* 148:541, 1987.

369. Neff CC, vanSonnenberg E: CT of diverticulitis: diagnosis and treatment, *Radiol Clin North Am* 27:743, 1989.

370. Matsumoto T et al: Ultrasonic and CT findings in penicillin-induced nonpseudomembranous colitis, *Gastrointest Radiol* 15:329, 1990.

371. Federle MP et al: Computed tomographic findings in bowel infarction, *AJR* 142:91, 1984.

372. Hoddick W, Jeffrey RB, Federle MP: CT differentiation of portal venous air from biliary tract air, *J Comput Assist Tomogr* 6:633, 1982.

373. Goldberg HI et al: Computed tomography in the evaluation of Crohn disease, *AJR* 140:277, 1983.

374. Alexander ES et al: Fistulas and sinus tracts: radiologic evaluation, management, and outcome, *Gastrointest Radiol* 7:135, 1982.

375. Frick MP et al: Evaluation of abdominal fistulas with computed body tomography (CT), *Comput Radiol* 6:17, 1982.

376. Colley DP, Farrell JA, Clark RA: Perforated colon carcinoma presenting as a suprarenal mass, *Comput Tomogr* 5:55, 1981.

377. Scatarige JC et al: CT abnormalities in right lower quadrant inflammatory disease: review of findings in 26 adults, *Gastrointest Radiol* 12:156, 1987.

378. Bates FT et al: Pneumatosis intestinalis in bone marrow transplantation patients: diagnosis on routine chest radiographs, *AJR* 152:991, 1989.

379. Adams GW et al: CT detection of typhlitis, *J Comput Assist Tomogr* 9:363, 1985.

380. Frick MP et al: Computed tomography of neutropenic colitis, *AJR* 143:763, 1984.

381. Guillaumin E et al: Perirectal inflammatory disease: CT findings, *Radiology* 161:153, 1986.

382. Donaldson JS, Gilsanz V: CT findings in rectal cuff abscess following surgery for Hirschsprung disease, *J Comput Assist Tomogr* 10:151, 1986.

383. Brown JJ et al: Ileal J pouch: radiologic evaluation in patients with and without postoperative infectious complications, *Radiology* 174:115, 1990.

384. Matsumoto T et al: *Yersinia* terminal ileitis: sonographic findings in eight patients, *AJR* 156:965, 1991.

385. Puylaert JBCM, Kristjánsdóttir S, Golterman KL et al: Typhoid fever: diagnosis by using sonography, *AJR* 153:745, 1989.

386. Puylaert JBCM: Acute appendicitis: US evaluation using graded compression, *Radiology* 158:355, 1986.

387. Silverstein FE, Kimmey MB: 20-MHz ultrasound system for imaging the intestinal wall, *Ultrasound Med Biol* 15:273, 1989.

388. Larson JM et al: Acute Meckel's diverticulitis diagnosis by ultrasonography, *J Clin Ultrasound* 17:682, 1989.

389. Townsend RR, Jeffrey RB Jr, Laing FC: Cecal diverticulitis differentiated from appendicitis using graded compression sonography, *AJR* 152:1229, 1989.

390. Puylaert JBCM: Mesenteric adenitis and acute terminal ileitis: US evaluation using graded compression, *Radiology* 161:691, 1986.

391. Vijayaraghavan SB: Sonographic features of pneumatosis of the small bowel, *J Clin Ultrasound* 18:579, 1990.

392. Kimmey MB et al: Diagnosis of inflammatory bowel disease with ultrasound: an in vitro study, *Invest Radiol* 25:1085, 1990.

393. Dinkel E et al: Real-time ultrasound in Crohn's disease: characteristic features and clinical implications, *Pediatr Radiol* 16:8, 1986.

394. Khaw KT et al: Ultrasonic patterns in inflammatory bowel disease *Clin Radiol* 43:171, 1991.

395. Limberg B: Diagnosis of ulcerative colitis and colonic Crohn's disease by colonic sonography, *J Clin Ultrasound* 17:25, 1989.

396. Limberg B: Sonographic features of colonic Crohn's disease: comparison of in vivo and in vitro studies, *J Clin Ultrasound* 18:161, 1990.

397. Verbanck JJ et al: Can sonography diagnose acute colonic diverticulitis in patients with acute intestinal inflammation? A prospective study, *J Clin Ultrasound* 17:661, 1989.

398. Wada M, Kikuchi Y, Doy M: Uncomplicated acute diverticulitis of the cecum and ascending colon: sonographic findings in 18 patients, *AJR* 155:283, 1990.

399. Wilson SR, Toi A: Value of sonography in the diagnosis of acute diverticulitis of the colon, *AJR* 154:1199, 1990.

400. Kaminsky S et al: Gadopentate dimeglumine as a bowel contrast agent: safety and efficacy, *Radiology* 178:503, 1991.

401. Mitchell DG: Comparison of Kaopectate with barium for negative and positive enteric contrast at MR imaging, *Radiology* 181:475, 1991.

402. Rubin DL et al: Intraluminal contrast enhancement and MR visualization of the bowel wall: efficacy of PFOB, *JMRI* 1:371, 1991.

403. Stehling MK et al: Gastrointestinal tract: dynamic MR studies with echo-planar imaging, *Radiology* 171:41, 1989.

404. Koelbel G et al: Diagnosis of fistulae and sinus tracts in patients with Crohn disease: value of MR imaging, *AJR* 152:999, 1989.

ADDITIONAL READINGS

Jones B, Abbruzzese AA: Obstructing giant pseudopolyps in granulomatous colitis, *Gastrointest Radiol* 3:437, 1978.

Munyer TP et al: Postinflammatory polyposis (PIP) of the colon: the radiologic-pathologic spectrum, *Radiology* 145:607, 1982.

Nelson JA et al: Ulcerative and granulomatous colitis: variation in observer interpretation and in roentgenographic appearance as related to time, *AJR* 119:369, 1973.

Simpkins KC, Stevenson GW: The modified Malmo double contrast barium enema in colitis: an assessment of its accuracy in reflecting sigmoidoscopic findings, *Br J Radiol* 45:486, 1972.

Slater G, Greenstein AJ, Aufses AH: Anal carcinoma in patients with Crohn's disease, *Ann Surg* 199:348, 1984.

30 *Small Bowel Neoplasms*

ROBERT E. KOEHLER

Neoplasms of the small bowel are rare, constituting only 2% to 3% of the tumors of the gastrointestinal (GI) tract.[1] For a variety of reasons, neoplasms of the small intestine present both the clinician and the radiologist with a formidable diagnostic challenge. They may cause acute bleeding, bowel obstruction, or a palpable mass. Symptoms and signs are often absent or are intermittent and nonspecific, consisting only of poorly localized abdominal pain, a vague feeling of flatulence, or chronic occult GI blood loss. With the exception of tumors metastatic to the small bowel, small bowel neoplasms tend to concentrate at the two ends of the bowel, in the duodenum and proximal jejunum and in the distal ileum.

RADIOGRAPHIC DETECTION
Barium studies

Barium studies remain the chief radiographic examination for detecting tumors of the small intestine. In some centers the time-honored method of administering a mixture of barium sulfate and water by mouth is being supplemented by the enteroclysis procedure, in which the barium mixture is administered through a tube passed through the nose or mouth into the jejunum. This allows greater control over the degree of small bowel distension and has been advocated as superior in detecting small bowel tumors.[2-4]

Tumors that are located proximally are usually easier to detect on barium studies because adjacent bowel segments tend to overlap less in this area, and fluoroscopy with palpation can thus be employed more effectively. Those occurring in overlapping loops of ileum in the pelvis can be very difficult to image unless enteroclysis is performed. Despite these difficulties, the radiographic patterns of small intestinal neoplasms are often quite distinctive and sometimes permit an accurate prediction of the histologic type.

Computed tomography

Computed tomography (CT) is playing an increasingly important role in the detection of small bowel neoplasms. This is not surprising in view of the fact that CT is more and more the first abdominal radiographic procedure used in patients with vague abdominal complaints, weight loss, and other nonspecific symptoms and signs that are sometimes the only clinical indications of small bowel tumors.

In a review of CT findings in 35 patients with small bowel neoplasms,[5] CT findings were considered abnormal in 34 cases (97%) and the neoplasm itself was seen in 28 (80%). Barium studies were interpreted as abnormal in 88% of the patients in whom they were done. CT scans in 63 patients with primary small bowel tumors seen at the Mayo Clinic were interpreted as showing the tumor in 73% of cases.[6] Of 17 undetected tumors, all were smaller than 3 cm, and most were 2 cm or smaller. No tumors seen on barium studies were missed on CT.

Small bowel tumors not infrequently present clinically with obstructive symptoms caused by intussusception. The CT appearance of intussusception is quite characteristic,[7] and its recognition is becoming routine.

BENIGN TUMORS

Benign tumors of a variety of types occur in the small bowel, but approximately 90% of benign tumors are leiomyomas, lipomas, adenomas, and hemangiomas. Of these, leiomyomas, lipomas, and adenomatous polyps are the most common and occur with roughly equal frequency. Although tumors of the small bowel are more often benign than malignant, the benign tumors are usually asymptomatic and commonly go undiscovered, except at autopsy. Symptomatic small bowel tumors found radiographically or at surgery are much more likely to be malignant.

When benign tumors of the small intestine are evident clinically, they usually present with abdominal pain, small bowel obstruction, bleeding, or a palpable mass. Obstruction is often caused by the intussusception of tumors that are intraluminal in location. Bleeding can occur when ulceration develops in an adenoma or in the mucosa covering a submucosal or intramural tumor.

Leiomyomas

Leiomyomas of the small intestine occur with slightly greater frequency in the jejunum than in the ileum. Often they occur in the subserosal layer of the bowel wall and show little protrusion into the lumen, in which case barium studies show only displacement of bowel loops by the extrinsic tumor. Leiomyomas that originate in the submucosa appear as smooth, oval or rounded filling defects or as pedunculated intraluminal defects. Intussusception may occur (Fig. 30-1). Dumbbell-shaped lesions occur, in which a bilobed tumor protrudes both outside the bowel and into the lumen.

The CT appearance of intestinal leiomyomas is fairly characteristic. These tumors average 5 cm in diameter, are smoothly marginated, and are spheric or ovoid.[8] Their char-

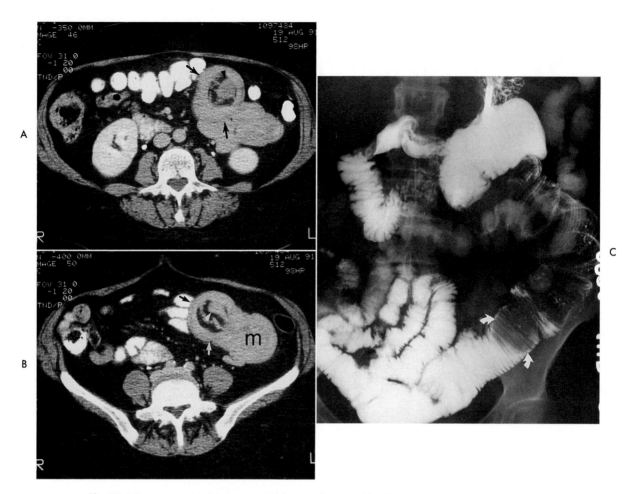

Fig. 30-1 Intussuscepting leiomyoma of jejunum discovered incidentally on CT scan done for other reasons. **A,** CT scan proximal to the tumor shows the dilated intussuscipiens *(arrows)* containing intussusceptum *(arrowhead)* and associated mesenteric fat. **B,** Scan at the level of the tumor shows intussuscipiens *(arrows)*, intussusceptum *(arrowhead)*, and leading mass *(M)*. **C,** Subsequent barium study shows a smooth, spherical, intraluminal filling defect *(arrows)* with associated intussusception that is not causing obstruction.

acteristic eccentric growth pattern is often more obvious on CT than on barium studies.[9] There is early enhancement with bolus injection of intravenous contrast material. The tumor may be uniform in CT attenuation or may show a central area of diminished attenuation.[5] There may be focal areas of calcification in the tumor.

Gastrointestinal bleeding in a young to middle-aged adult is the most likely clinical presentation of intestinal leiomyomas. The bleeding often occurs in repeated episodes with the passage of melena or dark red blood through the rectum. Slow, chronic, occult bleeding, such as may occur with an adenocarcinoma of the jejunum, is not as likely. Angiography is helpful in demonstrating small intestinal leiomyomas,[10] even if performed at a time when the patient is not actively bleeding (Fig. 30-2). These tumors are hypervascular and show intense opacification during the cap-

illary phase of the injection, and early opacification of mesenteric veins draining the tumor is usually seen.

Leiomyomas have been reported to show up as a focal area of increased uptake on technetium 99m (Tc 99m)–red blood cell scintigraphy done to detect the source of GI hemorrhage.[11] The same is true on radionuclide examinations with Tc 99m pertechnetate to detect Meckel's diverticulum.[12]

Rarely, leiomyoblastomas occur in the small intestine. In their clinical presentation and appearance on barium examinations, CT, radionuclide studies, and angiography, they resemble intestinal leiomyoma.

Lipomas

Lipomas occur somewhat less frequently in the small intestine than adenomas or leiomyomas, but when present

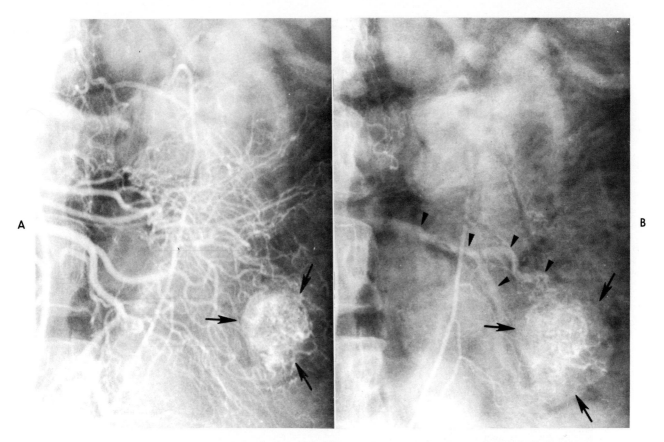

Fig. 30-2 Arteriographic demonstration of jejunal leiomyoma in 54-year-old woman with three major episodes of gastrointestinal bleeding in 2 years. Barium studies and endoscopic examinations were unrevealing. At surgery tumor was subserosal and did not protrude into lumen. **A,** Late arterial phase shows tumor stain *(arrows)* and irregular vessels within mass. **B,** Prominent veins *(arrowheads)* drain tumor *(arrows)*.

they usually arise in the ileum.[13] Symptoms are often absent, but as is the case with other benign small bowel tumors, bleeding or intussusception may occur. Like leiomyomas, lipomas appear on barium studies as smooth, round or oval filling defects with an appearance suggesting an intramural location. Manual pressure on the abdomen during fluoroscopy may cause sufficient change in the shape of a lipoma to indicate its soft, fatty nature[14] (Fig. 30-3). As with lipomas elsewhere in the body, their appearance on CT can be characteristic: a sharply demarcated round or ovoid mass with a uniform, low CT attenuation similar to that of normal fat.[5,15,16] One report[14] describes strands of soft tissue density extending into the fatty tumor from its pseudopedicle in cases in which the mucosal surface of the tumor is ulcerated.

Adenomas

Adenomas constitute about 25% of benign small bowel tumors.[1,17] They occur more frequently in the duodenum than in the jejunum and more frequently in the jejunum than in the ileum. The histologic pattern can be either tubular (glandular) or villous. Degeneration of adenomas into adenocarcinomas is unusual but can occur. Radiographically adenomas appear as intraluminal filling defects that are usually pedunculated and may have a lobulated surface (Fig. 30-4). The stalk can be several centimeters long, leaving the polyp free to move back and forth in a segment of duodenum or jejunum.

Hemangiomas

Hemangiomas occur predominantly in the jejunum and, when clinically detectable, involve gastrointestinal bleeding or anemia. Mechanical obstruction is rare but can occur in patients with hemangiomas that are sclerotic and cause luminal narrowing. Bleeding is thought to occur because of the absence of muscular and elastic tissue in the thin-walled vessels of the tumor. Small intestinal hemangiomas are not usually detected radiographically but may be evident as an intramural or intraluminal rounded polypoid mass. Calcified phleboliths are usually not seen. These tumors occur with an increased incidence in patients with Turner's syndrome, Sturge-Weber syndrome, tuberous

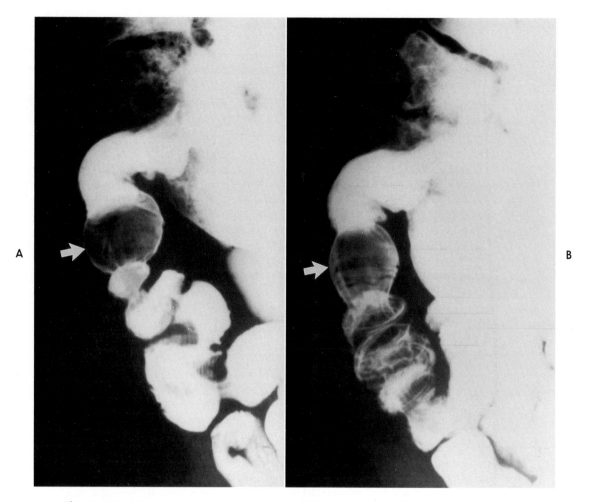

Fig. 30-3 Ileal lipoma in a 50-year-old woman with trace positive test for fecal occult blood. **A** and **B** show the change in shape of the lesion induced by manual palpation.

sclerosis, and the blue rubber-bleb nevus syndrome.[18] Patients with hereditary hemorrhagic telangiectasia (Osler-Weber-Rendu disease) may have cavernous hemangiomas of the small bowel in addition to the more characteristic telangiectatic lesions. The small bowel lesions in these patients may be evident angiographically but are not ordinarily visible on barium studies.

Uncommon tumors

Myoepithelial hamartoma, also called *ectopic pancreas* when it contains pancreatic acinar tissue, is a rare benign neoplasm occurring most often in the gastric antrum and proximal duodenum but occasionally in the jejunum or ileum.[13,17,19] It is thought to be a developmental abnormality rather than a true neoplasm and contains muscular and epithelial elements. Central umbilication of these lesions has been reported but is not often seen. Hamartomas of the Peutz-Jeghers type also occur in the small intestine and are discussed later in this chapter.

Inflammatory fibroid polyps, also referred to as *inflammatory pseudotumors,* are occasionally encountered in the ileum in patients in their fifties and sixties[13,20] and can be the leading focus of intussusception. Their cause is uncertain, but they are probably an inflammatory response to some form of injury. On barium studies they appear as single, smooth, rounded filling defects in the distal small intestine. They average 1 to 4 cm in size.

Neurofibromas and neurogenic tumors of other cell types also occur in the small bowel.[13,21,22] About 15% of patients with intestinal neurofibroma have generalized neurofibromatosis—von Recklinghausen's disease—and this diagnosis should certainly be considered in a patient with multiple intestinal neurofibromas. About 25% of patients with neurofibromatosis have neurofibromas of the small bowel, making it one of the more common organs to be involved.[23] The radiographic appearances on barium examination and angiography are similar to those of leiomyomas.[24] Degeneration into malignant neurofibrosarcoma can occur.

Fibromas, lymphangiomas, and other tumors can also occur, but all are rare.

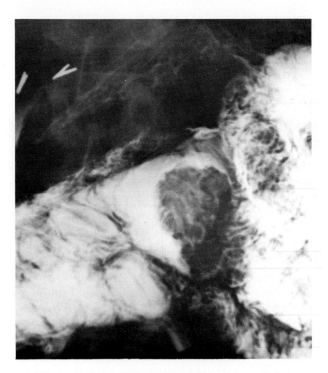

Fig. 30-4 Intraluminal polypoid filling defect, 3.5 cm in size, represents benign villous adenoma. Patient had previously undergone resection of colon carcinoma.
Courtesy of Dr. Andrew L. Tievsky.

POLYPOSIS SYNDROMES
Peutz-Jeghers syndrome

Peutz-Jeghers syndrome is inherited as an autosomal dominant trait, although in about half of patients the disease occurs without a family history.[25] The syndrome consists of hamartomatous polyps of the GI tract and characteristic brown pigmented lesions of the skin and mucous membrane of the lips and sometimes over the extensor surfaces of the joints of the hands and feet. Patients are often in their twenties at the time of diagnosis. They may be asymptomatic, but intussusception may occur, leading to signs of mechanical obstruction.[7] GI blood loss and anemia are common.

Some evidence suggests a minor increase in the risk of carcinoma developing in the stomach and duodenum, but epidemiologic data conflict on this point.[26-28] In one series 5% of female patients with Peutz-Jeghers syndrome developed sex cord tumors of the ovary.[29]

The polyps affect predominantly the small bowel, which is involved in nearly all cases, and approximately one fourth of patients with this syndrome have polyps in the colon and stomach as well. The polyps vary from tiny lesions that are undetectable radiographically to lesions as large as 4 cm (Fig. 30-5). The polyps in Peutz-Jeghers syndrome are also visible on CT[30] as intraluminal filling defects of soft tissue attenuation. Extensively involved segments can appear "carpeted" by innumerable tiny polyps.

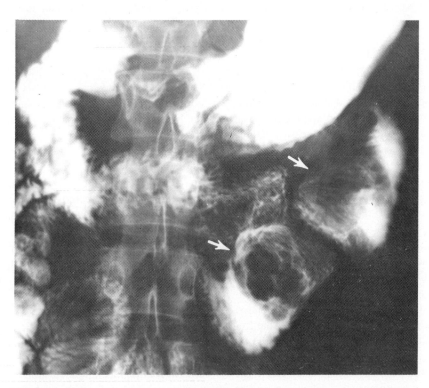

Fig. 30-5 Peutz-Jeghers syndrome in 24-year-old woman with typical mucocutaneous pigmented areas of lips. Two 3-cm hamartomas are seen in proximal jejunum *(arrows)*.

Cronkhite-Canada syndrome

Cronkhite-Canada syndrome[31] is a rare polyposis syndrome that involves the small bowel in approximately half of the cases, whereas polyps occur in the stomach and colon in virtually all affected patients. Histologically the polyps are inflammatory in nature and contain dilated interstitial glands that may be cystic. No true neoplastic tissue is present, and there is no increase in the risk of malignancy developing. The polyps develop after the age of 40 years, and no sexual, racial, familial, or geographic predilection is known.[32] Ectodermal changes are also a feature, consisting of alopecia, brownish hyperpigmentation of the skin, and dystrophic changes of the nails. Patients have abdominal pain and diarrhea that becomes chronic and unrelenting. Malabsorption and the GI loss of albumin and electrolytes can be severe, and the downhill course commonly ends in death. No cause has yet been determined.

Syndromes rarely affecting the small bowel

Familial polyposis coli is a hereditary polyposis syndrome affecting the colon, in which there is a great increase in the risk of colonic carcinoma developing. Most of the polyps are adenomas (some are hyperplastic), and they occur sometimes in the stomach and occasionally in the small bowel. In one series, nine patients developed adenomas of the ileum after colectomy for familial polyposis of the colon.[33,34] Patients with Gardner's syndrome, which may be a variant of familial polyposis, also develop small intestinal adenomas on occasion. These are concentrated in the ileum and consist of either adenomas or hyperplastic lymphoid polyps.[35] These patients are at risk for duodenal adenomas, and especially of malignant change to adenocarcinoma in periampullary villous adenomas.

Juvenile polyposis is another syndrome predominantly affecting the colon, in which small bowel polyps occasionally occur. The genetic nature of this syndrome is still uncertain, but it appears to be inherited in some cases. The polyps are hamartomatous and involve excessive lamina propria containing epithelial-lined tubules that may undergo cystic dilatation. They occur most often in children and can lead to clinically significant bleeding. Autoamputation of juvenile polyps is occasionally noted and is thought to result from ischemic necrosis of the polyp when its pedicle twists.[25]

Patients with multiple endocrine neoplasia syndrome— type IIB—develop medullary carcinoma of the thyroid, pheochromocytoma, diffuse ganglioneuromatosis of the GI tract, and other abnormalities. Most patients with this inherited condition have GI symptoms,[36] usually constipation and diarrhea. The syndrome may be recognized by the frequent occurrence of diffuse swelling of the lips caused by proliferation of neural tissue. Nodular proliferation of the myenteric neural plexus can affect the small and large bowel, and the resulting neuromuscular defect can lead to the formation of large diverticula and an adynamic megacolon.

The Ruvalcaba-Myhre-Smith syndrome[37,38] consists of macrocephaly, pigmented genital lesions, intestinal polyposis, and other abnormalities. The mode of inheritance is thought to be autosomal dominant. The polyps are hamartomas and occur anywhere in the alimentary tract including the small bowel.

CARCINOID TUMORS
Clinical features

Carcinoid tumors of the small intestine arise from enterochromaffin cells, and some are capable of producing a variety of hormones, including serotonin and kinin peptides. These tumors arise in a wide variety of sites within the body, but the majority originate in the GI tract.[39] The appendix is the most common site of origin, accounting for 40% of cases in an extensive review of the files of the National Cancer Institute.[40] Between 20% and 30% of carcinoid tumors arise in the small intestine, and of these the great majority occur in the ileum.[41-43] Overall, carcinoid tumors constitute approximately one third of the tumors originating in the small intestine.

Carcinoid tumors are somewhat unusual in that the standard histologic criteria of malignancy (anaplasia and frequency of mitosis) do not accurately predict their malignant behavior. Malignancy is best determined by the presence of local invasion or distant metastatic spread. Tumor stage, as judged by a modified Dukes' classification conventionally used to assess carcinoma of the colon, correlates well with survival rate.[44,45] Large tumors are more likely to behave in malignant fashion than are small tumors[46]; those under 1 cm in diameter rarely metastasize. Tumors that are symptomatic and those that exceed 2 cm in diameter are associated with distant spread at the time of diagnosis in about 90% of cases. The growth rate of the tumor is slow, and long survivals are often reported even with patients in whom there is spread to lymph nodes or the liver. Up to 36% of patients with carcinoid tumors are found to have other malignant neoplasms. These associated tumors are as likely to cause the patients' deaths as is the carcinoid tumor itself.[47,48]

When present, symptoms of a small intestinal carcinoid tumor are often nonspecific or are the same as those of small bowel obstruction. Crampy abdominal pain, distention, vomiting, and bleeding can all occur. Bleeding results from ulceration of the tumor itself or from portal-systemic collateral veins that form when the tumor obstructs the mesenteric venous outflow.[49]

Carcinoid syndrome

Carcinoid syndrome is a specific set of symptoms mediated by serotonin and other hormonally active compounds produced by the tumor.[46,50,51] The syndrome includes diarrhea, abdominal cramps, flushing of the skin, asthma, and cardiac valvular lesions, particularly of the right heart. Carcinoid tumors that are confined to the small bowel and mesentery do not produce the carcinoid syndrome, apparently because serotonin released by the tumor into the mesenteric veins is metabolized on passage through the liver. The presence of the syndrome is therefore a good indicator of the metastatic spread of a small intestinal carcinoid tumor to the liver. The syndrome can occur with primary carcinoid tumors of other organs such as those of bronchial or ovarian origin.

Radiographic features

The radiographic findings in cases of small intestinal carcinoid tumors vary considerably, depending on the stage of the illness at the time the radiographic study is performed. The majority are small mural nodules measuring less than 1.5 cm in diameter. If the tumor is detected at this stage, it appears as a small, sharply defined submucosal lesion, typically in the distal ileum. Mechanical obstruction is not usually present at this stage unless the tumor is large enough to cause intussusception (Fig. 30-6). As the carcinoid tumor grows outside the bowel lumen, it infiltrates the bowel wall, mesentery, and, eventually, adjacent lymph nodes (Fig. 30-7).

The bowel muscle may undergo hypertrophic thickening, presumably as a result of stimulation by serotonin or other hormones produced by the tumor. Even more striking is the fibroblastic proliferation induced in the adjacent mesentery. Together these effects combine to cause kinking, angulation, and narrowing of the bowel lumen and sometimes the appearance of a mesenteric mass. Affected bowel loops become fixed and appear to be separated from each other. The desmoplastic response in the mesentery puts tension on the bowel wall at certain points, causing focal areas of speculation and straightening of the mucosal fold pattern (Figs. 30-8 and 30-9). Occasionally, ischemia caused by the occlusion of mesenteric arteries or veins leads to intramural hemorrhage with the appearance of thumbprinting on barium studies.

Because the radiographic findings can mimic those of a number of other conditions, the diagnosis of a small intestinal carcinoid tumor cannot usually be made with certainty on the basis of the barium examination unless the carcinoid syndrome is also present. Fixation, kinking, and angulation of the small bowel may also be the result of postoperative adhesions or an inflammatory mass. The fibroblastic proliferation in the mesentery can simulate retroperitoneal fibrosis even to the point of appearing along with a ureteral obstruction.[52] Regional enteritis can occasionally produce a radiographic picture indistinguishable from that of carcinoid tumor. Patients with ileal carcinoid have been mistak-

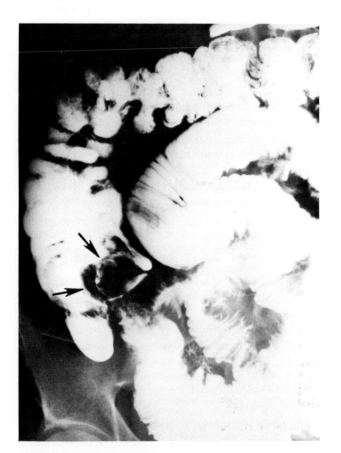

Fig. 30-6 Carcinoid tumor of terminal ileum with early intussusception into colon (*arrows*). Note partial small bowel obstruction.

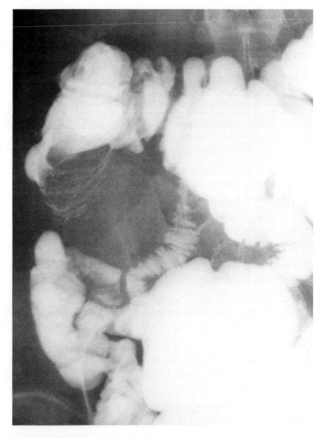

Fig. 30-7 Large intussuscepting carcinoid tumor of distal ileum with considerable mass effect on adjacent loops.

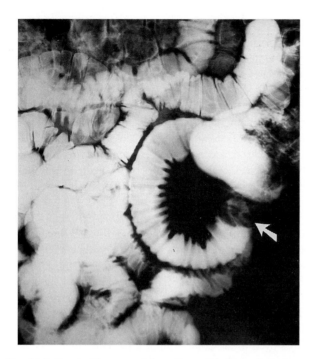

Fig. 30-8 Carcinoid tumor of the mid small intestine seen on enteroclysis in a 50-year-old man with recurrent abdominal pain relieved by vomiting. The tumor *(arrows)* partially obstructs the bowel. Spread into the adjacent mesentery is causing separation of bowel loops and fold thickening as a result of mesenteric venous and lymphatic obstruction.

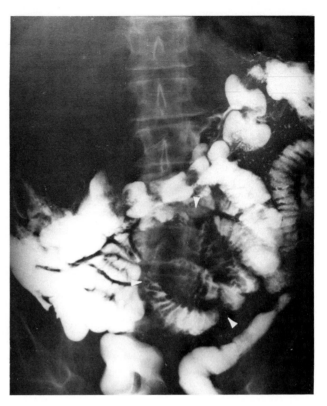

Fig. 30-9 Carcinoid tumor of ileum with mesenteric involvement *(arrowheads.)* Note large liver and straightened, spiculated appearance of small bowel folds, indicating hepatic metastasis.

enly treated for Crohn's disease for as long as 4 years before the correct diagnosis was revealed at operation.[53] Carcinoid tumor should be considered as a possibility in patients thought to have Crohn's disease but in whom the ileal disease progresses unusually rapidly or the age at onset is over 45 years.

CT is proving to be very helpful in detecting carcinoid tumors of the small intestine and in delineating the extent of their spread. The primary tumor is often not recognized, but in symptomatic patients, mesenteric spread and metastatic deposits in the liver and retroperitoneal lymph nodes are frequently detectable. Typically the carcinoid tumor appears on CT as a mass in the root of the mesentery with a diameter of 2 to 4 cm. The tumor may contain flecks of calcium but is otherwise of homogeneous CT attenuation. Thin, straight, or curvilinear fibrous strands sometimes radiate from the mass in a characteristic stellate pattern. A retractile effect on adjacent bowel loops may be recognizable. This mesenteric involvement has been reported to be visible on CT in 40% to 50% of cases.[6,54] Similar findings can be seen by magnetic resonance imaging (MRI).[55]

Angiography is useful in detecting and confirming the presence of small intestinal carcinoid tumors.[56] There is irregularity of medium-sized mesenteric arteries in the region of the tumor. Characteristically these vessels take on a stel-

late or sunburst appearance, radiating from the area of greatest tumor involvement. Draining veins are not usually seen, and an angiographic tumor stain may be visible but is not prominent. Sometimes the stellate arrangement of the mesenteric arteries is not noted, but arterial irregularity, kinking, and encasement can usually be seen. Angiography is also useful in demonstrating the presence of hepatic metastases that are almost uniformly hypervascular and therefore easy to demonstrate (Fig. 30-10). Epinephrine-assisted angiography has been shown to enhance the tumor stain in occasional cases of primary tumor and hepatic metastases.[57]

While radionuclide imaging has not played a prominent role in the detection of carcinoid tumors, some interesting work has been done with I-131 metaiodobenzylguanidine (MIBG). MIBG is a structural analogue to norepinephrine and has a high affinity for chromaffin cells in the adrenal medulla. MIBG scintigraphy has been shown to be capable of imaging intestinal carcinoids and their distant metastatic deposits.[58]

LYMPHOMAS
Clinical features

Malignant lymphomas constitute about 30% of all malignant tumors in the small bowel. They are less common than adenocarcinomas in most older series[1,17] but are as

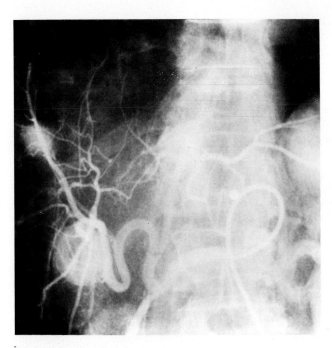

Fig. 30-10 Hypervascular deposits of metastatic carcinoid tumor in liver shown on celiac angiogram.

prevalent or more prevalent in recent reports.[5,6,41] The great majority are non-Hodgkin's lymphoma of B cell origin.[59] About 60% are of the diffuse histiocytic type, the second most common type being poorly differentiated lymphocytic lymphoma. In about half of patients the tumor occurs in the small intestine as a primary neoplasm and is confined to the GI tract. Another 20% to 30% have nodal involvement. The remainder show widespread dissemination at the time of diagnosis. Intestinal lymphoma that is localized at presentation is thought to originate from mucosa-associated lymphoid tissue (MALT).[60] It tends to respond well to surgical resection, with or without local radiotherapy, and long-term survival is common. This is in distinction to disseminated, peripheral non-Hodgkin's lymphoma with bowel involvement, which usually progresses relentlessly.

Intestinal lymphoma occurs over a wide age range but is usually found in adults, most commonly in the fourth to sixth decades of life. Some series show a male predominance.[61] Numerous deposits of lymphoid tissue that occur normally in the small bowel, particularly in the form of Peyer's patches in the distal ileum, probably are the site of lymphoma's origin, and their concentration in the ileum may explain the predominance of ileal over jejunal lymphomas.

The majority of patients found to have a malignant lymphoma involving the small bowel are symptomatic.[62] Abdominal pain, nausea, and vomiting are the most common complaints and are usually related to partial mechanical small bowel obstruction, sometimes associated with intussusception in the case of polypoid tumors. Constipation, di-

arrhea, and weight loss can occur.[61] Malabsorption is occasionally found. Patients with ulcerated lesions may experience melena. Perforation, so unusual in patients with ✳ adenocarcinoma of the small bowel, occurs in about 15% of patients with a small bowel lymphoma. In 10% to 20% of patients, multiple small bowel lesions are found.

Associated conditions

Gastrointestinal lymphomas, including those in the small bowel, occur with increased frequency in patients with acquired immunodeficiency syndrome (AIDS).[63] They are typically aggressive and of non-Hodgkin's type. They often present as large masses with central excavation and associated lymph node enlargement. Lymphoma may also be found in other sites at the time of diagnosis. Chronic pharmacologic suppression of the immune system to prevent organ transplant rejection, previous chemotherapy for malignancy, and systemic lupus erythematosus also predispose patients to lymphomas of the intestine and other sites.

As is the case of adenocarcinomas, lymphomas of the small bowel occur with an increased incidence in patients with celiac disease.[64-67] In this clinical setting the tumors are usually of T cell origin, and they tend to occur in the proximal small intestine. In patients with celiac disease, when an intestinal lymphoma develops it usually does so after many years of malabsorption,[68,69] but lymphoma can occasionally occur early in the illness. In a few elderly patients the two diseases have occasionally been diagnosed simultaneously.[67] The possibility of lymphoma should come to mind whenever a treated, asymptomatic patient with celiac disease develops new or worsening symptoms (Fig. 30-11).

There are reported cases of intestinal lymphoma developing in patients with Crohn's disease,[70,71] but a predisposition to lymphoma has not been definitely established. Complicating this issue is the fact that the radiographic features of Crohn's disease and intestinal lymphoma are occasionally similar enough to prevent the two being distinguished by radiographic means.[72]

Radiographic features

Malignant lymphomas of the small intestine have protean radiographic manifestations. These were classified in 1979 by Marshak et al.[73] into five different patterns: (1) multiple nodules (Figs. 30-12 and 30-13), (2) an infiltrating tumor (Fig. 30-14), (3) a polypoid mass, (4) an endoexoenteric form with excavation, fistula formation, or both, and (5) mesenteric involvement with extraluminal mass (Fig. 30-15). Although this morphologic classification was based primarily on the findings of barium small bowel examinations, it also applies well to the CT appearance of intestinal lymphoma. Recent reports[6,67,74] have reported the infiltrating, circumferential mass to be the most common appearance, and the cavitary, or endoexoenteric, form is next most commonly reported. In the descriptions that follow,

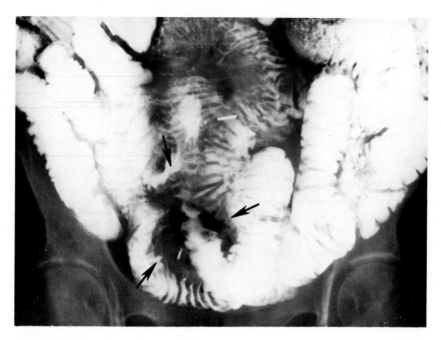

Fig. 30-11 Film of middle-aged woman with celiac disease of several years' duration, recently with poor response to gluten-free diet. In addition to dilatation typical of sprue, there is a localized area *(arrows)* of separation of loops and thickened mucosal folds in the right lower abdomen, which proved to be histiocytic lymphoma.

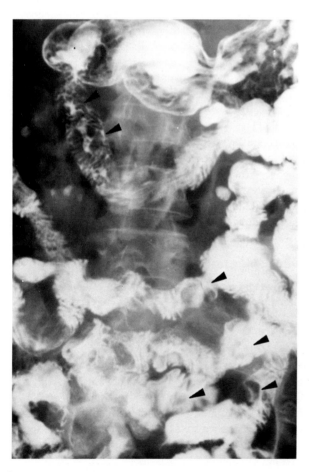

Fig. 30-12 Histiocytic lymphoma of small bowel. There are 1- to 2-cm mural nodules in the duodenum, jejunum, and ileum *(arrowheads)*. Those in the duodenum are ulcerated.

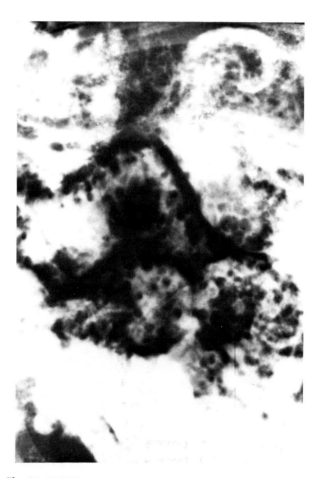

Fig. 30-13 Diffuse small intestinal lymphoma with nodular thickening of mucosal folds. Nodules range from 2 to 4 mm in size.

the various morphologic forms are described in descending order of occurrence.

In the infiltrating form, focal or diffuse thickening of the bowel wall takes place. When focal, the tumor forms a circumferential mass with discrete, shelflike margins. The <u>length of the involved intestine is typically 8 to 12 cm, longer than</u> the involved segment in <u>most intestinal adenocarcinomas</u>. Submucosal infiltration by lymphoma causes effacement of the mucosal fold pattern, and nodularity or ulceration may render the luminal surface irregular.[67] Luminal caliber may be narrowed, normal, or widened (aneurysmal dilatation) (Fig. 30-16). <u>When the lumen is narrowed, this is seldom sufficient to cause obstruction (again unlike adenocarcinoma)</u>.

When the tumor infiltration is more diffuse, the abnormal region may fade imperceptibly into adjacent normal bowel. Mucosal folds in the involved segment may appear thickened and irregular or flattened and effaced. Occasionally the involved segment of bowel appears featureless and devoid of any mucosal folds (Fig. 30-17). <u>One or more areas of narrowing of the lumen are often present</u>. The <u>separation of adjacent loops</u> of bowel may give further evidence of the mural thickening.

In the cavitary or so-called endoexoenteric form of in-

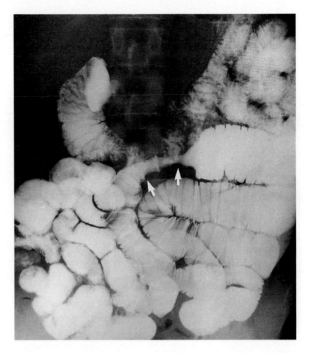

Fig. 30-14 Enteroclysis on a 52-year-old woman with lymphoma of the distal jejunum. Infiltration of the intestinal wall has caused a tapered stricture *(arrows)* with thickening of valvulae conniventes at the tumor margins. Proximal dilatation caused by low-grade mechanical obstruction as seen here is usually seen better on enteroclysis than on conventional peroral examination.

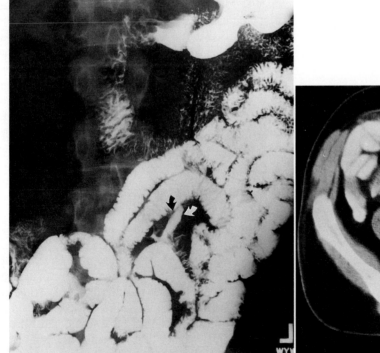

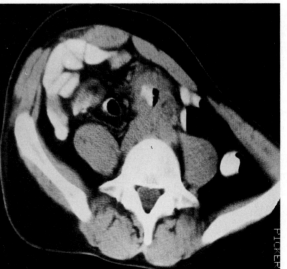

Fig. 30-15 Intestinal lymphoma in a 44-year-old man with abdominal pain and a palpable abdominal mass. **A,** Irregular ulcer *(arrows)* with thickening of adjacent mucosal folds seen on barium study. **B,** Follow-up CT scan (done in right lateral decubitus position) shows a mesenteric mass with extension to the retroperitoneum. A cavity within the mass communicates with the ileal lumen. At operation the right kidney was also involved.

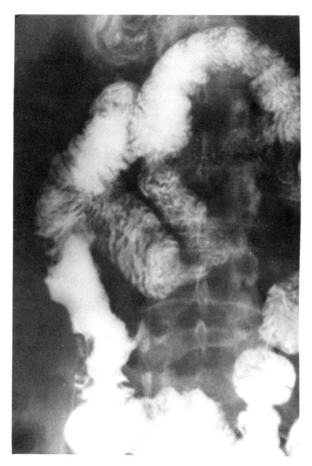

Fig. 30-16 Histiocytic lymphoma of small intestine. Widened irregular lumen represents excavation within tumor.

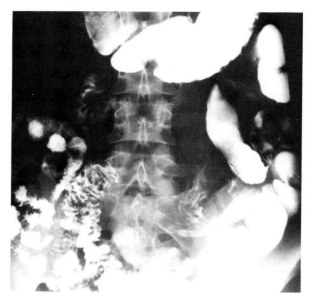

Fig. 30-17 Jejunal lymphoma. Involved portion of bowel is featureless and exhibits moulage phenomenon. Lack of dilatation distally enables differentiation from celiac disease.

testinal lymphoma, the tumor contains an ulceration or excavation that appears as an irregular collection that does not conform to the contour of a normal segment of bowel. When such a central excavation takes on the appearance of a widened area of the bowel lumen, the term *aneurysmal dilatation* is sometimes applied. The excavation can be as large as to occupy most of the volume of the mass, leaving only a shell of viable tumor. Adjacent bowel loops are displaced by the effect of the mass. There may be associated mesenteric abscess or fistulas between the tumor and nearby intestinal segments.

3) When the tumor is predominantly extraluminal it usually occupies and enlarges mesenteric lymph nodes. The adjacent retroperitoneum may also be filled with the tumor. The nodal mass indents the mesenteric border of the small intestine in a scalloped pattern that can be characteristic and striking on CT scans.[67] The fixation and angulation caused by adhesions that accompany some types of tumors metastatic to the mesentery are usually not seen.

4) Although listed first in Marshak's classification, the multiple nodular pattern of intestinal lymphoma is one of its less common radiographic patterns. This appearance is more often seen in patients with T cell lymphoma associated with celiac disease. In patients with the multiple-nodular form of the disease, nodules of varying size appear as intramural or intraluminal filling defects. Sometimes, particularly in the ileum, these are so numerous that they cause the contour of the involved segment of bowel to appear diffusely irregular. When the nodules are ulcerated, a central depression can sometimes be seen radiographically. Tiny nodules studding the valvulae conniventes may require enteroclysis to make them visible radiographically.[67] When the terminal ileum is involved, multiple nodules are often seen in the adjacent cecum. The bowel usually retains its normal caliber and is not fixed in position.

5) A discrete intraluminal polypoid mass can sometimes be seen. It is this form of intestinal lymphoma that is often associated with a mechanical obstruction caused by intussusception. As with the other patterns of intestinal lymphoma, the mass may achieve a large size.

CT is particularly useful in detecting, characterizing, and staging lymphoma of the small bowel.[45] It can demonstrate almost all of the features mentioned above. While enteroclysis is touted by some as a more sensitive method for detecting intestinal lymphoma, most would agree that radiographic characterization of the extent of disease is best done by CT. CT is especially adept at showing the bowel wall thickening that results from infiltration by lymphoma. Endogenous bowel gas or orally administered contrast material renders the lumen visible and shows areas of cavitation within the tumor. Enlargement of regional mesenteric lymph nodes and the finding of a large mass without mechanical bowel obstruction are features frequently seen in non-Hodgkin's lymphomas on CT scans.

Ultrasonography can also be useful in demonstrating small intestinal lymphomas. Like lymphomas elsewhere in the body, those arising in the bowel tend to be relatively sonolucent.[75] The typical picture is one of circumferentially thickened bowel wall forming a hypoechoic mass with strong central echoes emanating from mucus or gas within the bowel lumen.

Superior mesenteric arteriography has been studied in cases of small bowel lymphomas.[76] The tumors tend to be hypovascular, and, in general, arteriography has not been found to be diagnostically useful.

Lymphoma variants

Hodgkin's disease can produce some of the same radiographic findings that are seen in patients with non-Hodgkin's lymphomas. In Hodgkin's lymphoma, however, large excavations, fistulas, and aneurysmal dilatation are uncommon.[73] Mesenteric fibrosis along with resultant angulation and narrowing of the bowel is occasionally seen because Hodgkin's disease sometimes stimulates a desmoplastic response in tissues surrounding the tumor. Mesenteric lymph node enlargement, on the other hand, occurs in only 4% of patients with this form of intestinal lymphoma.[59]

Burkitt's lymphoma is a tumor of B lymphocytes that affects patients in the first three decades of life. American patients with Burkitt's lymphoma usually present with abdominal masses that grow rapidly and are often large at the time of diagnosis.[77] The malignant lymphocytes have an affinity for the Peyer's patches of the ileum. Mesenteric lymph nodes are often involved. Affected loops of small bowel may show narrowing and irregular thickening of folds.[78]

The primary jejunal lymphoma of the type known as Mediterranean lymphoma appears to be a clinically distinct entity.[79,80] It occurs predominantly among persons of Arabian and non-Ashkenazi Jewish descent. It is particularly prevalent in southern Iran, where it constitutes the majority of cases of intestinal lymphoma. Mediterranean lymphomas affect younger persons than the usual non-Hodgkin's lymphomas of the small intestine. The duodenum and jejunum are the areas primarily affected. The radiographic findings consist of marked, uniform, diffuse thickening of mucosal folds resulting from massive infiltration of plasma cells.[81] The portions of the small bowel that are uninvolved with lymphoma show a spruelike pattern, particularly in the ileum. In some patients there is a tendency to develop nodules superimposed on the thickened folds, and there may be separation of bowel loops by masses of enlarged lymph nodes in the mesentery. Clinical evidence of malabsorption is often accompanied by the radiographic signs of increased fluid in the small bowel lumen (i.e., flocculation, segmentation, and mild dilatation).

Differential diagnosis

Because of the protean radiographic manifestations of intestinal lymphomas, a variety of other conditions must be considered in the differential diagnosis. Intramural hematoma due to a coagulopathy or blunt abdominal trauma sometimes produces an appearance resembling the diffuse infiltrating form of lymphoma. Extrinsic inflammatory processes in the abdomen can produce a mass effect along with displacement and narrowing of adjacent bowel loops. Such an appearance can be caused by an abscess due to perforation of the appendix or a diverticulum. The inflammatory process of acute pancreatitis can dissect into the right lower abdomen, causing changes in the adjacent colon and ileum that mimic a lymphoma. Often the bowel loops overlying such inflammatory masses exhibit thickened, straight folds and kinking and fixation caused by adhesions—findings not typical of intestinal lymphomas.

Regional enteritis is sometimes difficult to distinguish radiographically from an intestinal lymphoma.[82,83] An inflamed mass of matted bowel loops can simulate mesenteric infiltration by a tumor, and the narrowing and thickening of folds can be seen in both conditions. The history of a chronic recurrent illness is more consistent with Crohn's disease, whereas the presence of nodules, polypoid masses, or aneurysmal dilatation should suggest the diagnosis of lymphoma.

Other types of tumors, particularly sarcomas and metastatic tumors, can simulate a lymphoma.[84] The nodules of metastatic melanoma can have an appearance indistinguishable from the multinodular form of intestinal lymphoma. An adenocarcinoma can usually be distinguished by its jejunal location and by the presence of marked localized narrowing.

ADENOCARCINOMAS
Clinical features

Adenocarcinomas constitute about one fourth of primary malignant tumors occurring in the small intestine.[41] Because the majority of carcinomas of the small bowel are symptomatic when detected, however, an adenocarcinoma is the most likely tumor to be found at surgery when a primary symptomatic small intestinal malignancy is discovered. These tumors are most common in the duodenum and proximal jejunum, and the likelihood of occurrence diminishes with increasing distance from the ligament of Treitz. Less than 15% of these tumors occur in the ileum, distinguishing them from carcinoid tumors, which are common in that region.

Small intestinal adenocarcinomas are somewhat more common in males than in females. Most probably arise from adenomas, and Sellner[85] has presented convincing evidence that the adenoma-carcinoma sequence takes place in the small intestine as it does in the colon. The 5-year survival rate is about 20%.[86] The survival rate is lower for patients with tumors of the duodenum than for patients with tumors arising in the jejunum, partly because of the complexity of surgical resection of duodenal tumors. The survival difference is also related to the fact that jejunal tumors are more likely than duodenal tumors to be infiltrative (rather than polypoid). For this reason, obstruction is likely to occur relatively earlier with adenocarcinomas in the jejunum than with those in the duodenum, and jejunal tumors are more likely to be detected early in the course of the disease.

Good[1] reported abdominal pain, obstruction, or both in 90% of patients with an adenocarcinoma of the small bowel; over half the patients in that series had bleeding or anemia as well. A small abdominal mass is palpable in only about 30% of cases.

Radiographic features

The radiographic appearance of adenocarcinoma of the small intestine is similar to that of a carcinoma of the esophagus or colon. Infiltrating tumors are the most common and appear as short, well-demarcated segments of narrowing with an irregular lumen indicating replacement of the mucosa by the tumor (Figs. 30-18 and 30-19). These tumors tend to have overhanging edges.[87] Not uncommonly there is ulceration within the mass (Fig. 30-20). Infiltrating tumors of this type incite a local scirrhous reaction in the bowel wall, and there is gradual mechanical obstruction of the bowel by the tumor. Prestenotic dilatation can be quite marked. Small plaquelike polypoid adenocarcinomas involving one wall of the jejunum have been detected by enteroclysis. With improvement in radiographic techniques for detecting early carcinomas in the small bowel, this pattern may be found to be more common than has previously been recognized. Adenocarcinomas have also been found

in the small intestine in the form of a pedunculated polyp, but this is rare.

CT shows the circumferential thickening of the bowel wall to best advantage (Fig. 30-21). It is good at demonstrating local invasion of the mesentery.[88] The tumor mass is typically 3 to 8 cm in diameter. It may be uniform in CT attenuation or may contain one or more areas of low attenuation.[5] Enlargement of regional mesenteric lymph nodes is seen in half of patients,[6] but the involved lymph nodes are not usually as large as those in cases of small bowel lymphoma.

Associated conditions

Small intestinal adenocarcinomas occur with a higher incidence in patients with adult celiac disease.[66,89] Characteristically there is a latent period of 20 years or more between the onset of malabsorption and the discovery of the tumor. For reasons that are not understood, the tumor is most likely to occur in patients who are unresponsive to a gluten-free diet.

Some evidence suggests a minor increase in the risk of a small bowel adenocarcinoma developing in patients with regional enteritis.[90-92] Recrudescence of symptoms of enteritis after a period of good disease control may herald the development of a carcinoma. Barium studies may show fistulas to the tumor, which rarely occurs in adenocarcinomas of the small bowel in patients without inflammatory bowel disease.

SARCOMAS

Sarcomas of spindle cell origin are another type of primary malignant tumor likely to be found in the small bowel. Although liposarcomas, schwannomas, and other tumors of

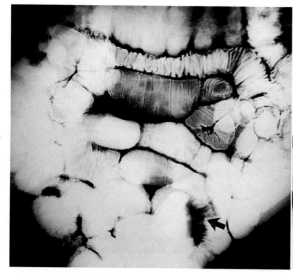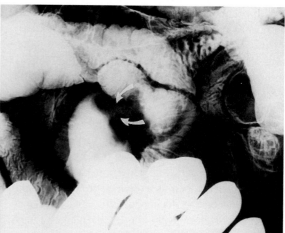

Fig. 30-18 Adenocarcinoma of the ileum that had escaped detection on prior small bowel series. **A,** Overhead film from enteroclysis shows short segmental narrowing *(arrow)* partially obscured by overlying loops. **B,** The lesion *(arrows)* was best seen by fluoroscopy with palpation.

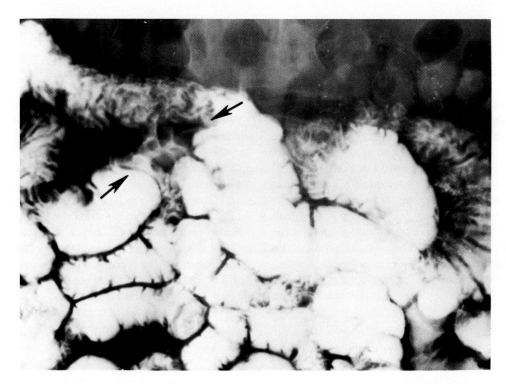

Fig. 30-19 Film of elderly man with unexplained gastrointestinal bleeding and previous small bowel series interpreted as normal. Narrowed, nodular segment 3 cm in size *(arrows)* in jejunum is causing slight obstruction. Adenocarcinoma was found at surgery.

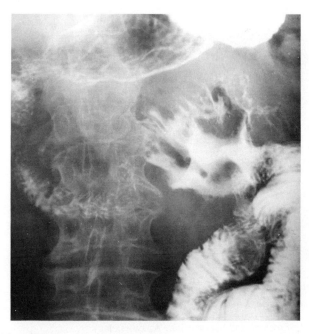

Fig. 30-20 Film of asymptomatic elderly man with anemia. There is an irregular 8-cm cavity communicating with jejunal lumen at the ligament of Treitz. Adenocarcinoma was found, although radiographic findings might also suggest lymphoma or sarcoma.

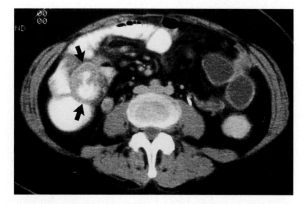

Fig. 30-21 Small jejunal adenocarcinoma *(arrows)* causing focal infiltration of bowel wall with irregular lumenal narrowing.

mesenchymal origin are found in rare instances,[93] the majority of primary sarcomas of the small intestine arise from smooth muscle. They almost always produce clinical signs and symptoms and rarely are encountered as incidental findings at autopsy. Melena and abdominal pain are common symptoms that tend to occur when the tumor has reached considerable size and has undergone necrosis or ulceration. Because these tumors grow slowly and extend outside the bowel lumen, mechanical obstruction is a relatively late manifestation. These tumors average 11 to 12 cm in size,[6,8] large enough to be palpable on abdominal examination in many patients at the time they are discovered.

Leiomyosarcomas can occur at any level in the small bowel but are rare in the duodenum. Radiographically the tumor appears as an extrinsic mass with the displacement of overlying intestinal loops that may be adherent. A prominent transverse stretching of parallel mucosal folds can indicate the site of the tumor. When necrosis and ulceration occur, an irregular cavity develops within the tumor and may fill with barium. Barium also outlines fistulous tracts

into the tumor mass in some cases. A distinction between a benign leiomyoma and a malignant leiomyosarcoma cannot be made reliably on radiographic grounds alone; however, smooth muscle tumors that are large or show significant central ulceration or fistula formation are usually malignant.[94] Radiographic criteria are ordinarily not helpful in distinguishing leiomyosarcomas from sarcomas of other cell types.

CT scans are useful in showing the extent of small bowel sarcomas, since they are largely extraluminal. The contrast-filled excavations within these tumors are readily detected on CT, and there may be necrotic regions of low CT attenuation within the tumor that do not communicate with the lumen of the bowel. CT may also display metastatic deposits in the liver, and these too may contain central, low-attenuation areas of necrosis. The dense, focal calcifications that occur in many gastrointestinal sarcomas of spindle cell origin show up well on CT.

As is the case with leiomyomas, these tumors are vascular, and arteriography can be useful in patients who are

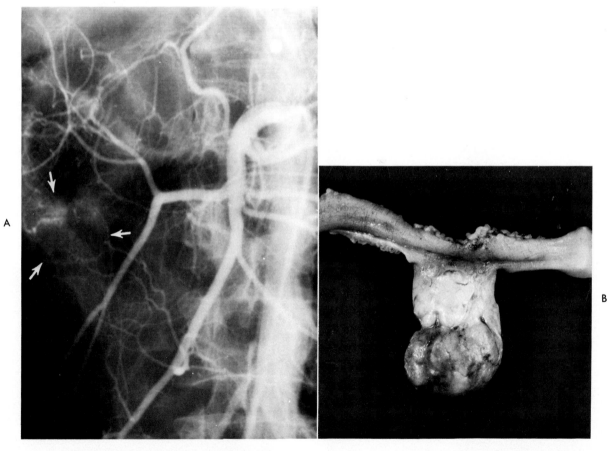

Fig. 30-22 Films of 44-year-old man with acute onset of melena and hypotension. **A,** Emergency superior mesenteric arteriogram showed fine arterial branches of the ileocolic artery outlining a 2.5-cm mass *(arrows)* containing irregularly dilated vessels, indicating vascular tumor. **B,** At surgery leiomyosarcoma was found arising from the serosal surface of the ileum. Tumor lay outside the lumen, but there was a small ulcer in the overlying mucosa.

bleeding[95] (Fig. 30-22). Tumor stain can be intense during the capillary phase of an arteriographic injection, and prominent feeding arteries and draining veins are characteristic. Uptake of Tc 99m pertechnitate Meckel's scans has also been reported.[12,96]

METASTATIC TUMORS
General features

A discussion of neoplasms of the small bowel would not be complete without consideration of the many forms of malignant tumors that can involve the small intestine secondarily. Patients with malignant disease often develop signs and symptoms of abdominal disease, and barium studies and CT are important in determining whether the symptoms indicate the presence of metastatic spread to the bowel or mesentery. Radiographic studies also play an important part in determining the stage of those tumors, such as melanoma, that have a propensity for spreading to the small bowel. Increasingly, enteroclysis is recommended as the technique of choice because it allows compression films to be made of well-distended bowel; these films are thought to be most sensitive in detecting small mural nodules and subtle pleating of folds, which may be the first radiographic manifestations of metastatic small bowel disease.[97]

The signs and symptoms of secondary neoplasms of the small bowel are not specific. Often patients are free of symptoms or have intermittent, poorly localized abdominal pain. GI bleeding and mechanical obstruction are the two most common specific signs. GI blood loss occurs in 20% to 30% of these patients and is most common in metastatic lesions that ulcerate or cavitate. Obstruction is most likely with tumors that stimulate a fibrotic reaction causing fixation, angulation, and narrowing of the bowel. Occasionally, perforation occurs, and rare instances of malabsorption are reported when the tumor replaces a large portion of the small intestine.[98]

Metastatic tumors reach the small intestine by several routes. Meyers and McSweeney[99] emphasized the importance of determining the route of spread because both the organ of origin and the tumor's radiographic appearance largely depend on it. Tumor cells can reach the small intestine through the blood (embolic), through intraperitoneal spread, through the lymphatic chain (Fig. 30-23), or by direct extension from an adjacent tumor mass. Of these four routes, the first two are the most common modes of tumor spread to the small bowel.

Intraperitoneal seeding occurs most often from tumors of GI origin in men and ovarian tumors in women (Figs. 30-24 and 30-25, *A*). The seeding of tumor cells into intraperitoneal fluid takes place, and the resultant secondary tumor deposits occur in predictable locations. The classic Blummer's shelf represents tumor in the prerectal pouch of Douglas, a dependent recess of the peritoneal cavity in the pelvis (Fig. 30-25, *B*). As many as half of the patients with intraperitoneal spread of a tumor to the GI tract have in-

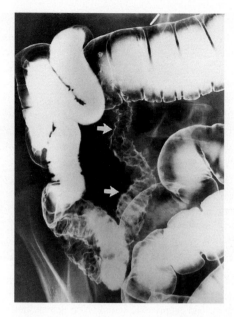

Fig. 30-23 Metastatic colon carcinoma after right hemicolectomy. Thickened, nodular ileal folds *(arrows)* result from encasement of bowel and from venous and lymphatic obstruction caused by tumor in mesentery and mesenteric lymph nodes.

volvement in this area. When a barium enema reveals the typical narrowing and irregularity of the rectum at the level of the upper sacrum, one should look carefully for evidence of intraperitoneal spread of tumor to the small intestine as well. Intraperitoneal fluid flows naturally along the root of the mesentery to the right lower quadrant, causing tumor nodules to grow in the wall and mesentery of the distal ileum, cecum, and ascending colon.

The hematogenous dissemination of tumor to the small intestine occurs most commonly in patients with melanoma or carcinoma of the lung. Mural nodules are evident and may be seen at any level in the small bowel (Fig. 30-26). The nodules are usually multiple and may be uniform or dissimilar in size. When their growth rate outstrips their blood supply, a central depression or ulceration may occur, giving the classically described bull's-eye, or target, appearance. These nodules tend to occur on the antimesenteric border of the bowel and sometimes grow into large polypoid masses that cavitate, particularly in patients with melanoma.

Metastatic melanoma

Although melanoma constitutes only about 3% of malignant neoplasms, its tendency to disseminate widely in most patients makes it one of the most common tumors to metastasize to the small bowel. Metastatic spread to the small bowel has been found by autopsy in 58% of patients with melanoma; however, small bowel involvement is detected less frequently in the clinical setting.[100] When the small bowel is involved, there is usually spread of the tumor to

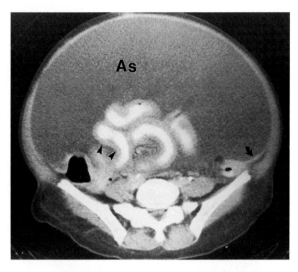

Fig. 30-24 Diffuse intraperitoneal spread of ovarian carcinoma. Thickening of small bowel wall *(arrowheads)* results from a thick layer of tumor laid evenly over serosa. Also note ascites *(As)* and parietal peritoneum thickened by tumor *(arrow)*.

other areas of the body as well. Dissemination is almost always borne by blood, and the generous arterial supply to the small bowel is probably the major factor accounting for the fact that this segment of the GI tract is more commonly involved than any other.

The radiographic manifestations of metastatic melanoma to the small intestine are many.[101] Most often, there are multiple nodules in the bowel wall (Fig. 30-27, *A*). These extend into the lumen as polypoid filling defects and may have a significant extraluminal component as well. In rare instances they are so numerous that they simulate the appearance of a polyposis syndrome. The bull's-eye, or target, appearance, caused by a depression in the center of the nodule, is less often noted in the jejunum and ileum, in contrast to the stomach and duodenum, where this appearance is common (Fig. 30-27, *B*). Intussusception occurs in 10% to 20% of patients with melanoma nodules in the small intestine, but the intussusception is sometimes transient and does not always cause clinically evident obstruction.

Another pattern commonly seen in patients with metastatic melanoma to the small intestine is that of an ulcerating mass (Fig. 30-28). This appearance can mimic that of

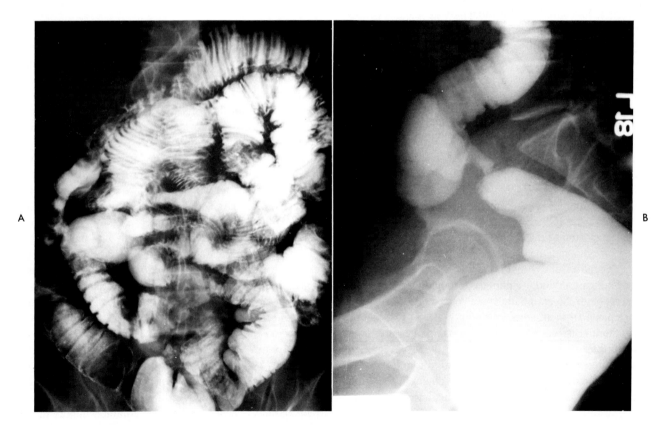

Fig. 30-25 Adenocarcinoma of stomach with diffuse intraperitoneal spread to small bowel and mesentery. **A,** Numerous intestinal loops are narrowed and draped over nodules of metastatic carcinoma. Note stretched, straightened mucosal folds in these areas. **B,** Lateral view of rectum on barium enema shows narrowing by tumor in the pouch of Douglas.

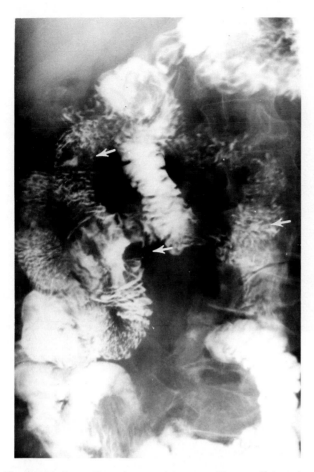

Fig. 30-26 Oat cell carcinoma of lung reaching small intestine via hematogenous route. Central ulcerations within mural nodules *(arrows)* give so-called bull's-eye appearance.

a necrotic sarcoma or that of an abscess or pseudocyst that drains spontaneously into the bowel. Significant widening of the bowel lumen may occur at the site of the excavation, and the cavity can occupy almost the entire volume of the mass. This appearance may also be seen with a lymphoma or leiomyosarcoma of the small intestine. Bleeding is common in patients with this sort of involvement and can either be occult or occur as an acute hemorrhagic episode.

About 15% of patients with melanoma develop mesenteric or omental metastases, probably also on a hematogenous basis. These cause extrinsic impressions on the small bowel as seen on barium studies. Nodules that originate in the mesentery may progress to invade adjacent bowel loops. Least commonly, melanoma can take an infiltrating form in the small bowel and can mimic the radiographic appearance of a primary adenocarcinoma.

Metastatic carcinoma

Carcinomas metastatic to the small bowel have a somewhat different appearance.[102] The colon and the ovary are common sites of origin of the primary tumor, and intraperitoneal seeding occurs with both.[81] Typically, nodules of tumor grow in the mesentery or peritoneum and may incite considerable fibrosis in the surrounding tissues. This leads to a fixation of bowel loops and stretching and fixation of the transverse mucosal folds, which take on a straightened or pleated appearance (Fig. 30-29). Angulation of the bowel may occur.

Metastatic tumors may have an annular appearance similar to that of typical primary adenocarcinoma.[103] Polypoid protrusions into the bowel may occur, and mechanical obstruction of one degree or another occurs in about one third of these patients. Hematogenous spread with the pattern of multiple mural nodules is less common. Diffuse thickening of the mucosal folds of a segment of ileum can result from metastatic spread to mesenteric lymph nodes with resultant lymphatic obstruction.[104] In patients with intraperitoneal spread of metastatic tumor, CT shows ascites and thickening of the parietal peritoneum. Thickening of the visceral peritoneum by serosal tumor gives the small intestine a thick-walled appearance (Fig. 30-23).

Kaposi's sarcoma

Kaposi's sarcoma is a skin tumor with a propensity to involve the GI tract. Formerly this unusual tumor was predominantly one of men over age 50 who were of northern Italian or eastern European ancestry. Nowadays, however, the epidemiology of the disease has changed significantly because of its strong association with AIDS. About 50% of homosexual men with AIDS and cutaneous Kaposi's sarcoma have GI involvement by the tumor. Hematogenous dissemination to the GI tract frequently occurs in the form of multiple nodules like those developing in patients with metastatic melanoma. Central ulceration of the nodules may occur. Contiguous nodules are sometimes so numerous that they resemble the appearance of thumbprinting[98] or irregular fold thickening.[105]

Germ cell tumors

Small intestinal metastatic lesions are noted in only about 4% of patients with germ cell tumors of the testes, but these deserve mention because the pattern of spread is somewhat different from that seen in cases of melanoma or metastatic carcinoma. The vast majority of testicular tumors metastatic to the small bowel are embryonal carcinomas, but many contain other malignant tissue elements as well.[106] Retroperitoneal lymph node involvement is present in virtually all patients in whom small bowel metastatic disease is detected, and involvement of the bowel is caused by direct extension from an adjacent retroperitoneal and mesenteric tumor in the majority of cases. Peritoneal seeding occurs rarely, and embolic or hematogenous spread can be seen in those tumors containing elements of a choriocarcinoma.

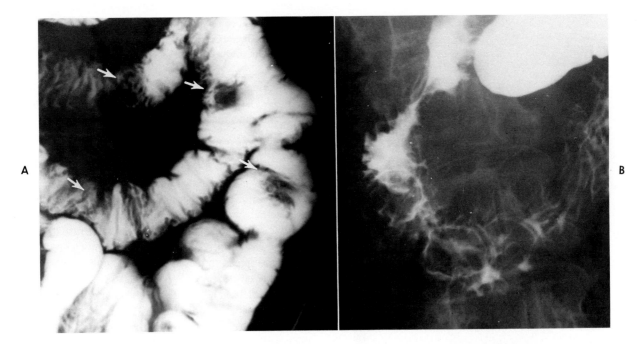

Fig. 30-27 Metastatic melanoma. **A,** Multiple mural nodules *(arrows)* in jejunum. **B,** Similar nodules in duodenum showed central ulcerations.

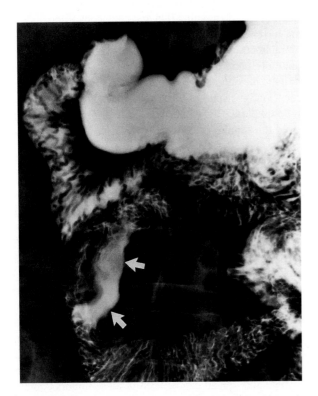

Fig. 30-28 Metastatic melanoma to jejunum. Note large ulcer *(arrowheads)* in the mass.

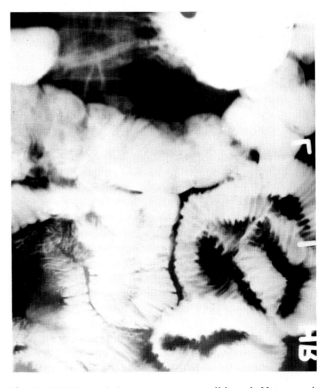

Fig. 30-29 Metastatic breast cancer to small bowel. Note prominent transverse stretching of mucosal folds over multiple masses.

REFERENCES

1. Good CA: Tumors of the small intestine, *AJR* 89:685, 1963.
2. Bessette JR et al: Primary malignant tumors in small bowel: a comparison of the small-bowel enema and conventional follow-through, *AJR* 153:741, 1989.
3. Maglinte DDT et al: Detection of surgical lesions of the small bowel by enteroclysis, *Am J Surg* 147:225, 1984.
4. Maglinte DDT et al: The role of the physician in the late diagnosis of primary malignant tumors of the small intestine, *Am J Gastroenterol* 86:304, 1991.
5. Laurent F et al: Diagnosis and categorization of small bowel neoplasms: role of computed tomography, *Gastrointest Radiol* 16:115, 1991.
6. Dudiak KM, Johnson CD, Stephens DH: Primary tumors of the small intestine: CT evaluation, *AJR* 152:995, 1989.
7. Bar-Ziv J, Solomon A: Computed tomography in adult intussusception, *Gastrointest Radiol* 16:264, 1991.
8. Megibow AJ et al: CT evaluation of gastrointestinal leiomyomas and leiomyosarcomas, *AJR* 144:727, 1985.
9. Merine D, Fishman EK, Jones B: CT evaluation of small bowel tumors, *Appl Radiol,* July:56, 1987.
10. Uflacker R et al: Angiography in primary myomas of the alimentary tract, *Radiology* 139:361, 1981.
11. McDonald KL: Technetium-99m RBC scintigraphy in the evaluation of small bowel leiomyoma, *Clin Nucl Med* 12:131, 1987.
12. Dunn EK et al: Ileal leiomyosarcoma and leiomyoma: false-positive scintiscans for Meckel's diverticulum, *Clin Nucl Med* 12:440, 1987.
13. Olmstead WW et al: Tumors of the small intestine with little or no malignant predisposition: a review of the literature and report of 56 cases, *Gastrointest Radiol* 12:231, 1987.
14. Taylor AJ, Stewart ET, Dodds WJ: Gastrointestinal lipomas: a radiologic and pathologic review, *AJR* 155:1205, 1990.
15. Ormson MJ, Stephens DH, Carlson HC: CT recognition of intestinal lipomatosis, *AJR* 144:313, 1985.
16. Yoshimitsu K et al: Computed tomography of ileocolic intussusception caused by a lipoma, *J Comput Assist Tomogr* 13:704, 1989.
17. Darling RC, Welch CE: Tumors of the small intestine, *N Engl J Med* 260:397, 1959.
18. Schey WL, Emanuel B, Raffensperger J: Benign neoplasia and pseudoneoplasia of the small bowel in children, *Gastrointest Radiol* 4:47, 1979.
19. Bracke PG et al: Polypoid hamartoma of the jejunum, *Gastrointest Radiol* 16:113, 1991.
20. LiVolsi VA, Perzin KH: Inflammatory pseudotumors (inflammatory fibrous polyps) of the small intestine: a clinicopathologic study, *Dig Dis Sci* 20:325, 1975.
21. Davis GB, Berke RN: The radiology corner: intestinal neurofibromas in von Recklinghausen's disease, *Am J Gastroenterol* 60:410, 1973.
22. Sivak MV, Sullivan BH, Farmer RG: Neurogenic tumors of the small intestine: review of the literature and review of a case with endoscopic removal, *Gastroenterology* 68:374, 1975.
23. Ginsburg LD: Eccentric polyposis of the small bowel, *Radiology* 116:561, 1975.
24. Uflacker R, Alves MA, Diehl JC: Gastrointestinal involvement in neurofibromatosis: angiographic presentation, *Gastrointest Radiol* 10:163, 1985.
25. Bussey HJR, Veale AMD, Morson BC: Genetics of gastrointestinal polyposis, *Gastroenterology* 74:1325, 1978.
26. Giardiello FM et al: Increased risk of cancer in the Peutz-Jeghers syndrome, *N Engl J Med* 316:1511, 1987.
27. Linos DA et al: Does Peutz-Jeghers syndrome predispose to gastrointestinal malignancy? *Arch Surg* 116:1182, 1981.
28. Matuchansky C et al: Peutz-Jeghers syndrome with metastasizing carcinoma arising from a jejunal hamartoma, *Gastroenterology* 77:1311, 1979.
29. Scully RE: Sex cord tumor with annular tubules: a distinctive ovarian tumor of the Peutz-Jeghers syndrome, *Cancer* 25:1107, 1970.
30. Sener RN et al: Peutz-Jeghers syndrome: CT and US demonstration of small bowel polyps, *Gastrointest Radiol* 16:21, 1991.
31. Cronkhite LW, Canada WJ: Generalized gastrointestinal polyposis: an unusual syndrome of polyposis, pigmentation, alopecia and onychotrophia, *N Engl J Med* 252:1011, 1955.
32. Koehler PR, Kyaw MM, Fenlon JW: Diffuse gastrointestinal polyposis with ectodermal changes, *Radiology* 103:589, 1972.
33. Beart RW, Fleming CR, Banks PM: Tubulovillous adenomas in a continent ileostomy after proctocolectomy for familial polyposis, *Dig Dis Sci* 27:553, 1982.
34. Hamilton SR et al: Ileal adenomas after colectomy in nine patients with adenomatous polyposis coli/Gardner's syndrome, *Gastroenterology* 77:1252, 1979.
35. Nayler EW, Lebenthal E: Gardner's syndrome: recent developments in research and management, *Dig Dis Sci* 25:945, 1980.
36. Barwick KW: Gastrointestinal manifestations of multiple endocrine neoplasia, type IIB, *J Clin Gastroenterol* 5:83, 1983.
37. Foster MA, Kilcyne RF: Ruvalcaba-Myhre-Smith syndrome: a new consideration in the differential diagnosis of intestinal polyps, *Gastrointest Radiol* 11:349, 1986.
38. Ruvalcaba RHA, Myhre S, Smith DW: Sotos syndrome with intestinal polyposis and pigmentary changes of the genitalia, *Clin Genet* 18:413, 1980.
39. Teitelbaum SL: The carcinoid, *Am J Surg* 123:564, 1972.
40. Godwin DJ: Carcinoid tumors—an analysis of 2837 cases, *Cancer* 36:560, 1975.
41. Desa LAJ et al: Primary jejunoileal tumors: a review of 45 cases, *World J Surg* 15:81, 1991.
42. Zeitels J et al: Carcinoid tumors, *Arch Surg* 117:732, 1982.
43. Nwiloh JO et al: Carcinoid tumors, *J Surg Oncol* 45:261, 1990.
44. Agranovich AL et al: Carcinoid tumor of the gastrointestinal tract: prognostic factors and disease outcome, *J Surg Oncol* 47:45, 1991.
45. Moesta KT, Schlag P: Proposal for a new carcinoid tumour staging system based on tumour tissue infiltration and primary metastasis; a prospective multicentre carcinoid tumour evaluation study, *Eur J Surg Oncol* 16:280, 1990.
46. Sax RE, Speck R, Cleveland JC: Analysis of thirty-one patients with carcinoid tumor of the gastrointestinal tract, *Am Surg* 36:511, 1970.
47. Beaton HL: Carcinoid tumors of the alimentary tract, *CA Cancer J Clin* 32:92, 1982.
48. Kothari T, Mangla JC: Malignant tumors associated with carcinoid tumors of the gastrointestinal tract, *J Clin Gastroenterol* 3 (suppl 1):43, 1981.
49. Margolies MN, Palmer EL, Geller SG: Case records of the Massachusetts General Hospital (Case 37—1985), *N Engl J Med* 313:680, 1985.
50. McDonald RA: A study of 356 carcinoids of the gastrointestinal tract: report of 4 new cases of the carcinoid syndrome, *Am J Med* 21:867, 1956.
51. Modlin IM: Carcinoid syndrome, *J Clin Gastroenterol* 2:349, 1980.
52. Morin LJ, Zuerner RT, Hanover NH: Retroperitoneal fibrosis and carcinoid tumor, *JAMA* 216:1647, 1971.
53. Mir-Madjlessi SH, Winkelman EI, Davis GA: Carcinoid tumors of the terminal ileum simulating Crohn's disease, *Cleve Clin J Med* 55:257, 1988.
54. Picus D et al: Computed tomography of abdominal carcinoid tumors, *AJR* 143:581, 1984.
55. Eastwood GL et al: Case records of the Massachusetts General Hospital (Case 20—1986), *N Engl J Med* 314:1369, 1986.
56. Kinkhabwala M, Balthazar EJ: Carcinoid tumors of the alimentary tract. II. Angiographic diagnosis of small intestinal and colonic lesions, *Gastrointest Radiol* 3:57, 1978.
57. Goldstein HM, Miller M: Angiographic evaluation of carcinoid tumors of the small intestine: the value of epinephrine, *Radiology* 114:23, 1975.

58. Adolf JMG et al: Carcinoid tumors: CT and I-131 meta-iodo-benzylguanidine scintigraphy, *Radiology* 164:199, 1987.

59. Brady LW, Asbell SO: Malignant lymphoma of the gastrointestinal tract, *Radiology* 137:291, 1980.

60. Hickish T, Cunningham D: Gastrointestinal non-Hodgkin's lymphoma, *Bailliere's Clin Gastroenterol* 4:191, 1990.

61. SenGupta SK, Sinha SN: Clinicopathological features of primary gastrointestinal lymphomas: a study of 42 cases, *Aust N Z J Surg* 61:133, 1991.

62. Loehr WJ et al: Primary lymphoma of the gastrointestinal tract: a review of 100 cases, *Ann Surg* 170:232, 1969.

63. Townsend R: CT in AIDS-related lymphoma, *AJR* 156:969, 1991.

64. Hodges JR et al: Malignant histiocytosis of the intestine, *Dig Dis Sci* 24:631, 1979.

65. Klingenstein RJ, Ferrucci JT, Lamarre LP: Case records of the Massachusetts General Hospital, Case 53-1987, *N Engl J Med* 317:1715, 1987.

66. Seaman WB, Galdabini JJ, Ferrucci JT: Case records of the Massachusetts General Hospital, Case 48-1976, *N Engl J Med* 295:1242, 1976.

67. Rubesin SE et al: Non-Hodgkin lymphoma of the small intestine, *Radiographics* 10:985, 1990.

68. Swinson CM et al: Coeliac disease and malignancy, *Lancet* 1:111, 1983.

69. Harris OD et al: Malignancy in adult celiac disease and idiopathic steatorrhea, *Am J Med* 42:899, 1967.

70. Glick SN et al: Development of lymphoma in patients with Crohn disease, *Radiology* 153:337, 1984.

71. Sartoris DJ et al: Small bowel lymphoma and regional enteritis: radiographic similarities, *Radiology* 152:291, 1984.

72. Megibow AJ: Gastrointestinal lymphoma: role of CT in diagnosis and management, *Semin Ultrasound CT MR* 7:43, 1986.

73. Marshak RH, Lindner AE, Maklansky D: Lymphoreticular disorders of the gastrointestinal tract: roentgenographic features, *Gastrointest Radiol* 4:103, 1979.

74. Gourtsoyiannis NC, Nolan DJ: Lymphoma of the small intestine: radiological appearances, *Clin Radiol* 39:639, 1988.

75. Georg C, Schwerk WB, Georg K: Gastrointestinal lymphoma: sonographic findings in 54 patients, *AJR* 155:795, 1990.

76. Lunderquist A et al: Selective superior mesenteric arteriography in reticulum cell sarcoma of the small bowel, *Radiology* 98:113, 1971.

77. Banks PM et al: American Burkitt's lymphoma: a clinicopathologic study of 30 cases: II. Pathologic correlations, *Am J Med* 58:322, 1975.

78. Cohen AM et al: Case records of the Massachusetts General Hospital, Case 45-1978, *N Engl J Med* 229:1121, 1978.

79. Ramos L et al: Radiological characteristics of primary intestinal lymphoma of the "Mediterranean" type: observations of 12 cases, *Radiology* 126:379, 1978.

80. Vessal K et al: Immunoproliferative small intestinal disease with duodenojejunal lymphoma: radiologic changes, *AJR* 135:491, 1980.

81. Smith SJ, Carlson HC, Gisvold JJ: Secondary neoplasms of the small bowel, *Radiology* 125:29, 1977.

82. Gallego MS et al: Primary adenocarcinoma of the terminal ileum simulating Crohn's disease, *Gastrointest Radiol* 11:355, 1986.

83. Millman PJ et al: Primary ileal adenocarcinoma simulating Crohn's disease, *Gastrointest Radiol* 5:55, 1980.

84. Nasr K et al: Primary upper small intestinal lymphoma: a report of 40 cases from Iran, *Dig Dis Sci* 21:313, 1971.

85. Sellner F: Investigations on the significance of the adenoma-carcinoma sequence in the small bowel, *Cancer* 66:702, 1990.

86. Sellink JL: Tumors. In *Radiologic atlas of common diseases of the small bowel*, Leiden, The Netherlands, 1976, HE Stenfert Kroese.

87. Ekberg O, Eckholm S: Radiology in primary small bowel carcinoma, *Gastrointest Radiol* 5:49, 1980.

88. Thompson WM, Halvorsen RA: Computed tomographic staging of gastrointestinal malignancies: Part II. The small bowel, colon, and rectum, *Invest Radiol* 22:96, 1987.

89. Petreshock EP, Pessah M, Menachemi E: Adenocarcinoma of the jejunum associated with nontropical sprue, *Dig Dis Sci* 20:796, 1975.

90. Kerber GW, Frank PH: Carcinoma of the small intestine and colon as a complication of Crohn disease: radiologic manifestations, *Radiology* 150:639, 1984.

91. Rubio CA et al: Crohn's disease and adenocarcinoma of the intestinal tract, *Dis Colon Rectum* 34:174, 1991.

92. Traube J et al: Crohn's disease and adenocarcinoma of the bowel, *Dig Dis Sci* 25:939, 1980.

93. Hansen D, Pedersen A, Pedersen K: Malignant intestinal schwannoma, *Acta Chir Scand* 156:729, 1990.

94. Starr GF, Dockerty MB: Leiomyomas and leiomyosarcomas of the small intestine, *Cancer* 8:101, 1955.

95. Hansen CP, Colstrup H, Mogensen AM: Recurrent gastrointestinal bleeding due to leiomyosarcoma of the small intestine, *Eur J Surg* 157:227, 1991.

96. Moote D, Ehrlich L, Martin RH: Detection of small bowel leiomyosarcoma during a Meckel's scan, *Clin Nucl Med* 12:440, 1987.

97. Oddson TA et al: The spectrum of small bowel melanoma, *Gastrointest Radiol* 3:419, 1978.

98. Byrk D et al: Kaposi's sarcoma of the intestinal tract: roentgen manifestations, *Gastrointest Radiol* 3:425, 1978.

99. Meyers MA, McSweeney J: Secondary neoplasms of the bowel, *Radiology* 105:1, 1972.

100. Goldstein HM, Beydoun MT, Dodd GD: Radiologic spectrum of melanoma metastatic to the gastrointestinal tract, *AJR* 129:605, 1977.

101. Plavsic B, Robinson AE: Variations in gastrointestinal melanoma metastases, *Acta Radiol* 31:493, 1990.

102. Chang SF et al: The protean gastrointestinal manifestations of metastatic breast cancer, *Radiology* 126:11, 1978.

103. Levine MS, Drooz AT, Herlinger H: Annular malignancies of the small bowel, *Gastrointest Radiol* 12:53, 1987.

104. Moffatt RE, Gourley WK: Ileal lymphatic metastases from cecal carcinoma, *Radiology* 135:55, 1980.

105. Wall SD, Friedman SL, Margulis AR: Gastrointestinal Kaposi's sarcoma in AIDS: radiographic manifestations, *J Clin Gastroenterol* 6:165, 1984.

106. Chait MM, Kurtz RC, Hajdu SI: Gastrointestinal tract metastasis in patients with germ-cell tumor of the testis, *Dig Dis Sci* 23:925, 1978.

31 *Vascular Disorders of the Small Intestine*

DANIEL J. NOLAN

MESENTERIC ISCHEMIA AND INFARCTION

Mesenteric vascular disease can be classified as arterial occlusion by embolus, thrombosis, compression, or trauma; nonocclusive ischemia and infarction; and mesenteric venous thrombosis.[1] Ischemia occurs when an organ receives insufficient oxygen-bearing blood to perform its normal function; infarction is death of part or all of an organ, resulting from ischemia.

Sudden interruption of the superior mesenteric arterial blood supply results in ischemic changes that frequently progress to infarction. Embolic occlusion of the superior mesenteric artery may be caused by mitral valve disease, thrombus formation after myocardial infarction, the onset of atrial fibrillation, or an embolus passing into the arterial circulation via a patent foramen ovale. Acute mesenteric ischemia may also be caused by displacement of atheromatous plaques at the origin of the superior mesenteric artery or by blunt or penetrating abdominal trauma severely damaging or transecting the superior mesenteric artery.

Nonocclusive ischemia occurs where there is inadequate perfusion of the intestine with oxygenated blood. Conditions that give rise to these low flow states include decreased cardiac output, mesenteric arterial to arterial steal, mesenteric arterial to venous shunting, and mesenteric arterial vasoconstriction.[2] Cardiac output may be reduced in primary cardiac disorders, arrhythmias, and hypovolemia. In patients with mesenteric arterial vasoconstriction, arterial vasospasm reduces the blood flow through the patent but acutely contracted arteries.[2-4] Mesenteric arterial vasoconstriction can result from the use of certain therapeutic agents, such as digitalis, vasopressin, and ergot preparations, and from abuse of agents such as cocaine.[5,6]

Mesenteric venous thrombosis is an uncommon cause of intestinal ischemia and infarction.[7] Conditions that may cause mesenteric venous occlusion are blunt or penetrating trauma, pelvic infection, diverticulitis, appendicitis, peritonitis, and parasitic infection. It may also be caused by pancreatitis, pancreatic carcinoma and metastases in the mesentery (especially carcinoid), internal hernias, closed-loop obstruction, portal hypertension associated with oral contraceptives, and pregnancy.[2,8]

Acute mesenteric ischemia presents with the sudden onset of cramping abdominal pain and vomiting. These presenting symptoms are nonspecific, so diagnosis and treatment are frequently delayed.[9] Diarrhea may develop and progress to hemorrhage. As the ischemia persists and progresses to infarction, an elevated white blood count, fever, and signs of peritonitis may develop.[2] Superior mesenteric occlusion from trauma, penetrating or blunt, is usually sudden, severe, and extensive.

Plain abdominal radiographs and computed tomography (CT), described in Chapter 107, play an important role in evaluating acute intestinal ischemia and infarction.

Barium studies occasionally have a role in the investigation of suspected acute intestinal ischemia. Characteristically, there is thickening of the valvulae conniventes (Fig. 31-1), which can be quite marked during or shortly after the acute ischemic episode. These changes frequently resolve, and a repeat examination 6 weeks later may show that the intestine has returned to normal. Occasionally an ischemic stricture may develop.

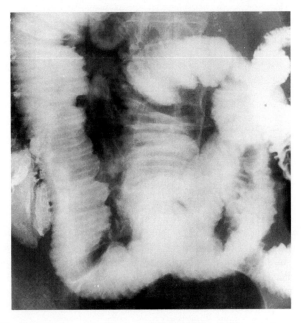

Fig. 31-1 Mesenteric ischemia. Thickened valvulae conniventes are seen in a long segment of small intestine.

The patient with mesenteric venous thrombosis may be investigated for nonspecific abdominal symptoms. It is therefore important to be aware of the radiologic appearances on barium studies. There is frequently a segment or segments of intestine showing marked thickening of the valvulae conniventes and intestinal wall with mesenteric thickening seen as separation of the loops of barium-filled intestine[10] (Fig. 31-2). A long zone of transition is seen between the uninvolved segments, and this is characterized by progressive thickening of the valvulae conniventes. Late findings include dilatation of the more proximal small intestine and evidence of ascites. Pseudotumors, "thumbprinting," caused by focal hemorrhages, are seen occasionally.

ISCHEMIC INTESTINAL STRICTURES

Ischemic strictures of the small intestine are uncommon. They may result from thrombosis or embolism of the mesenteric vessels or from mesenteric venous thrombosis in hemophiliacs and patients on anticoagulant therapy. Localized strictures after radiotherapy result from ischemia. Enteric-coated potassium tablets were formerly one of the most common causes of ischemic strictures of the small intestine,[11,12] but this is no longer the case. Strangulated hernia can result in ischemic stenosis with strictures up to 10 cm in length. Symptoms may develop within 7 to 10 days or present several years after strangulation.[12]

Blunt abdominal trauma may result in ischemic strictures.[13] Ischemia, localized to a short segment of intestine, occurs either as a result of a short mesenteric tear or by direct crushing of the intestine against the spine. It may be months or even years after the injury before the onset of symptoms. Barium examination shows the stricture as a short segment of narrowing, sometimes with dilatation of the more proximal intestine (Fig. 31-3).

INTRAMURAL HEMORRHAGE

Bleeding into the wall of the jejunum or ileum may occur in patients taking anticoagulant medications or in those with bleeding disorders.[14] Idiopathic thrombocytopenic purpura, leukemia, Henoch-Schönlein purpura, and, rarely, hemophilia predispose to intramural hemorrhage. Abdomi-

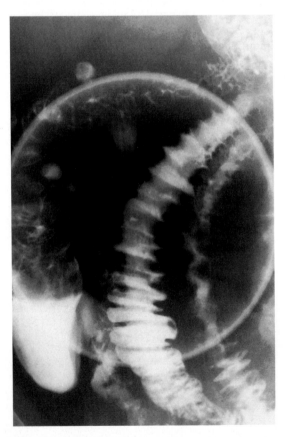

Fig. 31-2 Chronic ischemia caused by mesenteric venous thrombosis. Gross thickening of the valvulae conniventes with narrowing of the lumen and separation of the loops is seen in a segment of ileum. The patient, a 76-year-old woman, presented with abdominal pain, flatulence, and vomiting. At operation a mass of carcinoid tumor was found infiltrating the root of the mesentery, resulting in venous thrombosis.
From Nolan DJ: *Radiological atlas of gastrointestinal disease,* New York, 1983, John Wiley.

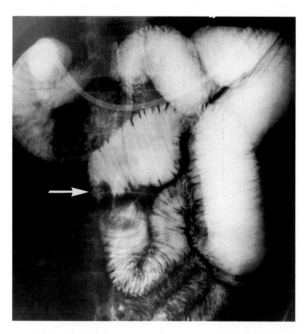

Fig. 31-3 Ischemic stricture resulting from trauma causing obstruction. A short, tight stricture is seen in the proximal jejunum *(arrow).* There is an abrupt transition in caliber between the dilated jejunum proximal to the stricture and the collapsed loops distally. The patient, a 33-year-old man, had been hospitalized 3 months earlier for 24 hours after blunt abdominal trauma. This examination was performed when he presented with anorexia, abdominal pain, vomiting, and weight loss. Histologic examination of the resected specimen showed ischemic damage of the circular muscle coat, with contraction and fibrosis.
From Nolan DJ: *Radiological atlas of gastrointestinal disease,* New York, 1983, John Wiley.

nal trauma is an occasional cause of intramural intestinal hemorrhage.

Abdominal pain, melena, an abdominal mass, or intestinal obstruction are the probable presenting features. On barium examination the changes in the small intestine may be localized, segmental, or diffuse. Localized intramural hemorrhage is seen as an intramural mass (Fig. 31-4). When the intramural hemorrhage is segmental or diffuse, uniform symmetric thickening of the valvulae conniventes with a symmetric spikelike configuration simulating a stack of coins is seen.[14]

CHRONIC RADIATION ENTERITIS

Chronic radiation enteritis, although an uncommon sequela of abdominopelvic radiation therapy, is a significant

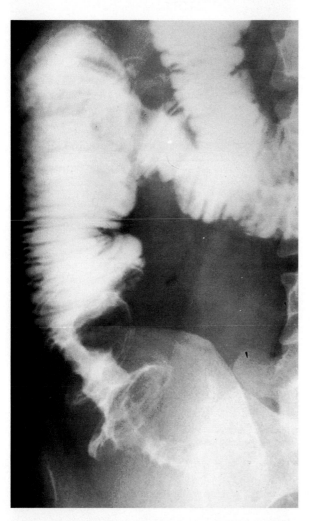

Fig. 31-4 Intramural hematoma. Large, concentric submucosal filling defects are seen in a short segment of small intestine, causing obstruction. The patient was receiving anticoagulant therapy and presented with intestinal obstruction.
Courtesy of Dr. WJ Norman, Shrewsbury, England; From Nolan DJ, Herlinger H: *Vascular lesions of the small bowel*. In Gore RM, Levine MS, Laufer I, eds: *Textbook of gastrointestinal radiology*, Philadelphia, WB Saunders (in press).

cause of morbidity in patients who survive malignant disease.[15] The majority of patients are women who have received radiotherapy for carcinoma of the genital tract.[15] The underlying pathologic process is endarteritis obliterans with compromise of the microvascular circulation.[16] There is a predisposition to the development of radiation enteritis in patients with hypertension or diabetes. Previous abdominal surgery or peritonitis before radiotherapy results in normally mobile loops of intestine being bound down in the pelvis within the radiotherapy field. The incidence of late radiation effects on the intestine is unknown, but the accepted figure is about 2% to 5%.[17]

There is considerable variation in the interval between radiation therapy and the onset of symptoms attributable to chronic radiation enteritis. The latent period varies from persistent diarrhea starting during therapy to 25 years later[15]; most patients present 2 to 10 years after therapy. Typical presenting symptoms include intermittent intestinal obstruction and malabsorption, which may be subclinical; abdominal pain; diarrhea; and weight loss.

Enteroclysis is excellent for evaluating the changes in the intestine caused by radiation enteritis. Characteristic radiologic signs include thickening of the valvulae conniventes, stenosis, mucosal tacking, mural thickening, effacement of the mucosal pattern, ulceration, sinuses, fistulas, and adhesions.[15,18]

Thickening of the valvulae conniventes caused by submucosal edema or fibrotic infiltration is a most frequently observed sign (Fig. 31-5). Valvulae are considered to be thickened if they are greater than 2 mm thick. The thickened folds tend to remain straight, unlike in Crohn's disease in which thickening is irregular with frequent fusion of valvulae.

Narrowing and stenosis are characteristic findings (Figs. 31-6, and 31-7). Stenosis may be single or multiple and

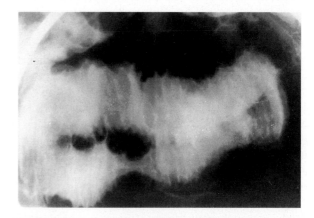

Fig. 31-5 Chronic radiation enteritis. A spot compression radiograph taken during enteroclysis shows thickening of the valvulae conniventes and mucosal tacking in a short segment of ileum.
From Mendelson RM, Nolan DJ: *Clin Radiol* 36:141, 1985.

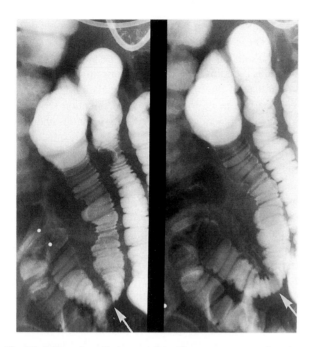

Fig. 31-6 Chronic radiation enteritis. Two spot compression views show a short stricture in the ileum *(arrows)*. The stricture was causing obstruction, but there was no dilatation of the immediately proximal segment because it was also involved in the disease process.

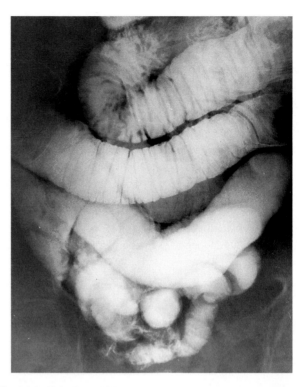

Fig. 31-7 Chronic radiation enteritis. A moderately long segment of narrowed ileum located in the pelvis is causing intestinal obstruction.

vary in length from a short segment to a stricture several centimeters in length. Dilatation proximal to the stenotic segment or segments indicates the presence of obstruction (Fig. 31-7).

Mural thickening (Fig. 31-8) is defined as a combined wall thickness of greater than 2 mm when adjacent loops are parallel for at least 4 cm under compression. On fluoroscopy, peristaltic activity is decreased or absent in the segment affected. Mucosal tacking (Fig. 31-5) is seen as angulation and distortion of the mucosal folds on the antimesenteric border of the intestine caused by adhesions between the intestine and the inflamed mesentery.

Complete effacement of the mucosal pattern gives a featureless outline. When a number of featureless segments are adherent, it is difficult to distinguish individual segments even with the use of compression. Then the characteristic "pool-of-barium" appearance may be seen[15,18] (Fig. 31-9). Ulceration is a recognized pathologic feature of radiation enteritis but is only occasionally seen when the ulcers are deep.[19] Ulcers are more likely to be associated with strictures. Sinuses and fistulas (Fig. 31-10), which may occur as complications after surgery for chronic radiation enteritis, are usually clearly outlined on barium examination.

On CT chronic radiation enteritis is seen as a masslike confluence of shortened loops of intestine with thickening of the intestinal wall, thickening of the adjacent mesentery, adherent adjacent loops, and increased density of mesenteric fat.[20]

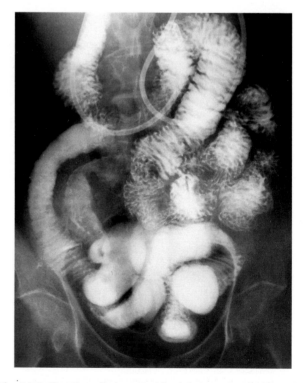

Fig. 31-8 Chronic radiation enteritis. A long segment of intestine is abnormal with almost complete effacement of the mucosal pattern. Characteristic mural thickening can also be seen.

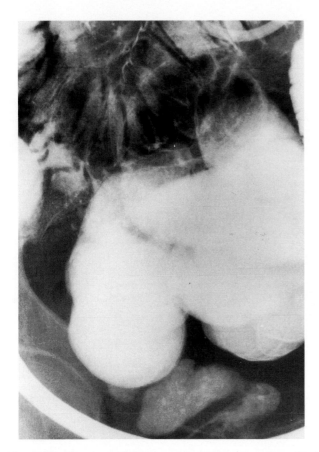

Fig. 31-9 Chronic radiation enteritis. Adherent, barium-filled loops in which the individual segments are barely discernible give the characteristic "pool-of-barium" appearance.
From Mendelson RM, Nolan DJ: *Clin Radiol* 36:141, 1985.

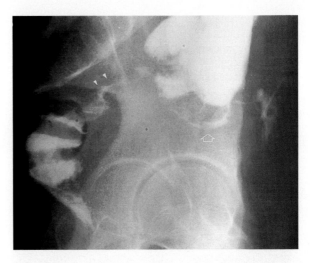

Fig. 31-10 Chronic radiation enteritis. Ileorectal *(arrowheads)* and ileocutaneous *(arrow)* fistulas are outlined with barium.

SYSTEMIC SCLEROSIS

The small intestine is frequently affected in patients with systemic sclerosis (scleroderma), often early in the course of the disorder.[21]

Thinning and fibrosis of the circular and longitudinal smooth muscle is the main finding on pathologic examination of the affected small intestine. Similar smooth muscle changes occur in visceral myopathy; the circular muscle is involved to a greater extent in systemic sclerosis, the longitudinal muscle in visceral myopathy.[22] Small artery occlusion is also a manifestation of systemic sclerosis, although there are no symptoms of chronic small intestinal ischemia.[21]

There is no correlation between the duration, severity, or frequency of other organ involvement and small intestinal involvement. Malabsorption caused by bacterial colonization of the small intestine results in steatorrhea, which is the characteristic mode of clinical presentation when the organ is involved. The radiologic examination is the only satisfactory method for diagnosis. Peroral jejunal biopsy specimens do not yield adequate histologic specimens. To make a histologic diagnosis it is necessary to have a full-thickness biopsy specimen of the small intestine.

The characteristic radiologic findings on barium examination are delayed intestinal transit caused by diminished peristalsis, dilatation of the duodenum and jejunum, sacculation (Figs. 31-11, 31-12, and 31-13), and the "wire-spring" or "hidebound" appearance. Duodenal dilatation can be quite marked. Sacculations, also called *pseudodiverticula,* have a characteristic appearance. They are large, broad-based outpouchings, often with a squared contour, and are usually located in the jejunum. Visceral myopathy is the only other condition in which sacculations are seen.

The "wire-spring"[21] or "hidebound" appearance[23] (Fig. 31-14) is characteristic of systemic sclerosis and is seen as an increased number of thin mucosal folds. The appearances are seen best in the mid and distal small intestine and result from the preferential thinning and fibrosis of the circular smooth muscle while the longitudinal smooth muscle remains mostly intact and contracts in the normal manner.

VASCULITIS
Henoch-Schönlein purpura

Henoch-Schönlein purpura frequently involves the small intestine. The disorder mostly affects young men and is characterized by a nontraumatic hemorrhagic diathesis with bleeding into the joints, skin, and viscera without a platelet abnormality. Increased capillary fragility is responsible for extravasation of serosanguineous fluid into the intestinal wall and results in edema of the mucosa and submucosa[24] (Fig. 31-15). There is a relatively high incidence of intussusception in children with Henoch-Schönlein purpura.

Polyarteritis nodosa

Only occasionally is the small intestine involved in polyarteritis nodosa. Craig[25] reported a case of multiple small

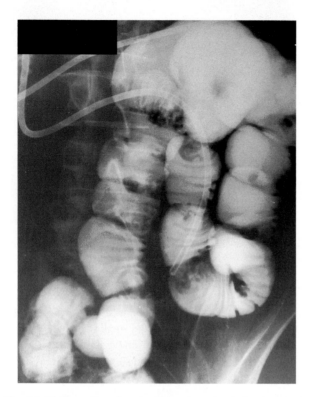

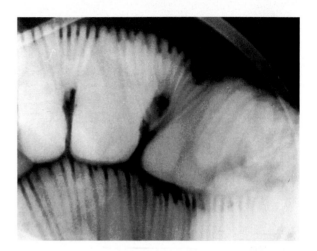

Fig. 31-12 Systemic sclerosis. A spot view of wide-necked sacculation.

Fig. 31-11 Systemic sclerosis. Extensive sacculation is seen in the jejunum.

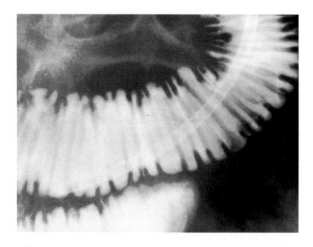

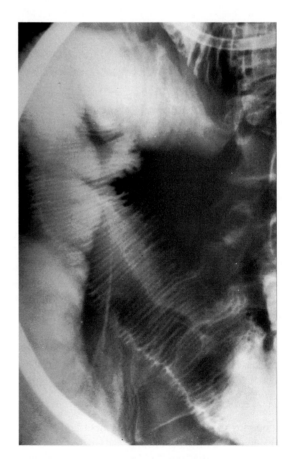

Fig. 31-13 Systemic sclerosis. Multiple small sacculations.

Fig. 31-14 Systemic sclerosis. A spot compression view shows the characteristic "hidebound" or "concertina" appearance.
From Nolan DJ, Cadman PJ: *Clin Radiol* 38:295, 1987.

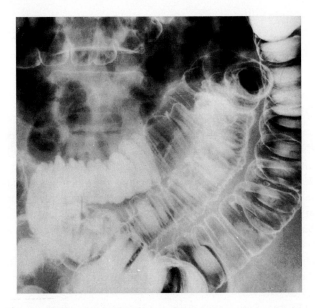

Fig. 31-15 View of midileum and adjacent descending colon during double-contrast barium enema. The 39-year-old woman had a sore throat followed by flitting arthralgia, an evanescent pruritic rash that came and went several times, and abdominal pain with mild diarrhea. A diagnosis of Henoch-Schönlein purpura was made. No treatment was given. A small bowel study 10 days later showed appearance almost back to normal.

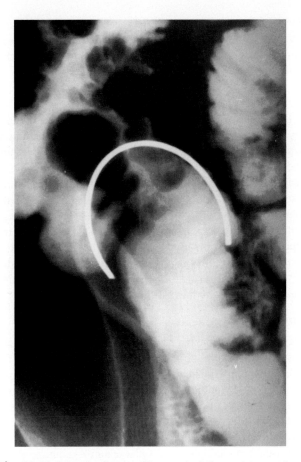

Fig. 31-16 Behçet's disease. The terminal ileum, just proximal to the ileocecal valve, is abnormal with narrowing of the lumen, irregularity, and slight proximal dilatation in a patient with Behçet's disease. Note that the ileocecal valve is also enlarged. Courtesy of Dr. DJ Allison, London.

intestinal perforations caused by polyarteritis nodosa and reviewed seven similar cases from the literature. Marshak and Lindner[26] illustrated a case of polyarteritis nodosa with marked thickening of the valvulae conniventes shown on barium examination.

Behçet's disease

Behçet's disease is a chronic systemic disorder with a diversity of symptoms. It mostly affects males aged between 10 and 30 years.[27] The histopathologic basis of the disorder is a nonspecific vasculitis. Patients characteristically present with orogenital ulceration, although many systems can be involved. Exacerbations and remissions frequently occur. Patients with gastrointestinal involvement may develop abdominal pain, vomiting, diarrhea, or constipation. Changes resembling Crohn's disease may be seen in the small and large intestines, mostly in the ileocecal area (Fig. 31-16).

Rheumatoid arthritis

Small intestinal involvement is rare in rheumatoid arthritis and is caused by a vasculitis.[28] Bienenstock and colleagues[29] reported a case of mesenteric arteritis and intestinal infarction in a patient with rheumatoid arthritis. A vasculitis-induced ischemic stricture was reported by Kuehne et al.[28]

Ehlers-Danlos syndrome

Ehlers-Danlos syndrome is an uncommon condition characterized by laxity and hypermotility of the joints, gross laxity of the skin, and wide thin scars that frequently overlie the bony prominences. The fragility of tissue that is characteristic of the dermal changes may also involve the gastrointestinal tract.[30] Extensive jejunal diverticulosis may be seen in young patients with this disorder.[31] Spontaneous perforation of the intestine and massive gastrointestinal hemorrhage are uncommon but potentially lethal complications.[30] Beighton et al.[30] reported intramural hematomas of the jejunum and intraperitoneal bleeding in a 19-year-old woman.

Thromboangitis obliterans

Rarely, thromboangitis obliterans involves the distal branches of the superior mesenteric artery, producing local ischemic changes in the intestine.[32,33] Irregular narrowing of the lumen with gross thickening of the valvulae conniventes of the ileum was seen in the case reported by Herrington and Grossman.[32] The changes may progress to ischemic stenosis.[26]

Systemic lupus erythematosus

Lupus gastrointestinal vasculitis is a more common entity than is generally recognized.[34] The most common symptoms are anorexia, abdominal pain, nausea, vomiting, and occasionally diarrhea or gastrointestinal bleeding. Exacerbations and remissions are characteristic features of intestinal involvement.[35] On barium examination the small intestine shows thickening of the valvulae conniventes, sometimes with narrowing of the lumen and spasm. The mucosa may slough, giving the lumen an amorphous appearance.[36] After treatment with steroids, the intestine usually returns to normal.[34,36] The ischemic changes in the small intestine may, however, progress to infarction.[37]

Cogan's syndrome

Cogan's syndrome is a rare disorder of young adults manifested by nonsyphilitic interstitial keratitis and audiovestibular symptoms, including bilateral deafness, vertigo, and tinnitus.[38,39] Symptoms occur in rapid succession; sequelae include deafness, vasculitis, aortic insufficiency, blindness, and death. Mucosal ulceration of the intestine has been described in a number of cases; in the case reported by Thomas[39] the terminal ileum showed a featureless outline (Fig. 31-17).

Cryoglobulinemia

An intestinal vasculitis may be seen in essential cryoglobulinemia.[40] A localized irregular narrowing of a segment of ileum was seen in the case reported by Reza et al.[40]

NONSTEROIDAL ANTIINFLAMMATORY DRUG–INDUCED ENTERITIS

Long-term use of nonsteroidal antiinflammatory drugs (NSAIDs) may lead to nonspecific ulceration of the small intestine with occult blood and protein loss. In a large postmortem study, evidence of nonspecific ulceration was found in 13.5% of patients who had been on long-term (daily for at least 6 months) NSAID therapy, whereas patients who had been on short-term NSAID therapy or aspirin had a prevalence of 6.3% of nonspecific ulceration.[41] These changes of nonspecific ulceration may develop anywhere in the small intestine, but the ileum is involved in the majority of patients.

In some patients, changes similar to Crohn's disease have been described,[42] and NSAIDs activate inflammatory bowel disease.[43] In other patients, NSAIDs produce a characteristic pathologic appearance of multiple concentric, circumferential, diaphragm-like strictures that can progress to marked lumenal stenosis.[44] Many of these patients present with symptoms of intermittent intestinal obstruction. Characteristically, the diaphragm-like lesions are a focus of submucosal fibrosis, and the adjacent muscularis mucosa is broken up and merges with the underlying fibrosis.

Most patients taking NSAIDs who require a barium ex-

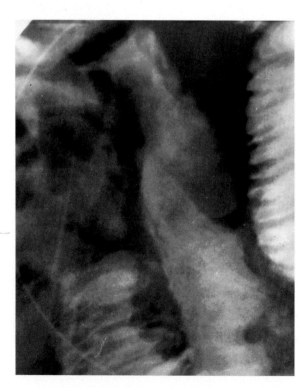

Fig. 31-17 Cogan's syndrome. A spot view of the terminal ileum from the case reported by Thomas[39] shows that the normal mucosal pattern has been replaced by a featureless outline.

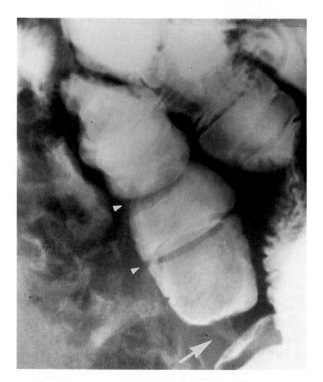

Fig. 31-18 NSAID enteritis. A short stricture *(arrow)* and the characteristic "diaphragm" *(arrowheads)* appearance shown in the terminal ileum on a spot compression view.

amination have suspected gastrointestinal blood loss or intermittent obstruction. On barium examination, changes in the terminal ileum similar to the appearances of Crohn's disease have been described.[45] Strictures may be seen, and it is possible to identify the characteristic diaphragm-like narrowing on barium examination, particularly when enteroclysis is used[46] (Fig. 31-18).

VASCULAR MALFORMATIONS

Vascular malformations may be congenital or acquired.[47] Arteriovenous malformations are mostly congenital in origin, and because it can be difficult to differentiate congenital vascular malformations from acquired angiomas, the term *angiomatous malformations* is suggested to include both types.

Angiomatous malformations are usually solitary and on angiography are shown as a meshwork of dilated vessels, often supplied by tortuous dilated arteries. Enlarged veins accompany these arteries, and venous filling may be rapid, with opacification in the arterial phase. Early venous filling and clearing may occur even when no other abnormality is detected.

Superselective angiography may be required to detect and pinpoint vascular malformations and hemangiomas.[48] This should be followed by intraoperative arteriography if there is doubt about the identification of the lesion at operation.[49] Hereditary hemorrhagic telangiectasia is characterized by multiple vascular malformations and involvement of multiple systems, including the skin and lips. It is transmitted by mendelian recessive inheritance. Mesenteric angiography shows multiple angiomatous malformations in the intestine.

Hemangiomas are tumorlike vascular lesions classified as capillary hemangiomas when the vascular channels are tightly packed and cavernous hemangiomas when they consist of larger vascular spaces.[50] They may be single or multiple and characteristically present with bleeding (Fig. 31-19).

INTESTINAL VARICES

Varices, which may develop in the small intestine in patients with portal hypertension, occasionally present with bleeding. These varices may be quite large and can be demonstrated on superior mesenteric angiography or by cathe-

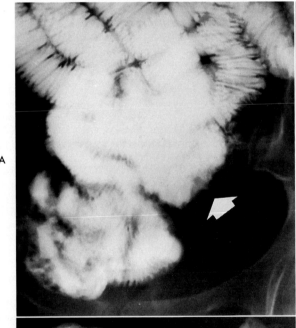

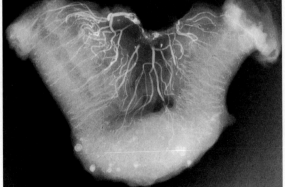

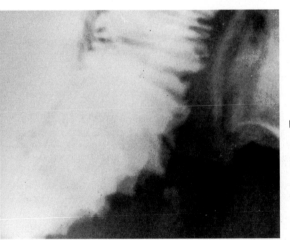

Fig. 31-19 Hemangioma shown on barium study. **A,** The wall of a short segment of the small intestine is distorted and irregular *(arrow).* **B,** Small phleboliths can be identified adjacent to the abnormal intestine. **C,** An angiogram of the resected specimen. The patient, a 26-year-old woman, presented with melena. Selective superior mesenteric angiography was the initial investigation and showed no abnormality or vascular pattern, but phleboliths were noted. After the barium examination the patient was operated on and the hemangioma resected.
Courtesy of Dr. Louise Shepherd, Kettering, England; From Nolan DJ: *Radiological atlas of gastrointestinal disease,* New York, 1983, John Wiley.

terizing the right ovarian vein via the inferior vena cava.[51] Intestinal varices may be seen on barium studies as submucosal serpiginous longitudinal filling defects.[52,53]

REFERENCES

1. Hildebrand HD, Zierler RE: Mesenteric vascular disease, *Am J Surg* 139:188, 1980.
2. Scholz FJ: Intestinal ischaemia, *Radiol Clin North Am* (in press).
3. Siegelman SS, Sprayregen S, Boley SJ: Angiographic diagnosis of mesenteric arterial vasoconstriction, *Radiology* 112:533, 1974.
4. Clark RA, Gallant TE: Acute mesenteric ischaemia: angiographic spectrum, *AJR* 142:555, 1984.
5. Nalbandian H, Sheth N, Dietrich R, Georgiou J: Intestinal ischaemia caused by cocaine ingestion: report of two cases, *Surgery* 97:374, 1985.
6. Freudenberger RS, Cappell MS, Hutt DA: Intestinal infarction after intravenous cocaine abuse, *Ann Intern Med* 113:715, 1990.
7. Abdu RA, Zakhour BJ, Dallis DJ: Mesenteric venous thrombosis 1911–1984, *Surgery* 101:383, 1987.
8. Grendell JH, Ockner RK: Mesenteric venous thrombosis, *Gastroenterology* 82:358, 1982.
9. Wilson C, Gupta R, Gilmour DC, Imrie CW: Acute superior mesenteric ischaemia, *Br J Surg* 74:279, 1987.
10. Clemett AR, Chang J: The radiological diagnosis of spontaneous mesenteric venous thrombosis, *Am J Gastroenterol* 63:209, 1975.
11. Kradjian RM: Ischaemic stenosis of small intestine, *Arch Surg* 91:829, 1965.
12. Raf LE: Ischaemic stenosis of small intestine, *Acta Chir Scand* 135:253, 1969.
13. Marks CG, Nolan DJ, Piris J, Webster CU: Small bowel strictures after blunt abdominal trauma, *Br J Surg* 66:663, 1979.
14. Khilnani MT, Marshak RH, Eliasoph J, Wolf BS: Intramural intestinal haemorrhage, *AJR* 92:1061, 1964.
15. Mendelson RM, Nolan DJ: The radiological features of chronic radiation enteritis, *Clin Radiol* 36:141, 1985.
16. Carr ND, Pullen BR, Hasleton PS, Schofield PF: Microvascular studies in human radiation bowel disease, *Gut* 25:448, 1984.
17. Galland RB, Spencer J: The natural history of clinically established radiation enteritis. In Galland RB, Spencer J, eds: *Radiation enteritis,* London, 1990, Edward Arnold.
18. Mason GR, Dietrich P, Friedland GW, Hanks GE: The radiological findings in radiation-induced enteritis and colitis. A review of 30 cases, *Clin Radiol* 21:232, 1970.
19. Halls JM: Radiation damage of the small intestine, *Clin Radiol* 16:173, 1965.
20. Fishman EK, Zinreich ES, Jones B, Siegelman SS: Computed tomographic diagnosis of radiation ileitis, *Gastrointest Radiol* 9:149, 1984.
21. Bluestone R, MacMahon M, Dawson JM: Systemic sclerosis and small bowel involvement, *Gut* 10:183, 1969.
22. Rohrmann CA Jr, Ricci MT, Krishnamurthy S, Schuffler MD: Radiologic and histologic differentiation of neuromuscular disorders of the gastrointestinal tract, visceral myopathies, visceral neuropathies, and progressive systemic sclerosis, *AJR* 143:933, 1984.
23. Horowitz AL, Meyers MA: The "hide-bound" small bowel of scleroderma: characteristic mucosal fold pattern, *AJR* 119:332, 1973.
24. Handel J, Schwartz S: Gastrointestinal manifestations of the Schönlein-Henoch syndrome, *AJR* 78:643, 1957.
25. Craig RDP: Multiple perforations of the small intestine in polyarteritis nodosa, *Gastroenterology* 44:355, 1963.
26. Marshak RH, Lindner AE: *Radiology of the small intestine,* ed 2. Philadelphia, 1976, WB Saunders.
27. Rosenberger A, Adler OB, Haim S: Radiological aspects of Behçet disease, *Radiology* 144:261, 1982.
28. Kuehne SE, Gauvin GP, Shortsleeve MJ: Small bowel stricture caused by rheumatoid vasculitis, *Radiology* 184:215, 1992.
29. Bienenstock H, Minick CR, Rogoff B: Mesenteric arteritis and intestinal infarction in rheumatoid arthritis, *Arch Intern Med* 119:359, 1967.
30. Beighton PH, Murdoch JL, Votteler T: Gastrointestinal complications of Ehlers-Danlos syndrome, *Gut* 10:1004, 1969.
31. Aldridge RT: Ehlers-Danlos syndrome causing intestinal obstruction, *Br J Surg* 54:22, 1967.
32. Herrington JL Jr, Grossman LA: Surgical lesions of the small and large intestine resulting from Buerger's disease, *Ann Surg* 168:1079, 1968.
33. Morson BC, Dawson IMP: *Gastrointestinal pathology,* ed 2, Oxford, 1979, Blackwell Scientific.
34. Shapeero LG, Myers A, Oberkircher PE, Miller WT: Acute reversible lupus vasculitis of the gastrointestinal tract, *Radiology* 112:569, 1974.
35. Bruce J, Sircus W: Disseminated lupus erythematosus of the alimentary tract, *Lancet* 1:795, 1959.
36. Train JS, Hertz I, Cohen BA, Samach M: Lupus vasculitis: reversal of radiographic findings after steroid therapy, *Am J Gastroenterol* 76:460, 1981.
37. Finkbiner RB, Dekker JP: Ulceration and perforation of the intestine due to necrotizing arteritis, *N Engl J Med* 268:14, 1963.
38. Cogan DG: Syndrome of nonsyphilitic interstitial keratitis and vestibuloauditory symptoms, *Arch Ophthalmol* 33:145, 1945.
39. Thomas HG: Case report: clinical and radiological features of Cogan's syndrome—nonsyphilitic interstitial keratitis, audiovestibular symptoms and systemic manifestations, *Clin Radiol* 45:418, 1992.
40. Reza MJ, Roth BE, Pops MA, Goldberg L: Intestinal vasculitis in essential mixed cryoglobulinemia, *Ann Intern Med* 81:632, 1974.
41. Allison MC, Allan G, Howatson MB, Torrance CJ, Lee FD, Russell RI: Gastrointestinal damage associated with the use of nonsteroidal antiinflammatory drugs, *N Engl J Med* 327:749, 1992.
42. Banerjee AK: Enteropathy induced by nonsteroidal antiinflammatory drugs, *Br Med J* 298:1539, 1989.
43. Kaufmann HJ, Taubin HL: Nonsteroidal antiinflammatory drugs activate quiescent inflammatory bowel disease, *Ann Intern Med* 107:513, 1987.
44. Lang J, Price AB, Levi AJ, Burke M, Gumpel JM et al: Diaphragm disease: pathology of disease of the small intestine induced by nonsteroidal antiinflammatory drugs, *J Clin Pathol* 41:516, 1988.
45. Saverymuttu SH, Thomas A, Grundy A, Maxwell JD: Ileal stricturing after long-term indomethacin treatment, *Postgrad Med J* 62:967, 1986.
46. Levi S, de Lacey G, Price AB, Gumpel MJ, Levi AJ et al: "Diaphragm-like" strictures of the small bowel in patients treated with nonsteroidal antiinflammatory drugs, *Br J Radiol* 63:186, 1990.
47. Fataar S, Morton P, Schulman: Arteriovenous malformations of the gastrointestinal tract, *Clin Radiol* 32:623, 1981.
48. Allison DJ, Hemingway AP, Cunningham DA: Angiography in gastrointestinal bleeding, *Lancet* 2:30, 1982.
49. Athanasoulis CA, Moncure AC, Greenfield AJ, et al: Intraoperative localisation of small bowel bleeding sites with combined use of angiographic methods and methylene blue injection, *Surgery* 87:77, 1980.
50. Nolan DJ, Herlinger H: Vascular lesions of the small bowel. In Gore RM, Levine MS, Laufer I, eds: *Textbook of gastrointestinal radiology,* Philadelphia, WB Saunders (in press).
51. Gray RK, Grollman JH Jr: Acute lower gastrointestinal bleeding secondary to varices of the superior mesenteric venous system, *Radiology* 111:559, 1974.
52. Fleming RJ, Seaman WB: Roentgenographic demonstration of unusual extra-esophageal varices, *AJR* 103:281, 1968.
53. Agarwal D, Scholz FJ: Small-bowel varices demonstrated by enteroclysis, *Radiology* 140:350, 1981.

32 *Malabsorption, Immunodeficiency, and Miscellaneous Disorders of the Small Bowel*

MAX RYAN
JAMES CARR

The importance of radiology in the diagnosis of the causes of malabsorption has declined with the advent of endoscopic methods for obtaining duodenal, jejunal, and ileal biopsy material, as these, together with stool and duodenal aspirate analysis, can often yield findings that establish a diagnosis. However, this is not always the case.[1] Many patients are still sent for a small bowel study early in their investigation, as it is considered a benign procedure and one that is often helpful in evaluating the results of treatment. For all these reasons, it is important to be familiar with the techniques, findings, and pitfalls of the radiology of the small bowel.

Malabsorption is the most common clinical presentation of most of the functional disorders of the small bowel. Its causes are myriad and, indeed, practically all of the conditions considered in this chapter can either present with symptoms of malabsorption, show some of its features radiologically, or both.[2] Although a specific radiologic diagnosis is often impossible, and can be achieved only in combination with biopsy and biochemical findings,[1] a useful differential list can often be generated, and occasionally a specific diagnosis can be made.

Moreover, endoscopy and biopsy cannot disclose anatomic abnormalities of the small bowel, such as fistulas or diverticula. These abnormalities may be nonspecific, and, in diseases such as lymphoma, lymphangiectasia, eosinophilic enteritis, mastocytosis, amyloidosis, and Crohn's disease, which typically exhibit a patchy distribution, the lesions may be missed.[1] Clinical and biochemical information must be available to the radiologist so that a clinically helpful and appropriate differential diagnostic list can be generated. The role of the radiologist is to conduct the most appropriate examination for the specific problem, produce outstanding images, analyze the various radiologic abnormalities, and finally attempt to correlate these with the many clinical conditions with which they may be associated.

The barium small bowel examination can be carried out using either the small bowel meal method or enteroclysis.[3] The conventional follow-through method, combined with a barium meal, is not recommended by some authors,[4,6] but is considered acceptable by others, if carried out in a dedicated manner.[3] A specifically tailored small bowel meal examination can be an excellent investigation.[4] Recommended concentrations of barium vary.[4,6] The administration of 500 ml of more dilute (25% weight per volume [w/v]) barium, supervised by the radiologist with screening and spot radiographs obtained using compression, is a satisfactory method in our experience. This technique has some limitations due to the presence of overlapping bowel loops, and, although malabsorption patterns are adequately shown, short strictures and tumors may be missed. To achieve a reasonably quick examination, the stomach should not be allowed to empty until the terminal ileum has been reached, and the administration of additional barium is usually required for this.[7] Whichever technique is used, it should be done in a meticulous manner and tailored to the clinical problem. If the follow-through meal proves technically unsuccessful, or if a specific disease process such as lymphoma complicating celiac disease is suspected, enteroclysis is indicated.

Enteroclysis, in which a peroral catheter is positioned beyond the duodenojejunal flexure and a dilute barium suspension (19% w/v) infused, is the more definitive investigation.[3,8] However, enteroclysis is invasive and requires good cooperation between the patient and operator. Sedation may be used, but, even so, some patients have difficulty tolerating intubation, and the small bowel meal method may have to be used instead.

MAIN RADIOLOGIC FINDINGS IN FUNCTIONAL DISEASES OF THE SMALL BOWEL

The main radiologic abnormalities that may be encountered are:

- Dilatation
- Increased amount of intestinal fluid
- Changes in the valvulae conniventes
- Nodulation
- Motility changes
- Narrowing

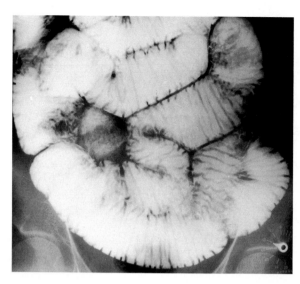

Fig. 32-1 Dilatation of the small bowel in a patient with celiac disease, the most common radiologic finding in this disease, although a nonspecific one. Note the squaring of the ends of the valvulae.

Dilatation

The caliber of the small intestine varies depending on the method of examination used. With enteroclysis, a diameter greater than 4.5 cm in the upper jejunum, 4 cm in the mid small bowel, and 3 cm in the ileum is considered abnormal. On a follow-through examination, the jejunal caliber should not exceed 3.5 cm, nor the ileal caliber 3 cm.[9] Dilatation in the presence of disease may be segmental or uniform and is the dominant radiologic feature in patients with gluten-induced enteropathy, scleroderma, and severe chronic pancreatic enzyme deficiency, as well as in patients taking various drugs—mainly narcotics and anticholinergics (Fig. 32-1).

Valvulae conniventes

The valvulae conniventes are considered to be thickened when they measure more than 2 mm.[9] The folds may be either uniformly swollen or distorted and nodular. Uniform thickening is seen in the presence of intestinal edema resulting from various causes, as well as in intestinal lymphangiectasia (Fig. 32-2). It also occurs in inflammations such as giardiasis and in infiltrations like amyloidosis. Irregular, distorted, and nodular thickening of the folds is seen in Whipple's disease, eosinophilic gastroenteritis, Crohn's disease, and lymphoma. Other conditions, such as giardiasis and Zollinger-Ellison syndrome, can exhibit a mixture of uniform swelling and distorted nodular thickening (Fig. 32-3).

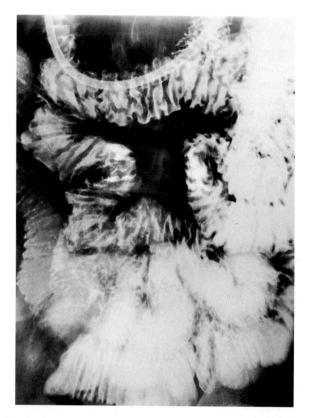

Fig. 32-2 Primary lymphangiectasia in a 21-year-old man with developmental anomalies. There is uniform swelling of the mucosal folds with dilution in the lower jejunal loops due to excessive secretions.
Courtesy of Dr. David Lintott.

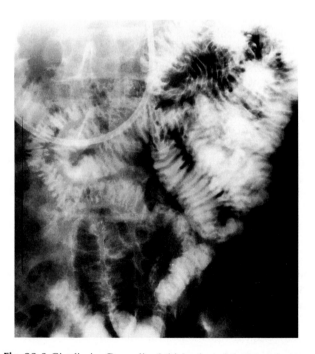

Fig. 32-3 Giardiasis. Generalized thickening of the jejunal mucosal folds with some dilution in the midjejunum due to the increased secretions. Intermittent spasm was also noted.
Courtesy of Dr. Dan Nolan.

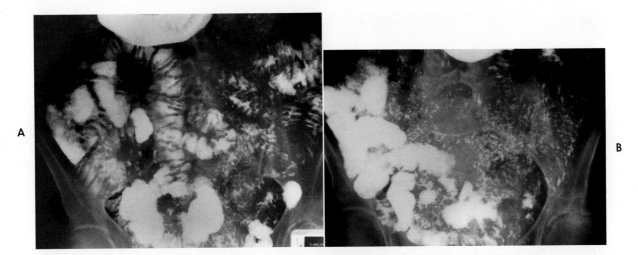

Fig. 32-4 Giardiasis. Thickening and distortion of the jejunal mucosal folds with some fragmentation of the barium. **A,** There was rapid transit through the jejunum due to the spasm and irritability. **B,** A half hour later, the ileum is reached but appears normal. Note the breakup of the residual barium in the jejunum caused by excess secretions.

Increased intestinal fluid

The so-called wet bowel is due to either diminished absorption of water, as in gluten-induced enteropathy with severe hypoalbuminemia, or increased secretions, as in hypoglobulinemia, lymphangiectasia/protein-losing enteropathy, giardiasis (Fig. 32-4), Zollinger-Ellison syndrome, and sometimes eosinophilic gastroenteritis.

Nodulation

Diffuse, punctate, sandlike nodulation is found in the presence of nodular lymphoid hyperplasia, which may be associated with hypogammaglobulinemia and lymphoma.[6] In Whipple's disease, it is more commonly seen in association with deformed valvulae conniventes. Sandlike nodulation may also occur in the presence of lymphangiectasia, Waldenstrom's macroglobulinemia, and mastocytosis. In Peutz-Jeghers syndrome and metastases, the nodules are usually larger and vary in size.

Motility changes

Increased or diminished transit time through the small intestine is difficult to evaluate because of the inherent variation in normals. The normal time for barium to travel through the small bowel to the cecum can range from 1 to 2 hours. If the stomach is allowed to empty and is not refilled, on occasion it may take several hours for the barium to reach the cecum in normal individuals. Rapid transit time, so-called *intestinal hurry,* may be seen in hyperkinetic states from any cause and is a typical feature in carcinoid syndrome and graft-versus-host disease. Delayed passage of barium is seen in patients with hypothyroidism; in association with certain drug therapies, especially tricy-

clic antidepressants[10] (clonidine); and in mural diseases such as scleroderma[11] and hollow visceral myopathy[12] (intestinal pseudoobstruction) (Fig. 32-5).

Narrowing

Strictures can arise in any malignancy and in inflammatory bowel disease and infections, as well as in ischemia and radiation enteritis. Focal or generalized narrowing is also seen in severe celiac disease (Fig. 32-6) milk and soybean sensitivity, graft-versus-host disease, and strongyloidiasis.

PRIMARY SMALL INTESTINAL DISEASE

The term *malabsorption* refers to a defect in the absorption of the main ingredients of food, that is, fat, proteins, and carbohydrates, from the small intestine.[2] This gives rise to the malabsorption syndrome, which is characterized by steatorrhea (the passage of bulky, fatty, and foul-smelling stools), weight loss, abdominal distention, skin pigmentation, and retarded growth and development. Malabsorption also produces deficiencies of other nutrients, such as folic acid, vitamin B_{12}, and B complex vitamins, vitamin K, iron, calcium, and magnesium. Osteomalacia is a late complication.

Celiac disease, herpetiform dermatitis, other protein-induced enteropathies, refractory celiac, unclassified celiac, and tropical sprue show similar histologic changes. The findings from transoral biopsy are invariably positive and allow differentiation into those diseases that produce a flat mucosa with an avillous appearance, and those that exhibit a variably patchy appearance. Each of these, in turn, may be divided into those with a nonspecific histologic appear-

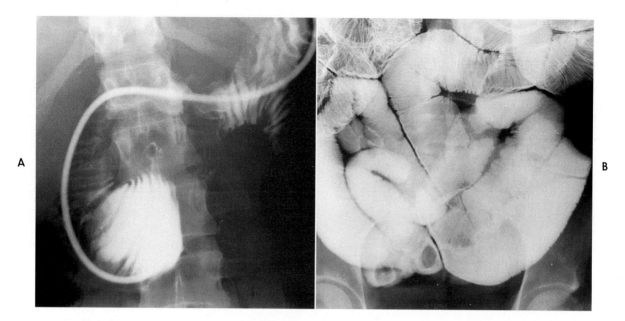

Fig. 32-5 Dilatation of the second part of the duodenum (**A**) noted during intubation for small bowel enema in a patient with scleroderma. Generalized dilatation of the small bowel was present with hypomotility (**B**).

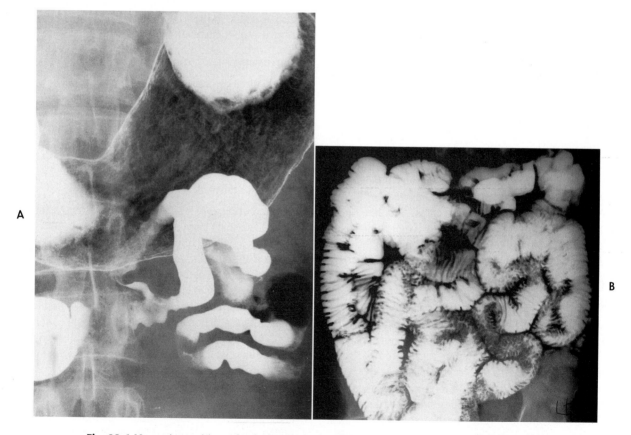

Fig. 32-6 Narrowing and loss of valvulae (**A**) in the jejunum of a patient with celiac disease who presented with heartburn. The jejunal abnormality was causing delayed gastric emptying. The follow-through (**B**) again shows the ileal appearance of the jejunum and the jejunal appearance of the ileal folds in the right lower quadrant, as well as dilatation and squaring of the ends of some of the valvulae.

ance and those with some features that permit a specific diagnosis.[13]

Celiac disease (gluten-induced enteropathy)

Celiac disease, also known as nontropical sprue and gluten-induced enteropathy, is the most common small bowel disease producing the malabsorption syndrome, with a high incidence in the populations of Ireland and Northern Europe. It is due to the sensitivity of the small intestine to alpha-gliadin, a component of gluten in certain grains. There is a familial susceptibility that has a genetic basis. There is also evidence suggesting the existence of an immune reaction in the intestinal mucosa.[14]

Clinical features

Celiac disease may present in childhood, but there is a second peak in the third and fourth decades. Although the classic presentation consists of steatorrhea and weight loss or failure to thrive, sometimes the disease is milder and the symptoms are related to one or more of the dietary deficiencies involved. The range of presentation is wide. It includes anemia (iron or folate deficiency), bleeding (vitamin K deficiency), mental changes (possibly due to folate deficiency), skin rashes, stomatitis, or an insidious general malaise that the patient does not realize exists until gluten is removed from the diet and they feel reborn. Osteomalacia with bone pain or fractures can be the presenting symptoms, as well as menstrual irregularities in women, impotence in men, and infertility in both.

Herpetiform dermatitis

Herpetiform dermatitis (Duhring's disease) is a skin disease that is closely associated with a celiac-like state. The enteritis is less severe than that in celiac disease, and the histologic lesion is often patchy. The disease is also complicated by lymphoma, and the skin lesions respond promptly with dapsone treatment and slowly with a strict gluten-free diet. The enteric aspect is usually subclinical, but steatorrhea occurs in 25% of the cases.[1]

Refractory celiac disease

Refractory celiac disease is seen in those patients with a diagnosed gluten-induced enteropathy who experience either only partial relief of their symptoms on a gluten-free diet, or recurrence of symptoms after a short period of improvement. Often no cause for their poor clinical response can be found, but some exhibit an additional hypersensitivity to other proteins.[13]

Unclassified celiac disease

Unclassified celiac disease is a rare type of malabsorption that neither responds to the withdrawal of gluten nor of other proteins from the diet. The cause is unknown.

Tropical sprue

The clinical and radiologic features of tropical sprue are similar to those of celiac disease but the etiology differs. Unlike celiac disease, tropical sprue is endemic in the tropics and there are occasional epidemics. Visitors to the tropics may acquire the disease, but it may not become manifest for months or even years after exposure. The cause is uncertain, but the bacterial flora of the bowel is disturbed, suggesting an infectious cause, and treatment with tetracycline and folic acid is effective, although not necessarily quick. It may take a year or more before an affected individual is completely cured. Multiple biopsy specimens show the lesion to be variable in severity, and unlike celiac disease, the proximal bowel is not the most severely affected.

RADIOLOGY OF CELIAC DISEASE

The changes typical of celiac disease depicted by barium examination are dilatation, hypersecretion, and alterations in the valvulae conniventes.[15] Approximately 10% of patients show no radiologic abnormality.

Dilatation

Dilatation of the small bowel is the most important sign and invariably affects the mid and distal jejunum (Fig. 32-7). It is practically always present in celiac disease and tropical sprue. The other main conditions causing nonobstructive dilatation are scleroderma and the ingestion of certain drugs.

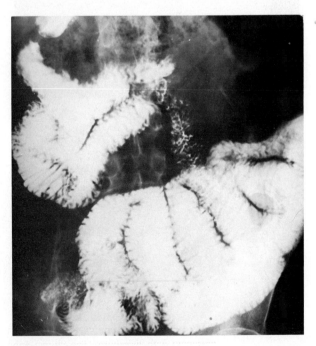

Fig. 32-7 Sprue. There is moderate dilatation of the proximal jejunum. The intestinal loops are pliable and flaccid.

The valvulae conniventes

In celiac disease the valvulae conniventes may exhibit five types of appearance: normal, squared ends, jejunoileal distribution reversed, absence, and thickening, listed in order of frequency. In most patients the valvulae look normal individually, but often the ends at the margin are squared off rather than rounded, probably due to the dilatation (Fig. 32-1). In all but the mildest disease, there are more folds than usual in the ileum and fewer in the jejunum. This reversal of distribution is a striking and common feature (Fig. 32-8).[16,17] Herlinger[18] found that the folds are best assessed by enteroclysis and are usually reduced in number. He suggested that adult celiac disease may be diagnosed if there are less than three folds per 2.5 cm in the distended proximal jejunum on enteroclysis examinations (Fig. 32-9). In the jejunum, loss of the jejunal folds produces colonlike haustrations, "colonization of the jejunum."[17] This may progress to the so-called moulage sign, described later, with complete absence of valvulae in the duodenum and jejunum[18] (see Figs. 32-6 and 32-10).

Finally, in those few patients with severe disease and hypoproteinemia, the valvulae may be thickened.[15]

Hypersecretion

Hypersecretion, or excessive fluid in the intestinal loops, is more likely due to a defect in the absorption of water by the diseased mucosa than to osmosis of fluid into the lumen. In the presence of hypersecretion, the barium appears diluted and may assume a granular appearance. Rarely, the fatty nature of the intestinal contents may allow malabsorption to be suspected on computed tomographic (CT) scans (Fig. 32-11).

Flocculation

Flocculation may occur and represents the precipitation of irregular clumps of barium mixed with intestinal secretions within dilated loops. As an isolated sign (i.e., without dilatation), it is not a reliable finding, and, with adequate amounts of modern barium preparations, it is very rarely seen. The faint irregular stippling of residual barium, normally seen in the small intestine, may be exaggerated,

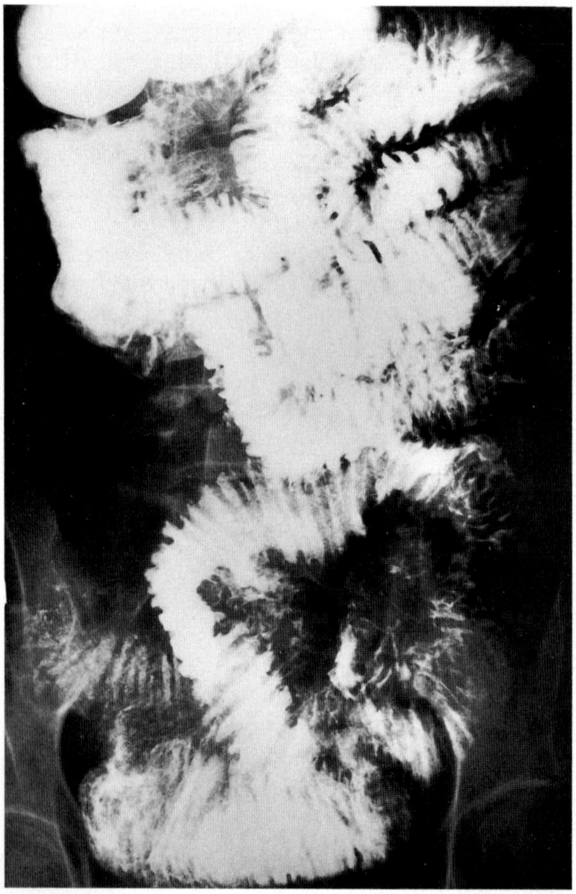

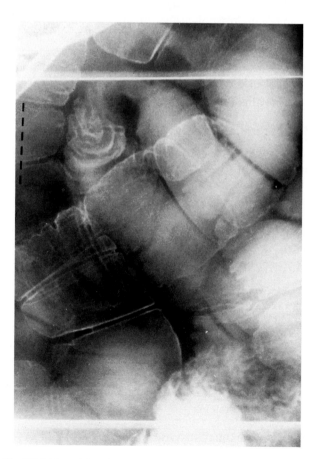

Fig. 32-8 Celiac disease. There is moderate dilatation of the jejunal loops with thickening of the valvulae conniventes. Some segmentation is seen, with dilution in the ileum and a "jejunal pattern" in the pelvis and right iliac fossa.

Fig. 32-9 Enteroclysis in adult patient with coeliac disease in the distended proximal jejunum. The folds are widely separated, with only two folds crossed by lines representing a distance of 25 mm. Courtesy of Dr. Hans Herlinger; from *Clin Radiol* 45:73, 1992.

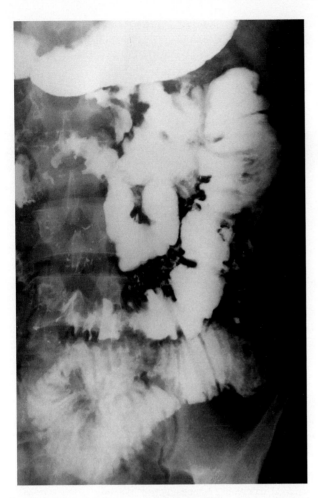

Fig. 32-10 Advanced case of untreated coeliac disease. There is absence of the jejunal pattern, which has been replaced by a featureless proximal jejunum—the moulage sign. There is dilution of the barium in the pelvic loops, where there is a jejunal pattern.

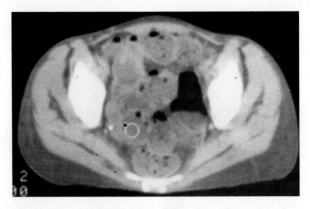

Fig. 32-11 CT scan in a patient with celiac disease who did not respond to a gluten-free diet. It was eventually discovered that she was receiving communion with a gluten-containing wafer twice a week while in the hospital. The CT scan shows the fatty content of the intestine, with a Hounsfield number of −32.

imparting a coarse appearance called *scattering* or *segmentation* (Fig. 32-8).

The moulage sign

The moulage sign (which is French in origin and means "cast" or "mould") is seen in advanced cases of celiac disease in which there is complete absence of valvulae, and there is otherwise a featureless appearance (see Figs. 32-6, *A*, and 32-10). The bowel may be dilated, but often there is some narrowing in these severe cases. It is an uncommon sign.

Intussusception

Transient enteroenteric intussusception is frequently seen, especially in the jejunum. This may be preceded by mural notches or filling defects due to intermittent coalescence of the walls[19] (Fig. 32-12).

COMPLICATIONS OF CELIAC DISEASE
Lymphoma

The main complications of celiac disease are the late development of intestinal or mesenteric lymphoma, now classified as malignant histocytosis, and carcinoma, especially in the small bowel and less frequently in the esophagus.[20] Because of this, regular follow-up of affected patients is advisable. If there is any alteration in the clinical condition, particularly the development of pyrexia, melena, or relapse while still on a gluten-free diet, enteroclysis should be performed, followed if necessary by ultrasonography and CT. Enteroclysis may reveal either mucosal irregularity with mural swelling or a local segment of narrowing with ulceration (Fig. 32-13). On CT an irregular soft tissue mass with nodular thickening of the intestinal wall and enlarged mesenteric nodes may be seen. Imaging is essential when pursuing a possible diagnosis of a complicating lymphoma, as it may be missed by biopsy.

Chronic ulcerative jejunoileitis

Ulcerative jejunoileitis is a rare nongranulomatous disease that may also cause malabsorption.[5] It now appears to be considered a rare complication of gluten-sensitive enteropathy, and not a distinct disease. It is not clear whether it represents a transition phase between celiac disease and lymphoma. Biopsy specimens show a variety of features, including malignant T cells. It affects the proximal jejunum and extends distally, and rarely affects the colon or stomach.

The radiologic findings encountered in a barium study are irregular luminal narrowing alternating with relatively dilated areas[21,22] (Fig. 32-14). There is no overall dilatation, as seen in celiac disease. Ulcers are rarely detected. There is a pathologic thickening of the bowel wall, which would probably be obvious on ultrasound or CT studies.

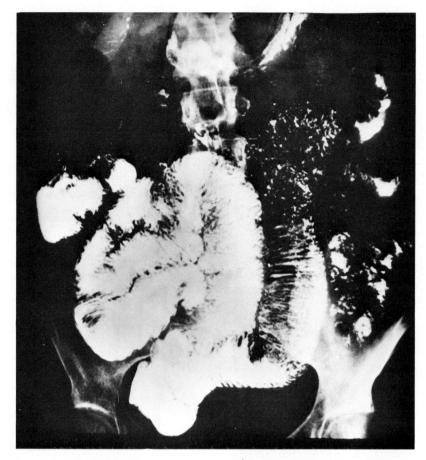

Fig. 32-12 Sprue. There is moderate dilatation of the entire jejunum, along with thinning of the valvulae conniventes, minimal fragmentation, and increased secretions. Nonobstructive intussusception is noted in the distal jejunum.

The prognosis is uncertain, both because of the rarity of the condition and because its nature has only recently been clarified.[23]

Collagenous sprue

Collagenous sprue is a rare disease that carries a poor prognosis. It is considered to be a complication rather than a variant of celiac disease. It is refractory to dietary control measures, and the diagnosis is established by small bowel biopsy, which show abnormal collagen deposition.[24]

COW'S MILK PROTEIN AND SOY PROTEIN ALLERGY

Enterocolitis in infancy due to cow's milk protein allergy or soy protein allergy is a well-recognized entity and is a common cause of malabsorption or inflammatory bowel disease in the first year of life. These children are usually diagnosed on the basis of the clinical history, but they often have a flat duodenal mucosa that is indistinguishable from that of celiac disease[25] and also have visible inflammatory changes on sigmoidoscopy. The ra-

diologic changes include duodenal and jejunal fold thickening, loss of valvulae with a moulage appearance in the mid and distal small bowel, and signs of a proctocolitis[26] (Figs. 32-15 and 32-16).

INTESTINAL LYMPHANGIECTASIA

Intestinal lymphangiectasia[27] may be congenital (rare) or acquired due to obstruction of lymphatics caused by an abdominal malignancy, chronic infection, retroperitoneal fibrosis, trauma, constrictive pericarditis, or irradiation. The congenital type is due to malformation of the lymphatics, often affecting many areas of the body. It may present at any time from birth to adulthood, often with asymmetric edema of an extremity or with more diffuse edema resulting from hypoproteinemia.[28] The acquired type arises later in life and often in conjunction with manifestations of the causative disease.[29] In both forms there is a loss of serum proteins stemming from the gross dilatation and rupture of the lymphatics of the lamina propria into the small intestine (protein-losing enteropathy). There is hypoglobulinemia mainly affecting the immunoglobulin G (IgG) level, which is associated with low levels of serum

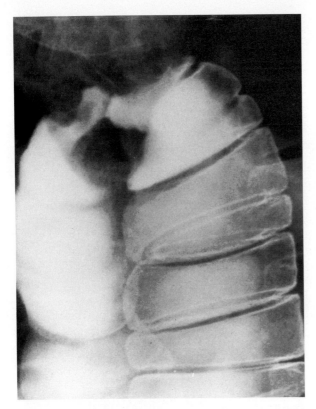

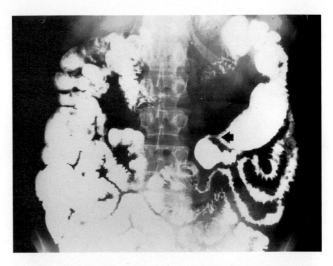

Fig. 32-14 Resected specimen shows ulcerative jejunitis. No granulomata, lymphomatous infiltration, or villous atrophy are seen. At autopsy, a year later, a mild villous atrophy was seen in the small intestine, and multifocal areas of colonic mucosal ulceration were evident. A diagnosis of celiac disease with subtotal villous atrophy had been made 20 years previously.

Fig. 32-13 An 81-year-old man with prolonged diarrhea and weight loss who did not respond to a gluten-free diet. Small bowel enema confirmed the diagnosis of celiac disease and demonstrated three short ulcerated segments with annular constriction. The most proximal jejunal lesion is illustrated here. Histologic studies showed diffuse areas of non-Hodgkin's lymphoma of B cell origin.
Courtesy of Dr. Hans Herlinger; from *Clin Radiol* 45:73, 1992.

albumin and to a lesser extent the levels of other proteins. As a result, there is peripheral and small intestine edema that causes diarrhea and steatorrhea. Chylous ascites may result from blockage of the serosal and mesenteric lymphatics, and pleural effusions from involvement of the thoracic duct.

The findings on barium studies consist of generalized thickening of the valvulae conniventes, similar to that encountered in small bowel edema resulting from other causes[30] (Fig. 32-17). The swelling of the mucosal folds is more extensive and uniform throughout the small intestine, sometimes imparting a "stacked coin" appearance.[18] Features associated with excessive secretions may also be seen, including flocculation and fragmentation, and this may obscure the fine nodules because of the presence of engorged villi, which may sometimes be seen. The findings may simulate gluten-induced enteropathy, but dilatation is minimal or absent.

The finding of increased fecal radioactivity after the intravenous injection of radioactive protein, usually chromium chloride, may help establish the diagnosis.[27] More recently, measurement of the alpha-antitrypsin level in the stools has been shown to be a good marker for protein-losing enteropathy without the need for radioactive labeling.[2]

Ultrasound and CT should be performed if secondary lymphangiectasia is suspected. Lymphangiography may show obstruction or hypoplasia of lymphatic channels, indicating that the congenital variety is a form of systemic lymphatic dysplasia.[17] The findings yielded by jejunal biopsy specimens that include the submucosa can confirm the presence of lymphangiectasia.

ABETALIPOPROTEINEMIA

Abetalipoproteinemia is a rare autosomal recessive disorder. The intestinal cells lack apoprotein B, and this interferes with fat absorption. The villi appear normal on biopsy specimens of the small intestine, but the absorptive epithelial cells are engorged with fat[31] and the red cells are abnormal and spiny.[2]

Clinically there is malabsorption in early life, suggesting the presence of celiac disease. The full syndrome, which develops by the time of adolescence, is the result of malabsorption of fat-soluble vitamins and consists of a progressive neurologic disorder in which there is retinopathy (retinitis pigmentosa) and spinocerebellar degeneration. These complications can be prevented by administering large doses of vitamin E. The radiologic picture is one of malabsorption.

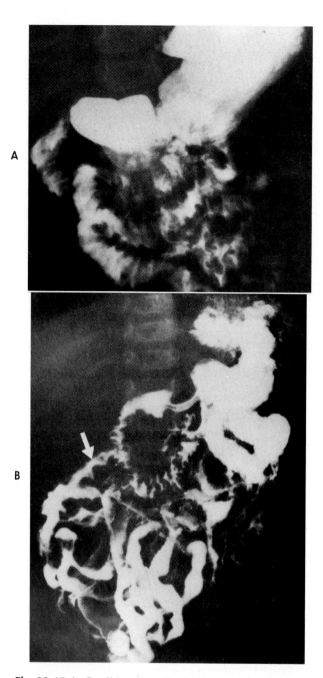

A

B

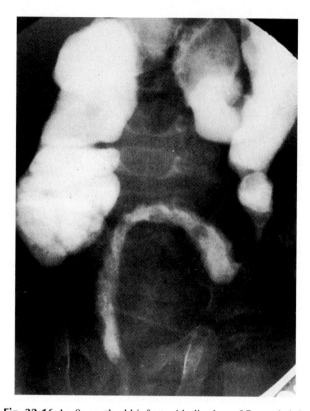

Fig. 32-15 A, Small bowel study obtained in an 8-month-old infant with generalized edema and diarrhea of 6 weeks' duration, showing thickening of the duodenal and jejunal valvulae with excess fluid. Replacement of cow's milk with soy formula led to rapid recovery. **B,** A 10-week-old infant with diarrhea of 2 weeks' duration that started when breast feeding was replaced with cow's milk. Deterioration continued after a switch to soy formula. Barium study shows thick valvulae in the jejunum, a ribbonlike ileum, and colonic thumb printing *(arrow).* Recovery occurred with parenteral nutrition and was maintained when goat's milk was substituted.
From Richards DG: *Radiology* 167:721, 1988.

Fig. 32-16 An 8-month-old infant with diarrhea of 7 months' duration, which had started as soon as cow's milk supplementation was introduced. Rectal ulceration was found by sigmoidoscopy, and water-soluble contrast enema shows a severe proctocolitis. Slow recovery occurred on an elemental hypoallergenic diet.
From Richards DG: *Radiology* 167:721, 1988.

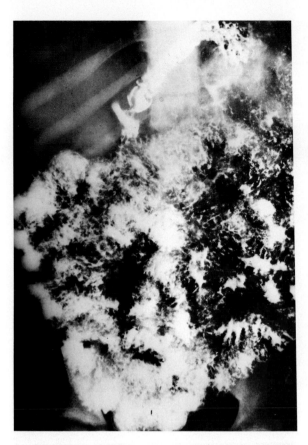

Fig. 32-17 Intestinal lymphangiectasia. The entire small bowel is involved. There is a moderate increase in secretions, with minimal segmentation, fragmentation, and diffuse thickening of the folds. There is no dilatation. The serum albumin level in this patient was 1 g/100 ml. Radiographic alterations result from the intestinal edema secondary to hypoproteinemia.

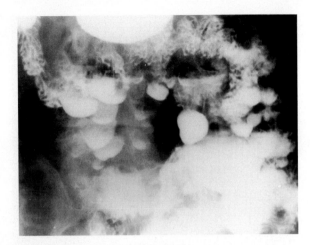

Fig. 32-18 Multiple jejunal diverticula demonstrated with the patient in the erect position. Such patients sometimes present with diarrhea due to bacterial overgrowth, causing malabsorption.

STASIS

A number of conditions can cause malabsorption as a result of stasis, because this permits bacterial overgrowth to take place. With an increase in the number of bacteria, the flora changes to one more characteristic of the cecum, consisting of *E. coli* and anaerobes. The bacteria compete with the host for the uptake of numerous nutrients, including vitamin B$_{12}$, thiamine, fat (and with fat also vitamins D, A, and E), and iron.

Conditions that may cause this include multiple diverticula (Fig. 32-18), blind loops, and chronic dilatation due to strictures, especially in Crohn's disease (Fig. 32-19). In addition, patients with scleroderma, amyloidosis, or hollow visceral myopathy may develop malabsorption on this basis. Scleroderma and amyloid are discussed later.

Hollow visceral myopathy (intestinal pseudoobstruction)

Primary idiopathic pseudoobstruction encompasses a variety of conditions that may present in childhood or adult life, or, in the more severe cases, in infancy. It includes neuropathies, the megacystis-microcolon-hypoperistalsis syndrome, and hollow visceral myopathy. The prognosis is poor when the disease presents in infancy, with only the rare child surviving to late childhood. In hollow visceral myopathy,[31] there is degeneration of the myenteric plexus in the longitudinal and circular layers without involvement of the nerves.

The condition may be familial, but random cases are found. In the familial variety the urinary system may be involved with dilatation of the renal pelvis and bladder due to the smooth muscle contraction in the bladder neck. The esophagus is usually affected, and detection of severely impaired esophageal peristalsis may be a helpful clue to the widespread nature of the problem. Aspiration and reflux esophagitis are common in affected infants as the result of gastric stasis.

In adults the conditions present with symptoms and signs of small intestine stasis but without evidence of obstruction, which must be excluded. Symptoms consist of pain and distention, early satiety, and diarrhea, with weight loss and malnutrition common. Barium studies show a marked delay in the passage of contrast through dilated fluid-filled small bowel loops, with poor or nonexistent peristalsis. Plain films often show distention and fluid levels (Fig. 32-20). In some children there is a modest response to cisapride treatment.

INFESTATIONS WITH MALABSORPTION PATTERNS
Giardiasis

Giardiasis[32,33] is found worldwide and is an important cause of travelers' diarrhea. It is most common in children. There is an infestation of the duodenum and proximal small intestine by a microscopic parasite, *Giardia lamblia*, which

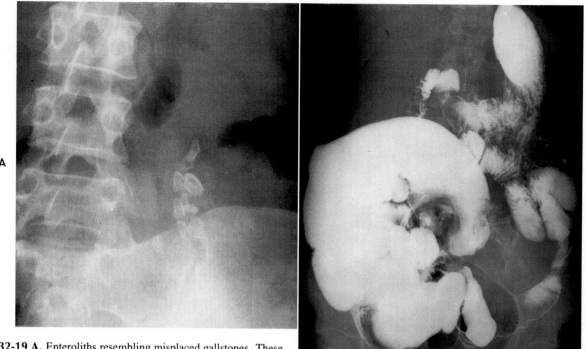

Fig. 32-19 A, Enteroliths resembling misplaced gallstones. These develop occasionally in a chronically obstructed bowel, as in this young woman with long-standing Crohn's disease and strictures **(B)** that have led to bacterial overgrowth and malabsorption.

is acquired by drinking unsanitary water. The illness is usually acute, and symptoms consist of abdominal pain, distention, and diarrhea with offensive foul-smelling yellow stools.[34] It may be prolonged and chronic and lead to malabsorption and growth retardation in children and severe weight loss in adults.

Radiologic examination of the small bowel shows hyperirritability, thickening of the valvulae conniventes, and hypersecretion (Fig. 32-21). Because of the spasm and irritability, barium transit through the jejunum is rapid, but the ileum appears normal (see Fig. 32-4). These are nonspecific changes, but a history of travel should raise suspicions and the organism is usually, although not always, found in the stools. Endoscopy and biopsy of the distal duodenum, as well as examination of duodenal washings, may be more fruitful. Giardiasis often affects patients with immunologic deficiency conditions and is frequently associated with immunoglobulin A (IgA) deficiency and lymphoma. In these instances the fine nodular changes typical of lymphoid hyperplasia may also be seen (Fig. 32-22).

Strongyloides stercoralis infection

Strongyloides stercoralis is found worldwide, particularly in warmer climates. It is discussed in more detail in Chapter 46. The disease may be either acute in onset or a serious chronic debilitating illness. The most common complaints are abdominal discomfort and pain, followed by

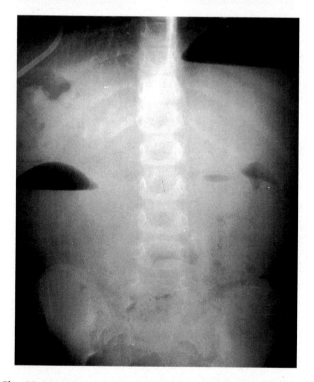

Fig. 32-20 A 5-year-old child with pseudoobstruction. She had delayed transit in the esophagus, stomach, small bowel, and colon. At this time the gastric emptying delay was causing the greatest problem, and the film shows the fluid levels in the gastric fundus and antrum. Cisapride had only a minimal effect in improving transit.

nausea, weight loss, vomiting, and diarrhea.[35] It is mentioned here because it can produce a spruelike syndrome in which there is malabsorption and flattened jejunal villi. It is a serious condition that may be fatal and can complicate any immunodeficiency state.

Barium studies may show dilatation or narrowing of the duodenum, with thickening or absence of the valvulae conniventes in the duodenum and proximal jejunum and delay in the passage of barium (Fig. 32-23; see also Fig. 46-58). In severe cases a rigid "pipe-stem" stenosis with irregular narrowing may be seen.[17] The disease may present in patients now living in a temperate climate, many years after the original infection was acquired in the tropics, often with an acute illness following years of poor health.

ENTEROPATHIC IMMUNOGLOBULIN DEFICIENCY STATES

The gastrointestinal (GI) tract may be affected by impairment of immune function resulting from any cause. Some of the conditions that affect GI function include cancer and its treatment, organ transplantation, chronic immunosuppressive drug therapy, congenital immunodeficiency syndromes, infections leading to immunodeficiency, old age, and a few other medical conditions such as diabetes, liver disease, and uremia.

The following are discussed in this section: (1) acquired immunodeficiency syndrome (AIDS) (see Chapter 47 for a fuller description); (2) graft-versus-host disease; and (3) the inherited immunodeficiency diseases with GI manifestations, particularly selective IgA deficiency, common variable hypoglobulinemia, and Bruton's X-linked hypogammaglobulinemia.

Patients with defective immune states may develop nonspecific GI symptoms such as diarrhea and malabsorption. These conditions may be primary or secondary to a known disease. Assigning diseases to this category is a somewhat arbitrary matter. For example, it may well be appropriate to place Mediterranean lymphoma in this category, and perhaps eventually Crohn's disease, as the links between infection, immunosuppression, and tumorogenesis become more clear.

Acquired immunodeficiency syndrome

Inflammatory changes similar to those found with giardiasis may also be induced by other small bowel infections and are mainly seen in opportunistic infections associated with AIDS, particularly cytomegalovirus, *Cryptosporidium,* and *Mycobacterium avium-intracellulare,* which are discussed in detail in Chapter 47. They are discussed briefly

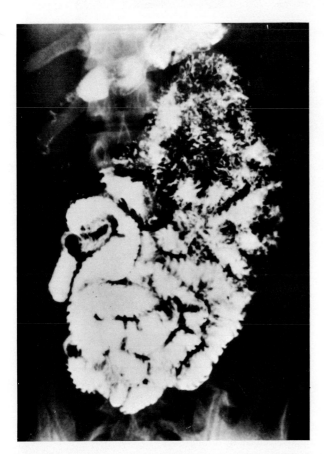

Fig. 32-21 Giardiasis. There is spasm and irritability of the jejunum associated with increased secretions and thickening of the valvulae conniventes. Findings are secondary to the inflammatory process. The distal ileum was normal.

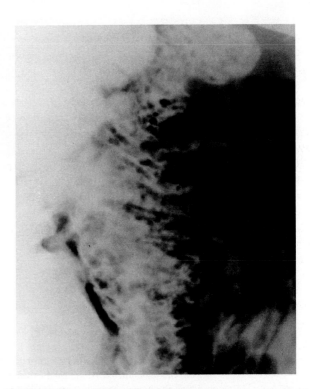

Fig. 32-22 Tiny nodules of lymphoid hyperplasia in a patient with hypogammaglobulinemia. Such nodules in the terminal ileum of a child or teenager are normal, but may be scattered throughout the small or large bowel in this condition.

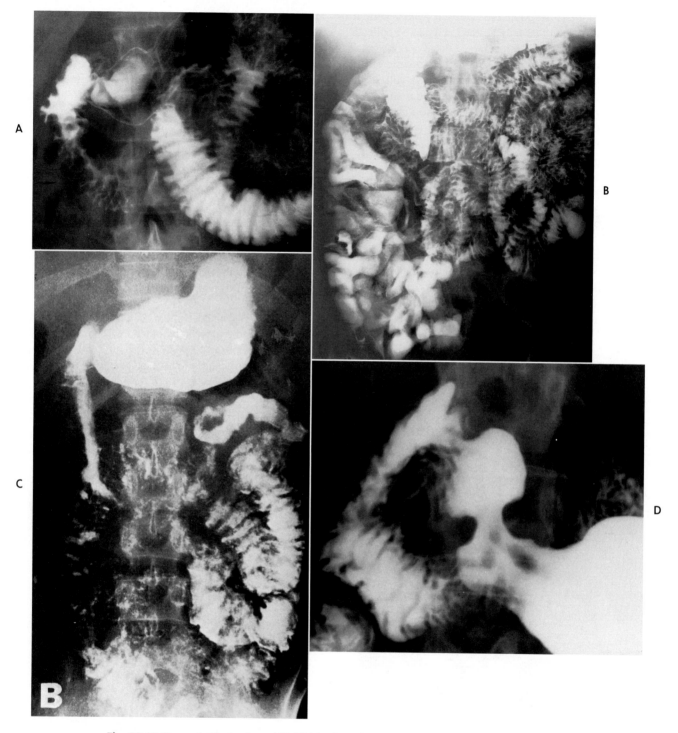

Fig. 32-23 Strongyloidiasis. **A,** and **B,** Thickening of the valvulae, spasm, and excess fluid in a patient from South America with weight loss, diarrhea, and abdominal pain. These signs can also be seen in giardiasis. **C,** More severe involvement of the duodenum and dilatation with thickened folds in the jejunum. **D,** An unusual example of gastric involvement by *Strongyloides stercoralis*, in which the biopsy findings were positive.
A and **B** courtesy of D. Nolan.

here, from the standpoint of their differentiation from other causes of malabsorption.

Malabsorption and diarrhea are common in human immunodeficiency virus (HIV) infections. Mucosal biopsy specimens from many of these patients show evidence of mucosal injury consisting of villous atrophy and mononuclear cell infiltrations infected with HIV.[36] A significant proportion of these patients also have *Cryptosporidium* and *Microsporidium* infections[37] (Fig. 32-24). Other organisms such as *Candida albicans* and *Strongyloides* can also cause diarrhea and malabsorption in immunocompromised patients.[38]

Kaposi's sarcoma and non-Hodgkin's lymphoma may also occur in the small intestine of AIDS patients and may not be distinguishable radiologically. In Kaposi's sarcoma[38] there may be blunting and thickening of the folds, as well as mural nodules that project into the lumen, thereby producing filling defects (Fig. 32-25). In lymphoma, there may be diffuse discrete thickening of the small intestinal folds with hypersecretion, and short ulcerated strictures resembling carcinoma may occur (Fig. 32-26). The thickened folds may become irregular, nodular, and coarse, with consequent thickening of the wall and separation of the loops (Fig. 32-27). In both types of malignancy there is a high

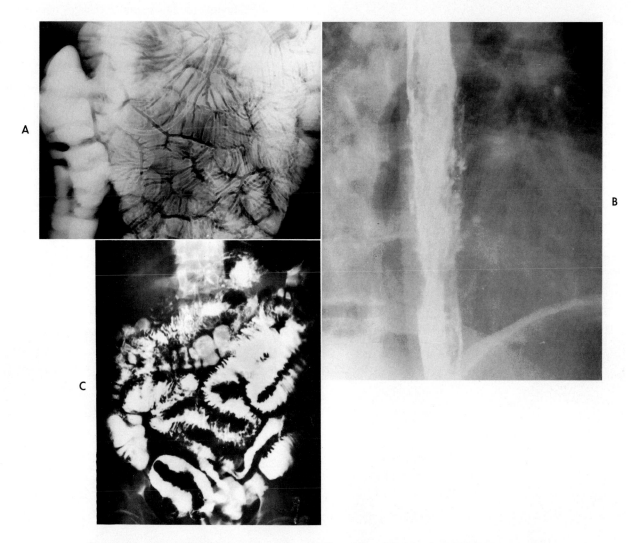

Fig. 32-24 A 26-year-old man with profuse diarrhea and weight loss. Colonoscopy had shown mild colitis with partial loss of the vessel pattern but no ulceration. The small bowel study **(A)** shows only mild fold thickening and haustral thickening. The swallow study **(B),** however, reveals a severe esophagitis, and the multiplicity of findings led to consideration of HIV infection. *Cryptosporidium* infection was confirmed but may not have been the only infecting agent. **C,** Cryptosporidiosis. Thickening of the folds of the jejunum and proximal ileum associated with increased secretions, spasm, and irritability, representing an inflammatory process. No discrete ulcerations are identified.
Courtesy of Dr. Emil Balthazar.

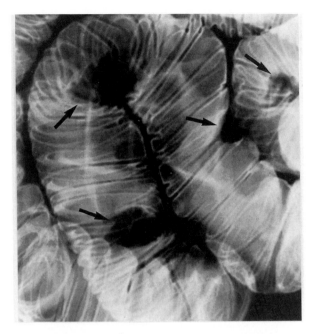

Fig. 32-25 Kaposi's sarcoma of the small bowel (shown by enteroclysis). Multiple submucosal nodules *(arrows)* with normal intervening jejunal mucosa.
Courtesy of Dr. Jacques Reeders.

incidence of retroperitoneal and mesenteric lymphadenopathy, and CT studies are helpful in assessing this. The diagnosis ultimately depends on the biopsy findings.

Mycobacterium involvement of the small bowel produces the clinical and histologic features of Whipple's disease and hence is sometimes called *pseudo-Whipple's disease*,[38,39] although this term is not universally accepted.[13,18] It causes irregular thickening of the valvulae conniventes in the proximal jejunum and occasionally nodulation. Ultrasound and CT may demonstrate enlargement of the peritoneal and mesenteric glands that is indistinguishable from the picture presented by AIDS-related Kaposi's sarcoma or lymphoma.[40]

Cytomegalovirus produces similar changes but also has a tendency to cause discrete ulcers (Fig. 32-28), which may become deep and perforate.

Graft-versus-host disease

Graft-versus-host disease may develop following allogenic bone marrow transplantation when there is an immunologic reaction to the donor lymphoid graft. The skin, liver, and GI tract of the host may be involved,[17,41] in conjunction with an overwhelming secretory diarrhea. The GI symptoms in a patient at risk, however, may be due to either graft-versus-host disease or to viral enteritis. Unfortunately, neither contrast studies nor CT examination can distinguish between these two entities.[42,43]

Radiologic examination of the alimentary tract shows the disease has three stages[41,44]:

1. In the acute phase, which often occurs 4 to 5 days after the onset of GI symptoms, there is simulta-

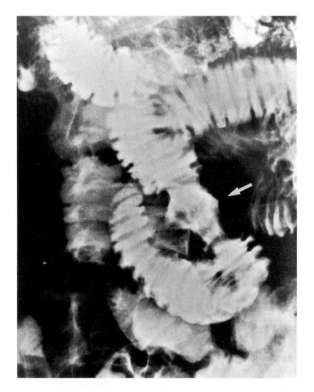

Fig. 32-26 AIDS-related lymphoma of the small bowel in which there is local scalloping of contour *(arrows)*.
Courtesy of Dr. Jacques Reeders.

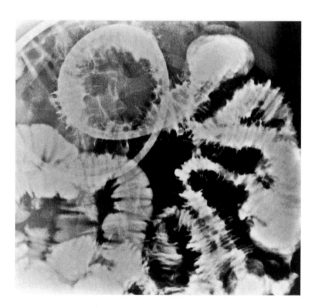

Fig. 32-27 AIDS-related B cell lymphoma of the proximal jejunum. There is irregular thickening of the folds and separation due to mesenteric infiltration.
Courtesy of Dr. Jacques Reeders.

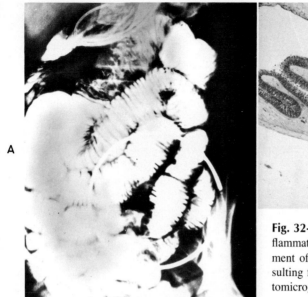

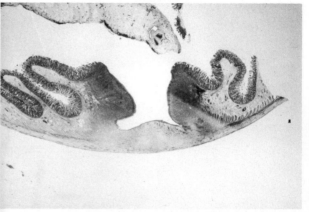

Fig. 32-28 A, Cytomegalovirus infection of the small bowel. Inflammatory changes consist of fold thickening, plus a short segment of narrowing caused by marked spasm and irritability, resulting from localized superficial ulceration. **B,** Low-power photomicrograph showing a small superficial ulceration.

neous and uniform thickening of the intestinal wall, rapid transit, and excess secretion. A ribbonlike narrowing of the lumen and thickening of the wall may be seen throughout most of the small intestine (Fig. 32-29).

2. In the subacute phase, which takes place 13 to 96 days after the onset of GI symptoms, radiologic studies show changes similar to those of the acute phase, often exhibiting a striking segmental distribution.

3. In the resolution phase, there is improvement with no abnormality or effacement of the mucosal folds but with mural thickening confined to the terminal ileum.

Plain film changes have also been described,[45] but do not establish the diagnosis, although the abdominal films are abnormal in 95% of the cases. The most alarming sign seen on plain films in patients with the disorder is pneumatosis coli.[46] The right colon is affected in most cases, and the radiologic appearance resembles that seen in patients with an infarcted bowel (Fig. 32-30). However, although intestinal disease contributed to the deaths of 7 of 18 patients with this sign in one series,[46] it can follow a benign course and may not even require colectomy. The radiologic findings of pneumatosis coli alert the clinician, but, whereas in many of these patients this indicates the need for immediate surgery, in patients who have received a bone marrow transplant the clinical state will also guide the approach to therapy. Even the development of retroperitoneal air is not an absolute indication for surgery. However, in the clinical context of systemic infection or shock, the finding of pneumatosis is a very poor prognostic sign.

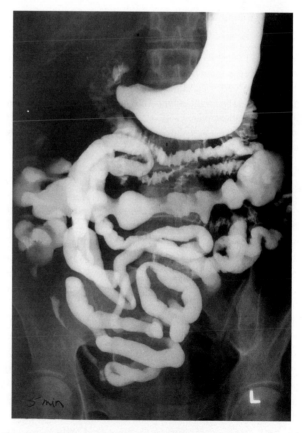

Fig. 32-29 Patient with severe diarrhea that developed 5 weeks after bone marrow transplantation. This is the 5 minute film, and contrast is already at the splenic flexure. The toothpaste-like appearance of the small bowel is characteristic of graft-versus-host disease, but the radiologic appearance does not permit differentiation from viral infection.

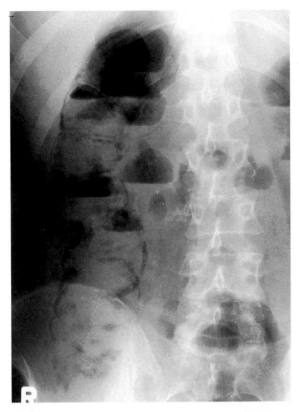

Fig. 32-30 Patient with diarrhea and mild abdominal pain that appeared 2 weeks after bone marrow transplantation, who did not appear to be very sick clinically. The plain film shows startling pneumatosis of the right colon. Although this is a worrisome finding, some of these patients do well when treated conservatively, and the need for surgery should be assessed on clinical rather than purely radiologic grounds.

Primary immunodeficiency syndromes

Selective IgA deficiency is common,[47] affecting up to 1 in 500 of the population, and most of these individuals are asymptomatic.[48] When infections do occur, they are usually recurrent bacterial and sinopulmonary disorders, and the GI tract is seldom involved. However, there is an association between celiac disease and pernicious anemia, although there is probably little if any increased incidence of giardiasis, and jejunal biopsy specimens appear normal when examined by light microscopy.

Common variable hypogammaglobulinemia is second to IgA deficiency as the most common primary immunodeficiency in adults, and represents a heterogeneous group of disorders that center on a defect in terminal B lymphocyte differentiation. It presents in the second or third decade of life with either respiratory infections or diarrhea and steatorrhea. Two thirds of the patients have diarrhea, and two thirds have malabsorption. Giardiasis is common and causes extensive mucosal damage, which leads to the malabsorption. Cryptosporidiosis and strongyloidiasis have also been reported to occur with the disorder.[47]

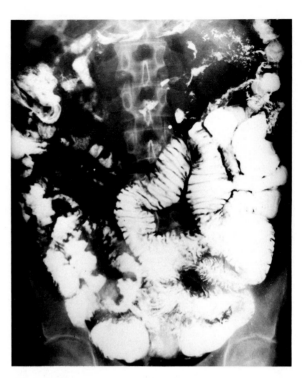

Fig. 32-31 Hypogammaglobulinemic sprue. The radiologic findings are indistinguishable from those of celiac sprue, and include dilatation with thinning of the folds, segmentation, fragmentation, and increased secretions.

Bruton's X-linked hypogammaglobulinemia is rarer and occurs almost exclusively in boys, typically with respiratory infections and, in 30% of the cases, with GI infections. *Campylobacter* infections are particularly common. Giardiasis causes severe damage and steatorrhea but responds readily to treatment. Perirectal abscesses and small bowel bacterial overgrowth occur, and there is an increased risk of lymphoma and leukemia in these patients.

Radiology in primary immunodeficiency disorders

Small bowel studies may reveal the features described in the following sections.

MALABSORPTION PATTERN

In common variable hypoglobulinemic states and selective IgA deficiency, the malabsorption pattern may simulate that of celiac disease, with dilatation of the small intestine and thinning of the folds (Fig. 32-31). Patients respond well to a gluten-free diet.

NODULAR LYMPHOID HYPERPLASIA

Nodular lymphoid hyperplasia may be due to congenital or acquired hypoglobulinemia, with depressed IgA levels revealed by serum immunoelectrophoresis. It is associated with an increased susceptibility to giardiasis. It is most often seen in patients with common variable immunoglobulin deficiency and less commonly in those with selective IgA deficiency and lymphoma. There is hypertrophy and enlargement of the submucosal lymphoid follicles throughout the entire small intestine, and the colon may also be involved.

Barium studies show multiple tiny 2 to 3-mm nodules on the submucosal surface throughout the entire small

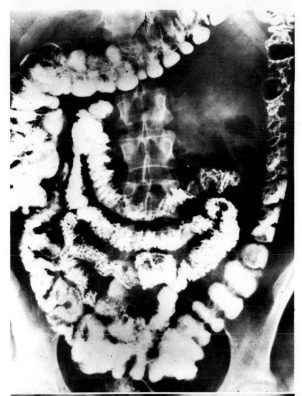

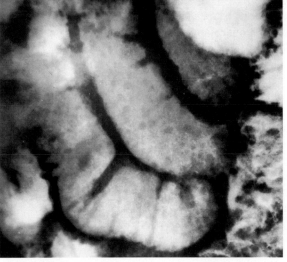

Fig. 32-32 Nodular lymphoid hyperplasia. Radiographic examination was performed because of diarrhea in a patient with markedly depressed IgA levels. There are numerous small circular nodules measuring 2 to 4 mm in diameter throughout the jejunum and ileum, without evidence of ulceration or a discrete mass.

bowel. This is often described as sandlike in appearance (Fig. 32-32). If a similar appearance is found throughout the small bowel, this may be a manifestation of mastocytosis. The mucosal folds are otherwise normal, but, if there is associated giardiasis, the tiny nodules may be superimposed on thickened folds.

Nodular lymphoid hyperplasia, which is restricted to the terminal ileum, may be seen in young people and is of no clinical significance.[50]

INFLAMMATORY CHANGES

Inflammatory changes are usually secondary to giardiasis (Fig. 32-21), campylobacteriosis, or, very rarely, cryptosporidiosis or strongyloidosis, as previously described.

Other intestinal inflammatory disorders that have been reported to occur with common variable hypoglobulinemia include Crohn's disease and ulcerative jejunitis.[47,51]

THICKENING OF FOLDS

Thickening of the folds is not a characteristic of primary enteropathic immunodeficiencies, except when there is a secondary infection such as giardiasis. Thickened folds are, however, a feature of secondary immunoglobulin disorders such as lymphoma, alpha chain disease, Waldenstrom's macroglobulinemia, intestinal lymphangiectasia, and amyloid disease (described later).

SYSTEMIC DISEASES
Mediterranean lymphoma (alpha-chain disease)

Mediterranean lymphoma[52,53] is also called *diffuse primary small bowel lymphoma* and *immunoproliferative small intestinal disease*. It is an unusual condition that begins as a benign-appearing, antibiotic-responsive immunoproliferative lesion, which usually slowly progresses to become fatal intestinal lymphoma.[54] There is good evidence that bacterial colonization of the small bowel is important in the etiology of the disease, which mainly affects young males from third world countries. There is extensive lymphatic infiltration of the mucosa and submucosa of the small intestine, mainly affecting the jejunum with extension into the duodenum and ileum.[55]

Initially the proliferating IgA-secreting lymphocytes, which derive from an expanded abnormal clone, produce an infiltrate made up of mature plasma cells. Later, dystrophic cells appear, and, eventually after some years, a frank lymphomatous proliferation ensues. Mesenteric lymph nodes may be involved. Clinically, there is abdominal pain, often with palpable masses, and clubbing and low-grade fever are common.[56] In addition, diarrhea, weight loss, and malabsorption are seen, as in tropical sprue.

Radiologic studies of the duodenum and small bowel[55] may reveal the existence of thickened folds (Fig. 32-33), with or without innumerable fine granular elevations but lacking ulcerations or luminal narrowing. In severe cases,

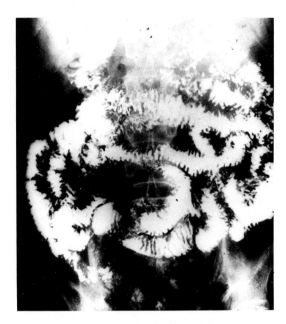

Fig. 32-33 Alpha chain disease. There is thickening of the folds throughout the jejunum and proximal ileum. Small bowel biopsy exhibited extensive infiltrates, with plasma cells and lymphocytes. The electrophoretic pattern was consistent with alpha chain disease.

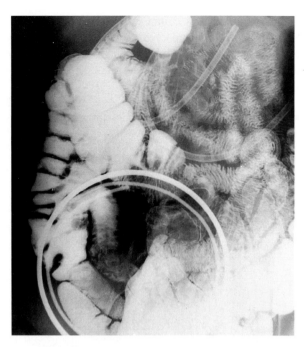

Fig. 32-34 This 27-year-old woman was seen after she had suffered multiple episodes of abdominal pain. She had undergone numerous investigations in two different hospitals, including upper and lower endoscopy, complete barium studies, CT, ultrasound, and angiography. All results were normal, as is this small bowel enema. The diagnosis of Mediterranean fever was made by a new physician who came to this conclusion after reviewing the patient's history. Her attacks are now well controlled by colchicine.

which include lymphatic obstruction, there may be features of lymphangiectasia. An additional malabsorption pattern makes radiologic differentiation from celiac disease very difficult, and the diagnosis is ultimately confirmed by characteristic biopsy findings. A further problem is that lymphoma may develop in patients with long-standing celiac disease. Intestinal loops may be displaced by an abdominal mass, and ultrasound or CT may be helpful in demonstrating lymphadenopathy.

The diffuse form of alpha heavy chain disease just described invariably develops into intestinal lymphoma.

Mediterranean fever

Mediterranean fever[57] should not be confused with Mediterranean lymphoma. It is a disease of unknown etiology that affects people of Sephardic Jewish, Arabic, and Armenian descent, but also those of Italian, Ashkenazic Jewish, and Anglo-Saxon ancestry. *Familial paroxysmal polyserositis* is another acceptable name for the disorder, and the disease usually presents between the ages of 5 and 15, although onset can range from infancy to the age of 52. Symptoms consist of acute and recurrent attacks of abdominal pain, almost always accompanied by fever. The pain spreads from its initial site and may splint the chest, with shoulder tip pain. Plain abdominal radiographs may show distention of the bowel, with fluid levels and bowel wall edema, with decreased peristalsis. Negative laparotomy findings are not uncommon. Chest pain, which may be

pleuritic, arthritis, and painful erythematous skin swellings on the lower legs or dorsum of the feet may occur. Amyloidosis is a feared, and common, complication in the Middle East, and is the cause of death in 25% of affected patients in Israel. Oddly, amyloidosis is almost unknown as a complication among patients living in the United States.

The importance of the disease for radiologists is twofold. First, patients may be seen in the emergency room with an acute abdomen, with positive findings, which, when combined with the clinical signs, may prompt unwarranted surgery. Second, after several attacks, many of these patients are referred for a GI workup that includes radiologic studies of the small bowel, colon, or both, which turn out to be normal (Fig. 32-34). An astute radiologist, on talking to the patient, may occasionally tumble to the diagnosis and save the patient much unnecessary investigation.

Colchicine is now an effective treatment that can control the disease, sometimes completely.[58,59]

Scleroderma

Scleroderma, or progressive systemic sclerosis, is a generalized disorder that often involves the GI tract.[60] The esophagus is invariably affected, and problems include impaired or absent smooth muscle peristalsis.

There is a patchy destruction of the muscularis propria in the small intestine, mainly involving the duodenum and jejunum. There is also degeneration of both the circular and longitudinal muscle layers and replacement by collagen tissue. Mesenteric vasculitis may be a contributory factor.

Impaired motility gives rise to bacterial overgrowth, with alterations in the bile acids and consequent malabsorption. Important clinical findings are skin changes, Raynaud's phenomenon, and arthropathy.

The following radiologic changes may be found:

1. Dilatation may occur that mainly affects the duodenum and proximal jejunum.[61,62] Gross dilatation of the duodenal loop may mimic an obstruction at the duodenojejunal flexure (Fig. 32-35). Occasionally there is uniform dilatation of much of the small bowel, with poor or absent peristalsis (Fig. 32-36).
2. The valvulae conniventes are straight and close together, producing a "pleating" or "hidebound" appearance[11,63,64] (Fig. 32-37).
3. Sacculation with the formation of pseudodiverticula possessing wide necks may be seen in the small intestine[65,66] and colon.
4. There is marked delay in the transit of barium through the small intestine due to diminished peristalsis, which may produce malabsorption[11,67] resulting from bacterial overgrowth (Fig. 32-36).

5. Occasionally, pneumatosis cystoides intestinalis may cause a chronic benign pneumoperitoneum.[61,68,69]

The differential diagnosis of scleroderma from other conditions is usually not difficult, as there is invariable involvement of the esophagus in scleroderma. Dilatation of the duodenal loop is usually a striking feature and, on direct questioning, many of the patients admit to having Raynaud's phenomenon.

Chronic intestinal pseudoobstruction may also be secondary to systemic diseases such as scleroderma and amyloidosis, in which the chronic stasis leads to bacterial overgrowth, malabsorption, and steatorrhea.[70]

Whipple's disease

Whipple's disease,[71,72] which is very rare, is also known as *intestinal lipodystrophy*. It is seen mainly, but not exclusively, in middle-aged white men and has been reported in both infants and octogenarians. Thirteen percent of the patients are female. The disease is possibly due to a bacteria-like organism and responds to antibiotic therapy (either penicillin plus streptomycin or trimethoprim/sulfamethoxazole), which should be continued for a year to minimize the chance of relapse. Relapse can be associated with irreversible dementia, which shows no response to antibiotics, and death. The Whipple's bacillus has not been

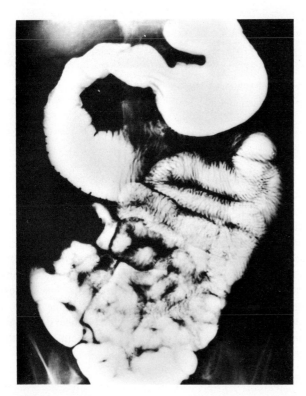

Fig. 32-35 Scleroderma. There is marked dilatation of the duodenum without organic obstruction at the ligament of Treitz. There is moderate hypomotility of barium through the small bowel.

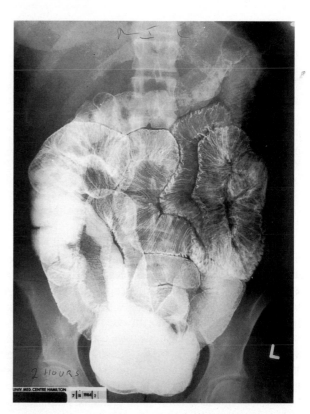

Fig. 32-36 Two-hour film of a small bowel enema study in a patient with hypomotility resulting from scleroderma. Initially she was seen because of malabsorption resulting from bacterial overgrowth. Esophageal motility was also impaired.

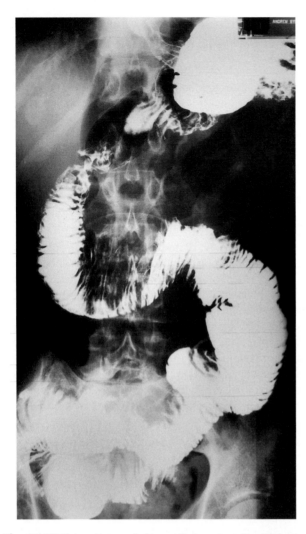

Fig. 32-37 Scleroderma of the small intestine showing rather straight valvulae, which are close together and thus produce the appearance described as "pleating." There is also mild dilatation.

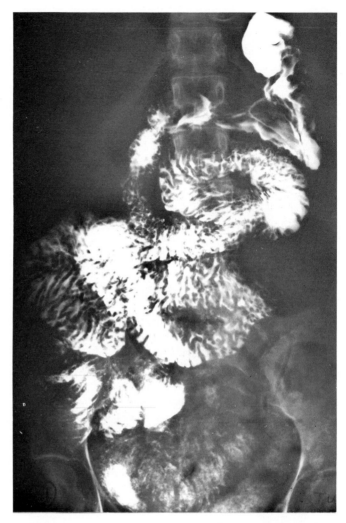

Fig. 32-38 Whipple's disease. There is thickening of the folds of the duodenum and jejunum.

cultured or reproduced in animal models, and there is evidence of a subtle defect in cellular immunity even in well patients, as well as an association with HLA-B27.[73]

Microscopy reveals the existence of massive infiltration of the lamina propria of the small intestine and lymph nodes by macrophages containing a glycoprotein that reacts to staining with periodic acid–Schiff. Electron microscopy shows the bacilli, but it is not an essential study.

Clinically, patients have diarrhea, crampy abdominal pain and distention, steatorrhea, weight loss, intermittent arthralgia, skin pigmentation, lymphadenopathy, and peripheral edema.

Small bowel studies show some dilatation with irregular thickening of the valvulae conniventes throughout the small intestine, which is more marked in the jejunum[74] (Figs. 32-38 and 32-39). Diffuse, tiny 1-mm nodules may be superimposed on the swollen folds and result from enlarged villi.[75]

The presence of lymphadenopathy may be confirmed by ultrasound and CT. The adenopathy is striking, and the lobulated nodes, which may be 3 to 4 cm in diameter, characteristically show low attenuation.[76,77] On ultrasound, a distinctive diffusely echogenic appearance has been noted.[78] The combination of an echogenic lymphadenopathy on ultrasound and low-attenuation lymphadenopathy on CT in a young adult man with arthralgia is very suggestive of Whipple's disease, although the CT appearance is not specific.[79] Endoscopic biopsy is the ultimate diagnostic tool, with the harvesting of four to six specimens, as the disease process is occasionally focal.

Differential diagnosis

The radiologic findings alone may be difficult to distinguish from those of lymphoma, lymphangiectasia, or amyloidosis. The irregular thickening of the folds, the absence of jejunoileal fold pattern reversal, and the minimal degree

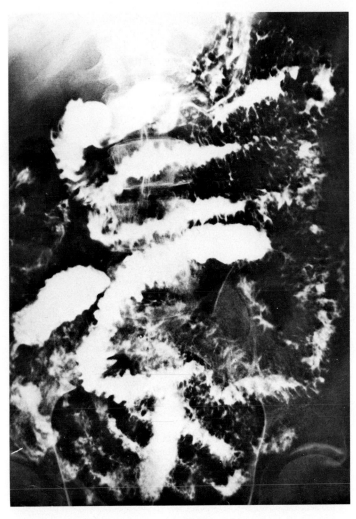

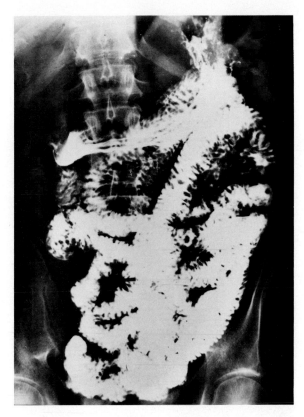

Fig. 32-40 Amyloidosis. There is diffuse, sharply demarcated symmetric thickening of the folds without significant dilatation. Segmentation and fragmentation are absent. There is no evidence of inflammation.

Fig. 32-39 Whipple's disease. The folds of the jejunum and proximal ileum are blunted, redundant, thickened, and slightly nodular. Fragmentation and segmentation are minimal.

of dilatation usually permit its differentiation from celiac disease. The clinical features and biopsy findings should establish the diagnosis.

Other rare conditions, such as mastocytosis and histoplasmosis, exhibit characteristic clinical findings and are discussed later. Sarcoidosis may be difficult to distinguish from Whipple's disease clinically, but the radiologic and histologic features are distinctive.

Amyloidosis

The small intestine may be involved in primary and secondary types of amyloidosis, and this is not an uncommon finding.[80] Amyloid is initially deposited in the vicinity of the mucosal and submucosal vessels and stains abnormally. Later, there is diffuse involvement of all layers. Clinically, patients have abdominal pain, diarrhea, melena, and malabsorption. The diagnosis is based on the results of rectal, small intestine, or gingival biopsy.

A small bowel study may show diffuse thickening of the folds throughout the entire small intestine[74,81] (Fig. 32-40). Fold enlargement in the ileum may produce an appearance resembling the feathery pattern of normal jejunum, which has been described as "jejunization" of the ileum[15,74] (Fig. 32-41). However, this should not be confused with celiac disease, because there is no loss of valvulae in the jejunum (only thickening) and there is no dilatation, segmentation, or fragmentation. A fine 1- to 3-mm nodular pattern has been demonstrated on double-contrast studies of the small intestine. Rarely, large deposits in the intestinal tract give rise to tumorlike nodules. The passage of the barium through the small intestine may be delayed, with diffuse intestinal infiltration. In severe cases, malabsorption may be found.[74]

The appearance presented by amyloidosis may be confused with that of Whipple's disease, which shows more severe involvement of the jejunum with more fold irregularity and usually some dilatation.

Waldenstrom's macroglobulinemia

Waldenstrom's macroglobulinemia is an IgM-secreting variant of multiple myeloma, the main feature of which is the high level of a monoclonal IgM macroglobulin fraction

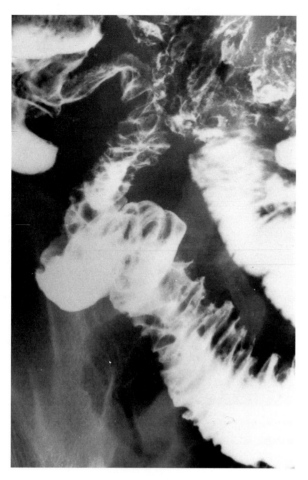

Fig. 32-41 Amyloidosis in which there is thickening of the ileal mucosal folds, imparting a rather jejunal appearance to the ileum. In this patient, however, the amyloidosis was a late complication of cystic fibrosis.

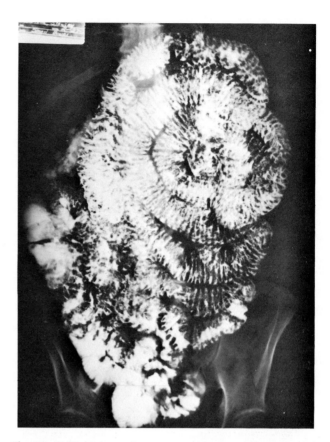

Fig. 32-42 Waldenstrom's macroglobulinemia. The folds of the jejunum and proximal ileum are disorganized and thickened and have a spikelike configuration. The changes result from massive infiltration of the bowel wall with plasma cells and lymphocytes.

of serum protein. Clinically, onset is insidious, and it is usually seen in men over 40 years of age. Patients typically complain of anemia, bleeding diathesis, lymphadenopathy, and massive hepatosplenomegaly. Diarrhea and steatorrhea are rarely found but, when present, may be associated with an abnormal small bowel resulting from the deposition of large amounts of IgM in the intestinal lamina propria and mesenteric lymph nodes, which impairs absorption.[82-84]

Radiologic examination shows that the folds of the small intestine are thickened and have a spiky outline (Figs. 32-42 and 32-43). The mucosal surface may have a tiny granular or nodular appearance. CT may be helpful in demonstrating the extent of disease and monitoring the effects of treatment.[85]

Mastocytosis

Mastocytosis is a disease consisting of mast cell proliferation and exists in two forms. The cutaneous form is urticaria pigmentosa. The systemic form causes headache,

pruritus, flushing, dizziness, wheezing, and tachycardia. GI complaints, which occur in 25% of affected patients, include abdominal pain, nausea, diarrhea, malabsorption, and gastritis. Both hepatosplenomegaly and gastroduodenal ulcers occur. The presence of bone sclerosis is often the clue to the diagnosis. Malabsorption is due to infiltration of the small bowel with mast cells and subsequent edema. The radiologic features comprise thickening of the valvulae conniventes and of mucosal nodules with a diameter of less than 5 mm, mainly located in the jejunum.[86]

Histoplasmosis

Histoplasmosis is caused by *Histoplasma capsulatum*, an intracellular organism that causes the formation of solitary lesions in the skin or bone, or it may be confined to the lung. Disseminated disease occurs and may involve the GI tract.[74] Liver involvement is a prominent feature. Anemia, thrombocytopenia, and pulmonary changes may also occur. Clinically patients have fever, malaise, anorexia, and weight loss. Twenty-five percent of the patients are immunosuppressed or have malignant disease.

Histoplasmosis causes an ulcerative enteritis, most com-

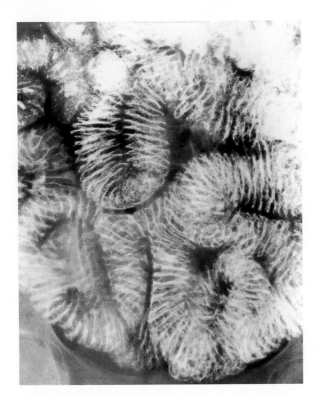

Fig. 32-43 Waldenstrom's macroglobulinemia. There is a diffuse uniform thickening of the mucosal folds, which have a typical spikelike outline. Nodulation of the mucosal surface is also noted. Courtesy of Dr. Evlogais.

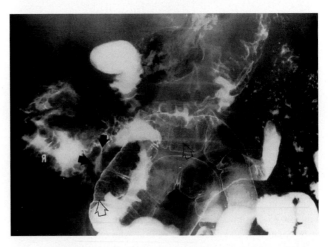

Fig. 32-44 Histoplasmosis. There is diffuse infiltration in the lower ileal loops and cecum with mucosal edema and ulceration. Ileocecal fistula is seen (*arrow*), and ileorectal fistulization is also present (not pictured). There is also extensive involvement of the duodenal loop with mucosal edema and ulceration. Aphthous ulceration is seen in the jejunum *(open arrow)*.

monly in the terminal ileum and cecum, where it may mimic Crohn's disease[87] (Fig. 32-44), and then involves the esophagus and contiguous organs. About one third of the patients have ulceration, and 20% have masses or strictures.[88] External compression resulting from inflammatory masses is also seen. Rarely, if there is extensive involvement of the small bowel, it may present with a protein-losing enteropathy simulating Whipple's disease.

GI PATHOLOGY AND BIOCHEMICAL CHANGES
Zollinger-Ellison syndrome

Gastrin-secreting tumors arising in the pancreas or elsewhere produce high acid states that may cause upper GI ulcerations and malabsorption.[89] They may be benign or malignant, and, when patients with Zollinger-Ellison syndrome die of the disease, it is more often due to malignancy than to peptic ulceration or its complications.

Thickening of the mucosal folds in the duodenum and proximal intestine may be seen, and this results from gastric hypersecretion. There is dilution of the barium, producing a granular appearance. Flocculation and a moulage effect may also be observed. Dilatation of the second part of the duodenum together with coarse thickened folds is a prominent finding. The diagnosis is suggested by the presence of multiple ulcers in the stomach, duodenum, and

proximal jejunum, although the diagnosis may not be obvious, as 25% of the patients have no peptic ulcer and two thirds have only a single, apparently simple, peptic ulcer.[11] Therefore, when the serum gastrin level is high, a more specific test is required. The secretin provocation test is currently favored for this purpose, and is positive in about 90% of patients with an active gastrinoma. The preferred procedure for demonstrating the tumor in or near the pancreas is now endoscopic ultrasound.

Eosinophilic gastroenteritis

The cause of eosinophilic gastroenteritis[47] is unknown. A history of allergy to certain foods, previously thought common, is found in less than 20% of the patients.[90] Spontaneous remissions may occur, and the disease responds to steroid therapy. There may be focal or diffuse lesions in the small intestine, but mainly in the latter. Gastric involvement is usually confined to the pyloric antrum. Histologically, there is infiltration of the small intestinal wall by inflammatory cells, especially eosinophils. Ulceration is occasionally seen, and there is often an associated fibrotic reaction. Ascites may occur if the subserosa is involved.

Clinically, patients experience recurrent abdominal pain, vomiting, diarrhea, and anemia. Small bowel involvement may produce malabsorption and hypoproteinemia, which are secondary to a protein-losing enteropathy.[74]

Barium studies disclose narrowing of the pyloric antrum in 90% of the cases, with a thick rigid wall simulating carcinoma.[91] In the small intestine there is irregular nodular thickening of the folds that is variably distributed over seg-

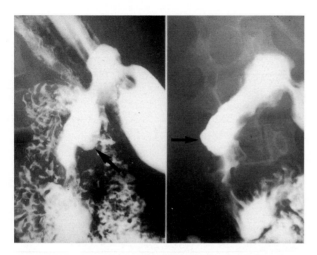

Fig. 32-45 Eosinophilic enteritis in a 7-year-old child who was seen because of abdominal pain. Ultrasound examination showed duodenal thickening, and a barium study showed the large ulcer in the second part *(arrow)*, which was confirmed at endoscopy. In the gastric antrum there was a small red patch of mucosa, and biopsy of this tissue revealed massive eosinophilic infiltration. Steroid therapy was effective, but the patient suffered relapse when they were withdrawn, thus necessitating maintenance therapy.

ments of the proximal small intestine. Ulceration may be seen occasionally (Fig. 32-45).

Ultrasonography may be helpful in differentiating eosinophilic gastroenteritis from Crohn's disease and lymphoma,[92] although major wall thickening may be seen. The diagnosis is confirmed by a full-thickness biopsy specimen showing eosinophilic infiltration and by a blood count revealing eosinophilia.

Chronic pancreatitis

Severe chronic pancreatitis[74] may cause malabsorption and produce radiologic changes. There may be moderate generalized dilatation of the small intestine, with some swelling of the folds due to edema associated with hypoalbuminemia. Pancreatic calcification may be seen.

Cystic fibrosis

In cystic fibrosis, barium studies may rarely depict narrowing of the duodenum, with thickened folds and sometimes a sacculated appearance to the outer border.[93] The jejunum may be normal, but irregular lacelike hazy filling defects with an almost haustral outline of the lumen may be seen in the ileum. These changes are believed to be due to inspissated mucus. Radiologic findings may suggest a late diagnosis of cystic fibrosis, which can be confirmed by the sweat test.

Intestinal lactase deficiency

Lactase is the enzyme responsible for hydrolysis of disaccharides, and deficiency may give rise to diarrhea and

malabsorption. Patients typically complain of abdominal cramps and diarrhea after the ingestion of milk or milk products. Radiologic findings may assist in the diagnosis, as the addition of 25 g of lactose to the barium provokes a marked decrease in the transit time and the secretion of excessive intraluminal fluid, which dilutes the barium.[94] If the test result is positive, the study can be repeated with regular barium, and the then normal appearance confirms the diagnosis. Intolerance to maltose and fructose can be tested in the same way. In practice, radiology is no longer used for confirming this diagnosis, which is now accomplished with the hydrogen breath test and the measurement of lactose activity in a jejunal biopsy specimen.

INFLAMMATORY DISEASES

Crohn's disease and tuberculosis, which are covered under inflammatory conditions, may occasionally, in severe cases, present as malabsorption.

SECONDARY CHANGES RESULTING FROM OTHER CAUSES
Short bowel syndrome

Short bowel syndrome results from an inadequate absorptive surface due to surgical resections or the formation of fistulas. Resection of the proximal small bowel reduces the area for absorption, and ileal resections cause a loss of bile salts, which are essential for the digestion of fat (Fig. 32-46). Fistulas may short-circuit the small bowel, effectively producing a shortened gut, and this will also alter the flora.

Radiologic studies are helpful in the investigation of suspected fistulas, and single-contrast techniques are preferred.

Small intestinal edema

When the serum albumin level falls below 2.5 mg/100 ml, the resultant reduced intracapillary osmotic pressure causes increased fluid accumulation in the extracellular spaces, producing edema of the small bowel. This can happen in hepatic cirrhosis, chronic renal failure, right ventricular failure, or malnutrition. Laënnec's cirrhosis is the most common cause.

Barium studies may show uniform thickening of the valvulae conniventes throughout the small intestine due to an increased fluid content in the mucosal and submucosal layers (Fig. 32-47). The folds may be club-shaped and closer together than normal. Hypersecretion may produce dilution of the barium. Separation of the loops may be seen if ascites is present.

Drugs

Certain narcotic and anticholinergic drugs may produce intestinal dilatation due to diminished peristalsis, but signs of malabsorption are absent. Other agents responsible for malabsorption are neomycin, cholestyramine, colchicine, paraaminosalicylic acid, and ethyl alcohol, as well as the biguanides (used as oral antidiabetic drugs), purgatives

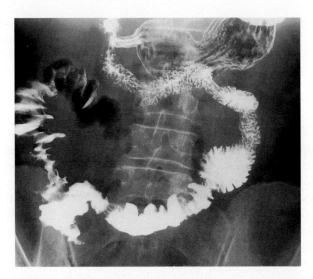

Fig. 32-46 A short bowel in a 62-year-old woman who had undergone resection for small bowel ischemia. Single-contrast studies are adequate for demonstrating the length of the residual intestine.

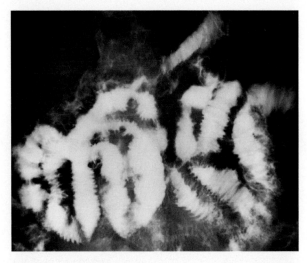

Fig. 32-47 Small intestinal edema in which there is uniform thickening of the valvulae conniventes throughout the small intestine, with some separation of the loops secondary to cirrhosis with hypoalbuminemia. Some of the mucosal folds are club shaped and close together.

(when there is chronic abuse), methotrexate (used in the chemotherapy of malignancy), and occasionally methyldopa.[2,26,74] Multiple mechanisms are involved, including structural damage to the mucosa, inhibition of enzymes, and precipitation of bile acids and fatty acids. Radiologic changes are rarely seen, but long-term ingestion of the offending agents may lead to a clinical picture of ileus or obstruction, especially in psychiatric patients. When psychiatric patients are admitted with symptoms and signs of obstruction, the question of ileus from drug intake should be seriously pursued, especially if the results of a barium enema are negative.

Ischemic enteritis

Ischemic enteritis may occur in elderly patients with atherosclerosis, in young women taking anovular medication, or secondary to trauma. Embolic phenomena from cardiac lesions are usually acute surgical emergencies. In the presence of subacute mesenteric arterial or venous occlusion, intramural edema and hemorrhage may arise in the affected ischemic segment of small intestine.

Clinically, patients complain of crampy abdominal pain of some months' duration, often after food intake. Angiographic findings may help when the disorder is suspected clinically, but if barium is given, it will show uniform thickening of the folds, which may have a segmental distribution. The folds are often close together, producing a "stacked coin" appearance.[74] In more seriously affected patients, the folds are thickened and blunted and, in some segments, a "rigid picket fence" appearance is seen, as occurs in Crohn's disease, with narrowing of the lumen.[95] "Thumb printing" may be seen and may result from either mucosal

edema or submucosal hemorrhage. These appearances may be mimicked by Schönlein-Henoch purpura, lymphoma, or Crohn's disease. The changes may resolve spontaneously, but, if severe, there is necrosis and ulceration and, after healing, possibly sacculation or pseudodiverticula on the antimesenteric border of the intestine. In very severe cases, a featureless narrow segment of small bowel may be produced[96] and strictures may develop (Fig. 32-48).

Radiation enteritis

Radiotherapy to the abdominal or pelvic organs may cause damage to the small bowel.[18,97,98] This is usually due to a reactive obliterative endarteritis and may present with acute, subacute, or chronic symptoms. The acute type is rare and usually appears in the weeks following treatment; symptoms consist of abdominal pain, distention, diarrhea, and vomiting. On barium examination, the affected segments exhibit changes characteristic of edema, with thumb printing, uniform thickening of the valvulae with a spiked appearance, and proximal bowel distention.

The subacute and chronic types are more common. The subacute form occurs in the months following treatment, whereas the chronic type may take years to develop. The clinical presentation is usually abdominal pain and frequently malabsorption, often with anemia or rectal bleeding. The small bowel changes are essentially ischemic and consist of areas of narrowing that involve the bowel in a patchy manner. The wall thickening may cause the loops to become fixed, angulated, and separated (Fig. 32-49). There is reduced peristalsis and pooling of barium within the loops.[5,95,96] Strictures and complications such as fistu-

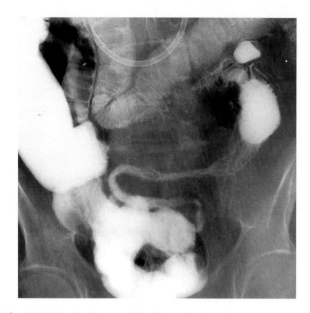

Fig. 32-48 Ischemic enteritis with residual stricture in a patient who had recovered from an episode of ischemia, but then developed colic after meals, which progressed to episodes of obstruction. The small bowel enema shows the dilatation proximal to the long strictured segments.

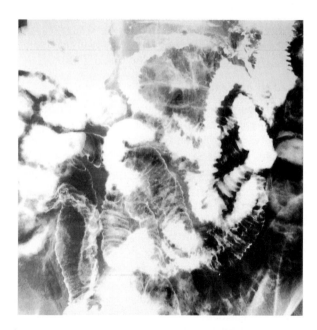

Fig. 32-49 Radiation enteritis. The jejunal folds show uniform swelling due to edema, with some separation of the loops, in a patient who had undergone radiotherapy for lymphoma.
Courtesy of Dr. Michael Daly.

las can alter the small bowel flora and cause malabsorption. The patient's history is an essential component of the examination in order to differentiate radiation enteritis from Crohn's and other inflammatory and neoplastic diseases.

Irritable bowel syndrome

A barium enema is usually done to exclude the existence of organic disease in patients with irritable bowel syndrome. Sometimes, colonic contractions are seen, which can be correlated with the site of pain. Occasionally, a barium meal examination and dedicated small bowel study may be requested to exclude small intestine disease in patients with clinical signs of irritable bowel syndrome. The small intestine may show segmental spasm and distention or an excessively rapid transit time, which is often a feature of functional diarrhea. This has been called *functional enterocolonopathy*,[99,100] but the evaluation is rather subjective and poorly validated.

REFERENCES

1. Powell DW: Approach to the patient with diarrhea. In Yamada T, ed: *Textbook of gastroenterology*, Philadelphia, 1991, JB Lippincott.
2. Losowsky MS: Malabsorption. In Leddingham DJ, Warrell DA, Weatherall DJ, ed: *Oxford textbook of medicine*, New York, 1987, Oxford University Press.
3. Maglinte DDT, Lappas JC, Kelvin FM et al: Small bowel radiography: how, when and why? *Radiology* 163:297, 1987.
4. Gilchrist AM, Mills JOM: Radiological examination of the small bowel, *Ulster Med J* 58:124, 1989.
5. Costello RW, Lyons DJ, Fielding JF: Ulcerative jejunitis: are we missing cases? *Ir J Med Sci* 160:342, 1990.
6. Federle MP, Goldberg HI: Radiography of the small intestine. In Sleisenger MH, Fordtran JS, eds: *Gastrointestinal disease*, ed 3, Philadelphia 1983, WB Saunders.
7. Richards DG, Stevenson GW: Laxatives prior to small bowel follow-through: are they necessary for a rapid and good-quality examination? *Gastrointest Radiol* 15:66, 1990.
8. Nolan DJ, Cadman PJ: The small bowel enema made easy, *Clin Radiol* 38:295, 1987.
9. Maglinte DDT, Herlinger H: Anatomy of the small intestine. In Herlinger H, Maglinte DDT, eds: *Clinical radiology of the small intestine*, Philadelphia, 1989, WB Saunders.
10. Anukas S, Chokhavatia S: Dysmotility of the small bowel. In Yamada T, ed: *Textbook of gastroenterology*, Philadelphia, 1991, JB Lippincott.
11. Olmsted W, Madewell J: The oesophageal and small bowel manifestations of progressive systemic sclerosis, *Gastrointest Radiol* 1:33, 1976.
12. Anuras S: Intestinal pseudo-obstruction syndrome, *Annu Rev Med* 39:1, 1988.
13. Small bowel mucosal disease. In Lewin KJ, Riddell RH, Weinstein WM, eds: *Gastrointestinal pathology and its clinical implications*. New York, 1992, Igaku-Shoin.
14. Shanahan F, Weinstein WM: Extending the scope in coeliac disease, *N Engl J Med* 429:782, 1988 (editorial).
15. Maklansky D, Lindner AE: Malabsorption and immune deficiencies. In Margulis AP, Burhenne HJ, eds: *Alimentary tract radiology*, ed 4, St. Louis, 1989, Mosby–Year Book.
16. Antes G, Eggemann F: *Small bowel radiology*, Berlin, 1988, Springer-Verlag.
17. Nolan DJ: The small intestine. In Grainger RG, Allison DJ, eds: *Diagnostic radiology*, New York, 1986, Churchill Livingstone.

18. Herlinger H: Radiology in malabsorption, *Clin Radiol* 45:73, 78, 1992.

19. Bret P, Cuche C, Schmutz G: *Radiology of the small intestine*, Paris, 1989, Springer-Verlag.

20. McCarthy CF: Malignancy in coeliac disease, *Eur J Gastroenterol Hepatol* 3:125, 1991.

21. Lamont CM, Adams FG, Mills PR: Radiology in idiopathic chronic ulcerative enteritis, *Clin Radiol* 33:283, 1982.

22. Brunton F, Guyer PB: Malignant histiocytosis and ulcerative jejunitis of the small intestine, *Clin Radiol* 34:291, 1983.

23. Sussman NL, Sutton FM: Miscellaneous diseases of the small intestine. In Yamada T, ed: *Textbook of gastroenterology*, Philadelphia, 1991, JB Lippincott.

24. Weinstein WM, Saunders DR, Tytgat GN et al: Collagenous sprue—an unrecognized type of malabsorption, *N Engl J Med* 283:1297, 1970.

25. Ament ME, Rubin CE: Soy protein—another cause of the flat intestinal lesion, *Gastroenterology* 62:227, 1972.

26. Richards DG, Somers S, Issenman RM: Cow's milk protein/soy protein allergy: gastrointestinal imaging, *Radiology* 167:721, 1988.

27. Shimkin PM, Waldmann TA, Krugman RL: Intestinal lymphangiectasia, *AJR* 110:827, 1970.

28. Vardy P, Lebenthal E, Shwachman H: Intestinal lymphangiectasia: a reappraisal, *Pediatrics* 55:842, 1975.

29. Pomeranz M, Waldman TA: Systemic abnormalities associated with gastrointestinal protein loss secondary to intestinal lymphangiectasia, *Gastroenterology* 45:703, 1963.

30. Donzelli F, Norberto L, Marigo et al: Primary intestinal lymphangiectasia. Comparison between endoscopic and radiological findings, *Helv Paediatr Acta* 35:169, 1980.

31. Wyngaarden JB, Smith LH Jr, Bennett JC: *Cecil's textbook of medicine*, ed 19, Philadelphia, 1992, WB Saunders.

32. Marshak RH, Ruoff M, Lindner AE: Roentgen manifestations of giardiasis, *AJR* 104:557, 1968.

33. Petri WA, Hill DR, Guerraat RL: Parasitic infections: protozoa. In Yamada T, ed: *Textbook of gastroenterology*, Philadelphia, 1991, JB Lippincott.

34. Wright SG, Tomkins AM, Ridley DS: Giardiasis: clinical and therapeutic aspects, *Gut* 18:343, 1977.

35. Cockshott P, Middlemiss H, eds. *Strongyloides* of the alimentary tract. In *Clinical radiology in the tropics*. Edinburgh, 1979, Churchill Livingstone.

36. Kotler PP, Francisco A, Clayton F, Scholes JV, Orentein JM: Small bowel intestinal injury and parasitic disease in AIDS, *Ann Intern Med* 13:444, 1990.

37. Peacock CS, Blanshard C, Tovey D, Ellis DS, Gazzard BG: Histological diagnosis of intestinal microsporidiosis in patients with AIDS, *J Clin Pathol* 44:558, 1991.

38. Reeders JWAW, Bartelsman JFWM, Antonides HR, Tytgat GNJ: The spectrum of gastrointestinal radiology in AIDS, *Eur J Radiol* 1:33, 1991.

39. Roth R, Owen RL, Keven DF: Acquired immunodeficiency syndrome with *Mycobacterium avium-intracellulare* lesions resembling those of Whipple's disease, *N Engl J Med* 309:1324, 1983.

40. Jeffrey RB Jr et al: Abdominal CT in acquired immunodeficiency syndrome, *AJR* 146:7, 1986.

41. Fisk JD et al: Gastrointestinal radiographic features of human graft-vs-host disease, *AJR* 136:329, 1981.

42. Jones B, Fishman EK, Kramer SS: Computed tomography of gastrointestinal inflammation after bone marrow transplantation, *AJR* 146:691, 1986.

43. Jones B, Kramer SS, Saral R: Gastrointestinal inflammation after bone marrow transplantation: graft versus host disease or opportunistic infection, *AJR* 150:277, 1988.

44. Patzik SB, Smith C, Kubicka RA et al: Bone marrow transplantation: clinical and radiologic aspects, *Radiographics* 11:601, 1991.

45. Belli AM, Williams MP: Graft-versus-host disease: findings on plain abdominal radiography. *Clin Radiol* 39:262, 1988.

46. Day DL, Ramsay NK, Letourneau JG: Pneumatosis intestinalis after bone marrow transplantation, *AJR* 151:85, 1988.

47. Shanahan F, Targan S: Gastrointestinal manifestations of immunologic disorders. In Yamada T et al, eds: *Textbook of gastroenterology*. Philadelphia, 1991, JB Lippincott.

48. Doe WF: Immunodeficiency and the gastrointestinal tract, *Clin Gastroenterol* 12:839, 1983.

49. Hodgson JR, Hoffman HN II, Huizenga KA: Roentgenologic features of lymphoid hyperplasia of the small intestine associated with dysgammaglobulinemia, *Radiology* 88:883, 1967.

50. Nagasako K, Takemoto T: Endoscopy of the ileocecal area, *Gastroenterology* 65:403, 1973.

51. Ament ME: Gastrointestinal manifestations of immunodeficiency diseases in infants, children and adults. In Targan S, Shanahan F, eds: *Immunology and immunopathology of the liver and gastrointestinal tract*, New York, 1989, Igaku-Shoin.

52. Seligmann M, Rambaud JC: Alpha-chain disease: an immunoproliferative disease of the secretory immune system, *Ann NY Acad Sci* 409:478, 1983.

53. Ramos L et al: Radiological characteristics of primary intestinal lymphoma of the "Mediterranean" type, observations on twelve cases, *Radiology* 126:379, 1978.

54. Khojasteh A: Immunoproliferative small intestinal disease: portrait of a potentially preventable cancer from the third world, *Am J Med* 89:483, 1990.

55. Matsumoto T, Iida M, Matsui T, Tanaka H, Fujishima M: The value of double-contrast study of the small intestine in immunoproliferative small intestinal disease, *Gastrointest Radiol* 15:159, 1990.

56. Neil GA, Weinstock JV: Gastrointestinal manifestations of systemic diseases. Yamada T et al, eds: *Textbook of gastroenterology*, New York, 1991, JB Lippincott.

57. Wolff SM: Familial Mediterranean fever. In Isselbacher KJ et al, eds: *Harrison's principles of internal medicine*, New York, 1980, McGraw-Hill.

58. Dinarello CA et al: Colchicine therapy for familial Mediterranean fever: a double-blind trial, *N Engl J Med* 291:934, 1974.

59. Wright DG et al: Efficiency of intermittent colchicine therapy in familial Mediterranean fever, *Ann Intern Med* 86:162, 1977.

60. Bluestone R, MacMahon M, Dawson JM: Systemic sclerosis and small bowel involvement, *Gut* 10:185, 1969.

61. Poirier T, Rankin G: Gastrointestinal manifestation of progressive systemic scleroderma, *Am J Gastroenterol* 58:30, 1972.

62. Anderson F: Megaduodenum, *Am J Gastroenterol* 62:509, 1974.

63. Horowitz AL, Meyers MA: The "hide-bound" small bowel of scleroderma: characteristic mucosal fold pattern, *AJR* 119:332, 1973.

64. Cohen S, Laufer I, Snape WJ et al: The gastrointestinal manifestations of scleroderma, *Gastroenterology* 79:155, 1980.

65. Quelz JM, Woloshin HJ: Sacculation of the small intestine in scleroderma, *Radiology* 105:513, 1972.

66. Hale C, Schatzki R: The roentgenological appearance of the gastrointestinal tract in scleroderma, *AJR* 51:407, 1944.

67. Stellaard F, Sauerbruch T, Luderschmidt CH et al: Intestinal involvement in progressive systemic sclerosis, *Gut* 28:446, 1987.

68. Gompels B: Pneumatosis cystoides intestinalis associated with progressive systemic sclerosis, *Br J Radiol* 42:701, 1969.

69. Miercort R, Merrill G: Pneumatosis and pseudo-obstruction in scleroderma, *Radiology* 92:359, 1969.

70. Schuffler MD, Deitch EA. Chronic idiopathic intestinal pseudo-obstruction: a surgical approach, *Ann Surg* 192:752, 1980.

71. Comer GM, Brandt LJ, Abissi CJ: Whipple's disease: a review, *Am J Gastroenterol* 78:107, 1983.

72. Philips RL, Carlson HC: The roentgenographic and clinical findings in Whipple's disease, *AJR* 123:268, 1975.

73. Dobbins WO, Klipstein: Chronic infections of the small intestine. In Yamada T et al, eds: *Textbook of gastroenterology,* New York, 1991, JB Lippincott.

74. Marshak RH, Lindner AE: Whipple's disease. In Marshak RH, Lindner AE, eds: *Radiology of the small intestine,* Philadelphia, 1970, WB Saunders.

75. Clemett AR, Marshak RH: Whipple's disease, Roentgen features and differential diagnosis, *Radiol Clin North Am* 7:105, 1969.

76. Li DBK, Rennie CS: Abdominal computed tomography in Whipple's disease, *J Comput Assist Tomogr* 5:249, 1981.

77. Rijke AM, Falke THM, de Vries RRP: Computed tomography in Whipple's disease, *J Comput Assist Tomogr* 7:1101, 1983.

78. Davis SJ, Patel A: Case report: distinctive echogenic lymphadenopathy in Whipple's disease, *Clin Radiol* 42:60, 1990.

79. Deutch SJ, Sandler MA, Alpern MB: Abdominal lymphadenopathy in benign disease: CT detection, *Radiology* 163:335, 1987.

80. Carlson HC, Breen JF: Amyloidosis and plasma cell dyscrasia: gastrointestinal involvement, *Semin Roentgenol* 21:128, 1986.

81. Seliger G, Krassner RL, Beranbaum ER, Miller F: The spectrum of roentgen appearance in amyloidosis in the small and large bowel: radiologic-pathologic correlation, *Radiology* 100:63, 1971.

82. Velosa FT, Fraga J, Saleiro JV: Macroglobulinemia and small intestinal disease. A case report with review of the literature, *J Clin Gastroenterol* 10:546, 1978.

83. Brandt LJ et al: Small intestinal involvement in Waldenstrom's macroglobulinemia: case report and review of the literature, *Dig Dis Sci* 26:174, 1981.

84. Bendine MS, et al: Intestinal involvement in Waldenstrom's macroglobulinemia, *Gastroenterology* 65:308, 1973.

85. Aspelin P et al: Abdominal computed tomography in macroglobulinemia (Waldenstrom's disease): report of a case, *Acta Radiol* 30:197, 1989.

86. Clemett AR et al: Gastrointestinal lesions in mastocytosis, *AJR* 103:405, 1968.

87. Parsons RJ, Jarafonatis CD: Histoplasmosis in man—report of seven cases and a review of 71 cases, *Arch Intern Med* 75:1, 1945.

88. Cappell MS, Mandell W, Grimes MM et al: Gastrointestinal histoplasmosis, *Dig Dis Sci* 33:353, 1988.

89. Wolfe MM, Jensen RT: Zollinger Ellison syndrome. Current concepts in diagnosis and management, *N Engl J Med* 317:1200, 1987.

90. Wilson JD et al: *Harrison's principles of internal medicine,* ed 12: New York, 1991, McGraw-Hill.

91. Schulman A, Morton PCH, Detrich BE: Eosinophilic gastroenteritis, *Clin Radiol* 31:101, 1980.

92. Pozniak MA et al: Current status of small bowel ultrasound, *Radiology* 30:597, 1990.

93. Rogers LF et al: Special report, *Radiology* 133:813, 1979.

94. Laws JW, Neale G: Radiological diagnosis of disaccharidase deficiency, *Lancet* 2:139, 1960.

95. Khilnani MT et al: Intramural intestinal haemorrhage, *AJR* 92:1061, 1964.

96. Nolan DJ: *Radiological atlas of gastrointestinal disease,* Chichester, 1983, John Wiley.

97. Mendelson RM, Nolan DJ: The radiological features of radiation enteritis, *Clin Radiol* 36:141, 1985.

98. Johnson RJ, Carrington BM: Pelvic radiation disease, *Clin Radiol* 45:4, 1992.

99. Moriarty KJ, Dawson AM: Functional abdominal pain: further evidence that the whole gut is affected, *Br Med J* 284:1670, 1982.

100. Corbet CL et al: Electrochemical detector for breath hydrogen determination: measurement of small bowel transit time in normal subjects and patients with the irritable bowel syndrome, *Gut* 22:836, 1981.

33 *Small Bowel Examination: Overview*

JOHN R. AMBERG

In considering the methods of examining the small bowel there is both good news and bad news. The good news is that disease in the small bowel is uncommon. This is particularly remarkable when one considers its length, a situation quite different from the one that prevails in the esophagus and rectum. The bad news is that it remains difficult to find these abnormalities when they occur.

Large randomized trials that compare the merits of the different methods of examining the small bowel have not been mounted. Because of the relative rarity of small bowel disease, it would take a long time to acquire significant data. This leaves us to consider the information contained in the preceding chapters prepared by practitioners who are expert in the small bowel examination, and to draw some conclusions from their work.

SMALL BOWEL FOLLOW-THROUGH METHOD

The conventional solid-column follow-through examination is still the most popular method for examining the small bowel and has been in use for many years. Despite some criticism, the method remains popular. Should we give it up? Does it give a false assurance? Has it endured only because there is so little small bowel disease? Reporting the small bowel as normal without actually examining it would lead to a remarkably high accuracy rate.

The small bowel follow-through examination has a number of things in its favor. The terminal ileum is often the site of an abnormality, and the routine method is adequate for studying this area. The addition of air to the colon (per-oral pneumocolon) produces a very good study of the ileocolic area. The ability of the conventional method to detect diffuse disease of the small bowel is satisfactory.

However, the conventional study falls short in the detection of localized disease, such as partially obstructive or nonobstructive neoplasia, Meckel's diverticula, and adhesions. It may be true that, with frequent fluoroscopy and filming, the accuracy of the follow-through examination can approach that of enteroclysis, as the more frequently the small bowel is examined, the closer the examination approaches enteroclysis. At times, rapid gastric emptying and strong small intestinal motility do produce images that rival those yielded by enteroclysis.

ENTEROCLYSIS WITH METHYLCELLULOSE

Enteroclysis, as developed by Maglinte, Herlinger, and Sellink, is an impressive technique. Dean Maglinte has been a hard-working practitioner of enteroclysis for many years, and his method reflects many refinements that were arrived at through trial and error. There is no absolute proof that all of these refinements are mandatory, however. For instance, I never use metoclopromide to aid passage of the tube, and it never seems to be needed. Besides that, I am a pharmacologic nihilist. It took me awhile to appreciate the need for an enteroclysis pump. Do not go without it if at all possible. I use peristaltic pumps discarded by the renal dialysis section. I do not measure the infusion rate, but instead watch the barium's progress through the small bowel, being careful that duodenogastric reflux is not occurring. I strongly believe the barium column should be watched *until* it reaches the colon. Although I would prefer to observe continuously during the entire procedure, this is poor radiation hygiene. Intermittent fluoroscopy does not mean that large gaps of time go by when the small bowel is not being observed. Enteroclysis, done sloppily and not according to the method described, contributes to diagnostic error. A well-done follow-through examination is preferable. It is not a passive radiographic-photo session but allows observation of small bowel dynamics.

Barium followed by the administration of methylcellulose is an appealing technique, in that it is a stress test of the small bowel. The large volume of the liquid facing a narrowed small bowel lumen presents a dramatic picture, and the narrowed area is accentuated as the proximal bowel dilates. It is usually impossible to duplicate this stress with the follow-through examination.

Recently I have found enteroclysis valuable in filling the Roux-en-Y jejunal loops created during jejunobiliary anastomoses (Figs 33-1 and 33-2). The ability to flood the small bowel with barium enhances reflux toward the biliary tract.

It is usually unnecessary to use enteroclysis to demonstrate diffuse small bowel disease. If a patient is known to have small bowel Crohn's disease, a regular small bowel follow-through study suffices. It permits accurate evaluation of the extent of disease, the sinus tracts, and fistulas.

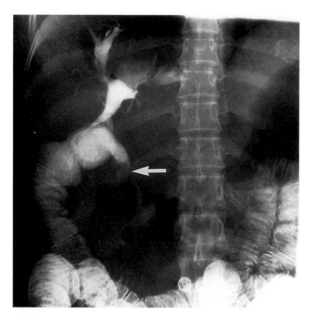

Fig. 33-1 Common duct stone (sump syndrome) visualized using enteroclysis in a patient with a Roux-en-Y choledochojejunostomy.

Maglinte has demonstrated the lack of yield from enteroclysis when it comes to finding bleeding sites in patients with end-stage renal disease.

ENTEROCLYSIS WITH AIR CONTRAST

Use of the air contrast technique in the performance of enteroclysis is interesting. It promises to make visualization of the small bowel mucosa comparable to that achieved for the colon. There is little argument over whether one can see small mucosal lesions better with the air contrast technique. Instead, the unsolved question is what patients would benefit from this approach. It might more accurately determine the extent of involvement in Crohn's disease. Currently it is not clear whether this knowledge would alter management. Its real benefit would be in finding abnormal areas missed with the other methods, but we need to know how often this occurs and in what clinical settings.

The argument against trying the barium-air technique is weak, when one realizes that Dr. Yao advocates watching the barium until it reaches the terminal ileum and then to add the air. After the air is introduced, glucagon or some other spasmolytic agent is given to paralyze the bowel. This allows evaluation of the small bowel that is comparable to that of the air contrast colon technique. Therefore it reaps all the benefits of the Maglinte technique plus superior mucosal visualization. This is the best method for showing mucosal detail of the small bowel.

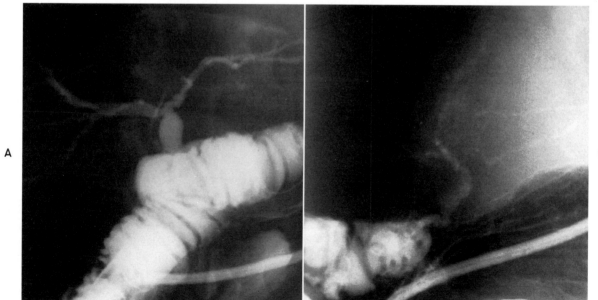

Fig. 33-2 A and **B,** Nonobstructed hepaticojejeunal anastomosis demonstrated using enteroclysis. This patient had episodes of fever following liver transplantation for primary sclerosing cholangitis.

GENERAL DISCUSSION

The usual indications for searching for an abnormality of the small bowel include the following:

1. Gastrointestinal bleeding unexplained after examination of the upper gastrointestinal tract and colon
2. A strong clinical suspicion of a partially obstructive small bowel process
3. Unexplained diarrhea
4. An abdominal mass, found by physical examination or one of the imaging methods, that is suspected to be in the small bowel

Given these indications, either primary enteroclysis or the follow-through method is an acceptable investigation.

When the findings yielded by the follow-through method are normal, I believe enteroclysis is then mandatory. Enteroclysis gives the best assurance that there is no lesion of the small bowel. This is the most frequent finding, and is important.

The enteroscope has not posed a serious challenge to the barium methods of examining the small intestine. Nevertheless, it is not wise to rest on our laurels. The various methods presented here should be part of the repertoire of all radiologists doing gastrointestinal examinations. The methods requiring intubation are not really difficult, and the lack of their more widespread use is appalling.

PART VII

COLON

34 *Normal Anatomy and Techniques of Examination of the Colon: Barium, CT, and MRI*

GILES W. STEVENSON

ANATOMY

The colon is attached to the posterior abdominal wall, either directly, as in the case of the ascending and descending colon, or indirectly by a mesentery (two leaves of peritoneum with enclosed fat, vessels, nerves, and lymphatics), as seen in the cecum, transverse colon, and sigmoid colon (Fig. 34-1).

The cecum usually lies in the right iliac fossa, inferior and anterior to the ascending colon, but its position can be quite variable because the entire ascending colon is not always fixed in a retroperitoneal manner. When the lower part of the small bowel mesentery extends to include the lower ascending colon, the cecum can move freely and may be found at different times low in the pelvis or upside down, high under the liver with the appendix above it. The appendix may normally contain air, which may be noted on computed tomographic (CT) scans. Fatty infiltration of the ileocecal valve is not rare, and both this and discrete lipomas of the colon can be confirmed when tissue with low attenuation is seen on CT scans.

Although the ascending colon usually has no mesocolon, both it and the descending colon may have one in 26% and 36% of cases, respectively.[1] These normally retroperitoneal portions of the colon pass anterolateral to the two kidneys (Fig. 34-2). However, when perirenal fat is deficient, as happens in some elderly women, the ascending and descending colon may be displaced lateral to the kidneys and may even lie behind them. Conversely, in some obese elderly men with abundant perirenal fat, these sections of colon may lie anteromedial to the kidney.[2] The unsuspected retrorenal position of the colon could thus pose a hazard during the performance of percutaneous diskectomy. One evaluation of 346 CT studies obtained with patients prone found only one patient with a retrorenal or retropsoas colon that might have been perforated at diskectomy, and

therefore routine pre-diskectomy prone CT was not recommended.[3] However, another study in which 1708 CT scans were evaluated revealed that the incidence ranged from 0.9 to 14%, depending on the vertebral level, with the highest figure found in women at the level of the lower calyces.[4]

The hepatic flexure has a fairly constant relationship to the liver and gallbladder, which can often be identified at colonoscopy. The transverse colon is attached to the posterior abdominal wall by the transverse mesocolon, which is extremely variable in length. The transverse colon may thus either run straight across the upper abdomen or dip deeply down into the pelvis.

The splenic flexure anatomically is formed at the point where the transverse mesocolon ceases and the descending colon becomes retroperitoneal. At this point the phrenicocolic ligament attaches the colon to the posterior lateral aspect of the left diaphragm. The radiologic and anatomic splenic flexures are, however, not the same. The highest point of the colon is actually in the transverse colon and quite mobile, so a tumor noted to be at the splenic flexure radiologically will be found in the left half of the transverse colon at surgery. Fixation of a short descending colon produces a transverse colon with a long and mobile left half, and this predisposes to the rare formation of a volvulus of the splenic flexure.

The sigmoid colon has a long mesentery and is variable in shape[5] (Fig. 34-3). These variations are relevant to the radiologist when performing a barium enema. About 60% of patients have a sigmoid loop, such that all the barium can be cleared from it during a double contrast barium enema (DCBE) by rotating the patient from the supine position to the left and into the prone position then back on the left side to the supine position, with variations in the de-

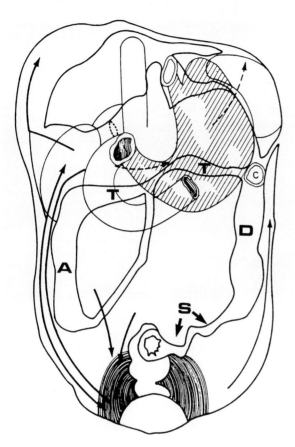

Fig. 34-1 Diagram of the pathways of flow of intraperitoneal exudates illustrates the posterior abdominal wall attachments of the ascending *(A)* and descending *(D)* colon, and of the sigmoid *(S)* and transverse *(T)* mesocolons.
From Churchill R, Meyers MA: Intraperitoneal fluid collections. In Myers MA, ed: *Computed tomography of the gastrointestinal tract,* New York, 1986, Springer Verlag.

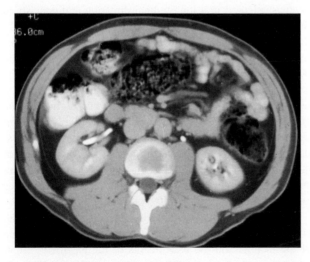

Fig. 34-2 CT scan shows the ascending colon filled with contrast and the descending colon filled with air and feces. Note the position anterolateral to the kidneys. The wall is more easily assessible against air than against dense contrast.

gree of head-up or head-down tilt (Fig. 34-4). However, more complex configurations occur, so one loop, or two sequential loops, may require turns to the right to clear them of barium puddles (Fig. 34-5).

The rectum starts in the midline at the level of the third sacral vertebra and follows the sacral curve, with the posterior mucosa not more than 1.5 cm from the bone except in the presence of disease or gross obesity. Anteriorly the peritoneal reflection forms the rectovesical pouch in males and the pouch of Douglas in females. The upper third of the rectum is covered with peritoneum laterally and anteriorly, and the middle third only anteriorly; the lower third

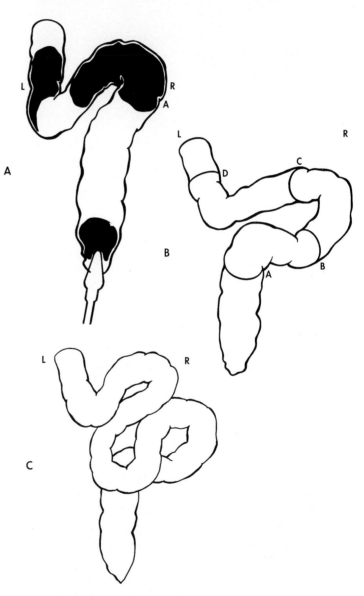

Fig. 34-3 Three configurations of the sigmoid colon. Almost 60% of patients have type A, from which barium puddles can be cleared without turning the patient on the right side. Types B and C require one or more turns to the right to achieve sigmoid clearing.
From Dobranowski J, Stringer DA, Somers S, Stevenson GW: *Procedures in gastrointestinal radiology,* New York, 1990, Springer Verlag.

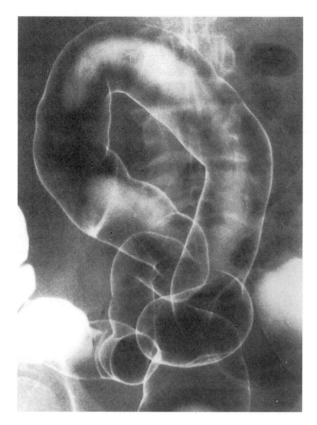

Fig. 34-4 This long but simple sigmoid loop has been completely cleared of barium puddles before the film was taken.

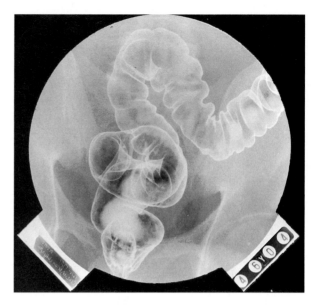

Fig. 34-5 A more complex sigmoid loop with almost complete clearing of barium puddles, although some remain in the rectum on this supine radiograph.

is subperitoneal. The rectum terminates in the anal canal, in which the external sphincter represents the continuation of the levator ani pelvic support muscles and the internal sphincter, the continuation of the muscularis propria of the rectum. These features can be shown well by endoscopic ultrasound (Chapter 48), as well as by CT and magnetic resonance imaging (MRI).

The vascular supply (Fig. 34-6) and major draining veins of the colon can be identified on CT sections in 87% to 100% of patients[6] (Fig. 34-7). The ileocolic artery is a late branch of the superior mesenteric and travels in the small bowel mesentery to supply the cecum. The right colic vessel crosses the retroperitoneum to supply the ascending colon. The middle colic artery arises early from the superior mesenteric and travels anteriorly in the transverse mesocolon to supply the transverse and much of the descending colon. The inferior mesenteric artery sends a branch to the left (the left colic), across the retroperitoneum, to supply the lower descending colon, and itself continues down and forward into the sigmoid mesocolon to supply the sigmoid. Its terminal branches continue distally along the rectosigmoid to anastomose with the inferior and middle hemor-

rhoidal arteries that arise from the pudendal and hypogastric arteries.

The wall of the colon contains the usual layers of serosa, muscularis, submucosa, and mucosa. A circular layer of the muscularis propria extends throughout the large bowel, and its thickness is even in all areas, except in the anal canal where it widens to form the internal anal sphincter. The orientation of its muscle fibers suggests that it is primarily responsible for the lumen-occluding contractions that regulate the flow of the luminal contents. A further muscular layer is oriented in a longitudinal direction and consists of three bundles called *taeniae*. At the colorectal junction, these broaden and fuse so that the rectum is evenly surrounded by longitudinal muscle. The taeniae are equidistant from each other and are located along the lines of the mesocolic insertions. They form longitudinal indentations, or folds, between which the walls of the colon bulge. The circular muscle layer is tonically contracted every few centimeters, and this indents the lumen and causes the formation of the haustral folds that produce saccular bulging of the bowel wall between the taeniae. The haustral folds are commonly seen in barium enema examinations, as well as on plain films and during ultrasound examination.

In the transverse colon there is a triangular shape to the colonic lumen, presumably due to the combined influence of the taeniae and the attachments of the gastrocolic ligament, the omentum, and the transverse mesocolon. This triangular shape is helpful during colonoscopy for indicating that the transverse colon has been entered. The haustra are less obvious in the sigmoid and are sometimes absent in the normal descending colon. The colon is widest in the cecum, and the caliber gradually decreases going toward the rectosigmoid, where it widens again as the rectum is entered. The ileocecal junction has a valve with two lips that project into the lumen of the cecum. It prevents reflux during a barium enema in over one half of the patients, but glucagon, given intravenously, will overcome this competence in all but about 25%.

The mucosa of the colon is usually covered by mucus, providing a smooth homogeneous surface. However, muscular spasm may transiently produce closely spaced circular folds. The surface may be nodular because of the prom-

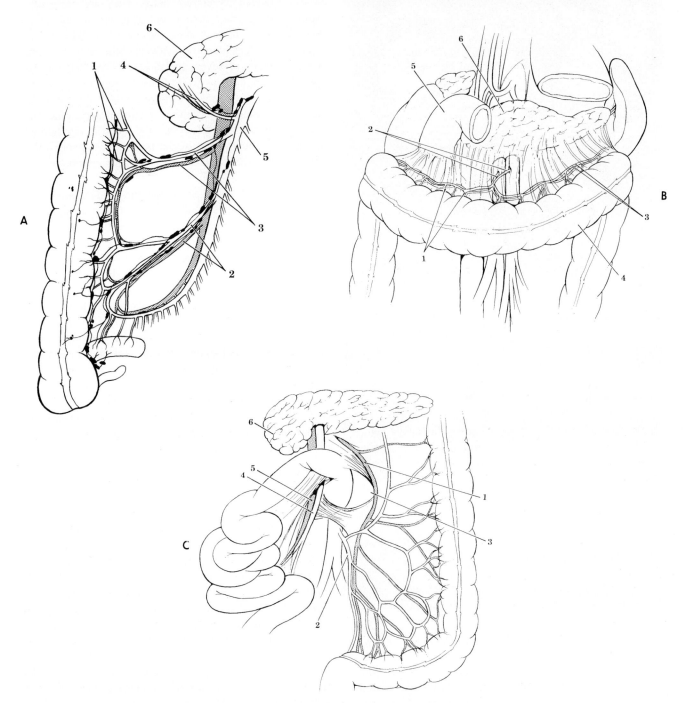

Fig. 34-6 A, The superior mesenteric artery (SMA) (*5*) and vein, with pancreaticoduodenal (*4*), right colic (*3*), and ileocolic (*2*), branches. **B,** The middle colic vessels (*2*) run anteriorly in the transverse mesocolon. **C,** The SMA and small bowel are retracted to the right to show the inferior mesentric artery (*2*) and vein (*1*) supplying the descending and sigmoid colon. Courtesy of Dr. Chusilp Charnsangavej.

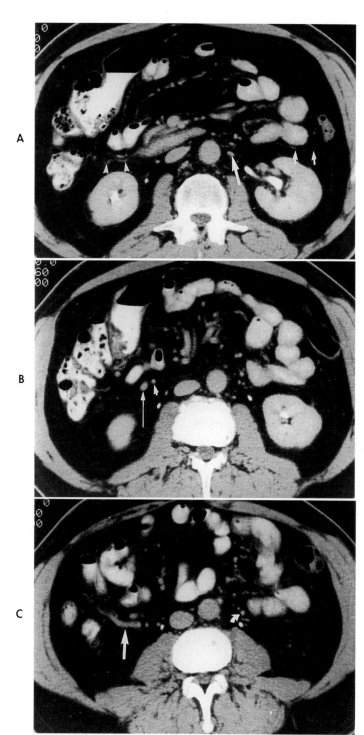

Fig. 34-7 A, The right colic vessels (*arrowheads*) cross the retroperitoneum. The inferior mesenteric artery (*large arrow*) and branches of the left colic (*small arrows*) are also shown. **B,** The ileocolic vein (*long arrow*) and artery (*short arrow*) can be seen in cross section. **C,** The terminal branch of the ileocolic is seen running along laterally (*long arrow*); also note the inferior mesentric artery (*curved arrow*).
Courtesy of Dr. Chusilp Charnsangavej.

inence of normal or enlarged lymphoid follicles, and, most rarely, the normal innominate grooves of the colon may be visible. These folds and their radiologic appearance have been described and explained over the past few years.[7-9] They are caused by thinning of the mucosa over the lymphoid follicles, and they form a fine network of lines, more or less arranged circumferentially. They are more often identified on barium enema studies in Japan than in the West. They can be seen at colonoscopy if a contrast agent is present, such as blood or methylene blue, and sometimes in the presence of severe melanosis. In this latter condition, they stand out as white lines because the mucosa is too thin over the grooves to become dark. In profile the grooves occasionally assume a spiculated appearance. Finally, in the presence of spasm, the mucosa may herniate transiently through the muscular layers, presumably alongside the vasa recta vessels, to produce transient diverticula[10] (see Fig. 3-19).

MRI is now being used to examine the anatomy of the anorectum, both at rest and dynamically during squeezing and straining maneuvers.[11] It has the advantage of multiplanar imaging, with the sagittal and coronal planes both being useful for this purpose. It also shows, better than defecography, the range of movement of the posterior rectal wall (using the posterior end of the plica of Kohlrausch or Houston's valve as a landmark), thereby permitting a reliable assessment of rectal descent on straining. However, many abnormalities on defecography are seen only during the actual process of straining during defecation. Nevertheless, it appears that measurements of the position, angle, and movement of the anorectal junction can be made with less inter- and intraobserver variation during an MRI examination with the patient prone than that possible with defecography, with the added advantages of no radiation and no need for vaginal opacification.

TECHNIQUES OF EXAMINATION

The history of alimentary tract radiology is discussed in Chapter 1. The past three decades have witnessed a resurgence in the popularity and accuracy of the DCBE, which has occurred simultaneous with the dramatic advances in endoscopy. With a few notable exceptions, the single contrast barium enema is no longer advocated as a routine examination for the colon. However, it remains the examination of choice in the very young, the very old, the seriously ill, and the very disabled.[12]

For most patients with large bowel symptoms who require investigation, the first imaging study may be a barium enema, flexible sigmoidoscopy, or colonoscopy. Although the total number of barium enemas has declined by 10% to 30% since 1982, large numbers of patients still receive barium enema examinations.[12,13] The well-performed examination is very accurate. A number of variations to the barium enema study exist and are described later in this chapter. Colonoscopy is also an accurate examination that has the added advantage of permitting biopsy and polypectomy. However, it has the disadvantages of greater price, a higher rate of complications, and less frequent complete examination of the cecum.

In the past decade CT has been well described as a method of examining the colon,[14,15] and is becoming the preferred examination in some clinical situations, such as for assessing acute diverticulitis and for staging rectal carcinoma, when this is necessary clinically. It can also play a major role in the management of complicated inflammatory bowel disease.

Ultrasound and MRI are both gaining importance in the assessment of patients with colorectal disease, but their roles are not yet well defined.

In the rest of this chapter, some of the technical aspects of these various imaging examinations of the colon are discussed. One of the challenges for radiologists and gastroenterologists is to revise their practices as the indications for each method of examination evolve and to integrate the use of the various techniques.

Radiographic contrast examinations

There are many methods and variations of each method for examining the colon, and no one "right way." Radiology residents should try out, and master, the techniques preferred in their own training hospital. They should then try out the variations described in the next few pages, as well as others described in the literature, before deciding on a routine method. Having settled on this routine method, the only certainty is then that it will require modification and improvement as the specialty makes more progress.

Equipment

There is great variation in the choice of equipment in different countries. Image intensifiers and television sets are now routine. In the United States 90% of the examination tables are "conventional," with an undercouch tube and overcouch intensifier. In Japan, over 90% of the examination tables are "remote" and have an overcouch tube. In Canada and Europe, the distribution is about half and half, although with some national variations. The remote units provide greater exposure to a table-side radiologist for doing interventional work but less exposure to the radiologist working from the safety of the control area. For the protection of the technologists, it is useful if they wear an audible radiation monitor or "chirper" while working in the room.

The radiographic images obtained with remote units are better, but those acquired with conventional ones are usually more than adequate. Excellent results are achieved with both types, and the choice comes down to personal preference. An exciting new development is the advent of digital technology in the fluoroscopy suite, together with work stations located outside the fluoroscopy room and connection to laser cameras. The initial impression is that these digital units allow greater patient throughput, with reduced radiation exposure to patients, and that the increased costs of the unit may be recouped by the reduction in film use.

Preliminaries

Some authors regard a preliminary abdominal radiograph, before starting a barium enema procedure, as an indispensable part of the procedure[16]; others suggest that it may be dispensed with,[17] unless there are concerns about an acute abdominal condition. It is not very useful in judging whether the bowel preparation has been successful. The author has abandoned it.

PREPARATION

Residual solid material (Fig. 34-8) interferes with the detection of polyps, cancers, and inflammation, and, conversely, may be mistaken for a neoplasm. Residual fluid dilutes the barium and diminishes the quality of the mucosal coating so that surface irregularities become more difficult or impossible to detect. Bowel preparation is therefore essential to ensure satisfactory imaging. The three components of preparation are dietary (and medication) restriction, initial removal of most solid material by a laxative, and final removal of smaller particles by liquid flushing, which may be administered orally or by enema.[17] There is such variation in the amount of stool in the human colon, and in its adherence to the mucosa, that a preparation that is 100% successful will be unnecessarily harsh for most patients. A strategy may therefore be adopted that produces an optimally clean colon in not less than 95% of the patients; the 5% that fail this approach should routinely be rescheduled for another examination.

Dietary restriction. One or two days of a restricted diet will reduce the amount of stool in the right colon in all but the most constipated of patients. In one approach, meat, fruit, and vegetables are avoided on the first day, with a high fluid intake. On the second day, only fluids are permitted. Miller[18] recommended 8 ounces (240 ml) of clear fluids taken on an hourly basis to a total of not less than 2 liters. On the day of the barium enema, only a single drink is permitted before the examination. Iron-containing medications are stopped two days before, as they make stool adhere to the mucosa.

Cathartics. Cathartics fall into two main groups: saline cathartics, which produce an osmotic load to suck fluid into the intestines (e.g., magnesium citrate and sodium phosphate), and irritant cathartics, which damage the small bowel mucosa and elicit increased peristalsis (e.g., castor oil and bisacodyl). Gelfand et al.[19] recommend a combination of the two. During the time that they are drinking 240 ml of water (a full glass) hourly, patients are given 300 ml of magnesium citrate at 4:00 P.M. and 60 ml of castor oil at 8:00 P.M. In Britain over the past decade, one preparation (Picolax) has gained widespread popularity; it is a mixture of magnesium citrate and sodium picosulfate.[17,20]

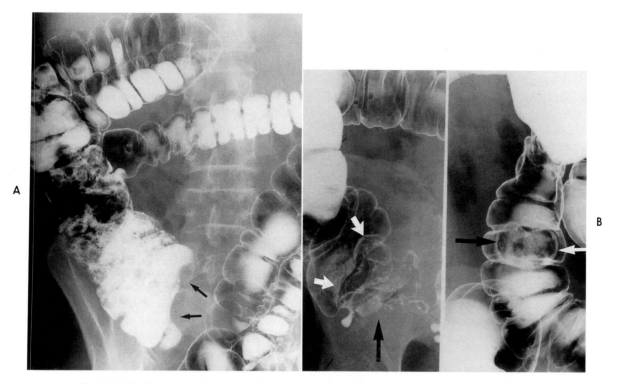

Fig. 34-8 The first barium enema in this patient (**A**) was reported to show no definite abnormality. A concavity in the lower pole of the cecum was misinterpreted *(arrow)*, and a second large tumor was hidden in retained stool in the ascending colon. **B,** After 9 months, and further anemia, the patient was referred to another institution, where the cecal and ascending colon carcinomas were found *(arrows).*
From Stevenson GW: *Cancer* 71(suppl):4198, 1993.

Final removal of small particles. Although many radiologists use the methods just described as the sole preparation, a completely clean colon is still not usually obtained, and this is the cause of a moderate failure rate, especially in the elderly. However, the colon is moderately dry, and good coating is obtained in the right colon in most patients. These preparations are acceptable only if attention is paid to detail, including the dietary restrictions and the large volumes of fluid to be consumed. Those 10% to 20% of the patients with failed preparation are rescheduled for further cleansing and reexamination.

To obtain a completely clean colon so that success rates over 95% can be achieved requires the final removal of fecal material, either by using a cleansing water enema[17,19] or by oral lavage.[21-23]

The cleansing enema should be administered in the radiology department using 1.5 or 2.0 liters of warm tap water administered slowly. The patient lies on the left side while receiving the first 500 ml, prone for the second 500 ml, and on the right side for the third 500 ml. At least 30 minutes should be allowed for evacuation, and preferably 60, especially if a DCBE study is to be performed. Lee and Bartram[24] recommend a minimum of 45 minutes.

If an oral flush is used, one of the polyethylene glycol

(PEG) mixtures is suitable and has the advantage of being satisfactory for colonoscopic, radiologic, and preoperative preparation. For a barium enema, the full 4 liters is consumed the evening before the examination, after the dietary restrictions have been observed and a contact laxative taken. For colonoscopy, the PEG is drunk on the morning of the examination to produce a sparkling clean, but very wet, bowel. If the PEG has been drunk the evening before colonoscopy, a surprising amount of mucus will be encountered in the right colon. This mucus does not appear to pose a problem for barium enema, and is presumably washed off and dissolved by the barium suspension.

There is no question that a water enema or orally administered PEG produces a wetter right colon than do oral cathartics alone, but there is less fecal residue. Sufficient time must be allowed to elapse between the colonic flush and the barium enema, and a sufficient quantity of barium must have flowed into the right colon to absorb any residual fluid and still produce good coating.

There is no convincing evidence as to which is the best preparation method, and the range of practice is wide.[12] However, there are certain basic principles that have been agreed upon, and the subject has been well reviewed by Gelfand and by Simpkins.[17,19] Both of these authors recommend a cleansing enema performed in the radiology department as the final component of bowel cleansing. Neither accepts that the simple laxative preparation is adequate for routine use, and generally the literature agrees with their contention.[25-29] The onus is on all radiologists to be able to document that their chosen technique is effective. A simple method[19] for doing this is to conduct regular quarterly reviews of 20 consecutive barium enemas: "If more than one or two examinations show any fecal material at all, the regimen should be changed, probably by instituting use of cleansing enemas." Similarly, those practitioners who make use of PEG or cleansing enemas should periodically review the adequacy of coating in the right colon.

Many attempts have been made to find a substitute for the cleansing enema. Only the oral PEG solutions have met the goals, and they prepare the bowel as well as the cathartic plus cleansing enema regimens, at a lower cost and at less inconvenience to the radiology department.[21-23] However, although they have become the standard preparation for colonoscopy, they have not gained widespread acceptance for use in the barium enemas. This is probably because of a perception that they produce an unacceptably wet colon with impaired coating, although this poses no more of a problem than do cleansing enemas[23] (Fig. 34-9). If facility constraints make it impossible to perform cleansing enemas, the alternatives are to use PEG, or to be willing to

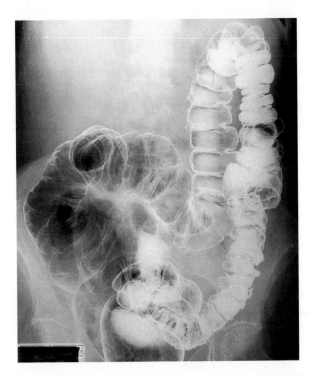

Fig. 34-9 Several technical errors can be seen here. The coating in the right colon is poor because not enough barium has been run into the right side to "mop up" the washout fluid, and the left colon is suboptimally distended because there is slight spasm and a relaxant has not been given.

stop examinations when significant stool is encountered and to repeat examinations when fecal residue is noted on films. To minimize the need for this in patients who are undergoing studies in departments not using a fluid cleansing method, the period of dietary restriction before the enema study should be lengthened to the limits of compliance, which, however, is unlikely to be more than 2 days.

It is not always possible to have 2 days for preparation, especially for inpatients, in whom a preparation that works in a few hours is often desirable. In this event, either oral PEG or cleansing enemas are absolutely necessary, after the usual laxatives have been given. If such facilities are not readily available in the department, the cleansing water enema can be administered on the fluoroscopic table.[19] Cleansing enemas performed on the ward are seldom adequate, as the nursing staff do not always have either the appropriate training that is necessary or the same vested interest in the final product—the radiograph. The oral PEG preparation is particularly useful before colonoscopy, which is being performed to investigate acute rectal bleeding, because the blood is all washed distally. It also allows the colonoscopist to determine at what point the area of bleeding has been passed, when clear yellow fluid is encountered.

REQUISITION FORM

The requisition form is a request for consultation from one health professional to another, and, in some jurisdictions, such a form signed by a physician is also a legal requirement before an x-ray examination can be performed. It is very much in the patient's best interest that a request form contain all relevant clinical information. This should include the question that is to be answered by the examination, any condition that is to be excluded, the likely clinical diagnosis, significant symptoms and signs, and description of any other conditions that may affect the conduct of the examination, the differential diagnosis, and ultimately the content of the report. Incomplete forms are not only a discourtesy to the radiologist, but, more important, they are also a discourtesy to the patient, lowering the quality of patient care. It is for this latter reason that radiologists should continue to insist throughout their careers on raising the standards of communication between themselves and the referring physicians. There are many strategies to adopt in pursuing this end, such as refusing to accept telephone bookings from problem practices and clinics, but to accept only properly completed faxed requisitions.

CONTRAST AGENTS

Barium. The major manufacturers now produce excellent-quality barium products that resist considerable dilution without flocculating, while maintaining their coating abilities. For DCBE studies, a high-density product of around 75% to 95% weight per volume (w/v) is preferred; for single-contrast enemas, a much lower density of between

15% to 20% w/v is required to promote a see-through effect with a high KV and compression. When choosing between rapid- and slow-flowing products for use in barium enemas, the slower-flowing (usually high-density) ones should be used by those radiologists who use colon-cleansing enemas or a PEG preparation, as they are likely to better withstand dilution. Products should not be diluted to achieve faster flow and save expense, as the coating properties will be destroyed.

Water-soluble contrast agents. Barium is dangerous in the peritoneum and passes slowly through the obstructed intestine. Hyperosmolar water-soluble contrast agents can absorb water and become dilute, safely demonstrate fistulas and sinus tracks, and pass rapidly through the intestine. This explains both the main indications and the risks associated with the use of Gastrografin (meglumine diatrizoate). It, or similar products, should be used as an enema whenever a leak from the colon to the peritoneum is suspected, such as in diverticulitis, perforated carcinoma, leaking anastomosis, and abdominal stab wounds communicating with the colon.[30] CT may now constitute a better initial approach to imaging the first two problems, and a diluted water-soluble contrast should be given first. Therapeutic water-soluble contrast enemas are discussed later.

The hyperosmolar nature of Gastrografin may provoke severe dehydration, shock, and death in hypovolemic infants, sick children, the very old, and the very ill. Therefore, the fluid and electrolyte status of such patients should be checked and monitored before the oral administration of this agent. Often, the decision will be made to use one of the nonionic agents. They are safer, and, because they do not become diluted, the images are often superior. This is discussed in more detail in the pediatric chapters.

Gas. Room air has been used traditionally for DCBEs. However, it has been clearly established that carbon dioxide works as well and is associated with much less pain after the procedure.[31] Coblentz et al.[31] found that 30% of the patients who underwent barium enema with room air experienced clinically significant pain, compared with only 11% of those in whom carbon dioxide was used; 74% of the patients reported no pain after carbon dioxide use and 38% after room air studies. No patient complained of very severe pain after carbon dioxide had been used, but 7% did so after the use of air. Similar dramatic differences have been noted with colonoscopy[32-35] (Table 34-1). Various

□ **TABLE 34-1**

Percentage of patients with and without pain after colonoscopy*

Grade†	During		6 hours postoperatively		24 hours postoperatively	
	Air	CO₂	Air	CO₂	Air	CO₂
0	26	17	50	97	56	95
1	22	25	32	3	24	—
2	22	21	7	—	8	—
3	19	29	11	—	12	5
4	11	8				
	$\chi^2 = 1.27$ NS		$\chi^2 = 17.6$ $p < 0.0005$		$\chi^2 = 12.35$ $p < 0.01$	

Comparing grade 0 (no pain) with all other grades:

	$\chi^2 = 0.64$ NS	$\chi^2 = 17.5$ $p < 0.0001$	$\chi^2 = 8.64$ $p = 0.003$

NS, not significant.

*Results were obtained by a patient questionnaire that was administered 1 hour after, 6 hours after, and 24 hours after colonoscopy, documenting the patient's perception of pain experienced during and after the procedure.

†*0*, None; *1*, mild; *2*, moderate; *3*, severe; *4*, extreme.

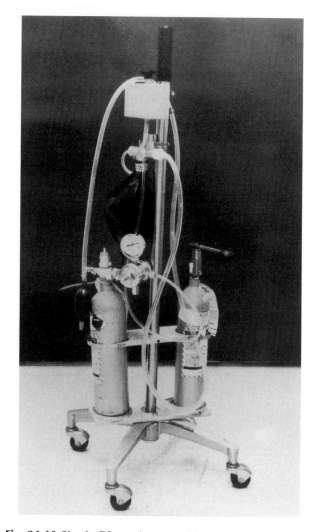

Fig. 34-10 Simple CO_2 equipment, with reducing valve and anesthetic bag for storing CO_2. Alternatively, several barium bags can be filled with CO_2 and used as a source of CO_2 for patients on the morning schedule.

simple devices have been devised for administering the carbon dioxide[36-39] (Fig. 34-10), and their cost is trivial. There is really little reason to continue using room air for these procedures, when carbon dioxide is so easy to use, so inexpensive, and so much more comfortable for the patients.

CONTRAINDICATIONS

Contraindications to performing a barium enema include suspected perforation, peritonitis, severe acute inflammatory bowel disease, toxic megacolon, and recent rectal biopsy using large forceps, such as that carried out during rigid sigmoidoscopy. In addition, the single-contrast examination is not indicated when searching for inflammatory bowel disease in mobile patients, nor as a primary examination in patients with either a history of rectal bleeding or a history or family history of polyps or colorectal cancer. The double-contrast examination is relatively contraindicated in infants, patients with limited mobility, or acute diverticulitis (CT is better for this purpose), or when looking for fistulas.

ADJUVANT DRUGS

Atropine, administered sublingually before a barium enema, used to be advocated to help dry out the colon and improve coating.[40] Although this is seldom done anymore, there have been no good studies that assess the merits of this or related approaches. The drug might work well after water-cleansing enemas, but less so after flushing with the nonabsorbable oral PEG solutions.

Both glucagon[41-44] and Buscopan[45] are used to relax the colon (Fig. 34-11). In 1987, 90% of centers were found to use some pharmacologic aids, and 83% of these used glucagon.[12] (Buscopan is currently unavailable in the United States.) Some centers routinely use relaxants to make the patient more comfortable, and thereby improve the quality of the films, while others give them only if spasm is seen (Fig. 34-12).

Glucagon is contraindicated in patients with pheochromocytomas and insulinomas, and very rarely there could be an anaphylactic reaction to the foreign protein. In addition, minor side effects are dose related, and are rare when the dose does not exceed 0.5 mg.[46] Buscopan (20 mg) causes dry mouth in most subjects, and blurred near vision on accommodation for 10 to 20 minutes in about 10% of the patients. It also causes tachycardia, and might cause hypertension in subjects taking beta-blockers. Glucagon should probably be used instead in patients taking beta-blockers, those on cardiac medication, and those who are suffering from heart failure or who have had a recent myocardial infarction. It could, in theory, precipitate an acute attack of glaucoma in patients with early closed-angle glaucoma. In general, it is sufficient to ask patients whether they have had any problem with their eyes, such as glaucoma, or any cardiac problem, and to use the more expensive glucagon when the answer to either question is "yes."

One other diagnostic application for glucagon (or Buscopan) in the colon is of interest. Radiologists have noted for years that some people have more spasm than others during barium enema study and also that some people experience more pain than others despite apparently similar spasm depicted on fluoroscopy. Ritsema and Thijn[47] examined 15 patients with irritable bowel syndrome (IBS) and 15 controls, both radiologically and manometrically, in a blinded prospective manner. Both groups exhibited sigmoid contractions, but there was no associated pain in the 15 controls and 2 patients with IBS, whereas 13 of the patients

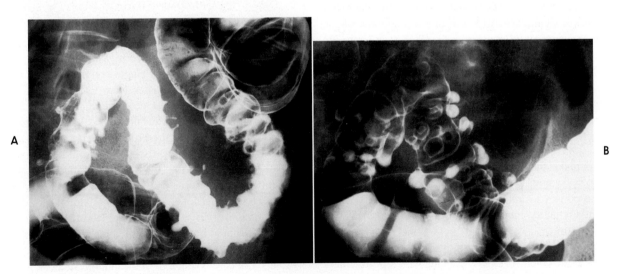

Fig. 34-11 The first film **(A)** shows poor distention and narrow necks to the diverticula due to some spasm. After the intravenous administration of Buscopan **(B),** the colon relaxes and mucosal detail is more easily examined.

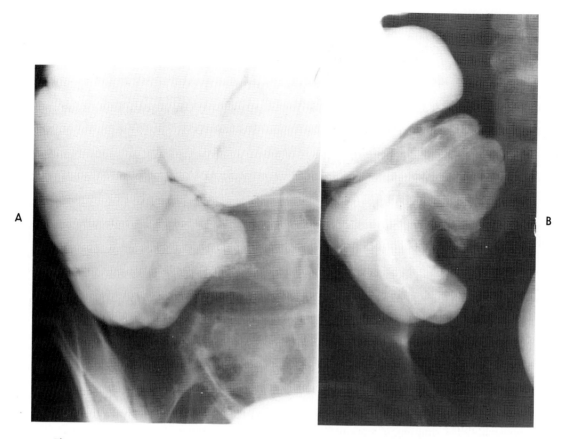

Fig. 34-12 A, It is occasionally difficult, particularly during fluoroscopic examination, to be sure that the cecum has been filled. Unless the appendix, terminal ileum, or ileocecal valve are positively identified, the examiner cannot assume that the cecum has been filled. **B,** Following intravenous administration of 1 ml glucagon, the cecum is visualized. There is no filling of the appendix; instead, there is an impression on the tip of the cecum caused by a periappendiceal abscess following perforation of appendix.

with IBS had pain at the time of the contractions. Both the pain and the contractions were relieved by glucagon. There was a significant difference in the amplitude of the painful and nonpainful contractions—28.2 ± 4.3 mm Hg and 12.3 ± 1.4 mm Hg, respectively ($p < 0.001$). This is an interesting study that merits confirmation. It has been traditional to make the diagnosis of IBS based on clinical findings and to use the barium enema in the expectation that a negative result is in keeping with the diagnosis of IBS. It appears as though a positive diagnosis of IBS may be possible in some patients by assessing their response to glucagon. To make the study more useful, a provocative test would be of value, as well as information on the specificity of responses to glucagon or provocative agents, since acute inflammatory conditions may also be associated with painful spasm.

In patients with inflammatory bowel disease or infection adjacent to the colon, in elderly patients with repeated mass action movements, or in the presence of severe spasm (Fig. 34-13) it may be essential to administer glucagon or Buscopan to achieve a diagnostically useful study.

ENEMA TIPS AND ADMINISTRATION SETS

Commercial enema tips are available with a medium (⅜-inch; 1 cm)-sized lumen, as well as the larger (half-inch; 1.25 cm)-bore air tips designed by Miller (Fig. 34-14). The smaller one is adequate for single-contrast studies, and the larger one promotes a faster flow for the more viscous double-contrast barium but costs more. They may be used with or without inflatable cuffs. The best way to judge whether an inflatable cuff is required is, as described by Stewart,[48] for the radiologist to perform a rectal examination just before inserting the tube. This detects any unusual anatomy and the occasional rectal tumor and allows an estimation of rectal tone. If there is any doubt raised by the rectal examination, then an inflatable cuff should be used. The cuff should be used with the manufacturer's inflater to avoid overinflation of the cuff, which can cause perforation. Extra care is required in the elderly, in those who have undergone pelvic irradiation, and in those who have had rectal inflammatory bowel disease or tumors. The air tube can be attached to a puffer for room air, to a puffer attached

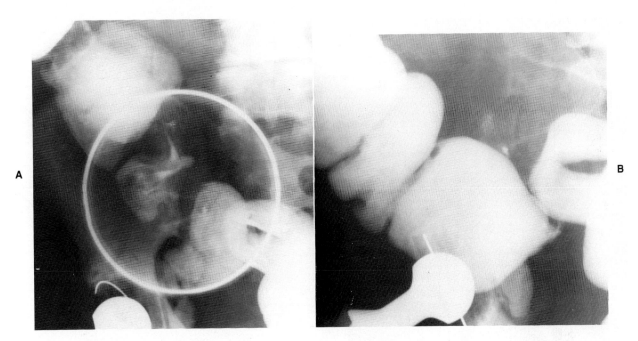

Fig. 34-13 A, Spastic cecum simulates a constricting lesion. **B,** Following the intravenous administration of 1 ml of glucagon, the cecum is distended.

to a pressure reduction device for carbon dioxide, as described by Coblentz, or to a puffer attached to another barium bag that has been prefilled with carbon dioxide instead of barium.

Single-contrast barium enema

The single-contrast barium enema is essentially a fluoroscopic examination in which, with the exception of the film obtained after evacuation, the radiographs simply record what has already been diagnosed. It really requires a radiologist at the table side because palpation and compression are integral. The barium is introduced slowly with the patient in the left lateral position, and the rectum and sigmoid are examined carefully as the contrast runs through them and before they have distended. Polyps may be seen well at this point, and the first film may be taken when the head of the column has just passed through the relatively underfilled sigmoid. Palpation and compression of each segment are performed as it fills, either using the lead glove or a compression device such as the Mayo spoon, the F spoon, or a balloon compression paddle (see Fig. 26-10). Spot radiographs of the uncoiled sigmoid, the two flexures, and the compressed cecum are usually obtained. Compression of the cecum is essential, as Miller has shown that a polyp 1 cm in diameter in a 10-cm-diameter cecum cannot be detected by any combination of barium density and KV. When the cecum or the flexures are inaccessible to palpation, this somewhat limits the ability of the single-contrast examination to detect small tumors. The rectum cannot be reliably examined by the technique. Overhead films are routinely taken, usually prone, supine, and posterior oblique films for

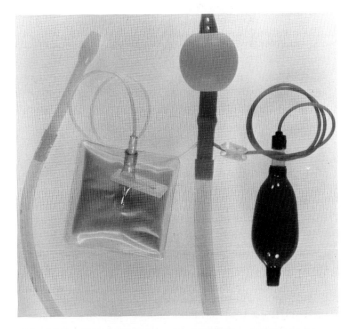

Fig. 34-14 *Left,* Plastic enema tip connected to wide-bore tubing. *Right,* Modern safe apparatus for the administration of a double-contrast enema. Bag with foam rubber cannot overinflate balloon. Inflation bulb connected to tubing is used to insufflate air after barium has been administered.

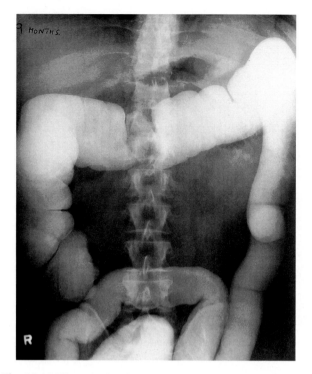

Fig. 34-15 Nine months after resection of a transverse colon carcinoma, this patient was found at colonoscopy to have an anastomotic recurrence, but the rest of the colon was clear. The surgeon wanted to visualize the amount of remaining colon in order to plan surgery. This single-contrast enema took 5 minutes and was adequate to answer the clinical question at hand, with little discomfort to the patient and minimal irradiation.

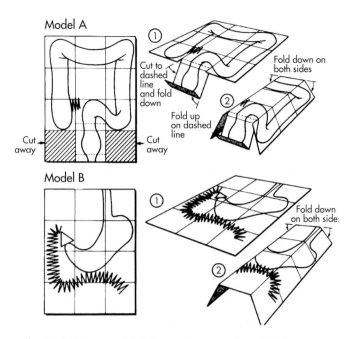

Fig. 34-16 Paper models illustrate the three-dimensional anatomy of the upper and lower GI tracts.
From Munro TG: *J Can Assoc Radiol* 40:162, 1989.

the flexures, a lateral film of the rectum, a prone-angled view of the sigmoid, and a postevacuation film. The last one is useful for occasionally showing small polypoid lesions and for showing mucosal edema in the presence of inflammatory bowel disease, although it is not as accurate for this purpose as double-contrast mucosal films.

The single-contrast examination can be quick and is not as arduous for patients as the double-contrast enema (Fig. 34-15). Although careful fluoroscopy is essential, not all authors totally rely on it. Gelfand,[49] for example, believes the first principle of the full-column enema to be ensuring that every portion of the column is radiographed in such a way as to be free of superimposition by other loops. He further recommends that it is desirable for each segment to be visible on two films so that any lesion suspected on one film can be confirmed on another.

Sometimes a complete colonic obstruction may be found on a single-contrast barium enema, without demonstrating the extent of the stricture. It is standard not to administer barium from above in this situation because of the risk of producing a complete clinical obstruction with inspissation of the barium.[50,51] It has been shown that water-soluble contrast may be safely administered after a complete obstruction has been revealed by a barium enema,[52] and also, in an experimental setting, that oral barium passes safely through a partial colonic obstruction in dogs.[53] More recently, Gotta et al.[54] have shown that it is safe to give barium orally after a DCBE has shown complete obstruction of the colon, and that the resulting films are helpful clinically in revealing additional lesions as well as in better characterizing the nature of the obstruction.[54] These investigators suggest three important criteria be met before oral barium is given: (1) no clinical signs or symptoms of mechanical obstruction; (2) upright and decubitus films showing no signs of obstruction; and (3) the colon preparation has been both well tolerated and effective.

Double-contrast barium enema

There are many different approaches to performing the barium enema, and they may be divided into those that are simple and those that are complex. The author prefers the complex as a normal routine, with attempts to sequentially clear barium puddles from all segments of the sigmoid. The method described first is a simple one that is appropriate to be learned as the initial technique by a radiology resident.

Once it has been mastered, the resident should try out the various simplified and complex methods described in the literature to develop an armamentarium of skills for dealing with the different problems that may arise and to arrive at a method that works well with an acceptable amount of effort on the part of both the patient and examiner. With patients of differing ages and physical stamina, varying examination goals dictated by different symptoms, and some patients having had sigmoidoscopy and others not, a variety of techniques will be required. An understanding of the three-dimensional anatomy is important, and a very simple cardboard model of it may be constructed (Fig. 34-16) that helps the neophyte to comprehend the three-dimensional principles involved in turning and positioning the patient during double-contrast examinations.[55]

BASIC COMPREHENSIVE TECHNIQUE

The routine examination should be started with the patient prone, and barium is introduced slowly until the head of the column reaches the mid transverse colon. This may take 500 to 600 ml of barium. Glucagon or Buscopan is given intravenously at the first sign of persistent spasm or poor distensibility. The head of the table is elevated 30 degrees, the barium bag is placed on the floor, and the rectum is then drained. The table is then placed flat, and gas (preferably carbon dioxide) is puffed in with slow squeezes of the puffer. Once air reaches the splenic flexure, the patient is turned onto the right side. As more air is introduced, the barium runs down into the right colon. Spot films are taken of the rectum and sigmoid (Fig. 34-17), usually a lateral, a prone, prone left-side-up oblique, and supine right-

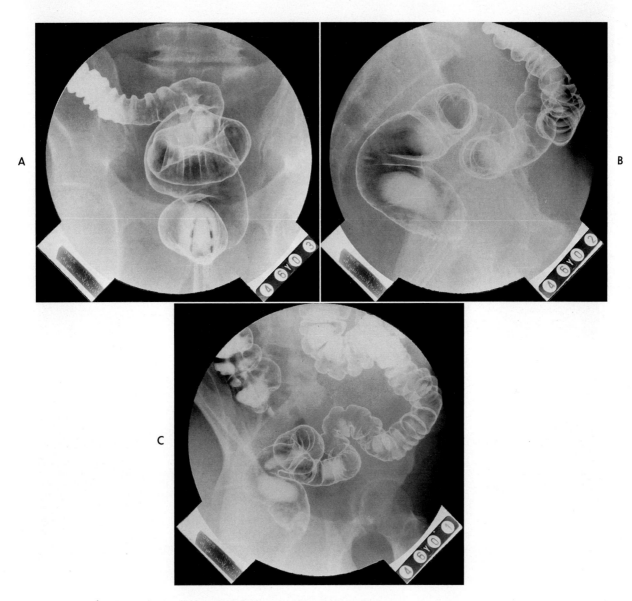

Fig. 34-17 Prone **(A)**, lateral **(B)**, and supine-oblique **(C)** double-contrast spot films of the sigmoid colon.

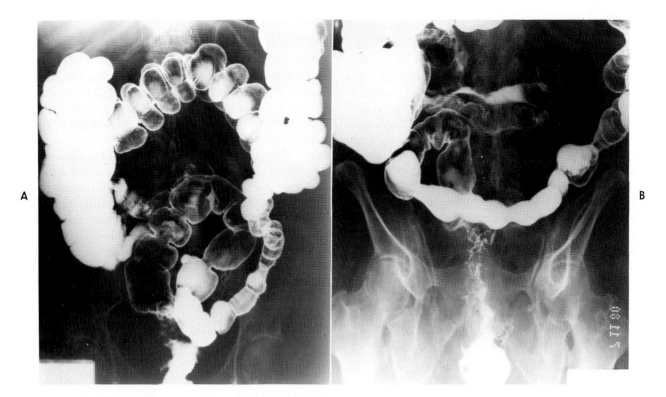

Fig. 34-18 A, Carcinoma of the rectosigmoid is not seen well. **B,** Lesion is well seen on an angled view.

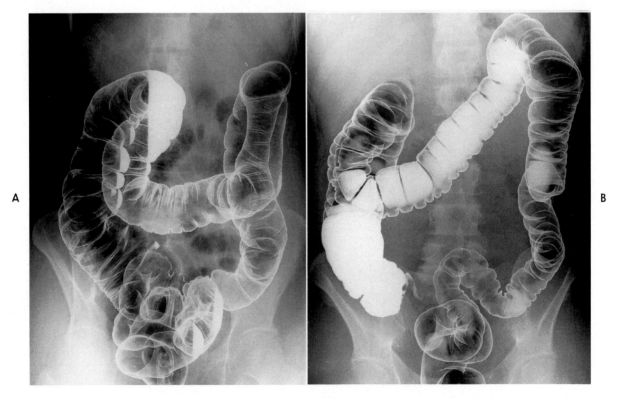

Fig. 34-19 Right-side-up decubitus **(A)** and prone **(B)** films showing the degree of distention and relaxation required.

side-up oblique view. For longer sigmoid colons, a supine left-side-up oblique film is also obtained. After this, the table is tipped upright so that barium can fill the cecum and then placed flat again. The patient is rotated completely twice, and enough gas is introduced to adequately distend the whole colon. Five overhead films are taken: a prone view, a 30-degree prone-angled film of the sigmoid (Fig. 34-18), plus a supine and both lateral decubitus films (Fig. 34-19). A sixth, a cross-table lateral view of the rectum, is added by some (Fig. 34-20). Apart from the decubitus film, all are taken by the radiologist in a remote room and by the technologist in a conventional room. The radiologist reviews the films as they come out of the processor, and then takes three more double-contrast spot films—of the two flexures with the patient erect and of the cecum with the patient usually supine oblique. Finally, a spot film of the rectum is obtained immediately after the rectal tube is removed (Fig. 34-21).

The spot films of the flexures and cecum (Fig. 34-22) may be taken before the overhead views, but coating is better if they are delayed. This also affords more opportunity for the first films to be reviewed to determine whether any areas need checking. It is important to obtain enough films to show all areas of the colon in double contrast in two projections.[56-58]

VARIATIONS

Simplified methods include the seven-step method originally outlined by Miller and Maglinte,[59] in which barium and air are introduced without fluoroscopy following a prescribed series of turns. This displays the colon well in a moderate proportion of patients, but, in many cases, further maneuvering is needed to fill the right colon.

An even simpler method that works very well has been described by Gelfand and Ott,[60] and makes the double-contrast enema procedure less arduous than most single-contrast examinations. With the patient prone and holding onto handles at the head of the table, and following the injection of glucagon (0.5 mg intravenously), the barium is introduced with the table tipped 15 to 20 degrees head down, until the barium reaches the distal transverse colon. Thirty pumps of air are next administered with a bulb type of puffer. The table head is then elevated, and the rectum and distal colon are drained of barium. The table is placed horizontally, and an additional 30 puffs of air are given. Fluoroscopy is used briefly to check that the entire colon is distended and that there is plenty of barium in the transverse colon. The enema tip is removed, and radiography is started. The first movement of the patient *must* be onto the right side and then onto the back so that all the barium in the transverse colon runs into the ascending colon. The initial films of the rectum and sigmoid are obtained during this maneuver. Provided a full range of films is taken, this technique yields excellent results. Sixty puffs of air are not always needed, or tolerated. In the author's experience, the intravenous relaxant is an important component of this technique, as air evacuated due to spasm cannot easily be replaced. Several rotations of the patient, after the cecum has been filled, considerably improves the coating. This simplified approach makes the double-contrast enema possible in many patients who could not tolerate the more complex

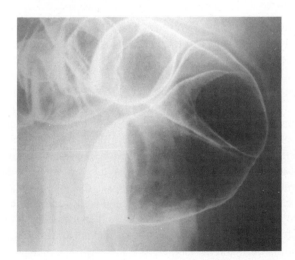

Fig. 34-20 Cross-table lateral film of rectum with double-contrast technique.

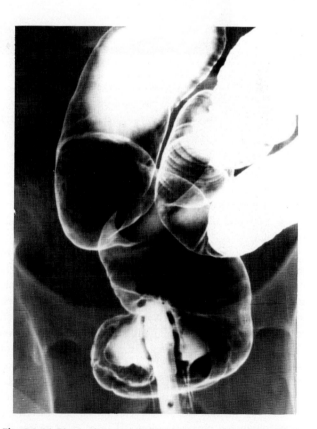

Fig. 34-21 Plastic tip remaining in the rectum distended with the double-contrast technique is obscuring rectal carcinoma.

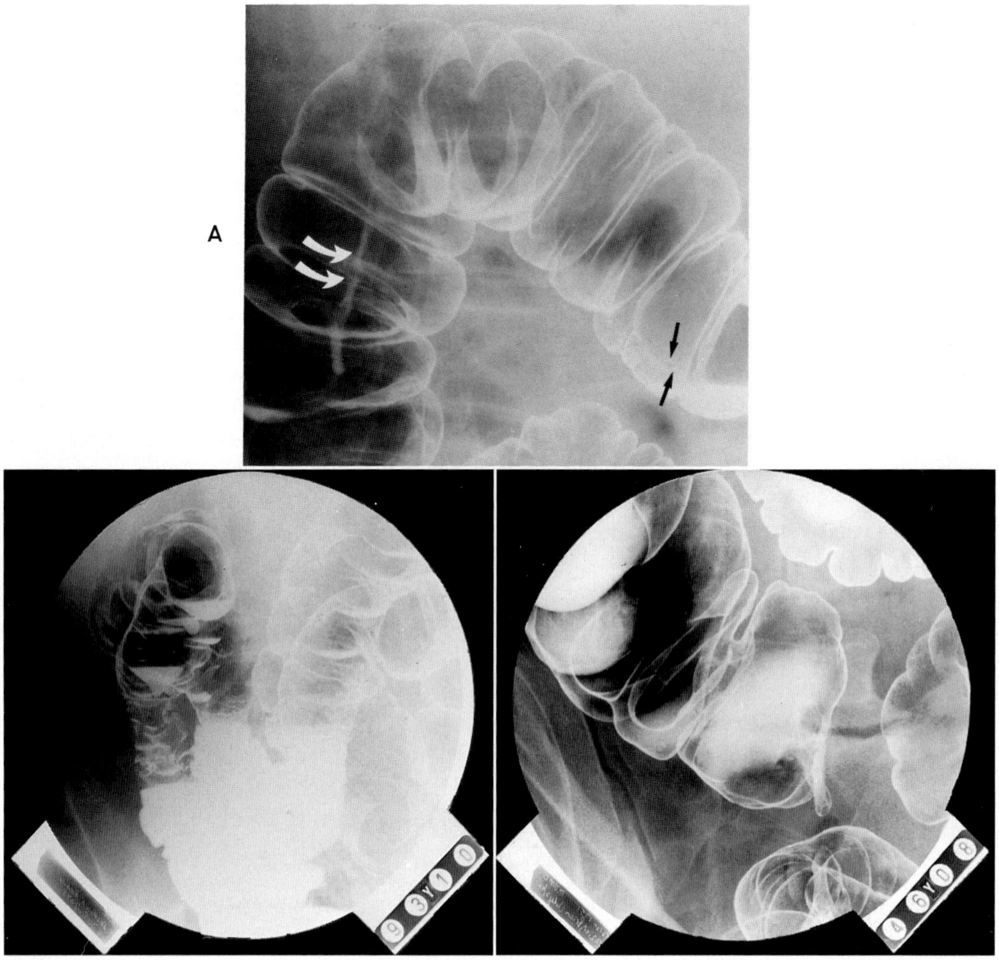

Fig. 34-22 Two films of the hepatic flexure showing adequate (**A**) and inadequate (**B**) distention. In **A,** a strand of mucus and a tiny transverse colon polyp were seen *(arrows)*. In **B,** there was insufficient gas and inadequate rotation, and serious disease could readily be missed. Finally, the cecum is shown with adequate but not optimal clearance of the barium puddle (**C**).

methods. If carbon dioxide is used, the enema tip should not be removed before filming because absorption of the gas is rapid and additional puffs would then be needed during filming.

More complex methods can be used when attempting to achieve complete drainage of the sigmoid before the right colon fills.[5] They depend on two principles. First is a thorough understanding of the three-dimensional anatomy of the sigmoid loops in its three basic configurations, described earlier. The second is realizing that gas only displaces barium downward and not along a flat horizontal segment of colon. The radiologist should therefore vertically position each segment of colon that is to be cleared by turning the patient and raising or lowering the head of the table, as necessary. This method can yield excellent images of even the most convoluted sigmoid colons, if there is no major diverticular disease. The justification for the extra effort and radiation exposure involved is that 90% of the overlooked polyps are in the sigmoid colon. Once films have been taken of the cleared sigmoid, the patient is turned from the supine Trendelenburg position onto the right side, to move the barium onward into the right colon. Often this allows the entire left colon to be filmed free of major barium puddles (Fig. 34-23). The table head is then elevated to promote the flow of barium down into the cecum, and, after further rotations to coat the right colon, the rest of the overhead films are taken. Spot films of the flexures are taken with the patient erect and with adequate distention. Finally, the cecum must be emptied to obtain double-contrast views. To do this, the patient is turned onto the *right* side (not the left, because the ileocecal valve will then trap barium in the cecum), and the table head is lowered. The patient may even have to be placed semiprone for the cecal barium to run up into the ascending colon, but, once it has done so, the cecum will remain clear as the patient returns from the right side down to the supine position required for the films to be taken.

If flexible sigmoidoscopy has been performed before the barium enema study, all this extra effort to completely clear the sigmoid, plus the added radiation exposure, may be redundant. In this event, the simplified method described by Gelfand may, in fact, be superior, as it focuses on the right colon where up to 40% of the cancers found by radiologists are located.[61]

Another variant of the double-contrast enema in patients with diverticular disease is the post double-contrast sigmoid flush. Between 500 to 700 ml of either water or very dilute barium is introduced after all the double-contrast films have been obtained (Fig. 34-24). Lappas et al.[62] found that water and dilute barium yielded better sigmoid images in 65% and 75% of the patients studied, respectively. In particular, it often allowed them to confirm polyps or exclude artifacts noted on the double-contrast films. Lunderquist achieved a similar aim by starting the examination with careful observation of the initial flow through the sigmoid, then taking one single-contrast sigmoid film before continu-

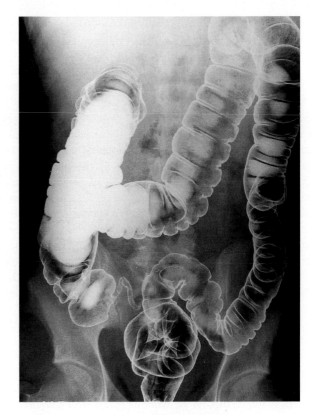

Fig. 34-23 After complete clearing of the sigmoid, almost all of the barium has been tipped into the right colon, and this permits an oblique film of the left colon to be obtained in double contrast. After further rotations, some of the barium will return to the left side.

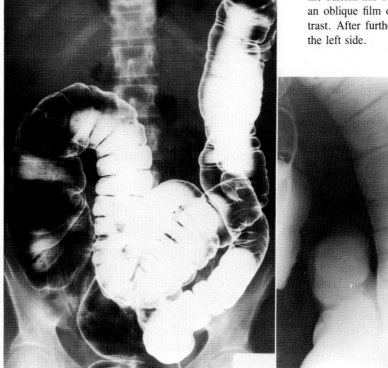

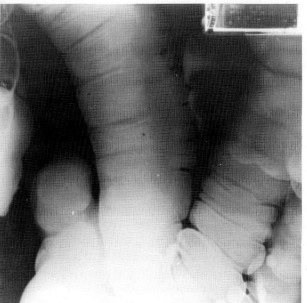

Fig. 34-24 Value of follow-up of double-contrast examination with single-contrast technique. **A,** Large defect is seen in proximal transverse colon. After patient evacuated barium and gas, barium was introduced into the rectum, and spot films and prone and supine overhead films were obtained. No lesion was seen. **B,** Spot film of single-contrast enema after double-contrast examination.

ing with the full double-contrast examination. He also found that occasionally carrying out this part of the study first avoids major uncertainty later on.

A final variation is to train the technologist in the gastrointestinal section to perform the double-contrast barium enema. This is an issue that arouses strong opinions.[63-65] Somers and Miller[66,67] have both shown that technologists can be trained to perform high-quality examinations, and, in Japan, routine upper and lower double-contrast studies are performed by technologists in many institutions. It is the normal course of events that complex procedures are introduced by the innovators, and, as in the case of lymphangiography, can for a few years be performed only by the originators and their immediate colleagues. The procedures then become simplified, are taken over by other specialists in related fields (radiologists from surgeons, and even neurologists from radiologists), and finally the technical aspect is delegated, under properly defined and controlled supervision, to trained technologists. Ultrasound is a good example. In Britain it remains the practice for radiologists to perform most ultrasound examinations themselves, although this is changing.[63] From the North American perspective this is a poor use of their time. Instead, in the North American scenario, one radiologist supervises, checks, and reports on the work of several technologists in an ultrasound department; the British counterpart, on the other hand, can traditionally achieve only one fifth the productivity. Moreover, the quality of routine images achieved by the dedicated technologist is frequently superior. The same principles may apply to the double-contrast barium enema, especially if close supervision and availability of the radiologist are ensured.

PROBLEM SOLVING

Inadequate bowel preparation. When fecal matter is noted as the colon is filling with barium, it is tempting to continue with the planned DCBE, to try to salvage the examination and save the patient the inconvenience of rescheduling. However, this is not usually in the patient's best interest. There are instead two reasonable courses of action.

The first is to stop the flow of barium at once and hang a 2-liter bag of water in its place. A fluoroscopically controlled cleansing enema can be administered and, if the amount of stool is not excessive and only a small amount of barium has been introduced, the patient can then be sent to evacuate the bowel contents. Then, after a delay of at least an hour, the procedure can be restarted. If the patient is old, and small lesions are unimportant, the examination can be restarted as a single-contrast study after only a few minutes, recognizing the compromise in quality.

Alternatively, the examination can be rescheduled. This is the best course of action when a large amount of stool is found or if a great deal of barium has been introduced in a patient in whom the detection of moderate-sized polyps would be a relevant finding.

Air lock. During double-contrast enemas, the gas may bypass the barium, and, especially if there is some redundancy of loops, the inexperienced radiologist will announce that there is an air lock and that barium cannot be advanced any further. In this situation, often too much barium has been drained or the head of the column has not reached the transverse colon. The situation can usually be rescued, provided it is dealt with quickly, because, after half an hour of struggle, the barium coating will start to crack and the patient will be exhausted. The examiner may have to decide in this situation whether to convert the study to a single-contrast examination or to reschedule the patient for either a peroral pneumocolon study or a repeat barium enema.

If the problem has been present only for a few minutes, and the patient is fit, enough barium should be run in below the kink so that there is sufficient fluid in the colon to reach the cecum. Next, as described by Thoeni,[16] and recommended by Miller, additional air should be introduced to unfold the flexures and fully distend the colon. At this point it is usually a straightforward matter to move the barium around to the right colon by using gravity and observing the direction that the barium has to take to run into the next segment.

Spasm and incontinence. Spasm may be overcome in most patients by administering Buscopan or glucagon, but sometimes only for a short while. In the elderly, or when spasm is seen early, barium should be introduced slowly, and injection of the hypotonic agent delayed for a while so that its effect will last until all the films have been taken. The limited duration of action of these drugs is the reason why the author prefers to give them selectively, and late in the examination, just before the first films are taken. Often, when the drugs are administered at the beginning of the examination, their effect wears off just as the films are about to be taken.

Problems with incontinence may be predicted by the preliminary rectal digital examination. However, leakage can also readily occur around a balloon catheter. Therefore, in those patients in whom leakage is likely, the barium should be given slowly, with gentle traction exerted on the catheter to hold the balloon against the anorectal junction. Care is then taken to drain the rectum completely of barium and to fill the rectum and rectosigmoid with air. From then on, provided no barium has drained back into the rectum, only air can leak.

In the very old, mass actions are a relatively frequent problem. The only safe maneuver to salvage the situation is to put the bag on the floor quickly and to open the tap in the hope that the contraction will drive the barium back into the bag instead of onto the table. There is no time to give a relaxant to abolish a mass action once it is under way, although this is worth doing in the hope of preventing or minimizing others.

Immobile patients. There is no patient too old to undergo a double-contrast enema, but immobility makes the procedure more difficult, and old age renders the detection of small polyps of less value. A simple method is needed for helping technologists decide who should have double-contrast and who should have single-contrast examinations. One rule of thumb that works is that any patient who can come into the room, climb onto the table, and turn prone unaided should undergo a double-contrast examination (P. Yoong, personal communication). The simplified method of performing a double-contrast study described by Gelfand and Ott[60] allows the procedure to be extended to more patients. Some authors prefer to do a careful single-contrast examination rather than risk a compromised double-contrast study if the patient cannot turn prone. Others prefer to do a limited double-contrast examination, but there is then more chance of missing lesions with a compromised double-contrast examination than with a carefully performed single-contrast study in the elderly or very immobile patient.

Sometimes a double-contrast examination is under way when it becomes apparent that the patient is actually unfit for the study. If this is recognized quickly, satisfactory results may still often be obtained by allowing the patient to evacuate the bowel contents and then switching to the single-contrast approach. If the patient is exhausted, the study should be stopped, the actual need for an examination reviewed, and the patient then scheduled for either endoscopy or a single-contrast enema.

Failure to fill cecum. Simpkins considers failure to fill the cecum the worst crime (apart from perforating the colon), as the patient has come so far, but not far enough, and the study must be rescheduled. Several maneuvers may be tried to salvage the situation, including abdominal massage with the patient on the right side while insufflating air, sitting up, and deep breathing. If all the films have been taken, a final method is to introduce water or very dilute barium, as this will often displace the denser initial barium to the cecum and allow surprisingly good cecal films to be obtained. If the examination is abandoned with the cecum unseen, but with the colon clean, the best course of action that is the least traumatic for the patient is to perform a peroral pneumocolon examination the following morning. When this approach is adopted, clear fluids may be taken up until midnight, but no food consumed until the pneumocolon has been finished. This administration of barium by mouth and air per rectum constitutes a less traumatic way of visualizing the cecum than to repeat the barium enema.

Choice of double versus single contrast

The radiopaque enema has been performed for almost 90 years,[68] and the double contrast for 70.[69] Problems with barium quality prevented acceptance of the air method until Welin[70] in Sweden perfected it in the 1950s. It then spread to England in the following decade.[71] The 1960s and 1970s saw the method further refined and popularized in Europe,[72,73] North America,[55-57] and Japan,[74-77] with the appearance of numerous outstanding publications. Controversy continued for awhile over the proper place for each technique, but the issues are very simple.

Both methods require a clean colon and meticulous technique. The essentials of the single-contrast method can be learned rapidly, but "to do the examination properly requires a mastery of the art of fluoroscopy."[17] Learning how to perform one of the simplified double-contrast methods properly can also be taught quickly, but the art then for the neophyte is in reading the radiographs, and supervision and double reading are very important. Indeed, the trainee should first review the films before leaving the department, then review them again briefly to acquire an overall impression before examining each film systematically from one end of the colon to the other, being sure that every segment of bowel has been well displayed on one or more radiographs. Finally the trainee should reexamine the danger areas of cecum, sigmoid, and rectum where lesions are most easily overlooked. The review process should then be repeated by the supervisor.

There is clear evidence that the double-contrast technique is superior for detecting small neoplasms[72,78-81] and inflammatory bowel disease.[73,82,83]

The aesthetic superiority of the double-contrast technique is also relevant. This provides a motivating force for both technologists and radiologists to do it well, as a lapse from the normal high standard is very obvious and invites critical comment that helps to maintain standards.

Although a few experts still use single-contrast enemas extensively,[84] most, and now the majority of general radiologists, routinely use the DCBE.[40,85,86] The 1987 survey of leading medical centers around the world revealed that the percentage of practitioners routinely using the double-contrast method had increased from 6% in 1976 to 56% in 1987.[87] Gelfand et al.[88] have suggested that, despite its increased cost, the additional accuracy it affords justifies DCBE in patients with gastrointestinal bleeding, early inflammatory bowel disease, or a history of a colon neoplasm, and in all patients over 40 who can tolerate the procedure. In general, the consensus is that the DCBE should be the routine radiographic approach, bearing in mind that there are some contraindications to its use. The single-contrast technique is excellent for use in these circumstances (the very young, very old, very ill, very disabled, and those with a suspected obstruction),[12] if performed with care, and it should continue to be taught in residency programs.

Other methods
WATER-SOLUBLE CONTRAST ENEMA

Patients who undergo a water-soluble contrast enema are often ill, and the examination is being performed to answer a very specific question, which guides the selection of the density of the contrast and the positioning of the patient.

Thus, for demonstrating a fistula, undiluted Gastrografin is used; to visualize an obstruction, it may be diluted. If a rectovaginal fistula is suspected, the examination is started with the patient in the lateral position, the contrast is run in slowly, and some early films are taken as soon as anything unusual is seen. Once contrast has flooded through a fistula, it is often difficult to sort out the anatomy. However, if a series of images have been recorded from the beginning, it is often possible to reconstruct the sequence of events in one's mind and to understand the pathology involved.

Vaginography may also be used for the detection of colovaginal fistulas.[89] Indeed, this is the best technique for this purpose. To perform it, a Foley catheter is used with a 30-ml balloon and Hypaque (meglumine diatrizoate or sodium) can be infused under gravity. The patient should be in the lateral position so that a fistula in the anteroposterior direction can be seen well.

Gastrografin is expensive and should be used judiciously. For example, when a moderate volume of Gastrografin has been introduced and it has only reached the hepatic flexure, rather than opening more bottles of Gastrografin at this point, a liter of water may be added to the bag. This will displace the dense Gastrografin into the cecum and distal ileum, but will clear and render invisible the overlying loops of sigmoid colon that would otherwise interfere with visualization of the cecum and distal small bowel that may lie in the pelvis. Avoiding problems with hyperosmolarity in pediatric patients is discussed in Chapters 100 and 101.

INSTANT AND GAS ENEMAS

With the advent of flexible endoscopy, the instant and gas enema studies are less often required but may occasionally be useful. The instant double-contrast enema examination is used only in patients with an established diagnosis of ulcerative colitis when the active disease extends farther than the proctoscope can reach and the clinician wants to know its extent.[90] The technique relies on the fact that the diseased colon contains no formed stool, which is held up in the more proximal normal colon. Thus the patient can go directly to the radiology department from the clinic, without bowel preparation. A single preliminary abdominal radiograph is taken to exclude the presence of severe disease or toxic megacolon, and barium is introduced until stool is encountered. The rectum and distal colon are then drained, and air (or carbon dioxide) is introduced to distend the colon. The patient rotates once through 360 degrees, and three large films are taken: prone, lateral, and erect. This examination reveals the extent of ulcerative colitis with minimal radiation exposure and inconvenience to the patient.

Because of the ease of colonoscopy in these patients, there is a tendency to use it rather than the instant enema, stopping when stool or normal mucosa is encountered. The examination has no place when looking for dysplasia or carcinoma in patients with long-standing colitis, as immacu-

late bowel preparation is required in such instances.

The air enema[91] supplements plain films and is helpful in demonstrating the state of the mucosa in patients when a barium enema is not desired. In very ill patients, carbon dioxide should be used instead of air, as it is absorbed rapidly and cannot exacerbate existing disease by increasing distention.

A technique for decompressing a toxic dilatation has been described and consists of simply rolling the patient, which moves gas distally and allows it to be passed rectally.[92] Part of the reason that gas remains in the transverse colon in sick patients is simply that it is anterior. Rolling, by placing the patient's left side up, then prone, and then the right side up, promotes the flow of gas distally in patients with toxic dilatation or Ogilvie's syndrome, and in those who have just undergone a DCBE or colonoscopy. When leaving the department after a DCBE with air, patients should be told how to do this positioning should they get severe cramps, as some of them will, as transverse colonic gas cannot be passed while patients are sitting.

REPEAT ENEMA VERSUS ENDOSCOPY

When a double- or single-contrast examination fails or yields equivocal results in some segment of the colon, the question then arises whether it should be repeated or whether the patient should undergo colonoscopy. The answer depends partly on the relative quality, expense, and safety of the two procedures in the local center, but two generalizations apply: (1) if the enema was well performed, or as well as could be achieved, and a question remains, then colonoscopy should be done; but (2) if the enema examination was a complete failure, for example, because of inadequate bowel preparation, then, if the indication was clear in the first place, the examination should be repeated.

COLOSTOMY ENEMAS

Upstream colostomy enemas are usually performed after abdominoperineal resection for cancer. In general, the first follow-up examination after such an operation should be colonoscopy rather than a barium enema because it is highly likely that polyps have formed that require removal. Furthermore, the examination is technically easy to perform and complications are correspondingly unlikely because the remaining colon is usually short with little or no sigmoid left. Once colonoscopy has successfully cleared the colon, regular follow-up is instituted. Both DCBE and colonoscopy are equally satisfactory for this purpose, unless the patient is severely obese or immobile, in which case colonoscopy is preferred by far. Since the task is to hunt for small neoplasms, any barium enema should be carried out using the double-contrast technique, after full bowel preparation.

A variety of methods are available for performing colostomy enemas, but they are divided into two approaches— use of either an internal balloon or a catheter with an external cone that is held pressed into the stoma by the patient. In one survey, 20% of the radiologists were found to use a balloon inflated inside the stoma.[12] Perforation of the bowel adjacent to a colostomy can have fatal consequences,[93] and therefore great care should be taken if a balloon is blown up inside a colostomy. The stoma should first be examined with a gloved finger to assess the direction and caliber of the lumen, and the catheter should be inserted gently but deeply. The balloon should be blown up only under direct fluoroscopic guidance after some contrast has been introduced to confirm that the balloon is within the intraperitoneal portion of the colon and that the colon is nondiseased. Not more than 20 ml of contrast should be used for this purpose.

The author does not recommend the balloon technique, even when the noted precautions are observed, and prefers instead the technique described by Goldstein and Miller.[94] In this, the balloon of a Foley catheter is cut with scissors and the balloon-side arm is cut and attached to an air (or carbon dioxide) puffer. The tip of a rubber nipple from a baby bottle is cut so that the Foley catheter can slide through it, but with a tight fit. The catheter is advanced some 6 inches (15 cm) beyond the nipple, and, after an initial digital examination of the stoma, the catheter is fed gently through the stoma until the nipple lies snugly in the colostomy. Two 4-inch (10-cm) square gauze pads, which are cut half-way through, are placed around the catheter, and the patient holds the gauze, nipple, and catheter in place, with the catheter between the fingers. It is best for them to use the right hand initially because the patient is usually first turned to the left. Barium is then introduced slowly, with an intravenous relaxant given when spasm is seen or at the latest possible moment before the first film is taken. Barium is allowed to flow to at least the mid transverse colon, and then gas is introduced. When gas bubbles pass the splenic flexure, the patient switches hands and rolls to the right. Once the right colon has filled, the table head is elevated to promote the passage of barium down into the cecum. A standard sequence of films is then taken, except that the prone films have to be prone oblique so that the patient can continue to hold the catheter.

Downstream colostomy enema. A downstream colostomy enema is usually done before closure of a colostomy. In an acute situation, it may be done to determine whether there is an anastomotic leak or whether a fistula has closed. In this situation, water-soluble contrast should be used, without dilution, and relaxants administered intravenously. In a study done before closure, either a water-soluble contrast agent or barium are satisfactory. It is more useful to introduce the contrast through the colostomy using a catheter and feeding nipple, since the anal sphincter provides resistance and allows good distention of the sigmoid colon to be achieved. If the enema is given from below, the contrast often spills out of the colostomy in an uncontrolled way, and distention is hard to achieve.

POSTRESECTION ENEMAS

In examining patients who have undergone resections of the sigmoid colon, the technique for DCBE is unchanged, except that a little less barium is used. If the right colon and ileocecal valve have been removed, however, the examination is more difficult because ileal flooding readily occurs and the sigmoid loops become hidden. Initially, therefore, the flow of barium should be stopped as soon as the descending colon is reached, and attempts should be made to obtain excellent images of the cleared sigmoid in double contrast before the barium passes around the splenic flexure. After this, the bag is rehung, and more barium can be introduced for filling the remainder of the colon.

PERORAL PNEUMOCOLON

The peroral pneumocolon examination is principally done to evaluate the terminal ileum (see Chapter 25). However, it is an excellent examination to use if difficulties have been experienced in filling the cecum during a barium enema study (Fig. 34-25, *A*) and may be considered after a failed colonoscopy if the hepatic flexure has been reached. The more usual approach in the latter circumstance is to do a barium enema an hour or so after the colonoscopy. This is a straightforward procedure without impairment of quality[95] but may be quite arduous if the patient has been very heavily sedated. The peroral pneumocolon approach should probably be reserved for those failed-colonoscopy patients who are heavily sedated, relatively old, or immobile, or in whom a good distal examination was achieved and only the cecum and ascending colon need to be examined.

Therapeutic examinations
CONSTIPATION

An apparent small bowel obstruction may develop in patients with severe constipation, and giving oral laxatives may only exacerbate rather than help the situations. In such patients, water enemas given at the bedside may prove sufficient for alleviating the problem. However, such enemas are often no more than repeated rectal washouts, and may therefore be ineffective. A water-soluble contrast agent such as the hyperosmolar Gastrografin may be given under fluoroscopic control, after first making sure that the patient's state of hydration and electrolyte balance are satisfactory. The examination should be conducted slowly to minimize discomfort, as the contrast may only creep around the inspissated and impacted stool, and it is important to get the contrast all the way to the cecum. In extreme cases, two or three such Gastrografin enemas may be necessary, performed on consecutive days, to clear the colon.

In some patients with cystic fibrosis, inspissation develops in both the colon and distal ileum, and similar therapeutic enemas may be required from time to time and greatly improve the patient's general health. Mucomyst (acetylcysteine) may be added to the Gastrografin and be refluxed into the terminal ileum to clear inspissated mucus in these teenagers.

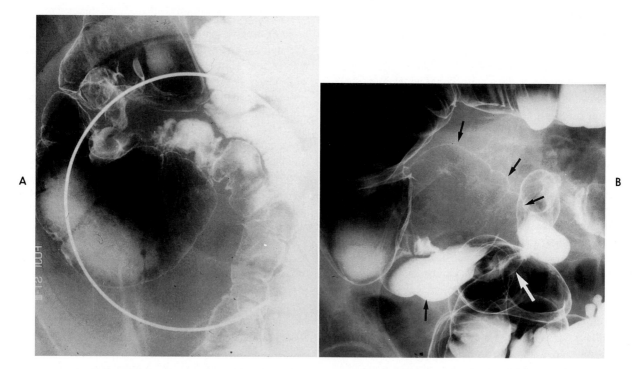

Fig. 34-25 A, This peroral pneumocolon study, obtained after colonoscopy that reached the cecum revealed negative findings, shows a large annular carcinoma in the ascending colon. The sulcus laterally was probably mistaken for the lower cecal pole. **B,** A large carcinoma of the cecum was missed originally. A malignant invasion of the hepatic flexure was detected, which turned out to be due to gallbladder carcinoma, and vigilance was relaxed. Although the outline of the cecum is not abnormal *(arrows),* the relative opacity of the large cecum compared with the dark ascending colon shows that the lumen is reduced in the anteroposterior diameter, and this was in fact due to a very large cecal carcinoma.
A from Stevenson GW: *Cancer* 71(suppl):4198, 1993.

INTUSSUSCEPTION

The diagnosis and radiologic management of intussusception are discussed in Chapter 100.

Complications

Perforation of the colon has been reported to occur in from 1 in 2500 to 1 in 12,500 examinations,[96-99] and the resulting mortality is reported to range from 13% to 80%, with 40% to 50% the most usual figure for intraperitoneal perforation and a lower fatality rate for retroperitoneal perforation of the rectum.[100] Thus the barium enema is not without risk, although it is safer than colonoscopy, which has perforation risks of approximately 1 in 500 to 1 in 1000 and a mortality ranging between 1 in 1958 to 1 in 5000.[101-103] Perforation during a barium enema may result from overinflation of balloons in the rectum,[104] inflation of balloons inside colostomies and ileostomies,[105] deep sigmoidoscopic biopsies,[106,107] or examination in an attack of acute severe inflammatory bowel disease. In acute diverticulitis or perforating carcinoma, the enema is simply demonstrating an existing fistula from the diverticulitis, but, when there is any suspicion of such a leak, water-soluble contrast should be used, or a CT study done instead. If the water-soluble contrast examination yields negative findings, a barium enema can be performed, if still necessary. Occasionally, an enema tip perforates the colon for no good reason.[108] A barium enema is probably safe after biopsy has been performed using the regular small colonoscopic forceps,[109] and there is no need to delay.

Other complications include constipation resulting from the inspissation of barium. This can be minimized by telling patients to drink plenty of fluids after a barium examination and by advising those with constipation to take laxatives until their stool returns to a normal color. The problem of constipation after barium meals was so common and so serious in one geriatric inpatient unit that the administration of 50 g of lactulose was recommended as a routine measure after any barium study.[110]

Transient bacteremia has been described as a complication of barium enemas and is probably very common. It is not customary to take any precautions for this, but it would be prudent to prescribe prophylactic antibiotics for those patients known to have mitral valve disease or for those who have undergone surgical valve replacements.

Anaphylactic reactions to the barium have been reported and can be fatal, but are very rare.[111-115] It was suggested that such reactions were becoming more common.[116] After this, however, came reports of sensitivity to the latex balloons used as retention cuffs on enema tips, and many of the reactions attributed to barium or glucagon may in fact have been due to the latex.[117] There was a great increase in the use of disposable balloon enema tips during the 1980s as high-quality products became available and as the popularity of the double-contrast enema study increased. During a 22-month period in 1988 to 1989, 158 barium-related incidents were reported to one company, 148 associated with a barium enema (nine of which were fatal). In five of the fatal cases, the reaction developed after insertion of the tip and before barium had been introduced. In another series, reactions developed in six patients during barium enema, with one death. The serum was examined in three patients, including the fatal case, and revealed latex-specific IgE antibodies.[118] Latex-based balloons were therefore recalled and have now been replaced by silicone-based products. During this same time period, allergies to latex gloves and condoms were also reported, but the enema tip reactions are striking for their speed and severity. The ability of the rectal mucosa to absorb large molecules almost instantaneously into the circulation probably plays a role in this.[117]

What can a radiologist do to minimize the risk of a complication during barium enemas?[17,107] The risk of perforation can be reduced by attention to the following six points:

1. Use rectal balloon catheters only when digital examination shows a lax sphincter and in the absence of known rectal pathology or previous pelvic irradiation.
2. Inflate such a balloon only with the manufacturer's recommended puffer and not to more than 50 ml.
3. Avoid balloon inflation inside colostomies and ileostomies.
4. Use water-soluble contrast initially in the presence of acute abdominal conditions.
5. Wait 7 days after a rectal biopsy has been performed with large forceps, and after polypectomy of sessile polyps over 10 mm in diameter.
6. Infuse contrast with caution in patients with obstruction, to avoid massive distention below an obstructing tumor.

In addition to these measures, advise patients to drink large quantities of fluids for 24 hours after the examination, and give laxatives or lactulose to constipated elderly patients. Antibiotic prophylaxis should be considered for those with mitral valve disease or prosthetic valves who are having enemas after full bowel cleansing. Certainly they should be used in any patient undergoing an emergency enema with an unprepared bowel. Finally, beware of using latex products in the rectum.

Reporting

An approach to the examination of radiographs has already been described. Simpkins[119] has also suggested a method of reporting barium enema findings that can help referring physicians make decisions regarding further investigations. Often the quality of the examination, and therefore the degree of the radiologist's confidence in a normal or abnormal finding, varies depending on the segment of the colon involved. A standard diagram of the colon can be printed on each DCBE report, and different-colored crayons used to indicate the degree of confidence in the findings for the various segments—*green* meaning confident; *yellow,* minor reservations; and *red,* poorly examined and serious pathology not excluded. Thus the sigmoid might be colored red and the rest of the colon green in a patient with complex sigmoid loops and marked diverticular disease. Alternatively the radiologist could simply dictate a line in the conclusion to indicate any reservations. This type of honesty is much more useful to the referring physician than the phrase "no major pathology detected on this examination," which is an example of that sturdy and enduring "plant," the radiologic hedge. Finally, there is ample evidence that double reading of the barium enema films increases the yield of important pathology,[120] since an error in perception is the source of most oversights[80] (Fig. 34-25, *B*). In one study double reading produced a 13% increase in the sensitivity of the examination and triple reading, 19%.[121] The price paid in terms of decreased specificity depended on where the threshold was set: With the inclusion of definite, probable, and possible lesions, the specificity dropped to 74%, but, with the exclusion of possible lesions, it was 91%, whereas the sensitivity dropped only from 83.3% to 81.8% when possible lesions were excluded. It is probably better, in general, to report only definite and probable polyps and to ignore "possible" lesions, as this then translates into a huge amount of colonoscopy performed for what ultimately turns out to have been fecal residue.

Endoscopy of the colon

The original large bowel endoscopes were straight metal tubes, optimistically called *sigmoidoscopes,* that allowed examination of the rectum. They were good for detecting inflammation but less accurate than DCBE for detecting neoplasms.[122] The advent of flexible fiberoptic endoscopes around 1970 represented a diagnostic and therapeutic revolution in the investigation and management of large bowel disease. This was further enhanced and expanded on by the subsequent development of videoendoscopes and the application of this technology to laparoscopy. For barium enemas, the usual scopes are now the 60-cm flexible sigmoidoscope and the 180-cm colonoscope. High-quality color printers are starting to be used with the videoscopes, so proper documentation of the endoscopic findings will soon be a standard expectation and requirement.

Flexible sigmoidoscopy is an outpatient procedure that is almost entirely safe.[123] It is usually carried out after limited preparation with one or two phosphasoda enemas. The appropriate techniques are easy to learn; indeed, seven training sessions is the average number required for learning how to use the shorter 35-cm sigmoidoscope, and twelve sessions for the 60-cm version. The 35-cm scope can examine the entire sigmoid in 13% of the cases, detects 80% of the polyps seen with the 60-cm instrument, and is preferred by patients. The examination takes 5 minutes compared with 8 to 10 minutes for the 60-cm scope. The longer instrument can examine the whole sigmoid in about 80% of patients, if the bowel is clean.[123]

Colonoscopy requires a scrupulously clean colon, but substantial fluid is not a problem. Oral lavage using the PEG solution, following a laxative, is therefore ideal. Experienced physicians can reach the cecum in 95% of the patients and examine the terminal ileum in 90% of these. In practice, success in reaching the cecum is achieved in 50% to 75% of patients in several series, so there is a wide range in ability.[124] Many patients prefer colonoscopy to barium enema probably because of the sedation and the usual immediacy of feedback regarding the findings. Because sedation is usually required, the patient has to be driven home.

Integration of endoscopy and radiology

Colonoscopy and barium enema studies are both accurate and useful. The DCBE has the advantages of less expense, less risk, and greater completeness of the examination. Endoscopy permits polypectomy, detects small polyps better, although these are clinically unimportant,[125-133] and yields more accurate findings in the sigmoid colon when there is diverticular disease.[134-136] Endoscopy is too expensive and dangerous to use, for example, as a routine screening tool, but DCBE is pointless for examining patients who have substantial polyps, as they only have to return for colonoscopy. Several authors have pointed out that, not only does flexible sigmoidoscopy provide a great increase in the yield of polyps detected in the sigmoid,[135,137-139] but also it can be performed immediately before a barium enema without impairing the quality of the barium enema.[135,140-142] Indeed, the combined examination is a very powerful diagnostic tool. Alternatively, when facilities and logistics permit, flexible sigmoidoscopy can be used to help physicians decide which patients should undergo barium enema and which (those with polyps) should instead undergo colonoscopy.[139,142] Such strategies can be adopted to ensure that the two techniques are used in their areas of strength[143-145] and that patients receive maximal benefit for the least cost and at the least risk.

Should endoscopy replace barium enema? Fork[146] has recently summarized the issues and came to the conclusion that, although he is usually more correct as a colonoscopist than as a radiologist, since for every lesion missed colonoscopically there are five to eight times as many overlooked radiologically. Very few lesions 10 mm in diameter or larger are actually missed by either technique, although some clearly are, and large tumors are sometimes over-

looked by both techniques[147] (Fig. 34-25). In countries where the procedures compete on equal terms without the influence of money, as in Scandinavia, barium enemas are still done before fiber endoscopy in most noncolitic patients. "This is justified by the sufficiently high sensitivity, the accurate documentation of any mucosal lesion, and the unchallenged ability to unveil extracolonic disorders otherwise hidden: endometriosis, pelvic and gynecological tumours, organ dislocations, skeletal metastases, kidney and gall bladder stones, aneurysms, fistulas, etc."[146] Fork quotes Simpkins, who contends that "there is no clinical, scientific, or economic justification for the wholesale replacement of barium radiology by endoscopy."[119]

Ultrasound

Transabdominal ultrasound is not usually considered a primary method of investigation of the alimentary tract, although the endoluminal techniques described in Chapters 11, 13, 23, 35, 40, and 44 are adding a new dimension. In addition, ultrasound colonoscopes are becoming available that will further extend the potential of this procedure.[148] Nevertheless, alimentary tract abnormalities are regularly detected with ultrasound (Fig. 34-26). There are several reports describing the ultrasound findings in various diseases (see Chapter 18), but there is little help from the literature when it comes to judging whether ultrasound or CT is the more useful. One exception is a report on the ultrasound findings in diverticular disease,[149] in which there were no false-negative sonographic findings, suggesting that ultrasound may be a useful screening tool for such patients when the availability of CT is limited.

To examine the wall of the alimentary tract, it must be distended with water, preferably degassed,[150] and a smooth muscle relaxant is usually required. In addition, a water enema may also be useful to help distinguish the presence of free fluid or a mass in the pelvis from gut contents.[151] The width of the normal colonic wall measures 3 mm or less, provided the colon is distended to a caliber of 5 cm.[152] Graded compression has proved to be a useful technique when examining patients for bowel wall thickening. It is also helpful in the diagnosis of appendicitis (Fig. 34-27) and in differentiating between appendicitis and *Campylobacter* ileitis.[153] It is a sensible first investigation in a patient suspected of having appendicitis, with a sensitivity just below and a specificity in excess of 90%,[154-156] based on the finding of a noncompressible appendix with a diameter of 6 mm. Bowel wall thickening can be visualized with enough reliability to detect Crohn's disease and ulcerative colitis, and frequently to tell them apart.[157] Antibiotic-induced colitis can be diagnosed in an appropriate clinical setting,[158] but perhaps not distinguished from ischemic colitis, nor is the demonstration of pathology in pseudomembranous colitis as clearly detailed as it is with CT.[159] Localized bowel wall thickening (i.e., polyps and small tumors) can also be detected with ultrasound, and the pre-

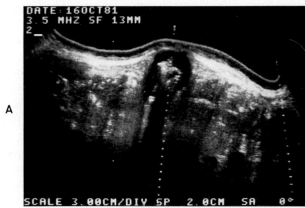
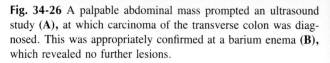
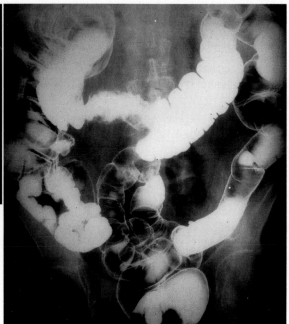

Fig. 34-26 A palpable abdominal mass prompted an ultrasound study (**A**), at which carcinoma of the transverse colon was diagnosed. This was appropriately confirmed at a barium enema (**B**), which revealed no further lesions.

liminary work by Limberg and others suggests that ultrasound may become the method of choice for colorectal screening.[160,161]

In summary, ultrasound can fairly reliably depict bowel wall thickening in a variety of diseases,[162] can sometimes distinguish between ulcerative colitis and Crohn's disease, can probably be used to rule out diverticulitis, and may be an excellent initial investigation for elucidating the nature of suspected alimentary tract disorders, on account of its ability to reveal so many other abnormalities and thereby to direct what other more invasive investigations should be carried out. The technique of graded compression, first described by Puylaert,[163] with careful search of all segments of the bowel, is very important, and should be supplemented on occasion with water enemas and relaxants. It is inevitable, and to be welcomed, that the use of abdominal ultrasound will expand dramatically over the next few years, far beyond the confines of the radiology department.[164] However, the greatest need with regard to improved transabdominal ultrasound of the colon is a superior contrast agent. Water does improve resolution, but air pockets remain a problem. Early results with cellulose suspensions show promise of their providing superior imaging; they appear to absorb gas and yield better images than does degassed water.[165]

Computed tomography

As for any examination of the colon, when performing a CT study it is necessary to appropriately prepare the bowel, and dietary restriction consisting of a clear fluid diet for 24 hours plus oral laxatives should be prescribed. When there is urgency, and there are no contraindications, either 4 li-

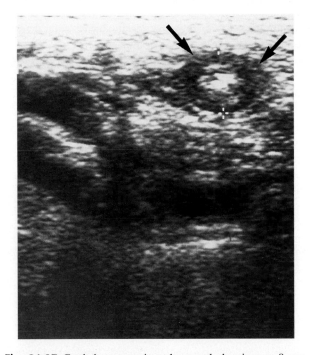

Fig. 34-27 Graded-compression ultrasound showing an 8-mm-thick and noncompressible appendix in a child, who was confirmed to have acute appendicitis.
Courtesy of Dr. Cathy Babcook.

ters of an oral PEG solution can be given or a 2-liter water-cleansing enema, to which 20 ml of liquid bisacodyl has been added.

In addition, contrast should be given orally, some 3 to 12 hours in advance, if colonic filling is desired, and a further 500 ml of oral contrast should be given approximately 45 minutes before scanning to opacify distal ileal loops. This oral contrast may be 2% to 3% solutions of Gastrografin or Hypaque, 2% barium suspensions,[166-168] or 12.5% fat emulsions.[169] These have been discussed in Chapter 25.[166-173] However, these agents do not produce good colonic distention. Some authors regard the main focus of CT as the "paraintestinal compartments"[146] and are content to have the colonic mucosa indicated by a small amount of oral contrast. Others prefer to include the evaluation of intramural and intraluminal pathology whenever possible and therefore desire colonic distention. This may be achieved with fluid enemas,[174] but air insufflation gives particularly good results (Fig. 34-28), both of the colonic wall[175] and for the documentation of fistulas.[176-178]

Air can be introduced with a soft rubber catheter using a bulb for insufflation. The air should be introduced slowly until the patient feels the urge to defecate. If glucagon or Buscopan are given first, more gas will be tolerated and with less discomfort.

A scout film is obtained first, and then the abdomen is scanned from the domes of the diaphragms to the anal canal. A convenient sequence is to obtain 10-mm sections at 15-mm intervals initially. Once ectopic air is shown, a detailed second look at a specific lesion using 10×10-mm contiguous sections, or rarely 5×5-mm sections, can be carried out and will show the density surrounding a fistulous tract representing the acute inflammatory response.[179] Contiguous sections are helpful to show small lesions, and occasionally a change in position may be helpful for disclosing these, or additional air may be required.[178]

Initial imaging may be carried out with a standard window of 300 to 500 HU, but careful review using 1000 to 2000 HU and -200 to -500 HU will help delineate intraluminal and small lesions.[178]

A compromise solution in a busy department is probably to use insufflated air, as described by Balthazar and Megibow,[178] when the colon is the region of primary interest, but to use a retrograde enema of contrast without bowel preparation,[180] or an oral contrast such as emulsified 12.5% corn oil given 12 hours before scanning, to opacify the colon for routine abdominal CT. Less attention to the colon than this may only lead to confusion stemming from the lack of distention and adherent feces.[181]

A water enema has also been recommended as an alternative to rectal air, and the images that have been published also show there is excellent detail of the bowel wall and of thickening due to tumors.[182,183] However, in one series, 7% of the patients could not retain the 1200 ml of liquid required, so the table had to be cleaned, and this will limit the appeal of the technique. Nevertheless, the relative densities of water, the bowel wall, tumor, and fat are such that the images are excellent, with less problems with artifacts than that encountered with air. This technique particularly lends itself to tumor staging, while air is probably more useful in the evaluation of acute disease and suspected fistula.

Metoclopramide has been demonstrated to provide more rapid and improved opacification of the distal ileum and proximal colon following its oral administration.[184] These authors recommended the routine administration of 10 mg of metoclopramide for outpatients if there are no plans to use rectal contrast, as well as in inpatients who are scheduled for emergency CT.[184]

In the scanning of patients with obstruction, oral contrast should be given, but it may not reach the level of obstruction. Vascular enhancement is important, as there may be rotation of vascular pedicles, in which case a rapid 50-ml bolus delivered at a rate of 1.5 to 2 ml per second, followed by a sustained infusion of 100 ml given at 0.8 ml per second, is convenient for accomplishing this in adult patients.[185] Rectal contrast should usually not be given, although the merits of carbon dioxide, which is rapidly absorbed, need to be evaluated. A complete abdominal scan is performed, and then the scan is reviewed going from the rectum proximally. Once dilated loops are encountered, the further acquisition of 5×5-mm sections through the area of interest may yield a diagnosis.[185]

The advent of fast rotational CT scanning is improving the resolution and revealing pathologic features not seen previously, such as intramural air in severe ulcerative colitis. In addition, a complete vascular study of the abdomen can now be obtained during a 30-second breath hold, and the resolution obtained is opening up the possibility that CT may replace abdominal angiography as a less expensive and less invasive method of evaluating, for example, vascular stenoses and occlusions.[186]

For further information on CT of the gastrointestinal tract, the reader is referred to the July 1989 issue of *Radio-*

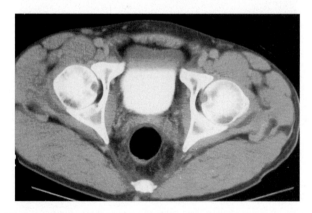

Fig. 34-28 The wall of the rectum can be visualized readily after distention with air, and against the surrounding fat.

logic Clinics of North America, and the discussion contained therein on technical principles.[187]

Magnetic resonance scanning

MRI has not really advanced very far in terms of the alimentary tract, and a recent text on MRI baldly states that, "with regard to the gastrointestinal system, the use of MRI is limited to the liver."[188] Nevertheless, a number of research reports have revealed that progress is being made. In vitro studies have shown that MRI can image three to five layers in the bowel wall with short TR and TE, and that use of long TR/TE images permits resolution into six or eight distinct layers, including adherent mucus on the mucosa and an external layer of pericolonic fat. There was good correlation with the degree of invasion found histologically, and these, and other results, suggest that MRI will, in due course, be very valuable in the evaluation of colorectal tumors.[189]

Rectal cleansing and intravenously administered glucagon are both helpful in improving the examination. Various contrast agents for use in MRI of the gut are discussed in Chapter 25.[190-193] In addition, Ros et al.[194] have evaluated the role of standard, slightly diluted (upper 60% weight per weight [w/w]; lower 66% w/w) barium sulfate preparations, and found they produced consistent and even imaging of both upper and lower gastrointestinal tracts, with par-

ticular improvements in the rectum and distal sigmoid, and in the stomach and duodenum, especially on T1 sequences. No artifacts were encountered, and the advantages of being able to scan shortly after a fluoroscopic study had been done were stressed.

Whole-body coils have been used so far for colorectal imaging, but endoluminal coils are being investigated for this purpose.[195] At this point, all that can be said is that it is feasible. There is no evidence yet as to how endoluminal MRI compares with either endoluminal ultrasound or spiral CT. Abdominal straps placed across the lower abdomen and pelvis are used by some to try to reduce respiratory artifacts.[196] A standard examination technique for the rectum[197] employs initial sagittal T2 scans with a spin-echo sequence and slice thickness of preferably 5 mm. This is followed by transverse T2 scans and T1 scans with a shorter TR and TE, and a slice thickness of 10 mm. These images are then assessed, and frequently coronal T2 scans are found to be needed, sometimes with gadolinium-DTPA–enhanced T1 scans. The use of T1 and T2 multiplanar examinations, with repeated T1 sequences after the injection of a contrast agent, makes this a time-consuming examination.[190] Balzarini therefore suggests that such a protocol be restricted to those cases most prone to diagnostic error, namely those patients with a suspected relapse occurring within 6 months of resection, but without definite proof of

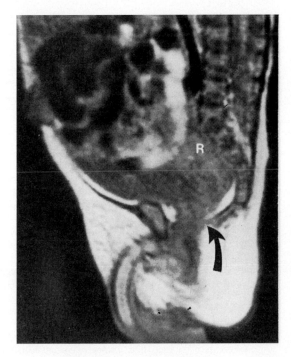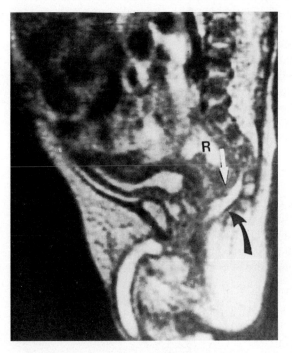

Fig. 34-29 Proton-density and T2 images in a child with rectal atresia. In the T2 image, the meconium in the blind-ending rectum is increased in intensity *(R),* allowing the muscular wall of the blind rectal pouch *(straight arrow)* to be seen well above the levator muscle *(curved arrow).*
From Demas BE, Hricak H, Wall SD: The rectum and anal canal. In Higgins CB, Hricak H, Helms CA, eds: *Magnetic resonance imaging of the body,* New York, 1992, Raven Press.

recurrence on other examinations or on a preliminary standard MRI study.

The first clinical indications for MRI of the large bowel will probably be in the pelvis. Already its possible applications in the assessment of congenital anal anomalies[197] (Fig. 34-29) and pelvic floor dysfunctions in adults[11] are being developed, as well as its use in the evaluation of pelvic inflammatory disease with fistulas and local tumor recurrence.[197-199] Coronal sections are particularly helpful for assessing perirectal inflammatory disease.[197]

Functional metabolic imaging of the colon

The era of functional biochemical imaging is tantalizingly close. With regard to colonic disease, two tools are of particular interest to clinical radiologists. The positron emission tomographic (PET) scanner can measure in vivo glucose consumption and therefore might conceivably be able to distinguish fibrosis from recurrent tumor. One such study of PET versus MRI showed that, of 15 patients with suspected recurrent tumor, all 11 with actual recurrence demonstrated increased uptake of FDG (fluorine-18-2-fluoro-2-deoxy-D-glucose) in the suspicious mass, while the four who proved to have only fibrosis did not.[200] Furthermore, FDG uptake may fall if therapy is successful, raising the possibility of PET scanning being used to monitor therapy. However, few hospitals will have a PET scanner and cyclotron, and those that do will have other priorities for a long while yet. Immunoscintigraphy offers a less expensive approach to the problem. Monoclonal antibodies labeled with indium 111 can be imaged using single-photon emission CT (SPECT) scanning, and some agents target colon cancer (one known as β-72.3 targets 95% of the colon cancers). The sensitivity of immunoscintigraphy in the liver at present is less than that of MRI or CTAP, but sensitivity for detecting peritoneal, pelvic, and serosal metastases is good (better than that of CT),[201] as is the specificity. One report cited showed a positive predictive value of 97% for identifying extrahepatic abdominal metastases. In 12% of the patients in one study, clinical decisions were affected by the results (e.g., the detection of occult metastasis).[201] The development of antibodies to the murine immunoglobulin is currently a problem (in 39% of the patients), and this restricts repetition of the test.[202]

Neither PET nor immunoscintigraphy are yet established clinical tools, but both may turn out to be useful in the functional imaging of colonic disease.

REFERENCES

1. Williams PL, Warwick R, eds: *Gray's anatomy*, ed 36, Philadelphia, 1980, WB Saunders.
2. Hadar H, Gadoth N: Positional relations of colon and kidney, determined by perirenal fat, *AJR* 143:773, 1984.
3. Helms CA, Munk PL, Witt WS et al: Retrorenal colon: implications of percutaneous diskectomy, *Radiology* 171:864, 1989.
4. Prassopoulos P, Goutsoyiannis N, Cavouras D, Pantelides N: A study of the variation of colonic positioning in the pararenal space as shown by computed tomography, *Eur J Radiol* 10:44, 1990.
5. Dobranowski J, Stringer DA, Somers S, Stevenson GW: *Procedures in gastrointestinal radiology*, New York, 1990, Springer Verlag.
6. Silverman PM, Kelvin FM, Korobkin M, Dunnick NR: Computed tomography of the normal mesentery, *AJR* 143:953, 1984.
7. Williams I: Innominate grooves in the surface of the mucosa, *Radiology* 84:877, 1965.
8. Matsuura K, Nakata H, Takeda N et al: Innominate lines of the colon, *Radiology* 123:581, 1977.
9. Cole FM: Innominate grooves of the colon: morphologic characteristics and etiologic mechanisms, *Radiology* 128:41, 1978.
10. Rawlinson J, Brunton FJ: Transient diverticula of the colon. *Br J Radiol* 62:27, 1989.
11. Kruyt RH, Delemarre JBVM, Doornbos J: Normal anorectum: dynamic MR imaging anatomy, *Radiology* 179:159, 1991.
12. Margulis AR, Thoeni RF: The present status of the radiologic examination of the colon, *Radiology* 167:1, 1988.
13. Thoeni RF, Margulis AR: The state of radiographic technique in the examination of the colon: a survey, *Radiology* 127:317, 1978.
14. Moss AA et al: The value of computed tomography in the detection and staging of recurrent rectal carcinoma, *J Comput Assist Tomogr* 5:870, 1981.
15. Thoeni RF: Detection and staging of primary rectal and rectosigmoid carcinoma by computed tomography, *Radiology* 141:135, 1981.
16. Thoeni RF: The colon: radiologic examination. In Margulis AR, Burhenne HJ, eds: *Alimentary tract radiology*, ed 4, St Louis, 1989, Mosby–Year Book.
17. Simpkins KC: Barium enema technique: the normal large bowel. In *A textbook of radiological diagnosis*, vol 4, The alimentary tract, ed 5, London, 1988, HK Lewis.
18. Miller RE: Examination of the colon, *Curr Probl Radiol* 5:5, 1975.
19. Gelfand DW, Chen MYM, Ott DJ: Preparing the colon for the barium enema examination, *Radiology* 178:609, 1991.
20. De Lacey G, Benson M, Wilkins R et al: Routine colonic lavage is unnecessary for double contrast barium enema in outpatients, *Br Med J* 284:1021, 1982.
21. Davis GR, Smith HJ: Double-contrast examination of the colon after preparation with Golytely (a balanced lavage solution), *Gastrointest Radiol* 8:173, 1983.
22. Girard CM, Rugh KS, DiPalmaa JA et al: Comparison of Golytely lavage with standard diet/cathartic preparation for double contrast barium enema, *AJR* 142:1147, 1984.
23. Fitzsimons P, Shorvon P, Frost RA, Stevenson GW: A comparison of Golytely and standard preparation for barium enema, *J Can Assoc Radiol* 38:109, 1987.
24. Lee SH, Bartram CI: Determining the minimum interval between cleansing water enema and double contrast barium enema examination, *Clin Radiol* 41:331, 1990.
25. Brouwers JRBJ, van Ouwerkerk WPL, de Boer SM et al: A controlled trial of senna preparations and other laxatives used for bowel cleansing prior to radiological examination, *Pharmacology* 20:58, 1980.
26. Present AJ, Jameson B, Burhenne HJ et al: Evaluation of 12 colon cleansing regimens with single contrast barium enema, *AJR* 139:855, 1982.
27. Fork FT, Ekberg O, Nilsson G et al: Colon cleansing regimens: a clinical study in 1200 patients, *Gastrointest Radiol* 7:383, 1982.
28. Hawes RH, Lehman GA, Brunelle RL et al: Comparative efficacy of colon cleansing methods: standard preparation vs. colimac lavage, *AJR* 142:309, 1984.
29. Bartram CI, Mootoosamy IM, Lim IKH: Washout versus nonwashout (picolax) preparation for double contrast barium enemas, *Clin Radiol* 35:143, 1984.
30. Margulis AR: Water-soluble contrast agents in the gastrointestinal tract. In Miller RE, Skucas J, eds: *Radiographic contrast agents*, Baltimore, 1977, University Park Press.

31. Coblentz CL, Frost RA, Molinaro V, Stevenson GW: Pain after barium enema: effect of CO_2 and air on double-contrast study, *Radiology* 157:35, 1985.
32. Stevenson GW, Wilson JA, Wilkinson J et al: Pain following colonoscopy: elimination with carbon dioxide, *Gastrointest Endosc* 38:564, 1992.
33. Hussein AM, Bartram CI, Williams CB: Carbon dioxide insufflation for more comfortable colonoscopy, *Gastrointest Endosc* 30:68, 1984.
34. Rogers BHG: CO_2 during colonoscopy for safety and comfort, *Gastrointest Endosc* 31:108, 1985.
35. Phaosawasadi K, Cooley W, Wheeler J, Rice P: Carbon dioxide–insufflated colonoscopy: an ignored superior technique, *Gastrointest Endosc* 32:330, 1986.
36. Bartram CI: A simple method for using carbon dioxide during double contrast barium enema, *Clin Radiol* 40:318, 1989.
37. Pochaczevsky R: Double contrast examination of the colon with carbon dioxide: the use of effervescent powder, *AJR* 149:502, 1987.
38. Bessette JR, Maglinte DD: Double-contrast barium enema study: simple conversion to CO_2, *Radiology* 162:274, 1987.
39. Bernier P, Coblentz C: CO_2 delivery system for double-contrast barium enema examinations, *Radiology* 159:264, 1986.
40. Laufer I: Double contrast enema: technical aspects. In *Double contrast gastrointestinal radiology,* Philadelphia, 1979, WB Saunders.
41. Ferrucci JR, Benedict KT: Anticholinergic aided study of the gastrointestinal tract, *Radiol Clin North Am* 9:2339, 1971.
42. Harned RK, Stelling CB, William S: Glucagon and barium enema examinations: controlled clinical trial, *AJR* 126:981, 1976.
43. Miller RE et al: Hypotonic colon examination with glucagon, *Radiology* 115:555, 1974.
44. Kreel L: Pharmacoradiology in barium examinations with special reference to glucagon, *Br J Radiol* 48:691, 1975.
45. Simpkins KC: Radiology now. The colon pacified, *Br J Radiol* 49:303, 1976.
46. Miller RE, Chernish SM, Brunelle RI: Gastrointestinal radiography with glucagon, *Gastrointest Radiol* 4:1, 1979.
47. Ritsema GH, Thijn CJP: Painful irritable bowel syndrome and sigmoid contractions, *Clin Radiol* 43:113, 1991.
48. Stewart ET, Dodds WJ: Predictability of rectal incontinence on barium enema examination, *AJR* 132:197, 1979.
49. Gelfand DW: Techniques for examining the colon. In *Gastrointestinal radiology,* New York, 1984, Churchill Livingstone.
50. Gelfand DW: Complications of routine gastrointestinal radiologic procedures: I. Complications of routine fluoroscopic studies, *Gastrointest Radiol* 5:293, 1980.
51. Killingback M: Acute large bowel obstruction precipitated by barium x-ray examination, *Med J Austr* 2:503, 1964.
52. Kory LA, Epstein BS: The oral use of iodinated water soluble contrast agents for visualising the proximal colon when barium enema examination reveals complete obstruction, *AJR* 115:355, 1972.
53. Grossman R, Miller W, Dann R: Oral barium sulphate in partial large bowel obstruction, *Radiology* 136:327, 1980.
54. Gotta C, Palau GA, Demos TC et al: Colonic stenoses: use of barium when retrograde flow is completely obstructed on barium enema studies, *Radiology* 177:703, 1990.
55. Munro TG: A simple model for teaching double contrast examinations of the gastrointestinal tract, *J Can Assoc Radiol* 40:162, 1989.
56. Miller RE: Examination of the colon, *Curr Probl Radiol* 5:1, 1975.
57. Gelfand DW: *Gastrointestinal radiology,* New York, 1984, Churchill Livingstone.
58. Laufer I: Double contrast enema: technical aspects. In *Double contrast gastrointestinal radiology,* Philadelphia, 1979, WB Saunders.
59. Miller RE, Maglinte DDT: Barium pneumocolon: technologist performed '7 pump' method. *AJR* 139:1230, 1982.
60. Gelfand DW, Ott DJ: Double-contrast enema: a simplified method for filling the colon, *AJR* 154:279, 1990.
61. Kelvin FM, Maglinte DDT, Stephens BA: Colorectal carcinoma detected initially with barium enema examination: site distribution and implications, *Radiology* 169:649, 1988.
62. Lappas JC, Maglinte DDT, Kopecky KK: Diverticular disease: imaging with post-double-contrast sigmoid flush, *Radiology* 168:35, 1988.
63. Saxton HM: Should radiologists report on every film, *Clin Radiol* 45:1, 1992.
64. Chapman AH: Should radiographers perform barium enemas, *Clin Radiol* 46:69, 1992.
65. Simpkins KC: Should radiologists perform and report every examination, *Clin Radiol* 46:69, 1992.
66. Campbell JA, Lieberman M, Miller RE: Experience with technician performance of gastrointestinal examinations, *Radiology* 92:65, 1969.
67. Somers S, Stevenson GW, Laufer I et al: Evaluation of double contrast barium enemas performed by radiographic technologists, *J Can Assoc Radiol* 32:227, 1981.
68. Schüle A: Ueber die Sondierung und Radiographie des Dickdarms, *Arch Verdauungskr* 10:111, 1904.
69. Fischer AW: A roentgenologic method for examination of the large intestine: combination of the contrast material enema with insufflation with air, *Klin Wochenschr* 2:1595, 1923.
70. Welin S: Modern trends in diagnostic radiology of the colon, *Br J Radiol* 31:453, 1958.
71. Young AC: The Malmo enema at St. Mark's hospital. A preliminary report, *Proc R Soc Med* 57:275, 1964.
72. Simpkins KC, Young AC: The radiology of colonic and rectal polyps, *Br J Surg* 55:731, 1968.
73. Simpkins KC, Stevenson GW: The modified Malmö double contrast barium enema in colitis: an assessment of its accuracy in reflecting sigmoidoscopic findings, *Br J Radiol* 45:486, 1972.
74. Ishikawa N, Shirakabe H, Ichikawa H: *Intestinal tuberculosis* (in Japanese). Tokyo, 1955, Kenehara Shuppan.
75. Maruyama M, Sugiyama N, Takekoshi T et al: Double contrast radiography of the colon and rectum by means of the universal gyroscopic x-ray television apparatus (in English), *Nippon Acta Radiol* 33:799, 1973.
76. Maruyama M: *Radiologic diagnosis of polyps and carcinoma of the large bowel,* Tokyo, 1978, Igaku Shoin.
77. Matsukawa M: Barium enema and polyp detection. In Maruyama M, Kimura K, eds: *Review of clinical research in gastroenterology,* Tokyo, 1988, Igaku Shoin.
78. Williams CB, Hunt RF, Loose HWC et al: Colonoscopy in the management of colon polyps, *Br J Surg* 61:673, 1974.
79. Thoeni RF, Menuck L: Comparison of barium enema and colonoscopy in the detection of small polyps, *Radiology* 124:631, 1977.
80. Ott DJ, Gelfand DW, Ramquist NA: Causes of error in gastrointestinal examinations. II: Barium enema examinations, *Gastrointest Radiol* 5:99, 1980.
81. Laufer I, Levine MS: *Double contrast gastrointestinal radiology,* ed 2, Philadelphia, 1992, WB Saunders.
82. Laufer I: Double contrast enema: myths and misconceptions, *Gastrointest Radiol* 1:19, 1976.
83. Bartram CI, Walmsley K: A radiological and pathological correlation of the mucosal changes in ulcerative colitis, *Clin Radiol* 29:323, 1978.
84. Johnson CM, Carlson HC, Taylor WF et al: Barium enemas of carcinoma of the colon: sensitivity of double- and single-contrast studies, *AJR* 140:1143, 1983.
85. Gelfand DW, Ott DJ: Single versus double contrast studies, *AJR* 137:523, 1981.
86. Fork FT, Lindström C, Ekelund GR: Reliability of routine double contrast examination of the large bowel: a prospective clinical study, *Gastrointest Radiol* 8:163, 1983.
87. Thoeni RF, Margulis AR: The state of radiographic technique in the examination of the colon: a survey in 1987, *Radiology* 167:7, 1988.

88. Gelfand DW, Ott DJ, Tritico R: Costs of gastrointestinal examinations: a comparative study, *Gastrointest Radiol* 3:135, 1978.

89. Arnold MW, Aguilar PS, Stewart WRC: Vaginography: an easy and safe technique for diagnosis of colovaginal fistulas, *Dis Colon Rectum* 33:344, 1990.

90. Young AC: The 'instant' barium enema in proctocolitis, *Proc R Soc Med* 56:491, 1963.

91. Preston D, Bartram CI, Thomas BM et al: Air introduced per rectum can be used to give radiological contrast in severe acute colitis, *Gut* 2:1914, 1980.

92. Present DH, Wolfson D, Gelernt IM et al: Medical decompression of toxic megacolon by "rolling": A new technique of decompression with favourable long term follow up, *J Clin Gastroenterol* 10:485, 1988.

93. Bettman RB, Richter HM, Drugas HT: Perforation of colostomy loop by soft rubber catheter, *JAMA* 151:206, 1953.

94. Goldstein HM, Miller MH: Air contrast colon examination in patients with colostomies, *AJR* 127:607, 1976.

95. Mark DG, Rex DK, Lappas JC: Quality of air contrast barium enema performed the same day as incomplete colonoscopy with air insufflation, *Gastrointest Endosc* 38:693, 1992.

96. Masel H, Masel JP, Casey KV: A survey of colon examination techniques in Australia and New Zealand, with a review of complications, *Australas Radiol* 15:140, 1971.

97. Gardiner H, Miller RE: Barium peritonitis: a new therapeutic approach, *Am J Surg* 125:350, 1973.

98. Han SY, Tishler JM: Perforation of the colon above the peritoneal reflection during the barium enema examination, *Radiology* 144:253, 1982.

99. Seaman WB, Wells J: Complications of the barium enema, *Gastroenterology* 48:728, 1965.

100. Ansell G: Alimentary tract. In Ansell G, ed: *Complications in diagnostic radiology,* Oxford, 1976, Blackwell.

101. Gilbert DA, Hallstrohm AP, Shaneyfelt SL et al: The national ASGE complications of colonoscopy survey, *Gastrointest Endosc* 30:156, 1984 (abstract).

102. Kronberg-Oddense (personal communication).

103. Rogers BHG, Silvis S, Nebel OT: Complications of flexible fibreoptic colonoscopy and polypectomy, *Gastrointest Endosc* 22:73, 1975.

104. Nelson JA, Davies AU, Dodds WJ: Rectal balloons: complications, causes and recommendations, *Invest Radiol* 14:48, 1979.

105. Spiro RH, Hertz RE: Colostomy perforation, *Surgery* 60:590, 1966.

106. Hemley SD, Kanick V: Perforation of the rectum: a complication of barium enema following rectal biopsy: report of two cases, *Am J Dig Dis* 8:882, 1963.

107. Williams SM, Harned RH: Recognition and prevention of barium enema complications, *Curr Probl Diagn Radiol* July/Aug 1991, p 123.

108. Pratt JH, Jackman RJ: Perforation of rectal wall by enema tip, *Mayo Clin Proc* 20:277, 1945.

109. Harned RK, Consigny PM, Cooper NB et al: Barium enema examination following biopsy of the rectum or colon, *Radiology* 145:11, 1982.

110. Prout BJ, Datta SB, Wilson TS: Colonic retention of barium in the elderly after barium meal examination, and its treatment with lactulose, *Br Med J* 4:530, 1972.

111. Feczko PJ, Simms SM, Bakirci N: Fatal hypersensitivity during a barium enema, *AJR* 153:275, 1989.

112. Schwartz EE, Glick SN, Foggs MB et al: Hypersensitivity reactions after barium enema examinations, *AJR* 143:103, 1984.

113. Javors BR, Applbaum Y, Gerard P: Severe allergic reaction: an unusual complication of barium enema, *Gastrointest Radiol* 9:357, 1984.

114. Gelfand DW, Sowers JC, DePonter KA et al: Anaphylactic and allergic reactions during double contrast studies. Is glucagon or barium suspension the allergen? *AJR* 144:405, 1985.

115. Harrington RA, Kaul AF: Cardiopulmonary arrest following barium enema examination with glucagon, *Drug Intell Clin Pharmacol* 21:721, 1987.

116. Feczko PJ: Increased frequency of reactions to contrast materials during gastrointestinal studies, *Radiology* 174:367, 1990.

117. Gelfand DW: Barium enemas, latex balloons, and anaphylactic reactions, *AJR* 156:1, 1991.

118. Ownby DR, Tomlanovich M, Sammons N et al: Anaphylaxis associated with latex allergy during barium enema examinations, *AJR* 156:903, 1991.

119. Simpkins KC: Annual oration: Bring out your barium, *J Can Assoc Radiol* 40:5, 1989.

120. Kelvin FM, Gardiner R, Stevenson GW: Colorectal carcinoma missed on double contrast barium enema study: a problem in perception, *AJR* 137:307, 1981.

121. Markus JB, Somers S, O'Malley et al: Double contrast barium enema studies: effect of multiple reading on perception error, *Radiology* 175:155, 1990.

122. Laufer I, Smith NCW, Mullens JE: The radiologic demonstration of colorectal polyps undetected by endoscopy, *Gastroenterology* 70:167, 1976.

123. Manier JW: Flexible sigmoidoscopy. In Sivak MV, ed: *Gastroenterologic endoscopy,* Philadelphia, 1987, WB Saunders.

124. Obrecht WF, Wu WC, Gelfand DW et al: The extent of successful colonoscopy: a second assessment using modern equipment, *Gastrointest Radiol* 9:161, 1984.

125. Waye JD, Frankel A, Braunfeld SF: The histopathology of small colon polyps, *Gastrointest Endosc* 26:80, 1980 (abstract).

126. Gottlieb LS, Winawer SJ, Sternberg S et al. National Polyp Study (NPS): the diminutive colonic polyp, *Gastrointest Endosc* 30:143, 1984 (abstract).

127. Stryker SJ, Wolff BE, Culp EE et al: Natural history of untreated colonic polyps, *Gastroenterology* 93:1009, 1987.

128. Atkin WS, Morson BC, Cuzick J: Long-term risk of colorectal cancer after excision of rectosigmoid adenomas, *N Engl J Med* 326:658, 1992.

129. Labayle D, Fischer D, Vielh P et al: Sulindac causes regression of rectal polyps in familial adenomatous polyposis, *Gastroenterology* 101:635, 1991.

130. Rigau J, Pique JM, Rubio E, Planas R, Tarrech JM, Bordas JM: Effects of long-term Sulindac therapy on colonic polyposis, *Ann Intern Med* 115:952, 1991.

131. Bussey HJR, DeCosse JJ, Deschner EE et al: A randomized trial of ascorbic acid in polyposis coli, *Cancer* 50:1434, 1982.

132. Nicholls RJ, Springall RG, Gallagher P: Regression of rectal adenomas after colectomy and ileorectal anastomosis for familial adenomatous polyposis, *Br Med J* 296:1707, 1988.

133. Vogelstein B, Fearon ER, Hamilton SR et al: Genetic alterations during colorectal-tumor development, *N Engl J Med* 319:525, 1988.

134. Baker SR, Alterman DD: False-negative barium enema in patients with sigmoid cancer and coexistent diverticula, *Gastrointest Radiol* 10:171, 1985.

135. Saito Y, Slezac P, Rubio C: The diagnostic value of combining flexible sigmoidoscopy and double-contrast barium enema as a one-stage procedure, *Gastrointest Radiol* 14:357, 1989.

136. Warden MJ, Petrelli NJ, Herrera L: Endoscopy versus double contrast barium enema in the evaluation of patients with symptoms suggestive of colorectal carcinoma, *Am J Surg* 155:224, 1988.

137. Vellacott KD, Hardcastle JD: An evaluation of flexible fibreoptic sigmoidoscopy, *Br Med J* 283:1583, 1981.

138. Vellacott KD, Amar SS, Hardcastle JD: Comparison of rigid and flexible fiberoptic sigmoidoscopy with double contrast barium enema, *Br J Surg* 69:399, 1982.

139. Warden MJ, Petrelli NJ, Herrera L, Mittelman A: The role of colonoscopy and flexible sigmoidoscopy in screening for colorectal carcinoma, *Dis Colon Rectum* 30:52, 1987.

140. Eckardt VF, Kanzler G, Willems D: Same-day versus separate-day

sigmoidoscopy and double contrast barium enema: a randomized controlled study, *Gastrointest Endosc* 35:512, 1989.

141. Marshall JB, Hoyt TS, Seger RM, Reid JC, Beyer KL, Butt JH: Air-contrast barium enema studies after flexible proctosigmoidoscopy: randomized controlled clinical trial, *Radiology* 176:549, 1990.

142. Stevenson GW, Hernandez C: Single visit screening and treatment of first degree relatives: colon cancer pilot study, *Dis Colon Rectum* 34:1120, 1991.

143. Ott DJ, Gelfand DW, Wu WC, Kerr RM: Sensitivity of double contrast barium enema: emphasis on polyp detection, *AJR* 135:327, 1980.

144. Reference deleted in galleys.

145. Farrands PA, Vellacott KD, Amar SS, Balfour TW, Hardcastle JD: Flexible fiberoptic sigmoidoscopy and double-contrast barium enema examination in the identification of adenomas and carcinoma of the colon, *Dis Colon Rectum* 26:725, 1983.

146. Fork FT: Fibre endoscopy versus radiology. In Lunderquist A, Pettersson H, eds: *Gastrointestinal and urogenital radiology* (Nicer Series on Diagnostic Imaging), London, 1991, Merit Communications.

147. Glick SN, Teplick SK, Balfe DM et al: Large colonic neoplasms missed by endoscopy, *AJR* 152:513, 1989.

148. Rosch T, Lorenz R, Classen M: Endoscopic ultrasonography in the evaluation of colon and rectal disease, *Gastrointest Endosc* 36:s33, 1990.

149. Wilson SR, Toi A: The value of sonography in the diagnosis of acute diverticulitis of the colon, *AJR* 154:1199, 1990.

150. Hirooka N, Ohno T, Misonoo M et al: Sono-enterocolonography by oral water administration, *J Clin Ultrasound* 17:585, 1989.

151. Rubin C, Kurtz AB, Goldberg BB: Water enema: a new ultrasound technique in defining pelvic anatomy, *J Clin Ultrasound* 6:28, 1978.

152. Fleischer AC, Muhletaler CA, James AE: Sonographic assessment of the bowel wall, *AJR* 136:887, 1981.

153. Puylaert JBC, Lalisang RI, van der Werf SDJ et al: *Campylobacter* ileocolitis mimicking acute appendicitis: Differentiation with graded compression, *Radiology* 166:737, 1988.

154. Jeffrey RB, Laing FC, Lewis FR: Acute appendicitis: high resolution real time ultrasound findings, *Radiology* 163:11, 1987.

155. Gaensler EHL, Jeffrey RB, Laing FC et al: Sonography in patients with suspected acute appendicitis: value in establishing alternative diagnosis, *AJR* 152:49, 1989.

156. Abu-Yousef MM, Bleicher JJ, Maher JW et al: High resolution sonography of acute appendicitis, *AJR* 149:53, 1987.

157. Limberg B: Diagnosis of acute ulcerative colitis and colonic Crohn's disease by colonic sonography, *J Clin Ultrasound* 17:25, 1989.

158. Matsumoto T, Iida M, Matsui T et al: Ultrasonic and CT findings in penicillin induced nonpseudomembranous colitis, *Gastrointest Radiol* 15:329, 1990.

159. Letourneau JG, Day DL, Steely JW et al: CT appearance of antibiotic induced colitis, *Gastrointest Radiol* 12:257, 1987.

160. Limberg B: Diagnosis of large bowel tumours by colonic sonography, *Lancet* 335:144, 1990.

161. Price J, Metreweli C: Ultrasonic diagnosis of clinically nonpalpable primary colonic neoplasms, *Br J Radiol* 61:190, 1988.

162. Khaw KT, Yeoman LJ, Saverymuttu SH et al: Ultrasonic patterns in inflammatory bowel disease, *Clin Radiol* 43:171, 1991.

163. Puylaert JBCM: Acute appendicitis: US evaluation using graded compression, *Radiology* 158:355, 1986.

164. Mittelstaedt CA: Ultrasound. In Yamada T et al, eds: *Textbook of gastroenterology,* Philadelphia, 1991, JB Lippincott.

165. Lund PJ, Fritz TA, Unger EC et al: Cellulose as a gastrointestinal US contrast agent, *Radiology* 185:783, 1992.

166. Hatfield KD, Segal SD, Tait K: Barium sulphate for abdominal computer assisted tomography, *J Comput Assist Tomogr* 4:570, 1980.

167. Carr DH, Banks LM: Comparison of barium and diatrizoate bowel labelling agents in computed tomography, *Br J Radiol* 58:393, 1985.

168. Mitchell DG, Bjorgvinsson E, terMeulen D et al: Gastrograffin vs

dilute barium for colonic CT examination: A blind randomised study, *J Comput Assist Tomogr* 9:451, 1981.

169. Raptopoulos V, Davis MA, Davidoff A et al: Fat density oral contrast agent for abdominal CT, *Radiology* 164:653, 1987.

170. Bach DB: Telebrix: a better tasting oral contrast agent for abdominal computed tomography, *J Can Assoc Radiol* 42:98, 1991.

171. Tannous WN, Azouz EM: Bowel opacification for abdominal computed tomography in children: a clinical trial of oral Telebrix 38, *J Can Assoc Radiol* 42:102, 1991.

172. Aronberg DJ, Lee JKT, Sagel SS et al: *Techniques in computed body tomography,* New York, 1983, Raven Press.

173. Mitchell DG, Bjorgvinsson E, terMeulen D et al: Comparison of Telebrix-Gastro and Gastrograffin in abdominal computed tomography, *Eur J Radiol* 9:179, 1989.

174. Desai RK, Tagliabue JR, Wegryn SA, Einstein DM: CT evaluation of wall thickening in the alimentary tract, *Radiographics* 11:771, 1991.

175. Solomon A, Michowitz M, Papo J, Yust I: Computed tomographic air enema technique to demonstrate colonic neoplasms, *Gastrointest Radiol* 11:194, 1986.

176. Megibow AJ, Zerhouni H et al: Air insufflation of the colon as an adjunct to computed tomography of the pelvis, *J Comput Assist Tomogr* 4:797, 1984.

177. Megibow AJ, Zerhouni EA, Hulnick DH et al: Air contrast techniques in gastrointestinal computed tomography, *AJR* 145:418, 1985.

178. Balthazar EJ: The colon: In Megibow AJ, Balthazar EJ, eds: *Computed tomography of the gastrointestinal tract,* St. Louis, 1986, Mosby–Year Book.

179. Balthazar EJ, Megibow AJ, Schinella RA et al: Limitations in the CT diagnosis of acute diverticulitis: comparison of CT, contrast enema, and pathologic findings in 16 patients, *AJR* 154:281, 1990.

180. Baron RL: Application of computed tomography to the gastrointestinal tract. In Yamada T, ed: *Textbook of gastroenterology,* Philadelphia, 1991, JB Lippincott.

181. Megibow AJ: Diverticulitis. In Myers MA, ed: *Computed tomography of the gastrointestinal tract,* New York, 1986, Springer Verlag.

182. Angelelli G, Macarani L: CT of the bowel: use of water to enhance depiction, *Radiology* 169:848, 1988.

183. Gossios KJ, Tsianos EV, Kontogiannis DS: Water as contrast medium for computed tomography study of colonic wall lesions, *Gastrointest Radiol* 17:125, 1992.

184. Thoeni RH, Filson RG: Abdominal and pelvic CT: use of oral metoclopramide to enhance bowel opacification, *Radiology* 169:391, 1988.

185. Megibow AJ, Balthazar EJ, Cho KC et al: Bowel obstruction: evaluation with CT, *Radiology* 180:313, 1991.

186. Rubin GD, Dake MD, Napel SA et al: Three dimensional spiral CT angiography of the abdomen: initial clinical experience, *Radiology* 186:147, 1993.

187. Raptopoulos V: Technical principles in CT evaluation of the gut, *Radiol Clin North Am* 27:631, 1989.

188. Saini S, Stark DD: Magnetic resonance imaging. In Yamada T et al, eds: *Textbook of gastroenterology,* Philadelphia, 1991, JB Lippincott.

189. Imai Y, Kressel HY, Saul SH et al: Colorectal tumours: an in vitro study of high-resolution MR imaging, *Radiology* 177:695, 1990.

190. Balzarini L, Ceglia E, D'Ippolito G et al: Local recurrence of rectosigmoid cancer: What about the choice of MRI for diagnosis? *Gastrointest Radiol* 15:338, 1990.

191. Tait RP, Li KCP, Storm BL et al: Enteric MRI contrast agents: comparative study of five potential agents in humans, *Magn Reson Imaging* 9:559, 1991.

192. Balzarini L, Aime S, Barbero L et al: Magnetic resonance imaging of the gastrointestinal tract: investigation of baby milk as a low cost contrast agent, *Eur J Radiol* 15:171, 1992.

193. Biset GS: Evaluation of potential practical oral contrast agents for

pediatric magnetic resonance imaging. Preliminary observations, *Pediatr Radiol* 20:61, 1989.

194. Ros PR, Steinman RM, Torres GM: The value of barium as a gastrointestinal contrast agent in MR imaging: a comparison study in normal volunteers, *AJR* 157:761, 1991.

195. Chan TW, Kressel HY, Milestone B et al: Rectal carcinoma: staging at MR imaging with endorectal surface coil, *Radiology* 181:461, 1991.

196. de Lange EE, Fechner RE, Spaulding CA et al: Rectal carcinoma treated by preoperative radiation: MR imaging and histopathologic correlation, *AJR* 158:287, 1992.

197. Demas BE, Hricak H, Wall SD: The rectum and anal canal. In Higgins CB, Hricak H, Helms CA, eds: *Magnetic resonance imaging of the body,* New York, 1992, Raven Press.

198. Waizer A, Powsner E, Russo I et al: Prospective comparison study of magnetic resonance imaging versus transrectal ultrasound for preoperative staging and follow up of rectal cancer, *Dis Colon Rectum* 34:1068, 1991.

199. Hodgman CG, MacCarty RL, Wolff BG et al: Preoperative staging of rectal carcinoma by computed tomography and 0.15T magnetic resonance imaging, *Dis Colon Rectum* 29:446, 1986.

200. Ito K, Kato T, Tadokoro M et al: Recurrent rectal cancer and scar: differentiation with PET and MR imaging, *Radiology* 182:549, 1992.

201. Doerr RJ, Abdel-Nabi H, Krag D: Radiolabelled antibody imaging in the management of colorectal cancer: results of a multicenter clinical study, *Ann Surg* 214:118, 1991.

202. Collier BD, Abdel-Nabi H, Doerr RJ et al: Immunoscintigraphy performed with an In[111] labelled CYT-103 in the management of colorectal cancer: comparison with CT, *Radiology* 185:179, 1992.

35 *Normal Anatomy and Techniques of Examination of the Colon and Rectum: Endosonography*

JOSE F. BOTET
CHARLES J. LIGHTDALE

The colon and rectum, although in reality part of a single continuum, are considered here as two discrete entities because the techniques and instruments used in both examinations differ.

COLON
Normal anatomy

The colon lies between the ileocecal valve and the junction with the rectum, and measures approximately 100 cm long. Anatomically, it is divided into the ascending, transverse, descending, and sigmoid segments. Each segment is separated from the other by a flexure: the hepatic flexure separating the ascending from the transverse colon; the splenic flexure separating the transverse from the descending colon; and the sigmoid flexure separating the descending from the sigmoid colon. The colon is an easily distended organ, but, in pathologic conditions, it may be either narrowed or grossly distended. The diameter of the normal colon decreases going from the cecum to the sigmoid. It may be extremely redundant or it may be foreshortened in certain pathologic conditions.

From an ultrasonographic perspective, it is a difficult organ to evaluate because the relationships at each level are difficult to reproduce and the position of the transducer is difficult to determine, unless aided by direct visualization of the lumen or the use of fluoroscopy.

Cecum and ascending colon

The position of the cecum is difficult to ascertain endosonographically. The ileocecal valve, when identifiable medially, is one of the few landmarks to help orient the positioning of the scope. Usually the abundance of gas from surrounding small bowel loops renders it difficult to determine what is anterior and posterior. As the hepatic flexure is approached, the right hepatic lobe and right kidney can be visualized. No major vessels can be visualized consistently, although the right renal artery and vein in the hilum of the right kidney may sometimes be seen. The lymphatic drainage of the colon is toward the mesentery (Fig. 35-1).

Transverse colon

As the transducer moves over the hepatic flexure, there is a dramatic change in the ultrasound images. As the axis tilts 90 degrees horizontally, the plane of imaging is sagittal. The close relationship of the hepatic flexure to the gallbladder fossa can be appreciated in most cases. The inferior vena cava and aorta are far posterior to the colon and, depending on the distance and air present in the intervening stomach and duodenum, may or may not be visualized. The relationship of the splenic flexure to the spleen and left kidney can be appreciated in most cases. The lymphatic drainage of the transverse colon is toward the mesocolon posteriorly (Fig. 35-2).

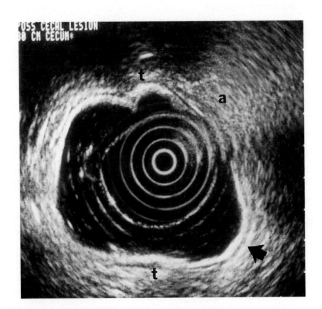

Fig. 35-1 Cecum. Note the taenias *(t)*. The five-layered wall is well demonstrated *(black arrowhead)*. Technical artifact *(a)* is due to the forward-viewing channel overlying the transducer (7.5 MHz).

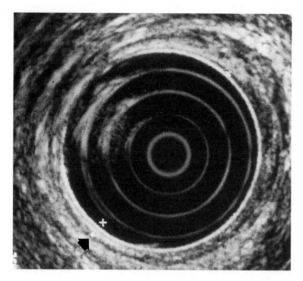

Fig. 35-2 Transverse colon. Few landmarks can be seen due to the surrounding bowel air. The five layers of the wall are well depicted *(arrowhead)*.

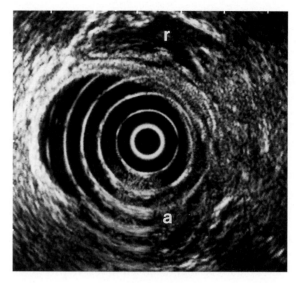

Fig. 35-3 Sigmoid. The sigmoid reflexion *(r)* can be imaged through the lower sigmoid. *a,* Technical artifact.

Descending colon

The transition at the splenic flexure can be observed by tilting the axis of the scope, and thereby reversing the observed images. The spleen and left kidney are two constant landmarks at the splenic flexure. Below this level, it is difficult to ascertain the position of the endoscope unless aided by fluoroscopy. Again, the transition from the descending colon can be identified endoscopically by the change in the relative position of the surrounding structures as the axis of the scope changes.

Sigmoid

The curvature of the sigmoid is extremely variable, making it difficult to ascertain relationships, especially because the angle of the transducer can be complex in that it may be angled inferiorly and posteriorly. The most constant orienting relationships are to the distended bladder and, in females, to the uterine fundus and body. Depending on how posterior the sigmoid is and how close to the uterus, it may be possible to observe the left iliac vessels and, if close enough, the uterine vessels. It is important not to confuse vessels with lymph nodes in this area (Fig. 35-3).

Examination technique
Preparation

Patients undergoing colonic endosonography go through the same preparation as for a colonoscopy or double-contrast barium enema. As is done for upper gastrointestinal tract evaluations, on arrival, the patient undergoes a pre-procedure interview in which a short clinical history is obtained, vital signs are recorded, and the results of pertinent prior studies and laboratory tests are reviewed. Patients are

then transferred to a procedure room, where informed consent is obtained. An intravenous line is started. The patient's vital signs, including pulse oximetry, are measured, and the patient is placed in the lithotomy position. Oxygen, given through a nasal cannula, is routinely administered at the rate of 2 liters per minute. A preliminary digital examination of the rectum is performed. The use of intravenous sedation, usually a combination of meperidine acting benzodiazepine, is an elective aspect of the procedure, with the dosage titrated on an individual basis.

Procedure

The usual procedure consists of two parts. Because the endosonographic scope used for the evaluation of the colon (Olympus CF UM20) is a forward-viewing scope, it can also be used to perform a preliminary colonoscopy. The examination should be carried out to the cecum, and any observed or suspected abnormalities should be noted for later endosonographic evaluation. The instrument is introduced again under visual control and advanced to the cecum. The balloon overlying the transducer is then filled with water, the cecum is filled with water, and air is suctioned. Using the previously described landmarks, the evaluation takes place as the instrument is slowly withdrawn. The colonic wall layers are identical to those seen in the upper gastrointestinal tract, and any disruption can be observed. The water can be maneuvered into the area of interest by rotating the patient. The authors routinely do not use a tilt table, although it may be helpful in cases of significantly redundant colon. It is helpful to position the scope visually over any suspected abnormality, as this greatly simplifies the procedure.

There are several common difficulties that can be encountered in examinations of the colon. One is difficulty in advancing the scope to the cecum. This is a common problem during conventional colonoscopies in patients with significantly redundant colon. Poor preparation is a second problem. The presence of residual fecal material or a large amount of mucus or blood will interfere with the quality of the images. A third difficulty is poor patient tolerance. Because sedation is elective, and the endosonographic colonoscope is far more rigid than a conventional endoscope, a patient who tolerated a conventional colonoscopy without intravenous sedation may become uncomfortable or agitated during endosonography. Another common pitfall in the examination is the presence of large amounts of air in the colon that either defy suction or remain despite the use of large amounts of water. This is especially common in the cecum. Decompression, done over a period of minutes, using a rectal tube may be necessary.

As mentioned previously, the examination is tailored to evaluate the specific suspicious findings that prompted the procedure, including any originally unsuspected findings discovered in the preliminary colonoscopy.

RECTUM

The endosonographic evaluation of the gastrointestinal tract began in the rectum. Wild and Reid [1] first reported its use in the rectum in a landmark article published in 1956. They used a bistable probe to differentiate between solid and cystic lesions. The first modern systems were investigated by DiMagno et al. [2] at the Mayo Clinic. This early instrument consisted of an endoscope with a liner array attached to its side. In developing this technology, the cardinal principles of intraluminal ultrasound took shape. The need for good acoustic contact between the transducer and the rectal wall was solved by the placement of a water-filled balloon. Further developments in ultrasound equipment led to the advent of the rigid transrectal probes, which were originally developed with other organs such as the prostate and female pelvis in mind. Because these structures can be imaged quite well with sector scanners, most of the rigid transducers use this technology. Few manufacturers offer the full 360-degree field of view used in endoscopic sonographic equipment. The frequencies used in this area are the result of a compromise. High frequencies allow evaluation of the rectal wall but have little penetration, thus furnishing limited information on the pelvic structures and nodes. Conversely, low frequencies provide a deeper view into the pelvic anatomic structures, but the resolution of the rectal layers is diminished. This has spawned two different imaging strategies. The rigid probes tend to use lower-frequency transducers (5 to 7.5 MHz) because they are mainly used in the evaluation of other pelvic structures such as the prostate in males and uterus and ovaries in females, although they have also been used in the staging of rectal tumors.[3-12] The flexible endoscopes use higher frequencies

(7.5 to 12 MHz), because their main focus is on the bowel wall.[13-15]

Normal anatomy
Rectum

From a surgical standpoint, the rectum extends superiorly from the sacral promontory, follows the sacrum and coccyx, and ends in the anal canal after passing through the levator ani muscles. It measures between 12 and 15 cm in length. There are three infoldings, also called *transverse folds of Houston,* that correspond to the three lateral curvatures. The rectum is divided into three parts by peritoneal reflections. The cranial portion is intraabdominal and retroperitoneal and is covered by the peritoneum anteriorly and laterally. The midportion is covered by the peritoneum anteriorly. The lower third is not covered by the peritoneum and lies outside the abdominal cavity. The peritoneal reflection varies according to sex, and ranges between 7 and 9 cm in males and between 5 and 7.5 cm from the anal verge in females. This reflection corresponds in position to that of the middle valve of Houston.

There are other important anatomic relationships. In males the prostate is anterior to the rectum and above it are the seminal vesicles (Fig. 35-4 and 35-5). It is separated from these structures by the fascia of Denonvilliers. The bladder lies superiorly and anteriorly to the prostate. In females the anterior relationship is to the vagina and cervix inferiorly and anteriorly, respectively. Above the rectum is

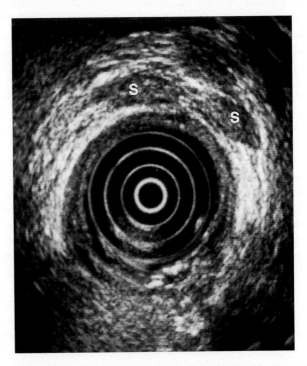

Fig. 35-4 Seminal vesicles. Endoscopic sonographic imaging of the seminal vesicles *(S)*. Note the 360-degree field of view. A 7.5-MHz transducer was used.

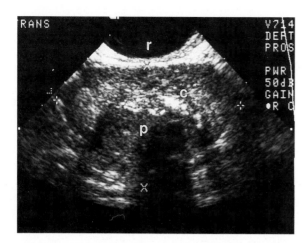

Fig. 35-5 Prostate. Ultrasound images of the prostate *(p)* using a conventional transrectal 5-MHz transducer. Note the 90-degree field of view in the transverse plane. Some calcifications *(c)* are noted within the substance of the prostate. *r,* Rectal lumen.

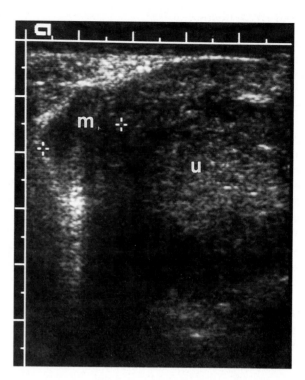

Fig. 35-6 Uterus. Ultrasound images of an enlarged uterus *(u)*. Small superficial myomas *(m)* are noted in the periphery. Image taken in the longitudinal plane with a conventional transrectal 5-MHz transducer. The ability of these transducers to obtain images in the longitudinal and transverse planes is an asset when imaging pelvic structures.

located the uterus (Fig. 35-6), but this depends on the rotation of the uterus. In the female pelvis the uterus is located between the rectum and the bladder.

There are three levels to the blood supply of the rectum. All interconnect freely through functional anastomoses. The upper level is formed by a terminal branch of the inferior mesenteric artery, the rectal artery. Paired branches of the hypogastric arteries, the middle rectal arteries, constitute the middle level, and the inferior rectal arteries constitute the lower level. They also arise from the hypogastric arteries. The venous drainage is accomplished through the hemorrhoidal plexus to the hypogastric veins or middle sacral vein. The lymphatic drainage of the upper rectum follows the superior rectal vein into the paraaortic lymph nodes. The middle level drainage follows the hypogastric vessels.

Anus

The anal canal represents the distal portion of the large bowel and extends from the dentate line formed by the columns of Morgagni, of which there are between six and fourteen. It typically measures 3 to 4 cm in length. Below the dentate line the columnar epithelium changes into squamous epithelium, with a transition area between 6 and 12 mm above the dentate line. Relationships at this level are few, but the tip of the coccyx may allow differentiation of anterior from posterior (Fig. 35-7).

No major vessels can be identified in this area, except for the hemorrhoidal plexus. However, this is usually not identifiable in normal subjects because the veins are compressed by the water-filled balloon.

The lymphatic drainage of the upper anus follows the hypogastric vessels, whereas the lower end drains into the inguinal lymph nodes.

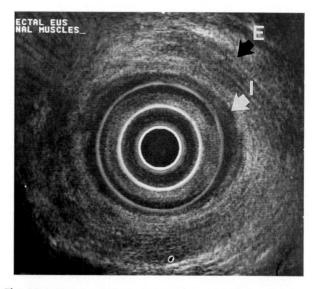

Fig. 35-7 Rectal sphincters. Endosonography of the anal canal demonstrates two muscle layers surrounding the anus. These are the internal sphincter muscle *(i)* and the external sphincter muscle *(e)*.

Examination technique
Preparation

Patients receive the same preparation as for colonic examination.

Procedure

There are two different techniques for the evaluation of the rectum and anus. A conventional ultrasound machine with a rigid probe may be used for this purpose, of which there are multiple designs and as many manufacturers. Two main types of transducers are used: mechanical or electronic transducers permitting a 360-degree field of view or variations of sector scanning, which can be fired in a longitudinal, transverse, or in a forward direction. Either rigid or flexible probes are currently available for both systems. The flexible probes are available with or without optical guidance.

In keeping with the variety of equipment used for this purpose, different techniques have evolved. The authors describe the one currently used at their institution when flexible, optically guided transducers are used. The endoscope we use for the evaluation of the colon (Olympus CF UM20) is forward-viewing with a 7.5-MHz transducer at its end. Using the previously described landmarks for orientation, the evaluation is carried out as the instrument is slowly withdrawn. The rectal wall layers are identical to those in the colon. Any disruption can be observed. The water can be maneuvered into the area of interest by rotating the patient. It is helpful to position the scope visually over any suspected abnormality, as this greatly simplifies the procedure.

REFERENCES

1. Wild JJ, Reid JM: Intrarectal ultrasound, *Br J Phys Med* 19:248, 1956.
2. DiMagno EP, Regan PT, Clain JE et al: Human endoscopic ultrasonography, *Gastroenterology* 83:824, 1982.
3. Saitoh N, Okui K, Sarashina H et al: Evaluation of echographic diagnosis of rectal cancer using intrarectal ultrasonic examination, *Dis Colon Rectum* 29:234, 1986.
4. Romano G, DeRosa P, Vallon G et al: Intrarectal ultrasound and computed tomography in the pre- and post-operative assessment of patients with rectal carcinoma, *Br J Surg* 72(suppl.):S117, 1985.
5. Konishi F, Muto T, Takahashi H et al: Transrectal ultrasonography for the assessment of invasion of rectal carcinoma, *Dis Colon Rectum* 28:889, 1985.
6. Beynon J, Mortensen NJM, Foy DMA et al: Pre-operative assessment of local invasion in rectal cancer: digital examination, endoluminal sonography or computed tomography? *Br J Surg* 73:1015, 1986.
7. Anderson R, Aus G: Transrectal ultrasound-guided biopsy for verification of lymph-node metastasis in rectal cancer: case report, *Acta Chir Scand* 156:659, 1990.
8. Lorentzen T, Torp-Pedersen S, Nolsoe C: Transrectal ultrasound findings of prostate cancer mimicking primary rectal tumor, *Acta Radiol* 31:625, 1990.
9. Hinder JM, Chu J, Bokey EL et al: Use of transrectal ultrasound to evaluate direct tumor spread and lymph node status in patients with rectal cancer, *Aust NZ J Surg* 60:19, 1990.
10. Dershaw DD, Enker WE, Cohen AM, Sigurdson ER: Transrectal ultrasonography of rectal carcinoma, *Cancer* 66:2336, 1990.
11. Waizer A, Zitron S, Ben-Baruch D et al: Comparative study for preoperative staging of rectal cancer, *Dis Colon Rectum* 32:53, 1989.
12. Waizer A, Powsner E, Russo I et al: Prospective comparative study of magnetic resonance imaging versus transrectal ultrasound for preoperative staging and follow-up of rectal cancer: preliminary report, *Dis Colon Rectum* 34:1068, 1991.
13. Goldman S, Arvidsson H, Norming U et al: Transrectal ultrasound and computed tomography in preoperative staging of lower rectal adenocarcinoma, *Gastrointest Radiol* 16:259, 1991.
14. Beynon J, Roe AM, Foy DM et al: Preoperative staging of local invasion in rectal cancer using endoluminal ultrasound, *J R Soc Med* 80:23, 1987.
15. Berdov BA, Slesarev VI, Fedlaev JB: Transrectal and transvaginal ultrasonic diagnosis of rectal cancer, *Radiol Diagn* (Berl) 31:529, 1990.

36 *Diverticular Disease of the Colon: Conventional Radiology*

PIERRE SCHNYDER
BERTRAND DUVOISIN

Diverticular disease has been diagnosed with increasing frequency during the twentieth century, becoming a disease that now carries great economic consequences. One estimate puts the number of affected Americans at 30 million and the health-care costs at more than $300 million a year.[1,2]

The introduction of the barium enema led to the demonstration of symptomless diverticula. In the 1960s pathologists, radiologists, and surgeons, in the process of measuring intraluminal pressures, produced new evidence that focused attention on a muscular abnormality always known but largely ignored, but now thought to be of fundamental importance. This muscular abnormality is responsible for the complex distorsions of the colon that can occur and is of prime interest to the radiologist.

The 1970s saw the development of the epidemiologic study, sparked by the enthusiasm of Painter and Burkitt,[3] who showed an inverse relationship between the incidence of diverticular disease and the amount of roughage in the diet of each population. This discovery prompted work on treatment and ways in which to prevent the problem. During this period the diagnostic capabilities improved, with the advent of better enemas, angiography, and colonoscopy, but research into two basic problems has hardly started. No one has yet identified the cause of inflammation, a dangerous but uncommon complication of diverticulosis, nor has any progress been made toward understanding the underlying muscular abnormality, possibly because smooth muscle physiology[4] and the way in which the human colon functions are little understood. Vague words like *spasm* and *contracture* remain acceptable descriptions but reflect our lack of understanding.

METHOD OF EXAMINATION

It is valuable to examine the plain film of the abdomen with great care, not so much to look for diverticulosis, but to search for diverticulitis. Sacs can occasionally be recognized as a row of appropriately sized gas-filled shadows that run parallel to the line of the colon, but a poorly contoured soft tissue mass and obliteration of the peritoneal fat lines suggest the presence of inflammation. An irregular gas shadow may point to the existence of an abscess. Although this is often not a reliable diagnostic sign, suspicions based on clinical findings may influence the direction that further investigations take.

Demonstrating diverticular sacs and the distorted lumen typical of diverticular disease is easy, requiring no more than a well-performed enema in a well-prepared patient. The left posterior oblique view is a worthwhile component. Spasm of the sigmoid and lower descending colon is very common, and films taken at an early filling stage show a narrowed lumen, which, at a later stage, relaxes and assumes the characteristic deformity. Careful spot films of any suspicious areas, obtained with the colon in maximal distention, are essential. There is a good case[5-7] for the frequent use of smooth muscle relaxants such as glucagon, which both abolishes spasm and allows full distention without pain or discomfort to the patient. Full distention reduces the number of overlapping lines in any picture, making the visual recognition of an abnormality easier.

Inflammation usually occurs in the form of microperforations that rapidly seal[8] (see Fig. 36-9), leading to the formation of small intramural or subserous abscesses; however, large abscesses and free perforation are also familiar problems.

When the clinical picture indicates acute inflammation, the radiologist is asked to perform an enema study for diagnostic purposes. Current thinking rejects the concept that the radiologist should delay this enema for as long as possible to allow a thick-walled barrier to form around any leak. However, because free barium in the peritoneal cavity will only worsen the prognosis in an already severely ill patient, the enema must be carried out using any of the numerous water-soluble contrast materials available. Furthermore, diverticular perforation is an emergency that should not require a barium enema study for the diagnosis of colonic mucosal derangements, even if the coexistence of diverticula and carcinoma is common.[9,10] In these instances, a double-contrast barium enema or colonoscopy should be performed in a thoroughly clean colon, 2 or 3 weeks after the acute episode. During the acute phase a "gentle" low-pressure water-soluble contrast enema should be performed. This study should be carefully monitored by fluoroscopy and stopped at the first sign of a leak.[11]

Isotope scanning and ultrasonography[12-14] (see Fig. 36-3, *C*) have proved their worth in the detection of abscesses in the abdomen. Computed tomography (CT) performed in the acute phase of the disease[15,16] is currently the most sensitive and specific test for diagnosing the complications of acute diverticulitis. It should be considered early in the course of the disease when a diverticular abscess or fistula is suspected so that immediate and appropriate therapy can be instituted, consisting of percutaneous drainage, surgery, or conservative therapy[17-19] (see Fig. 36-3, *B* and *D*).

Magnetic resonance imaging (MRI) promises to be an alternative approach in studying the relationship of the abscess to the urinary bladder and colon (Fig. 36-1). MRI offers direct coronal and sagittal views, besides transverse ones and a variety of other sequences that can furnish information about the nature of the soft tissue consistency.

INCIDENCE

The thesis of Painter and Burkitt,[3] that the epidemiology of diverticular disease would supply clues to its pathogenesis, has led to the study of its incidence in many parts of the world. There are now several reports of its worldwide distribution,[3,20-22] and only the generally agreed-upon conclusions are cited here. As the authors of these various accounts all stress, the numbers in published series are all derived from selected groups of patients, such as hospital admission figures, x-ray department records, and autopsy findings. Therefore the true incidence remains a matter of guesswork.

For Western industrial nations, diverticular disease was rare during the nineteenth century[3] but has steadily become more common during the past 80 years. Autopsy figures for the elderly in the early part of the century yield an incidence of 5% to 10%, but recently an incidence of 50% has been cited.[23-25] This constitutes striking evidence that diverticulosis is very much a disease of the twentieth century. In Western countries, at least one person out of two can expect to acquire colon diverticula by the age of 60.[24,25] The sex incidence is changing, in that initially twice as many men as women were affected, but series collected over the past 20 years now reveal a slight preponderance of women.[24,26]

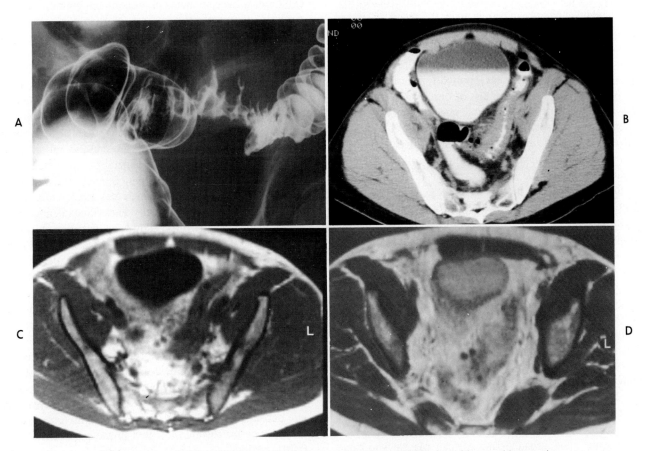

Fig. 36-1 Diverticulitis with abscess impinging on the urinary bladder in a 66-year-old man. **A,** Spot film from a barium enema study showing spasm and the impression made by the abscess. **B,** Transverse CT section shows abscess impinging on the urinary bladder. Small bubbles are seen within the abscess. There is contrast material in both the colon and bladder. **C,** T1 MRI image. **D,** In a T2 MRI image, the abscess and its effect on the surrounding organs are well seen. Both T1 and T2 images provide information equivalent to that yielded by contrast-enhanced CT scans.

In a large series consisting of 102 patients, Johnson et al.[18] showed in 1987 that a contrast enema yielded true-positive results in 77%, false-negative results in 50%, and indeterminate findings in 7%. The CT accuracy was much lower; true-positive results at that time were obtained in only 38%, false-negative results in 21%, and uncertain results in 38% of the patients. The authors' concluded from this that the contrast enema should remain the initial routine examination in patients with suspected diverticulitis. One year later, similar conclusions were published by Feczko et al.[27] and Lappas et al.,[28] this latter group having compared CT scans and double-contrast images of the large bowel followed by a single-contrast sigmoid flush. More recent papers[2,15,17] cite much higher CT sensitivities and specificities, probably attributable to better CT technology, the intravenous injection of iodinated contrast material, improved CT parameters such as slice thickness and interscan distances, and the use of large amounts of oral and rectal contrast material. Based on our experience, we share the opinions of these authors and prefer CT for diagnosing the complications of acute diverticulitis.

There are no known congenital forms of diverticular disease, and it is very rare in people under the age of 25. Based on the findings of autopsy studies conducted in the United States, a steady increase, from a 10% incidence in the third decade to a 50% incidence over the age 75,[26] has been noted, and similar figures are reported for Australia.[24] For all symptomatic patients the age of onset was under 29 in less than 1% of the patients and under 49 in only 11%, whereas 56% of the patients were between 50 to 70 years old at the time of onset. Series of surgical patients have been reported describing diverticulitis as a diagnosis to be considered in patients under the age of 40.[27,29,30] It may be that the disease is now affecting a younger age group than was the case at the beginning of the century. Such figures are based on those patients who come to the attention of physicians, but, as Almy and Howell[20] point out, many cases remain symptomless and thus go unrecorded.

The contrast between these figures and the frequency of the disease in those populations that consume a high-roughage diet is very striking. The disease is virtually unknown in the native population of Africa.[3] It is very rare in the Indian subcontinent, the Middle East, the Far East,[31] and Japan.[22,32] The hospital admission rate for diverticulitis per 100,000 population is 80 times higher in Scotland than it is in Malaysia.[32] In other words, the incidence is low in those people who eat a large amount of roughage. That the factor responsible is an environmental one is made more likely by the fact that Japanese who have emigrated to Hawaii[33] and urban South African blacks who have adopted a Western diet are now acquiring the disease in greater numbers.[34] Two matched groups from the city of Oxford in England have been compared.[35] A vegetarian group, which exhibited a 12% incidence of diverticula, ate more dietary fiber than did the control subjects, 33% of whom had diverticula. The rise of the disease in England[3] is believed to follow by 40 years the change from coarse, unrefined bread to that made from roller-milled flour, from which much of the fiber is removed. A majority of clinicians now believe that the addition of bran to the diet alleviates the symptoms. The results of the Oxford study, among others, have encouraged some practitioners to think in terms of prophylaxis. However, as yet, how bran brings about this effect remains unexplained,[36] even though bran and dietary fiber preparations were recently shown to have a preventive effect on diverticular disease in rats[37] and humans.[38] Smits et al.,[38] in a recent prospectively randomized limited series consisting of 21 patients, found that the efficacy and tolerance of lactulose (Duphalac), in the treatment of diverticular disease were slightly increased over those associated with a high-fiber diet.

PATHOGENESIS

The presence of a muscular abnormality, already clear from radiologic and pathologic observations, has also been explored by measurements of intraluminal pressures and recordings of myoelectric activity. Earlier work, in which pressure measurements were combined with cineradiology, led to an attractively simple concept that the pressure was raised in small local segments and forced out pulsion diverticular through weak spots in the muscle wall.[39] However, more recent papers that include symptomless patients have shown that increased motility is not always found in patients with diverticula and that, if present, it correlates better with symptoms than with the presence of sacs.[40,41] Connell himself,[21] who has considerable experience in this field, has warned against arguing too much from intraluminal pressure measurements, which may largely reflect only a narrowed lumen. A potentially more fundamental observation is that a myoelectric slow-wave pattern occurring at an abnormal frequency of 12 cpm has been observed in the sigmoid of patients with symptomatic diverticular disease. This phenomenon largely disappears after a bran diet is instituted.[42] The distorted lumen shown by the barium enema examination can be the sole evidence of a muscular dysfunction, with all other investigations yielding normal results.

Cortesini and Pantalone[41] recently confirmed the association between asymptomatic diverticular disease and high intraluminal pressure. Indeed, they demonstrated that the colonic motility index was significantly higher in symptomatic patients with diverticular disease than in asymptomatic ones during the resting ($p < 0.001$) and postprandial ($p < 0.001$) periods.

Diverticulitis has been reported at a very young age in patients with a number of rare syndromes, including Marfan's syndrome,[43,44] the Ehlers-Danlos syndrome,[45] and intestinal ganglioneuromatosis.[46]

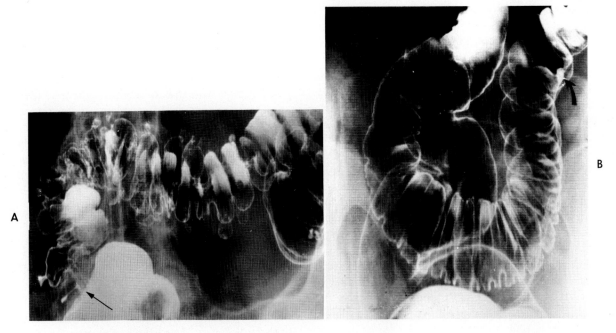

Fig. 36-2 A, Diverticular disease in Hampton's view. This picture, in which the x rays roughly parallel the mesentery, exhibits an alternating pattern of infolding and diverticula along the surface of the lumen. Note local contraction has deformed one diverticulum *(arrow)*. Some sacs are slightly irregular, but there was no basis in the patient's history for suspecting previous diverticulitis. Because this patient was not operated on, it is impossible to prove the actual nature of this tiny defect. **B,** A fully distended sigmoid colon in Hampton's view. This pattern of numerous transverse folds that imparts a crenated appearance persisted throughout the examination. A solitary sac is visible in the proximal sigmoid *(arrow)*. This is an example of diverticular disease without diverticula.

Diverticula

Common colonic diverticula represent acquired herniations of the mucosa and muscularis mucosae,[47] and some at least are reducible hernias. Most radiologists have seen sacs at the early filling stage that disappear on full distention. Sacs seen easily on one enema may never appear on a subsequent one. In size, they vary from tiny spikes to 2-cm spheres, but most commonly they are 5 to 10 mm in diameter. In full distention they are spherical or ovoid and rarely bilobed. The radiologic appearance is altered by the amount of feces within the cavity. When empty, they are flask shaped, but a large scybalum can occlude the outer edge of the opening, leaving only a short stubby neck filled with barium. Small pieces of retained feces produce an irregular outline (Figs. 36-2, 36-3, *A*, and 36-4, *A*).

Diverticula are found in all zones of the colon, although by far the most common site is the sigmoid. Some patients may have a small number of sacs confined to one part, but Hughes,[24] in a study of autopsy cases, could not confirm a separate subgroup of sacs that are confined to the right colon. The upper half of the rectum is rarely a site of sac formation.[48,49]

The circular muscle is fasciculated[50] and arranged in small packets, roughly like washers around a bolt. The mucosa protrudes between the fasciculi, but this causes no local damage to the muscle, which is pushed up into small hillocks on each side of the opening (Fig. 36-5). Between the taeniae is a fine layer of longitudinal muscle organized into a network, and fibers from this are carried into the convexity of the sac.[51] The details of this condition and its radiologic picture are depicted in Figs. 36-5 and 36-6.

In the left half of the colon the sacs emerge in four rows, one on each side of the mesenteric taenia and one on the mesenteric side of each antimesenteric taenia (Fig. 36-7). The close relationship of these sites to the penetrating blood vessel has been known for half a century, but two investigations[52-54] have explored the problem thoroughly and very similar conclusions were reached. The investigators propose that the rectal arteries have long and short branches, and these are responsible for the formation of the rows of sacs down the length of the colon (see Fig. 36-6, *A*). Each penetrating vessel divides rapidly after it has passed through the muscular wall to form a submucosal plexus. The view of Tagliacozzo and Virno[53,54] on the exact nature of this mechanism is shown in Fig. 36-8. An increase in the intraluminal pressure in turn raises the pressure in the submucosa, and this forces out the artery and the loose connective tissue around it, raising a small mound

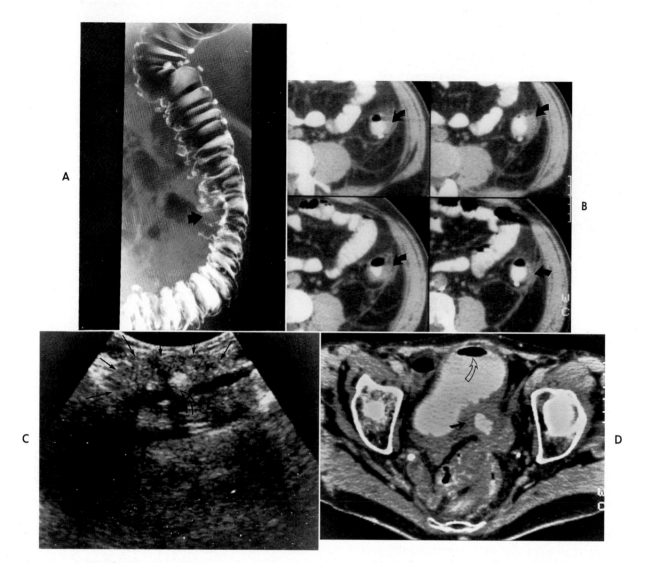

Fig. 36-3 A, An abscess. An extrinsic-pressure defect is seen *(arrow)* in conjunction with two deformed sacs. This was not visible on routine films but only on oblique spot films taken at the site of an easily palpable mass. **B,** Diverticulitis of the sigmoid colon. These 4-mm-thick CT sections show a 15 × 5–mm ill-defined abscess *(arrows)* arising from a diverticulum of the mesenteric aspect of the left colon. The abscess involves the lateroconal fascia and extends along the lower portion of the anterior and posterior perirenal fascia. The lesion was treated conservatively with antibiotics. **C,** Diverticulitis of the sigmoid colon. This ultrasonographic view was obtained parallel to the axis of the intestinal lumen *(L),* which has a tubular appearance. Both walls of the colon are thickened. The 8-mm hyperechogenic round mass *(open arrow)* represents a diverticulum surrounded by a heterogeneous ill-defined mass *(arrows)* that involved the mesenteric fat and corresponded to a peridiverticular abscess. The lesion was treated conservatively. **D,** Peridiverticular abscess *(arrow)* and sigmoid colon, in close contact with the left lateral wall of the bladder, displayed on 4-mm-thick CT sections. The left bladder wall is markedly thickened and irregular, mimicking a malignant tumor. The lumen of the diverticulum is filled with rectal water-soluble contrast material, although the vesical lumen contains iodinated contrast that was injected intravenously and an air fluid level *(open arrow)* responsible for pneumaturia.

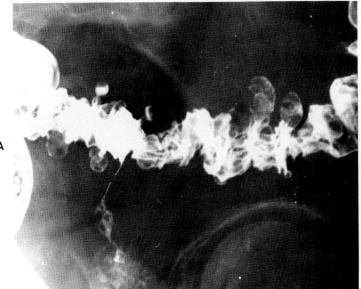

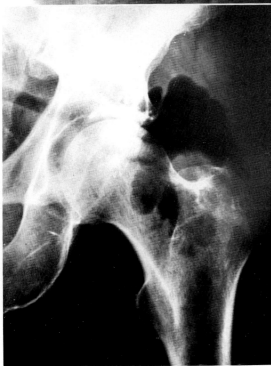

Fig. 36-4 A, Transperitoneal spread of inflammation. This woman's first symptom was urinary infection with pneumaturia. In this depiction of a partially contracted sigmoid, diverticular disease is obvious. A pencil-thin track, which needed some enhancement to demonstrate it in print, channels barium to the bladder via a small abscess cavity. Note the minimal deformity of colon at the point where the fistula to the bladder originates. **B,** Retroperitoneal spread of inflammation. This man consulted orthopedic surgeons because of pain in his hip and swelling posteriorly. A barium enema revealed the presence of a track through the sacrosciatic notch that connected an air-filled posterior abscess with a diverticular abscess.
Courtesy of Dr. A. Moss.

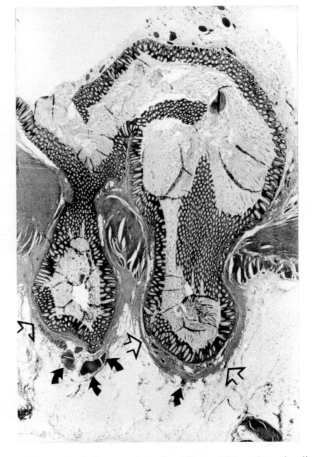

on the serosal surface.[55] The emerging artery then pulls the mucosa into the gap, and, as the diverticulum moves outside the wall, it remains covered by a netlike collection of blood vessels that were originally lying in the submucosa (see Fig. 36-5).

This explains the usual finding of sacs in four rows, but it is not complete. Occasional sacs are found in the lateral wall and in the antimesenteric zone (see Figs. 36-1, *A*, and 36-7, *A*) where there are no penetrating vessels. Williams[55] postulated that persistent shortening of the bowel crumples

Fig. 36-5 Longitudinal sections through two folds and nearby diverticula. Note the structure of the folds which is bending the whole wall inward, and a diverticulum pushing aside fasciculated circular muscle. Vessels *(curved arrows)* run over the top of sacs. Covering the sacs is a fine layer of longitudinal muscle mixed with fibrous tissue *(open arrows).*

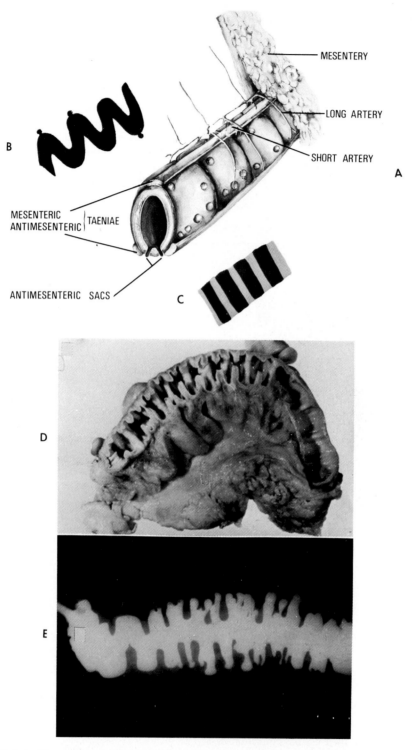

Fig. 36-6 A, The anatomy of the sigmoid colon. **B,** A radiograph obtained in line with the mesentery shows the saw-tooth sign and sacs on the horizon. **C,** Radiograph taken at right angles to the mesentery, and approximating an oblique view of the sigmoid, shows half-shadow bars with sacs that are largely hidden. **D,** The sigmoid has been fixed, distended, and cut to show the interhaustral folds, which have an alternating pattern down the length of the gut. **E,** Preoperative radiograph of the specimen shown in **D,** taken in line with the mesentery to show the anatomy of the zigzag lumen.

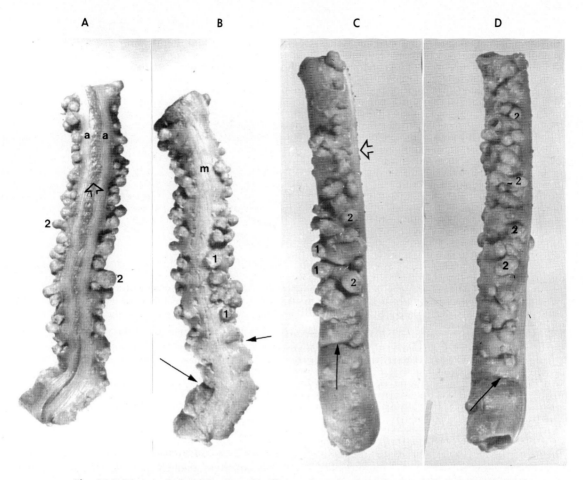

Fig. 36-7 Diverticulosis of the sigmoid. The specimen has been fixed and distended, with the fat dissected away. **A,** View from the antimesenteric side, with two taeniae visible *(a)*. **B,** View from the mesenteric side with a single taenia visible *(m)*. **C** and **D,** Views of each side. Note the diverticula emerge from the longer lateral walls in two rows, one close to the mesenteric taenia *(1)* and the other close to each antimesenteric taenia *(2)*. Much smaller sacs are seen in the antimesenteric zone in **A** and on the horizon in **C** *(open arrowheads)*. Infoldings *(arrows)* are seen on the horizon in the mesenteric line in **A** and **B** and en face on the lateral wall in **C** and **D**.

the circular layer in the same way that a coat sleeve wrinkles when it is pulled up the arm. This can crack the circular muscle in a circumferential fashion and give rise to weak areas through which diverticula emerge. This is especially true of the short antimesenteric zone where the cracking can lead to a ridge-shaped herniation.

SIGNIFICANCE AND RADIOLOGY OF A MUSCULAR ABNORMALITY

The striking feature[56] noted on surgical specimens of diverticular disease is the thickness of the muscle in the affected area. The taeniae are prominent and tough, and may even be white, resembling the state of the pyloric muscle in congenital hypertrophic stenosis. The circular muscle is thick and convoluted, and the lumen is filled with an excess of normal mucosa. The nearby mesentery is firm and thick, giving an impression of the existence of additional

fat. However, these findings can be present in the absence of inflammation and occasionally even without a single diverticulum.[56]

The key to understanding the nature of this radiographic mass is to realize that the sigmoid is an asymmetric structure and cannot be regarded as a simple cylinder. The taeniae are arranged as an isosceles triangle, with the apex located under the mesentery. The other two, the antimesenteric taeniae, lie opposite and close together to form the base of the triangle and enclose a short length of antimesenteric wall (see Figs. 36-6 and 36-7). The lateral walls, each between the mesenteric taeniae and one antimesenteric taenia, are flexible and bend inward to form the interhaustral folds. These folds are deep on one lateral wall but lose height as they travel around the circumference, so the haustrum opposite is smooth and distended. Seen from the lumen, they are crescent shaped, and each is composed of

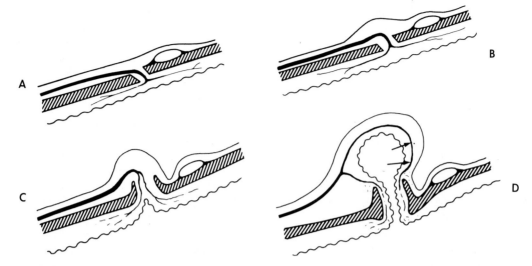

Fig. 36-8 Relationship of diverticula to blood vessels. **A,** A penetrating branch of a long artery, which is piercing the circular muscle close to the antimesenteric taenia and dividing immediately. **B,** Pressure in the lumen raises the pressure in the submucosal space and forces out the artery and submucosa, while the mucosa stays in the lumen. **C,** With further expulsion of the vessels, the mucosa extrudes and finally comes to lie outside **(D),** enclosed in a net of what were originally submucosal vessels. Arrows mark the common sites of arterial damage in severe cases of diverticular bleeding.
Modified from Tagliacozzo S, Virno F: *Ann Ital Chir* 38:420, 1961; and Meyers MA, Alonzo DR, Baer JW: *AJR* 127:901, 1976.

two layers of muscle with an inner mucosal cover (see Fig. 36-5). Inspection of these figures reveals the difficulty in giving measurements for the "thickness" of the wall, without carefully specifying the end points of such measurements. The diverticula arise from the lateral walls, and the interhaustral folds assume an alternating pattern from side to side as one moves down the length of the bowel. A radiograph taken in the line of the mesentery will show the folds and diverticula on the horizon, whereas in one obtained at right angles in single contrast the filled lumen hides the sacs and shows the folds as half-shadow bars (see Fig. 36-6, *A*).

American radiologists were the first to suggest the reason for this picture, arguing that the primary fault was that the colon had failed to elongate fully, and this prevented the folds from moving apart and flattening out as they do normally. Since then, some secondary evidence has come to light in support of this postulate.[55] The sigmoid can be compared to a fan that has failed to open fully in the affected segment. Thus this segment contains within each centimeter of its length more muscle, nerve cells, mucosa, and blood vessels than would the normal segment,[57] whereas the related mesentery is bunched up to form part of the palpable thickening. As a result, the longitudinal muscle is shorter than normal in the resting state and cannot elongate fully. It can still contract and relax,[58] but histologists can offer no explanation for this. The best term for describing this set of observations is *contracture*, which

was defined for striated muscle by Gasser[59] as a "term without definition, convenient in its vagueness for various states of muscle shortening, themselves not well understood." Although a contracture of the longitudinal muscle is responsible for causing the zigzag lumen, the circular muscle may, on inspection with the naked eye, vary from a normal width, as seen at autopsy in diverticulosis of the elderly, to a state in which the bowel feels as swollen and hard as a tumor mass. The shortening persists, at least in part, after the administration of smooth muscle relaxants and is found in autopsy specimens. There is no histologic explanation for this feature, which is summarized in Fleischner et al.'s phrase[60] "spasm which persists becomes permanent," or put vaguely by the term *myostatic contracture*. Some pathologists consider hypertrophy to be the cause of the muscle thickening, but there is only a single paper supporting this view.[61]

Radiologists became interested in the variants, in which one wall had a spiky or crenated outline, and in patterns in which the infolding was not as regular, as just described. Noting the association with diverticulosis elsewhere in the colon, they called this a *prediverticular state* when it was found in the absence of sacs, and some work has been done on elucidating the nature of the underlying pathology. Arfwidson[61] has described several examples, all compatible with a failure to elongate in conjunction with an irregular crumpling of the haustral walls. Where the folds from each lateral wall cross the antimesenteric zone, they are short but numerous and disrupt the outline to produce a unilateral palisade sign. In severe cases the whole zone is cracked circumferentially and a ridge-shaped herniation occurs, leading to a castellated edge. Williams[55] discusses these patterns in detail; they are only a problem when they occur in the absence of sacs (see Fig. 36-1, *B*). In this instance, they are best described as *diverticular disease without diverticula*. All radiologists know that they are seen transiently during a normal enema, and that they must persist in maximal distention before the diagnosis is even contemplated.

DIVERTICULITIS

The term *diverticulitis* is used here to mean the presence of inflammation, not merely diverticular disease exhibiting symptoms, and it is beneficial to consider first the clinical diagnosis of this complication. In some patients this is easy, because they have a painful mass and local signs of peritoneal irritation, as well as fever and leukocytosis. Many of this group require surgery, which proves the diagnosis; however, in a larger number of patients, there is pain and tenderness, but not collateral evidence of inflammation.[30] The patient gets better on conservative treatment, and the diagnosis remains uncertain. It is likely that the pain and a mass can result from the muscular dysfunction alone,[56] and these cannot be held to be absolute evidence of inflammation. Conversely, inflammation can occur without symptoms. Hughes,[24] in a series made up of 200 hospital autopsies, found that 3% had had diverticulitis but never complained of relevant symptoms, including one patient with an abscess 1 cm in diameter. In patients with colovesical fistulas, the first symptom may not be the pain and fever of an original infection, but the painless pneumaturia resulting from its extension. Except for the severe cases, the clinical diagnosis of inflammation preoperatively can be very uncertain. The radiologic diagnosis of diverticulitis is based on three findings: (1) deformed sacs, (2) demonstration of an abscess, and (3) extravasation of water-soluble contrast material.

Deformed sacs

Two groups of authors[8,56] have agreed that the earliest pathologic change is a focal inflammation in the lymph follicle within the mucosa of the diverticulum. This leads to a microperforation and the formation of a small abscess outside it (Fig. 36-9, *A*), which then deforms the general smooth outline of the sac (Fig. 36-9, *B*). The surgical specimen may show three or four sacs that are affected simultaneously (Fig. 36-9). Diverticulitis is now an established cause of deformed sacs, although no exact radiopathologic correlation in an individual diverticulum has been found. What is much less certain is whether the reverse of this situation is true, because there are other causes of deformity. Obviously, if a small quantity of retained feces is stuck to the wall, this will alter the barium outline (see Fig. 36-4, *A*). The sacs, which have a thin layer of longitudinal mus-

cle over them, often look irregular or flattened when the colon is fully or partially contracted (see Fig. 36-1, *A*). It is possible that an irregularity represents old fibrous scarring and not an active abscess. Nevertheless, if such a minor deformity is detected in a fully distended zone, this serves as a useful indication of the common form of inflammation, microperforations. The only paper[62] reporting on a double-blind study using the authors' present criteria consisted of a group of 13 patients. Eight of them were found to have deformed sacs, and five of these eight had severe deformities. The pathologist identified diverticulitis in only four, and diverticulosis in the remaining nine.

There are certainly cases in which inflammation prevents the affected sac from filling with barium and, when this occurs around a solitary sac, the colon can look normal or, at the most, show a prediverticular state. When this happens on the right side, the clinical diagnosis is usually appendicitis or cholecystitis. This situation has given rise to the notion of a separate subdivision of right-sided sacs.

Demonstration of abscess

The etiology of perforation is not clear. Significant inflammation of the perforated diverticulum is very infrequent.[63] This suggests that a transient surge of intraluminal pressure may more often be responsible for the rupture. Concomitant or other etiologic factors include ischemia, stercoral ulcerations, and foreign bodies.[64] A pericolic abscess can assume the appearance of a pressure defect on the filled colon (see Fig. 36-3, *A*). Multiple spot films may be needed to demonstrate an otherwise easily palpable abscess. It is not uncommon for the abscess to produce a small, difficult-to-find deformity on the colon, and even large abscesses may go undetected.[10]

In the correct clinical setting, other techniques can be used to demonstrate the abscess. Isotope scanning with gallium 67[65] as well as ultrasonography[66] (Fig. 36-3, *C*) have both proved useful for this purpose. However, these are now being increasingly replaced by CT examinations,[17,19,64,67-69] which can display subtle peridiverticular changes, such as a discrete increase in the attenuation value of the mesenteric fat, thickening of the colonic wall,[15,64,70-75] slight enlargement of the peritoneal fascia (Fig. 36-3, *B*), or minute fluid collections in the paracolic spaces. Such abnormalities are disclosed by 63% of the CT scans obtained during the acute episodes.[64] CT is also the best and the most reliable device for guiding the drainage of large diverticular abscesses[73,76-80] and for demonstrating fistulas[81] (Fig. 36-3, *D*).

Extravasation of contrast material

The most reliable sign of diverticulitis, mimicked only by a perforated carcinoma, is the presence of contrast material outside the lumen. This sign is usually easy to recognize (Fig. 36-10). A characteristic extravasation takes on the appearance of a track running parallel to the bowel wall

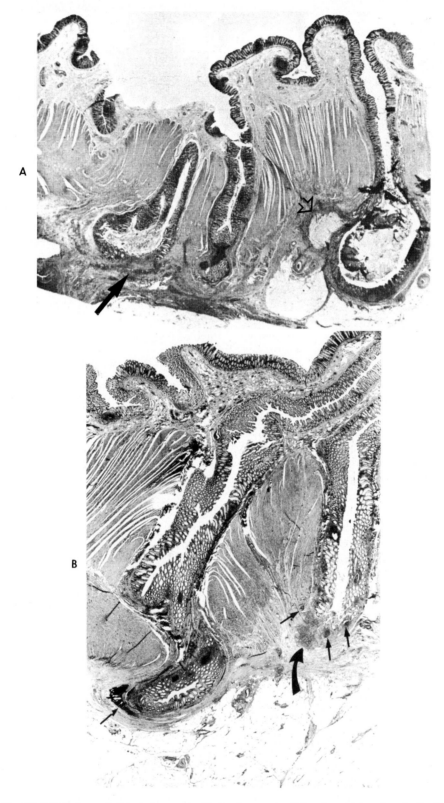

Fig. 36-9 Pathology of distorted sacs. **A,** Photomicrograph of the sigmoid in a longitudinal section. Outside the diverticulum on the right is a small thick-walled abscess *(open arrow)*. At the apex of the diverticulum on the left is a fibrous scar, with thickening of the nearby serosa *(arrow)* indicating previous inflammation. **B,** Photomicrograph showing a healed perforation of a diverticulum on the right side *(curved arrow)*, with evidence of fibrous scar tissue. On the left side, the diverticulum is distorted and partially circumscribed by fibrous tissue that infiltrates the thin layer of longitudinal muscle. Numerous veins and arteries, possessing marked wall thickening *(straight arrow)*, course in the vicinity of both sacs' bottoms.

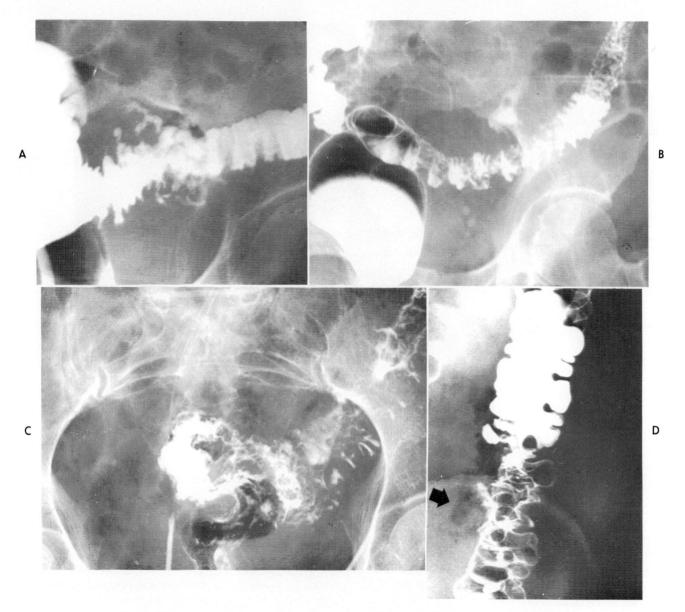

Fig. 36-10 Leakage of barium outside the lumen. **A,** Obvious leak. **B,** Leak into a circumscribed abscess cavity. **C,** Barium collection seen as a triangular area in an en face view. This did not appear except in a film obtained after evacuation. **D,** The medial edge of the mid–descending colon is distorted, and an arrow points to an air-filled abscess. A tiny leak of barium has occurred from a distorted diverticulum.

in the region of the sigmoid and pelvic portions of the colon (Fig. 36-11). It is a long abscess located in the subserosal layer and communicates with several sacs. This, with the original lumen, produces a double-track sign that can be up to 15 cm long. It is also present when Crohn's disease is superimposed on diverticular disease.

Accuracy of diagnosis

Estimates of the radiologic success rates in diagnosing diverticulitis are hard to find, for the reasons already dis-

cussed. In patients with the severe form of inflammation, that is, those requiring surgery, Schnyder et al.[62] found blind rereading of the films by two experienced observers yielded an 80% accuracy, although one suspects that, in the general run of patients, this success would not be repeated. Parks,[82] who based his study on a large series of hospital admissions, made the clinical diagnosis of diverticulitis in 426 patients using 1969 criteria. The radiologists, on the other hand, diagnosed inflammation in only 231 cases. In the clinical setting of a gynecologic mass subsequently

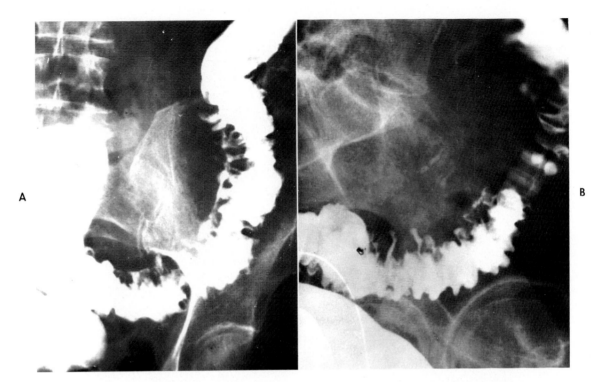

Fig. 36-11 A, A long-tracking subserous abscess. A long track of barium runs beside the sigmoid and pelvic colon, giving the impression of a second channel situated alongside the main lumen. Note at the proximal end the localized low-filling defect caused by submucosal edema, which resembles a flat carcinoma. **B,** A short linear subserous abscess found in a woman who had suffered a single attack of clinical diverticulitis. Note the 2-cm-long line of barium running parallel to the lumen. It took several films to prove its separation from a nearby area of arterial calcification. Distally are seen several deformed sacs. The symptoms, which were never severe, resolved without operation.

shown to result from diverticulitis, the radiologists made the correct diagnosis in only 2 of the 19 enema studies.[83] Considerable improvement in the accuracy of the radiologic diagnosis since the early 1980s stems from the use of CT and ultrasonography. According to Morris and Tudor,[64] who studied a series of 41 patients, plain films of the abdomen demonstrated abnormalities in only 33%. The barium enema examinations yielded positive findings in 60%, and the CT examinations accomplished this in 63% of the patients.

More recently, Labs et al.[17] showed that CT had a sensitivity of 100% for the detection of diverticular abscess in a series of 10 patients subsequently proved by surgery to have the abnormality, although a contrast enema identified this correctly in only two of them. Similarly, Kyunghee et al.[85] prospectively evaluated the diagnostic value of CT and the barium enema study in 27 patients with diverticulitis, subsequently confirmed either at surgery (11 cases) or by the patient's clinical response to medical therapy (16 cases). CT correctly identified diverticulitis in 93% (25/27) of the patients. These results were encouraging when compared with barium enema results, of which only 80% (20/25) correctly detected the disease.

DIFFERENTIAL DIAGNOSIS
Carcinoma

The apple-core stricture with shouldered ends contrasts with the tapered ends, the intact mucosa, and the variability typical of the diverticular strictures. When there is a solitary sac in the midst of the narrowed area, this is strong evidence against a carcinomatous narrowing (Fig. 36-12, *A*). Neoplastic narrowings tend to be less than 7 cm long, but this is not a reliable guide.[62] The appearance of a low, flat carcinoma involving only one side of the lumen must be distinguished from that due to extrinsic pressure.[84]

Polyps

Diverticula seen projecting beyond the lumen pose no problem in detection, but, when viewed en face, they appear as a white circle, which resembles the ring of barium trapped around the base of a polyp.[85] The distinction is discussed and illustrated in Chapter 38. The white rim of the diverticulum is sharp on its outer border and fuzzy on its inner border, and the reverse is true for a polyp. This is a useful but not always easy sign to spot. The infolded muscular walls can also mimic a polyp on a single-contrast

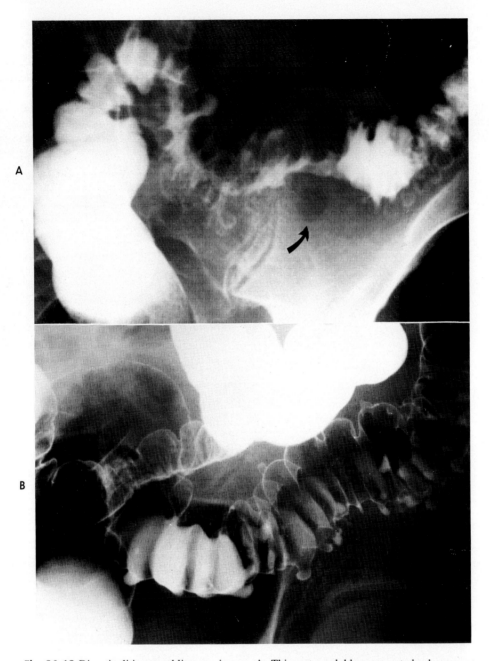

Fig. 36-12 Diverticulitis resembling carcinoma. **A,** This water-soluble enema study shows a partial obstruction and a circumferential mass effect with shouldered ends resembling an encircling carcinoma. The presence of a gas collection *(arrow)* on the antimesenteric side of the colon was of value here because it pointed to the existence of a diverticular abscess. A single sac opens off the middle of the narrowed area. **B,** Seven weeks later, after antibiotic treatment, a formal double-contrast study with barium shows resolution of the abscess, leaving a picture of simple diverticulosis.

view. The detection of polyps in the distorted lumen is unquestionably difficult, but the diagnosis must always be borne in mind whenever there is bleeding. Antifoaming agents are now contained in most barium preparations to prevent the formation of air bubbles, which tend to generate confusing shadows.

Other causes of extrinsic-pressure defects *which may mimic a pericolic abscess*

Ovarian tumors and pelvic metastases are among the most frequent causes of extrinsic-pressure defects on the distal colon. Differentiating them from diverticular abscesses is now very possible with ultrasonography and CT.

Ischemic colitis

Pain, fever, and rectal bleeding can be the initial symptoms of segmental colitis, to which the sigmoid is not immune, although not commonly affected. Some of the individual radiologic signs resemble the distortions characteristic of diverticular disease, but the papers that have been published on the topic do not represent it as a difficult problem in differential diagnosis.

COMPLICATIONS
Obstruction

Complete or almost complete clinical obstruction is seen in the presence of diverticulitis, but sigmoid carcinoma is a more common cause. Smooth muscle relaxants may be helpful for widening the lumen and allowing enough contrast to pass into it, thus permitting the actual pathology to be depicted and the exact diagnosis established (see Figs.

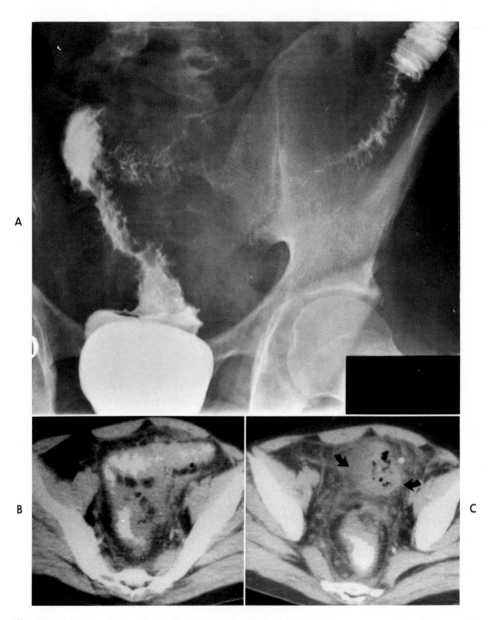

Fig. 36-13 A, A contrast-enhanced enema study obtained in the emergency room in a 26-year-old man with fever who was seen after a 2-day history of abdominal pain in the left lower quadrant. Despite the intravenous administration of glucagon, the lumen of both the sigmoid colon and rectosigmoid junction failed to open. The mucosal folds are distorted but preserved. The necks of several diverticula can be identified in the distal colon. **B** and **C,** These 8-mm-thick CT sections obtained at 16-mm intervals display marked concentric thickening of the sigmoid wall, a 5-cm peritoneal gas-containing mass *(arrows)*, and widespread infiltration of the pelvic fat.

36-2 and 36-13, *A*). This does not always happen, and, interestingly enough, complete retrograde obstruction can be found in a patient who is having normal bowel action.[86]

Bleeding

Small amounts of blood in the feces are common, even in patients who are eventually diagnosed as having diverticulosis. In the elderly patient, who radiologically manifests typical diverticulosis with numerous sacs, a specific type of blood loss can arise that is unheralded, painless, and profuse enough to be exsanguinating. Although often treated in the past by the blind excision of either a part of or the entire colon, the advent of arteriography and colonoscopy has now made it possible to localize the bleeding area and carry out limited resection (Fig. 36-14). These techniques have given rise to two unexpected results. First, in up to half of the cases,[87,88] the source of the bleeding has been found not to be a diverticulum, but an angiomatous malformation located in the submucosa. These may be multiple, and any remaining after resection can be a source of recurrent bleeding. Second, the identification of the actual bleeding diverticulum in the surgical specimen has prompted a reassessment of the pathologic conditions, and this has revealed that the damage to the blood vessel is not actually a consequence of inflammation.[89] Instead, at the point where the penetration artery passes the neck of the

sac (see Fig. 36-8, *D*), there is a peculiar change in this small artery, consisting of intimal thickening, reduplication of the internal elastic lamina, and atrophy of the media. This histologic picture is not specific to diverticulosis, but has also been found at other sites and as the result of other causes, these being mechanical, thermal, or chemical trauma, and immunologic disease. It is not clear why the blood always enters the lumen and never spreads into the subserous layer. Such bleeding has been treated with vasopressin or selective arterial embolization.[88,90-93]

Spread of inflammation and fistula formation

Although often well contained, the infection in diverticulitis can cause widespread peritonitis and free gas to form in the peritoneal cavity. Pus can then be subsequently localized in any of the well-known sites. The initial symptoms, which are referable to the colon, may be minimal, and the first evidence of diverticulitis may be discovered some distance from the left iliac fossa. Transperitoneal spread can cause fistula formation to most organs in the lower half of the abdomen, including the bladder,[81] vagina, fallopian tubes, and other parts of the colon, the small intestine, and the ureter. In the large series of patients studied at the Lahey Clinic,[94] the only common sites were found to be the bladder, the vagina, and the skin. With colovesical fistulas, the contrast enemas revealed the track in only 5 of 17 cases (see Fig. 36-4, *A*), and it was fully outlined in all of these. Cystoscopy detected the lesion in 16 of 17 ✳ cases.

More difficult to diagnose is the spread of pus in the retroperitoneal space, where it may first be recognized in a perinephric site, then track down to the pararectal region to mimic Crohn's disease or pass through the sacrosciatic notch to present as an abscess in the buttock or thigh (Fig. 31-4, *B*). Currently, ultrasonography[12-14] (Fig. 36-3, *C*), CT[7,8] (see Figs. 36-1, *B* and 36-3, *B*), and MRI (see Fig. 36-1, *C* and *D*) are the best means for diagnosing in their early stages the peritoneal and extraperitoneal abscesses arising from a diverticular origin.

When spread takes place via the mesenteric veins and causes liver abscesses or gas to form in the portal veins, these changes are also optimally demonstrated by ultrasonography.[95-97]

DISEASES COEXISTING WITH DIVERTICULA

With perhaps half of the people in their retirement years afflicted with diverticula, the presence of a second unrelated disease is not unlikely, and such patients pose diagnostic problems.

Diverticular disease with neoplasm

The symptoms of diverticular disease and a neoplasm in the distal colon can be very similar, and, their simultaneous occurrence makes radiologic interpretation difficult.[62,98,99] Obstruction, perforation, and fistula are seen in both. Di-

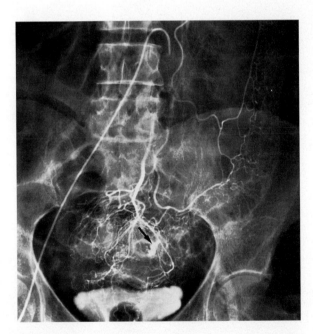

Fig. 36-14 This superselective angiogram of the inferior mesenteric artery obtained in a 60-year-old patient who was admitted because of massive rectal bleeding displays a leak of iodinated contrast material *(arrow)* arising from a diverticulum in the mesenteric aspect of the distal sigmoid colon. Bleeding was successfully controlled and treated with repeated arterial injections of vasopressin.

verticular disease characteristically involves long lengths of colon, but the pattern of involvement can vary along that length; the problem then is deciding whether one small part of the total deformity represents an added carcinoma. There are no hard-and-fast rules that apply here. Air contrast films obtained with the colon in maximal distention, with spot films obtained with the patient in various positions, are used to achieve a three-dimensional visual synthesis. With care, it is possible to eliminate the spasm that can produce an apple-core narrowing, but local submucosal or mucosal edema can look like a flat neoplasm, especially in the cases that exhibit the double-track sign (see Fig. 36-11, *A*). It is certainly possible to make a confident double diagnosis (Fig. 36-15, *A*), but the published findings give no cause for self-congratulation on this score. The authors of older papers suggest that the diagnosis is difficult or impossible in up to half of the cases.[62] Schnyder et al.[62] provided a selection of illustrative radiographs to prove this point.

They reported that, in the blind assessment of 73 enema studies done in patients with diverticular disease, 13 cases were ultimately found to have additional neoplasms. The observers failed to find half the neoplasms and made a significant number of false-positive diagnoses in cases of diverticulitis. Analysis of individual radiologic signs also did not yield a useful guide. Boulos,[9] in a study of 105 patients with symptomatic sigmoid diverticular disease, reported that colonoscopy revealed an associated carcinoma in 6.6% of the patients and adenoma in 27.6%, with a peak incidence occurring between 60 and 79 years of age and an equal sex distribution. Extensive diverticulosis was shown to constitute an important factor that limited the sensitivity of barium enema in the evaluation of sigmoid masses.[98] Indeed, 3.1% of the lesions are missed in patients with less than 15 diverticula, while in those with more than 15 diverticula, 20.4% of the tumors go undetected.[98]

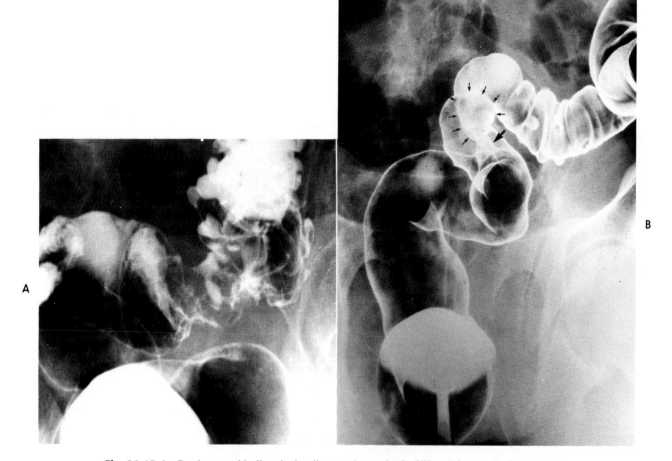

Fig. 36-15 A, Carcinoma with diverticular disease. A neoplastic filling defect encircling perhaps two thirds of the lumen in an area of diverticulosis (compare with Fig. 36-9, *A*). **B,** Diverticulosis and polyp. This pedunculated polyp was responsible for causing recurrent rectal bleeding in a 71-year-old man. An area of diverticulosis in the nearby sigmoid is an additional finding that was not relevant in this patient. This is an example of the degree of colonic distention that is possible after glucagon administration, without the production of pain. *Small arrows,* Polyp; *larger arrow,* stalk.

Diverticular disease with Crohn's disease

An initial assertion,[100] that a long subserous abscess which exhibits the double-track sign very likely represents Crohn's disease, has not been substantiated,[101] but there are now sufficient cases which confirm that Crohn's disease can arise in a sigmoid affected with diverticular disease.[102] The pathologic characteristics of 21 cases have been described.[103] In 11 cases, the granulomatous disease was confined to the lumen, but, in the remainder, the mucosa of the sacs was involved, leading to pericolic inflammation. For the radiologist, this added type of inflammation must always be borne in mind, and a routine search should be made for aphthous ulcers, transmural ulcers, and lesions elsewhere in the colon.

The difficulty in discerning between colonic diverticulitis and Crohn's disease is well demonstrated in a recent paper published by Petros et al.[104] These authors report on their own findings in 10 patients and those in another 15 patients from the literature.[102,105,106] They demonstrated that the diagnosis of simultaneous colonic diverticulitis and Crohn's disease was established in 71% (43/60) of the cases by pathologic examination, in 33% (20/60) by sigmoidoscopy and biopsy, and in 3.3% (2/60) by barium enema.

Diverticular disease with ulcerative colitis

Ulcerative colitis, commonly a disease of young people, shows a second peak incidence in the elderly at a time in life when diverticular disease is common. Jalan et al.[107] found a 25% incidence of diverticular disease in their patients with ulcerative colitis who were over 60. The diagnosis is easy and based on finding superficial ulceration over a length of rectum and colon.[108,109] Diverticulitis with ulcerative colitis is not as common as might be expected, but, when it occurs, the prognosis is poor.[110]

Diverticular disease with angiodysplasia

The significance of combined diverticular disease and angiodysplasia was discussed under the complications of bleeding.

CLASSIFICATION

The terms *diverticulosis* and *diverticulitis* are deeply embedded in the literature, but today the radiologic interpretations and pathologic conditions must be described in terms of three elements: sacs, muscular abnormality, and inflammation, which occur in varying proportions in each patient at any given time. No classification approaches perfection. For the radiologist, assessment of the muscular thickening is the most difficult. The classification that embraces most clinical settings follows.

Scattered diverticula

A small number of sacs are visible in cases of scattered diverticula, but no muscular hypertrophy can be recognized.

Diverticulosis

Diverticulosis is a common radiologic picture. There are many sacs and there is shortening of the sigmoid and pelvic portions of the colon. The exact course of the lumen indicates the existence of a muscular hypertrophy. It is not obviously narrowed, however, and there is no evidence to indicate inflammation.

Diverticular disease without diverticula

When there are no diverticula, the muscular abnormality is mild and assumes a serrated appearance along the inside surface of the distal colon with no visible sacs. This is the "prediverticular state," and, in its pure form, is rare; however, the pelvic colon may show this appearance in the presence of obvious diverticulosis of the sigmoid.

Diverticular disease

The term *diverticular disease* is applied to avoid specifying whether inflammation is present or not. It is valuable in view of the proved inaccuracy of clinical and radiologic techniques in detecting inflammation. This term embraces diverticulosis with symptoms. At one end of the spectrum is the finding of gross zonal narrowing of the lumen, which pathologic examination reveals is a very thick muscle wall.

Diverticulitis

Any of the patterns mentioned, when they occur in conjunction with clear evidence of inflammation and diverticular perforation, represent diverticulitis.

REFERENCES

1. U.S. Department of Health, Education and Welfare: *Report to the Congress of the United States of the National Commission on Digestive Diseases,* vol 4, part 4, Washington, DC, 1979, (NIH) 79-1887.
2. Chappuis CW, Cohn I Jr: Acute colonic diverticulitis, *Surg Clin North Am* 68:301, 1988.
3. Painter NS, Burkitt DP: Diverticular disease of the colon: a deficiency disease of Western civilisation, *Br Med J* 2:450, 1971.
4. Bulbring E, Bolton TB: Smooth muscle, *Br Med Bull* 35:209, 1979.
5. Ferrucci JT et al: Double tracking in the sigmoid colon, *Radiology* 120:307, 1976.
6. Harned RK et al: Glucagon and barium enema examinations: a controlled clinical trial, *AJR* 126:981, 1976.
7. Miller RE et al: Hypotonic colon examination with glucagon, *Radiology* 113:555, 1974.
8. Fleischner FG, Ming SC: Revised concepts on diverticular disease of the colon. II. So-called diverticulitis: sigmoiditis and peridiverticulitis: diverticular abscess, fistula and frank peritonitis, *Radiology* 84:599, 1965.
9. Boulos PB et al: Diverticula, neoplasia, or both? Early detection of carcinoma in sigmoid diverticular disease, *Am Surg* 202:607, 1985.
10. Stein GN: Radiology of colonic diverticular disease, *Postgrad Med* 60:95, 1976.
11. Marshak RH, Lindner AE, Marlansky D: Diverticulosis and diverticulitis of the colon, *Mount Sinai J Med* 46:261, 1979.
12. Wilson SR, Toi A: The value of sonography in the diagnosis of acute diverticulitis of the colon, *AJR* 154:1199, 1990.
13. Verbanck J et al: Can sonography diagnose acute colonic diverticu-

litis in patients with acute intestinal inflammation? A prospective study, *J Clin Ultrasound* 17:661, 1989.

14. Wada M, Kikuchi Y, Doy M: Uncomplicated acute diverticulitis of the cecum and ascending colon: sonographic findings in 18 patients, *AJR* 155:283, 1990.

15. Neff CC, van Sonnenberg E: CT of diverticulitis. Diagnosis and treatment, *Radiol Clin North Am* 27:743, 1989.

16. Kyunghee CC et al: Sigmoid diverticulitis: diagnostic role of CT— comparison with barium enema studies, *Radiology* 176:111, 1990.

17. Labs JD et al: Complications of acute diverticulitis of the colon: improved early diagnosis with computerized tomography, *Am J Surg* 155:331, 1988.

18. Johnson CD et al: Diagnosis of acute colonic diverticulitis: comparison of barium enema and CT, *AJR* 148:541, 1987.

19. Lieberman JM, Haaga JR: Computed tomography of diverticulitis, *J Comput Assist Tomogr* 7:431, 1983.

20. Almy TP, Howell DA: Diverticular disease of the colon, *N Engl J Med* 302:324, 1980.

21. Connell AM: Pathogenesis of diverticular disease of the colon, *Adv Intern Med* 22:377, 1977.

22. Chia JG et al: Trends of diverticular disease of the large bowel in a newly developed country, *Dis Colon Rectum* 34:498, 1991.

23. Hackford AW, Veidenheimer MC: Diverticular disease of the colon, *Surg Clin North Am* 65:347, 1985.

24. Hughes LE: Postmortem survey of diverticular disease of the colon, *Gut* 10:336, 1969.

25. Parks TG: Natural history of diverticular disease of the colon, *Clin Gastroenterol* 4:53, 1975.

26. Parks TG: Natural history of diverticular disease of the colon: a review of 521 cases, *Br Med J* 4:639, 1969.

27. Feczko PJ et al: Acute diverticulitis in patients under 40 years of age: radiologic diagnosis, *AJR* 150:1311, 1988.

28. Lappas JC et al: Diverticular disease: imaging with post-double-contrast sigmoid flush, *Radiology* 168:35, 1988.

29. Evans WE, Dawson RG: Diverticulitis in the young adult, *Am Surg* 36:518, 1970.

30. Homer MJ, Danford RO: Acute diverticulitis in the young adult, *Radiology* 125:623, 1977.

31. Coode PE, Chan KW, Chan YT: Polyps and diverticula of the large intestine: a necropsy survey in Hong Kong, *Gut* 26:1045, 1985.

32. Kyle J, Davidson A: Incidence of diverticulitis, *Scand J Gastroenterol* 2:77, 1967.

33. Stemmermann GN, Yatani R: Diverticulosis and polyps of the large intestine. A necropsy study of Hawaii Japanese, *Cancer* 31:1260, 1973.

34. Segal I, Solomon A, Hunt JA: Emergence of diverticular disease in the South African Black, *Gastroenterology* 72:215, 1977.

35. Gear JSS et al: Symptomless diverticular disease and intake of dietary fibre, *Lancet* 1:511, 1979.

36. Thompson WG: Do colonic diverticula cause symptoms: *Am J Gastroenterol* 81:613, 1986.

37. Berry CS et al: Dietary fibre and prevention of diverticular disease of the colon: evidence from rats, *Lancet* 4:294, 1984.

38. Smits BJ, Whitehead AM, Prescott P: Lactulose in the treatment of symptomatic diverticular disease: a comparative study with high-fibre diet, *Br J Clin Pract* 44:314, 1990.

39. Painter NS et al: Segmentation and localisation of intraluminal pressures in the human colon, with special reference to the pathogenesis of colonic diverticula, *Gastroenterology* 49:169, 1965.

40. Eastwood MA et al: Colonic function in patients with diverticular disease, *Lancet* 1:1181, 1978.

41. Cortesini C, Pantalone D: Usefulness of colonic motility study in identifying patients at risk for complicated diverticular disease, *Dis Colon Rectum* 34:339, 1991.

42. Taylor I, Duthie HL: Bran tablets and diverticular disease, *Br Med J* 1:988, 1976.

43. Cook JYM: Spontaneous perforation of the colon: report of two cases in a family exhibiting Marfan's stigmata, *Ohio Med J* 64:73, 1968.

44. Miekle JE, Becker KL, Gross JB: Diverticulitis of the colon in a young man with Marfan's syndrome, *Gastroenterology* 48:379, 1965.

45. Beighton PH, Mudoch JL, Votteler T: Gastrointestinal complications of the Ehlers Danlos syndrome, *Gut* 10:1004, 1969.

46. Lucaya L et al: Syndrome of multiple mucosal neuromas, medullary thyroid carcinoma and pheochromocytomas: cause of diverticular disease in children, *AJR* 133:1186, 1978.

47. Damron JR, Leiber A, Simmons T: Rectal diverticula, *Radiology* 115:599, 1979.

48. Fields SI, Haskell L, Libson E: CT appearance of giant colonic diverticulum, *Gastrointest Radiol* 12:71, 1987.

49. Smith TR, Tyler IM: CT demonstration of a giant colonic diverticulum, *Gastrointest Radiol* 12:73, 1987.

50. Pace L, Williams I: The organisation of the muscular wall of the human colon, *Gut* 10:352, 1969.

51. Whiteway J, Morson BC: Pathology of the ageing—diverticular disease, *Clin Gastroenterol* 14:829, 1985.

52. Meyers MA et al: The angioarchitecture of colonic diverticula, *Radiology* 108:249, 1973.

53. Tagliacozzo S, Virno F: The vascularisation of the colon wall: morphological study, *Ann Ital Chir* 38:301, 1961.

54. Tagliacozzo S, Virno F: Vascular relationships of diverticula of the colon, *Ann Ital Chir* 38:420, 1961.

55. Williams I: Diverticular disease of the colon without diverticula, *Radiology* 89:401, 1967.

56. Morson BC, Dawson IMP: *Gastrointestinal pathology*, ed 2, Oxford, London, 1979, Blackwell.

57. Lumb GD, Protheroe RHB: Mucosal inflammatory spread in diverticulitis and ulcerative colitis, *Arch Pathol* 62:185, 1956.

58. Williams I: The resemblance of diverticular disease of the colon to a myostatic contracture, *Br J Radiol* 40:2, 1967.

59. Gasser HS: Contractures of skeletal muscle, *Physiol Rev* 10:35, 1930.

60. Fleischner FG, Ming SC, Henken EM: Revised concepts on diverticular disease of the colon. I. Diverticulosis: emphasis on tissue derangement and the irritable colon syndrome, *Radiology* 83:859, 1964.

61. Arfwidson F: Pathogenesis of multiple diverticula of the sigmoid colon in diverticular disease, *Acta Chir Scand* 342(suppl):1, 1964.

62. Schnyder P, Moss A, Thoeni R, Margulis A: A double-blind study of radiological accuracy in diverticulitis, diverticulosis and carcinoma of the sigmoid colon, *J Clin Gastroenterol* 1:55, 1979.

63. Ryan P: Changing concepts in diverticular disease, *Dis Colon Rectum* 26:12, 1983.

64. Morris DL, Tudor RG: The management of inflammatory complications of colonic diverticular disease, *Br J Hosp Med* 37:36, 1987.

65. Lindahl J et al: 99m-Technetium-HmPAO-labelled leucocytes in the diagnosis of acute colonic diverticulitis, *Acta Chir Scand* 155:479, 1989.

66. Wilson SR, Toi A: The value of sonography in the diagnosis of acute diverticulitis of the colon, *AJR* 154:1199, 1990.

67. Gore RM, Goldberg HI: Computed tomographic evaluation of the gastrointestinal tract in diseases other than primary adenocarcinoma, *Radiol Clin North Am* 20:781, 1982.

68. Morris J et al: The utility of computed tomography in colonic diverticulitis, *Ann Surg* 204:128, 1986.

69. Pillari G et al: Computed tomography of diverticulitis, *Gastrointest Radiol* 9:263, 1984.

70. Butch RJ et al: Drainage of pelvic abscesses through the greater sciatic foramen, *Radiology* 158:487, 1986.

71. Fisher JK: Abnormal colonic wall thickening on computed tomography. *J Comput Assist Tomogr* 7:90, 1983.

72. Hulnick DH et al: Computed tomography in the evaluation of diverticulitis, *Radiology* 152:491, 1984.
73. Mueller PR et al: Sigmoid diverticular abscesses: percutaneous drainage as an adjunct to surgical resection in 24 cases, *Radiology* 164:321, 1987.
74. Neff CC et al: Diverticular abscesses: percutaneous drainage, *Radiology* 163:15, 1987.
75. van Sonnenberg E, Mueller PR, Ferrucci JT Jr: Percutaneous drainage of 250 abdominal abscesses and fluid collections. I. Results, failures and complications, *Radiology* 151:337, 1984.
76. Feldberg MAM, Hendriks MJ, van Waes PFGM: Role of CT in diagnosis and management of complications of diverticular disease, *Gastrointest Radiol* 10:370, 1985.
77. Kleinhaus U, Rosenberg A: Computed tomography–guided percutaneous drainage of right upper abdominal abscess, *Cardiovasc Intervent Radiol* 5:8, 1982.
78. Mueller PR, van Sonnenberg E, Ferrucci JT Jr: Percutaneous drainage of 250 abdominal abscesses and fluid collections: II. Current procedural concepts, *Radiology* 151:343, 1984.
79. Saini S et al: Percutaneous drainage of diverticular abscess: an adjunct to surgical therapy, *Arch Surg* 121:475, 1986.
80. Stabile BE, Puccio E, van Sonnenberg E, Neff CC: Preoperative percutaneous drainage of diverticular abscesses, *Am J Surg* 159:99, 1990.
81. Goldman SM et al: CT demonstration of colovesical fistulae secondary to diverticulitis, *J Comput Assist Tomogr* 8:462, 1984.
82. Parks TG et al: Limitations of radiology in the differentiation of diverticulitis and diverticulosis of the colon, *Br Med J* 2:136, 1970.
83. Walker JD, Gray LA Sr, Polk HC Jr: Diverticulitis in women: an unappreciated clinical presentation, *Ann Surg* 185:402, 1977.
84. King DW, Lubowski DZ, Armstrong AS: Sigmoid stricture at colonoscopy—an indication for surgery, *Int J Colorectal Dis* 5:161, 1990.
85. Keller CE et al: Radiologic recognition of colonic diverticula simulating polyps, *AJR* 143:93, 1984.
86. Williams I: Mass movements (mass peristalsis) and diverticular disease of the colon, *Br J Radiol* 40:2, 1967.
87. Talman EA, Dixon DS, Gutierrez FE: Role of arteriography in rectal haemorrhage due to arteriovenous malformations and diverticulosis, *Ann Surg* 190:203, 1979.
88. Welch CE: Catheter drainage of abdominal abscesses, *N Engl J Med* 305:694, 1981.
89. Meyers MA, Alonzo DR, Baer JW: Pathogenesis of massively bleeding colonic diverticulosis: new observations, *AJR* 127:901, 1976.
90. Athanasoulis CA et al: Mesenteric arterial infusions of vasopressin for hemorrhage from colonic diverticulosis, *Am J Surg* 129:212, 1975.
91. Goldberger LE, Bookstein JJ: Transcatheter embolism for the treatment of diverticular hemorrhage, *Radiology* 122:613, 1977.
92. Britt LG, Warren L, Moore OF 3rd: Selective management of lower gastrointestinal bleeding, *Am Surg* 49:121, 1983.
93. Browder W, Cerise EJ, Litwin MS: Impact of emergency angiography in massive lower gastrointestinal bleeding, *Ann Surg* 204:530, 1986.
94. Colcock BP, Stahmann FD: Fistula complication diverticular disease of the colon, *Ann Surg* 175:838, 1972.
95. Cambria RP, Margolies MN: Hepatic portal venous gas in diverticulitis, *Arch Surg* 117:834, 1982.
96. Fataar S, Cadogan E, Spruyt O: Ultrasonography of hepatic portal venous gas due to diverticulitis, *Br J Radiol* 59:183, 1986.
97. Laing CF, Rego JD, Jeffrey RB: Ultrasonographic identification of portal vein gas, *J Clin Ultrasound* 12:512, 1984.
98. Baker SR, Alterman DD: False-negative barium enema in patients with sigmoid cancer and coexistent diverticula, *Gastrointest Radiol* 10:171, 1985.
99. Miller WT et al: Bowler-hat sign: a simple principle for differentiating polyps from diverticula, *Radiology* 173:615, 1989.
100. Marshak H, Janowitz HD, Present D: Granulomatous colitis in association with diverticula, *N Engl J Med* 283:1080, 1970.
101. Ferrucci JT Jr, Jaffer F, Seidler R: Muscle spasm in diverticulosis: evaluation of retrograde colon obstruction by hypotonic barium enema, *J Can Assoc Radiol* 25:269, 1974.
102. Schmid GT et al: Crohn's disease of the colon and its distinction from diverticulitis, *Gut* 9:7, 1968.
103. Meyers MA et al: Pathogenesis of diverticulitis complicating granulomatous colitis, *Gastroenterology* 74:24, 1978.
104. Petros JG, Happ RA: Crohn's colitis in patients with diverticular disease, *Am J Gastroenterol* 86:247, 1991.
105. Berridge FR, Dick AP: Effect of Crohn's disease on colonic diverticula, *Br J Radiol* 49:926, 1976.
106. McCue J et al: Coexistent Crohn's disease and sigmoid diverticulosis. *Postgrad Med J* 65:636, 1989.
107. Jalan DN et al: Faecal stasis and diverticular disease of the colon in ulcerative colitis, *Gut* 11:688, 1970.
108. Beranbaum SL, Beranbaum ER: Small polypoid lesions associated with spastic diverticulosis, *Dis Colon Rectum* 8:78, 1965.
109. Beranbaum SL, Yagmai M, Beranbaum ER: Ulcerative colitis in association with diverticular disease of the colon, *Radiology* 85:880, 1965.
110. Bates T, Kaminsky V: Diverticulitis and ulcerative colitis, *Br J Surg* 61:293, 1974.

37 *Cross-Sectional Imaging in the Evaluation of Acute Diverticulitis*

MARK E. BAKER

Over the past 10 years cross-sectional imaging has played an increasingly important role in the diagnosis and treatment of bowel disorders. Cross-sectional imaging is ideally suited to evaluate diverticulitis because the disease and its complications involve the wall and surrounding tissues, regions obscure to luminal studies. Indeed, in several centers, computed tomography (CT) is the preferred imaging modality in the evaluation of any patient with suspected diverticulitis.

The purpose of this chapter is to review the pathophysiology, clinical presentation, and treatment of the disease process; the CT examination techniques necessary for assessing acute diverticulitis; the CT findings and differential diagnosis of acute diverticulitis; and the respective roles of contrast enema studies and CT in a patient with suspected acute diverticulitis. Sonography is mentioned briefly, but this is covered more extensively in Chapter 109.

PATHOPHYSIOLOGY

Diverticular disease represents an important medical problem in the Western world. It has been estimated that, by the age of 80 years, 50% of the population of the United States will have diverticular disease.[1] Although it is impossible to determine the actual incidence of diverticulitis, it has been estimated that acute inflammation will develop during the lifetime in between 10% and 25% of such patients.[2] In a series in which 503 patients were followed for a certain length time, diverticulitis developed in 16.8%.[3] Strict criteria were used to define an episode of diverticulitis, and consisted of left lower quadrant pain and local tenderness, acute constipation or diarrhea, fever, and leukocytosis. Diverticulitis was suspected in another 12.9%, who did not meet these strict criteria. In another series, this one from the Lahey Clinic, where 294 patients were followed for 10 to 30 years, 8.5% suffered an episode of acute diverticulitis, with 18% of these patients experiencing at least one attack.[4] It has been calculated that 1% to 3% of those patients with diverticulosis face an annual risk of developing diverticulitis.[5] Thus, although many patients sustain attacks of acute inflammatory disease, a significant portion of those with diverticulosis do not.

Fortunately, less than 20% of the patients with diverticulitis require hospitalization for their first attack,[2] with the percentage increasing with repeated attacks.[6] The actual number of patients who undergo colonic resection for the management of acute diverticulitis is unknown, but the number is probably relatively low when considered in terms of the overall population. In the Lahey Clinic series, only 16 of 294 (5.4%) patients with diverticulosis underwent surgical therapy.[4] In a retrospective review of 673 cases collected over the course of 10 years, only 93 (14%) patients underwent resection.[7] Therefore, for many patients, an attack of acute diverticulitis is relatively mild and does not require extensive or expensive diagnostic or therapeutic interventions.

Complications such as abscess formation, perforation, bowel obstruction, and fistula formation occur in from 20% to 30% of the patients during their first attack,[8,9] with the number increasing to 60% for repeated attacks.[10] The recurrence rate of attacks has been estimated to be 30% (most taking place within 5 years of the previous attack).[2] For patients under the age of 40, the rate increases to approximately 50%.[11]

There has been a precipitous rise in the frequency of diverticular disease during this century.[12,13] The cause appears to be related to the dietary habits of the Western population.[14] In modern Western society, the amount of nondigestible fiber in food is relatively low,[12,13] and low-volume, hard stools result from this. These require high-pressure, propulsive efforts on the part of the colonic musculature to pass through the colon.

The colon normally functions as segments that create localized areas of high pressure, a process called *segmentation*.[15] The combination of segmentation and the presence of thick, inspissated stool presumably causes pulsion pseudodiverticula to form at weak points in the colon where intramural blood vessels penetrate. The process is most intense where the lumen of the bowel narrows (Laplace's law)—the sigmoid colon. In addition, the stool is at its hardest in the sigmoid, as most of the fluid has been resorbed at this point. Unfortunately, this theory does not entirely explain the disease, as motility is normal in many asymptomatic patients with diverticulosis and abnormal in symptomatic patients.[16]

Diverticulitis occurs when an operculum of one of these pseudodiverticula becomes occluded. The exact cause of this is unknown, but it causes feces to become entrapped and inspissated. The hardened stool then is the source of

mechanical irritation and subsequent ulceration.[16] The inflammatory process starts in the lymphoid tissue of the diverticular apices, often in only a single diverticulum.[17] Because the wall of the diverticulum (really a pseudodiverticulum) is thin, perforation into the paracolic fat is common. Thus, the term *acute diverticulitis* is actually a misnomer, as it is truly a peridiverticular inflammatory process. Inflammation in the paracolic fat is almost always present. Occasionally, the perforation occurs longitudinally into or immediately outside the adjacent wall, creating a dissecting, intramural, or paramural abscess with little to no paracolic inflammatory changes.[17] Diverticula that perforate along the mesenteric border protrude between the mesenteric leaves, and the resultant inflammation and abscess are confined between these leaves.[18] Diverticula that perforate along the antimesenteric border are often adjacent to the pelvic floor, and the resultant inflammation and abscess are often confined by the floor itself.[18] Free peritoneal perforation is uncommon. Fistulization can also extend to any adjacent structure, including the urinary bladder, vagina, small bowel, and even the skin. Other complications resulting from the inflammatory process include peritonitis arising from free perforation, plus small bowel and colonic obstruction.

Another important morphologic and pathologic process that occurs in the context of diverticular disease is muscular hypertrophy, and this is found in 50% to 70% of the resected specimens.[13] Acute diverticulitis may be incorrectly diagnosed in many patients (usually those with mild signs and symptoms) who exhibit these muscular changes. In a series of resected specimens, Morson[19] found no evidence of inflammation in one third of the patients with symptomatic disease. He considered the cause of the symptoms in these patients to be the muscular abnormality, not diverticulitis. Nonetheless, muscular hypertrophy thickens the wall of the colon, and this constitutes a major CT sign of acute diverticulitis.

CLINICAL PRESENTATION

The clinical presentation of acute diverticulitis is quite variable, and depends on many factors. Typically, the patient complains of the rapid onset of left lower abdominal pain and fever, accompanied by an abrupt change in bowel habits (either diarrhea or constipation). Most patients hospitalized have had symptoms for less than a month.[20] In one series, the presenting feature was abdominal pain in 71% and constipation or diarrhea, or both, in 41%.[8] The pain most commonly arises in the lower abdomen, and is more severe on the left.[9]

Typical physical examination findings consist of tachycardia, fever, and left lower quadrant tenderness and guarding. There is often abdominal distention, and a mass may be palpated during either an abdominal or rectal examination. Leukocytosis is often present, although, in one series, 64% of 130 patients with complicated diverticular disease

found at surgery had had a white count less than 12,000 cells per cubic millimeter.[21]

At presentation, the differential diagnosis includes a localized perforated colon carcinoma, ischemic colitis, infectious or inflammatory colitis, and diverticular disease without inflammation and perforation. In patients less than 40 years of age, diagnosis is usually delayed or incorrect because the disease is uncommon in this age group.[2,22] In these patients, the preoperative diagnosis is usually acute appendicitis, inflammatory bowel disease, pelvic inflammatory disease, or acute cholecystitis.

In recent years, there have been dramatic changes in the makeup of the patient population with acute inflammation.[23] More patients with immune system impairment (diabetes, steroid therapy, postsplenectomy, post–organ transplant, chemotherapy, and alcoholism) as well as the elderly are seen with the disease. Objective signs and symptoms are often absent in these patients, especially in those on corticosteroid therapy. In these cases, there is often a large discrepancy between the objective clinical data and the radiographic information, and free perforation is a common event.[24,25]

TREATMENT

The therapy for acute diverticulitis is controversial. It is often individualized and is usually based on the physician's preference and the patient's state. In general, those patients with mild signs and symptoms are managed medically. Most patients recover within 48 hours on oral antibiotic treatment. Conservative therapy is ineffective in some, especially those with a local or distant abscess, or both. For those patients with more serious disease, hospitalization is mandatory, with treatment consisting of bowel rest, intravenous fluids, and antibiotics.

The indications for surgery include the complications of sepsis, free perforation, obstruction, fistula formation, recurrent attacks of inflammation (more than two), a persistent painful mass (usually an abscess), marked narrowing of the sigmoid colon, diverticulitis presenting in young patients, and the question of a possible carcinoma.[12,13] In many centers, percutaneous drainage of a diverticular abscess may obviate surgery or at least alter the timing.[26-28] When there is perforation, obstruction, or fistula formation, surgery is often unavoidable. Patients under the age of 40 usually undergo resection of the affected segment because of the otherwise high percentage of recurrence. Other types of patients who routinely undergo resection include those who have had repeated attacks and those who are immunocompromised (including diabetics, patients on steroids, alcoholics, and so on).[25] What is unclear is whether a patient with an abscess requires colonic resection if the abscess can be effectively treated with percutaneous and medical management.

The preferred surgical approach is a one-stage procedure, and consists of the elective resection of the affected seg-

ment with a primary anastomosis done 6 to 8 weeks after the attack and after appropriate medical therapy has been carried out.[12,13] When infection and pus are found in the surgical bed, or obstruction or perforation mandates non-elective surgery, either a two-stage or three-stage procedure is performed. The most commonly used two-stage approach is the Hartmann's procedure. In the first stage, the sigmoid is resected, the rectum is closed, and any abscess is drained. Reanastomosis of the colon with the rectum constitutes the second stage of the approach. In the first part of the three-stage procedure, only a transverse colostomy is performed, leaving the diseased colon in place. After appropriate medical therapy, the diseased segment is then resected. Closure of the colostomy is the last stage of this approach.

Obviously, the single-stage surgical procedure is preferred, as it is elective and requires only one recovery pe-

riod. This approach is reserved only for those patients who do not have generalized fecal or purulent peritonitis or extensive paracolic inflammation and abscess formation, as the primary anastomosis of the single-stage procedure is more likely to break down if there is extensive inflammation or abscess formation in the paracolic fat.

The advantage of the one-stage procedure is the major impetus behind the percutaneous drainage of a paracolic diverticular abscess[26-28] (Fig. 37-1). If there is an abscess that is technically drainable under radiographic guidance, the surgical bed can then be sterilized and, in many cases, this makes possible the one-stage surgical procedure. The data to support this protocol are limited but encouraging. In a recent series consisting of 19 patients with diverticular abscess, 14 of 19 (74%) of the abscesses were successfully drained and the patients subsequently underwent a single-

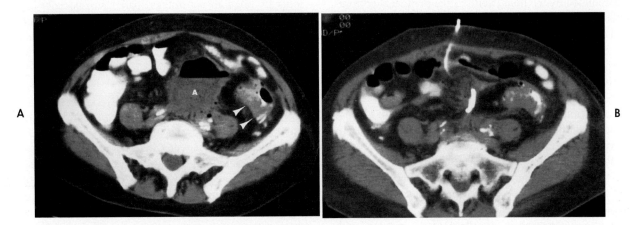

Fig. 37-1 A, Diverticular abscess that was successfully drained with a percutaneous catheter. **B,** After 4 days of drainage, the abscess has completely resolved. The patient subsequently underwent a one-stage surgical procedure. The wall of the sigmoid colon is asymmetrically thickened by the inflammatory process (**A,** *arrowheads*).

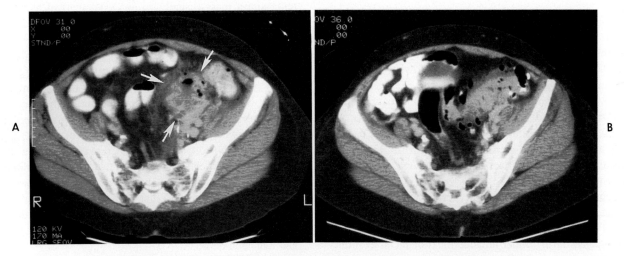

Fig. 37-2 A, Small (<5 cm) diverticular abscess *(arrows)* that was successfully treated with intravenous antibiotics alone. **B,** After 8 days of treatment, the abscess has resolved.

stage sigmoidectomy and primary anastomosis without complications.[28] However, appropriate patient selection is critical for such percutaneous management. Patients with obstruction, free perforation, or generalized peritonitis are not candidates for percutaneous catheter management. Further, according to Stabile et al.,[28] small abscesses (<5 cm) should not be drained percutaneously because they are usually rendered sterile with modern intravenous antibiotics and can then be resected en bloc with the colon (Fig. 37-2).

In the author's evolving experience, if a diverticular abscess is evident on a CT scan and is technically drainable, it is almost always drained percutaneously at the surgeon's request, including the small abscesses. Almost all such patients experience an uncomplicated clinical course and often do not later have to undergo resection. What is not known is the eventual outcome if the abscess had not been drained percutaneously. The author has seen several patients with abscesses up to 5 cm in diameter that were effectively treated with antibiotics alone (see Fig. 37-2).

COMPUTED TOMOGRAPHY
Technique

Proper technique in the CT evaluation of bowel disorders is essential to ensure an accurate diagnosis.[29] To assess the bowel with CT, there must be appropriate lumen preparation plus lumen opacification and distention in order to visualize both the mucosa and the bowel wall. Further, the intravenous administration of contrast media is essential in many cases, and, finally, slice collimation and intervals must be adequate to portray the pathology.

The most sensitive and specific diagnoses can be made in the presence of a clean colon.[29] Unfortunately, in cases of acute diverticulitis, this is almost always impossible to achieve. Therefore, every effort should be made to ensure proper lumen opacification and distention. The goal is to accurately determine the thickness of the wall and the state of the mucosa, and to differentiate mural from extramural processes.

An oral contrast agent is always used in patients with acute diverticulitis to ensure opacification of the stomach, small bowel, and, in most cases, the right colon. Either dilute water-soluble iodine or barium solutions can be used for this purpose, with equal success. Some practitioners use metoclopramide to hasten bowel motility and opacification.[29] In most cases, though, after 800 to 1000 ml of contrast is ingested over 1 to 2 hours, this will produce adequate opacification of the small bowel and right colon. During that time, though, especially if there is an ileus, there will be inadequate opacification and distention of the sigmoid colon. In many instances, the diagnosis of a colonic abnormality can be made without distention, especially if pericolonic abnormalities exist. Nonetheless, even in these cases, it is necessary to opacify and distend the colon so that a more specific diagnosis can be rendered.

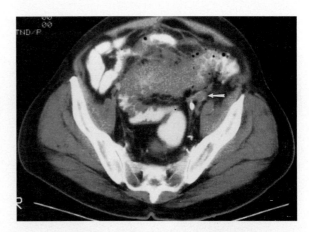

Fig. 37-3 Diverticulitis involving a long segment of the sigmoid colon. Positive (dilute water-soluble) rectal contrast outlines and distends the lumen. The colon wall is symmetrically thickened and there is soft tissue stranding in the adjacent fat. A small pus collection *(arrow)* is present just anterolateral to the left ureter.

Traditionally, a positive rectal contrast agent is given to distend the colon and allow the lumen to be easily identified (Fig. 37-3). Air insufflation or the use of a negative contrast agent affords the added advantage of mucosal evaluation and reduces lesion obscuration[29,30] (Fig. 37-4). Most of the time, air rather than dilute radiopaque contrast should be used. In general, most patients can tolerate either the rectal administration of 10 to 15 puffs of air using an barium enema insufflation bulb or 200 to 300 ml of a dilute positive contrast agent. Patient comfort is the usual measure of the maximum volume that should be administered. Regardless of the contrast agent used, if gentle and judicious care is taken during rectal instillation, no complications should result.[30,31]

The use of intravenous contrast is somewhat controversial. When used, scanning in the arterial phase more clearly portrays the colonic wall and the interface between the wall and pericolonic fat.[29] Further, intravenous contrast optimizes hepatic abscess detection. Some, however, do not administer contrast when trying to detect colovesical fistulas.[32] In acutely ill patients, fistula detection is a secondary priority. Therefore, most patients receive intravenous contrast media.

For proper evaluation, it is essential to scan in a contiguous fashion, using at least 8- to 10-mm-thick slices. Further, selective reexamination using a 4- to 5-mm slice thickness after additional lumen distention has been achieved, the patient's position has been changed, or both measures, often enhances the diagnosis.[29,30]

Some investigators scan from the pubic symphysis cephalad to the iliac crest, and continue through the liver only if the findings are positive.[30] This focused approach is probably best for determining whether there is acute *sigmoid* diverticulitis. Unfortunately, many of the author's acutely

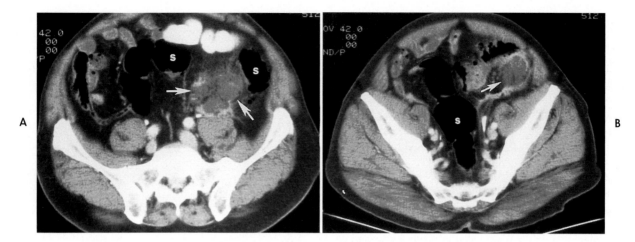

Fig. 37-4 A and **B,** A diverticular inflammatory process *(arrows)* involving the paracolic fat anterior to the left psoas and iliopsoas muscles. Negative contrast (air) has been used to distend the sigmoid colon *(S).* The inflammation is becoming confluent and is developing an enhancing wall. Only a small amount of fluid could be aspirated.

ill patients are being evaluated for generalized abdominal pain and fever, and acute diverticulitis is only one possible diagnosis. Therefore, the entire abdomen is scanned.

At the author's institution, the standard CT routine for a patient with an acute abdomen is incremental, dynamic scanning with the acquisition of rapid contiguous, 10-mm scans through the liver and 15-mm scans of the pubic symphysis during the rapid intravenous administration of 150 ml of contrast medium. Selective 10- and 5-mm slices are then obtained at the appropriate levels, usually after the instillation of air in the rectum. Occasionally, the patient is placed in the prone or decubitus position to facilitate distention and wall delineation.

CT diagnosis of acute diverticulitis and differential diagnosis

The CT diagnosis of acute diverticulitis is based on several findings, including wall thickening, paracolic fat changes, local and distant abscess, fistulas, bowel and ureteric obstruction, and peritonitis (see box below). Localized wall thickening (>3-5 mm) is the hallmark of acute diverticulitis; in one series, it was present in 70% of the patients[29,33] (Figs. 37-1, 37-3, and 37-5). The lumen must be adequately distended to ensure accurate determination of wall thickness. Wall thickening may either be focal and eccentric or, more commonly, circumferential and symmetric.

Unfortunately, wall thickening *alone* is a nonspecific and unreliable finding.[29,34] A focally thickened colon wall occurs in the context of muscular hypertrophy resulting from diverticulosis, carcinoma, Crohn's disease, ischemia, irradiation, pseudomembranous colitis, infectious colitides, inflammation of the appendices epiploicae, and a perforated foreign body. Some consider focal sigmoid wall thickening associated with pericolic changes to be diagnostic of acute diverticulitis.[34] In other areas of the colon, where other diseases are more common, these findings are much more nonspecific.

□ **CT FINDINGS IN ACUTE DIVERTICULITIS** □

Focal colonic wall thickening (>3-5 mm)
Linear to confluent paracolic fat soft tissue changes
Paracolic abscess
Fluid or contrast within a thick-walled colon
Distant abscess
Evidence for fistula formation (vesicular air or contrast)

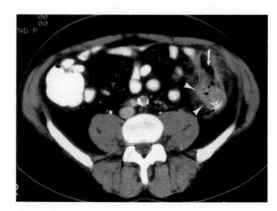

Fig. 37-5 Diverticulitis involving the distal descending colon. The wall is asymmetrically thickened *(arrowheads)* and there is extraluminal, paracolic air *(arrow)* indicating a localized perforation.

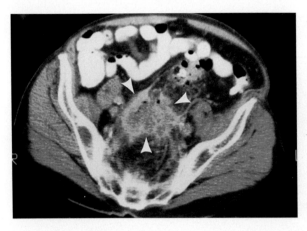

Fig. 37-6 A diverticular inflammatory process *(arrowheads)* containing a small amount of extraluminal air. Although a small amount of pus is present, the process is primarily solid and not amenable to drainage.

Pericolic fat inflammatory changes are the most common CT finding in the presence of acute diverticulitis; in one series they were noted in 98% of the patients[33] (Figs. 37-3 to 37-6). The normally homogeneous fat attenuation is altered by linear soft tissue stranding or more poorly defined areas of hazy soft tissue opacity. As the inflammation progresses, the areas become more confluent (see Fig. 38-4). There can be areas of water attenuation interspersed between the confluent areas of soft tissue density (see Fig. 37-6). In these cases, liquid pus coexists with indurated, inflamed mesenteric fat.

Local abscess formation is also a common finding (present in 35% to 59% of the patients[30,33]; however, the proportion of patients presenting with an abscess depends on the population studied. Abscesses appear on CT scans as localized collections with a water-density or near–water-

density attenuation, which may or may not have a well-defined wall (see Figs. 37-1 and 37-2). Air can exist within the abscess (see Figs. 37-1 and 37-2) and may be the dominant finding[34] (Fig. 37-7). Occasionally, large air-filled abscess cavities can assume the appearance of an unopacified colon. In these cases, contiguous slices and careful tracing of the course of the colon is essential in differentiating the colon from the abscess. In such instances, a positive rectal contrast agent may be more helpful than air insufflation, as an abscess may contain gas but will not contain contrast unless there is a connection between the bowel and the abscess (see Fig. 37-7).

CT can also identify other complications of diverticulitis. Distant abscesses are uncommon,[33] but their identification is critical in planning and mounting appropriate patient care. Colovesical fistulas also occur, and the presence of air in the urinary bladder in the absence of prior instrumentation is a diagnostic sign.[32] If intravenous contrast has not been given, but oral or rectal positive contrast has been, the presence of contrast in the urinary bladder is also a diagnostic finding. Bowel and ureteric obstruction can also be identified with CT. It has been claimed that the presence of ascites is diagnostic proof of peritonitis, but the evidence for this is weak.[34,35] There can be small amounts of pelvic fluid found in patients with acute diverticulitis who do not have peritonitis. Free air and localized pericolic air may also be seen (Figs. 37-5 and 37-8). Although diverticula are often identified in patients with acute diverticulitis, their presence does not establish the diagnosis.[33,34]

The CT findings noted in cases of diverticulitis are nonspecific.[29,31,34] A focally thickened sigmoid colon wall associated with soft tissue paracolic changes, an abscess, or both findings, are almost always due to acute diverticulitis (see Figs. 37-1 to 37-3). Nonetheless, the differential diagnosis is extensive, and includes appendicitis, Crohn's disease, foreign body perforation, tuboovarian abscess involv-

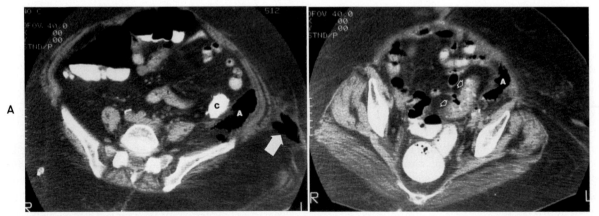

Fig. 37-7 **A,** Extraperitoneal perforation of diverticulitis in an immunocompromised patient (diabetes). The perforation consists entirely of air *(A)* and extends into the subcutaneous fat *(arrow).* **B,** The sigmoid colon is only minimally thickened *(open arrows).* Positive contrast opacifies the colon *(C).*

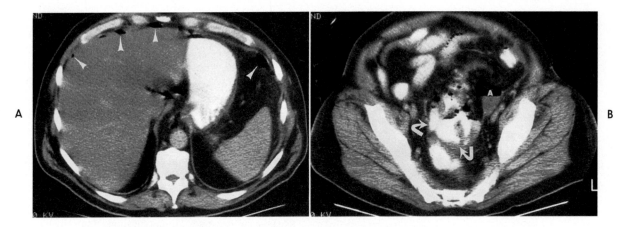

Fig. 37-8 Intraperitoneal perforation of diverticulitis. **A,** Free peritoneal air is present underneath the diaphragm *(arrowheads).* **B,** In the pelvis, there is extravasation of the rectally administered positive contrast (Gastrografin) *(curved arrows).* In addition, there is a small air-containing abscess *(A)* in the left pelvis.

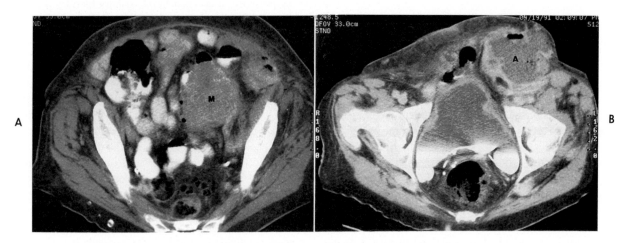

Fig. 37-9 A and **B,** A perforated colon carcinoma with a left groin abscess. The sigmoid colon wall is asymmetrically thickened by a bulky mass *(M).* The abscess *(A)* involves the left groin due to extraperitoneal extension of the perforation. Pathologically, extensive sigmoid diverticulosis was also present.

ing the sigmoid colon, infarction of the appendices epiploicae, ischemic colitis (especially outside the sigmoid colon), pelvic inflammatory disease, and colon carcinoma, with or without perforation.[30,31,34] Appendicitis is usually a right lower quadrant process, but if it has involved the pelvis and sigmoid colon, differentiating it from these other disorders can occasionally be difficult. Crohn's disease can mimic diverticulitis. Nonetheless, the clinical aspects of the disease and other radiographic signs almost always distinguish it from diverticulitis.

Unless a radiopaque object can be identified, foreign body perforation is indistinguishable from diverticulitis, as is infarction of the appendices epiploicae.[36] Fortunately, these are uncommon events, and, in fact, their treatment

may be similar to that adopted for acute diverticulitis. Pelvic inflammatory disease rarely mimics diverticulitis, and, in most cases, the clinical presentation establishes the diagnosis. Rarely, these patients do exhibit confusing signs and symptoms, and therefore undergo CT scanning.

The most troublesome problem in the differential diagnosis is posed by colon carcinoma, especially when the carcinoma has perforated.[29,31,34,37-39] Colon carcinoma and diverticular disease commonly affect the sigmoid colon, and may even coexist[40,41] (Fig. 37-9). Further, some patients with acute diverticulitis exhibit symptoms of colonic obstruction. On CT scans, colon carcinoma is more commonly seen to thicken the colon eccentrically and asymmetrically[29,34,38] and to cause more bulky wall thickening (Fig.

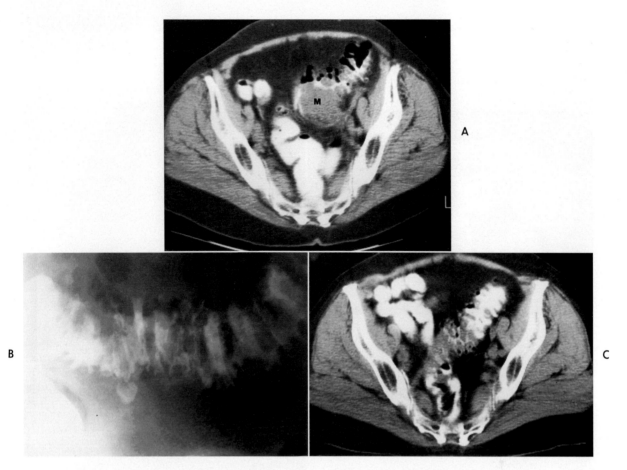

Fig. 37-10 Acute diverticulitis mimicking a colon carcinoma. **A,** An initial CT scan shows an asymmetric mass *(M)* involving the wall of the sigmoid colon. **B,** A contrast enema study shows only diverticula without mucosal ulceration or mass. **C,** A follow-up CT scan obtained 4 months later shows complete resolution of the mass.

37-9). However, diverticulitis can present similar findings (Fig. 37-10). The paracolic fat changes found in both diseases are often indistinguishable.[34] Despite published data to the contrary,[38] the author and others have discovered that the combination of a perforated carcinoma and abscess formation may be impossible to distinguish from diverticulitis[27,34,37] (Fig. 37-11). Further, a chronically inflamed, indurated colonic wall in conjunction with a large inflammatory mass resulting from diverticulitis cannot be distinguished from a carcinoma[29,39] (Figs. 37-10 and 37-12). Although the finding of mild symmetric wall thickening involving a short segment of colon favors the diagnosis of diverticulitis, early colon carcinoma can present the same appearance.[29] The contrast enema can be very helpful in differentiating between these two entities (Figs. 37-10 to 37-12), although the conclusions drawn from several clinical series have challenged the use of this investigation in patients with colonic lumenal narrowing.[41,42] In these series, a significant number of tumors were missed on both prospective and retrospective examinations, and the authors

instead recommend the use of flexible sigmoidoscopy or colonoscopy in the evaluation of these patients.

The sensitivity of CT in detecting diverticulitis has also been questioned.[31,39] There is a small subset of patients who have acute diverticulitis, either with intramural involvement alone or with minimal, radiographically undetectable pericolic inflammatory changes.[31,39] In these cases, the CT findings are falsely negative. Changes above or below certain segments of the horizontally positioned sigmoid colon may be especially difficult to visualize with axial scanning.[29,34,39] In these cases, narrow collimation and air insufflation may be helpful for divulging their presence.

CT versus the contrast enema study

Traditionally, the radiographic diagnosis of acute diverticulitis has been made using the contrast enema examination.[34] The findings indicating diverticulitis are often secondary, however, and include diverticula associated with luminal narrowing, spasm, tethering, intramural sinus tract formation, a mass effect, or extravasation of the contrast

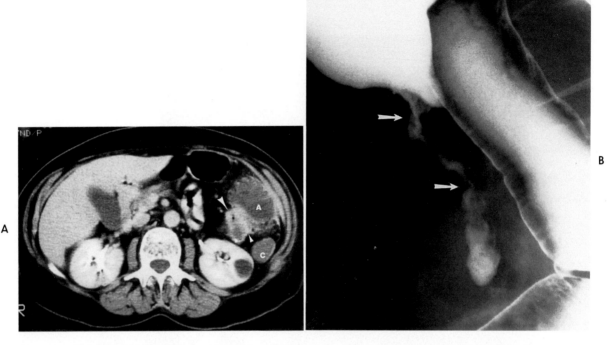

Fig. 37-11 Perforated colon carcinoma with abscess formation mimicking acute diverticulitis. **A,** A CT scan shows only mild wall thickening *(arrowheads)* of the ascending limb of the splenic flexure. An abscess *(A)* is adjacent to the affected colon, and anterior to the fluid-filled descending colon *(C)*. **B,** A contrast enema study shows a classic annular carcinoma with mucosal ulceration *(arrows)*.

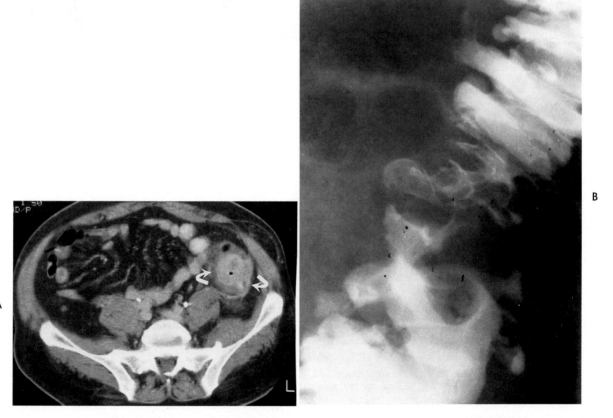

Fig. 37-12 Acute diverticulitis mimicking colon carcinoma. **A,** The CT scan shows symmetric, marked wall thickening of the sigmoid colon *(curved arrows)*. The differential diagnosis includes diverticulitis and carcinoma. **B,** The contrast enema study shows diverticular disease and luminal narrowing, but no loss of the mucosa.

agent. Clinicians have been reluctant to use the contrast enema in acute situations for fear of the presence of perforation and because of the discomfort involved. In a series from the author's institution, no complications arose as the result of an enema performed in the acute setting.[31] Further, rectal contrast agent is commonly used in CT examinations.[29,30]

Recently, there has been considerable controversy over the relative roles of the contrast enema versus CT in the evaluation of acute diverticulitis.[27,30-32,43-48] In many centers, CT is now the procedure of choice.[27,30,33] The contrast enema is limited because only the lumen and the mucosa are visualized, and diverticulitis is an extramucosal process. Further, CT's ability to visualize the colonic wall and extracolonic structures make it ideal for detecting some of the most serious complications of diverticulitis—local and distant abscesses.

Understanding the role of radiology in the diagnosis and treatment of diverticulitis lies in understanding the disease process. As previously noted, when first seen, a large cohort of patients with acute diverticulitis have mild disease and do not need imaging. In a recently presented prospective series comparing the contrast enema study with CT, 42% of the patients had a minor form of diverticulitis that did not require percutaneous drainage.[47] In these patients, neither the CT nor the contrast enema findings altered the therapy that was instituted.

Most series evaluating the merits of CT in the detection of acute diverticulitis are composed of acutely ill, hospitalized patients, with the majority ultimately requiring surgery, making this an obviously preselected and skewed population.[30,33] In other series that comprise a less severely affected population, the CT findings did not alter the management of patients; instead the ultimate management decisions were made on clinical grounds.[31,46] Most of these series are now somewhat dated, and document an outdated management approach in patients with acute diverticulitis. The most recent series in which the contrast enema study was compared with CT was conducted in patients with acute sigmoid diverticulitis, and showed CT is clearly superior to the contrast enema in this setting.[30] However, in this series, not all patients with the disease were evaluated.

The role for CT in the evaluation of acute diverticulitis is now much clearer (see box above). Its main advantage in patients with acute diverticulitis is in the detection of extracolonic manifestations, primarily an abscess. In most cases, percutaneous drainage is performed when an abscess is detected. CT may also correctly identify disease in patients with suspected diverticulitis in the presence of another process.[30] Finally, because the clinical assessment is limited and the findings often misleading, CT can provide vital information in immunocompromised patients with a suspected abdominal disorder. Therefore, the appropriate use of CT requires the application of appropriate preselection criteria (see box above).

□ INDICATIONS FOR CT EVALUATION OF ACUTE DIVERTICULITIS □

Acutely ill patients with signs and symptoms suggesting acute diverticulitis with abscess formation
Signs and symptoms of diverticulitis unresponsive to medical treatment
Immunocompromised patients
  Diabetes
  Steroid use
  Chemotherapy
  Organ transplant
  Alcoholic
  Elderly
Acute abdominal condition in a patient when diverticulitis is a possible diagnosis

---

Acutely ill patients with suspected diverticulitis clearly need to undergo CT scanning to detect a possible abscess. Further, CT scanning is necessary in any patient who has already received medical treatment for diverticulitis but not responded. Unless free air has been detected on plain radiographs, a CT scan is also extremely useful in immunocompromised patients with a suspected abdominal disorder. Finally, CT is very useful in evaluating patients with an acute abdominal condition when the signs and symptoms are nonspecific and acute diverticulitis is part of the differential diagnosis.

The detection of an abscess does not always alter the course of therapy. In fact, some practitioners often do not percutaneously drain abscesses less than 3 to 5 cm in diameter, but treat them medically[27,28] (see Fig. 37-2). There is also no evidence to support the contention that the presence of a pericolic abscess alone mandates surgical resection. Therefore, using CT as a means to determine whether the patient requires colonic resection has no scientific basis.

The author no longer recommends the routine use of a contrast enema as the initial radiographic investigation in a patient with suspected acute diverticulitis. However, it can be used to complement CT and is very helpful when the CT findings are equivocal.[34,39] In those instances when CT cannot distinguish diverticulitis from carcinoma, the enema often provides the necessary information (Figs. 37-10 to 37-12). Further, when the CT findings are negative and diverticulitis is still suspected, the contrast enema findings may correctly identify the process.[39]

RIGHT-SIDED DIVERTICULITIS

Right-sided diverticulitis is an uncommon disease that is more commonly reported from the Orient, accounting for less than 2% of the cases of acute diverticulitis in Western

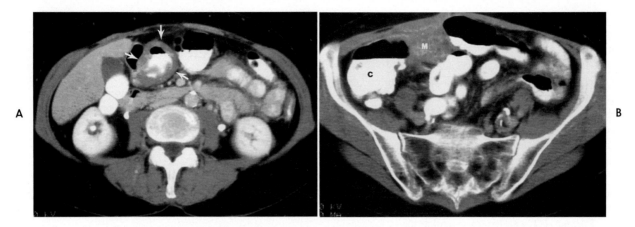

Fig. 37-13 Right-sided diverticulitis misdiagnosed as a perforated gastric ulcer. The patient initially exhibited right upper quadrant pain. **A,** A CT scan taken through the antrum shows thickening of the gastric wall *(arrows)*. **B,** A scan obtained through the pelvis shows a soft tissue "mass" *(M)* medial to the cecum *(C)* that was thought to represent the inferior extent of an inflammation resulting from a perforated antral ulcer. At surgery, right-sided diverticulitis was diagnosed. The thickened antral wall was secondary to the colonic inflammatory process.

series[49,50] and less than 5% of all cases worldwide.[51] Because of its location and presentation, it is commonly misdiagnosed preoperatively (Fig. 37-13), usually as acute appendicitis. Because the initial therapy for this disorder is conservative, an accurate preoperative diagnosis is desirable.

Two series suggest that CT may be helpful in the appropriate diagnosis of this entity.[52,53] If a pericolic soft tissue process exists above the ileocecal valve, and diverticula are present, these findings suggest the diagnosis. Crohn's disease and carcinoma can present similar appearances. Because other diseases are more common in this region of the bowel, the problem of nonspecificity is further compounded. If a pericolic soft tissue process is present below the ileocecal valve, the diagnosis then becomes very difficult. In these cases, a contrast enema or graded-compression ultrasound may be helpful in the differentiation.[54,55] A normal appendix should exclude the possibility of acute appendicitis.

SONOGRAPHY IN THE DIAGNOSIS OF ACUTE DIVERTICULITIS

The use of sonography in the evaluation of patients with colonic diverticulitis is not new,[56] and has recently been emphasized.[57] In at least one center, sonographic evaluation has proved to be both sensitive and specific for detecting acute diverticulitis of the left colon, especially for identifying paracolic abscesses.[57] Sonography may provide a quick and easy screening examination, as it can depict colonic wall thickening, inflammatory diverticula, and paracolic fat changes. The high cost of a CT examination could be avoided if ultrasound were used as the screening examination. Further, theoretically, sonography would not be be-

set by the limitations of the contrast enema study. This subject is covered in more detail in Chapter 109.

In the author's opinion, more experience is necessary before a strong recommendation can be made on behalf of sonography. The limitations of sonography, such as in the detection of interloop abscesses, the differentiation of gas-filled abscesses from normal bowel, and technically inadequate scans resulting from severe ileus, should be determined and documented. Nonetheless, at least in the United States, sonography is underutilized in the investigation of this and other diseases, and further work in this area is warranted.

REFERENCES

1. Connell AM: Pathogenesis of diverticular disease of the colon, *Adv Intern Med* 22:377, 1977.
2. Parks TG: Natural history of diverticular disease of the colon, *Clin Gastroenterol* 4:53, 1975.
3. Horner JL: Natural history of diverticulosis of the colon, *Am J Dig Dis* 3:343, 1958.
4. Boles RS, Jordan SM: The clinical significance of diverticulosis, *Gastroenterology* 35:579, 1958.
5. Schwartz JT, Graham DY: Diverticular disease of the large intestine. In Kirsner JB, Shorter RG, eds: *Diseases of the colon, rectum, and anal canal,* Baltimore, 1988, Williams & Wilkins.
6. Kyle J, Davidson AL: The changing pattern of hospital admissions for diverticular disease of the colon, *Br J Surg* 62:537, 1975.
7. Alexander J, Karl RC, Skinner DB: Results of changing trends in the surgical management of complications of diverticular disease, *Surgery* 94:683, 1983.
8. Zollinger RW: The prognosis in diverticulitis of the colon, *Arch Surg* 97:418, 1968.
9. Parks, TG: Reappraisal of clinical features of diverticular disease of the colon, *Br Med J* 4:642, 1969.
10. Marshall SF: Earlier resection in one stage for diverticulitis of the colon, *Am Surg* 29:337, 1963.
11. Ourial K, Schwartz SI: Diverticular disease in the young patient, *Surg Gynecol Obstet* 156:1, 1983.

12. Steinhagen RM, Aufsas AH: Diverticular disease. In Moody FG, ed: *Surgical treatment of digestive disease,* ed 3, Chicago, 1990, Mosby–Year Book.
13. Roberts PL, Veidenheimer MC: Diverticular disease. In Zuidema GD, ed: *Surgery of the alimentary tract,* vol IV, ed 3, Philadelphia, 1991, WB Saunders.
14. Painter NS, Burkitt DP: Diverticular disease of the colon, a 20th century problem, *Clin Gastroenterol* 4:3, 1975.
15. Painter NS et al: Segmentation and the localization of intraluminal pressures in the human colon, with special reference to the pathogenesis of colonic diverticula, *Gastroenterology* 49:169, 1965.
16. Almy TP, Howell DA: Diverticular disease of the colon, *N Engl J Med* 302:324, 1975.
17. Morson BC: Pathology of diverticular disease of the colon, *Clin Gastroenterol* 4:37, 1975.
18. Nicholas GG el al: Diagnosis of diverticulitis of the colon: role of barium enema in defining pericolic inflammation, *Ann Surg* 176:205, 1972.
19. Morson BC: The muscle abnormality in diverticular disease of the colon, *Br J Radiol* 36:385, 1963.
20. Parks TG: Natural history of diverticular disease of the colon: a review of 521 cases, *Br Med J* 4:639, 1969.
21. Hackford AW, Schoetz DJ, Coller JA, Veidenheimer MC: Surgical management of complicated diverticulitis: The Lahey Clinic experience, 1967-1982, *Dis Colon Rectum* 28:317, 1985.
22. Feczko PJ et al: Acute diverticulitis in patients under 40 years of age: radiologic diagnosis, *AJR* 150:1311, 1988.
23. Rodkey GV, Welch GE: The changing patterns in the surgical treatment of diverticular disease, *Ann Surg* 200:466, 1984.
24. Perkins JD, Shield CF, Chang FC, Farha GJ: Acute diverticulitis: comparison of treatment in immunocompromised and nonimmunocompromised patients, *Am J Surg* 148:745, 1984.
25. Tyau ES et al: Acute diverticulitis: a complicated problem in the immumocompromised patient, *Arch Surg* 126:855, 1991.
26. Mueller PR et al: Sigmoid diverticular abscesses: percutaneous drainage as an adjunct to surgical resection in 24 cases, *Radiology* 164:321, 1987.
27. Neff CC, van Sonnenberg E: CT of diverticulitis: diagnosis and treatment, *Radiol Clin North Am* 27:743, 1989.
28. Stabile BE, Puccio E, van Sonnenberg E: Preoperative percutaneous drainage of diverticular abscesses, *Am J Surg* 159:99, 1990.
29. Balthazar EJ: CT of the gastrointestinal tract: principles and interpretation, *AJR* 156:23, 1990.
30. Cho KC et al: Sigmoid diverticulitis: diagnostic role of CT comparison with barium enema studies, *Radiology* 176:111, 1990.
31. Johnson CD et al: Diagnosis of acute colonic diverticulitis: comparison of barium enema and CT, *AJR* 148:541, 1987.
32. Labs JD et al: Complications of acute diverticulitis of the colon: improved early diagnosis with computerized tomography, *Am J Surg* 155:331, 1988.
33. Hulnick DH et al: Computed tomography in the evaluation of diverticulitis, *Radiology* 152:491, 1984.
34. Cho KC: Computed tomography in colonic diverticulitis. In Herlinger H, Megibow AJ, eds: *Advances in gastrointestinal radiology,* vol 1, St Louis, 1991, Mosby–Year Book.
35. Megibow AJ, Balthazar EJ: *Computed tomography of the gastrointestinal tract,* St Louis, 1986, Mosby–Year Book.
36. Ghahremani GG et al: Appendices epiploicae of the colon: radiologic and pathologic features, *Radiographics* 12:59, 1992.
37. Evans SJJ et al: Can CT distinguish between diverticulitis and perforated colon cancer? Presented at the 17th Annual Meeting of the Society of Gastrointestinal Radiologists, Nassau, Bahamas, January 1988.
38. Hulnick DH et al: Perforated colorectal neoplasms: correlation of clinical, contrast enema and CT examination, *Radiology* 164:611, 1987.
39. Balthazar EJ et al: Limitations in the CT diagnosis of acute diverticulitis: comparison of CT, contrast enema and pathologic findings in 16 patients, *AJR* 154:281, 1990.
40. Krukowski ZH, Koruth NM, Matheson NA: Evolving practice in acute diverticulitis, *Br J Surg* 72:684, 1985.
41. Boulos PB, Cowin AP, Karamanolis DG: Diverticula, neoplasia or both? *Ann Surg* 202:607, 1985.
42. Schnyder P, Moss AA, Thoeni RF, Margulis AR: A double-blind study of radiologic accuracy in diverticulitis, diverticulosis and carcinoma of the sigmoid colon, *J Clin Gastroenterol* 1:55, 1979.
43. Pillari G et al: Computed tomography of diverticulitis, *Gastrointest Radiol* 9:263, 1984.
44. Feldberg MAM, Hendriks MJ, van Waes PFGM: Role of CT in diagnosis and management of complications of diverticular disease, *Gastrointest Radiol* 10:370, 1985.
45. Raval B et al: Role of computed tomography in diverticulitis, *J Comput Assist Tomogr* 11:144, 1987.
46. Morris J et al: The utility of computed tomography in colonic diverticulitis, *Ann Surg* 204:128, 1986.
47. Schiau R, Mirescu D, Ambrosetti P: Acute diverticulitis of the descending colon: role of CT in the pretherapeutic workup, *Radiology* 181(P):123, 1991.
48. Welch CE: Computerized tomography scans for all patients with diverticulitis, *Am J Surg* 155:336, 1988 (editorial comment).
49. Magness LJ, Van Heerden JA, Judd ES: Diverticular disease of the right colon, *Dis Colon Rectum* 27:454, 1984.
50. Fischer MG, Farkas AM: Diverticulitis of the cecum and ascending colon, *Surg Gynecol Obstet* 140:30, 1975.
51. Asch MJ, Markowitz AM: Cecal diverticulitis: report of 16 cases and a review of the literature, *Surgery* 65:906, 1969.
52. Balthazar EJ et al: Cecal diverticulitis: evaluation with CT, *Radiology* 162:79, 1987.
53. Scatarige JC et al: Diverticulitis of the right colon: CT observations, *AJR* 148:737, 1987.
54. Townsend RR, Jeffrey RB, Laing FC: Cecal diverticulitis differentiated from appendicitis using graded-compression sonography, *AJR* 152:1229, 1989.
55. Wada M, Kikuchi Y, Doy M: Uncomplicated acute diverticulitis of the cecum and ascending colon: sonographic findings in 18 patients, *AJR* 155:283, 1990.
56. Parulekar SG: Sonography of colonic diverticulitis, *J Ultrasound Med* 4:659, 1985.
57. Wilson SR, Toi A: The value of sonography in the diagnosis of acute diverticulitis of the colon, *AJR* 154:1199, 1990.

38 *Neoplastic Colonic Lesions*

EDWARD T. STEWART
WYLIE J. DODDS

Because colonic polyps may harbor a malignant tumor or lead to a malignancy, the detection of polypoid colonic lesions is an important diagnostic challenge for the radiologist. In this chapter, sporadic isolated colonic polyps, colonic polyposis syndromes, and malignancies are discussed.

DEFINITIONS

The word *polyp* is derived from the Greek *polypus,* meaning "many footed." Although the term *polyp* is often used to mean an epithelial adenoma, the word really signifies any bump or outgrowth that projects into the bowel lumen. Thus the generic usage of *polyp* is not specific for the histologic features of the lesion. In practice the word is generally used to describe an intraluminal colonic lesion that is usually less than 3 to 4 cm in size. Larger lesions are ordinarily referred to as a *mass* or *tumor*. Clearly, however, some overlap exists among the meanings and usages of these different terms.

CLASSIFICATION

A classification of polypoid colonic lesions is shown in the box at right. Colonic polyps include nonneoplastic lesions as well as benign and malignant neoplasms. The most common colonic polyps are small hyperplastic excrescences of epithelial metaplasia, generally only a few millimeters in size.[1] Lesions greater than about 0.5 cm are usually neoplasms. Benign epithelial adenomas are the most common neoplasm in the colon, followed by carcinomas. Carcinoid tumors are classified as malignant tumors because these lesions have considerable potential for malignancy, especially when greater than 2 cm in size. Primary colonic sarcomas, such as lymphomas and leiomyosarcomas, are rare. Metastatic lesions may occur by hematogenous spread, direct invasion, or peritoneal seeding.

PATHOLOGY
Histology

The histologic characteristics of colon polyps allow the pathologist to categorize most polypoid lesions of the colon with considerable accuracy.[2] Hyperplastic polyps contain mucosal glands lined by a single layer of columnar epithelium with infoldings arranged in a coiled fashion.[1] Hamartomas represent a malformation of cellular elements indigenous to the colonic mucosa.[3] Juvenile polyps are classified as cystic hamartomas by some pathologists and as in-

---

☐ **CLASSIFICATION OF POLYPOID COLONIC LESIONS** ☐

I. Polypoid colonic lesions of epithelial origin
  A. Neoplastic
    1. Benign lesions
      a. Tubular adenoma
      b. Tubulovillous adenoma
      c. Villous adenoma
    2. Malignant lesions
      a. Carcinoma
      b. Carcinoid tumor
  B. Nonneoplastic
    1. Hyperplastic metaplasia
    2. Inflammatory pseudopolyp
    3. Hamartomas
      a. Cystic (juvenile polyp)
      b. Cellular (Peutz-Jeghers)
    4. Lymphoid tissue
    5. Barium granuloma
    6. Heterotopia (for example, gastric)
    7. Ameboma, tuberculoma
    8. Malakoplakia
II. Polypoid colonic lesions of subepithelial origin
  A. Neoplastic
    1. Benign lesions
      a. Lipoma
      b. Leiomyoma
      c. Neurofibroma
      d. Hemangioma
      e. Lymphangioma
      f. Endothelioma
      g. Myeloblastoma
    2. Malignant lesions
      a. Lymphoma
      b. Sarcoma
      c. Metastases
  B. Nonneoplastic
    1. Endometriosis
    2. Enteric cyst
    3. Duplication
    4. Pneumatosis
    5. Hematoma
    6. Varix

flammatory retention cysts by others. The only polyps with significant malignant potential are neoplastic polyps. Therefore these polypoid lesions are the focus of attention. Neoplastic polyps are either benign or malignant. This distinction is essential. Benign neoplastic polyps are either simple tubular adenomas or have varying amounts of villous components.[4] A tubular adenoma can therefore contain areas with villous architecture that may or may not dominate the histologic appearance of the polyp. When malignant degeneration occurs in a tubular adenoma, tubulovillous adenomas, or villous adenomas, the malignant process can either occupy a portion of the polyp or replace the entire polyp. Villous architecture appears to be more premalignant than simple tubular epithelium. Carcinoma in situ is limited to the lamina propria. Because lymphatics in the wall of the colon do not extend into the lamina propria but only to the muscularis mucosae, tumors limited to the lamina propria have a good prognosis. It is important to emphasize that the majority of polypoid lesions more than a centimeter in diameter will in fact be neoplastic polyps that are potentially malignant. Thus the emphasis is on polyp detection.

Morphology

Polypoid colonic lesions show different morphologic characteristics. The three general morphologic forms are (1) sessile plaques, (2) sessile hemispheres, and (3) pedunculated spheres (Fig. 38-1). Flat polypoid lesions (Fig. 38-1, A) are raised plaques of variable shape that are generally smooth when small but often have a lobulated or irregular surface when larger than 1 to 2 cm. The intermediate sessile lesions tend to be roundish mounds or hemispheres (Fig. 38-1, B) but may be oval or smoothly lobulated. Such lesions have a broad base, and their vertical height is about

50% to 80% of their transverse diameter. Pedunculated polyps are usually more than 0.5 cm in size and may have either a short pedicle (Fig. 38-1, C) or long pedicle (Fig. 38-2). The polyp head is generally spherical. On gross examination, both pedunculated and sessile adenomas tend to have a slightly convoluted surface contour. Juvenile and submucosal polyps usually have a smooth contour. Ulceration of a polyp, tenting at its margin, or irregularity of its stalk suggests the presence of malignancy. Traction on a polyp by endoscopic biopsy forceps can produce a "pseudostalk," which frequently leads to a discrepancy in the way a polyp is described by a radiologist and endoscopist.

Distribution

Although sporadic colonic polyps may occur as solitary lesions, they are commonly multiple.[5] About half of the patients with an index lesion harbor one or more additional synchronous polyps.[6] The presence of multiple polyps should raise the possibility of a polyposis syndrome. A bona fide polyposis syndrome, however, is uncommon in patients with fewer than a dozen polyps. In patients with more than a dozen polyps, a polyposis syndrome is likely. Many patients with a sporadic colonic adenoma or carcinoma subsequently develop one or more metachronous polypoid lesions. In some instances, however, polyps classified as metachronous lesions are undoubtedly polyps that were missed in the initial examination.

Some studies report that polyps are distributed evenly throughout the colon,[6,7] but the bulk of evidence indicates that adenomas congregate in the rectosigmoid region.[8,9] Carcinomas have a similar distribution.[8] Although most neoplastic polyps are located within the rectum and sigmoid, recent studies show that about 50% of adenomas and carcinomas are beyond the reach of the rigid sigmoido-

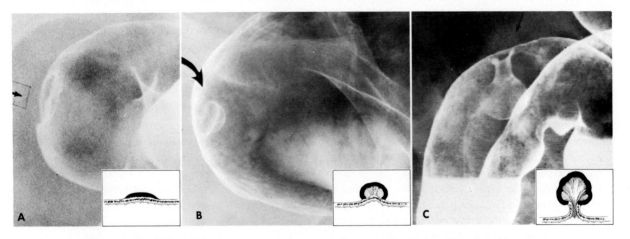

Fig. 38-1 Morphologic forms of polypoid colonic lesions. **A,** Sessile plaque seen tangentially. **B,** Sessile hemispheric moundlike lesion seen obliquely. Slight undercutting at margins traps ring of barium that overlaps coated dome of polyp to create hat sign. **C,** Pedunculated sphere. Pedunculated polyp on short stalk is seen in profile.
From Youker JE, Welin S: *Radiology* 84:610, 1965.

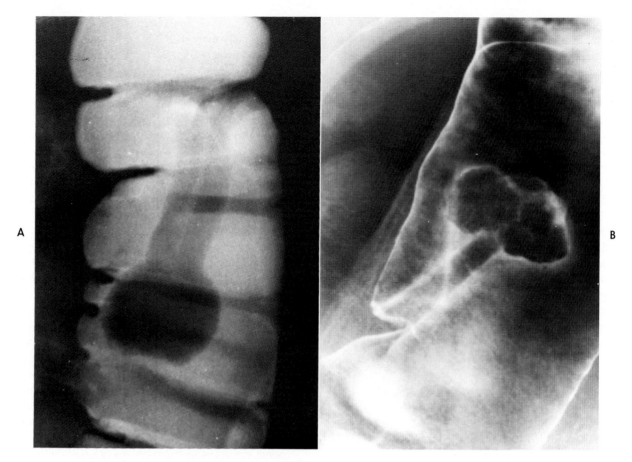

Fig. 38-2 Pedunculated polyps on long stalk. Both lesions were located in distal left colon. **A,** Adenoma shown in single-contrast examination with thick tubular stalk with roundish polyp head. **B,** Juvenile polyp shown in double-contrast examination. Tubular stalk is slightly flared at its origin and exerts traction on colonic wall.

scope.[10] Some evidence suggests that there are more polyps proximal to the rectosigmoid in older patients (more than 60 years).[11] Therefore radiographic examination or fiberoptic endoscopy is needed to diagnose lesions proximal to the rectosigmoid.

Cancer origin

There is strong evidence to support the influence of environmental factors on the incidence of colorectal neoplasms. Worldwide, the incidence of neoplasms is higher in the industrialized countries, and, in the United States, the incidence of colorectal carcinoma approaches 160,000 new cases per year. The evidence supporting the environmental hypothesis is the rapid increase in the incidence of colorectal neoplasms in individuals who have moved from low-risk environments to the industrialized world. Naturally occurring carcinogens, such as bile acids, may be a contributing etiologic factor, but diet is a major consideration, including the possible impact of red meat and a high fat intake. Additionally, the effect of the transit time on bowel contents probably plays a major role. The consumption of

refined grains and sugars promotes lengthy transit times, and therefore encourages the prolonged contact of either naturally occurring or ingested carcinogens with the colonic mucosa. These environmental factors may be modified by genetic characteristics, an area that is currently receiving a great deal of interest. We now know that some families have much higher rates of colon neoplasms, and it has been postulated that 5% to 6% of the cases of colorectal carcinoma may occur in these families.[12]

There are two major theories on the origin of colon carcinomas. One suggests that the malignancy develops mainly de novo as a primary colon cancer.[13,14] The second theory, favored currently by most researchers, suggests that colon cancer arises from adenomas, especially villous adenomas.[15-17] Subsequently the cancer may obliterate all evidence of the antecedent adenoma.[1] The following evidence is marshalled to support this hypothesis: (1) documented small colon cancers less than 0.5 cm in size are uncommon,[1] (2) cancers can be demonstrated in some adenomas,[17] (3) a high percentage of patients with colon cancer have synchronous polyps, (4) colon cancer has the same distribution as adenomas, and (5) the vigorous removal of rectal polyps is associated with a decreased incidence of rectal carcinomas.[18,19] Although the adenoma theory is widely accepted at present, the two theories of pathogenesis are not mutually exclusive. Some colon cancers might arise de novo, whereas others may develop from a preexisting adenoma.

Although the genesis of colon carcinomas is an important question, the precise origin does not affect the role of radiology in evaluating patients with possible colonic polyps. The main function of the radiologic examination is to accurately identify polypoid colonic lesions. Once a polypoid lesion is demonstrated, histologic assessment is usually necessary to determine the presence or absence of carcinoma.

HIGH-RISK GROUPS

The incidence of polyps in patients undergoing a sigmoidoscopy, a contrast enema examination, or both ranges from about 8% to 24%.[20-23] The prevalence of polypoid colonic lesions increases progressively with age. The increase in incidence of neoplastic polyps beyond the age of 40 years has prompted recommendations for the routine surveillance of the colon in an effort to detect neoplastic polyps in older patients. After the age of 50 years, more than 10% of individuals have colonic polyps, and by age 70 years the incidence may reach 50% or more.[24] In addition to the patient's age, risk factors for both colonic adenomas and carcinomas include Hemoccult-positive stool, previous history of a polyp, and family history of colon polyps or carcinoma. Patients with chronic ulcerative colitis have a high risk for developing a colon carcinoma. Screening programs for high-risk groups incorporate various diagnostic procedures, such as Hemoccult stool testing, positive contrast enema examination, endoscopy, and either flexible sigmoidoscopy or pancolonoscopy. Guidelines for the use of these modalities change from time to time but are generally available in the American Cancer Society recommendations. The weight of evidence supports the use of screening procedures to detect lesions at early stages: a higher number of Dukes' A lesions are detected in asymptomatic patients whose tumor is detected by screening than in patients who initially have clinical findings.

CLINICAL SYMPTOMS

The majority of patients with sporadic colon polyps or small carcinomas do not have clinical symptoms. The most common clinical feature is rectal bleeding. Occult blood loss may produce symptoms caused by anemia. Occasionally, polypoid colonic lesions cause intussusception[25] or rarely prolapse through the rectum.[26] Large polypoid masses, especially those in the left colon and sigmoid, cause overt colonic obstruction. Villous tumors of the rectosigmoid occasionally lead to clinical complaints resulting from hypokalemia or protein loss. In cases of carcinomas, a variety of initial clinical symptoms may be caused by local or distant metastases.

DETECTION
Contrast enema

At present radiographic examinations and endoscopy are the two major methods for detecting polypoid lesions of the colon. The radiographic examination may be either a single-contrast barium enema or double-contrast pneumocolon examination. In the past much controversy existed over which of the two examinations was preferable for detecting colonic polyps. In 1967 Welin[23] in Sweden reported that the pneumocolon examination detected colonic polyps in about 13% of the patients examined, a figure equivalent to the incidence of polyps in autopsy reports in that country. American researchers reported an 8% incidence of colonic polyps detected by single-contrast examination.[27] The difficulty with these early studies was that a reliable method did not exist at the time for identifying false-negative radiographic findings. Possibly for this reason, the single-contrast examination remained the major examination method in North America.

With the introduction of colonoscopy in North America in 1969, a diagnostic yardstick became available against which radiographic findings could be evaluated. During the 1970s and 1980s, comparison studies of radiographic and colonoscopic findings suggested that colonic polyps were missed more commonly with the single-contrast barium enema than with the pneumocolon examination[5,24,28-33] (Table 38-1). Analysis of the available data suggests that the barium enema misses about 25% of polyps 1 cm or larger in size and 40% to 45% of lesions less than 1 cm in size. Some investigators[34] advocate single-contrast examination coupled with direct proctoscopic examination as a satisfac-

☐ **TABLE 38-1**

Polypoid colonic lesions undetected by radiographic examination

Examination	Total	Missed lesions (%)	
		1 cm	0.5 to 0.9 cm
Barium enema examination			
Sugarbaker et al.[30]	17	2	5
Williams et al.[32]	48	23	40
Wolff et al.[33]	42	14	73
Leinecke et al.[29]	36	15	54
Ott et al.[36]	17	10	28
Pneumocolon examination			
Williams et al.[32]	15	2	13
Laufer et al.[28]	5	0	0
Ott[36]	14	4	12
Hogan et al.[5]	22	18	48

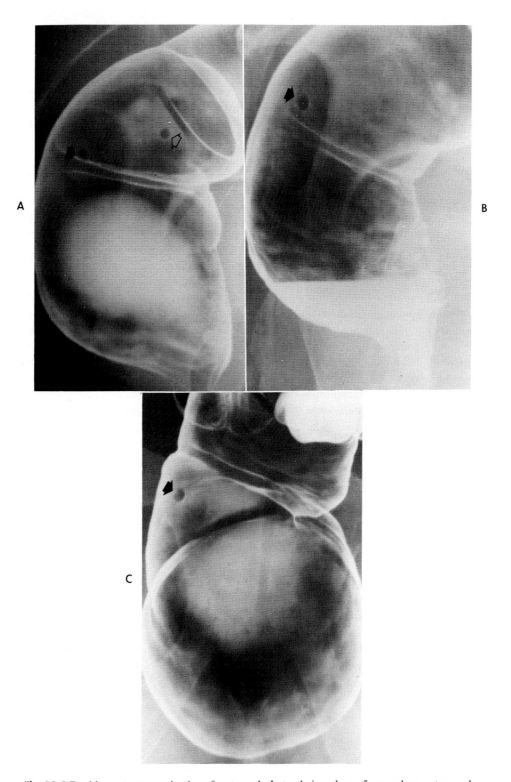

Fig. 38-3 Double-contrast examination of rectum. **A,** Lateral view shows 5-mm adenomatous polyp *(closed arrow)* and 4-mm air bubble *(open arrow)*. **B,** In upright lateral view taken subsequently, air bubble has disappeared but small polypoid lesion *(arrow)* remains unchanged. This lesion, located immediately proximal to a rectal fold (Houston's valve), was not seen at initial proctoscopy. **C,** Posteroanterior projection confirms presence of small sessile polyp *(arrow)* that was located on the posterolateral wall of the proximal rectum.

tory method of screening for colonic polyps. In contrast, other published studies suggest that a smaller percentage of polyps are missed with the pneumocolon examination than with the barium enema.[35,36] The published evidence, however, is largely circumstantial in that many of these studies were retrospective and the barium enema and pneumocolon examinations were rarely performed on the same patient.[37] An optimal study comparing the two radiographic methods has yet to be conducted. Nonetheless, on the basis of the evidence available, the pneumocolon examination is now being used much more in the United States than it was in the past.[38] Several North American researchers have championed and improved the examination.[39-42] Another reason for the increased use of the pneumocolon is the increased interest in the detection of diminutive polyps (no greater than 5 mm in diameter). Despite the earlier statements that diminutive polyps are most likely hyperplastic in origin, recent evidence indicates that at least half of these diminutive polyps are in fact adenomas and therefore important lesions.[2,43] The sensitivity of single- and double-contrast examinations decreases dramatically when studying diminutive polyps.[44] The detection levels for these small polyps may be as low as 20%. Although many radiologists have disregarded diminutive polyps in the past, we believe that any diminutive polyp should be mentioned in the radiographic report. Although tiny polyps rarely harbor malignancy at the time of biopsy, the identification of the presence of a diminutive adenoma would affect the subsequent surveillance of the patient. Surveillance schemes are based on the presence of adenomas in the colon and not on the size of the adenoma.

From our review of the medical literature and from our own experience, we believe that the pneumocolon examination is more sensitive than the conventional barium enema for detecting colonic polyps, but either method may miss lesions. In our experience, based on prospective and retrospective comparisons with endoscopic findings, the pneumocolon examination misses about 5% to 10% of polyps 1 cm or more in size and about 30% to 40% of smaller lesions. Counting the number of polyps missed, however, may be misleading. Because many patients have synchronous lesions,[24] the colon is commonly evaluated successfully, even though individual polyps may be overlooked. Approximately half of patients harboring adenomatous polyps will have one or more additional polyps. For example, it is common to find two or three polyps a centimeter or more in size and overlook an additional polyp of similar size. Analyzed from this perspective, the pneumocolon examination is 90% accurate in identifying index polyps in patients with one or more polyps at least 0.5 cm in size. It may be as high as 97% accurate in identifying index polyps in patients with one or more polyps at least 1 cm in size. Considered in this manner, the pneumocolon examination is an excellent screening method for selecting patients for colonoscopy.[45] At present the pneumocolon is our standard examination for patients with suspected colonic polyps or lower intestinal bleeding. We deviate liberally from the strategy, however, with uncooperative, debilitated or immobile patients and patients with massive diverticulosis. Patients who are unable to stand are not good candidates for double-contrast examinations in an effort to detect polyps. A good single-contrast barium enema examination is preferable to a poor pneumocolon examination.

Before the use of pneumocolon examinations, rectal polypoid lesions were almost exclusively relegated to the domain of the proctosigmoidoscope. The double-contrast examination, however, is especially well suited for evaluating the rectum (Fig. 38-3). A relatively common occurrence is the demonstration of a rectal polyp with a pneumocolon examination that is not detected with protoscopy.[46] The polyps missed by proctoscopy are commonly hidden from view, because they are located on the proximal surface of rectal valves (Fig. 38-3). To maximize the efficacy of the double-contrast examination of the rectum, it is desirable to avoid inflated rectal balloons that may obscure low-lying lesions[47] as well as cause injury (Fig. 38-4).[48] Digital examination of the anus and rectum before administering contrast enemas of the colon provides important useful information for the radiologist.[49] Assessment of anal tone helps minimize the use of rectal balloons, because the probability of rectal continence can be predicted from the quality of anal tone, irrespective of the patient's age.[50] Furthermore, polypoid rectal lesions not detected by the referring clinician are occasionally palpated.

Colonoscopy

Fiberoptic colonoscopy has substantially altered the diagnosis and management of polypoid colonic lesions. The colonoscopic method not only detects colonic polyps but also allows histologic diagnosis and therapeutic excision. In our opinion, colonoscopy has served an important function by stimulating improvements in colon radiology.

Although most researchers agree that colonoscopy is more sensitive than radiography for detecting colonic polyps, some lesions are clearly missed by colonoscopy.[46] The results of earlier studies suggested that colonoscopy seldom missed polypoid lesions and was far superior to radiography. These earlier claims, however, were exaggerated. Because the colonoscopist generally already knew the radiographic findings, colonoscopy was taken as the yardstick for detection, lesion size was not always specified, and a method was not used to discover false-negative colonoscopic findings.[37] In our experience with both retrospective[29] and prospective studies, colonoscopy fails to detect about 5% of polypoid lesions 1 cm or more in size (Fig. 38-5) and about 10% to 15% of lesions smaller than 1 cm. Similar observations have been made in England by Williams.[51] Specific results in a given locale, however, vary depending on numerous factors, including the patient population, the examiner's expertise, and the adequacy of co-

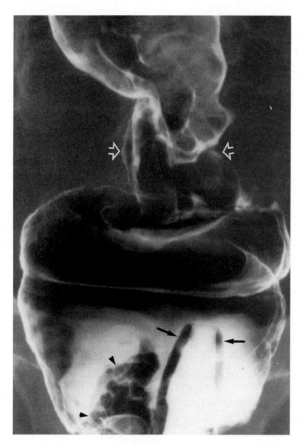

Fig. 38-4 Rectal carcinoma. Two independent lesions in the rectum are demonstrated in this patient. The barium enema tip *(arrows)* lies immediately adjacent to a nodular infiltrating carcinoma just inside the anal verge *(closed arrowheads)*. The second, much more infiltrating, carcinoma is seen just proximal to this area, just above the first valve of Houston *(open arrowheads)*. The double-contrast examination is uniquely suited to examine the rectum. However, the use of a balloon retention catheter might well obscure the lower-lying lesion. Films of the rectum obtained without the enema tip in place avoid the artifacts produced by either the enema tip or its inflatable balloon.

lon cleansing. An optimal pneumocolon examination should compare favorably with colonoscopy in identifying polypoid colonic lesions 1 cm or larger in size.

Although colonoscopy is a more sensitive method than radiographic examination for detecting colonic polyps, we believe the radiographic examination accompanied by proctosigmoid endoscopy should remain the major initial screening method for detecting colonic polyps. In particular, the double-contrast pneumocolon examination is especially well suited for detecting colonic polyps. We favor the continued widespread use of the radiographic method because (1) it nearly invariably examines the whole colon, whereas many colonoscopies fail to reach the right side of the colon; (2) the radiographic method requires less time and is much less expensive; (3) the radiographic examina-

tion is generally well tolerated by most patients; and (4) the capability for high-volume colonoscopy is not available in most areas.

Although many researchers agree that the colonoscopic and radiologic examinations are complementary rather than competitive,[32,33] others advocate substituting colonoscopy for positive-contrast studies. For the above reasons we disagree with this approach. We believe that colonoscopy is used most effectively in high-risk patients, in patients with known polyps, or for follow-up. The routine replacement of sigmoidoscopy and radiographic examinations by colonoscopy would not be cost-effective, because a high percentage of patients examined radiographically do not have a pathologic condition. Second, although the radiographic method may miss individual polyps, it identifies index lesions with high accuracy. Such patients can then undergo endoscopy. Many colonoscopists prefer a radiographic examination antecedent to colonoscopy, because the radiographic findings provide a map of the colon and identify most of the polyps present. Furthermore, the radiographic findings tend to improve the accuracy of colonoscopy. The colonoscopist often must make several passes through a region reported to contain a polyp before the lesion is found. In contrast to selective colonoscopic examinations, routine colonoscopy is efficacious in high-risk patients with negative radiographic findings. For example, colonoscopy detects a high yield of benign polyps and small carcinomas in patients with a Hemoccult-positive stool who have had negative findings on sigmoidoscopy and radiography.[52,53] A clean colon is essential for both the contrast enema and colonoscopic examinations.[54,55] Most polypoid lesions missed by either radiography or colonoscopy tend to be in areas of redundant colon, especially the rectosigmoid area, which has the highest incidence of lesions.[29,45,46] Colonoscopy is especially prone to miss lesions on the inner margin of bowel curvatures. For these reasons, the examiner should give extra attention to the sigmoid and colonic flexures. We routinely take multiple spot films of the sigmoid. The reasons for false-negative findings in the radiographic examination other than redundant bowel include retained feces, a suboptimal radiographic technique, clustered diverticula (Fig. 38-6), and observer error.[45,56,57] Interpreting the pneumocolon examination is more difficult than interpreting the single-contrast barium enema examination (Fig. 38-7). On the second viewing of an air contrast study, it is not unusual to identify a polyp that was overlooked during the initial interpretation.[57]

Two serious potential errors can occur when comparing the radiologic examination with the colonoscopic examination. The first of these involves location. Judgment about the location of the colonoscope tip can be extremely inaccurate.[58] The length of the scope introduced into the patient often has no relationship to its actual position within the colon. At times virtually the entire scope can be coiled within the sigmoid colon. At other times the colon tele-

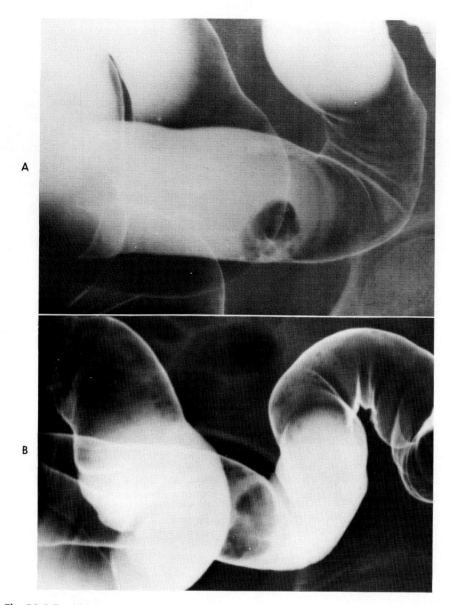

Fig. 38-5 Double-contrast examination shows sigmoid adenoma, 2 cm in diameter, not observed at colonoscopy. **A,** Initial pneumocolon study demonstrates sizable lesion in midsigmoid. Lesion appears sessile because polyp head obscures the crumpled stalk that was several centimeters in length. **B,** Repeat pneumocolon examination 1 week later was performed because of negative colonoscopic findings. Sigmoid polyp is again demonstrated. On repeat colonoscopy, only single glimpse of lesion was obtained during repeated passage of scope. Alpha maneuver was required to negotiate the sigmoid. Simultaneous fluoroscopy showed that the coiled sigmoid repeatedly sprung off the scope during its withdrawal, just as the scope head neared the lesion. Subsequently, the pedunculated polyp was removed at laparotomy.

scopes over the colonoscope, and the cecum is reached with less than 60 to 70 cm of scope. Thus inaccuracies in locating lesions can lead to serious errors in surgical planning. In addition, polyps identified at the time of double-contrast examination may or may not in fact correspond to the polyps identified at the time of colonoscopy, depending on the technique. It is not unusual for an endoscopist to incorrectly identify the location of a polyp that is seen to much better

advantage on the radiographic examination. False-positive radiographic findings should be verified by a repeat positive-contrast examination. In our experience, the number of radiologic false-negative findings greatly exceeds the number of false-positive findings. A second area of concern is the sizing of polyps. The inherent errors caused by magnification during radiographic examination can lead to inaccurate assessment of polyp size.[59] By the same token,

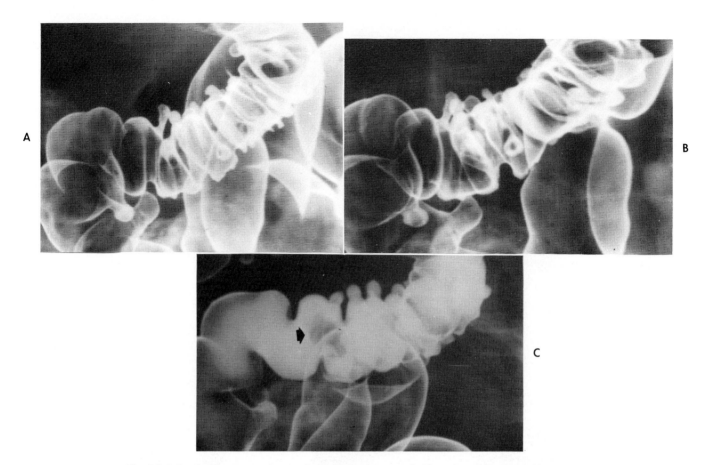

Fig. 38-6 On double-contrast images in pneumocolon examination. **A** and **B,** A sessile sigmoid polyp is completely obscured by a cluster of diverticula, despite films of excellent technical quality. Polyp *(arrow)* was visualized only on a single-contrast image, **C,** when barium flooded the loop.

the endoscopic assessment of polyp size can also be highly inaccurate. Because malignant potential is closely correlated with polyp size, major errors in size assessments from radiographs and colonoscopy can affect the clinical outcome and published statistics. To avoid this problem, the polyps should be removed in toto and measured before fixing to avoid the 15% shrinkage at fixation.[59]

Confidence level

A number of variables affect the interpretation of contrast colon examinations. Although radiographic images are often considered positive or negative, a considerable borderline area exists as well. Consequently the radiologic report should convey a confidence level for any given study. Studies featuring a clean colon, good barium coating, and optimal anatomy elicit a high level of confidence. In contrast, studies with suboptimal colon cleansing, poor barium coating, and suboptimal display of redundant loops often result in a low confidence level in the presence or absence of colonic polypoid lesions. Depending on the specific circumstances, suboptimal radiographic studies of the colon

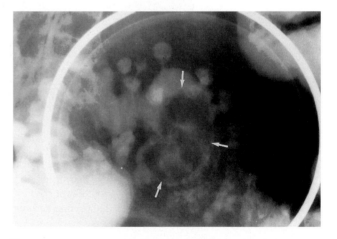

Fig. 38-7 Sigmoid carcinoma. This single-contrast examination of the sigmoid colon demonstrates a deformity due to extensive diverticulosis. A compression film nicely demonstrates a large intraluminal polypoid lesion *(arrows),* which in this case turned out to be adenocarcinoma. A compression film, coupled with a single-contrast examination, of a deformed sigmoid colon such as this is an integral part of the assessment of this area. When sigmoid deformity is marked, a double-contrast examination is less useful in the detection of intraluminal polypoid filling defects.

may be repeated or the needed information obtained by other methods. With the evaluation of individual colonic filling defects, a confidence level can be readily transmitted to the referring physician. We suggest that the diagnosis of a polypoid lesion requires a confidence level of greater than 95%. Confidence limits of 50% to 95% merit an interpretation of a probable polyp, and a possible polyp is said to be present when the examiner's confidence is less than 50%. Persistence and skill enable the radiologist to minimize the number of diagnoses in the probable and possible categories. A variety of maneuvers, such as the supplemental use of glucagon, compression techniques, additional films, and colon refilling, generally determine whether a filling defect is an artifact or a true lesion. In cases of equivocal polypoid lesions, additional studies are needed to resolve the issue.

In our experience, the major error committed by experienced radiologists is overlooking polypoid colonic lesions rather than making false-positive diagnoses. Perceptive errors seem to account for the majority of mistakes.[60] Even large lesions can be misinterpreted on double-contrast examinations because of perceptive errors. This occasional shortcoming has prompted the use of single-contrast exam-

inations to supplement double-contrast examinations that are negative in very high-risk patients, especially those with significant blood loss. Perceptive errors with regard to larger lesions may be lessened when using the single-contrast technique. When the radiologist has a high confidence level that a polypoid lesion is present, the likelihood of a real lesion is high, even when the findings from an initial colonoscopy are negative. The possibility of a real lesion should not be dismissed on the basis of negative colonoscopic findings; rather, an additional radiographic or colonoscopic examination should be performed to resolve the conflict (Fig. 38-8). When a filling defect of identical location, size, and configuration is shown on two different radiographic examinations, a real lesion is nearly always present, regardless of the colonoscopic findings (see Figs. 38-5 and 38-8). We have encountered only a few exceptions to this principle.

RADIOLOGIC FEATURES
Differentiation from artifacts

Polypoid colonic lesions must be distinguished from intraluminal and extraluminal artifacts.[61] Polyps may be simulated by intraluminal fecal material, gas bubbles (see Fig.

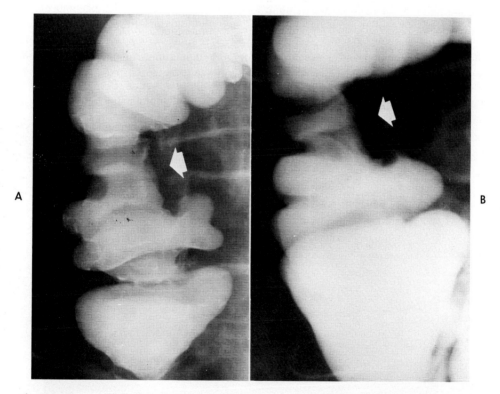

Fig. 38-8 Sessile carcinoma of the right colon not seen at colonoscopy. **A,** Plaquelike carcinoma *(arrow)* about 3 cm in length is seen along the medial margin of the proximal right colon, several centimeters above the ileocecal valve. Colonoscopy was performed for tissue diagnosis. Despite passage of the scope to the cecum, no lesion was observed. **B,** Repeat barium enema 1 week later demonstrates lesion *(arrow)* of identical size, shape, and location as that shown on initial radiographic examination. Infiltrating carcinoma was resected at subsequent laparotomy.

38-3, *A*), oil droplets, mucus, and foreign bodies.[62,63] Generally such intraluminal artifacts change location with shifts in the patient's position; however, fecal material may adhere to the mucosa. Adherent feces usually have an irregular shape, uneven barium coating, and fuzzy margins, but in some instances may simulate a sessile polyp. Air bubbles less than 1 cm in size are generally perfectly round, whereas larger accumulations trapped within the dome of a bowel loop tend to be ovoid. Bubbles often occur in pairs or clusters. Wetting agents, such as simethicone, minimize trapped bubbles. The appearance of oil droplets from lubricating agents is similar to that of bubbles. Mucus may appear in strands or globs. The latter form may simulate a polypoid lesion, especially when anchored in a diverticulum and projecting into the bowel lumen. Ingested foreign bodies, such as seeds, occasionally simulate colonic polyps but often have a typical ovoid, elongated, or slightly triangular shape with very smooth margins.

Structures intrinsic to the bowel wall, such as diverticula, mucosal plications, and haustral folds or knuckles at angulations, may also simulate true polypoid lesions. On pneumocolon examination diverticula seen face on may simulate sessile polyps. With multiple films, however, the diverticula may be seen to fill with barium, to have an air-fluid level, or to project clear of the bowel lumen. The ring projected by the barium lining of an air-filled diverticulum tends on face-on views to have a smooth outer margin and a hazy inner margin, whereas the reverse is the case for a barium-coated polyp. This distinction, however, is not very reliable. Manual pressure over a diverticulum may change its size and shape or result in some filling with barium.[64] Occasional stool-filled diverticula can project into the colon lumen, simulating a polyp. Mucosal plications or haustral folds seen end on may mimic a polyp. These filling defects tend to have a slightly teardrop shape, and their identity is generally evident on multiple views. Pseudotumors produced by angulations at flexures may be confused with polyps.[61] An inverted appendiceal stump (Fig. 38-9) or plump ileocecal valve containing fat (Fig. 38-10) must also be differentiated from polypoid neoplasms.[65,66]

Occasionally, extraluminal compression from an abscess, neoplasm, or mucocele may indent the bowel wall and simulate an intrinsic polypoid lesion. Additionally, extraluminal densities caused by a vertebral spinous process, vertebral pedicle, or vascular calcification may project over the bowel and simulate a polyp. These artifacts, however, generally project clear of the bowel on other views.

Morphologic findings

On radiographs, polypoid colonic lesions appear either sessile or pedunculated. Sessile lesions have a broad base and are either moundlike protuberances or flattened plaques. Pedunculated polyps may have a long or short stalk. They may be attached at a point on a spherelike head. The specific radiographic findings differ somewhat between the barium enema and pneumocolon examinations and among en face, tangential, and oblique views.

Flat sessile lesions have a vertical height that is less than 50% of their transverse diameter (Fig. 38-11). The marginal contour may be tapered or squarish, but undercutting is

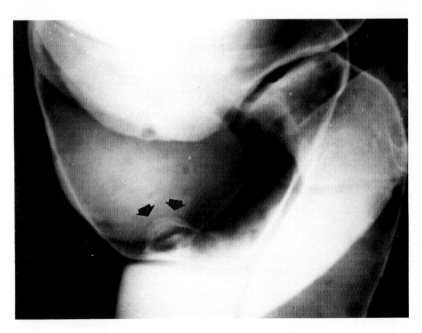

Fig. 38-9 Inverted appendiceal stump *(arrows)* appears as a sessile cecal polyp. Identity of the abnormality was suggested by its location, accompanied by a history of appendectomy. Biopsy material obtained at colonoscopy showed normal colonic mucosa.

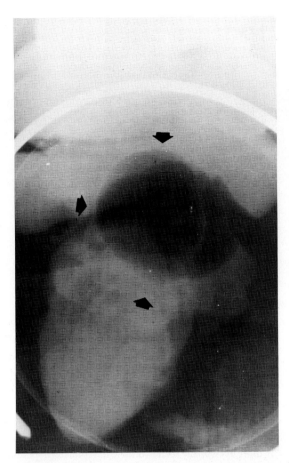

Fig. 38-10 Prominent ileocecal valve enlarged by fat deposition may masquerade as a cecal neoplasm *(arrows).* Identity of the prominent valve is determined by its location, smooth margins, and symmetry. Fatty valves are soft and often splay on compression. Barium in the valve orifice reveals identity of the tumor defect as the ileocecal valve; this finding is not shown well here. Additional cecal filling or use of glucagon may promote frank reflux of barium into the terminal ileum and further define the valve contours. In some cases, small bowel follow-through is necessary to confirm the identity of an enlarged ileocecal valve. Any contour irregularity or rigidity of valve suggests neoplastic infiltration and requires additional diagnostic evaluation.

rare. Polypoid lesions 0.5 cm or less in size are commonly flat, occasionally rounded, and seldom pedunculated. On en face projections, flat sessile polyps commonly escape detection in single-contrast examinations. Their shallow vertical height does not result in sufficient radiographic attenuation to project through the barium column. In contrast, with the pneumocolon examination such lesions are often identified face on as ringlike densities that are generally round or ovoid. The surface of the lesion may appear reticular, mamillated, or granular. When viewed tangentially, flat sessile lesions project into a barium or air column as a plaquelike filling defect. In cases of larger lesions, the margin of the colonic wall may lose its normal curved contour and appear as a flat, rigid area.

In the single-contrast examination, protuberant sessile polyps have a vertical height that is 50% or more of their width. The base is broad with either flared or undercut margins. In the barium enema examination sessile lesions seen en face appear as a roundish or slightly oval filling defect. Thin barium (15% to 20% weight per volume [w/v]) and high photon penetration (120-kV technique) are needed to image such lesions through the barium column. Manual palpation is useful for demonstrating the lesion and should be done routinely for the whole colon.[34] In the tangential view, protuberant sessile polyps project as hemispheric defects into the contour of the barium column. In some instances, undercutting at the margins can be appreciated.

In pneumocolon examinations, protuberant sessile polyps are seen face on as a ringlike density that represents the side walls of the barium-coated lesion. Visualization requires a good coating with high-density barium (90% to 100% w/v). In addition to overhead and decubitus films, multiple spot films taken with the patient recumbent and erect help detect such lesions. A tangential view reveals the hemispheric configuration of the polyp. When undercutting is present, barium fills the crevice and may be seen as a crescent or oval ring if the lesion is viewed obliquely. In this circumstance the second barium ring from the undercut margin projected onto the barium outline of the mound-like contour of the polyp may produce the hat sign (see Fig. 38-1, *B*)—the appearance simulates a bowler hat. The barium-coated body of the polyp represents the crown, and the barium around the undercut base, the brim.[67]

With pedunculated lesions the polyp head is always seen more or less en face, because the spherical head does not have a broad attachment with the colonic mucosa. On barium enema, the head of a polypoid polyp is usually identified by a roundish filling defect, whereas on the pneumocolon examination it appears as a coated sphere. In many instances, the stalk is not clearly visualized, and thus the polyp may be judged to be a sessile lesion (see Fig. 38-5). In tangential views, the polyp head often lies against the colonic wall, simulating a protuberant sessile lesion.

Pedunculated polyps generally shift in position during the radiographic examination. If the stalk is long (2 to 5 cm), the polyp head may move axially a distance of 4 to 10 cm along the bowel lumen. Polyps on short stalks move a shorter distance, and polyps attached to a point may be seen to jiggle back and forth. These phenomena are best seen with manual compression during the barium enema examination but may also be appreciated during the fluoroscopic portion of the pneumocolon examination. In upright or decubitus views, pedunculated polyps may hang suspended within the bowel lumen. On barium enema views, long pedicles may be seen as straight tubular filling defects that flare slightly at their base (see Fig. 38-2, *B*). When not stretched, the stalk is serpiginous and may mimic a lobulated broad-based lesion. On tangential views, a polyp lying limp on a short stalk may simulate a flat sessile lesion.

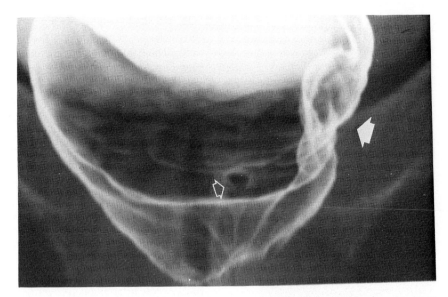

Fig. 38-11 Malignant carcinoid tumor of the rectum. A lobulated flat lesion, 2.5 cm in diameter, is seen on the lateral wall of the rectum *(closed arrow)*. A hyperplastic polyp, 5 mm in diameter *(open arrow)*, is also present.
Courtesy of Dr. Harvey M. Goldstein.

When the stalk attachment to the polyp head is seen en face along its longitudinal axis, the pedicle may appear as a circle within the larger circle of the polyp head. This appearance gives a "bull's eye" or "target sign" in both the barium enema and pneumocolon examinations. The appearance varies with the angle of viewing. Occasionally, a false target sign occurs when a sessile polyp contacts the opposite colonic wall, which results in a "touch" artifact on pneumocolon examinations.

Potential for malignancy

With individual colonic polyps the distinction between benign and malignant lesions generally depends on histologic diagnosis and is seldom possible using radiographic criteria. Nonetheless, estimates of the probability of malignancy can be made on the basis of radiologic findings. In such assessments several variables require consideration. In general, the radiographic findings correspond to the gross morphologic characteristics of the polypoid lesion.

Size

The single most important feature for estimating the probability of malignancy is the polyp's size.[51,67] With polypoid lesions of any shape, the incidence of histologic malignancy is directly related to the polyp's diameter. Polyps less than 0.5 cm in diameter are rarely malignant, whereas polyps 1 cm or less in diameter have about a 1% to 2% incidence of malignancy.[4,67] Above a diameter of 1 cm, the incidence of polyp malignancy rises sharply. About 10% of polyps between 1 and 2 cm in diameter harbor malignancy,[68] and 20% to 46% of polyps greater than 2 cm in size are cancerous.[7,68]

Pedunculation

Polyps with a well-defined pedicle have a substantially lower incidence of malignancy than sessile lesions of comparable diameter.[69,70] Protuberant sessile lesions with undercut margins appear to be in an early phase of pedunculation. A smooth pedicle 2 cm or more in length almost always indicates a benign lesion (see Fig. 38-2). The adenoma is confined to the polyp head, and the stalk represents an elongation of normal mucosa, possibly caused by repeated tugging on the polyp by colonic contractions. The implication of a long, smooth stalk therefore is that the neoplasm is not fixed to the submucosal layers of the bowel wall,[13] and consequently malignancy is unlikely. Even when a focus of carcinoma exists in the head of a well-defined pedunculated polyp, metastases to regional nodes or distant sites are rare.[71] In cases of frank polypoid cancers, the pedicle is usually thick, short, and irregular.

Surface contour

In some instances, the outline and surface contour of colonic polyps may provide clues to the underlying histologic condition, but radiographic findings in this category are usually unreliable. Although many adenomas have a lobular surface, much like a raspberry, this feature is rarely identifiable on radiographs. The presence of a reticular or filiform surface pattern (see Fig. 38-12) suggests a villous tumor,[72,73] but these findings are seldom present when villous tumors are less than 2 to 3 cm in size.

Generally adenomas have a roundish or ovoid shape, but they may show asymmetry or gross lobulation. Triangular, squarish, trapezoid, polyhedral, or bizarre configurations increase the probability of malignancy.[69] Stool adherent to

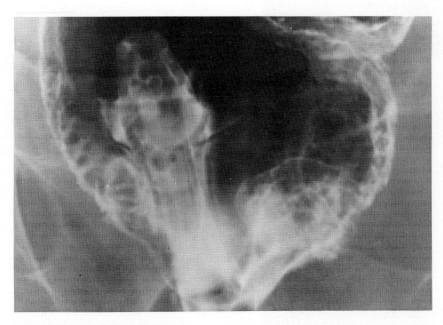

Fig. 38-12 Flat carpet villous adenoma has spread 270 degrees around the distal rectum without compromising the lumen. Irregular, reticular surface appearances of the lesion are characteristic of villous tumor. Extensive rectal lesions such as this villous tumor may be obscured by inflated rectal balloon.

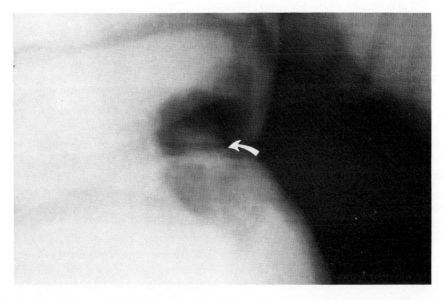

Fig. 38-13 Sessile adenocarcinoma with central ulceration. A sessile filling defect, 2.5 cm in diameter, is located on the lesser curvature of the hepatic flexure. Central ulceration *(arrow)* indicates a high probability of malignancy.

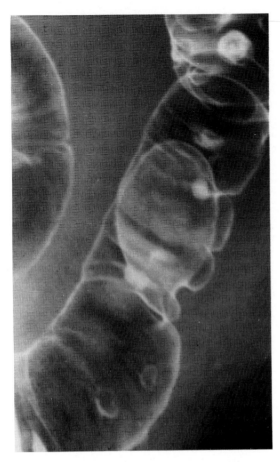

Fig. 38-14 Lipoma in the proximal sigmoid. Smooth-walled, oval lesion has short, broad pedicle. Exquisitely sharp margins of the lesion are characteristic of lipoma. Scattered diverticula are present.

bowel wall may exhibit similar features. A discrete surface ulceration is highly suggestive of a carcinoma (Fig. 38-13). Another contour finding suggesting malignancy is an indentation of the polyp base when the lesion is seen in the tangential view. This finding suggests infiltration and invasion of the mucosa adjacent to the lesion.

With polyps greater than 1 cm in size, an exquisitely sharp contour (Fig. 38-14) with smooth tapering margins seen on tangential views suggests a benign submucosal tumor or carcinoid tumor. The presence of uniformly pleated or scalloped margins (Fig. 38-15) suggests an endometrioma.[74]

Location

Polyp location generally does not help in distinguishing benign from malignant lesions. In some instances, however, the location of polypoid lesions may weight the diagnostic probabilities. For example, polypoid lesions at the cecal tip are likely to be related to the appendix—an inverted stump (see Fig. 38-9), prolapse, abscess, or muco-cele. The ileocecal valve may simulate a polypoid neoplasm. Fatty infiltration of the valve may cause a pronounced filling defect. Even when prominent, however, the normal valve is smooth and symmetric (see Fig. 38-10). In en face projections, barium extending into the valve orifice often has a characteristic stellate appearance. Any nodularity or asymmetry suggests malignancy.

Although sessile filling defects located low in the rectum may be caused by internal hemorrhoids, such rectal lesions suggest the possibility of a villous tumor, squamous carcinoma, or cloacogenic carcinoma. Carcinoid tumors and leiomyomas also have a high predilection for the rectum. Barium granulomas and benign lymphoid tissue[74] may cause polypoid rectal lesions. Sessile polypoid lesions located adjacent to Douglas' pouch or along the attachment of the sigmoid mesentery raise the possibility of metastatic seeding from malignant tumor or endometriosis (see Fig. 38-15).

A sessile polypoid filling defect located along the lateral margin of the distal splenic flexure raises the possibility of the extension of neoplasm or inflammation through the phrenocolic ligament. Similarly, an extension of a neoplastic or inflammatory process through the gastrocolic ligament tends to involve the superior margin of the transverse colon, whereas an extension through the transverse mesocolon can cause tumorlike lesions along the inferior margin of the transverse colon.[76] Although such processes generally involve a relatively long colonic segment, they occasionally simulate an intrinsic polypoid tumor.

Growth rate

Another useful factor in the evaluation for malignancy is the polyp's growth rate. In a study conducted in Malmö, Sweden, a group of patients with 375 polypoid colonic tumors were followed with serial double-contrast enemas.[67] Of the 375 tumors, 135 were excised, and the histologic findings were compared with the rates of growth. Results of the study were expressed as both the absolute linear growth rate and the doubling time.[67] Carcinomas predominated among lesions, showing the most rapid growth rates, with doubling times from 138 to 1155 days. This doubling rate corresponded to a linear rate of increased diameter between 0.0003 and 0.025 mm a day. Thus the colonic carcinomas had a very slow growth rate. Even the most rapidly growing cancer required 100 days to increase its diameter by 2.5 mm. At this rate of growth, a tumor 1 mm in diameter would require 6 to 8 years to attain a diameter of 6 cm. Adenomatous polyps tended to grow more slowly than carcinomas; however, the growth rate of some adenomas was as rapid as that of cancer.

Analysis of the Malmö study results showed that a doubling time of more than 1155 days was associated with a 1% to 2% probability of cancer. With a doubling time of 300 to 1155 days, the probability of cancer increased to 19% to 29%, and with a doubling time less than 300 days

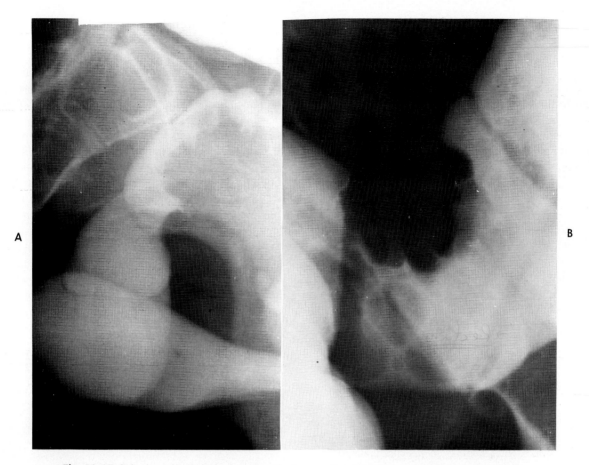

Fig. 38-15 Colonic endometriosis. In two patients an endometrioma is seen, **A,** along the anterior wall of the rectosigmoid adjacent to Douglas' pouch and, **B,** along the superior margin of the sigmoid adjacent to its mesenteric junction. Both lesions are excentric and show scalloping or pleating of the mucosa, findings typical of endometrioma.

the cancer probability was 35%. These results suggest that any increase in the size of a colonic polyp should be considered an indication for removal.

SPECIFIC POLYPOID LESIONS
Adenomas

Adenomatous polyps are the most common neoplasm of the colon. Most adenomatous polyps are sessile or pedunculated tubular adenomas. However, the remaining lesions are either tubulovillous adenomas or pure villous adenomas. About 10% of adenomatous polyps are probably completely villous in architecture, and these tend to be sessile lesions, which have a predilection for the rectum and the cecum.[72,73] For a given size, villous tumors have a likelihood of harboring carcinoma 10 times as great as that of tubular adenomas. In some instances villous tumors greater than 1 cm in size can be identified on radiographs by a fine or coarse reticular pattern of barium on their surface that gives the lesion a wartlike appearance. The more proximal the lesion, the less likely it is to have a typical villous appearance.[73] In some cases villous tumors appear as annular plaques or spreading carpet lesions (see Fig. 38-12) with surface irregularity or mamillation. Large rectal lesions are often seen as broad-based tumors that may have a soft consistency on the digital rectal examination. The extensive surface area of villous tumors may cause diarrhea with excessive loss of potassium or less commonly of albumen.

Lipomas

Among benign colonic tumors, lipomas are second in prevalence to adenomas. About two thirds of alimentary tract lipomas occur in the colon. They are common in elderly women. Although patients with a colonic lipoma are commonly asymptomatic, symptoms when present include abdominal pain, constipation, rectal bleeding, and diarrhea. Most colonic lipomas are submucosal, and about 10% are subserosal. About 40% are located in the right side of the colon and 20% in the sigmoid. The lesions usually range in size from 1 to 10 cm. The submucosal variety is usually sessile but occasionally may be pedunculated (see Fig. 38-14) and lead to intussusception.[77,78] The usual radiographic appearance is one of a smooth, sharply outlined hemispheric mass. Because the tumors are soft, their contour is often altered by peristalsis or compression.[79]

Juvenile polyps

Most juvenile polyps occur as isolated colonic lesions in children less than 10 years old. The lesion is solitary in about 75% of cases. When multiple, the lesions seldom number more than two or three.[80] The family history is usually negative for colonic polyps. Rectal bleeding is the most common symptom. Other symptoms include rectal prolapse, abdominal pain, and diarrhea.[81] On the barium enema examination, juvenile polyps are identified as roundish filling defects, often pedunculated (see Fig. 38-2, *B*), that are located most commonly in the rectum or sigmoid. Because the lesions are benign and have a tendency toward autoamputation or regression, their removal is not mandatory in the absence of significant bleeding or intussusception. However, their true nature is usually not known before removal and examination.

Carcinoid tumors → *Rectum*

Approximately 15% of alimentary tract carcinoid tumors occur in the large bowel, and nearly all of these are in the rectum.[82] Rectal carcinoid tumors constitute about 1% to 2% of rectal polyps greater than 0.5 cm in size. Carcinoid tumors arise from Kulchitsky's cells deep in the epithelium and generally appear as submucosal nodules. These lesions are generally incidental findings in patients undergoing a routine proctoscopic examination.[83] On contrast enema examinations, rectal carcinoid tumors usually appear as sessile hemispheric lesions with sharp margins. Occasionally, they are bulky or annular.

Colonic carcinoid tumors should be considered malignant lesions. About 15% of rectal carcinoids are accompanied by metastases. This figure soars to 75% to 90% for lesions 2 cm or more in size[84] (see Fig. 38-11). The 5-year survival rate is nearly 100% for patients with lesions less than 2 cm in size but decreases to 40% for those with lesions 2 cm or larger.[84] Metastatic rectal carcinoid tumors rarely cause the carcinoid syndrome.

Endometriosis

After adenomas and lipomas, endometriomas are the third most common benign tumor of the rectum and colon.[85] Intestinal implants of endometriosis are estimated to occur in about 4% of women,[86] with rectosigmoid involvement in 85% of such cases.[87] Most patients have evidence of pelvic endometrial involvement on pelvic examination.

Although intestinal involvement in cases of endometriosis is common, intestinal symptoms occur in only a small percentage of women with intestinal endometrial implants. The usual age for the appearance of symptoms is 20 to 40 years, but intestinal symptoms may present initially in postmenopausal women. The more common complaints caused by intestinal endometriosis include tenderness, constipa-

tion, diarrhea, and pelvic or rectal pain. Rectal bleeding is relatively uncommon.[74] The symptoms often wax and wane in severity during the menstrual cycle.

On barium enema examination, endometrial implants to the large bowel are generally seen (1) along the superior anterior rectal wall near the rectosigmoid junction from seeding into Douglas' pouch (see Fig. 38-15, *A*) or (2) along the superior margin of the sigmoid from implants at the attachment of the sigmoid mesentery (see Fig. 38-15, *B*). Involvement of the appendix and terminal ileum is an occasional finding. Endometrial implants invade the muscular and submucosal layers of the bowel wall but generally spare the mucosa, thereby accounting for the low incidence of bleeding. The implants generally appear as smooth, eccentric submucosal lesions that project for a variable distance into the bowel lumen. In some instances, the implants evoke a hypertrophic response of the muscularis mucosae that causes pleating or transverse ridging of the

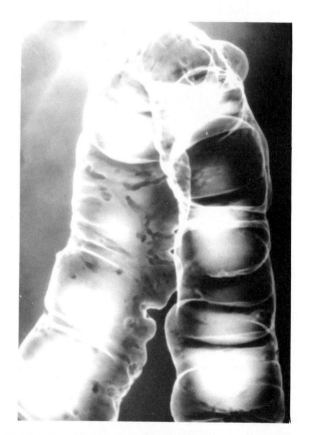

Fig. 38-16 Filiform pseudopolyposis in patient with chronic ulcerative colitis. Filiform pseudopolyps can be misconstrued as multiple adenomatous polyps. Typically, filiform polyps are long and pedunculated and sometimes even wormlike in appearance. The colon characteristically exhibits normal length and haustration. These latter features can lead to misinterpretation that these patients have multiple adenomatous polyps. Simple biopsy and excision should confirm the true nature of postinflammatory pseudopolyps.

overlying mucosa,[74] giving the lesion a characteristic scal- ✳
✳ loped appearance (see Fig. 38-15). Most lesions are eccentric and cause only mild to modest luminal narrowing. Occasionally, the lesions encircle the bowel and cause a significant obstruction. The differential diagnosis includes benign submucosal tumors, malignant serosal implants, diverticulitis, and carcinomas.

Other tumors

In addition to the more common benign tumors described, a number of unusual or rare benign polypoid lesions of the colon may occur. These include leiomyoma, fibroma, neurogenic tumor, hemangioma, lymphangioma, endothelioma, granular cell myoblastoma, cysts, and duplication. In most cases these tumors are located submucosally, the mucosa is intact, and their radiographic appearance suggests a benign lesion. Occasionally, postinflammatory pseudopolyps mimic a polyposis syndrome (Fig. 38-16).

MANAGEMENT
Treatment

Before the widespread use of colonoscopy during the past 2 decades, the only option for removing colonic polyps above the reach of a sigmoidoscope was laparotomy. Consequently, the risk of a malignant polyp had to be weighed against the 0.5% to 1% mortality of operative therapy. For this reason, polyps 1 cm or less in diameter were commonly observed, whereas larger lesions were generally removed surgically. Colonoscopy has substantially altered this traditional strategy because of its minimal mortality and morbidity compared with those of surgery.

Because even diminutive polyps less than 5 mm have about a 50% chance of being an adenoma,[43] endoscopic biopsy has become routine, and such lesions are generally removed at the time of biopsy. The preferred current management of polyps in the colon is endoscopic removal if possible or at least biopsy to confirm the histologic condition. A rationale for the routine removal of all colonic polyps greater than 0.5 cm in size is suggested by Gilbertsen's study[19] of rectal lesions. When rectal polyps were routinely excised or fulgurated in a large series of patients, the occurrence of rectal carcinomas was lower than that anticipated in the general population. The evidence available strongly suggests that colonic polyps greater than 1 cm in size should be removed, except in exceptional circumstances, such as in patients with severe debilitation or a short life expectancy. Current practice is to remove all polyps, whether sessile or pedunculated. On rare occasions, colonic polyps in adults may undergo spontaneous autoamputation.[88] *Every 3 yrs. after age of _____*

Surveillance *- 1, 3, 3, 3, ... following polyp removal.*

Another important consideration is patient follow-up and surveillance.[57] Patients who have had a colonic adenoma

✳ or carcinoma are at risk for the subsequent development of additional large bowel neoplasms. Such patients are generally considered to have a "tumor-prone" colon, and follow-up surveillance is indicated. At present, however, the optimal interval and modality for follow-up examination have not been clearly established. Most researchers in the field believe that a number of factors should influence the timing of surveillance. Factors such as the multiplicity of polyps, recurrence rate, histologic architecture (tubular versus villous), and presence of dysplasia may dictate some variations in follow-up. Surveillance schemes include Hemoccult testing, positive-contrast radiographic examination, and colonoscopy. At present a follow-up examination, usually endoscopic, should be done 1 year after removal of a neoplastic polyp to detect any synchronous lesions missed initially or to search for new lesions. Thereafter, follow-up examinations are dictated by the biologic activity in any given patient. For most patients surveillance examinations can be done every 3 years. Guidelines based on epidemiologic data will be forthcoming in the near future.

POLYPOSIS SYNDROMES

Although the prevalence of gastrointestinal polyposis syndromes is low, most radiologists during their careers encounter patients with intestinal polyposis. More than 300 cases each of multiple familial polyposis and the Peutz-Jeghers syndrome and about 200 cases of Gardner's syndrome have been documented in the literature. Undoubtedly many patients with these syndromes are not reported. The results of two independent studies suggest that the incidence of multiple familial polyposis in the United States is about 1 in 7000 to 8000 live births.[89,90] The Peutz-Jeghers syndrome has been estimated to occur at about the same incidence as familial multiple polyposis.[91] Multiple colonic juvenile polyps may develop in young adults as well as in children. Turcot's syndrome and the Cronkhite-Canada syndrome, although rare, are well-defined clinical entities. Several recent reviews discuss these syndromes in detail.[92,93]

The radiologist plays an important role in the diagnosis and evaluation of the polyposis syndromes. Many patients with unsuspected alimentary tract polyposis are referred for a radiographic examination for unrelated gastrointestinal symptoms. The polyposis syndrome should be considered when (1) a gastrointestinal polyp is identified in a young patient, (2) multiple polyps are demonstrated in any patient, or (3) a colon carcinoma is present in a patient less than 40 years old. A strong suspicion is imperative in these cases, because the failure to recognize polyposis coli syndromes associated with the development of malignancy almost inevitably results in tragedy for the patient and other afflicted family members. Elective colon resection results in clinical cure for these patients. It is equally important that other polyposis syndromes, such as the Peutz-Jeghers syndrome and the Cronkhite-Canada syndrome, are diagnosed accu-

---

□ **POLYPOSIS SYNDROMES INVOLVING THE COLON** □

1. Hereditary polyposis syndromes
   a. Familial multiple polyposis
   b. Gardner's syndrome
   c. Peutz-Jeghers syndrome
   d. Ruvalcaba-Myhre-Smith syndrome
   e. Turcot syndrome
   f. Muir-Torre syndrome
   g. Cowden's disease
2. Nonhereditary polyposis syndromes
   a. Cronkhite-Canada syndrome
   b. Juvenile polyposis (sometimes hereditary)

---

rately so that appropriate management may be rendered for the patient.

Gastrointestinal polyposis syndromes that affect the colon may be classified as hereditary or nonhereditary types, as shown in the box above. The three major hereditary syndromes—familial multiple polyposis, Gardner's syndrome, and the Peutz-Jeghers syndrome—have autosomal dominant inheritance. Consequently about half the offspring of individuals with these syndromes will be afflicted; no sex predilection occurs. Turcot's syndrome appears to be transmitted by an autosomal homozygous recessive gene. The Cronkhite-Canada syndrome is nonfamilial. The majority of patients with juvenile polyposis have a negative family history.

Familial multiple polyposis

Familial multiple polyposis is characterized by hereditary transmission, polyposis coli, and the eventual development of a colon carcinoma. The disease, recognized since Cripps' description[94] in 1882, is the best known hereditary gastrointestinal polyposis syndrome and serves as a prototype with which other polyposis syndromes can be compared. Patients with multiple polyposis, studied by Dukes[95] and Veal,[96] reveal an autosomal dominant mechanism of inheritance. The abnormal gene has high penetrance, estimated to be about 80%. About two thirds of afflicted individuals have a positive family history of colonic polyps or carcinoma, and about one third are sporadic cases.[96]

The onset of clinical symptoms usually occurs during the third or fourth decade of life, these patients having an average age of about 30 years. The clinical symptoms include vague abdominal pain, diarrhea, bloody stools, weight loss, and prolapse of a polyp through the rectum. Occasionally, the disorder is associated with an electrolyte depletion significant enough to cause weakness or a protein-losing enteropathy that results in hypoalbuminemia and edema. A high percentage of individuals with clinical symptoms have

an existing colon carcinoma or develop a large bowel malignancy within 2 years.[96]

The colonic polyps are numerous, ranging from pin-head lesions to those 1 cm or more in size, and may be sessile or pedunculated. The rectum and left side of the colon are more commonly involved than the right side of the colon, but often the entire colonic mucosa is carpeted with myriads of polyps, such that normal mucosa is not seen. A generalized form of adenomatous polyposis has been termed *diffuse familial polyposis*.[97] In the past, polyps in the stomach, small bowel, or both were believed to occur in fewer than 5% of cases, but recent reports, primarily from Japan, claim a high incidence of gastric, duodenal, and small bowel polyps in patients with familial multiple polyposis.[98-100] The increased prevalence of gastric polyps in Japanese patients may be partially explained by better detection methods with the routine use of double-contrast examinations and by hereditary or dietary factors. Although Japanese patients with multiple familial polyposis might have a predilection to develop gastric and perhaps small bowel polyps, extracolonic polyps still appear to be uncommon in North American and European patients. Biopsies showed that most of the gastric and duodenal polyps were hyperplastic rather than adenomatous. Hyperplastic gastric polyps have been reported in Japanese patients without a polyposis syndrome.[102] An association between these gastric lesions and carcinomas has not been established. Outside Japan, only one case of gastric cancer in a patient with adenomatous polyposis coli has been reported.[103] However, patients with familial multiple polyposis do have some increased risk for developing carcinoma of the duodenum.

The colonic polyps in patients with familial multiple polyposis generally arise during the first or second decade of life but are not usually evident until after puberty. Occasionally, the polyps develop for the first time in afflicted individuals when they are older than 40 years of age. Histologically, the polyps are indistinguishable from the common solitary adenomatous polyps found in the general adult population. Occasionally, villous adenomas or inflammatory polyps may also be present. Colon cancers arise about 15 years after the onset of polyposis, a time interval similar to that recorded for the development of colon cancer after the onset of chronic ulcerative colitis. As a rule, colon cancers develop in patients with familial multiple polyposis between the ages of 20 to 40 years and rarely occur below the age of 20 years.[104] A colon carcinoma develops in nearly 100% of untreated patients. The natural history of the disease in untreated patients is death from metastatic diseases by the age of 45 years, the average age being 40 years.[96]

Although sigmoidoscopic findings are nearly always positive when a colon radiographic examination shows polyps,[104] a radiographic examination should be performed in all suspected patients to document the size, number, and distribution of the polyps and to search for a carcinoma

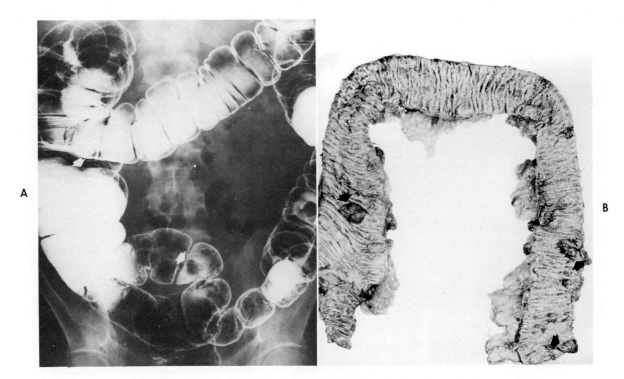

Fig. 38-17 Familial multiple polyposis. **A,** Pneumocolon examination demonstrates numerous 2- to 5-mm polyps and three 1.5- to 2-cm polypoid carcinoma *(arrows)*. **B,** Gross specimen of resected colon. Myriads of small polyps are seen along with three polypoid carcinomas *(arrows)*.

(Fig. 38-17). The polyps may be identified as multiple punctate eminences that impart a serrated to saw-tooth contour to the intraluminal column of barium or as larger filling defects 1 to 2 cm in diameter.[105] Some of the lesions may have pedicles. In many instances the polyps are most numerous in the left colon. Small, elusive polyps 1 to 2 mm in diameter may be hidden by barium but are often clearly shown in the pneumocolon examination. Carcinomas may appear as polypoid filling defects, areas of symmetric segmental narrowing, or typical annular lesions with overhanging margins. Multiple carcinomas are common (Fig. 38-18).

Because a colon carcinoma eventually develops in virtually all patients with familial multiple polyposis, the need for early diagnosis in affected individuals and subsequent family screening cannot be overemphasized. Familial multiple polyposis should be regarded as a curable disease. The colon is a dispensable organ, not necessary for useful life, and a colon carcinoma is entirely preventable if afflicted patients are identified when they are young and a prophylactic total colectomy is performed.[106] Generally surgery can be deferred until the patients are in their late teens or early twenties. Colectomy with an ileorectal anastomosis is a suitable operation for reliable patients who will return for follow-up proctoscopy.[107] In some patients the rectal polyps regress following colectomy.[108] Recurrent rectal polyps may be eradicated by cautery.

Gardner's syndrome

In a series of articles published between 1950 and 1953, Gardner and Richard[109] described a syndrome featuring an autosomal dominant inheritance, multiple soft tissue tumors, osteomatosis, polyposis coli, and a potential for colon malignancy. About 20% of afflicted patients have the complete triad of soft tissue tumors, osteomatosis, and polyposis.[110]

Patients with Gardner's syndrome may seek medical treatment for cosmetic deformities caused by soft tissue or bony lesions, dental abnormalities, or abdominal symptoms. Symptoms referable to the colon are similar to those described for patients with familial multiple polyposis. In some instances, these patients have complaints of excessive scar formation (keloids) or symptoms of bowel obstruction caused by peritoneal adhesions.

The cutaneous lesions consist of sebaceous or inclusion cysts that are most numerous on the scalp and back, but may be present on the face or extremities. Benign mesenchymal tumors include fibromas, lipomas, lipofibromas, leiomyomas, and neurofibromas.[111] Malignant sarcomas, such as fibrosarcomas and leiomyosarcomas, are unusual but do occur. The fibrous tissue in patients with Gardner's syndrome often has a pronounced tendency toward proliferation, thereby resulting in desmoid tumors, keloids, hypertrophied scars, mammary fibromatosis, peritoneal adhesions, mesenteric fibrosis, and retroperitoneal fibrosis. Fi-

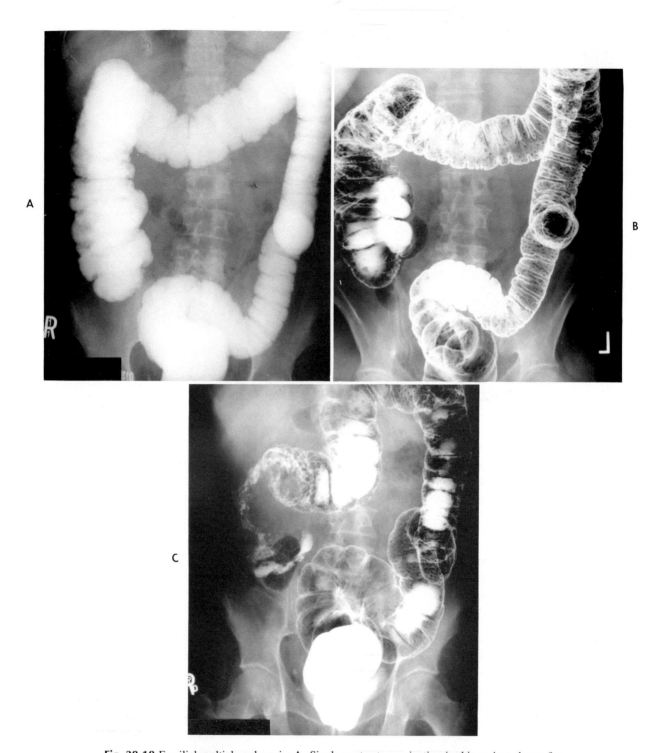

Fig. 38-18 Familial multiple polyposis. **A,** Single-contrast examination in this patient shows fine marginal contour irregularities caused by multiple polyposis. Myriads of small polyps are not well seen on the overhead film. **B,** Double-contrast examination nicely demonstrates the myriad of small polyps of varying sizes, from several millimeters up to 1 cm. They involve the entire colon. **C,** Patient refused colectomy and 4 years later returned with a large fungating, infiltrating adenocarcinoma on right side of colon.

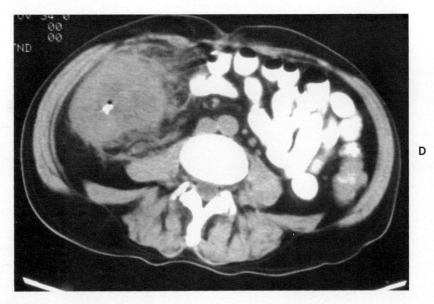

Fig. 38-18 cont'd D, CT scan done at this time demonstrates large, bulky tumor that encompasses the entire circumference of the right side of the colon with extension into the mesentery. Patient had numerous liver metastases by this time as well.

brous tissue proliferation may arise either spontaneously or in response to injury or surgery.

Localized areas of dense bone (osteomas), appearing as exostoses or enostoses, are commonly present in the maxilla, mandible, or skull (Fig. 38-19, *A* and *B*). Localized bony overgrowth may cause a cosmetic deformity.[112] The long bones, particularly the femur and tibia, are commonly abnormal and demonstrate localized cortical thickening (Fig. 38-19, *C*), wavy cortical thickening, or exostoses.[113] The long bones may also be slightly shortened and bowed. Dental abnormalities commonly present include odontomas, unerupted supernumerary teeth, hypercementosis, and a tendency toward numerous caries. The bone and soft tissue lesions often appear before or during puberty and may precede the development of polyps.

The polyps in Gardner's syndrome tend to be limited to the colon. Extracolonic polyps are believed to occur in 5% or less of the patients.[93] Recent reports, however, suggest that a higher incidence exists for polyps in the stomach, duodenum, and small bowel.[114-116] There is a considerably increased incidence of carcinoma of the duodenum and a slight increase for stomach and small bowel. Lymphoid hyperplasia of the terminal ileum, commonly present in cases of Gardner's syndrome, may cause a cobblestone appearance that simulates multiple adenomas. The polyps generally appear during the teens and increase in number during the third and fourth decades of life, often resulting in carpeting of the entire colon (Fig. 38-20, *A*). The polyps do not differ from the adenomatous polyps present in patients with familial multiple polyposis. Further, virtually all patients with Gardner's syndrome eventually develop a colon carcinoma

if the colon is not removed (Fig. 38-20, *B*). In patients with a colon carcinoma, the average age at death is 41 years, which is essentially identical to that of patients with familial multiple polyposis dying from large bowel cancer.[117]

McKusick[117] has suggested that the genes causing Gardner's syndrome and familial polyposis may be alleles occurring at the same chromosomal locus. Other researchers believe that Gardner's syndrome and familial multiple polyposis represent opposite poles of a disease spectrum produced by a single pleotrophic gene with varying expressivity.[118] Contrary to earlier opinions,[119] the colonic polyps associated with the two syndromes do not differ in growth pattern, distribution, number, histologic features, or malignant potential. Incomplete manifestations of Gardner's syndrome occur in individual patients or some families. Polyposis coli may be accompanied by only the soft tissue or bony lesions. Conversely, patients with familial multiple polyposis have a tendency to develop desmoid tumors and small bowel adhesions.[93,118] Whatever the relationship between Gardner's syndrome and familial polyposis, the threat of colon malignancy is identical, and prophylactic colectomy should be performed when patients afflicted with either syndrome are about 20 years of age.

Peutz-Jeghers syndrome

In 1921 Peutz[120] described the association of mucocutaneous pigmentation and gastrointestinal polyposis in members of a Dutch family. The syndrome remained generally unrecognized, however, until 1949 when Jeghers et al.[121] reported 10 patients with the syndrome and documented an autosomal dominant mode of inheritance. The Peutz-

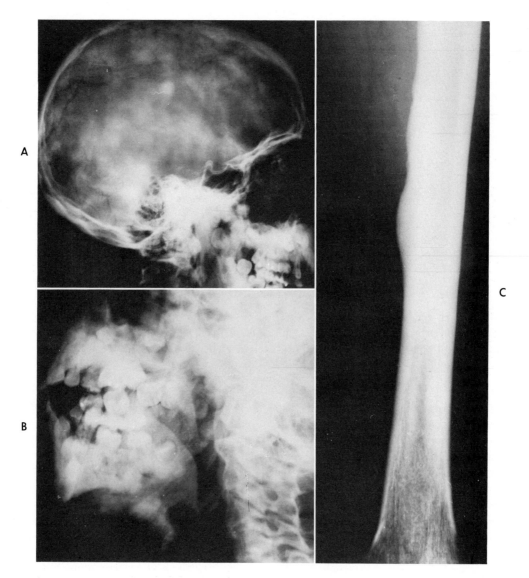

Fig. 38-19 Bony abnormalities associated with Gardner's syndrome. **A,** Multiple osteomas of skull. **B,** Osteomatosis of mandible. **C,** Localized cortical thickening of femur.

Jeghers syndrome is worldwide in its distribution and has no racial predilection. About 50% of the reported cases have a positive family history, whereas the remaining 50% are sporadic.[122] The characteristic mucocutaneous pigmented lesions usually develop during infancy or early childhood[123] and are present in nearly all patients with the Peutz-Jeghers syndrome.[124,125] Unless the lesions are specifically looked for, however, they often are not noticed by either the patient or physician. The mucocutaneous lesions appear as brown or black, oval or slightly irregular macules 1 to 5 mm in diameter. The lesions are most common on the lips, particularly the mucosal surface of the lower lip and the buccal mucosa. Pigmentation occurs less commonly on the face or volar aspect of the hands and feet.

The clinical symptomatology is usually related to gastro-intestinal polyposis. The most common clinical symptom is cramping abdominal pain caused by small bowel intussusception.[126] Most of the intussusceptions are transient,[127] but some persist and cause a significant small bowel obstruction. Rectal bleeding, or melena, occurs in about 30% of the patients, but massive gastrointestinal bleeding is rare. Chronic anemia caused by low-grade intestinal blood loss is commonly present. In some instances colonic intussusception[128] or prolapse of a rectal polyp brings the patient to clinical attention.

The polyps in cases of the Peutz-Jeghers syndrome occur predominantly in the alimentary tract but are occasionally located in the urinary or respiratory tract. The small bowel is involved in more than 95% of the patients, the colon and rectum in about 30%, and the stomach in about

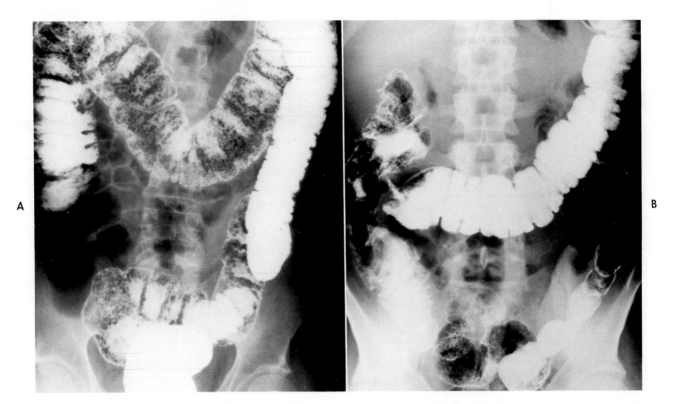

Fig. 38-20 Colon examinations in two individuals with Gardner's syndrome from same family. **A,** Myriads of small polyps carpet colon. **B,** Annular hepatic flexure carcinoma is present. Numerous small polyps are seen in sigmoid.
Courtesy of Dr. Alvin A. Watne.

25%. The polyps are multiple and range in size from 0.1 to 3 cm. Myriads of 1- to 2-mm nodules may be present in the small bowel, but carpeting has not been observed in the stomach or colon. The small bowel and gastric polyps, once considered precancerous adenomas, are currently regarded as benign hamartomatous malformations without malignant potential.[122,125] Most colonic polyps in cases of the Peutz-Jeghers syndrome, however, are proliferative mucosal lesions that are indistinguishable from adenomatous polyps.[3] The overall incidence of alimentary tract carcinomas in these patients is estimated to be about 2% to 3%.[126] Most of the gastrointestinal carcinomas in these patients have been reported to occur in the stomach, duodenum, and colon.[126,129] Carcinomas are rare in the jejunum and ileum.[126] Jejunal or ileal polyps are usually shown during a carefully performed small bowel examination using compression and spot films.[127] Colonic polyps, when present, number from two to a dozen or more (Fig. 38-21, *A*). Diffuse carpeting of the colon has not been observed. The colonic lesions are often pedunculated. Sessile lesions greater than 1 to 1.5 cm in diameter, lesions demonstrating rapid growth, and annular lesions (Fig. 38-21, *B*) should be regarded as suspicious for carcinoma.

Patients with the Peutz-Jeghers syndrome benefit from supportive, conservative treatment. Indiscriminate prophylactic resection of intestine may cause death from malabsorption. Surgery should be reserved for patients with a persistent obstruction, severe bleeding, or a suspected malignancy, and during the operation the surgeon should sacrifice as little bowel as possible.[125]

Ruvalcaba-Myhre-Smith syndrome

In 1980, Ruvalcaba, Myhre, and Smith[130] described a syndrome consisting of macrocephaly, pigmented genital lesions in males, and intestinal polyposis. Although only a few cases have been reported, the syndrome appears to be transmitted by autosomal dominant inheritance.[131] Other features of the syndrome include mental retardation, lipid storage myopathy, and subcutaneous lipomas.

The genital skin lesions consist of hyperpigmented macules that are present on the glans and shaft of the penis. Pigmented macules are absent on the scrotum or the genitalia of female patients. The intestinal lesions involve the bowel, with reports of multiple scattered polyps involving the gastric antrum, duodenum, small bowel, and colon.[131] Available biopsy material from the colonic polyps indicates that the lesions are hamartomas.[130,131] There has been no evidence of malignant potential.

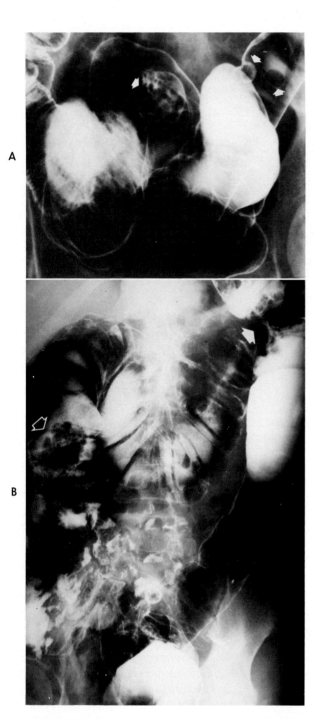

Fig. 38-21 Colon lesions in two patients with Peutz-Jeghers syndrome. **A,** Three benign sigmoid polyps *(arrows)* but no other colon lesions are present. **B,** Constricting carcinoma *(arrow)* is seen in splenic flexure; resected colon also demonstrated about 1 dozen benign polyps scattered throughout the large bowel. Sessile hamartoma *(open arrow)* is present in cecum.

Turcot syndrome

An association between polyposis coli and central nervous tumors was suggested by Turcot et al.[132] in 1959. To date, about 15 patients (10 from four families) with the syndrome have been documented.[133,134] The fact that neither brain tumors nor colonic polyps appeared in parents of affected individuals suggests an autosomal recessive mode of inheritance.[135] Brain tumors may occasionally occur in patients with multiple familial polyposis or Gardner's syndrome, perhaps as an isolated coincidental occurrence.[135,136]

In each of these patients, clinical symptoms developed during the second decade and consisted predominantly of either diarrhea caused by colonic polyps or seizures caused by a brain tumor. Most of the patients died as a result of their central nervous system malignancy. The polyps are multiple, range in diameter from 0.1 to 3 cm, and are limited to the rectum and colon. The polyps appear to be benign adenomas,[135] but the histologic description has often been incomplete. A colon carcinoma was present in four of the reported patients.[132,135] The majority of central nervous system tumors have been supratentorial glioblastomas.

Muir-Torre syndrome

The Muir-Torre syndrome was first described in the mid-1960s by Muir and later by Torre.[137,138] There are now at least 40 reported cases of this familial syndrome.[139] The syndrome is characterized by multiple sebaceous neoplasms of the skin, with or without keratoacanthomas, which are associated with multiple visceral neoplasms. So far the syndrome has shown no sex predilection, generally presents in the fifth and sixth decades, and has a strong family history. Skin lesions may precede the other manifestations. Although about 40% of these patients have benign intestinal polyps, over 90% have some gastrointestinal visceral malignancy. Eighty percent of the patients have colon carcinoma, with 5% afflicted with gastric and 8% with duodenal carcinoma. In 50% of the reported cases, the patients have some urogenital malignancy, usually endometrial, bladder, or renal carcinoma. Twelve percent of the patients have lung or laryngeal carcinoma. There may be some overlap with the family cancer syndrome described by Lynch et al.[140]

Cowden's disease: multiple hamartoma syndrome

Cowden's disease was described in 1963 by Lloyd and Dennis[141] and is named after the original family affected by it. It is characterized by questionable autosomal dominant inheritance with equal male and female incidence. The age of onset is reported to range from 4 to 75 years of age.[142]

Affected patients have verrucose skin lesions on the feet and papillomas of the lips and pharynx. Mandibular and maxillary hypoplasia may also be seen. Polyps are scattered throughout the gastrointestinal tract and may be either inflammatory or hamartomatous. There is no known increase in the frequency of visceral neoplasms in patients with the syndrome, although breast and thyroid carcinoma have been associated with the disease.

Cronkhite-Canada syndrome

In 1955, Cronkhite and Canada[143] described two patients with generalized gastrointestinal polyposis associated with ectodermal abnormalities. Since that time, more than 20 additional isolated case reports have appeared in the literature.[134,144,145] The disorder develops during middle or old age (ranging from 42 to 75 years of age, the average being 60 years) and shows no sexual, familial, racial, or geographic predilection.

The most common initial symptom is diarrhea of several months' or more duration. The stools are watery and often contain blood, mucus, or both. The diarrhea is usually accompanied by anorexia, vomiting, abdominal pain, and severe weight loss. Marked weakness results from electrolyte loss, and hypocalcemia often causes tetany. Protein is also lost in the stool, and most patients develop peripheral edema as the result of hypoalbuminemia. The ectodermal abnormalities invariably present include alopecia, brownish hyperpigmentation, and atrophy of the fingernails and toenails.

Radiographic examinations demonstrate multiple gastric and colonic polyps (Fig. 38-22). More than half the patients have evidence of small bowel polyps that may be accompanied by thickened mucosal folds and increased intraluminal fluid. Esophageal polyps have been described in two patients.

In the histologic examination, the polyps once regarded as adenomas[143] reveal inflammatory changes of the juvenile type.[134,146] Villous atrophy or a cystlike dilatation of glands, also seen in Menetrier's disease, may be present. The lesions do not appear to be associated with any potential for gastrointestinal malignancy.

In women, the disease generally has an inexorable downhill course resulting in death from inanition and cachexia within 6 to 18 months after the onset of diarrhea. In men, there is a tendency for remission.

Juvenile polyposis

Juvenile polyps, although occasionally present in adults, are so named because they generally develop during childhood. These polyps, also called *retention* or *inflammatory polyps,* have typical gross and histologic features that distinguish them from adenomatous polyps and cellular hamartomas. The juvenile polyp usually has a smooth, round contour, whereas adenomatous polyps often have a fissured, lobulated appearance. The polyps are soft in consistency and in a cut surface reveal many cystic spaces filled with mucin. The main histologic feature is abundant connective tissue stroma that contains cystic structures lined with epithelium. Numerous inflammatory cells may be

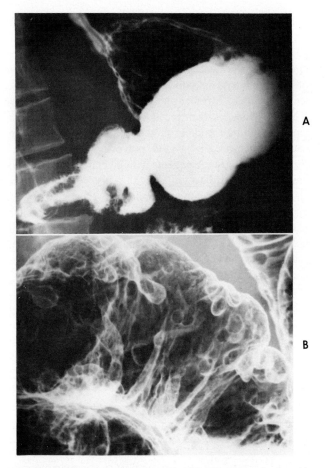

Fig. 38-22 Cronkhite-Canada syndrome. **A,** Hundreds of polypoid lesions, pinhead in size, mamillate the distal half of the stomach. Several larger polypoid lesions are also present in the antrum. **B,** In spot film of the splenic flexure, numerous polypoid lesions are well shown.

present. The lesions are nonneoplastic and have no potential for malignancy.

Juvenile polyps are seen in several different clinical conditions. Most juvenile polyps occur in children as isolated colonic lesions that are either solitary or few in number. This type of nonhereditary, isolated colonic polyp has been discussed earlier. Less commonly, colonic juvenile polyps may develop as multiple lesions referred to as *juvenile polyposis coli.* Multiple juvenile colonic polyps may (1) exist without extracolonic lesions in cases of juvenile polyposis coli, (2) involve the stomach and small bowel in cases of generalized juvenile polyposis, (3) occur as numerous lesions carpeting the colon in infants, (4) coexist with adenomatous polyps in some patients with familial multiple polyposis or Gardner's syndrome, and (5) develop in the colon in patients with the Cronkhite-Canada syndrome.

Occasionally, numerous juvenile polyps develop in the colon[147] and, in some instances, also in the stomach or small bowel or both.[148] These forms of intestinal juvenile polyposis may be encountered in teenagers and adults as well as in children. A positive family history is commonly present. In hereditary forms an autosomal dominant pattern appears to be present. The most common clinical symptom of juvenile polyposis coli is mild rectal bleeding that may lead to anemia. Juvenile rectal polyps are thought to have a greater tendency than rectal adenomas toward anal prolapse. In the past, radical surgery has been considered unnecessary because the juvenile polyps have negligible risk for malignancy. Some patients with juvenile polyposis coli, however, come from families with a history of colon carcinoma.[147] Rarely colonic juvenile polyps and a carcinoma may coexist.[149] Veale et al.[147] suggest that a genetic allele may modify the expression of the gene in order for familial multiple polyposis to cause juvenile rather than adenomatous polyps; however, the risk of colon cancer may be retained in some families.

A rare, nonfamilial juvenile polyposis syndrome has been described in infants.[150-152] Clinical symptoms generally appear during the first few months after birth. Numerous juvenile polyps are present in the colon, but may occur also in the stomach or small bowel, or both. Intraluminal loss of blood and protein lead to bleeding, diarrhea, anemia, hypoproteinemia, and edema. Most of the afflicted children have died before 17 months of age.

HEREDITARY NONPOLYPOSIS COLORECTAL CARCINOMA

Early recognition of genetic influences in the incidence of colonic polyps led to the descriptions of the previously mentioned well-defined syndromes. Recent interest in genetic factors and the recognition of families exhibiting high incidences of colorectal malignancy have resulted in the description of a new group of patients, referred to as *hereditary nonpolyposis colorectal cancer* (HNPCC) *families*.[12,176,177] In these families, there is an autosomal predisposition for carcinoma of the colorectum. The tumors usually appear early in life and are often multiple. At this time, no chromosomal abnormalities have been identified, unlike familial multiple polyposis in which a genetic defect in the long arm of chromosome 5 has been described[178] (see Chapter 41). It is estimated that these HNPCC families may account for up to 5% or 6% of the cases of colorectal malignancy.

Two forms of HNPCC have been described by Lynch et al.,[12,176,179] the Lynch I and II; both forms are inherited autosomal syndromes. Families with the Lynch I are characterized by the early onset of colorectal cancer, the proximal location of the tumors in the right colon, and multiple primary colon cancers. Families with the Lynch II exhibit the same features, but additionally have a high incidence

---

☐ **DIFFERENTIAL DIAGNOSIS OF MULTIPLE COLONIC FILLING DEFECTS** ☐

1. Foreign material
   a. Fecal material
   b. Gas bubbles
   c. Ingested foreign bodies[62]
2. Inflammatory pseudopolyps
   a. Ulcerative colitis[105]
   b. Granulomatous colitis[153]
   c. Amebiasis[154]
   d. Schistosomiasis[155]
   e. Antibiotic colitis[156]
   f. Ischemic colitis
   g. Radiation
3. Pneumatosis[157]
4. Lymphoid tissue
   a. Benign lymphoid hyperplasia[158]
   b. Lymphonodular hyperplasia[159]
   c. Lymphangiectasis[160]
5. Nonneoplastic processes
   a. Cystic fibrosis[161]
   b. Tuberous sclerosis[162]
   c. Amyloidosis[163]
   d. Urticaria[164]
   e. Herpes zoster[165]
   f. Ischemic thumbprints[166]
   g. Cowden's disease[167]
   h. Giant hyperplastic polyposis

6. Benign neoplasms
   a. Lipomatosis[168]
   b. Hemangiomatosis
   c. Lymphangiomatosis
   d. Neurofibromatosis[169]
   e. Ganglioneuromatosis[170]
7. Malignant tumors
   a. Lymphoma[171]
   b. Leukemia[172]
   c. Kaposi's sarcoma[173,174]
   d. Metastases[175]
8. Polyposis syndromes
   a. Familial multiple polyposis
   b. Gardner's syndrome
   c. Peutz-Jeghers syndrome
   d. Ruvalcaba-Myhre-Smith syndrome
   e. Turcot syndrome
   f. Cowden's disease
   g. Muir-Torre syndrome
   h. Cronkhite-Canada syndrome
   i. Juvenile polyposis

☐ **TABLE 38-2**
Summary of the features characterizing gastrointestinal polyposis syndromes

| Syndrome | Usual age at symptom onset (yr) | Hereditary transmission | Distribution (%) | | | Histology | Additional features | Prognosis |
			Stomach	Small bowel	Colon			
Multiple polyposis	15 to 30	Dominant	<5	<5	100	Adenomas	—	Colon carcinoma
Gardner's syndrome	15 to 30	Dominant	~5	~5	100	Adenomas	Soft tissue tumors, osteomatosis	Colon carcinoma
Peutz-Jeghers syndrome	10 to 30	Dominant	25	95	30	Cellular hamartomas	Pigmented skin lesions	Occasional GI tract carcinoma
Ruvalcaba-Myhre-Smith syndrome	Variable	Dominant	100	100	100	Hamartomas	Macrocephaly, penile macules, mental retardation	Occasional GI tract pain
Muir-Torre syndrome	50 to 70	Dominant		Scattered		Adenomas	Sebaceous neoplasms of the skin with or without keratoacanthomas	Multiple visceral malignancies: 80% colon cancer, 50% urogenital cancer
Cowden's disease	40	May be familial		Scattered		Hamartomas or inflammation	Verrucose skin and oropharyngeal lesion	Breast and thyroid cancer
Turcot syndrome	Teens	Recessive	—	—	100	Adenomas	Central nervous system tumors	Central nervous system tumors
Cronkhite-Canada syndrome	40 to 70	None	100	<50	100	Inflammation, glandular dilatation	Alopecia, onychia, hyperpigmentation, diarrhea, protein and electrolyte losses	Often die of cachexia
Juvenile polyposis	<10	May be familial	>5	>5	100	Inflammatory	Diarrhea with protein loss may occur	GI tract carcinoma

of endometrial cancer, ovarian cancer, and, occasionally, pancreatic, small bowel, stomach, laryngeal, or urogenital cancer.[140,180,181]

It is important to initiate screening of family members because of the early onset of tumors. Screening should begin very early, some advocating as early as age 25. The syndrome should have expressed itself by age 65.

Differential diagnosis

Generally the gastrointestinal polyposis syndromes are readily distinguished from each other. Once the radiologist suspects the diagnosis of a polyposis syndrome, the specific syndrome can usually be established by obtaining a family history and examining the patient for soft tissue tumors or mucocutaneous lesions. Radiographic examination of the entire gastrointestinal tract is needed to determine the number, size, and distribution of polyps and to identify any associated gastrointestinal malignancy. This information is helpful not only in making the differential diagnosis but also in planning therapy.

In some patients, the findings overlap between the established polyposis syndromes, such as those described between familial multiple polyposis and Gardner's syndrome. Additionally, some families may demonstrate a familial modification of the general features of a given syndrome. For example, some families with the Peutz-Jeghers syndrome may have a distribution of polyps that differs from the average values shown in Table 38-2. In one family, polyps were located predominantly in the small bowel and stomach,[123] whereas in other families the polyps were located primarily in the small bowel and colon.[124]

In addition to the differentiation of the polyposis syndromes that affect the colon, the polyposis coli syndromes must also be distinguished from other conditions that may cause multiple filling defects in the colon (see box on p. 788). Full knowledge of the clinical, laboratory, and radiologic findings for a given patient usually permits an accurate diagnosis of the underlying condition. Precise differentiation between the diagnostic possibilities, however, often depends on endoscopy and a histologic examination of tissue material.

MALIGNANCIES OF THE COLON

The previous text dealt with the concepts pertaining to the evolution and detection of adenomatous polyps and carcinoma, and how they may be influenced by environmental and genetic factors. As previously stated, the confirmation of malignancy usually awaits the findings yielded by endoscopic or surgical biopsy, or the results from histologic examination of the surgical specimen following complete removal.

Radiologic findings that reliably suggest malignancy include (1) lesions greater than 2 cm in diameter, (2) a rapid change in size, (3) infiltration and fixation, and (4) ulceration. These features of tumor growth can present variably

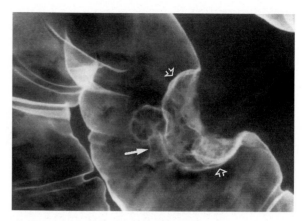

Fig. 38-23 Polyploid colonic lesions. A pedunculated polypoid lesion *(arrow)* lies immediately adjacent to the second larger sessile lesion *(arrowheads),* with tenting of its serosal surface. The size and morphologic characteristics of the larger lesion are suspicious signs indicating malignancy. In this case, the larger lesion contained carcinoma and the pedunculated lesion was a benign neoplastic polyp.
Courtesy of Dr. Arunas E. Gasparaitis.

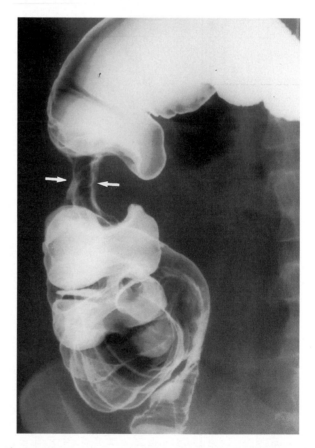

Fig. 38-24 Carcinoma of the right colon. Carcinoma is present in the ascending colon above the ileocecal valve. The tumor *(arrows)* has an annular appearance. Notice the overhanging margins on the distal ends of the tumor. Adequate distention is necessary to clearly demonstrate the radiographic features of this large, bulky annular lesion.

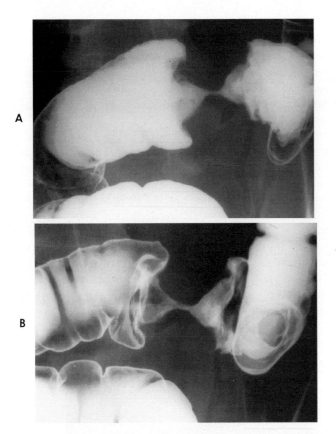

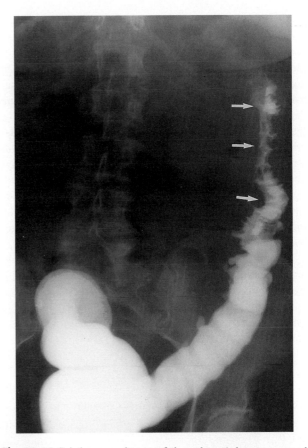

Fig. 38-25 Carcinoma of the sigmoid colon. **A,** During the single-contrast phase of this double-contrast enema examination, barium outlines the annular infiltrating sigmoid adenocarcinoma very nicely. **B,** The same features are also shown during the double-contrast phase of the examination. Although the features are similar in both studies, often the significance of this narrowed area is confirmed by the single-contrast phase of the study. Smaller polyps are much better seen during the double-contrast portion of the examination.

Fig. 38-26 Scirrhous carcinoma of the colon. A long, narrowed segment of the left colon *(arrows)* also exhibits a nodular appearance. The differential characteristics of this lesion include both benign and malignant disease. However, in this case, the infiltrating process is due to primary adenocarcinoma of the colon that is infiltrating the left colon for a very long distance. Occasionally, scirrhous tumors are encountered and can be confused with segments affected by inflammatory bowel disease.

as a (1) polypoid or intraluminal mass, (2) annular or constricting mass, or (3) infiltrating or scirrhous mass (Figs. 38-23 to 38-26). Although adenocarcinoma is, by far, the most common malignancy, other malignancies are encountered, including histologic variants of adenocarcinoma such as colloid carcinoma, signet-ring cell carcinoma, adenosquamous carcinoma, squamous carcinoma, and small cell carcinoma. The term *cloacogenic carcinoma* refers to the low-lying rectal malignancies arising from cells thought to derive from primitive cloaca. Although histologic characteristics may identify these tumors, they are morphologically and radiologically indistinct from other malignancies.

When adenocarcinoma arises on the dysplastic epithelium that forms in *ulcerative colitis,* it often presents the morphologic appearance of a stricture, with little evidence of an intraluminal mass to suggest the existence of a tumor. Because of this, strictures occurring in patients with chronic ulcerative colitis should be biopsied to exclude the possibility of infiltrating adenocarcinoma. In these patients, if severe dysplasia is found at the time of colonic endoscopic biopsy, this may prompt total colectomy, hopefully before the evolution of carcinoma.

Primary lymphoma of the colon is a rare malignancy, occurring in less than 1% of the cases of large bowel tumors. Occasionally, it is superimposed on long-standing ulcerative colitis, and is now occurring in patients with AIDS. Primary colonic lymphoma, as described by Dawson et al.[182] is limited to those cases that do not have an abnormal chest film, hepatosplenomegaly, superficial lymphadenopathy, or an abnormal peripheral blood smear. There may be local or associated adenopathy adjacent to the colon in patients with these tumors. Using this strict criterion, the number of primary large bowel lymphomas encountered in any given practice is quite small. There are three forms of primary lymphoma: either low-grade or high-grade polymorphic *B*-cell lymphoma, or malignant lymphoma polyposis.[183,184] The findings from most published series indicate that primary lymphoma occurs more often in the cecum and rectum than elsewhere. Morphologically, these tumors are indistinct from adenocarcinoma, although occasional features may suggest lymphoma. Lymphomatous polyposis is characterized by numerous nodular filling defects in the colon, which are often diffuse and involve the entire colon[185] (Figs. 38-27 to 38-30). One must discriminate this morphologic appearance from familial polyposis or other benign disease, such as lymphonodular hyperplasia, postinflammatory pseudopolyposis, and pneumatosis cystoides intestinalis. Aneurysmal ulceration occurring in large, bulky, primary lymphomas also suggests the diagnosis, as this type of ulceration is unusual for adenocarcinoma.

Secondary neoplasms of the colon, as defined by Meyers,[186] can involve the colon as the result of (1) direct invasion from contiguous tumors, or spread by means of fascial or lymphatic pathways from noncontiguous tumors, (2) intraperitoneal seeding, or (3) hematogenous metastases from distant primary sites.

Secondary involvement of the colon can be due to a variety of primary tumors, including stomach, pancreas, ovary, uterus, prostate, kidney, melanoma, breast, and lung. Benign disease, such as inflammatory disease of the pancreas and tuboovarian structures, may involve the colon and produce findings indistinguishable from those of malignancy.

The morphologic appearance of secondary neoplasms often depends on the mechanism of spread. Typically, hematogenous metastases are multiple and begin as submucosal deposits. These may go on to ulcerate and, generally, present as polypoid filling defects. Peritoneal implants are frequently desmoplastic and produce fixation and spiculation as the tumor grows on the serosal surface. Tumor extending from nearby or contiguous organs produces fixation, infiltration, and a mass effect. Knowledge of the anatomy and relationship of organs in the fascial pathway ensures not only a better understanding of the disease process, but also improves the differential considerations.

Kaposi's sarcoma, when seen in patients with AIDS, is an aggressive malignancy.[187,188] The visceral manifestation

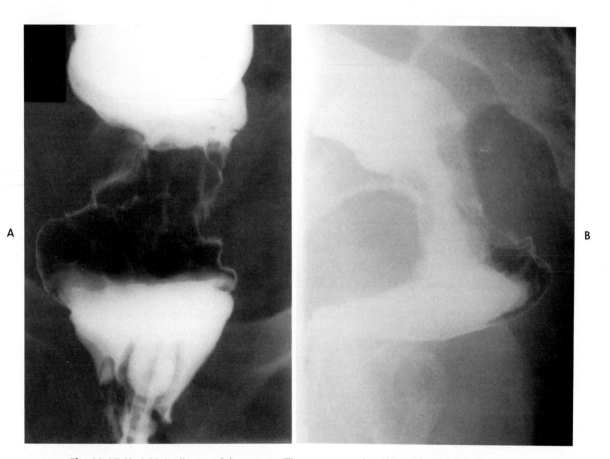

Fig. 38-27 Hodgkin's disease of the rectum. The anteroposterior (**A**) and lateral (**B**) views of infiltrating Hodgkin's disease of the rectum are indistinguishable from carcinoma morphologically. As is often the case, the morphologic distinction between various types of tumors can be extremely difficult.
From Harned R: *Radiology* 120:319, 1976.

of Kaposi's sarcoma is the same no matter where it is found, and usually consists of numerous nodules, which are often umbilicated or associated with thickened folds (Fig. 38-31). Its superimposition on an opportunistic infection of the bowel is a frequent finding.

The role of CT is primarily in the staging of carcinoma of the colon, as it is most accurate when evaluating extraluminal disease such as adenopathy, peritoneal dissemination, or distant metastases (i.e., hepatic metastases). In practice, CT is most often employed in the postoperative follow-up of these patients, rather than in the initial staging of invasive carcinoma. Although occasional suture-line recurrence does occur, most recurrent disease is outside of the colon in regional nodes or peritoneum, or takes the form of distant metastases. Direct examination of the colon during follow-up is primarily directed at detecting metachronous lesions, which should be removed.

Complications of carcinoma of the colon

Obstruction may be the initial complaint. The small-diameter left colon and sigmoid colon is the more likely site of obstruction as tumors grow, than is the much larger right colon.

Hemorrhage is a common feature of ulcerated carcinomas. Slow blood loss leading to iron deficiency anemia is very common, but severe hemorrhage is a rare event. Massive colonic bleeding should instead raise suspicion of other causes, including diverticulitis, an arteriovenous malformation, or inflammatory bowel disease.

Ulceration and necrosis can occasionally cause *perforation,* and symptoms are then often more suggestive of diverticulitis than carcinoma. Perforated tumors are usually walled off; however, *fistulization* to the bladder, vagina, or adjacent bowel may occur. Because similar complications can also arise from diverticulitis, this benign disease is always part of the differential diagnosis and must be excluded. However, this is often difficult, even with positive-contrast studies or CT scanning. Direct visualization is often compromised by severe narrowing of the colon, resulting in inadequate visualization and biopsy; therefore, surgery may be the only way to establish the correct diagnosis.

An unusual type of *colitis* may occasionally be seen proximal to a high-grade obstruction (Fig. 38-32). It has been

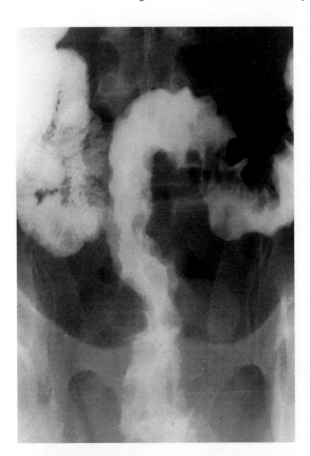

Fig. 38-28 Lymphoma of the rectosigmoid colon. Extensive infiltrative nodular lesions involving the rectum, rectosigmoid, and sigmoid are due to infiltrating lymphoma. Nodular infiltration is a characteristic feature of lymphoma. Notice the overlap in this case with findings that might be seen in acute ulcerative colitis or ischemic bowel disease.

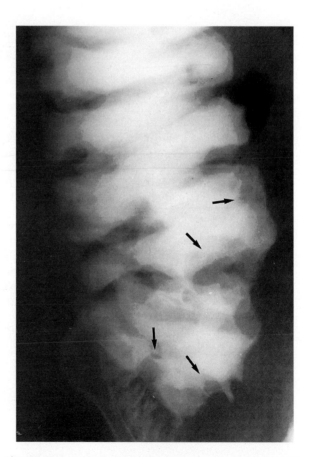

Fig. 38-29 Lymphoma of the colon. Notice the multiple nodules involving the right colon *(arrows)*. In this case, the lesions are due to diffuse involvement with primary colonic lymphoma.

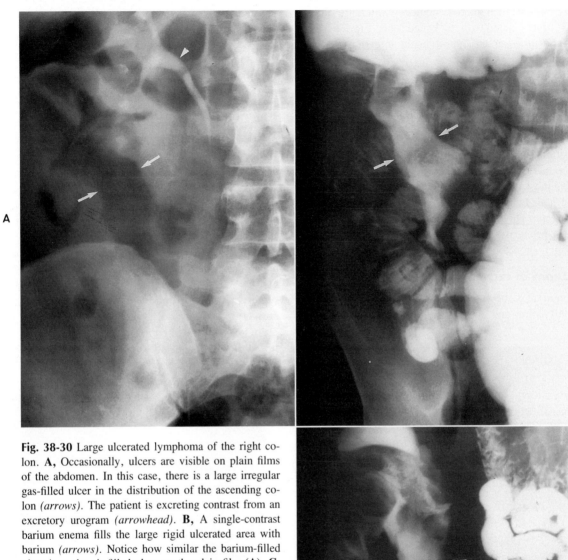

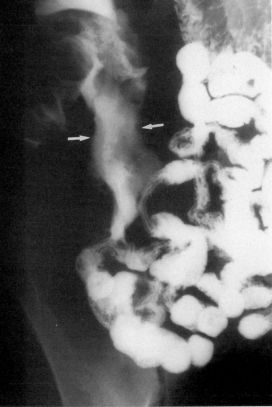

Fig. 38-30 Large ulcerated lymphoma of the right colon. **A,** Occasionally, ulcers are visible on plain films of the abdomen. In this case, there is a large irregular gas-filled ulcer in the distribution of the ascending colon *(arrows)*. The patient is excreting contrast from an excretory urogram *(arrowhead)*. **B,** A single-contrast barium enema fills the large rigid ulcerated area with barium *(arrows)*. Notice how similar the barium-filled ulcer is to the air-filled ulcer on the plain film **(A)**. **C,** A small bowel examination is followed through to the right colon. Once again, a large ulcerated area is demonstrated on the small bowel follow-through that possesses features identical to those seen in **A** and **B** *(arrows)*. Occasionally, large and sometimes small ulcers are very nicely demonstrated on plain films. This lesion is almost certainly malignant, and the large "aneurysmal" ulceration should suggest lymphoma, which was the diagnosis in this case.

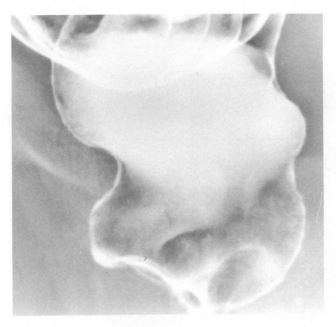

Fig. 38-31 Kaposi's sarcoma of rectum. The smooth margins of multiple defects indicate extramucosal origin.

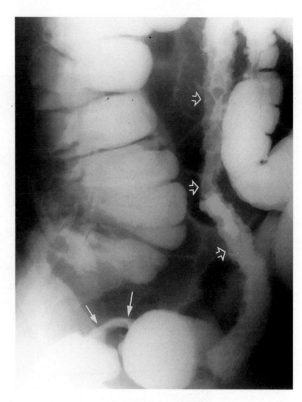

Fig. 38-32 Colitis proximal to an obstruction. An annular sigmoid colon *(arrows)* is associated with pseudomembranous colitis proximal to the obstruction *(arrowheads)*. This peculiar form of pseudomembranous colitis may rarely be related to partial obstruction.

termed variously as *inflammatory, ischemic,* or *urticarial*. The etiology of this type of colitis is unclear, but it resembles pseudomembranous colitis radiographically and may well be the result of some as yet unexplained vascular phenomenon.

Intussusception of tumor, especially originating in the cecal area, may occasionally be encountered (Fig. 38-33). Both benign and malignant masses may serve as the point of origin for colocolo or ileocolic intussusception. Following reduction of the intussusception, the morphologic features of the mass may allow differentiation of benign from malignant disease.

Caveats pertaining to radiologic examination of carcinoma of the colon

1. Complete filling of the colon should be documented, either by visualization of the cecal tip, appendix, or both, or by reflux into the terminal ileum. The haustral pattern of the right colon may mimic the cecum, giving the false impression that the cecum has been filled despite complete obstruction by adenocarcinoma. Because of this perceptive error, even very large tumors of the right colon are occasionally overlooked.

2. When complete obstruction by carcinoma of the colon at any location is encountered, the remaining colon proximal to the obstruction is not examined. Following resection, the remainder of the colon must be examined to exclude the possibility of synchronous lesions. This can be done via a colostomy or following primary reanastomosis, either endoscopically, radiologically, or both. Synchronous carcinomas can be expected in approximately 5% of the patients. Additional benign adenomatous polyps occur with an even higher frequency, in approximately 50% of such patients, and these should all be removed.

3. High-grade narrowing of the colon may take on the appearance of complete obstruction during a retrograde barium enema examination. However, the patient may have no clinical symptoms or radiographic evidence of obstruction (Fig. 38-34). This phenomenon of obstruction is probably due to mucosal prolapse into the narrowed lumen. In this instance, a small bowel examination will usually permit a very adequate examination of the proximal colon, thereby allowing visualization of the true extent of the obstructing lesion.

4. In the presence of complete obstruction of the colon by tumor, it is better to perform a water-soluble contrast examination, which allows for the subsequent performance of endoscopy and biopsy without the delay required for barium to clear from the colon. This facilitates the rapid evaluation of these patients.

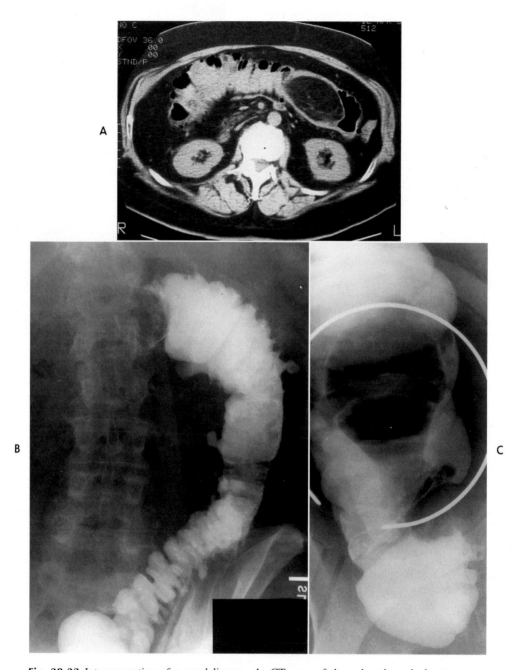

Fig. 38-33 Intussusception of a cecal lipoma. **A,** CT scan of the colon through the transverse colon demonstrates a large intraluminal mass in the distal transverse colon. The CT numbers are characteristic of fat. This is a large cecal lipoma that is causing intussusception, with the point of origin now in the distal transverse colon. **B,** A single-contrast barium enema study outlines the smooth-surface contour of the lipoma. **C,** Following complete reduction of the intussusception, the large, pedunculated lipoma is now clearly visible in its entirety. In this case, not only are the morphologic features consistent with a benign lipoma, but the CT appearance is also characteristic of a fatty tumor.

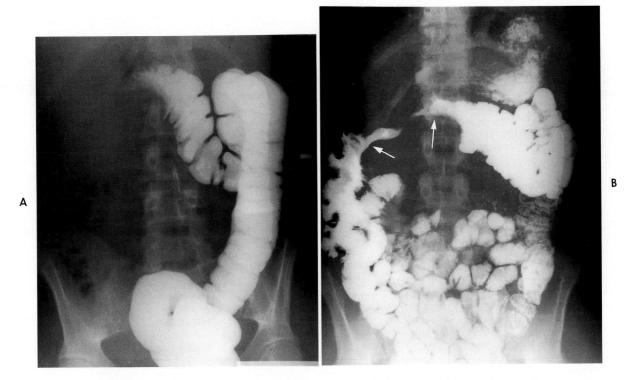

Fig. 38-34 Carcinoma of the colon. **A,** A single-contrast barium enema demonstrates complete obstruction of the retrograde flow of contrast in the proximal transverse colon. Notice the otherwise absence of evidence of colonic obstruction. The patient was asymptomatic other than having anemia and Hemoccult-positive stool. **B,** A small bowel follow-through into the colon confirms the presence of a large infiltrating annular carcinoma of the transverse colon *(arrows).* This examination gives additional information as to the cause and extent of the obstruction. Notice how barium traverses the narrowed colon despite the apparent obstruction during retrograde filling.

REFERENCES

1. Lane N, Fenoglio CM: Observations on the adenoma as precursor to ordinary large bowel carcinoma, *Gastrointest Radiol* 1:111, 1976.

2. Olmstead WW et al: The solitary colonic polyp: radiologic-histologic differentiation and significance, *Radiology* 160:9, 1986.

3. Morson BC: Some peculiarities in the histology of intestinal polyps, *Dis Colon Rectum* 5:337, 1962.

4. Grinnell RS, Lane N: Benign and malignant adenomatous polyps and papillary adenomas of the colon and rectum: an analysis of 1,856 tumors in 1,335 patients, *Int Abstr Surg* 105:519, 1958.

5. Hogan WJ et al: A prospective comparison of the accuracy of colonoscopy vs air-barium contrast exam for detection of colonic polypoid lesions (abstract), *Gastrointest Endosc* 23:230, 1977.

6. Arminski TC, McLean DW: Incidence and distribution of adenomatous polyps of the colon and rectum based on 1,000 autopsy examinations, *Dis Colon Rectum* 7:249, 1964.

7. Welch CE, Hedberg SE: *Polypoid lesions of the gastrointestinal tract,* ed 2, Philadelphia, 1975, WB Saunders.

8. Gillespie PE et al: Colonic adenomas: a colonoscopy survey, *Gut* 20:240, 1979.

9. Wolff WI, Shinya H: Endoscopic polypectomy: therapeutic and clinicopathologic aspects, *Cancer* 36:683, 1975.

10. Snyder DN et al: Changes in site distribution of colorectal carcinoma in Connecticut, 1940-1973, *Am J Dig Dis* 22:791, 1977.

11. Bernstein MA et al: Distribution of colonic polyps: increased incidence of proximal lesions in older patients. *Radiology* 155:35, 1985.

12. Lynch HT et al: Hereditary nonpolyposis colorectal cancer (Lynch syndromes I and II), *Cancer* 56:934, 1985.

13. Castleman B, Krickstein HZ: Do adenomatous polyps of the colon become malignant? *N Engl J Med* 267:469, 1962.

14. Spratt JS Jr, Ackerman LV, Moyer CA: Relationship of polyps of the colon to colonic cancer, *Ann Surg* 148:682, 1958.

15. Appel MF, Spjut HJ, Estrada RG: The significance of villous component in colonic polyps, *Am J Surg* 134:770, 1977.

16. Fenoglio CM, Lane N: The anatomical precursor of colorectal carcinoma, *Cancer* 34:819, 1974.

17. Morson BC: The polyp-cancer sequence in the large bowel, *Proc R Soc Med* 67:451, 1974.

18. Gilbertson VA: Proctosigmoidoscopy and polypectomy in reducing the incidence of rectal cancer, *Cancer* 34:936, 1974.

19. Gilbertson VA et al: Invasive carcinoma of the large intestine: a preventable disease? *Surgery* 57:363, 1965.

20. Enquist IF: The incidence and significance of polyps of the colon and the rectum, *Surgery* 42:681, 1957.

21. Rosensweig J, Horwitz A: Adenomatous tumours of the colon and rectum: the importance of early detection and treatment, *Am Surg* 24:515, 1958.

22. Walske B, Hamilton J, Kisner P: From benign polyp to carcinoma, *Arch Surg* 70:318, 1955.

23. Welin S: Results of the Malmö technique of colon examination, *JAMA* 199:369, 1967.

24. Ott DJ, Gelfand DW: Colorectal tumors: pathology and detection, *AJR* 131:691, 1978.

25. Dodds WJ, McGlaughlin PS: Intestinal intussusception in adults, *Am J Gastroenterol* 55:284, 1971.

26. Youker JE, Dodds WJ: Colon and rectum. In Steckel RJ, Kagan AR, eds: *Diagnosis and staging of cancer*, Philadelphia, 1976, WB Saunders.

27. Jarre HA, Figiel SJ: Refinements in radiologic diagnosis of colonic disease. In Rajewsky B, ed: *Proceedings of Ninth International Congress of Radiology,* vol 1, Stuttgart, 1961, Georg Thieme.

28. Laufer I, Smith NCW, Mullens JE: The radiological demonstration of colorectal polyps undetected by endoscopy, *Gastroenterology* 70:167, 1976.

29. Leinicke JL et al: A comparison of colonoscopy and roentgenography for detecting polypoid lesions of the colon, *Gastrointest Radiol* 2:125, 1977.

30. Sugarbaker PH et al: Colonoscopy in the management of diseases of the colon and rectum, *Surg Gynecol Obstet* 139:341, 1974.

31. Thoeni RF, Menuck L: Comparison of barium enema and colonoscopy in the detection of small colonic polyps, *Radiology* 124:631, 1977.

32. Williams CB et al: Colonoscopy in the management of colon polyps, *Br J Surg* 61:673, 1974.

33. Wolff WI et al: Comparison of colonoscopy and the contrast enema in five hundred patients with colorectal disease, *Am J Surg* 129:181, 1975.

34. Teefey SA, Carlson HC: The fluoroscopic barium enema in colonic polyp detection, *AJR* 141:1279, 1983.

35. Gelfand DW, Ott DJ: Single vs. double contrast gastrointestinal studies: critical analysis of reported statistics, *AJR* 137:523, 1981.

36. Ott DJ et al: Single-contrast vs. double-contrast barium enema in the detection of colonic polyps, *AJR* 146:993, 1986.

37. Dodds WJ, Stewart ET, Hogan WJ: The role of colonoscopy and roentgenology in the detection of polypoid colonic lesions, *Am J Dig Dis* 22:646, 1977.

38. Thoeni RJ, Margulis AR: The state of radiographic technique in the examination of the colon: a survey, *Radiology* 127:317, 1978.

39. Evers K et al: Double-contrast enema examination for detection of rectal carcinoma, *Radiology* 140:635, 1981.

40. Laufer I: The double-contrast enema: myths and misconceptions, *Gastrointest Radiol* 1:19, 1976.

41. Miller RE: Barium enema examination with large-bore tubing and drainage, *Radiology* 82:905, 1964.

42. Miller RE, Lehman GE: The barium enema: is it obsolete? *JAMA* 235:2842, 1976.

43. Feczko PJ et al: Small colonic polyps: a reappraisal of their significance, *Radiology* 152:301, 1984.

44. Rex DK et al: Sensitivity of double-contrast barium study for left-colon polyps, *Radiology* 158:69, 1986.

45. Ott DJ et al: Sensitivity of double-contrast barium enema: emphasis on polyp detection, *AJR* 135:327, 1980.

46. Miller RE, Lehman G: Polypoid colonic lesions undetected by endoscopy, *Radiology* 129:295, 1978.

47. Dodds WJ, Stewart ET, Nelson JA: Rectal balloon catheters and the barium enema examination, *Gastrointest Radiol* 5:277, 1980.

48. Nelson JA, Daniels AU, Dodds WJ: Rectal balloons: complications, causes and recommendations, *Invest Radiol* 14:48, 1979.

49. Stewart ET, Dodds WJ, Nelson JA: Value of digital rectal exam before barium enemas, *Radiology* (in press).

50. Stewart ET, Dodds WJ: Predictability of rectal incontinence on barium enema examination, *AJR* 132:197, 1979.

51. Williams C: Personal communication, 1986.

52. Teague RH et al: Colonscopy for investigation of unexplained rectal bleeding, *Lancet* 1:1350, 1978.

53. Tedesco FJ et al: Colonoscopic evaluation of rectal bleeding: a study of 304 patients, *Ann Intern Med* 89:907, 1978.

54. Dodds WJ et al: An evaluation of colon cleansing regimens, *AJR* 128:57, 1977.

55. Miller RE: The cleansing enema, *Radiology* 117:483, 1975.

56. Dodds WJ: Roentgen examination of the colon: relevant questions, *Invest Radiol* 7:63, 1972.

57. Kelvin FM, Maglinte DT: Colorectal carcinoma: a radiologic and clinical review, *Radiology* 164:1, 1987.

58. Frager DH et al: Problems in the colonoscopic localization of tumors: continued value of the barium enema, *Gastrointest Radiol* 12:343, 1987.

59. Rose CP et al: Inaccuracy of radiographic measurements of colon polyps, *J Can Assoc Radiol* 32:21, 1981.

60. Kelvin FM et al: Colorectal carcinoma missed on double contrast barium enema study: a problem in perception, *AJR* 137:307, 1981.

61. Gohel VK, Kressel HY, Laufer I: Double-contrast artifacts, *Gastrointest Radiol* 3:139, 1978.

62. Press HC Jr, Davis TW: Ingested foreign bodies simulating polyposis: report of six cases, *AJR* 127:1040, 1976.

63. Youker JE, Welin S: Differentiation of true polypoid tumors of the colon from extraneous material: a new roentgen sign, *Radiology* 84:610, 1965.

64. Friedland GW, Pooler GJ: False-positive "eccentric target sign" on barium-air contrast enema examination, *Radiology* 99:67, 1971.

65. Hulten J: Lipomatosis of the ileocaecal valve, *Acta Chir Scand* 129:104, 1965.

66. Mylärniemi H, Perttala Y, Peltokallio P: Tumor-like lesions of the cecum following inversion of the appendix, *Am J Dig Dis* 19:547, 1974.

67. Welin S, Youker J, Spratt JS: The rates and patterns of growth of 375 tumors of the large intestine and rectum observed serially by double contrast enema study (Malmö technique), *AJR* 90:673, 1963.

68. Muto T, Bussey HJR, Morson BC: The evolution of cancer of the colon and rectum, *Cancer* 36:2251, 1975.

69. Marshak RH, Lindner AE, Maklansky D: Adenomatous polyps of the colon: a rational approach, *JAMA* 235:2856, 1976.

70. Youker JE, Welin S, Main G: Computer analysis in the differentiation of benign and malignant polypoid lesions of the colon, *Radiology* 90:794, 1967.

71. Smith TR: Pedunculated malignant colonic polyps with superficial invasion of the stalks, *Radiology* 115:593, 1975.

72. Delammare J et al: Villous tumors of the colon and rectum: double-contrast study of 47 cases, *Gastrointest Radiol* 5:69, 1980.

73. Kaye JJ, Bragg DG: Unusual roentgenologic and clinicopathologic features of villous adenomas of the colon, *Radiology* 91:799, 1968.

74. Zimmer G et al: Colonic endometriosis: roentgen studies with a five-year followup, *Am J Gastroenterol* 64:410, 1975.

75. Stout AP: Tumors of the colon and rectum (excluding carcinoma and adenoma). In Turell, R, ed: *Diseases of the colon and anorectum,* vol 1, Philadelphia, 1959, WB Saunders.

76. Meyers MA et al: Haustral anatomy and pathology: a new look. I. Roentgen identification of normal patterns and relationships, *Radiology* 108:497, 1973.

77. Deeths TM, Dodds WJ: Lipoma of the colon, *Am J Gastroenterol* 58:326, 1972.

78. Ginzburg L, Weingarten M, Fischer MG: Submucous lipoma of the colon, *Ann Surg* 148:767, 1958.

79. Wolf BS, Melamed M, Khilnani MT: Lipoma of the colon, *J Mt Sinai Hosp NY* 21:80, 1954.

80. Silverberg SG: "Juvenile" retention polyps of the colon and rectum, *Am J Dig Dis* 15:617, 1970.

81. Holgersen LO, Miller PE, Zintel HA: Juvenile polyps of the colon, *Surg* 69:288, 1971.

82. Tumacder OC et al: Carcinoid tumors of the rectum: a review of 40 cases, *Arch Surg* 97:261, 1968.

83. Postlethwait RW: Gastrointestinal carcinoid tumors: a review, *Postgrad Med* 40:445, 1966.

84. Orloff MJ: Carcinoid tumors of the rectum, *Cancer* 27:175, 1971.

85. Ferguson EF Jr, Houston CH: Benign and malignant tumors of the colon and rectum, *South Med J* 65:1213, 1972.

86. Ecker JA, Doane WA, Dickson DR: Endometriosis of the gastrointestinal tract, *Am J Gastroenterol* 41:405, 1964.

87. Macafee CH, Greer HL: Intestinal endometriosis: report of 29 cases and survey of the literature, *J Obstet Gynecol Br Emp* 67:539, 1960.

88. Paul RE Jr, Gherardi GJ, Miller HH: Autoamputation of benign and malignant colonic polyps: report of two cases, *Dis Colon Rectum* 17:331, 1974.

89. Pierce ER: Some genetic aspects of familial multiple polyposis of the colon in a kindred of 1,422 members, *Dis Colon Rectum* 11:321, 1968.

90. Reed TE, Neel JV: A genetic study of multiple polyposis of the colon (with an appendix deriving a method of estimating relative fitness), *Am J Hum Genet* 7:236, 1955.

91. McConnell RB: *The genetics of gastrointestinal disorders,* London, 1966, Oxford University Press.

92. Dodds WJ: Clinical and roentgen features of the intestinal polyposis syndromes, *Gastrointest Radiol* 1:127, 1976.

93. Dodds WJ, Lydon SB: Intestinal polyposis syndromes, *CRC Crit Rev Clin Radiol Nucl Med* 5:295, 1974.

94. Cripps H: Two cases of disseminated polyps of the colon, *Trans Pathol Soc Lond* 33:165, 1882.

95. Dukes CE: Familial intestinal polyposis, *Ann R Coll Surg Engl* 10:293, 1952.

96. Veale AMO: *Intestinal polyposis,* Cambridge, 1965, Cambridge University Press.

97. Yonemoto R et al: Familial polyposis of the entire gastrointestinal tract, *Arch Surg* 99:427, 1969.

98. Denzler TB, Harned RK, Pergam CJ: Gastric polyps in familial polyposis coli, *Radiology* 130:63, 1979.

99. Itai Y et al: Radiographic features of gastric polyps in familial adenomatosis coli, *AJR* 127:73, 1977.

100. Ohsato K et al: Small-intestinal involvement in familial polyposis diagnosed by operative intestinal fiberscopy: report of four cases, *Dis Colon Rectum* 20:414, 1977.

101. Ushio K et al: Lesions associated with familial polyposis coli: studies of lesions of the stomach, duodenum, bones and teeth, *Gastrointest Radiol* 1:67, 1976.

102. Iida M et al: Spontaneous disappearance of fundic gland polyposis: report of three cases, *Gastroenterology* 79:725, 1980.

103. Murphy FS, Mireles M, Beltran A: Familial polyposis of the colon and gastric carcinoma: concurrent conditions in a 16-year-old boy, *JAMA* 179:1026, 1962.

104. Lockhart-Mummery HE: Intestinal polyposis, *Practitioner* 203:620, 1969.

105. Marshak RH, Mosely JE, Wolf BS: The roentgen findings in familial polyposis with special emphasis on differential diagnosis, *Radiology* 80:374, 1963.

106. Kennedy B et al: Familial multiple polyposis: a "curable" disease, *Wis J Med* 70:230, 1971.

107. Harvey JC, Quan SHQ, Stearns MW: Management of familial polyposis with preservation of the rectum, *Surgery* 84:476, 1978.

108. Cole JW, McKalen A, Powel J: The role of ileal contents in the spontaneous regression of rectal adenomas, *Dis Colon Rectum* 4:413, 1961.

109. Gardner EJ, Richard RC: Multiple cutaneous and subcutaneous lesions occurring simultaneously with hereditary polyposis and osteomatosis, *Am J Hum Genet* 5:139, 1953.

110. Watne AL et al: The diagnosis and surgical treatment of patients with Gardner's syndrome, *Surgery* 82:327, 1977.

111. Coli RD et al: Gardner's syndrome: a revisit to the previously described family, *Am J Dig Dis* 15:551, 1970.

112. Ziter MH: Roentgenographic findings in Gardner's syndrome, *JAMA* 192:158, 1965.

113. Chang CH et al: Bone abnormalities in Gardner's syndrome, *AJR* 103:645, 1968.

114. Grosberg SJ: Gardner's syndrome and villous adenoma of jejunum, *Am Surg* 41:177, 1975.

115. Hamilton SR et al: Ileal adenomas after colectomy in nine patients with adenomatous polyposis coli/Gardner's syndrome, *Gastroenterology* 77:1252, 1979.

116. Keshgegian AA, Enterline HT: Gardner's syndrome with duodenal adenomas, gastric adenomyoma and thyroid papillary-follicular adenocarcinoma, *Dis Colon Rectum* 21:255, 1978.

117. Watne AL, Johnson JG, Chang CH: The challenge of Gardner's syndrome, *Cancer* 19:266, 1969.

118. Smith WG: Multiple polyposis, Gardner's syndrome and desmoid tumors, *Dis Colon Rectum* 1:323, 1958.

119. McKusick VA: Genetic factors in intestinal polyposis, *JAMA* 182:271, 1962.

120. Peutz JLA: Ober een zeer merkwaardige, geocombineerde familaire Polyposis van de Slymvliezen van den Tractus intestinalis met die van de Neuskeelholte en Gepaard met eigen aardige Pigmentaties van Huiden Slijmvlieze, *Ned Maandschr Geneeskd* 10:134, 1921.

121. Jeghers H, McKusick VA, Katz KH: Generalized intestinal polyposis and melanin spots of the oral mucosa, lips and digits: a syndrome of diagnostic significance, *N Engl J Med* 241:933, 1949.

122. Bartholomew LG et al: Intestinal polyposis associated with mucocutaneous pigmentation, *Surg Gynecol Obstet* 115:1, 1962.

123. Burdick D, Prior J, Scanlon GT: Peutz-Jeghers syndrome: clinicalpathologic study of a large family with a 10-year follow-up, *Cancer* 16:854, 1963.

124. Dodds WJ et al: Investigation of a large Negro family with Peutz-Jeghers syndrome, *Gastroenterology* 60:657, 1971.

125. Dormandy TL: Gastrointestinal polyposis with mucocutaneous pigmentation (Peutz-Jeghers syndrome), *N Engl J Med* 256:1093, 1957.

126. Dozois RR et al: The Peutz-Jeghers syndrome: is there a predisposition to the development of intestinal malignancy, *Arch Surg* 98:509, 1969.

127. Godard JE et al: Peutz-Jeghers syndrome: clinical and roentgenographic features, *AJR* 113:316, 1971.

128. McAllister AJ, Richards KF: Peutz-Jeghers syndrome: experience with twenty patients in five generations, *Am J Surg* 134:717, 1977.

129. Dodds WJ et al: Peutz-Jeghers syndrome and gastrointestinal malignancy, *AJR* 115:374, 1972.

130. Ruvalcaba RHA, Myhre S, Smith DW: Sotos syndrome with intestinal polyposis and pigmentary changes of the genitalia, *Clin Genet* 18:413, 1980.

131. Foster MA, Kilcoyne RF: Ruvalcaba-Myhre-Smith syndrome: a new consideration in the differential diagnosis of intestinal polyposis, *Gastrointest Radiol* 11:349, 1986.

132. Turcot J, Després J, St Pierre F: Malignant tumors of the central nervous system associated with familial polyposis of the colon: report of two cases, *Dis Colon Rectum* 2:465, 1959.

133. Baughman FA Jr et al: The glioma-polyposis syndrome, *N Engl J Med* 281:1345, 1969.

134. Johnson GK et al: Cronkhite-Canada syndrome: gastrointestinal pathophysiology and morphology, *Gastroenterology* 63:140, 1972.

135. Itoh H et al: Turcot's syndrome and its mode of inheritance, *Gut* 20:414, 1979.

136. Binder MK et al: Colon polyps, sebaceous cysts, gastric polyps, and malignant brain tumor in a family, *Am J Dig Dis* 23:460, 1978.

137. Muir EG et al: Multiple primary carcinomata of the colon, duodenum, and larynx associated with kerato-acanthomata of the face, *Br J Surg* 54:191, 1967.

138. Torre D et al: Society transactions, *Arch Dermatol* 98:549, 1968.

139. Schwartz RA et al: The Muir-Torre syndrome: a disease of sebaceous and colonic neoplasms, *Dermatologica* 178:23, 1989.

140. Lynch HT et al: Tumor variation in three extended Lynch syndrome II kindreds, *Am J Gastroenterol* 83:741, 1988.

141. Lloyd KM, Dennis M: Cowden's disease: a possible new symptom complex with multiple system involvement, *Ann Intern Med* 58:136, 1963.

142. Weinstock JV, Kawanishi H: Gastrointestinal polyposis with orocutaneous hamartomas (Cowden's disease), *Gastroenterology* 74:890, 1978.

143. Cronkhite LW Jr, Canada WJ: Generalized gastrointestinal polyposis: an unusual syndrome of pigmentation, alopecia, and onychotrophia, *N Engl J Med* 252:1011, 1955.

144. Ali M et al: Cronkhite-Canada syndrome: report of a case with bacteriologic, immunologic, and electron microscopic studies, *Gastroenterology* 79:731, 1980.

145. Rubin M et al: Cronkhite-Canada syndrome: report of an unusual case, *Gastroenterology* 79:737, 1980.

146. Diner WC: The Cronkhite-Canada syndrome, *Radiology* 105:715, 1972.

147. Veale AMO et al: Juvenile polyposis coli, *J Med Genet* 3:5, 1966.

148. Sachatello CR, Pickren JW, Grace JT: Generalized juvenile gastrointestinal polyposis: a hereditary syndrome, *Gastroenterology* 58:699, 1970.

149. Goodman ZD, Yardley JH, Milligan FD: Pathogenesis of colonic polyps in multiple juvenile polyposis: report of a case associated with gastric polyps and carcinoma of the rectum, *Cancer* 43:1906, 1979.

150. Ruymann FB: Juvenile polyps with cachexia: report of an infant and comparison with Cronkhite-Canada syndrome in adults, *Gastroenterology* 57:431, 1969.

151. Schwartz AM, McCauley RGK: Juvenile gastrointestinal polyposis, *Radiology* 121:441, 1976.

152. Soper RT, Kent TH: Fatal juvenile polyposis in infancy, *Surgery* 69:692, 1971.

153. Freeman AH et al: Pseudopolyposis in Crohn's disease, *Br J Radiol* 51:782, 1978.

154. Berkowitz D, Berstein LH: Colonic pseudopolyps in association with amebic colitis, *Gastroenterology* 68:786, 1975.

155. Nebel OT et al: Schistosomal disease of the colon: a reversible form of polyposis, *Gastroenterology* 67:939, 1974.

156. Stanley RJ, Melson GL, Tedesco FJ: The spectrum of radiographic findings in antibiotic-related pseudomembranous colitis, *Radiology* 111:519, 1974.

157. Calne RY: Gas cysts of the large bowel simulating multiple polyposis, *Br J Surg* 47:212, 1959.

158. Capitanio MA, Kirkpatrick JA: Lymphoid hyperplasia of the colon in children, *Radiology* 94:323, 1970.

159. De Smet AR, Tubergen DG, Martel W: Nodular lymphoid hyperplasia of the colon associated with dysgammaglobulinemia, *AJR* 127:515, 1976.

160. Schaefer JW, Griffen WO Jr, Dubilier LD: Colonic lymphangiectasis associated with a potassium depletion syndrome, *Gastroenterology* 55:515, 1968.

161. Grossman H, Berdon WE, Baker DH: Gastrointestinal findings in cystic fibrosis, *AJR* 97:227, 1966.

162. Devroede G, Herman P: Multiple polyposis of the colon as a sign of systemic hamartomatosis (tuberous sclerosis) (abstract), *Gastroenterology* 66:A-30/684, 1974.

163. Pear RL: The radiographic manifestations of amyloidosis, *AJR* 111:821, 1971.

164. Johnson TH, Caldwell KW: Angioneurotic edema of the colon, *Radiology* 99:61, 1971.

165. Menuck LS et al: Colonic changes of herpes zoster, *AJR* 127:273, 1976.

166. Wittenberg J et al: Ischemic colitis: radiology and pathophysiology, *AJR* 123:287, 1975.

167. Nuss DD et al: Multiple harmartoma syndrome (Cowden's disease), *Arch Dermatol* 114:743, 1978.

168. O'Connell DJ, Shaw DG, Swain VAJ: Epiploic lipomatosis and lipomatous polyposis of the colon, *Br J Radiol* 49:969, 1976.

169. Lukash WM et al: Gastrointestinal neoplasms in von Recklinghausen's disease, *Arch Surg* 92:905, 1966.

170. Anderson TE, Spackman TJ, Schwartz SS: Roentgen findings in intestinal ganglioneuromatosis: its association with medullary thyroid carcinoma and pheochromocytoma, *Radiology* 101:93, 1971.

171. Pochaczevsky R, Sherman RS: Diffuse lymphomatous disease of the colon: its roentgen appearance, *AJR* 87:670, 1962.

172. Cornes JS, Jones TG: Leukaemic lesions of the gastrointestinal tract, *J Clin Pathol* 15:305, 1962.

173. Byrk D et al: Kaposi's sarcoma of the intestinal tract: roentgen manifestations, *Gastroenterol Radiol* 3:425, 1978.

174. Rose HS et al: Alimentary tract involvement in Kaposi sarcoma: radiologic and endoscopic findings in 25 homosexual men, *AJR* 139:661, 1982.

175. Sacks BA, Joffe N, Antonioli DA: Metastatic melanoma presenting clinically as multiple colonic polyps, *AJR* 129:511, 1977.

176. Lynch HT et al: Natural history of colorectal cancer in hereditary nonpolyposis colorectal cancer (Lynch syndromes I and II), *Dis Colon Rectum* 31:439, 1988.

177. Vasen HFA et al: The tumour spectrum in hereditary non-polyposis colorectal cancer: a study of 24 kindreds in The Netherlands, *Int J Cancer* 46:31, 1990.

178. Bodmer WF et al: Localization of the gene for familial adenomatous polyposis on chromosome 5, *Nature* 328:614, 1987.

179. Lynch HT et al: Phenotypic variation in colorectal adenoma/cancer expression in two families, *Cancer* 66:909, 1990.

180. Lynch HT et al: The Lynch syndrome II and urological malignancies, *J Urol* 143:24, 1990.

181. Lynch HT et al: Variable gastrointestinal and urologic cancers in a Lynch syndrome II kindred, *Dis Colon Rectum* 34:891, 1991.

182. Dawson IMP, Cornes JS, Morson BC: Primary malignant lymphoid tumours of the intestinal tract, *Br J Surg* 49:80, 1961.

183. Shepherd NA et al: Primary malignant lymphoma of the colon and rectum. A histopathological and immunohistochemical analysis of 45 cases with clinicopathological correlations, *Histopathology* 12:235, 1988.

184. Henry CA, Berry RE: Primary lymphoma of the large intestine, *Am Surgeon* 54:262, 1988.

185. Cornes JS: Multiple lymphomatous polyposis of the gastrointestinal tract, *Cancer* 14:249, 1961.

186. Meyers MA: *Dynamic radiology of the abdomen,* New York, 1982, Springer-Verlag.

187. Wall SD et al: Multifocal abnormalities of the gastrointestinal tract in AIDS, *AJR* 146:1, 1986.

188. Frager DH et al: Gastrointestinal complications of AIDS: radiologic features, *Radiology* 158:597, 1986.

ADDITIONAL READINGS

Järvinen HJ: Familial cancer: a review on hereditary cancer traits with special regard to colorectal carcinoma, *Acta Oncol* 27:783, 1988.

Winawer SJ et al: Feasibility of fecal occult-blood testing for detection of colorectal neoplasia: debits and credits, *Cancer* 40:2616, 1977.

39 *Computed Tomography and Magnetic Resonance Imaging in Colorectal Carcinoma: Staging and Detection of Postoperative Recurrence*

ALEC J. MEGIBOW

Colorectal carcinoma is currently the second most common internal malignancy in the population of the United States. Approximately 1 in 25 Americans will incur this disease during their lifetime, and 1 in 37 Americans will die of it.[1] Advances in surgical and diagnostic techniques have led to improvements in the stage-corrected 5-year survival rate of from 43% in 1960 to 54% in 1979. Survival in patients with colorectal carcinoma varies depending on the depth of tumor penetration through the colonic wall; the presence of metastatic disease to regional lymph nodes, both in terms of the number of positive nodes as well as the proximity of these nodes to the primary lesion; and the presence of distant organ metastases, with the liver, peritoneal cavity, and lung parenchyma the most common sites.[2]

There are three distinct areas in which radiologists are involved in the management of patients with colorectal carcinoma. The first is in the detection of the tumor within the bowel lumen and consists of a properly performed barium enema examination. The second is in the preoperative staging of the tumor, and the third is in the postoperative follow-up, with the object to detect local recurrence or distant metastases. This chapter deals with the role of computed tomography (CT) and magnetic resonance imaging (MRI) in both the preoperative staging and postoperative surveillance of patients with known colorectal cancer.

The use of transrectal ultrasound in patients with colorectal carcinoma is discussed elsewhere in this text. The evaluation of the liver is also critical in the initial investigation of these patients, and the techniques of liver imaging are also detailed in other chapters in this text.

GOALS OF IMAGING STUDIES

The goals of imaging studies in patients with colorectal carcinoma are to provide the surgeon and oncologist with a complete and accurate assessment of the important morphologic features of the primary tumor, to detect and document local and distant spread of the disease, and to elucidate the nature of clinically occult complications. Thus the ideal procedure should furnish a true measure of the depth of tumor penetration into or through the bowel wall, detect any metastases in adjacent or distant lymph nodes or in other sites, and identify any key prognostic features that would have an impact on patient survival. This information can then be used to facilitate a safe and complete abdominal surgical exploration and the extirpation of accessible disease, as well as to identify those patients who would benefit from adjuvant therapy. Imaging also plays an important role in patient follow-up, for it can detect the presence and extent of postoperative recurrent or persistent disease, as suggested by changes in the patient's clinical status or laboratory values, such as the levels of carcinoembryonic antigen (CEA) and the results of liver function studies.[3]

Currently, no single imaging procedure can provide all of this information. Realization of the true value of imaging in patients with colorectal carcinoma awaits improvements in both radiologic technology and in the therapeutic options. Until that time, clinicians and surgeons will depend on imaging procedures to provide them with specific, albeit limited, information. In many institutions, patients with colorectal carcinoma are not routinely imaged preoperatively. In others, including the author's, however, surgeons who specialize in colorectal surgery often request preoperative imaging studies so that they can obtain an estimate of the extent of extraluminal local disease or an idea of other possible complications, such as the perforation or involvement of contiguous organs, and so they can know in advance whether there are distant metastases, particularly to the liver.

COMPUTED TOMOGRAPHY
Techniques

Clinically relevant information can be yielded by CT only through careful adherence to appropriate techniques that al-

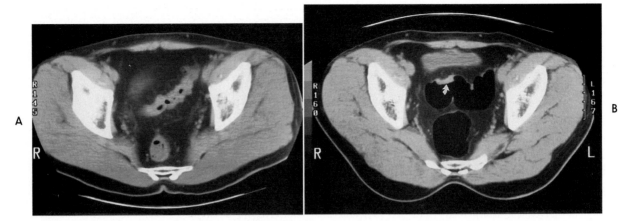

Fig. 39-1 Value of distention of lumen. **A,** Normal-appearing sigmoid. **B,** Repeat scan obtained at same time as **A,** following air insufflation. Obvious lesion seen in the distal sigmoid *(arrow).*

low visualization of the significant diagnostic features of colorectal cancer. Specifically, accurate depiction of the extent of tumor within or through the bowel wall, detection of any metastatic disease to regional or distant lymph nodes, and identification of distant metastases are imperative.

Colon preparation and rectal contrast material

Lack of bowel distention and remaining fecal debris limit the ability of CT to detect a colorectal neoplasm (Fig. 39-1, *A*). Patients undergoing a preoperative evaluation of colorectal cancer at our institution are asked to undergo a thorough bowel preparation before the CT examination. We have found that using a negative contrast agent to distend the lumen has substantially improved our appreciation of the presence and nature of the lesion (Fig. 39-1, *B*).

There are two mediums that can be used in negative-contrast evaluations of bowel lesions—air or water.[4,5] Each technique has its own advantages, and the final choice is left to the examining radiologist. Air is easy to administer, and there is an inherent lower risk of damage to the equipment if the patient cannot tolerate the insufflation. The disadvantages of air are that it may be necessary to reposition the patient to maximize distention of the segment of colon in question, and to alter routine "soft tissue windows" to optimally visualize the thickness of the bowel wall. When water contrast is used, both excellent negative contrast and depiction of the thickness of the normal versus abnormal bowel wall can be achieved using routine windowing; however, the colon must be distended with at least 2000 ml of water to obtain optimal diagnostic conditions, thus stressing patient tolerance. Regardless of the technique chosen, the administration, either of glucagon 0.5 mg given intravenously or 1.0 mg given intramuscularly, facilitates hypotonia and improves image quality, not to mention patient acceptance.

Patient positioning and CT techniques

Patient positioning for the CT examination is dictated by the location of the tumor. At the author's institution, we generally perform the initial dynamic scan of the upper abdomen with the patient in a standard supine position, and then obtain scans with the patient in other positions that optimize detection of the primary lesion. To evaluate a carcinoma in the right colon, it is best to scan the air-filled colon with the patient in a left-side-down decubitus position. For investigating rectosigmoid lesions, it is best to obtain scans with the patient prone, to allow the insufflated air to rise into the relatively posterior rectosigmoid. Once the technologists become familiar with the repositioning routine, the CT examination time is only minimally prolonged.

The use of 4- to 5-mm slice collimation increases the level of confidence when assessing the serosal margins of the tumor, and this usually permits more accurate tumor staging. Furthermore, the ability to recognize pericolic changes, such as perforation or local peritoneal seeding, is also enhanced. The mechanisms responsible for the improved image quality are the reduction in partial volume averaging and a more precise pixel representation. True spatial resolution is not altered. Although the decreased collimation results in increased noise, this can be overcome by increasing the milliampere level, thus maintaining consistent image quality.

Intravenous contrast

The proper administration of intravenous contrast is integral to the success of a CT examination. Aside from its importance in the detection of hepatic metastases, contrast material is essential for outlining the retroperitoneal and pelvic blood vessels, which allows the recognition of abnormal lymph nodes, and for enhancing the primary neoplasm, thus making the tumor more conspicuous and accentuating the mural features, such as low attenuation in mucinous lesions or submucosal edema in obstructing lesions.

The value of intravenous contrast agents can be maximized by using a double-bolus technique for the examination of the upper abdomen and liver and the lower abdomen and pelvis. An initial volume of 100 to 120 ml can be injected at a rate of 1.5 to 3 ml per second for dynamic CT scanning of the upper abdomen and a second bolus of 50 to 80 ml delivered at a rate of 1.5 ml per second for examination of the lower abdomen and pelvis.

Appearance of primary colorectal carcinoma

The typical morphologic patterns of colorectal carcinoma shown on barium studies, which include polypoid, annular constricting, infiltrating or stenosing, and ulcerative features, can also be depicted by CT.

Colorectal carcinoma is most often recognized as an area of focal, irregular thickening of the wall of the colon. When the colon is distended with air, irregularities of the mucosal surface of the lesion and other surface features can also be visualized in many cases. Ulcerative tumors assume the appearance of large masses possessing excavated cavities, and both polypoid (Fig. 39-2) and annular lesions (Fig. 39-3) can be depicted accurately. Colorectal tumors are most often slightly hyperdense on intravenous contrast–enhanced scans. Occasionally, the tumor mass may have calcifications within it, particularly in mucin-secreting neoplasms. Areas of low attenuation may also be seen within portions of the mass, indicating necrosis or focal areas of mucin collection.

Squamous cell tumors of the anal canal are most commonly seen as low-attenuation masses.[6] However, it is unusual to observe a complete ring of low attenuation within the thickened bowel wall; this finding more often represents nonneoplastic wall thickening. Villous adenomas have occasionally been reported to exhibit a water density.[7]

Penetration of colorectal carcinomas into the pericolic fat is suggested by the presence of projections with a soft tissue density that emanate from the serosal surface (Fig. 39-4). The thickness and size of the mucosal portion of the lesion do not necessarily correlate with the exact point of transmural extension, however. Thus identification of the entire luminal portion of the tumor is necessary to ensure that the entire serosal aspect of the tumor is visualized. A surrounding inflammatory reaction may simulate transmural tumor extension. However, secondary signs of penetration, such as an ill-defined clouding of the pericolic fat and thickening of contiguous fascial reflections, are often seen, and this clarifies the picture.

Lymph node metastases

If there are lymph node metastases from colorectal carcinoma, this forecasts a significant decrease in survival rate. In a series of 2037 patients with rectal cancers who under-

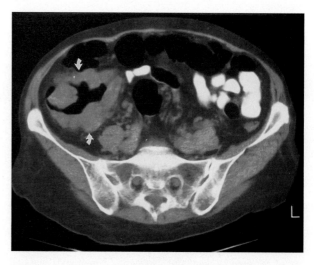

Fig. 39-2 Polypoid cecal tumor. A lobulated lesion is clearly seen that involves the entire cecum *(arrows)*.

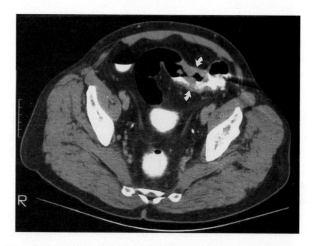

Fig. 39-3 Annular carcinoma of the sigmoid colon. An abrupt region of wall thickening is seen in the air-filled lumen *(arrows)*. Note the lack of pericolic inflammatory changes.

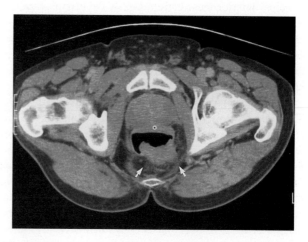

Fig. 39-4 Invasive rectal carcinoma. Bulky tumor is seen posteriorly with obvious extension into the perirectal fat *(arrows)*.

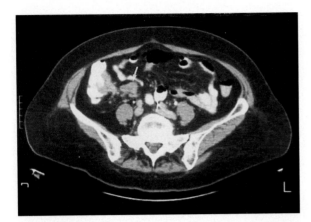

Fig. 39-5 Cecal carcinoma with local adenopathy. An irregular soft tissue attenuation is seen along the medial cecal wall, indicative of the primary neoplasm. Notice the lymph node mass adjacent to the tumor *(arrow)*.

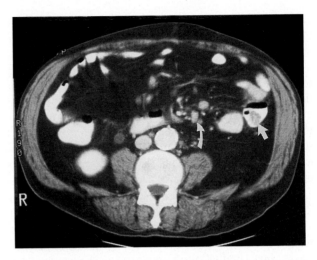

Fig. 39-6 Apparent intraluminal tumor with lymph node metastases. A nonpenetrating intraluminal tumor is seen in the descending colon *(arrow)*. Note the multiple discretely enlarged nodes in the adjacent mesentery *(curved arrow)*.

went resection, the corrected 5-year survival rate was 84% in patients without nodal metastases, but was 32% in the presence of nodal metastases.[8] Therefore any preoperative "staging" study must be able to accurately determine the presence of lymph node metastases.

The likelihood of lymph node metastases is directly related to the degree of penetration through the bowel wall and the grade of the lesion. However, even some low-grade cancers can present with lymph node metastases (Fig. 39-5). Preoperative knowledge of this is important; otherwise, incomplete treatment, such as only a simple fulguration, might be carried out in these patients.

Knowledge of the normal drainage pathways allows one to predict the approximate location of abnormal nodes. Four groups of lymph nodes drain the left colon and rectum: the epicolic nodes within the peritoneal covering of the colon; the paracolic nodes accompanying the marginal vessels; the intermediate mesocolic nodes within the mesocolon; and the principal inferior mesenteric nodes at the origin of the inferior mesenteric vein (Fig. 39-6). Rectal cancer can additionally spread laterally along the middle and inferior hemorrhoidal vessels toward the pelvic side wall, and thus to the obturator nodes. This permits retrograde dissemination into the paraaortic nodes.[9]

Cross-sectional imaging techniques are limited by their ability to diagnose lymph node metastases only on the basis of node size. In general, retroperitoneal nodes greater than 2 cm in cross section, intraabdominal nodes greater than 1 to 2 cm in cross-section, or clusters of more than three intraabdominal nodes are all considered to indicate metastases. In addition, nodes in patients with colorectal cancer may be enlarged as the result of either metastatic disease or reactive hyperplasia (sinus histiocytosis). Interestingly, the prognosis is better for those patients with the latter finding, than it is even for those patients with no

lymph node metastases or sinus histiocytosis.[10] This is believed to reflect an improved balance between tumor aggression and host resistance. In a series comparing survival of patients with Dukes stage B and C colon carcinoma, those with lymph node sinus histiocytosis exhibited a 5-year survival of 77%, compared to 59% in those without histiocytosis.[10]

The sensitivity of CT in the detection of lymph node metastases using the standard size criteria just noted was only 26%.[11] However, the sensitivity increases to 73% when different size criteria are used—1 cm for retroperitoneal and intraabdominal nodes or clusters of three or more 1-cm intraabdominal nodes, although the specificity and positive predictive values are then only 58% and 79%, respectively.[12] Thus, CT is inadequate for the detection and classification of lymph nodes in patients with colorectal carcinoma.[11,12]

Distant metastases

In 30% of the cases of colorectal cancer, patients are first seen when the disease is in an advanced and metastatic stage. Hepatic and pulmonary metastases are the most common. Other forms of dissemination include direct invasion of contiguous organs, such as the liver and spleen, occurring in about 10% of the cases, and peritoneal seeding. The radiologic appearances of these sites of tumor spread and invasion are not unique to colon cancer, and these are discussed elsewhere in this text.

In females, colorectal carcinoma can metastasize to the ovaries, and some patients may actually present with an adnexal mass. The CT appearance is virtually identical to that of primary ovarian cancer. A colorectal carcinoma metastasis should be suspected whenever an "adnexal mass" is encountered in elderly women over 65 years old or in those who have coexisting hepatic metastases. Careful attention to the colonic cleansing regimen before CT scanning, the use of air insufflation or water distention, and dynamic contrast-enhanced scans are helpful for identifying the underlying primary colonic neoplasm.[13]

Accuracy of CT staging

Two large published series have addressed the accuracy of CT in the staging of colorectal carcinoma.[11,12] The first series consisted of 103 patients who underwent surgical resection, and compared CT staging with the Dukes classification.[11] CT-based staging was correct in only 48% of the patients when compared with the Dukes staging system, which interestingly downstaged 83% of the cases and upstaged only 17%. CT could not distinguish between Dukes stage A and B1, but could correctly show that the lesion was confined to the bowel wall. CT showed a sensitivity of 61% in the detection of local extension (invasion of pericolonic fat), 26% for nodal metastases, and 73% for hepatic metastases.

In the second study, 90 preoperative CT scans from patients with colorectal carcinoma were compared with the surgical findings.[12] CT-based staging was correct in 64% of the patients. Similar to the first study, the overwhelming number of errors were due to downstaging local extension (accounting for 94% of the errors) and not to upstaging it. The overall sensitivity of CT in determining local tumor extension was 55%. Its sensitivity for detecting regional lymph node metastases was 73%, and for detecting hepatic metastases, 79%. Comparing the results of CT with the Dukes system, CT was correct in 57% of Dukes' A lesions, 17% of Dukes' B lesions, 68% of Dukes' C lesions, and 81% of the Dukes' D lesions.

Based on the findings yielded by both these studies, CT is not sufficiently accurate to warrant its routine preoperative use. However, CT is highly sensitive for identifying advanced disease, and was most useful in those instances when clinically advanced disease was unsuspected, in that it made possible specific definition of the extent of tumor spread, and hence the preoperative planning of rational therapy.

Complications of colorectal cancer

Colorectal cancer may produce several complications, which may manifest a variable spectrum of radiologic appearances. The most significant of these are colonic obstruction and perforation. The presence of either of these complications can significantly affect patient survival. In a Gastrointestinal Tumor Study Group analysis, obstruction was found to be an independent prognostic feature, separate from Dukes' stage, and the presence of tumor perforation was important in determining the duration of disease-free survival.[14]

Most patients with bowel obstruction are not referred for imaging, because prompt surgical decompression is critical and the cause of the obstruction can be determined at the time of surgery. However, in those instances when the cause of the obstruction is equivocal, or even when colorectal carcinoma is suspected as the cause, CT may be appropriately utilized to confirm the diagnosis and to assess the remainder of the abdominal cavity. CT has proved to be 95% accurate in the diagnosis of bowel obstruction and to correctly predict the nature of the obstruction in 78% of the patients[15] (Fig. 39-7). Furthermore, CT has been shown to be accurate in the detection of intussusception (Fig. 39-8). When there is evidence of colonic obstruction distal to a colon carcinoma, one must suspect a second primary neo-

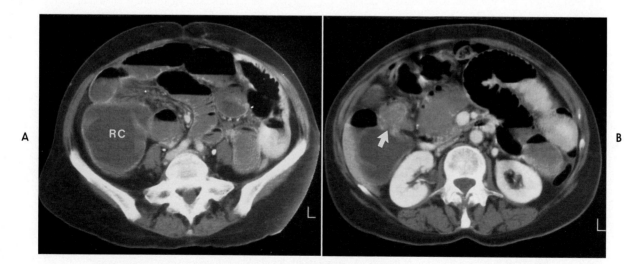

Fig. 39-7 Obstructing right colon carcinoma. **A,** Dilated small bowel loops and a dilated right colon *(RC)* are noted. **B,** Scan obtained at the transition point reveals stenotic carcinoma proximal to the hepatic flexure *(arrow).*

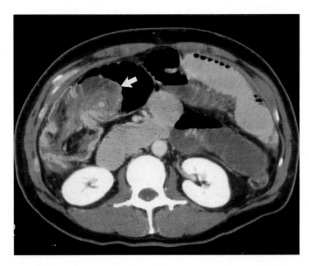

Fig. 39-8 Colocolic intussusception. Note the leading polypoid tumor *(arrow)*. Proximally, there are signs of bowel obstruction.

plasm (Fig. 39-9). However, intraperitoneal spread of the tumor with secondary adhesions or kinking of the bowel may also be responsible for the distal obstruction.

Perforation of colorectal carcinoma is a relatively uncommon event. Furthermore, a significant percentage of patients with perforated tumors do not manifest the clinical symptoms of toxicity, further reducing clinical suspicion of this complication. In addition, contrast studies of the colon often cannot detect colorectal carcinoma perforation. However, tumor perforation is relatively easy to recognize on CT scans. Thus, CT should be performed in patients whenever the contrast examination findings do not fully explain the clinical findings or whenever they suggest extramucosal disease.

In our series, it was possible to identify and correctly classify the disease in 36 of 38 patients with perforated colonic neoplasms, based on the CT findings.[16] The most common finding was a colonic mass with an associated phlegmon or abscess. Distant metastases were found in 11 of the 38 cases. On the basis of our findings, one might conclude that a colonic perforation has resulted from an underlying carcinoma when the degree of bowel wall thickness in the region of the perforation is greater than one would expect from diverticulitis, a more common cause of perforation. Diverticulitis is usually associated with only mild to moderate wall thickening (4-5 mm), although it can vary from 1 to 3 cm.[17] There is, therefore, a significant overlap in the degree of colonic wall thickening in the presence of diverticulitis and colon carcinoma, particularly when wall thickening is between 1 and 3 cm, and the CT findings in this setting have been shown to be indeterminate approximately 11% of the time.[16,17] In these cases, direct luminal investigation, either with endoscopy or barium, should be performed to help establish the diagnosis.[17] However, even these studies may not yield diagnostic findings in many of these patients.

MAGNETIC RESONANCE IMAGING

Magnetic resonance imaging can provide cross-sectional images of the colon that are similar to CT images in the information they provide. However, the technique has additional promise because it can detect mild changes in soft tissue contrast, which might both improve the detection of local tumor spread and provide more specifics concerning lymph node metastases. In other words, because of the MR signal differences between fat and soft tissue, it may be easier to perceive local tumor extension. Similarly, one *might* be able to recognize signal alterations in unenlarged lymph nodes, which may reflect intranodal metastases. MRI can

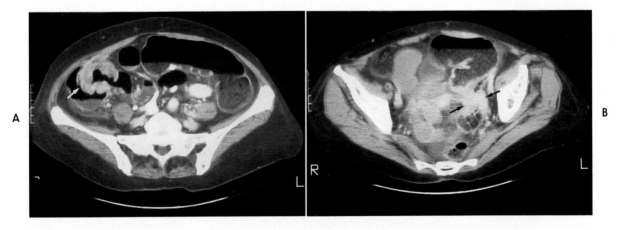

Fig. 39-9 Synchronous primary tumors. **A,** A polypoid, lobulated cecal neoplasm is seen *(arrow)*. The colon distal to this lesion is dilated, raising the suspicion of an obstructing lesion. **B,** A second soft tissue attenuation neoplasm is seen in the sigmoid colon *(arrows)*. This lesion resulted in clinical obstruction. Endoscopy and contrast studies were unable to visualize the proximal colon.

detect hepatic metastases with a sensitivity at least equal to that of CT, and thus MRI should be ideal for preoperative evaluation.

So far, most of the clinical experience with MR imaging of colorectal carcinoma has been with spin-echo techniques utilizing a full-body coil. The primary tumors can be visualized as regions of focal wall thickening and enhance with intravenously administered gadolinium-DTPA.[18] Not surprisingly, good colonic cleansing preparation and luminal distention using either contrast material or balloon inflation facilitate detection of the primary tumor.[19,20] The signal from the lesion depends on the choice of pulse sequence as well as the histologic nature of the tumor (Fig. 39-10). On conventional T1 sequences (short TR/TE), the neoplasms are uniformly hypointense with respect to perirectal fat, which makes this sequence useful for assessing gross extramural extension. Using T2 sequences (long TR/TE), the lesions become progressively brighter as the echo time increases, which limits the utility of extramural assessment (Figs. 39-10 and 39-11). However, with the use of balloon distention and small field-of-view (FOV) imaging, T2 sequences can depict the bowel wall layers.[21] Thus, these sequences seem useful for assessing the intramural spread of tumor.

Significant advances in the evaluation of local extension of disease are resulting from modifications in surface-coil technology. Local staging has been considerably improved with the use of dual external surface coils. Further improvements in the evaluation of rectal cancer can be realized with the use of endorectal coils. Excellent correlation with pathologic specimens has been demonstrated.[22] On T2 images, infiltrating carcinoma takes on the appearance of localized intramural thickening with hypointense and intact muscle layers, while intramuscular infiltration is recognized as a discontinuity or interruption of the muscle layer by isointense or relatively hyperintense tumor[23] (Fig. 39-12). The clinical impact of this increased ability to locally "stage" lesions destined for surgical removal (and thereby make them amenable to exact pathologic staging) has yet to be determined.

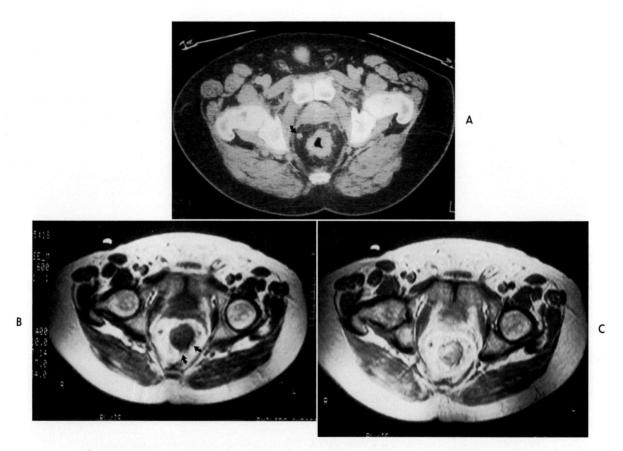

Fig. 39-10 CT and MR studies depicting rectal cancer. **A,** CT scan shows a circumferential, locally invasive rectal neoplasm along with a solitary enlarged perirectal lymph node *(arrow)*. **B,** A T1 MR image reveals an abnormal node and shows tumor penetration into the perirectal fat *(arrows)*. **C,** A T2 MR image reveals the abnormal node. As the signal from the tumor brightens, the ability to recognize penetration into the fat is diminished.

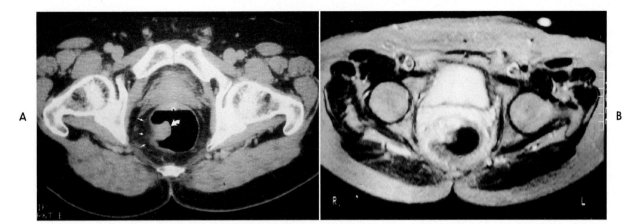

Fig. 39-11 CT and MR studies depicting rectal cancer. **A,** A CT scan reveals polypoid rectal cancer *(arrow)*. Local invasion is depicted by the presence of subtle soft tissue strands extending into the perirectal fat *(small arrows)*. **B,** A T2 MR image reveals signal brightening from the tumor with loss of ability to visualize local extension.

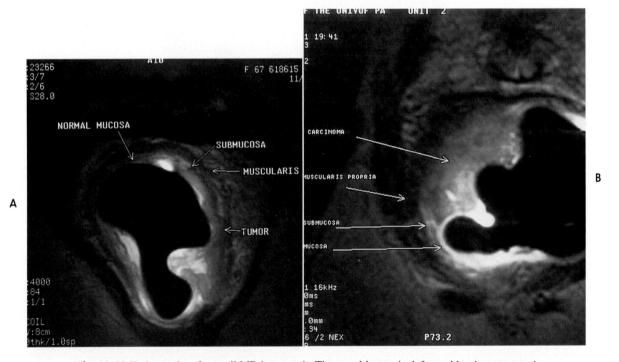

Fig. 39-12 Endorectal surface-coil MR images. **A,** The rectal lumen is deformed by the tumor and the intermediate-signal neoplasm is seen. Note the hypointense signal indicating the muscularis is intact, although the tumor has invaded the submucosa. **B,** In a different patient, the muscularis is thickened and its signal slightly increased compared to that in the uninvolved portion. This tumor has extended well into the wall of the rectum.
Courtesy of Drs. Mitchell Schnall and Herbert Kressel.

FOLLOW-UP IMAGING OF COLORECTAL CARCINOMA

As treatment options evolve, an expanding number of patients with recurrent disease can be cured, or the disease significantly palliated.[24] However, follow-up protocols have not been clearly defined, although most clinicians agree that the interval of follow-up should be dictated by the stage and grade of the primary tumor at initial presentation. Although controversy exists, most oncologists observe the postoperative cause of colorectal cancer patients by taking serial measurements of the CEA levels, supplemented by imaging tests when these are elevated. In an NIH study, 67% of the patients manifested a progressive rise in their CEA level as the first indication of recurrence, followed by changes brought to light by physical examination. CT detected early recurrence in only two patients before the CEA level was abnormal. Thus, imaging is called on to localize the site of tumor recurrence predicted by abnormal laboratory values.[25] Colorectal carcinoma can recur in multiple sites, and detection of disease at any of these levels requires organ-specific techniques, particularly in the liver. Discussion of proper imaging techniques in these different regions is beyond the scope of this chapter, and the following discussion centers instead on imaging of locoregional failure.

Interest in imaging locoregional colorectal carcinoma recurrence was ignited by reports of the ability of CT to evaluate the patient following abdominoperineal resection.[26,27] Up to this point, there was no other method available for examining this clinically inaccessible region. On CT images, recurrent tumor masses appear as bulky infiltrating lesions. They can be locally invasive into the tip of the coccyx or into the greater sciatic foramen. When prescribing the scanning protocol for these patients, it is critical to be sure that the slices are programmed to cover the entire region of potential recurrence (the ischial tuberosities can serve as a useful caudal landmark). One must also bear in mind that normal pelvic viscera will descend into the previous rectal fossa. In the female, the uterus may be seen to lie against the sacral promontory. In the male, the prostate gland and seminal vesicles are not removed during surgery, and these structures may be confused for recurrent disease. Thus, an initial baseline CT scan should be obtained soon after surgery. This study can show the postoperative reorientation of the pelvic viscera as well as postoperative soft tissue "stranding," thus allowing for a more sensitive appreciation of subsequent serial changes. Fine-needle aspiration biopsy should be carried out in any regions where a suspicious mass is found.

As experience has accumulated, it has become apparent that extensive masslike fibrotic deposits develop in some patients, which are indistinguishable from neoplastic masses on CT scans. Obviously, normal aspiration biopsy findings do not rule out recurrence, because, even though they may truly reflect a disease-free state, they may also be falsely negative due to sampling errors. In the presence of heterogeneous masses, biopsy results are often more likely positive when tissue is obtained from regions of lower attenuation.[28]

MRI can also display cross-sectional information, and, furthermore, through analysis of signal changes, it is possible to assess cellularity. This particular property has been exploited in the analysis of perineal masses in the rectal fossa. Because T2 spin-echo imaging is sensitive to fluid content, progressive lengthening of the echo and repetition times can display signal changes that can discriminate between acellular scar (fibrosis) and recurrent tumor.[29,30] The basis for this is the lack of signal brightening in fibrotic masses as the echo time increases (Fig. 39-13).

The value of MRI is limited in those patients who have

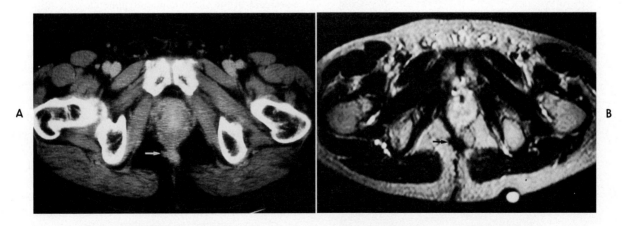

Fig. 39-13 MR differentiation of fibrosis. **A,** CT study reveals a small mass *(arrow)* along the perineal crease in a patient who had undergone abdominoperineal resection for rectal cancer. **B,** Long TR/TE MR image shows the mass remains "dark" *(arrow),* indicating fibrosis and not tumor.

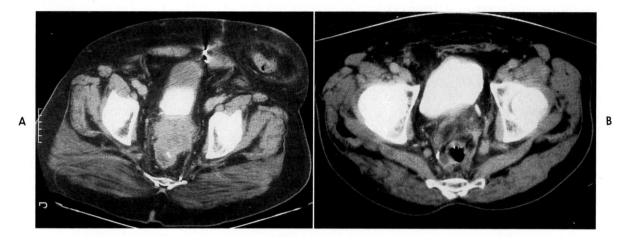

Fig. 39-14 Anastomotic (suture-line) recurrences in two cases. **A,** A bulky heterogeneous mass extends from the anterior rectal wall and engulfs the prostate gland. The patient had undergone a low anterior resection for rectal cancer. **B,** A mixed-attenuation mass is seen at the level of the low anterior resection. Note the preservation of the luminal contour of the rectum. Needle biopsy results confirmed the suture-line recurrence.

undergone radiation therapy because edema in the tissues can produce signal brightening when no neoplastic tissue exists. The length of time it takes for MR findings to become reliable following irradiation has not yet been defined precisely. In one study, recurrent masses following radiation treatment were correlated with histologic findings.[31] In this study, false-positive masses (a bright signal on long TR/TE MRI scans) resulting from acellular edema and false-negative scans (a dark signal on long TR/TE MR scans) resulting from extensive desmoplasia were encountered.[31]

Anastomotic (suture-line) recurrences form along the serosal aspect of the bowel wall and can be detected with

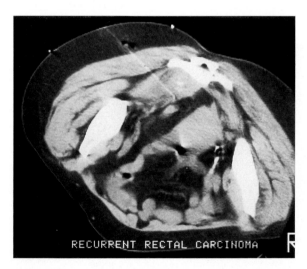

Fig. 39-15 Fine-needle aspiration biopsy of recurrent rectal carcinoma. CT-guided biopsy shows 21-gauge needle in right lower pelvis.

cross-sectional imaging (Fig. 39-14). Segmental colectomies will result in anastomoses at predictable levels. Thin-section (5-mm) scans obtained over the region of the suspected anastomosis are helpful in excluding serosal disease at these levels. Other complications, such as hydronephrosis or bowel obstruction, also can be detected by imaging studies.

In general, a combination of CT and biopsy or MRI and CT can be used to detect recurrent tumor and to differentiate tumor recurrence from scar. Liberal use of fine-needle aspiration biopsy is recommended for assessing suspected local recurrence (Fig. 39-15).

OTHER IMAGING MODALITIES

There has been considerable interest in the use of positron emission tomography (PET) and monoclonal antibody measurement in the surveillance of patients with suspected recurrent colonic carcinoma, because, by detecting abnormal metabolic activity, biochemical markers are potentially more sensitive for identifying the existence of neoplastic tissue than is morphologic imaging. So far, these techniques are not generally available; however, the results from initial studies appear promising.

Experience with PET scanning is limited. ^{18}F-fluorodeoxyglucose (FDG) uptake is an indicator of glucose metabolism, and as such can indicate the presence of viable cancer cells.[32] In one small study consisting of 15 patients with suspected recurrent tumor (focal soft tissue masses demonstrated by CT), the respective capabilities of PET and MRI were compared.[33] PET was able to demonstrate increased FDG uptake in all 11 patients with proved recurrence and MRI was able to distinguish 10 of the 11 patients with recurrent tumor from those with scar.

Monoclonal antibody measurement may provide the most

sensitive and specific method of detecting occult disease. This is especially true in settings where the findings from conventional radiographic methods like CT are equivocal, or in the setting of elevated serum markers. Detection rates of 87% for 100% for local recurrences have been reported with the use of indium 111 FO23C5.[34] In the patient with elevated serum markers and negative results from a conventional workup, including CT, radiolabeled antibodies have been shown to be very valuable for localizing recurrent or metastatic tumor. Patt et al.[35] studied 20 patients with elevated CEA levels and no radiographic evidence of disease. They were able to correctly identify tumor in 19 of these patients, and were able to confirm 52% of all scanpositive sites as cancer.

As experience with immunoscintigraphy grows, it becomes apparent that CT and immunoscintigraphy are complementary, and that immunoscintigraphy will identify tumor in those instances when CT cannot, and vice versa. The combination of these two modalities may yield even more definitive diagnostic information. For example, when an equivocal soft tissue density is seen on CT or possible blood pool transmission CT, single-photon-emission CT (SPECT) or immunoscintigraphy can serve as a direct method of comparison.[36] At the author's institution, we have used CT plus SPECT fusion techniques to identify the nature of an anatomic structure on CT images shown to contain increased activity on antibody SPECT examinations. This has been helpful in identifying false-positive uptake in normal activity–containing structures, such as blood vessels, and has been helpful in locating the site of tumor recurrence when the CT findings were negative. As computer software programs are developed and more volumetric data sets are acquired, it is likely that use of this technology will increase.

REFERENCES

1. Silverberg E, Lubera J: Cancer statistics, *Cancer* 38:5, 1988.
2. Cohen AM, Shank B, Friedman MA: Colorectal cancer. In de Vita DT, Hellman S, Rosenblum SA, eds: *Cancer: principles and practice of oncology,* ed 3, Philadelphia, 1989, JB Lippincott.
3. Thoeni RF: Colorectal cancer: cross-sectional imaging for staging of primary tumor and detection of local recurrence, *AJR* 156:909, 1991.
4. Gossios KJ, Tsianos EV, Kontogiannis DS, Demou LL, Tatsis CK et al: Water as contrast medium for computed tomography study of colonic wall lesions, *Gastrointest Radiol* 17:125, 1992.
5. Megibow AJ, Zerhouni EA, Hulnick DH, Balthazar EJ, Beranbaum ER: Air opacification of the colon as adjunct in CT evaluation of the pelvis, *J Comput Assist Tomogr* 8:797, 1983.
6. Cohan RH, Silverman PM, Thompson WM, Halvorsen RA, Baker ME: Computed tomography of epithelial neoplasms of the anal canal, *AJR* 145:569, 1985.
7. Coscina WF, Arger PH, Herlinger H, Levine MS, Coleman BG et al: CT diagnosis of villous adenoma, *J Comput Assist Tomogr* 10:764, 1986.
8. Dukes CE, Bussey HJR: The spread of rectal cancer and its effect on prognosis, *Br J Cancer* 12:309, 1958.
9. Granfield CAJ, Charnsangajev C, Dubrow RA, Varma DGK, Curley SA et al: Regional lymph node metastases in carcinoma of the left side of the colon and rectum. CT demonstration, *AJR* 159:757, 1992.
10. Murray D, Hreno A, Dutton J et al: Prognosis in colon cancer: a pathologic reassessment, *Arch Surg* 110:908, 1975.
11. Freeny PC, Marks WM, Ryan JA, Bolen JW: Colorectal carcinoma evaluation with CT: preoperative recurrence, *Radiology* 158:347, 1986.
12. Balthazar EJ, Megibow AJ, Hulnick D, Naidich DP: Carcinoma of the colon: detection and preoperative staging by CT, *AJR* 150:301, 1988.
13. Megibow AJ, Hulnick DH, Balthazar EJ, Bosniak MA: Ovarian metastases: computed tomographic appearances, *Radiology* 156:161, 1985.
14. Steinberg SM, Barkin JS, Kaplan RS et al: Prognostic indicators of colon tumors: The Gastrointestinal Tumor Study Group experience, *Cancer* 57:1866, 1986.
15. Megibow AJ, Balthazar EJ, Cho KC, Medwid SW, Birnbaum BA et al: Bowel obstruction: evaluation with CT, *Radiology* 180:313, 1991.
16. Hulnick DH, Megibow AJ, Balthazar EJ et al: Perforated colorectal neoplasms: correlation of clinical, contrast enema and CT examination, *Radiology* 164:611, 1987.
17. Balthazar EJ, Megibow AJ, Schinella RA, Gordon R: Limitations in the CT diagnosis of acute diverticulitis: comparison of CT, contrast enema, and pathologic findings in 16 patients, *AJR* 154:281, 1990.
18. Balzarini L, Ceglia E, D'Ippolito G, Petrillo R et al: Local recurrence of rectosigmoid cancer: what about the choice of MRI for diagnosis, *Gastrointest Radiol* 15:338, 1990.
19. Neuerburg JM, Klose KC, Bohndorf K, Guenther RW: Rectosigmoid malignancies; evaluation with contrast enhanced MR imaging, *Radiology* 181:209, 1991.
20. deLange EE, Fechner RE, Edge SB, Spaulding CA: Preoperative staging of rectal carcinoma with MR imaging: surgical and histopathologic correlation, *Radiology* 176:623, 1990.
21. Okizuka H, Sugimura K, Omoto Y et al: Assessment with MR imaging of local staging of rectal cancer, *Radiology* 181:209, 1991.
22. Imai Y, Kressel HY, Saul SH, Chao PW et al: Colorectal tumors: an in vitro study of high resolution MR imaging, *Radiology* 177:695, 1990.
23. Chan TW, Kressel HY, Milestone B, Tomachefski J, Schnall M et al: Rectal carcinoma: staging at MR imaging with endorectal surface coil, *Radiology* 181:461, 1991.
24. August DA, Ostrow RT, Sugarbaker PH: Clinical perspective of human colorectal cancer metastasis, *Cancer Metastasis Rev* 3:303, 1984.
25. Sugarbaker PH, Gianola FJ, Dwyer A, Neuman NR: A simplified plan for follow-up of patients with colon and rectal cancer supported by prospective studies of laboratory and radiologic test results, *Surgery* 102:79, 1987.
26. Lee JKT, Stanley RJ, Sagel SS et al: CT appearance for rectal carcinoma, *Radiology* 141:737, 1981.
27. Kelvin FM, Korobkin M, Heaston DK et al: The pelvis after surgery for rectal carcinoma. Serial CT observations with emphasis on nonneoplastic features, *AJR* 141:959, 1983.
28. Butch RJ, Wittenberg J, Mueller PR, Simeone JF, Meyer JE et al: Presacral masses after abdominoperineal resection for colorectal carcinoma: the need for needle biopsy, *AJR* 144:309, 1985.
29. Johnson RJ, Jenkins JP, Isherwood I, James RD, Schofield PF: Quantitative magnetic resonance imaging in rectal carcinoma, *Br J Radiol* 60:761, 1987.
30. Krestin VG, Steinrich W, Friedmann G: Recurrent rectal cancer: diagnosis with MR imaging versus CT, *Radiology* 168:307, 1988.
31. deLange EE, Fechner RE, Wanebo HJ: Suspected recurrent rectosigmoid carcinoma after abdominoperineal resection: MR imaging and histopathologic findings, *Radiology* 170:323, 1989.
32. Kim EE, Haynie TP: Positron emission tomography of ^{18}F-fluorodeoxyglucose in the evaluation of gastrointestinal tumors. In Herlinger H, Megibow AJ, eds: *Advances in gastrointestinal radiology,* vol 2, St Louis, 1992, Mosby–Year Book.
33. Ito K, Kato T, Tadokoro M, Ishiguchi T, Oshima M et al: Recurrent

rectal cancer and scar: differentiation with PET and MR imaging, *Radiology* 182:549, 1992.

34. Gasparini, Riva RP, Moscatelli G, Paganelli G, Benini S et al: Antibody-guided diagnosis: an Italian experience of CEA-expressing tumors, *Int J Cancer* 2(suppl):1144, 1988.

35. Patt YZ, Lamki LM, Shanken J et al: Imaging with indium-111 labeled anticarcinoembryonic antigen monoclonal antibody: ZCE-025 antigen–producing cancer in patients with rising serum carcinoembryonic antigen levels and occult metastases, *J Clin Oncol* 8:1246, 1990.

36. Kramer EL, Noz ME, Sanger JJ, Megibow A, Maguire GQ: CT/SPECT fusion to correlate radiolabeled monoclonal antibody uptake with abdominal CT findings, *Radiology* 172:861, 1989.

40 *Endosonographic Staging of Rectal Cancer*

CLIVE I. BARTRAM
JOHN BEYNON

Wild and Reid[1] pioneered the technique of rectal endosonography (RES) in the 1950s. However, it was not until the early 1980s that the full diagnostic potential of this examination was realized, when the technical development of endoluminal probes had progressed sufficiently to give really detailed views of the bowel wall layers. The first reports of the use of endoluminal scanning in the evaluation of rectal cancer appeared in 1983.[2,3]

Low rectal cancer has traditionally been assessed by digital examination,[4] with a reported accuracy of 60% to 80%[5-7] for predicting tumor confinement to the wall. The Dukes[8] classification, based on the meticulous examination of surgical specimens, reveals the detrimental effect on patient survival when there is tumor penetration of the muscularis propria and lymph node involvement (Table 40-1). This reflects the underlying relationship between the degree of infiltration and the risk of lymphatic spread. For example, there is only a 10% risk of metastasis to lymph nodes when the cancer is limited to the rectal wall, and then only with poorly differentiated tumors; this contrasts with a 70% risk when the cancer has spread into the perirectal tissues.[9] Other pathologic determinants that can be used to predict survival include the histologic grade of the cancer and the extent of lymphocytic infiltration.[10]

The extent of tumor infiltration is therefore only one of several factors in the staging of rectal cancer. Although it may be true that the present surgical management of the majority of rectal cancers will not be influenced significantly by preoperative staging, there are situations in which accurate staging may influence management. For instance, adjuvant therapy may be considered for large tumors, or for those invading local structures. Local excision may be appropriate in selected patients if the tumor is small (<3 cm), mobile, well differentiated, in the low rectum, and there is no lymph node involvement.[11,12]

The value of RES therefore rests on the extent to which clinicians consider it to be more accurate in determining rectal wall infiltration or lymph node involvement than other investigations and whether the information obtained will alter patient management.[4]

TECHNIQUE AND APPARATUS

A number of different types of probes are available for RES. Both authors have used the Brüel & Kjær rectal endoprobe (Fig. 40-1) almost exclusively. This probe can be inserted through a rectoscope (length, 20 cm; internal diameter, 19 mm), which is really essential when examining lesions above the main rectal fold, locating small tumors, and passing the probe through an anastomosis. Inserting a probe blindly through an anastomosis is potentially dangerous, and it is difficult to negotiate the probe around the rectal fold without direct vision and air insufflation. Blind insertion therefore effectively limits RES to the examination of tumors in the distal 12 cm of the rectum.[13]

The plane for scanning is usually either transverse or longitudinal, although some multiplanar probes are now available. The radial view generated by a mechanically rotating probe may be preferred,[13] but requires a water-filled latex

□ **TABLE 40-1**
The Dukes[8] classification of rectal cancer

Group	Definition	5-year survival
A	Spread by continuity into submucosa or muscularis propria but not beyond; no lymph node involvement	90%-100%
B	Tumor has penetrated muscularis propria; no lymph node involvement	50%-70%
C	Lymph node involvement irrespective of tumor extent	25%-35%
Subdivisions		
C1	Nodes not involved at surgical ligature	
C2	Nodes involved at ligature	

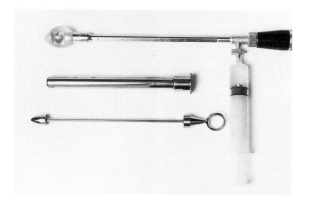

Fig. 40-1 The type 1850 Brüel & Kjaer endoprobe with a water-filled balloon and 7-MHz transducer attached. With the balloon deflated, this may be passed through the short rectoscope shown.

balloon for achieving acoustic contact and for preventing damage to the rectal wall. Linear arrays still require a water-filled rectum for acoustic transmission, but this does not have to be contained within a latex balloon. A disadvantage of balloons is that the balloon presses the lesion into the bowel wall, which may lead to an overestimation of the degree of penetration of the tumor (Fig. 40-10).

The Brüel & Kjær rectal probe (type 1850) is 24 cm in length and 17 mm in maximum diameter. A 5.5- or 7-MHz endoprobe may be fitted to it. For most applications, the 7-MHz probe is preferred. This has a focal length of 2 to 4.5 cm, with a minimum beam width of 1.1 mm. The endoprobe is mechanically rotated, and the speed of rotation can be varied between 1.9 and 2.8 cycles per second. Specially designed latex balloons are secured over the probe by two retaining rings. The entire assembly may be covered with a condom, with some gel first applied over the balloon to prevent any air interface. Only limited cleaning of the assembly is then necessary between cases; otherwise, the probe must be dismantled, cleaned, and disinfected in glutaraldehyde for 20 minutes.

It is important that the rectum is cleared of all fecal matter before the examination, and standard bowel preparations may be used for this purpose. A disposable enema, however, may leave a semifluid layer on the mucosa. Instead, the use of two glycerin suppositories has been recommended, as no fluid residue is left.[5] Patients are examined in the left lateral position. If the lesion is easy to palpate, the probe may be inserted blind; otherwise, the rectoscope should be inserted first, the lesion identified, and then the probe inserted so that it lies above the lesion. When the balloon has been distended with 40 to 60 ml of degassed water, the transducer can be switched on. If this is done before balloon distention, the balloon may tear. The probe and rectoscope are then moved slowly down over the area of interest. The position of the probe and volume of water in the balloon should be varied to obtain optimum images

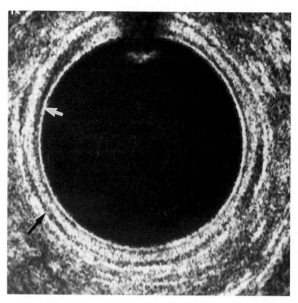

Fig. 40-2 Normal sonographic five-layer appearance of the rectal wall. The inner bright echo *(white arrow)* is formed from the balloon and mucosa interfaces. Immediately deep to this is the inner hypoechoic ring, representing the deep mucosa and muscularis mucosae. The outer hypoechoic ring *(black arrow)* is the muscularis propria. Between these lies the hyperechoic submucosa. Outside the muscularis propria is another hyperechoic layer possessing a poorly defined outer border. This represents the adventitia of the rectum as it merges into the perirectal fat. A gas bubble within the water-filled balloon creates an acoustic shadow superiorly.

of the lesion. This is usually accomplished with the probe lying centrally in the water-filled balloon, which places the rectal wall in the middle of the probe's focal range. In the presence of high rectal lesions (>12 cm from the anal canal), the probe cannot be moved back over the lesion and the rectoscope must be reinserted.

NORMAL ENDOSONOGRAPHIC ANATOMY OF THE RECTAL WALL

Using the Brüel & Kjær 7-MHz probe, five layers should be visible in the rectal wall, consisting of three hyperechoic layers interspersed with two hypoechoic layers[5,13] (Fig. 40-2). There has been much discussion in the literature as to whether some of these layers actually represent true anatomic layers of the bowel wall or simply acoustic reflections at anatomic interfaces, as the thickness of the layers is less or close to the axial resolution of the probe.[14] The number of layers reported varies between two and seven,[15-20] although all authors agree that the outer hypoechoic layer represents the muscularis propria. Using higher-frequency probes (7.5-MHz linear or 12-MHz rotating), this layer may be seen to be separated by a narrow echogenic band (Fig. 40-3), representing the division be-

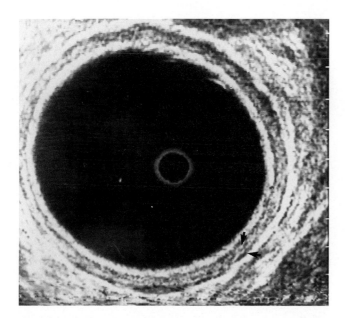

Fig. 40-3 In part of the wall it is possible to see the muscularis propria divided into two layers *(arrows),* an inner circular and an outer longitudinal.

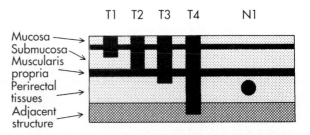

Fig. 40-4 The TNM classification of colorectal carcinoma,[21] slightly modified for application to rectal cancer. The prefix "u" is often used to denote ultrasound staging. *T1,* Tumor invasion into the submucosa; *T2,* invasion of the muscularis propria; *T3,* invasion through the muscularis propria into the perirectal tissues; *T4,* tumor directly invades local organs or structures; *N0,* no regional lymph node involvement; *N1,* metastasis to perirectal lymph nodes.

tween the inner circular and outer longitudinal muscle layers of the rectum.[13,20]

When scanning is done with the probe in a water bath, the balloon creates a thin bright reflection. However, when resected specimens were suspended in a water bath,[18,19] the initial hyperechoic reflection was still present, even without the interposition of a balloon. Stripping the mucosa left the inner hypoechoic layer, which disappeared when the muscularis mucosae was removed. Stripping the submucosa eliminated the intervening echogenic layer, and the outer hypoechoic layer was abolished when the muscularis propria was detached. The findings from such in vitro experiments have confirmed that the mucosal interface is the source of the inner hyperechoic reflection, with the balloon merely adding to the strength of this reflection. The inner hypoechoic layer represents a combination of the mucosa and muscularis mucosae. The next hyperechoic layer is the submucosa, and the outer hypoechoic layer, the muscularis propria.

Peripheral to the muscularis propria is an nonhomogeneous echogenic layer made up of perirectal fat, vessels, and lymph nodes. The superior rectal artery divides at the S3 vertebral level, and its divisions on either side of the rectum may sometimes be visible. The venous pattern is irregular, and veins may be seen running obliquely in and out of view as the probe is moved. Normal mesorectal lymph nodes are small, with a maximum diameter of 3 mm; they are isoechoic with the fat.

Anteriorly, the bladder is visible in both sexes. In males, the seminal vesicles, prostate, and bulbourethral glands can be observed, and, in females, the vagina and uterus are seen superiorly. Sometimes the fallopian tubes and ovaries can be seen.

Common artifacts are caused by air bubbles in the balloon (see Fig. 40-2), which create an arc of reverberation echoes, and fecal residue between the balloon and the rectal wall, which imparts an irregular speckled texture.

ASSESSMENT OF DEPTH OF TUMOR PENETRATION

Rectal cancer, in keeping with most gastrointestinal cancer, is relatively uniformly hypoechoic, and is staged endosonographically by assessing tumor penetration of the bowel wall and lymph node involvement according to the TMN classification[21] (Fig. 40-4). The prefix "u" may be added to denote staging by ultrasound.

T1 tumors are confined to the submucosa, with no interruption to this bright middle interface (Fig. 40-5). A 7-MHz probe does not seem to provide sufficient resolution to permit a benign lesion to be distinguished from an early T1 carcinoma. A T2 cancer is still confined to the rectal wall. The hypoechoic muscularis propria is not breached, and, although it may be thinned or distorted, the outer edge remains intact (Figs. 40-6 and 40-7). T3 tumors penetrate the wall and invade the perirectal fat. The edge of the tumor is often irregular with small peglike projections (Fig. 40-8). Penetration may be quite localized, so that the lesion must be scanned carefully throughout its length. Invasion of an adjacent structure places the tumor in the T4 category (Fig. 40-9).

The reported accuracy for TMN staging, when the endosonographic findings are compared with histologic findings in resected specimens, varies from 81% to 93%, with a mean of 88.2%[3,7,14,17,22-28] (Table 40-2). In a study of 38 cases of rectal cancer,[19] invasion beyond the muscularis propria was predicted with a sensitivity of 96%, specificity of 92%, and positive predictive value of 96%. Tumors may be understaged when there are localized 1- to 2-mm exten-

☐ **TABLE 40-2**

Accuracy of rectal endosonography in the assessment of tumor penetration

Reference	No. of cases	% Correct
Dragstedt and Gammelgaard[3]	13	85
Hildebrandt and Feifel[22]	25	92
Konishi et al.[17]	38	84
Romano et al.[23]	23	91
Saitoh et al.[16]	88	90
Hildebrandt et al.[14]	76	88
Rifkin and Wechsler[24]	81	84
Beynon et al.[25]	100	93
Goldman et al.[26]	32	81
Candio et al.[27]	55	90
Glaser et al.[28]	117	88
Konishi et al.[20]	49	90
Dershaw et al.[7]	38	90
		(mean, 88.2%)

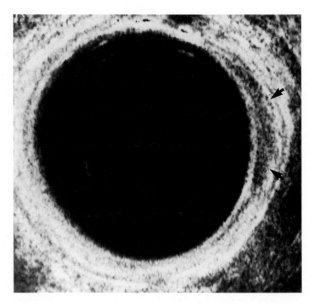

Fig. 40-5 A uT1 tumor. The submucosa is invaded but intact *(arrows).*

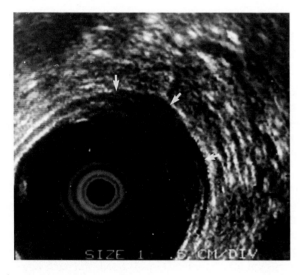

Fig. 40-6 A uT2 tumor. The submucosa has been breached and the muscularis propria invaded, though intact *(arrows).*

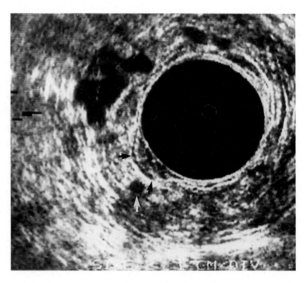

Fig. 40-7 A uT2 tumor. The muscularis propria is intact *(small black arrows).* A hypoechoic lymph node is seen *(white arrow),* which, after resection, was found to be inflammatory.

sions into the muscle or perirectal fat, which are either not recognized or below sonographic resolution. In practice, overstaging lesions as T3 tumors represents more of a problem, and again depends on the acoustic resolution for ascertaining whether the muscularis propria is breached. Two other technical problems may contribute to the problem of overstaging associated with radial scanning. In the first, when a lesion is not at right angles to the beam, as is frequent in the rectal ampulla, the angled view of the tumor with regard to the bowel wall may give a exaggerated impression of tumor penetration. The second is a general point, in that, as the balloon is distended, it tends to press a polypoid lesion into the wall. The lumen may look circular but the outer aspect of the wall bulges out where the lesion has been pressed into it, and this may make it more difficult to trace the muscularis propria throughout (Fig. 40-10).

The maximum thickness of the tumor may also be re-

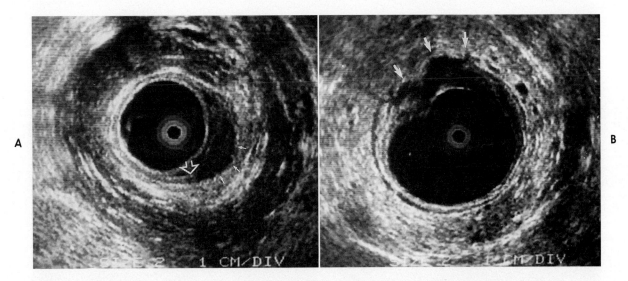

Fig. 40-8 Two examples of uT3 tumors. **A,** The invaded end of the submucosa and muscularis propria is clearly seen *(open arrow),* with irregular peglike extensions into the perirectal fat *(small white arrows)* indicating early penetration of the muscularis propria. **B,** More obvious infiltration of the perirectal fat *(arrows).*

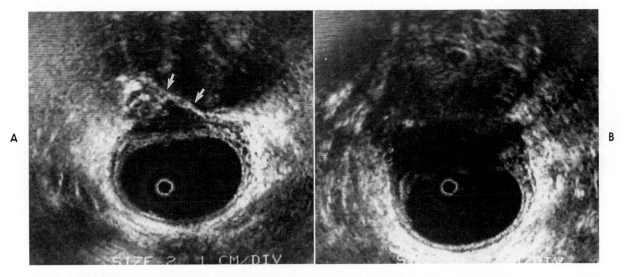

Fig. 40-9 A uT4 tumor. **A,** At this level, the small anterior carcinoma has not breached Denonvillier's fascia, which is seen as a bright interface *(arrows)* between the rectum and the prostate. **B,** At a slightly higher level, the interface is no longer visible and the tumor has infiltrated the prostate.

corded, to indicate its lateral extent and to furnish some estimate of the circumferential involvement based on how many quadrants are affected (Fig. 40-11). When there is extramural spread, infiltration of the pelvic structures, notably of the prostate or vagina, must be excluded. Loss of the echogenic capsular reflection indicates prostatic invasion (see Fig. 40-9). Invasion of the rectovaginal septum may also be assessed by endovaginal scanning. Involve-

ment of more peripherally placed structures within the pelvic cavity is more accurately determined by computed tomography.

Ultrasound staging is complicated in patients who have undergone preoperative radiotherapy, as the resulting edema and fibrosis obliterate normal tissue planes[7,29] (Fig. 40-12). All tumors may appear to be transmural. Acute perirectal changes may also suggest infiltration of adjacent

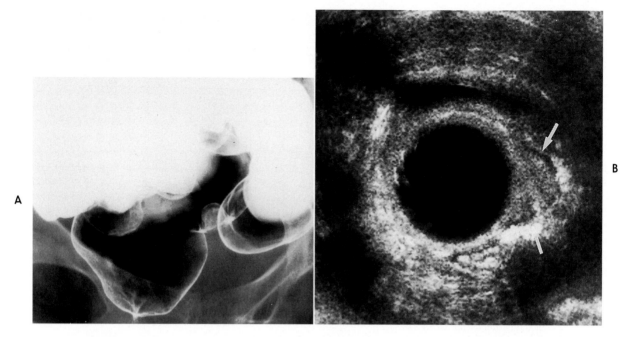

Fig. 40-10 Balloon pressure on a lesion has deformed the wall, and led to misdiagnosis. **A,** The barium enema shows an 11-mm sessile polyp in the distal rectum, which proved to be benign when the excisional biopsy specimen was examined histologically. **B,** On a rectal endosonographic image, the lesion *(arrows)* seems to have invaded the muscularis propria, suggesting a uT2 lesion, when in reality was a uT0 polyp.

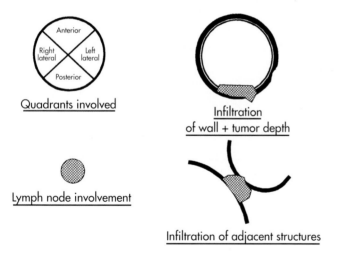

Fig. 40-11 An overview of the rectal endosonographic assessment of rectal cancer. The tumor may be defined by the quadrant, or quadrants, involved, the depth of bowel wall infiltration (uTMN staging), lymph node involvement, and the infiltration of adjacent structures.

structures, such as the prostate. Such problems may be resolved by obtaining a delayed repeat scan when the acute radiotherapy-induced changes have subsided.[7] In one study,[29] rectal cancer was accurately staged in 86%, but this figure was only 47% in those patients who had undergone irradiation (Fig. 40-13). Experience with this problem is limited, but it seems prudent to remain critical of endosonographic staging following radiotherapy.

LYMPH NODE INVOLVEMENT

Visualization of the side wall of the pelvis is limited with the equipment currently available, and only the lymph nodes in the mesorectum are effectively scanned. These perirectal lymph nodes are small, usually less than 3 mm in diameter, and are seldom visualized because they are isoechoic with perirectal fat.

An in vitro study of perirectal lymph nodes has revealed that there is a significant difference in the attenuation coefficients between nonspecific inflamed nodes and ones with metastatic replacement.[30] In reactive changes the normal tissue architecture is preserved but is destroyed by tumor, and the homogeneous cellular mass creates few reflections. Reactive nodes therefore tend to have internal echoes and metastatic nodes none. Reactive nodes may be homogeneously isoechoic with fat, and visualized only by the presence of a thin peripheral hypoechoic ring, or they may be slightly hypoechoic relative to fat but with internal echoes (Fig. 40-14). By comparison, involved nodes are uniformly hypoechoic with no internal echo, well defined, and either round or oval (Fig. 40-15). Unfortunately, because of variations in inflammatory patterns, about 17% of nodes with mainly edematous changes appear hypoechoic, simulating involvement.

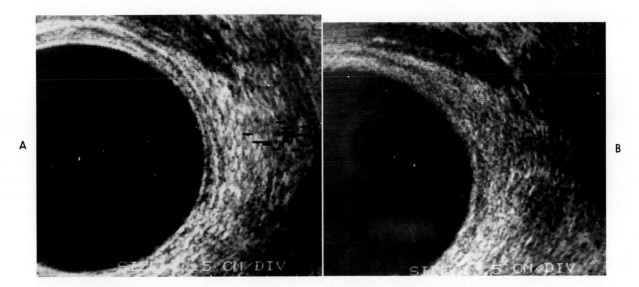

Fig. 40-12 Radiation-induced changes in the bowel wall. **A,** In a female patient who underwent radiotherapy for cervical cancer, the low rectal wall appears normal anteriorly. All the layers are visible. **B,** At a higher level, in which the rectum was within the radiotherapy field, the wall has become thickened and indistinct. Only one hypoechoic layer is identified.

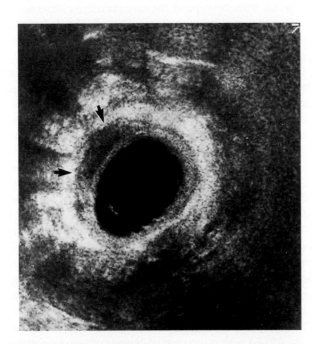

Fig. 40-13 This small rectal cancer had been treated by radiotherapy. The rectum shows quite marked narrowing, thickening of the submucosa, and very echogenic perirectal fat. The normal sonographic layers of the rectal wall have been lost, and it is difficult to determine the extent of penetration of the residual tumor *(arrows).*

Size does not help when it comes to distinguishing reactive from metastatic nodes. Both exceed 3 mm in diameter. In one series, histologically involved nodes ranged from 2 to 13 mm and noninvolved nodes from 0.5 to 12 mm.[31] Although involved nodes were statistically larger than noninvolved nodes, there was sufficient overlap such that size alone is not a reliable criterion for differentiation (Fig. 40-16).

If tumor involvement is assumed for any visible hypoechoic node, a 73% to 86% accuracy may be achieved. In 100 cases of rectal cancer, the sensitivity for predicting involvement was 88%; the specificity, 79%; the positive predictive value, 78%; and the negative predictive value, 89%.[31] By averaging the figures from several reports, an overall accuracy figure of 80% was arrived at (Table 40-3). Earlier studies in which a 5.5-MHz transducer was used

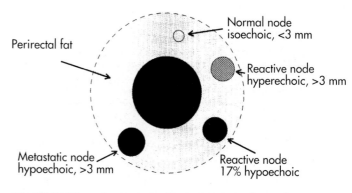

Fig. 40-14 The various sonographic appearances of normal, reactive, and metastatic lymph nodes in the perirectal fat.

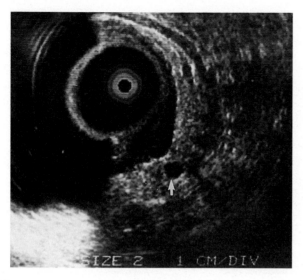

Fig. 40-15 A typical metastatic node *(arrow)* that is 7 mm in diameter, rounded, and uniformly hypoechoic. A uT3 carcinoma is visible just above it.

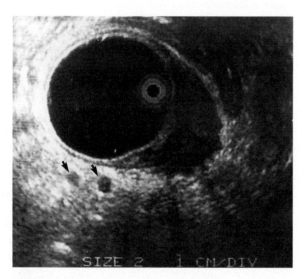

Fig. 40-16 A uT3 carcinoma. Note the peglike projections of tumor infiltration into the perirectal fat. There are also two 5-mm lymph nodes *(arrows)*, which are both reactive and of varying echogenicity.

☐ **TABLE 40-3**

Accuracy of rectal endosonography in assessing perirectal lymph node involvement

Reference	No. of cases	% Correct
Rifkin and Wechsler[24]	81	86
Saitoh et al.[16]	71	73
Beynon et al.[31]	95	83
Hildebrant et al.[30]	113	78
Glaser et al.[28]	117	79
		(mean, 79.8%)

revealed lower sensitivities in the 50% to 60% range, confirming that at least 7 MHz is required to resolve with any accuracy the acoustic changes in perirectal nodes.

Only generalizations regarding lymph node involvement can be made from the endosonographic findings, using the current technology. If no node is seen, the probability of lymph node involvement is low, but high if hypoechoic nodes are present. Hyperechoic nodes are almost certainly due to reactive changes. Those with a mixed pattern are probably inflammatory. A further limitation to RES is the extent to which the lymph node chain can be interrogated. The vascular pedicle in a resection specimen contains nodes well out of the scanning field, so that perhaps only about half the nodes examined pathologically have been scanned.

LOCAL RECURRENCE

Local recurrence is defined as the presence of cancer at or close to the anastomotic site, in the wound or drain site, after primary resection. Recurrence rates of 5% to 20% may be expected within 2 years of surgery, but are even higher with longer follow-up and in autopsy studies.[32] Local recurrence is attributed to inadequate extirpation of the primary tumor at the resection margin, laterally or in the mesorectum,[33] or to the implantation of viable tumor cells shed at the time of surgery. The most important factor is probably residual primary tumor in its lateral extent. Local recurrence may lead to a remorseless, painful death, so early diagnosis with the hope of curative surgery is important.

Recurrent tumor is hypoechoic and clearly defined against the echogenic perirectal fat, so that very small impalpable lesions may be detected by endosonography (Fig. 40-17). Endovaginal ultrasonography can be performed in females after abdominoperineal resection, or to assess an anteriorly located recurrence.

The sonographic appearance of the anastomosis is variable and depends on the method of construction. Some luminal narrowing and irregular thickening of the submucosa and muscle layer are common (Fig. 40-18). If the anastomosis has been stapled, the staples create a composite ring of short linear reflections with minimal acoustic shadowing (Fig. 40-19), or a double hyperechoic row.[34]

Granulomas that form at the anastomosis may be detected and biopsied endoscopically. Sonographically these usually involve only the submucosa (Fig. 40-20), and further extension suggests recurrence (Fig. 40-21). Fluid collections in the pelvic cavity are quite common postoperatively (Fig. 40-22). Small bowel loops, the uterus, and the ovaries lie deeper in the pelvic cavity after resection, and should not be confused with a recurrence. Biopsy of any focal lesion is feasible under ultrasound guidance to achieve histologic confirmation of recurrence.[5,13]

A recurrence rate of 14% was reported for 120 patients. Of the 17 patients with recurrence, six were asymptomatic and the recurrence was detected only by endosonography.

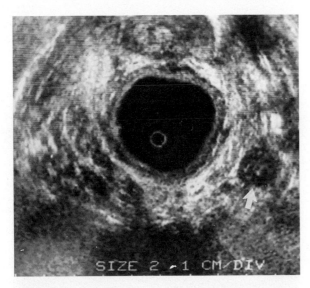

Fig. 40-17 A 12-mm recurrence in the perirectal tissues *(arrow)*.

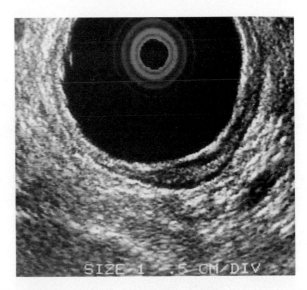

Fig. 40-18 A hand-sewn anastomosis, with the muscle and submucosal layers showing an irregular appearance.

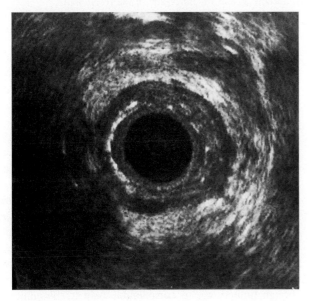

Fig. 40-19 A stapled anastomosis. The staples are visible as highly reflective lesions within the wall.

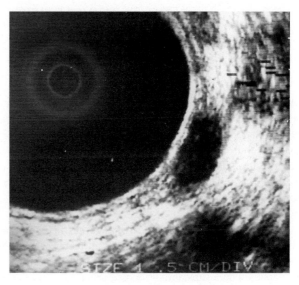

Fig. 40-20 There is a well-defined, 1.5-cm hypoechoic mass near the rectal wall, though it is difficult to ascertain what level it arises from. A granuloma was confirmed in the biopsy specimen.

All six were localized to the pelvis and less than 3 cm, and a "curative" resection was possible.[34] Once the recurrence became symptomatic and detectable by other means, such as digital examination, in many cases, only palliative surgery was then possible.

Endoscopic follow-up is also of value, and, if intraluminal tumor is found, endoscopic biopsy is the obvious investigation. However, most recurrence starts extramurally, with mural infiltration a late phenomenon, so that endoscopy is unlikely to afford diagnosis of recurrence in its early stages, and, when it does, the bulk of the tumor will be extraluminal. In this respect, it is as important to perform

CT following anterior resection, as it is after an abdominoperineal excision. RES combines the advantages of both, plus has the additional benefits of low cost and nonionizing radiation. As with CT, postoperative fibrosis or granulation tissue may pose diagnostic problems. Biopsy is recommended for confirmation, but, to reduce unnecessary biopsies, the lesion may be monitored by repeat studies.[28]

THE ROLE OF ENDOSONOGRAPHY IN RECTAL CANCER

Findings from a number of studies comparing RES to CT in the staging of rectal cancer[5,22-25,35-37] have confirmed

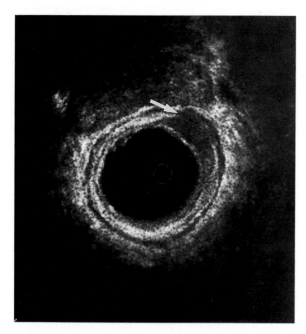

Fig. 40-21 A nodule was palpable within the rectum after local excision of a small rectal cancer. The lesion is seen to have just invaded through the muscularis propria *(arrow)*, and was a uT3 recurrence.

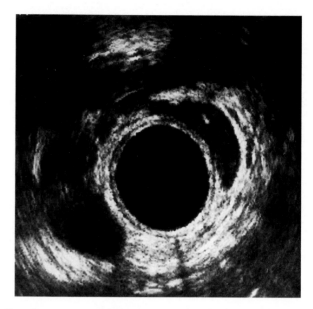

Fig. 40-22 Two large mucous retention cysts create well-defined hypoechoic lesions on either side of the rectal wall.

that RES is more sensitive for predicting perirectal infiltration, and, although capable of demonstrating small perirectal lymph nodes, both techniques fail to distinguish between reactive and involved nodes. CT gives a clearer picture of the pelvic side wall, and would be the examination of choice for assessing large fixed tumors, with RES preferred for smaller mobile lesions being considered for local resection.

Unfortunately, no practical advantage has been demonstrated for the routine RES staging of all rectal cancer. As Dukes showed, spread of tumor outside the rectal wall is associated with a substantially worse prognosis, correlating with lymph node involvement. RES assessment of lymph node involvement is inadequate, however, both in terms of the completeness of the lymphatic pathway examined and in its ability to distinguish early involvement from reactive changes. It also depicts cancers with uniform echogenicity, irrespective of the degree of differentiation, which is another factor that is important in determining prognosis.

However, despite these limitations, the technique has definite value in several clinical situations:

1. To assess small (<3 cm) well-differentiated cancers that are being considered for local resection. RES can reveal the degree of penetration of the bowel wall and whether any lymph node is visible. Penetration through the wall, visualized lymph nodes, or both, would be factors militating against local resection.
2. To reveal the nature of large villous adenomas, be-

cause it may be difficult to exclude clinically a small focus of malignancy. Submucosal resection would be contraindicated if there was invasion of the muscularis propria. RES is an effective method to exclude local invasion.
3. To evaluate low rectal cancers with possible invasion of adjacent structures, such as the prostate.
4. To examine the anastomosis and perirectal tissue for local recurrent disease.
5. To investigate any mass palpable per rectum. As with possible local recurrence, biopsy may be performed under ultrasound guidance for histologic confirmation.

In conclusion, RES is a safe and rapid examination with defined roles in the investigation of rectal cancer, which, although limited, are of considerable help to the clinician in the evaluation and subsequent care of these patients. Experience in this technique is a valuable accomplishment for the radiologist working with coloproctologists.

REFERENCES

1. Wild JJ, Reid JM: Diagnostic use of ultrasound, *Br J Phys Med* 19:248, 1956.
2. Alzin HH, Kohlberger E, Schwaiger R, Allousi S: Valeur de l'échographie endorectale dans la chirurgie du rectum, *Ann Radiol* 26:334, 1983.
3. Dragstedt J, Gammelgaard J: Endoluminal ultrasonic scanning in the evaluation of rectal cancer, *Gastrointest Radiol* 8:367, 1983.
4. Hawley PR: Commentary: does rectal endosonography influence rectal cancer treatment? *Int J Colorect Dis* 1:224, 1986.
5. Beynon J: An evaluation of the role of rectal endosonography in rectal cancer, *Ann R Coll Surg Engl* 71:131, 1989.
6. Nicholls RJ, York Mason A, Morson BC, Dixon AK, Kelsey Fry A: The clinical staging of rectal cancer, *Br J Surg* 69:404, 1982.

7. Dershaw DD, Enker WE, Cohen AM, Sigurdson ER: Transrectal ultrasound of rectal cancer, *Cancer* 66:2336, 1990.

8. Dukes CE, Bussey HJR: The spread of rectal cancer and its effect on prognosis, *Br J Cancer* 12:309, 1958.

9. Morson BC: Factors influencing the prognosis of early cancer of the rectum, *Proc R Soc Med* 59:607, 1966.

10. Jass JR, Atkin S, Cuzick J, Bussey HJR, Morson BC et al: The grading of rectal cancer: historical perspectives and a multivariate analysis of 447 cases, *Histopathology* 10:437, 1986.

11. Whiteway J, Nicholls RJ, Morson BC: The role of surgical local excision in the treatment of rectal cancer, *Br J Surg* 72:694, 1985.

12. Biggers OR, Beart RW, Duane M, Ilstrup MS: Local excision of rectal cancer, *Dis Colon Rectum* 29:374, 1986.

13. Beynon J, Feifel G, Hildebrandt U, Mortensen NJMcC: *An atlas of rectal endosonography,* Vienna, New York, 1991, Springer-Verlag.

14. Hildebrandt U, Fiefel G, Schwartz HP, Scherr O: Endorectal ultrasound: instrumentation and clinical aspects, *Int J Colorectal Dis* 1:212, 1986.

15. Rifkin MD, Marks GJ: Transrectal US as an adjunct in the diagnosis of rectal and extrarectal tumours, *Radiology* 157:499, 1985.

16. Saitoh N, Okui K, Sarashina H, Suzuki M, Arai T et al: Evaluation of echographic diagnosis of rectal cancer using intrarectal ultrasonic examination, *Dis Colon Rectum* 29:234, 1986.

17. Konishi F, Muot T, Takahashi H, Itoh K, Kanazawa K et al: Transrectal ultrasonography for the assessment of invasion of rectal carcinoma, *Dis Colon Rectum* 28:889, 1985.

18. Beynon J, Mortensen NJMcC, Foy DMA, Channer JL, Virjee J et al: Endorectal sonography: laboratory and clinical experience in Bristol, *Int J Colorectal Dis* 1:212, 1986.

19. Beynon J, Foy DMA, Channer JL, Temple LN, Virjee J et al: The ultrasonographic anatomy of the normal colon and rectum, *Dis Colon Rectum* 29:810, 1986.

20. Konishi F, Ugajai H, Ito K, Hanazawa K: Endorectal ultrasonography with a 7.5MHz linear array scanner for the assessment of invasion of rectal cancer, *Int J Colorect Dis* 5:15, 1990.

21. UICC, Hermanek P, Sobin LH, eds: *TMN classification of malignant tumours,* ed 4. New York, 1987, Springer.

22. Hildebrandt U, Feifel G: Pre-operative staging of rectal cancer by intrarectal ultrasound, *Dis Colon Rectum* 28:42, 1985.

23. Romano G, De Rosa P, Vallone G, Rotondo A, Grassi R et al: Intrarectal ultrasound and computed tomography in the pre- and postoperative assessment of patients with rectal carcinoma, *Br J Surg* 72(suppl):S117, 1985.

24. Rifkin MD, Wechsler RJ: A comparison of computed tomography and endorectal ultrasound in staging rectal caner, *Int J Colorectal Dis* 1:219, 1986.

25. Beynon J, Mortensen NJ, Foy DMA, Channer JL, Virjee J et al: Preoperative assessment of local invasion in rectal cancer: digital examination, endoluminal sonography or computed tomography? *Br J Surg* 73:1015, 1986.

26. Goldman S, Arvidsson H, Norming U, Lagerstedt U, Magnusson I et al: Transrectal ultrasound and computed tomography in preoperative staging of lower rectal adenocarcinoma, *Gastrointest Radiol* 16:259, 1991.

27. Candio G, Mosca F, Campatelli A, Cei A, Ferrari M et al: Endosonographic staging of rectal carcinoma, *Gastrointest Radiol* 12:289, 1987.

28. Glaser F, Schlag P, Herfarth C: Endorectal ultrasonography for the assessment of invasion of rectal tumours and lymph node involvement, *Br J Surg* 77:883, 1990.

29. Napoleon R, Pujol B, Berger F, Valette PJ, Gerard JP et al: Accuracy of endosonography in the staging of rectal cancer treated by radiotherapy, *Br J Surg* 78:785, 1991.

30. Hildebrandt U, Klein T, Schwarz H-P, Koch B, Schmitt RM: Endosonography of perirectal lymph nodes, *Dis Colon Rectum* 33:863, 1990.

31. Beynon J, Mortensen NJMcC, Foy DMA et al: Preoperative assessment of mesorectal lymph node involvement in rectal cancer, *Br J Surg* 76:276, 1989.

32. Carlsson U, Lasson A, Ekelund G: Recurrence rates after curative surgery for rectal carcinoma, with special reference to their accuracy, *Dis Colon Rectum* 28:413, 1985.

33. Quirke P, Durdey P, Dixon MF, Williams NS: Local recurrence of rectal adenocarcinoma due to inadequate surgical resection: histopathological study of lateral tumour spread and surgical excision, *Lancet* 2:996, 1986.

34. Mascagni D, Corbellini L, Urciuoli P, Di Matteo G: Endoluminal ultrasound for the early detection of local recurrence of rectal cancer, *Br J Surg* 76:1176, 1989.

35. Waizer A, Ziron S, Ben-Baruch D, Baniel J, Wolloch Y et al: Comparative study for preoperative staging of rectal cancer, *Dis Colon Rectum* 32:53, 1989.

36. Holdsworth PJ, Johnston D, Challmers AC, Chennels B, Dixon HF et al: Endoluminal ultrasound and computed tomography in the staging of rectal cancer, *Br J Surg* 75:1019, 1988.

37. Krammann B, Hildebrant U: Computed tomography versus endosonography in the staging of rectal carcinoma: a comparative study, *Int J Colorectal Dis* 1:216, 1986.

41 *Colorectal Cancer Screening*

F. T. FORK
GILES W. STEVENSON

INCIDENCE OF COLORECTAL NEOPLASIA
Colorectal cancer

The incidence of colorectal cancer (CRC) varies greatly throughout the world. The lowest rates are found in the populations of Africa, Asia, and Latin America. However, in northwestern Europe and North America, CRC ranks as one of the three most common fatal malignancies, along with lung and breast cancer, and members of these populations face a lifetime risk of developing the disease of 5% to 6%.[1,2] Moreover, because the survival statistics in patients who undergo surgical treatment for symptomatic CRC have improved only marginally over the last four decades,[3] the calculated risk of dying of CRC is 2% to 3%.[4,5] The major risk arises after the age of 40.[4] A three to five times increase in the incidence of CRC has been observed in population studies conducted in migrants who have moved from low-risk to high-risk countries. The reasons for the geographic differences are unknown, but are likely to involve environmental factors, including diet.[6]

The chances of cure in patients with CRC depend on the stage at which it is diagnosed. Treatment at an early stage allows 50% of patients to survive 5 years and 29% for 10 years, while, of those with advanced disease, 91% are dead within 5 years, and 97% of those patients who receive only symptomatic treatment die within 5 years.[7] However, almost 25% of the cases of CRC are incidental findings at autopsy,[8] and only 6% of the deaths attributable to CRC occur before the age of 65, so that the main impact of screening for CRC is in preventing death in the elderly.

Colorectal adenoma

Almost all CRC develops from adenomatous polyps, and the risk of malignancy becomes greater with an increase in the size and number of adenomas and the amount of villous component.[9,10] Part of the evidence for this adenoma-to-carcinoma sequence has come from the study of families with familial adenomatous polyposis, in whom affected individuals all develop CRC due to genetic defects in the mucosal epithelium.[11] The prevalence of adenomas increases with age, ranging from 8% to 30% at age 50 and from 34% to 55% at age 80. However, most of these adenomas are small, and the prevalence of adenomas 10 mm or more across is only 3% at the age of 50 and 5.5% at the age of 80.[12,13]

Markers

The genetic defect responsible for familial adenomatous polyposis has been localized to chromosome 5, and its position has been ascertained.[14] The gene itself has also been identified and characterized, thereby allowing much better evaluation of families at risk (Fig. 41-1). Other genetic changes have been found in tissue obtained from sporadic cases of CRC, including changes in the DNA content, mutations in the *ras* oncogenes, and deletions involving chromosomes 5, 17, and 18. Such investigations are providing interesting sidelights that are suggesting, for example, that proximal and distal colon cancers may differ in the genetic mechanisms responsible for their initiation, and offer hope that a simple test may ultimately be developed that would indicate whether an individual faces a high or low risk of acquiring CRC.[15] Very soon it may be possible, as a routine measure, to establish whether an individual in an affected family does, or does not, possess the relevant gene.

RISK FACTORS FOR CRC
Age and sex

CRC is uncommon before the age of 40, but, after 50, the age-specific incidence rate doubles with every decade, with no sex predominance for colon cancer but a male predominance for rectal cancer. The median age at which rectal carcinoma is diagnosed is 67.6 years, and, for colon carcinoma, it is 69.6 years.

Adenoma patient

A patient who has had a single adenoma removed, but no further treatment, faces an 85% risk of developing another metachronous adenoma over the next 25 years,[9] and probably a 12% risk of developing colon cancer over the next 25 years, as well; that is, the risk in these patients is at least doubled compared with that in the general population. The chance of an adenoma containing carcinoma also increases with the size of the lesion; it is around 1% in lesions less than 10 mm, 10% in lesions between 10 and 20 mm, and 30% to 50% in lesions over 2 cm, especially in those with a villous component. The risk of an adenoma degenerating into a carcinoma is approximately 5%, and this risk also becomes greater when the number of adenomas is increased, the size exceeds 2 cm, and villous and tubulovillous components are present[16,17] (Fig. 41-2). Ad-

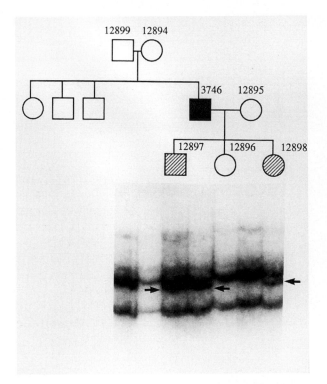

Fig. 41-1 Pedigree and DNA analysis in a family with adenomatous polyposis coli (APC). APC developed in the patient *(#3746)*, although his parents did not have it. DNA analysis shows that he and two of his three children have a unique conformer *(arrows)* that represents a 2-base deletion in the gene DP2.5 (the APC gene), which interferes with its function. This deletion has thus arisen as a spontaneous mutation in this enormous protein; it is heterozygous and has been transmitted to some of his children. (The DNA strip of each individual is directly below the same individual in the pedigree.)
Courtesy of Groden J et al: *Cell* 66:589, 1991.

enomas adjacent to a carcinoma are more likely to be dysplastic or invasive than are solitary adenomas.[18]

Carcinoma patient

A patient with CRC has a 1.5% to 5% chance of having a simultaneous (synchronous) second lesion, and a 5% to 10% chance of a later (metachronous) colon cancer developing.[19] In one series that included a 35-year follow-up, the chance of a second cancer developing rose as high as 19% (four times the average risk). The number of adenomas and cancers present initially seems an important determinant of risk.[9,20]

Cancer family syndromes

It is clear that, in general, relatives of patients with CRC are themselves at increased risk of developing the disease,[21-25] although the actual risk varies from family to family and is often hard to predict for an individual.[26,27] The risk appears to be about two and a half to three times greater for first-degree relatives when only a single family member has CRC,[28,29] but around four to five times greater

when two members have CRC,[30] or if the index case is under 55.[29,31] Although epidemiologic studies have not proved the value of screening the first-degree relatives of a patient with sporadic CRC, some authorities do recommend such screening, starting a little younger than that done in the general population.[32]

Analyses of these families has revealed that they can be subdivided into three groups. In the first are families with no preponderance of cancer in general, but with one or two members who have CRC. The second group consists of those families with defined genetic disorders possessing the hallmark of multiple polyps (the polyposis syndromes). The third group comprises those families who are prone to develop carcinomas at a young age, and CRC in these families has been called *hereditary nonpolyposis colon cancer*.

Hereditary nonpolyposis colon cancer

Hereditary nonpolyposis colon cancer represents the most important group of familial CRC, as it is probably where screening can have its greatest impact on colon cancer mortality, for the least cost. This familial cancer syndrome was first reported by Warthin in 1913, and has been characterized in some detail by Lynch and others.[28,33] Its main features include (1) an autosomal dominant mode of genetic transmission of the liability to colorectal and some other adenocarcinomas, (2) a tendency for the colorectal tumors to be proximal in location,[34] (3) early age of onset, and (4) multiple primary malignancies.

In some families, the risk appears to be limited to CRC (Lynch I), whereas, in others, there is an excess of other cancers, especially endometrial, ovarian, and breast, but also bladder, stomach, skin, pancreas, and brain (Lynch II)[12,35,36] (Fig. 41-3). Although the mode of inheritance follows an autosomal dominant pattern, penetrance is incomplete, and is around 27% for the men and 78% for the women of affected families.[37] The risk of developing colon cancer in an individual from such a family is increased sevenfold over that faced by the general population, and is not less than 35%. In addition, the risk of breast cancer developing in the women of such families is five times greater (1.0 in 3.7).[38] The Lynch syndromes are the source of from 4% to 10% of all cases of CRC, while the inherited polyposis syndromes and inflammatory bowel disease account for only 0.2% and 0.6%, respectively.[39] Thus, focusing screening efforts on families with the Lynch syndrome could make a small but real dent in the mortality from CRC, and, moreover, accomplish this in a younger age group than that usually affected by CRC.

Because flat adenomas in the right colon may be more common in these syndromes (they are usually quite uncommon), their detection requires that both the coating and quality of examination be optimal. If the radiology is not optimal, a high incidence of flat adenomas might warrant an increased indication for performing colonoscopy, though these lesions are also quite easily overlooked endoscopically.

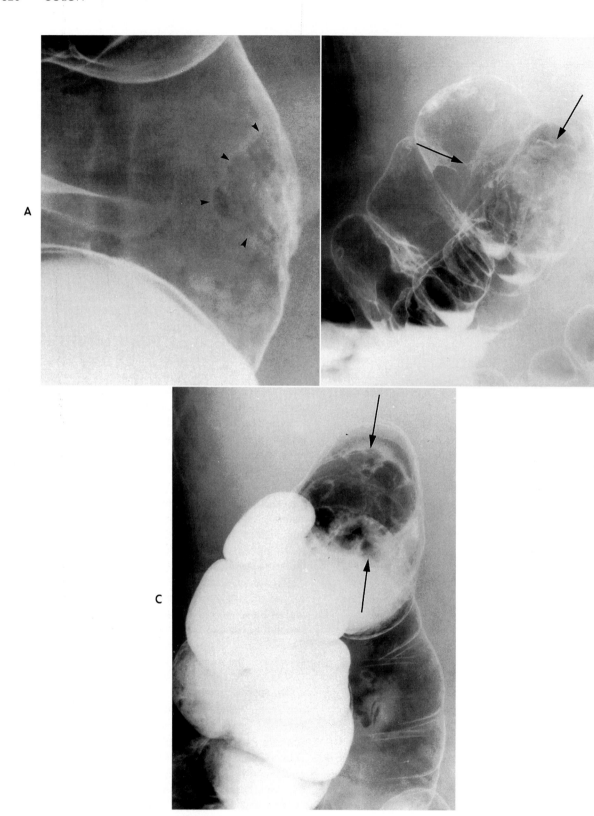

Fig. 41-2 Villous lesions. These tumors may be either sessile (**A**) or polypoidal (**B** and **C**). The flat ones are easy to overlook radiologically and colonoscopically. They often secrete mucus and coat poorly. The lesion in **B** was overlooked at fluoroscopy, but, on review of the film, some large fecal residue was suspected *(arrows)*. Review of an enema study obtained 2 years before (**C**) revealed "feces" at the same spot; colonoscopy subsequently revealed a 5-cm-diameter benign villous adenoma that was resected.

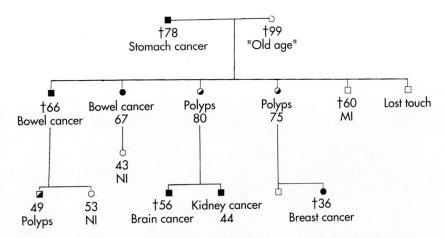

Fig. 41-3 Family tree of a Lynch II family. In the youngest adult generation, the only patient screened underwent adenoma removal, two declined screening, and one is untraceable; two have already died of cancer and the last has survived a renal carcinoma. In Lynch I families, the tumors tend to be limited to the colon. Screening of these families could probably eliminate about 5% of the mortality from colorectal carcinoma in the overall population. *MI*, Myocardial infarction; †, time of death.

Inherited polyposis syndromes

There are several polyposis syndromes, of which familial polyposis coli and Gardner's syndrome are the best known and most common,[34,40,41] occurring in about 1 in 7,000 to 10,000 people. These are inherited as an autosomal dominant trait, and are thought to be either different expressions of the same genetic defect or very closely related. The gene, which has recently been identified on the long arm of chromosome 5, is called *DP 2.5*. It is a huge protein with a molecular weight of around 2 million, which may explain why up to one third of the cases of familial polyposis coli are sporadic[42] (see Fig. 41-1). Many of the mutations discovered in the adenomatous polyposis coli (APC) gene would be expected to inactivate it, and this supports the hypothesis that the normal function of the APC gene is to serve as a tumor suppressor, analogous to the retinoblastoma gene. Clinically, familial polyposis coli constitutes a syndrome of colorectal adenomas, and, in decreasing order of frequency, duodenal, gastric, and small bowel adenomas. Gardner's syndrome, on the other hand, includes multiple soft tissue tumors and osteomatosis,[40,43,44] in addition to the adenomatous polyps. Recent genetic studies have shown that there are more than a dozen distinct variants of the disorder, all of which breed true within a family.

The adenomatous polyps in the colon are very numerous, in excess of a hundred and often as much as in the thousands. They usually start to appear during childhood, though rarely in adult life, and there is about an 80% penetrance of the gene. In those patients in whom adenomas do appear, transformation to carcinoma is inevitable, most often in the left colon.[34,45] Recently, an odd feature in the eye was discovered to be associated with the colon adeno-

mas. This consists of chronic hypertrophy of the retinal pigment epithelium, which can be observed on slit lamp examination. The combination of normal retinas, normal sigmoidoscopic findings, and negative gene markers effectively reduces the likelihood of acquiring the condition to 0.02 at age 20 and to 0.01 by age 30, so that screening may not have to be lifelong.[14,46,47]

Other inherited polyposis syndromes with some risk for malignancy include the Peutz-Jeghers syndrome, Turcot syndrome, and multiple juvenile polyposis, but the risk of malignancy is small for all of these.[48,49]

It is not quite clear where patients with the Muir-Torre syndrome should be classified, as the characteristic features (sebaceous hyperplasia, basal cell cancer, and/or keratoacanthoma with visceral cancers with improved survival) may be found in patients who also fit into the Lynch II category.[38]

Chronic ulcerative colitis

The complication of ulcerative colitis by CRC was described by Crohn and Rosenburg[50] in 1925. There is a geographic variation in the risk, ranging from as low as 9% over the course of 25 years[51] to up to a cumulative incidence of 0.5% to 2% *per year* after the first 10 years.[52-54] However, there is virtually no increased risk of CRC developing in patients with left-sided colitis that has lasted for less than 10 years.[54-58] Screening is more complicated in these patients, as the development of cancer does not progress through the adenomatous polyp stage, but instead through a dysplasia stage,[55,59-62] usually without coexistent cancer.[61]

The dysplastic epithelium is almost flat initially, although, in a certain proportion of cases, a substantial mac-

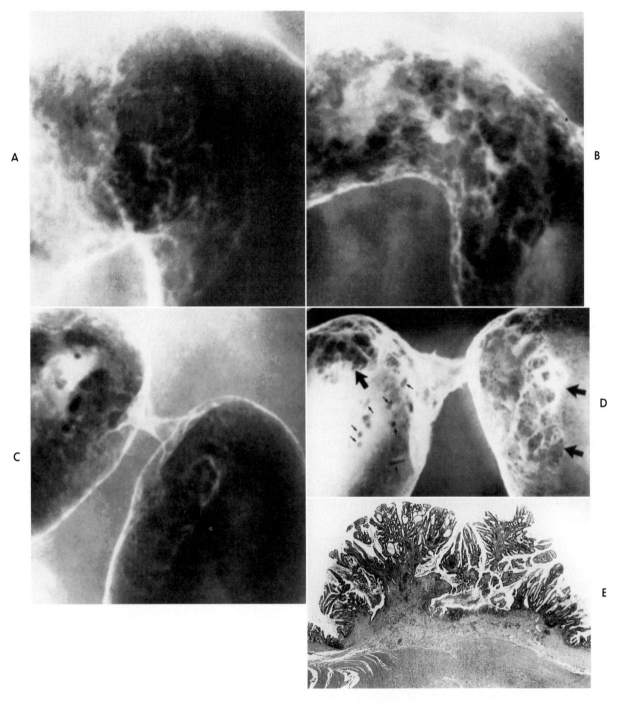

Fig. 41-4 A, Splenic flexure seen on a barium enema study 18 years after the onset of severe ulcerative colitis. **B,** Same region at 20 years showing the development of macroscopically visible dysplasia and slight narrowing. **C,** At 21.5 years, there is a stricture and dysplastic masses on the mucosa on either side, better seen on the resected specimen (**D** and **E**). The stricture was due to adenocarcinoma, which was still limited to the colon, and the patient is still alive 10 years later. The tiny arrows in **D** point to benign postinflammatory polypoidal tags.
From Stevenson GW et al: *AJR* 143:108, 1984.

roscopically visible mass of dysplastic tissue appears, known as *DALM* (the dysplasia-associated lesion or mass), and carcinoma is commonly also present in such cases[63] (Fig. 41-4). Detection of dysplasia requires analysis of biopsy tissue obtained by colonoscopy.[56,64] It is difficult to recognize it in the presence of active inflammation or epithelial regeneration, but the criteria for histologic diagnosis are now well established.[59] The detection of dysplasia is important, as there is an associated increased danger of cancer in the colon, oftentimes remote from the dysplastic mucosa that has been sampled.[65,66]

Flow cytometry DNA analysis is not yet useful as a routine screening tool.[67,68] A barium enema study has little role, although both dysplasia and DALM may be demonstrated if excellent technique is used[69-71] (Fig. 41-4), and this examination may be useful in those patients who have a distal stricture that prevents complete colonoscopy.

Surveillance in patients with chronic ulcerative colitis has not proved beneficial. A review of four surveillance studies revealed that one in five carcinomas was missed by screening,[55,56,61,72-74] and results were no better among those who complied with the protocol than in those who did not. The current results yielded by some continuing trials suggest that those who undergo screening are not likely to live longer than those who do not.[75] The value of such programs has therefore been questioned,[76-78] and early surgery may in fact be safer in the long term in cases of total ulcerative colitis, thereby ensuring a greater likelihood of sustained good health.[62,79] Finally, if the money spent on colonoscopic surveillance in patients with ulcerative colitis were instead spent on screening for occult blood–positive individuals over 50 years of age, this would yield at least ten times as many patients with CRC as are now detected.[80]

Nevertheless, for radiologists, involvement in this problem will be limited to the occasional opportunity to try to demonstrate dysplasia, DALM, or flat infiltrating carcinomas in patients with chronic ulcerative colitis, often when colonoscopy is not possible.

Crohn's enterocolitis

There is a small increase in the incidence of colonic cancer in patients with long-standing Crohn's colitis,[81] and also an increased incidence of cancer in segments of bowel that have been subjected to surgical bypass. There is no evidence of any benefit from screening, although it has been recommended.[82]

PREVENTION OF CRC

The primary prevention of CRC by eliminating its cause through the identification of predisposing genetic or environmental factors is not yet feasible, although some genetic markers have been identified and individuals on high-fat, low-fiber diets show a 1.5 times increase in the incidence of the disease.[6,83]

Secondary prevention is defined as the early detection and removal of premalignant lesions, the adenoma, and can be carried out either by mass screening or case finding.[84,85]

General principles of screening

To put matters into perspective, it is worth noting that the overall increase in life expectancy, if all mortal cancers were eradicated in a given population, would only be 2.5 years.[84] The objective of screening for cancer is to reduce mortality, and an ideal program uses a simple and inexpensive test to identify that small subgroup of a population that is at risk for acquiring a common serious disease at a young age. To accomplish this, there should be a precursor that can be identified, whose simple and inexpensive treatment would eliminate all risk of the disease.[32]

Colon cancer meets some of these criteria, but not all. There is a benign precursor (adenoma) that takes at least 3 years to become detectable,[86] and 5 to 20 years to become cancerous. The characteristics of the adenoma allow some estimation of its malignant potential.[87] Only 42% of the patients, when they present clinically, have curable disease,[88] and surgery before the cancer has spread beyond the bowel substantially improves the chance of cure.[9,16,85,89,90] However, factors that do not meet these criteria are that the precursor exists in 35% of the population, the greatest risk is in the elderly who have the least to gain from screening, the results of simple tests are unreliable, and those tests that are reliable are both expensive and not without risk.

Test acceptability

For a screening test to be effective, it must be acceptable to patients to ensure a high degree of compliance. The main concern of those who undergo screening is whether it will increase their survival.[75] The number and stages of cancers detected in a screening program is irrelevant information in the patient's estimation.

Test validity

The validity of a medical test is described in terms of its sensitivity, specificity,[91] false positives, and false negatives. The prevalence of the disease has an important bearing on the validity. When the vast majority of a population is not afflicted by the disease, the specificity tends to be high for the test, even when screening for a rather common disease such as CRC with a prevalence of 50 per 100,000. As all positives must be further examined to either confirm or exclude the disease screened for, the number of false positives must be kept low. A specific test should entail no unnecessary physical and mental distress on the part of asymptomatic patients, and the costs to the individual and society should be kept to a minimum.

Compliance

A screening program will be unsuccessful if it is not acceptable to those who are offered the test, and will fail unless most of the target population is screened. Low compliance makes it unlikely that any reduction in mortality will be realized,[1] and screening programs should ideally be "consumer oriented and service initiated." This means that the invitation to undergo the test must explain the health benefits, and comment on its acceptability, relevance, and efficacy. The screening service should also provide subsequent repeat tests at appropriate intervals, and be capable of dealing both with those in whom the disease is found and the attendant fears and anxieties.[92] The low compliance rates noted for the ongoing randomized trials for CRC are partly due to public ignorance of the CRC threat, and probably also to the unpleasantness of having to provide fecal samples demanded by the screening test.

Principles in evaluating screening programs
Lead-time bias

The aim of screening for CRC is to find lesions in asymptomatic patients. At the time when such a lesion is detected, it will be many months before it would have caused symptoms. Thus, if it is detected 10 months earlier, without really affecting survival, there will be an apparent 10-month improval in survival after diagnosis.[1] Thus, at its worst, an unsuccessful screening program will simply afford subjects a longer time to live with the knowledge that they have cancer, without any actual prolongation of life (Fig. 41-5).

Length-time bias

Tumors that grow slowly are more likely to be detected by screening, whereas rapidly progressing abnormalities are missed and become symptomatic between screenings; these are called *interval cancers*. The importance of length-bias diminishes with subsequent screenings, but may account for the high survival figures associated with a single episode of screening, due to the less aggressive character of the lesions discovered (Fig. 43-6). Length-time bias partly accounted for the findings in the 1960s concerning patients with lung cancer. Chest x-ray screening was considered responsible for a 23% 5-year survival in asymptomatic patients, versus 5% for those who presented with symptoms.

Selection bias

The probabilities of developing disease differ between screened subjects and controls. Patients with advanced disease will seek out routine medical care, whereas those with vague symptoms may take advantage of a screening program instead. In addition, individuals who participate in a screening program tend to be healthy and they have intrinsically better survival rates for all diseases than do the less healthy and less health-conscious individuals, who tend to refuse screening and are referred to as *nonresponders*.[91] This selection bias is eliminated in randomized trials.

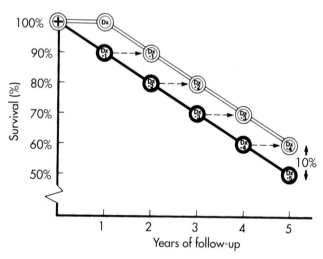

Fig. 41-5 Lead-time bias. Clinical diagnosis and usual survival are represented by the solid line, for a condition in which half the patients are dead after 5 years. If a screening test is used that detects the disease 1 year earlier, and if treatment is actually no more effective when applied earlier, a fictitious 10% improval in survival is achieved, as shown by the open line. This occurs because the starting point for counting survivors has been shifted back 1 year.
From Sackett DL, Haynes RB, Tugwell P: *Clinical epidemiology: a basic science for clinical medicine*, Boston, 1985, Little, Brown.

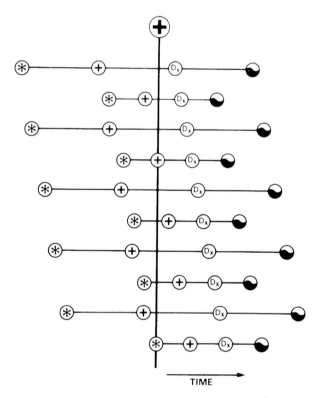

Fig. 41-6 Screening tests tend to detect preferentially the most slowly growing tumors, a phenomenon called *length-time bias*. Tumors that progress rapidly through the phases are less likely to be detected than are those with a lengthy preclinical phase, and adjustment for lead time bias does not correct for this error. Cancer inception; +, the earliest possible detection by the screening test, *Dx*, the usual clinical diagnosis; *yin/yang*, the outcome.
From Sackett DL, Haynes RB, Tugwell P: *Clinical epidemiology: a basic science for clinical medicine*, Boston, 1985, Little, Brown.

Screening intervals

The effectiveness of a screening program also depends on how well and how frequently screening is performed.[92] When planning screening strategies, it is important not to exceed the mean detection lead times gained, because the screening would then detect only the slow-growing tumors. In this situation, extended screening intervals will not result in any earlier detection than that afforded by routine clinical investigations, but instead yield a large number of interval cancers in less favorable stages. As the value of a screening program may only be expressed in terms of reduced mortality rates, not prolonged survival, too long a screening interval will jeopardize the screening results. If the ratio of slow-to-fast–growing cancers in less favorable stages is high, the effect of length bias is increased.[93]

Further bias

It is not known whether the sensitivity of the screening test and the growth rate of CRC varies in different age groups, but, if it were so, this would influence the screening intervals. It is also unknown how many of the screen-detected adenomas or early cancers would never have been lethal. Large autopsy studies show that many CRCs are actually diagnosed after death.[8] In elderly patients, adenomas under 1 cm are also unlikely to produce clinical disease, but, when detected, these patients must then endure the discomfort and risk inherent to the treatment. It seems sensible therefore to regard 75 years as the upper age limit for CRC screening.

In summary, three different types of bias (lead, length, and volunteer selection) can cause a screening program to appear to bring about improved survival, even when it is actually worthless. In addition, three types of harm may be inflicted as the result of an ill-advised screening program. First, the test result may be wrong, in that a positive result may not ultimately indicate the presence of the target disorder. In our experience, only some 8% of those individuals with a positive occult blood test result turn out to have a neoplasm. Second, the treatment may do more harm than good. The lipid-screening program and subsequent clofibrate treatment was responsible for the deaths of at least 5000 asymptomatic Americans.[91] Colonoscopic screening of all Americans starting at age 40, and every 5 years thereafter, would lead to not less than 200 procedure-related deaths a year, with this figure doubling every 5 years. Finally, screening programs can prompt individuals to become overly aware that they are sick or at risk, and some will then modify their lives to their detriment. For these reasons, it is imperative to be sure that a net benefit will result before implementing a general population screening program.[20]

Screening methodology

At present there are no ideal markers for CRC, and the only feasible methods for CRC screening currently available are fecal occult-blood tests (FOBT), endoscopic procedures, and barium enema studies. In the future, genetic screening methods may identify high-risk individuals, who may then proceed to undergo a diagnostic workup.

The efficacy of a screening program is exposed to irrational influences. Its clinical accuracy is reduced by false results, stemming from either random, technical factors, such as fecal residue and incomplete exploration of the colon, or from nonrandom, biologic features, that is, whether a lesion is bleeding at the time of the screen.

False-positive results cause needless anxiety,[94] but are unfortunately encountered with all diagnostic procedures. They are more common with barium enema studies than with endoscopy.

Carcinoembryonic antigen

The carcinoembryonic antigen (CEA) assay is unsuitable for mass screening. Results are negative in the presence of early, localized colon cancers, and levels are sometimes elevated in the presence of cancers from diverse sites as well as nonneoplastic diseases.[95,96]

Fecal occult-blood tests

Since 1901, when Boas first proposed the possible value of FOBT, numerous chromogenic tests have been designed that capitalize on the oxidizing ability of hemoglobin or its derivatives to cause a shift in color.[97]

The ideal test should have a low sensitivity for upper gastrointestinal bleeding and should not register the normal gastrointestinal blood loss of about 0.6 to 2.0 ml per day, but react only to the increased blood loss resulting from a neoplasm.[15,98] The test is reliably positive when the blood loss in stool ranges from 10 to 15 ml per day. The mean blood loss from a CRC depends on its size and location, but is unrelated to Dukes staging.[99] Even though early cancers and premalignant adenomas bleed little and sporadically, tests for occult blood in stool are widely used in CRC screening today because of their relative simplicity and low initial cost.

There are three types of tests for occult blood on the market: the guaiac, the heme-porphyrin, and the Hemselect. The guaiac tests depend on the detection of peroxidase activity of intact heme, with a relatively high sensitivity for identifying bleeding arising from the lower gastrointestinal tract. Haemoccult is the most popular of these tests, and the blood concentration in the stool must be between 500 and 1500 μg per gram for the test to be positive. The guaiac tests are inexpensive, but subjects have to adhere to a no-meat diet and avoid taking vitamin C, aspirin, and other NSAIDs.[94,100,101]

The heme-porphyrin tests such as Hemoquant measure heme and heme-derived porphyrins in stool.[102] This means that blood coming from the right colon, and which has completely broken down to porphyrin, may be detected more reliably by the Hemoquant than by the Hemoccult test, which tends to detect left colon cancers better than those on the right side. This test is very sensitive to the presence of blood, with considerable overlap between normal subjects and patients with CRC. Any blood loss less than 2000 μ per gram is considered normal, which means that the test cannot detect low-grade colonic bleeding.

Hemselect is another new product,[103] and also detects hemoglobin before it breaks down to hematin. The test is said to detect all cases of rectal cancer. Hemselect has been shown in at least one study to be more sensitive than Hemoquant, which in turn was more sensitive than Hemoccult. Therefore, Hemselect is claimed to be the current preferred test, with a specificity of 98%[104]; however, this is a premature claim, as there is still very much more experience with Hemoccult, which is a much simpler test to use. The immunochemical tests are expensive laboratory tests, but have the advantage of not requiring any change in diet or medication. In a series of patients with symptomatic CRC and adenomas, Hemeselect showed a greater sensitivity compared to that observed for other tests of occult blood, especially for adenomas, including those less than 10 mm in diameter.[104] The manufacture of these tests in a simple nonlaboratory form would represent a substantial breakthrough in improving the specificity of occult blood testing.

Diagnostic follow-up procedures

Fecal occult-blood tests will detect some of the cancers in a population survey, but will miss many. They are therefore unsuitable for *excluding* cancer in high-risk subjects. To exclude cancer or adenomas, or to follow up on a positive occult-blood test, a barium enema study, endoscopy, or both are necessary in order to examine the entire large bowel.

Flexible sigmoidoscopy

In 1973, Dale et al.[105] published data from a randomized trial indicating that periodic screening with proctosigmoidoscopy over a 7-year period led to a decrease in the mortality from CRC. Results from other screening programs in which flexible sigmoidoscopy was used have not shown such a reduction in mortality, although the results of one controlled study suggest this.[106] However, its large yield of 40% of benign and malignant neoplastic lesions located in the distal colon and rectum[107] has established flexible sigmoidoscopy as a worthwhile examination in the periodic health checkup, and it is not ineffective as a case detection tool.[108] It has no role as the only imaging method in patients at high risk, or in those with positive occult-blood findings, as the whole colon should be examined in such patients. The perforation rate for flexible sigmoidoscopy in one report was as high as 1 in 2200,[109] but several reports of series have been published that cite no perforations.[107]

Kelvin et al.[110] have recently emphasized that radiolo-

gists need to take increased note of the possibility of lesions in the right colon. He noted that 19% to 24% of colon cancers are on the right side, compared with 8% to 14% in the 1940s. Now that so many lesions in the left colon are being diagnosed by flexible sigmoidoscopy, and these patients then undergo colonoscopy or resection, radiologists may find that up to 40% of the cancers in patients scheduled for barium enema studies are in the right colon.[110]

Diagnostic procedures of the total large bowel

The method used for imaging the entire large bowel depends on the preference of the examiner. The procedures are inconvenient, may cause discomfort and pain, and are also potentially hazardous to the patient. The morbidity figure for the double-contrast barium enema (DCBE) is 0.04% and 1.7% for diagnostic colonoscopy; the mortality rates are one tenth of these.[111-113] As examination of the entire large bowel requires a substantial staff and expensive equipment, neither radiology nor endoscopy is suitable for use in mass screening programs of the general population, especially while these are still of no proven benefit.

RADIOLOGY

The DCBE examination has the advantage of being able to image well even loops and areas beyond an obstruction. The risk of overlooking significant malignant lesions in optimally performed DCBE studies[114,115] is very low, especially if they are double read.[116,117] At 85% to 90%, the sensitivity of such studies for identifying significant polyps approaches that of colonoscopy.[115,118-120] A positive DCBE result may thus identify those patients who should undergo therapeutic colonoscopy. It has been dogma that patients with positive FOBT results should always undergo colonoscopy,[2] even if DCBE findings are negative. However, an increasing amount of data suggests the combination of flexible sigmoidoscopy and a DCBE study is a sufficient compromise for these patients.[121-123] On the other hand, patients in whom colonoscopy was difficult or incomplete, and also those at very great risk for CRC, should undergo both radiographic and colonoscopic examinations.[124] Most series in which the merits of DCBE and colonoscopy have been compared have regarded the colonoscopic results as the gold standard, taking no account of endoscopic false negatives, 39% of which in one series were in the cecum[125] (Fig. 41-7). The endoscopic-based belief that the cecum has been reached is not always true.[126] Both air contrast barium enema studies and colonoscopy are highly sensitive for detecting CRC and can complement each other in this objective. However, colonoscopy is more sensitive for detecting adenomas, especially in the sigmoid colon.[118,122] In our institution, we have found that usually eight to ten adenomas are overlooked on radiographic studies for every lesion missed colonoscopically. The missed lesions are usually small, less than 10 mm in diameter.[124,126,127]

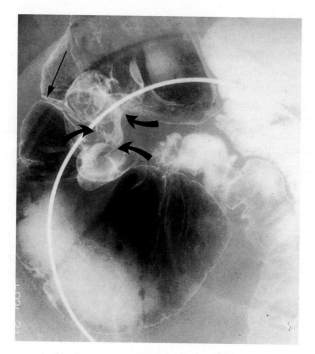

Fig. 41-7 Ascending colon cancer missed by colonoscopy. Colonoscopy was believed to reach the cecum in this patient, but, as anemia remained unexplained, a small bowel meal study was performed. This examination, with carbon dioxide administered per rectum, reveals the tumor *(curved arrows)*. The sulcus above the tumor laterally was presumably mistaken for the cecum, although the appendix and ileocecal valve cannot have been identified. Such errors are becoming more common as the use of colonoscopy becomes widespread. A barium enema study should always be performed after colonoscopy if the ileocecal valve orifice and cecal pole have not been identified with certainty.

COLONOSCOPY

The morbidity and mortality rates associated with diagnostic colonoscopy are small when it is performed by experts. However, if colonoscopy were to be the diagnostic tool in a mass screening program to detect CRC, a large number of new endoscopists would then have to devote themselves to performing it. This would probably translate into an increase in the death rate to up to 0.1%. If the number of lives saved by the early diagnosis of CRC were substantially greater than the number of iatrogenic deaths, this risk might be acceptable. However, those individuals who participate in a screening program are not patients, but asymptomatic subjects who have agreed to take part in a program with the expectation of benefit. Under these circumstances, it is inappropriate to use a screening tool for the general population with a risk of death as high as that associated with colonoscopy.

In the absence of a colonic obstruction, an expert can perform complete colonoscopy 98% the time.[128] If such trained personnel are available, colonoscopy may be regarded as the initial method of choice in high-risk subjects.

In most situations, however, it is more sensible to use the approach suggested by Warden et al.,[129,130] which is to use flexible sigmoidoscopy to determine whether to proceed to a barium enema or colonoscopy study. Those patients shown by flexible sigmoidoscopy to have polyps of 5 mm or greater should then undergo colonoscopy for polypectomy, and those with negative sigmoidoscopic findings should have a barium enema study. Using this protocol, Warden noted that a barium enema study found a polyp in only 1.8% of those patients with negative sigmoidoscopy findings, which was later confirmed (though there were also a few false-positive barium enema results), but that, in 34% of those with adenomas detected by sigmoidoscopy, additional tumors were found by colonoscopy further round the bowel. It has been shown that flexible sigmoidoscopy can be performed immediately before the barium enema (with a considerable increase in the diagnostic yield),[122] and that this does not impair the quality of the radiologic examination.[131] This approach has also been assessed as part of a screening program for high-risk subjects, and it made possible a one-day screen, with most subjects who had polyps undergoing polypectomy at this initial visit. Those without polyps have the benefit of both barium enema and sigmoidoscopic examinations,[132] which ensures added security in the sigmoid, where most radiologic errors occur.

Results of screening programs to date

A reduction in mortality was reported in 1979 for a group screened with sigmoidoscopy, compared with a control group.[105,133] These results have not yet been confirmed by any other studies. Gilbertsen and Nelms[134] showed that the use of rigid sigmoidoscopy led to a reduction in the expected incidence of rectal cancer, but this study was not designed in a way that could demonstrate an effect on mortality.[134]

Clinical trials with FOBT

The sensitivity of the Hemoccult test in the prospective detection of large adenomas and early cancers is approximately 20%, and this is due to the fact that only adenomas more than 20 mm across may lose more than 2 ml of blood per day. The corresponding figure in the detection of all cancers is 25% to 50%, with some patients already in an advanced stage and symptomatic at the time of detection.[99,135] The limited sensitivity of the Hemoccult test for detecting CRC may be explained by the fact that the tumors do not bleed enough or not at all.[136] As a consequence, they show up as interval cancers in the controlled population-based trials.[121,137]

Based on available statistics, the positive predictive value of a positive Hemoccult test result for early stage cancer is calculated to be less than 10%. Not surprisingly, total colonoscopy in 210 asymptomatic individuals who faced an average risk for having CRC, despite negative FOBT results, revealed neoplasms in 53 (25%). Two of these lesions were cancers and the rest were adenomas, all located above the sigmoid colon.[86]

UNCONTROLLED TRIALS

The findings from some uncontrolled trials of three guaiac test kits were reported in the 1970s. A positive rate of 1% to 5% was cited, along with a positive predictive value for CRC of 8% to 12% and for adenoma of up to 47%. Compliance was low, and false-negative results were encountered in 15% of the colon cancer patients and 44% of those with polyps. However, most of the cancers found were Dukes' stage A and B.

CONTROLLED TRIALS

Two major trials are under way in the United States. The first was started in 1974 and consisted of 22,000 asymptomatic patients over the age of 40. Both screened and control groups underwent sigmoidoscopy, and the study group had FOBT, which led to the detection of 45 adenomas and 59 cancers. Of the cancers detected by FOBT, 65% were staged as early, whereas only 33% of those detected by sigmoidoscopy were early.[127] A 43% reduction in mortality was observed over the course of a decade in the screened group, but this did not prove statistically significant.

In the second trial, consisting of 48,000 patients and randomized into groups, 183 cancers were discovered and 22 were missed.[138] Of the cancers, 78% were Dukes' stage A and B.[139] The compliance in both these studies was high at 75% to 80%.

In an attempt to prove a reduction in mortality from screening, three European studies are under way, one in Sweden,[137] one in Denmark,[121] and one in England.[140] Two are using colonoscopic surveillance and one, flexible sigmoidoscopy and barium enema (Table 41-1). Favorable results of the studies have included a high proportion of Dukes' A cancers detected in all three studies; this was 51% for the two Scandinavian studies and 61% for the English one. No decrease in mortality has yet been shown, and, in fact, the sizes of all the present study populations are insufficient to detect a reduction in the mortality rates of 15% to 25%.[141] Given the present screening methods and the realities of compliance, between 250,000 and 380,000 subjects will have to be entered into each arm of a controlled trial and followed for over a decade for meaningful mortality statistics to be realized.[142] Many studies show an interim hope of benefit, in that more cancers have been found among the screened subjects, the histologic staging has been favorable, and the interval cancers have been both fewer and less advanced. However, the results of only two studies have demonstrated longer survival and fewer deaths,[121,143] and these figures are not yet statistically significant.

No reduction in mortality has so far been demonstrated as a consequence of screening for CRC with FOBT, although the compiled data from ongoing studies probably will show this.[121,137,140,143,144] Based on these results, the magnitude of the mortality benefit may reach somewhere between 10% to 30%.[1]

Metaanalysis is a technique that pools results from a number of studies in a statistically valid manner, and might increase the power of the various studies to demonstrate reduced mortality. A serious attempt to do this, however, has yielded data showing that screening of the general population is not yet justified.[136]

Economy

There is no question that the detection of CRC at Dukes' stage A and B improves the 5-year survival from the current 42% to around 80%.[145] However, quite apart from the need to prove reduced mortality, there are a number of other factors that must be considered when assessing the merits of screening a population. Physicians as well as politicians increasingly have to be concerned with the optimum allocation of financial resources in the community.[145] A positive FOBT is inexpensive,[146,147] but costs will be incurred from radiology and endoscopic investigations as well as in

---

☐ **TABLE 41-1**

European randomized screening trials for colorectal cancer*

				No. of cases				
				Screen-detected cancer				
Study	No. of subjects	Compliance	Pos FOBT	Adenoma	Cancer	Interval cancer	Nonresponders	Controls
Kerwenter[137] 1988	13,759	65%	882	154	51	16	10	20
Kronberg[121] 1989	30,970	67%	215	221	50	40	39	115
Hardcastle[140] 1989	53,464	53%	618	367	76	22	83	123

Data from Ekelund G, Lindström C: *Gut* 15:654, 1974; Stower MJ, Hardcastle JD: *Eur J Surg Oncol* 11:119, 1985.

*Interim results of some major fecal occult-blood test (FOBT) trials. Note that, although there is a good yield of cancer, compliance is not high, interval cancers are not uncommon, and there are many cancers in nonresponders. It is likely that mortality reduction will be demonstrated soon, but better tests and strategies are needed to identify those who need detailed examination.

terms of time lost from work, and curative surgery may be more expensive than palliative treatment.[148] The costs of mounting and maintaining a screening program for an entire country are huge, and constitute some billions of dollars in the United States.[1] The costs would be substantially reduced if screening were instead directed only to the small groups of subjects who are at high risk, but this will not appreciably influence the mortality from CRC in the population as a whole, as less than 10% of CRC patients actually fall into such high-risk groups.

Summary and screening guidelines

The primary aim of screening programs is to reduce mortality,[84] and, although CRC tends to affect an older population that is also at risk for death from other causes, the early detection and curative treatment of CRC in a *young* patient would mean many years gained in life expectancy. It may well be, however, that the major benefit from screening will not be in terms of a reduction in mortality, but stem from a reduction in morbidity through the need for less extensive treatment.

Screening programs are a source of mental stress for the participants, especially that due to false-positive results, and this has to be considered in the overall harm-to-benefit ratio of a program. However, this may be less of a concern in CRC screening than in breast cancer screening. The perceived stress level resulting from a Hemoccult screening program was found to be similar for both those with negative results and those with false-positive ones, and both groups deemed the test worthwhile.[149] Those in whom no cancer was found, but an adenoma removed, considered themselves saved from a potentially mortal disease, rather than the "victims of a false alarm."

Average-risk individual

Several organizations recommend a screening protocol consisting of annual fecal occult-blood testing and flexible sigmoidoscopy performed every 3 to 5 years, while others do not advocate any screening for average-risk individuals.[1] It is clear that there is still no evidence of decreased mortality from CRC screening, and there is not yet any justification for the use of public resources to screen average-risk individuals. However, if screening is to be carried out beyond simple occult-blood testing, a combined approach consisting of an initial flexible sigmoidoscopy examination followed by an air contrast barium enema study is recommended. This allows the radiologist to focus more attention on the cecum, where cancer is common and endoscopy often difficult. A DCBE study, however, fails to detect half of the polyps in the rectosigmoid area, whereas flexible sigmoidoscopy overlooks almost one fifth.[122] There is a 50% probability that a 5-mm polyp is an adenoma, and this is 93% for those larger than 5 mm.[122,150-153] The chance that an adenoma under 5 mm is an invasive cancer is almost nil[153] (Table 41-2). Flexible sigmoidoscopy by itself pro-

□ **TABLE 41-2**

Incidence of cancer in colon polyps*

Size (mm)	Status	Incidence	Status	Incidence
<5	In situ	2 (0.4%)		
6-9	Early	15 (4.9%)	Advanced	1 (0.3%)
10-19	Early	38 (20%)	Advanced	3 (1.6%)
20-30	Early	15 (28%)	Advanced	21 (39%)
>31	Early	2 (0.3%)	Advanced	254 (99%)

Modified from Matsukawa M: Barium enema and polyp detection. In Maruyama M, Kimura T, eds: *Review of clinical research in gastroenterology*, New York, 1988, Igaku Shoin.
*Only dysplasia (cancer in situ) was found in adenomas under 5 mm, and even in polyps (6-9 mm) there was only a single tumor (0.3%) invading beyond the submucosa. Only very safe procedures can be justified to detect lesions of this size, bearing in mind the slow growth rate of such tumors.

vides almost as great a benefit from a statistical standpoint as it does when performed in combination with DCBE, even though it cannot examine the proximal colon.[107]

Previous CRC

Because the risk of a second carcinoma rises steadily to a cumulative 20% after 25 years in patients who have had CRC, such patients should undergo a thorough check of the whole colon around the time of their treatment, and, then, for those who survive, regular follow-up. This should consist of either barium enema studies combined with flexible sigmoidoscopy or of colonoscopy, and both this choice and the interval between examinations depends on the nature of the initial lesion, whether there were other polyps, and, if so, their size and histologic type. Once two consecutive examinations have confirmed that the colon is clear, follow-up every 5 years is sufficient.

A similar regimen is appropriate after the removal of a significant adenoma (>9 mm), but there is no information on how often, or even if, follow-up is required after the removal of tiny (<5 mm) adenomas.[90] Although it is current practice to do so,[2] others have expressed reservations because of the excessive cost involved and because the risk associated with the procedures is actually higher than the risk from disease.[154]

Familial CRC

FAMILIAL POLYPOSIS SYNDROME

Patients with familial polyposis syndrome should be screened yearly beginning in adolescence, and those who do not have colectomy should be screened at 3-year intervals after the age of 35. Because of the documented excess of right colon tumors in this disorder, which may be flat adenomas, a case can be made for the selection of colonoscopy as the screening tool.[15,31] It may be acceptable to discontinue screening after the age of 25 in those with negative sigmoidoscopy findings, no evidence of chronic retinal pigment hypertrophy, and no gene markers for the disease.[14,46,47]

HEREDITARY NONPOLYPOSIS COLON CANCER

Members of families affected by hereditary nonpolyposis colon cancer (Lynch I and II) face a risk of up to 40% of acquiring the disease, which is at least seven times that of the general population.[1,37,38] They should be screened either from the age of 40, or 10 years younger than the earliest age at which colon cancer was diagnosed in their family, whichever is younger. Either flexible sigmoidoscopy combined with barium enema studies or colonoscopy should be the screening method. After the results of two consecutive examinations are negative, screening every 5 years is probably sufficient. Particular care should be taken to achieve an excellent examination of the right colon.

FIRST-DEGREE RELATIVES OF COLON CANCER PATIENTS

This is a difficult group to come to any definite conclusions about. The numbers of subjects involved is often large, and the increased risk that they face is only modest. If a decision is made to screen only the relatives of patients whose disease appeared when they were younger than 55, and those with two members of the family with colon cancer, this will reduce the numbers to about 10%, and will include almost all the families with hereditary nonpolyposis colon cancer. Compliance is also much greater among the relatives of these younger colon cancer patients.

☐ HOW TO DECIDE WHEN TO SEEK AN EARLY DIAGNOSIS* ☐

1. Does early diagnosis really lead to improved clinical outcomes (in terms of survival, function, and quality of life)?
2. Can you manage the additional clinical time required to confirm the diagnosis and provide long-term care for those who screen positive?
3. Will the patients in whom an early diagnosis is achieved comply with your subsequent recommendations and treatment regimens?
4. Has the effectiveness of individual components of a periodic health examination or multiphasic screening program been demonstrated prior to their combination?
5. Does the burden of disability from the target disease warrant action?
6. Are the cost, accuracy, and acceptability of the screening test adequate for your purpose?

From Sackett DL, Haynes RB, Tugwell P: *Clinical epidemiology: a basic science for clinical medicine*, Boston, 1985, Little, Brown.
*Questions that should be satisfied before embarking on screening programs. The answer is still "no" for 4 and 6, while 2 and 3 are problematic. That 1 and 5 deserve an emphatic "yes" encourages further work on colorectal screening.

Finally, having constructed some guidelines, it is possible to apply a simple test to check whether they are based on reasonable and sound evidence. Sackett has formulated six questions that should be considered before deciding to seek an early diagnosis for a disease (see box below).

For CRC, the answers to questions 1 and 5 are a definite "yes." For questions 2 and 3, the response has to be "only for those who are not very old and are at seriously increased risk," while, for questions 4 and 6, the answer is "no." It is frustrating not to be able to screen for, and prevent, a disease that has such a long and macroscopically visible premalignant phase, but simple tools for identifying only those who need treatment are not yet available, and it is important to avoid doing more harm than good in the wake of the enthusiasm to screen.

REFERENCES

1. Ransohoff DF, Lang CA: Screening for colorectal cancer, *N Engl J Med* 325:37, 1991 (current concepts).
2. Fleischer DE, Goldberg SB, Browning TH et al: Detection and surveillance of colorectal cancer, *JAMA* 261:580, 1989.
3. Bailar JC III, Smith EM: Progress against cancer? *N Engl J Med* 314:1226, 1986.
4. Schottenfeld D, Winawer SJ: Large intestine. In Schottenfield D, Fraumeni JF, eds: *Cancer epidemiology and prevention*, Philadelphia, 1982, WB Saunders.
5. Seidman H, Mushinski MH, Gelb SK et al: Probabilities of eventually developing or dying of cancer—United States 1985, *CA Cancer J Clin* 35:36, 1985.
6. West DW, Slattery ML, Robinson LM et al: Dietary intake and colonic cancer: sex and anatomic site–specific associations, *Am J Epidemiol* 130:883, 1989.
7. Berge T, Ekelund G, Mellner C et al: Carcinoma of the colon and rectum in a defined population, *Acta Chir Scand* [Suppl] 438:1,1973.
8. Berge T, Lundberg S: Cancer in Malmö 1958-1969. An autopsy study, *Acta Pathol Microbiol Scand* [Suppl] section A, 1977.
9. Morson BC: Genesis of colorectal cancer. *Clin Gastroenterol* 505, 1976.
10. Winawer SJ, Zauber AG, Stewart E et al: The natural history of colorectal cancer. Opportunities for intervention, *Cancer* 67:1143, 1991.
11. Bodmer WF, Bailey CJ, Bodmer J et al: Localization of the gene for familial adenomatous polyposis on chromosome 5, *Nature* 328:614, 1987.
12. Chapman I: Adenomatous polypi of large intestine: incidence and distribution, *Ann Surg* 157:223, 1963.
13. Vatn MH, Stalsberg H: The prevalence of polyps of the large intestine in Oslo: an autopsy study, *Cancer* 49:819, 1982.
14. Tops CMJ, Wijnem JT, Griffoen G et al: Presymptomatic diagnosis of familial adenomatous polyposis by bridging DNA markers, *Lancet* 2:1361, 1989.
15. Hardcastle JD, Winawer SJ, Burt RW et al: Screening for colorectal neoplasia, *Working Party Reports* 1990, pp 27-35.
16. Morson BC: The evolution of colorectal carcinoma, *Clin Radiol* 35:425, 1984.
17. Lambert R, Sobin LH, Waye JD et al: The management of patients with colorectal adenomas, *CA Cancer J Clin* 34:167, 1984.
18. Ekelund G, Lindström C: Histopathological analysis of benign polyps in patients with carcinoma of the colon and rectum, *Gut* 15:654, 1974.
19. Schottenfeld D: Patient risk factors and the detection of early cancer, *Prev Med* 1:335, 1972.
20. Schottenfeld D, Berg JW, Virsky B: Incidence of multiple primary

cancers. II. Index cancers arising in the stomach and lower digestive system, *J Natl Cancer Inst* 43:77, 1969.

21. Fraumeni JF: Clinical patterns of family cancer. In Mulvihill JJ, Miller RW, Fraumeni JF, eds: *Genetics of human cancer,* New York, 1977, Raven Press.

22. Cannon-Albright LA, Skolnick MH, Bishop DT et al: Common inheritance of susceptibility to colonic adenomatous polyps and associated colorectal cancer, *N Engl J Med* 319:533, 1988.

23. Li FF: Investigative approach to familial cancer: clinical studies. In Mulhivill JJ, Miller RW, Fraumeni JF, eds: *Genetics of human cancer,* New York, 1977, Raven Press.

24. Rozen P, Fireman Z, Terdiman R et al: Selective screening for colorectal tumours in the Tel-Aviv area: relevance of epidemiology and family history, *Cancer* 47:827, 1981.

25. Lovett E: Familial factors in the etiology of carcinoma of the large bowel, *Proc R Soc Med* 67:21, 1974.

26. Grossman S, Milos ML: Colonoscopic screening of persons with suspected risk factor for colon cancer. 1. Family history, *Gastroenterology* 94:395, 1988.

27. Armitage NC, Farrands PA, Mangham CM et al: Faecal occult blood screening of first degree relatives of patients with colorectal cancer, *Int J Colorect Dis* 1:248, 1986.

28. Lynch HT, Lynch PM, Albana WA et al: Hereditary cancer: ascertainment and management, *CA Cancer J Clin* 29:216, 1979.

29. Lovett E: Family studies in cancer of the colon and rectum, *Br J Surg* 63:13, 1976.

30. Rozen P, Ron E: A cost-effective analysis of using colonoscopy for screening family members of colon cancer patients, *Gastrointest Endosc* 34:219, 1988.

31. Rozen P, Fireman Z, Figer A et al: Family history of colorectal cancer as a marker of potential malignancy within a screening program, *Cancer* 60:248, 1987.

32. Winawer SJ, Prorok P, Macrea F et al: Surveillance and early diagnosis of colorectal cancer, *Cancer Detect Prev* 8:373, 1985.

33. Cannon-Albright LA, Thomas TC, Bishop DT et al: Characteristics of familial colon cancer in a large population data base, *Cancer* 64:1971, 1989.

34. Anderson DE: Familial predisposition. In Schottenfeld D, Fraumeni JR, eds: *Cancer epidemiology and prevention,* Philadelphia, 1982, Saunders.

35. Lynch HT, Lynch PM, Lynch JF: Analysis of genetics of inherited colon cancer. In Winawer SJ, Schottenfield D, Sherlock P, eds: *Colorectal cancer, prevention, epidemiology, and screening,* New York, 1980, Raven Press.

36. Heinzelmann R: A cancer prone family. Discussion of the question of inheritability of colonic carcinoma, *Helv Chir Acta* 31:316, 1964.

37. Itoh H, Houlston RS, Harcopos C et al: Risk of cancer death in first-degree relatives of patients with hereditary nonpolyposis cancer syndrome (Lynch type II): a study of 130 kindreds in the United Kingdom, *Br J Surg* 77:1367, 1990.

38. Lynch HT, Watson P, Kreigler M et al: Differential diagnosis of hereditary nonpolyposis colorectal cancer (Lynch syndrome 1 and Lynch syndrome II), *Dis Colon Rectum* 31:372, 1988.

39. Mecklin J-P: Frequency of hereditary colorectal carcinoma, *Gastroenterology* 93:1021, 1987.

40. Gardner EJ, Richards RC: Multiple cutaneous and subcutaneous lesions occurring simultaneously with hereditary polyposis and osteomatosis, *Am J Hum Genet* 5:139, 1953.

41. Erbe RW: Inherited gastrointestinal polyposis syndrome, *N Engl J Med* 294:1101, 1976.

42. Groden J, Thliveris A, Samowitz et al: Identification and characterization of the familial adenomatous polyposis coli gene, *Cell* 66:589, 1991.

43. Coli RD et al: Gardner's syndrome: a revisit to the previously described family, *Am J Dig Dis* 15:551, 1970.

44. Ziter MH: Roentgenographic findings in Gardner's syndrome, *JAMA* 192:158, 1965.

45. Lynch PM, Lynch HT, Herns RE: Hereditary proximal colon cancer, *Dis Colon Rectum* 20:661, 1977.

46. Houlston R, Slack J, Murday V: Risks estimates for screening adenomatous polyposis coli, *Lancet* 335:484, 1990.

47. Chapman PD, Church W, Burn J et al: The detection of congenital hypertrophy of retinal pigment epithelium (CHRPE) by indirect ophthalmoscopy: a reliable clinical feature of familial adenomatous polyposis, *Br Med J* 298:353, 1989.

48. Kussin SZ, Lipkin M, Winawer SJ: Inherited colon cancer, state of the art, *Am J Gastroenterol* 72:448, 1979.

49. Bussey HJR, Veale AMO, Morson BC: Genetics of gastrointestinal polyposis, *Gastroenterology* 74:1325, 1978.

50. Crohn BB, Rosenberg H: The sigmoidoscopic picture of chronic ulcerative colitis (non-specific), *Am J Med Sci* 170:220, 1925.

51. Hughes RG, Hall TJ, Block GE et al: The prognosis of carcinoma of the colon complicating ulcerative colitis, *Surg Gynecol Obstet* 146:46, 1978.

52. Devroede G: Risk of cancer in inflammatory bowel disease. In Winawer SJ, Schottenfield D, Sherlock P, eds: *Progress in cancer research and therapy,* New York, 1980, Raven Press.

53. Lennard-Jones JE, Morson BC, Ritchie JK et al: Cancer in colitis: assessment of the individual risk by clinical and histological criteria, *Gastroenterology* 73:1280, 1977.

54. Greenstein AJ, Sachar DD, Smith H et al: Cancer in universal and left-sided ulcerative colitis: factors determining risk, *Gastroenterology* 77:290, 1979.

55. Rosenstock E, Farmer RG, Petras R et al: Surveillance for colonic carcinoma in ulcerative colitis, *Gastroenterology* 89:1342, 1985.

56. Nugent FW, Haggitt RC: Results of a long-term prospective surveillance program for dysplasia in ulcerative colitis, *Gastroenterology* 86:1197, 1986.

57. Granqvist S, Gabrielsson N, Sundelin P et al: Precancerous lesions in the mucosa in ulcerative colitis, *Scand J Gastroenterol* 15:289, 1980.

58. Gyde SN, Prior P, Allan RN et al: Colorectal cancer in ulcerative colitis: a cohort study of primary referrals from three centres, *Gut* 29:206, 1988.

59. Ridell RH, Goldman H, Ransohoff DF et al: Dysplasia in inflammatory bowel disease: standardized classification with provisional clinical applications, *Hum Pathol* 14:931, 1983.

60. Kerwenter J, Ahlman H, Hultén L: Cancer risk in extensive ulcerative colitis, *Ann Surg* 15:824, 1978.

61. Lennard-Jones JE, Melville DM, Morson BC et al: Precancer and cancer in extensive ulcerative colitis: findings among 401 patients over 22 years, *Gut* 31:800, 1990.

62. Ekbom A, Helmick C, Zack M et al: Ulcerative colitis and colorectal cancer: a population-based study, *N Engl J Med* 323:1228, 1990.

63. Löfberg R, Broström O, Karlén P et al: Colonoscopic surveillance in long-standing total ulcerative colitis—a 15-year follow-up study, *Gastroenterology* 99:1021, 1990.

64. Lennard-Jones JE, Morson BC, Ritchie JK et al: Cancer surveillance in ulcerative colitis: experience over 15 years, *Lancet* 2:149, 1983.

65. Ransohoff DF, Riddell RH, Levin B: Ulcerative colitis and colonic cancer: problems in assessing the diagnostic usefulness of mucosal dysplasia, *Dis Colon Rectum* 28:383, 1985.

66. Ehsanullah M, Filipe MI, Gazzard B: Mucin secretion in inflammatory bowel disease: correlation with disease activity and dysplasia, *Gut* 23:485, 1982.

67. Löfberg R, Tribukait B, Öst Å et al: Flow cytometric DNA analysis in longstanding ulcerative colitis: a method of prediction of dysplasia and carcinoma development? *Gut* 28:1100, 1987.

68. Fozard JBJ, Quirke P, Dixon MF et al: DNA aneuploidy in ulcerative colitis, *Gut* 28:1414, 1987.

69. Frank P, Riddell R, Feczko P et al: Radiological detection of colonic dysplasia (precarcinoma) in chronic ulcerative colitis, *Gastrointest Radiol* 3:209, 1978.

70. Kelvin F, Woodward B, McLeod M et al: Prospective diagnosis of dysplasia (precancer) in chronic ulcerative colitis, *AJR* 138:347, 1982.

71. Stevenson GW, Goodacre R, Jackson R et al: Dysplasia to carcinoma transformation in ulcerative colitis, *AJR* 143:108, 1984.

72. Nugent FW, Haggitt RC: Long-term follow-up, including cancer surveillance for patients with ulcerative colitis, *Clin Gastroenterol* 9:459, 1980.

73. Collin RH, Feldman M, Fordtran JS: Colon cancer, dysplasia, and surveillance in patients with ulcerative colitis, *N Engl J Med* 316:1654, 1987.

74. Blackstone MO, Riddell RH, Rogers BHG et al: Dysplasia associated lesion or mass (DALM) detected by colonoscopy in longstanding ulcerative colitis. An indication for colectomy, *Gastroenterology* 80:366, 1981.

75. Gyde S: Screening for colorectal cancer in ulcerative colitis: dubious benefits and high costs, *Gut* 31:1089, 1990.

76. Jones HW, Grogono J, Hoare AM: Surveillance in ulcerative colitis: burdens and benefit, *Gut* 29:325, 1988.

77. Thirlby RC: Colonoscopic surveillance for cancer in patients with chronic ulcerative colitis: is it working? Selected summaries, *Gastroenterology* 100:570, 1991.

78. Fozard JBJ, Dixon MF: Colonoscopic surveillance in ulcerative colitis—dysplasia through the looking glass, *Gut* 30:285, 1989.

79. Lennard-Jones JE: Cancer risk in ulcerative colitis: surveillance or surgery, *Br J Surg* 72(suppl):S84, 1985.

80. Miller MP, Stanley TV: Results of a mass screening program for colorectal cancer, *Arch Surg* 123:63, 1988.

81. Lightdale CJ, Sherlock P: Cancer in Crohn's disease: Memorial Hospital experience and review of the literature. In Winawer SJ, Schottenfeld D, Sherlock P, eds: *Progress in cancer research and therapy,* New York, 1980, Raven Press.

82. Winawer SJ, Schottenfeld D, Flehinger BJ: Colorectal cancer screening, *J Natl Cancer Inst* 84:243, 1991.

83. Zedeck MS: Experimental colon carcinogenesis. In Lipkin M, Good RA, eds: *Gastrointestinal tract cancer,* New York, 1978, Plenum.

84. Miller AB: Principles of screening and of the evaluation of screening programs. In Miller AB, ed: *Screening for cancer,* Toronto, 1985, Academic Press.

85. Winawer SJ: Detection and diagnosis of colorectal cancer, *Cancer* 51:2519, 1983.

86. Rex DK, Lehman GA, Hawes RH et al: Screening colonoscopy in asymptomatic average-risk persons with negative fecal occult blood tests, *Gastroenterology* 100:64, 1991.

87. Morson BC: The polyp-cancer sequence in the large bowel, *Proc R Soc Med* 67:451, 1974.

88. Stearns MW Jr: Adenocarcinoma. In Stearn MW Jr, ed: *Neoplasms of the colon, rectum and anus,* New York, 1980, John Wiley.

89. Stower MJ, Hardcastle JD: The results of 1115 patients with colorectal cancer treated over an 8-year period in a single hospital, *Eur J Surg Oncol* 11:119, 1985.

90. Stryker SJ, Wolff BG, Culp CE et al: Natural history of untreated polyps, *Gastroenterology* 93:1009, 1987.

91. Sackett DL, Haynes RB, Tugwell P: *Clinical epidemiology: a basic science for clinical medicine,* Boston, 1985, Little, Brown.

92. Hobbs P: Factors affecting population participation in breast cancer screening. In Ziant G, ed: *Practical modalities of an efficient screening for breast cancer in the European community,* Amsterdam, 1989, Excerpta Medica.

93. Moskowitz M: Breast cancer screening: all's well that ends well, or much ado about nothing, *AJR* 151:659, 1988.

94. Knight K, Fielding J, Battista R: Occult blood screening for colorectal cancer, *JAMA* 261:587, 1989.

95. LoGerfo P, Krupey J, Hansen HJ: Demonstration of an antigen common to several varieties of neoplasia, *N Engl J Med* 285:138, 1971.

96. Constanza ME, Das S, Nathanson L et al: Carcinoembryonic antigen: report of a screening study, *Cancer* 33:583, 1974.

97. Gregor DH: Diagnosis of large-bowel cancer in asymptomatic patients, *JAMA* 201:943, 1967.

98. Stroehlein JR, Fairbanks VF, McGill DB et al: Hemoccult detection by fecal occult blood quantitated by radioassay, *Am J Dig Dis* 21:841, 1976.

99. Macrae FA, St John DJB: Relationship between patterns of bleeding and Haemoccult sensitivity in patients with colorectal cancer or adenomas, *Gastroenterology* 82:891, 1982.

100. Fleisher M, Schwartz MK, Winawer SJ: Fecal occult blood testing. In Miller AB, ed: *Screening for cancer,* Toronto, 1985, Academic Press.

101. Macrae FA, St John DJ, Caligiore P et al: Optimal dietary conditions for Haemoccult testing, *Gastroenterology* 82:899, 1982.

102. Ahlquist DA, McGill DB, Fleming JL: Patterns of occult bleeding in asymptomatic colorectal cancer, *Cancer* 63:1826, 1989.

103. Va'ananan P, Tenhunen R: Rapid immunochemical detection of faecal occult blood by use of a latex agglutination test, *Clin Chem* 34:1763, 1988.

104. St John DJB, Young GS, Alexeyeff M et al: Most large and medium colorectal adenomas can be detected by immunochemical occult blood tests, *Gastroenterology* 98(suppl A):312, 1990.

105. Dale LG, Friedman GD, Ramcharan S et al: Multiphasic checkup evaluation study: 3. Outpatient clinic utilization, hospitalization, and mortality experience after 7 years, *Prev Med* 2:221, 1973.

106. Selby JV, Friedman GD, Collen MF: Sigmoidoscopy and mortality from colorectal cancer: the Kaiser Permanente Multiphasic Evaluation study, *J Clin Epidemiol* 41:427, 1988.

107. Eddy DM: Screening for colorectal cancer, *Ann Intern Med* 113:373, 1990.

108. Eddy DM, Nugent FW, Eddy JF et al: Screening for colorectal cancer in a high-risk population, *Gastroenterology* 92:682, 1987.

109. Gupta TP, Silverman AL, Desai TK et al: Prevention of colon cancer in primary care practice, *Primary Care* 16:157, 1989.

110. Kelvin FM, Maglinte DDT, Stephens BA: Colorectal carcinoma detected initially with barium enema examination: site distribution and implications, *Radiology* 169:649, 1988.

111. Ott DJ, Gelfand DW, Yu MC et al: Colonoscopy and barium enema: a radiologic viewpoint, *South Med J* 78:1033, 1985.

112. Frühmorgen P, Demling L: Complications of diagnostic and therapeutic colonoscopy in the Federal Republic of Germany. Results of an inquiry, *Endoscopy* 11:146, 1979.

113. Lörinc P, Brahme F: Perforation of the colon during examination by the double contrast method, *Gastroenterology* 37:770, 1959.

114. Beggs I, Thomas BM: Diagnosis of carcinoma of the colon by barium enema, *Clin Radiol* 34:423, 1983.

115. Fork FT, Lindström, Ekelund GR: Reliability of routine double contrast examination of the large bowel in polyp detection: a prospective clinical study, *Gastrointest Radiol* 8:163, 1983.

116. Kelvin FM, Gardiner R, Vas W, Stevenson GW: Colorectal carcinoma missed on double contrast barium enema study: a problem in perception, *AJR* 137:307, 1981.

117. Markus JB, Somers S, O'Malley BP et al: Double contrast barium enema studies: effect of multiple reading on perception error, *Radiology* 175:155, 1990.

118. Ott DJ, Gelfand DW, Wu WC et al: Sensitivity of double contrast barium enema: emphasis on polyp detection, *AJR* 135:327, 1980.

119. Williams CB, Macrae FA, Bartram CI: A prospective study of diagnostic methods in adenoma follow up, *Endoscopy* 143:74, 1982.

120. Waye J, Braunfield S: Surveillance intervals after colonoscopic polypectomy, *Endoscopy* 14:79, 1982.

121. Kronberg O, Fenger C, Olsen J et al: Repeated screening for colorectal cancer with fecal occult blood test. A prospective randomized study at Funen, Denmark, *Scand J Gastroenterol* 24:599, 1989.

122. Saito Y, Slezak P, Rubio C: The diagnostic value of combining flexible sigmoidoscopy and double-contrast barium enema as a one-stage procedure, *Gastrointest Radiol* 14:357, 1989.

123. Farrands PA, Vellacott KD, Amar SS et al: Flexible fiberoptic sig-

moidoscopy and double contrast barium enema in the identification of adenomas and carcinomas of the colon, *Dis Colon Rectum* 26:725, 1983.

124. Macrae FA, Williams CB: Sigmoidoscopy and other tests for colorectal cancer. In Miller AB, ed: *Screening for cancer,* New York, 1985, Academic Press.

125. Glick SN, Teplick SK, Balfe DM et al: Large colonic neoplasms missed by endoscopy, *AJR* 152:513, 1989.

126. Fork F-T: Radiographic findings in overlooked colon carcinomas. A retrospective analysis, *Acta Radiol* 29:331, 1988.

127. Winawer SJ, Andrews M, Flehinger B et al: Progress report on controlled trial of fecal occult blood testing for the detection of colorectal neoplasia, *Cancer* 45:2959, 1980.

128. Waye JD, Bashkoff E: Total colonoscopy: is it always possible? *Gastrointest Endosc* 37:152, 1991.

129. Warden MJ, Petrelli NJ, Herrera L et al: The role of colonoscopy and flexible sigmoidoscopy in screening for colorectal carcinoma, *Dis Colon Rectum* 30:52, 1987.

130. Warden MJ, Petrelli NJ, Herrera L et al: Endoscopy versus double contrast barium enema in the evaluation of patients with symptoms suggestive of colorectal carcinoma, *Am J Surg* 155:224, 1988.

131. Eckardt VF, Kanzler G, Willems D: Same day versus separate day sigmoidoscopy and double contrast barium enema: a randomized controlled study, *Gastrointest Endosc* 35:512, 1989.

132. Stevenson GW, Hernandez C: Single visit screening and treatment of first degree relatives: colon cancer pilot study, *Dis Colon Rectum* 34:1120, 1991.

133. Dales LG, Friedman GD, Collen MF: Evaluating periodic multiphasic health checkups: a controlled trial, *J Chron Dis* 32:385, 1979.

134. Gilbertsen VA, Nelms J: The prevention of invasive cancer of the rectum, *Cancer* 41:1137, 1978.

135. Bang KM, Tillett S, Hoar A et al: Sensitivity of fecal occult blood testing and flexible sigmoidoscopy for colorectal cancer screening, *J Occup Med* 28:709, 1986.

136. Windeler J, Köbberling J: Colorectal carcinoma and Haemoccult. A study of its value in mass screening using meta-analysis, *Int J Colorect Dis* 2:223, 1987.

137. Kerwenter J, Björk S, Haglind E et al: Screening and rescreening for colorectal cancer. A controlled trial of fecal occult blood testing in 27,700 subjects, *Cancer* 62:645, 1988.

138. Mandel JS, Bond JH, Bradley M et al: Sensitivity, specificity, and positive predictivity for the Hemoccult test in screening for colorectal cancer, *Gastroenterology* 97:597, 1989.

139. Gilbertsen VA, McHugh R, Schuman L et al: The earlier detection of colorectal cancers. A preliminary report of the results of the occult blood study, *Cancer* 45:2899, 1980.

140. Hardcastle JD, Armitage NC, Chamberlain J et al: Fecal occult blood screening for colorectal cancer in the general population. Results of a controlled trial, *Cancer* 58:397, 1986.

141. Carlsson U, Ekelund G, Eriksson R et al: Evaluation of possibilities for mass screening for colorectal cancer with Hemoccult (R) fecal blood test, *Dis Colon Rectum* 29:553, 1986.

142. Lindgren B: Screening for cancer: the economic perspective. Paper presented at the 21st Berzelius Symposia, University of Lund. Malmö, 1991, The Swedish Institute for Health Economics.

143. Flehinger BJ, Herbert E, Winawer SJ et al: Screening for colorectal cancer with fecal occult blood test and sigmoidoscopy: preliminary report of the colon project of Memorial Sloan-Kettering Cancer Center and PMI-Strang Clinic. In Chamberlain J, Miller AB, eds: *Screening for gastrointestinal cancer,* Toronto, 1988, Huber.

144. Enke WE, Laffer UT, Block GE: Enhanced survival of patients with colon and rectal cancer is based upon wide anatomic resection, *Ann Surg* 190:350, 1979.

145. Simpson P: Economic aspects of screening. In: Prorok PC, Miller AB, eds: *Screening for cancer* (UICC Technical Report Series), vol 78, Geneva, 1984, pp 81-93.

146. Walker A, Whynes DK, Chamberlain JO et al: The cost of screening for colorectal cancer, *J Epidemiol Commun Health* 45:220, 1991.

147. Woodward A, Weller D: Colorectal cancer: implications of mass screening for public health, *Med J Austr* 153:81; 564, 1990.

148. Tuck J, Walker A, Whynes DK et al: Screening and the costs of treating colorectal cancer: some preliminary results, *Public Health* 103:413, 1989.

149. Mant D, Fitzpatrick R, Hogg A et al: Experiences of patients with false positive results from colorectal cancer screening, *Br J Gen Pract* 40:423, 1990.

150. Ott DJ, Gelfand DW, Ramquist NA: Causes of error in gastrointestinal radiology. II. Barium enema examination, *Gastrointest Radiol* 5:99, 1980.

151. Maxfield RG, Maxfield CM: Colonoscopy as a primary diagnostic procedure in chronic gastrointestinal tract bleeding, *Arch Surg* 121:401, 1986.

152. Laufer IG, Smith NCW, Mullens JE: The radiological demonstration of colorectal polyps undetected by endoscopy, *Gastroenterology* 70:167, 1976.

153. Matsukawa M: Barium enema and polyp detection. In Maruyama M, Kimura T, eds: *Review of clinical research in gastroenterology,* New York, 1988, Igaku Shoin.

154. Ransohoff DF, Lang CA, Kuo HS: Colonoscopic surveillance after polypectomy: considerations of cost effectiveness, *Ann Intern Med* 114:177, 1991.

42 Defecography: Techniques and Normal Findings

FREDERICK M. KELVIN
GILES W. STEVENSON

In the past decade, there has been an explosion of interest in anorectal physiology and disorders of defecation. These disorders fall into two main categories: those involving impaired or incomplete evacuation (obstructed defecation) and those resulting in anal incontinence. There is a wide range of investigative methods for the assessment of anorectal dysfunction, including anorectal manometry, electromyography, and nerve stimulation studies. Defecography (evacuation proctography) has assumed a prominent role within this spectrum of techniques.

It demonstrates the anorectal anatomy and serves as a method of observing and recording the act of rectal evacuation. It furnishes a unique assessment of anorectal function. It is, therefore, appropriate to review some of the basic anatomic and physiologic features of the anorectal region before discussing the technique itself.

ANATOMIC AND PHYSIOLOGIC CONSIDERATIONS

The anal canal, which is approximately 4 cm long, extends from the anorectal junction to the anal verge. Two strong muscular sphincters surround the anal canal so that, at rest, it is completely collapsed and forms an anteroposterior slit. Anal endosonography can directly image these two sphincters, and is particularly useful for demonstrating sphincteric defects in the setting of anal incontinence.

The deeper of the two sphincters (that closest to the lumen) is the internal anal sphincter (IAS), which is a direct continuation of the circular muscle of the rectum. This smooth muscle sphincter is responsible for supplying about 80% of the resting tone of the anal sphincter complex. Acute distention of the rectum leads to relaxation of the IAS, a response referred to as the *rectoanal inhibitory reflex.*

The voluntary external anal sphincter (EAS) is the more superficial sphincter (the one farthest from the lumen and nearest the skin) (Fig. 42-1). Despite being composed of striated muscle, the EAS exhibits resting electrical activity. Its main action, however, is to squeeze the anal canal tightly shut when it is voluntarily contracted. This causes the anal canal to both lengthen and constrict. The main nerve supply of the EAS originates from the pudendal nerve.

The third muscle involved in maintaining continence is the puborectalis. It arises from the pubic symphysis and passes backward to form a sling around the distal rectum. When the puborectalis contracts, it draws the rectum forward, and thereby maintains the anorectal angle (Fig. 42-1). The puborectalis is the most anterior component of the levator ani, which forms the posterior part of the pelvic diaphragm. The main function of the levator ani is to help support the pelvic viscera (Fig 42-2).

The puborectalis and contiguous portion of the EAS form the anorectal ring at the upper end of the anal canal; on rectal examinations, the posterior part of this ring is easily palpated as the puborectalis shelf. Although the puborectalis is usually considered a component of the levator ani, recent evidence suggests that it is also an integral part of the EAS. It appears to be innervated by both the pudendal

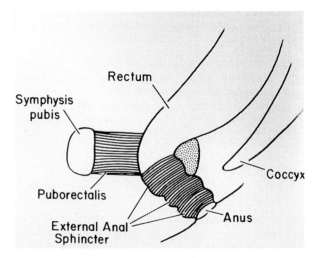

Fig. 42-1 The anal sphincter and puborectalis. The puborectalis arises from the pubic symphysis and forms a sling around the lower rectum. Contraction of the puborectalis pulls the lower rectum forward, producing an angle between its axis and that of the anal canal, the anorectal angle. The anal canal is enveloped by the voluntary external anal sphincter, deep to which is the internal sphincter (not shown).
From Sleisinger MH, Fordtran JS, eds: *Gastrointestinal disease: pathophysiology, diagnosis, management,* ed 4, Philadelphia, 1989, WB Saunders.

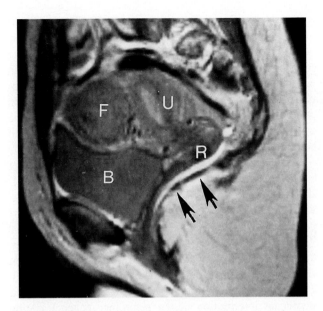

Fig. 42-2 Normal levator ani muscle. A sagittal magnetic resonance image (TR, 2400 msec; TE, 25 msec) of the pelvis. The normal levator ani *(arrows)* is seen as an almost horizontally oriented curvilinear structure that is supporting the rectum *(R)* and posterior aspect of the bladder *(B)*. It also supports the uterus *(U)* and the vagina. A uterine fibroid *(F)* is present.

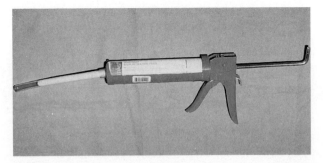

Fig. 42-3 A commercially available caulking gun, together with the tube of thick barium paste contained in the kit. Note the plastic, partially filled rectal tube, which is attached to one end of the caulking gun.

nerve and branches of S3 and S4. The pudendal nerve is particularly vulnerable to stretch injury stemming from repeated straining during defecation. The resulting pudendal neuropathy may impair EAS and puborectalis function and, thereby, lead to anal incontinence.

A number of factors are thought to be involved in the maintenance of anal continence.[1] The high-pressure zone in the anal canal is mainly a function of the IAS at rest, and the squeezing-down action of the EAS and puborectalis. Maintenance of the anorectal angle by the continuous contraction of the puborectalis is important, although how this works is the subject of much dispute. Sensory receptors in the rectum or surrounding pelvic floor muscles can discriminate between a gas, liquid, and solid content. However, acute sensory discrimination appears to be a function of the anal mucosa, which probably samples contents once the rectoanal inhibitory reflex is triggered. Rectal distensibility (compliance) is also important; as distention proceeds, the intraluminal pressure normally remains low, and this permits normal individuals to accommodate approximately 400 ml of rectal content. When large volumes are infused into the rectum, some refluxes into the sigmoid colon, suggesting that it too is involved in maintaining continence.

TECHNIQUES OF DEFECOGRAPHY

Defecography can dynamically assess the process of defecation by recording the rectal expulsion of a thick barium paste, which approximates the consistency of feces. In ad-

dition, it provides information concerning the function of the pelvic floor muscles (puborectalis and levator ani). In essence, the technique consists of filling the rectum with appropriate contrast material, seating the patient on a radiolucent commode, obtaining a series of lateral films of the anorectal region, and finally recording the process of rectal evacuation. It is customary to take these films with the patient at rest, as well as during voluntary contraction of the anal sphincter and pelvic floor muscles (squeezing), straining down, and defecation.

The examination is usually extremely well tolerated by patients, and is considerably less uncomfortable than a barium enema study, as large bowel filling is limited to the rectum and sigmoid colon. The entire study generally takes 15 minutes.

Defecographic equipment

Although defecography can be performed using standard barium suspensions and without a special commode, most centers utilize a viscous barium paste for opacifying the rectum and a specially constructed radiolucent commode. It is also essential to have a method for the continuous or rapid-sequence recording of the process of rectal evacuation.

Contrast media

Viscous barium pastes for use in defecography are available commercially (e.g., Anatrast; (E-Z-EM Co., Westbury, NY), or can be prepared from barium powder and potato starch.[2] Because of the high viscosity of these media, a caulking gun is attached to the rectal tube to facilitate introduction of the material into the rectum. This caulking gun comes with some of the commercially available contrast agents such as Anatrast (Fig. 42-3), or can be obtained from a hardware store. An alternative, but much more expensive, option is an orthopedic cement gun.

Vaginal opacification

In women, the vagina is routinely opacified to aid in the recognition of an enterocele (prolapsed small bowel) that has descended into the rectovaginal space. Many radiologists use a tampon soaked in contrast material for this purpose, but this may act as a splint and limit movement of the anterior rectal wall.[3] In view of this, it is preferable to opacify the vagina by introducing liquid barium via a foreshortened Foley catheter, and then to place a folded gauze square in the introitus to limit vaginal loss of barium. Alternatively, a water-soluble contrast formulated with an appropriate low-pH gel may be used.[4] Some investigators routinely use orally ingested barium to opacify the pelvic small bowel in women, so that enteroceles are more readily recognizable.

Special commode

A specially designed commode is generally used for defecographic examinations (Fig. 42-4). Besides providing a comfortable seat, it should be possible to easily and safely attach the commode to the fluoroscopic table. The seat is made of a radiolucent material; both wood[5] and Perspex[6] have been used for this purpose. The commode incorporates a radiographic filtration device that compensates for the marked difference in density between the widest part of the pelvis and the perineal region below the line of the buttocks. Adequate filtration may be achieved with either copper filters or one or more large plastic bottles filled with water (Fig. 42-5).[5] Disposable plastic bags or plastic receptacles are generally used to collect the evacuated barium paste. A radiopaque ruler is incorporated into the midline of the commode so that distances in the sagittal plane can be directly measured.

Suitable commodes can be constructed by enterprising hospital engineers,[5,6] but commercial ones are also available (e.g., the Brunswick defecography chair; E-Z-EM Co., Westbury, NY).

Recording of rectal evacuation

The process of evacuation is most frequently recorded on videotape. This may be supplemented with 105-mm spot films or larger-sized films, but care should be taken to avoid significant interruption of the recording sequence during defecation. Cineradiography is an alternative, but subjects the patient to a high dose of radiation and is not widely

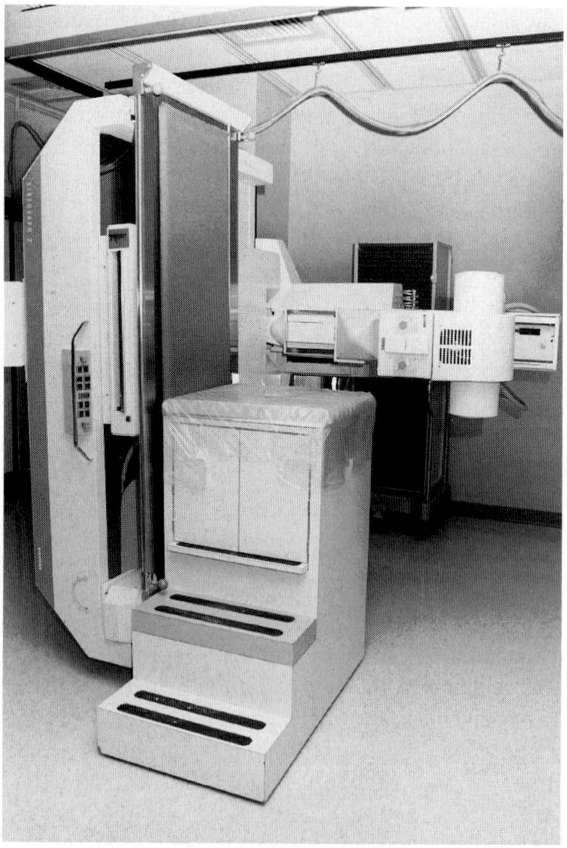

Fig. 42-4 A specially designed commode for defecography, which is anchored to the adjacent upright fluoroscopic table. Steps are incorporated into its structure, and an egg-crate foam pad is placed on top of the commode for patient comfort.

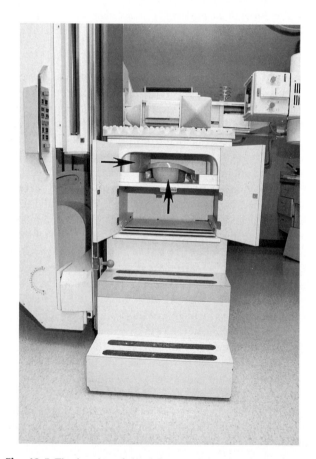

Fig. 42-5 The interior of the defecography commode. A disposable plastic receptacle (*vertical arrow*) collects the evacuated barium paste. A water-filled bottle (*horizontal arrow*) is placed inside the commode, so that the density of the perineum more closely approximates that of the more cephalad pelvis.

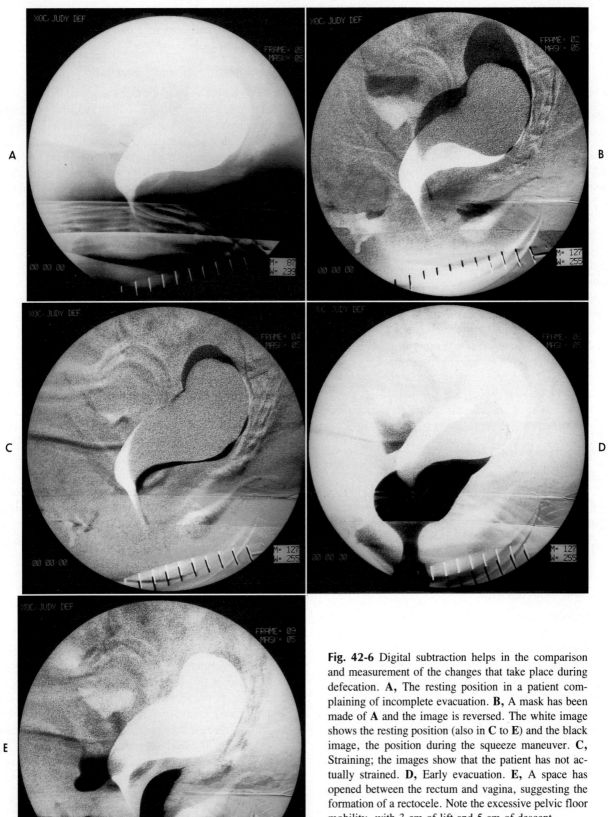

Fig. 42-6 Digital subtraction helps in the comparison and measurement of the changes that take place during defecation. **A,** The resting position in a patient complaining of incomplete evacuation. **B,** A mask has been made of **A** and the image is reversed. The white image shows the resting position (also in **C** to **E**) and the black image, the position during the squeeze maneuver. **C,** Straining; the images show that the patient has not actually strained. **D,** Early evacuation. **E,** A space has opened between the rectum and vagina, suggesting the formation of a rectocele. Note the excessive pelvic floor mobility, with 3 cm of lift and 5 cm of descent.

available. Digitization of the fluoroscopic image may be utilized increasingly in the future. The edge-enhancement features show bony landmarks more clearly, the radiation dose, which is a concern,[7] may be reduced, and subtraction techniques may prove helpful (Fig. 42-6).

VARIATIONS OF DEFECOGRAPHIC TECHNIQUE
Balloon proctography

Balloon proctography is a relatively simple study in which a deflated balloon is introduced into the rectum, the balloon is filled with a barium suspension, and lateral sitting films of the anorectum are taken at rest and on straining.[8] The Lahr balloon,[9] which also measures anal sphincter pressures, represents a modification of this technique. To reduce the radiation dosage, a scintigraphic version of balloon proctography has also been developed.[10] Balloon proctography has several disadvantages compared to defecography. Most importantly, it does not record the process of rectal evacuation. The balloon also does not accurately reflect the rectal contour, so that any alterations in configuration, such as intussusception, cannot be recognized. In addition, the degree of balloon insertion may change the anorectal angle, thereby confusing its measurement.[3] For these reasons, balloon proctography is now rarely used as a radiographic study in clinical practice, and has been largely replaced by defecography.

The balloon expulsion test

The balloon expulsion test is a derivative of balloon proctography, and is widely used by colorectal surgeons as a test of obstructed defecation. In this nonradiographic procedure, the patient is asked to expel a rectal balloon filled with 50 to 60 ml of water. Most patients with normal defecatory function can do this without difficulty, but those with obstructed defecation cannot do so spontaneously.[11]

Simplified defecography

A simplified form of defecography, which avoids the need for a commode or specialized contrast media, has been described by Poon et al.[12] In this method, the rectum is opacified with a standard high-density liquid barium suspension introduced via a urinary catheter syringe. The study is then performed with the patient lying in the lateral position on the radiographic table. The authors have found that this technique was able to demonstrate approximately 90% of the findings subsequently shown on standard defecography using a commode and the same type of barium suspension. Many investigators consider relatively liquid barium suspensions to be unsuitable, however, because they can be evacuated with relatively little muscular force. In addition, many subjects augment contraction of their pelvic floor muscles when the rectum is filled with liquid, thereby altering the appearances at defecography. To date, no studies of defecography have been performed that compared the type of recumbent examination carried out by Poon et al. with "commode defecography" utilizing a viscous barium paste.

Quantification of rectal evacuation

It is possible to quantify rectal evacuation using a procedure referred to as *rectodynamics,*[13] which is analogous to the urodynamic method used to assess bladder emptying. In this technique, the patient is asked to evacuate as rapidly and completely as possible 100 ml of barium paste into a disposable plastic bag lying on a weight transducer. In this way, several aspects of defecation can be quantified, including the maximum emptying rate, the time it takes to achieve maximum emptying, and the proportion of barium evacuated. This method may ultimately be useful both diagnostically and for monitoring the response to treatment.

EXAMINATION PROCEDURE

Bowel preparation is unnecessary when performing defecography, as the rectum is usually empty. In women, the small bowel is often filled initially, and the vagina is routinely opacified. Following this, contrast material is introduced into the rectum. If, as is customary, a viscous barium paste is employed, 30 to 50 ml of liquid barium is introduced first, because this improves the coating of the rectal mucosa and aids in the visualization of changes in the rectal wall configuration, such as intussusception. Introduction of the barium paste is continued until the patient experiences discomfort due to rectal distention, or until about 250 ml has been instilled. As the tube is withdrawn, a small amount of contrast can be injected to better delineate the anal canal. Finally, a small amount of barium or barium-impregnated petroleum jelly is smeared on the patient's skin immediately next to the anal orifice so that the length of the anal canal can be measured.

The patient then sits on the specially constructed commode in the lateral projection beside the upright fluoroscopic table. Lateral films are obtained with the patient at rest and squeezing down. Some investigators also take a film as the patient is straining without evacuating. The patient is then asked to evacuate, and this process is recorded, usually on videotape. Unless evacuation is unusually rapid, at least one or two films can be obtained during emptying. Finally, a postevacuation film is taken with the patient straining maximally. Patients with difficulty in emptying should be asked if they normally use additional maneuvers to aid evacuation, such as applying digital pressure on the perineum or posterior vaginal wall. If so, they should be told to perform these maneuvers so that their respective effect on defecation can be assessed.

Anteroposterior or oblique views may be useful, especially if unusual or confusing findings are seen in the lateral position. Anteroposterior films obtained at rest and on straining in the erect position after evacuation (anteroposterior stress proctography) have been found useful for demonstrating rectal fold prolapse into the anal canal (rectoanal intussusception) that is not evident in the lateral projection.[14]

Aiding mechanisms

Some patients with outlet obstruction devise methods for overcoming the problem, and the radiologist should ask about this beforehand. It is sometimes useful to have the patient demonstrate the aiding maneuver during proctography. Common methods include pressing the anal canal posteriorly to increase the anorectal angle, lifting the perineum, pressing the posterior wall of the vagina posteriorly to reduce a rectocele, and reducing a prolapsing intussusception.

NORMAL APPEARANCES

Knowledge of the spectrum of normal appearances observed at defecography is largely based on the findings from three studies.[14-16] Bartram et al.[15] described their radiographic findings in patients without a history of defecatory abnormality who were referred for barium enema study. Goei et al.[16] used similar selection criteria in their study; all subjects were older than 41 years of age. Shorvon et al.[17] performed defecography in normal volunteers who had no history of a defecatory abnormality; all were under the age of 35 and all women were nulliparous. The subjects' age is an important factor, as anorectal and pelvic floor function is known to deteriorate with age,[18] and, for this reason, most symptomatic patients referred for defecography are middle-aged or elderly. In essence, the subjects in these three studies were selected on the basis of an absence of anorectal symptoms. However, it should not be automatically assumed that asymptomatic individuals are normal. With progressive impairment of pelvic floor function, a previously asymptomatic finding may well become clinically significant. This is particularly likely to occur in women as a consequence of progressive pelvic neuropathy.

A variety of measurable parameters can be assessed from the films obtained during the study. These include the length of the anal canal, the position of the anorectal junction, the anorectal angle, the width of the rectovaginal space, and the rectosacral gap.

Anal canal

At rest, the anal canal is usually closed, so that, at most, only its fold pattern is visible (Fig. 42-7, *A*). In Shorvon et al.'s series, three of the asymptomatic women had an open anal canal at rest; all three became incontinent on coughing and straining.[17] Such findings support the contention that some asymptomatic individuals have an abnormal proctographic appearance, thus placing them at risk for subsequent clinical dysfunction, in this instance, anal incontinence. The rectum normally shows a smooth outline, and its volume can be roughly assessed. Rectal volume usually cannot be equated with the volume of injected contrast material, as there is generally some reflux into the sigmoid colon (Fig. 42-7, *A*).

The anal canal length is measured as the distance between the anal orifice and the point where the parallel straight sides of the anal canal meet the cone-shaped walls of the distal rectum (Fig. 42-8). This latter point constitutes the anorectal junction (Figs. 42-7 and 42-8). The mean radiographic length of the anal canal in men is 2.2 cm and in women, 1.6 cm.[17] The anal canal length may be an important predictor of surgical outcome in incontinent patients, as those with a relatively short anal canal tend to be unimproved following postanal repair.[20] The radiographic length of the anal canal is considerably less than the manometrically derived measurement, which averages 4 cm for men and 3.7 cm for women.[21] The manometric high-pressure readings are obtained from the cone-shaped area of the distal rectum, suggesting that it is actually part of the anal canal. This probably explains the discrepancy between the anal canal lengths determined manometrically and those obtained at defecography. With the rectum empty, as it is during manometry, the entire anal canal is closed. However, when the rectum is full during the early phase of defecography, the upper part of the anal sphincter relaxes, and physiologically this is probably part of the inhibitory reflex. This reflex also activates the "sampling zone," which transmits information centrally concerning the nature of the material in the lower rectum and upper canal, whether it is air, which may be safely voided, or liquid or solid, which may not be.

Anorectal junction level

The level of the pelvic floor has traditionally been defined by the pubococcygeal line.[7] This line is difficult to identify at defecography, and most workers prefer to use the more readily visible ischial tuberosity instead. The position of the pelvic floor at rest is then defined by the position of the anorectal junction with respect to the inferior margin of the ischial tuberosity (see Fig. 42-7, *A*). In young subjects, the anorectal junction at rest usually lies close to this bony landmark. Shorvon et al.[17] found that the mean resting position of the anorectal junction was 0.4 cm above the ischial tuberosity in women (with one standard deviation of 1.3 cm) and 1.6 cm above this point in men (with one standard deviation of 0.9 cm).[17] In elderly women, its mean resting position is 1.3 cm lower,[18] probably because of progressive denervation. A variety of configurations is seen at the anorectal junction. Even though the puborectalis has resting tone, it is relatively unusual to see an impression attributable to this muscle in the resting position (Fig. 42-9).

Anorectal angle

Because the anorectal angle is thought to be important for maintaining normal continence, considerable attention has been devoted to its measurement. The angle is most commonly measured between the axis of the anal canal and a line drawn along the posterior border of the distal rectum

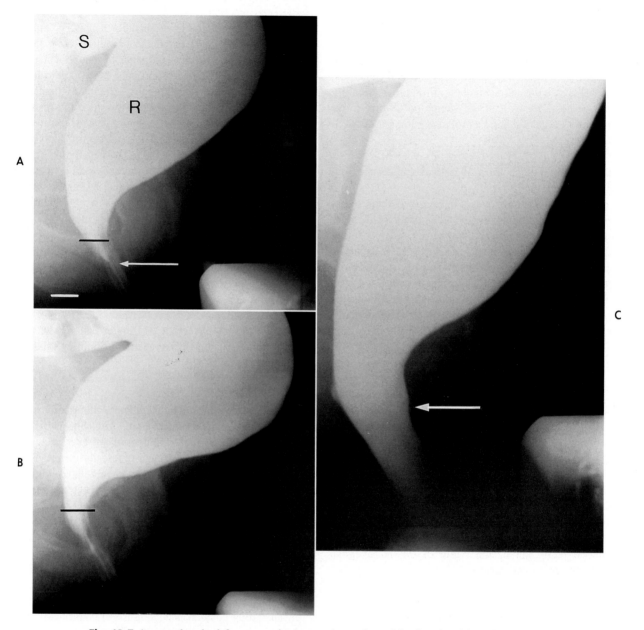

Fig. 42-7 A normal male defecogram. **A,** At rest the anal canal is closed and its collapsed fold pattern is visible *(arrow)*. The rectum *(R)* is well distended and exhibits a smooth outline. Reflux into the distal sigmoid colon *(S)* is discernible. The anorectal junction is indicated *(horizontal black line),* and lies approximately 2 cm above the inferior margin of the ischial tuberosity *(horizontal white line)*. **B,** On squeezing down, the posterior wall of the lower rectum has elevated and the anal canal has increased in length. There is an associated elevation of the anorectal junction *(horizontal black line)*. **C,** During evacuation, there is widening of the anorectal angle, and the lower rectum and anal canal form an uninterrupted funnel-shaped lumen *(arrow)*.

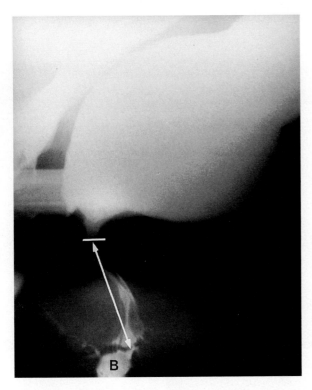

Fig. 42-8 Measurement of anal canal length. Defecogram film obtained at rest. The length of the anal canal *(oblique arrowed line)* is measured as the distance between the collection of barium *(B)* at the anal orifice distally and the anorectal junction proximally *(horizontal line).*

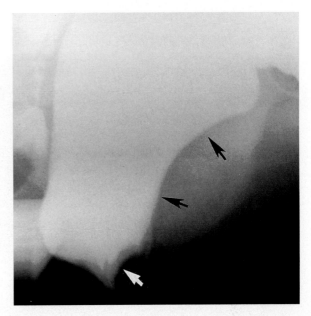

Fig. 42-9 A normal defecogram, in which the puborectalis and levator ani impressions are distinct. In this film taken at rest, there is a generalized broad impression on the posterior rectal wall *(black arrows),* which is attributable to the levator ani. In addition, there is a more inferior, shorter impression at the anorectal junction *(white arrow),* which probably represents the effect of the puborectalis sling. A puborectalis impression is more commonly seen when the patient squeezes down.

(Fig. 42-10, *A*); this is sometimes referred to as the *posterior anorectal angle.* An alternative method is to draw the rectal line through the central axis of the distal rectal lumen (Fig. 42-10, *A*). When this central rectal angle is used rather than the posterior anorectal angle, the mean measurement of the angle is approximately 20 degrees greater.[15,22] Regardless of the method of measurement, the range of the normal resting anorectal angle is very wide. For example, the posterior anorectal angle varies between 65 and 125 degrees in men, and between 70 and 135 degrees in women, with a mean of approximately 95 degrees for both sexes.[17] In most normal subjects, however, the posterior anorectal angle does not exceed 120 degrees. There is considerable interobserver variation in the measurement of the angle.[22] When the posterior anorectal angle is used, placement of a line along the posterior margin of the rectum is frequently arbitrary because of the curvature of this part of the bowel wall (see Fig. 42-9). A microcomputer has been used to derive the central axis of the distal rectal lumen when the central rectal angle is measured.[23] This axis is particularly difficult to determine in women when a large rectocele is present.[22,23] Considerable caution should therefore be exercised when assessing the significance of the anorectal an-

gle, both because of its inexactness and its wide range of normal values.

Rectovaginal septum

The relationship of the rectum to the vagina and the sacrum should also be noted. The opacified vagina is normally closely apposed to the anterior wall of the rectum, and the rectosacral gap at the S3 level is usually less than 1 cm (see Fig. 42-10, *A*).

Changes during defecography
On squeezing

The pelvic floor muscles and the voluntary external anal sphincter contract during squeezing. Levator ani contraction causes the posterior wall of the distal rectum to elevate and the anorectal angle to become more acute because of the increased contraction of the puborectalis sling (see Figs. 42-7 and 42-10, *B*). The mean decrease in the anorectal angle from its resting value is approximately 20 degrees and some decrease is observed in virtually all normal subjects.[16,17] Failure to decrease the anorectal angle on squeezing is therefore reliable evidence of impaired pelvic floor contraction. Contraction of the external anal sphincter augments the length of the anal canal[24]; this can almost invariably be demonstrated in men (see Fig. 42-7, *B*), but

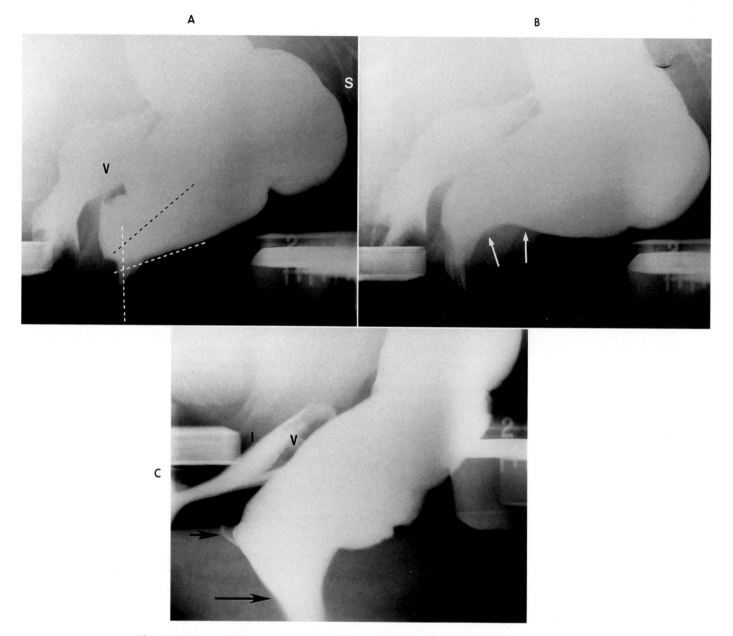

Fig. 42-10 A normal female defecogram. **A** In this film taken at rest, the vertical dotted line is superimposed on the axis of the anal canal. The anorectal angle may be measured either between this line and a line drawn through the posterior rectal margin *(oblique white dotted line),* or between the anal canal and a line placed along the central axis of the rectal lumen *(black dotted line).* The opacified vagina *(V)* is closely apposed to the anterior rectal margin. The rectosacral gap is less than 1 cm. Note the midline centimeter marker which permits corrections of measurements for magnification. S, Sacrum. **B,** On squeezing down, the distal rectum has elevated *(arrows)* and the anorectal angle is smaller, though accurate measurement is hampered because the posterior rectal margin no longer forms a straight line. **C,** On evacuation, the continuous funnel-shaped configuration of the lower rectum and anal canal is evident *(long arrow).* Precise placement of the anorectal junction is difficult, but there has been significant descent below the level of the ischial tuberosity *(I).* Note the presence of a small, virtually empty rectocele *(short arrow).* The vagina *(V)* remains closely apposed to the anterior wall of the rectum.

is only evident in two thirds of normal women.[17] Elevation of the anorectal junction is seen in almost all normal subjects (see Fig. 42-7); and the mean elevation is of the order of 1 to 2 cm.[16,17] This is probably brought about by the combination of both pelvic floor contraction and lengthening of the anal canal. The findings described here indicate the value of the squeeze film as a test of pelvic floor function; if the anorectal angle does not decrease or the anorectal junction does not elevate, these are almost always abnormal findings.

On straining

When a subject strains down without defecating, the puborectalis and levator anus muscle should relax, thereby stressing the continence mechanism. Relaxation of the pelvic floor muscles should lead to an increase in the anorectal angle and descent of the anorectal junction. However, on straining down, up to 30% of normal subjects show a paradoxical increase in the anorectal angle,[16,17] and, less often, the anorectal junction may also be elevated.[16] These paradoxical changes probably reflect contraction of the pelvic floor muscles stemming from the subject's fear of possible incontinence when trying to strain but not defecate. For this reason, the straining film obtained before defecation is the least reliable of the films. Straining after defecation is probably more informative, and we usually defer this maneuver to the end of the examination.

Defecation

Defecation is initiated in response to the sensation of rectal distention. Initially the subject bears down, thereby raising the intraabdominal pressure and causing the pelvic floor to descend. The pelvic floor muscles and internal anal sphincter relax, the latter probably triggered by the rectoanal inhibitory reflex. Relaxation of the puborectalis effaces the anorectal angle. The distal rectum and upper anal canal then assume a continuous funnel-shaped configuration as evacuation ensues (see Figs. 42-7, *C,* and 42-10, *C*). Evacuation is probably a passive phenomenon, in which the raised intraabdominal pressure squeezes the rectum against the levator ani.[15] Peristaltic contraction is not observed at defecography.

In many normal subjects, there is a temporary delay before defecation commences. Using a relatively thin barium suspension, Bartram et al.[15] found that the average time for the anal canal to open fully was 4.5 seconds, and rectal emptying was usually completed within 30 seconds, with an average of 11 seconds. Evacuation is more prolonged when a more viscous barium paste is used. The maximal width of the anal canal averages 1.5 cm, and seldom exceeds 2 cm.[15] Complete emptying of the rectum is seen in only half the normal population.[2,16]

Pelvic floor descent

Pelvic floor descent on defecation is measured as the distance the anorectal junction descends from its resting posi-

tion. In normal subjects, pelvic floor descent usually averages 2 to 3 cm and generally does not exceed 4.5 cm.[15-17] Thus, with an elevation of 1 to 2 cm and descent of 2 to 3 cm, the total excursion of the pelvic floor in normal individuals is around 3 to 5 cm, although the range in normals is large; in one series it ranged from 1.8 to 5.4 cm in men and from 0.7 to 5.9 cm in women.[17] Pinho et al.[18] have shown that the extent of pelvic floor descent decreases in the elderly, probably because the resting position is lower and the muscles are already a little stretched. The pelvic floor descent, as measured at defecography, is greater than the clinically determined perineal descent, which is measured with the patient lying down and only straining.

Changes in rectal wall configuration

A variety of changes in the rectal wall configuration may be seen during normal defecation. Small folds, mainly on the posterior wall of the lower rectum, are common, and probably represent pleating of redundant mucosa as the rectum collapses.[15] Infoldings greater than 3 mm in width probably represent the full thickness of the rectal wall rather than merely mucosal prolapse or redundancy. Such infoldings, if they are circumferential and show evidence of distal excursion, indicate the presence of rectal intussusception (Fig. 42-11). Rectal intussusception, or intussusception that extends to the anorectal junction, appears to be relatively common in normal subjects, but actual extension into the anal canal is almost never seen.[17]

Rectoceles are an almost ubiquitous finding in asymptomatic women and may also be seen in asymptomatic males, though less frequently.[15,17] However, asymptomatic rectoceles are generally small (less than 2 cm in depth) and rarely retain barium (see Fig. 42-10, *C*). Both during (see Fig. 42-10, *C*) and after evacuation, the rectum and upper vagina should remain closely apposed. Rectovaginal separation is uncommon in normal subjects.[17] Widening of the rectovaginal space by 2 cm or more suggests the presence of an enterocele; less often, this is caused by a sigmoidocele or uterine prolapse.[25] Prior opacification of the pelvic small bowel usually eliminates the need for a repeat examination when rectovaginal separation is seen, as an enterocele is the most common cause.[25] The subject should always be asked to strain repeatedly at the end of defecation. This aids in demonstrating the extent of pelvic floor descent, and may reveal an otherwise undetected enterocele.[25]

As has been pointed out, defecography is not an exact reproduction of the act of defecation.[15] Even a thick barium paste does not necessarily approximate the consistency of stool, which itself varies both from subject to subject and from time to time within the same individual. The method of rectal distention is also not entirely physiologic, as filling is carried out in a retrograde fashion. Defecography, however, does provide dynamic and reproducible information about anorectal and pelvic floor function that currently cannot be readily obtained by any other radiographic techniques. Although advances in magnetic resonance im-

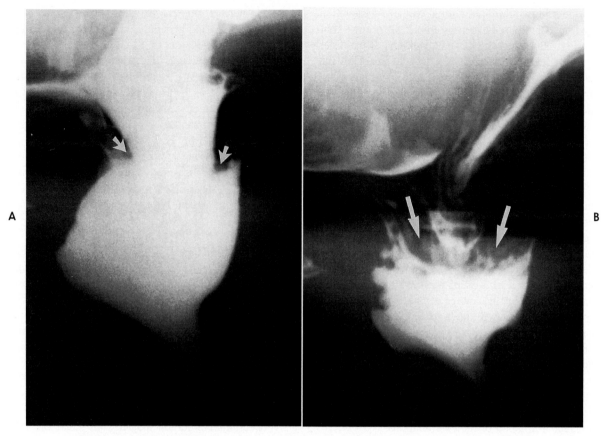

Fig. 42-11 Intrarectal intussusception in a symptomatic patient. **A,** During the early stage of evacuation, infoldings have developed on the anterior and posterior walls of the rectum *(arrows)* approximately 6 cm above the anorectal junction. This circumferential infolding constitutes the beginning of a rectal intussusception. **B,** At a later stage of evacuation, the intussusception is deeper and wider *(arrows),* as it has descended farther into the rectum. Note, however, that the intussusception has not reached the anorectal junction.

aging[26] and ultrasonography may ultimately assign defecography to a lesser role (see Chapters 43 and 44), the technique currently remains a pivotal test of anorectal function.

REFERENCES

1. Pemberton JH: Anatomy and physiology of the anus and rectum. In Zuidema GD, ed: *Shackelford's surgery of the alimentary tract,* Philadelphia, 1991, WB Saunders.
2. Mahieu P, Pringot J, Bodart P: Defecography: I. Description of a new procedure and results in normal patients, *Gastrointest Radiol* 9:247, 1984.
3. Kelvin FM, Stevenson GW: Radiologic investigation: the anorectum and vagina. In Benson JT, ed: *Female pelvic floor disorders: investigation and management,* New York 1992, WW Norton.
4. Archer BD, Somers S, Stevenson GW: Contrast medium gel for marking vaginal position during defecography, *Radiology* 182:278, 1992.
5. Bernier P, Stevenson GW, Shorvon P: Defecography commode, *Radiology* 166:891, 1988.
6. Ginai AZ: Technical report: evacuation proctography (defecography). A new seat and method of examination, *Clin Radiol* 42:214, 1990.
7. Goei R, Kemerink G: Radiation dose in defecography, *Radiology* 176:137, 1990.
8. Preston DM, Lennard-Jones JE, Thomas BM: The balloon proctogram, *Br J Surg* 71:29, 1984.
9. Lahr CJ et al: Balloon topography. A simple method of evaluating anal function, *Dis Colon Rectum* 29:1, 1986.
10. Barkel DC et al: Scintigraphic assessment of the anorectal angle in health and after ileal pouch–anal anastomosis, *Ann Surg* 208:42, 1988.
11. Pemberton JH, Rath DM, Ilstrup DM: Evaluation and surgical treatment of severe chronic constipation, *Ann Surg* 214:403, 1991.
12. Poon FW, Lauder JC, Finlay IG: Technical report: evacuating proctography. A simplified technique, *Clin Radiol* 44:113, 1991.
13. Kamm MA, Bartram CI, Lennard-Jones JE: Rectodynamics—quantifying rectal evacuation, *Int J Colorect Dis* 4:161, 1989.
14. McGee S, Bartram CI: The value of anteroposterior stress proctography in the diagnosis of intra-anal intussusception of the rectum, *Clin Radiol* 45:66, 1992 (abstract).
15. Bartram CI, Turnbull GK, Lennard-Jones JE: Evacuation proctography: an investigation of rectal expulsion in 20 subjects without defecatory disturbance, *Gastrointest Radiol* 13:72, 1988.
16. Goei R et al: Anorectal function: defecographic measurement in asymptomatic subjects, *Radiology* 173:137, 1989.
17. Shorvon PJ et al: Defecography in normal volunteers: results and implications, *Gut* 30:1737, 1989.

18. Pinho M et al: The effect of age on pelvic floor dynamics, *Int J Colorect Dis* 5:207, 1990.

19. Shorvon PJ, Stevenson GW: Defaecography: setting up a service, *Br J Hosp Med* 41:460, 1989.

20. Yoshioka K, Hyland G, Keighley MRB: Physiological changes after postanal repair and parameters predicting outcome, *Br J Surg* 75:1220, 1988.

21. McHugh SM, Diamant NE: Anal canal pressure profile: a reappraisal as determined by rapid pull-through technique, *Gut* 28:1234, 1987.

22. Penninckx F et al: Observer variation in the radiological measurement of the anorectal angle, *Int J Colorect Dis* 5:94, 1990.

23. Yoshioka K et al: How reliable is measurement of the anorectal angle by videoproctography? *Dis Colon Rectum* 34:1010, 1991.

24. Shorvon PJ, Henry M: The clinical value of defecography. In Herlinger H, Megibow AJ, eds: *Advances in gastrointestinal radiology,* St Louis, 1991, Mosby–Year Book.

25. Kelvin FM, Maglinte DDT, Hornback JA, Benson JT: Pelvic prolapse: assessment with evacuation proctography (defecography), *Radiology* 184:547, 1992.

26. Yang A et al: Pelvic floor descent in women: dynamic evaluation with fast MR imaging and cinematic display, *Radiology* 179:25, 1991.

43 *Investigation of Constipation and Incontinence*

PHILIP J. SHORVON
MICHAEL HENRY

CONSTIPATION

Constipation is a common complaint that is frequently treated indifferently by physician and lay person alike. However, it may indicate either a serious underlying disorder or else be the cause of such suffering to patients that it significantly affects their life-style and sense of well being.

Patient history and definition

It is important to find out precisely what a patient means by *constipation* and to obtain a full history to determine the correct investigational pathway. Some patients may simply be describing infrequency of defecation or the passing of hard or small stools. Others may be alluding to difficulties in evacuation, such as straining to evacuate, feelings of incomplete evacuation, or difficulties in initiating evacuation—all of which may reflect *outlet obstruction*. Others may refer to feelings of abdominal bloating, which may be completely unrelated to colonic or anorectal function. Clearly, associated symptoms such as weight loss or passing blood or mucus per rectum are also important to elicit, and in adulthood a change in frequency of defecation must always be considered suspicious for malignancy. Finally, it can be useful to enquire directly if patients are employing any mechanisms to assist with defecation.

Some attempts to define constipation have been based on population surveys of individuals not seeking health care. In the United Kingdom less than 1% of the population defecate less than once per week, as compared with 4% in the United States.[1,2] Similarly 10% of Britons and 17% of Americans report the need to strain to pass stool. The definition of constipation offered by Drossman and colleagues[2]—straining to pass stool 25% or more of the time and/or two or less acts of defecation per week—is now generally accepted.

Investigation

Constipation is such a common complaint that it is important not to overinvestigate. Furthermore, because of the large number of possible investigations (see the box above), it is important to choose according to the clinical presentation.[3]

Symptoms suggestive of onset in childhood

A number of conditions present in adulthood, although symptoms can be traced back into childhood. In particular Hirschsprung's disease and megarectum and megacolon need to be differentiated because both may be present as gross fecal loading of the rectum and all or part of the colon on a plain-film. (Fig. 43-1). Chronic idiopathic constipation may commence in childhood (see later discussion).

☐ **INVESTIGATIONS FOR CONSTIPATION** ☐

RADIOLOGIC

Plain film
Plain film as part of transit study (shapes study)
Barium enema
   Single contrast
      With unprepared colon
      With prepared colon
   Double contrast
Defecogram (evacuation proctogram)
Integrated EMG/proctography
Balloon proctography

ISOTOPIC

Isotope transit studies
Isotope evacuation studies

ULTRASONOGRAPHIC

Anal endosonography

ENDOSCOPIC

Colonoscopy
Flexible sigmoidoscopy
Flexible sigmoidoscopy and barium enema combined

ANORECTAL MANOMETRY
ANORECTAL ELECTROPHYSIOLOGY
COLONIC MANOMETRY

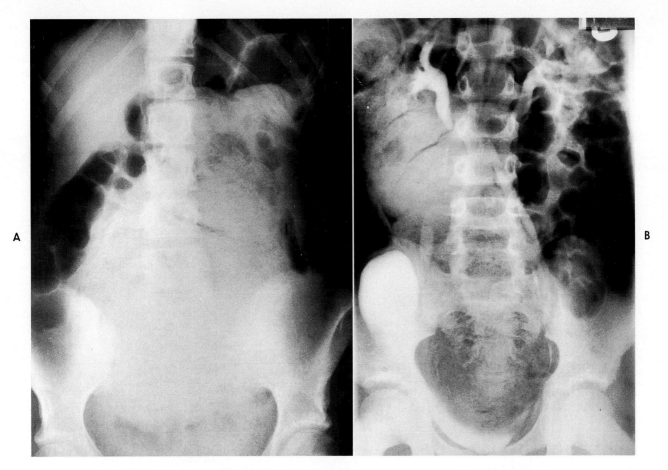

Fig. 43-1 Idiopathic megacolon. **A,** Plain abdominal film demonstrates a grossly dilated and fecally loaded rectum and distal colon in this young patient. **B,** Intravenous urography. The dilated rectum is causing partial obstruction of the left ureter. The bladder is markedly compressed.

Hirschsprung's disease and megarectum and megacolon

Hirshsprung's disease is a familial disease, although it is not inherited in a simple Mendelian fashion. It occurs in about 1 in 4500 live births with a male preponderance of 4:1.[4] Pathologically there is a loss of ganglion cells in the neural plexus of the bowel wall extending for a variable distance proximally from the anorectal junction.[5] Occasionally only a very short segment is involved; conversely, very rarely the small bowel may be involved as well. Clinically there is a wide spectrum of presentation, from acute obstruction in neonates to chronic constipation in adults. The vast majority are diagnosed during infancy and childhood. Soiling is uncommon.

Idiopathic megarectum and idiopathic megacolon can be regarded as the same disease. The rectum is grossly dilated, and this can extend a variable length proximally. The cause is uncertain; some cases appear to be related to painful anorectal conditions in childhood such as fissures. Patients usually present in early childhood or late adolescence, and the

sex incidence is equal. Defecation is usually irregular and infrequent, and soiling is common.

Differentiation between Hirschsprung's disease and idiopathic megacolon is important because the treatment strategy differs, but this cannot be confidently achieved radiologically. Both diseases can cause a megarectum, which is defined on a contrast study as a lateral diameter of the rectum of >6.5 cm at the pelvic inlet.[6] If a megarectum is suspected, then a limited unprepared enema should be administered to confirm the diagnosis and rule out any stricturing lesion. A lateral view of the rectum is essential. Water-soluble contrast is usually recommended to prevent barium impaction. Hirschsprung's disease is suggested if a narrow segment and transition zone are seen, but this is often absent in adults because the affected segment is very short. Once the diagnosis is suggested on a radiograph, further investigation is necessary.

The simplest screening investigation for detection of Hirschsprung's disease is the rectosphincteric inhibitory reflex, which is safe and relatively noninvasive. Reflex inhibition of internal anal sphincter tone in response to mechanical distension of the rectum was first described by Gowers[7] in 1877, and then by Denny-Brown and Robertson in 1935.[8] It would appear to be a neurogenic response elicited by mechanoreceptors situated mostly in the rectum and to a lesser extent in the sigmoid colon. The reflex is preserved when the rectum is fully mobilized and its extrinsic nerve supply disrupted, yet it is abolished after myotomy[9]; this

confirms that the pathway for conduction of the reflex is facilitated by intrinsic intramural nerve pathways. This reflex is abolished in patients with Hirschsprung's disease and can be tested by measuring internal sphincter pressure while distending a previously inserted rectal balloon with air. The air is introduced rapidly, and a reflex fall in pressure is a normal observation after inflation of as little as 30 ml of air into the balloon. In patients with a megarectum it is im-

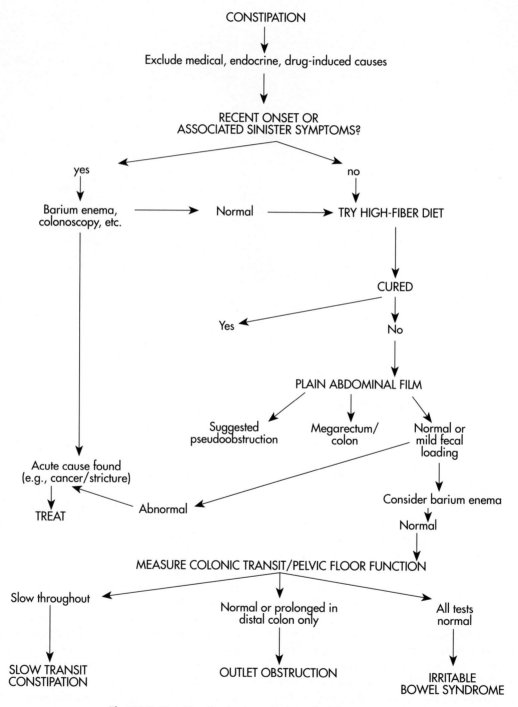

Fig. 43-2 Algorithm for the investigation of adult constipation.

portant to introduce large volumes of air (up to 300 ml) to cause rectal distension, otherwise a false-negative result is obtained.

In a study of 94 adult patients with a megacolon, 29 had Hirschsprung's disease and 65 an idiopathic megacolon.[11] The rectosphincteric inhibitory reflex was absent in 18 of 19 patients with Hirschsprung's disease. In the non-Hirschsprung group of patients the reflex was present in 34 of 41 patients tested but was absent in 7. It is clear there-fore that the diagnosis of Hirschsprung's disease ultimately depends on histologic demonstration of the absence of gan-glion cells and requires deep biopsy of the rectum, usually 2 to 3 cm above the dentate line.[12] An interesting observa-tion is that patients with idiopathic childhood megacolon tend to have paradoxic contraction of the external sphinc-ter on attempted expulsion of an intrarectal balloon.

Onset of symptoms in adulthood

A wide spectrum of diseases can result in constipa-tion in adulthood (Fig. 43-2) either as a direct compli-cation or as a consequence of drug treatment (see the boxes below). It behoves the physician not to send all patients for colonic imaging, and normally a diagnostic algorithm is used.

The wide variety of drug-induced endocrine and meta-bolic disorders that can be responsible are initially excluded by an appropriate physical examination and blood tests, al-though the cause of constipation remains unexplained in many patients. Patients with recent onset of constipation re-quire colonic imaging. Young adults with long-standing constipation without symptoms or signs are often treated with a high-fiber diet, and if this is successful no further investigation is necessary.

Pseudoobstruction

The term *pseudoobstruction* refers to disorders in which there are symptoms and signs of intestinal obstruction but no mechanical cause can be identified.[13,14] Initially it was intended to refer to an acute situation (ileus) but was later broadened to incorporate a chronic process (chronic pseu-doobstruction).[15] Christensen[16] later recommended that the term refer only to the chronic forms and that the acute forms be simply termed *ileus;* for the purposes of this discussion only the chronic forms are considered.

Chronic intestinal pseudoobstruction presents with a spectrum of symptoms from constipation to malabsorption and diarrhea. It is usually divided into primary (cause un-

---

☐ CAUSES OF ADULT CONSTIPATION ☐

PHYSIOLOGIC

Lack of fiber in diet
Pregnancy
Old age

COLORECTAL AND ANAL PHYSICAL ABNORMALITIES

Hirschsprung's disease
Anal fissure
Colonic stricture
Chagas' disease

ENDOCRINE AND METABOLIC DISORDERS

Hypothyroidism
Hypercalcemia
Hypopituitarism
Heavy metal poisoning
Porphyria

NEUROLOGIC

Autonomic neuropathies
Spinal cord lesions (particularly lumbar sacral/cauda
    equina)
Specific neurologic diseases (multiple sclerosis, myotonia
    dystrophica, and Parkinson's disease)
Sacral nerve damage

PSYCHIATRIC

Depression
Schizophrenia
Anorexia nervosa
Purgative abuse

DRUG INDUCED (See the box at right)

OTHER

Amyloidosis
Systemic sclerosis

UNKNOWN CAUSE

Pseudoobstruction (some forms)
Idiopathic megacolon
Idiopathic chronic constipation
Irritable bowel syndrome

☐ DRUGS IMPLICATED IN CAUSING CONSTIPATION ☐

DRUG CATEGORY	EXAMPLE
Opiates	Morphine
Opiate derivatives	Dihydrocodeine
Anticonvulsants	Phenytoin
Anticholinergics	Atropine
Monoamine oxidase inhibitor	Phenelzine
Antacids	Aluminum hydroxide
Psychiatric drugs	Phenothiazines/tricyclics
Hematinics	Ferrous sulfate
Cytotoxics	Vincristine

☐ **SECONDARY CAUSES OF CHRONIC INTESTINAL PSEUDOOBSTRUCTION** ☐

SMOOTH MUSCLE DISORDERS

Systemic sclerosis

NEUROLOGIC DISORDERS

Chagas' disease
Hirschsprung's disease
Parkinson's disease

ENDOCRINE DISORDERS

Hypothyroidism
Hypopituitarism
Hypoparathyroidism
Diabetes

PHARMACOLOGIC

Phenothiazines
Tricyclics
Anticholinergics
Cathartics
Opiates

OTHER

Amyloidosis

---

known), familial, and secondary forms. The secondary causes are listed in the box above.

Plain abdominal films usually give the first clue to pseudoobstruction. In a radiologic and histologic correlative study of 40 patients with chronic intestinal pseudoobstruction, the patients were divided into those with systemic sclerosis, visceral neuropathies, and visceral myopathies. A third of those patients with systemic sclerosis had normal plain films; the rest showed an obstruction pattern in the small bowel. Half the patients with visceral neuropathies had a small bowel obstruction pattern, and the rest had dilatation of both the small and large bowel. A pattern indicative of large bowel obstruction alone was rare. Esophageal involvement was common in all categories, gastric involvement was uncommon, and duodenal dilatation occurred in half of the patients with systemic sclerosis and in virtually all the rest. Patients with myopathies commonly lacked colonic haustra, whereas this was rare in those with neuropathies. Occasionally, benign pneumatosis intestinalis or pneumoperitoneum may accompany pseudoobstruction.

A barium enema or small bowel study may be required to rule out mechanical obstruction. In general a single-contrast enema is preferred to a double-contrast study and is performed on an unprepared colon. A conventional barium follow-through to exclude small bowel obstruction will

often prove a frustrating and inadequate study because of bowel dilatation and slow passage of barium; a small bowel study with intubation is preferable in ruling out a stricture.

A number of clues into the cause of obstruction may emerge from these studies. Packing of valvulae conniventes is seen in systemic sclerosis but rarely in other conditions. Dilatation, atony, and lack of haustra are common in visceral myopathies, whereas neuropathies often show dysmotility rather than atony, particularly in the esophagus. More elaborate tests of esophageal, gastric, and small bowel motility may help confirm plain film and barium findings.

Constipation in the elderly

Constipation is common in the elderly and has been shown to be multifactorial, although it is only infrequently caused by slow transit. Immobility, medication causing constipation, and impaired rectal sensation are of more importance in elderly patients than in younger ones.

Chronic idiopathic constipation

Some patients have chronic constipation without any obvious cause found by basic clinical assessment. The constipation is often severe and intractable, and the majority of patients are young women.

Labeling a patient as having chronic idiopathic constipation is largely a diagnosis of exclusion. However, because of the age and relative fitness of many of these patients, some physicians make the diagnosis without employing the full gamut of possible biochemical and imaging tests. Nevertheless, many clinicians find a barium enema examination (as opposed to colonoscopy) useful, since this usually rules out megacolon/megarectum or Hirschsprung's disease, as well as identifies unexpected strictures. A colon of normal caliber, although often long, is typical in these patients.

Many patients with chronic idiopathic constipation have suffered for many years and may harbor some hostility toward the medical profession. Many complain of pain and bloating, and some have undergone unnecessary laparotomies. Their symptoms are often exacerbated rather than improved by high-fiber diets. Although there is some evidence of psychologic factors contributing to this condition,[18,19] intensive investigation of this relatively small group of patients over the last 15 years has indicated that additional pathophysiologic mechanisms are almost certainly involved.

Two major factors have been identified as contributing to this disorder: colonic slow transit and outlet obstruction. Some individuals show a clear separation of these factors, but for the most part radiologic and physiologic testing reveal a combination of both. This is not surprising, since precise measurement of either entity is not possible, and each affects the other. For instance, slow transit leads to hard stools that are difficult to evacuate and results in chronic straining, simulating an outlet disorder. Conversely, severe outlet obstruction may result in infrequent defecation and retention of markers.

Recent studies have also indicated that a sensory neuropathy may be a contributing factor in these patients[20] and that anismus (see later) appears to be one part of the multifactorial but common problem of constipation in patients with multiple sclerosis.[21,22]

Even in preselected groups of patients sent to referral centers for investigation of constipation, a number show no abnormality in all objective testing, and such patients are often labeled as suffering from irritable bowel syndrome. In one recent study at the Mayo Clinic this category actually comprised 70% of all referrals.[23]

Measurement of colonic transit

Colonic transit is complicated, and considerable mixing of colonic contents occurs in normal subjects. Markers given sequentially may appear in the stool together, and heavier markers tend to move more slowly than light markers. The effect of the size of marker is unknown. Forward and backward movement of colonic contents occurs at the haustral level. A mass movement can occur, and this is occasionally observed after filling the colon with barium during a barium enema, especially in the very old. Defecation empties the rectum and distal colon; occasionally, contents as far proximal as the transverse colon may be evacuated.

Although simple analysis of fecal residue on the plain film can be well correlated with colonic transit,[24] there are two main quantifiable and acceptable ways of measuring transit. Patients may take an oral form of a variety of different radiopaque markers, and these can be followed on their transit through the bowel by plain film radiography. The advantage of this method is its simplicity and availability,[25] and there is potential for some quantification. The main disadvantage is the radiation dose; it is acceptable if only a single film is taken but is more problematic if multiple films are necessary, as in some regimens. Ingestion of radioisotopes attached to a suitable carrier and subsequent observation of transit with a gamma camera is an alternative method. Such isotope methods allow continuous monitoring without the need to increase an already small isotope load; they are quantifiable and can distinguish between solid and liquid transit if required. These methods are not as satisfactory as the well-established gastric emptying techniques because of the prolonged periods of observation, the necessity for an isotope with a longer half-life than technetium, and the difficulties with separating activity from overlapping small and large bowel. Some groups have instilled isotope directly into the cecum by either colonoscopy or orocecal intubation, but clearly this is invasive.[26] For these reasons most departments use radiopaque marker systems with the isotope methods confined to research units or specialized centers. Methods that release isotope in the ileum by use of pH-sensitive polymers show promise.[27]

When measuring transit, most centers discontinue any laxative the patient is taking for at least 48 hours before the study. Some units supplement the diet with bran, but this can be unacceptable to patients with chronic idiopathic constipation because it can exacerbate symptoms such as bloating. Most centers now use short segments of cut up polyethylene tubing as radiopaque markers. Many different approaches have been described. At the simplest level a number of markers can be ingested on day 1, and a single abdominal radiograph taken at a fixed interval a number of days later. Both Hinton et al.[28] and Martelli et al.[29] administered 20 markers. The former group demonstrated that if all markers were present on day 4 or four or more markers were still present on day 6, then slow transit existed. The latter group stated that more than 20% of the markers retained at day 5 was abnormal, and this simple criterion has been widely adopted (Fig. 43-3).

Transit measurements are further complicated by by the fact that transit varies in different segments of the colon.[30] Logically, patients with outlet obstruction as opposed to generalized colonic slow transit (colonic inertia) may fail to excrete the markers by day 5, since these are retained in the distal colon. Segmental assessment can be refined in a number of different ways. The most logical method of taking markers, and following with 12 hourly films until they are passed, exposes the patient to unacceptable doses of ra-

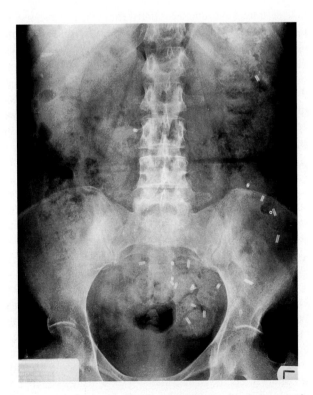

Fig. 43-3 Shapes study. Twenty radiopaque polyethylene markers were taken 5 days before. All are still retained in the colon, indicating slow transit.

diation. Different-shaped markers can be taken on three successive days, and then a film taken on day 4 and subsequent days until the first markers have passed. This reduces the number of films and still differentiates segmental transit.[31] Perhaps more elegant are methods where markers are given on successive days for at least 5 days to reach a steady state, whereby an equal number of markers are theoretically entering the colon as are leaving it. If 24 markers are given each day, and a film is taken on day 6, then simply counting the number of markers provides an estimate of the colonic transit time in hours; counting the number of markers in each segment furnishes a similar estimate of the segmental transit time. Using such methods, the total colonic transit time has been shown to have a mean of 35 hours with an upper limit of normal of 72, this being evenly split between the right, left, and rectosigmoid segments. One practical point: it is clearly essential to know the number and timing of markers ingested in relation to any film taken before a sensible report is issued.

Slow transit constipation

Patients with "pure" slow transit constipation tend to retain radiographic markers throughout the colon, and some of these patients are offered surgery. Lane[32] described subtotal colectomy and ileorectal anastomosis for severe idiopathic constipation as long ago as 1908, and the condition is sometimes named after him. Although this operation is successful in some patients, many have recurrent constipation or intractable diarrhea afterward. Others have recurrent severe abdominal pain, and a proportion of all patients ultimately need an ileostomy. Some of the failures may be due to poor selection criteria, but even when careful physiologic testing is performed to ensure that slow transit is the relevant pathophysiologic mechanism, results of colectomy are not always satisfactory. Experience with newer "prokinetic" agents such as cisapride[33] as an alternative to surgery is limited and disappointing.

Outlet obstruction

Study of pelvic floor mechanisms is technically easier and more accessible than motility of the colon as a whole, and much of the ingenuity in investigation has been in the study of rectal evacuation.

Anal physiology and constipation

An assessment of anal physiology can occasionally be helpful in the investigation of the constipated patient. Of the 801 patients referred for examination of anal physiology to the Sir Alan Parks Unit at St Mark's Hospital in London, 103 patients (13%) were referred because of their constipation.[34] In practice we have found that physiologic studies rarely affect the management of these patients except in the exclusion of Hirschsprungs's disease by the demonstration of the rectosphincteric inhibitory reflex and the assessment of sphincter function in a patient under consideration for total colectomy and ileorectal anastomosis.

The normal sequence of events that allow rectal emptying has been described in an earlier chapter. Outlet obstruction refers to a failure of these mechanisms resulting in difficulty in or incompleteness of emptying of the rectum.

Anismus

During normal defecation or straining a reflex inhibition of electrical activities (action potentials) occurs in the pelvic floor musculature. Some patients apparently have either failure of relaxation or inappropriate contraction of the puborectalis, anal sphincter, or both on attempted defecation. This can be tested using defecography, balloon sphincterography, balloon expulsion tests, anorectal manometry, and electromyography (EMG), although concordance does not always exist between these various methods. On EMG recordings in these patients (and in some with solitary rectal ulcer syndrome) it was shown that these patients not only displayed failure of inhibition of electrical activity in the pelvic floor but also recruitment of motor unit activity occurred in some instances.[35] The condition has been dubbed *anismus*,[36] but others favor terms such as *puborectalis syndrome, spastic pelvic floor*, and *rectal floor dyssynergia*.

During normal defecation or straining there is reflex inhibition of the puborectalis accompanied by flattening of the anorectal angle. On proctography the typical indicators of anismus are failure to efface (or even accentuation of) the puborectalis impression during straining, poor anal canal opening, and often incomplete or intermittent evacuation (Fig. 43-4). Sometimes the impression is overcome only by extreme straining and excessive pelvic floor descent. In fact, it is important to check at defecography that at least some pelvic floor descent occurs, since this is an indication of raised intraabdominal pressure and therefore a serious attempt at evacuation. Even if this is seen, it is difficult to rule out voluntary contraction of the pelvic floor despite straining, and this is a criticism of the diagnosis of anismus that applies to any method of testing.

Although proctographic appearances can be highly suggestive, attempts are usually made to confirm the diagnosis by nonproctographic methods.[37] Few studies are available to validate proctographic studies. Wald et al.[38] demonstrated a poor correlation between proctographic diagnosis of anismus compared with anorectal manometry but did not include electrophysiology. Wexner et al.[39] found a poor correlation between EMG-diagnosed paradoxic contraction of the puborectalis and proctographic demonstration of the same, although incomplete relaxation, excessive pelvic floor descent, and rectocele formation were common. EMG studies are invasive, however, and cannot be assumed to be the gold standard because patients may voluntarily contract the puborectalis more readily in the laboratory situation. Indeed it has been shown that failure of relaxation of pelvic floor musculature or recruitment of additional motor units on straining is nonspecific and can be demonstrated in a wide range of proctologic disorders.[40] In Wexner et al.'s study 35% of the patients with paradoxic puborectalis

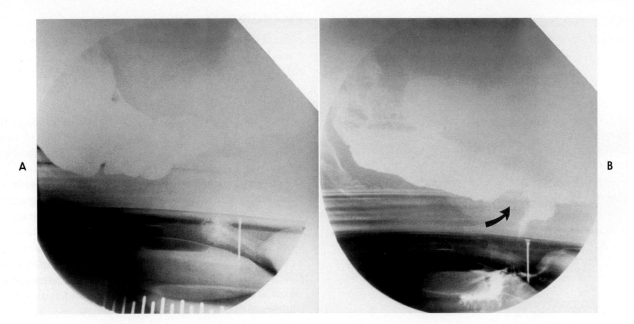

Fig. 43-4 Evacuating proctogram in anismus. **A,** At rest a normal configuration of the colon is seen. **B,** On attempted defecation there is a normal amount of descent of the pelvic floor, but the puborectalis impression has accentuated *(arrow).*

contraction diagnosed with EMG had rapid and complete emptying of the rectum at defecography, tending to confirm that EMG may produce false-positive results. Furthermore, failure to efface the puborectalis impression during straining, rather than actual accentuation, may still be a sign of inappropriate contraction of the muscle. It is our belief that radiologic methods of diagnosis of anismus are more reliable than electrophysiology.

Treatment of anismus is unsatisfactory. Internal sphincterotomy or myomectomy have been tried, [41,42] as have posterior[43] and lateral division[44] of the puborectalis, but none with reliable improvement and always at the risk of incontinence. On the basis that anismus is a "learned response" many groups are now looking at the effectiveness of biofeedback methods to relax the puborectalis and sphincter mechanisms during defecation.

Other causes of outlet obstruction

In some patients with symptoms of obstructed defecation, paradoxic contraction of the puborectalis is not encountered, but, at defecography, an internal intussusception is observed[45] that 'plugs' the internal anal orifice (Fig. 43-5). The patient may then strain excessively and ineffectively as the intussusception stimulates receptors in the anal canal and simulates stool. These patients typically report straining for prolonged periods when defecating and incomplete or intermittent defecation. In some patients a variant of this is seen when the anterior wall of the rectum prolapses into the anal canal. Anterior wall prolapse and intussusception may be manifestations of the solitary rectal ulcer syndrome.[46] This is often associated with increased intrarectal

pressure during straining. The results of rectopexy to prevent intussusception in these patients are variable. Radiographic improvement is not always accompanied by resolution of symptoms.[47,48]

Chronic straining is thought to lead to excessive ballooning of the perineum (pelvic floor descent). This may be associated with rectocele and intussusception formation and is more common in females.[49] Care must be taken in attributing these radiologic findings to straining alone because they may be found in young, healthy (largely female) volunteers without any history of a defecatory disorder. Nevertheless, some subjects complain of ineffective and incomplete defecation and produce large rectoceles at proctography and retain significant amounts of contrast in the rectocele at the end of evacuation (Fig. 43-6). It is easy to surmise that retention of hard stool in such a rectocele could produce symptoms; in normal volunteers rectoceles were common, but significant retention of barium did not occur. Surgical correction of rectoceles may relieve symptoms.[52]

Some patients with prolonged histories of straining produce pouches of mucosa through the pelvic floor musculature—the *posterolateral rectal pouch*[53] (Fig. 43-7). These normally occur only during straining and are therefore seen only at defecography. They may be missed on standard lateral projections and require oblique or anteroposterior views for confirmation. With time they may become permanent and can be quite large. It is postulated that these can be a cause of pelvic floor discomfort and feelings of incomplete defecation.

Many patients with outlet obstruction will evolve aiding

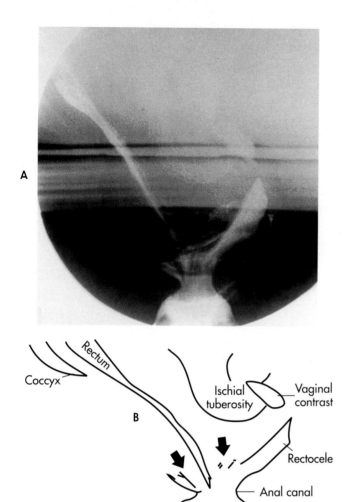

Fig. 43-5 Evacuating proctogram in a patient with obstructed defecation. An intussusception has impacted in the anal canal preventing any further evacuation. Note the gap between the vagina and anterior rectal wall indicating an enterocele.

mechanisms to help in achieving defecation. Asking patients to demonstrate these at proctography often helps to confirm that an observed radiologic abnormality is relevant to the patient's symptoms; for example, some patients with anismus insert a gloved finger into the rectum and press down on the puborectalis impression to achieve defecation, saying they can feel a "bar" or "ridge" that they must overcome. Others press on a rectocele by applying pressure on the perineum or posterior vaginal wall to try to empty a rectocele, and patients with an obstructing intussusception may demonstrate attempts to disimpact it.

INCONTINENCE

Fecal incontinence is a surprisingly common disorder but a less common complaint. It is particularly common in the elderly[54]; in residential homes for the elderly the incidence was found to be 10%.[55] Another study demonstrated a prevalence of fecal or double incontinence of 4.2/1000 in men 15 to 64 years of age and 10.9/1000 in men of 65 years and over. The corresponding rates in women were 1.7/1000 in those 15 to 64 years of age and 13.3/1000 in those over 65 years.[56]

Anal incontinence can be a source of considerable morbidity and embarrassment; hence a sympathetic approach to management and investigation is of particular importance in these patients. The causes of this condition can be classified simply as enteric, neurologic, or muscular. However, a combination of factors are commonly involved in any one patient, and it is best to consider the entire defecation mechanism as a whole when unravelling the mechanism of incontinence except in simple enteric causes.

Enteric causes

Any cause of severe diarrhea can so stress the normal continence mechanisms that incontinence may develop. Some individuals are likely to be more prone to this than others; both physiologic[57] and proctographic studies[50] have shown a wide range of normal values, with some young patients apparently possessing only marginal anorectal function.

Physiologic components of the mechanisms of fecal continence and their testing

Anal continence is the summation of a complex and poorly understood series of factors; those currently recognized are enumerated in the following sections.

Internal sphincter

The internal sphincter is a condensation of the internal circular muscle layer of the rectum and is approximately 5 mm thick and 30 to 50 mm long. The muscle is in a state of continuous contraction that is significantly greater than that developed by isolated colonic circular muscle.[58] Surgical division of the internal sphincter (sphincterotomy) rarely leads to significant loss of continence, indicating that the muscle does not play a major function in continence. It would appear that the sphincter's main role is to provide a fine-tuning mechanism that maintains continence to flatus and liquid stools.

External sphincter and pelvic floor

The muscles of the external sphincter and pelvic floor display the phenomenon, unusual in skeletal muscle, of continuous electrical tone that is maintained during sleep and without conscious effort.[59] The resting electrical activity is facilitated by means of a spinal reflex arc that increases electrical tone during changes in posture and other acts

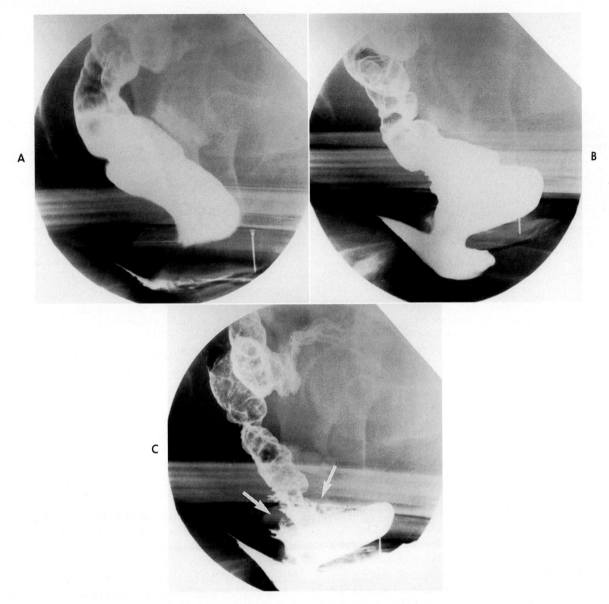

Fig. 43-6 Evacuating proctogram in a patient with incomplete evacuation. **A,** At rest there is abnormal pelvic floor descent. The anal canal is closed. **B,** During evacuation further descent has occurred, and a rectocele is forming. **C,** At the end of defecation marked perineal floor descent is seen, a rectocele has trapped barium, and a late intussusception *(arrows)* is forming. The rectocele was emptied by the patient applying pressure to the posterior vaginal wall.

(e.g., coughing and sneezing) that raise intraabdominal pressure and thereby threaten anal continence. The external sphincter is capable of strong voluntary contraction that can be maintained for approximately 60 seconds. This probably acts as a safety mechanism propelling stool back into the rectum if it enters the proximal anal canal as a consequence of the rectosphincteric inhibitory reflex. Contraction of the puborectalis component of the pelvic floor is essential for maintaining normal control. Contraction of this muscle creates an acute angle between the anus and lower rectum (the anorectal angle). It is not known why this anatomic angle is important or how it functions, but gross incontinence commonly occurs if the angle becomes markedly oblique.[60]

Anorectal sensation

At a level approximating to the dentate line is a profusion of sensory receptors that are more densely packed than at the anal margin. Most of these receptors consist of Meissner's corpuscles, Krause's end bulbs, Golgi-Mazzoni bod-

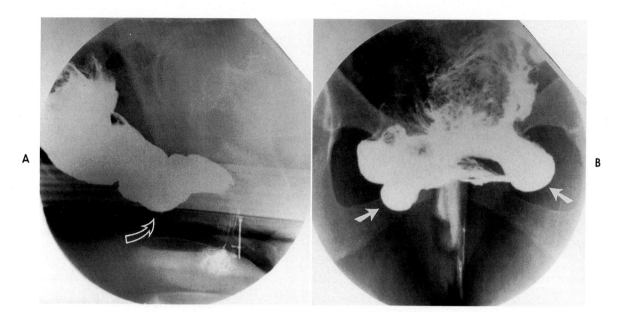

Fig. 43-7 Posterolateral rectal pouch. This condition is hard to appreciate on the conventional lateral proctogram (**A**), but its position is shown by the arrow. These pouches, which are secondary to chronic straining, are much more evident on the anteroposterior views (**B**).

ies, and genital corpuscles. Any disease or abnormality developing in this region, such as an anal fissure or intersphincteric abscess, is hence a source of considerable pain. The sensation of a full rectum is an important component of continence, since it provides a warning to the brain of impending defecation or, if the moment is not propitious, of the need to institute protective mechanisms by vigorous contraction of the pelvic floor. Since the sensation of rectal fullness is preserved even after subtotal rectal excision and coloanal anastomosis, it has become apparent that the sensory receptors reside in the nearby pelvic floor musculature that cradles the rectum.[61]

Another important component of sensation is the discrimination between flatus and feces, which has been demonstrated to be a function of the rectosphincteric inhibitory sampling reflex.[62] When the rectum fills at the completion of a peristaltic wave in the sigmoid, rectal distension occurs. This in turn causes a reflex relaxation of the internal anal sphincter and so permits a small sample of rectal contents to intrude into the upper anal canal where they make contact with the sensory-rich zone at the dentate line. A message is then related to the sensory cortex indicating the presence of feces or flatus; if feces are determined, vigorous contraction of the external sphincter follows, propelling it back into the rectum.

It is evident that all these factors play a role in concert in the maintenance of normal continence. Hence, if the internal sphincter is damaged but the pelvic floor muscles remain intact, the patient is usually grossly continent with

perhaps a slight disability precipitated by diarrhea or flatus. On the other hand, if both sphincters are weak in combination with sensory loss, severe incontinence is inevitable.

Defecation

Once the need for defecation is perceived, and if it is convenient, the mental processes interact to cause reflex inhibition of electrical tone in the pelvic floor. This increases the obliquity of the anorectal angle and facilitates the passage of the fecal bolus. The rectosphincteric inhibitory reflex similarly eases the passage of rectal contents. The propulsive force is probably provided by a combination of rising intraabdominal pressure and rectal peristalsis. The evidence in favor of the latter remains fairly scant. At the completion of defecation there is a burst of electrical activity within the pelvic floor as tone (and the anorectal angle) is restored; this phenomenon is sometimes referred to as the *closing reflex*.[63]

Neurologic pathways involved in the continence mechanism

The visceral component of the anorectum is innervated by the autonomic nervous system. The parasympathetic system innervates by way of the S1 and S2 splanchnic nerves and the sympathetic system by way of the L1 and L2 ganglions. Sympathetic activity is excitatory and parasympathetic activity inhibitory to the internal anal sphincter, and both sets of nerves carry sensory information. The somatic supply is different. The motor supply to the puborectalis is through a branch of the S4 nerve root, and the supply to the external anal sphincter as well as the sensory supply to the lower anal canal is through the pudendal nerve (S2-S3). The exact pathways in the higher centers are not fully understood but may be more fully worked out with correlations of neurologic deficits and anatomic lesions as detected by magnetic resonance imaging. Conscious control of the anorectal region is through the frontal cortex. Communication is through the parasagittal motor cortex through the oligosymptomatic pathway to the Onuf nucleus in the ventral gray matter of the S2-S3 region of the spinal cord. This nucleus carries the lower motor neurons innervating both the urinary and fecal continence mechanisms.

Physiologic tests of anorectal function

As a consequence of the developing interest in the treatment of functional disorders of the anorectum, more accurate methods of studying the function of this region have been attempted. Although progress has been made, no gold standard test of function has yet been developed.

Manometry

Traditionally, manometry is the simplest and most accurate method for measuring anal function. A variety of devices for recording anal pressure have been described, ranging from the simple and inexpensive to the extraordinarily complex and costly. In practice, reliable data can be obtained by simple methods. At St Mark's Hospital in London, we attach a small balloon (diameter 4 mm) to a ureteric catheter. The system is filled with water and connected to a pressure transducer. The probe is introduced into the rectum and then withdrawn into the anus at 1-cm intervals. Pressures are recorded in the resting state and repeated during a period of maximal voluntary contraction. This provides a crude but valuable assessment of internal sphincter (resting tone) and external sphincter (squeeze tone) function. In general, no better method of assessing internal sphincter function exists, since smooth muscle electromyography in vivo is notoriously unreliable. However, as a measure of external sphincter/pelvic floor function, the technique is less reliable because it depends on patient cooperation and understanding, which cannot be guaranteed. In addition, squeeze pressure can be achieved in some patients by vigorous contraction of the adductor muscles, giving rise to the false impression that the external sphincter is functioning normally.

Electromyography
CONVENTIONAL

The application of conventional concentric needle electrodes as a means of studying external sphincter function[64] has been superseded by the more accurate method of single-fiber EMG (see next section). Conventional EMG provides gross information on the presence of active skeletal muscle and therefore has been employed to identify the site of di-

vided muscle ends in patients with sphincter division who are being considered for sphincter repair. The advent of anal ultrasound techniques, which are less invasive and much less painful, has rendered this approach obsolete. Sometimes this method has been used to identify constipated patients with anismus and paradoxic contraction of the pelvic floor. Radiologic techniques have generally proved more reliable and informative.

SINGLE FIBER

With concentric needle electrodes (conventional technique), individual muscle fiber action potentials cannot usually be recognized reliably within the motor unit action potential. Single muscle action potentials can be recorded extracellularly by using an electrode with a small leading-off surface. Recordings are made with the cannula of the electrode as a reference electrode and with a separate surface ground electrode. An amplifier with a 500-Hz low-frequency filter setting and a trigger-delay line are required, and recordings are made with the time base of the amplifier set at 2 to 5 mS per division.

With this technique it is possible to identify and quantify denervation in the skeletal muscle under investigation. In normal circumstances axonal firing is responsible for one or two muscle action potentials. Where denervation has occurred the usual physiologic response is for reinnervation to occur. Hence, in a patient with denervated muscle, the single-fiber EMG demonstrates polyphasic action potential that can be quantified and averaged for different areas in that muscle. This concept is referred to as the fiber density of the muscle and approximates the number of muscle fibers supplied by one axon. In patients with anal incontinence due to nerve damage (e.g., as sustained during a traumatic vaginal delivery), fiber density is increased.[65]

Techniques of nerve stimulation

Having established that the cause of the functional deficit in the external sphincter/pelvic floor is neurogenic in origin, it is sometimes important to identify whether the anatomic site of the injury sustained is central (spinal cord/cauda equina) or peripheral (pudendal nerves) in origin.

The most important component of neurologic injury is localized damage to the pudendal nerves. Function in these nerves can be accurately assessed by measuring the pudendal nerve terminal motor latency (PNTML). Pudendal nerve stimulation is performed transrectally with a rubber-finger stall containing two stimulating electrodes at the tip and two recording electrodes at the base.[66] Square wave stimuli, 0.1 mS long and 50 V are administered through the tip, which is placed over the ischial tuberosity through the rectum. The external anal sphincter contraction is detected with the surface electrodes and the oscilloscope tracing then analyzed. The latency is measured as the interval between onset of the stimulus and first dissociation of the tracing from the isoelectric line corresponding with external sphincter contraction. In patients with incontinence due to pudendal nerve damage the latency is significantly increased.

Central components of the neurogenic pathway may be tested either by spinal stimulation[67] or by stimulation of the cerebral cortex.[68] These studies may be important in the investigation of the patient with a short history of symptoms, which may be the consequence of a tumor affecting the central nervous system. These studies are highly specialized and are not employed in the routine assessment of patients referred for anal incontinence.

Anorectal sensation tests

Testing a function that requires a subjective response (i.e., conscious perception of a stimulus) necessarily lacks objectivity. Previously the only method for testing sensation consisted of inserting a Miller-Abbott balloon into the rectum and filling it until the patient first became aware of the balloon and, later, the point at which the sensation became distinctly uncomfortable.[69] Such techniques are a crude but valuable means of assessing rectal capacity, which may be reduced in ulcerative colitis and may be a factor militating against ileorectal anastomosis.

More recently, anal canal sensation has been measured with greater accuracy by employing the electrosensitivity method.[70] This method involves incrementally increasing the electrical current delivered to a platinum probe inserted into the anal canal until the patient first becomes aware of the electrical stimulus. The method gives reproducible and reliable data. With this method it has been confirmed that the middle portion of the anal canal is the most sensitive and that sensation is blunted in patients with neurogenic anal incontinence.

Neurologic causes
Upper motor neuron disorders

A wide range of neurologic disorders affecting the brain can result in fecal incontinence. These include diseases affecting neuronal function diffusely, such as dementias, cerebrovascular disease, and hydrocephalus, and those with more focal processes, such as intracranial neoplasms and multiple sclerosis. Similar processes affecting the spinal cord and diseases causing spinal compression also can cause incontinence.

With disease solely affecting the upper motor neuron pathways, reflex induction of both micturition and defecation are usually possible. Resting anal pressures may be normal, but voluntary inhibition of the continence mechanism can be absent. Patients with multiple sclerosis, for instance, often have severe constipation.[21] Although the cause can be multifactorial, failure of the puborectalis and sphincter mechanism to relax (anorectal dyssynergia) can contribute to this complication. These patients also may be incontinent because of impaired sensation, increased reflex to rectal filling, and poor control of voluntary contraction of the pelvic floor muscles and external sphincter.

Lower motor neuron disorders

Disorders of the lower motor neuron are the most important because they are relatively common and potentially avoidable. Damage to the lower motor neuron axis results in weakness and atrophy of the pelvic floor musculature and the sphincter muscles.[71] The perineal floor then bulges excessively when the intraabdominal pressure is increased such as during straining (perineal floor descent).

Two major factors are thought to be responsible for pudendal nerve neuropathy: chronic straining at stool and childbirth.[72] Reversible changes in pudendal nerve latency have been demonstrated after even a single episode of straining.[73] Once established, a vicious circle can ensue. Perineal floor descent results in inefficient evacuation and further straining, thereby increasing neuropathy and further descent. This ultimately leads to incontinence.

Even normal childbirth is suspected of producing neuropathic changes in the pudendal nerve, and such changes are compounded by long labor, instrumentation, and multiparity.[72] Physical damage to the sphincters also can occur during childbirth.[74]

Although most instances of lower motor neuron incontinence are believed to result from these factors, a small proportion are caused by more specific focal diseases affecting Onuf's nucleus or the cauda equina, such as multiple sclerosis, lumbar disc disease, lumbar canal stenosis, and ankylosing spondylitis. The peripheral nerves can also be affected by local pelvic tumors, trauma, and peripheral neuropathies (e.g., diabetes mellitus), as well as by more specific autonomic neuronal disorders.

Sensory deficits

Although rarely isolated, many neurologic causes of incontinence may be accompanied by sensory deficits.[75] Such patients may not be aware of a full rectum or anal filling until it is too late, and defecation occurs.

Complex lesions

Clearly, many patients have complex neurologic disorders with upper and lower motor neuron components as well as sensory deficits and actual sphincter damage. Physiologic, electromyographic, sensory, manometric, and morphologic tests identify to some extent the various components of the problem.[76]

Radiologic value in investigation of incontinent patients

Various radiologic procedures have been used to investigate incontinence per se, but currently radiology does not have a major role and should always be considered in conjunction with clinical and physiologic data.

Appropriate radiologic studies may be required to demonstrate an enteric cause of incontinence, for example, to discover the cause of chronic diarrhea. When diarrhea is absent, examinations are tailored to the clinical problem.

Severe constipation resulting in excessive straining may in time cause incontinence through pelvic floor descent and associated pudendal neuropathy, and therefore investigation may be directed paradoxically to the cause of constipation. The importance of neurologic damage in so-called idiopathic incontinence, whether due to such factors as prolonged labor or chronic straining, cannot be overemphasized. In addition, morphologic studies of the sphincter mechanisms using intraanal ultrasound and, more recently, MRI are playing an increasingly important role.

Role of defecography

Defecography, apart from its role in the identification of mechanisms leading to chronic constipation and subsequent incontinence, has a limited role in assessing the anorectal angle, pelvic floor musculature, and associated morphologic abnormalities (such as rectal intussusception, prolapse, enteroceles, and sigmoidoceles) in patients with incontinence. Methodologically it is important to use a barium paste; liquid barium places stress on even a normal continence mechanism and leads to an unnecessarily messy examination in incontinent patients. By the time imaging is commenced, the rectum may already be empty, and, in any event, no effort is needed from the patient to expel the barium, which may prevent the formation of some important structural abnormalities. A contrast-soaked tampon may inhibit rectocele formation, and alternative methods of vaginal opacification (e.g., contrast-soaked gauze or contrast gel)[77] are to be preferred. Finally, enteroceles, which are an important component in some patients with prolapse, are best demonstrated with prior opacification of the small bowel.

A strong correlation exists between major incontinence and a nonfunctioning puborectalis muscle, and quite possibly the anorectal angle may be a very important parameter in the assessment of incontinence. However, most investigations have found this measurement of limited value.[78]

It is difficult to reach consensus as to where to measure the rectal axis component of this angle. If standardized, wide intraobserver and interobserver variation exists in its measurement even among experts.[79-81] Measurement is particularly difficult when the puborectalis impression is indistinct—a common situation when measurement seems clinically desirable. Even if the anorectal angle could be reliably measured, its value depends on the activity of the puborectalis and on the amount of pelvic floor descent; with descent, the angle naturally becomes more obtuse. A recent study confirmed that both in chronic constipation and incontinence the position of the anorectal junction was low and the anorectal angle large in comparison with controls, but that constipated patients tended to retain their ability to raise the pelvic floor and narrow the anorectal angle on squeeze as compared with those who are incontinent (unpublished observations).

Certain patterns of proctographic appearance are common in incontinent patients. The patient often has a pudendal neuropathy and is usually female. The pelvic floor tends to show some descent and often balloons on straining. The anorectal angle tends to be obtuse with limited change on squeeze. The anal canal is short (or even nonexistent radiologically) and may be open at rest. Even if the canal is closed, contrast may be lost involuntarily on coughing. Closure or lengthening of the anal canal is variable on squeeze depending on the integrity of the external sphincter. On straining to evacuate, rectal emptying is often rapid, and an enterocele (or other organ prolapsing into the pouch of Douglas) may develop (Fig. 43-8). In patients with marked descent, a rectocele is common, as is a late intussusception, which may progress to become intraanal or even external (procidentia).

Incontinent patients may demonstrate some or all of the above features. Demonstration of such features, when combined with manometric, electrophysiologic, and endosonographic data, is important for surgical planning. The surgeon must decide whether an operation to restore the anorectal angle (e.g., postanal repair)[82] is all that is necessary, or whether some form of rectopexy (fixation of the rectum to the sacral curve) alone or in addition is required. A sphincter repair may be necessary, or it may be decided that any restorative procedure is unlikely to succeed, thus making colostomy the best option. Careful analysis of the proctogram can be crucial in this planning.

RECTAL PROLAPSE

Rectal prolapse is slightly out of the domain of this chapter, since it can occur in a patient with an intact continence mechanism. Rectal prolapse is just one part of pelvic floor prolapse as a whole. Traditionally the various components of pelvic floor prolapse have been considered separately by different specialties (bladder by urologists, uterus and vagina by gynecologists, and rectum by coloproctologists), and it is only now that these artificial barriers are being dismantled.[83,84]

Rectal prolapse tends to occur at the extremes of life. In very young children it is more common in boys and tends to respond to conservative management. In adults it is more common in women, although not to the same degree as idiopathic incontinence; its etiology is different, and it occurs as frequently in nulliparous as multiparous women.[85]

The many theories relating to rectal prolapse all fall short in distinguishing cause from effect in patients with established prolapse. A weak anal sphincter may be a primary event or secondary to repeated stretching of the pelvic floor by the prolapsing rectum, and a few patients with prolapse do have normal sphincter pressures. Interestingly, one study found no difference in sphincter pressures between a group of patients with rectal prolapse and age-matched controls.[86] A deep rectovaginal pouch (of Douglas) may be an initiating event, as suggested by Moschcowitz,[87] but most think it is a result of stretching following repeated prolapse. Sim-

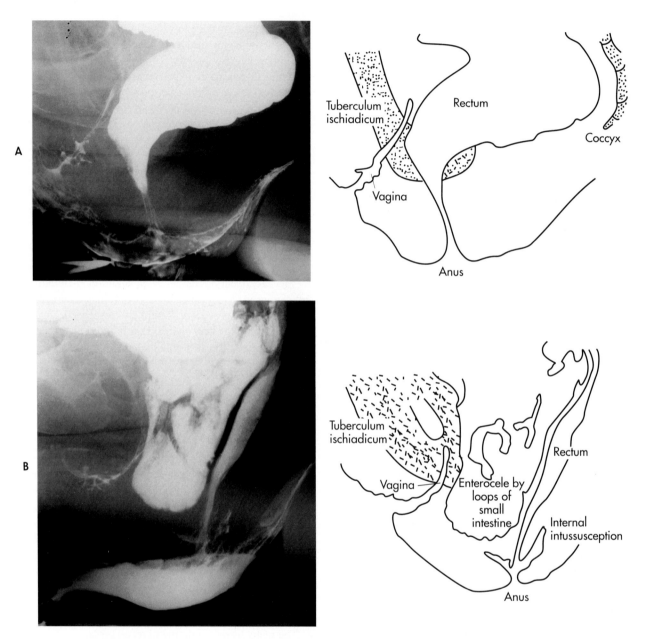

Fig. 43-8 A and **B,** Proctograms. **A,** At rest the configuration of the rectum and anal canal is normal. **B,** At the end of defecation, an intrarectal intussusception has formed down to the level of the anal canal. An opacified small bowel confirms the presence of an associated enterocele between the anterior wall of the rectum and the posterior wall of the vagina. **C** and **D,** Dynamic MRI scans.

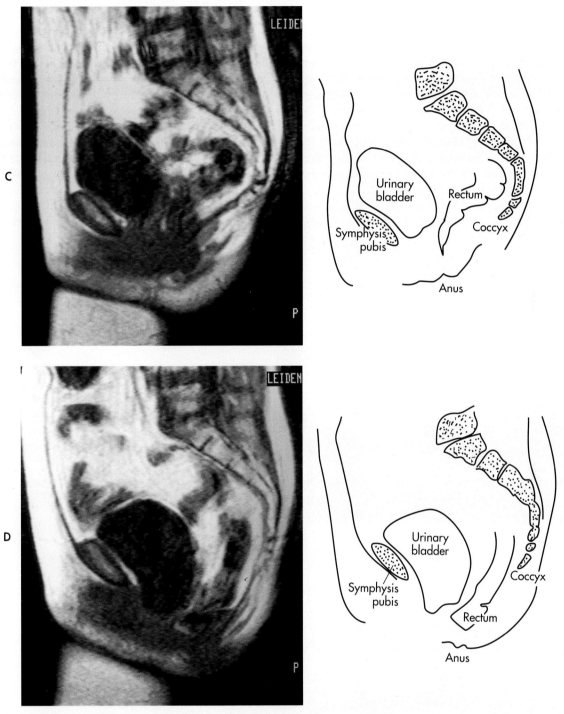

Fig. 43-8, cont'd C, At rest this confirms no abnormality. **D,** During straining there is marked descent of the anterior compartment (bladder) and posterior compartment (rectum). The middle compartment (uterus) cannot be assessed because of previous hysterectomy. The intussusception and enterocele clearly shown on the proctogram are not visualized.
Courtesy of Dr. R.H. Kruyt.

ilarly, poor fixation of the rectum to the presacral tissues may facilitate intrarectal intussusception and subsequent prolapse or be secondary to it.

Role of proctography in prolapse

Prolapse may seem to be such a dramatic symptom that radiologic demonstration is unnecessary. However, patients may only complain of incontinence, pruritis ani, bleeding, feelings of incomplete evacuation, or other symptoms. Even if a history of "something prolapsing" is given, the patient's description may be unclear. Physical examination may reveal only associated clinical signs, and patients may be inhibited from demonstrating prolapse on the examination couch. In one study rectal prolapse was clinically occult in 27 of 127 patients with the condition.[88]

Evacuation proctography can be invaluable in the investigation of prolapse.[89] It may demonstrate occult prolapse in those patients with suspicious symptoms or who are being investigated for a variety of other presentations such as incontinence and perineal discomfort. It also demonstrates the mechanism of prolapse, which can be helpful in surgical planning. A number of anatomic associations of prolapse are seen at proctography. The rectum may be poorly fixed to the sacrum, and this is evidenced either by it being entirely separate from the sacrum, its place taken by sigmoid colon, or by the rectosacral gap being greater than 1 cm. The rectovaginal pouch (or rectovesicle pouch in males) is often deep, which is usually evident only on evacuation, and the pelvic floor often shows abnormal descent.

Most rectal prolapse commences as a midrectal intussusception that progresses toward the anus, as shown on elegant early studies using rectal markers attached to the rectal mucosa.[90] Individual cases demonstrate different mechanisms such as commencement of the prolapse in the distal

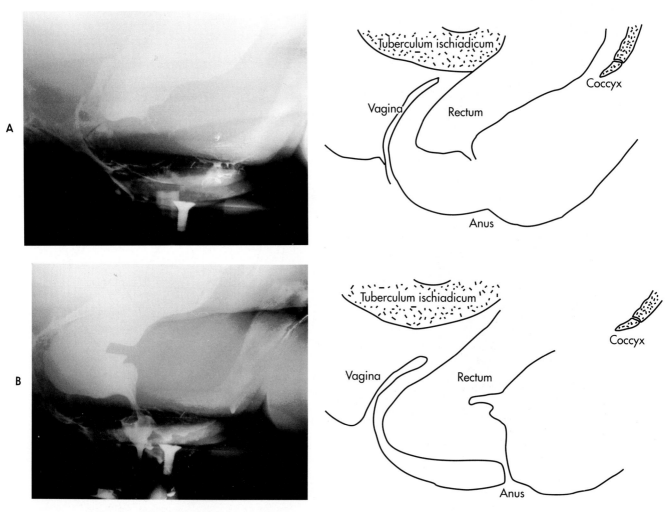

Fig. 43-9 A and **B,** Proctograms. **A,** Pelvic floor descent is evident at rest, and a small rectocele is present. **B,** On straining there is further pelvic floor descent and marked enlargement of the rectocele.

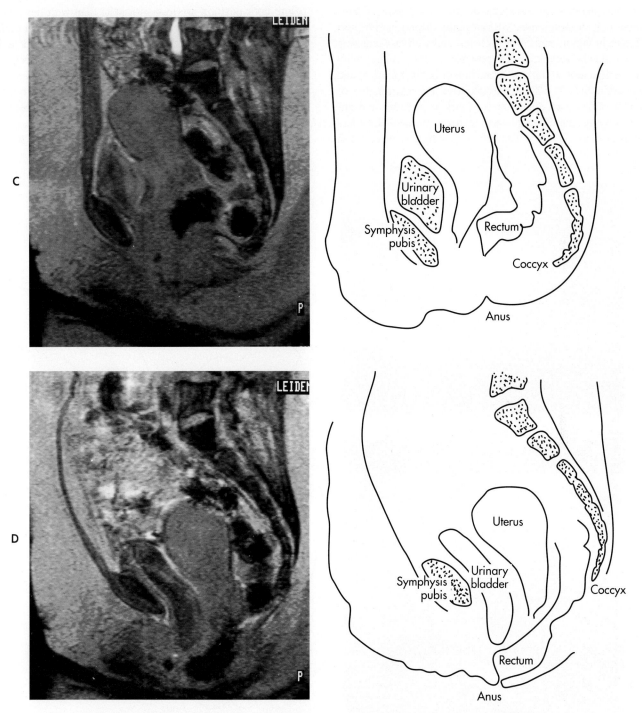

Fig. 43-9, cont'd C and **D,** MRI scans. **C,** The MRI study is normal at rest. **D,** On straining, the marked descent of the posterior compartment (rectum) is seen, accompanied by prolapse of the anterior compartment (bladder) but not the middle compartment (uterus), which has remained essentially stationary. The rectocele is not visualized.
Courtesy of Dr. R.H. Kruyt.

rectum; careful analysis of the videotapes prove necessary. Sometimes the mechanisms seem to defy analysis, with the prolapse occurring swiftly between very few video frames.

Magnetic resonance imaging

Magnetic resonance imaging has recently been used in the investigation of anorectal disorders, particularly prolapse in its widest sense. MRI elegantly displays pelvic soft tissues in sagittal and coronal planes, and with fast-scanning gradient echo techniques it is possible to obtain images with the patient at rest, during contraction of pelvic muscles, and on straining.[91,92] MRI has emphasized the interrelation of rectal prolapse to other forms of pelvic prolapse and encourages the multidisciplinary approach to these disorders (Figs. 43-8 to 43-10). The relative movement of one soft tissue to another can be analyzed with MRI, particularly if a landmark such as the plica of Kohlrausch on the posterior rectal wall can be identified. This, for instance, may make assessment of the fixation of the rectum to the sacrum more reliable and aid surgical planning. Early impressions are that interobserver variations in measurements of pelvic floor position are less with MRI than with defecography. Morphologic changes in the rectum are not well seen on MRI. Certain other features are missed because the act of defecation cannot be visualized on MRI, and therefore it is unlikely to replace defecography. However, there is no doubt that MRI will become more pivotal in the investigation of anorectal disorders because of its multiplanar ability, lack of gonadal irradiation, and complete imaging of the pelvic organs. MRI also is showing promise in iden-

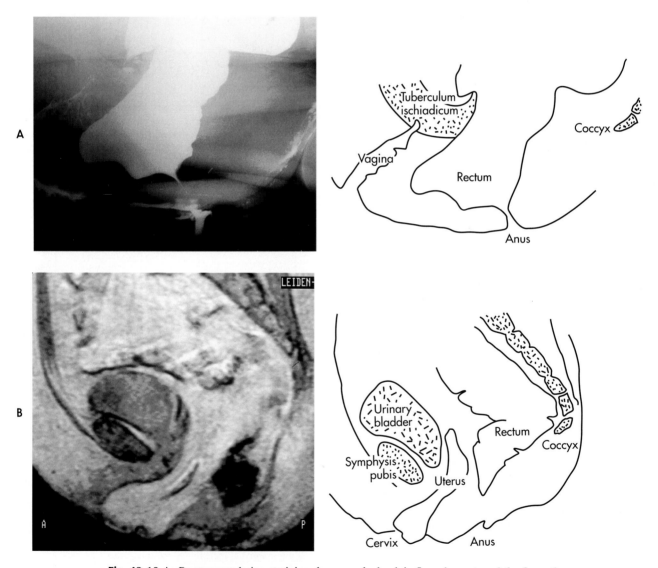

Fig. 43-10 A, Proctogram during straining shows marked pelvic floor descent, and the formation of a large rectocele. **B,** MRI scan during straining shows a prolapsed uterus with some descent of the posterior compartment but none of the anterior compartment. The rectocele is not visualized. Courtesy of Dr. R.H. Kruyt.

tifying the precise anatomy in patients with anorectal anomalies, both before[93] and after surgery.[94]

REFERENCES

1. Connell AM, Hilton C, Irvine C et al: Variation of bowel habit in two population samples *Br Med J* 2:1095, 1965.
2. Drossman DA, Sandler RS, McKee DC, Lovitz AJ: Bowel habits amongst subjects not seeking health care, *Gastroenterology* 83:529, 1979.
3. Berman IR, Manning DH, Harris MS: Streamlining the management of defecation disorders, *Dis Colon Rectum* 33:778, 1990.
4. Orr JD, Scobie WG: Presentation and incidence of Hirschsprung's disease, *Br Med J* 287:1671, 1983.
5. Meier-Ruge W: Hirschsprung's disease: its aetiology, pathogenesis, and differential diagnosis, *Curr Topics Pathol* 59:131, 1970.
6. Preston DM, Lennard-Jones JE, Thomas BM: Towards a radiological definition of idiopathic megacolon, *Gastrointest Radiol* 10:167, 1985.
7. Gowers WR: The autonomic action of the internal anal sphincter in man, *Proc R Soc Lond* 26:77, 1877.
8. Denny-Brown D, Robertson EG: An investigation of the nervous control of defecation, *Brain* 58:256, 1935.
9. Lubowski DZ, Nicholls RJ, Swash M, Jordan MJ: Neural control of internal anal sphincter function, *Br J Surg* 74:668, 1987.
10. Callaghan RP, Nixon HH: Megarectum: physiological observation, *Arch Dis Childhood* 39:153, 1964.
11. Barnes PRH, Lennard-Jones JE, Howley PR, Todd IP: Hirschsprung's disease and idiopathic megacolon in adults and adolescents, *Gut* 27:534, 1986.
12. Ikawa H, Kim SH, Hendren H, Donahoe PK: Acetyl cholinesterase and manometry in the diagnosis of the constipated child, *Arch Surg* 121:435, 1986.
13. Dudley HA, Sinclair IS, McLaren et al: Intestinal pseudoobstruction, *J R Coll Surg Edin* 3:206, 1958.
14. Dudley HA, Patterson-Brown S: Pseudoobstruction, *Br Med J* 292:1157, 1986.
15. Faulk DL, Anuras S, Christensen J: Chronic intestinal pseudoobstruction, *Gastroenterology* 92:786, 1978.
16. Christensen J: Intestinal pseudoobstruction and paralytic ileus. In Moody FG, Carey LC, Jones RS et al: *Surgical treatment of digestive disease,* Chicago, 1986, Mosby–Year Book.
17. Rohrmann CA, Ricci MT, Krishnamurthy S, Schuffler MD: Radiologic and histologic differentiation of neuromuscular disorders of the gastrointestinal tract, *AJR* 143:933, 1984.
18. Whitehead WE, Schuster MM: Behavioural approaches to the treatment of gastrointestinal motility disorders, *Med Clin North Am* 65:1397, 1981.
19. Preston DM, Pfeffer J, Lennard-Jones JE: Psychiatric assessment of patients with severe constipation, *Gut* 25:A582, 1984.
20. Kamm MA, Lennard-Jones JE: Rectal musocal electrosensory resting: evidence for a rectal sensory neuropathy in idiopathic constipation, *Dis Colon Rectum* 33:419, 1990.
21. Chia YW, Gill KP, Jameson JS et al: Paradoxical puborectalis contraction is a feature of constipation in multiple sclerosis patients, *Dis Colon Rectum* (submitted for publication).
22. Hinds JP, Wald A: Colonic and anorectal dysfunction associated with multiple sclerosis, *Am J Gastroenterol* 84:587, 1989.
23. Pemberton JH, Rath DM, Ilstrup DM: Evaluation and surgical treatment of severe chronic constipation, *Ann Surg* 214:403, 1991.
24. Starreveld JS, Pols MA, Van Wijk HJ et al: The plain abdominal radiograph in the assessment of constipation, *Z Gastroenterol* 28:335, 1990.
25. Krevsky B, Malmud LS, D'Ercole F et al: Colonic transit scintigraphy: a physiological approach to the quantitive measurement of colonic transit in humans, *Gastroenterology* 91:1102, 1986.
26. Spiller RC, Brown ML, Phillips SF: Decreased fluid tolerance, ac-

celerated transit, and abnormality of the human colon induced by oleic acid, *Gastroenterology* 91:100, 1986.
27. Proano M, Camillieri M, Phillips SF et al: Transit of solids through the human colon: regional quantification on the unprepared bowel, *Am J Physiol* 258:G856, 1990.
28. Hinton JM, Lennard-Jones JE, Young AC: A new method for studying gut transit times using radiopaque markers, *Gut* 10:842, 1969.
29. Martelli H, Devroede G, Arhan P et al: Some parameters of large bowel motility in normal man, *Gastroenterology* 75:612, 1978.
30. Metcalf AM, Phillips SF, Zinsmeister AR et al: Simplified assessment of segmental colonic transit, *Gastroenterology* 92:40, 1987.
31. Abrahamsson H, Antov S, Bosaeus I: Gastrointestinal and colonic segmental transit time evaluated by a single abdominal x-ray in healthy subjects and constipated patients, *Scand J Gastroenterol* 23(suppl 152):72, 1988.
32. Lane WA: Chronic intestinal stasis, *Br Med J* 2:1125, 1912.
33. Krevsky B, Malmud LS, Maurer AH et al: Cisapride accelerates colonic transit in constipated patients with colonic inertia, *Gastroenterology* 94:A293, 1988.
34. Speakman CTM, Henry MM: The work of an anorectal physiology laboratory. In Henry MM, ed: *Bailliere's clinical gastroenterology: anorectal disorders* London, 1992, Bailliere Tindall.
35. Rutter KRP: Electromyographic changes in certain pelvic floor abnormalities, *Proc R Soc Med* 67:53, 1974.
36. Preston DM, Lennard-Jones JE: Anismus in chronic constipation, *Dig Dis Sci* 30:413, 1985.
37. Turnbull GK, Lennard-Jones JE, Bartram CI: Failure of rectal expulsion as a cause of constipation: why fibre and laxatives sometimes fail, *Lancet* 2:767, 1986.
38. Wald A, Caruana BJ, Freimanis M et al: Contribution of evacuation proctography and anorectal manometry to evaluation of adults with constipation and defecatory difficulties, *Dig Dis Sci* 35:481, 1990.
39. Wexner SD, Marchetti F, Salanga V et al: Neurophysiologic assessment of the anal sphincters, *Dis Colon Rectum* 34:606, 1991.
40. Jones PN, Lubowski DZ, Swash M, Henry MM: Is paradoxical contraction of puborectalis muscle of functional importance? *Dis Col Rectum* 30:667, 1987.
41. Martelli H, Devroede G, Arhan P et al: Mechanisms of idiopathic constipation: outlet obstruction *Gastroenterology* 75:623, 1978.
42. Yoshioka K, Keithley MRB: Anorectal myectomy for outlet obstruction, *Br J Surg* 74:373, 1988.
43. Barnes PRH, Hawley PR, Preston DM, Lennard-Jones JE: Experience of posterior division of the puborectalis muscle in the management of chronic constipation, *Br J Surg* 72:475, 1985.
44. Kamm MA, Hawley PR, Lennard-Jones JE: Lateral division of the puborectalis muscle in the management of severe constipation, *Br J Surg* 75:661, 1988.
45. Goei R, Baeten C: Rectal intussusception and rectal prolapse: detection and postoperative evaluation with defecography, *Radiology* 174:124, 1990.
46. Goei R, Baeten C, Arends JW: Solitary rectal ulcer syndrome: findings at barium enema and defecography, *Radiology* 168:303, 1988.
47. Orrom WJ, Bartolo DCC, Miller R et al: Rectopexy is an ineffective treatment for obstructed defecation, *Dis Colon Rectum* 34:41, 1991.
48. Berman IR, Manning DM, Dudley WK, Wright K: Anatomic specificity in the diagnosis and treatment of internal rectal prolapse, *Dis Colon Rectum* 28:816, 1985.
49. Parks AG, Porter W, Hardcastle JD: The syndrome of the descending perineum, *Proc R Soc Med* 89:477, 1966.
50. Shorvon PJ, McHugh S, Diamant NE, Somers S, Stevenson GW: Defecography in normal volunteers: results and implications *Gut* 30:1737, 1989.
51. Freimanis MG, Wald A, Caruana B, Bauman DH: Evacuation proctography in normal volunteers, *Invest Radiol* 26:58, 1991.
52. Sehapayak S: Transrectal repair of rectocele: an extended armamentarium of colorectal surgeons: a report of 355 patients, *Dis Colon Rectum* 28:422, 1985.

53. Shorvon PJ, Stevenson GW: Defaecography: setting up a service, *Br J Hosp Med* 41:460, 1989.

54. Brocklehurst JC: Management of anal incontinence, *Clin Gastroenterol* 4:479, 1975.

55. Tobin GW, Brocklehurst JC: Faecal incontinence in residential homes of the elderly: prevalence, aetiology, and management, *Age Ageing* 15:41, 1986.

56. Thomas TM, Egan M, Walgrove A et al: The prevalence of faecal and double incontinence, *Comm Med* 6:216, 1984.

57. McHugh SM, Diamant NE: Effect of age, gender, and parity on anal canal pressures: contribution of impaired anal sphincter function to fecal incontinence, *Dig Dis Sci* 32:726, 1987.

58. Burleigh DE, D'Mello A, Parks AG: Responses of isolated human internal anal sphincter to drugs and electrical field stimulation, *Gastroenterology* 77:484, 1979.

59. Floyd W, Walls EW: Electromyography of the sphincter ani externus in man, *J Physiol* 122:599, 1953.

60. Hardcastle JD, Parks AG: A study of anal incontinence and some principles of surgical treatment, *Proc R Soc Med* 63:116, 1970.

61. Lane RHS, Parks AG: Function of the anal sphincters following coloanal anastomosis, *Br J Surg* 64:596, 1977.

62. Miller R, Lewis GT, Bartolo DCC et al: Sensory discrimination and dynamic activity in the anorectum: evidence using a new ambulatory technique, *Br J Surg* 75:1003, 1988.

63. Porter NH: Physiological study of the pelvic floor in rectal prolapse, *Ann R Soc Med* 286:379, 1962.

64. Adrian ED, Bronck DW: The discharge of impulses in motor nerve fibre, *J Physiol* 67:119, 1929.

65. Neill ME, Swash M: Increased motor unit fibre density in the external sphincter muscle in anorectal incontinence: a single fibre EMG study, *J Neurol Neurosurg Psych* 43:343, 1980.

66. Kiff ES, Swash M: Slowed conduction in the pudendal nerves in idiopathic (neurogenic) faecal incontinence, *Br J Surg* 71:614, 1984.

67. Snooks SJ, Swash M, Henry MM: Abnormalities in central and peripheral nerve conduction in patients with anorectal incontinence, *J R Soc Med* 78:294, 1985.

68. Merton PA, Hill DK, Morton HB, Marsden CD: Scope of a technique for electrical stimulation of human brain, spinal cord, and muscle, *Lancet* 2:597, 1982.

69. Roe AM, Bartolo DCC, Mortensen NJM: New methods for assessment of anal sensation in various anorectal disorders, *Br J Surg* 73:310, 1986.

70. Rogers JJ, Henry MM, Misiewicz JJ: Combined sensory and motor deficit in faecal incontinence, *Gut* 29:5, 1988.

71. Snooks SJ, Barnes PR, Swash M, Henry MM: Damage to the innervation of the pelvic floor musculature in chronic constipation, *Gastroenterology* 89:977, 1985.

72. Snooks SJ, Swash M, Henry MM, Setchell M: Risk factors in childbirth causing damage to the pelvic floor innervation, *Int J Colorectal Dis* 1:20, 1986.

73. Lubowski DZ, Swash M, Nicholls RJ et al: Increase in pudendal nerve terminal motor latency with defecation straining. *Br J Surg* 75:1095, 1988.

74. Law PJ, Kasmm MA, Bartram CI: Anal endosonography in the investigation of faecal incontinence, *Br J Surg* 78:312, 1991.

75. Lubowski DZ, Nicholls RJ: Faecal incontinence associated with reduced pelvic sensation, *Br J Surg* 75:1086, 1988.

76. Pescatori M, Ravo B: Diagnostic anorectal functional studies, *Surg Clin North Am* 68:1231, 1988.

77. Archer BD, Somers S, Stevenson GW: Contrast medium gel for marking vaginal position during defecography, *Radiology* 182:27, 1992.

78. Felt Bersma RJF, Klinkenberg-Knol EC, Meu Wissen SGM: Anorectal function investigations in incontinent and continent patients: differences and discriminatory value, *Dis Colon Rectum* 33:479, 1990.

79. Ferrante SL, Perry RE, Schreiman JS et al: The reproducibility of measuring the anorectal angle in defecography, *Dis Colon Rectum* 34:51, 1991.

80. Penninckx F, DeBruyne C, Lestar B, Kerremans R: Observer variations in the radiological measurement of the anorectal angle, *Int J Colorectal Dis* 5:94, 1990.

81. Goei R, Van Engelshoven J, Schouter H et al: Anorectal function: defecographic measurement in asymptomatic subjects, *Radiology* 173:137, 1989.

82. Hunter RA, Saccone GTP, Sarre R et al: Faecal incontinence: manometric and radiological changes following postanal repair, *Aust N Z J Surg* 59:697, 1989.

83. Benson JT, ed: *Female pelvic floor disorders,* New York, 1992, Norton.

84. Wall LL, De Lancey JOL: The politics of prolapse: a revisionist approach to disorders of the pelvic floor in women, *Perspect Biol Med* 34:486, 1991.

85. Wassef R, Rothenberger DA, Goldberg SM: Rectal prolapse, *Curr Probl Surg* 23:402, 1986.

86. Keithley MR, Makuria T, Alexander-Williams J et al: Clinical and manometric evaluation of rectal prolapse and incontinence, *Br J Surg* 67:54, 1980.

87. Moschcowitz AV: The pathogenesis, anatomy, and cure of prolapse of the rectum, *Surg Gynecol Obstet* 15:7, 1912.

88. Failes D, Killingback M, Stuart M et al: Rectal prolapse, *Aust N Z J Surg* 49:72, 1979.

89. Kuijpers JHC, De Morree H: Toward a selection of the most appropriate procedures in the treatment of complete rectal prolapse, *Dis Colon Rectum* 31:355, 1988.

90. Broden B, Snellman B: Procidentia of the rectum studied with cineradiography: a contribution to the discussion of causative mechanisms *Dis Colon Rectum* 11:330, 1968.

91. Kruyt RH, Delamarre JBVM, Doornbos J, Vogel HJ: Normal anorectum: dynamic MR imaging anatomy, *Radiology* 179:159, 1991.

92. Yang A, Mostwin JL, Rosenshein NB, Zehouni EA: Pelvic floor descent in women: dynamic evaluation with fast MR imaging and cinematic display, *Radiology* 179:25, 1991.

93. Sato Y, Pringle KC, Bergmasn RA et al: Congenital anorectal anomalies: MR imaging, *Radiology* 168:157, 1988.

94. Vade A, Reyes H, Wilbur A et al: The anorectal sphincter after rectal pull-through surgery for anorectal abnormalities: MRI evaluation, *Pediatr Radiol* 19:179, 1989.

44 *Anal Endosonography*

CLIVE I. BARTRAM

Endosonography of the anal canal is a simple technique that provides detailed resolution of sphincter anatomy. This morphologic evidence about the internal and external sphincters complements the functional information derived from anorectal physiology and defecography. In combination these three form a powerful and complete clinical investigative system for anorectal disorders.

Most endoluminal probes have been designed for prostatic or rectal imaging, and they usually have a balloon system to couple the probe to the compliant rectal wall. The inherent tone of the anal sphincters compresses and deforms any balloon, and a hard cone is required to provide a minimal stand-off. The walls of the cone should be parallel to minimize anatomic distortion of the canal. As the sphincters are basically circular structures around the canal, a mechanically rotating probe, which gives a complete cross-sectional image, probably provides the easiest image for evaluation of sphincter abnormalities.[1-3] Multiplanar imaging also has been advocated to improve visualization of the anorectal junction on longitudinal scanning.[4]

TECHNIQUE

The equipment currently used in anal endosonography has been a Brüel & Kjær ultrasound scanner type 1486 with endorectal probe type 1850 and a 7-MHz endoprobe. A hard plastic cone with an outer diameter of 1.7 cm (Fig. 44-1) was substituted for the rectal balloon system and filled with degassed water. The probe is small enough to be well tolerated, and the walls are parallel so that the canal is not distorted. The transducer is rotated mechanically at 1.9 to 2.8 cycles per second. The 7-MHz endoprobe has a focal length of 2.0 to 4.5 cm with a minimal beam width of 1.1 mm. The beam is emitted at a right angles so that a 360-degree radial swept image is obtained.[1,2]

Patients are examined in the left lateral position. No preparation is required. The probe is covered by a condom with ultrasound gel over the cone to prevent any air interface. The probe should be inserted just into the rectum, and the canal is imaged as the probe is slowly withdrawn. The length of the canal may be judged from where acoustic contact starts in the distal ampulla to its loss exteriorly. Between cases the probe may be wiped with industrial spirit. For full sterilization it has to be dismantled, washed, and soaked in glutaraldehyde for 20 minutes.

In practice it has been found easier to keep the probe in the same plane as the patient so that anterior would be on the right of the field. However, to prevent confusion all the images are presented in the normal ultrasound orientation with anterior uppermost.

NORMAL ANATOMY

The endosonographic anatomy of the anal canal corresponds to that of the rectum, with the superimposition of the two sphincter mechanisms. The basic pattern consists of the following four layers (Fig. 44-2):

1. Subepithelium (hyperechoic)

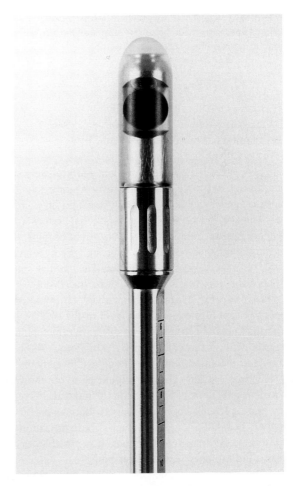

Fig. 44-1 The hard cone modification to the Brüel & Kjær endorectal 1850 probe for use in the anal canal.

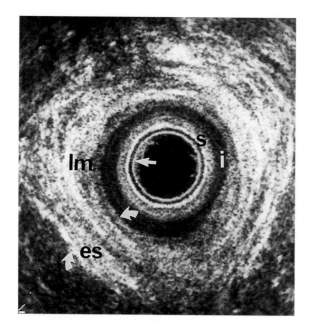

Fig. 44-2 Normal sonographic anatomy of the anal canal. The cone creates two bright reflections *(straight arrow)*. The subepithelium *(s)* is hyperechoic, and the internal sphincter *(i)* hypoechoic. The longitudinal muscle *(lm)* and external sphincter *(es)* form two indistinguishable hyperechoic layers *(curved arrows)*. Anterior is uppermost with the patient's right on the left side, conforming to normal cross-sectional orientation.

2. Internal sphincter (hypoechoic)
3. Longitudinal muscle (hyperechoic)
4. External sphincter (hyperechoic)

The cone creates a double reflection, unfortunately often strong enough to form a distracting reverberation echo. The mucosa is rarely visible as a thin hypoechoic layer immediately outside the cone. The subepithelial tissues (often called *submucosa*, although this is incorrect because there is no muscularis mucosae in the anal canal) are hyperechoic and thicker than the rectal submucosa. The circular smooth muscle of the muscularis propria can be traced down from the rectum into the internal sphincter, which is uniformly hypoechoic and terminates at the level of the dentate line.

The thickness and echogenicity of the internal sphincter increases with age[5] as the proportion of fibrous tissue increases and the smooth muscle atrophies.[6] In patients less than 55 years old the sphincter should be hypoechoic and 2.4 to 2.7 mm thick (95% confidence interval). Over 55 years the sphincter becomes more inhomogeneous in echogenicity and 2.8 to 3.4 mm thick. These measurements apply to a probe diameter of 1.7 cm. It is possible for it to appear a little thinner with a larger probe.

The conjoined longitudinal coat, or longitudinal muscle, surrounding the internal sphincter is a continuation of the outer longitudinal muscle coat of the rectum, augmented by an extensive fibroelastic component from the pelvic fascia. The connective tissue within this layer permeates the sphincters and invests the entire perianal region. This anchors the rectum and sphincters within the pelvic floor and perineum and provides fibroelastic support for the sphincters.[7] It forms a prominent hyperechoic circular layer between the internal and external sphincters in both sexes and terminates in multiple septal extensions, which pass through the subcutaneous external sphincter to insert into the perianal skin. The echogenicity of this layer, as with each layer, is a function of its fibrous content. The longitudinal muscle layer is not sonographically always uniform, and thin short hypoechoic arcs within it may be due to segments of smooth muscle devoid of connective tissue.

The anatomy of the external sphincters is complex and still a subject of debate. Generally a trilaminar arrangement is accepted with deep, superficial and subcutaneous divisions. The relationship of the deep part to the puborectalis remains controversial. As the probe is withdrawn from within the rectum, the puborectalis comes into view as a hyperechoic U-shaped sling at the level of the levators, with the arms of the sling diverging slightly as they run forward to the posterior aspect of the pubic bones (Fig. 44-3). The external sphincter is recognized by a change in direction of the fiber bundles anteriorly, which, instead of diverging, start to converge into an annular ring. The deep part of the external sphincter may be separated from the puborectalis by a thin hypoechoic layer or appear confluent with it. In females there is little external sphincter anteriorly high in the canal, as the muscle bundles from the deep, superficial, and subcutaneous parts combine anteriorly to form a single muscle bundle low in the canal.[8] As the probe is withdrawn, the ends of the deep external sphincter may appear truncated (Fig. 46-3) as the cross-sectional ultrasound beam cuts through the fibers sloping down to the anterior bundle. There is often some variation as to how the fibers cross over anteriorly. It is not uncommon to see a slip of external sphincter crossing the midline.[9] However, the external sphincter should fuse into a complete ring at some point low in the canal. In males the external sphincter is more symmetric and annular at all levels, usually with an outer hypoechoic ring in the superficial and subcutaneous parts (Fig. 44-4). This is sometimes seen in females down low in the canal. In both sexes the longitudinal muscle layer seems contiguous with the external sphincter. In females the echogenicity is identical, and the layers are difficult to differentiate.

Lateral to the external sphincter ill-defined linear reflections arise from fibrous septa within the ischiorectal fossae. Posteriorly a well-defined triangular shadow is created by the coccyx and anococcygeal ligament. Anteriorly in females is the vagina and membranous urethra. In males the bulbar urethra is seen below the prostate. The perineal body is not clearly defined and is represented by an area of relatively amorphous hypoechoic tissue immediately anterior

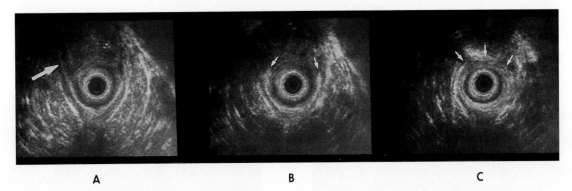

Fig. 44-3 Normal anatomy of the external sphincter in a female. **A,** At a high level the divergent puborectalis is visible *(arrow)*. **B,** Slightly lower down the external sphincter is turning in but appears cut off *(arrows)*. **C,** At the midlevel of the canal the external sphincter is now a complete ring *(arrows)*.

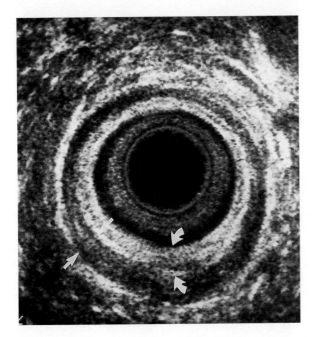

Fig. 44-4 At the midlevel of the canal the external sphincter in this male patient is clearly defined as a hypoechoic ring *(straight arrows)* around the longitudinal muscle *(curved arrows)*.

to the external sphincter. The superficial transverse perineal muscles may be seen converging into it.

The radial position of any abnormality is best described by viewing the canal as a clock face, with 12 o'clock anteriorly, and localizing the lesion by the hour it corresponds to in position. The longitudinal position of a lesion within the canal is more difficult to define with a purely cross-sectional view. The canal length may be estimated on withdrawal of the probe, but this is difficult to measure accurately. Lesions are best related to high, mid, or low positions in the canal, according to their relationships to the sphincters:

High: puborectalis and upper external sphincter
Mid: below puborectalis at the terminal portion of the internal sphincter
Low: caudal to the termination of the internal sphincter

INTERNAL SPHINCTER ABNORMALITIES

Damage to the sphincter, of either traumatic or surgical origin, manifests sonographically as either an actual break or irregular thinning. Surgical incision of the sphincter, as in lateral sphincterotomy, leaves a clearly defined break with the cut edges of the sphincter rounded and well defined. The sphincter tends to spring apart a little and bunch up, so the defect is wider than the surgical incision, and the remaining sphincter a little thicker than normal (Fig. 44-5). Forcible dilatation of the anal canal, either surgically or traumatically induced, may tear the sphincter in single (Fig. 44-6) or multiple areas (Fig. 44-7), giving a fragmented appearance[10] (Fig. 44-8). Even if the sphincter is not actually torn, damage may still be visible as abnormal thinning (Fig. 44-9).

The thickness of the internal sphincter varies with age, but a sphincter ≥ 4 mm thick is abnormal at any age. This may be associated with anal pain of proctalgia fugax nature, constipation (Fig. 44-10), solitary rectal ulcer syndrome, or prolapse. With rectal prolapse the subepithelial tissues are thickened. The underlying histopathology is not yet understood. Wedge resection of a very grossly thickened internal sphincter in a patient with crippling proctalgia fugax revealed a gross smooth muscle myopathy on electron microscopy.[11] Conversely an internal sphincter of ≤ 2 mm in elderly patients is abnormal (Fig. 44-11), suggesting atrophy of the smooth muscle and may be associated with low resting pressures.[12]

EXTERNAL SPHINCTER ABNORMALITIES

Traumatic damage to the striated muscle of the external sphincter heals with granulation tissue and fibrosis. These

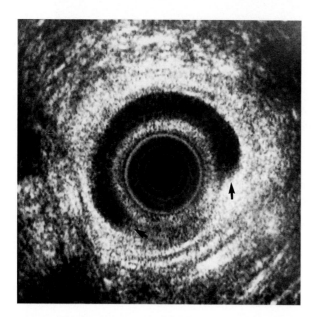

Fig. 44-5 Lateral sphincterotomy defect in the internal sphincter between the 3 o'clock and 7 o'clock positions. Note the rounded ends *(arrows)* and that the residual sphincter is of normal hypoechogenicity but has bunched up.

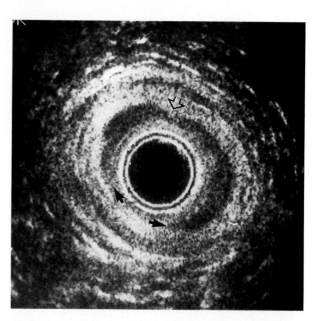

Fig. 44-6 A 56-year-old man with poor sphincter control after an anal stretch for fissure. There is a defect at the 6 o'clock to 9 o'clock positions in the internal sphincter *(solid arrows)* with a smaller thinned segment at 12 o'clock *(open arrow)*.

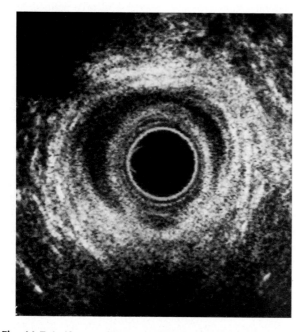

Fig. 44-7 A 43-year-old woman with fecal incontinence after an anal stretch. Internal sphincter defects are present between the 3 o'clock and 5 o'clock and 7 o'clock and 8 o'clock positions.

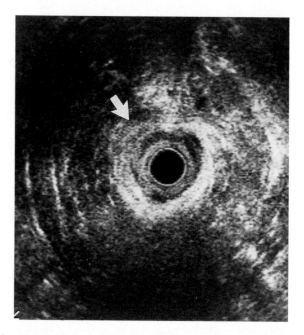

Fig. 44-8 A 28-year-old woman who became incontinent after an assault that involved a bottle being forcibly inserted into the rectum. The internal sphincter has been fragmented, and the external sphincter is partially fragmented between the 9 o'clock and 12 o'clock positions *(arrows)*.
From Bartram CI, Burnett SJD: *Atlas of anal endosonography,* Oxford, 1991, Butterworth-Heinemann.

scars may be referred to as defects, which really dates back to their initial description by electromyographic mapping, in which the electrically inert scar was seen as a defect compared with normal muscle activity.[13]

Defects in the external sphincter require careful assessment.[12-14] It is important to remember individual variation as well as the essential difference in the configuration of the external sphincter between the sexes. A rule to follow is that the posterolateral aspects of the sphincter should be intact at all levels in both sexes, deficient anteriorly in females at a high level, but intact at mid and low levels (Fig. 44-3).

INCONTINENCE

Continence is complex and multifactorial. It depends on the neuromuscular integrity of the pelvic floor and anal sphincters. Eighty-five percent of the resting tone of the anal canal is considered to be due to the internal sphincter, with the rise in pressure on voluntary contraction, or squeeze, a function of the external sphincter. Damage to the pudendal nerve is revealed by prolonged motor nerve latencies.

In the elderly a thin internal sphincter (≤ 2 mm) is abnormal and may be found in some patients with idiopathic incontinence (Fig. 44-11). This may indicate smooth muscle atrophy and be a contributory factor to fecal incontinence by lowering the resting pressure in the anal canal. A direct relationship between the thickness of the internal sphincter and the resting pressure has been suggested.[12]

Dilatation of the anus, from a stretch procedure with the

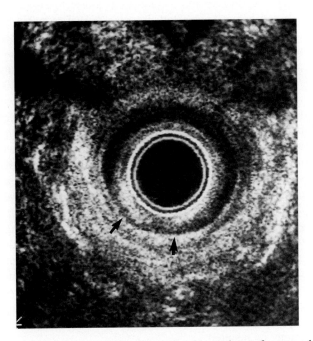

Fig. 44-9 A 42-year-old woman rendered incontinent after an anal stretch. Note the extreme thinning of the internal sphincter posteriorly between the 5 o'clock and 9 o'clock positions *(arrows).*

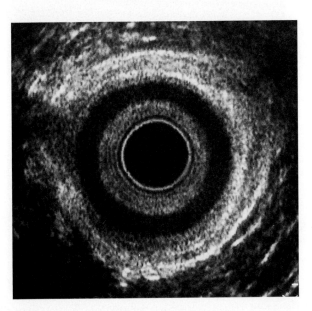

Fig. 44-10 A 32-year-old women with constipation and anal pain. The internal sphincter is slightly thickened (4 mm), and the subepithelial tissues are prominent secondary to intraanal intussusception.

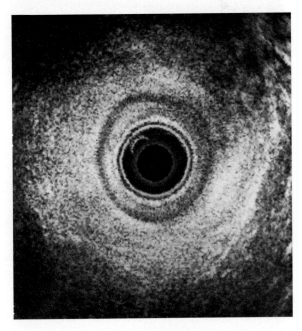

Fig. 44-11 A 70-year-old woman with fecal incontinence and an abnormally thin internal sphincter (<2 mm).

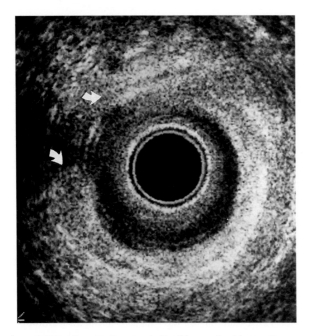

Fig. 44-12 Defects in the external and internal sphincters between the 9 o'clock and 11 o'clock positions in the external sphincter *(arrows)* and in the 9 o'clock and 1 o'clock positions in the internal sphincter after obstetric trauma.

patient under general anaesthesia, or any traumatic cause may cause irreparable damage to the internal sphincter. Anal dilatation remains a common treatment for fissure-in-ano and hemorrhoids, with the objective of reducing the resting pressure of the anal canal. A number of studies have indicated that continence may be compromised. In a review of 14 patients with fecal incontinence after anal stretch, disruption of the internal sphincter was found in 13 (93%) (Figs. 44-6 to 44-9). Rather than a single break the sphincter was fragmented with irregular thinning and several breaks in 12 (86%). Remnants of the sphincter were noted to be hyperechoic in 4 (29%), suggesting fibrotic replacement. In 5 (36%) defects also were seen in the external sphincter.[10] By contrast, lateral sphincterotomy produces a clean break in the sphincter (Fig. 44-5). The ends are well defined and rounded. The sphincter tends to spring apart a little when cut, although the fibrous mesh from the longitudinal muscle helps hold it in place. It has been noted that after limited sphincterotomies the internal sphincter may seem relatively normal some months later. Whether this represents true regrowth of the internal sphincter or hypoechoic granulation tissue is not known. Repair of a surgically divided sphincter is feasible. A fragmented sphincter cannot be repaired.

External sphincter defects are seen as an amorphous segment interrupting the continuity of the sphincter.[1] The echogenicity of the scarred area varies but is usually hypoechoic relative to the normal sphincter (Fig. 44-12). Some-

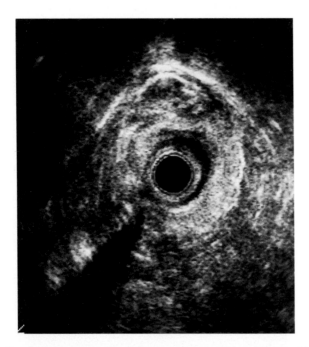

Fig. 44-13 Perineal trauma from a knife wound in a 30-year-old man with an external sphincter defect at the 6 o'clock to 8 o'clock positions and acoustic shadowing from part of this.
From Bartram CI, Burnett SJD: *Atlas of anal endosonography,* Oxford, 1991, Butterworth-Heinemann.

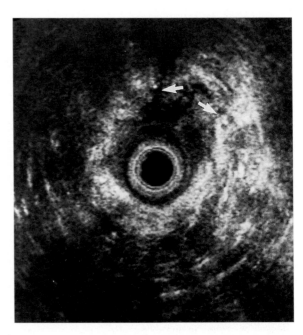

Fig. 44-14 There is a large anterior external sphincter defect *(arrows)* after rotational forceps were applied during labor and delivery. The patient was fecally incontinent immediately postpartum.

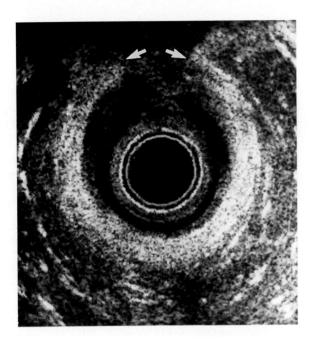

Fig. 44-15 A 37-year-old woman still incontinent after an anterior repair for sphincter damage after forceps delivery 11 years previously. A large gap *(arrows)* remains between the 11 o'clock and 12 o'clock positions.

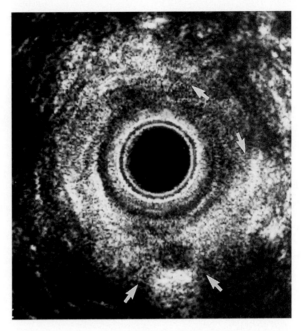

Fig. 44-16 A postanal repair had been performed on this 54-year-old woman who was incontinent after a forceps delivery. There is a typical deformity secondary to the postanal repair posteriorly at the 6 o'clock position *(arrows)*, but a well-defined external sphincter defect at the 12 o'clock to 3 o'clock position remains *(arrows)*.

times a strong reflection from a fibrous tissue interface close to the probe produces a large reverberation echo with posterior acoustic shadowing (Fig. 44-13). Changes may extend into the ischiorectal fossae where hemorrhage has become organized adjacent to the damaged sphincter. The defect usually extends through the full thickness of the sphincter but may be only partial (Fig. 44-10).

Obstetric trauma is a significant factor in the development of incontinence in females (Figs. 44-12 and 44-14). A review of 62 patients with incontinence of flatus or feces revealed that 90% had defects of the external sphincter and 65% of the internal sphincter.[15] In a prospective study of 121 women examined 6 weeks before and after vaginal delivery all primiparous women (63) had a normal sphincter before delivery, and after delivery 35% had an internal sphincter defect, 16% an external sphincter defect, and 14% had damage to both sphincters.[16] In total, 37% had evidence of sphincter damage; 49% of the 37 multiparous women had preexisting sphincter defects—46% internal and 22% external. After delivery these worsened in 37%, and 5% developed new external sphincter defects. Sphincter damage was most frequent when forceps had been applied.

External sphincter defects are often difficult to palpate, and endosonography in one series of 44 consecutive patients with fecal incontinence revealed external sphincter defects in 4/11 (36%) when clinically the patients were considered to have idiopathic neurogenic incontinence.

Anal endosonography also has a role assessing the sphincters after repair operations for incontinence. In a successful repair no gap should remain between the sphincter ends, which are either overlapped or opposed. Endosonography may show that the repair is unsatisfactory or that damage to other parts of the sphincter has been overlooked (Figs. 44-15 and 44-16).

CONSTIPATION

In 13 of 47 patients with constipation a slightly thickened internal sphincter in the 4- to 5-mm range was found (unpublished data). Anecdotally a few of these patients have had lateral sphincterotomy with benefit. The incidence of internal sphincter abnormality in solitary rectal ulcer may be higher, although this is not fully documented. If repeated straining has led to prolapse, a thickened subepithelium is seen (Fig. 44-10).

CONCLUSION AND INDICATIONS

Anal endosonography has an important role in determining the presence and extent of sphincter defects in patients with fecal incontinence, and the findings complement those from physiologic studies. Its role in constipation is less clear, as the overall incidence and significance of changes in the internal sphincter is as yet undetermined. The main clinical signs to look for during anal endosonography may be summarized as follows:

I. *Incontinence*

A. Internal sphincter
   1. ≤2 mm thick
   2. Defects
   3. Fragmentation, anal stretch (?)
B. External sphincter
   1. Defects, obstetric trauma (?)

II. *Constipation*

A. Internal sphincter
   1. ≥4 mm thick
   2. Thickened subepithelium, prolapse (?)

REFERENCES

1. Law PJ, Bartram CI: Anal endosonography: technique and normal anatomy, *Gastrointest Radiol* 14:349, 1989.

2. Bartram CI, Burnett SJD: *Atlas of anal endosonography,* Oxford, 1991, Butterworth-Heinemann.

3. Bartram C, Law P: Anal endosonography: technique and applications. In Herlinger H, Megibow AJ, eds: *Advances in gastrointestinal radiology,* Chicago, 1991, Mosby–Year Book.

4. Nielsen MB, Pedersen JF, Hauge C, Rasmussen O, Christiansen J: Endosonography of the anal sphincter: findings in healthy volunteers, *AJR* 157:1199, 1991.

5. Burnett SJD, Bartram CI: Endosonography variations of the normal internal anal sphincter, *Int J Coloproctol* 6:2, 1991.

6. Klosterhalfen B, Offner F, Topf N, Vogel P, Mittermayer C: Sclerosis of the internal sphincter—a process of aging, *Dis Colon Rectum* 33:606, 1990.

7. Haas PA, Fox TA: The importance of the perianal connective tissue in the surgical anatomy and function of the anus, *Dis Colon Rectum* 20:303, 1977.

8. Oh C, Kark AE: Anatomy of the external anal sphincter, *Br J Surg* 59:717, 1972.

9. Gorsch RV: *Proctologic anatomy,* ed 2, Baltimore, 1955, Williams & Wilkins.

10. Speakman CTM, Burnett SJD, Kamm MA, Bartram CI: Sphincter injury following anal dilatation demonstrated by anal endosonography, *Br J Surg* 78:1429, 1991.

11. Kamm MA, Hoyle CHV, Burleigh DE, Law PJ, Swash M et al: Hereditary internal anal sphincter myopathy causing proctalgia fugax and constipation, *Gastroenterology* 100:805, 1991.

12. Law PJ, Kamm MA, Bartram CI: Anal endosonography in the investigation of faecal incontinence, *Br J Surg* 78:280, 1991.

13. Browing GGP, Motson RW, Henry MH: Combined sphincter repair and postanal repair for the treatment of complicated injuries to the anal sphincters, *Ann R Coll Surg* 70:324, 1988.

14. Burnett SJD, Speakman CTM, Bartram CI: Confirmation of endosonographic detection of external anal sphincter defects by simultaneous electromyographic mapping, *Br J Surg* 78:448, 1991.

15. Burnett SJD, Spence-Jones C, Speakman CTM, Kamm MA, Hudson CN et al: Unsuspected sphincter damage following childbirth revealed by anal endosonography, *Br J Radiol* 64:225, 1991.

16. Sultan AH, Kamm MS, Hudson CN, Bartram CI: Vaginal delivery causes anal sphincter disruption in 37% of patients (prospective ultrasound study)—a major determinant for the development of faecal incontinence (abstract) American Gastroenterology Association meeting, San Francisco, May 1992,

45 Applications and Limitations of Imaging in Staging and Follow-up of Gastrointestinal Neoplasms

DAVID J. BRAGG
WILLIAM M. THOMPSON
EDWARD W. HUMPHREY

From a surgical viewpoint the value of an imaging procedure depends on three possible results. It must contribute directly to the decision of whether to operate on the patient, it must guide the surgeon in the performance of the operation, or it must provide staging information that the surgeon cannot readily obtain during the course of the operation or from the pathologists. The negative consequences of not operating on a patient who could benefit from surgery usually exceed those of surgical exploration of a patient for whom nothing can be done. The specificity of preoperative imaging procedures is more important than sensitivity.

The reason for operating on patients with carcinoma of the esophagus, stomach, or colon is not primarily to stage the tumor nor is it only to cure the disease. If a patient can be expected to live 6 months or more and if the primary tumor can be resected and gastrointestinal (GI) continuity restored, not withstanding the presence of incurable disease, considerable palliation can be offered to the patients even if their lives are not prolonged.

The following discussion is intended to place the current role of imaging in patients with tumor of the hollow GI tract in a clinical perspective. Imaging procedures play a small role in the preoperative staging of patients with GI malignancies. Because of the current limitations of imaging, this role should be focused on the recognition of distant metastatic disease and on the earlier recognition of recurrence following initial treatment, particularly in colon cancer patients. This effort must be coordinated with the oncologists to maximize the staging yield for each patient.

The fundamental issue in the staging of hollow organ GI tract malignancies is the determination of the depth of tumor invasion through the bowel wall and the accurate detection of regional and distant lymph node involvement. Detection of distant metastases is also critical. In each of the three major sites—esophagus, stomach, and colon—none of our imaging techniques provide accurate enough evaluation of the bowel wall for establishing fundamental therapeutic options. Also the detection and analysis of abnormal regional lymph nodes are insufficiently accurate with any of our existing imaging techniques to provide useful pretreatment information that would alter the therapeutic approach.

Currently the main applications for imaging in the patient with hollow organ GI tract malignancy should be focused on the recognition of distant metastatic disease, particularly hepatic involvement, complications of the primary tumor (perforation, fistulization, and the like), and in the posttreatment follow-up of the patient.

ESOPHAGEAL CANCER

The staging of esophageal cancers is based on the TNM (tumor, node, metastasis) system, modified in 1988 and recently republished in 1992[1] (see the box on p. 882). The basis for staging esophageal cancer, as with more distal, hollow organ cancers, depends on the depth of invasion of the primary tumor, the presence or absence of regional lymph nodes, and distant metastatic disease. The contrast esophagram more accurately defines the oral and anal limits of the cancer but fails to assess depth of invasion, the fundamental criteria for defining T.

The surgical approach to squamous cell carcinoma of the esophagus has changed over the past several years. Most centers perform a transabdominal esophagectomy and gastric pull-up with a cervical anastomosis (the M.B. Orringer approach). A thoracotomy is then avoided; however, visual inspection and dissection of mediastinal lymph nodes is not possible. Such an approach is usually preceded by combined radiation and chemotherapy. Some centers still use the surgical approach popularized by David Skinner—a mediastinal esophagectomy, en-bloc lymph node dissection, and colonic interposition.

The critical need for imaging procedures in staging assumes a different role with the two differing surgical approaches. With the Skinner procedure, imaging procedures may identify those patients with unresectable cancers. With the Orringer approach, imaging procedures form the basis for stage grouping and treatment planning but seldom influence a decision to proceed with the procedure.

Some reports of the use of magnetic resonance imaging (MRI) and computed tomography (CT) convey a disap-

---

□ TNM STAGING SYSTEM FOR THE ESOPHAGUS □

PRIMARY TUMOR (T)

TX   Primary tumor cannot be assessed
T0   No evidence of primary tumor
Tis   Carcinoma in situ
T1   Tumor invades lamina propria or submucosa
T2   Tumor invades muscularis propria
T3   Tumor invades adventitia
T4   Tumor invades adjacent structures

REGIONAL LYMPH NODES (N)

NX   Regional lymph nodes cannot be assessed
N0   No regional lymph node metastasis
N1   Regional lymph node metastasis

DISTANT METASTASIS (M)

MX   Presence of distant metastasis cannot be assessed
M0   No distant metastasis
M1   Distant metastasis

STAGE GROUPING

Stage 0	Tis	N0	M0
Stage 1	T1	N0	M0
Stage IIA	T2	N0	M0
	T3	N0	M0
Stage IIB	T1	N1	M0
	T2	N1	M0
Stage III	T3	N1	M0
	T4	Any N	M0
Stage IV	Any T	Any N	M1

From Beahrs OH, Henson DE, Hutter RVP, Kennedy BJ: *Manual for staging of cancer*, ed 4, Philadelphia, 1992, JB Lippincott.

---

pointing accuracy in staging cancers, primarily because of the inability of these techniques to gauge depth of invasion.[2] Other reports suggest the accuracy exceeds 90%.[3] Less enthusiastic reviews suggest significant variations in staging accuracy with CT.[4,5] These variations reflect the problems not only in assessing transmural invasion of the tumor, the absence of a well-defined outer limit of the esophageal wall since the esophagus lacks a serosal margin, but also in defining extraesophageal invasion confidently.

The hallmark of extraesophageal invasion is the obliteration of fat planes, often a difficult task in a cachectic patient (Fig. 45-1). Several articles have defined criteria for the assessment of aortic invasion; however, this is an uncommon feature with esophageal cancer.[6] Recently, CT and MRI were used to evaluate the presence or absence of aortic or tracheobronchial invasion, which is an important surgical criterion for nonresectability. Both techniques allowed

recognition of invasion of these critical structures in six instances, with one false-positive instance. Again, both of these sites of tumor extension are important to define, but they were uncommon in Takashima et al.'s experience.[7]

Very few reports have compared the accuracy of modern MRI and CT in the staging of patients with esophageal carcinoma. It is currently presumed the two technologies share equal sensitivity and specificity.[8]

Currently, transluminal esophageal ultrasound (EUS) appears to hold promise as a technique to assess not only transmural invasion but also regional lymph node involvement. Initial reports, primarily from centers in Asia and Europe, indicate the greater accuracy of EUS and compare the results of EUS with CT in the preoperative staging of patients with esophageal carcinoma. EUS can analyze the individual esophageal layers and more accurately define depth of tumor penetration. In addition, a potential exists for lymph node staging, reported to be more accurate than CT.[9-11] The fundamental technical limitation of EUS in its current stage of development is the inability of the instrument to traverse incompletely obstructing or stenotic esophageal cancers. With current instrumentation, the device is unable to traverse the tumor in nearly 20% of the patients, limiting its application in these individuals. The liver and abdomen cannot be evaluated by EUS.

Another application of ultrasound is cutaneous scanning of the neck and upper thorax to detect supraclavicular lymph node involvement. Sonography was more accurate than CT in a recent report, suggesting its application in patients with proximal thoracic esophageal cancer locations. Obviously, histologic verification of the abnormal lymph nodes must be obtained.[12]

Neither CT nor MRI appears to be sufficiently accurate to justify their routine application in the preoperative assessment of the patient with esophageal cancer, other than in the assessment of complications and distant metastatic disease, primarily to the liver and the lung. Quite possibly, EUS may become more flexible and accurate to traverse narrowed segments of the involved esophagus and provide more accurate staging data.

The accurate assessment of regional lymph node involvement remains frustrating, in part because of the complex network of lymphatics within the esophagus and the variability in which flow tends to occur along the longitudinal axis of the esophagus. Skip areas of involvement by tumor in these complex lymphatics have been known to occur for years.[13]

After the patient is treated with surgery, radiation therapy, or both, cross-sectional imaging techniques do provide a useful role in the recognition of recurrent cancer. Unfortunately, few series have stratified patients and analyzed them with CT and MRI to determine procedural accuracy and which, if either, is superior. The criteria for the recognition of recurrence is based on the performance of a baseline study some 3 to 4 months after initial therapy. The rec-

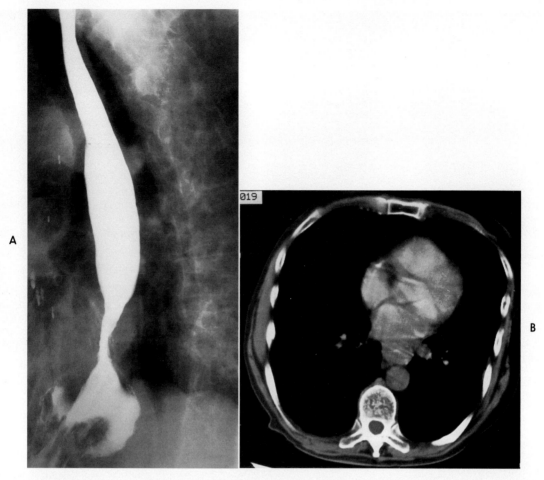

Fig. 45-1 Unresectable esophageal squamous cell cancer not predicted by CT. **A,** Contrast esophagram revealing a typical distal third cancer proven on biopsy to be a squamous cell cancer. **B,** Noncontrast-enhanced CT scan showing transmural extension but no evidence of cardiac invasion found at surgery at this level.

ognition of an enlarging boundary and detection of a local mass, plus extension to critical mediastinal structures—liver and lung metastatic disease—form the criteria for the recognition of recurrent tumor. Unfortunately, no current therapy can salvage the patient once these events are detected (Fig. 45-2).

In summary, in the patient with esophageal carcinoma EUS forms the cornerstone for preoperative assessment of the depth of wall penetration and recognition of regional lymph node disease. If the tumor site cannot be traversed by EUS, CT is the second staging option of choice. Although CT can be helpful in the preoperative evaluation, it should be reserved to answer specific questions. If the surgeon is looking for a reason not to operate, CT can determine the presence of large tumors invading the mediastinum, liver metastases, and the like. Also, CT can prove useful in evaluating patients receiving radiation therapy and those in nonoperative protocols. Follow-up of the patient

after definitive treatment should include a baseline examination between 3 and 4 months after completion of primary therapy. Again, CT forms the cornerstone for evaluation and recognition of recurrences, with plain chest radiographs sufficient to detect metastatic lung disease. Abnormal results from laboratory studies should suggest the need for evaluation of liver metastatic disease (see the box on p. 885).

GASTRIC CANCER

The application of imaging procedures to the staging process for gastric cancer has been even less successful. The primary use of cross-sectional imaging examinations should be in the recognition of distant metastatic disease before and after definitive treatment. Metastases appear first in the liver, since it is the initial organ receiving venous drainage from the stomach, with less frequent metastatic involvement found in the lungs, brain, or skeletal system. Regional

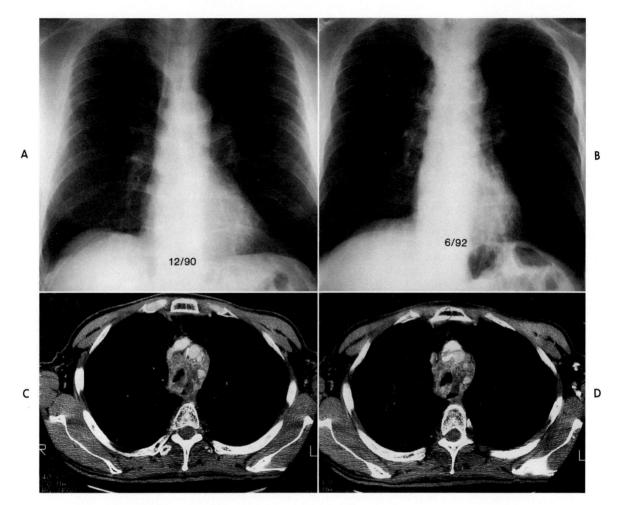

Fig. 45-2 Recurrent inoperable squamous cell cancer of the esophagus 2 years after initial treatment. **A,** Frontal chest radiograph at the time of initial diagnosis. **B,** Frontal chest radiograph 14 months after radiation therapy showing widening of the superior mediastinum. CT studies should be performed to confirm tumor recurrence in this setting. **C** and **D,** Contrast-enhanced CT scan showing mediastinal tumor and tumor deforming the patulous esophagus.

metastases, either through direct extension to the pancreas or omentum are difficult to identify with certainty and accuracy. Neither CT nor MRI can accurately reflect the depth of tumor penetration through the gastric wall nor the involvement of regional lymph nodes.

The surgeon, confronted with a patient with an aggressive gastric neoplasm, is interested primarily in information regarding distant metastases to the liver or thorax, since skeletal and brain metastases from gastric cancers are far less commonly seen early in the course of the disease.

The history and current debate as to the role of CT and MRI in the staging of gastric carcinoma is thoroughly discussed in Chapter 21. CT does not possess sufficient accuracy to nonoperatively stage the patient with gastric carcinoma in terms of defining the T or N staging components of the TNM staging system[14,15] (see the box on p. 885).

Quite possibly, EUS may provide some useful information, as has been summarized for esophageal cancers. The problem relates to the more difficult challenge of distending the gastric wall in contrast to the narrower lumen of the esophagus. In addition, anatomically accurate recognition of the regional lymph nodes is a difficult challenge with EUS in contrast to the esophagus.[16]

Screening for metastatic liver disease is best accomplished with either contrast-enhanced CT or MRI. MRI enjoys equal accuracy to CT but adds an increment of specificity beyond the capability of the contrast-enhanced CT. Future improvements in both CT and MRI will provide faster scanning times, allowing image acquisition during single breath–holding maneuvers, which should provide sensitivity gains, complemented further by improvements in contrast materials. Intraoperative hepatic ultrasound adds

---

□ STAGING AND FOLLOW-UP
RECOMMENDATIONS FOR
ESOPHAGEAL CANCER □

STAGING

Contrast esophagram—upper GI series
Chest radiographs (posteroanterior and lateral)
Contrast-enhanced CT of mediastinum, liver, upper
    abdomen
Endoscopic ultrasound

FOLLOW-UP

Chest x-ray studies (posteroanterior and lateral)
3 to 4 months after treatment:
    Contrast esophagram
    CT if abnormalities found on chest x-ray or esopha-
        gram

---

yet an additional complement to palpation at the time of surgical exploration.[17]

Standard posteroanterior and lateral chest radiographs are sufficient to screen the patient before surgery for metastatic intrathoracic disease. The pattern of metastatic spread to the lungs usually is lymphangitic. Although chest radiographs are nonspecific, they should serve as a rather sensitive screen in the presence of patient symptoms to suggest the presence of lymphangitic metastatic lung involvement. Brain and skeletal metastatic disease should be heralded by symptoms suggesting specific imaging procedures appropriate to their detection.

In summary, imaging procedures have a relatively small yet specific role in the preoperative staging of the patient with gastric carcinoma. Characterization of the gastric carcinoma is best performed with traditional double-contrast upper GI series, with CT or MRI reserved for regional assessment of the tumor and, most importantly, screening of the liver for metastatic disease. Intraoperative ultrasound of the liver adds an additional edge of sensitivity to operative inspection and palpation.

In the follow-up of the patient, after primary intervention, imaging procedures should be prompted by specific symptoms or abnormal laboratory findings, rather than a specific formula of imaging procedures applied during any temporal sequence after surgery.

COLORECTAL CANCER

Colorectal cancers are a much more common neoplasm. They share a similar staging shortfall with cancers of the esophagus and stomach. The TNM staging system (see the box above) is based on the depth of wall penetration by the cancer, spread to extracolonic neighboring tissues, lymph node metastases, and distant spread primarily to the liver

---

□ TNM STAGING SYSTEM FOR THE
STOMACH □

PRIMARY TUMOR (T)

TX   Primary tumor cannot be assessed
T0   No evidence of primary tumor
Tis Carcinoma in situ; intraepithelial tumor without in-
     vasion of lamina propria
T1   Tumor invades lamina propria or submucosa
T2   Tumor invades muscularis propria or subserosa
T3   Tumor penetrates serosa (visceral peritoneum) with-
     out invasion of adjacent structures
T4   Tumor invades adjacent structures

LYMPH NODE (N)

NX   Regional lymph node(s) cannot be assessed
N0   No regional lymph node metastasis
N1   Metastasis in perigastric lymph node(s) within 3 cm
     of edge of primary tumor
N2   Metastasis in perigastric lymph node(s) more than 3
     cm from edge of primary tumor, or in lymph nodes
     along left gastric, common hepatic, splenic, or ce-
     liac arteries

DISTANT METASTASIS (M)

MX   Presence of distant metastasis cannot be assessed
M0   No distant metastasis
M1   Distant metastasis

STAGE GROUPING

Stage 0	Tis	N0	M0
Stage IA	T1	N0	M0
Stage IB	T1	N1	M0
	T2	N0	M0
Stage II	T1	N2	M0
	T2	N1	M0
	T3	N0	M0
Stage IIIA	T2	N2	M0
	T3	N1	M0
	T4	N0	M0
Stage IIIB	T3	N2	M0
	T4	N1	M0
Stage IV	T4	N2	M0
	Any T	Any N	M1

From Beahrs OH, Henson DE, Hutter RVP, Kennedy BJ: *Manual for staging of cancer,* ed 4, Philadelphia, 1992, JB Lippincott.

---

and lung. Current imaging technologies fail to possess the accuracy to define either wall penetration or regional involvement.[18]

The role of MRI is unclear as it applies to staging the patient with colorectal carcinoma. The development of endorectal coils may enhance the visualization of the T compartment but is made difficult by the endoluminal location

---

□ TNM STAGING SYSTEM FOR THE COLON AND RECTUM □

PRIMARY TUMOR (T)

TX　Primary tumor cannot be assessed
T0　No evidence of primary tumor
Tis　Carcinoma in situ; intraepithelial tumor or invasion of lamina propria
T1　Tumor invades submucosa
T2　Tumor invades muscularis propria
T3　Tumor invades through muscularis propria into sub-serosa or into nonperitonealized pericolic or perirectal tissues
T4　Tumor directly invades other organs or structures, and/or perforates visceral peritoneum

LYMPH NODE (N)

NX　Regional lymph node(s) cannot be assessed
N0　No regional lymph node metastasis
N1　Metastasis in 1 to 3 pericolic or perirectal lymph nodes
N2　Metastasis in 4 or more pericolic or perirectal lymph nodes

DISTANT METASTASIS (M)

MX　Presence of distant metastasis cannot be assessed
M0　No distant metastasis
M1　Distant metastasis

STAGE GROUPING

Stage	T	N	M	DUKES
Stage 0	Tis	N0	M0	
Stage I	T1	N0	M0	A
	T2	N0	M0	
Stage II	T3	N0	M0	B
	T4	N0	M0	
Stage III	Any T	N1	M0	C
	Any T	N2	M0	
	Any T	N3	M0	
Stage IV	Any T	Any N	M1	

From Beahrs OH, Henson DE, Hutter RVP, Kennedy BJ: *Manual for staging of cancer,* ed 4, Philadelphia, 1992, JB Lippincott.

□ STAGING AND FOLLOW-UP RECOMMENDATIONS FOR COLORECTAL CANCER □

STAGING

Double contrast barium enema
Contrast-enhanced CT of regional area of tumor and liver
Chest radiograph (posteroanterior and lateral)

FOLLOW-UP

Contrast-enhanced CT of regional area and liver
CEA levels (if elevated, repeat CT scans)

---

of the tumor, not dissimilar to the circumstance with esophageal cancers. More recently, EUS has been applied to the regional staging of colorectal carcinomas with limited initial results.[19]

A strategy for the application of imaging in the assessment of metastatic disease should recognize the initial location of the tumor. If the colorectal tumor is within the peritoneal reflection, the distribution of metastatic disease will follow a regional course through the lymph nodes to the liver. If the cancer lies outside the peritoneal reflection, venous drainage may bypass the portal system with a potential for direct metastatic disease to the thorax or osseous system, bypassing the liver.

Recent articles have suggested a potential application of preoperative staging of colon cancer using hydrocolonic sonography—filling the colon with water and transabdominally scanning the abdomen. An improved staging yield suggests a potential application of this new technique.[20]

Over a decade has passed since the first applications of labeled antibodies were applied to colon cancer imaging. No useful technique has yet emerged, primarily because of technical difficulties (signal-to-noise problems) and lack of specific affinity of the antibody to tumors and regional lymph nodes, in addition to distant metastatic sites in the liver. Nonetheless, improved specificity and sensitivity may result from future improvements in monoclonal antibody developments.[21]

Cross-sectional imaging techniques provide an opportunity for the early recognition of recurrences after primary treatment for colorectal tumors. It is essential to perform a baseline study 3 to 4 months after surgery to determine the appearance of the operative site. Since most rectosigmoid recurrences appear within 2 years, subsequent studies in patients with rectosigmoid cancers should be performed every 6 months for 2 years and then yearly and should be compared with this baseline study in the monitoring of change in the operative site. Even though there is not as much data, the same is true for more proximal colon carcinomas. To date, it has not been possible to detect characteristic signal changes on MRI to allow for distinguishing recurrent tumor from operative changes or complications.[22] It is therefore currently recommended that contrast-enhanced CT be the imaging technique of choice in monitoring the patient with colorectal carcinoma for recurrence after primary therapy.[23] Carcinoembryonic antigen (CEA) levels should serve as the monitor for tumor status change, together with appropriate laboratory values and patient symptoms. Changing CEA and laboratory values or new symptoms should prompt repeat abdominal CT scanning (see the box above).

REFERENCES

1. Beahrs OH, Henson DE, Hutter RVP, Kennedy BJ, eds: *Manual for staging of cancer,* ed 4, Philadelphia, 1992, JB Lippincott.
2. Quint LE, Glazer GM, Orringer MB: Esophageal imaging by MR and CT: study of normal anatomy and neoplasms, *Radiology* 156:727, 1985.
3. Halvorsen RA Jr, Thompson WM: Primary neoplasms of the hollow organs of the gastrointestinal tract: staging and follow-up, *Cancer* 67:1181, 1991.
4. Botet JF et al: Preoperative staging of esophageal cancer: comparison of endoscopic ultrasound and dynamic CT, *Radiology* 181:419, 1991.
5. Sharma OP, Subnani S: Role of computerized tomography imaging in staging oesophageal carcinoma, *Semin Surg Oncol* 5:355, 1989.
6. Postlethwait R: *Surgery of the esophagus,* ed 2, East Norwalk, Conn, 1985, Appleton-Century-Crofts.
7. Takashima S, Takeuchi N, Shiozaki H et al: Carcinoma of the esophagus: CT vs MR imaging in determining resectability, *AJR* 156:297, 1991.
8. Halvorsen RA, Thompson WM: Carcinoma of the gastrointestinal tract. Categorical course on imaging of cancers, American College of Radiology: Syllabus for categorical course on oncologic imaging, 1992.
9. Tio TL, Coene PP, Schouwink MH, Tytgat GN: Esophagogastric carcinoma: preoperative TNM classification with endosonography, *Radiology* 173:411, 1989.
10. Rice TW, Boyce GA, Sivak MV: Esophageal ultrasound and the preoperative staging of carcinoma of the esophagus, *J Thorac Cardiovasc Surg* 101:536, 1991.
11. Vilgrain V, Mompoint D, Palazzo L et al: Staging of esophageal carcinoma: comparison of results with endoscopic sonography and CT, *AJR* 155:277, 1990.
12. Overhagen H, Lameris JS, Berger MV et al: Supraclavicular lymph node metastases in carcinoma of the esophagus and gastroesophageal junction: assessment with CT, ultrasound, and US-guided fine-needle aspiration biopsy, *Radiology* 179:155, 1991.
13. DeVita VT, Hellman S, Rosenberg SA: *Cancer: principles and practice of oncology,* ed 3, Philadelphia, 1989, JB Lippincott.
14. Sussman SK, Halvorsen RA Jr, Illescas FF et al: Gastric adenocarcinoma: CT vs surgical staging, *Radiology* 167:335, 1988.
15. Botet JF, Lightdale CJ, Zauber AG et al: Preoperative staging of gastric cancer: comparison of endoscopic ultrasound and dynamic CT, *Radiology* 181:426, 1991.
16. Ferrucci JT: Liver tumor imaging: current concepts. Categorical course on imaging of cancers, American College of Radiology, Syllabus for categorical course on oncologic imaging, 1992.
17. Balthazar EJ, Megibow AJ, Hulnick D et al: Carcinoma of the colon: detection and preoperative staging by CT, *AJR* 146:301, 1988.
18. Moss AA: Imaging of colorectal carcinoma, *Radiology* 170:308, 1989.
19. Tio TL, Coene PP, van Delden OM et al: Colorectal carcinoma: preoperative TNM classification with endosonography, *Radiology* 179:165, 1991.
20. Limberg B: Diagnosis and staging of colonic tumors by conventional abdominal sonography as compared with hydrocolonic sonography, *N Engl J Med* 327:65, 1992.
21. Davidson BR, Young H, Waddington WA et al: Preoperative imaging of colorectal cancers: targeting the epithelial membrane antigen with a radiation-labeled monoclonal antibody, *Cancer* 69:625, 1992.
22. Rafto SE, Amendola MA, Gefter WB: MR imaging of recurrent colorectal carcinoma vs fibrosis, *J Comput Assist Tomogr* 12:521, 1988.
23. Thoeni RF: Colorectal cancer: cross-sectional imaging for staging of primary tumor and detection of local recurrence, *AJR* 156:909, 1991.

PART VIII

MISCELLANEOUS DISORDERS OF THE GASTROINTESTINAL TRACT

46 *Infections and Infestations*

MAURICE M. REEDER
PHILIP E. S. PALMER

The gastrointestinal infestations and infections[1-17] that afflict humankind, many of which are relatively uncommon in the developed countries of the Western world, are nonetheless becoming more prevalent in the West as people travel throughout the world and as increasing numbers of affected people emigrate to nonendemic areas. This chapter considers the spectrum of these disorders and their radiologic and clinical characteristics.

BACTERIAL INFECTIONS
Gastrointestinal tuberculosis

Tuberculosis of the alimentary tract[18-44] is now a rare disease, although it is clear from the radiologic, surgical, and pathologic literature published before 1950 that it used to be far more common than it now is. Although the general decrease in tuberculosis must in part be attributable to the advent of adequate chemotherapy, other factors are probably contributory. Tuberculosis of the lungs and skeleton is still extremely common in many parts of the world, and, yet, with few exceptions, tuberculosis of the alimentary tract has become very uncommon. Significant series have been reported only from India in the past 20 years (400 cases were reported for one hospital in 5 years, which amounted to 15% of all gastrointestinal studies). In North America and Europe, it is a very rare disease. Whenever it occurs, it most commonly affects the lower small bowel, cecum, and ascending colon. It is much less common in the esophagus, stomach, and upper small bowel. In this respect, there has been little change over the years; the ileocecal region has always been the most common site of infection. However, both previously and currently, peritonitis is a common manifestation of tuberculosis within the abdomen.

As it does elsewhere in the body, tuberculosis in the alimentary tract causes the formation of granulomas. Clinically and radiologically these may be manifested as ulcers, masses, or hypertrophic tumors (tuberculomas). If the infection is chronic or the patient's immunity is sufficient, there will be fibrosis, leading to a stricture or malfunction of the normal alimentary peristalsis.

Apart from symptoms and signs similar to those of tuberculosis anywhere in the body, that is, loss of weight, general malaise, and "feeling unwell," there are no specific findings that may point to the clinical diagnosis of alimentary tract tuberculosis. Nausea, vomiting, diarrhea, or, in some cases, constipation can occur. Distention due to intestinal obstruction may be the presenting symptom when there is a stricture or adhesions. The clinical findings in a patient with peritonitis may be helpful, but this is the only time when the clinical diagnosis is likely to be correct. In fact, depending on the site of the lesion, the initial clinical impression will nearly always suggest malignant disease. When the esophagus or stomach is involved, benign peptic ulceration may occasionally be suspected, and, when the small bowel is affected, the clinical findings may suggest acute or chronic low-grade gastroenteritis. Any pattern of colitis may be suggested when the large bowel is involved. The whole clinical picture is essentially vague and ill defined. Wherever the lesion and whatever the findings, only histologic evaluation will establish the diagnosis.

There are no specific laboratory tests that can be used in the diagnostic workup. It is difficult to recover the mycobacteria from gastric washings when there is tuberculous esophageal or gastric ulceration. It is equally difficult to recover them from feces when the colon or rectum is involved, but should *Mycobacterium tuberculosis* be detected in the stool, it represents an important finding. Most patients will be anemic, and some will have blood in the stool. Many will be underweight. The vast majority of patients will have a positive tuberculin skin reaction (Mantoux or purified protein derivative [PPD]), but the laboratory findings will be of little guidance to the correct diagnosis.

Much has been written about the incidence of pulmonary tuberculosis in patients with alimentary tract infection, and vice versa, but the reports are conflicting. Although it is not unusual to find a pulmonary tuberculous lesion associated with alimentary tract tuberculosis (in one series 20% of such patients had active pulmonary tuberculosis), it is by no means a consistent finding.[18,31,39] Many patients who have tuberculosis of the alimentary tract will have normal chest radiograph findings, and the absence of pulmonary infection should not in any way negate the diagnosis.[34] On the other hand, many thousands of patients have active pulmonary tuberculosis and repeatedly swallow sputum containing active mycobacteria but never develop clinical alimentary tract infection. Nevertheless, the finding of pulmonary tuberculosis may sway the diagnosis. For example, when proctoscopy reveals an unusual ulcer in the rectum in a patient with pulmonary tuberculosis, this must raise suspicion that the rectal ulceration is also tuberculous. Yet, if the chest radiograph findings are normal, tuberculosis cannot be excluded, and suspicion of a tuberculous ulcer must remain.

It is not difficult to demonstrate most alimentary tract tuberculous lesions radiologically, but it is much more difficult, if not impossible, to identify their cause. The histologic findings will almost always be a surprise and will often spark a sense of relief that the lesion is not malignant.

Tuberculosis of the esophagus

Tuberculosis of the esophagus initiates an inflammatory reaction that results in ulceration, thickening of the esophageal wall, or least commonly, a tumor. Direct spread from caseating tuberculous lymph nodes in the mediastinum may involve the esophagus. All these varieties may cause fistulas to form between the esophagus and the mediastinum, or occasionally into the trachea or a bronchus. Almost all heal by fibrosis, so a stricture is the most common manifestation (Fig. 46-1).

The upper half of the esophagus is most frequently affected, and no age group is exempt. Patients typically complain of difficulty in swallowing, which may be slow or relatively acute in onset. When there is an obvious stricture or ulcer, the clinical history and appearance mimic those associated with malignancy. Tuberculous ulcers are usually flat and partially surround the esophagus, and, when there is intramural thickening, normal peristalsis is disrupted.

Although the upper part of the esophagus is most frequently affected, tuberculous ulceration and strictures can also arise in the lower third of the esophagus. The differential diagnosis in this instance is the same and consists of benign or malignant stricture or ulceration. In some cases, the narrowing in the region of the cardia may produce a dilated esophagus that resembles achalasia, the stricture of peptic esophagitis, or a neoplasm.

Tuberculosis of the stomach

Tuberculosis may cause the stomach to ulcerate or become fibrotic and resemble malignant infiltration (as in linitis plastica); less commonly, tuberculosis may occur as a

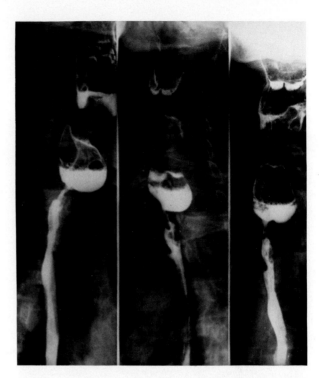

Fig. 46-1 Tuberculous stricture in the upper third of the esophagus with marked proximal dilatation above a narrow, elongated, and irregular stricture. Histologic confirmation would be necessary to distinguish this from inflammatory strictures resulting from other causes and from carcinoma.
From Reeder MM, Palmer PES: *The radiology of tropical diseases,* Baltimore, 1981, Williams & Wilkins.

hypertrophic "mass" (Fig. 46-2). The radiologic and pathologic variations are considerable. Even an erosive tuberculous gastritis has been reported in which there were numerous small mucosal defects, almost like a type of miliary disease.

The clinical symptoms are those of peptic ulceration or neoplasm and cannot be distinguished. If there is active pulmonary tuberculosis, the disease may at least be suggested. The most common site for a tuberculous ulcer is near the pylorus. Some tuberculous ulcers are very shallow but can be quite extensive.[29,41] These are unlikely to be mistaken for malignancy. In other cases, there is induration around the ulcer, the edge of which is undermined; this cannot be mistaken for benign peptic ulceration. A not infrequent presentation is pyloric obstruction, which may be due to tuberculous ulceration, fibrosis subsequent to such an ulcer, severe submucosal thickening, or, in some cases, extrinsic pressure exerted by tuberculous lymphadenopathy. If these lymph nodes caseate, the pylorus or greater curve of the stomach may become directly involved. However, as with most cases of marked pyloric obstruction, the true cause cannot be diagnosed radiologically.

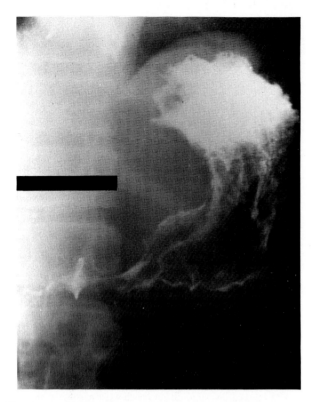

Fig. 46-2 Tuberculous gastritis causing thickening of the wall of the stomach and narrowing of the pyloric antrum in an African patient. The duodenal bulb and C loop are also distorted and narrowed.
From Reeder MM, Palmer PES: *The radiology of tropical diseases,* Baltimore, 1981, Williams & Wilkins.

Tuberculosis of the duodenum and small bowel

Tuberculosis affects all parts of the small bowel, the jejunum very infrequently, the duodenum occasionally, and the lower part of the ileum most commonly. There may be ulceration, granulomatous thickening, or, occasionally, hyperplastic nodules or tuberculoma. Any part of the small bowel, but particularly the duodenum, can be distorted by tuberculous lymphadenopathy (Fig. 46-3). It is unlikely that the correct diagnosis will be made on either clinical or radiologic grounds, but ultrasound or computed tomography (CT) will depict the enlarged lymph nodes.

The common clinical presentation in patients with tuberculosis of the duodenum and small bowel is obstruction, either high in the duodenum or jejunum or, most commonly, in the lower part of the ileum.

Tuberculosis of the duodenum most commonly takes the form of either ulceration or strictures, both most frequently in the third part of the duodenal loop. A thick, hypertrophic mucosa, almost resembling polyps, has been reported; granulomatous infiltration along short lengths of the duodenum may abolish peristalsis or even cause narrowing of the lumen. Isolated tuberculous involvement of the duodenum is uncommon; it will be associated either with lesions

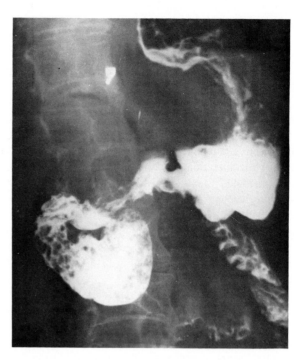

Fig. 46-3 Tuberculosis involving the stomach and duodenum. Infiltration along the lesser curvature has narrowed the stomach, and the duodenal bulb is deformed. A nodular mucosal contour is evident in the duodenum. Partial obstruction of the third portion of the duodenum is caused by tuberculous celiac lymph nodes.

elsewhere in the small bowel or, quite frequently, with gastric tuberculosis. In one series, 11% of the patients with gastric tuberculosis were also found to have duodenal infection.[27] When there is ulceration, the ulcers are frequently multiple and associated with considerable thickening of the duodenal wall. Perforation with fistula formation can occur. As healing takes place, this almost always results in contraction and stenosis, leading to duodenal obstruction.

In the ileum, tuberculosis causes the formation of transverse ulcers in Peyer's patches, typically with undermined edges. This is usually a chronic condition, and may be accompanied by considerable dilatation of the small bowel above the narrow areas. The accurate demonstration of lower small bowel tuberculosis can be enhanced by use of a small bowel enema study, which can show the exact site and the characteristics of the stricture, or strictures. However, even using this technique, radiologic differentiation from Crohn's disease is very difficult (Fig. 46-4). Tuberculosis may cause the formation of fistulas similar to those seen in patients with regional ileitis. They may arise at multiple levels and can be insidious in onset and chronic. Because Crohn's disease is rare in many parts of the world, for instance, India, a knowledge of geography may be more helpful than the radiologic findings in establishing the diagnosis.

A small bowel obstruction stemming from tuberculous

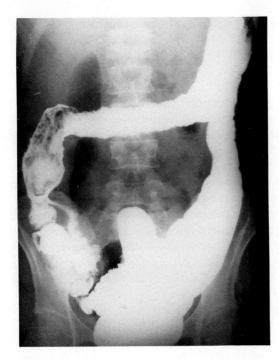

Fig. 46-4 Tuberculous ileocolitis manifested by a narrowed ileum and cecum, narrowing of the right and transverse portions of the colon with loss of haustra, and extensive ulceration. The left portion of the colon is normal. Crohn's disease and occasionally amebiasis may produce this radiographic pattern.

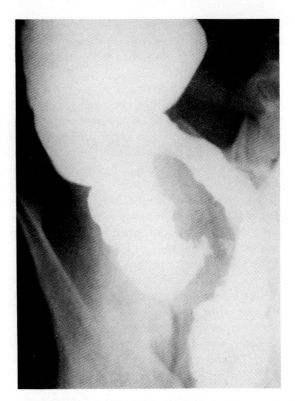

Fig. 46-5 Narrowed, shrunken, conical cecum and narrowed, ulcerated terminal ileum typical of ileocecal tuberculosis. Note the gaping ileocecal valve.

peritonitis is not uncommon. Adhesions may also result from tuberculous enteritis.[34]

Pressure on the duodenal loop exerted by tuberculous lymphadenopathy may cause extrinsic distortion and even obstruction. This may arise in the acute stage or, as the lymphadenopathy heals, may be a consequence of the subsequent fibrosis. It is impossible to differentiate the distortion from malignant lymphadenopathy, or in some cases from enlargement of the pancreas, even using CT or ultrasound. The clinical and radiologic diagnosis is likely to be lymphoma or malignancy, since tuberculous lymphadenopathy in the abdomen is uncommon and unrecognizable unless there is generalized tuberculous peritonitis.

Ileocecal tuberculosis

The ileocecum is and always has been the most common site for gastrointestinal tuberculosis, and, because of the marked local reaction, has also been called *hyperplastic tuberculosis of the gastrointestinal tract*[10,11] (Fig. 46-5). In some series, it is said to account for 80% to 90% of all the cases of gastrointestinal tuberculosis, although this figure is probably high as an overall average.

The classic radiographic appearance of ileocecal tuberculosis on barium enema examinations is that of a conical, shrunken, retracted cecum combined with a narrow ulcerated terminal ileum[19] (Fig. 46-5). The cecal deformity is

the result of spasm that occurs early in the disease and of a transmural infiltrate with fibrosis that takes place in the more advanced phases. Narrowing of the terminal ileum may be caused by persistent irritability, with rapid emptying of the narrowed segment when filling retrogradely or antegradely (Stierlin's sign) during a barium enema study. This narrowing corresponds to the acute inflammatory phase of the disease. It may also stem from stricture accompanied by thickening and ulceration of the bowel wall in advanced ileocecal tuberculosis. The ileocecal valve has been described as "gaping,"[30] similar to that seen in chronic ulcerative colitis (Fig. 46-5). In the more advanced ileal lesions, deep fissures and ulcers develop, as well as enterocutaneous fistulas. Circumferential deep ileal ulcers may eventually perforate when a clinical and pulmonary response to antitubercular drugs is seen. Most perforations, however, are of the walled-off type rather than of the free intraperitoneal type. Ultrasound and CT will demonstrate the mass of inflammatory tissue, but there are no characteristic findings on which to base a diagnosis of tuberculosis.

Because the mesocolon contracts, the cecum may be pulled out of the iliac fossa, and at the same time be reduced in size by fibrosis. Similarly, the hepatic flexure may be pulled downward. There may be a partial stricture of the ileocecal junction, also resulting from fibrosis. The terminal ileum therefore dilates and, as viewed on a barium enema, may seem to be suspended and hanging from the cecum (Fig. 46-6). Both clinically and radiologically, movement of the cecum is restricted in every direction. Spontaneous sinus formation is not common, but fistulas may form between various loops of bowel, particularly after surgical interference, if the correct diagnosis has not been recognized at the time of surgery. Pericecal abscesses are not common, but, when they do occur, may resemble an appendiceal or an amebic abscess.

Although it is essential to use a barium enema when examining the large bowel in a patient with tuberculosis, a small bowel study should also be performed. The lower part of the cecum may appear to be obliterated, and reflux of an enema into the ileum may not be achieved or may be incomplete. The small bowel study helps in excluding other sites of small bowel infection and in delineating the exact involvement of the terminal ileum and the ileocecal junction. In about 20% of the cases of ileocecal tuberculosis, there are other small bowel strictures, particularly in the distal ileum. In other patients, the granulomatous infiltration

of the bowel wall may assume an appearance similar to the rigid "tube" seen in Crohn's disease. When these occur in combination with the granulomatous cecal mass and the overall fibrosis, the distortion at the ileocecal region may be considerable.

In the hypertrophic variety (or perhaps "stage" is a better term, because most hypertrophic tuberculous infections will eventually fibrose), the hypertrophic masses may be observed on barium studies to project into the lumen of the cecum and ascending colon. Because there is almost always some associated contraction, it may be possible to deduce the correct (tuberculous) cause in this instance. As the hypertrophic granulomas progress, the cecum assumes a conical shape on radiologic studies and stenosis occurs, both at the ileocecal junction and in the ascending colon.[19] Eventually, only a strip of barium may outline the affected area, particularly at the junction of the cecum and ascending colon (Fig. 46-7).

Radiologically, the differential diagnosis of such a distortion includes an appendiceal or an amebic abscess (Fig. 46-8). Other cases resemble Crohn's disease. In many reports, reflux from the cecum into the ileum is a relatively uncommon finding in tuberculosis, as compared to amebiasis or a malignancy. However, at some stages, a patulous ileocecal valve is seen,[30] particularly in India. This may reflect the slower development of fibrosis when the infection is more acute and overwhelming. To further complicate the differential diagnosis, amebiasis can also occasionally be a fibrosing condition. However, amebiasis

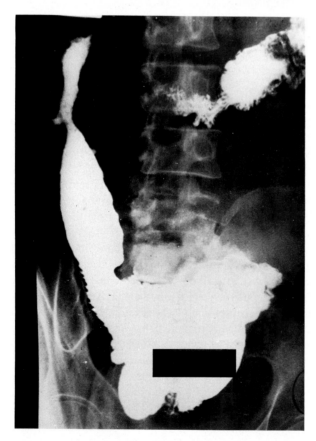

Fig. 46-6 Contracted cecum typical of tuberculosis. There is ulceration of the terminal ileum and minimal obstruction. The ileum is dilated and seems to hang from a small contracted cecum. From Reeder MM, Palmer PES: *The radiology of tropical diseases,* Baltimore, 1981, Williams & Wilkins.

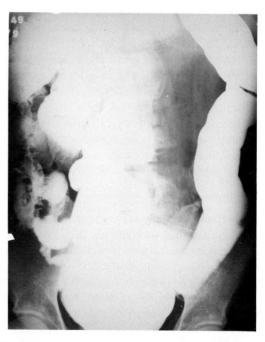

Fig. 46-7 Deep penetrating ulcers and fissures of the cecum and ascending colon cause extensive narrowing and deformity of the right portion of the colon in a patient with ileocecal tuberculosis.

seldom affects the small bowel above the terminal ileum. Finding amebae in the stool may resolve the radiologic dilemma.

Bone infection in the ilium has resulted from a tuberculous abscess in the region of the cecum. As with other tuberculous infections, it tends to be chronic and may even be mistaken for actinomycosis.

Tuberculosis of the colon

Below the cecum, tuberculous granulomas occur in the colon either as colitis or strictures, and either may be multifocal.[6,16] Ulceration also takes place, usually in the early stages, but is seldom seen radiologically. Tuberculous infection usually spreads over short distances, 5 to 7 cm, and seldom involves extensive areas of the colon.

The clinical presentation of the strictures usually consists of incomplete obstruction without severe pain. The most likely clinical diagnosis will be malignant disease or, in appropriate geographic areas, an ameboma. Making the differential diagnosis based on the radiologic findings can be extremely difficult. Similarly, tuberculous colitis may resemble amebiasis, in that it can affect short lengths of bowel and occasionally involve several sites. Perforation and fistulas are not often seen in tuberculosis, but both may occur, and a pericolic abscess may form.

A barium enema will show the constricted and often edematous area of bowel and only occasionally will reveal the involvement of other lengths of bowel. The stricture is seldom as marked as the "apple-core" narrowing characteristic of malignancy, and seldom is as extensive as an ameboma. However, tuberculosis of the colon is not a diagnosis made with great accuracy on radiologic grounds.

Tuberculosis of the rectum

Tuberculous infection seldom involves the rectum, but it may rarely present as an ulcerating proctitis (Fig. 46-9). Fistulas may form, and rectal strictures have been reported. Chronic sciatic-rectal abscesses may be tuberculous in origin. There are no distinguishing radiologic characteristics.

Enteroliths

Intestinal calculi are not common but may form above any bowel stricture. When the stricture is high within the

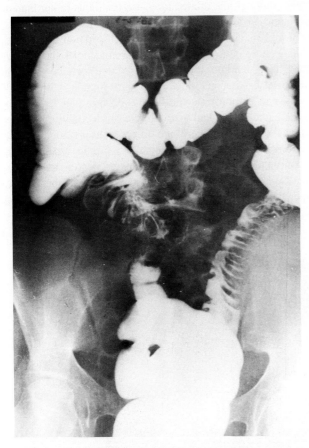

Fig. 46-8 Tuberculosis of the cecum and colon. The cecum is displaced upward by lymphadenopathy; the mucosa is edematous and swollen. A mass was palpable and the clinical findings suggested malignancy. Marked mucosal changes in the sigmoid colon prompted an alternative diagnosis of amebiasis or lymphoma, and tuberculosis was not considered. The combination of matting and adhesions of the small bowel, fixation of the ileocecal junction, and a contracted cecum suggests the correct diagnosis of tuberculosis. The massive lymphadenopathy seen here is unusual when tuberculosis is the single problem.
From Reeder MM, Palmer PES: *The radiology of tropical diseases,* Baltimore, 1981, Williams & Wilkins.

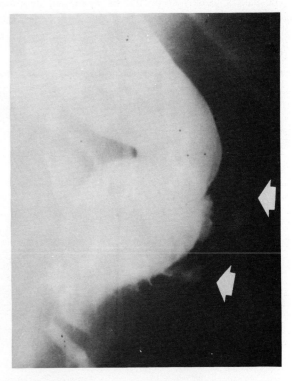

Fig. 46-9 Deep penetrating rectal ulcers and fissures along with perirectal strictures *(arrows)*—a result of tuberculosis. This patient also had pulmonary tuberculosis.

small bowel, the enteroliths are usually nonopaque, as they are then composed of choleic acid. In the lower small bowel, which possesses a more alkaline medium and a higher concentration of calcium salts, enteroliths are often opaque. Some are completely opacified, whereas others have translucent centers with only a ring of calcification. In some countries, such calcified enteroliths may be found in the lower ileum or colon in 3% to 4% of cases with intestinal tuberculosis. They vary from multiple small stones to single large lamellated calculi. They must be differentiated from renal stones or gallstones and, less commonly, from vesical stones. It is seldom difficult to distinguish them radiologically from calcified granulomas within the lymph nodes, although ultrasound may sometimes provide more accurate information. Tuberculosis is not the only cause of enterolithiasis, and, in the industrialized world, Crohn's disease is the more frequent finding. However, the possibility of tuberculosis should be considered whenever such calculi are seen.

Peritoneal tuberculosis

Peritonitis is the most common presentation of tuberculosis within the abdomen. In some countries the peritoneum may be the most common single nonpulmonary site of infection. In every case, there is associated abdominal lymphadenopathy, and in most there is ascites. It is seldom possible, even histologically, to locate the primary tuberculous focus.

The patient usually complains of abdominal distention and pain, but many of the findings are nonspecific, con-

sisting of weight loss, tiredness, and ill health. About one third of the patients are afebrile. The tuberculous skin reaction (either Mantoux or PPD) is usually positive, but can be negative. Chest radiograph findings are usually normal. A thorough clinical examination may bring to light lymphadenopathy outside the abdomen, most commonly in the neck. Within the abdomen, the liver and spleen may be enlarged but difficult to palpate, and the abdomen will be doughy to palpation and often tender. Abdominal distention may be due to ascites or, in some cases, to subacute obstruction. In some patients, it is possible to palpate a mass of enlarged lymph nodes, particularly in the right iliac fossa.

Routine supine and erect radiographs of the abdomen can confirm the clinical suggestion of ascites, and often depict distended loops of small bowel, with thickened intestinal walls, although the dilated loops suggest ileus rather than a mechanical obstruction. As healing progresses, adhesions form and may later cause subacute obstruction at various levels. There is no indication for barium studies during the acute stage, but later they can be used to determine whether the bowel has become fixed or remains mobile. Ultrasound or CT can demonstrate the fluid collection and loculation in the acute stage, and also allow early recognition of the lymphadenopathy. There are three types of tuberculous peritonitis: a wet-ascitic type, a dry-plastic type, and a fibrotic-fixed type. The first exhibits ascites or pockets of loculated fluid with a thickened mesentery. In the plastic type, the mesenteric lymph nodes are enlarged and there is central caseation necrosis and adhesions, while the fibrotic-

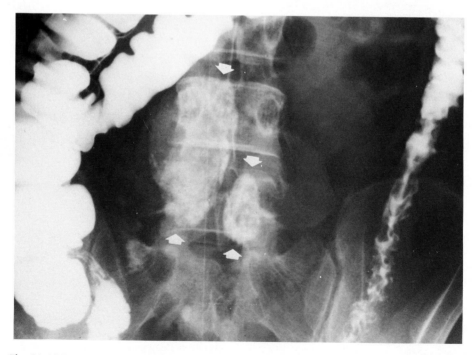

Fig. 46-10 Irregular patchy calcifications distributed throughout large tuberculous mesenteric lymph nodes (arrows). This patient had an inactive case of pulmonary tuberculosis.

fixed type presents with a thickened omentum and a mass. There is seldom any intrinsic abnormality in the small bowel in cases of tuberculous peritonitis, but the lymphadenopathy may cause distortion.

The typical calcified tuberculous lymph nodes tend to cluster, with lobulated contours and spotty calcification throughout (Fig. 46-10). These nodes vary in size from 0.5 to 10 cm. Calcification of the mesenteric lymph nodes 1 to 2 years after the onset of intestinal infection has been reported.

Differential diagnosis

Gastric tuberculosis must be differentiated radiographically from gastric carcinoma, lymphoma, and syphilis.

Intestinal tuberculosis is a granulomatous disease that involves all layers of the bowel wall. Crohn's disease must be the first entity considered in the differential diagnosis, particularly when the ileocecal region is involved. These two processes may be indistinguishable radiographically. However, when active pulmonary tuberculosis is associated with a typical ileocecal deformity, this makes a tuberculous etiology a little more likely than Crohn's disease. Periappendiceal abscess may also cause the cecal deformities and narrowing of the terminal ileum that are suggestive of tuberculosis. Cecal diverticulitis or typhlitis rarely produces similar cecal narrowing. Although amebiasis may produce the typical shrunken cecum seen in tuberculosis, small bowel involvement is rarely associated with this infection. Lymphoma and carcinoma of the cecum may produce a short truncated cecal tip. However, cecal carcinoma that crosses the ileocecal valve and involves the ileum is rare, and the margins of a carcinoma do not ordinarily taper but tend to be sharply demarcated.

More extensive tuberculosis that involves the colon must be differentiated from ulcerative colitis, Crohn's disease, the colitis of bacillary dysentery, amebic colitis, ischemic colitis, and pseudomembranous colitis. However, idiopathic ulcerative colitis does not lead to the formation of deep ulcerations and fistulas, as does tuberculous colitis. Nevertheless, the other forms of ulcerating colitis may be indistinguishable radiographically from tuberculous colitis.

Salmonella infections[45-55]

Many species of *Salmonella* may be responsible for food poisoning that originates from the ingestion of contaminated foods.[48,50] This infectious type of food poisoning, in which the salmonellae produce a thermostabile endotoxin that irritates the mucosa of both the stomach and the small and large bowels, must be differentiated from the toxin type of food poisoning, which is caused by enterotoxin-producing organisms such as staphylococci.[51]

Infected carrier animals or their by-products, such as eggs, meat, and milk, are the principal sources of *Salmonella* infections in humans. Chronic or temporary human carriers, especially those engaged in food handling, can play an important role in the transmission of the disease, as can flies, cockroaches, and other insects.[12,51]

Once ingested, *Salmonella* incubates for 7 to 30 hours before gastroenteritis ensues. Infected persons may suffer headaches, pyrexia, nausea, vomiting, and diarrhea with fluid stools that contain mucus and occasionally small amounts of blood. Patients with *Salmonella* food poisoning usually recover in about 5 days, but occasionally they may become extremely toxic and advance into a typhoid state. The mortality from this fulminant form of the disease is about 1%.[51]

When necropsy has been performed in the rare individuals who die of *Salmonella* food poisoning, the mucosa of the stomach and small and large bowels has been found to be inflamed and hyperemic, and covered with a slimy exudate, small hemorrhages, and superficial ulcers, especially in the colon.[51] Peyer's patches are usually swollen, and the spleen may be enlarged and soft in patients with septicemia. In infants, and rarely in adults, complications such as osteomyelitis, purulent arthritis, tendinitis, intraperitoneal abscesses, subacute bacterial endocarditis, aortitis, and meningitis may result from the septicemia. An outbreak of such food poisoning may affect a large number of people, as happened recently when an academic department of radiology was temporarily devastated by such an event.

Reports on the radiologic evaluation of patients with *Salmonella* gastroenterocolitis are rare[12] (Figs. 46-11 and 46-12).

Typhoid fever

Typhoid fever,[45-55] which is caused by *Salmonella typhi,* and the paratyphoid fever, which is caused by the paratyphi A, B, and C bacilli of the *Salmonella* species, are specifically human diseases. They are transmitted via the excreta from one infected person to another, usually through polluted drinking water. Occasionally, organisms are transmitted by means of dairy products or other food items that are contaminated by chronic carriers of the organism. Although flies and contaminated shellfish may also act as intermediaries, the enteric fevers are primarily water-borne diseases. This fact explains the explosive onset of epidemics in military or civilian populations.[51]

After the bacilli enter the gastrointestinal tract, they invade the intestinal lymphatic system and multiply, eventually entering the blood stream, where they are phagocytized by the reticuloendothelial cells, liver, and spleen. A secondary bacteremia develops when the bacilli are released from the liver and spleen, and this event coincides with the incipient clinical manifestations of the disease.[51] The incubation period for typhoid fever is usually 10 to 15 days. Characteristic lesions develop in the intestinal lymphatic tissues, especially in the terminal ileum. The colon is involved in only one third of the patients, although not extensively,[51] and includes hyperplasia of Peyer's patches, hyperemia and edema of the follicles, and mucosal inflammation. The inflammatory changes are maximal at about the tenth day, after which they may resolve, or, more commonly, necrosis of the hyperplastic lymphoid tissue ensues. This necrosis results in the sloughing of the overlying mucosa, leaving behind ulcers of various extent and depth.[45,51] The oval-shaped ulcers situated on the long axis of the intestinal lumen on the antimesenteric margin of the distal ileum coincide with the distribution of Peyer's patches.[12,45] The ulcers are deepest near the ileocecal valve, where perforation is most frequent. Toward the end of the second week or dur-

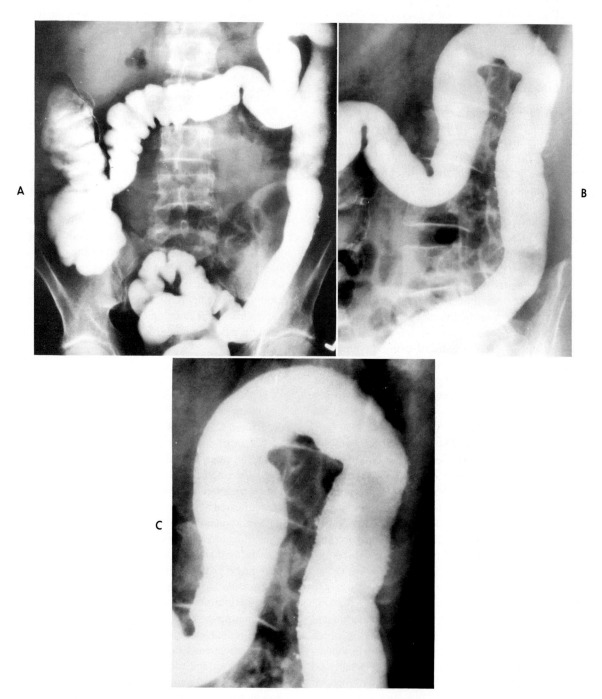

Fig. 46-11 *Salmonella* colitis. **A, B,** and **C,** Numerous collar-button ulcerations are seen along both borders of the descending colon and sigmoid. Sigmoidoscopy revealed a friable, ulcerated mucosa. *Salmonella* organisms were cultured from both the feces and scrapings of the rectal mucosa. The radiographic findings in this type of colitis are indistinguishable from those of idiopathic ulcerative colitis.
Courtesy of Dr. Leslie Reyer.

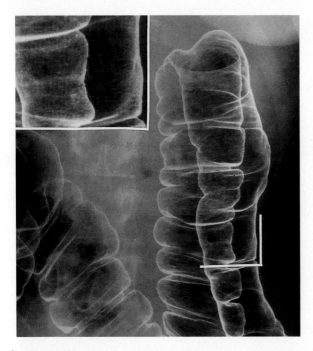

Fig. 46-12 This 26-year-old woman suffered the sudden onset of persistent watery diarrhea, nausea, and vomiting. After 2 weeks, a double-contrast barium enema was performed, showing numerous tiny ulcers that were evenly distributed throughout the whole colon. Stool cultures confirmed the growth of *Salmonella*. She made a complete recovery.
Courtesy of Dr. T. Fork.

ing the third week of illness, further sloughing of necrotic ulcerating tissue may lead to intestinal perforation and hemorrhage.[45]

Radiologic findings

Because the pathologic anatomy and clinical course of typhoid and paratyphoid fevers are well known, radiographic examination is rarely indicated, except when perforation of a typhoid ulcer is suspected. Such perforation in the distal ileum is a complication in 2% to 4% of all such ulcers and is the cause of 25% to 40% of the deaths from typhoid fever.[45] Most investigators agree that perforation occurs between the end of the second week and the fourth week of the clinical illness,[49,55] though others have noted perforation to take place earlier in the course, sometimes after only 3 to 7 days of clinical symptoms.[45,49] The clinical severity of the typhoid illness is apparently not related to the occurrence of perforation.[45]

The main radiographic finding in patients with typhoid fever, but *without* intestinal perforation, is the accumulation of gas, which is produced by a paralytic ileus in distended loops of bowel, especially in the small bowel.[45,49] Fluid levels are uncommon in this instance. By contrast, peritonitis resulting from other diseases typically produces a generalized paralytic ileus that includes gaseous disten-

tion of the entire intestine, with the colon more distended than the small bowel. Kinking, edema, and adhesions may cause mechanical obstruction that further distends the small bowel after perforation.[45,49]

The presence of free intraperitoneal gas in typhoid patients *with* perforation is considered uncommon by some investigators,[47] but others have reported that up to 65% of patients with free perforation have evidence of free gas.[45] Segments of the distal small bowel may be irregularly narrowed and fixed, as depicted by the outline of the intraluminal gas[45] (Fig. 46-13). When combined with paralytic ileus resulting from generalized peritonitis, inflammatory hyperplasia of the ileocecal valve may add to the radiographic appearance of a mixed paralytic and obstructive ileus.[45]

The large amounts of free intraperitoneal gas that appear after perforation in some patients may be explained by the excessive amount of gas that has distended the small bowel before perforation. The absence of free intraperitoneal gas in other instances may be the result of insidious perforations that have been walled off by adhesions before radiographic examination.[45]

Published descriptions of barium study findings in the small intestine and colon of patients with typhoid fever are rare. Chèrigiè et al.[46] reported on their observations gleaned from examinations of the small bowel performed in 32 patients studied during a typhoid epidemic that occurred in France in 1950. They found the caliber of the jejunum was dilated to two or three times its normal size, with enlargement and edema of the valves of Kerckring that looked like "stacked plates." Small pea-sized mucosal nodules were found in the distal ileum, which was found to represent hypertrophy of the Peyer's patches. Small ulcerations of the distal ileum were seen in only three of their patients. Transit of barium through the small intestine took about 5 hours, with delay noted in the dilated areas.

Schinz et al.[47] noted that, as in tuberculosis, typhoid bacilli tend to invade the lower ileum because of the greater abundance of lymphatic tissue there. In the initial stages, the dominant pathologic and radiographic appearances consist of mucosal edema, with thickening of the folds, narrowing of the lumen, and mural rigidity. During the advanced stage of typhoid fever, the extensively ulcerated intestinal surface assumes the appearance of a ragged and ill-defined contour on radiographs[12] (Fig. 46-14). Healing of ulcers by the formation of granulation tissue may begin about the fourth week of the disease. When healing is complete, a slightly depressed, smooth scar remains, which does not cause stricture or intestinal obstruction.[51]

A chronic typhoid infection of the intestinal tract of 4 years' duration has been described.[52] Serial radiographs of the small bowel in this patient revealed extensive segmentation and puddling of barium throughout the ileum, with loss of the normal mucosal folds and dilatation of the bowel loops. Hypermotility of the intestine was observed, with barium reaching the cecum in 1 hour. Similar findings have

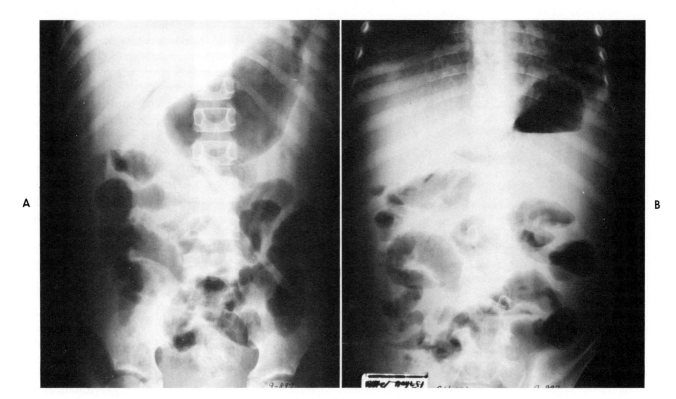

Fig. 46-13 Typhoid fever with perforation. **A,** Note the multiple loops of distended, gas-filled small bowel on this supine view. **B,** In an upright projection, multiple resting fluid levels are seen. The properitoneal fat lines are lost, and several of the small bowel loops, especially those in the right lower quadrant, appear fixed on two projections. Free gas can be seen below the liver margin on both views. A radiograph of the chest obtained in the erect position showed free air beneath the right hemidiaphragm.
Courtesy of Dr. Stanley Bohrer.

been reported to result from paratyphoid fever caused by *Salmonella schottmuelleri* (paratyphi B).[53] Paratyphoid fevers usually do not produce extensive lymphatic invasion and ulceration, as does typhoid fever. More often, postmortem studies of intestinal specimens from patients with paratyphoid fever reveal that little or no change has taken place, although the entire intestine may be acutely inflamed.[55] In the paratyphoid fevers and some other forms of salmonellosis, ulceration of the large intestine is more common than it is in typhoid fever.

The differential diagnosis in patients with terminal ileal spasticity and ulceration and later luminal rigidity, includes regional enteritis, tuberculous ileitis, histoplasmosis, lymphosarcoma, radiation vasculitis, ischemia, and periarteritis nodosa. Regional enteritis and tuberculosis, in particular, may resemble the radiographic findings of typhoid fever.

Bacillary dysentery

Bacillary dysentery,[56-62] or shigellosis, is an acute or chronic inflammatory disease that involves the colon and occasionally the distal ileum. Epidemics of dysentery have occurred throughout recorded history whenever large groups of people living in crowded communities such as armies, prisons, or mental institutions have neglected the cardinal rules of sanitation. Great wars have been won or lost as a result of outbreaks of dysentery among the opposing armies. The disease is worldwide in distribution but is most frequent and severe in the inhabitants of those developing countries in the wet, humid tropics, where poor sanitation and primitive conditions prevail.

The disease is named for members of the genus *Shigella*, the dysentery bacilli, which vary markedly in terms of their antigenicity and pathogenicity. *Shigella dysenteriae*, the Shiga bacillus, produces a potent endotoxin and is responsible for the epidemics of severe diarrhea in the tropics and subtropics. *Shigella* of the Flexner, Sonne, and Boyd subgroups are not endotoxin producers and are generally less pathogenic, causing less serious disease and a lower incidence of chronic dysentery. The Flexner and Sonne subgroups are the most common causes of bacillary dysentery in the United States, England, Europe, Egypt, and the Ori-

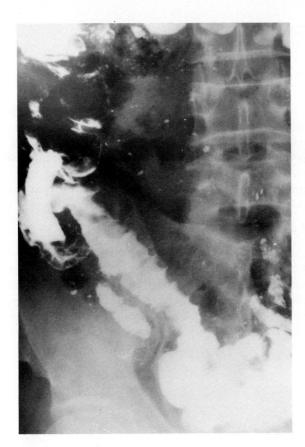

Fig. 46-14 Straightening and rigidity of the terminal ileum with pronounced edema and irregularity of the lumen, a result of typhoid fever. Numerous ulcers that project from both sides of the ileum produce a spiked, ragged bowel contour. There are several lucent areas near the ileocecal area that represent hypertrophied Peyer's patches. The cecum and ascending colon are incompletely filled.

ent. The Boyd subgroup is found in India and Egypt. However, strains of any of the four *Shigella* subgroups may be encountered in North America, where bacillary dysentery is primarily an institutional disease and arises in nursery schools, mental institutions, prisons, and military compounds. Sonne dysentery has been prevalent in America, England, and Europe in recent winters, especially afflicting children.[12]

Bacillary dysentery occurs almost exclusively in humans. Human carriers are common where the disease is prevalent and are the only important reservoir of shigellosis. Pollution of the water supply by feces, contamination of food by infected food handlers, and transfer of the bacilli by flies are the principal modes of transmission.[56,60] Epidemics commonly occur after mild cases and are often overlooked. In epidemics, positive cultures may be obtained in up to 25% of the apparently healthy contacts. About 3% of those who recover from an attack of shigellosis become asymptomatic carriers and for variable periods.[60]

Clinically, the incubation period varies from 24 hours to

a week. The disease may begin suddenly or insidiously, but commonly occurs as a simple diarrhea that may be quite varied in its severity, such that cases can be classified into the following clinical types: mild (catarrhal), acute, fulminating, relapsing, and chronic.

The chief clinical symptoms are the manifestations of the colitis and include gripping abdominal pain, tenesmus, and frequently the passage of loose stools that may vary greatly in number and character. The abdomen is often rigid early in the disease. Patients may suffer high fever that rises to 104° F, vomiting, and leukocytosis. In severe cases of shigellosis, the stools may eventually consist only of frequently evacuated blood-stained mucus containing a characteristic purulent, cellular exudate, and great numbers of dysentery bacilli. There may be 20 to 40 involuntary evacuations per day, accompanied by intense tenesmus and abdominal pain, such that the patient must remain literally "glued" to the toilet.

A swollen, diffusely inflamed rectal mucosa, often covered with mucus and pus, may be seen through the proctoscope. Underlying this exudate is a granular mucous membrane that freely oozes blood. Shallow ulcerations, which are irregular in size and shape and covered with pus, may be present.

Pathologically, shigellosis is characterized by an acute, diffuse inflammation of the colon with initial hyperemia of the mucosa, followed by edema, hemorrhage, and leukocytic infiltration. This process often extends into the submucosa and causes marked thickening of the intestinal wall. Epithelial necrosis and desquamation with the formation of a diphtheritic membrane is followed by ulceration that may extend deep into the submucosa and occasionally into the muscularis[59,60]; perforation is rare. Inflammation is usually not distributed uniformly throughout the colon, but is most severe in the rectosigmoid and descending colon. The terminal ileum is occasionally involved. Secondary bacterial infection occurs once ulcerative lesions have developed, and may be important in the transition to the chronic stage of the disease, in which adjacent lesions may be joined by ulcerating channels beneath bridges of hyperplastic mucosa. Mucosal retention cysts may harbor *Shigella* bacilli, which are intermittently discharged in the chronic carrier state.[60]

In patients with chronic bacillary dysentery, there is typically extensive scarring and fibrosis of the colon, indolent ulceration, and a continued subacute or chronic inflammation that periodically becomes acute. The disease resembles chronic idiopathic ulcerative colitis, both clinically and pathologically, including a tendency to undergo exacerbation and remission. During periods of active disease, the patient may have fever and diarrhea with varying amounts of blood, mucus, and a cellular exudate in the stools.[60]

Radiologic findings

The radiographic findings are determined by the severity and stage of the disease. Many radiographic features of bacillary dysentery resemble those seen in other inflammatory diseases of the small and large bowel. Plain films of the abdomen may show a considerable amount of gas in the small intestine and colon. Barium examination of the small intestine may show mucosal edema, segmentation, loss of the normal fold pattern, hypersecretion, and especially hypermotility with a rapid transit time.[58,61]

Many patients with bacillary dysentery exhibit no radiologic changes in the colon on barium enema examinations. However, in active, moderately advanced disease, there may be edema of the mucosa with spasm and an irregular outline to the bowel wall.[62] Complete filling of the colon and distal ileum is difficult to accomplish because of spasmodic contractions and tenesmus. Postevacuation films usually show complete elimination of the barium.[58]

In more severe cases of *Shigella* dysentery, focal ulcerations may exist, which usually are not deep and rarely extend into the muscularis. These superficial ulcers are most prevalent in the rectosigmoid colon, but may be found throughout the colon in advanced cases[12] (Figs. 46-15 and 46-16). At this stage, the ulcerated appearance of the colon radiologically may resemble acute ulcerative colitis, with an irregular bowel contour, marked spasm, and eventual partial cicatricial stenoses.[61,62]

In chronic cases, transient spasmodic emptyings and reflux fillings may take place, and the colon may be rigid and tubelike in some segments with a loss of haustrations.

Postevacuation films show segmental puddling of the barium with a lack of haustral markings.[58]

The radiographic differential diagnosis of bacillary dysentery includes acute and chronic idiopathic ulcerative colitis, *Salmonella* enterocolitis, pseudomembranous enterocolitis, and amebiasis. All are inflammatory diseases that produce edema, spasm, and ulceration of the small bowel or colon. Crohn's disease and tuberculosis may also produce similar radiologic findings, although these inflammatory diseases tend to be more segmental and eccentric in distribution, and show deeper ulcerations and, at times, fistula formation and stenoses.

Campylobacter infection

Only since 1977 have improved culture techniques permitted the recognition that *Campylobacter* is a major cause of dysentery worldwide, accounting for up to 20% of positive stool cultures in patients with acute bacillary dysentery. It is primarily a disease of children and young adults[63] and is the most common cause of acute infectious colitis in

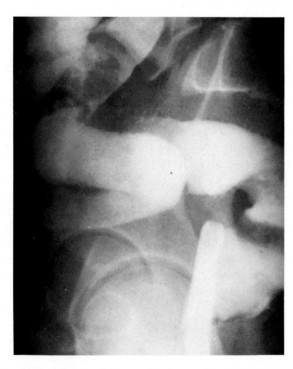

Fig. 46-15 Multiple, shallow, collar-button ulcerations are present in the sigmoid colon of this patient with bacillary dysentery (shigellosis). The presacral space is widened and the rectal valves are thickened because of inflammation in the rectosigmoid colon.

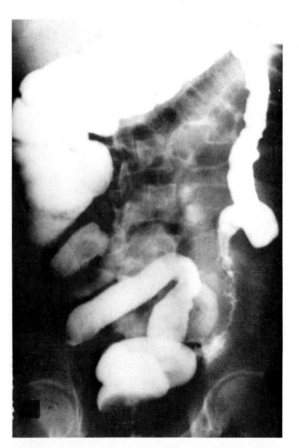

Fig. 46-16 Bacillary dysentery. There is tubular narrowing of the descending and proximal sigmoid colon, with multiple small ulcerations and irregularity of the mucosal pattern. The rectum and distal sigmoid colon appear normal.
From Reeder MM, Palmer PES: *The radiology of tropical diseases,* Baltimore, 1981, Williams & Wilkins.

children. The diarrhea may be watery or bloody, but pain and tenderness are typical, so that appendicitis is often suspected. Sigmoidoscopy, however, will reveal the presence of proctocolitis in up to 80% of the cases. Patients with either ulcerative colitis or Crohn's disease may be affected, and this may pose a diagnostic problem, which is resolved by the isolation of *Campylobacter jejuni* from stool, as well as by the patient's response to therapy and long-term follow-up. Most patients require no specific therapy apart from fluid and electrolyte support, but erythromycin is the most frequently recommended antibiotic. Radiologic features range from none to a picture of toxic dilatation. A barium enema in a patient with moderate disease may reveal ulceration with a widespread distribution, as occurs in ulcerative colitis, but with discrete small ulcers, as seen in Crohn's disease.[64]

Pseudomembranous enterocolitis

Pseudomembranous enterocolitis[65-75] is a disease that involves both the small and large bowel. It derives its name from the fact that a pseudomembrane forms, which is composed of necrotic debris that adheres to the superficially ulcerated mucosa. Of the many causes, the one most frequently implicated is an antibiotic-induced change in the intestinal flora.[69] Penicillin,[71] lincomycin,[65] streptomycin,[68] chlortetracycline, and chloramphenicol[74] have all been known to alter the normal *Escherichia coli* and *Bacteroides* flora of the intestine. The consequence may be an overgrowth of pathogenic organisms. Until the past decade, the most common offending organism was thought to be *Staphylococcus aureus*,[68,71] but now mixed gram-positive and gram-negative rods have also been reported, as well as *Proteus* infections.[65,68] However, in 1978 Bartlett identified *Clostridium difficile* as the source of the cytotoxin that had been isolated a year earlier in the stool of patients with antibiotic-associated pseudomembranous colitis. It is now clear that this organism is the major cause of antibiotic-associated colitis and diarrhea.[72,73]

The carrier state is rare in outpatients, but not uncommon in hospital patients. In one study, stool cultures were positive for *Clostridium difficile* on admission in 7% of the patients, and a further 21% acquired infection in the hospital, although diarrhea developed in only one third of these.[73] The organism produces two cytotoxins, and diagnosis is made more often, and more reliably, by a stool cytotoxin assay than by culture of the organism.

An attack of pseudomembranous enterocolitis is usually heralded by the onset of diarrhea, with or without blood, typically during the first week of antibiotic therapy.[72] Abdominal cramps and tenderness, and sometimes signs of peritonitis,[68,71] are associated with the diarrhea. Hypoproteinemia with peripheral edema and ascites has also been reported.[71]

Proctoscopic examination discloses a friable and erythematous mucosa with a yellow-green exudate or patchy, adherent, elevated yellow mucosal plaques, which may become a confluent purulent pseudomembrane.[65,68,71]

In the gross specimen of a bowel affected by pseudomembranous colitis, the bowel wall is markedly thickened, a yellow-green patchy or confluent pseudomembrane has formed, and the mucosa is ulcerated.[71] Shallow mucosal ulcerations are present, although occasionally ulceration may extend into the submucosa. Goblet cell hypertrophy of the mucosa may be seen. The lamina propria and submucosal area are edematous and filled with a cellular infiltrate. These histologic changes are nonspecific, however, and may be seen in many other forms of enteritis, such as typhoid fever, bacillary dysentery, septicemia, and uremia.

Radiologic findings

Plain radiographs of the abdomen are usually first obtained in patients with a sudden onset of severe diarrhea. An adynamic ileus pattern with distention of the small and large bowel may be seen at this time.[68] The ileus may be caused by associated peritonitis, by electrolyte disturbances caused by the severe diarrhea, or possibly by the release of enterotoxin from the offending bacteria. Frequently, the colon is greatly distended and its contour is irregular. Thumbprint-like indentations in the gas-filled transverse colon may simulate the appearance of the toxic megacolon typical of chronic ulcerative colitis[67,68] and ischemic colitis. Indeed, in the adult inpatients of many hospitals, particularly in those hospitals with a large number of immunocompromised patients taking antibiotics, pseudomembranous colitis is now the most common cause of a toxic dilatation pattern on plain films, with thickened haustra or thumbprinting. In the presence of severe advanced colitis, air in the bowel wall may be seen.[68]

If plain x-ray is abnormal, extreme caution should be exercised before a barium enema study is performed. A markedly dilated colon with an irregular contour in a febrile patient with bloody diarrhea contraindicates a barium enema examination because the high pressure involved could cause perforation of the necrotic megacolon. Once the acute colonic dilatation somewhat resolves, however, and there is a change in symptoms for the better, a barium enema examination may be performed with caution under low pressure, although flexible sigmoidoscopy is more commonly employed for this purpose and is more useful. Extensive vascular involvement with occlusion of small vessels and lymphatics has been reported in cases of pseudomembranous colitis, and may be reversible.[68] An irregular, ragged, polypoid contour to the colon wall is seen on barium enema studies.[65] The pseudomembrane itself often covers a vast area of the mucosa and accounts for the irregular appearance on these studies[65] (Fig. 46-17). Ulcerations, although present, are usually shallow and are often covered by a pseudomembrane. These findings are similar, both histologically and radiographically, to those exhibited by isch-

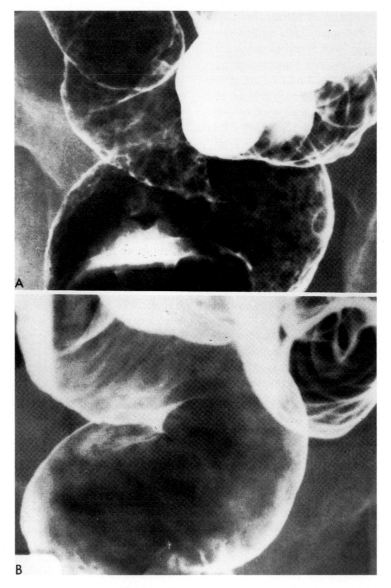

Fig. 46-17 Pseudomembranous colitis in a 66-year-old man that was due to infection with *Clostridium difficile*. **A,** Mucosal plaques produce filling defects varying in shape from oval to square. **B,** After treatment with vancomycin for 2 weeks, the rectal mucosa has returned to normal. From *Radiol Clin North Am* Dec 1982.

emic colitis. In milder cases, the pseudomembranes are more discrete and may be seen on barium enema studies as small nodules, which disappear after therapy.

The small bowel may also be involved,[70,71] and this is indicated by the presence of edema in the valvulae conniventes and the bowel wall, with accompanying thickening and separation of the loops. Ulceration and complete loss of the fold pattern may be seen in more severely affected areas.

In many cases, the diarrhea stops if the antibiotics are discontinued promptly. However, because of the significant morbidity and mortality from the disease, it is customary to initiate treatment. The initial drug of choice, vancomy-

cin, is effective but very expensive. Metronidazole is equally effective, one tenth the price of vancomycin, and has a similar relapse rate of around 16%.[75]

Pseudomembranous enterocolitis may resolve completely, or cause the formation of a smooth atrophic-appearing colon without haustra, which simulates inactive chronic ulcerative colitis.[67] Stenosis and strictures of both the large and small bowel may also arise.

Differential diagnosis

Many other diseases may produce a radiographic picture similar to the one encountered in pseudomembranous colitis. Ulcerative colitis, both in its active and healed phases, may resemble pseudomembranous enterocolitis on both plain radiographs (toxic megacolon) and barium enema examination,[70] though the distribution of pseudomembranous enterocolitis may be more patchy than that of ulcerative colitis. Identifiable pseudopolyps, as seen in some cases of ulcerative colitis, rarely occur in pseudomembranous enterocolitis. However, any form of ulcerating colitis may take on a radiographic appearance similar to that of pseudomembranous enterocolitis. These possibilities include Crohn's disease, amebiasis, *Salmonella-Shigella* colitis, and particularly ischemic colitis. When the small bowel is involved, ischemia, radiation enteritis, regional enteritis, periarteritis nodosa, and lymphoma should be considered in the differential diagnoses.

Acute gastroenteritis

Acute nonspecific gastroenteritis[76-78] is the most frequent gastrointestinal disease, and yet one in which a cause is rarely proved. So-called traveler's diarrhea, acute epidemic gastroenteritis, or "mal de turista" may be caused by *Shigella*, *Giardia*, or *Entamoeba histolytica*, but 70% of all cases are due to enterotoxigenic *E. coli*.[76,77] The disease is a self-limiting pathophysiologic process and is characterized by altered water and electrolyte absorption, increased intestinal motility, or, in some instances, ileus of the small and large bowel.

The radiographic findings in patients with acute gastroenteritis are nearly always confined to the plain radiographs of the abdomen. Air-fluid levels may be seen in dilated loops of the small and large bowel (Fig. 46-18). Dilatation and fluid may become so prominent as to simulate a mechanical obstruction of the large bowel. The outpouring of large amounts of water and electrolytes into the small bowel results in dilatation, air-fluid levels, and increased but often incoordinated motor activity. Electrolyte loss may also produce an adynamic ileus pattern. Air-fluid levels in a distended large and small bowel, coupled with a history of diarrhea of acute onset, permit differentiation from mechanical obstruction.

On those rare occasions when barium meal studies or a barium enema examination is performed in patients with acute diarrhea, no specific radiographic findings are noted. The small bowel is found to be dilated, but the mucosal pattern is normal. A fluoroscopic examination may disclose increased motility, which causes rapid changes in the location and extent of the air-fluid levels. When ileus is pronounced, little activity is noted. On a barium enema examination, mucosal edema is best demonstrated on a postevacuation radiograph but is of no diagnostic value because such changes may occur in acute diarrhea from any cause, such as food poisoning, bacillary dysentery, cholera, and ulcerative and amebic colitis.

Antibiotic prophylaxis will inevitably spawn an increase in the incidence of resistant strains of *E. coli* and is therefore an antisocial practice, except in those individuals for whom even a mild attack would be disastrous.[77] Bismuth subsalicylate at a dose of 524 mg a day can reduce the attack rate by 65%,[78] and doxycycline and Cotrimoxazole

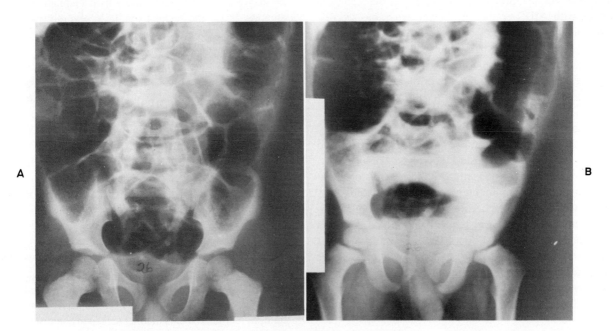

Fig. 46-18 Acute gastroenteritis in a child who suffered the sudden onset of diarrhea and abdominal cramps with only one episode of vomiting. Although acute gastroenteritis was epidemic in the community at the time, no specific etiologic agent was isolated in this child. Note the dilatation (**A**) and the air-filled levels (**B**) in the small and large bowel.

(sulfamethoxazole), among other antibiotics, can shorten the duration of the illness from as much as 5 days down to 1 or 2 days if taken at the first sign of diarrhea.[77]

Helicobacter pylori

Because of its relationship to peptic ulceration, *Helicobacter pylori* is discussed in Chapters 16 and 24. Suffice it to say here that the discovery that duodenal ulcer disease, and much gastric ulceration, is an infectious disease is one of the more remarkable developments of the past decade and carries implications that have not yet been fully implemented into medical therapeutics.[79-81]

CHLAMYDIAL INFECTIONS

Lymphogranuloma venereum

Lymphogranuloma venereum (LGV),[82-92] also known as *lymphopathia venereum,* is a venereal disease that is especially common in the tropics.[82-84] The disease has been reported for all races and in most countries, and those most at risk of acquiring it are prostitutes, people practicing unprotected anal intercourse, and those who engage in sexual intercourse with multiple partners. It is frequently found in the inhabitants of seaports of Africa, South India, Indonesia, the southern United States (for example, New Orleans), Latin America, Jamaica, and other Caribbean islands. In some areas it has assumed epidemic proportions and constitutes an important public health problem. The disease must be considered in the differential diagnosis of any inflammatory process or stricture involving the rectosigmoid colon. The various infections that can affect the rectum in patients with AIDS or the gay bowel syndrome are discussed in Chapter 47.

LGV is caused by a species of the genus *Chlamydia,* long considered to be viruses and previously designated *Bedsonia.* These obligate intracellular organisms measure 300 μm in their infectious stage and are now morphologically classified as bacteria, occupying a position between the rickettsiae and viruses. LGV is acquired almost exclusively through sexual contact. The organisms can be recovered from the primary genital lesions, involved lymph nodes, and the inflammatory lesions of the rectosigmoid colon and pelvic soft tissues. The initial herpetiform lesion develops about 2 weeks after infection, and is usually a tiny, painless papule, vesicle, or ulcer which is located on the penis in men and on the vulva, posterior vaginal wall, or cervix in women, where it usually escapes detection. Because *Chlamydia trachomatis* is markedly lymphotropic, the regional lymph nodes are rapidly invaded, producing an acute purulent lymphadenitis (bubo formation) 4 to 8 weeks after infection.

In men the secondary stage of the disease develops insidiously and pursues a chronic indolent course in which the inguinal lymph nodes become enlarged, matted together, and fluctuant, with draining sinuses. In women there are usually no localizing symptoms until the pelvic lymph nodes (especially the anorectal group) are invaded, with subsequent involvement of the rectum and discharge of blood and pus in the stools.[82,87] The difference in the lymphatic drainage between the two sexes is responsible for the much greater involvement of the rectosigmoid colon in women and its relative rarity among men, except when the organism has been implanted directly into the rectum.

The pathologic changes that take place in the rectum stem from the invasion and blockage of the rectal lymphatics by *Chlamydia.* There is subsequent lymphangitis, lymphatic stasis, rectal edema, cellular infiltration into the submucosa and muscularis, endarteritis and phlebitis, and eventually mucosal destruction.[85,87] The sequence of pelvic lymphadenitis, lymphatic stasis, and secondary infection leads to ulcerative proctocolitis, elephantiasis of the genitalia, and the formation of perirectal fistulas and abscesses. Examination of rectal biopsy specimens may reveal the presence of granulomas in the rectal wall. Later in the disease, fibrosis leads to the development of rectal or rectosigmoid strictures. In women, involvement of the rectovaginal septum often causes a large rectovaginal fistula to form in the center of the posterior vaginal wall above the anorectal ring and distal to the stricture.[82-84]

The third stage of LGV is most striking in women and is characterized by chronic proctitis and extensive fibrosis with the development of a rectosigmoid stricture. Rectal pain, tenesmus, constipation, and narrow stools are then the dominant clinical features. A rectovaginal fistula with the passage of feces through the vagina frequently develops, as may a perianal abscess and vulvar elephantiasis. In this stenotic phase the rectal ampulla is severely narrowed by scarring, and proctoscopy often shows a friable, bleeding, ulcerated mucosa overlying the stricture. The perianal skin is thickened and edematous, and there may be a characteristic lymphorrhoid present. The lower edge of the stricture can usually be palpated 2.5 to 5 cm from the anal orifice but is never farther than 12.5 cm from the anus. The stricture varies in diameter, from a slight narrowing to an almost complete stenosis of the rectal lumen.

The diagnosis of LGV may be confirmed by the complement fixation test, by the Frei intradermal test, or by the recovery of *Chlamydia* organisms from the blood, feces, or buboes.

Radiologic findings

The radiographic features of LGV have been well documented by several investigators,[82-86,88-91] especially Annamunthodo and Marryatt[82,83] in their review of 144 black patients from Jamaica, 90% of whom were female. These authors recognized two distinct stages of the disease, in that 34 of their cases had generalized proctocolitis and 113 chronic cases had anorectal stricture. Thus the findings encountered in barium enema examinations depend largely on the phase and activity of the disease.

In the prestenotic phase the rectal ampulla is narrowed and spasm is present, with accompanying loss of the normal haustral and mucosal pattern in the rectum and occasionally in the sigmoid colon.[82,85] The contour of the narrowed rectum is irregular and ulcerated (Fig. 46-19). Fistulous tracts and perirectal abscesses may be present, as well as widening of the presacral space, with anterior displacement of the rectosigmoid colon[85,90] (Fig. 46-20). The fistulas may extend to the buttocks and occasionally upward to involve the parametrium, peritoneum, sigmoid colon, and rarely the small bowel.[89]

As the disease progresses to fibrosis, strictures of varied lengths may develop.[82] The strictures of LGV are usually long and tubular with a tapering proximal (and sometimes distal) edge (Fig. 46-21). They may involve the anorectal area, the entire rectum and sigmoid colon, or occasionally areas higher in the colon. Strictures as long as 25 cm have been noted.[85] Many are palpable within 3 to 5 cm of the

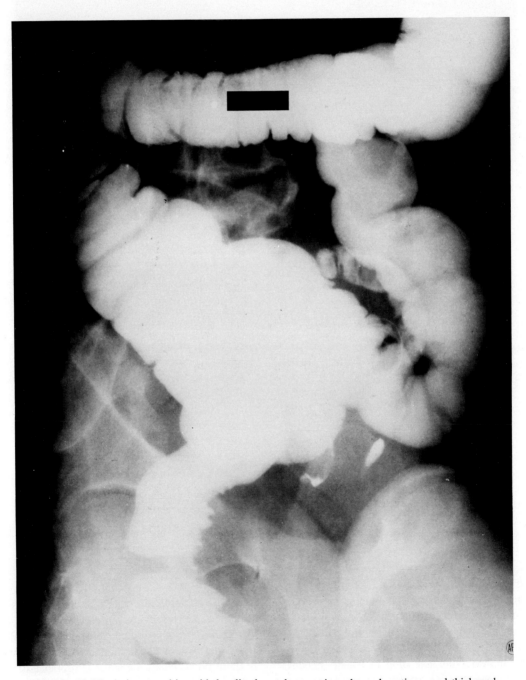

Fig. 46-19 Ulcerative proctitis, with localized rectal narrowing, deep ulcerations, and thickened rectal valves caused by lymphogranuloma venereum.

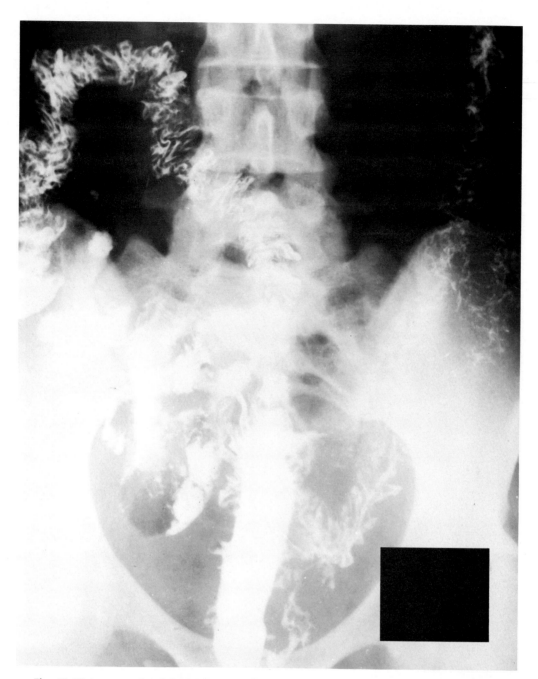

Fig. 46-20 A narrowed and rigid rectosigmoid colon resulting from lymphogranuloma venereum. The rectosigmoid junction is straightened because of a large perirectal abscess. Multiple deep and shallow perirectal sinuses extend laterally and downward to the perineum.
From Reeder MM, Palmer PES: *The radiology of tropical diseases,* Baltimore, 1981, Williams & Wilkins.

anus and are readily identified on a barium enema examination. Distal rectal strictures arising just above the anorectal junction may extend to narrow the entire rectal ampulla[87] (Fig. 46-22).

The strictures of the rectum and colon are usually in continuity with each other but occasionally skip areas with apparently normal colon intervening, similar to the strictures seen in Crohn's disease and tuberculous colitis.[82] The rectal lumen may be severely narrowed and take on a string-like or filiform appearance, resulting in obstruction. Dilatation and loss of haustration of the bowel proximal to a stricture often impart a conical appearance to the rectosigmoid colon.

The contour of the narrowed rectosigmoid colon may be

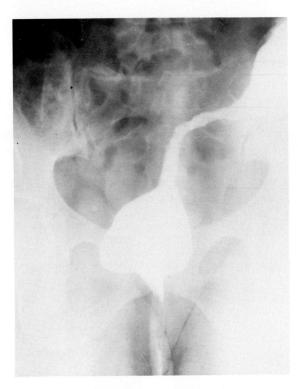

Fig. 46-21 A woman with a rectosigmoid stricture caused by lymphogranuloma venereum. Note the sparing of the distal rectum and the ulcerated appearance of the stricture. Both the proximal and distal margins taper smoothly. Dilatation and loss of haustration above the stricture impart a conical appearance to the cecum.

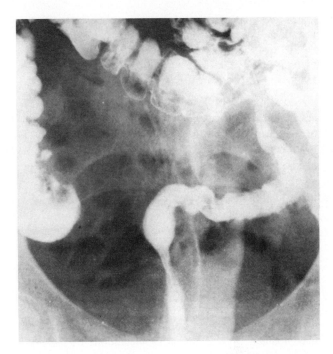

Fig. 46-22 Lymphogranuloma in a South African man. There is marked narrowing of the entire rectum and an irregular ulcerated contour to the moderately narrowed and shortened sigmoid colon. The rectal wall is considerably thickened, rigid, and fibrotic. From Reeder MM, Palmer PES: *The radiology of tropical diseases,* Baltimore, 1981, Williams & Wilkins.

smooth but frequently is irregular because of mucosal ulceration and the occasional formation of fistulous tracts.[85] In Annamunthodo and Marryatt's series,[82,83] the major complications encountered were rectovaginal fistulas (34 patients), perianal sinuses, fistulas and abscesses (26 patients), and elephantiasis of the vulva (9 patients). Short or long perirectal sinuses may extend outward at right angles or downward from the rectum to the perineum, always at or below the site of the stricture. These fistulous tracts may extend into large perirectal abscesses, reenter the bowel, or connect with the vagina, perineum, or anterior surface of the abdomen. Lateral and oblique radiographs of the rectum are most helpful in demonstrating rectovaginal fistulas and retrorectal sinuses.[12]

Differential diagnosis

When a rectal stricture is disclosed radiographically, many inflammatory diseases of the colon must be considered, such as idiopathic chronic ulcerative colitis and, especially, the granulomatous diseases such as Crohn's disease, tuberculosis, schistosomiasis, amebiasis, and actinomycosis, because they may all produce radiographic findings similar to those of LGV.[12] In many of these diseases,

rectal biopsy specimens may exhibit granulomas similar to those seen in LGV.

Amebiasis and tuberculosis can cause proctocolitis, rectal narrowing, and perianal fistulas. Actinomycosis, although rare, can cause the formation of fistulous tracts. All can occasionally mimic LGV. Schistosomiasis may cause diffuse irregular narrowing and ulceration of the rectosigmoid colon, sometimes in conjunction with a large pelvic abscess. However, fistulous tracts, which are so common in LGV, do not form in schistosomiasis. Conversely, colonic granulomatous polyps may be seen in schistosomiasis, especially in cases encountered in Africa and the Orient, but they do not occur in LGV.

Posttraumatic strictures, caused by foreign bodies or by the sclerosing agents used in hemorrhoid treatment, may be smooth and radiographically may resemble those of LGV; however, they seldom cause fistulas or ulceration. Colitis cystica profunda may cause nodular rectal lesions, but the rectal narrowing does not extend into the sigmoid colon in this instance; sigmoidoscopy and rectal biopsy findings can easily differentiate between the two diseases. A perirectal abscess or tumor may cause rectal narrowing, but in these instances the mucosa overlying the narrow rectal wall is usually not ulcerated.

A scirrhous infiltrating type of carcinoma can also produce a lengthy rectal stricture, but the mucosa is usually not ulcerated as it so often is in LGV, and sinus tracts and fistulas do not often develop in cancer.

FUNGAL INFECTIONS
Gastrointestinal candidiasis

Gastrointestinal candidiasis,[93-101] or moniliasis, is caused by the fungus *Candida albicans.* This commensal organism is found in the mouth and upper respiratory and gastrointestinal tracts of many normal persons. It may become pathogenic but only in the presence of underlying debilitating states, such as those brought about by prolonged antibiotic therapy[101,102] that alters the nature of the gastrointestinal flora, by AIDS, malignancy, or chemotherapy for a neoplastic disease (immunosuppressive agents, steroids, and antimetabolites). Blood dyscrasias, such as sickle cell disease[100] and especially leukemia,[94] advanced tuberculosis or diabetes, drug addiction, and malnutrition (either dietary or resulting from abnormal intestinal absorption) are other underlying causes. Candidal infections of the gastrointestinal tract are frequently accompanied by oral thrush or ulcerations of the buccal mucosa, but this relationship is not absolute.[99] Although all sites in the gastrointestinal tract may be invaded by *C. albicans,* the oral cavity, pharynx, and esophagus are the most commonly involved. Dysphagia is therefore the most common presenting symptom.

In children, vomiting and dehydration resulting from esophagitis is common and may lead to aspiration and pulmonary infection.[102] Plaquelike white patches on the gums and pharyngeal mucosa indicate oral involvement.

In the esophagus the lesions are ulcerative or membranous and can extend deep into the muscular coat. Both yeast and pseudohyphal fungal colonies arise. The yeast form produces surface granulomas and membranes, whereas the hyphal form penetrates into the esophageal layers and causes deep microabscesses and ulcers to form. Similar changes take place in other affected mucosal surfaces. Esophagoscopy may reveal an erythematous and ulcerated esophageal mucosa, sometimes with a visible pseudomembrane. When these plaques or membranes are removed, they leave a raw, granulating base.

The diagnosis of candidal gastrointestinal lesions is difficult. Identification of mycelia in the feces is an important finding, and they are thought to represent evidence of invasion of the mucosa rather than of simple saprophytic activity, as may be the case when only yeast cells are found in the feces.[102] The ultimate diagnosis is established by the demonstration of mycelia in material obtained from the gastrointestinal ulcerations or on histologic sections. Gram's and periodic acid–Schiff staining are necessary to show the fungi in the caseating foci or abscesses. Invasion of the gastrointestinal tract by *Candida* organisms may be followed by septicemia.[101] Ulcerating gastrointestinal lesions provide a portal of entry for *Candida* organisms into the intestinal venules and thus into the circulation. Specific antibody ti-

tes have been found in the blood and are of diagnostic value.[101]

Radiologic findings

Radiographic abnormalities resulting from *C. albicans* are most frequently seen in the esophagus.[98] A long segment, particularly in the lower half of the esophagus, is often involved, although short plaquelike lesions also appear. The esophageal lumen may be wide and remain distended because of the involvement of deeper layers. The tone is partially lost, and both primary and secondary peristalsis are sluggish because of the muscular involvement. On the

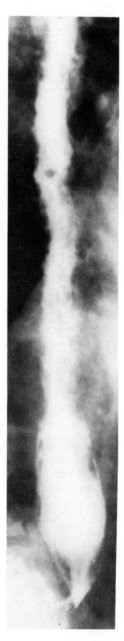

Fig. 46-23 An irregular, shaggy, esophageal contour, the result of ulcerating candidal esophagitis.

other hand, esophageal spasm as well as atony have been noted in the presence of candidal esophagitis.[12,100]

Because of the granulomas and ulceration, the mucous membrane seen on barium studies is irregular, ragged, and shaggy, like a carpet (Fig. 46-23). This appearance is produced by mucosal ulceration and by a pseudomembrane that covers areas of ulceration.[12,95,96] The pseudohyphae trap the barium and retain it for a long period, whereas normally the mucosal coating is lost soon after the bolus travels down the esophagus. In milder cases, multiple small smooth nodules are seen; these are caused by edema and a cellular infiltrate accompanied by granuloma formation, but without ulceration of the esophagus[95] (Fig. 46-24). The radiographic findings reverse rapidly when antibiotics and steroids are stopped and antifungal drugs are administered.

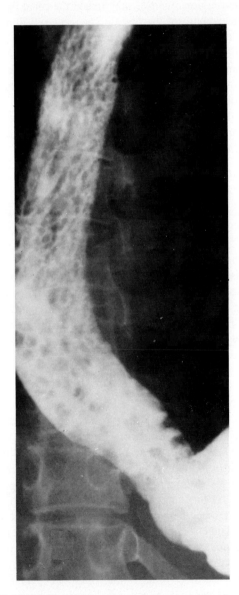

Fig. 46-24 Small nodular contour defects resulting from a candidal invasion without ulceration (cobblestone esophagus). From Goldberg HI, Dodds WJ: *AJR* 104:608, 1968.

C. albicans esophagitis must be differentiated from esophagitis stemming from other causes, such as that due to caustic agents and reflux esophagitis. A history of the ingestion of caustic agents or of long-standing heartburn is helpful in the differentiation. Reflux esophagitis is usually not as extensive, and the ulcerations are not as prominent as they are in candidal esophagitis. When herpes simplex involves the esophagus it may mimic a candidal infection, especially when severe. In mild cases, when there are discrete ulcers on otherwise normal mucosa, the differentiation from the nodules and plaques of mild candidiasis is easy. In more severe disease, in which there is edema, thickened folds, ulcerations, and extensive necrotic debris, the distinction may be impossible radiologically. At times, esophageal varices may be confused with candidal esophagitis, but the contour irregularity is smooth and not ragged, and varices will be most prominent in the lower third of the esophagus.

Upper gastrointestinal candidal infection most frequently afflicts very ill infants or the aged.[12,102] Both groups of patients pose technical difficulties radiologically, and it may be impossible to obtain the mucosal studies that are required for diagnosis. Candidiasis in the stomach and small bowel is thus usually revealed only at autopsy, without signs having been observed radiographically. In one large series,[93] no specific gastrointestinal radiographic abnormality below the esophagus was reported.

When seen, changes in the stomach and small bowel result from extensive ulceration and invasion by the fungus. Peristalsis is sluggish. The main mucosal folds are partly preserved, but the minor folds are effaced, with prolonged retention of the barium in a shaggy, carpetlike pseudomembrane covering the mucosal lining. This secondary pseudomembranous formation may result in a ragged, irregular-appearing ulcer with associated edema. The pseudomembrane may be proliferative and contain many mycelia that produce irregular intraluminal filling defects (Fig. 46-25). A repeat gastrointestinal study after treatment shows the restoration of peristalsis and normal mucosa and no retention of contrast on the mucosa, a process that takes several weeks.

There are no specific changes in the small intestine attributable to candidiasis, but an irritable colon pattern may be observed in the large bowel.[12]

Gastrointestinal histoplasmosis

Gastrointestinal involvement by the fungus *Histoplasma capsulatum*[103-110] produces clinical and radiographic findings similar to those of tuberculosis. As in tuberculosis, the lung is the main portal of entry and the site of primary infection.[108] Occasionally, a primary intestinal infection has been reported.[103] More often, however, there is radiographic evidence of pulmonary histoplasmosis in patients with gastrointestinal involvement.[108,110]

The swallowing of organism-laden sputum results in mu-

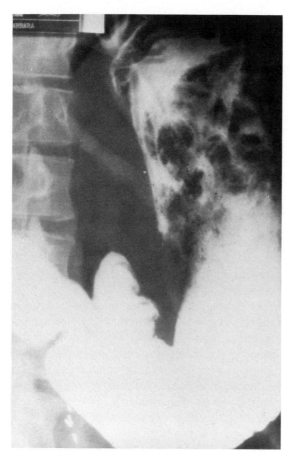

Fig. 46-25 Amorphous, irregular, filling defects that persisted in their location and appearance—the result of a massive candidal invasion that included ulceration and pseudomembranous formation.
Courtesy of Dr. Harold Jacobson.

cosal involvement, whereas hematogenous spread brings about involvement of the submucosa of the bowel.[110] Dissemination to the gastrointestinal tract produces symptoms in only 20% of the patients, and these include weight loss, anorexia, abdominal pain, and watery diarrhea with involvement of the colon. Gastrointestinal hemorrhage with perforation, peritonitis, and intestinal obstruction have also constituted initial manifestations.[108]

Histoplasmosis has been encountered in nearly all areas of the gastrointestinal tract. Ulcerating granulomatous lesions of the pharynx[110] and anus have been noted, as have lesions in more common sites of the disease, such as the ileum, cecum, jejunum, and colon.[104-108] The esophagus may be involved after spread from involved mediastinal lymph nodes.

Radiologic findings

Plain radiographs of the abdomen in patients with gastrointestinal histoplasmosis may frequently depict small,

round, calcified granulomas in the spleen. Because of the frequent involvement of the reticuloendothelial system by histoplasmosis, hepatosplenomegaly may also exist.[110]

Gastrointestinal histoplasmosis involves lymphoid aggregates in the submucosa and causes a granulomatous infiltrate with transmural involvement. A radiographic pattern is produced, similar to that of tuberculosis, and takes three different forms:

1. The mucosal pattern may be distorted by either small nodules or ulcerations resulting from the underlying granulomatous reaction[104,107-109] (Fig. 46-26). The ulcers are generally shallow and difficult to see radiographically.
2. A mass in the area of the terminal ileum and cecum, which results from the involvement of Peyer's patches and regional nodes, may indent the cecal tip.[104] In a later phase of the disease, scarring and fibrosis may cause stricture and deformity.[104,108]
3. Generalized widening of the mucosal folds of the small bowel by edema stemming from the protein-losing enteropathy, with underlying intestinal histoplasmosis, has been reported.[103]

The differential diagnosis is identical to that of tuberculosis, and consists of Crohn's disease, tuberculosis, periappendiceal abscess, carcinoma, and lymphoma.

UNKNOWN ETIOLOGY
Tropical sprue

Depending largely on the geographic area in which the patient lives, or comes from, there are two varieties of sprue.[111-121] There is little to distinguish the nontropical from the tropical variety, and it is not possible for the radiologist to differentiate among the various causes that may produce the spruelike syndrome. Both varieties of sprue are usually classified under the heading of "idiopathic steatorrhea." However, abnormalities of the pancreas or of biliary flow, or changes in the bowel wall or mesentery due to amyloidosis, scleroderma, mesenteric thrombosis, and the effects of various poisons such as arsenic and some antibiotics, can all produce the radiologic appearance of sprue. Many intestinal parasites, particularly *Giardia, Ancylostoma, Capillaria,* and *Strongyloides,* produce similar pictures, and there has been much debate whether the parasites are the cause or the result of the intestinal disturbance.

Malabsorption through the small bowel can therefore occur in many different diseases. The clinical symptoms are similar and the radiologic findings almost identical. The main difference between nontropical and tropical sprue is that the latter is almost always megaloblastic and responds to antibiotic and vitamin therapy; nontropical sprue is difficult to treat and seldom is associated with a megaloblastic bone marrow. Most authorities believe that tropical sprue is at least in large part infectious in etiology, although the organism has not yet been isolated. Both varieties of sprue result in malabsorption, alteration of the bacterial

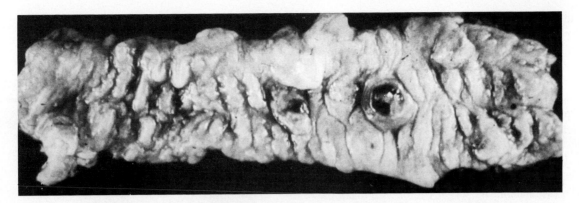

Fig. 46-26 Section of colon from a child with disseminated histoplasmosis, showing thickened indurated mucosal folds. The nodular lesions resulted from microabscesses in the colon wall, which were filled with fungi and had become necrotic and ulcerated.
From Silverman FN et al: *Am J Med* 19:410, 1955.

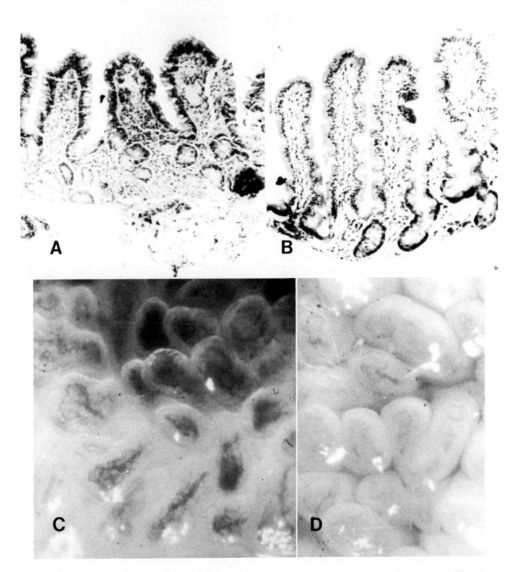

Fig. 46-27 Tropical sprue. A jejunal biopsy specimen before **(A)** and after **(B)** therapy. The endoscopic view before **(C)** and after **(D)** therapy.
From Reeder MM, Palmer PES: *The radiology of tropical diseases,* Baltimore, 1981, Williams & Wilkins.

flora of the gut, and dysfunction of normal bowel movement. However, correlation of the pathologic with the radiologic findings is not consistent. In some patients there are remarkably few histologic abnormalities, whereas in others there is edema of the bowel wall, atrophy of the villi or other layers of the mucosa, and degeneration of the intramural plexus. In tropical sprue there is almost always a chronic inflammatory reaction in the lamina propria accompanied by a varying degree of edema; this may be followed by atrophy. Eventually, all layers of the small bowel may become atrophic and thin, and the full length of the gastrointestinal tract, including the tongue (filiform papillae), may be affected. In both varieties of sprue, there may be some regeneration, but this is most marked in tropical sprue, in that there is often a dramatic response to antibiotic therapy plus folate and vitamin B_{12} replacement (Fig. 46-27).

Clinically, the disease may be very mild and almost asymptomatic, or it may become severe and exhibit all the complications of malabsorption. Diarrhea is almost always present, accompanied by fatigue and lassitude. Remissions and exacerbations are frequent, with patients experiencing progressive ill health, steatorrhea, and eventually abdominal pain, with the explosive defecation of bulky, foul-smelling stools. Bleeding may occur, and evidence of vitamin deficiency, particularly of the vitamin B complex, becomes evident in the skin, tongue, mouth, and eyes. There may be a peripheral neuropathy. The severity of the illness and the enteric disturbance may lead to loss of appetite with dehydration, which can progress to cardiac and adrenal failure.

Radiologic findings

The radiologic evidence of sprue depends on the duration and severity of the disease. In mild or moderate cases, plain films of the abdomen depict normal findings. As the disease becomes more severe, there may be evidence of mild ileus with air-fluid levels scattered throughout the abdomen on the erect film.

Barium studies must be carried out using modern non-flocculating barium, and the diagnosis of a "sprue" pattern is invalid unless this type of barium is used. Abnormalities have been reported in the esophagus, stomach, and occasionally the large bowel, but these findings are minimal and play no part in the diagnosis.

There are four radiologic groups of findings, related to alterations in peristalsis, caliber, secretions, and mucosa.

Variable peristalsis is the hallmark, with segments of bowel that are hypotonic and others exhibiting rapid peristalsis. Overall, this leads to segmentation of the barium and an increased transit time. The variable peristalsis occasionally leads to intussusception, which may be transient as the part of the bowel that is moving actively proceeds into an inactive segment.

Dilatation of some segments is seen in 80% of the patients; it is usually persistent and involves a lengthy seg-

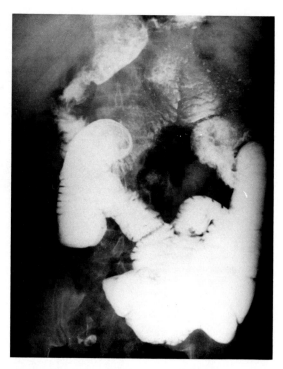

Fig. 46-28 Tropical sprue. There is generalized dilatation of the proximal small bowel loops as well as smudging and dilution of barium in the left upper quadrant caused by the collection of excess fluid in several loops of the proximal jejunum. The moulage sign appears when the barium reaches these dilated, fluid-filled, hypotonic segments. Note the normal-sized, but widely spaced and therefore sparser, folds in the jejunum.
From Reeder MM, Palmer PES: *The radiology of tropical diseases,* Baltimore, 1981, Williams & Wilkins.

ment of bowel, especially in the midsmall bowel. It is associated with stagnation (Fig. 46-28).

An increased content of poorly saturated fatty acids and mucin causes dilution and, if severe, may overcome the ability of the barium to remain in even suspension. This leads to coarse clumping of the barium that fragments into various sections, with associated stasis (Fig. 46-29).

The mucosa is often edematous, and this causes the valvulae conniventes to thicken and assume a characteristic cogwheel pattern (Fig. 46-30), instead of their normal feathery pattern. Later, atrophy may occur and the mucosal folds disappear altogether. This may be associated with considerable thinning of the bowel wall and lessened intervals between the bowel loops, which may heighten the risk of perforation during a peroral capsule biopsy. Endoscopic biopsy, which involves obtaining smaller specimens limited to the mucosa, is preferred in such patients and has, in any event, largely superseded capsule biopsy.

There is some inconstancy of these various findings, with variation in the appearance during the course of an examination (Fig. 46-31) that is rather characteristic of the disease. After successful treatment, radiologic documentation

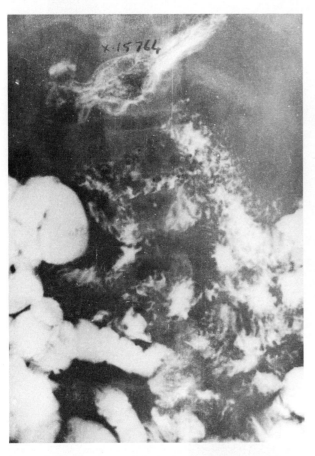

Fig. 46-29 Segmentation of the barium column is noted in a patient from India who had tropical sprue. Scattered boli of barium remain in the same loops for a long time. There is also coarse clumping and fragmentation of the barium within affected loops. From Reeder MM, Palmer PES: *The radiology of tropical diseases*, Baltimore, 1981, Williams & Wilkins.

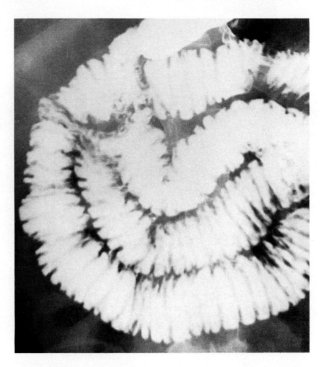

Fig. 46-30 Tropical sprue. Thickening of the valvulae conniventes (primary and secondary mucosal folds, valves of Kerckring) produces a cogwheel appearance in the mucosa of the proximal small bowel. There is also an increase in the caliber of these loops due to loss of tone and slowed peristalsis. From Reeder MM, Palmer PES: *The radiology of tropical diseases*, Baltimore, 1981, Williams & Wilkins.

of improvement tends to lag behind the histologically confirmed healing by up to several months.

PARASITIC DISEASES
Parasitic infections[122-129]

Parasites vary as widely as the human primates and other animals they inhabit. They are not a new problem. Alimentary worms were a recognized condition in ancient Egypt (recorded in the Ebers Papyrus about 1500 BC), and it is probable that the biblical description of the plague of fiery serpents (in the book of Numbers) refers to guinea worms. In fact, we have not improved upon the method of extraction recommended then—winding the worm around a piece of stick. The best of the early descriptions of worms was that of Avicenna (980 to 1037 AD), who wrote about the symptoms produced by tapeworms, roundworms, and threadworms and the different ways of treating affected patients. References to roundworms have been found in Greek

texts and in the writings from Mesopotamia, Rome, and China. Yet, despite their ancient lineage, the facts about their life cycle were not unraveled until 1916.

The history of parasitic infections is as diverse as the life cycles and pathologic characteristics of the parasites themselves; whereas echinococcosis (hydatid disease) was well known to Hippocrates and Galen, intestinal capillariasis was discovered only in 1963. It is not only their histories that vary, but their sizes as well: tapeworms may be 30 feet (9 meters) long, but even more harmful parasites can be seen only with a high-power microscope.

War has always been a stimulus for medical research. Strongyloidiasis was first recognized in 1876 in French soldiers who had been stationed in Cochin China (now Vietnam). New knowledge about filariasis, malaria, paragonimiasis, amebiasis, and other parasitic diseases was gained in World War II and during the Korean and Vietnam conflicts. In war or peace, parasites continue to plague mankind and are an enormous source of morbidity, mortality, and economic distress.

Parasites are found worldwide—they are not just confined to the tropics or to the poor. They flourish where sanitation and hygiene are inadequate and may easily be acquired, even by fastidious travelers. Although geography, social status, cultural practices, and education play a large

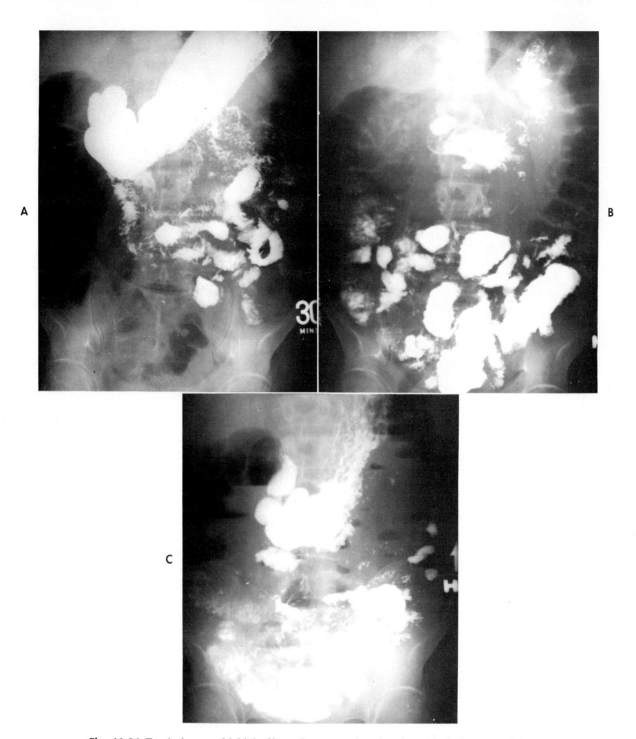

Fig. 46-31 Tropical sprue. Multiple films taken at varying time intervals during a small bowel series in a patient with tropical sprue illustrate the changing patterns that can occur during a single examination. **A,** At 30 minutes, there is no dilatation of the proximal small bowel loops, but the normal feathery mucosal pattern in the duodenum and proximal jejunum is lost, whereas many of the midjejunal loops show sparse or absent valvulae conniventes. There is also some flocculation and segmentation of the barium column. **B,** At 1 hour, there is marked segmentation and the barium is stagnant in multiple hypotonic and dilated loops of the distal jejunum and ileum. Some coarse clumping of barium is also noted, and no normal mucosal folds are seen. **C,** At 1 hour, an erect film of the abdomen shows multiple air-fluid levels in the small bowel and colon. Rather marked early flocculation and segmentation of the barium column are undoubtedly related to the presence of excessive fluid within the bowel, as well as disordered motility. Involvement of the colon, with slightly dilated hypotonic loops of large bowel containing air-fluid levels, is well demonstrated in this patient.

From Reeder MM, Palmer PES: *The radiology of tropical diseases,* Baltimore, 1981, Williams & Wilkins.

part in parasitic epidemiology, outbreaks of giardiasis have occurred in sophisticated ski resorts, and gourmet diners in Japan have been infected with anisakiasis from the consumption of raw fish—a gastronomic taste and therefore risk that is now being acquired throughout the world.

The number of people infected with parasites throughout the world is almost unimaginable, but a few examples will suffice. Perhaps 25% of the world's population harbor roundworms, and in many parts of the tropics the incidence may be well over 90%.[128] In 1968 it was estimated that 10% of the world's population harbored the ameba. In 1978 the estimate was revised to 20%, although perhaps only 5% or 6% of these people suffer invasive and therefore clinical amebiasis.[129] The number of patients with schistosomiasis is difficult to assess, but in 1981 600 million were thought to be infected,[125] although other estimates place the incidence at somewhat over 200 million. Figures for ancylostomiasis (hookworm) suggest that 900 million people, almost one fifth of the world's population, are infected,[128] although this estimate may be high.

There is wide variation in the prevalence of parasitic diseases among countries, particularly in the tropics. Because parasites can be found in the most unlikely patients, whose clinical states may vary from normal health to severe illness, physicians must always be aware of the possibility of parasites in the alimentary tract, even in the seemingly least likely of candidates. Knowledge of where patients have lived or traveled is as important to the diagnosis as laboratory tests and radiologic images. The manifestations of those with chronic infection may differ considerably from the often acute picture typical of a first infection. Parasites and the diseases they cause tend to be unpredictable.

Parasites are not confined to humans, and many wild animals die of their parasitic infections. The king of beasts, the lion, who survives the territorial imperatives and lives to fight another day, will often die ignominiously of worms. Many animals are an essential part of the life cycle of parasites, so that eating infected animals, walking on contaminated ground, and swimming in contaminated water are the most common of the many ways in which parasites enter their hosts.

In many parts of the world and in many immigrants who come to the United States or Europe, multiple parasitism will be the rule rather than the exception. Three or four different infections may lie hidden, and either go unnoticed or even be accepted as normal by the patient. In many cases the parasite will not be the reason the patient seeks a doctor's case, and finding a parasite does not always mean that the cause of the patient's ill health has been discovered. There may well be yet another problem. The opposite is also true, particularly in immigrants and those from poorly developed rural areas. Finding a positive cause for ill health, such as tuberculosis, should not end the search for concomitant parasites in the alimentary tract or elsewhere.[123]

Protozoal infections

AMEBIC DYSENTERY (AMEBIASIS)

Amebiasis[130-137] is an infection caused by a pathogenic protozoan *Entamoeba histolytica*. Many other strains or species of amebas occur in humans, but very few are pathogenic. Even *E. histolytica* can be nonpathogenic until combined with bacteria, in which case some amebas produce strong proteolytic enzymes, and lysis of the intestinal epithelium occurs. Only then does the patient change from being a carrier to having clinical amebiasis. After invasion, significant antibodies can be found.

A person becomes infected by consuming either contaminated food or water, and the disease is usually transmitted by human cyst carriers. In the tropics, transmission may also take place through the consumption of water from polluted wells or food contaminated by human night soil, or from coming into contact with vectors such as cockroaches and flies. Animals do not appear to be a frequent source of human infection. The infection is found throughout the world, even in nontropical countries. It is not a disease of adults only; in West Africa, more than 60% of all victims are under the age of 10 years, and most of these are under the age of 5. Even infants in the first year or two of life can be infected. The diagnosis is established by the finding of amebae in the stools. A single negative examination, even when a careful technique is used, is not sufficient, and a rectal biopsy may be necessary. It is essential that stool specimens be examined while still warm and fresh. Numerous serologic tests are not all completely reliable, but if both immunosorbent assay and immunoelectrophoresis are performed, there will be no false-negative results. Test results can remain positive for up to 2 years after the disease is eradicated and are therefore less reliable as a therapeutic index.

The clinical spectrum is very wide, ranging from relatively good health to severe illness. The patient's history is quite unreliable, and there may be no episode of dysentery. Symptoms usually develop within 8 to 11 days after invasion, but they sometimes take months or even years to appear. There can be acute dysentery with gripping abdominal pain, tenderness, and fever, but there may be alternating constipation and diarrhea or no bowel symptoms whatsoever. The first attack may subside spontaneously or, alternatively, persist for weeks. Recurrent remission and exacerbation occur in the chronic form of amebic dysentery. Because the amebae spread either directly or by embolism, liver abscesses are common and often extend through the diaphragm and pleura to the lungs. Hematogenous spread may be responsible for causing pulmonary or brain abscesses. The skin can be infected, particularly when there is a fistula, and abscesses can form in the perineum, genitourinary tract, and pelvis.

When there is direct extension through the wall of the large bowel, with associated bacterial infection, a large and sometimes hard tumor (an ameboma) may develop in or ad-

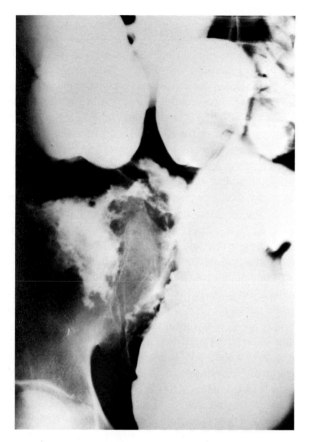

Fig. 46-32 An ameboma adjacent to the cecum possessing a cavity that connects with the bowel lumen.

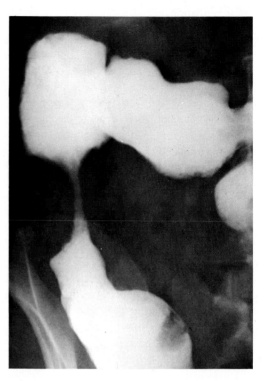

Fig. 46-33 Stricture in the ascending colon with severe alteration in the mucosal pattern of the right half of the colon in a patient with amebiasis.

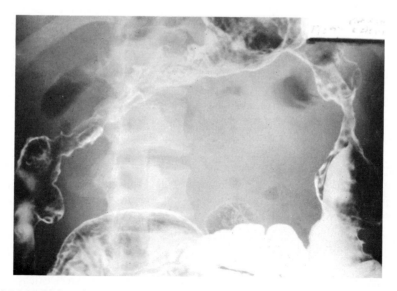

Fig. 46-34 Multiple strictures and complete distortion of the mucosal pattern in the ascending, transverse, and descending colon in a patient with amebiasis.

jacent to the bowel (Fig. 46-32). This is common around the cecum but can occur anywhere in the colon and may strongly resemble a neoplasm with an "apple-core" lesion.[135] Differentiation may not be possible in some patients, but the smooth tapering edge of the lesion and the presence of amebiasis elsewhere in the colon are the most useful indicators. If there is a reasonable doubt of an amebic infection, the patient should be treated for amebiasis before surgery, and the "malignancy" often then changes or even disappears.

The radiologic findings in amebiasis are as numerous and varied as the clinical presentation, and a high index of suspicion is needed.[132] The earliest findings occur around the cecum and ascending colon and are due to the edema and ulceration of the bowel. There is also rigidity and thickening of the bowel wall with an irregular mucosa and multiple tiny ulcers (Figs. 46-33 and 46-34). Normal areas may intervene, as in Crohn's disease, and, if amebiasis is suspected in any part of the bowel, very careful examination of the bowel elsewhere is called for. There can be so much spasm and edema that it is difficult to distend any part of the colon. As the ulcers deepen, the edges become undermined, and the characteristic flask-shaped ulcer can be demonstrated radiologically. At this stage, the outline of the cecum is often hazy and indistinct, perhaps suggesting inadequate bowel preparation before the examination. The cecum eventually becomes less mobile and rather rigid but usually can be distended with a barium enema, which is not possible with a malignancy. The transition from normal to abnormal is very gradual, and, again, this differs from the more abrupt change typical of a neoplasm. Such areas can arise throughout the bowel, and, if the edema is severe, there will be "thumb printing" (Fig. 46-35). The whole colon may be involved, and it may give the appearance of acute ulcerative colitis.[133] Occasionally the terminal ileum becomes infected because it is common for the ileocecal valve to be incompetent, and reflux then takes place. In very severe and often fatal cases, an acute toxic megacolon may be seen. In children the symptoms in general are often more acute: one or more amebic ulcers may perforate and generalized peritonitis may occur. Even in children, an ameboma may cause intussusception and obstruction with transmural peritonitis.[130]

When the disease is chronic, the picture is that of contraction and rigidity with fixed deformity (Fig. 46-36). The cecum often becomes conical and the terminal ileum rigid and tubular. Multiple fistulas with surrounding abscesses can form, and late in the disease the bowel wall may be quite smooth, as ultimately occurs in ulcerative colitis.

Abscesses can form anywhere in the liver, although most frequently they arise in the right lobe. They may be solitary or multiple. When close to the diaphragm, there is first

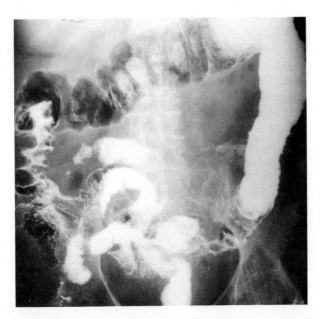

Fig. 46-35 Severe ulcerative colitis in a patient with amebiasis with marked "thumb printing" in the ascending colon. There are widespread mural spicules and ulceration in the descending and sigmoid colon, and the terminal ileum is also involved.
From Reeder MM, Palmer PES: *The radiology of tropical diseases*, Baltimore, 1981, Williams & Wilkins; Armed Forces Institute of Pathology, No. 67-10134-2 229498-233.

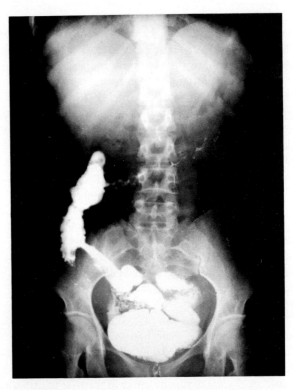

Fig. 46-36 A fixed, contracted, rigid, and ulcerated cecum caused by chronic amebiasis. The ileocecal valve is fixed and incompetent, and the terminal ileum is tubular. There are fistulas extending from the tip of the cecum.
From Reeder MM, Palmer PES: *The radiology of tropical diseases*, Baltimore, 1981, Williams & Wilkins.

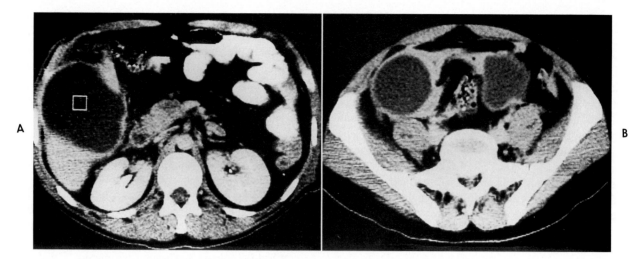

Fig. 46-37 CT scan showing an amebic abscess in the right lobe of the liver **(A),** and two separate intraperitoneal abscesses in the lower abdomen and pelvis of the same patient **(B).**
Courtesy of Dr. Michael Federle.

loss of movement and then a pleural reaction and edema appear in the nearby lung. Perforation of the abscess through the diaphragm and into the chest may account for the finding of amebae in the sputum. Perforation into the pericardium can be a very dangerous event. The liver abscesses are best demonstrated by CT (Fig. 46-37), ultrasonography (Fig. 46-38), or magnetic resonance imaging (MRI), and are frequently peripheral.[131,134] Angiography shows displacement of the vessels and a ring of increased vascularity around the abscess. Larger abscesses can also be identified on radionuclide scans (Fig. 46-39). With regard to CT and ultrasound examinations, it must be remembered that, early in the infection, some abscesses are isodense and may be totally or partially hyperechoic.[124] When abscess is suspected on clinical grounds but the ultrasound examination yields negative findings, the examination should be repeated within a day or two because liquefaction occurs centrally and the sonic findings will change. Alternatively, CT scanning with contrast enhancement may reveal the hyperemic wall and an otherwise isodense abscess a little earlier on. Despite the existence of many different descriptions, there is no method of imaging that can reliably differentiate an amebic from a pyogenic liver abscess.

An hepatic abscess can rupture into the biliary tract and may cause jaundice. Plain films may show gas within the liver. Perforation can occur into the peritoneum, around the kidneys, or directly into the stomach or gut. Trauma can cause an abscess to rupture either in the liver or elsewhere, and this may be the way in which the abscess is first discovered. After treatment, a liver abscess may disappear entirely, leave some scarring, or occasionally calcify. Healing may take many months, and the central cavity may persist for years, although it will be sterile.

Amebiasis mimics many diseases, including ulcerative colitis, with or without megacolon; the narrow areas, deep ulcers, fistulas, and skip areas characteristic of Crohn's disease; or the tight stricture or mass typical of malignancy. A serologic check is easy and not only may avoid surgery but may literally be lifesaving. Radiologists need to maintain a high index of suspicion for amebiasis.

Chagas' disease

Although Chagas' disease[138-153] (American trypanosomiasis) is found only in the central and southern half of the American continent, from Texas to Argentina, the World Health Organization estimated in 1960 that there were at least 7 million infected individuals and another 35 million exposed to the infection.[153] It thus represents an important public health problem in many South American nations, especially in rural eastern Brazil where more than 30% of all adults with clinical evidence of chronic Chagas' disease die of the infection.[139,143,146]

Despite research conducted since 1909, when the disease was first described by Carlos Chagas, it remains a baffling disorder with many unresolved problems and a multitude of different manifestations in both its acute and chronic stages. In the acute phase it may lead to extensive myocarditis and encephalitis; in its chronic form, besides the severe myocardiopathy, there is a decrease in the number of ganglion cells in the central and peripheral autonomic nervous system, which may cause marked enlargement of the heart, esophagus, colon, and other hollow viscera. The heart is the most commonly involved organ, and, in both the acute and chronic phases, myocarditis accounts for greater morbidity and mortality than does the involvement of all other organs combined. Chronic Chagas' disease accounts for thousands of cases of cardiomyopathy in hyper-

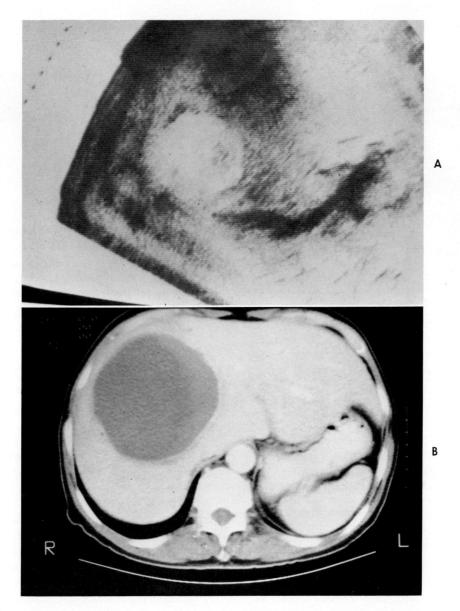

Fig. 46-38 Ultrasonographic (**A**) and CT (**B**) appearances of amebic abscesses in the liver. The findings are very nonspecific, as an amebic abscess cannot be distinguished from any other type of liver abscess.

endemic areas such as in Argentina, Uruguay, Chile, and Venezuela, and is a special problem in eastern Brazil, where megaesophagus and megacolon are commonly seen in addition to the cardiac involvement.

Chagas' disease primarily afflicts children and young adults who live in mud huts in rural areas. The causative organism, *Trypanosoma cruzi,* is a tiny pleomorphic protozoon that inhabits the blood and tissues of humans and animals. It is transmitted by several species of reduviid or *Triatoma* bugs, which become infected after feeding on humans, or on armadillos or other animal hosts. These blood-sucking bugs have a predilection for biting sleeping chil-

dren on the face at night. Infection results from contamination of the punctured skin by the insect's feces, which are loaded with trypanosomes. Once introduced into the body, the protozoa travel within the bloodstream as flagellated trypanosomal C- or U-shaped forms. Once they invade tissue cells, especially the reticuloendothelial cells, muscle, and glia, they undergo transformation to leishmanial forms. These divide by binary fission to form intracellular colonies that fill and rupture the invaded cells. The fact that *T. cruzi* multiplies within the host cell's cytoplasm and not in the blood makes Chagas' disease especially difficult to treat.

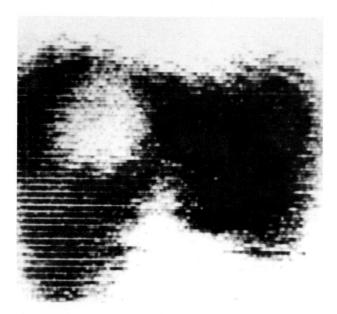

Fig. 46-39 A radionuclide scan (enhanced with Tc 99m–sulfur colloid) shows a large amebic abscess in the right lobe of the liver, spreading toward the upper surface. The diaphragm in this patient was involved, and there was a right-sided pleural effusion with edema in the right lower lobe.
From Reeder MM, Palmer PES: *The radiology of tropical disease*, Baltimore, 1981, Williams & Wilkins.

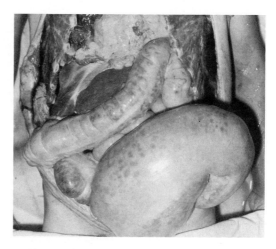

Fig. 46-40 Megacolon at necropsy in a patient with chronic Chagas' disease. Note the massive distention and elongation of the rectosigmoid colon, with less marked dilatation of the more proximal portion.
Courtesy of Dr. Clovis Simão.

Once the cell has ruptured, the liberated organisms either invade adjacent cells or are destroyed by macrophages, which release a neurotoxin that attacks and over time destroys the ganglion cells in the myenteric plexi of the affected organ.[143,145] The heart, brain, esophagus, and colon are the principal sites of involvement, although the spleen, liver, lymph nodes, bronchi, ureters, and salivary glands may also be affected.

In the acute phase of the infection, which is most commonly seen in children, there may be fever, edema, anemia, lymphadenitis, meningoencephalitis, and especially myocarditis.[150] The mortality rate from acute myocarditis or meningoencephalitis varies from 2% to 10%.

The pathogenesis of Chagas' disease involves at least three distinct phases, each with its own pathologic processes. Once defense mechanisms have developed during the acute phase, the disease passes into a latent phase of many years' duration, during which the parasites are difficult to demonstrate either in the blood or in body tissues.

The third, or chronic (late), stage of the disease gives rise to the Chagas' syndromes that are the end result of the destruction of ganglion cells in the central or peripheral nervous system that took place during the acute phase. The lesions may be widespread but are most severe in the heart, muscles, nervous system, and gastrointestinal tract, particularly the esophagus and colon.

The three stages of the disease, although originating from one cause, are clinically and radiologically distinct. The middle or latent period is clinically silent, whereas the acute and late stages can be severe and dramatic in their clinical and radiologic manifestations.

Thus, after a period of as many as 10 to 20 years, and probably after repeated infections with the trypanosome, the systemic changes of the chronic stage may develop, especially involving the heart, esophagus, and rectosigmoid colon. Several Brazilian investigators[140,143-146] have clearly established that aperistalsis and dilatation of the esophagus and colon are common late sequelae of *T. cruzi* infection, in addition to the more common chronic chagasic cardiomyopathy. In Ferreira-Santos's large series,[143] the complement fixation text for trypanosomiasis was positive in 95% of the members of a large group of autopsied or surgically treated patients with esophageal and colonic aperistalsis. The age range in this series was 2 to 75 years, with an average of 33 years. Brasil[140] suggested that the term *aperistalsis* be applied to the chronic form of Chagas' disease to denote the pathophysiologic disturbances, consisting of motor incoordination, defective esophageal and colonic motility, and disturbed or absent peristalsis without propulsive efficiency, that characterize the advanced cases. Koberle[145,146] demonstrated that the quantitative and qualitative reduction in the number of ganglia throughout the entire gastrointestinal tract is responsible for causing the aperistalsis and atony, which in turn results in the dilatation of the hollow viscera. Although ganglia deficiency may be seen throughout the entire gastrointestinal tract, both clinically and radiographically, the esophagus and the rectosigmoid colon exhibit the greatest distention, probably because they are subjected to the greatest mechanical pressure and stasis (Fig. 46-40).

RADIOLOGIC FINDINGS

The earliest radiographic manifestations of Chagas' disease in the esophagus relate only to motor dysfunction. Tone is maintained in the early stage, and there may be little or no dilatation. Gradually increasing disturbances in tone, rhythm, and motility over the course of several years give rise to the bizarre, dysrhythmic contractions observed on barium swallow. Hypercontractility, increased tone, and hypertrophy of the circular muscle layers are manifestations of motor dysfunction that often result in dysphagia. Later, as denervation progresses, hypotonia, aperistalsis, stasis, and dilatation occur. The transverse diameter of the flaccid esophagus may reach 7 cm or more, and contractions may be weak and uncoordinated, or even absent[143] (Fig. 46-41).

The appearance of an advanced megaesophagus on plain films of the chest and on barium swallow is remarkably similar to that of achalasia. In both entities the dilated esophagus appears on frontal films as a vertical density located along the entire right paramediastinal border; it is usually distended with air and sometimes shows an air-fluid level if the patient has recently ingested liquids. Often there is tapering of the distal esophageal segment down to the cardiac sphincter, and the radiologic picture may be indistinguishable from that of achalasia, although the cause is quite different. The passage of food or barium through this area may be delayed because of failed relaxation and motor in-

coordination at the level of the sphincter, as well as a lack of propulsive peristalsis throughout the esophagus. Food may become lodged in the esophagus and cause local irritation, leading to inflammation, ulceration, bleeding, perforation, and fistulas. Carcinoma develops in 7% of patients with megaesophagus, sometimes involving rupture into the mediastinum and abscess formation[143,150] (Fig. 46-42).

In most cases of advanced chronic Chagas' disease, there is a generalized enlargement of the heart, resulting from chronic myocardiopathy[138,146,148,150] (Fig. 46-43). The lungs are clear, and no pleural fluid is present until the end-stages of cardiac failure. In rare cases the bronchi, ureters, and gallbladder may be dilated.

There are usually no radiographic changes in the stomach or small bowel, other than occasional cases of megastomach, megaduodenum, or megajejunum (Fig. 46-44).

In patients with megacolon the predominant symptom is chronic obstipation, with bowel movements occurring at intervals ranging from 8 days to several months. Large boluses of desiccated feces may become impacted in the di-

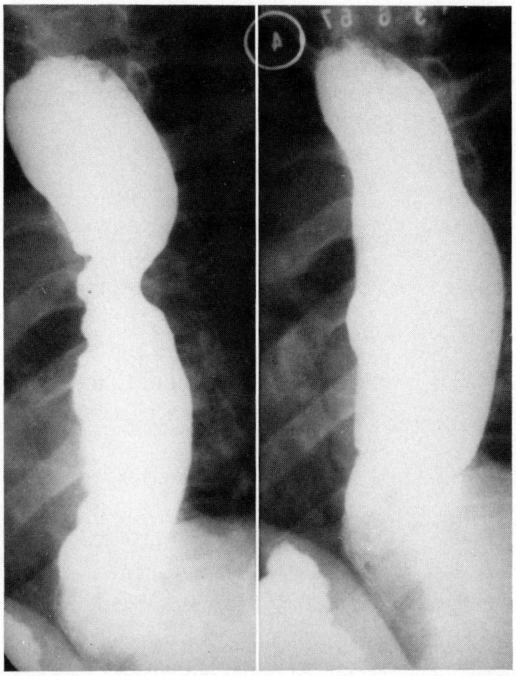

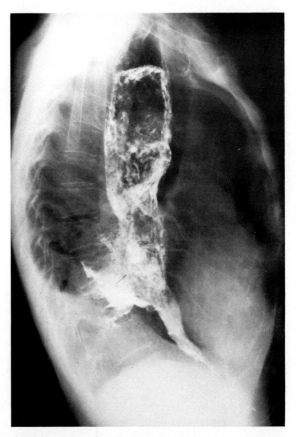

Fig. 46-42 Megaesophagus in an adult Brazilian man with Chagas' disease in whom carcinoma developed in the distal third of the esophagus, with perforation to form a large abscess extending into the right lower lobe and pleural space.
From Reeder MM, Palmer PES: *The radiology of tropical diseases,* Baltimore, 1981, Williams & Wilkins.

Fig. 46-41 Megaesophagus in a Brazilian patient with chronic Chagas' disease. The considerable esophageal dilatation and altered peristalsis denote advanced disease. Local, incoordinate, nonpropulsive contractions are present.
From Reeder MM, Hamilton LC: *Semin Roentgenol* 3:62, 1968.

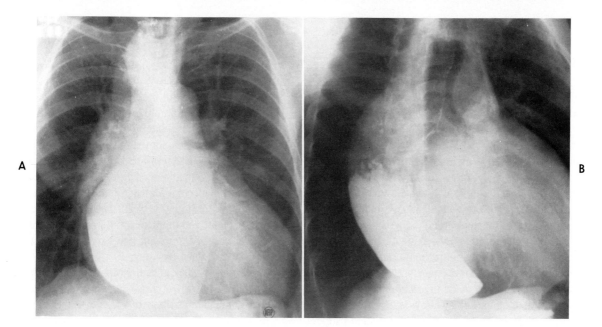

Fig. 46-43 Megaesophagus and myocardiopathy in a 58-year-old Brazilian man with Chagas' disease. A, Posteroanterior view shows a prominent soft tissue density along the entire right mediastinal border, caused by a greatly dilated esophagus that was partially filled with barium. Convexities of the right and left sides of the heart are prominent because of enlargement of the two sides. The left atrial enlargement produces a bulge along the left upper cardiac border and upward displacement of the left main bronchus. No pulmonary vascular congestion is noted. B, A right oblique view shows posterior displacement of the megaesophagus by a grossly dilated left atrium. From Reeder MM, Simäo C: *Semin Roentgenol* 4:374, 1969.

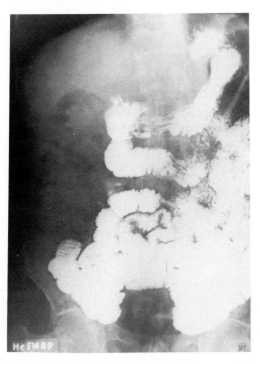

Fig. 46-44 Megaduodenum and megajejunum in a 57-year-old Brazilian man with Chagas' disease. At surgery the duodenum was found to be dilated throughout its length. Neither ulcers nor obstruction by aortic mesenteric vessels was present.
Courtesy of Dr. Clovis Simäo.

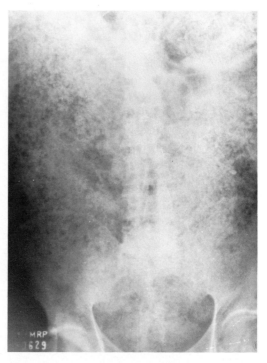

Fig. 46-45 Megacolon with a massive amount of retained feces throughout a grossly dilated colon, opacifying virtually the entire abdomen, in this 51-year-old Brazilian man with chronic Chagas' disease. The patient had suffered progressive intestinal constipation for more than 14 years, despite two previous partial resections of the colon. Following this examination, the entire colon was removed after it was emptied of fecalomas. The colon measured 10 cm in diameter and contained numerous small mucosal ulcers and secondary inflammation. The wall was not thickened uniformly; instead, it was thin in some places and thick in others.
Courtesy of Dr. Clovis Simäo.

lated, atonic rectosigmoid colon, leading to inflammation and stasis ulceration. Sigmoid volvulus, which occurs in 10% of the patients, is often the reason for the patient finally seeking medical attention.[144]

On plain radiographs of the abdomen, multiple large coproliths may be seen, along with a dilated and often redundant colon[148-150] (Fig. 46-45). A dilated splenic flexure or elongated sigmoid colon may sometimes be seen beneath an elevated left hemidiaphragm, simulating the splenic flexure syndrome.[150] The striking elongation and dilatation of the rectosigmoid and descending colon are best illustrated by a barium enema examination (Fig. 46-46). The haustral markings of the colon are diminished or absent, and colonic contractility and evacuation are poor, with most of the barium and retained feces still present on postevacuation films.[144] A cobblestone mucosal pattern is occasionally seen within a portion of the dilated distal colon or rectum, and this pattern is similar to that seen in the presence of mucosal hives caused by a hypersensitivity phenomenon[144] (Fig. 46-47). Rarely a diffusely ulcerated distal colon may be seen.[144]

Occasionally the dilatation of the colon is not uniform throughout. A less distended, short segment of the colon, where the loss of ganglia and subsequent dilatation are less pronounced than in the dilated adjacent bowel, may predispose to the formation of a sigmoid volvulus. A massively dilated loop of sigmoid colon is seen, often with a promi-nent air-fluid level on the erect view (Fig. 46-48). A barium enema may show the typical beaklike or twisted appearance of the colon at the site of the volvulus (Fig. 46-49).

Giardiasis

Giardia lamblia is one of the most common intestinal parasites that afflict humans and is worldwide in distribution.[154-172] It is found in 4% to 16% of the inhabitants of tropical countries and in 3% to 20% of the children living in parts of the southern United States.[168] The organism is found most often in children, especially those from large families or living in institutions such as schools and orphanages. The reported incidence of infection in institutionalized people ranges from 2% to 50%. Occasional epidemics have occurred in cities such as Aspen, Colorado, where leakage of sewage into part of the town's water supply was responsible for the outbreak. Until two decades ago, it was thought that this ubiquitous organism did not invade the mucosa of the duodenum and jejunum (its usual habitat), and that there were no specific radiologic manifestations of giardiasis.[161] Recent studies have shown that neither of these prior assumptions is true, and giardiasis is now recognized as an important cause of diarrhea, malabsorption, and inflammatory changes in the proximal small bowel in many patients throughout the world, especially in children and in individuals with immunoglobulin deficiencies.[158,170] It must be remembered, however, that the vast

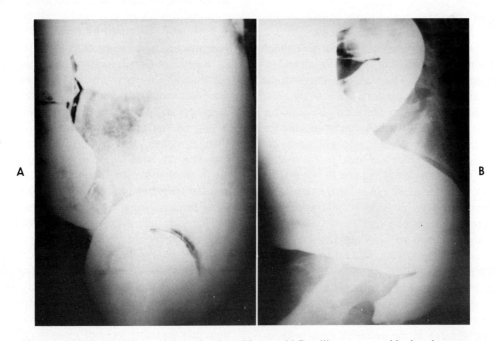

Fig. 46-46 Chagas' disease of the colon in a 56-year-old Brazilian woman with chronic trypanosomiasis. Anteroposterior (**A**) and lateral (**B**) views show massive dilatation of the entire left colon. Note the large fecaliths within the colon. The rectum is not dilated to the same extent as the sigmoid and descending colon because of the action of the pelvic musculature. A follow-up radiograph obtained 47 days later showed marked retention of the barium from this examination.
From Reeder MM, Hamilton LC: *Semin Roentgenol* 3:62, 1968.

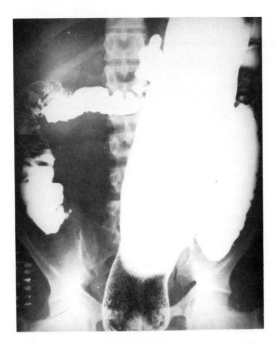

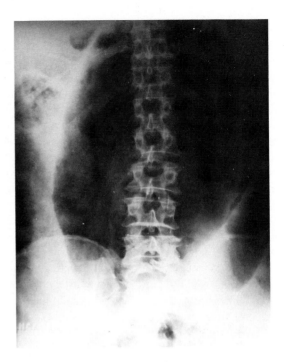

Fig. 46-47 Chagas' disease of the colon. There is severe distention and elongation of the rectum plus the sigmoid and descending colon in this Brazilian man. The caliber of the proximal portion of the colon is normal. A cobblestone mucosal pattern is seen in the rectum, similar to that seen in the presence of mucosal hives resulting from a hypersensitivity phenomenon.
From Reeder MM, Hamilton LC: *Semin Roentgenol* 3:62, 1968.

Fig. 46-48 Volvulus of the sigmoid colon in a 59-year-old Brazilian man with Chagas' disease, who had suffered abdominal colic, distention, and obstipation for 15 days. A 180-degree torsion of the mesosigmoid colon was discovered at surgery.
From Reeder MM, Hamilton LC: *Semin Roentgenol* 3:62, 1968.

majority of people infected with *G. lamblia* exhibit no clinical or radiographic manifestations of the disease.

The organisms are usually harmless protozoa that attach themselves to the mucosal surface of the duodenum and jejunum by their sucking disks. There are two stages in the life cycle of *G. lamblia:* the trophozoite (an actively moving flagellated form) and the cyst, which may be passed in the stool. Humans acquire giardiasis by ingesting contaminated food or water containing viable cysts, which pass unharmed through the gastric juices and undergo excystation in the duodenum, with each cyst giving rise to two trophozoites. These flagellates are usually found in the mucus between the intestinal villi and rarely in intestinal crypts. They may attach to the mucosal epithelium of the duodenum and jejunum and rarely the ileum and may actually invade the mucosa and occasionally produce a mild inflammatory reaction in the lamina propria of the crypts.

In a number of patients with symptomatic giardiasis, electron microscopy study of small bowel biopsy specimens can disclose acute and chronic inflammatory changes, abnormal villi, and damage to the epithelial cells with increased mitoses.[163,172] The villi are short and thickened, with an increased cellular infiltrate in the lamina propria.

Malabsorption is often associated with giardiasis, and is thought to result from the irritation, inflammatory reaction, and altered epithelial function caused by cellular damage and disturbed epithelial cell maturation. Other theories propose that there may be a mechanical barrier to the absorption of nutrients caused by the massive numbers of parasites attached to the mucosal surface, or that an overwhelming number of *Giardia* organisms compete with the host for nutrients.[169] However, the exact mechanism responsible for the malabsorption in giardiasis remains unproved because there appears to be no direct correlation between the malabsorption and the severity of the underlying mucosal changes in many patients.[164] The diagnosis of giardiasis may be established by the discovery of cysts or trophozoites in stool specimens or in duodenal aspirates. In some cases examination of serial sections and impression smears made from intestinal biopsy specimens may be necessary.

The vast majority of people infected with *G. lamblia* have no symptoms, but, in a minority, usually children or persons with suppressed immunologic systems, there may be a variety of symptoms, ranging from mild abdominal discomfort to nausea, anorexia, fever, weight loss, flatulence, recurrent diarrhea, malabsorption, and steatorrhea.[155,159] The stools and clinical manifestations in children may resemble those of sprue or celiac disease.[159] The individual response of a patient infected with *G. lamblia* varies, depending on the number of organisms present, the patient's age and nutritional status, the existence of an associated bacterial infection or immunoglobulin deficiency.[164,172]

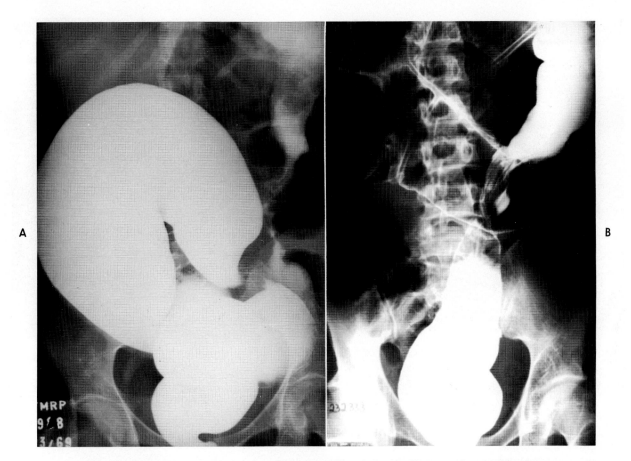

Fig. 46-49 Sigmoid volvulus in two different Brazilian patients with megacolon resulting from Chagas' disease. **A,** There is a typical beaklike appearance to the barium column as it reaches the volvulus in the proximal sigmoid colon. **B,** The classic twisted appearance of the sigmoid colon is well seen, with a slight amount of barium passing beyond the area of the volvulus in the midsigmoid colon. Note the considerable distention of the entire large bowel caused by underlying chagasic aganglionosis.
From Reeder MM, Palmer PES: *The radiology of tropical diseases,* Baltimore, 1981, Williams & Wilkins.

RADIOLOGIC FINDINGS

Until the mid-1960s, reports of radiographic changes linked to giardiasis were rare. In 1944 Welch[171] described irritability of the duodenal cap with coarsening of the mucosal pattern in 22 of 29 patients with giardiasis. Later, Peterson[166] described a deficiency pattern in patients with *G. lamblia* infection that consisted of pronounced segmentation, moderate dilatation of the small bowel loops, coarsening of the mucosal folds in the midportion of the small bowel, and prolonged transit time. Since those early reports, Marshak et al.,[164] Reeder et al.,[168,169] and Basu[156] have described radiographic changes of an inflammatory nature, usually localized to the duodenum and jejunum, in patients with giardiasis. The proximal ileum is rarely involved; the lower ileum and the colon appear normal.

The changes in the mucosa may be quite marked, with thickening, blunting, distortion, and spiking of the folds (Fig. 46-50). There is marked spasm and irritability of the bowel, resulting in a rapid change in the configuration of the valvulae conniventes[165,169] (Fig. 46-51). There is rapid transit of the barium through the affected area, with narrowing of the bowel lumen because of the spasm. Owing to the resultant poor filling of the duodenum and jejunum with barium, fluoroscopic spot filming is difficult, unless the patient is given large amounts of barium. Secretions are often increased, causing blurring of the mucosal folds that is sometimes associated with fragmentation and segmentation. Cure or clinical improvement is associated with a restoration of the normal intestinal pattern. This takes place after the organisms have been eradicated by quinacrine hydrochloride (Atabrine) therapy, usually within a month.[164]

In addition to these inflammatory changes, there may also be a small bowel malabsorption or deficiency pattern, especially in children as part of a spruelike syndrome.[159] Although malabsorption may be observed clinically and to some extent radiographically, the radiographic appearance

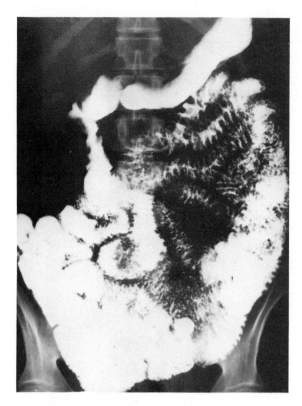

Fig. 46-50 Giardiasis. The second portion of the duodenum is markedly irregular, and considerable spasm is noted within the duodenal sweep and proximal jejunum. These loops are poorly filled because of irritability and are separated from each other. The mucosal folds are thickened, and secretions are increased. The bowel lumen is slightly rigid and narrowed. The changes suggest an inflammatory reaction rather than a malabsorption pattern. They disappeared after quinacrine hydrochloride therapy for the giardiasis.
Courtesy of Dr. Richard H. Marshak.

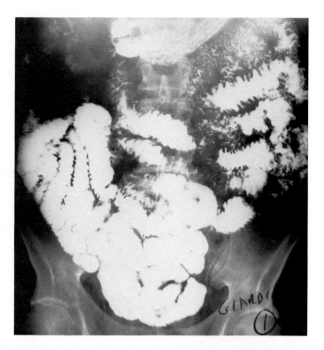

Fig. 46-51 Giardiasis. There is spasm and irritability of the proximal small bowel and a normal-appearing ileum. The mucosal folds in the duodenum and jejunum are thickened and spiked, and there is segmentation and fragmentation of the barium column, resulting from a combination of irritability, mucosal edema, and increased secretions.
Courtesy of Dr. Richard H. Marshak.

in giardiasis (as well as that in some patients with strongyloidiasis and hookworm disease) is chiefly the result of inflammation, at least in the proximal small bowel[165,169]; a spruelike pattern may also exist in the distal jejunum and ileum of some of these patients.[169]

There is an unusually high incidence of giardiasis in patients with the syndrome of dysgammaglobulinemia, nodular lymphoid hyperplasia, recurrent respiratory and urinary tract infections, chronic spruelike diarrhea, and other clinical and radiographic evidence of malabsorption[161,162,167] (Fig. 46-52). The generally lowered resistance of these patients seems to permit the usually innocuous *Giardia* organisms to flourish in the small bowel. The innumerable, tiny, uniform 2- to 3-mm nodular lesions found throughout the small intestine are not related to giardiasis but represent hypertrophy of the lymphoid follicles (Fig. 46-53).

Localization of the pathologic and radiologic changes that occur in giardiasis to the duodenum and jejunum is of great importance in the differential diagnosis, because many other gastrointestinal diseases are thereby excluded. The principal differential considerations include other parasitic diseases, such as strongyloidiasis and hookworm disease, as well as other inflammatory diseases of the proximal small bowel, such as Whipple's disease and eosinophilic enteritis.[169] Intestinal lymphangiectasia, lymphoma, amyloidosis, vascular diseases, and pancreatitis are unlikely to be confused with giardiasis, as they are associated with more pronounced changes in the mucosal fold pattern but less extensive spasm, fragmentation, and secretions than are seen in giardiasis. In cases of giardiasis in which the "deficiency pattern" is prominent, the differential diagnosis includes other causes of malabsorption, but these only rarely simulate the overall radiographic pattern seen in giardiasis, especially when the prominent inflammatory changes and spasm in the duodenum and jejunum are recognized.

When the disease is suspected, endoscopy is the best diagnostic test, both for biopsy of the distal duodenum and for the collection of duodenal fluid aspirate for histologic examination.

Helminthic infections
Nematodes (roundworms)
ASCARIASIS[173-183]

Ascaris lumbricoides is the most common roundworm, particularly in children; infections by *Toxocara canis* and

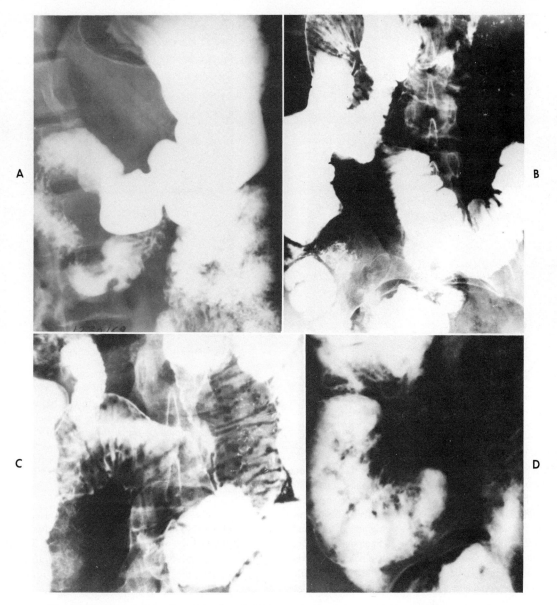

Fig. 46-52 Giardiasis and nodular lymphoid hyperplasia of the small intestine in a 24-year-old woman with dysgammaglobulinemia, recurrent respiratory infections, and a constant spruelike diarrhea. **A,** The mucosal pattern within the duodenal bulb and C loop is coarse, and the folds are somewhat edematous. A duodenal sweep failed to fill out normally, as seen on multiple spot films; this indicated slight spasm. **B,** Abnormal motor activity with dilatation of multiple loops of the jejunum and ileum, together with segmentation of the barium column and coarsening of the mucosal folds, is seen in some areas. **B and C,** The mucosa of the entire jejunum and ileum is uniformly studded with numerous tiny, round polypoid lesions 1 to 3 mm in diameter. These nodules are especially well outlined in areas of air-barium contrast. **D,** Nodules are also present in the terminal ileum and right portion of the colon.
From Reeder MM: *Radiology* 93:427, 1969.

T. cati and by *Ascaris suum* are rare. In 1979 it was estimated that between 800 million and 1 billion persons were infected with *Ascaris,* making it third among the 10 most common human infections.[129] Whereas the infection is most common where temperatures are warm and there is high humidity, any area where there is overpopulation and poor sanitation is at risk, and there are probably several million hosts to this parasite in North America. *Ascaris* infection is acquired by ingesting food, water, or soil that has been contaminated with embryonated eggs. Self-contamination, particularly among children, is common. Uncooked vegetables (particularly in areas where night soil

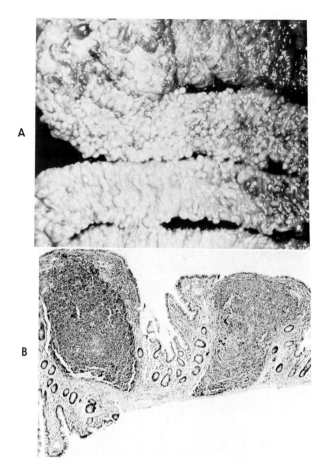

Fig. 46-53 A, Gross specimen of small intestine from a patient with nodular lymphoid hyperplasia, in which innumerable small uniform polypoid lesions studded the mucosal surface. These tiny nodules account for the multiple round filling defects noted on radiographs of the small bowel. **B,** Photomicrograph of a jejunal biopsy specimen from a patient with dysgammaglobulinemia and nodular lymphoid hyperplasia. The lymphoid follicles within the lamina propria are greatly enlarged and elevate the mucosal surface to produce a polypoid appearance. Overlying villi appear flattened. (Hematoxylin- eosin; ×50.)
From Reeder MM, Palmer PES: *The radiology of tropical diseases,* Baltimore, 1981, Williams & Wilkins.

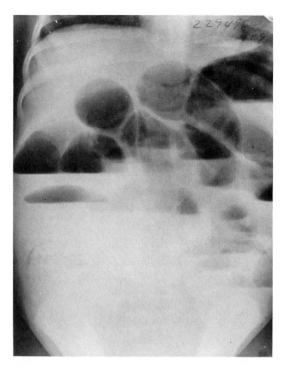

Fig. 46-54 Ascariasis can cause mechanical small bowel obstruction because of the large number of worms, usually forming a bolus in the ileum. Sometimes a worm can be recognized, but because this is a common cause of obstruction in childhood, possible ascariasis should be borne in mind even if worms cannot be seen.
From Reeder MM, Palmer PES: Armed Forces Institute of Pathology, photographic negative No. 67-10130-1.

is used for a fertilizer) and polluted drinking water are other important sources of infection.

The *Ascaris* eggs become infective within about 3 weeks in shady, moist soil. A minimum temperature exceeding 70° F is necessary for this. When swallowed, the outer shell of the ova is digested by the gastric juices, and the ova hatch in the small bowel to become free tiny larvae, which then penetrate the epithelium of the intestinal mucosa. They then pass either through the portal system into the liver or via the intestinal lymphatics to the thoracic duct. By either route, they can reach the lungs via the right heart, and a few days later perforate the alveoli. After molting twice and growing in the lungs, they travel up the bronchi and tra-

chea and are then swallowed. They mature as worms within the lumen of the small intestine, reaching 35 cm in about 2 months. Copulation occurs in the small intestine, and a single female may produce millions of eggs in 6 months. A new generation of ova appears in the feces at the end of the 2- to 3-month cycle.

The clinical symptoms first appear as the larvae lodge in the lungs, and they include those of bronchitis or pneumonia, particularly in children. Pyrexia ranging from 99° to 105° F with chills and vomiting, coughing, and even hemoptysis can occur. There is usually a pronounced eosinophilia during this stage (50% or more for a short period). Asthma may result, particularly in Asian Indians. In the next stage, as the worms mature in the intestinal tract, there may be few or even no symptoms. Sometimes there is nausea, vomiting or abdominal discomfort, or perhaps colicky pain. Distention and tenderness and, surprisingly, constipation may result. Some patients become hypersensitive and present with meningism, idiopathic epilepsy, or febrile convulsions. Then, as the worm population grows, there may be partial or complete intestinal obstruction. Children may harbor more than 2000 worms, which can be entwined and form a large bolus; this is not an uncommon complication.[180] The most common site of obstruction is the ileocecal region, but blockage can occur anywhere in the small or large bowel; gastric outlet obstruction is also reported (Fig. 46-54). Intussusception and volvulus can take place, but much less commonly. In one series 13% of all acute abdominal emergencies in children were due to ascariasis.[183]

The worms may find their way into the biliary tract, and this is one of the most common causes of jaundice in children, particularly in the populations of China, South Africa, and South America. When the infection is chronic,

cholecystitis, cholangitis, pancreatitis, and even liver abscess may develop. Biliary ascariasis has been found in persons of all ages, and most respond to conservative treatment. Reports from China, Japan, and Colombia suggest an etiologic relationship in the development of gallstones.[177]

The laboratory diagnosis depends on the identification of adult worms or eggs in the stool, vomit, sputum, or small bowel aspirates, aided by very characteristic radiologic or ultrasound findings. The eosinophilia fluctuates and is especially high in the pulmonary phase. When the worms are in the intestine, it usually ranges from 5% to 12%. Immunodiagnostic tests are unreliable because there is a cross reaction with antigens from other helminths. Immunoglobulin E may be found in fecal extracts.

Radiologic diagnosis. Large collections of worms are often identifiable on a plain film of the abdomen, contrasted against the gas in the bowel and resembling a tangled group of thick cords. They can also be seen on ultrasonograms. In addition, there may be evidence of partial or complete mechanical intestinal obstruction. After the patient swallows the barium, the outline of the individual worm can be seen as an elongated radiolucent filling defect that is most common in the jejunum and ileum but may be anywhere in the alimentary tract from the esophagus to the rectum (Figs. 46-55 and 46-56). If the patient has not eaten for about 12 hours, the worms ingest the barium. In this event, a thin white thread can be seen running the length of the worm's body, which is itself outlined by the surrounding barium in the bowel. The position and shape of the worm may indicate which way it is moving or if it is reacting favorably to an anthelmintic agent. There may be an associated disordered pattern of the small bowel mucosa, with thickening

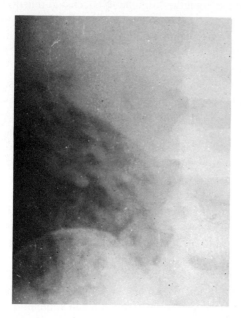

Fig. 46-55 Soft tissue film of the abdomen in a child shows multiple ascarides in a loop of bowel.

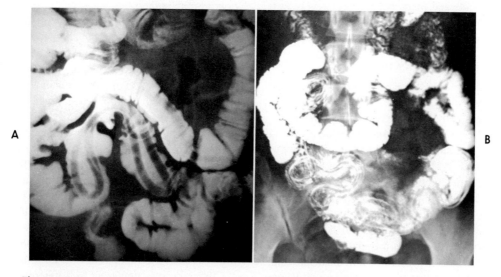

Fig. 46-56 **A,** *Ascaris* in the mid–small bowel outlined with barium. **B,** *Ascaris* in the small bowel with the alimentary tract of *Ascaris* worms demonstrated.
Courtesy of Dr. J.P. Balikian.

of the mucosal folds. The mass of worms can be well demonstrated by ultrasonography and, if there are sufficient numbers, by CT (it is hoped, as a chance finding, however).

Ultrasonography is the easiest way to demonstrate the worm in the biliary tract, where it may be seen either in cross section or lengthwise.[177] If ultrasound is not available, the worm can be revealed by endoscopic retrograde cholangiopancreatography and also by T-tube or transhepatic cholangiograms. In the pancreatic duct the worm can be seen on ultrasonograms.

Rarely the worm escapes from the bowel and forms a "tumor." This may lie free in the peritoneal cavity, and the differential diagnosis, as well as the operation, can be very difficult (see the section on helminthoma later in this chapter).

In the larval stage, particularly in children, the chest radiograph may show soft, patchy, ill-defined asymmetric densities that are often transient (Löffler's pneumonia). These are due to a localized pulmonary reaction or even necrosis and hemorrhage, and they may develop into bronchopneumonia. If the adult worm is aspirated into the lung, this can lead to collapse of the lobe or the entire lung. Eventually, pulmonary granulomas and fibrosis may form where the larvae die, and this can even appear as a solitary pulmonary nodule.

Differential diagnosis. The appearances of the gastrointestinal and biliary tracts are so characteristic, either on barium studies or ultrasonograms, that they are not likely to be misinterpreted. On the chest radiograph, the most important factor in diagnosis is to remember the possibility. The transient nature of the lung densities is very helpful because seldom does an ordinary bacterial infection change so rapidly in size, position, and shape. However, the pulmonary changes are very nonspecific. When *Ascaris* infection is highly likely and eosinophilia is demonstrated, examination of the stools and treatment for worms may produce a remarkable cure in the patient with suspected bronchopneumonia or pulmonary tuberculosis.

ANCYLOSTOMIASIS (HOOKWORM DISEASE)

Ancylostomiasis[4,12,128,129,184] is an infection with one or more species of the Ancylostomidae, most commonly *Ancylostoma duodenale* and *Necator americanus,* which may occur together. Geographically, *Ancylostoma* is found throughout the Mediterranean, the Middle East, Eastern Europe, Pakistan, and northern India. *Necator* extends throughout Central and South America, the West Indies, sub-Saharan Africa, India, and Sri Lanka. Mixed infections are found in Asia, particularly in Burma, Malaysia, Vietnam, Laos, Cambodia, Taiwan, China, and Japan. In the United States, *Necator* is found in the south and in Puerto Rico. Thus *N. americanus* is predominant in the tropics and *A. duodenale* in the temperate climates. Intensive efforts have brought about a reduction in the incidence of infection during the past 50 years, particularly in North America, but infection is still extremely common in the tropics, exceeding 90% in the populations of some parts of Latin America, Asia, and Africa.[128,129] An agricultural environment is important in the spread of hookworm, particularly in areas such as coffee and cocoa plantations, where there is high humidity in the shade and a very fertile soil. The use of human night soil for fertilization maintains the disease in many parts of the Orient; indeed humans themselves may be the primary factor in the epidemiology. It is common in workers in mines and tunnels, and wherever people walk unshod. Hookworms are also found in other primates and animals, ranging from the rhinoceros to rodents. Those ancylostomes (*A. braziliense, A. caninum,* and *A. malayanum*) that inhabit animals only occasionally invade humans, in whom they seldom undergo full development but can cause a localized skin eruption.

The small hookworms, measured in millimeters, firmly attach themselves to the intestinal mucosa in humans, sucking blood, tissue, and intestinal juices to obtain nourishment. They may live for 6 or more years within the intestine, and produce 50 million eggs per female during that time. The eggs develop as they travel in the intestine, and, if deposited in warm, moist soil, the embryos become visible within 24 hours, double their size within the next 48 hours, and become infective within another week. They are active and can swim, wriggle, or climb a moist surface, being capable of traveling through as much as 1 meter (3 feet) of light soil. They remain viable for up to 6 weeks.

The larvae usually enter humans through the skin of the foot or ankle and occasionally through the mouth. The normal site of penetration is through a hair follicle. They then move into the lymphatic or blood circulation. From the lung capillaries and alveoli they migrate up the bronchi and are then swallowed, to mature again in the small intestine, usually the jejunum. Other more complex methods of infection are uncommon but can occur.

Although there may be intraalveolar and interstitial hemorrhage in the lungs, most of the pathologic changes take place in the second and third portions of the jejunum, where there are minor mucosal changes that can disappear with therapy. Examination of intestinal biopsy specimens reveals a marked eosinophilia along with other findings resembling those of sprue. Laboratory findings can establish diagnosis when eggs are found in a fresh sample of feces, but at least 20 eggs are needed to distinguish between a clinical and a subclinical infection, and differentiation from *Strongyloides* infection may be difficult. A skin test antigen is available for screening large populations. Anemia can result from the loss of as much as 100 ml of blood per day in the event of a heavy infection. The anemia is usually hypochromic and microcytic, but there may also be a hypoplastic bone marrow. Peripheral eosinophilia is often found.

Clinically, it is important to differentiate between hookworm carriers and those with hookworm disease; the former are asymptomatic, but those with the disease exhibit anemia and symptoms that result from malnutrition and concomitant illness. There are two clinical phases. In the first, during migration and development of the larvae, there can be pruritus and vesiculation where the larvae have penetrated the skin, and these sites may become infected. Pulmonary symptoms develop within 2 weeks and are often mild and transient. The chest x-ray findings are normal. At this stage, there will be a marked peripheral eosinophilia. When *A. duodenale* reaches the small bowel, this can precipitate severe diarrhea with foul-smelling stools. Thereafter, the patient often has no symptoms for prolonged periods, although dyspepsia, nausea, and pain may occur. As the anemia worsens, the general symptoms of tiredness, weakness, and palpitations develop. Hemoglobin levels of 1 g/100 ml have been reported, as well as an eosinophilia of between 90% to 100%. Concomitant cardiac disease and nephritis can occur.

The most common finding on a chest radiograph is mild cardiac enlargement from the anemia and hypoproteinemia. In most patients the results of barium examinations are normal. In others the small intestine pattern may be somewhat abnormal, resembling a deficiency pattern with coarsening and irregularity of the mucosa. The changes are usually proportional to the severity of the infection, and the ileum is usually normal unless infection is severe. In the radiologic examination, attention should be focused on the jejunum, where there is likely to be thickening of the mucosal folds and distortion of the loops, with either dilatation or contraction. The differential diagnosis includes other parasitic infections, particularly giardiasis and strongyloidiasis, and any other cause of the malabsorption pattern. The differentiation between hookworm disease and steatorrhea from another cause may be very difficult. There seems to be some geographic variation in the incidence of steatorrhea-like findings.

Hookworms have rarely been found in bone and soft tissues, especially in fibrosarcomas.[12]

STRONGYLOIDIASIS

Immunosuppression is of particular importance in *Strongyloides* infection.[185-188] Although some patients may have no symptoms, the immunosuppressed patient may develop very severe disease. Until recently, strongyloidiasis was considered to be a disease of the small bowel, but very acute ulcerating colitis can occur in severe cases.[185]

Strongyloides stercoralis occurs worldwide, but it is most common in the tropics. No age group is exempt, although it is more common in adults. Humans are the major host, but dogs and chimpanzees can be infected. The female parasite, usually residing in the duodenum or upper jejunum, can reproduce without a male parasite and may deposit 30 to 50 eggs per day for several months. When discharged in the feces, the larvae feed on the soil and require 4 months to develop. In tropical countries multiplication can occur on the ground, which becomes heavily contaminated.

Where conditions are unfavorable, filariform larvae develop, and these remain mobile and can infect humans, penetrating the skin on contact. However, in this form the larvae die within a few days unless they come in contact with a host. Penetration in humans is usually through the sole of the foot or hands and causes a mild local reaction. The larvae travel through blood vessels and lymphatics to the heart, then into the lungs, where they enter the alveolar sacs and then molt to become worms. At this stage there may be a bleeding inflammatory response in the lungs and some eosinophilia. If there is a very heavy infestation, pulmonary hemorrhage, eosinophilic nodules, and bronchopneumonia with consequent damage to the pulmonary tissue can result.

Further migration through the bronchial tree and down the esophagus allows the worms to reach the duodenum and jejunum, where they burrow into the mucosa and establish themselves. Invasion can occur in any other part of the gastrointestinal tract, from the stomach to the anus, but usually the female parasites mature in the crypts of the small intestine and invade only the superficial layers of the mucosa without penetrating the muscularis. Some filariform larvae penetrate the mesenteric venules and start the cycle again through the process of endoautoinfection. Autoinfection can also take place through the anal and perianal skin, so the cycle of infection can persist for 10 years or more, even despite a change of environment and no external reinfection.

In the bowel, there may be only a catarrhal enteritis, with increased mucosal congestion and mucous secretion, but this may progress to an edematous phase, with thickening of the intestinal wall, swelling of the folds, and then flattening and atrophy of the mucosa. At this stage, the clinical appearance may resemble that of sprue, and, by then, parasites will infest all layers of the intestinal wall. The most severe stage is ulcerative enteritis, with thickening of the intestinal wall caused by edema and fibrosis; this causes the formation of a rigid tubelike intestine. The mucosa will then be atrophied and ulcerated, with granulomas in the mucosa and submucosa and marked eosinophilic infiltration. Ulcers of up to 7 mm in diameter may be seen in the large bowel, and when the patient is immunosuppressed, there may be severe paralytic ileus clinically.

These three varieties of pathologic response (catarrhal, edematous, and ulcerative) are responsible for causing a wide variation in the gastrointestinal symptoms and radiologic findings. In the first two phases, reversal can be complete, but residual fibrosis will result from the ulcerative stage. The hyperinfective stage, with involvement of the colon, almost always occurs in patients who are immunosuppressed for natural or therapeutic reasons.[184] Histologically, it can be difficult to identify the *Strongyloides* organisms or ova in the mucosa of the colon, but larvae may be seen throughout the intestinal wall and lymphatics, and in the mesenteric lymph nodes in severe cases. Jaundice can result when the biliary tract has been invaded, but it is more commonly due to obstruction resulting from edema and spasm of the ampulla of Vater. The damage to the gut can be so severe that septicemia from *E. coli* or other organisms can develop, with metastatic abscesses forming in almost any part of the body.

Laboratory diagnosis is accomplished by the identification of the larvae or adult worms in fresh stools or sometimes by stool culture. Multiple stool specimens may have to be examined and it is not usual to find ova. The larvae can also be found on duodenal aspirates, and this probably represents a more accurate method than stool examination; the findings in duodenal or jejunal biopsy specimens can often confirm the diagnosis. There is a complement fixation test that is nonspecific and is of little help in making the diagnosis. There is usually a pronounced eosinophilia, but, if this starts to fall during an infection, it may indicate a suppressed immune reaction and a poor prognosis.

Clinically, patients may complain of irritation at the site of skin penetration or around the anus during autoinfection, and, if the larvae move under the skin, there can be a severe pruritus. Pulmonary symptoms vary from an innocuous cough and mild hemoptysis to frank pneumonia and asthma; bronchopneumonia can develop, as it can in other parasitic infections. However, the changes in the chest are usually less than might be expected. Abdominal symptoms depend on the intensity of the infection; some patients may have no complaints, and others may have gastritis or mild crampy abdominal pain. Food ingestion tends to exacerbate the problem. Later the pain becomes more diffuse and the abdomen more distended. Diarrhea, often watery and with mucus, can develop. As the infection becomes more chronic, patients suffer weight loss and anorexia and exhibit a clinical picture that may resemble that of peptic ulceration, other parasitic infections, or sprue. When the host is immunosuppressed, overwhelming rapid malnutrition and death, with gross abdominal distention, may ensue.

Radiologic findings. The correct diagnosis may be suspected on a radiologic basis in patients who are referred with a clinical diagnosis of peptic ulceration or other gastrointestinal disease because barium studies characteristically show prominent mucosal folds with an irritable, tender duodenum.[185,187] There may be excess mucous secretion, with rapid peristalsis and irritability, and the transit may be so rapid that the proximal small intestine is difficult to evaluate. The ileum may be widened and show a coarse mucosal pattern. At this stage, the findings are fully reversible. In the more severe cases the inflammatory process is much more widespread in the duodenum and jejunum, with a malabsorption (Fig. 46-57) or spruelike pattern, delayed gastric emptying, hypomotility with slow transit times, and an increase in the diameter of the small intestine. Return to normal is still possible at this stage. However, in the third and most severe stage of infection, plain films of the abdomen show multiple dilated small

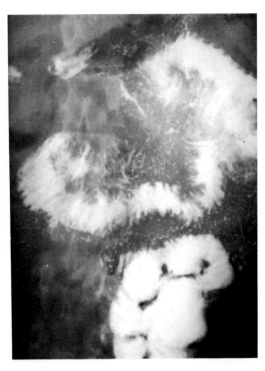

Fig. 46-57 Malabsorption pattern in the upper jejunum seen in severe cases of strongyloidiasis.
Courtesy of Prof. P. Cockshott.

bowel loops, suggesting paralytic ileus or even partial obstruction. If either of these is mistakenly diagnosed, a laparotomy may have an unfortunate outcome, as surgery should be avoided. There is marked hypotonia and rigidity of multiple segments of the small bowel stemming from the severe inflammatory and fibrotic response to the larvae. The stomach may be small with mucosal atrophy. Peristalsis in the duodenum and proximal jejunum may be absent; the appearance lower in the bowel may suggest regional ileitis, with alternating segments of constriction and dilatation. There is complete loss of the mucosa, where a narrow pipestem segment eventually develops (Fig. 46-58), with thickening of the bowel wall and mesenteric lymphadenopathy. In the presence of immunosuppression, severe *Strongyloides* colitis can develop and result in hemorrhage, sepsis, and death. A barium examination in these cases shows an extensive ulcerating colitis, with both small and large ulcers and sinus formation, especially in the left colon. The bowel may be nodular from the cecum to the rectum, with almost complete loss of haustration. This constitutes a very severe state, which is irreversible and often fatal.[185]

The differential diagnosis includes other parasitic infections, especially giardiasis, but, as the disease progresses, malabsorption and regional ileitis are added to the considerations. In the severe cases, ulcerative colitis (from any cause) may be suspected. In most cases, the challenge is to exclude small bowel obstruction and thereby to avoid per-

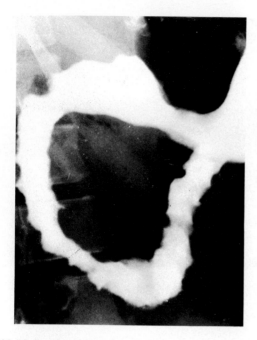

Fig. 46-58 Duodenal loop in a severe case of strongyloidiasis shows pipe-stem rigidity.
Courtesy of Dr. J. Barton.

forming surgery during the course of the severe infection. In the chest the pattern may be indistinguishable from that associated with Löffler's syndrome, presenting with patchy areas of pneumonia as is the case in other parasitic diseases. An immunosuppressed patient may also have pulmonary edema, hemorrhage, and generalized infection.

OESOPHAGOSTOMIASIS (HELMINTHOMAS)

A helminthoma is an inflammatory tumor of the bowel wall resulting from penetration of the wall of the cecum or colon by an intestinal worm.[184,189-191] In theory this is possible for many of the intestinal parasites and can be encountered in any part of the world, but, although penetration of the gut does occur occasionally, particularly in heavy *Ascaris* infections, the usual result is peritonitis rather than the marked inflammatory reaction known as *helminthoma*. Such "tumors" have been reported most commonly from West and East Africa[177] but have also been reported from South America; one case was reported from Indonesia.

The parasites most commonly responsible are the strongyli: *Oesophagostomum apiostomum, Oesophagostomum stephanostomum*, and, rarely, the hookworm *Ancylostoma duodenale* and *Oesophagostomum brumpti*. Although it is difficult to assess the frequency of oesophagostoma infection in humans, they are common parasites in the colon of many animals, particularly sheep, goats, pigs, cattle, apes, and monkeys, in which they cause serious illness with dysentery, peritonitis, and malnutrition. The worms are found throughout Africa and in Brazil, Indonesia, the Phil-

ippines, and parts of China. The ova resemble those of the hookworm. In many patients, the worms cause relatively little general reaction until the bowel wall is entered. Then there is abdominal pain, which is usually localized to the affected bowel segment, most commonly in the right lower quadrant. Seldom is there nausea, dysentery, or vomiting. There may be a low-grade fever, but this is not a constant finding. The history is usually vague, nonspecific, and brief, often of only 2 to 5 days' duration. Children may have a somewhat longer attack, lasting 2 or 3 weeks and simulating intussusception. Clinical examination usually reveals an easily palpated, tender mass, often smooth and well localized but sometimes more diffuse. The white blood cell count is elevated, and there may be some eosinophilia. The usual clinical diagnosis is an appendiceal or pericecal abscess, or amebiasis. In children the cecal wall can be penetrated anteriorly, and an abdominal wall abscess may be the presenting finding.

What happens next is variable. After the acute phase, the mass may subside, with subsequent resolution and absorption of the inflammatory reaction and calcification of the worm. This may become visible on plain films of the abdomen, and may even be an incidental finding at some later date. Alternatively, the abscess may perforate into the bowel lumen or into the peritoneal cavity and cause peritonitis, or the abscess may become adherent to the abdominal wall. In many cases the whole process is more chronic, resulting in the formation of a large granulomatous mass in which specific identification of the worm is now impossible. In this setting there may be extensive adhesions to neighboring structures and central caseous necrosis or calcified fibrotic nodules. Both clinically and histologically the infection must be differentiated from amebiasis, tuberculosis, and schistosomiasis. Surgical resection is usually required, and it is probable that the actual cause of many of these cases has been missed once they have entered the chronic stage. (There are only some 50 cases recorded in the literature.)

Seldom has a radiologic investigation been carried out in such cases because the patients usually have an obvious indication for surgery. The essential finding on a barium enema is a mass within the wall of the bowel. The helminthoma seldom encircles the bowel lumen but narrows it eccentrically, since the mass is partially intramural and largely extramural. Extrinsic pressure and the mass within the bowel wall cause distortion (Fig. 46-59). The most common location of the mass is in the region of the cecum or ascending colon, but helminthomas have also been found in the transverse and descending colon. Air contrast studies show that the mucosa is intact but stretched over the underlying intramural tumor, the edge of which is usually reasonably well defined. There is usually too much edema for the tiny perforation that marks the route of the worm to be seen. As the tumor enlarges and nearby tissue becomes involved, the bowel wall becomes thick. Contraction,

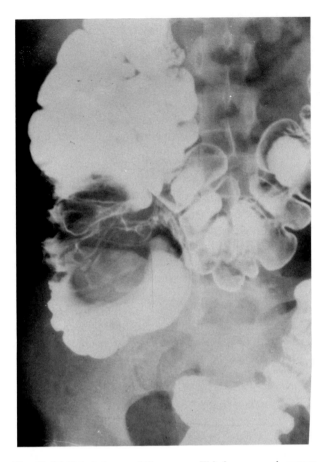

Fig. 46-59 Helminthoma of the cecum. This large granulomatous tumor, caused by a worm burrowing into the wall of the cecum, must be distinguished from ameboma, tuberculosis, and carcinoma in patients coming from the tropics.
From Reeder MM, Palmer PES: *The radiology of tropical diseases,* Baltimore, 1981, Williams & Wilkins.

which is so common in amebiasis and tuberculosis, is unlikely.

The tumor is most likely to be mistaken for a colon carcinoma, which partially encircles the bowel wall (Fig. 46-60). However, the helminthoma differs, in that it seldom produces mucosal ulceration or destruction (and there is seldom melena clinically). In addition, the outline of the mass is often well defined. In the more acute cases, the most likely diagnosis will be an appendiceal abscess or even an amebic abscess of the ileocecal region. A high index of suspicion is *most important* so that the diagnosis can be made preoperatively.

Localized bowel granulomas have been caused by other parasites. *Anisakiasis* may occasionally cause ileal or cecal nodules or masses to form. Similarly, *Angiostrongylus costaricensis* has been known to deposit eggs in the cecal and ileal wall, causing nodular granulomas. Parasitic embolism resulting from *Spiruroidea physalopteridae,* has also been reported from Australia; it led to the development of eosinophilic granulomas in the distal small bowel. None of

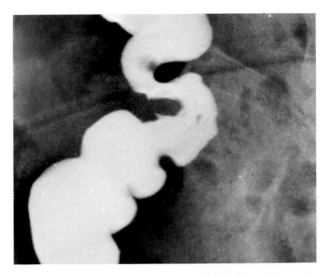

Fig. 46-60 Crypt in a narrow segment of colon in a patient infected with *Oesophagostomum apiostomum.*
Courtesy of Dr. M. Welchman.

these findings appear to have been documented radiologically, and, if they were seen, it would still be impossible to make the correct diagnosis.

When considering the differential diagnosis of helminthoma, it is helpful to remember that malignant disease of the bowel is very rare in many parts of the world, as is diverticulitis. Amebiasis, which is common in such countries, instead poses the principal problem in the differential diagnosis. A high index of suspicion is the examiner's most important single asset.

ANISAKIASIS

The full name of the parasite responsible for anisakiasis,[192-195] *Anisakis marina,* indicates its habitat. The adult form is found in whales and dolphins, whereas the larvae are found in many species of fish, including herring, mackerel, cod, salmon, and squid. Humans become infected when they eat raw fish because the larvae, which are normally in the peritoneum of the fish, may migrate into the muscles.[192]

In humans the larvae burrow into the gastric mucosa and cause ulceration, but they have also been found in the small bowel, colon, and rectum. Perforation into the human peritoneum is possible, with consequent irritation, fluid formation, and associated lymphadenopathy. Histologically there is a marked eosinophilic reaction in the tissue around the site of perforation, suggesting that the ulcer is actually a local, presensitized reaction to the parasite, although the reaction is far more than would be expected if it were due merely to the burrowing of the parasite. There is some geographic variation in terms of the site of the lesion. In patients from Holland who had eaten lightly salted herring, the ulcers were mainly in the ileum. In 92 Japanese patients,

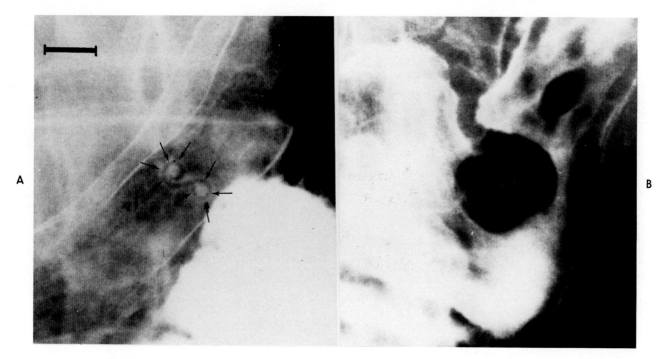

Fig. 46-61 A, *Anisakis* worm outlined in a double-contrast barium meal study in the stomach of an adult patient. **B,** A well-defined antral phlegmon causes an intramural inflammatory mass. Courtesy of Dr. Masayoshi Namiki.

mainly the stomach was involved, with the ileum affected in only 30%. In another Japanese series, 12 small bowel infections were reported.[195]

A history of eating raw fish is very important, and symptoms may arise in 24 hours. These usually resemble those of subacute peptic ulceration, but when the small bowel is infected, the complaints suggest gastroenteritis or even appendicitis. In some patients there may be severe pain and evidence of ileus. Laboratory examinations are not helpful, and stool findings are usually negative. Specific antibodies for the larvae can be detected within 1 to 60 days after they have been ingested. Radiologically, a carefully performed double-contrast barium study of the stomach may show a submucosal mass, and even the worm may be seen[193] (Fig. 46-61). It can also be revealed by endoscopy and sometimes removed in this way. In the small bowel the appearance simulates that of Crohn's disease.[194] There is irregular thickening of the jejunum, ileum, or colon, with mucosal edema, luminal narrowing, and dilatation of the proximal intestine. In some cases, threadlike filling defects suggesting the presence of tiny worms can be seen on the barium study. The plain radiographs may show evidence of ileus. Surgery is seldom indicated.

TRICHURIASIS (WHIPWORM INFECTION)[196-205]

Millions of people in the tropics, more than 350 million in 1947, are infected with *Trichuris trichiura,* often in association with *Ascaris.* In the United States trichuriasis is found chiefly in inhabitants of the southern Appalachian Mountains and rural Louisiana, where fecal pollution, dense shade near the houses, and heavy rainfall favor growth of the parasite. In Brazil it is the most common parasite affecting residents of the large cities, with an incidence of up to 40%; in Costa Rica, it is found in almost all patients suffering from chronic diarrhea.[202-204] Yet, radiologic demonstration is extremely rare. One female worm may produce up to 10,000 ova daily; these can develop in warm soil within 2 to 4 weeks, or remain latent for 5 or more years. Humans become infected when they ingest contaminated soil, food, or water, and small children are affected more often than adults. Within the bowel, the ovum is softened by intestinal juices, and the larva escapes and gains nourishment from the small bowel. It migrates to the cecum, or sometimes lower in the large bowel, and takes 2 or 3 months to assume full adult form. In severe *Trichuris* infections, the entire colon, including the rectum and appendix, may be infected, but the organism is uncommon in the ileum and may be totally unsuspected clinically. If there is no reinfection, the cycle completes itself within 3 years.

The adult *T. trichiura* organism has a characteristic whiplike shape; the anterior three fifths of the worm is long and threadlike and contains the mouth and esophagus. The broader posterior portion, or "handle," of the whip contains the reproductive organs and is spirally coiled in the male parasite but describes a semilunar arc in the female. The parasites are attached to the cecum and colon by means of

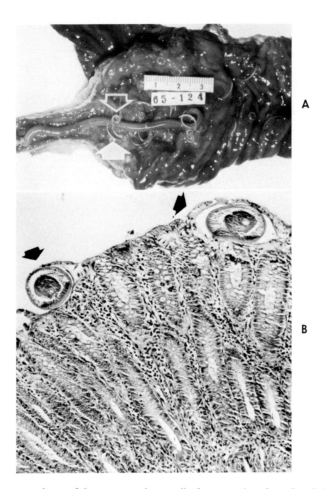

Fig. 46-62 A, Gross specimen of the cecum and appendix from a patient from San Salvador shows coexistent whipworm and *Ascaris* infection, a frequent combination. The glistening mucosal surface is not inflamed or ulcerated, but coated with a thick mucus secreted in the vicinity of the numerous whipworms, especially near the appendix. Note the typical coiled appearance of the male parasites *(open arrow)* and the curved semilunar configuration of the female worms *(solid arrow),* as their posterior portions protrude into the bowel lumen. **B,** The anterior portions of two whipworms are seen in cross section as they lie embedded in their typical location beneath the surface epithelium of the colonic mucosa *(arrows).* Note the lack of any significant inflammatory reaction in the vicinity of the worms. (Hematoxylin-eosin; ×40.)
From Reeder MM, Astacio JE, Theros EG: *Radiology* 90:382, 1968.

their slender anterior ends, which transfix superficial folds of mucosa. They lie embedded beneath the surface epithelium between intestinal villi amid considerable mucus; their blunt posterior portions are either coiled or project freely into the bowel lumen as semilunar arcs (Fig. 46-62). There is usually no inflammatory reaction at the site of attachment, although liquefaction necrosis of adjacent cells, ulcerations, and some bleeding may occur in severe infections.

The diagnosis depends on the identification of the worms during sigmoidoscopy or on stool concentration studies. Eosinophilia is common in the presence of a heavy whipworm infection, and there may be an iron-deficiency ane-

mia. Heavily infected children may have severe chronic diarrhea lasting for years, with resulting ill health[199]; however, even in patients with diarrhea, trichuriasis may be a coincidental finding.

Occasional deaths resulting from profuse hemorrhage or intussusception have been reported.[198,202] *T. trichiura* has also been associated with appendicitis in the tropics; in one series from Colombia, a parasite was found in 16 of 20 patients with appendicitis.[204] Allergic manifestations such as urticaria, rhinitis, and eosinophilia are frequent. Radiology rarely plays a significant role in the diagnosis of trichuriasis, and published case reports in which radiologic investigations were carried out are rare.[197,202] However, the

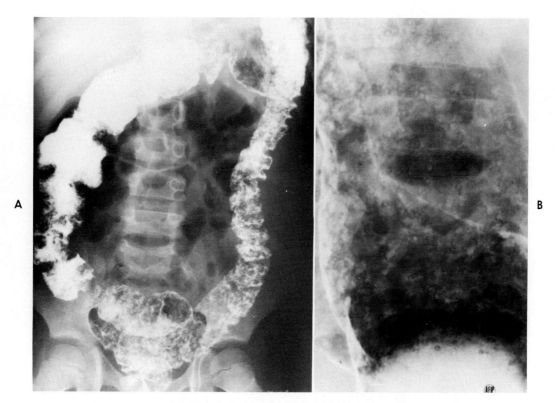

Fig. 46-63 A, Trichuriasis in a 7-year-old boy with profuse rectal bleeding. Innumerable whipworms were found attached to the rectal mucosa at proctoscopy. A granular mucosal pattern was noted on the barium enema examination, similar in appearance to cystic fibrosis. Flocculation of the barium and poor mucosal coating are due to the excessive mucous secretions surrounding the numerous whipworms. **B,** This magnified view of the rectosigmoid colon on an air contrast barium enema examination shows the outlines of many tiny whipworms attached to the mucosa, with their posterior portions either tightly coiled or unfurled in a whiplike configuration.
From Reeder MM, Astacio JE, Theros EG: *Radiology* 90:382, 1968.

worms may be found during a barium enema examination as part of an investigation for rectal bleeding or other colon disease.

The radiographic appearance of the colon in trichuriasis was described in 1968 by Reeder et al.,[202] who based their findings on the barium enema examination performed in a 7-year-old boy from San Salvador (Fig. 46-63). A routine barium enema may be unremarkable or may show a granular mucosal pattern throughout the colon. An air contrast barium enema is definitive and can demonstrate clearly the wavy radiolucent outlines of numerous small trichurids against the air and barium background of the colon and rectum.[197,202-204] The characteristic uncurled, crescentic, or whiplike pattern of the female parasite and the tightly coiled "pinwheel" or "target" pattern of the male worm can be recognized[197] (Fig. 46-64). Subsequently, patients from South Africa, Brazil, and elsewhere have been shown to exhibit identical findings on air contrast examinations. These pathognomonic radiographic features should be kept in mind whenever patients from endemic areas and poor socioeconomic backgrounds are examined (Figs. 46-62 and 46-65).

DRACUNCULUS MEDINENSIS (GUINEA WORM INFESTATION)

Dracunculus medinensis infection deserves only brief mention because it is not an alimentary tract disease, even though infection occurs through the oral ingestion of the larvae. The adult dead worm frequently calcifies and assumes a typical long linear serpiginous or whorled appearance that may be found anywhere in the soft tissues, and thus superimposed on films of the abdomen or pelvis. Such calcified worms are much more common in the limbs, however[12] (Fig. 46-66).

INTESTINAL CAPILLARIASIS

A small hairlike nematode, *Capillaria philippensis,* is responsible for a disease that occurs in outbreaks and starts

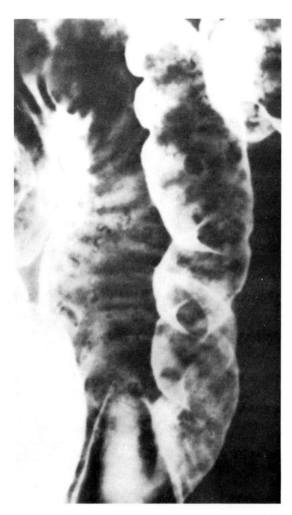

Fig. 46-64 Massive *Trichuris* infection in a Brazilian child. An air contrast examination of the colon depicts the typical wavy outlines of innumerable trichurids in the rectosigmoid colon; some are tightly coiled in the "target" pattern typical of male parasites, whereas others are unfurled in the whiplike configuration characteristic of female parasites.
From Reeder MM, Palmer PES: *The radiology of tropical disease*, Baltimore, 1981, Williams & Wilkins.

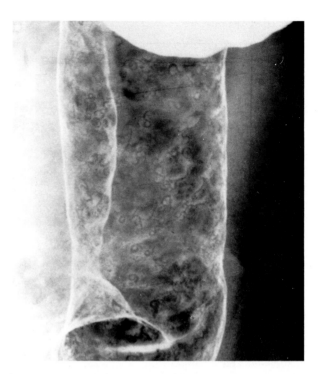

Fig. 46-65 This double-contrast enema study shows *Trichuris trichiura* worms outlined in the descending colon.
Courtesy of Prof. B.J. Cremin.

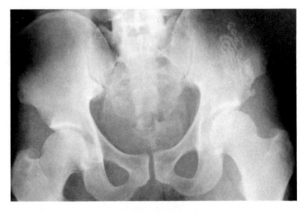

Fig. 46-66 A calcified (dead) adult female *Dracunculus* in the soft tissues overlying the left ilium. This was a chance finding in a patient being examined because of an injury. Faint calcification, caused by schistosomiasis, can be seen in the bladder, another unexpected finding.
From Reeder MM, Palmer PES: *The radiology of tropical diseases*, Baltimore, 1981, Williams & Wilkins.

with vague pain and borborygmus, progressing through profuse diarrhea, to weight loss, anorexia, protein-losing enteropathy, and emaciation, with death in up to 35% of the males in some outbreaks.[205,206] For some reason, the disease is both more common and more severe in males, with a usual mortality of around 10%. Thiabendazole can bring about improvement.[205]

No natural animal reservoir has been found. All forms of the parasite (ova, larvae, and adult worms) are found at the same time in the intestine, suggesting that autoreinfection occurs. The adult worms burrow into the mucosa of the distal jejunum and proximal ileum.

Radiologic findings include variable dilatation of segments of the small bowel, with some nonspecific segmentation and flocculation. The most characteristic radiologic finding appears to be thickening of the valvulae conniventes of the distal jejunum and proximal ileum.[206] The disease is seen predominantly in inhabitants of the Philippines and Thailand.

ANGIOSTRONGYLIASIS

One species of the *Angiostrongylus* parasite can set up residence in the distal branches of the human superior mesenteric artery, but most species colonize the vascular system of the rat. *A. costaricensis* may produce symptoms by causing thrombosis, and hence ischemia and infarction, or its eggs may be deposited in the wall of the distal ileum and cecum, producing nodular granulomas.[205] Such masses may bring about subacute intestinal obstruction or infarction of the bowel after the death of the parent intravascular parasite. As the name implies, this organism is most frequently seen in Costa Rica and Honduras and is most common in children. In a report from Australia, Spiruroidea physalopteridae was reported to cause infarcts and eosinophilic granulomas in the distal small bowel. Vascular embolization is also the mechanism.[205]

Cestodes (tapeworms)

Tapeworms are among man's oldest companions and may grow to 30 feet in length. Their existence has been known for millennia. The two most common ones are *Taenia saginata* and *T. solium*. Although many other tapeworms can infect humans, most do not have any radiologic significance; among these, heavy infestation of the fish tapeworm, *Diphyllobothrium latum* (found in freshwater fish and crustaceans), may cause mechanical intestinal obstruction and a background eosinophilia and anemia. None of the others has gastrointestinal significance.

The beef tapeworm, *T. saginata* (Figs. 46-67 and 46-68), is found throughout the world, sometimes in a high proportion of the population, as in Ethiopia. The pork tapeworm, *T. solium,* although also widespread, is much less common. Mixed infections may occur. The life cycles of the worms are similar, but the intermediate host of *T. saginata* is cattle and that of *T. solium* is pigs. The adult worm lives in the alimentary tract of humans, attached by its scolex to the mucosa, usually in the mid–small bowel. The worms have no alimentary tract, and they absorb nutrients through their surfaces from the content of the intestine. The eggs are passed in the feces and are then ingested by grazing cattle or pigs, where they hatch in the intestine of the intermediate host. Burrowing through the intestinal wall to reach a blood vessel or lymph channel, they enter striated muscles. There the larva develops into *Cysticercus bovis* in cattle and *C. cellulosae* in pigs. If the meat is eaten either raw or insufficiently cooked, the life cycle in humans starts again. Cysticerci are also found in cats, rats, monkeys, dogs, giraffes, buffaloes, llamas, and some antelope.

The laboratory diagnosis depends on the discovery of the ova, or proglottids, in the stools. Eosinophilia is common. Clinically, many patients show no significant illness. Others may complain of abdominal discomfort, loss of weight and appetite, indigestion, or diarrhea. The presence of multiple worms may occasionally cause obstruction, and pruritus ani is not uncommon.

The adult *T. saginata* organism is very seldom demonstrated radiologically[207,208] because it does not ingest contrast material. When seen, there is a long and gradually widening radiolucent line within the barium pattern, usually in

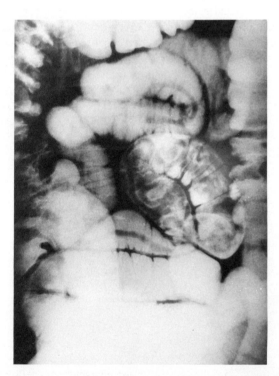

Fig. 46-67 The negative shadow produced by an adult *Taenia saginata* worm in the ileum of a 25-year-old Lebanese patient complaining of acute abdominal pain. When the worm was passed after treatment, it was 210 cm long.
Courtesy of Dr. Lawrence E. Fetterman.

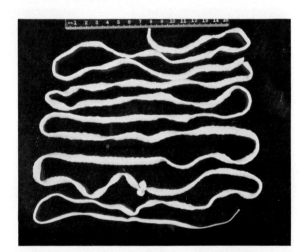

Fig. 46-68 Adult *Taenia saginata* worm. The head is at the bottom of the picture, and the worm gradually widens into hundreds of individual segments (proglottids). Worms 20 to 30 feet (6-9 meters) long have been recorded.
From Reeder MM, Palmer PES: *The radiology of tropical diseases,* Baltimore, 1981, Williams & Wilkins.

the jejunum or ileum. At its neck, it may be 1 to 2 mm wide, but distally it may be 12 mm or more.[207] It is often folded and reduplicated but is always continuous and may reach 20 or more feet in length.

The eggs of *T. solium* may accidentally be ingested by humans, who then unwittingly become the intermediate host for cysticercosis. The *C. cellulosae* cyst is an irritant to the host; it becomes encapsulated and surrounded by fibrous tissue and may eventually calcify, a process that can take 5 years. Whether it ultimately affects the host depends on the number and the location of the cysts. They are very common in muscle and usually produce no related symptoms, but cysts in the brain may cause epilepsy, and those in the spinal canal may obstruct the flow of cerebrospinal fluid. There are no gastrointestinal symptoms, but the typical calcified linear or oval cyst, which is 4 to 10 mm in length, may be found superimposed on the abdomen, particularly when the muscles of the back, flanks, or abdominal wall are heavily infested.[12,205]

Other tapeworms may affect humans, especially children in the tropics. These include *Hymenolepis nana,* as well as *Raillietina celebensis* in the Far East and Western Australia, and *Inermicapsifer madagascarensis* in East and Central Africa.[205]

ECHINOCOCCOSIS (HYDATID DISEASE)

There are two types of *Echinococcus* infections[209-240]: *E. granulosus* is the more common, and *E. multilocularis* the less common, though much more invasive and frequently resembling malignancy. *E. granulosus* infection causes the formation of large cysts and is found worldwide but is more common in temperate climates. The life cycle requires two hosts—a dog and a grazing animal, usually sheep, cattle, or pigs. It can also be found in wolves and some deer. The adult parasite is a tiny tapeworm, usually found by the hundreds or thousands in the small intestine of dogs. Excreted in the feces, the eggs contaminate wide areas of pasture and are subsequently ingested by the grazing animals. Humans become accidentally infected, either through direct contact with infected dogs or by ingesting food, water, or soil containing the eggs. Occasionally, the infection may be transmitted through the consumption of uncooked foods, such as salads.

In the human host, the external layers of the eggs are digested and the larvae migrate through the intestinal mucosa into the mesenteric veins and lymphatics, then to be carried to many different parts of the body. Because the liver acts as an effective filter, this is the most common site for cysts, exceeding 90% in some series. However, the larvae may lodge anywhere in the body, including the peritoneum, spleen, kidneys, brain, bones, heart, and muscles. Many larvae are overcome by the host reaction, but those that survive develop into tiny cysts containing a small amount of clear fluid. The cyst grows steadily until it becomes clinically evident. The average rate of growth is 1 to 3 cm a year but varies depending on the type of tissue surrounding it. Thus, the cysts grow more rapidly in the lung than in the liver. Each cyst has two walls—a thick outer laminated ectocyst and a more delicate inner membrane, the endocyst. As the cyst grows, a reaction takes place around it in the compressed host tissue, and this forms the third layer, the pericyst. The active part of the cyst is

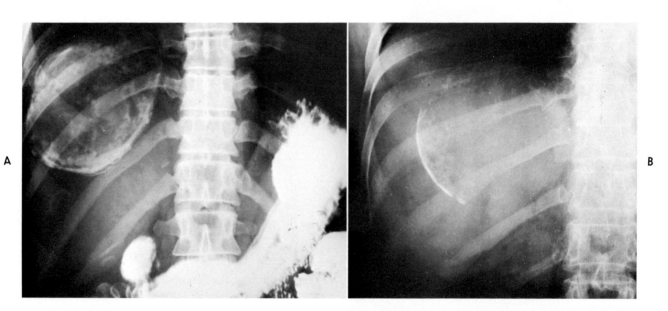

Fig. 46-69 Calcified *Echinococcus* cysts in the liver. **A,** A calcified cyst containing multiple daughter cysts found in a 37-old-year Basque woman. **B,** A segmentally calcified *Echinococcus* cyst in a young Greek woman.

the inner germinal epithelium with its brood capsules and scoleces, from which the new worms develop. The brood capsules usually detach from the germinal layer and may be found as "hydatid sand" at the bottom of the cyst, recognizable on ultrasonographic or CT scans. "Daughter" cysts may develop within the original cyst (Fig. 46-69, *A*), but they are usually thought to result from mechanical, chemical, or bacterial insult. CT scanning and ultrasonography have shown multiple septa, caused by these daughter cysts, within the overall hydatid outline.

Provided the hydatid cyst is contained within the pericyst, there are few local symptoms other than those due to the size of the cyst itself. Once the pericyst is damaged, infection nearly always ensues, and there may be a severe host reaction and sometimes fatal anaphylaxis. About 30% of the cysts die and may become partially or completely calcified, but a partially calcified cyst should not be regarded as harmless (Fig. 46-69).

Within the liver, most cysts are 10 cm or more in diameter before they are recognized clinically, but eventually there may be pressure on the biliary tract, with indigestion, nausea, or vomiting, and sometimes pain. Rupture can represent an acute emergency if the cysts break through into the lung or peritoneal cavity, sometimes causing anaphylaxis. On the other hand, hydatid infection can remain latent for many years and be discovered only accidentally. Although there are various serologic tests to detect the disease, none is 100% accurate, and multiple methods of detection may be necessary.

On plain films, these cysts may be seen to cause generalized enlargement of the liver or a localized bulge in the hepatic outline, with a hump in the diaphragm in some cases. They are usually spherical and sometimes distorted by the rib cage. In more than 50% of the cases, partial or crescentic calcification occurs in the cyst wall, or, if the cyst has been damaged, the calcification may depict a collapsed and amorphous state.[212] Angiography shows that the cysts are avascular, sometimes with a hypervascular rim in the capillary phase, but the findings are nonspecific, as are the scintigraphic findings. Ultrasonography, CT scanning, and MRI have made it possible to recognize small cysts and show that they are usually multiple (Fig. 46-70). The ultrasound appearances have been divided into various categories[213,215,233]:

1. Pure fluid. The cyst is sonolucent in this setting, with marked enhancement of the back wall echoes. The cysts are round and well defined. The small cysts are "punched out" and sonolucent, and the actual cyst wall may not be easily distinguished.

2. Fluid with a split wall. In this instance the cyst is less well rounded and sags. A floating membrane may be seen internally that is very characteristic of hydatid disease and suggests lowered intracystic pressure.

3. Both fluid and septa. When there are both fluid and septa, the cyst is usually well defined but divided into

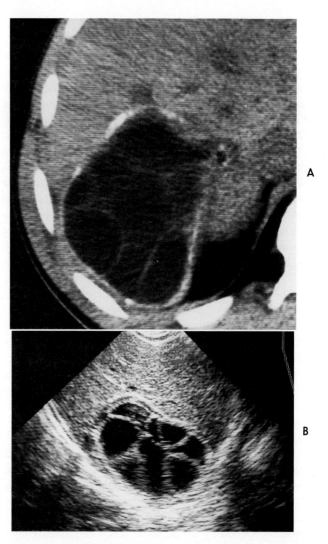

Fig. 46-70 A hydatid cyst in the liver with numerous daughter cysts. Calcification can be seen in the wall of the loculated cyst on this CT scan **(A),** and many germinal membranes and brood capsules of the individual daughter cysts can be seen on the ultrasound scan **(B).**
Courtesy of Dr. John R. Haaga.

sections of varying shapes, usually oval or rounded. The back echoes are enhanced, and there is a honeycomb image.

4. Irregular shape. Irregularly shaped cysts have a variable echo pattern and are usually round but rough in outline. They can be hypoechoic with irregular echoes, hyperechoic and solid without back wall shadows, or in an intermediate phase that may include both of these findings, often in clustered nodular groups.

5. Hyperechoic. Some cysts are very hyperechoic with a cone-shaped shadow, and only the thick reflecting front wall may be seen.

When there are multiple cysts, there may be considerable overlap. Most hydatid cysts are simple sonolucent cysts that are difficult to distinguish from simple liver cysts, hematoma, or abscess. If the collapsed membrane and septa are recognized, diagnosis is simplified. Sometimes the hydatid sand can be seen at the bottom, and, if this moves, it may account for a variation in appearance. Once the cyst is infected, recognition can be very difficult. Differentiating a hydatid cyst from a hepatoma based on the ultrasonographic findings is not easy. In countries where hepatomas are common, such tumors often appear as a large irregular echogenic mass with ill-defined and irregular margins, and often there are strong echoes within the mass. The European and North American variety of hepatoma is more homogeneous and more closely resembles a metastasis; differentiation from some hydatid cysts can then be difficult.

The CT findings are diagnostically very accurate (Fig. 46-71). The cysts are round, oval, or flattened if they are on the edge of the liver. The attenuation is similar to that of water. About 80% of the cysts have marginal calcification, and more than half have daughter cysts within them. The endocystic membrane can usually be recognized, and the contents are not always homogeneous, probably because of the hydatid sand. Contrast material seldom enhances the cysts unless there is marked compression of the host tissue.

On MRI studies the cysts are well demonstrated with spin-echo pulse sequences, and are equally well seen on both T1 and T2 images, so it is probably best to use both. A thin, low-intensity rim may surround the hydatid cysts and can be helpful in the differential diagnosis. This rim is probably caused by the pericyst, which is primarily composed of collagen.

The appearance of a hydatid cyst changes with treatment.

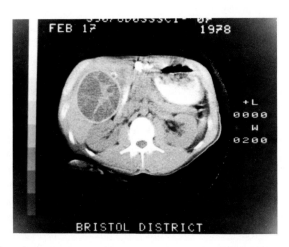

Fig. 46-71 Hydatid cyst within the liver, demonstrated by CT. The capsule is well seen, and loculations within the cyst are well demonstrated.

After drug therapy, the cyst may collapse or slowly shrink, with a decrease in tension within the cyst and a transonic halo. Daughter cysts tend to lose their clarity and even disappear. Changes can also happen when there is trauma and the cyst ruptures, in which case numerous daughter cysts may develop. At surgery, cysts may either be removed or invaginated in the residual space, which may then be filled with omentum. Serial ultrasonography or CT scanning is needed to watch the shrinkage and resulting fibrosis, which may take up to 2 years. Although ultrasonograms may show a decrease in cyst size, detachment of the cyst membrane, and other signs of regression, the effect of drug therapy is widely variable, and some cysts will continue to grow despite treatment. Initial regression may be followed by further progression. Therefore, prolonged observation is needed.

Hydatid cysts may form in the pancreas and show round, partially calcified cystic lesions. Solitary or even multiple cysts in the spleen or kidney may calcify and have to be differentiated from other cysts, few of which have septa or calcify to the same extent. Cysts elsewhere cause pressure symptoms; some present as achalasia resulting from pressure exerted near the cardia, and others press on the rectum or cause symptoms elsewhere in the alimentary tract.

E. multilocularis is a very different disease.[12] It is probably most common in eastern Europe and Turkey but is found in Canada, Alaska, and parts of China and central Asia. It is particularly prevalent in areas of cold and high altitude. The life cycle is much the same as that for *E. granulosus,* with dogs, cats, or foxes usually involved. Although in the beginning it is a benign and afebrile infection, the outcome is usually fatal. Macroscopically it is very difficult to distinguish from malignancy, particularly in the liver, kidney, or bone. There are multiple cystic spaces, about 0.5 cm in diameter, that produce a honeycomb or spongy appearance (alveolar echinococcosis). Histologically, there is necrosis, a granulomatous inflammatory reaction, and membranes around the multiple small cysts. Clinical signs are those of an enlarging mass within the liver and consist of portal hypertension, splenomegaly, jaundice, and then ascites.

The radiologic picture of the chronic granulomatous reaction and the multiple small cysts is characteristic. In nearly 70% of the infections, there are numerous small calcified spheres with radiolucent centers, ranging from 2 to 4 mm in diameter. Recognition on ultrasonograms is not always easy because the small cysts are inhomogeneous and may not be easily distinguished from liver tissue. There may be a great variation in the attenuation on CT scans ranging from +5 to +60 Hounsfield units. Calcification can be observed around the edges of cysts, but sometimes there is an amorphous, plaquelike, racemose pattern throughout. This combination of clustered microcalcification with necrosis is very suggestive of *E. multilocularis* infection, but it is not an easy diagnosis. In one series reported from Turkey, 60% of the cases were diagnosed as liver malignancy.

Both varieties of hydatid disease can be diagnosed by endoscopic retrograde cholangiopancreatography, which is most commonly performed when the presenting symptom is jaundice. However, CT scanning and ultrasonography are the preferable imaging investigations unless the plain radiographs show a typical calcified cyst or group of cysts. When found during an abdominal examination, it is essential to remember that hydatid disease can occur anywhere in the body. One cyst is unlikely to be the end of the patient's problems.

Trematodes (flukes)

LIVER FLUKES

Of the flukes that infect the biliary tract, three are most important. The Oriental liver fluke, *Clonorchis sinensis,* occurs throughout East Asia, Japan, Korea, coastal China, Taiwan, and Southeast Asia. The liver fluke, *Fasciola hepatica,* is found in Europe, the one-time U.S.S.R., the Middle East, Asia, Africa, Australia, and Central and South America. *Opisthorchis felineus* occurs in central, eastern, and southern Europe, with isolated cases reported from India, Vietnam, North Korea, Japan, and the Philippines. *O. viverrini* is important in northeast Thailand and in Laos, where it is surprisingly common.

Clonorchiasis. *Clonorchis sinensis* inhabits the bile ducts of humans, mammals, and birds. It is about 10 to 20 mm long, flat, and somewhat pointed. Its eggs are laid in the small biliary ducts and pass through the common bile duct into the duodenum and then the colon. Excreted in the feces, hatching occurs when the eggs are ingested by a snail of the family Buliminae. Further development of the miracidia within the snail takes 4 or 5 weeks. The resulting free-swimming cercariae penetrate the muscles of freshwater fish, particularly carp, and, after several weeks of further development, are once again infective when the fish is eaten raw or poorly cooked. The larvae then move up to the biliary tree in the host, using their suckers to do so, and mature into adult flukes. Secondary bacterial infection is common, but the clinical significance of clonorchiasis depends entirely on the extent of the infection. The flukes can persist for up to 20 years, and more than 21,000 have been found in some patients. It is not surprising that the pancreatic duct also becomes infected and that the flukes may be found in the stomach and duodenum or gallbladder.

So much irritation within the biliary tract leads to the development of calculi, acute suppurative cholangitis, recurrent pyogenic cholangitis, and acute pancreatitis. It is a major cause of cholangiocarcinoma. Biliary stasis and incomplete obstruction occur, and infection with *E. coli* or salmonellae is not uncommon. Multiple abscesses that originate in the biliary system may progress and cause a severe febrile illness with jaundice. Secondary infection with *Ascaris* is uncommon.

Clonorchiasis should be considered in any patient with liver disease, particularly anyone coming from the endemic areas of the Far East. The laboratory diagnosis is accomplished by the detection of the eggs either in feces or in bile or fluid after incubation. There is often an associated leukocytosis (over 30,000) and an eosinophilia of up to 40%. Surprisingly, the majority of infections are asymptomatic at first. Fever, indigestion, and pain in the right upper quadrant may then develop. This may progress to diarrhea, anorexia, and liver tenderness and enlargement. In the more advanced cases, the liver becomes cirrhotic, and there may be ascites and marked jaundice. The cause of death is usually the result of severe repeated infection or cholangiocarcinoma.

The flukes can be demonstrated by operative or transhepatic cholangiography, and occasionally by intravenous cholangiography, appearing as 1 to 2 cm curved or crescentic filling defects within dilated bile ducts.[12] Far more easily recognized are the features of severe cholangitis with biliary stasis, sludge, and stones accompanying dilatation and constriction of the bile ducts. These features, as well as the often associated hepatic abscesses, may be demonstrated by ultrasonography, CT, and MRI.[241] There are no findings specific to the abscess, except the associated cholangitis. In chest studies, nonspecific pulmonary alveolar densities have been described but exhibit no diagnostic characteristics.

Fascioliasis. Another live fluke, *Fasciola,* although it is common and causes clinical symptoms, has not been recognized reliably on radiologic examinations. However, the changes in the liver on CT have been described as characteristic.[242-244] There are nodular intrahepatic lesions with diminished attenuation, ranging in size from 4 to 10 mm but sometimes as large as 2 cm. In addition, branching lesions are sometimes seen. A contrast-enhanced CT examination furnishes better definition of the nodules. After treatment the lesions may either partially or completely disappear; however, there has also been a report of a spontaneous decrease in the size of one low-density area on a scan that occurred before treatment, despite the patient's continuing symptoms. CT scanning is therefore useful, not only for diagnosis but for the follow-up of patients with fascioliasis. There is no proved relationship between fascioliasis and carcinoma of the liver.

Opisthorchiasis. The *Opisthorchis* liver flukes are usually found in cats or fish-eating animals. *O. felineus* is the most common, but infection with *O. viverrini* is more readily recognized radiologically—especially in the population of Southeast Asia, where it is so prevalent. Similar infections have been reported in New Guinea and Ecuador. Humans are an accidental host and probably acquire it by eating infected pigs or fish. The life cycle is the same as that of *C. sinensis* and lasts about 4 months. The irritation in the biliary tract is more severe, with hypertrophy and thickening of the mucosa and duct walls, and considerable dilatation of the bile ducts up to 5 to 6 mm. There may be numerous parasites (8000 flukes), and these can cause mechanical obstruction and biliary stasis. Large cysts may develop, with a diameter of up to 7 cm or more, depending very much on the severity of the infection. Ascending cholangitis may often develop, spreading to cause hepatitis or multiple abscesses.[245] Rupture of such an abscess has been described. There is little doubt that opisthorchiasis predisposes to the development of cholangiocarcinoma, but, somewhat surprisingly, there is no further evidence that there is an increased incidence of cirrhosis of the liver in affected patients. Chronic cholecystitis does occur, but opisthorchiasis does not predispose to the development of biliary calculi. Jaundice is common and is especially likely when there is an hepatic malignancy.

Cholangiography, ultrasonography, or CT scanning may show multiple small dilatations of the intrahepatic bile ducts, with diffuse saccular changes appearing as the condition progresses. Eventually, there is marked cystic dilatation, and this combination of large areas of cystic dilatation with the presence of multiple small cysts is pathognomonic.[245] When there is cholangiocarcinoma, there is likely to be massive hepatomegaly, and such tumors are frequently multiple.[246] Although cholangiography can show long, slender filling defects in the bile ducts, the differential diagnosis of the actual parasite can be made only when the flukes have been recovered and examined.

Vascular flukes (schistosomiasis). Four species of *Schistosoma* cause significant infection in humans[247-262]: *S. haematobium, S. mansoni,* and *S. japonicum* are the most common and *S. intercalatum* is less so. Other schistosomes are parasitic for cattle or birds and occasionally are found in humans, though seldom cause significant symptoms in these instances and have not been described radiologically.

Bilharziasis, one of the synonyms for schistosomiasis, has been known for 5000 years and infects about 200 million persons worldwide. Strict hygiene would eliminate the infection within a generation. *S. haematobium* is common throughout Africa, the Mediterranean, and Southwest Asia; *S. mansoni* (Fig. 46-72) is more prevalent in North Africa, Arabia, the West Indies, and the northern parts of South America; and *S. japonicum* occurs in China, Japan, Taiwan, the Philippines, and the Celebes. Concomitant infection with *S. haematobium* and *S. mansoni* is not uncommon, particularly in North Africa. *S. intercalatum* is found only in central and equatorial Africa. Because there are many different reactions to the different species, parasitologists have tried to divide them into separate subcategories, but this is of no importance to radiologists. Infection with schistosomes is so common in many parts of the world that it is part of normal existence, reinfection is usual, and local people disregard many of the symptoms.

The pattern of development is similar for all varieties. The flukes live in pairs and copulate in the portal vein or in its mesenteric tributaries (or the vesical plexus for *S.*

haematobium). They are strictly intravenous parasites. Females leave the male after 1 to 20 years and swim upstream to reach the smallest venule possible, where the eggs are deposited. This is in the wall of the bladder or ureter for *S. haematobium,* the rectum or large intestine for *S. mansoni,* and the small intestine, proximal colon, or rectum for *S. japonicum* and *S. intercalatum.* This division is not absolute, in that *S. haematobium* can infect the intestines. The cycle then depends on the eggs reaching water and finding suitable snail hosts, with the subsequent development of cercariae, which penetrate the unbroken skin or buccal mucous membrane to reenter the host. Then, carried through the lymphatics and veins, the larvae eventually reach the portal system and liver, where they mature. The flukes may live for 10 to 15 years and, although there is variation for each species, may produce an enormous number of eggs. It is the eggs or cercariae that are responsible for most of the clinical problems. Seldom do liver flukes cause any symptoms or radiologic findings unless they embolize during treatment and produce an inflammatory reaction when dead. The clinical disease is much more commonly due to the presence of eggs or miracidia. The characteristic histologic lesion is a severe granuloma with the formation of a nodular scar, inside which is usually a calcified egg. There are many factors in the host tissue reaction, but all lead to significant fibrosis, and, if this occurs in a vessel, particularly in the lungs, the intima and wall can be damaged. Because recanalization of the granuloma can occur, small arteriovenous fistulas or even an aneurysm may develop.

S. mansoni and *S. japonicum* parasites mainly affect the alimentary tract, and the discharge of hundreds of eggs through the intestinal mucosa causes a marked fibrotic reaction. If the eggs cannot escape, more inflammation forms around them, which causes the eggs to die and yet further granuloma tissue to form. This may develop into polyps, strictures, or ulceration. Unfortunately, not all the eggs are trapped in the mesenteric venules of the colon or small bowel, or the urinary tract. Many are forced back into the portal venous system, then penetrate the walls of the small portal veins and lodge in the periportal connective tissue. Once again there is a marked inflammatory reaction, which causes multiple granulomas of the liver and fibrous tissue to form, followed by obstruction of the small portal veins, before the eggs enter the hepatic sinusoids and produce a presinusoidal block. Portal hypertension therefore occurs long before there is any change in liver function. The vascular changes consist of a combination of granulomas, sclerosis, narrowing, and thrombophlebitis, with the development of new capillary networks that form intrahepatic shunts. Extensive portal systemic collaterals may also form outside the liver, with resultant increased pressure in the hepatic artery. Late in the disease, the fibrosis becomes more generalized and the liver becomes smaller.

The earliest radiographic findings in the colon consist of an edematous mucosa, with mural spicules and tiny ulcers.

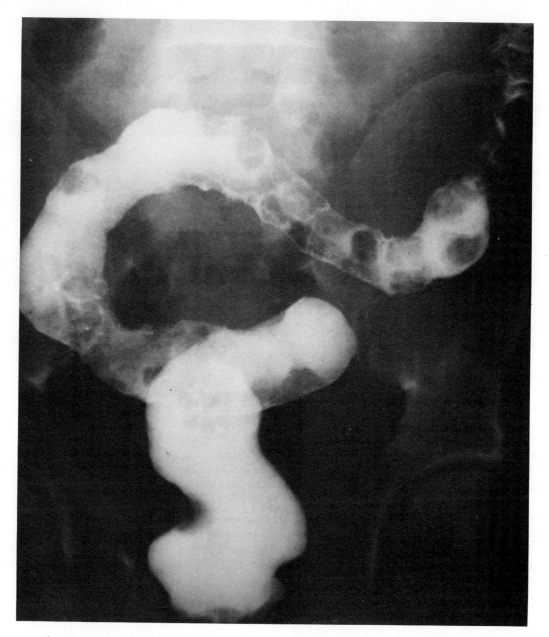

Fig. 46-72 Multiple small filling defects in the rectum and sigmoid colon in a patient infected with *Schistosoma mansoni*.

There is often marked spasm and then loss of haustration, particularly in the descending and sigmoid colon. If there is heavy and chronic infection, multiple polyps may develop, particularly in the rectum and sigmoid and descending colon. They start as submucosal granulomas, which lift the overlying mucosa and are very friable and liable to bleed. They may become quite large and even cause obstruction or intussusception.[256] The extent of polyp formation varies significantly in different countries, being fairly common in Egypt and Arabia, particularly when there are combined *S. mansoni* and *S. haematobium* infections. Polyps are much less common in the Americas, in whom ste-

nosing granulomas with pericolic infiltration and strictures are more likely. A pericolic schistosomal abscess (a schistosoma or bilharzioma) may appear in the bowel wall or the mesentery and simulate carcinoma.[261]

S. japonicum causes similar changes in the small bowel. The flukes live in the superior mesenteric veins and deposit their ova within the small bowel. The changes are very widespread and result from the submucosal granulomas (which can be seen on biopsy specimens) and enlarged lymph nodes. As elsewhere the end result is fibrosis and constriction, and, because this affects the mesentery, the duodenal loop may be deformed, not only by intrinsic granulomas but also by the adhesions. In the early stages the mucosa is edematous, coarse, and irregular, particularly in the upper jejunum. There is decreased motility because of the thickening, and then relaxation occurs and dilatation ensues. There is often excess mucus.[262]

The changes in the portal system that lead to portal hypertension, marked splenomegaly, and ascites are similar for both *S. mansoni* and *S. japonicum* infections. Esophageal and gastric varices develop and may be very prominent. They are easily demonstrated by barium swallow studies, splenoportography, or endoscopy.

CT scanning has occasionally depicted calcification around the rectum and presacral tissues. It is important to remember that this calcification is within the ova and not in the fibrous tissue or granulomas. Similar calcification develops in multiple areas throughout the colon, which is most easily seen when the colon is distended; it assumes a laminar pattern, which becomes more amorphous as the bowel collapses. Under experimental conditions it has been found to appear about 60 days after infection, but it is neither an indicator of severity nor of the activity of the parasite. It is only an incidental finding.

Schistosomiasis is a complex and multifocal disease and is best understood if one realizes that it is primarily a disease of the vascular system that causes a severe granulomatous reaction at various stages in its development. This occurs when the fluke or ova are dead but seldom while either is alive.[12] This is one of the many ways the schistosome is unique and contradictory.

Other flukes. Four other flukes cause disease in humans, but there are no descriptions of their radiologic characteristics. *Fasciolopsis buski, Echninostoma ilocanum, Metagonimus yokogawi,* and *Gastrodiscoides hominis* affect the duodenum, jejunum, and right colon, respectively, and are found in countries from Southeast Asia and the Pacific to Egypt.

Pentastomida

Two-tongue worms infect humans, gaining entry through the alimentary tract but causing no gastrointestinal symptoms. When dead, they often become calcified within the peritoneum, liver, or spleen, and should be easily recognized and differentiated from calculi or calcified lymph nodes.

Armillifer armillatus and *A. moniliformis* cause porocephaliasis or pentastomiasis in humans. These parasites live in the trachea and bronchi of snakes, particularly pythons, adders, and cobras. *A. armillatus* infections are most common in West Africa and much less common on the continent. *A. moniliformis* occurs in the python and other snakes of India, Malaysia, Southeast Asia, China, Indonesia, and the Philippines. The eggs may be ingested in contaminated water or from the eating of snake meat. The larvae are then freed in the intestine and come to lie under the peritoneum, molting to become nymphs. They may mi-

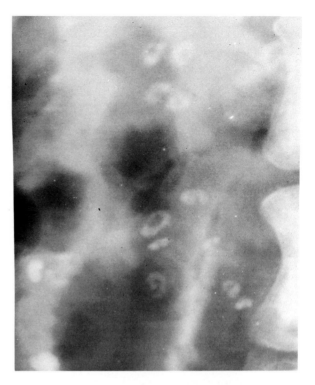

Fig. 46-73 Calcified *Armillifer armillatus* nymphs in the peritoneum.

grate across the diaphragm to the pleural cavity. They can also be found within the liver or spleen, but their route is not understood.

The presence of *Armillifer* may be of some diagnostic significance if there is a heavy infection because the larvae may cause such an acute peritoneal irritation that an abdominal emergency such as appendicitis or a perforated viscus may be suspected. The organisms have been seen at laparotomy moving beneath the peritoneum. The radiologic finding of curved, calcified nymphs, which are scattered throughout the peritoneum, pleura, liver, and spleen, is characteristic[263,264] (Fig. 46-73). They are not found in muscle and should be easily distinguished from cysticercosis, which predominantly affects peripheral muscles.

REFERENCES
General references

1. Berk RN, Lasser EC: *Radiology of the ileocecal area*, Philadelphia, 1975, WB Saunders.
2. Binford CH, Connor DH, eds: Pathology of tropical and extraordinary diseases, Washington, DC, 1976, Armed Forces Institute of Pathology.
3. Calder JF, DeCock K, Stass B: Diagnostic ultrasound in abdominal disease. First experiences in Kenya, *E Afr Med J* 57:607, 1980.
4. Cockshott P, Middlemiss H: *Clinical radiology in the tropics*, London, 1979, Churchill Livingstone.
5. Davey WW, ed: *Companion to surgery in Africa.* Edinburgh, 1986, E&S Livingston.
6. Eisenberg RL: *Gastrointestinal radiology*, ed 2, Philadelphia, 1989, JP Lippincott.

7. Farman J, Rabinowitz JG, Meyers MA: *Roentgenology of infectious colitis,* AJR 119:375, 1973.

8. Palmer PE: Diagnostic imaging in parasitic infections, *Pediatr Clin North Am* 32(4):1019, 1985.

9. Reeder MM: Parasitic diseases. In Marshak RH, Lindner AE, Maklansky D, eds: *Radiology of the colon,* Philadelphia, 1980, WB Saunders.

10. Reeder MM, Hamilton LC: Radiologic diagnosis of tropical diseases of the gastrointestinal tract, *Radiol Clin North Am* 7:57, 1969.

11. Reeder MM, Hamilton LC: Tropical diseases of the colon, *Semin Roentgenol* 3:62, 1968.

12. Reeder MM, Palmer PES: *The radiology of tropical diseases with epidemiological, pathological and clinical correlations,* Baltimore, 1981, Williams & Wilkins.

13. Stoll, NR: This wormy world, *J Parasitol* 33:1, 1947 (updated by WHO under the same title, 1984).

14. Strickland GT: *Hunter's tropical medicine,* ed 7, Philadelphia, 1991, WB Saunders.

15. Tedesco R, Moore S: Infectious diseases mimicking inflammatory bowel disease, *Am Surg* 48:243, 1982.

16. Thoeni RF, Margulis AR: Radiology in inflammatory disease of the colon: an area of increased interest for the modern clinician, *Invest Radiol* 4:281, 1980.

17. Wilcocks C, Manson-Bahr PEC: *Manson's tropical disease,* ed 17, Baltimore, 1972, Williams & Wilkins.

Bacterial infections

18. Abrams JS, Holden WD: Tuberculosis of the gastrointestinal tract, *Arch Surg* 89:282, 1964.

19. Anscombe AR, Keddie NC, Schofield PF: Caecal tuberculosis, *Gut* 8:337, 1967.

20. Ball PAJ: Abdominal tuberculosis. In Davey WW, ed: *Companion to surgery in Africa,* Edinburg, 1968, E&S Livingstone.

21. Balthazar EJ, Bryk D: Segmental tuberculosis of the colon: radiographic features in seven cases, *Gastrointest Radiol* 5:75, 1980.

22. Bhansali SK: Abdominal tuberculosis. Experiences with 300 cases, *Am J Gastroenterol* 67:324, 1977.

23. Black GA, Carsky EW: Duodenal tuberculosis, *AJR* 131:329, 1978.

24. Brenner SM, Annes G, Parker JG: Tuberculosis colitis simulating nonspecific granulomatous disease of the colon, *Am J Dig Dis* 15:85, 1970.

25. Burke GJ, Zafar SA: Problems in distinguishing tuberculosis of bowel from Crohn's disease in Asians, *Br Med J* 4:395, 1975.

26. Carrera GF, Young S, Lewicki AM: Intestinal tuberculosis, *Gastrointest Radiol* 1:147, 1976.

27. Chazan BI, Aitchison JD: Gastric tuberculosis, *Br Med J* 2:1288, 1960.

28. El Masri SH et al: Abdominal tuberculosis in Sudanese patients, *East Afr Med J* 54:319, 1977.

29. Gaines W, Steinbach HL, Lowenhaupt E: Tuberculosis of the stomach, *Radiology* 58:808, 1952.

30. Gershon-Cohen J, Kremens V: X-ray studies of the ileocecal valve in ileocecal tuberculosis, *Radiology* 62:251, 1954.

31. Granet E: Intestinal tuberculosis: a clinical, roentgenological and pathological study of 2086 patients affected with pulmonary tuberculosis, *Am J Dig Dis* 2:209, 1935.

32. Gupta SK et al: Duodenal tuberculosis, *Clin Radiol* 39:159, 1988.

33. Herlinger H: Angiography in the diagnosis of ileocecal tuberculosis, *Gastrointest Radiol* 2:371, 1978.

34. Hughes HJ, Carr DT, Geraci JE: Tuberculous peritonitis: a review of 34 cases with emphasis on the diagnostic aspects, *Dis Chest* 38:42, 1960.

35. Kolawole TM, Lewis EA: Radiologic study of tuberculosis of the abdomen, *AJR* 123:348, 1975.

36. Lee DH, Lim JH, Ko YT, Yoon Y: Sonographic findings in tuberculous peritonitis of wet-ascitic type, *Clin Radiol* 44:306, 1991.

37. Marshak RH, Lindner AE: *Radiology of the small intestine,* ed 2, Philadelphia, 1976, WB Saunders.

38. McDonald JB, Middleton PJ: Tuberculosis of the colon simulating carcinoma, *Radiology* 118:293, 1976.

39. Mitchell RS, Bristol LJ: Intestinal tuberculosis: an analysis of 346 cases diagnosed by routine intestinal radiography in 5,529 admissions for pulmonary tuberculosis, 1924-1949, *Am J Med Sci* 227:241, 1954.

40. Paterson DE: Tuberculosis of the upper alimentary tract. In Middlemiss H, ed: *Tropical radiology,* London, 1961, William Heinemann.

41. Pinto RS, Zausner J, Beranbaum ER: Gastric tuberculosis. Report of a case with discussion of angiographic findings, *AJR* 110:808, 1970.

42. Thoeni R, Margulis A: Gastrointestinal tuberculosis, *Semin Roentgenol* 14:283, 1979.

43. Vaidya MG, Sodhi JS: Gastrointestinal tract tuberculosis: a study of 102 cases including 55 hemicolectomies, *Clin Radiol* 29:189, 1978.

44. Werbeloff L et al: The radiology of tuberculosis of the gastrointestinal tract, *Br J Radiol* 46:329, 1973.

45. Bohrer SP: Typhoid perforation of the ileum, *Br J Radiol* 39:37, 1966.

46. Chèrigiè E et al: Aspect radiologique du grêle chez les typhiques, *J Radiol Electrol* 34:522, 1953.

47. Cockshott WP: Typhoid. In Schinz HR, ed: *Roentgen diagnosis,* ed 2, vol 3, New York, 1969, Grune & Stratton.

48. Elegbeleye OO: Typhoid fever in Lagos, Nigeria, *West Indian Med J* 25:39, 1976.

49. Huckstep RL: *Typhoid fever and other salmonella infections,* Edinburgh, 1962, E & S Livingstone.

50. Hunter GW III, Swartzwelder JC, Clyde DF: *Tropical medicine,* ed 5, Philadelphia, 1976, WB Saunders.

51. Pontes JF: Disorders of the small intestine, *Ciba Clin Symp* 12:107, 1960.

52. Rappaprot EM, Rappaport EO: Typhoid enterocolitis simulating chronic bacillary dysentery: report of a case with cure by chloromycetin, *N Engl J Med* 242:698, 1950.

53. Silverman DN, Leslie A: Simulation of chronic bacterial dysentery by paratyphoid B infection, *Gastroenterology* 4:53, 1945.

54. Slomic AM, Rousseau B: *Salmonella* colitis: two cases of a milder form, *Ann Radiol* 19:431, 1976.

55. Wilcocks C, Manson-Bahr PH: *Manson's tropical diseases: a manual of diseases of warm climates,* ed 17, London, 1976, Baillière Tindall.

56. Christie AB: Bacillary dysentery, *Br Med J* 2:285, 1968.

57. Dammin GJ: Shigellosis. In Binford CH, Connor DH, eds: *Pathology of tropical and extraordinary diseases,* Washington, D.C., 1976, Armed Forces Institute of Pathology.

58. DeLorimier AA et al: *Clinical roentgenology,* vol 4, Springfield, IL, 1956, Charles C Thomas.

59. Farman J et al: Roentgenology of infectious colitis, *AJR* 119:375, 1973.

60. Hunter GW III et al: *Tropical medicine,* ed 5, Philadelphia, 1976, WB Saunders.

61. Schinz HR et al: *Roentgen-diagnostics,* vol 4, New York, 1954, Grune & Stratton.

62. Teplick JG, Haskin ME: *Roentgenologic diagnosis,* ed 2, Philadelphia, 1974, WB Saunders.

63. Kollitz JPM, Davis GB, Berk RM: *Campylobacter* colitis: a common form of infectious colitis, *Gastrointest Radiol* 6:227, 1981.

64. Gardiner R, Stevenson G: The colitides, *Radiol Clin North Am* 20(4):797, 1982.

65. Benner EJ, Tellman WH: Pseudomembranous colitis as a sequel to oral lincomycin therapy, *Am J Gastroenterol* 54:55, 1970.

66. Birnbaum D, Laufer A, Freund M: Pseudomembranous enterocolitis: a clinicopathologic study, *Gastroenterology* 41:345, 1961.

67. Brown CH, Ferrante WA, Davis WD Jr: Toxic dilatation of the colon complicating pseudomembranous enterocolitis, *Am J Dig Dis* 13:813, 1968.
68. Ecker JA et al: Pseudomembranous enterocolitis—an unwelcome gastrointestinal complication of antibiotic therapy, *Am J Gastroenterol* 54:214, 1970.
69. Gildenhorn HL, Springer EB, Amromin GD: Necrotizing enteropathy: roentgenographic features, *AJR* 88:942, 1962.
70. Goulston SJ, McGovern VJ: Pseudomembranous colitis, *Gut* 6:207, 1965.
71. Groll A et al: Fulminating noninfective pseudomembranous colitis, *Gastroenterology* 58:88, 1970.
72. LaMont JT: Bacterial infections of the colon. In Yamada ed:, *Textbook of gastroenterology*, Philadelphia, 1991, JB Lippincott.
73. McFarlan D, Mulligan RE, Kwok RY et al: Nosocomial acquisition of *Clostridium difficile* infection, *N Engl J Med* 320:340, 1989.
74. Reiner L, Schlesinger MJ, Miller GM: Pseudomembranous colitis following aureomycin and chloramphenicol, *AMA Arch Pathol* 54:39, 1952.
75. Teasley DG, Olson MM, Gebbhard RL, et al: Prospective randomized trial of metronidazole and vancomycin against *Clostridium difficile*–associated diarrhoea and colitis, *Lancet* 2:1043, 1983.
76. Gorbach SL et al: Travellers' diarrhea and toxigenic *E. coli*, *N Engl J Med* 292:933, 1975.
77. Preventing travellers diarrhea, *Lancet* 2:144, 1988 (editorial).
78. Dupont HL, Ericsson CD, Johnson PC et al: Prevention of traveller's diarrhea by the tablet formulation of bismuth subsalicylate, *JAMA* 257:1347, 1987.
79. Graham DY: *Helicobacter pylori:* its epidemiology and its role in duodenal ulcer disease, *J Gastroenterol Hepatol* 6:105, 1991.
80. Rauws EA, Tytgat GN: Cure of duodenal ulcer associated with eradication of *Helicobacter pylori*, *Lancet* 335:1233, 1990.
81. Marshall BJ, Goodwin CS, Warren RJ et al: Prospective double blind trial of duodenal ulcer relapse after eradication of *Campylobacter pylori*, *Lancet* 2:1437, 1988.

Chlamydial infections

82. Annamunthodo H: Rectal lymphogranuloma venereum in Jamaica, *Dis Colon Rectum* 4:17, 1961.
83. Annamunthodo H, Marryatt J: Barium studies in intestinal lymphogranuloma venereum, *Br J Radiol* 34:53, 1961.
84. Davey WW: *Companion to surgery in Africa*, London, 1968, E & S Livingstone.
85. Helper M, Szilagyi DE: Venereal lymphogranulomatous rectal stricture, *AJR* 48:179, 1942.
86. Klein I: Roentgen study of lymphogranuloma venereum: report of 24 cases, *AJR* 51:70, 1944.
87. Pessel JF: Lymphogranuloma venereum. In Bockus HL, ed: *Gastroenterology*, ed 2, vol 2, Philadelphia, 1967, WB Saunders.
88. Reeder MM, Palmer PES: *The radiology of tropical diseases, with epidemiological, pathological and clinical correlation*, Baltimore, 1981, Williams & Wilkins.
89. Rendich RA, Poppel MH: Lymphogranuloma of the colon, *Radiology* 33:472, 1939.
90. Spiesman MG et al: Lymphogranuloma inguinale: rectal stricture and prestricture, *Am J Dig Dis* 3:931, 1937.
91. Steinert R: Stricture of the rectum in lymphopathia venerea and its roentgenologic aspects, *Acta Radiol* 21:368, 1940.
92. Wright LT et al: Lymphogranulomatous strictures of the rectum: rèsumè of 476 cases, *Arch Surg* 53:499, 1946.
93. Brabander JO et al: Intestinal moniliasis in adults, *Can Med Assoc J* 77:478, 1957.
94. Craig JM, Farber S: The development of disseminated visceral mycosis during therapy for acute leukemia, *Am J Pathol* 29:601, 1953.
95. Goldberg HI, Dodds WJ: Cobblestone esophagus due to monilial infection, *AJR* 104:608, 1968.

96. Kaufman SA et al: Esophageal moniliasis, *Radiology* 75:726, 1960.
97. Reeder MM, Palmer PES: *The radiology of tropical diseases, with epidemiological, pathological and clinical correlation*, Baltimore, 1981, Williams & Wilkins.
98. Roberts L, Gibbons R, Gibbons G, Rice R, Thompson W: Adult esophageal candidiasis: a radiographic spectrum, *Radiographics* 7:289, 1987.
99. Rogers KB: Candida infections in paediatrics. In Winner HI, Hurley R, eds: *Symposium on* Candida *infections*. London, 1966, E & S Livingstone.
100. Sanders E et al: Monilial esophagitis in a patient with hemoglobin SC disease: demonstration of esophageal motor abnormality by cineradiofluorography, *Ann Intern Med* 57:650, 1962.
101. Smith JM: Mycoses of the alimentary tract, *Gut* 10:1035, 1969.
102. Winner HI, Hurley R: *Candida albicans*, London, 1964, J & A Churchill.
103. Bank S et al: Histoplasmosis of the small bowel with "giant" intestinal villi and secondary protein losing enteropathy, *Am J Med* 39:492, 1965.
104. Dietz MW: Ileocecal histoplasmosis, *Radiology* 91:285, 1968.
105. Henderson RG et al: *Histoplasma capsulatum* as cause of chronic ulcerative enteritis, *JAMA* 118:885, 1942.
106. Lee KR et al: The radiology corner. Gastrointestinal histoplasmosis, roentgenographic, clinical and pathological correlation, *Am J Gastroenterol* 63:255, 1975.
107. Negroni P: *Histoplasmosis: diagnosis and treatment*, rev ed, Springfield, IL, 1965, Charles C Thomas.
108. Perez CA et al: Some clinical and radiographic features of gastrointestinal histoplasmosis, *Radiology* 86:482, 1966.
109. Shull HJ: Human histoplasmosis: disease with protean manifestations often with digestive system involvement, *Gastroenterology* 25:582, 1953.
110. Silverman FN et al: Histoplasmosis, *Am J Med* 19:410, 1955.

Unknown etiology

111. Caldwell WI et al: The importance and reliability of the radiographic examination of the small bowel in patients with tropical sprue, *Radiology* 84:227, 1965.
112. Cockshott WP: Tropical sprue. In Rigler LG, ed: *Textbook of roentgen diagnosis*, ed 2, vol 3, New York, 1969, Grune & Stratton.
113. Floch MH, Caldwell WL, Sheehy TW: Histopathologic interpretation of small bowel roentgenography in tropical sprue, *AJR* 87:709, 1962.
114. Laws JW et al: Correlation of radiological and histological findings in idiopathic steatorrhea, *Br Med J* 1:1311, 1963.
115. Marshak RH, Lindner AE: Malabsorption syndrome, *Semin Roentgenol* 1:138, 1966.
116. Marshak RH, Lindner AE: *Radiology of the small intestine*, ed 2, Philadelphia, 1976, WB Saunders.
117. Misra RC et al: Correlation of clinical, biochemical, radiological, and histological findings in tropical sprue, *J Trop Med Hyg* 70:6, 1967.
118. Palmer ED: *Functional gastrointestinal disease*, Baltimore, 1967, Williams & Wilkins.
119. Paterson EE et al: Radiodiagnostic problems in malabsorption, *Br J Radiol* 38:181, 1965.
120. Reeder MM, Palmer PES: *The radiology of tropical diseases, with epidemiological, pathological and clinical correlation*, Baltimore, 1981, Williams & Wilkins.
121. Thomas G, Clain DJ: Endemic tropical sprue in Rhodesia, *Gut* 17:877, 1976.

Parasitic diseases

122. Binford MC, Connor DM: *Pathology of tropical and extraordinary diseases*, Washington, DC, 1976, The Armed Forces Institute of Pathology.

123. Chunge CN et al: Other parasitic diseases found in patients with visceral leishmaniasis, *E Afr Med J* 62:118, 1985.

124. Dalrymple RB et al: Hyperechoic liver abscesses. Unusual ultrasonic appearances, *Clin Radiol* 33:541, 1982.

125. Iarotski LS, Davis A: The schistosomiasis problem in the world: the results of a WHO questionnaire survey, *Bull WHO* 114:59:1981.

126. Manson-Bahr PH: *Manson's tropical diseases*, ed 15, London, 1960, Cassell.

127. Ralls WP et al: Pattern of resolution in successfully treated hepatic abscesses. Sonographic evaluation, *Radiology* 149:541, 1983.

128. Walsh JA, Warren KS: Selective primary health care: an interim strategy for disease control in developing countries, *N Engl J Med* 301:967, 1979.

129. World Health Organization: *Intestinal protozoan and helminthic infections,* technical report series 666, Geneva, 1981, World Health Organization.

130. Barker EM: Colonic perforations in amebiasis, *S Afr Med J* 32:634, 1958.

131. Boultbee JE, Simjee AE, Rooknooden F, Engelbrecht ME: Experiences with grey scale ultrasonography in hepatic amoebiasis, *Clin Radiol* 30:683, 1979.

132. Cardoso JM, Kimura K, Stoopen M et al: Radiology of invasive amebiasis of the colon, *AJR* 182:935, 1977.

133. Juniper K Jr: Acute amebic colitis, *Am J Med* 33:377, 1962.

134. Kern P et al: Hepatic amoebic abscess. Ultrasonographic and clinical follow up studies in 20 patients, *Ultraschall Med* 3:7, 1982.

135. Recio PM: Ameboma of the colon, *Dis Colon Rectum* 8:205, 1965.

136. Rogers LF, Ralls PW, Boswell WD et al: Amebiasis: unusual radiographic manifestations, *AJR* 135:1253, 1980.

137. Weinfeld A: Roentgen appearance of intestinal amebiasis, *AJR* 96:311, 1966.

138. Anselmi A et al: Cardiovascular radiology in acute and chronic Chagas' myocardiopathy. Morphologic and dynamic study of the cardiac contour correlated with the histologic changes observed in myocardiopathies attributed to *Schizotrypanum cruzi, Am Heart J* 73:626, 1967.

139. Atias A et al: Megaesophagus, megacolon, and Chagas' disease in Chile, *Gastroenterology* 44:433, 1963.

140. Brasil A: Aperistalsis of the esophagus, *Rev Bras Gastroenterol* 7:21, 1955.

141. Dantas RO: Idiopathic achalasia and chagasic megaesophagus, *J Clin Gastroenterol* 10:13, 1988.

142. de Rezende JM, Moreira H: Chagasic megaesophagus and megacolon. Historical review and present concepts. *Arq Gastroenterol* 25:32, 1988.

143. Ferreira-Santos R: Aperistalsis of the esophagus and colon (megaesophagus and megacolon) etiologically related to Chagas' disease, *Am J Dig Dis* 6:700, 1961.

144. Ferreira-Santos R, Carril CF: Acquired megacolon in Chagas' disease, *Dis Colon Rectum* 7:353, 1964.

145. Koberle F: Megaesophagus, *Gastroenterology* 34:460, 1958.

146. Koberle F: Enteromegaly and cardiomegaly in Chagas' disease, *Gut* 4:399, 1963.

147. Lopes ER: Megaesophagus, megacolon and cancer, *Rev Soc Bras Med Trop* 21:91, 1988.

148. Reeder MM, Hamilton LC: Tropical diseases of the colon, *Semin Roentgenol* 3:62, 1968.

149. Reeder MM, Hamilton LC: Radiologic diagnosis of tropical diseases of the gastrointestinal tract, *Radiol Clin North Am* 7:57, 1969.

150. Reeder MM, Palmer PES: *The radiology of tropical diseases, with epidemiological, pathological and clinical correlation*, Baltimore, 1981, Williams & Wilkins.

151. Reeder MM, Simäo C: Chagas' myocardiopathy, *Semin Roentgenol* 4:374, 1969.

152. Villanova MG, Meneghelli UG, Dantas RO: Gallbladder motor function in chagasic patients with megacolon and/or megaesophagus, *Digestion* 36:189, 1987.

153. World Health Organization: *Chagas' disease: report of a study group,* technical report series 202:1, Geneva, 1960, World Health Organization.

154. Amini F: Giardiasis and steatorrhea, *J Trop Med Hyg* 66:190, 1963.

155. Antia FP et al: Giardiasis in adults, *Indian J Med Sci* 20:471, 1966.

156. Basu SP: Radiological appearance of duodenal bulb in giardiasis, *Bull Calcutta Sch Trop Med* 13:64, 1965.

157. Bloch C, Tuchman LR: Diffuse small intestine abnormality due to *Giardia lamblia* with roentgen and clinical reversibility after therapy: case report, *J Mt Sinai Hosp* 34:116, 1967.

158. Brandberg LL et al: Histological demonstration of mucosal invasion by *Giardia lamblia* in man, *Gastroenterology* 52:143, 1967.

159. Cortner JA: Giardiasis, a cause of celiac syndrome, *Am J Dis Child* 98:311, 1959.

160. Gupta DN et al: Adult giardiasis. Incidence and absorption studies, *J Assoc Physicians India* 13:477, 1965.

161. Hermans PE et al: Dysgammaglobulinemia associated with nodular lymphoid hyperplasia of the small intestine, *Am J Med* 40:78, 1966.

162. Hodgson JR et al: Roentgenologic features of lymphoid hyperplasia of the small intestine associated with dysgammaglobulinemia, *Radiology* 88:883, 1967.

163. Hoskins LC et al: Clinical giardiasis and intestinal malabsorption, *Gastroenterology* 53:265, 1967.

164. Marshak RH et al: Roentgen manifestations of giardiasis, *AJR* 104:557, 1968.

165. Marshak RH, Lindner AE: *Radiology of the small intestine,* ed 2, Philadelphia, 1976, WB Saunders.

166. Peterson GM: Intestinal changes in *Giardia lamblia* infestation, *AJR* 77:670, 1957.

167. Reeder MM: RPC of the mouth from the AFIP, *Radiology* 93:427, 1969.

168. Reeder MM, Hamilton LC: Radiologic diagnosis of tropical diseases of the gastrointestinal tract, *Radiol Clin North Am* 7:57, 1969.

169. Reeder MM, Palmer PES: *The radiology of tropical diseases, with epidemiological, pathological, and clinical correlation*, Baltimore, 1981, Williams & Wilkins.

170. Takano J, Yardley JH: Jejunal lesions in patients with giardiasis and malabsorption: an electron microscopic study, *Bull John Hopkins Hosp* 116:413, 1965.

171. Welch PB: Giardiasis with unusual findings, *Gastroenterology* 3:98, 1944.

172. Yardley JH, Bayless TM: Giardiasis, *Gastroenterology* 52:301, 1967.

173. Baird JK, Mistrey M, Pimsler M, Connor DH: Fatal human ascariasis following secondary massive infection, *Am J Trop Med Hyg* 35:314, 1986.

174. Choudhuri G, Saha SS, Tandon RK: Gastric ascariasis, *Am J Gastroenterol* 81:788, 1986.

175. Clarke WFB, Hagley KE: Ultrasonography in the diagnosis and management of biliary ascariasis, *Wis Med J* 34:265, 1985.

176. Cremin BJ: Real time ultrasound in paediatric biliary ascariasis, *S Afr Med J* 61:914, 1982.

177. Cremin BJ: Ultrasonic diagnosis of biliary ascariasis: "a bulls-eye in the tripe O." *Br J Radiol* 55:683, 1985.

178. Kamath PS, Joseph DC, Chandran R et al: Biliary ascariasis: ultrasonography, endoscopic retrograde cholangiopancreatography, and biliary drainage, *Gastroenterology* 91:730, 1986.

179. Lloyd DA: Massive hepatobiliary ascariasis in childhood, *Br J Surg* 68:468, 1981.

180. Okumura M et al: Acute intestinal obstruction by *Ascaris*. Analysis of 455 cases, *Rev Inst Med Trop Sao Paulo* 16:292, 1975.

181. Radin DR, Vachon LA: CT findings in biliary and pancreatic ascariasis, *J Comput Assist Tomogr* 10:508, 1986.

182. Ramos CCF, Ramos AMdeO, Carhalho ARL: Pseudotumourous form of ascariasis, *Am J Trop Med Hyg* 29:795, 1980.

183. Wynne JM, Ellman BAH: Bolus obstruction by *Ascaris lumbricoides, S Afr Med J* 63:644, 1983.

184. Elmes BGT, McAdam IW: Helminthic abscess, a surgical complication of oesophagostomes and hookworm, *Ann Trop Med Parasitol* 48:1, 1954.

185. Dallemand S, Waxman M, Farman J: Radiological manifestations of *Strongyloides stercoralealis,* Gastroradiol 8:45, 1983.

186. Drasin GF, Moss JP, Cheng SH: *Strongyloides stercoralis* colitis: findings in four cases, *Radiology* 126:619, 1978.

187. Louisy CL, Batrton CJ: The radiological diagnosis of *Strongyloides stercoralis* enteritis, *Radiology* 98:535, 1971.

188. Scully RE, Mark EJ, McNeely BU: Case records of the Massachusetts General Hospital. *Strongyloides stercoralis* hyperinfection, *N Engl J Med* 314:903, 1986.

189. Ashby BS et al: Eosinophil granuloma of the gastrointestinal tract caused by the herring parasite, *Eustoma rotundatum, Br Med J* 1:1141, 1964.

190. Davey WW: Helminthoma. In Davey WW, ed: *Companion to surgery in Africa,* Edinburgh, 1968, E & S Livingstone.

191. Reeder MM, Palmer PES: *The radiology of tropical diseases, with epidemiological, pathological and clinical correlation,* Baltimore, 1981, Williams & Wilkins.

192. Kuipers FC: Eosinophilic phlegmonous inflammation of the alimentary canal caused by a parasite from the herring, *Pathol Microbiol* 27:925, 1964.

193. Matsui T, Iida M, Murakami M et al: Intestinal anisakiasis: clinical and radiologic features, *Radiology* 157:199, 1985.

194. Richman RH, Lewicki AN: Right ileo-colitis secondary to anisakiasis, *AJR* 119:329, 1973.

195. Yokogawa M, Yoshimura H: Clinico-pathologic studies on larval anisakiasis in Japan, *Am J Trop Med Hyg* 16:723, 1967.

196. Boon WH, Hoh TK: Severe whipworm infestation in children, *Singapore Med J* 2:34, 1961.

197. Fisher RM, Cremin BJ: Rectal bleeding due to *Trichuris trichiura, Br J Radiol* 43:214, 1970.

198. Getz L: Massive infection with *Trichuris trichiura* in children: report of four cases with autopsy, *Am J Dis Child* 70:19, 1945.

199. Hunter GW III, Swartzwelder JC, Clyde DF: *Tropical medicine,* ed 5, Philadelphia, 1976, WB Saunders.

200. Jung RC, Beaver PC: Clinical observation on *Trichocephalus trichiurus* (whipworm) infestation in children, *Pediatrics* 8:548, 1952.

201. Marcial-Rojas RA: *Pathology of protozoal and helminthic diseases,* Huntington, NY, 1975, Robert Krieger.

202. Reeder MM, Astacio JE, Theros EG: Case of the month from the AFIP: massive *Trichuris* infestation of the colon, *Radiology* 90:382, 1968.

203. Reeder MM, Hamilton LC: Tropical diseases of the colon, *Semin Roentgenol* 3:62, 1968.

204. Reeder MM, Palmer PES: *The radiology of tropical diseases, with epidemiological, pathological and clinical correlation,* Baltimore, 1981, Williams & Wilkins.

205. Cockshott WP, Middlemiss H: *Clinical radiology in the tropics,* New York, 1979, Churchill Livingstone.

206. Paulino GN, Wittenberg J: Intestinal capillariasis—a new cause of a malabsorption patterns, *AJR* 117:340, 1973.

207. Gold BM, Meyers MA: Radiologic manifestations of *Taenia saginata* infestation, *AJR* 128:493, 1977.

208. Geahavoc Z, Joanes JF, Chew FM: The radiological diagnosis of tapeworms: two cases of *Taenia saginata* infestation, *Can Med Assoc J* 102:967, 1970.

209. Acunas B, Rozanes I Acunas G: Retroperitoneal hydatic cyst presenting as a thigh mass: computed tomographic findings, *Clin Radiol* 44:285, 1991.

210. Akhan O, Dincer A, Saatci I et al: Spinal intradural hydatid cyst in a child, *Br J Radiol* 64:465, 1991.

211. Alltree M: Scanning in hydatid disease, *Clin Radiol* 30:691, 1979.

212. Beggs I: The radiological appearances of hydatid disease, *Clin Radiol* 34:555, 1983.

213. Bezzi M, Teggi A, De Rosa F et al: Abdominal hydatid disease: US findings during medical treatment, *Radiology* 162:91, 1987.

214. Bonakdarour A: *Echinococcus* disease. Report of 112 cases from Iran and a review of 611 from the United States, *AJR* 99:660, 1967.

215. Gharbi HA, Hassine W, Brauner MW et al: Ultrasound examination of the hydatid liver, *Radiology* 139:459, 1981.

216. Gonzalez LR, Marcos J, Illanas M et al: Radiologic aspects of hepatic echinococcosis, *Radiology* 130:21, 1979.

217. Grabbe HA et al: Ultrasound examination of the hydatid liver, *Ultrasound* 139:459, 1981.

218. Grabbe E, Kern P, Heller M: Human echinococcosis: diagnostic value of computed tomography, *Trop Med Parasitol* 32:35, 1981.

219. Gupta SK, Tandon SC, Khanna S et al: Multiple intracranial hydatid cysts with post-operative dissemination, *Clin Radiol* 44:203, 1991.

220. Haaga JR, Alfidi RJ: *Computed tomography of the whole body,* ed 2, St Louis, 1988, Mosby–Year Book.

221. Hendaoui L, Siala M, Fourati A et al: Hydatid cyst of the aorta, *Clin Radiol* 43:423, 1991.

222. Hoff FL, Aisen AM, Walden ME et al: MR imaging in hydatid disease of the liver, *Gastrointest Radiol* 12:39, 1987.

223. Kirschner LP, Ferris RA, Mero JH et al: Hydatid disease of the liver evaluated by computed tomography, *J Comput Assist Tomogr* 2:229, 1978.

224. Kotoulas G, Gouliamos A, Kalovidouris A et al: Computed tomographic localization of pelvic hydatid disease, *Eur J Radiol* 11:38, 1990.

225. Missas S, Gouliamos A, Kourias E et al: Primary hydatid disease of the pancreas, *Gastrointest Radiol* 12:37, 1987.

226. Mittelstaedt CA: *Abdominal ultrasound,* New York, 1987, Churchill Livingstone.

227. Morris DL, Skene-Smith H, Haynes H et al: Abdominal hydatid disease. Computed tomographic and ultrasound changes during albendazole therapy, *Clin Radiol* 35:297, 1984.

228. Mousa AM, Rudwan MA, Marafi AA et al: Human cystic hydatid disease: treatment with interrupted courses of mebendazole, *J Trop Med Hyg* 89:257, 1986.

229. Niron EA, Ozer H: Ultrasound appearances of liver hydatid disease, *Br J Radiol* 54:335, 1981.

230. Niron EA, Ozer H, Dolunay H: Encysted peritoneal hydatodosis: unusual ultrasonographic and clinical presentation of liver echinococcosis, *Br J Radiol* 54:339, 1981.

231. Rudwan MA, Mousa AM, Muhtaseb SA: Abdominal hydatid disease: follow-up of mebendazole therapy by CT and ultrasounography, *Intern Surg* 71:22, 1986.

232. Scherer U, Weinzierl M, Sturm R et al: Computed tomography in hydatid disease of liver, *J Comput Assist Tomogr* 2:612, 1978.

233. Schulman A et al: Pseudo-solid appearance of simple and echinococcal cysts on ultrasonography, *S Afr Med J* 63:905, 1983.

234. Singcharoen T, Machanonda N, Powell LW et al: Sonographic changes of hydatid cyst of the liver after treatment with mebendazole and albendazole, *Br J Radiol* 58:905, 1985.

235. Taylor KJW: *Atlas of ultrasonography,* ed 2, New York, 1985, Churchill Livingstone.

236. Todorov T, Vutova K, Mechkov G et al: Evaluation of response to chemotherapy of human cystic echinococcosis, *Br J Radiol* 63:523, 1990.

237. Uysal V, Paksoy N: Echinococcosis multilocularis in Turkey, *J Trop Med Hyg* 89:249, 1986.

238. von Sinner WN: New diagnostic signs in hydatid disease; radiography, ultrasound, CT and MRI correlated to pathology, *Eur J Radiol* 12:150, 1991.

239. von Sinner WN: Successful treatment of disseminated hydatid disease using albendazole monitored by CT, *Eur J Radiol* 11:232, 1990.

240. von Sinner WN: Ultrasound, CT and MRI of ruptured and disseminated hydatid cysts, *Eur J Radiol* 11:31, 1990.

241. Choi TK, Wang KP, Wong J: Cholangiographic appearances in clonorchiasis, *Br J Radiol* 57:681, 1984.

242. Pulpeiro JR, Armesto V, Varela J et al: Fascioliasis: findings in 15 patients, *Br J Radiol* 64:798, 1991.

243. Serrano MAP, Vega A, Ortega E et al: Computed tomography of hepatic fascioliasis, *J Comput Assist Tomogr* 11:269, 1987.

244. Takeyama N, Okumura N, Sakai Y et al: Computed tomography findings of hepatic lesions in human fascioliasis: report of two cases, *Am J Gastroenterol* 81:1078, 1986.

245. Upatham ES, Viyanant V, Kurathong S et al: Relationships between prevalence and intensity of *Opisthorcis Viverrini* infection and clinical symptoms and signs in northeast Thailand, *Bull WHO* 62:451,1984.

246. Kurathong S, Lerdverasirikul P, Wongpaitoo V et al: *Opisthorcis viverrini* infection and cholangiocarcinoma: a prospective case-controlled study, *Gastroenterology* 89:151, 1985.

247. Araki T, Hayakawa K, Okada J et al: Hepatic schistosomiasis japonica identified by CT, *Radiology* 157:757, 1985.

248. Chait A: Schistosomiasis mansoni: roentgenologic observations in a nonendemic area, *AJR* 90:688, 1963.

249. Dimmette RM, Sproat HF: Rectosigmoid polyps in schistosomiasis, *Trop Med* 4:1057, 1955.

250. El-Afifi S: Intestinal bilharzia, *Dis Colon Rectum* 7:1, 1964.

251. El-Masry NA, Farid Z, Bassily S et al: Schistosomal colonic polyposis: clinical, radiological and parasitological study, *J Trop Med Hyg* 89:11, 1986.

252. Fataar S, Bassiony H, Satyanath S et al: CT of schistosomal calcification of the intestine, *AJR* 144:75, 1985.

253. Fataar S, Bassiony H, Hamed MS et al: Radiographic spectrum of rectocolonic calcification from schistosomiasis, *AJR* 142:933, 1984.

254. Garcia-Palmieri MR, Marcial-Rojas RA: The protean manifestations of schistosomiasis mansoni: a clinicopathological correlation, *Ann Intern Med* 57:763, 1962.

255. Kojiro M, Kakizoe S, Yano H et al: Hepatocellular carcinoma and schistosomiasis japonica: a clinicopathologic study of 59 autopsy cases of hepatocellular carcinoma associated with chronic schistosomiasis japonica, *Acta Pathol Jpn* 36:525, 1986.

256. Larotski LS, Davis A: The schistosomiasis problem in the world: the results of a WHO questionnaire survey, *Bull WHO* 59:114, 1981.

257. Medina JT et al: The roentgen appearance of Schistosomiasis mansoni involving the colon, *Radiology* 85:682, 1965.

258. Nagata O, Uto K, Sugihara H et al: Ultrasonic and x-ray tomographic findings of schistosomiasis japonicum, *Kurume Med J* 32:301, 1985.

259. Owor R, Madda JP: Schistosomiasis causing tumorlike lesions, *East Afr Med J* 54:137, 1977.

260. Pagan Saez H: *Schistosoma mansoni:* its radiographic manifestations, *Bol Assoc Med P Rico* 77:195-201, 1985.

261. Saad AMA, El Masri SH, Omer AHS et al: A clinico-pathological study on intestinal bilharziasis in the Sudan, *East Afr Med J* 62:397, 1985.

262. Sobrinho J, Kelsch F: Asbectos tumorais de sequistosomose do colon, *Rev Bras Radiol* 2:1, 1959.

263. Wang C et al: Roentgenologic changes of small intestine in Schistosomiasis japonica, *Chin J Radiol* 6:247, 1958.

264. Ardran GM: *Armillifer armillatus, Br J Radiol* 21:342, 1948.

265. Chartres JC: Radiological manifestations of parasitism by the tongue worms, *Br J Radiol* 38:503, 1965.

47 *Gastrointestinal Manifestations of the Acquired Immunodeficiency Syndrome*

PETER J. FECZKO

More than a decade has passed since the first reports of an illness that has come to be known as the acquired immunodeficiency syndrome (AIDS). In its first ten years the illness was responsible for over 100,000 deaths, with a gradual increase in this number with each ensuing year.[1-3] At its current rate of growth, AIDS will soon rank as the leading cause of death in men aged 25 to 44 and will be among the leading causes of death in women aged 15 to 44 and children aged 1 to 5.[2] It is estimated that over one million Americans are now infected with the human immunodeficiency virus (HIV), the pathogen responsible for the illness. The World Health Organization estimates that 10 million individuals worldwide are now infected with HIV, and that number may climb to 40 million by the year 2000.[1-3] Obviously, this disease has already had a major impact on the health-care industry, and this situation will undoubtedly continue to worsen as we move into the 21st century.

At one time the patients with AIDS were predominantly confined to major metropolitan centers, but recent findings now indicate a leveling off of the incidence of new cases among homosexual men and a decrease in the number of transfusion-related cases. At the same time there has been an increase in incidence among women and newborns. It is not surprising, therefore, that the HIV infection and clinical cases of AIDS are now being encountered with greater frequency outside the major urban areas.[4] Considering these data, it is becoming ever more likely that radiologists will encounter patients with HIV infection or AIDS regardless of where their practice is located. This means changes in the way in which procedures are performed as well as in the diagnostic considerations in patients.

HUMAN IMMUNODEFICIENCY VIRUS

Soon after the initial descriptions of the AIDS infection, it became apparent that the disease was caused by a communicable agent. Because of the selective loss of the helper T cells in these patients, researchers began to consider a human retrovirus as the etiologic agent, since these viruses are known to deplete the number of helper T cells. Two types of human retroviruses, HTLV-I and HTLV-II, had already been discovered to be the causative agents in a type of human leukemia. Thus, when the AIDS virus was found

to be a retrovirus, it was initially termed *HTLV-III* or the *lymphadenopathy virus*.[5-7] By convention, it is now called *HIV*, of which two forms have been found, HIV-1 and HIV-2.[5] HIV belongs to the subfamily of retroviruses called *lentivirus*, named for their slow course of infection. It is a single-stranded RNA virus, containing reverse transcriptase, surrounded by a lipid envelope. When the virus enters its target cells, it is translated into DNA, which is then incorporated into the host nucleus.[5-7]

A hallmark of the retroviruses is their latency period and their persistence despite an immune response. The inciting event that triggers the development of diffuse infection from the latency phase is uncertain, but it may be other viral infections.[5-7] The attachment sites for HIV exist not only on the helper T cells but also on macrophages, monocytes, crypt and enterochromaffin cells in the bowel epithelium, and certain glial cells, all of which may contain the virus.[6] In addition, the mechanism by which HIV destroys the host cells is uncertain, but it may be mediated by an immune response.[5,6] During their prolonged time in the body, HIV undergoes genetic variation, which makes the development of a vaccine difficult.[7]

A second immunodeficiency virus, HIV-2, has been encountered mainly among Africans but has also been found in patients in the United States. It is more closely related to the simian immunodeficiency virus, and its long-range biologic consequences have not yet been determined, although it appears less cytopathic than HIV-1.[5,6]

CLINICAL PRESENTATION AND STAGING OF HIV INFECTION

The patient with HIV infection may exhibit clinical symptoms during the primary viral infection, as well as secondarily during the immunodepleted stage.[8,9] Because of this, classification systems have been designed in order to categorize patients in terms of both treatment and prognosis. At present there are two such systems, one from the Centers for Disease Control (CDC) (see box on p. 953) and another from the Walter Reed Army Institute of Research.[10,11] The CDC system most closely approximates the clinical state and is the one described here.

Some patients are asymptomatic after their initial HIV

Adapted from CDC: Classification system for human T-lymphotropic virus type III/lymphadenopathy-associated virus infections, *MMWR* 35:334, 1986.

exposure. Others suffer an acute viral-like illness that may manifest various symptoms, including fever, pharyngitis, anorexia, nausea and vomiting, diarrhea, encephalitis, neuropathy, rashes, urticaria, and gingival ulceration.[8,9] The incubation period from the time of the initial exposure to that of the acute clinical illness varies from days to months. In the second phase the patient is an asymptomatic carrier. The third phase consists of a persistent (longer than 3 months) adenopathy at two or more sites. The last stage consists of secondary infections, secondary cancers, neurologic disease, or other life-threatening complications. This last stage is what most physicians categorize as AIDS.

Gastrointestinal (GI) symptoms such as diarrhea, nausea and vomiting, weight loss, anorexia, and even oral ulceration may arise at both the initial and late stages of HIV infection.[8-10] It is not uncommon to encounter a patient with AIDS and find out during their evaluation that they underwent an extensive GI evaluation several years before, probably during the initial HIV infection. Thus, the radiologist must consider the possibility of HIV infection whenever they encounter a young patient with this clinical picture.

EPIDEMIOLOGY AND NATURAL HISTORY

Much has been written about those who are at high risk for contracting the HIV infection. However, HIV infection is now a true pandemic and is seen in all demographic groups and ages, with a prevalence now believed to be several million.[1,3] Homosexual men have been the hardest hit in the United States, although the rate of infection appears to be leveling off in this group. Intravenous drug abuse as well as heterosexual transmission of the virus now account for increasing numbers of cases. In Africa, heterosexual spread is the primary route of infection, and this will undoubtedly account for a continued increase in the incidence

in this population. In utero transmission accounts for most of the pediatric cases, and it has even been reported to be transmitted through breast milk. Transmission by means of blood transfusion, the medical use of other body fluids, or organ transplantation has actually decreased.[1,3,7,12,13] Medical personnel are at risk of acquiring the disease from coming in contact with infected body fluids, and there have been sporadic reports of doctors and dentists transmitting the infection to their patients. Spread by arthropods or other vectors has not been proved.

Contraction of HIV infection after exposure depends on the route of exposure, the size of the inoculum, any predisposing diminished immunocompetence, and other unknown factors. Once a person is infected, there is an incubation period lasting from days to months, but averaging 2 to 4 weeks.[14,15] During this time, individuals may remain asymptomatic or suffer an acute viral-like illness. These seropositive individuals can then remain free of symptoms for months to many years. The reported rate of progression from an HIV-positive status to full-blown clinical AIDS varies greatly among studies, and somewhat depends on the population analyzed. Study findings have indicated that the median time from seroconversion to the appearance of AIDS varies greatly, ranging from 2 years in pediatric patients to as much as 11 years in one study.[14,15] The factors that influence this picture are the subject of controversy, but a prolonged primary viral illness, repeated infections, and environmental factors (drug use) have all been proposed to play a role. An important laboratory marker is the level of the T-helper (CD4) lymphocytes in the peripheral blood. CD4 levels below 200/mm^3 indicate immunosuppression, and these individuals usually face an imminent risk of developing AIDS.[16]

CLINICAL TESTING

A variety of serologic tests have been developed for the purpose of detecting HIV infection, and generally they have a sensitivity and specificity approaching 99%.[7,14] In most individuals, seroconversion takes place within 2 weeks of the primary illness, which itself also appears several weeks after the viral inoculation.[6,14] Thus a seronegative latency period can last from several weeks to months. Although there are conflicting data on this, most individuals probably seroconvert within 12 weeks of inoculation.[15] Rarely, a second seronegative period occurs in the terminal stages, and this is believed to indicate the extreme immunosuppression present at that time.[14,15]

Although other hematologic and antigenic abnormalities are detectable, the other important laboratory measurement is the peripheral lymphocyte level. There are two major groups of T-lymphocytes: T-helper (CD4) and T-suppressor (CD8). T-helper lymphocytes are the primary target of HIV, but T-suppressor lymphocytes are rarely infected. Active infection with HIV causes a depression of the CD4 level, and it is this level that most closely reflects the patient's immune status. Levels less than 400/mm^3 are significant, and those less than 200/mm^3 reflect severe depression. Conversely, the CD8 cells may actually increase in number, and this inversion of the normal CD4/CD8 ratio is emphasized in some studies. Although no single laboratory value is critical, the absolute CD4 level is currently the most important criterion for treatment.[16]

IMAGING OF THE PATIENT WITH HIV INFECTION

Most individuals with AIDS and some with HIV infection exhibit a variable degree of GI symptoms. Because of this, and because of some reluctance on the part of endoscopists to perform procedures in these patients, they are often referred for diagnostic studies of the GI tract. For these reasons, radiologists are frequently called upon in the evaluation of complications of this disease.

Conventional barium radiography remains an important modality in evaluating AIDS patients, with abnormalities encountered in up to 80% of them.[17] Much of the pathology encountered is superficial, involving the mucosal surfaces, and double-contrast studies are the preferred method for demonstrating such abnormalities. It has been reported that the yield of abnormalities is higher in these patients on double-contrast rather than single-contrast studies.[17] However, AIDS patients can be quite ill, and the type of examination must sometimes be geared to the clinical state of the patient.

In those patients with adenopathy or suspected malignancy, CT is the preferred method for evaluating the abdomen.[18-20] Its primary role is in the detection of adenopathy, liver or splenic abnormalities, and other extraintestinal masses. Often bowel pathology is apparent on CT scans as well, and this is important when the patient's condition does not permit an optimal barium study. In addition, CT-guided biopsy is frequently employed in obtaining tissue from lymph nodes or masses to help in differentiating disease. Certain diseases can be pathognomonic on CT, as will be discussed later.

The role of ultrasound is predominantly confined to the evaluation of the gallbladder and biliary system. When this system is involved, there can be subtle intraluminal and mural changes that can be most easily assessed by ultrasound. So far, magnetic resonance imaging (MRI) has found little use in the evaluation of these patients, but it may eventually possess increased sensitivity in the detection of solid organ lesions, and perhaps increased specificity in the evaluation of adenopathy. More than likely, however, MRI will continue to have a very limited role in the evaluation of abdominal pathology in AIDS patients.

OPPORTUNISTIC INFECTIONS OF THE GI TRACT

Chronic diarrhea plagues a majority of patients with AIDS, and other symptoms such as dysphagia and odynophagia, nausea and vomiting, anorexia, GI bleeding, and abdominal pain are common. The underlying cause for many of these problems is secondary infection by enteric pathogens. The gut is a major component of the immune system and possesses a substantial amount of lymphoid tissue. After the major insult to the patient's immunologic competency caused by HIV, the GI tract is particularly susceptible to these opportunistic infections.

Unfortunately, despite the number of abnormalities discovered during radiographic procedures, evaluation of these findings is exceedingly difficult for several reasons:

1. Infections can be multifocal and involve separate portions of the GI tract.
2. Multiple pathogenic organisms frequently involve the GI tract simultaneously. These may either affect separate portions of bowel, or only a part of the GI tract may be infected by several organisms (i.e., the small bowel).
3. The GI tract manifests only a limited spectrum of abnormalities in the disease, and it is difficult to distinguish these diseases radiographically, with a few exceptions.
4. Pathogens can be recovered in only approximately half of the patients with symptoms.[17] On the other hand, a patient may be symptomatic, with pathogens isolated, but still exhibit few radiographic abnormalities.

Enteric pathogens

A variety of pathogens can be isolated from the GI tract in AIDS patients, and more will likely be encountered in the years to come.[21,22] This constellation of organisms is more extensive than that seen in other immunosuppressive conditions, and some of these organisms are discussed in the following sections.

Fungal infection

Candida albicans is probably the most frequent and most symptom-producing mucosal infection in patients with AIDS. It is believed that *Candida* infection ultimately affects all patients with AIDS and can be seen even in the early stage of the HIV infection. Most infections involve the oropharynx. When the esophagus is affected, dysphagia and odynophagia may occur. The radiographic appearances have been well described.[23,24] Early changes may consist of small discrete plaques or nodules; in advanced disease, there is confluence of these plaques, thickening of the longitudinal folds, the formation of pseudomembranes, and ulceration (Figs. 47-1 and 47-2). A variety of motility disturbances have also been reported. Double-contrast esophagography is the most sensitive method for detecting early esophageal disease.[23,24] Rarely, *Candida* may also involve the upper GI tract or rectum and produce ulceration; it has even been known to infect the biliary system.

Other fungal diseases such as *Coccidiodes immitis* and *Histoplasma* rarely affect the GI tract, but when this does happen, it is usually during diffuse dissemination.

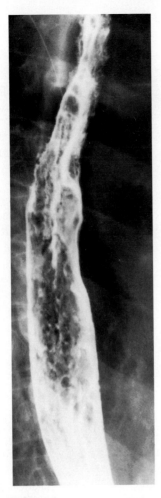

Fig. 47-1 Severe, diffuse esophagitis is evident secondary to *Candida* infection.

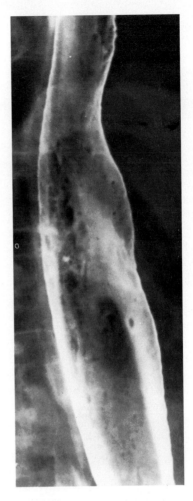

Fig. 47-2 There are a few plaquelike lesions in the midesophagus of this AIDS patient with mild *Candida* infection.

Viral diseases

Cytomegalovirus (CMV) is commonly found in humans, even in the immunocompetent. It is considered to be one of the most common pathogens in AIDS patients, and, unlike *Candida,* can contribute considerably to the mortality in these patients.[25] It is also one of the few organisms that can infect any portion of the GI tract, from the mouth to the anus. In the esophagus it can produce large flat ulcers (Fig. 47-3) that can become quite large, and this can be a distinguishing feature from herpes.[24-26] In the stomach and duodenum, CMV infection can bring about both focal and large confluent ulcerations, as well as markedly thickened folds (Fig. 47-4). The small bowel changes caused by CMV infection are nonspecific, with fold thickening the most evident. CMV is one of the major causes of diarrhea in AIDS patients. The colon changes can also be variable, ranging from discrete ulcers to diffuse ulceration and mucosal edema[27] (Fig. 47-5). CMV infection should be considered in the differential diagnosis of any GI tract abnormality in

AIDS patients; it can even mimic the characteristics of a neoplasm.

Herpes species is another pathogen frequently encountered not only in AIDS patients but also in the context of other forms of immunosuppression. Herpes simplex is a common cause of esophagitis in AIDS patients. It may be manifested as small, discrete ulcers against a background of normal mucosa, which may occasionally collect in clusters (Fig. 47-6), but in more severe forms these become confluent and impart a shaggy appearance to the esophagus, similar to that seen in *Candida* infections.[24,28] Herpes can also cause proctitis and colitis and take on a similar radiographic appearance of discrete or confluent ulceration (Fig. 47-7).

Protozoan infections

A variety of protozoa exist as enteric pathogens in the HIV patient. Cryptosporidiosis, although only recently discovered to be a pathogen in humans, is now recognized as

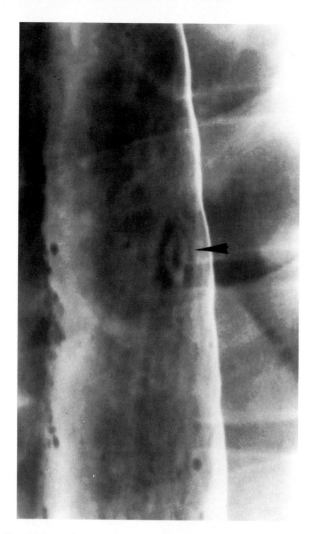

Fig. 47-3 A discrete ulcer *(arrowhead)* with surrounding edema is evident in the esophagus due to cytomegalovirus infection.

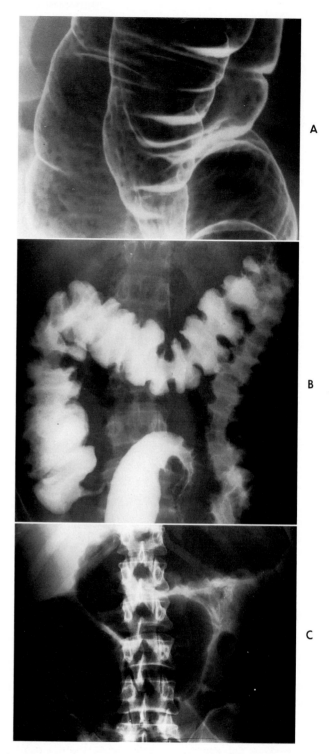

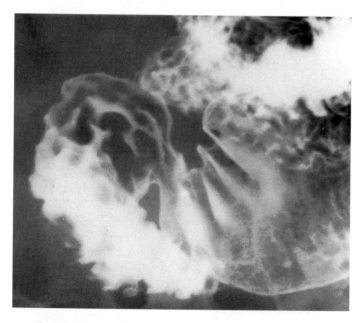

Fig. 47-4 Nonspecific inflammatory changes with fold thickening, secondary to cytomegalovirus infection, are present in the duodenal bulb of this AIDS patient.

Fig. 47-5 A, Numerous aphthous ulcers were scattered throughout the colon in this patient with cytomegalovirus (CMV) colitis. These changes are indistinguishable from those of Crohn's disease, and AIDS patients may often be misdiagnosed early in the disease. **B,** A single-contrast barium enema study demonstrates thickened haustral folds and ulcerated mucosa resulting from the CMV infection. This is a more advanced infection, but the radiographic abnormalities are nonspecific. **C,** An abdominal film reveals a dilated transverse colon and nodular folds. Toxic megacolon developed as the result of the CMV colitis, which eventually perforated and led to death in this patient.

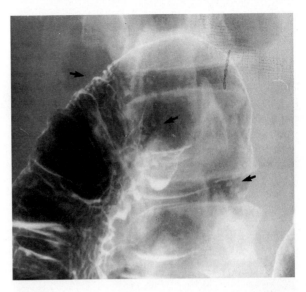

Fig. 47-7 A mixed type of ulceration in the colon with both discrete *(arrows)* and confluent ulceration secondary to herpes colitis.

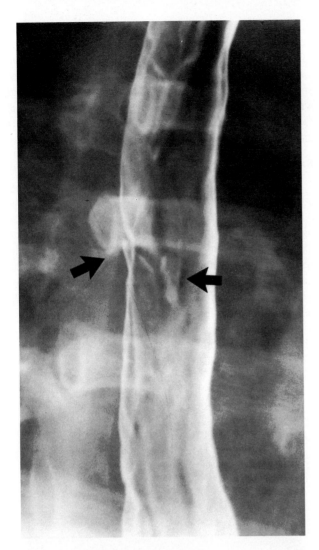

Fig. 47-6 Several discrete, amorphous ulcers *(arrows)* are evident in the esophagus of this AIDS patient and are the result of herpes esophagitis.

an important cause of a debilitating watery diarrhea in AIDS patients. It is a coccidial protozoon that stains with acid-fast agents and can be isolated from the stool. It is relatively resistant to treatment.[29] Infection predominantly involves the small bowel, particularly the proximal aspect, and leads to the formation of thickened folds and occasionally increased secretions and dilatation (Fig. 47-8). It has also been known to involve the biliary system and assume a cholangitic appearance.

Isospora belli and Microsporida are other coccidial protozoa that produce abnormalities similar to those of *Cryptosporidium*. They are encountered more frequently in the Haitian AIDS population and respond better to treatment than does *Cryptosporidium*.

Giardia lamblia is a flagellated protozoon that occurs in both a limited epidemic fashion and among the immuno-

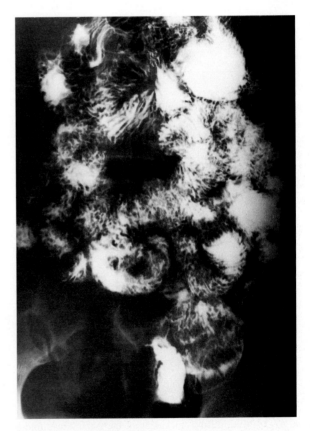

Fig. 47-8 Cryptosporidiosis of the small bowel. Note the thickened folds and mild segmentation of the barium column. These changes can be seen in many of the small bowel infections and are not specific for cryptosporidiosis.

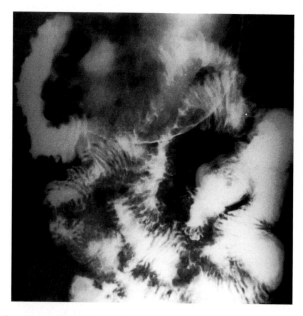

Fig. 47-9 Marked thickening of the folds of the proximal small bowel is evident, along with increased secretions, resulting from a *Giardia* infection of the small bowel. Again, these changes of thickened folds, increased secretions, and mild dilatation are seen in the presence of many of the small bowel infections.

suppressed.[30] It is infrequently encountered in AIDS patients. Radiographically, it produces thickened, irregular folds, with a predilection for the jejunum (Fig. 47-9). *Entamoeba histolytica* has also been reported in these patients, and typically it involves the colon and distal small bowel with inflammatory changes. The greatest frequency of infection with both these pathogens occurs among patients in the United States.

Bacteria

Mycobacterium avium-intracellulare (MAI) and other atypical mycobacteria occur with increased frequency in the AIDS patient.[31] The *Mycobacterium* species that principally involves the gut in these patients is MAI. It affects the small bowel and duodenum, producing thickened folds, with some increased secretions (Fig. 47-10). CT scans often reveal the presence of an associated lymphadenopathy, which may exhibit decreased density.[19,20] An important differential consideration whenever abdominal adenopathy is found in the AIDS patient is MAI infection. A small bowel biopsy specimen can demonstrate pathologic changes that

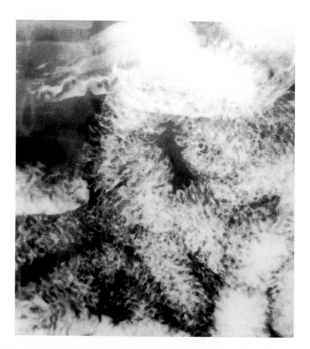

Fig. 47-10 Mild, diffuse thickening of the small bowel fold pattern is all that is present in this patient with *Mycobacterium avium-intracellulare* (MAI) infection of the small bowel. MAI can also produce adenopathy, which is a relatively pathognomonic finding due to its low density.

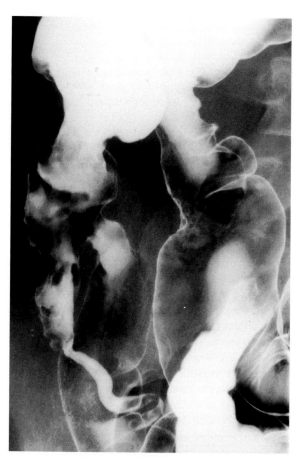

Fig. 47-11 Irregular stricturing of the cecum, ascending colon, and transverse colon resulting from *Mycobacterium tuberculosis* infection. This resulted from the reactivation of a pulmonary infection in this AIDS patient.

may mimic those of Whipple's disease. MAI has also been known to involve the biliary tract. *Mycobacterium tuberculosis* may also involve the bowel, but through a reactivation of the pulmonary disease (Fig. 47-11).

Other bacterial species that infect the gut with somewhat greater frequency in AIDS patients are *Salmonella, Shigella,* and *Campylobacter.* They can produce an acute inflammatory diarrhea, and nonspecific inflammatory changes may be evident in the large bowel. Also to be considered in homosexual men are sexually transmitted diseases that involve the bowel, particularly the rectum.[32] Diseases such as *lymphogranuloma venereum, Chlamydia, Neisseria gonorrhoeae,* and *Treponema pallidum* may cause a proctitis that is indistinguishable from that caused by the other previously described infectious agents. The frequency of *Clostridium difficile* colitis may also be increased in these patients.

Other enteric pathogens

Other unusual entities may beset the immunocompromised host. Intestinal spirochetes have been identified in the stool of AIDS patients. As with the other pathogens, the radiographic changes are nonspecific, and superficial ulceration is the most prominent finding (Fig. 47-12). Helminthic infection, resulting from *Strongyloides stercoralis,* has been reported as well. It is likely that, with time, other rare organisms will be isolated from these patients. However, from a radiologic perspective, they will undoubtedly be indistinguishable from the picture presented by the pathogens already described.

AIDS and HIV enteropathy

It is well recognized that a large number of patients with HIV infection suffer from a chronic diarrhea, but no identifiable enteric pathogen is ever isolated. The clinical symptoms may be quite severe and accompanied by malabsorption and weight loss. In the African population, this has even been termed "slim disease" by the World Health Organization.[9] Small bowel biopsy specimens from these patients show a gamut of changes, from normal small bowel mucosa to blunting of the villi, epithelial damage with decreased mitoses in the crypts, and chronic intestinal inflammation with intraepithelial lymphocytes.[9,12,14] Close evaluation of the mucosal cells has also revealed the existence of spherical, intracellular, viruslike particles as well as intranuclear inclusions, indicating that the intestinal mucosa is affected by some type of virus.

There is increasing evidence that these changes are due to primary HIV infection of the intestinal mucosa, or perhaps to some as yet identified virus. Electron microscopy examination of these gut tissues has disclosed the presence of tuboreticular structures that are also found in the lymphocytes and monocytes of AIDS patients.[9,12] Some authors believe that the crypt cells and enterochromaffin cells of the bowel epithelium are the target cells of the HIV vi-

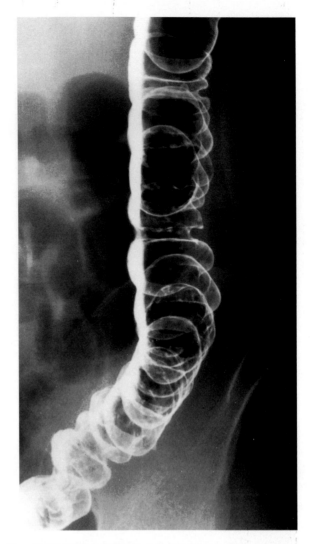

Fig. 47-12 Mild superficial ulceration in the colon caused by a spirochete infection.

rus, along with lymphocytes, monocytes, and glial cells.[6,9,33] Thus, a primary HIV infection of the intestinal mucosa can produce clinical symptoms in several ways. The first is by directly damaging the mucosa through interference with crypt cell growth. It has been noted that the enzyme activity in the brush border is diminished in these patients as well. In a second scenario, because the enterochromaffin cells have an endocrine function in the gut and help control motility and digestive functions, interference with this mechanism may contribute to the diarrhea.[6]

Early in the course of this condition, there may be few if any radiographic changes. Patients with more intense symptoms can exhibit an irregular small bowel mucosal pattern with thickening of the valvulae (Fig. 47-13). However, this appearance is indistinguishable from the small bowel changes produced by many of the enteric pathogens. In later stages, the small bowel abnormalities may include dilatation and increased secretions, but this is relatively uncom-

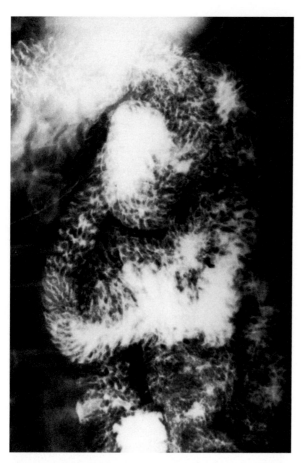

Fig. 47-13 Irregularity and mild prominence of the mucosal pattern in this patient with AIDS. This was considered secondary to a primary HIV enteropathy.

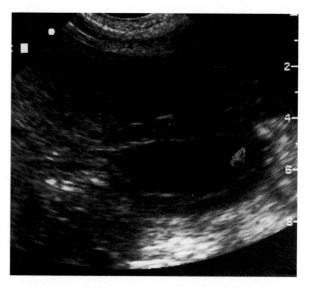

Fig. 47-14 Ultrasound of the gallbladder in an AIDS patient who had right upper quadrant pain shows a thickened gallbladder wall with no calculi, compatible with acalculous cholecystititis. This is usually due to cytomegalovirus or cryptosporidiosis.

mon. It has been postulated that CT may be helpful in differentiating AIDS enteropathy from intestinal opportunistic infections because in the former, the bowel wall is thin on CT scans, while many of the infections produce a thickened bowel wall.[17-19] Treatment of these patients is usually palliative, with emphasis on proper nutritional support.

Hepatobiliary abnormalities

There is a high incidence of both hepatic and biliary disease in the AIDS population. Clinically, over half the AIDS patients have hepatomegaly, and liver abnormalities are found in most patients at autopsy.[34-38] Several factors are responsible for this. First, liver disease is ubiquitous in the high-risk groups of intravenous drug abusers and male homosexuals. Second, the immunosuppression makes the liver and biliary tract vulnerable to a variety of infections. Finally, the liver is at risk for secondary involvement from other neoplasms, such as Kaposi's sarcoma and lymphoma. Despite this, hepatobiliary studies are not performed frequently in these patients because the hepatobiliary abnormalities have little actual impact on the mortality of the pa-

tient, and other problems encountered in AIDS tend to dominate the clinical management of these patients.

Liver

At some time during the course of the AIDS illness the liver is affected in most patients. The most common abnormality is a viral hepatitis, usually hepatitis B. Other viruses, including Epstein-Barr, can also produce hepatitis in these patients, but usually the clinical course is mild in these instances. Another viral hepatitis peculiar to AIDS patients is CMV hepatitis. This is seen when the CMV infection is widespread. Usually the extrahepatic abnormalities dominate the clinical picture, and jaundice is rare.[34]

Another diffuse infection of the liver can be caused by *Mycobacterium* organisms, particularly MAI. This appears to be the most common opportunistic infection of the liver in AIDS. Clinically it produces little morbidity but is the source of scattered intrahepatic granulomas in these patients.[34] Fungal infections due to *Cryptococcus* and other fungi have also been reported, but the liver changes in these instances are usually nonspecific. On rare occasions, focal large abscesses may develop within the liver resulting from fungous or bacteria infection, and these could be detected radiographically.

Neoplastic involvement of the liver is commonly seen at autopsy, when it also exists elsewhere in the body, but is rarely diagnosed premortem. Kaposi's sarcoma frequently metastasizes to the liver, but the lesions are tiny and widespread and often not detected radiographically. Lymphoma is more likely to produce focal large lesions in the liver, but this is relatively uncommon.

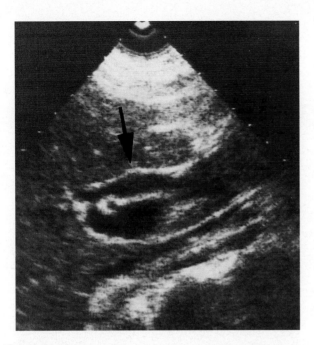

Fig. 47-15 Ultrasound study from a patient with right upper quadrant symptoms demonstrates a mildly dilated common bile duct *(arrow)* containing some nonechogenic debris, secondary to infectious cholangitis.

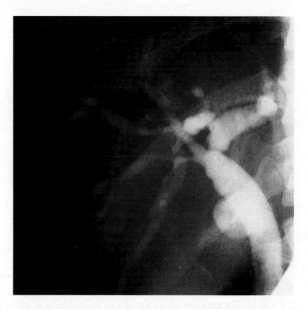

Fig. 47-16 This endoscopic retrograde cholangiopancreatographic study of the biliary system reveals irregular stricturing and dilatation of the intrahepatic ducts secondary to cholangitis resulting from cryptosporidiosis in this AIDS patient.

Biliary tract

Both the gallbladder and biliary tract are prospective sites of opportunistic infections, and more commonly produce clinical symptoms than does liver disease. The development of acalculous cholecystitis is being seen with increasing frequency in these patients. The clinical picture is typical and includes right upper quadrant pain and fever. Ultrasound can depict a thickened gallbladder wall without stones (Fig. 47-14). This is often attributable to CMV infection, but other fungal and protozoal parasites have also been implicated.[35-37]

Another commonly seen condition is AIDS-related cholangitis. Affected patients exhibit the classic symptoms of the region and sometimes jaundice.[36,37] This is usually secondary to an opportunistic infection stemming from cryptosporidiosis or CMV, although other agents have also been implicated. Cross-sectional imaging frequently shows dilated extrahepatic and even intrahepatic ducts, with occasional thickening of the walls and nonshadowing debris within the lumen (Fig. 47-15). Direct cholangiography, usually employing endoscopic retrograde cholangiopancreatography (ERCP), is more sensitive for this purpose. This can disclose abnormalities consistent with typical sclerosing cholangitis, including irregular ductal mucosa, focal stricturing and beading of the ducts, pruning of the ducts, and sometimes papillary stenosis (Fig. 47-16).

Imaging of hepatobiliary disease

Ultrasound should be the initial screening modality for evaluation of the right upper quadrant in AIDS patients because it is inexpensive, sensitive, and noninvasive. If biliary abnormalities are apparent, ERCP can be used for further evaluation. CT may be indicated if masses and adenopathy or some other abdominal pathology is evident. It is uncertain whether MRI is more sensitive for delineating the nature of intrahepatic pathology in AIDS patients, but this may represent one area where it may be of some benefit.

NEOPLASTIC DISEASE IN AIDS

The development of neoplasms is a well-recognized complication in immunosuppressed patients, particularly transplant recipients, and it is one of the first recognized complications of AIDS. In fact, it was the finding of certain rare tumors in young males that first alerted the world to the oncoming AIDS epidemic.[38] Even now, however, our understanding of why these tumors develop remains limited, and these secondary neoplasm continue to be a significant source of mortality in the AIDS population.

Kaposi's sarcoma

Kaposi's sarcoma was initially described in 1872 as a pigmented sarcoma of the skin. Histologically the tumor is characterized by irregular, endothelial-lined vascular channels, spindle-shaped cells, and varying degrees of mononuclear inflammatory infiltrates in the surrounding tissues.

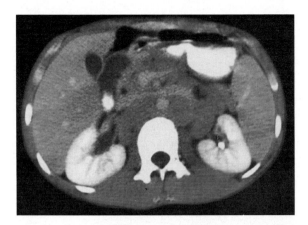

Fig. 47-17 Marked retroperitoneal adenopathy secondary to Kaposi's sarcoma. The patient was a hemophiliac who had no skin manifestations of the disorder.

Until the AIDS epidemic, Kaposi's sarcoma was considered a rare neoplasm, found mainly among elderly males living in Europe and the Mediterranean region, and following a slow, indolent clinical course with skin lesions predominating.[38-40] Interestingly, a more endemic and aggressive form was observed in Central Africa starting around 1950. Kaposi's sarcoma was also noted in renal transplant recipients starting around 1970.[38]

The development of Kaposi's sarcoma in AIDS patients is considered multifactorial. The cellular immunity characteristics of AIDS predisposes to the development of neoplasms. In addition, some tumor-stimulating virus, perhaps CMV, may be the inciting factor for Kaposi's sarcoma.[38,39] Interestingly the incidence of Kaposi's sarcoma in homosexual patients is several-fold greater than that in patients who acquire AIDS through intravenous drug use or other causes.[38-40] Because of the changing demographics of the AIDS epidemic, the proportion of AIDS patients with Kaposi's sarcoma has shown a steady decline over the past several years.

The type of Kaposi's sarcoma seen in the AIDS population differs clinically from the classic type, necessitating a new classification of the neoplasm.[38,39] The various clinical forms described are an aggressive form with cutaneous lesions and bone involvement, another aggressive type with cutaneous and visceral involvement, and a lymphadenopathic type with marked lymph node involvement but no cutaneous disease that afflicts young adults and children (Fig. 47-17). The clinical course in these patients is quite variable, but Kaposi's sarcoma does cause significant morbidity and some mortality in this group.

Involvement of the GI tract or abdomen is one of the most frequent manifestations of Kaposi's sarcoma. Lesions can be seen from the mouth to the anus and are multifocal, though the oropharynx is one of the most common sites (Fig. 47-18). Kaposi's sarcoma assumes a variable appearance in the GI tract but is predominantly a superficial le-

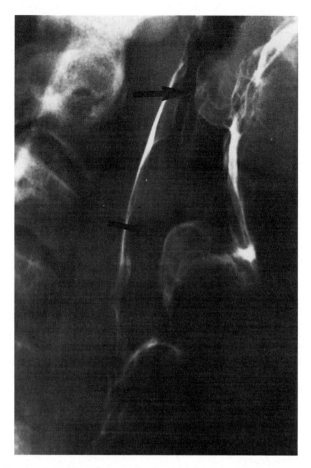

Fig. 47-18 Two discrete nodules arising from the base of the tongue and epiglottis in this AIDS patient with dysphagia. Analysis of biopsy specimens confirmed Kaposi's sarcoma.

sion. Often, a discrete nodule or a mass projecting into the lumen is seen, sometimes with a central ulceration that gives it a so-called bull's eye or target appearance (Fig. 47-19). In another variety, there is a diffuse infiltrating submucosal process that produces thickened folds and radiographically may appear similar to hemorrhage in the bowel wall (Fig. 47-20). Kaposi's sarcoma can also produce massive adenopathy. This may appear somewhat hypodense and can be difficult to distinguish from the adenopathy seen in the presence of MAI infection, or even lymphoma. The GI manifestations of Kaposi's sarcoma and abdominal adenopathy sometimes precede the cutaneous lesions.[41] Kaposi's sarcoma can also metastasize to other organs, particularly the liver. Occasionally, CT is able to demonstrate the liver metastases as low-density lesions and can also be helpful in the evaluation of other lesions in the GI tract and abdomen.

AIDS-related lymphoma

The lymphoma encountered in AIDS patients is a non-Hodgkin's lymphoma, usually the B-cell type. Occasion-

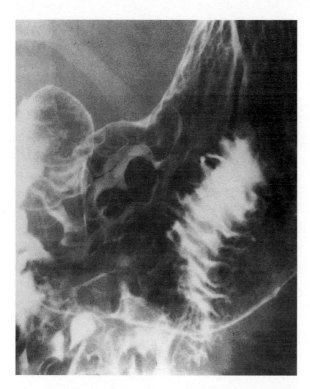

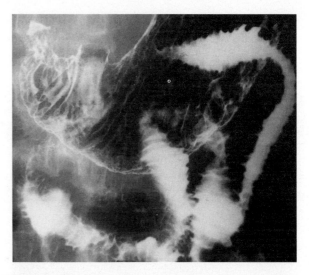

Fig. 47-20 Thickening and near effacement of the valvulae conniventes of the small bowel. This was secondary to Kaposi's sarcoma that had metastasized to the small bowel. The radiographic pattern resembles that of hemorrhage into the small bowel. This pattern is secondary to diffuse infiltration by Kaposi's sarcoma and is relatively unique to AIDS patients.

Fig. 47-19 Gastric polyps resulting from Kaposi's sarcoma that metastasized to the stomach. This is the more classic form, with discrete polyps and occasional central ulceration.

ally Hodgkin's lymphoma is also encountered in these patients. The distinctive clinical features of the AIDS variety include its highly aggressive nature, high-grade histologic subtypes, and an extremely high proportion of extranodal involvement, particularly in the central nervous system and GI tract.[38,39] Some think that Ebstein-Barr virus may serve as a lymphogenic stimulus in AIDS patients. The development of lymphoma may be one of the first manifestations of AIDS, and a history of the lymphadenopathy syndrome has been noted in these instances. With the advent of drug therapy, which is now prolonging the lives of HIV-infected individuals, some speculate that the incidence of AIDS-related lymphoma may increase with time. There is some controversy concerning this point, but a substantial increase in this complication has not yet been witnessed.[42]

The radiographic appearance of lymphoma is typically quite variable and remains so in the AIDS patient as well. Lesions of the bowel may assume the appearance of mucosal fold thickening of varying degrees, discrete nodules or masses, or infiltrating neoplasms with mucosal destruction (Figs. 47-21 and 47-22).[43-44] Conventional barium radiography is usually helpful for identifying these lesions, but the possible existence of multifocal lesions and extraintestinal disease must be sought. This is why CT examination of these patients is necessary to help demonstrate the extent of disease. AIDS-related lymphoma may be apparent

only as an adenopathy and may be indistinguishable from the adenopathy due to Kaposi's sarcoma or MAI infection[19,20,41,44] (Fig. 47-23). It may be necessary to obtain tissue by CT-guided biopsy to help in distinguishing among these entities.

Other neoplasms

There have been scattered reports of the development of other neoplasms in AIDS patients. One of these is squamous cell carcinoma of the anus, which is also more frequently seen among transplant recipients. The development of this unusual tumor may be related to a viral oncogenic stimulus in that region, which triggers the formation of condylomas.[38] It is not often evaluated radiographically but can sometimes be seen as an irregular infiltrating tumor at the anorectal junction (Fig. 47-24). CT may be used to further evaluate the area, although it is usually not warranted.

There have also been reports of squamous cell carcinoma of the oropharynx and esophagus.[45] Again, these lesions may also be inducted by other viral infections in the region. It is uncertain whether there will be a progressive increase in the incidence of these lesions with time. However, the possibility of further intestinal malignancies must be considered, particularly as HIV-infected patients survive longer. Intestinal malignancies are now being encountered increasingly among transplant recipients.[46]

RADIOLOGIC PRACTICE IN AN HIV ENVIRONMENT

As the extent of the HIV epidemic increases, along with the number of patients with actual AIDS, this will have a

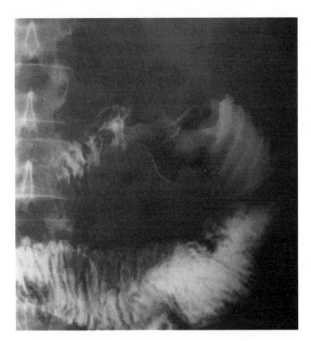

Fig. 47-21 An annular tumor of the proximal small bowel at the ligament of Treitz in this AIDS patient was secondary to non-Hodgkin's lymphoma.

dramatic impact on almost all radiologic practices, regardless of their type and location. There is an ever-increasing likelihood that radiologists will come into contact with HIV-infected patients on a routine basis. Thus the implementation of safety precautions for all radiologic procedures is mandatory to guard against transmission to health-care workers in the radiology department.

The virus is not only found in the blood; it can also be recovered from semen, vaginal fluid, cerebrospinal fluid, saliva, and even breast milk.[12,13] Therefore safeguards must be taken whenever contact with any of these patient fluids is possible. There have been numerous reports of HIV transmission to health-care workers, most involving accidental needle puncture. However, there have also been several reports of transmission occurring when contaminated blood has been splattered on the skin or face, with subsequent viral entry occurring through minor breaks in the skin or mucous membranes.

To reduce the risk of hospital personnel infection, particularly in the radiology department where little may be known about the patient's HIV status, several precautions must be taken.[47]

1. All members of the department should be educated in universal blood and body fluid precautions. Essentially, all body fluid from any patient must be considered a potential source of HIV.
2. Because inadvertent needle-stick injury remains the most likely source for accidental transmission, the proper use and disposal of all needles and sharp instruments should be taught and rigorously enforced.

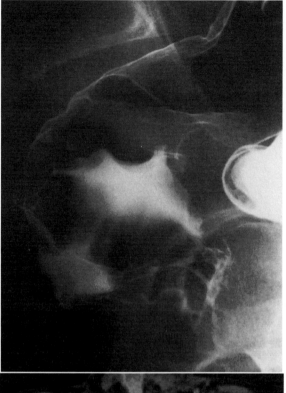

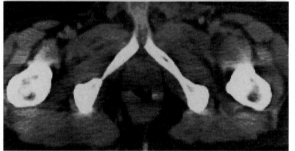

Fig. 47-22 A, Infiltrating tumor of the rectum secondary to lymphoma. **B,** CT scan of the same patient obtained through the rectum demonstrates diffuse thickening of the rectal wall. Similar changes may also be seen in conjunction with rectal infections in AIDS patients. Bowel wall thickening in AIDS may be due to either infection or tumor, and biopsy is often necessary for differentiation.

3. Any personnel who have direct contact with patients should wear some type of protective gloves. If the potential exists for the splashing or spraying of body fluids (i.e., angiography), masks or goggles and gowns should also be worn. Hand washing must be done after all procedures, even if gloves are worn.
4. Health-care workers with breaks in their skin or any of the many types of dermatitis should not assist in procedures when contact with body fluids may occur, even if they are wearing gloves.
5. Any clothing or devices that are contaminated with patient body fluids must be disposed of properly or

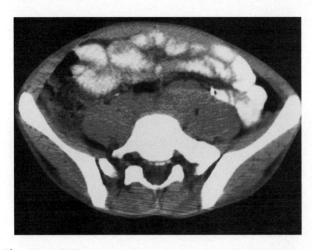

Fig. 47-23 Diffuse retroperitoneal adenopathy was secondary to a non-Hodgkins lymphoma. Kaposi's sarcoma and sometimes even *Mycobacterium avium-intracellulare* infection can produce extensive abdominal adenopathy.

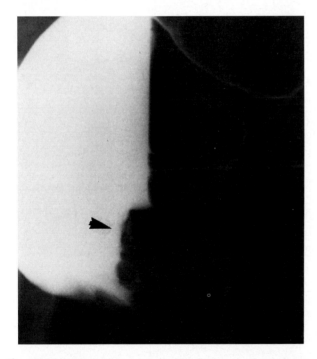

Fig. 47-24 A flat, rigid lesion in the distal rectum at the anal verge in this AIDS patient *(arrow)* was due to an infiltrating squamous cell carcinoma of the rectum.

properly sterilized. All personnel handling this material should wear gloves. The surfaces of equipment (e.g., table tops) can be easily disinfected using a dilute bleach solution, which is inexpensive and viricidal.

REFERENCES

1. CDC: The HIV/AIDS epidemic: the first 10 years, *MMWR* 40:357, 1991.
2. CDC: Mortality attributable to HIV infection/AIDS—United States, 1981-1990, *MMWR* 40:41, 1991.
3. CDC: HIV prevalence estimates and AIDS case projections for the United States: report based on a workshop. Recommendation and report #16, 11-30-90, *MMWR* 39:1, 1990.
4. Gardner LI et al: Evidence for spread of the human immunodeficiency virus into low prevalence areas of the United States, *J Acquir Immune Defic Syndr* 2:521, 1989.
5. Shaw GM, Wong-Staal F, Gallo RC: Etiology of AIDS: virology, molecular biology, and evolution of human immunodeficiency viruses. In DeVita VT et al, eds: *AIDS,* ed 2, Philadelphia, 1988, JB Lippincott.
6. Levy JA: Features of HIV and the host response that influence progression to disease. In Sande MA, Volberding PA, eds: *The medical management of AIDS,* ed 2, Philadelphia, 1990, WB Saunders.
7. Solinger AM, Hess EV: Acquired immune deficiency syndrome—an overview, *Semin Roentgenol* 22:9, 1987.
8. Tindall B et al: Primary HIV infection: clinical, immunologic and serologic aspects. In Sande MA, Volberding PA, eds: *The medical management of AIDS,* ed 2, Philadelphia, 1990, WB Saunders.
9. Yarchoan R, Pluda JM: Clinical aspects of infection with AIDS retrovirus: acute HIV infection, persistent generalized lymphadenopathy, and AIDS-related complex. In DeVita VT et al, eds: *AIDS,* ed 2, Philadelphia, 1988, JB Lippincott.
10. CDC: Classification system for human T-lymphotropic virus type III/lymphadenopathy–associated virus infections, *MMWR* 35:334, 1986.
11. Redfield RR, Wright CD, Tramont EC: The Walter Reed staging classification for HTLV-III/LAV infection, *N Engl J Med* 314:131, 1986.
12. Castro KG, Hardy AM, Curran JW: The acquired immunodeficiency syndrome: epidemiology and risk factors of transmission, *Med Clin North Am* 70:635, 1986.
13. Curran JW et al: Epidemiology of HIV infection and AIDS in the United States, *Science* 239:610, 1988.
14. Phair JP: Natural history of HIV infection. In Sande MA, Volberding PA: *The medical management of AIDS,* ed 2, Philadelphia, 1990, WB Saunders.
15. Moss AR, Bacchetti P: Natural history of HIV infection, *J Acquir Immune Defic Syndr* 3:55, 1989.
16. Taylor JM et al: CD4 percentage, CD4 number, and CD4:CD8 ratio in HIV infection: which to choose and how to use, *J Acquir Immune Defic Syndr* 2:114, 1989.
17. Wall SD et al: Multifocal abnormalities of the gastrointestinal tract in AIDS, *AJR* 146:1, 1986.
18. Federle MDP: A radiologist looks at AIDS: imaging evaluation based on symptom complexes, *Radiology* 166:553, 1988.
19. Jeffrey RB et al: Abdominal CT in acquired immunodeficiency syndrome, *AJR* 146:7, 1986.
20. Jones B, Fiskman EK: CT of the gut in the immunocompromised host, *Radiol Clin North Am* 27:763, 1989.
21. Quinn TC: Clinical approach to intestinal infections in homosexual men, *Med Clin North Am* 70:611, 1986.
22. Frager DH et al: Gastrointestinal complications of AIDS: radiologic features, *Radiology* 158:597, 1986.
23. Roberts L et al: Adult esophageal candidiasis: a radiographic spectrum, *Radiographics* 7:289, 1987.
24. Levine MS et al: Opportunistic esophagitis in AIDS: radiographic diagnosis, *Radiology* 165:815, 1987.
25. Teixidor HS et al: Cytomegalovirus infection of the alimentary canal: radiologic findings with pathologic correlation, *Radiology* 163:317, 1987.
26. Balthazar EJ et al: Cytomegalovirus esophagitis in AIDS: radiographic features in 16 patients, *AJR* 149:919, 1987.
27. Frager DH et al: Cytomegalovirus colitis in acquired immune defi-

ciency syndrome: radiologic spectrum, *Gastrointest Radiol* 11:241, 1986.

28. Levine MS et al: Herpes esophagitis, *AJR* 136:863, 1981.
29. Berk RN et al: Cryptosporidiosis of the stomach and small intestine in patients with AIDS, *AJR* 143:549, 1984.
30. Brandon J, Glick SN, Teplick SK: Intestinal giardiasis: the importance of serial filming, *AJR* 144:581, 1985.
31. Nyberg DA et al: Abdominal CT findings of disseminated *Mycobacterium avium-intracellulare* in AIDS, *AJR* 145:297, 1985.
32. Surawicz CM et al: Spectrum of rectal biopsy abnormalities in homosexual men with intestinal symptoms, *Gastroenterology* 91:651, 1986.
33. HIV-associated enteropathy, *Lancet* 2:777, 1989.
34. Schneiderman DJ: Hepatobiliary abnormalities of AIDS, *Gastroenterol Clin North Am* 17:615, 1988.
35. Blumberg RS et al: Cytomegalovirus- and Cryptosporidium-associated acalculous gangrenous cholecystitis, *Am J Med* 76:1118, 1984.
36. Romano AJ et al: Gallbladder and bile duct abnormalities in AIDS: sonographic findings in eight patients, *AJR* 150:123, 1988.
37. Dolmatch BL et al: AIDS-related cholangitis: radiographic findings in nine patients, *Radiology* 163:313, 1987.
38. Friedman SL: Gastrointestinal and hepatobiliary neoplasms in AIDS, *Gastroenterol Clin North Am* 17:465, 1988.

39. Nyberg DA, Federle MP: AIDS-related Kaposi sarcoma and lymphomas, *Semin Roentgenol* 22:54, 1987.
40. Rose HS et al: Alimentary tract involvement in Kaposi sarcoma: radiographic and endoscopic findings in 25 homosexual men, *AJR* 139:661, 1982.
41. Moon KL et al: Kaposi sarcoma and lymphadenopathy syndrome: limitations of abdominal CT in acquired immunodeficiency syndrome, *Radiology* 150:479, 1984.
42. CDC: Opportunistic non-Hodgkin's lymphomas among severely immunocompromised HIV-infected patients surviving for prolonged periods on antiretroviral therapy—United States, *MMWR* 40:591, 1991.
43. Rubesin SE et al: Non-Hodgkin lymphoma of the small intestine, *Radiographics* 10:985, 1990.
44. Townsend RR et al: Abdominal lymphoma in AIDS: evaluation with US, *Radiology* 171:719, 1989.
45. Frager DH et al: Squamous cell carcinoma of the esophagus in patients with acquired immunodeficiency syndrome, *Gastrointest Radiol* 13:358, 1988.
46. Feczko PJ, Mezwa DG: Gastrointestinal carcinomas in renal transplant recipients, *Gastrointest Radiol* 16:351, 1991.
47. Heller RM et al: AIDS awareness in the conduct of radiologic procedures: guidelines to safe practice, *Radiology* 166:563, 1988.

48 Gastrointestinal Bleeding: Endoscopy and Diagnostic Approach

D. E. BECKLY

Those conditions in which bleeding is the main clinical problem or a major problem demanding treatment in its own right are considered in this chapter. The many other conditions in which bleeding is a coincidental event are discussed elsewhere in this volume. Because the diagnosis and treatment of gastrointestinal (GI) tract bleeding poses both clinical and purely technical problems, some discussion is also focused on the clinical setting in which endoscopy is performed.

CLINICAL ASPECTS

GI bleeding may be either acute or chronic. Most of the conditions in which bleeding is the main problem trigger acute rather than chronic bleeding. From a practical point of view, cases can be classified as presenting a clinical picture of upper, lower, or indeterminate GI bleeding. Thus a patient with hematemesis, melena, or both is usually bleeding from a lesion proximal to the ligament of Treitz. A patient with bright red rectal bleeding is usually bleeding from the colon or rectum. If bleeding is torrential, red blood is passed per rectum no matter where the site of origin. When the clinical findings point to a bleeding site in the upper GI tract, or this is indeterminate, the upper tract should be the first investigated, normally using upper GI endoscopy. If this is negative the next investigation carried out depends on the rate of bleeding. If the bleeding is profuse and continuous, angiography can virtually always reveal the cause. If bleeding is intermittent, an isotope scan should be performed, as angiography has a lower yield in this setting. However, it is best not to rely on isotope scans as the sole method of localization.[1]

TIMING OF ENDOSCOPY

Early controversy over the value of emergency endoscopy has largely been overtaken by developments in endoscopic therapy. It is clear that, if endoscopy is to influence mortality, it will do so by enhancing the ability to predict the risk of rebleeding, and by allowing the timely implementation of endoscopic therapy to prevent it. Logically, this requires that endoscopy be performed as soon as possible after hospital admission. The risk of a peptic ulcer re-

bleeding is related to the presence or absence of certain visual features of the ulcer, as seen endoscopically. Thus active arterial bleeding, adherent clot, or the presence of a so-called visible vessel, all indicate a high risk of rebleeding, particularly when the last finding is associated with evidence of a patent underlying artery, as shown by Doppler ultrasound (see later discussion). The incidence of observed active bleeding varies according to the timing of the endoscopy.[2,3] An American Society of Gastrointestinal Endoscopy survey showed that bleeding was active in 41.5% patients who underwent endoscopy within 12 hours of admission, as opposed to 22.2% in those who underwent endoscopy 37 to 48 hours after admission.[4] The visible vessel may also be an evanescent phenomenon that disappears within 24 hours (Fig. 48-1), probably as the result of spontaneous thrombosis of the underlying artery. Thus it would appear that to obtain the most pessimistic, albeit accurate, prognosis, endoscopy should be performed early, as the signs may be more favorable later on. Another disadvantage of delaying endoscopy is that some patients may rebleed before endoscopy can be undertaken, thus not only possibly compromising them clinically but also resulting in a higher mortality. Furthermore, the absence of stigmata may make it impossible to know which of several observed lesions was responsible for the bleed. However, this is of more academic than practical interest, because the rebleeding risk is low when stigmata are lacking. Early endoscopy could result in the implementation of therapeutic endoscopic measures in some patients whose condition might have otherwise resolved spontaneously, but this may be an acceptable price to pay for a reduction in the rebleeding incidence.

A further problem with the early endoscopy approach is a practical and organizational one. Diagnostic endoscopy in the patient with GI bleeding is one of the more technically demanding forms of endoscopy, especially if it is combined with endoscopic therapy. For this reason it cannot be delegated to the less experienced endoscopists. The provision of a 24-hour emergency endoscopy service therefore requires the immediate availability of senior staff members. In large academic centers there are likely to be enough

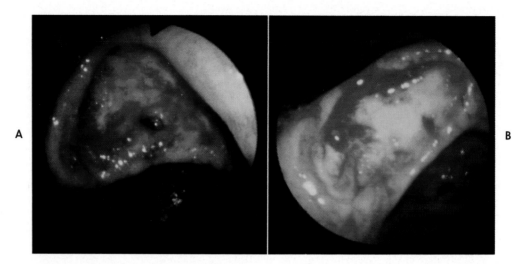

Fig. 48-1 A, Gastric ulcer, which has bled recently, showing a visible vessel located centrally in the ulcer crater. Doppler examination revealed negative findings. **B,** Same ulcer 24 hours later. Further bleeding has occurred, and the centrally placed visible vessel is now barely detectable. A new bleeding point is seen in the top left margin of the ulcer.

senior staff endoscopists to provide such a rota without undue difficulty. In smaller centers, however, there may be only one or two such staff members, and, under these circumstances, some compromise is probably required.

From a practical standpoint, it is probably best to perform endoscopy in patients as soon after initial assessment and stabilization of their condition as possible, when this is during the daytime. If a patient admitted at night is hemodynamically stable, it is reasonable to wait until the next convenient daytime slot. However, if the patient is actively bleeding after admission, endoscopy should not be delayed, regardless of the time of day.

TECHNIQUE OF UPPER GI ENDOSCOPY IN ACUTE BLEEDING

The actively bleeding patient presents a challenge, both clinically and endoscopically. The initial assessment should be made and resuscitation started before the patient is transferred to the endoscopy department. However, it is a mistake to delay endoscopy too long, as transfusion can be just as easily carried out in the endoscopy room as at the bedside, and, in many cases, it may be possible to achieve hemostasis using endoscopic methods (see later discussion). The endoscopy room must therefore be properly equipped for the resuscitation and monitoring of bleeding patients, and the endoscopy staff suitably trained.

Most acutely bleeding lesions of the upper GI tract are obvious endoscopically, but occasionally bleeding may be so profuse that it renders endoscopic diagnosis difficult. The key to this situation is an unhurried and systematic approach. It is usually possible to exclude an esophageal lesion during the initial intubation. If a stomach full of blood is then encountered, a good method is to pass the scope immediately to the pylorus. If a bright red plug of clot is

seen emerging from the pylorus into the stomach, this indicates a bleeding site in the duodenum or, rarely, in the proximal jejunum. Regardless of whether such a plug is seen, the endoscope is passed to the first part of the duodenum and the mucosal surface examined carefully using a wash catheter to remove any surface blood or clot. The second part of the duodenum is examined in the same fashion. Next, the instrument is withdrawn into the stomach, with particular care taken to examine the junction of the first and second parts of the duodenum, the fornices of the duodenal bulb, and the rim of the pylorus itself. A lesion can be easily overlooked in all these areas. Even if the stomach contains large amounts of blood, it is usually possible to see the antrum and lesser curve quite adequately because they are uncovered when the patient is in the left lateral position. Care must be taken during inversion of the endoscope not to allow the shaft of the instrument to overlie and obscure a small lesion high on the lesser curve. As in the duodenum, the mucosa should be carefully washed wherever there is adherent blood or clot. Large amounts of luminal blood tend to obscure the greater curve and posterior wall of the stomach, but these areas can be revealed by turning the patient supine and then into the right lateral position. Both during inversion and while the instrument is withdrawn, the whole lesser curve from the angulus up to and including the cardia is carefully examined. The fundus is examined with the scope inverted. Finally, the esophagus is reexamined during withdrawal of the instrument.

COMMON CONDITIONS AND THEIR TREATMENT
Esophageal varices

Acutely bleeding esophageal varices present a clinical picture that is often both dramatic and alarming. However, although the rate of bleeding may be quite rapid, few varices actually bleed faster than an intravenous (IV) drip will run with a wide-bore cannula inserted into the vein. Diagnosis is rarely a problem, but it should be remembered that small varices may collapse and disappear if the esophagus is overdistended with air. Management in the face of profuse bleeding may be a problem. Metoclopramide (20 mg IV) has been shown to be effective in arresting active variceal bleeding, and has the advantages of ready availability and simplicity of use.[5] If this fails to bring the bleeding under control, it may be necessary to insert a Minnesota tube, and this can allow time for adequate resuscitation and correction of the clotting abnormality. The first-line treatment of varices should be injection sclerotherapy, and this can either be performed immediately, or, in the event of profuse bleeding, after initial control has been achieved. Sclerotherapy can be carried out with a Minnesota tube still in situ, provided the esophageal balloon is deflated.

Technique and complications of injection sclerotherapy

A variety of sclerosants exists, and which one is used often depends as much on local preference as on any demonstrable superiority of one agent over another. Commonly used agents are ethanolamine oleate, 3% sodium tetradecyl sulfate, polidocanol, and dehydrated alcohol.[6] The chosen agent is injected through a sheathed needle, arranged so that the needle can be withdrawn into its sheath during insertion of the endoscope down the biopsy channel. The volume of sclerosant injected at any one site is important, as too great a volume can cause extensive ulceration of the mucosa, which may lead to deep necrosis and perforation. No more than 2 ml of 3% sodium tetradecyl sulfate should be injected at any one site, and, if the injection is paravariceal rather than intravariceal, 1 ml is enough. There is evidence that intravariceal injection produces more rapid thrombosis of varices than does paravariceal injection, and it is the practice of the author's institution to always attempt intravariceal injection. One injection is made into each varix as close to the cardia as practicable, and then a second injection is made 3 to 4 cm higher up in the same vein. No attempt is made to inject isolated fundal varices.

How often sclerotherapy should be repeated is open to argument.[7,8] Ideally, any ulceration stemming from the first set of injections should be allowed to heal before any further injections are performed. However, recurrent bleeding may necessitate earlier intervention. The risk is that, in the minority of cases in which sclerotherapy fails to control bleeding, repeated injections performed at too closely spaced intervals may so damage the esophagus as to render surgical esophageal transection impossible. It is the author's practice to limit injection sessions to a maximum of two per week. Any patient still bleeding significantly after two sclerotherapy sessions in 1 week undergoes transection. Such a policy has been advocated by others,[9] and is the

logical one when transection is readily available; but this protocol may need to be varied in other circumstances, or if the patient presents an intolerable surgical risk. The aim should be to continue with sclerotherapy until all significant varices are thrombosed. Sometimes it may be difficult to determine whether a varix is thrombosed or not. A Doppler ultrasound device passed via the endoscope biopsy channel may be helpful for determining this. Once all varices have been thrombosed, the patient is followed up to ensure that new varices are detected and treated in a timely fashion.

Unless specific contraindications exist, all patients with varices should be receiving propranolol in sufficient doses to lower their pulse rate by 25%, as this can help reduce the incidence of bleeding[10] and aid in preventing recurrence of varices.[11,12]

Complications of sclerotherapy

Besides effecting the desired thrombosis of varices, sclerosant injections may also produce superficial and deep necrosis of the esophageal wall as well as inflammation of the periesophageal tissues.[13,14] This, in turn, causes esophageal ulceration.[15] The symptoms of this complication are chest pain, fever, dysphagia, and pleural effusion. Chest pain was found to occur after 23% of sclerotherapy sessions, and a fever greater than 37.5° C after 40%. About half of all patients had pleural effusions, but most were small and most symptoms and signs resolved spontaneously.[16] Esophageal perforation following sclerotherapy has been reported to occur in 1% of the cases, and abscess formation in 0.3%. Strictures form in less than 10% of the cases, and pulmonary infiltrates in 9%. Atelectasis, pleural effusion, and mediastinal widening occur quite frequently, and respiratory insufficiency was encountered in 14 out of 390 sclerotherapy procedures.[17] A rare but frequently fatal complication of sclerotherapy is portal or mesenteric vein thrombosis.[18,19] Peritonitis may be a consequence of sclerotherapy,[20] and has been reported to occur in 3% of cases.[21] Other reported complications include cerebral abscess, meningitis,[22] pericarditis,[23] and carcinoma of the esophagus.[24]

Gastric varices

Gastric varices may be junctional or fundal. Junctional varices are continuous with distal esophageal varices and do not extend into the fundus. Fundal varices, on the other hand, are confined to the fundus. The response of junctional varices to sclerotherapy is similar to that of varices farther up the esophagus. This is not surprising, because flow in varices is frequently bidirectional and may vary with the respiratory phase, thus allowing the sclerosant to move both cephalad and caudad from the injection site. However, sclerotherapy for fundal varices is associated with poor results, in that there are high rates of rebleeding, increased complications, and lowered patient survival.[25,26] Splenic vein thrombosis may give rise to the syndrome of sinistral portal hypertension, which causes gastric varices but with a patent portal vein and normal liver function. The underlying splenic vein thrombosis may be caused by pancreatic carcinoma, pancreatitis, or a pancreatic pseudocyst. The diagnosis may be confirmed by ultrasound or angiography.[27] Some success in the treatment of fundal varices has been reported for injections of N-butyl-2-cyanoacrylate (Histoacryl).[28]

Prophylactic injection of varices

When varices are discovered but have not bled, this raises the question of whether prophylactic sclerotherapy is beneficial. Current wisdom dictates that it is not.[29,30] Indeed, in one recent multicenter trial, there was an unexplained increase in mortality in the sclerotherapy group, compared with that in a control group, despite a lower incidence of variceal bleeding in the former.[31] Propranolol may be a better option for this group of patients.[10,32]

Varices and pregnancy

Fortunately, it is quite uncommon for varices to arise in pregnant women, and most such patients are likely to have extrahepatic portal hypertension. The increase in circulating blood volume that takes place in pregnancy can cause previously stable, small varices to enlarge dramatically during the first trimester. Sclerotherapy can be performed safely in pregnant women,[33,34] and vaginal delivery is not contraindicated, as the pressure gradient across the variceal wall during straining is not substantially increased.[35]

Bleeding peptic ulcer
Epidemiology

Upper GI bleeding accounts for between 50 and 150 hospital admissions per 100,000 population.[36-39] The incidence of hospital admission for bleeding gastric ulcers in the United States has shown an upward trend, reaching 25 per 100,000 population in 1983, whereas that for duodenal ulcers has remained level at 22 per 100,000.[40] The age of patients with upper GI bleeding has increased dramatically from 6% to 17% over 60 years of age during the period 1921 to 1936 to 40% to 48% in the same age group during 1953 to 1973.[41] This is important, as nearly all the mortality occurs in this age group.[42] In an ASGE survey of 2225 patients with upper GI bleeding conducted in 1978 and 1979, 45.2% patients were found to be over 60 years old. Peptic ulcers were the cause of bleeding in 47.5%. Endoscopic findings were diagnostic in 91.9% of the cases, with 0.9% of the complications ascribed to the endoscopy. The overall mortality in this large series was 10.8%, but, of those who died, the cause of death in 69.7% was due to underlying disease, while 43.6% died as the result of bleeding and 13.7% of surgical complications. The mortality in patients without underlying disease was only 2.16%. Emergency surgery was associated with a threefold increase in mortality, compared with elective surgery.[43-45] Currently, overall mortality in the range of

3% to 5% is typical of the best centers,[46] with 95% of the deaths occurring in those over 65 years old.[47] Better teamwork between physicians and surgeons in the management of these cases is undoubtedly responsible for some of the improvement in mortality.[48] However, given the close links between mortality on the one hand and age and the need for surgery on the other, it seems likely that the greatest improvements will result from the use of nonsurgical methods of hemostasis when possible, and better operative and postoperative care when surgical intervention is unavoidable.

Pathophysiology of bleeding peptic ulcer

Ulcers bleed when a vessel in the ulcer base or edge erodes. This vessel is usually an artery, and a study in patients with gastric ulcers requiring resection for bleeding has shown the mean outside diameter of such arteries is 0.7 mm, and this ranges from 0.1 to 1.8 mm. An arteritis that includes polymorph infiltration and fibrinoid necrosis, predominantly involving the side of the artery nearest the ulcer base, has been recognized.[49] The fact that the process caused a hole to form in the side of the artery rather than complete transection may explain why normal hemostatic mechanisms fail to work in these cases when rebleeding occurs. The so-called visible vessel in the ulcer base has been shown to be a true vessel in some cases, but to be a plug of clot in a hole in the side of a vessel or a pseudoaneurysm in others. Another interesting finding is the discovery of recanalized thrombus in 24% of the bleeding vessels.[49] These findings accord well with the results of a study in which 49 recently bleeding ulcers were examined using an endoscopic Doppler probe. There was no underlying arterial flow in all 20 ulcers with nonraised dark stains in the base, and none of these rebled. Of the 29 ulcers with visible vessels or adherent fresh clot, 18 (62%) showed no flow and only two (11%) of these rebled. Eleven ulcers (38%) showed arterial flow immediately adjacent to the visible vessel or fresh clot, and eight (72%) of these rebled.[50] It would appear therefore that, for most bleeding ulcers, the pathologic process does indeed lead to thrombosis in the underlying artery, and these ulcers do not rebleed unless recanalization takes place or a new vessel is eroded. Those arteries in which flow persists are the ones at risk for rebleeding, and these represent only 38% to 50% of those ulcers with a visible vessel.[50,51]

Endoscopy

The aims of endoscopy in patients with bleeding peptic ulcers are threefold: (1) identification of the bleeding ulcer; (2) assessment of the rebleeding risk; and (3) endoscopic treatment of those ulcers that carry a high risk of rebleeding.

Identifying the ulcer responsible for the bleeding is not usually a problem, as discussed earlier, but multiple lesions may be found in up to one third of the cases.[43,44]

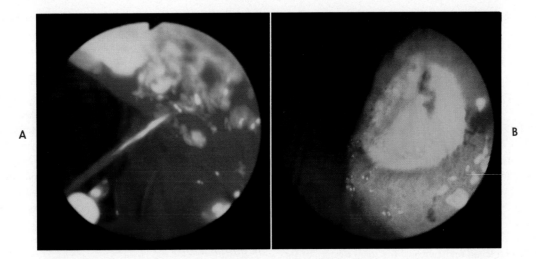

Fig. 48-2 A, Jetting arterial hemorrhage from a gastric ulcer. This was controlled by the injection of a total of 6 ml of 1:10,000 epinephrine and 3 ml of 3% sodium tetradecyl sulfate. The injection needle is seen in the lower left margin. **B,** Same ulcer 3 days later. The ulcer crater now shows only dark stains. There was no further bleeding.

Rebleeding risk

In 1978 the prognostic importance of certain endoscopic appearances characteristic of ulcers that had recently bled was recognized.[52] Since that time, numerous other investigators have confirmed the importance of these stigmata, in particular the so-called visible vessel.[53-55] The reported rebleeding rates associated with visible vessels have varied widely, ranging from 100%[53] to less than one third,[56,57] but some of these differences may actually be due to variations in the definition of the endoscopic features. If active arterial bleeding is found at the time of endoscopy, this carries an even higher risk of ongoing bleeding or rebleeding (Fig. 48-2). Despite some fairly wide variations in the literature, it has been suggested that the prevalence of arterial bleeding is 5%, and this carries an 80% to 100% ongoing or rebleeding rate. For the nonbleeding visible vessel, the prevalence is 15% to 20% and the rebleeding risk is 40% to 50%.[51] In this latter instance, the use of Doppler ultrasound, as already described, allows further segregation of the patients into a large (62%) low-risk group with an 11% chance of rebleeding and a smaller (38%) high-risk group that carries a 72% likelihood of rebleeding.[50]

Endoscopic hemostasis

The mortality associated with emergency surgery performed to arrest bleeding from peptic ulcer may be nearly three times that for elective surgery (23.7% versus 8.5%, respectively).[58] The elderly and those with serious coexisting disease are particularly at risk. Endoscopic methods for achieving hemostasis have proved to be both effective and safe.[59] However, no method of endoscopic hemostasis is entirely free of complications, and these methods should not be applied indiscriminately. Only those patients with a high rebleeding risk should be treated. The methods fall into two categories: thermal methods, which include lasers, heater probes, and diathermy; and injection therapy, which includes simple tamponade and the administration of vasoconstrictors and sclerosants.

Thermal methods
THEORETICAL CONSIDERATIONS

The exact mechanism by which heating brings about hemostasis is not known, but it is likely that it is through a combination of edema, which precipitates vascular tamponade, and a direct effect of protein denaturation in the vessel wall. Heating also causes collagen to contract, and this may be an important factor. Protein denaturation occurs at 57° C and collagen contraction at 80° C. At 250° C, carbonization takes place, with burning away of tissue. The aim of any hemostatic method should, therefore, be to achieve a temperature of over 80° C, but under 250° C, in order to prevent perforation of the vessel wall. It may indeed be advisable to keep the temperature under 100° C to prevent miniexplosions in the vessel due to the generation of steam.[60] Furthermore, it is almost certainly advantageous if the vessel walls can be pressed together during heating by applying direct coaptive pressure. This may aid closure of the vessel by facilitating protein bonding between the vessel walls. In addition, the heat sink effect of rapid blood flow is abolished.[60,61] Tissue heating can be accomplished by the application of laser light. The depth to which the heating process penetrates depends on the wavelength of the light, as well as on the total amount of energy applied. In this respect, the argon laser is inferior to the neodymium-YAG (Nd:YAG) laser. Contact tips are available but have not been widely used in the setting of peptic ulcer bleeding.

The heater probe consists of a heating element (diode) inside a Teflon-coated probe tip with a capability for the forceful irrigation of the target area as well as direct-vessel tamponade. Controlled amounts of thermal energy can be preset for delivery at the probe tip. The depth of coagulation depends on the amount of thermal energy applied.

Monopolar or multipolar diathermy can also be used to achieve tissue heating. Its heating effect is proportional to the current density. In monopolar diathermy, the current flows from the point where a single electrode is applied to exit the patient via a wide flat plate. The current density and therefore the heating effect are maximal near the electrode tip, but penetration is somewhat unpredictable, as it depends on the electrical resistance of the local tissue. With multipolar diathermy, the current passes between two or more electrodes at the probe tip. Penetration is more predictable in this instance because heat penetration is by thermal conduction, as it is for the heater probe. A disadvantage of this method is that the desiccation of local tissue increases the electrical resistance between the electrodes and diminishes the heating effect that can be achieved.

CLINICAL AND PRACTICAL CONSIDERATIONS

The results of randomized trials that compared Nd:YAG therapy with the results in a control group have demonstrated an improvement in the rebleeding rate, a reduced need for surgery, and reduced mortality associated with Nd:YAG laser treatment.[55,62-64] Reduced rebleeding rates and need for surgery have also been observed for the heater probe,[65,66] monopolar electrocoagulation,[67,68] and multipolar electrocoagulation.[69,70] When the merits of the Nd:YAG laser, heater probe, and bipolar electrocoagulation were compared, no significant differences were found in the rebleeding rates (10%, 19.4%, and 10%, respectively) or need for emergency surgery (7%, 13%, and 7%, respectively). It appears therefore that in expert hands all the thermal methods can accomplish worthwhile hemostasis, and no single method has yet emerged as the clear winner. Complications have been reported for all methods. Perforation is rare, occurring in approximately 1%. Bleeding may be induced in a nonbleeding vessel in up to 20% of the cases, but can usually be controlled by further hemostatic therapy.[59]

Injection therapy

Hemostasis can be achieved by the injection of varicoconstrictor or sclerosant agents, or both, into the bleeding artery, or close to it, using the same endoscopic injectors as used in the sclerotherapy of varices. Japanese workers have reported success with the use of concentrated alcohol.[71-73] Others have used polidicanol, either alone[74] or mixed with 1:10,000 epinephrine.[75] Initial hemostasis is achieved in 90% to 100% of the cases using this approach,

and rebleeding, although affecting nearly a quarter of the patients, is frequently stopped permanently by a second injection. Randomized controlled trials have shown both a reduced rebleeding rate[76,77] and need for emergency surgery[77,78] in patients who underwent injection therapy, compared to medically treated control groups. No difference was found in the rebleeding rate, requirement for surgery, or mortality when epinephrine injection therapy was compared with heater probe treatment.[79] However, less rebleeding was associated with heater probe treatment than with alcohol injection therapy.[80] Two trials have shown a significant improvement in the results of treatment from the combination of Nd:YAG laser treatment with epinephrine injections.[81,82]

Complications

The most frequently reported complication of injection therapy is perforation, and this appears to occur in 1% to 2% of the patients.[71,83] Fatal gastroduodenal necrosis was reported to occur in a previously hypoxemic patient who acquired a clostridial infection after injection of 5 ml of 1:10,000 epinephrine and 6 ml of 3% sodium tetradecyl sulfate.[84] Antral necrosis requiring surgery was also observed after the injection of 12 ml of 5% ethanolamine into a bleeding antral ulcer,[85] and pancreatoduodenal necrosis requiring surgery developed after the injection of cyanoacrylate in the treatment of a bleeding duodenal ulcer.[86] Although the incidence of complications is low, some of those associated with sclerotherapy may be serious, or even life threatening, and caution is therefore required. In particular, candidates for treatment should be carefully selected (see previous discussion), and the volumes of sclerosant used should be the minimal required to achieve hemostasis. The use of Doppler ultrasound may greatly facilitate both these aspects of sclerotherapy.

Other common causes of upper GI bleeding
Esophagitis

Esophagitis is a very common cause of minor upper GI bleeding and may cause profuse hemorrhage if coagulation is also impaired. It is commonly secondary to a hiatus hernia, but may also be due to gastric outflow obstruction, as seen in pyloric obstruction, or to the edema associated with a duodenal ulcer. Esophagitis is probably also responsible for the coffee-ground vomiting that accompanies organoaxial volvulus of the stomach.

Mallory Weiss tear

The Mallory Weiss tear is classically caused by violent vomiting, resulting in a mucosal laceration at the cardia, but may also occur in the absence of vomiting[87] (Fig. 48-3). Although the initial bleeding may be quite brisk, it is unusual for bleeding to continue or recur in the absence of a coagulopathy. The treatment adopted can therefore be conservative, but it is important to exclude the existence of

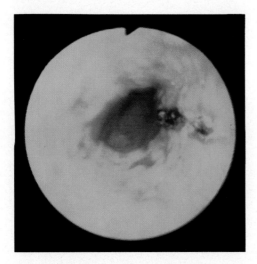

Fig. 48-3 A Mallory Weiss tear.

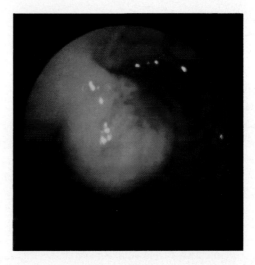

Fig. 48-4 Gastric leiomyoma. Bleeding is occurring from an ulcerated area of the fundus of the tumor. Endoscopic biopsy specimens are often normal, and the tumor may assume a dumbbell shape, penetrating through the gastric wall.

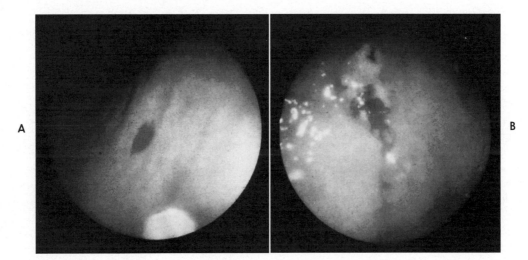

Fig. 48-5 A, Isolated gastric telangiectasia in a patient with chronic anemia. The white object in the lower half of the photograph is the tip of a laser light guide. **B,** Same patient after laser coagulation was performed using an Nd:YAG laser.
From Simkins KC: *A textbook of radiological diagnosis,* vol 4, ed 5, London, 1988, HK Lewis.

other bleeding lesions in the upper GI tract. This lesion must be distinguished from Boerhaave's syndrome, in which all the layers of the esophageal wall rupture, with free perforation into the mediastinum. This is a rare event and is usually caused by active resistance to vomiting.

Esophageal and gastric tumors

Carcinoma of the esophagus or stomach is common, but only rarely is manifested clinically by GI bleeding. The diagnosis is usually easy. Gastric or duodenal leiomyomas not infrequently present with bleeding, and exhibit a characteristic endoscopic appearance (Fig. 48-4). The initial symptom of gastric carcinoids may also be bleeding. In all these cases, treatment is directed at the underlying lesion.

Telangiectasia

Isolated gastric or duodenal telangiectasias are quite common and may be the cause of chronic anemia (Fig. 48-5). Only rarely does the patient prove to have the hereditary Osler-Weber-Rendu disease.

Gastritis

Subepithelial hemorrhage is quite common in alcoholic patients but is rarely a source of serious blood loss.[88]

Uncommon or infrequently recognized causes of upper GI bleeding
Dieulafoy lesion

The Dieulafoy lesion was probably first described by Gallard in 1884,[89] although it was not until a description by Dieulafoy, published in 1898,[90] that it was recognized to be a distinct entity. This lesion, which is most commonly found in the fundus of the stomach, consists of a bleeding artery surrounded by normal or near-normal mucosa. Although early descriptions implied the cause was peptic erosion, subsequent authors suggested the artery itself was aneurysmal. However, recent studies have shown that neither view is correct. There is no evidence of peptic ulceration, and all three layers of the vessel wall are normal without aneurysmal dilatation or vasculitis.[91,92] The abnormality is thought to be in the degree of proximity of a relatively large artery to the mucosal surface. There is subintimal fibrosis in affected arteries, but the exact mechanism responsible for the erosion and rupture is unclear.

The disease is more common in males[92,93] and is associated with alcoholism in 15% of the cases. It is also associated with peptic ulcer disease and with recent surgery. Although the fundus of the stomach is by far the most common site for these lesions to form, they have also been found in the duodenum,[94-96] jejunum,[97,98] and colon[99,100] (Fig. 48-6). The condition is probably more unrecognized than rare. Veldhuyzen Van Zanten et al.[101] published a review of 101 cases from the literature in 1986, plus six new cases. In 1988 Saueracker et al.[102] collected 156 cases from the world literature and added seven cases of their own. The age range in Veldhuyzen Van Zanten et al.'s review spanned 20 months to 93 years, with a mean of 52 years.

The importance of the Dieulafoy lesion is that it may be difficult if not impossible to diagnose when not actively bleeding, but it has a high tendency to recurrent massive hemorrhage, which is nearly always fatal if untreated. Furthermore, the common site of the lesion is on the high lesser curve and fundus of the stomach, an area that is surgically inaccessible, unless a long gastrotomy is created. Numerous reports have emphasized the difficulty in diagnosing the lesion. Angiography has been helpful,[103,104] but most authors advocate emergency repeat endoscopy.[94,95,101,105] Only rarely is the lesion correctly diagnosed in its nonbleeding state (Fig. 48-7).

The consensus is that, if a patient presenting with a hemodynamically significant upper GI bleed proves to have no identifiable lesion at the initial endoscopy examination, then Dieulafoy's lesion is one of the conditions that must be seriously considered. Endoscopy should be repeated immediately if rebleeding occurs, as this is the best time to

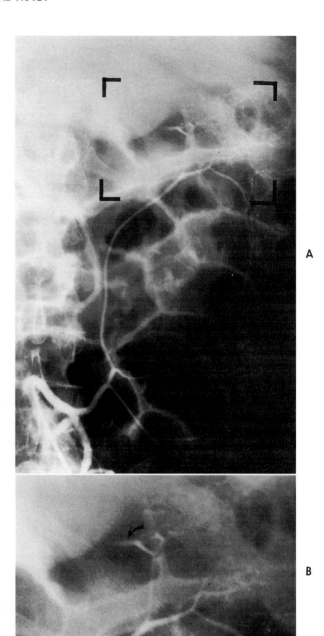

Fig. 48-6 A and **B,** Inferior mesenteric angiograms obtained in a 67-year-old man with massive rectal bleeding. There is a jetlike extravasation from a branch in the distal transverse colon *(arrow).* At operation, bleeding from a mucosal punctum typical of a Dieulafoy lesion was found.
Courtesy of Dr. I. P. Wells.

detect the lesion in its actively bleeding state. If the rapid rate of bleeding from the stomach does not permit identification of the bleeding site at endoscopy and emergency surgery is required, it is vital that a long gastrotomy be made so that the fundus can be adequately inspected. The mucosa should be carefully wiped to try to provoke rebleeding if active bleeding has stopped by then. If the Dieulafoy lesion can be identified at endoscopy, usually as an arterial

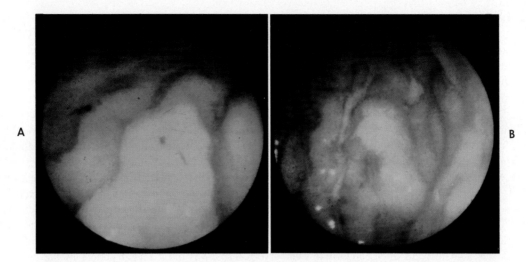

Fig. 48-7 A, Tiny brown stain at the site of a Dieulafoy lesion before laser coagulation. **B,** Same lesion after laser coagulation using an Nd:YAG laser. The immediate effect of laser coagulation was to produce bright red bleeding, but this stopped with subsequent coagulation.
From Simkins KC: *A textbook of radiological diagnosis,* vol 4, ed 5, London, 1988, HK Lewis.

jet coming from normal or near-normal mucosa, then endoscopic hemostasis should be attempted. Pointner et al.[105] successfully treated 18 of 22 patients using either sclerotherapy with polidocanol or bipolar electrocoagulation, or the two combined. Other authors have reported success in treating gastric Dieulafoy lesions using bipolar coagulation either alone[106] or in combination with epinephrine injections.[96] The heater probe has been used successfully in the treatment of both gastric lesions[107] and duodenal Dieulafoy disease.[94] The main problem has always been to establish the diagnosis, however.

Diffuse gastric antral telangiectasia: watermelon stomach

Watermelon stomach is another condition, which, like the Dieulafoy lesion, is probably more unrecognized than rare. The term *watermelon stomach* was first used by Jabbari et al. in 1984.[108] Raised bright red longitudinal folds in the gastric antrum radiating from the pylorus are characteristic features (Fig. 48-8) and somewhat resemble the longitudinal stripes in the skin of a watermelon. The condition is probably quite frequently mistaken for a florid form of hemorrhagic antral gastritis. However, biopsy specimens exhibit specific features, including mucosal hyperplasia, dilated mucosal capillaries, focal thrombosis, and fibromuscular hypertrophy in the lamina propria. There is no chronic inflammatory change. Furthermore, the condition does not resolve spontaneously and typically chronic anemia develops, which may be severe and require multiple blood transfusions. If the antral lesions are closely inspected using endoscopy, leashes of minute blood vessels can be seen that are similar in size to those seen in isolated telangiectasias. The lesions invariably stop abruptly at the pylorus and are usually confined to the antrum, although the author has ob-

served one case in which identical lesions existed in the antrum and at the cardia, but the latter were much less extensive.

Although the characteristic appearance is that of bright red raised folds that radiate from the pylorus, small detached satellite lesions are common. Variants of the disease in which antral involvement is more patchy or diffuse are also seen.[108-114]

A blood loss of 163 ml per day has been reported,[115] and losses of between 400 and 500 ml per week have been

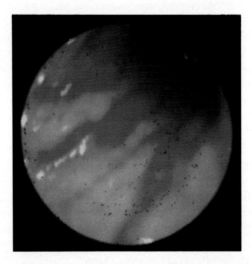

Fig. 48-8 Diffuse antral telangiectasia, or "watermelon stomach." The raised bright red ridges extending from the pylorus are typical of this condition, which may be mistaken for florid antral gastritis. Close endoscopic inspection shows that the redness is due to extensive telangiectasia. The histologic appearance is characteristic. The diagnosis is important, as the condition causes severe chronic anemia.

typical in the author's experience. Serum B_{12} levels are commonly low, or at the lower limit of normal, and, in some cases, there is a macrocytic anemia. The results of the Schilling test, when performed, are normal. In many cases, achlorhydria is provoked by a pentagastrin fast. This condition is associated with chronic liver disease and cirrhosis, and it has been observed in chronic active hepatitis,[108,116] primary biliary cirrhosis,[117,118] and alcoholic liver disease.[119] Treatment has traditionally consisted of antrectomy, which yields excellent results in fit patients.[108,109] However, the operative mortality may be as high as 7.4%.[112] Many of the patients are elderly, and endoscopic treatment by laser has proved very successful.[110,113,119,120,121] The heater probe has been used successfully,[122] as has sclerotherapy with alcohol.[123]

The telangiectasias tend to recur after endoscopic therapy, but typically treatment is effective for several years, and repeat treatment is also effective.

Hemobilia

The triad of GI blood loss, biliary colic, and jaundice suggests the presence of hemobilia, although both pain and jaundice may be absent.[124] Fifty percent of the cases of hemobilia are due to blunt trauma to the liver, and, under these circumstances, the diagnosis is suggested by the patient's history. However, bleeding may often be delayed by 3 to 4 weeks, and even by as much as 12 weeks after liver injury.[124-126]

Apart from blunt trauma, the most common causes of hemobilia are iatrogenic injury, incurred either during percutaneous biliary drainage or as a result of surgery or liver biopsy.[127,128] Again, the history can suggest the diagnosis in these cases. Hepatic artery aneurysms account for some 10% of the cases of biliary bleeding, and these are usually a consequence of atherosclerosis, trauma, or infection. They may be multiple and have been reported in patients with autoimmune disease.[129] Other rare causes of hemobilia include cystic artery aneurysm or pseudoaneurysm,[130,131] liver abscess,[132] the gallbladder vasculitis that occurs in mixed connective tissue disorders,[133] gallbladder metastases,[134] and cystadenocarcinoma of the bile duct.[135]

Bleeding may originate from the pancreatic duct and can be torrential if a pancreatic pseudocyst erodes the splenic artery. The diagnosis of hemobilia is easy if endoscopy reveals that active bleeding is coming from the major papilla, but, when the bleeding is intermittent, the diagnosis may be elusive. Angiography is helpful for excluding hepatic artery aneurysm, and angiographic embolization is probably the preferred treatment in most cases.[129,136,137]

Arterioenteric fistula

Although aortoenteric fistulas may arise from an otherwise uncomplicated aortic aneurysm, or even from an undilated aorta,[138] most cases appear after aortic graft operations. Other arterioenteric fistulas may arise as a result of malignant disease[139] or trauma.[140] When a patient with a history of an arterial graft presents with GI bleeding, the possibility of a graft enteric fistula must be entertained. Characteristically, there is a warning episode of bleeding before catastrophic hemorrhage takes place.

If endoscopy is performed in such a patient, it should be done as soon as possible and should include the third part of duodenum, which is the most common site of a proximal graft enteric fistula. If the endoscopy findings are negative, urgent laparotomy is advocated as the next step, because of the very high mortality associated with the delay in diagnosing and treating graft enteric fistulas. However, in a study of 74 bleeding episodes that occurred in 253 patients with aortic grafts, there was only one instance of an aortoenteric fistula. This patient had a positive preoperative CT scan, as did a recent patient of the author's (Fig. 48-9). Six patients underwent laparotomy, including the one with the fistula, and, of these, three were found to have intrinsic GI lesions. Another 30 patients were found to have intrinsic GI lesions during the diagnostic workup.[141]

Although the role of CT in the diagnosis of graft enteric fistula is not yet established, it appears promising.[142] However, it is vitally important not to delay laparotomy while waiting to perform endoscopy or CT when a graft enteric fistula is suspected. Angiography has generally been unrewarding in the identification of graft enteric fistulas,[138] but certainly has a place in the investigation of other arterioenteric fistulas, such as those associated with malignant disease or trauma, in which it may also have a therapeutic role. The diagnosis of aortoenteric fistula as the cause of bleeding in patients without a history of aneurysm or graft is difficult, because it is frequently not considered until too late. Perhaps the only clue to this diagnosis is the occurrence of back pain in conjunction with GI bleeding.[138,143]

Lower GI bleeding

Clinically, lower GI bleeding can take the form of acute or chronic red rectal bleeding, which can be continuous or intermittent, and vary from slight to massive. It may also take the form of either black or plum-colored melena. Slight to moderate chronic rectal bleeding may be associated with a wide variety of inflammatory or neoplastic conditions, in which the underlying condition is actually more important than the rectal bleeding itself. These conditions are discussed elsewhere in this volume.

Occasionally, rectal bleeding may pose a problem in its own right, either because it is severe enough to cause shock or because it is continuous and necessitates repeated blood transfusion. The method of investigation depends both on the rate of bleeding and the age of the patient. If the blood loss is so rapid that continuous transfusion is required to maintain hemodynamic stability, angiography can virtually always show the causative lesion, and in some cases allow therapy, either by the infusion of vasoconstrictors or by embolization. Colonoscopy under these conditions may be dif-

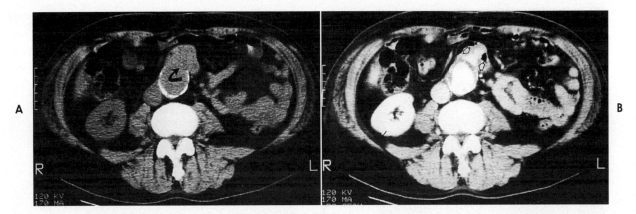

Fig. 48-9 A, Graft enteric fistula. A haematoma is seen extending from the anterior aspect of the proximal end of an aortic graft into the small bowel *(curved arrow)*. **B,** Same case after the intravenous administration of contrast medium showing active leakage of the agent into the small bowel *(open arrows)*.
Courtesy of Dr. N. J. Ring.

ficult, but intraoperative colonoscopy using antegrade colonic irrigation is claimed to be quicker and more effective than angiography.[144] More often the bleeding will have stopped by the time the patient reaches the hospital, or slowed to a non-life-threatening rate. Colonoscopy can be practical under these circumstances, and reveals the causative lesion in 50% to 70% the cases.[145,146] Whether colonoscopy should be performed as an emergency procedure depends on the individual circumstances of the case. Thus a single episode of bright red bleeding in an elderly patient that stops within 24 hours of hospital admission is likely due to diverticular disease and can be investigated in a routine manner. If bleeding continues beyond 24 hours or starts again after stopping, then colonoscopy should be performed on an urgent basis. Angiodysplasias, although only half as common a cause of bleeding as diverticula, are more likely to rebleed and rarely resolve without treatment.[147] When colonoscopy shows an actively bleeding angiodysplasia, endoscopic treatment is frequently successful[148] (Fig. 48-10). If colonoscopy reveals a nonbleeding angiodysplasia, this must be regarded with some skepticism, as these lesions are common and can therefore easily coexist with other causes of hemorrhage. Vascular ectasias in the colon afflict up to 70% of the patients with portal hypertension and have been successfully treated using a heater probe.[149] Colonic varices are common in patients with portal hypertension, and the rectum is the most frequent site.[150] Colonic varices in the absence of portal hypertension are a rare cause of frank rectal bleeding and may involve the entire colon[151,152] (Fig. 48-11). They may be familial.[153] Another very rare cause of acute severe rectal bleeding is the colonic Dieulafoy lesion (discussed earlier) (see Fig. 48-6). Finally, both occult bleeding or, more rarely, frank rectal bleeding may occur in runners.[154,155]

Indeterminate or occult GI bleeding

In some cases of GI bleeding, both upper GI tract endoscopy and colonoscopy studies yield negative findings, as do small bowel barium studies. Sometimes the bleeding is clearly in the upper GI tract; in other patients, it is unclear whether it is from the small bowel or the colon. The urea-to-creatinine ratio may be of some help in differentiating between the two, with ratios of more than 98 suggesting an upper GI tract lesion. If the evidence suggests an upper GI cause, then the first response should be to repeat the upper GI endoscopy, preferably during an episode

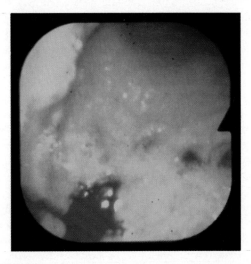

Fig. 48-10 Angiodysplasia in the cecum of a patient who had recently bled briskly per rectum. This was successfully treated by monopolar diathermy coagulation. Lesions no larger than the head of a pin may occasionally be the source of massive hemorrhage.
From Simkins KC: *A textbook of radiological diagnosis,* vol 4, ed 5, London, 1988, HK Lewis.

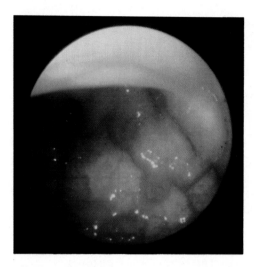

Fig. 48-11 Idiopathic colonic varices. Serpiginous dilated veins were present throughout the colon of this 17-year-old boy who had a long history of rectal bleeding. There were no esophageal or gastric varices, liver enzyme levels were normal, and Doppler ultrasound showed normal portal vein flow.

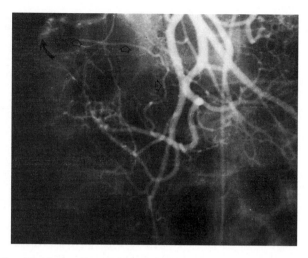

Fig. 48-12 Superior mesenteric angiogram from a 23-year-old man with massive rectal bleeding. There is extravasation of contrast medium in the upper right abdomen *(curved arrow)*. This is fed by a long ileocolic branch *(open arrows)*. At operation, bleeding was found to be coming from a Meckel's diverticulum lying in the right upper quadrant.

of active bleeding. The differential diagnosis in this setting consists of the Dieulafoy lesion, hemobilia, an arterioenteric fistula, and vascular anomalies. A push type enteroscopy using a pediatric colonoscope permits examination of the proximal jejunum and may reveal the cause of bleeding in up to 38% of the patients. Most of these patients are found to be bleeding from vascular malformations, and these may be successfully managed endoscopically.[156] If these examinations yield negative findings, angiography should be the next step. This has the highest yield if performed during the active bleeding phase, but may still reveal an abnormality in the nonbleeding phase.

When the results of upper endoscopy, colonoscopy, isotope studies, and angiography are all negative, a Sonde type of enteroscopy can disclose the lesion in a third of the cases. In most instances, this will be a vascular anomaly.[157] These same authors found that, in 22 of 37 patients with occult GI bleeding and negative enteroscopy findings, the eventual cause was found in the upper GI tract.

If Sonde-type enteroscopy is not available, or the findings are negative, then a planned laparotomy has a definite diagnostic as well as therapeutic role and should be combined with peroperative enteroscopy. This gives results comparable to those observed for Sonde-type enteroscopy[158] and was found to yield useful information in up to 13 of 14 such patients in one series.[159] It may, however, be associated with operative or postoperative complications.[160] In a series of 37 patients who were investigated by Thompson et al.[161] because of obscure GI bleeding, 46% had lesions shown only at laparotomy, even though all but two had undergone prior selective angiography. Half of the

14 vascular anomalies were not shown by angiography, as these were predominantly venous lesions. There were eight patients with Meckel's diverticulum in this series; five had technetium 99m pertechnetate scans, and all findings were negative in spite of confirmed ulcerated ectopic gastric mucosa in four. Only one of these cases was revealed by barium studies, which were performed in four. Meckel's diverticulum was suggested angiographically in two patients by the presence of an anomalous artery, and this was also the case in one of our own patients (Fig. 48-12). Seven patients had smooth muscle tumors, of which six were shown by angiography and one by surgery. Eight cases fell into a miscellaneous group, and these included duodenal reduplication, ulcerated duodenal diverticulum, ulcerated jejunal diverticulum, secondary deposits, solitary jejunal ulcer, multiple ischemic ulcers of the small bowel, and an ulcerated ileal lymphoma. The authors make the point that, in this series, only one patient under 50 years of age had a lesion that would not have been found by careful laparotomy, whereas, in those patients over the age of 50, there was a much higher incidence of vascular anomalies, which are difficult, if not impossible, to detect at laparotomy.[161]

Other rare causes of small bowel bleeding not represented in this series include small bowel ulcers due to vasculitis in polyarteritis nodosa, systemic lupus erythematosus, or rheumatoid arthritis,[162] tuberculosis,[163] and Crohn's disease.[164] GI bleeding may occur in the Ehlers-Danlos syndrome, stemming from abnormalities in the vessel walls,[165] and it may also complicate amyloidosis.[166]

49 *Scintigraphic Evaluation of Gastrointestinal Hemorrhage*

ALAN SIEGEL
ABASS ALAVI

EXTENT OF THE PROBLEM AND CAUSES OF BLEEDING

The morbidity and mortality in the patient with gastrointestinal (GI) hemorrhage can be decreased through the rapid localization of the bleeding site and the prompt institution of therapeutic interventions.[1] The mortality rate for major GI episodes is about 10%, and this has remained unchanged for the past 30 to 40 years.[2,3] About 15% of the patients require surgery. Several factors are associated with increased mortality in patients with upper GI bleeding, including age older than 60 years, rapid bleeding, and concurrent illnesses such as emphysema, coronary artery disease, stroke, congestive heart failure, or cirrhosis.[4-6]

GI hemorrhage can be divided into two major categories: upper and lower GI tract bleeding. The symptomatology and etiology of these entities, as well as the diagnostic and therapeutic approaches for each, tend to differ. The upper and lower GI tracts are divided by the ligament of Treitz, a fibromuscular band that extends from the left diaphragmatic crus to the antimesenteric border of the distal duodenum.

It may be possible to localize the site of bleeding to the upper or lower GI tract before performing any diagnostic studies. For instance, hematemesis indicates an upper GI tract source, whereas hematochezia points to the lower GI tract as the site of bleeding. However, rapid upper GI bleeding may also cause hematochezia. Melena usually indicates the source of bleeding is in the upper GI tract but can also arise from a source in the small bowel. When the aspirate from a nasogastric tube is bloody, this establishes the site of bleeding as proximal to the ligament of Treitz. However, if the nasogastric tube aspirate shows no blood, this does not rule out the upper GI tract as the bleeding site.

Because the causes of upper and lower GI bleeding are generally distinct, the patient's medical history may also give clues to the site of bleeding.

The most common causes of upper GI bleeding are erosive gastritis and duodenal ulcers, each accounting for 20% to 30% of the cases.[7] Other notable causes include gastric and esophageal varices, gastric ulcers, Mallory Weiss tears, and esophagitis. As much as 30% of the cases of upper GI bleeding may originate in the esophagus.[8] Tumors account for only about 3% of the cases,[3] and, in as many as 10% of the cases, no diagnosis can be made.[9]

Acute lower GI bleeding episodes are less common.[2] Frequently, the age of a patient can aid in the diagnosis. Among the most common causes of lower GI bleeding in elderly patients are angiodysplasia and diverticulosis. Angiodysplasia, also called *vascular ectasia,* is an acquired lesion that commonly afflicts patients over 60 years of age.[2] About 80% of these malformations occur in the cecum and the ascending colon.[10] It is estimated that 40% of the severe hemorrhages seen in elderly patients are caused by angiodysplasia and that 25% of the patients with GI bleeding who are over 60 years of age have these lesions.[9]

Diverticulosis is one of the most common causes of massive lower GI bleeding. About half of the patients over the age of 60 years have colonic diverticuli, and 20% of these will eventually bleed.[9] Although diverticuli predominate in the left side of the colon, 75% of the bleeding diverticuli are located on the right side. Diverticular bleeding is arterial in origin and tends to be more severe than angiodysplastic hemorrhage.[11]

There is an extensive list of other causes of lower GI bleeding, and these include carcinoma, polyps, hemorrhoids, radiation proctitis, and ischemic bowel disease. In younger patients, inflammatory bowel disease, Meckel's diverticuli, polyps, and intussusception must be considered.[9,12]

SURGERY FOR THE TREATMENT OF GI HEMORRHAGE

Most bleeding episodes (at least 80%[13,14]) stop spontaneously, and thus conservative management is a more common approach than surgical intervention. Surgery in patients with GI bleeding carries a high risk. The mortality in patients with upper GI bleeding is approximately 35%, and, in cases of lower GI bleeding when the bowel is not prepared, the mortality averages 28% but can be as high as 47%.[15-17] The mortality is also significantly higher if the surgery is emergent rather than elective; in cases of bleeding peptic ulcers, the death rate associated with emergency surgery is almost ten times that of elective surgery.[6] When surgery must be performed before the exact site of bleeding can be localized, there is a high incidence of rebleeding, with the accompanying additional morbidity and mortality.[17]

Every effort should be made to localize bleeding sites using scintigraphic, endoscopic, or angiographic means before performing surgery. If conservative management fails, the use of endoscopic or angiographic therapeutic maneuvers may preclude the need for surgery.

NONSCINTIGRAPHIC MODES OF EVALUATION

Barium studies have not proved useful in the evaluation of a patient with GI hemorrhage, especially if it is acute.[18] Study findings have shown that barium examination of both the upper and lower GI tracts is inferior to endoscopy in localizing the source of bleeding.[7,19-24] Barium studies may help in detecting structural lesions such as carcinoma, polyps, and diverticuli; in fact, the combination of flexible sigmoidoscopy and barium enema studies is actually superior to colonoscopy in the detection of diverticuli.[24] However, detection of these lesions does not necessarily mean that the bleeding site has been found. Additionally, the presence of barium in the colon may actually hinder the reading of angiograms obtained afterward. In the bleeding patient, barium studies should not be used routinely as the initial diagnostic modality.

Endoscopy can also be used as a therapeutic as well as a diagnostic tool in the bleeding patient, and has been successful in bringing about a reduction in the need for emergent surgery in instances of upper GI bleeding.[25,26] When combined with gastric lavage, a bleeding site in the upper GI tract may be identified 90% of the time.[27] It is more difficult for the scope to clear the lower GI tract, however, and endoscopy has been generally less successful in detecting lower GI bleeding.[18] Using the endoscope to gain entrance to the bleeding site, thermal coagulation of bleeding sites can then be achieved with lasers, monopolar or dipolar electrodes, and heater probes. Sclerotherapy can be carried out using such agents as ethanolamine oleate and sodium tetradecyl sulfate. Vasoconstriction is achieved with the topical application of epinephrine, and bleeding vessels can be obliterated with alcohol.[28]

The advantages of performing angiography in the patient with GI bleeding are its superior spatial resolution, plus it affords the opportunity to implement therapeutic maneuvers. Angiographic studies may reveal the actual bleeding vessel, and angiography is more precise and accurate in localizing the bleeding site than is scintigraphy.

Once the site is identified, several angiographic techniques may be used and are frequently successful in stopping the bleeding.[29-33] Vasopressin, which may be infused subselectively into the bleeding branch vessel to bring about vasoconstriction, is the most commonly used means of angiographic bleeding control.[34] Embolization can be performed with several materials, either temporarily using such agents as autogenous clot or Gelfoam, or permanently using Ivalon (polyvinyl alcohol) or steel coils.[35-38] Angiography has several drawbacks, however. It is an invasive procedure and involves the use of iodinated contrast material, which is nephrotoxic and may provoke allergic reactions,

some of which may be severe. Angiography also exposes the patient to a large dose of radiation. Furthermore, its sensitivity in detecting bleeding is much less than that of scintigraphy. The minimal rate of bleeding that angiography can detect is greater than 0.5 ml/min.[39] Angiography is often unsuccessful in detecting venous bleeding.[40]

SCINTIGRAPHIC MODES OF EVALUATION

Scintigraphic detection of GI bleeding can be approached in two ways. The first is based on the intravenous administration of radiolabeled particles or solutions that are then cleared from the vascular space through the influence of certain mechanisms. Particles present in blood that extravasate into the GI tract are not available for normal clearance. These substances include sulfur colloid, which is cleared by the liver, spleen, and bone marrow; heat-damaged red blood cells, which are extracted by the spleen; and diethylenetriaminepentaacetic acid (DTPA), which is filtered by the kidneys. All of these agents can be labeled with technetium 99m.

The second technique utilizes intravascular markers, including circulating red blood cells and serum albumin labeled with technetium 99. Such agents are not cleared from the bloodstream and allow imaging for an extended period, which is limited only by decay of the labeled radionuclide.

Radionuclide techniques do not possess the anatomic resolution of angiographic studies nor do they have a therapeutic application. The advantage of these studies is that they are highly sensitive (more so than angiography), can be performed quickly, and involve a relatively low radiation burden on the patient. If needed, the study can be repeated at short intervals. They are noninvasive, in that an arterial puncture is not needed and no iodinated contrast is used. There is also no danger of nephrotoxicity or allergic reactions.

However, for reasons explained later, these studies are not well suited for evaluating upper GI bleeding, and often endoscopy is the first-line examination in these circumstances. Scintigraphic studies are also excellent screening studies in patients with lower GI hemorrhage and are frequently the initial study of choice.

Sulfur colloid

Sulfur colloid is composed of small particles measuring from 1 to 2 μm. This agent has been used in liver spleen scans because, following intravenous administration, it is phagocytized by the macrophages of the reticuloendothelial system of the liver, spleen, and bone marrow. About half of the injected amount is removed from the intravascular space within 2.5 to 3 minutes.[41] Most of the activity is cleared from the vascular system within 10 to 15 minutes. If the patient is bleeding during the first few minutes after injection, the sulfur colloid particles extravasate with the blood into the bowel lumen, and thus are not picked up by the liver, spleen, or bone marrow.

Sulfur colloid may be labeled by technetium 99m by

means of a fairly simple process using a standard kit. The procedure does require boiling of the reagents, but this can usually be completed in less than 20 minutes. The labeling efficiency is high, and free technetium rarely poses a problem. Greater than 98% of the pertechnetate is labeled to the sulfur colloid particles.[42] Approximately 370 to 555 megabecquerel (MBq) (10 to 15 millicurie [mCi]) of technetium 99m can yield high-quality images. For children, 7.4 MBq/kg (200 μCi/kg) is an adequate dose.

To perform scintigraphy in the setting of GI hemorrhage, the patient should be positioned supine, with the gamma camera located anteriorly over the abdomen. The camera should be set for the 140-keV photopeak of technetium with a 20% window. A low-energy, all-purpose collimator is appropriate. The dose should be administered intravenously and immediate images obtained. When the activity can be identified on the persistence scope, the patient's position should be adjusted so that the lower edge of the liver is in the upper portion of the field of view. Images of the abdomen should be obtained for approximately 500,000 or 750,000 counts. Sequential images may be obtained for 20 or 30 minutes (Fig. 49-1). If abnormal activity that may represent a bleeding site is noted, additional images can be obtained as needed to identify transit through the bowel and to aid in localization (Figs. 49-2 and 49-3). If no abnormalities are seen, a left anterior oblique view of the upper abdomen may be taken so that bleeding sites superimposed over the left lobe of the liver and spleen are not missed. This also permits a more inferior image to be obtained in the event that the bleeding site is in the lower rectum (Fig. 49-4). This is a particular problem in instances of hemorrhoidal bleeding. Finally, if the patient has a bowel movement during the study, the bedpan can be imaged to obtain counts that can confirm whether the bleeding has occurred during the study in the rectal region. Likewise, a rectal examination followed by imaging or counting of the glove may give the same information.

Because activity is so completely cleared from the intravascular space, sulfur colloid bleeding scans provide an exquisite target-to-background ratio. Potentially confusing activity resulting from intravascular markers, such as from the kidneys, aorta, inferior vena cava, mesenteric vasculature, or bladder, is rarely a problem. This technique is highly sensitive for detecting slow bleeding rates, in that patients bleeding as slowly as 0.05 ml/per minute may have positive studies.[18,41] Rates such as these are far below the threshold for angiographic detection.

Scanning with technetium 99m sulfur colloid exposes patients to a low radiation dose. The liver, which is the critical organ, receives about 4 rads during the study,[43] and the total body dose is about 2 rads.

Because of the rapid clearance of sulfur colloid, the patient undergoing such a bleeding scan must be bleeding during the injection of the agent, or very shortly thereafter.

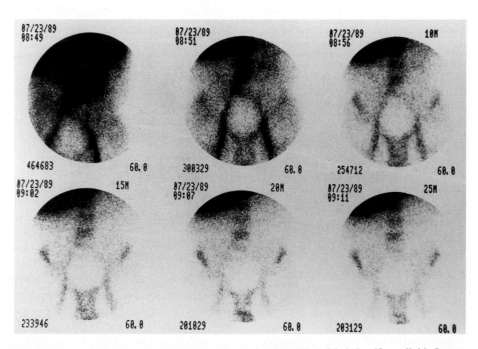

Fig. 49-1 Normal bleeding scan obtained using technetium 99m–labeled sulfur colloid. Images were taken for 1 minute each, acquired over 20 minutes. Note the intense activity in the vascular structures, including the aorta and iliac vessels, in the first two images. The intensity of this activity gradually fades and, at 20 minutes, is difficult to discern. This is an easy way to differentiate sulfur colloid from labeled red blood cell studies. At 20 minutes, activity is seen in the bone marrow and in the visualized portion of the liver, in its inferior aspect. No abnormal activity is noted. The clearance of sulfur colloid from the blood pool has left little background activity.

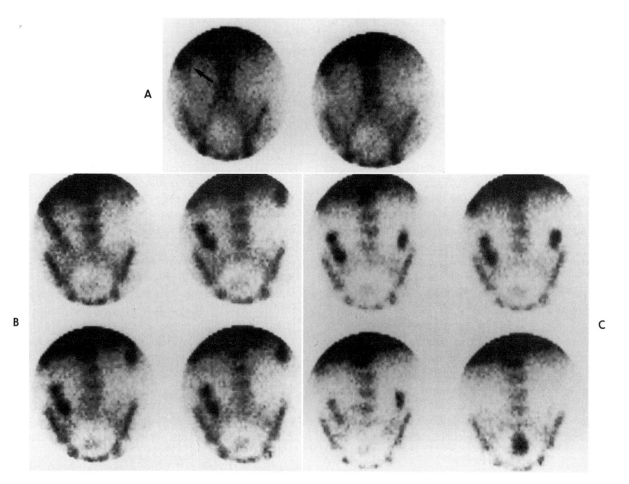

Fig. 49-2 Bleeding in the hepatic flexure as depicted by technetium 99m–labeled sulfur colloid scans **A,** At 7 and 8 minutes, **B,** At 25 to 28 minutes, **C,** At 33 to 36 minutes. The 7-minute image exhibits an abnormal area of activity in the right upper quadrant of the abdomen *(arrow),* inferior to the right lobe of the liver and corresponding to a site of bleeding in the hepatic flexure. Over the course of the study, the activity moves in both an antegrade (into the splenic flexure at 26 minutes and the rectum at 36 minutes) and a retrograde (activity can be seen progressing toward the cecum at 26 and 27 minutes) manner. It is extremely important to determine where the abnormal activity first appears. Because the blood moves rapidly through the bowel, viewing only delayed images may lead to incorrect localization.

This can be a problem, as GI bleeding is by nature intermittent. Bleeding will have stopped in a majority of patients by the time the bleeding scan is begun. If, after the study, rebleeding occurs, the scan can be repeated at any time. The only drawback to this is an increase in the radiation exposure to the patient, although that associated with this study is not high and, on the other hand, GI bleeding can be a life-threatening situation. In addition, most patients with lower GI bleeding are elderly and the delayed effects of radiation exposure are not then such a serious concern.

Sulfur colloid bleeding scans are of limited use in patients with upper GI bleeding, primarily because of the intense activity in the liver and spleen that obscures the upper abdomen. At times, the liver may also obscure portions of the transverse colon.

To identify a bleeding site, it is important for the abnormal activity to change its configuration during the imaging procedure. Blood moves rapidly in the bowel, both antegrade and retrograde. If the activity does not move, it is unlikely that what is seen is actual bleeding. In this instance, what is seen may represent an ectopic or accessory spleen or an abnormal focus of marrow (Fig. 49-5). Potentially confusing uptake can also arise in a transplanted kidney, the male genitalia, and arterial grafts.[44] Furthermore, it is often necessary to observe the configuration of the activity and the direction in which it travels to determine the exact site of the bleeding. For example, it may not be possible to differentiate a bleed in the small bowel from one in the colon until its course of travel is discerned (Fig. 49-6).

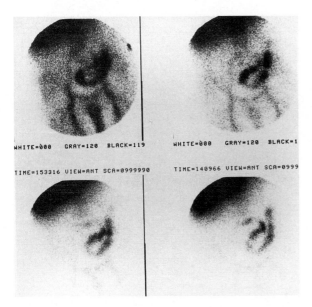

Fig. 49-3 Bleeding in the transverse colon as seen on technetium 99m–labeled sulfur colloid scans (25 through 29 minutes). Due to anatomic variations, even an obvious bleeding site can, at times, be difficult to localize. The bleeding site in this patient is located in a markedly redundant transverse colon. Knowledge of the patient's anatomy (such as may be acquired from prior barium studies) and frequently obtained delayed images may resolve the problem.

Albumin, heat-damaged red blood cells, and DTPA

Initial studies for the detection of GI bleeding used chromium 51–labeled red blood cells. This technique was limited by the inferior physical characteristics of chromium and did not yield optimal imaging.[45] Some of the earliest imaging studies used iodine 131– and technetium 99m–labeled albumin for the localization of bleeding sites,[46,47] but bleeding rates of only 2 to 3 ml per minute were detected.

Bleeding studies have also been performed with technetium 99m–DTPA.[48-52] Although this agent is not cleared from the intravascular space as rapidly as sulfur colloid (its half-life is 20 minutes), its primary route of extraction is through glomerular filtration, not into the liver and spleen. This gives DTPA an advantage in the investigation of bleeding in the upper abdomen. In addition, because of its slower excretion, bleeding may be detected as long as 1 hour after injection, and bleeding rates as low as 0.1 ml per minute have been detected.

The mechanism by which technetium 99m–labeled heat-damaged red blood cells can be used for the localization of GI bleeding is similar to that of sulfur colloid. Heat-damaged red blood cells are quickly removed from the intravascular space by the spleen. This method has reportedly detected bleeding rates of 0.12 ml per minute.[53] Although visualization of the upper abdomen is better when liver uptake is eliminated, the technique for the preparation of the red blood cells is tedious.

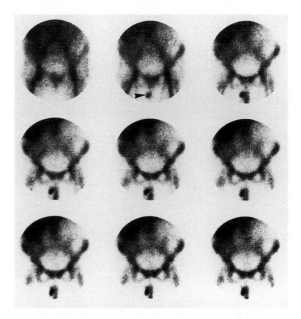

Fig. 49-4 Rectal bleeding as depicted on technetium 99m–labeled sulfur colloid scans (images from the first 9 minutes of the study). The bleeding site is first noted 1 minute into the examination *(arrow head)*. If the camera had been positioned slightly higher over the abdomen, this site would not have been visualized. A negative study should not be concluded until an image taken over the rectum is obtained. If the patient has a bowel movement during the examination, it should be determined whether there is activity in the feces, melena, or blood. If there is, this indicates active bleeding, and the radiologist should look further for the bleeding site.

Labeled red blood cells

Technetium 99m–labeled red blood cells is the most frequently used agent for the detection of GI bleeding. Red blood cells labeled with the radionuclide remain in the intravascular space until they are extravasated into the bowel lumen at a site of hemorrhage. This requires that the normal pattern of uptake be identified on the images from these studies.

There are three basic techniques for the labeling of red blood cells with technetium. All require reduction of the technetium from a valence state of +7 to +4. In the reduced state, the technetium blinds to the beta chain of hemoglobin. The most frequently used reducing agent is tin, in the form of stannous pyrophosphate, stannous chloride, stannous fluoride, and the like.

The in vivo technique is the simplest to perform.[54] The reducing agent, such as 7.5 mg of stannous pyrophosphate, is administered intravenously to the patient, which should be done by direct venipuncture and not through plastic tubing, to which it will bind. The reducing agent is then allowed to circulate for approximately 20 minutes and 740 to 925 MBq (20 to 25 mCi) of technetium 99m pertechnetate is next administered intravenously. The technetium

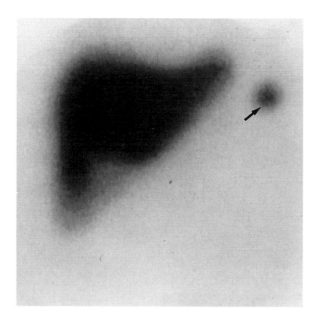

Fig. 49-5 An accessory spleen as shown on a technetium 99m–labeled sulfur colloid scan. This image was obtained in a patient who had undergone a splenectomy in the treatment of idiopathic thrombocytopenic purpura. The focus of activity in the left upper quadrant *(arrow)* represents an accessory spleen and did not move over time. It is essential for the intensity or configuration of a suspected site of bleeding to change to distinguish it from nonhemorrhagic sites of activity, such as an accessory or ectopic spleen or ectopic foci of bone marrow.

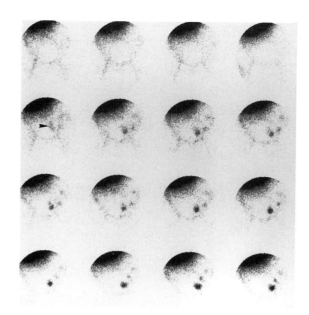

Fig. 49-6 Small bowel bleeding as shown on technetium 99m–labeled sulfur colloid scans. (Images were obtained from 6 to 22 minutes following administration of the contrast agent. Again, it is often necessary to observe the course of the activity through a series of delayed images to determine whether bleeding is in the large or small bowel. In addition, bleeding in the small bowel characteristically fades and then reappears *(arrowhead)*.

then crosses the membrane of the red blood cell and is bound. The main drawback of this technique is that only about 70% of the technetium ends up bound to the red blood cells. The free technetium is trapped by the thyroid gland and excreted by the kidneys, gastric mucosa, and choroid plexus.

The method of red blood cell labeling that is most efficient is also the most time consuming, and this is the in vitro technique.[55] Approximately 3 ml of the patient's blood is withdrawn into a syringe containing the technetium 99m pertechnetate, stannous pyrophosphate, and an anticoagulant. This sample is then agitated and centrifuged to separate the red blood cells from the plasma. The red blood cells are then washed in normal saline to remove any free pertechnetate and readministered to the patient. This method achieves a labeling efficiency of about 95% and greatly reduces the problems caused by the free pertechnetate inherent in the in vivo technique.

The modified in vitro, or "in vivtro," technique has been introduced to simplify the in vitro labeling procedure but to maintain its superior labeling efficiency.[56] Again, a reducing agent such as stannous pyrophosphate is administered, and, after equilibration, several milliliters of blood is withdrawn from the patient into a syringe containing technetium 99m pertechnetate and an anticoagulant. The sy-

ringe is then gently inverted for about 10 minutes and the contents readministered to the patient. Although the labeling efficiency is not equivalent to that of the in vitro method, about 85% of the pertechnetate binds to the red blood cells, and the technique is quite easy to perform.

More recently, commercial kits for performing modified in vitro labeling have been introduced (Ultratag RBC; Mallinkrodt, St. Louis, Mo). These are also quite simple to use and the labeling efficiency exceeds 90%.

After the labeling procedure, the patient is placed in the supine position under a gamma camera equipped with a low-energy, all-purpose collimator. The pulse-height analyzer should be set for the 140-keV peak of technetium with a 20% window. Sequential images of the abdomen should be acquired with the images taken either for time or count determinations, depending on the preference of the physician. The duration of the study depends on several factors. Because labeled red blood cells are not removed from the intravascular space, the interval during which useful images can be obtained depends on the half-life of the radionuclide, which is 6 hours in this setting. Images can usually be obtained for 24 hours. The condition of the patient, how long the camera is available for that case, and whether the study findings become positive also determine the duration of the study.

In these studies, the normal vasculature can be visualized, including the aorta, inferior vena cava, iliac vessels, portal and splenic veins, kidneys, liver, spleen, and heart.[57] As with studies utilizing sulfur colloid, a positive red blood cell bleeding scan is recognized by the appearance of activity within the bowel lumen. To be detected confidently and localized, the site of bleeding should conform to a bowel loop and change in configuration over time (Fig. 49-7 to 49-9). False-positive findings may be due to the presence of free technetium in the renal collecting systems or bladder, or to its excretion by the gastric mucosa and subsequent progression down into the more distal portions of the GI tract.[57] Because of the gastric excretion, imaging of upper GI tract bleeding is difficult and often not recommended. Vascular tumors, especially hemangiomas, may be visualized, as well as areas of hyperemia, such as the bowel in patients with inflammatory bowel disease, and nongastrointestinal sites of bleeding.[58] Imaging of the GI tract also is difficult in patients with varices.[59]

The rate of bleeding that can be detected by red blood cells labeled using the in vitro technique is similar to that possible with sulfur colloid scanning, though its ability to detect delayed bleeding may be an advantage over sulfur colloid studies because bleeding is, by nature, intermittent. However, due to the rapid transit of blood in the bowel, if delayed images of the abdomen are obtained during a labeled red blood cell study, it is possible that the blood in the bowel lumen may actually be remote from the site of bleeding. It is best to image a patient under the camera for as long as possible so as to capture the beginning of the bleeding. This may be difficult in patients in unstable conditions and in departments with a heavy workload. The use of late images must be regarded with extreme caution. If findings are equivocal, a second dose of labeled red blood cells may be successful in localizing the bleeding site.[60]

In a review of 175 consecutive sulfur colloid bleeding scans performed at the Hospital of the University of Pennsylvania, a bleeding site was localized in 24% of the cases. When the patient's condition and the demand for camera time allowed, negative studies were then followed by labeled red blood cell scanning with delayed imaging. Of these additional 50 studies, 14% yielded positive results (Table 49-1).

In summary, the appropriate technique to adopt in performing bleeding scintigraphy varies from institution to institution and should be tailored to the needs of each department.

Meckel's scans

Bleeding from a Meckel's diverticulum is an important cause of hemorrhage in the pediatric population, although it may occur in adults as well. Meckel's diverticula are congenital remnants of the omphalomesenteric duct that form on the antimesenteric border of the distal small bowel. In approximately 15% to 25% of the patients, these diverticula may contain gastric mucosa.[61,62] The acid produced from this ectopic gastric mucosa leads to erosions of the

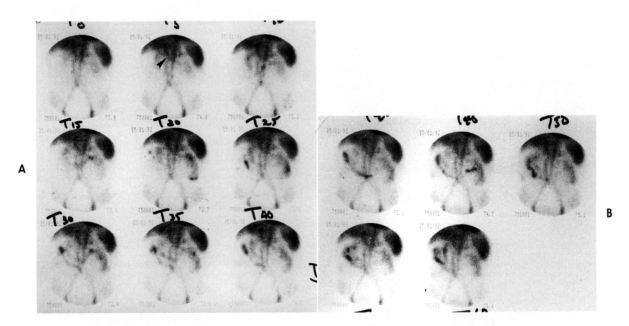

Fig. 49-7 Small bowel bleeding as shown on scans using technetium 99m–labeled red blood cells **A,** At 0 through 40 minutes. **B,** At 40 through 60 minutes. In this study the intravascular activity does not disappear with time. The aorta, inferior vena cava, and iliac vessels can be seen clearly 1 hour after the beginning of the study. Abnormal activity is first noted in the region of the sweep of the duodenum in the 5-minute image *(arrowhead)*. This site of bleeding was localized to a duodenal ulcer discovered at endoscopy.

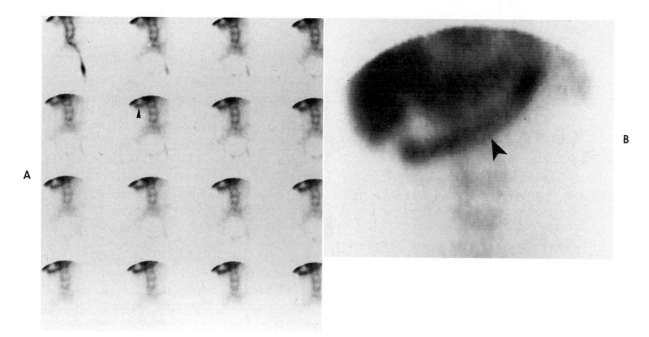

Fig. 49-8 Bleeding in the transverse colon as depicted on technetium 99m–labeled red blood cell scans. **A,** The first 16 minutes of the study. **B,** At 20 minutes. The transverse colon fills with activity during the course of this study. The 20-minute image demonstrates this portion of the colon, which is outlined inferior to the liver *(arrowhead)*. The liver in this patient is small. In patients with enlarged livers or spleens or with portions of the colon superimposed on the liver or spleen, bleeding sites in the superior aspects of the colon can be difficult to detect. In these instances, oblique views may help to reveal the location of the hemorrhage.

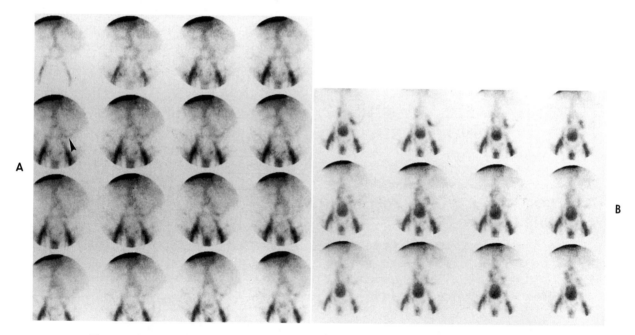

Fig. 49-9 Bleeding in the sigmoid colon as shown on technetium 99m–labeled red blood cell scans. **A,** The first 16 minutes of the study. **B,** At 21 through 33 minutes. Bleeding is first noted about 15 minutes into the study *(arrowhead)* and can be seen to more clearly fill the sigmoid colon in later images. Activity is also noted in the bladder at about 15 minutes and becomes more intense with time **(B)**. This is due to the existence of free technetium 99m pertechnetate, which is being filtered by the kidneys. Visualization of activity in the renal collecting systems or ureters can cause false-positive findings. Activity in the bladder may obscure a bleeding site. In addition, free pertechnetate is excreted by the gastric mucosa and, again, may cause false-positive results. This is why it is important to achieve high efficiency with the labeling procedure. The in vitro technique is best.

mucosa of the surrounding ileum and subsequent hemorrhage. The Meckel's diverticulum in approximately 95% of the patients with resultant GI bleeding contains gastric mucosa.

The Meckel's scan is used to localize ectopic gastric mucosa and not to detect hemorrhage. Technetium 99m pertechnetate is concentrated and then excreted by the mucus-producing cells of the gastric mucosa.[61,63] This

takes place whether it is located in the stomach or in ectopic foci.

Meckel's scans are thus performed following the intravenous administration of technetium 99m pertechnetate in a dose of 370 to 555 MBq (10 to 15 mCi) for adults and 7.4 MBq/kg (200 μCi/kg) for children. Images should be obtained sequentially, starting immediately after the injection (Fig. 49-10). The study may continue for as long as 1

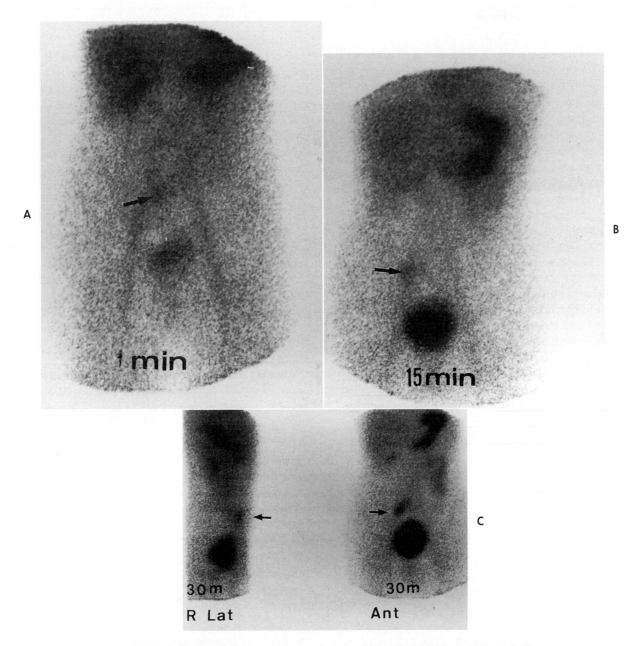

Fig. 49-10 Meckel's diverticulum shown on technetium 99m-pertechnetate scans. **A,** At 1 minute. **B,** At 15 minutes. **C,** At 30 minutes. An area of abnormal uptake is noted medial to the right iliac vessels at 1 minute *(arrow)*. The uptake is faint and can barely be distinguished from the background. By 15 minutes the intensity of uptake has increased considerably, and at 30 minutes the site of abnormal activity is distinctly seen *(arrows)*. On the right lateral view, the site of uptake is noted to be anterior *(arrow)*. These findings are considered typical for Meckel's diverticulum.

☐   **TABLE 49-1**

Breakdown of TcRBC bleeding scan results

Result	At first study		After negative study		After positive study	
	Positive	Negative	Positive	Negative	Positive	Negative
Number	5	6	7	43	4	2
Percentage	45	55	14	86	67	33
Percentage of total	7	9	10	64	6	3

TcRBC, technetium ^{99m} labeled red blood cells.

hour. It may be necessary to obtain right lateral and postvoid films to discern a diverticulum from overlying activity (Fig. 49-10). It is important not to confuse activity secreted by the stomach and moving down through the bowel for ectopic gastric mucosa. Activity in a Meckel's diverticulum should appear at approximately the same time as that in the stomach. The sensitivity for this study is stated to be as high as 75% to 85%.[64,65]

Several premedications have been used in patients in conjunction with these studies in an attempt to improve their accuracy. Pentagastrin is the 5–amino acid N-terminal of gastrin, a hormone produced in the gastric antrum that stimulates blood flow to the gastric mucosa and increases acid secretion. Results from animal studies have shown that pentagastrin may augment the gastric mucosal uptake of technetium 99m by 40%.[66,67] Because the amount of gastric mucosa in a Meckel's diverticulum, when it is present, is often small and its ability to concentrate pertechnetate is frequently limited, pentagastrin can increase the uptake and secretion of pertechnetate by this ectopic gastric mucosa and thus aid in the detection of the diverticulum. A major drawback of this method is that the pertechnetate secreted by the stomach also increases, and this could lead to false-positive results. Pentagastrin may be combined with intravenously administered glucagon, a smooth muscle relaxant that decreases peristalsis.

Another approach to Meckel's scanning has been pretreatment with cimetidine. Cimetidine is an H$_2$-receptor blocker that decreases the acid production by the stomach. Cimetidine will not affect the concentration of pertechnetate in the gastric mucosa but can suppress its secretion into the lumen of the stomach or diverticulum.[68] More recently, Meckel's scans have been performed with ranitidine premedication; this agent has potentially fewer side effects than cimetidine.[62]

CONCLUSIONS

The workup of the patient with GI hemorrhage depends on several factors. The findings from the history and physical examination plus the nature of the nasogastric tube aspirate frequently indicate whether the bleeding site is in the upper or lower GI tract. Further evaluation for localization depends on the patient's condition. If the patient's state is unstable and the bleeding cannot be controlled, it may be necessary to take the patient directly to surgery—a high-risk procedure in this setting. In the stable patient with upper GI tract bleeding, endoscopy is often the preferred test. If the bleeding is from the lower GI tract, scintigraphy is preferred.

Performing scintigraphic bleeding scans before angiography or surgery is carried out has several advantages. Angiographic findings are rarely positive when the results of the bleeding scan are negative. The bleeding scan, unlike the angiogram, is noninvasive and exposes the patient to much less radiation. Because the angiogram provides superior anatomic information and allows therapeutic maneuvers to be carried out, it would be ideal to confirm that the patient is bleeding by scintigraphy before proceeding further. The scan can also help guide the angiographer in locating the bleeding site.

Patients who require surgery to control a GI hemorrhage fare much better if a bleeding site is localized beforehand rather than undergoing a blind procedure.

Bleeding scintigraphy has also proved useful in the evaluation of therapy for hemorrhage. Scans can be performed after the infusion of vasopressin or the conclusion of other techniques to determine whether the intervention has been successful.

REFERENCES

1. Law DH, Watts HD: Gastrointestinal bleeding. In Sleisenger MH et al, eds: *Gastrointestinal disease,* Philadelphia, 1983, WB Saunders.
2. Sullivan BH: Gastrointestinal bleeding. In Farmer RG, Achkar E, Fleshler B, eds: *Clinical gastroenterology,* New York, 1983, Raven Press.
3. Silverstein FE et al: The national ASGE survey on upper gastrointestinal bleeding, *Gastrointest Endosc* 27:73, 1981.
4. Venables CW: Advances in the management of gastrointestinal bleeding, *Br J Hosp Med* 23:338, 1980.
5. Schiller KFR, Truelove SC, Williams DG: Haematemesis and melena, with special reference to factors influencing the outcome, *Br Med J* 2:7, 1970.
6. Brandt LG: *Gastrointestinal disorders of the elderly,* New York, 1984, Raven Press.
7. Earnest D: Stomach emergencies. In Gitnick G, ed: *Handbook of gastrointestinal emergencies,* New York, 1987, Medical Examination.
8. Ippoliti AF, Zamost BJ: Esophageal emergencies. In Gitnick G, ed: *Handbook of gastrointestinal emergencies,* New York, 1987, Medical Examination.

9. Bogoch A: Bleeding. In Berk JE, ed: *Gastroenterology,* Philadelphia, 1985, WB Saunders.

10. Meyer CT et al: Arteriovenous malformations of the bowel: an analysis of 22 cases and a review of the literature, *Medicine* 60:36, 1981.

11. Sun EA, Snape WJ Jr: Colon emergencies. In Gitnick G, ed: *Handbook of Gastrointestinal Emergencies,* New York, 1987, Medical Examination.

12. Eisenberg RL: *Gastrointestinal radiology,* Philadelphia, 1983, JB Lippincott.

13. Griffiths WU, Neumann DA, Welsh JD: The visible vessel as an indicator of uncontrolled or recurrent gastrointestinal hemorrhage, *N Engl J Med* 300:1411, 1979.

14. Behringer GE, Albright NL: Diverticular disease of the colon: a frequent cause of massive rectal bleeding, *Am J Surg* 125:419, 1973.

15. Kim U, Rudick J, Aufses AH: Surgical management of acute upper gastrointestinal bleeding: value of early diagnosis and prompt surgical intervention, *Arch Surg* 113:1444, 1978.

16. Bookstein JJ, Naderi MJ, Walter JF: Transcatheter embolization for lower gastrointestinal bleeding, *Radiology* 127:345, 1978.

17. Taylor FW, Epstein LI: Treatment of massive diverticular hemorrhage, *Arch Surg* 98:505, 1969.

18. Alavi A, McLean GK: Radioisotopic detection of gastrointestinal bleeding: an integrated approach with other diagnostic and therapeutic modalities. In Freeman LM, Weissman HS, eds: *Nuclear medicine annual 1980,* New York, 1980, Raven Press.

19. Gilbertsen VA et al: Colonoscopy in the detection of carcinoma of the intestine, *Surg Gynecol Obstet* 149:877, 1979.

20. Rosen AM, Fleischer DE: Upper GI bleeding in the eelderly: diagnosis and management, *Geriatrics* 44:26, 1989.

21. Dronfield MW et al: A prospective, randomised study of endoscopy and radiology in acute upper-gastrointestinal-tract bleeding, *Lancet* 1:1167, 1977.

22. Keller RT, Logan GM Jr: Comparison of emergent endoscopy and upper gastrointestinal series radiography in acute upper gastrointestinal haemorrhage, *Gut* 17:180, 1976.

23. Morris DW et al: Prospective, randomized study of diagnosis and outcome in acute upper-gastrointestinal bleeding: endoscopy versus conventional radiography, *Am J Dig Dis* 20:1103, 1975.

24. Irvine EJ et al: Prospective comparison of double contrast barium enema plus flexible sigmoidoscopy v colonoscopy in rectal bleeding: barium enema v colonoscopy in rectal bleeding, *Gut* 29:1188, 1988.

25. Laine L: Multipolar electrocoagulation in the treatment of active upper gastrointestinal hemorrhage, *N Engl J Med* 26:1613, 1987.

26. Fleischer D: Etiology and prevalence of persistent upper gastrointestinal bleeding in humans, *Gastroenterology* 90:217, 1986.

27. Massive upper gastrointestinal bleeding, *Br Med J* 1:403, 1974 (Editorial).

28. Gostout CJ: Acute gastrointestinal bleeding—a common problem revisited, *Mayo Clin Proc* 63:596, 1988.

29. Nussbaum M, Baum S, Blakemore WS: Clinical experience with the diagnosis and management of gastrointestinal hemorrhage by selective mesenteric catheterization, *Ann Surg* 170:506, 1969.

30. Conn HO, Ramsby GR, Storer EH: Selective intraarterial vasopressin in the treatment of upper gastrointestinal hemorrhage, *Gastroenterology* 63:634, 1972.

31. Rosch J et al: Selective arterial drug infusions in the treatment of acute gastrointestinal bleeding, *Gastroenterology* 59:341, 1970.

32. Baum S, Nussbaum M: The control of gastrointestinal hemorrhage by selective mesenteric arterial infusion of vasopressin, *Radiology* 98:497, 1974.

33. Baum S et al: Selective mesenteric arterial infusions in the management of massive diverticular hemorrhage, *N Engl J Med* 288:1269, 1973.

34. Baum S et al: Gastrointestinal hemorrhage. Angiographic diagnosis and control. In Hardy JD, Zollinger, eds: *Advances in surgery,* Chicago, 1973, Mosby–Year Book.

35. Bookstein JJ et al: Transcatheter hemostasis of gastrointestinal bleeding using modified autogenous clot, *Radiology* 113:277, 1974.

36. Barth KH, Strandberg JD, White RI: Long-term follow-up of transcatheter embolization with autologous clot, Oxycel and Gelfoam in domestic swine, *Invest Radiol* 12:273, 1977.

37. White RI et al: Therapeutic embolization with long-term occluding agents and their effects on embolized tissues. *Radiology* 125:677, 1977.

38. Gainturco C, Anderson JH, Wallace S: Mechanical devices for arterial occlusion, *AJR* 124:428, 1975.

39. White RI: *Fundamentals of vascular radiology,* Philadelphia, 1976, Lea & Febiger.

40. Athanasoulis CA: Angiography: its contribution to the emergency management of gastrointestinal hemorrhage, *Radiol Clin North Am* 14:265, 1976.

41. Alavi A, Dann RW, Baum S, Biery DN: Scintigraphic detection of acute gastrointestinal bleeding. *Radiology* 124:753, 1977.

42. Alavi A: Detection of gastrointestinal bleeding with ^{99m}Tc-sulfur colloid, *Semin Nucl Med* 12:126, 1982.

43. Summary of current radiation dose estimates to humans with various liver conditions from 99mTc-sulfur colloid. MIRD/Dose estimate report no. 3, *J Nucl Med* 16:108A-B, 1975.

44. Lecklitner ML: Pitfalls of gastrointestinal bleeding studies with ^{99m}Tc sulfur-colloid, *Semin Nucl Med* 16:155, 1986.

45. Ariel IM: The site of upper gastrointestinal bleeding. Detection by radioactive-tagged red blood cells. *JAMA* 180:212, 1962.

46. D'Addabbo A, Fersini M: Detection of intra-abdominal bleeding by radioisotope scanning after experimental extravasation, *J Nucl Biol Med* 18:170, 1974.

47. Winzelberg GG et al: Evaluation of gastrointestinal bleeding by red blood cells labeled in vivo with technetium-99m, *J Nucl Med* 20:1080, 1979.

48. Abdel-Dayem HM et al: Scintigraphic detection of acute gastrointestinal bleeding using Tc-99m DTPA, *Nucl Med Commun* 5:633, 1984.

49. Owunnane A et al: An experimental model for detection and localisation of gastrointestinal bleeding using Tc-99m DTPA, *Nuklearmedizin* 25:117, 1986.

50. Owunnane A et al: An experimental model for measuring gastrointestinal bleeding rate using Tc-99m DTPA in rabbits, *Comp News Nucl Med* 18:134, 1987.

51. Owunnane A et al: Development of an animal model using a closed system to study the sensitivity of a radiopharmaceutical for the detection of gastrointestinal bleeding, *Nuklearmedizin* 26:126, 1987.

52. Al-Suhaili AR et al: Upper gastrointestinal bleeding from the biliary tract (hematobilia), *Clin Nucl Med* 12:791, 1987.

53. Som P et al: Detection of gastrointestinal blood loss with ^{99m}Tc-labeled heat-treated red blood cells, *Radiology* 138:207, 1981.

54. Pavel DG, Zimmer AM, Patterson VN: In vivo labeling of red blood cells with ^{99m}Tc: a new approach to blood pool visualization, *J Nucl Med* 18:305, 1977.

55. Alavi A: Scintigraphic detection and localization of gastrointestinal bleeding sites. In Gottschalk A, Hoffer PB, Potchen EJ, eds: *Diagnostic nuclear medicine,* Baltimore, 1988, Williams & Wilkins.

56. Froelich LW et al: Time course of in vivo labelling of red blood cells, *J Nucl Med* 21:44, 1980, (abstract).

50 *Angiographic Diagnosis and Therapy of Gastrointestinal Tract Bleeding*

FREDERICK S. KELLER
ROBERT E. BARTON
JOSEF ROSCH

It was in 1960 that angiography was first reported to be useful in demonstrating a lesion responsible for recurrent gastrointestinal (GI) tract bleeding that had not been detected by conventional radiologic studies.[1] Since that time, angiography has played an important role in both the diagnosis and therapy of patients with GI hemorrhage.[2,3] In fact, the investigation of acute or chronic GI bleeding is now one of the more common indications for performing visceral angiography.

ACUTE GI HEMORRHAGE

In the early 1960s, after it was initially introduced for the localization of an acute GI hemorrhage, angiography was often the first procedure performed. However, this practice did not take into account the fact that approximately 75% to 80% of the patients with an acute GI hemorrhage cease bleeding with bedrest and medical therapy consisting of blood and fluid replacement and the correction of any coagulation defects. Today, endoscopy is the primary diagnostic and therapeutic modality for the investigation of upper GI tract bleeding. Arterial bleeding can be treated through the endoscopic application of a heater probe or electrocoagulation, and varices may be sclerosed or banded transendoscopically. Arteriography is therefore required only if medical therapy is unsuccessful in controlling hemorrhage. In most patients who continue to bleed from the upper GI tract, the diagnosis has usually already been established by endoscopy and the arteriography is performed in order to perform catheter hemostasis. Endoscopy is less effective in the diagnosis of lesions responsible for acute lower GI tract hemorrhage, especially during an episode of active bleeding, and angiography is performed to localize as well as treat the bleeding lesion (Fig. 50-1).

DIAGNOSIS OF ACUTE ARTERIAL BLEEDING

The angiographic diagnosis of acute arterial bleeding is based on visualization of the direct extravasation of contrast material into the GI lumen (Fig. 50-2). When bleeding is originating from a large artery, such as in patients with peptic ulcers or colonic diverticuli, it is readily demonstrated by selective arteriograms (Fig. 50-3). If, however, bleeding is from a minor source or multiple capillary sites, such as in the event of erosive gastritis or multiple stress ulcers, selective studies may not adequately demonstrate the hemorrhage and superselective studies are then needed, with injection into secondary and tertiary branches.

Acute GI bleeding is frequently intermittent, and, for the angiogram to yield positive findings, the patient must be bleeding actively at the time contrast material is injected into the artery that supplies the bleeding lesion.[4] Therefore proper timing is crucial for the successful localization of the hemorrhage site and subsequent therapy. If the rate of bleeding has decreased below 0.5 ml/per minute when the contrast material is injected, the arteriographic findings will be negative.

In the upper GI tract, hemorrhage activity is fairly easy to assess by means of lavage using a large-bore nasogastric tube. Bleeding is active if lavage returns bright red or pink fluid after the evacuation of clots. Other signs indicating active hemorrhage are tachycardia, hypotension, and a falling hematocrit after initial resuscitation.

In patients with acute lower GI tract bleeding, it is more difficult to confirm active bleeding at the time of angiography. Radionuclide scanning using technetium-labeled red blood cells or technetium sulfur colloid can indicate active hemorrhage occurring at a rate of 0.1 ml/per minute.[5-7] Therefore, if the radionuclide scan findings are negative, emergency arteriography need not be done. Isotope scanning thus has the potential to decrease the number of negative arteriograms and substantially increase the efficiency of angiography in patients with lower GI tract bleeding. If, however, the nuclear scan reveals the presence of acute hemorrhage, emergency arteriography is indicated to determine the exact site and nature of the lesion responsible and to institute some form of catheter therapy.

PHARMACOANGIOGRAPHY

Because of its intermittent, minute-to-minute nature, acute lower GI tract bleeding often stops or diminishes be-

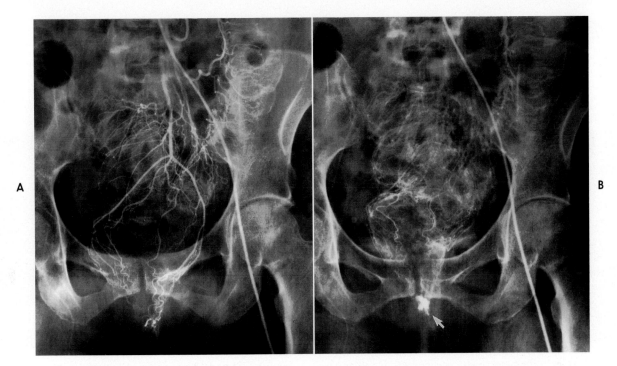

Fig. 50-1 Acute lower GI hemorrhage from the distal rectum. **A,** Early arterial phase of inferior mesenteric arteriogram. **B,** Venous phase shows active bleeding and extravasation of contrast *(arrow)*. During such an episode, blood travels both proximally and distally in the alimentary tract. Flexible sigmoidoscopy performed during acute bleeding failed to localize this lesion on two separate occasions, and each time fresh blood was reported to be visualized as high as the splenic flexure.

tween the time a positive radionuclide scan is obtained and arteriography is performed, or during the angiography itself. In these situations, recurrent active bleeding can sometimes be deliberately induced by the injection of vasodilators, anticoagulants, or fibrinolytics.[8,9] These aggressive diagnostic interventions should be reserved only for patients who pose severe diagnostic problems, and when the risk of prolonging or reactivating hemorrhage is outweighed by the potential diagnostic benefits. Interventions that either prolong or reactivate bleeding should be carried out only after discussion with the patient's gastroenterologist or surgeon, and only in those patients who are hemodynamically stable and for whom replacement blood is available.

ANGIOGRAPHIC CONTROL OF ACUTE GI HEMORRHAGE

Precise localization of the bleeding artery is the first step in the catheter therapy of acute GI hemorrhage. It has been shown that the bleeding lesion in patients with gastric hemorrhage was supplied by the left gastric artery in 85% of cases.[10] The right gastric and short gastric arteries each supplied the bleeding site in 5% of cases. The supply in the remaining 5% of the cases was from the gastroepiploic arteries (3%), gastroduodenal artery (1%), and phrenic artery (1%).[10] Duodenal bleeding may be supplied by the gastroduodenal artery, the inferior pancreaticoduodenal artery, or both of these. Small bowel and colonic hemorrhage orig-

inates from various branches of the superior and inferior mesenteric arteries that supply the area of the bleeding lesion. Distal rectal or anal bleeding may have a dual supply; the superior hemorrhoidal branches of the inferior mesenteric artery or the middle hemorrhoidal branches of the internal iliac arteries, or both.

Vasoconstrictive infusion therapy

Vasopressin, an octopeptide produced in the neurohypophysis, has a variety of pharmacologic actions. One of these, smooth muscle contraction, is most important for controlling GI bleeding. Vasopressin induces smooth muscle contraction in both the walls of arterioles, thereby causing vasoconstriction, and in the bowel wall, which compresses the penetrating blood vessels. The vasopressin infusion is prepared by mixing 200 U of vasopressin in 500 ml of 5% dextrose in water. The ultimate concentration of this solution is 0.4 U/ml and an infusion rate of 30 ml per hour results in a dose of 0.2 U/per minute. Vasopressin is infused selectively into the bleeding artery at a dose ranging from 0.1 to 0.4 U/per minute, depending on the rate of bleeding and arterial size. Infusion is continued for 12 to 36 hours, while the dose is gradually tapered. If there is no recurrence of bleeding, the catheter is kept open and normal saline or a 5% dextrose solution is infused for an additional 12 hours before its removal.

Vasopressin infusion is frequently successful in control-

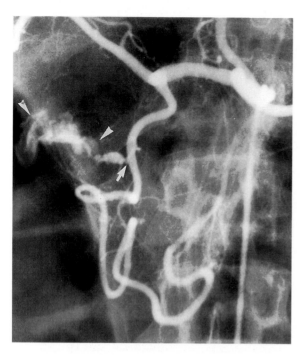

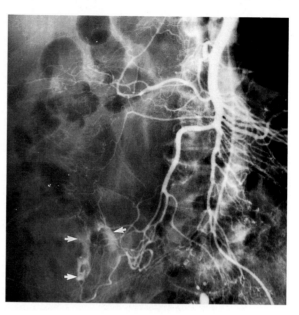

Fig. 50-2 Acute GI bleeding from a peptic ulcer. The ulcer has eroded into the gastroduodenal artery *(arrow)*, resulting in extravasation of contrast material into the lumen of the duodenum *(arrowheads)*.

Fig. 50-3 Acute GI bleeding from a colonic diverticulum. Superior mesenteric arteriography demonstrates acute extravasation of contrast material *(arrows)* from the diverticulum.

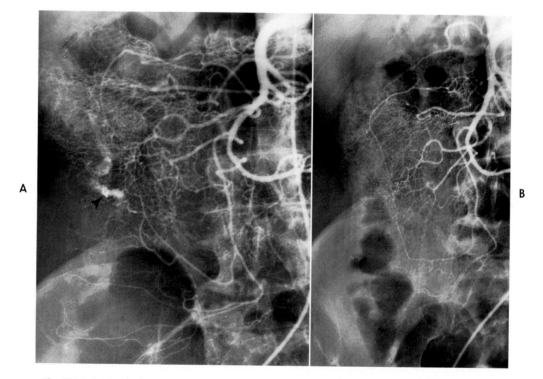

Fig. 50-4 A, Active hemorrhage can be seen on the initial arteriogram *(arrowhead)*. **B,** After the infusion of 0.3 U of vasopressin over 20 minutes, no hemorrhage is evident. Branches of the superior mesenteric artery are constricted.

ling bleeding from superficial gastric lesions, such as Mallory Weiss tears, hemorrhagic gastritis, and stress ulcers.[11-14] Diverticuli and angiodysplasias, the most common lesions responsible for massive acute colonic hemorrhage, are both quite responsive to vasopressin infusion[11,13,14] (Fig. 50-4). Once hemorrhage from a bleeding diverticulum has been brought under control, it is unlikely to recur and surgery can often be avoided. Angiodysplasias tend to rebleed periodically, and therefore resection is usually indicated after hemorrhage has been controlled and the patient's condition stabilized. If the bleeding lesion is near the splenic flexure, its blood supply may come from both the superior mesenteric and inferior mesenteric arteries. In such instances, infusions of both arteries may be required to control active bleeding.

Vasoconstrictive infusion therapy is substantially less effective in controlling hemorrhage from the duodenum than that from the stomach, small bowel, or colon.[15] Three reasons have been proposed to account for this. In the first, because of the dual blood supply to the duodenum from the celiac and the superior mesenteric arteries, infusion of only one limb of the arcade is frequently ineffective because the lesion continues to bleed from the opposite side. In the second, although vasopressin has its greatest effect on small vessels, duodenal hemorrhage often stems from the erosion of larger arteries that do not constrict when exposed to vasopressin. Finally, chronic inflammation secondary to peptic disease limits the ability of arteries near the ulcer to constrict, plus impairs the contractility of the adjacent duodenal wall.

If control of bleeding using either electrocoagulation or the heater probe has been unsuccessful, the vascular contractility in the area of the lesion will be impaired, rendering vasopressin infusion ineffective. The radiologist who performs visceral angiography for the diagnosis and management of GI bleeding should also know the potential side effects and complications of vasopressin therapy. These include hyponatremia, oliguria, hypertension, fluid overload, arrhythmias, and ischemia of the myocardium, bowel, or distal extremities.

Arterial embolotherapy

Since its introduction as a therapeutic modality in the management of GI bleeding 20 years ago, the indications for embolization have broadened.[16-18] Originally reserved as a last-ditch measure in high-risk patients, embolization, without an initial trial of vasoconstrictive therapy, is now preferred by many radiologists.[17] The goal of embolotherapy is to decrease the blood pressure at the site of the bleeding lesions and thereby allow a stable clot to form without causing tissue ischemia or necrosis. Compared with vasopressin infusion, embolotherapy has the advantages of being completed rapidly, plus avoiding the problems of long-term arterial catheterization and the multiple undesirable pharmacologic side effects of vasopressin (Fig. 50-5). Em-

bolization is, however, not without risk, and, unlike vasopressin, which can be decreased or discontinued at the first signs of untoward side effects, embolic particles, once injected, cannot be retrieved.

Embolic materials vary, and the ultimate selection depends on the preference of individual radiologists. Because GI hemorrhage is usually secondary to benign, self-limiting lesions, surgical gelatin or Gelfoam, a temporary vasoocclusive agent, is widely used to control or stop the bleeding. Recanalization usually takes place in 1 to 3 weeks. Cut into small pieces and mixed with contrast, the Gelfoam is slowly injected under fluoroscopic control. Permanent embolic materials are usually reserved for controlling hemorrhage resulting from invasion of the GI tract by primary or secondary malignancies.

Until recently, embolotherapy for the management of acute GI hemorrhage was limited to the upper GI tract (gastroesophageal junction, stomach, and duodenum). Because of its rich collateral supply, individual branches can be occluded with an almost negligible risk of ischemic complications. However, if the collateral blood supply has been compromised by previous surgical ligations or severe atherosclerotic obstructive disease, the risk of gastric or duodenal ischemia is increased.

Most gastric bleeding comes from the left gastric artery, which, fortunately, is usually not difficult to catheterize.[10] Originating as the first major branch of the celiac artery, it can readily be engaged using a Rösch left gastric or a Waltman loop type of catheter.[19,20] Once the vessel has been engaged, a stable, secure catheter position can be achieved by slightly withdrawing the catheter at the puncture site in the groin. In about 1% of the patients, the left gastric artery originates directly from the aorta just proximal to the origin of the celiac artery. In the presence of favorable arterial anatomy, the right gastroepiploic artery, which is occasionally the source of gastric bleeding, can be catheterized. However, selective catheterization of the short gastric and left gastroepiploic arteries is usually not feasible. When selective catheterization of the artery supplying the bleeding lesion is not possible, embolization should not be undertaken.

For embolization of the left gastric artery, tiny pledgets of Gelfoam are first introduced to achieve a more distal occlusion, and then larger pieces are introduced. If only proximal embolization of the left gastric artery is attempted with a large piece of Gelfoam or coil springs, hemorrhage may not be controlled because the rich collateral circulation can maintain sufficient arterial pressure at the bleeding site to prolong the bleeding.

The dual blood supply and large arteries involved in duodenal bleeding make successful embolotherapy more difficult.[21] Occasionally, simple embolization of the gastroduodenal artery is sufficient to control bleeding. However, whenever peptic erosion has caused large defects in the gastroduodenal artery, small particles of Gelfoam are fre-

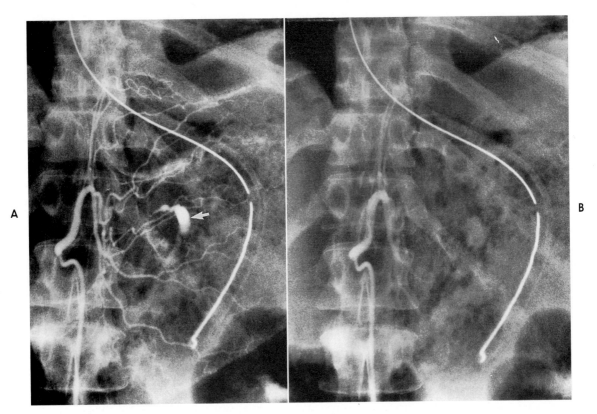

Fig. 50-5 Control of an acutely bleeding gastric ulcer by embolization. **A,** The initial left gastric arteriogram demonstrates acute hemorrhage from an ulcer on the posterior gastric wall *(arrow)*. **B,** Follow-up arteriography after embolization with Gelfoam particles shows occlusion of the major branches of the left gastric artery. Bleeding has ceased.

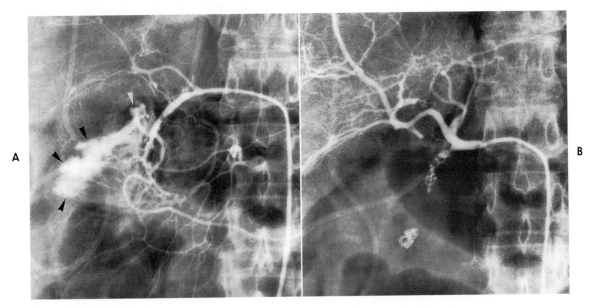

Fig. 50-6 Control of acute hemorrhage from a duodenal ulcer: **A,** Marked extravasation of contrast material *(arrowheads)* due to massive bleeding is visible on the initial gastroduodenal arteriogram. At this time, the patient was in hypovolemic shock, as evidenced by the intense vasoconstriction of the common hepatic artery. **B,** Follow-up arteriogram obtained after the placement of coil spring occluders both distal and proximal to the peptic erosion of the gastroduodenal artery reveals control of hemorrhage. Clinically, bleeding had ceased, and the caliber of the hepatic artery is now normal.

quently ineffective because they pass directly through the hole in the artery into the duodenal lumen. When this occurs, placing coil springs distal and proximal to the arterial defect or sealing it with cyanoacrylate is often successful in stopping hemorrhage (Fig. 50-6). Successful embolization of bleeding duodenal ulcers often requires treatment of both limbs of the pancreaticoduodenal arcade.[21] This necessitates selectively catheterizing the gastroduodenal and inferior pancreaticoduodenal arteries, and this can vary in the degree of difficulty, depending on the arterial anatomy. The use of coaxial microcatheters with fine steerable platinum-tipped guidewires can usually achieve rapid and safe subselective catheterization of almost all arteries.

In the mesenteric circulation, collateral pathways are less well developed than in the upper GI tract. Thus embolization has traditionally been reserved for life-threatening lower GI tract hemorrhage in high-risk surgical patients who do not respond to vasopressin therapy. However, in the past decade the careful embolization of lesions responsible for lower GI tract bleeding has been advocated by some radiologists.[22-24] Good results have been achieved in this setting especially in the presence of diverticuli that have not rebled after embolization.[22] Because the incidence of

ischemic complications after mesenteric embolization is significantly greater than it is after embolization in the upper GI tract, the procedure must be as superselective as possible. Coaxial catheter systems with platinum-tipped torquable guidewires permit precise catheterization of the bleeding artery itself. Patients are then closely monitored for several days afterward. If signs of peritoneal irritation develop, suggesting probable transmural infarction, surgery is required.[25] However, in this event, at least the patient is now hemodynamically stable and the operation can be done on an elective, and therefore safer, basis.

Chronic GI hemorrhage

Unlike acute GI bleeding, with its dramatic presentations of hematemesis, hematochezia, or melena, patients with chronic GI hemorrhage present with occult fecal blood and iron deficiency anemia. Occasionally, there are recurrent brief episodes of massive hemorrhage. Usually some type of tumor is diagnosed in these patients on barium or endoscopic examinations of the upper GI tract and colon. Angiography is performed only in those patients who continue to bleed despite negative barium and endoscopic findings. In patients with chronic GI bleeding, a positive angiogram

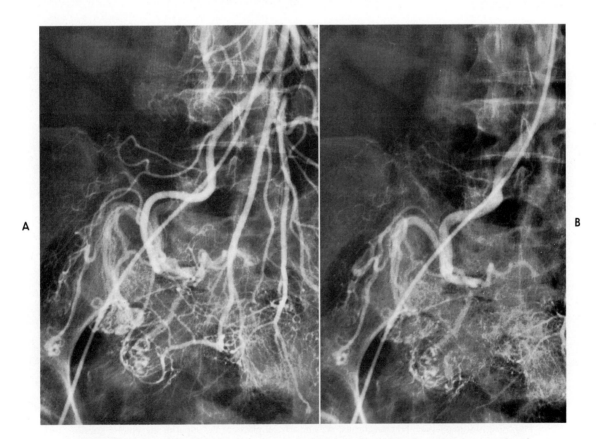

Fig. 50-7 Large angiodysplasia in the cecum. **A,** Early arteriographic phase shows a vascular nidus supplied by a large feeding artery. **B,** In the late arteriographic phase. Although the remainder of the vessels are in the late arteriographic phase, a large and densely opacified vein is seen exiting from the angiodysplasia.

usually reveals some form of hypervascular lesion rather than extravasation of contrast material into the lumen of the GI tract. The diagnosis in a significant number of patients with chronic or recurrent lower GI tract bleeding remains unknown even after competently performed arteriography.[26]

Angiodysplasia

Known variously as *telangiectasias, angiomas, vascular ectasias, angiodysplasias,* and *arteriovenous malformations,* these lesions are commonly responsible for lower GI tract bleeding, especially in the elderly[27-29] (Fig. 50-7). They are seen more frequently in patients with aortic and mitral valve disease or with hereditary hemorrhagic telangiectasia. Pathologically, angiodysplasias are clusters of ectatic submucosal vascular spaces. These lesions are not visible on barium examinations, although they can occasionally be seen during colonoscopy. Their angiographic appearance varies with their size. The appearance of slight dilatation of the distal portion of the feeder with a minimally enlarged early draining vein may be quite subtle and the only findings in the presence of smaller lesions (Fig. 50-8). Larger angiodysplasias have a tangle of vessels, the vascular tuft or nidus, which is opacified in the early arterial phase of the angiogram and empties into a prominent, early and dense-filling draining vein (Fig. 50-9).

Discovery of an angiodysplasia does not imply that it is the source of recurrent hemorrhage because this type of lesion often exists in elderly nonbleeding patients and may be an entirely coincidental finding in patients with chronic hemorrhage. The entire angiogram should therefore be carefully examined for the existence of any other lesion that might be the source of bleeding; if none is found, the area containing the angiodysplasia should be resected.

Precise preoperative localization of angiodysplasias is required, as these lesions can neither be seen nor palpated at surgery. The diagnostic angiogram is usually sufficient for localizing colonic angiodysplasias because the colon is a fixed structure. However, jejunal and ileal angiodysplasias are often difficult to find at surgery because, once the bowel is eviscerated for inspection, the spatial relationships between individual bowel loops are altered drastically (Fig.

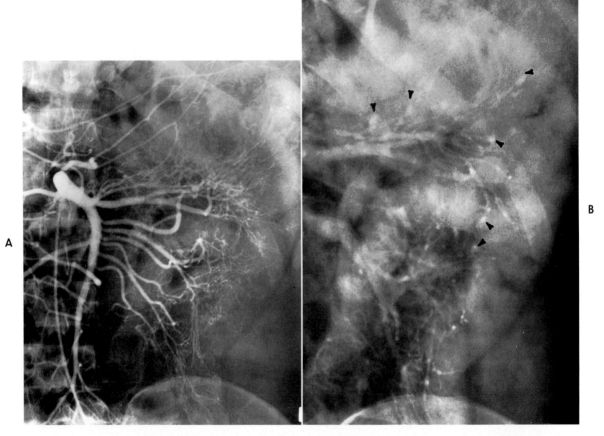

Fig. 50-8 Multiple jejunal telangiectasias. **A,** The arterial phase of the superior mesenteric arteriogram is normal. **B,** In the late arterial phase there is early venous drainage from jejunal branches, with multiple small telangiectasias (some marked by *arrowheads*) present in the distribution of the proximal jejunum. After segmental jejunal resection, this patient's chronic lower GI bleeding was cured.

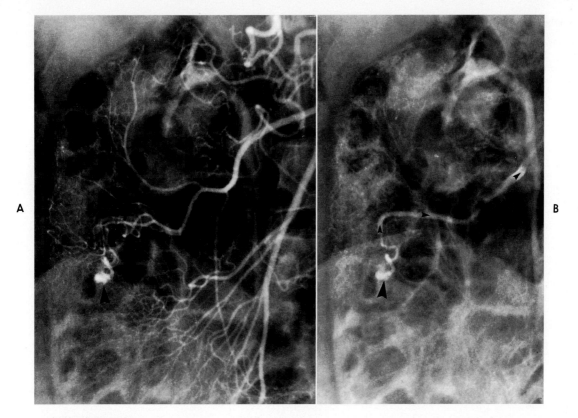

Fig. 50-9 Angiodysplasia of the right colon. Early **(A)** and middle **(B)** phases of a superior mesenteric arteriogram reveal the vascular tuft *(large arrowhead)* of the angiodysplasia. Prominent and intense venous drainage *(small arrowheads)* can be seen coming from the angiodysplasia, while the remainder of the colon is still in the late arterial phase.

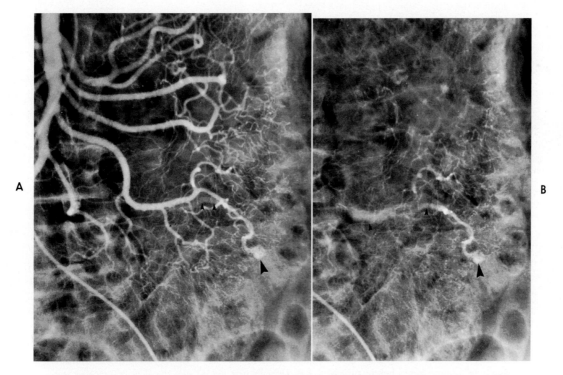

Fig. 50-10 Small bowel angiodysplasia. Early **(A)** and middle **(B)** arterial phases of a superior mesenteric arteriogram reveal the vascular tuft *(large arrowhead)* of the angiodysplasia. An early draining vein is visible in the early arterial phase *(small arrowheads)* but seen to better advantage in the midarterial phase. Incidentally noted are standing waves in several jejunal branches.

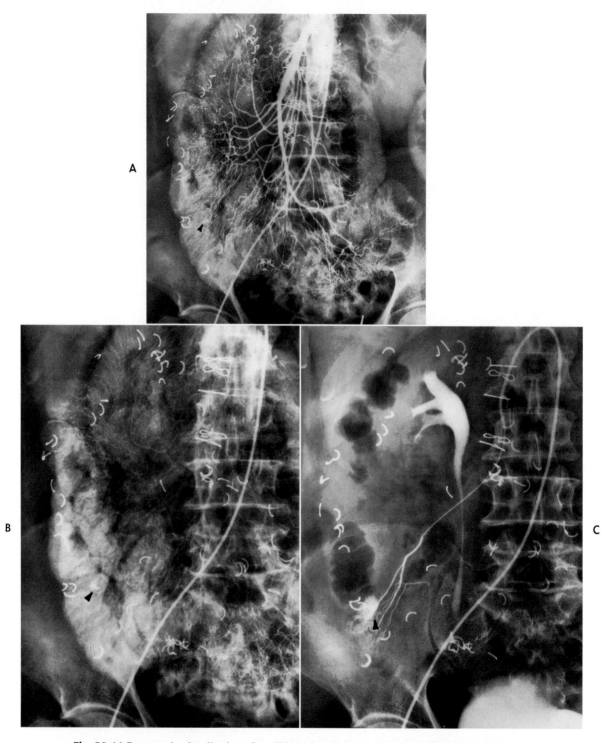

Fig. 50-11 Preoperative localization of small bowel angiodysplasia in a patient with chronic lower GI tract bleeding after a right and left hemicolectomy. Early **(A)** and late **(B)** arterial phases of the superior mesenteric arteriogram reveal a small angiomatous lesion *(arrowhead)* that is bleeding slowly. **C,** Immediately before surgery a 3-Fr catheter was placed into the ileal branch that supplied the area of the bleeding lesion.

50-10). Therefore, for these small bowel angiodysplasias, intraoperative localization is usually necessary so that the resection of long segments of uninvolved bowel is prevented. The angiodysplasia is localized just before surgery by placing a small 3-Fr catheter into the main feeding artery of the angiodysplasia. After angiography confirms the correct positioning of this small catheter, the patient is taken to surgery. With the bowel exposed, 1 ml of methylene blue is injected into the catheter to stain the segment of bowel containing the angiodysplasia[30] (Fig. 50-11).

Surgical resection is the primary form of therapy for angiodysplasias causing recurrent GI bleeding. Although acute bleeding episodes can almost always be controlled with vasopressin infusion, bleeding usually recurs. Embo-

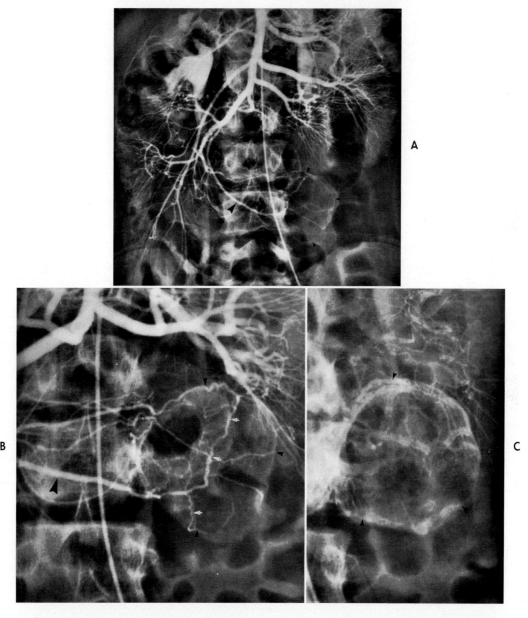

Fig. 50-12 Meckel's diverticulum in a young patient with chronic lower GI hemorrhage. **A,** A selective superior mesenteric arteriogram demonstrates an enlarged nonbranching embryonic ileal artery *(large arrowhead)* leading to the Meckel's diverticulum *(small arrowheads)*. **B,** The early phase of a superselective magnification arteriogram of the ileal artery supplying the diverticulum reveals irregular arteries in the wall of the Meckel's diverticulum *(small white arrows),* which are remnants of vitelline arteries. **C,** In the late phase there is an increased parenchymal blush in the wall of the Meckel's diverticulum *(small arrowheads)* due to the accumulation of contrast material in the gastric mucosa that lines it.

lization treatment for the control of rebleeding from angiodysplasias has also been reported.[31]

Meckel's diverticulum

Meckel's diverticulum is a common cause of both chronic and acute lower GI tract bleeding in young patients.[32] Because of the ectopic gastric mucosa contained in many Meckel's diverticuli, melena is frequently the initial symptom, even though the lesion is in the distal ileum. Arteriography, performed during an episode of acute hemorrhage from Meckel's diverticulum, shows extravasation of the contrast material in the distal bowel. If the angiogram is performed in the absence of active bleeding, an enlarged, long, nonbranching, embryonic ileal artery leading to the diverticulum is often seen. Additional angiographic findings include irregular arteries in the wall of the diverticulum, remnants of vitelline arteries, and an increased parenchymal blush arising from the lining of gastric mucosa[33] (Fig. 50-12).

GI BLEEDING FROM EXTRAALIMENTARY TRACT SOURCES
Hemobilia

Once considered an extremely rare cause of GI hemorrhage, hemobilia, bleeding into the biliary tract, has been encountered more frequently in recent years.[34,35] Trauma, either remote or recent, including iatrogenic injuries, is the most common cause. Although blunt trauma with liver laceration and penetrating stab wounds were well-known sources of hemobilia in the past, invasive diagnostic and therapeutic procedures, such as liver biopsy and percutaneous transhepatic biliary drainage, probably account for the largest percentage of cases today. Hemobilia also rarely results from fistulous erosion between an hepatic blood vessel and the adjacent biliary system secondary to a malignant, inflammatory, or degenerative disease.

The classic clinical triad of right upper quadrant colicky pain, jaundice, and GI bleeding constitutes the presentation in only one third of the patients.[34] Although GI bleeding is always part of the clinical picture, it varies in severity, ranging from massive hemorrhage to chronic, low-grade blood loss. The clinical diagnosis depends on the degree of suspicion that the GI blood loss is due to hemobilia, and may be difficult, especially if a long time has elapsed since the initial hepatic injury. The results of various tests can suggest the diagnosis of hemobilia. Ultrasonography and computed tomography (CT) may reveal the existence of blood clots in the gallbladder and a dilated biliary tree.[36] If there is a large pseudoaneurysm, it may be visualized by these modalities. Percutaneous transhepatic cholangiography may also show thrombus inside the biliary system. Endoscopy, if performed during an episode of active hemorrhage, can demonstrate blood issuing from the papilla. However, angiography or arterial portography, with direct visualization of the arterial or venous lesion that communicates with the bile duct, is required to confirm the diagnosis.

Angiographic findings associated with hemobilia include extravasation of contrast material into the biliary tree, arterial pseudoaneurysm, and an hepatic artery-to-portal vein fistula.[37,38] Of these, pseudoaneurysm is the most common and can be seen on hepatic arteriograms in about 65% of the patients with hemobilia.

Either surgical resection of the hepatic lobe containing the offending lesion or ligation of either the right or left hepatic artery, depending on the location of the lesion, has been the traditional form of therapy.[34] Currently, percutaneous transcatheter superselective occlusion of the artery (or portal venous branch) that supplies the pathologic lesion responsible for the hemobilia is now the therapy preferred both by surgeons and interventional radiologists.[37-39] When a large pseudoaneurysm exists in a proximal portion of a major hepatic artery, the angiographer should try to isolate it by bracketing it with coil springs placed just proximal and distal to the lesion (Fig. 50-13). For the treatment of peripheral arterial injuries, subselective embolization of the feeding artery as close as possible to the lesion itself is the best approach (Fig. 50-14). Nonselective, peripheral hepatic arterial occlusion with small particulate emboli is not recommended in the management of hemobilia.

Pancreatic hemorrhage

Although an uncommon complication of pancreatitis, massive hemorrhage is the major cause of death in greater than 50% of the fatalities attributed to the disease.[40] Digestion of the arterial walls by enzymes released as the result of the pancreatic inflammatory process causes the formation of pseudoaneurysms that may communicate with the lumens of various segments of the alimentary tract, the pancreatic duct (hemosuccus pancreaticus), or pseudocysts. Patients may present with either massive GI hemorrhage or a large expanding retroperitoneal hematoma.

Pancreatitis is usually suspected on clinical grounds and confirmed by CT findings, which often consist of a large pseudoaneurysm or pseudocyst filled with blood. Because even very tiny pseudoaneurysms may be responsible for significant hemorrhage, meticulously performed angiography is often necessary to identify and localize the offending lesion (Fig. 50-15). Surgical intervention, which is frequently necessary to manage the complications in patients with hemorrhagic pancreatitis, may be extremely difficult and can precipitate fulminant bleeding.[41] Preoperative embolization reduces the chances of serious blood loss during surgery, and may even obviate the need for surgery. Once identified, the pseudoaneurysm should be isolated by placing coil springs in the normal segments of artery both proximal and distal to the lesion. When manipulating the angiographic catheter close to such a pseudoaneurysm, all maneuvers should be done gently and with extreme care, as these lesions are fragile and known to rupture even with only the minimal pressure encountered during embolotherapy.[42]

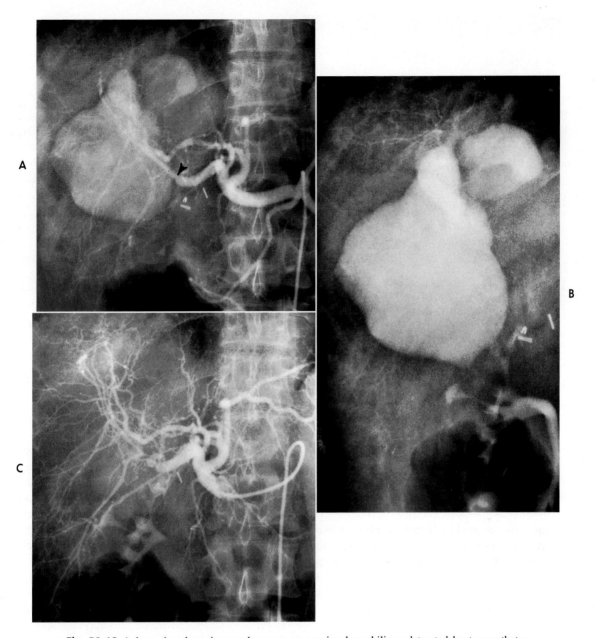

Fig. 50-13 A large intrahepatic pseudoaneurysm causing hemobilia and treated by transcatheter embolization. **A** and **B,** The early and late phases of an hepatic arteriogram show a large pseudoaneurysm in the right liver lobe. It originates from the right hepatic artery *(arrowhead)* and was the result of a machete wound inflicted in the right upper quadrant. **C,** Following transcatheter embolization with a coil spring, the pseudoaneurysm no longer fills, and afterward the patient had no further recurrence of hemobilia.

Aortoenteric and arterioenteric fistulas

Vascular graft anastomoses, pseudoaneurysms, and aneurysms that lie near and eventually erode into a portion of the alimentary tract as the result of continuous pulsations against them are unusual causes of GI bleeding. If the patient is bleeding actively at the time of angiography, extravasation is evident. However, for the angiogram to show the nature of the bleeding, the vessel responsible for the hemorrhage must be injected. This is especially important in patients with aortoenteric and arterioenteric fistulas, because usually only the visceral vessels—the celiac, superior mesenteric, and inferior mesenteric arteries—are examined in this setting. If there is a history of aortic graft or surgical repair of the iliac arteries, the angiographer must be aware of the possibility of a major vessel-to-enteric fistula and accordingly study the aorta and iliac arteries.

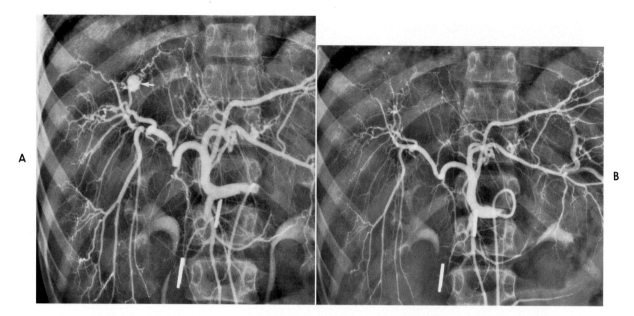

Fig. 50-14 Hepatic injury resulting in hemobilia treated by transcatheter embolotherapy. This 10-year-old girl suffered a liver laceration when the horse she was riding rolled on top of her. During the ensuing 6 weeks she had four episodes of upper GI tract hemorrhage. **A,** An hepatic angiogram demonstrates a pseudoaneurysm *(arrow)* in the superior portion of the right liver lobe that was responsible for the hemobilia. **B,** Follow-up arteriogram 6 weeks after the occlusion of the pseudoaneurysm confirms that it has been successfully obliterated. During the 13 years since the accident, the patient has had no further hemobilia.

The angiographic findings found in the context of aortoenteric and arterioenteric fistulas include some type of arterial abnormality such as a pseudoaneurysm or aneurysm, and, if bleeding is active, extravasation of contrast.[43] Because these lesions are always infected, surgery is required. If bleeding is massive, an occlusion balloon catheter can be inserted in the aorta or offending artery and inflated to tamponade the hemorrhage, thus stabilizing the patient's condition for emergency operation. If the patient is not a surgical candidate, endovascular stent grafting, which is now in an experimental phase, coupled with lifetime antibiotic coverage, may prove to be an acceptable alternative form of therapy.

GI HEMORRHAGE OF VENOUS ORIGIN
Diagnosis of venous bleeding

The diagnosis of acute variceal hemorrhage is usually based on the endoscopic findings, and most patients with bleeding varices only undergo visceral angiography before a contemplated surgical portosystemic shunt or transjugular intrahepatic portosystemic shunt (TIPS) procedure. In the unusual instance, when endoscopy cannot be performed, acute upper GI tract bleeding from esophageal varices can be diagnosed by angiography. Because extravasation of contrast material cannot be demonstrated by simple arterial portography, the angiographic diagnosis of variceal hemorrhage is based on the following two criteria: (1). visualization of varices during the venous phases of splenic angiography or on superior mesenteric or left gastric phar-

macoangiograms after the administration of tolazoline; and (2) exclusion of arterial or capillary bleeding sites[44] (Fig. 50-16). The latter is important, as approximately 40% of bleeding episodes in cirrhotic patients with known varices can be due to arterial or capillary sources such as Mallory Weiss tears, gastritis, or peptic ulcers.

Therapy for variceal hemorrhage
Vasopressin infusion

The selective infusion of low doses (0.2 to 0.4 U/min) of vasopressin into the superior mesenteric artery was an effective measure for decreasing portal pressure and blood flow and was also successful in stopping hemorrhage in a significant number of patients with portal hypertension and bleeding esophageal varices.[45] Several years later it was confirmed, both in experimental animals and in randomized clinical trials consisting of patients bleeding from esophageal varices, that low-dose peripheral intravenous infusions of vasopressin are as effective in reducing portal pressure and blood flow as is selective superior mesenteric arterial infusion.[46] Therefore, selective arterial vasopressin therapy has now been replaced by the simpler, less invasive intravenous administration.

Transhepatic embolization of gastroesophageal varices

Transhepatic obliteration of bleeding gastroesophageal varices was introduced in 1974 as a better measure than emergency portosystemic shunting to stop variceal hemor-

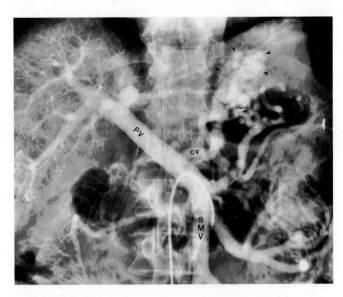

Fig. 50-16 Demonstration of portal hypertension and esophageal varices in a patient with upper GI tract hemorrhage. The venous phase of a superior mesenteric pharmacoangiogram, with tolazoline administered to produce vasodilation, reveals hepatopetal flow in the superior mesenteric vein *(SMV)* and portal vein *(PV)*, with hepatofugal flow in the coronary vein *(CV)* leading to gastroesophageal varices *(arrowheads)*.

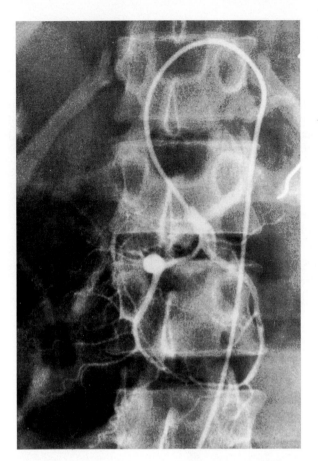

Fig. 50-15 Inferior pancreaticoduodenal arteriogram. A small pseudoaneurysm secondary to chronic pancreatitis is seen on the superselective arteriogram. This aneurysm had caused mass retroperitoneal hemorrhage and was not visible in the selective celiac arteriogram.

rhage when medical therapy has failed.[47-49] This technique involves transhepatic portal vein catheterization and venographic demonstration of the portal anatomy. All branches feeding the gastroesophageal varices are then selectively catheterized and occluded. The rationale underlying transhepatic variceal obliteration is that occlusion of the life-threatening portosystemic collaterals, the esophageal varices, can promote the formation of new portosystemic pathways or the enlargement of preexisting, beneficial, and less ominous ones.

Before transhepatic variceal obliteration is carried out, visceral arteriography should be performed to exclude a possible portal vein occlusion or a hypervascular liver lesion in the proposed catheter tract. If occlusion of the portal vein is seen during the venous phase of splenic or superior mesenteric arteriography, this rules out transhepatic variceal obliteration, as the catheter cannot then be advanced from the intrahepatic into the extrahepatic portal venous system.

Although, transhepatic variceal obliteration has been shown to be successful in controlling variceal hemorrhage in 85% to 100% of affected patients, technical difficulties involved in its performance and a high incidence of recurrent variceal hemorrhage has hindered its widespread use. Endoscopic sclerosis of esophageal varices, and more recently the TIPS procedure, have now replaced transhepatic variceal obliteration.

Transjugular intrahepatic portosystemic shunting

Although there are several therapeutic modalities, including sclerotherapy, surgical shunting and devascularization procedures, and liver transplantation, for the treatment of hemorrhage resulting from gastroesophageal varices, none is ideal. The shortcomings of these currently accepted therapies have prompted a search for additional treatment options. TIPS represents a new alternative in the management of portal hypertension. Early results suggest that its use may improve the outcomes in high-risk patients with variceal bleeding.

History

The idea of TIPS was conceived by Rösch et al.[50] in 1969 (Fig. 50-17). They created a tract between the portal and hepatic veins in dogs using long, coaxial dilators and stented it with plastic tubing to create a shunt; however, these small-diameter shunts invariably occluded after a short time.[51] Interest in TIPS was renewed with the development of the angioplasty balloon catheter. Colapinto et al.[52] reported the first use of TIPS in a human patient in 1982. In their technique, after embolization of the gastroe-

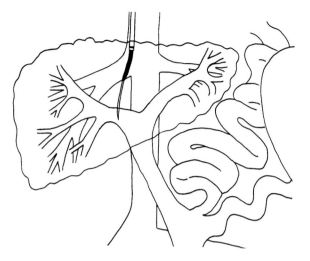

Fig. 50-17 Depiction of the puncture of the portal vein for creating a transjugular intrahepatic portosystemic shunt.

sophageal varices using a transjugular approach, a portosystemic shunt was created by inflating an angioplasty balloon in the tract between the hepatic and portal veins. No stent was used. This technique was eventually used to treat 15 patients and produced a mild decrease in the portal venous pressure averaging only 5.9 mm Hg. Although hemorrhage was controlled for a short time, recurrent variceal hemorrhage occurred in more than half of the patients, and all but two patients died within 6 months of the procedure.[53]

The advent of expandable stents was the final technologic development that brought TIPS to its current state. After the initial successful work on animals conducted by Palmaz, who used dogs, and Rösch, who used pigs, which involved expandable metallic stents placed in the shunt track, Richter et al.[54-57] performed the first TIPS procedure using metallic stents in a human patient in Freiberg, Germany, in January 1988.

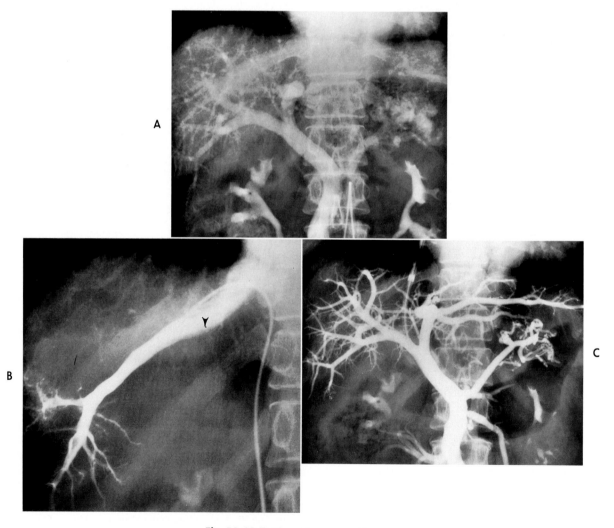

Fig. 50-18 For legend see opposite page.

Indications

Initially TIPS was performed only on an emergency basis in patients with massive bleeding and severe liver disease when sclerotherapy had failed, and who were not considered candidates for emergency surgical portosystemic shunts. Indications for the procedure were expanded after early results showed TIPS to be effective in the control of variceal hemorrhage. Currently, TIPS is performed quite often in patients who are candidates for liver transplantation when bleeding refractory to sclerotherapy develops before a donor liver becomes available (Fig. 50-18). In this setting, TIPS is preferable to shunt surgery, which only makes subsequent liver transplantation more difficult.[58] TIPS can effectively control variceal hemorrhage without complicating subsequent transplantation because the entire shunt is intrahepatic and no laparotomy is required.[59] We and other investigators are also performing TIPS electively as an alternative to shunt surgery in higher-risk patients who

rebleed after sclerotherapy or who have varices inaccessible to sclerotherapy, particularly gastric and duodenal varices or varices around an ileostomy or colostomy. TIPS has also been used to relieve intractable ascites.

The applications for TIPS may ultimately be expanded even further. Its ultimate role depends on the results of prospective, randomized trials that compare its merits to those of other treatment modalities.

Technique

Before TIPS is carried out, it is essential to confirm the patency of the portal vein and to evaluate the portal venous anatomy. Some now use ultrasound to document portal vein patency and to guide the puncture.[60] We routinely use arterial portography to demonstrate the anatomy. Injection of both the splenic and superior mesenteric arteries can provide a complete view of the portal venous system and may reveal unsuspected causes of variceal hemorrhage, such as

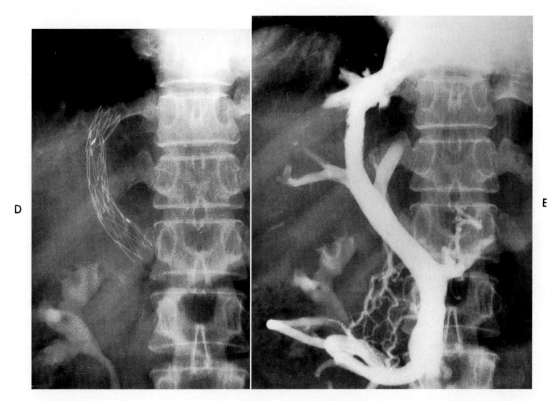

D   E

Fig. 50-18 A transjugular intrahepatic portosystemic shunt (TIPS) in a 48-year-old woman with Child type C cirrhosis and recurrent bleeding from gastroesophageal varices despite several sclerotherapy treatments. Since the procedure she has not had any bleeding, and, at a recent 3-month follow-up, she was doing well and ultrasound study documented shunt patency. **A,** Venous phase of a superior mesenteric angiogram demonstrates patency of the portal vein, the anatomy of its bifurcation, and filling of the gastroesophageal varices. **B,** An hepatic venogram demonstrates the anatomy of the right hepatic vein. Arrowhead indicates puncture site for the TIPS. **C,** A portal venogram after entrance into the right portal vein shows retrograde filling of gastic varices. The portal pressure was 40 mm Hg. **D,** An open film of the expanded Z-stent placed into the shunt tract and extending into the portal vein. **E,** Follow-up portogram after TIPS formation reveals excellent shunting with minimal filling of the hepatic portal radicles. There is no filling of the varices. The portal pressure decreased to 16 mm Hg.

splenic vein occlusion. Arterial portography may not demonstrate the portal vein in patients with well-advanced liver disease and hepatofugal portal venous flow. In this event, wedged hepatic venography should be performed at the time of the TIPS procedure so that the portal vein can be visualized (Fig. 50-19). We prefer to perform the angiographic study on the day before TIPS, but, in emergencies, it is combined with the TIPS procedure.

Little specific patient preparation is required. Patients are given broad-spectrum antibiotics beforehand. When patients have massive ascites, it has proved helpful to drain the ascites before the TIPS procedure, when feasible. This facilitates hepatic vein catheterization and the portal venous puncture by decreasing the angle between the hepatic veins and the inferior vena cava. In addition, a higher-quality fluoroscopic image can be obtained if the volume of ascites is decreased.

The TIPS procedure itself is performed with the patient under intravenous sedation, but it is important that the patient be alert enough to cooperate, particularly when breath-holding is called for. The right internal jugular vein is entered high in the neck, and a large vascular sheath is placed.

If the right internal jugular vein cannot be used, the procedure can be performed through the left internal jugular vein with minimal discomfort to the patient. TIPS has also been done via the right external jugular and right common femoral veins.[61,62] The right hepatic vein is then catheterized and a test injection of contrast is administered to confirm its suitability for creation of the TIPS. A puncture site is then selected in the hepatic vein cephalad to the level of the portal bifurcation. The catheter with a needle inside is rotated anteriorly in the proximal hepatic vein and wedged against the wall of the vein. The needle is then advanced with a forceful thrust to puncture the liver and portal vein. Ideally the right portal vein should be entered about 2 cm from its bifurcation. A more central puncture carries an added risk, because the portal vein bifurcation might then be entered outside the liver, and creation of a TIPS could cause massive intraperitoneal hemorrhage. A more peripheral puncture is safe but may make catheterization of the portal vein more difficult. Entry into the portal vein is usually the most difficult part of the procedure, with success greatly determined by the operator's experience.

Once the portal vein is accessed, a pigtail catheter is in-

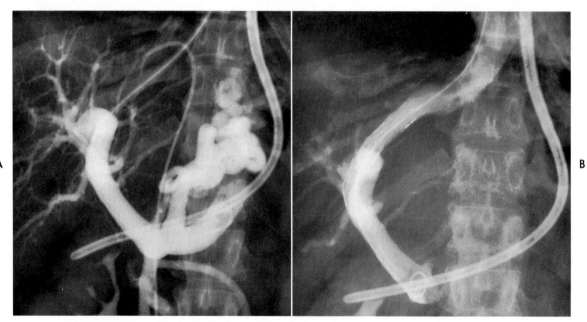

Fig. 50-19 A transjugular intrahepatic portosystemic shunt (TIPS) in a 63-year-old woman with idiopathic cirrhosis and recurrent massive bleeding from large gastric varices. Her bleeding ceased immediately after the procedure and did not recur during the 4 months before she received a liver transplant. The shunt was noted to be patent and well endothelialized at the time of surgery. **A,** A portal venogram after puncture of the portal branch reveals extensive gastric varices and retrograde filling of the mesenteric veins. The portal pressure was 43 mm Hg. **B,** A portal venogram after creation of the TIPS reveals almost complete shunting of the portal flow into the inferior vena cava. The portal pressure was 29 mm Hg; the patient had marked splenomegaly.

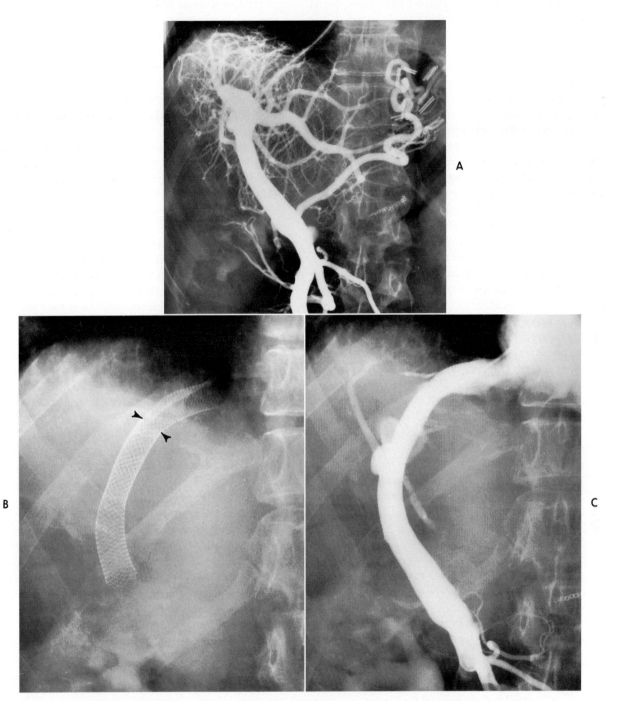

Fig. 50-20 A transjugular intrahepatic portosystemic shunt (TIPS) in a patient with chronic hepatitis, sclerosing cholangitis, and status post colectomy. He was having problems with recurrent bleeding from large varices in the area of ileostomy. After the procedure no bleeding recurred, and a recent ultrasound study confirmed continued shunt patency 6 months later. **A,** A portal venogram obtained after puncture of the left portal branch reveals gastric varices and retrograde filling of an enlarged superior mesenteric vein, which fed varices around the ileostomy. The portal pressure was 33 mm Hg. **B,** An open film of the stent placed into the shunt tract and extending into both the portal and hepatic vein. **C,** A portal venogram obtained after TIPS formation reveals almost complete shunting into the inferior vein cava, no filling of the gastric varices, and no retrograde flow to the superior mesenteric vein. The portal pressure had decreased to 14 mm Hg.

troduced and pressure measurements and direct portal venography performed. An angioplasty balloon catheter is introduced for dilation of the intrahepatic track. The hepatic parenchyma usually dilates easily; however, the hepatic vein wall, and particularly the portal vein wall, resist dilation. The patient usually experiences considerable discomfort during this maneuver, and should be given additional analgesia at this point.

After dilation of the hepatic parenchymal tract, it is ready for stenting. Three types of stents are currently used for TIPS: the Gianturco-Rosch Z-stent (Cook Incorporated, Bloomington, Ind.), the Palmaz stent (Johnson & Johnson Interventional Systems, Warren, NJ, and the Wallstent (Schneider, Minneapolis, Minn.), which were all originally developed for biliary stenting. It is extremely important that the entire length of the parenchymal tract be covered with stents. If the first stent does not completely cover the tract, an additional stent must be placed to achieve adequate long-term portal decompression (Fig. 50-20). Following stent placement, a multi-sidehole catheter is again advanced into the splenic vein, and followup portal venography is performed to ascertain patency and to obtain portal venous pressure measurements. If the portogram shows filling of the varices and the reduction in portal venous pressure is not adequate, the stents can be dilated to their maximal diameter with a balloon catheter. Most investigators advocate reducing the portosystemic gradient to 10 mm Hg. Should filling of varices persist even after maximal expansion of the stents, transcatheter embolization of varices can be performed.

Afterward, patients are observed for evidence of additional variceal bleeding, intraperitoneal hemorrhage, or encephalopathy. The duration of the hospitalization is determined by the patient's overall clinical condition. About half of the patients are discharged within 3 days of the TIPS procedure. Should recurrent variceal bleeding develop, the shunt should be recatheterized from the jugular or femoral approach to permit diagnostic portal venography and pressure measurements. Any stenosis in the shunt can be dilated at this time, additional stents placed, and any persistent varices embolized.

Results and discussion

Because TIPS has been performed clinically for only a very short time, little data have yet been published regarding it, especially the long-term results. Early experience clearly shows that TIPS can be performed successfully in nearly all patients,[57-60,63] with most investigators reporting a 100% success rate. However, the success of any shunt procedure depends on its ability to adequately reduce portal pressure. Most investigators performing TIPS have sought to reduce the portosystemic gradient to approximately 10 mm Hg, and this has been accomplished with near uniform success.

TIPS appears to be quite effective in controlling acute variceal hemorrhage. LaBerge et al.[64] successfully performed TIPS procedures in 30 of 32 patients who were actively bleeding at the time of the procedure. Of these, 28 patients stopped bleeding immediately and one of the two who did not respond was found to be bleeding from an ulcer at followup endoscopy. Hemorrhage has ceased immediately in all patients who were actively bleeding whom we have treated.

Rebleeding from varices after a TIPS procedure is reported to occur in 5% to 10% of the patients, and almost invariably stems from problems with the intrahepatic shunt. The low incidence of rebleeding is due in large part to the relatively high patency rates that have been achieved (Fig. 50-21). LaBerge et al.[64] have reported an overall shunt patency rate of 98%. All their surviving patients had patent shunts at the time of their report and all patients undergoing transplantation had patent shunts at the time of transplantation. In 2 of 20 patients in their series who died, the shunts had occluded. Eleven patients in their series, however, required some further intervention to maintain or restore shunt patency, yielding an ultimate primary patency of 86%. Others report primary patency rates of about 90%.

TIPS can be of particular benefit in prospective liver transplant patients with variceal bleeding uncontrolled by sclerotherapy because it requires no laparotomy or alteration in the extrahepatic portal venous anatomy. Iwatsuki et al.[58] have shown a trend toward an adverse outcome when surgical portosystemic shunting precede liver transplantation.[58] Surgical shunt procedures can cause the formation of intraabdominal adhesions, which can impede subsequent liver transplantation. In addition, the surgical shunt must be taken down at the time of transplantation, which further lengthens the operation. A properly performed TIPS procedure avoids both of these problems. However, the stents placed during TIPS should not extend into the extrahepatic portal vein or the suprahepatic inferior vena cava where they could complicate a subsequent transplant operation. Early results using TIPS in pretransplant patients have been quite encouraging.[59]

Besides controlling variceal hemorrhage, a couple of additional benefits of TIPS have come to light. These include the resolution of ascites, an increase in the platelet counts in approximately 50% of the patients with severe thrombocytopenia, and an increase in the hematocrit.[64,65]

Few serious complications attributable to the procedure have arisen. Intraperitoneal hemorrhage is the most feared complication, but it occurs only rarely. Procedure-related mortality has been remarkably low considering the status of the patient populations treated. Thirty-day mortality is as low as 2.4%. The 14% mortality cited by LaBerge et al.[64] is the highest reported and reflects the severity of disease in their patients. Fifty-five percent of their patients were in Child's class C and 32% were actively bleeding at

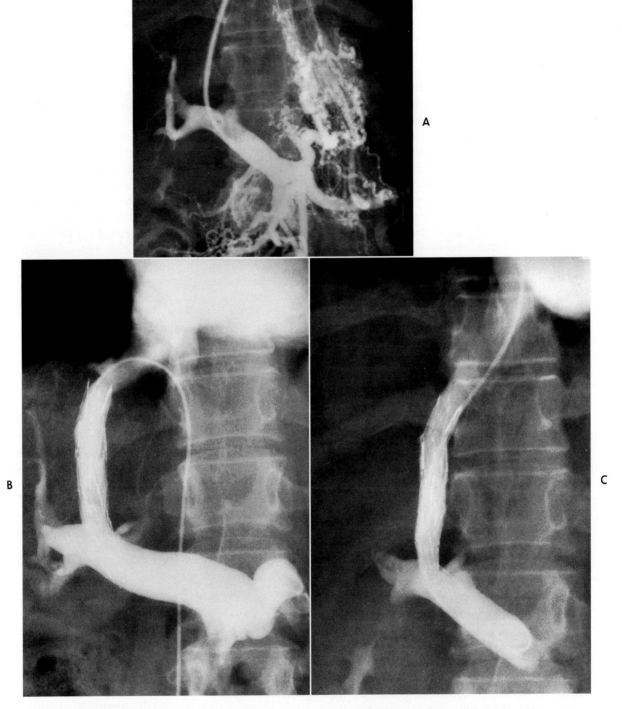

Fig. 50-21 A transjugular intrahepatic portasystemic shunt (TIPS) in a 55-year-old woman with alcoholic cirrhosis, ascites, and recurrent bleeding from gastroesophagal varices. She had undergone sclerotherapy of her esophageal varices. Her ascites disappeared after the procedure, and she has not had any bleeding recurrence. At the 6-month follow-up she was doing well without evidence of encephalopathy. **A,** A portal venogram obtained after puncture of the right portal vein reveals multiple gastric varices and poor filling of the intrahepatic portal radicles. The portal pressure was 41 mm Hg. **B,** A portal venogram obtained after TIPS formation reveals almost complete shunting of the portal circulation into the inferior vena cava and no filling of the varices. The portal pressure had decreased to 25 mm Hg. **C,** At 6-month follow-up this portal venogram revealed continued excellent shunting with no filling of the varices. The portal pressure was 16 mm Hg.

the time of the procedure. The two patients who died early in our series were moribund when the procedure was performed and received shunts in a last ditch effort to stop the variceal hemorrhage. Both patients stopped bleeding after an uncomplicated TIPS procedure, only to succumb to acute respiratory distress syndrome and liver failure.

Hepatic encephalopathy and liver failure have been major problems in patients after nonselective surgical portosystemic shunting,[66,67] and total diversion of the portal venous flow has been blamed for these complications.[68] It has recently been suggested that partial portal decompression may decrease the incidence of encephalopathy and liver failure. Sarfeh et al.[69] created progressively smaller portocaval H-grafts in patients over the course of several years. In their patients with small (8 to 10 mm) grafts, there was a 16% incidence of encephalopathy compared with 39% in those with large-caliber grafts. Residual portosystemic gradients of 17 and 12 cm H_2O for 8- and 10-mm grafts, respectively, resulted from the small grafts, whereas the large grafts brought about complete portal decompression. Johanson[70] reported encephalopathy in 6% and liver failure in 6% of the patients receiving small-caliber H-grafts, with resultant portosystemic gradients of 10.4 mm Hg. TIPSs resemble these small-caliber shunts in their hemodynamic effects, and therefore the rates of encephalopathy and liver failure should be similar.

The incidence of encephalopathy in patients undergoing a TIPS procedure appears to be relatively low. LaBerge et al.[64] encountered encephalopathy in 24 of their 96 patients; however, only nine of these patients did not have encephalopathy before the procedure. Among the other published series, only Darcy et al.[71] report a rate of encephalopathy exceeding 10%. Patients in this series underwent detailed psychometric testing to search for encephalopathy after the procedure, whereas patients in other series were assessed on more subjective clinical grounds. Differences in the criteria used to determine whether a patient was encephalopathic account for some of the varying results. Besides encephalopathy, there have been a few reports of liver failure following TIPS, but the actual incidence of this complication is uncertain.

Although the data concerning TIPS are preliminary, the following conclusions can be drawn from them: (1) intrahepatic portosystemic shunts can be created reliably and safely through a percutaneous approach; (2) the TIPS technique is effective in controlling variceal hemorrhage by lowering portal pressure; (3) the incidence of encephalopathy and liver failure is relatively low; and (4) creation of a TIPS does not hinder subsequent liver transplantation. Conclusions regarding the long-term efficacy of this treatment require further study.

The potential advantage of TIPS over surgical shunts is that the TIPS technique is essentially an angiographic procedure that does not require general anesthesia or laparot-omy and, in experienced hands, can be completed in less than 2 hours. This may lengthen survival in critically ill patients and certainly shortens the hospitalization as well as reduces the cost of treatment. The TIPS procedure is technically quite challenging, however. Considerable expertise in angiographic techniques and familiarity with the transjugular approach are both important to success.

Despite encouraging early results, TIPS is still a new and experimental procedure. Many questions regarding it remain unanswered and require further study. For example, it is unknown which stent performs best and what the long-term patency rates are. The best end point for the procedure also remains to be established. Is partial portal decompression adequate or should the varices be embolized concomitantly? Finally, how will the rates of hepatic encephalopathy, liver failure, and survival in patients undergoing TIPS compare with those in similar patients treated by sclerotherapy or surgery? The ultimate role of TIPS in the management of portal hypertension and its complications rests on the answers to these questions.

REFERENCES

1. Margulis AR, Heinbecker P, Bernard HR: Operative mesenteric arteriography in the search for the site of bleeding in unexplained gastrointestinal hemorrhage, *Surgery* 48:534, 1960.
2. Athanasoulis CA: Therapeutic applications of angiography, *N Engl J Med* 302:1117, 1980.
3. Rösch J, Antonovic R, Dotter CT: Current angiographic approach to diagnosis and therapy of acute gastrointestinal bleeding, *Fortschr Röntgenstr* 125:301, 1976.
4. Sos TA, Lee JG, Wixson D, Sniderman KW: Intermittent bleeding from minute to minute in acute massive gastrointestinal hemorrhage: arteriographic demonstration, *AJR* 131:1015, 1978.
5. Alavi A: Scintigraphic demonstration of acute gastrointestinal bleeding, *Gastrointest Radiol* 5:205, 1980.
6. Alavi A, Ring EJ: Localization of gastrointestinal bleeding: superiority of ^{99m}Tc sulfur colloid compared with angiography, *AJR* 137:741, 1981.
7. McKuscik KA, Froelick J, Callahan JR, Winzelberg GG, Strauss WH: ^{99m}Tc red blood cells for detection of gastrointestinal bleeding: experience with 80 patients, *AJR* 137:1113, 1981.
8. Rösch J, Keller FS, Wawrukiewicz AS et al: Pharmacoangiography in the diagnosis of recurrent massive lower gastrointestinal bleeding, *Radiology* 145:615, 1982.
9. Rösch J, Kozak BE, Keller FS et al: Interventional angiography in the diagnosis of lower gastrointestinal hemorrhage, *Eur J Radiol* 6(2):136, 1986.
10. Kelemouridis V, Athanasoulis CA, Waltman AC: Gastric bleeding sites: an angiographic study, *Radiology* 149:643, 1983.
11. Athanasoulis CA, Waltman AC, Novelline RA, Krudy AG, Sniderman KW: Angiography: its contribution to the emergency management of gastrointestinal hemorrhage, *Radiol Clin North Am* 14:265, 1976.
12. Eckstein MR, Kelemouridis V, Athanasoulis CA et al: Gastric bleeding: therapy with intraarterial vasopressin and embolization, *Radiology* 152:563, 1984.
13. Kadir S, Athanasoulis CA: Angiographic management of gastrointestinal bleeding with vasopressin, *Fortschr Röntgenstr* 127:111, 1977.
14. Keller FS, Rösch J: Angiography in the diagnosis and therapy of acute upper gastrointestinal bleeding, *Schweiz Med Wochenschr* 109:586, 1979.

15. Waltman AC, Greenfield AJ, Novelline RA et al: Pyloroduodenal bleeding and intraarterial vasopressin: clinical results, *AJR* 133:643, 1979.

16. Rösch J, Dotter CT, Brown MS: Selective arterial embolization, *Radiology* 102:303, 1972.

17. Gomes AS, Lois JF, McCoy RD: Angiographic treatment of gastrointestinal hemorrhage: comparison of vasopressin infusion and embolization, *AJR* 146:1031, 1986.

18. Lieberman DA, Keller FS, Kato RM, Rösch J: Arterial embolization for massive upper gastrointestinal tract bleeding in poor surgical candidates, *Gastroenterology* 86:876, 1984.

19. Rösch J, Grollman JH Jr: Superselective angiography in the diagnosis of abdominal pathology: technical considerations, *Radiology* 92:1008, 1969.

20. Waltman AC, Courey WR, Athanasoulis CA, Baum, S: Technique for left gastric artery catheterization, *Radiology* 109:732, 1973.

21. Ring EJ, Oleaga JA, Freeman D et al: Pitfalls in angiographic management of hemorrhage: hemodynamic consideration, *AJR* 129:1007, 1977.

22. Goldberger LE, Bookstein JJ: Transcatheter embolization in the treatment of diverticula hemorrhage, *Radiology* 122:613, 1977.

23. Palmaz JC, Walter JF, Cho KJ: Therapeutic embolization of small bowel arteries, *Radiology* 152:377, 1984.

24. Bookstein JJ, Naderi JJ, Walter JR: Transcatheter embolization for lower gastrointestinal bleeding, *Radiology* 127:345, 1978.

25. Mitty HA, Efremidis S, Keller RJ: Colonic stricture after transcatheter embolization for diverticular bleeding, *AJR* 133:519, 1979.

26. Sheedy PF, Fulton RE, Atwell DT: Angiographic evaluation in patients with chronic gastrointestinal bleeding, *AJR* 123:338, 1975.

27. Sprayregen S, Boley SJ: Vascular ectasias of the right colon, *JAMA* 239:962, 1977.

28. Baum S, Athansoulis CA, Waltman AC, Galdabini J, Shapiro RH et al: Angiodysplasia of the right colon: a cause of gastrointestinal bleeding, *AJR* 129:789, 1977.

29. Scully RE, Mark EJ, McNeely BU: Case records of the Massachusetts General Hospital, *N Engl J Med* 305:391, 1981.

30. Athanasoulis CA, Moncure AC, Greenfield AJ et al: Intraoperative localization of small bowel bleeding sites with combined use of angiographic methods and methylene blue injection, *Surgery* 87:77, 1980.

31. Sebrechts C, Bookstein JJ: Embolization in the management of lower gastrointestinal hemorrhage, *Semin Intervent Radiol* 5(1):39, 1988.

32. Meyerovitz MF, Fellows KE: Angiography in gastrointestinal bleeding in children, *AJR* 143:837, 1984.

33. Routh WD, Lawdahl RB, Lund E, Garcia JH, Keller FS: Meckel's diverticula: angiographic diagnosis in patients with non-acute hemorrhage and negative scintigraphy, *Pediatr Radiol* 20:152, 1990.

34. Sandblom P: *Hemobilia (biliary tract hemorrhage): history, pathology, diagnosis, treatment*, Springfield, Ill, 1972, Charles C Thomas.

35. Hoevlls J, Nelsson U: Intrahepatic vascular lesions following nonsurgical percutaneous transhepatic bile duct intubation, *Gastrointest Radiol* 5:127, 1980.

36. Krudy AG, Doppman JL, Bissonette MB et al: Hemobilia: computed tomography diagnosis, *Radiology* 148:785, 1983.

37. Mitchell SE, Shuman, LS, Kaufman SL et al: Biliary catheter drainage complicated by hemobilia: treatment by balloon embolotherapy, *Radiology* 157:645, 1985.

38. Vaughan R, Rösch J, Keller FS et al: Treatment of hemobilia by transcatheter vascular occlusion, *Eur J Radiol* 4:183, 1984.

39. Sclafani SJA, Shaftan GW, McAuley J: Interventional radiology in the management of hepatic trauma, *J Trauma* 24:256, 1984.

40. Kirby CK, Howard KM, Rhoades JE: Death due to delayed hemorrhage in acute pancreatitis, *Surg Gynecol Obstet* 100:458, 1955.

41. Frey F: Hemorrhagic pancreatitis, *Am J Surg* 137:616, 1979.

42. Lina JR, Jaques P, Mandell V: Aneurysm rupture secondary to transcatheter embolization, *AJR* 132:553, 1979.

43. Thompson WM, Jackson DC, Johnsrude IS: Aortoenteric and paraprosthetic-enteric fistuals: radiologic findings, *AJR* 127:235, 1976.

44. Reuter SR, Atkin TW: High dose left gastric angiography for demonstration of esophageal varices, *Radiology* 105:573, 1972.

45. Nusbaum M, Baum S, Blakemore WS et al: Pharmacologic control of portal hypertension, *Surgery* 62:299, 1967.

46. Barr, WE, Lakin PC, Rösch J: Similarity of arterial and intravenous vasopressin on portal and systemic hemodynamics, *Gastroenterology* 69:13, 1975.

47. Lunderquist A, Vang J: Transhepatic catheterization and obliteration of the coronary vein in patients with portal hypertension and esophageal varices, *N Engl J Med* 291:646, 1974.

48. Keller FS, Rösch J, Dotter CT, Jendrzejewski JW: Embolization in the treatment of bleeding gastroesophageal varices, *Semin Roentgenol* 16:103, 1981.

49. Viamonte M Jr, Pereireas R, Russell E, LaPage J, Huston D: Transhepatic obliteration of gastroesophageal varices: results in acute and nonacute bleeders, *AJR* 129:237, 1977.

50. Rösch J, Hanafee WN, Snow H: Transjugular portal venography and radiologic portacaval shunt: an experimental study. *Radiology* 1969; 92:1112-1114.

51. Rösch J, Hanafee W, Snow H, Barenfus M, Gary R: Transjugular intrahepatic portacaval shunt, *Am J Surg* 121:588, 1971.

52. Colapinto RF, Stronell TD, Birch SJ et al: Creation of an intrahepatic portosystemic shunt with a Gruntzig balloon catheter, *Can Med Assoc J* 126:267, 1982.

53. Gordon JD, Colapinto RF, Abecassis M et al: Transjugular intrahepatic portosystemic shunt: a nonoperative approach to life-threatening variceal bleeding, *Can J Surg* 30:45, 1987.

54. Palmaz JC, Sibbitt RR, Reuter SR, Garcia F, Tio FO: Expandable intrahepatic portacaval shunt stents: early experience in the dog, *AJR* 145:821, 1985.

55. Palmaz JC, Garcia F, Sibbitt RR et al: Expandable intrahepatic shunt stents in dogs with chronic portal hypertension, *AJR* 147:1251, 1986.

56. Rösch J, Uchida BT, Putnam JS: Experimental intrahepatic portacaval anastomosis: use of expandable Gianturco stents, *Radiology* 162:481, 1987.

57. Richter GM, Noeldge G, Palmaz JC et al: Transjugular intrahepatic portacaval stent shunt: preliminary clinical results, *Radiology* 174:1027, 1990.

58. Iwatsuki S, Starzl TE, Todo S et al: Liver transplantation in the treatment of bleeding esophageal varices, *Surgery* 104:697, 1988.

59. Ring EJ, Lake JR, Roberts JP et al: Percutaneous intrahepatic portosystemic shunts to control variceal bleeding prior to transplantation, *Ann Intern Med* 116:304, 1992.

60. Richter GM, Noeldge G, Palmaz JC, Roessle M: The transjugular intrahepatic portosystemic stent-shunt (TIPPS): results of a pilot study, *Cardiovasc Intervent Radiol* 13:200, 1990.

61. LaBerge JM, Ring EJ, Gordon RL: Percutaneous intrahepatic portosystemic shunt created via a femoral vein approach, *Radiology* 181:679, 1991.

62. Ring EJ; Personal communication.

63. Zemel G, Katzen BT, Becker GJ, Benenati JF, Sallee DS: Percutaneous transjugular portosystemic shunt, *JAMA* 266:390, 1991.

64. LaBerge JM, Gordon RL, Ring EJ: Transjugular intrahepatic portosystemic shunts with use of the Wallstent endoprosthesis: midterm results, Paper presented at the 17th Annual Meeting of the Society of Cardiovascular and Interventional Radiology, Washington, DC, April 1992.

65. Rösch J, Barton RE, Keller FS: Unpublished data, Charles Dotter Institute, Portland, Oregon.

66. Warren WD, Millikan WJ, Henderson JM et al: Ten years of portal hypertensive surgery at Emory, *Ann Surg* 195:530, 1982.

67. Villeneuve JP, Pomier-Layrargues G, Duguay L et al: Emergency portacaval shunt for variceal hemorrhage, *Am J Surg* 206:48, 1987.

68. Warren WD: Control of variceal bleeding: reassessment of rationale, *Am J Surg* 145:8, 1983.

69. Sarfeh IJ, Rypins EB, Mason GR: A systematic appraisal of portocaval H-graft diameters, *Ann Surg* 204:356, 1986.

70. Johansen K: Partial portal decompression for variceal hemorrhage, *Am J Surg* 157:479, 1989.

71. Darcy MD, Picus D, Hicks ME, Burns MA, Burton KE et al: Transjugular intrahepatic portosystemic shunts with use of the Wallstent, Paper presented at the 17th Annual Meeting of the Society of Cardiovascular and Interventional Radiology, Washington, DC, April 1992.

Index

A

A cells, 87, 1167
A$_2$ cells, 1167
A-mode ultrasound, history of, 16
A ring, 168
  in hiatus hernia, 219
Abdomen
  abscess in
    plain films and contrast studies in,
      2035-2042
    technetium 99m–labeled white blood
      cells in, 1531
  acute; *see* Acute abdomen
  angiography and; *see* Angiography
  computed tomographic survey of, 1463
  contrast media and; *see* Contrast agents
  esophageal trauma and, 216-218
  ligaments in, 1808
  liver transplantation complications of,
    1747-1748, 1749
  plain films of; *see* Abdominal radiography
  trauma to; *see* Abdominal trauma
Abdominal aortic aneurysm, leaking,
  2071-2073
Abdominal binder test, scintigraphic, 184
Abdominal esophagus, anatomy of, 28
Abdominal fluid, sonography of, 2100-2101
Abdominal great vessels, 65
Abdominal radiography
  of colon, 697
  in inflammatory bowel disease, 564-565
  spleen in, 1751, 1752
  techniques for, 2021
Abdominal trauma, 2120-2154
  abdominal aortography of, 2144, 2145
  algorithm for triage and management of,
    2152
  arteriography and therapeutic embolization
    in, 2143-2154
    bowel and, 2153
    complications of, 2146
    cut-film technique in, 2149
    diagnostic, 2143-2144
    diaphragmatic rupture and, 2153
    in hepatic vascular injury, 2147-2148
    initial evaluation in, 2143
    lumbar arteries and, 2153
    materials and techniques for, 2144-2146
    pancreas and, 2153
    in pelvis, 2150-2152
    pleural space and, 2153
    in renal vascular injury, 2149
    in spleen, 2146-2147
    superselective, 2149
  blunt
    algorithm for management of, 2152
    mechanism and pattern of injury in, 2120
  computed tomography of, 2094-2097
    bladder, 2136-2138
    bowel, 2138-2139

Abdominal trauma—cont'd
  computed tomography of—cont'd
    diagnostic peritoneal lavage versus,
      2120-2121
    diaphragmatic rupture and, 2141
    duodenal, 2133-2134
    hepatic, 2123-2130
    intraperitoneal fluid and, 2120-2121
    logistics and technique for, 2121-2122
    mesenteric, 2138-2139
    pancreatic, 2133
    patient management in, 2122-2123
    pelvic, 2140
    penetrating injury and, 2140-2141
    renal, 2135, 2136
    spinal fracture and, 2139, 2140
    splenic, 2130-2133
    vascular injury and, 2139
  gastric rupture in, 369
  ischemic intestinal strictures and, 650
  penetrating, computed tomography of,
    2140-2141
Abdominal wall
  defects in, pediatric, 1890-1891
  gas in, 334
    in gastric volvulus, 364
    plain films and contrast studies in,
      2068-2070
  gastroenteric cyst and, 1843
  hemorrhage in, 2089-2091
Abdominoperineal resection, 712
Aberrant hepatic artery, 1605, 1606, 1608
Aberrant left subclavian artery, 1845
Aberrant pancreas; *see* Ectopic pancreas
Aberrant thyroid gland, 122
Abetalipoproteinemia, 668
Ablation
  of cystic duct, 1382-1383
  in liver neoplasms, 1719
Abscess
  abdominal
    after liver transplantation, 1748
    candidal, 2083
    computed tomography of, 2082-2084
    plain films and contrast studies in,
      2035-2042
    technetium 99m–labeled white blood
      cells in, 1531
  after obesity surgery, 459-460
  amebic; *see* Amebic abscess
  appendiceal, 1802, 1926
    computed tomography of, 613, 614
    percutaneous drainage of, 2006-2007
  in colorectal carcinoma, 806
  in Crohn's disease, 591, 1893, 1894
  crypt, 573
  diverticular, 752-753, 759
    formation of, 755
    percutaneous drainage of, 2005-2006
    sonography of, 2105
  fungal

Abscess—cont'd
  fungal—cont'd
    abdominal, 2083
    in child, 1937, 1960-1961
  of gallbladder
    in carcinoma, 1331
    in gangrenous cholecystitis, 2087
  gas bubbles in, sonography of, 2100
  in gastrointestinal perforation, 2079
  helminthoma and, 934
  hepatic, 2039
    after liver transplantation, 1748
    amebic; *see* Amebic abscess
    arterial embolization and, 1729
    in child, 1975
    computed tomography of, 2082
    hepatic arterial embolization and, 1729
    magnetic resonance imaging of, 1493,
      1494
    percutaneous drainage of, 2001-2002
    rupture of, 918
    scintigraphy of, 1519, 1531
    ultrasonography of, 1475, 1476
  lesser sac, 2040
    plain films and contrast studies of,
      2037-2039
  of mediastinum, percutaneous abscess
    drainage of, 2009
  nonpyogenic, 2083
  obesity surgery and, 458-459
  pancreatic, 2034, 2039
    after transplantation, 1198, 1217-1221
    in child, 1952
    percutaneous drainage of, 2002-2004
    retroperitoneal, 2039
  paracolic, 2039
    percutaneous drainage of, 752
    plain films and contrast studies of, 2035,
      2039
  parapharyngeal, 120
  in pararenal space, 1818
  pelvic, 1801-1803
    appendicitis with, 1802
    Crohn's disease in, 612
    percutaneous abscess drainage of, 2006
    plain films and contrast studies of, 2039,
      2041
  percutaneous drainage of, 1998-2010
    in anastomotic leaks, 2007-2009
    barium examination and, 2007
    cholecystostomy in, 1381-1382
    computed tomography and, 1999, 2004,
      2006, 2007, 2009
    in Crohn's disease, 2005
    diagnostic aspiration in, 1999
    in enteric tumors, 2007
    in esophageal drainage, 2009
    follow-up care in, 2000-2001
    fundamentals of, 1998-2001
    in hepatic abscess, 2001-2002
    imaging for, 1998-1999

Abscess—cont'd
  percutaneous drainage of—cont'd
    magnetic resonance imaging in, 1998,
      1999
    in pancreatic abscess and fluid collections,
      2002-2004
    in periappendiceal abscess, 2006-2007
    in peridiverticular abscess, 2005-2006
    plain films in, 1998
    scintigraphy in, 1998-1999
    in splenic abscess, cysts, and tumors,
      2004-2005
    technique and materials in, 1999-2000
    ultrasonography in, 1998, 1999, 2001,
      2007, 2009
  pericholecystic, in cholecystitis, 1285-1286,
    1287
  pericolonic
    computed tomography of, 2085
    magnetic resonance imaging of, 618
  in perirenal space, 1810, 1818
  peritoneal, 1801-1802
    computed tomography of, 2081-2084
  pharyngeal, 1834-1835
  in psoas space, 1818
  pyogenic
    in child, 1936-1937, 1959
    computed tomography of, 2082
    of spleen, 1936-1937
  rectal, 614
  retroperitoneal, 1818-1819
    plain films and contrast studies of,
      2039-2042
  splenic; see Spleen, abscess of
  subhepatic, 2036-2037
  subphrenic, 2036-2037, 2038
Absence
  of cystic duct, 1262
  of diaphragm, total, 1858
  of pancreatic duct, 1261
  of portal vein, 1622
Absorption
  colonic, 89
  in duodenum and small bowel; see also
    Gastrointestinal tract, physiology of
  in esophageal endosonography, 187
Acalculous cholecystitis, 2110-2111
Acanthoma of gallbladder, 1326
Acanthosis of esophagus, 171, 172
Accessory bile ducts, 1256-1257
Accessory duct of Santorini, 1047
Accessory gallbladder, 1252-1254
Accessory hepatic vein, 31, 1444, 1445
Accessory papilla of Santorini, 285
Accessory spleen, 1763-1764
  anatomy of, 28
  in child, 1933, 1934, 1935
Accessory stomach, 318
Acetic acid, mucus and, 77
Acetylcholine, 75, 77
Acetylcysteine, 713
Acetylsalicylic acid
  in drug-induced enteritis, 656
  endoscopic sphincterotomy hazards of, 1345
  esophagitis from, 231
  in gastritis, 327
  in gastritis, in child, 1869
  as hazard in percutaneous transhepatic
    cholangiography, 1236
  as lithotripsy contraindication, 1359
  prostaglandins and, 72
  in tracheoesophageal fistula and atresia, 212
Achalasia
  amyl nitrite test in, 181
  in child, 1828, 1838-1839

Achalasia—cont'd
  in diffuse esophageal spasm, 204
  esophageal distention in, 187, 210
  in esophageal rupture, 217
  plain x-ray film of, 176
  vigorous, 203
Acid
  amino, 79-80
  esophageal, neutralization of, 73-75
  gastric, 75-76
    hypersecretion of, 352
Acid barium in fluoroscopy, 181
Acinar cell carcinoma, 1153-1154
  multiloculated cystic variant of, 1153
Acinar cell cystadenocarcinoma, 1155
Acinar cell giant cell tumor, 1153
Acoustic coupling gel, 1246
Acquired immunodeficiency syndrome,
    952-966
  bacterial infections in, 958-959
  CDC classification for, 953
  cholangitis in, 961
  clinical presentation and staging of, 952-953
  clinical testing for, 953-954
  duodenal disease in, 477
    sarcomatous, 492
  enteropathy in, 959-960
  epidemiology and natural history of, 953
  esophagitis in, 226, 228-229
  gastritis in, 326, 333
  hepatobiliary abnormalities in, 960-961
  imaging with, 954
  Kaposi's sarcoma in, 961-962, 963
    gastric, 435
    retroperitoneal, 1814
  lymphoma in, 962-963, 964
  neoplastic disease in, 961-963
  opportunistic infections in, 954-961
  precautions to prevent transmission of,
    964-965
  radiologic practice and, 963-965
  small bowel and
    enteropathy in, 671-674, 675
    functional diseases of, 671-674, 675
    infections in, 553, 554
    Kaposi's sarcoma of, 645
    lymphomas in, 635
  splenic infection in, 1780
  ulcerative colitis versus, 604
Acquisition time sequences, 1488-1489
Actinomycosis
  lymphogranuloma venereum versus, 907
  ulcerative colitis versus, 604
Acute abdomen, 2020-2119
  barium examination of
    in appendicitis, 2029-2030
    with computed tomography, 2076
    in diverticulitis, 2034
    in intussusception, 2054
    in obstruction, 2059
  chest conditions mimicking, 2021
  computed tomography of, 2076-2098
    in abdominal trauma, 2094-2097
    in gastrointestinal perforation, 2077-2081
    hemorrhage and, 2087-2091
    in inflammatory gastrointestinal lesions,
      2084-2087
    in intestinal ischemia, 2089-2091
    in intraabdominal hemorrhage, 2087-2089
    in intramural hemorrhage, 2089-2091
    in intraperitoneal abscess, 2081-2084
    in ischemia, 2087-2089
    in peritonitis, 2077-2081
    in strangulating small bowel obstruction,
      2091-2094

Acute abdomen—cont'd
  computed tomography of—cont'd
    technical considerations in, 2076-2077
  definition of, 2076
  obstruction in; see Obstruction
  overview of, 2118-2119
  pancreatitis in; see Pancreatitis, acute
  plain films and contrast studies in,
      2020-2075
    in abscesses, 2035-2042
    in ascites, 2028-2029
    in calcifications, 2023, 2073
    in colitis, 2065-2068
    in conditions simulating
      pneumoperitoneum, 2027-2028
    in diverticulitis, 2034, 2035
    in gynecologic disorders, 2073
    in inflammatory conditions, 2029-2032
    in intestinal obstruction, 2042-2063; see
      also Intestinal obstruction
    in intramural gas, 2068-2070
    in intraperitoneal fluid collections,
      2028-2029
    in leaking abdominal aortic aneurysm,
      2071-2073
    normal appearances in, 2022-2023
    in pancreatitis, 2032-2034
    in pneumoperitoneum, 2023, 2024, 2025,
      2026-2027
    in postoperative abdomen, 2028,
      2063-2065
    in pseudopneumoperitoneum, 2027-2028
    in renal colic, 2070-2071
    in suspected perforation, 2026, 2034
    techniques for, 2020-2022
  trauma in, 2120-2154; see also Abdominal
    trauma
  ultrasonography of, 2099-2117
    in appendicitis, 2102-2104
    approach in, 2099-2101
    in bile duct calculi, 2111-2112
    in biliary colic, 2111-2112
    in biliary parasites, 2112
    biliary tract and, 2108-2112
    in cholecystitis, 2109-2111
    in diverticulitis, 2104-2106
    in epidermoid cysts of spleen, 2115, 2116
    in extraintestinal manifestations of hollow
      gut disease, 2101-2102
    in hemobilia, 2112, 2113
    in hepatitis, 2114-2115
    hollow viscera and, 2101-2108
    in intussusception, 2054
    in ischemic bowel, 2108
    in liver, 2114-2115
    in mechanical bowel obstruction,
      2106-2108
    pancreas and, 2112-2113
    in pancreatitis, 2112-2113
    in peptic ulcer, 2108
    in splenic infarction, 2115
    in splenic rupture, 2115
    in splenic torsion, 2115
    in terminal ileitis, 2104
    in typhlitis, 2104
Adenocarcinoma
  Barrett's esophagitis and, 224, 226
  of biliary tract, 1266, 1267
  of breast in hepatic metastases, 1710
  cholangiocarcinoma as, 1333
  choledochal cyst and, 1266, 1267
  clinical features of, 639-640
  of colon, 775, 776; see also Carcinoma, of
    colon
    radiologic findings in, 791

Adenocarcinoma—cont'd
of colon—cont'd
surface contour of, 775, 776
conditions associated with, 640
duodenal, 488-492, 493, 495
esophageal, 243
of gallbladder, 1326, 1327, 1328, 1329, 1330
magnetic resonance imaging in, 1332
of liver
metastatic, 1496
mucin-producing, 1714
of mesentery, 1596
of pancreas; *see* Carcinoma, of pancreas; Pancreatic adenocarcinoma
retroperitoneal fibrosis in, 1816
of small bowel, 639-640, 641
of small bowel mesentery, 1823
of stomach
endosonography of, 451-454
in Europe, 387-398; *see also* Gastric carcinoma, in Europe
incidence of, 437
intraperitoneal spread of, 644
lymph node metastasis of, 440, 441
of uterus metastatic to liver, 1712
Adenoid, nasopharyngeal, 139
in child, 1827
Adenoid cystic carcinoma
of floor of mouth, 153
hypoglossal nerve and, 155
maxillary, 152
of nasopharynx, 160
of palate, 149
perineural spread of, 142, 150, 155
salivary gland, 139
Adenoma
adrenal gland, 1992-1993
of Brunner's gland, 488
of colon, 777
in average-risk person, 835
bias in screening for, 831
carcinoma contained in, 824
classification of, 762
colonoscopy in, 832
in elderly, 831
hereditary nonpolyposis cancer and, 825
malignant potential of, 763, 824, 825
origin of, 764
in rectosigmoid region, 763, 824-825, 835
risk factors for, 824-825
surveillance of, 779
of crypts of Lieberkühn, 488
of duodenum
tubular, 488, 492, 495
tubulovillous, 488
fecal occult-blood tests in, 833
gastric, 374-375, 376
carcinoma and, 406-407
villous, 435
hepatocellular; *see* Hepatocellular adenoma
Lieberkühn's, 488
of liver; *see also* Hepatocellular adenoma
in child, 1967
rupture of, 1475
ultrasonography of, 1476, 2114, 2115
in pancreatic duct, 1133, 1134-1135
small bowel, 629, 631
Adenomatous hyperplasia of liver
in hepatocellular carcinoma, 1691
nodular, 1480
magnetic resonance imaging of, 1494, 1543

Adenomatous malformation of lung, cystic, 1856
Adenomatous papilloma of duodenum, 488
Adenomatous polyp
of colon
detection of, 767
growth rate determination of, 776
screening for, 824, 827
of stomach, 406
Adenomatous polyposis, familial; *see* Familial adenomatous polyposis
Adenomatous polyposis coli; *see* Adenomatous polyp, of colon
Adenomyoma
cholecystokinin infusion in, 1230
congenital gallbladder septa and, 1255
in hyperplastic cholesteroses, 1289, 1290, 1291
in stomach, 318, 377
Adenopathy
in cecal carcinoma, 804
in gastric carcinoma, 442, 443
negative percutaneous abscess drainage and, 2007
retroperitoneal, 1819
Adenosquamous carcinoma
of gallbladder, 1326, 1330
of pancreas, 1152
Adhesions
after laparotomy, 2028
in Gardner's syndrome, 781
mesenteric, 1599, 1600
pelvic, enteroclysis and, 533
in small bowel obstruction, 2045, 2046, 2049, 2051
Adnexal mass, 804
Adrenal gland
anatomy of, 29, 30, 31, 61
computed tomography of, 53
fibrolamellar hepatic carcinoma metastatic to, 1679
hemorrhage of, after liver transplantation, 1748
magnetic resonance imaging of, 45, 53
metastases to, 1679, 1992-1993
percutaneous interventional radiology and, 1992-1993
sagittal section of, 44, 45
Adrenal vein, 31
Adrenocorticosteroids, 72
Adrenocorticotropic hormone
benign gastric carcinoid and, 384
in islet cell tumors, 1168, 1172, 1180
Adriamycin; *see* Doxorubicin
Adventitia
in esophageal endosonography, 265, 266
of gastrointestinal wall, 187
in percutaneous transhepatic cholangiography, 1238
venous plexus of liver and, 1610
Adynamic ileus, 2057
plain films and contrast studies of, 2028, 2063, 2064
Aflatoxins, 1663
Aganglionosis of colon, total, 1914-1915
Agastria, 1865, 1866
Age
esophageal motility and, 196
gastric endoscopy and, 302
pharyngeal function and, 137
Agenesis
of extrahepatic bile duct, 1259
of gallbladder, 1251-1254
of pancreas, 1045-1046, 1946, 1947
AIDS-related complex, 953

Air as contrast agent
in colon examination, 700, 713
in computed tomography, 718, 753-754, 755, 759, 802
for diverticular abscess, 755
for diverticulitis, 753-754
in endosonography, 727
in intussusception, 1901-1902
in small bowel examination, 690
in double-contrast enteroclysis, 548
in inflammatory bowel disease, 616
Air bubbles
in acute abdomen
extraperitoneal, 2078-2079
in gastric lumen, 2076
intraperitoneal, 2077-2078
in colon as artifact, 772
in gallbladder, 1242
in liver, 1493
Air-dome sign, 2025
Air lock in barium examination, 710
Airway closure in swallowing, 129
Alagille's syndrome, 1320
Albers-Schönberg, HE, 3
Albumin
in gastrointestinal scintigraphy, 987
in hepatic magnetic resonance imaging, 1499
Alcian blue mucin staining, 1134, 1145
Alcohol; *see also* Ethanol
in *Echinococcus* hepatic abscess drainage, 2002
in gastric ulcer injection therapy, 972, 973
in percutaneous injection for hepatocellular carcinoma, 1701, 1702
polyvinyl, 1728, 1729
in transcatheter hepatic embolization, 1728
Alcohol abuse
in chronic pancreatitis, 1091
in cirrhosis, 1534, 1549
angiosarcoma and, 1683
foamy degeneration of cells and, 1548
focal fatty infiltration and, 1519
malignant neoplasms with, 1477
vascular changes in, 1628
in erosive gastritis, 329
esophageal motor function and, 209
in hemochromatosis, 1560, 1561, 1562, 1563
in hemorrhagic gastritis, 330
in hepatitis, 1549
fatty liver and, 1547
in hepatocellular carcinoma, 1663
in injury gastropathy, 357
liver diseases and, 1548-1549
pharyngeal malignancies and, 139
in small bowel malabsorption, 684-685
in steatosis, 1548
Alfentanil, 1359
Alimentary tract; *see* Gastrointestinal tract
Alkaline agents
in corrosive gastropathy, 357
in esophagitis, 229
in child, 1847
Alkaline phosphatase in gallbladder carcinoma, 1325, 1334
Allergy, cow's milk, 1925
Allogeneic bone marrow transplant, 674
Alpha$_1$-antitrypsin
in hepatocellular adenoma, 1663
pancreatic tumor and, 1132
acinar cell carcinoma as, 1154
cystic, 1150
pancreatoblastoma as, 1156
Alpha cells, 1167

Alpha-chain disease, 677-678
Alpha fetoproteins
    in cholangiocarcinoma, 1333
    in hepatic carcinoma, 1463, 1478, 1678
    in hepatocellular carcinoma, 1665, 1666
Alpha-gliadin, 663
α-hCG; see Human chorionic gonadotropin
Alzheimer's disease, 133
Amebiasis
    ameboma and, 915-917
    colitis in
        plain films and contrast studies of,
            2067-2068
        radiologic follow-up in, 609
        ulcerative, 581, 607
    dysentery and, 915-919, 920
    inflammatory bowel disease versus, 603
    lymphogranuloma venereum versus, 907
    toxic megacolon in, 603
    ulcerative colitis versus, 607
Amebic abscess, 917-918
    in child, 1961
    computed tomography of, 2083
    percutaneous drainage in, 2001-2002
    ultrasonography of, 1475
Amebic dysentery, 915-919, 920
Ameboma, 915-917
American trypanosomiasis, 918-923, 924, 925
Amine precursor uptake and decarboxylation,
    67, 1167
Amino acids, 79-80
Aminocaproic acid, 1791
Amoxicillin, 478
Ampicillin, 1236
Amplatz superstiff catheter and guidewire,
    1407
Ampulla
    biliary duct, stenosis of, 1318-1319
    duodenal, 284-285
        anatomy of, 1227
        in child, 1946
        cholangiocarcinoma versus carcinoma in,
            1336
        computed tomography of, 1110, 1299,
            1300
        diverticula of, 469
            choledocholithiasis versus, 1300
        in endoscopy, 315, 317
        islet cell tumors and, 1190
        pancreatic endosonography of, 1127,
            1128
        pancreaticobiliary duct union and, 1262
        papillary carcinoma of, 1432
        ultrasonography of, 1298
    pancreatic duct, 1039
    phrenic, 168, 196
    of Vater; see Ampulla, duodenal
Ampullary pouch of gallbladder, 1226, 1227
Amsterdam stent, 1430
Amyl nitrite
    in esophageal fluoroscopy, 181, 202
    esophageal rings and, 234
    in pseudoachalasia, 188, 204
Amylase
    after endoscopic retrograde
        cholangiopancreatography, 1346
    after lithotripsy, 1105
    in pancreatic transplantation, 1197, 1198,
        1207, 1214
    in saliva, 73
Amyloidosis
    in Crohn's disease, 589
    in duodenum, 508
    esophageal motor function and, 209, 211
    versus fatty liver, 1554

Amyloidosis—cont'd
    small bowel, 678-679, 681, 682
        in Mediterranean fever, 678
    splenic, 1788
    in stomach, 360
Amyotrophic lateral sclerosis, 133, 211
Anaerobes in small bowel stasis, 669
Anal agenesis, 1912
Anal canal
    anatomy of, 694, 840
    in defecography, 845, 846, 847, 848
    length of, 845, 847
    squamous cell carcinoma of, 803
Anal dimple, percutaneous injection of contrast
        media through, 1912
Anal incontinence, 845
Anal sphincter
    external, voluntary, 840
    internal, 840
    obstruction of, 845
Analgesia
    in percutaneous interventional radiology
        in abdominal masses, 1988
        in biliary tract malignancy, 1401
    transcatheter hepatic embolization and, 1725
Anaphylaxis
    in barium reactions, 714
    ulcerative colitis versus, 604, 607
Anaplastic carcinoma of pancreas, 1152
Anastomosis
    after obesity surgery, leaking, 459-460
    after pancreatic transplantation, leaking,
        1198, 1221
    bile duct
        extrahepatic, to intestine, 1981
        leaks from, 1739-1740, 2007-2009
        in liver transplantation, 1736-1737,
            1739-1740
        percutaneous abscess drainage of,
            2007-2009
        percutaneous dilation of, 1383, 1384,
            1387, 1388-1389
        Roux-en-Y, 455, 456, 1414-1416
        strictures and obstruction in, 1383, 1384,
            1387, 1388-1389, 1740, 1741
    cervical esophagogastric, 277
        strictures and, 228
    choledochoenteric, 1426
    in diverticulitis resection, 750, 751
    duodenal, postoperative study of, 297, 300
    of esophagus, 212, 1841
    gastric, postoperative study of, 297, 300,
        453-454
    ileoanal, 585
        retrograde study of, 567
    ileocecal, 596
    ileocolic, 593
    ileorectal
        in familial multiple polyposis, 781
        in ulcerative colitis, 584-585
    jejunal, 1414
    jejunobiliary, 689, 690
    rectal, sonographic appearance of, 820
    recurrent colorectal carcinoma in, 810
    Roux-en-Y
        in malignant biliary tract disease,
            1414-1416
        in obesity surgery, 455, 456
Anatomy, 28-66
    of abdominal great vessels, 65
    of adrenal glands, 61
    of anus, 728
    of biliary system, 83-84, 85, 1223-1227
        common duct in, 33-34
        intrahepatic duct in, 1223-1224

Anatomy—cont'd
    of cecum, 725
    of colon, 35, 692-696, 725-726
        in child, 1907
        models of, 692-696
    of diaphragm, 32, 255
    of duodenum, 35, 284-285
        in endosonography, 314-316
        variants in, 285-286
    of esophagus, 168-176
        in child, 1836-1838
        cross-sectional, 173-176
    of gallbladder, 34
    of hepatic veins, 33
    of intraperitoneal compartments, 35, 54
    of kidneys, 61-63
    of liver; see Liver, anatomy of
    of mesentery, 1820-1822
    models of, 692-696
    of oral cavity, 144-146
    of pancreas, 47-61
        in adenocarcinoma, 1107-1109
        angiography and, 1023-1025
        in child, 1944
        endoscopic retrograde
            cholangiopancreatography and, 1020
        magnetic resonance imaging and, 1018
        percutaneous transhepatic
            cholangiography, 1022
    of peritoneum, 1795-1800
    of pharynx, 94-98
        of child, 1826-1828
    physiology and, 67
    of porta hepatis, 1224-1225
    of portacaval space, 34
    of portal veins, 33
    of rectum, 727-728, 814-815
    retroperitoneal, 63, 1807-1812
    of small bowel, 512-514
    of spleen, 34, 1760-1762
        in child, 1932
        variants in, 1763-1771
    of stomach, 31, 34-35, 282-284
        computed tomography and, 306-307
        endosonography and, 311
        gastric carcinoma and, 438-439
        variants in, 285
Anatrast, 841
Ancylostomiasis, 930-931
Anemia
    pernicious, 77
        in gastritis, 330
    sideroblastic, 1560
Anesthesia
    in esophageal motility disorders, 210
    for gastric endoscopy, 302
    in percutaneous intervention
        in dilation of biliary strictures, 1386
        in malignant biliary tract disease, 1401
Aneurysm
    aortic
        in esophageal compression, 270
        leaking abdominal, 2071-2073
        ruptured, 2088, 2089
    in colon ulceration, 792
    hepatic artery, 1615-1616
        in child, 1975
    inflammatory retroperitoneal, 1819
    as lithotripsy contraindication, 1359, 1364
    mycotic, 1772
    of portal vein, 1623, 1624
    pseudoaneurysm versus; see
        Pseudoaneurysm
    in small bowel lymphoma, 638
    splenic calcifications and, 1772

Anexate; *see* Flumazenil
Angiocath, 2076-2077
Angiodysolaria, 501
Angiodysplasia
  angiography of, 1000-1004
  in cecum, 977, 978
  portal hypertension and, 1598, 1599
Angiography, 994-1016
  of abdominal trauma, 2144, 2145
  in angiodysplasia, 1000-1004
  in arterial hemorrhage
    acute, 994-999
    chronic, 999-1004
  celiac; *see* Celiac angiography
  of duodenal vessels
    in congenital abnormalities, 467
    in ulcer hemorrhage, 486
  embolotherapy in, 997-999
  in gastrointestinal bleeding, 994-999
    from extraalimentary sources, 1004-1006
    scintigraphy versus, 984
    from venous origin, 1006-1014
  hepatic; *see* Liver, angiography of
  history of, 15, 24
  in intestinal varices, 657
  in ischemic enteritis, 685
  in islet cell tumors, 1179, 1182-1187, 1189
    in localization procedures, 1192
    venous sampling and, 1188
  in Meckel's diverticulum, 1004
  mesenteric, in rectal bleeding, 978, 979
  pancreatic, 1023, 1024
    in adenocarcinoma, 1110, 1123-1124
    in cystic neoplasms, 1152
    in hemangioma, 1160
    in mucinous adenomas, 1147
    in serous adenomas, 1141, 1142
    in transplantation, 1206
  pelvic, in trauma, 2150-2152
  pharmacodynamics and, 994-995
  of portal vein, 1610
  with scintigraphy in pancreatic
    transplantation; *see*
    Angioscintigraphy in pancreatic
    transplantation
  small bowel
    in arteriovenous malformation, 657
    in carcinoid, 634, 635
    in leiomyoma, 628, 629
    in sarcoma, 642
  of spleen, 1759-1760, 1761
  vasoconstrictive infusion therapy in,
    995-997
Angioma
  of esophagus, 251
  gastric, 383
  of liver in child, 1966
  of small bowel vessels, 657
Angiomyolipoma, hepatic, 1658, 1659
Angioplasty, percutaneous transluminal, 1628
Angiosarcoma
  of liver, 1480, 1683-1684
    scintigraphy in, 1528
  of spleen, 1787
    in child, 1937
Angioscintigraphy in pancreatic
    transplantation, 1202, 1203
  in arterial occlusion, 1219
  in occlusive disease, 1216-1217
  in pancreatitis, 1214
Angiostrongyliasis, 939
Anisakiasis, 934-935
Ankylosing spondylitis
  in Crohn's disease, 588
  in ulcerative colitis, 575

Anlage, pancreatic, 467-468
Annular carcinoma of sigmoid colon, 803
Annular pancreas, 467-468, 1046-1048
  in child, 1946, 1947
    in small bowel, 1884-1885
Anorectal agenesis, 1912
Anorectal angle, 841
  in defecography, 845-847, 848
Anorectal junction, 845
  elevation of, 845, 847, 849
  magnetic resonance imaging of, 696
Anorectal malformations, 1909-1912
Anorectal ring, 840
Anovestibular fistula, 1912
Anovulvar fistula, 1912
Antacids in Barrett's esophagitis, 226
Antegrade percutaneous fluoroscopically
    guided gastrostomy, 2018
Antegrade transhepatic sphincterotomy in
    percutaneous interventional
    radiology, 1426
Anterior fusion space, 1812
Anterior perineal anus, 1912
Antibiotics
  after barium enema, 714
  after endoscopic retrograde
    cholangiopancreatography, 1345
  in cholecystitis, 1281
  colitis from, 901
    appendicitis versus, 716
  in diverticulitis, 751
  in pancreatic transplantation, 1198
  for percutaneous biliary stricture dilation,
    1386
  in pericholecystic abscess, 1285
  in sigmoidectomy for diverticular abscess,
    753
  therapeutic embolization and
    splenic, 2147
    transcatheter hepatic, 1724-1725
Antibodies
  desmin, 555
  insulin, 1169
  monoclonal
    in colorectal carcinoma, 810
    in small bowel fine-needle aspiration
    cytology, 559
  S-100 protein, 555
  vimentin, 555
Anticholinergics
  esophagus and
    foreign bodies in, 216
    motility in, 211
    rings in, 234
    varices of, 242
  in small bowel dilatation, 660
Anticoagulants
  in esophageal mucosal tears, 218
  in intramural hemorrhage, 650-651
  as lithotripsy contraindication, 1359
Antidepressants
  small bowel motility and, 661
  xerostomia and, 73
Antidiarrhea agents in enteroclysis, 535
Antifoaming agent, 289
Antigens
  carcinoembryonic; *see* Carcinoembryonic
    antigen
  histocompatibility, in hemochromatosis,
    1560
Antihypertensives, 73
Antiinflammatory agents
  esophagitis from, 230
  nonsteroidal; *see* Nonsteroidal
    anti-inflammatory agents

Antimetabolites in ischemic bowel, 614
Antipyretics, 330
Antispasmodic agents
  in double-contrast enteroclysis with air, 548
  in toxic dilatation of colon, 565
Antiulcer drugs, 76
Antrum, gastric; *see* Gastric antrum
Anus
  anatomy of, 728
  congenital malformations of, 1909-1912
  defecography and, 840; *see also*
    Defecography
  mucosa of, 841
Aorta
  anatomy of, 28, 42
  in angiography for abdominal trauma, 2144,
    2145
  esophageal carcinoma in, 274, 275, 277,
    279
  in esophageal endosonography, 189, 190
  pigtail flush catheter in, 2144
  retroperitoneal diseases and, 1819
  sagittal, 42
  ultrasonography of, 42, 43
Aortic aneurysm
  in esophageal compression, 270
  leaking
    computed tomography of, 2088, 2089
    plain films and contrast studies in,
    2071-2073
Aortoduodenal fistula, 501
Aortoenteric fistula, 1005-1006
Aortography
  in hepatic artery disease, 1606
  in trauma, 2144, 2145
Aperistalsis
  in Chagas' disease, 920
  in esophagus, 194
Aphthous ulcer; *see* Ulcer, aphthous
Apoprotein B deficiency, 668
Appendiceal stump in colon as artifact, 772
Appendicitis
  in child, 1925-1926
  computed tomography of, 613, 614, 2080,
    2084-2085
  in Crohn's disease, 596
  differential diagnosis in, 716
  with pelvic abscess, 1802
  plain films and contrast studies of,
    2029-2031
  retrocecal, 2030
  ultrasonography of, 2102-2104
Appendicolith
  in child, 1925-1926
  computed tomography of, 2084, 2085
  percutaneous abscess drainage of, 2007
  ultrasonography of, 2102, 2103
Appendix
  calculi in, 2022, 2023, 2029
  inflammatory reaction around, 2085
  percutaneous abscess drainage of,
    2006-2007
  ultrasonography of, 1926
Apple-peel appearance in jejunum or ileum,
    1885
APUD; *see* Amine precursor uptake and
    decarboxylation
APUDomas, 1167; *see also* Islet cell tumor
ARA; *see* Anorectal angle
Arabinogalactin, 1501
ARC; *see* AIDS-related complex
Arcuate vessels, 28
Areae gastrica
  absent or small, 330
  computed digital radiography of, 402

Areae gastrica—cont'd
  enlargement of, 329
  normal appearance of, 283, 304
Armillifer, 946
Arsenical exposure
  angiosarcoma from, 1683
  hepatic scintigraphy in, 1528, 1640
Arterial catheterization, hepatic, 1725-1726
Arterial embolization, hepatic, 1723-1729
Arterial portography, 1567-1572, 1606-1607
  in cirrhosis, 1545, 1567-1572
  computed tomography with, 1447-1449
    in hepatocellular carcinoma, 1688-1690
  magnetic resonance imaging with, 1499
  in varices, 1585
Arterioduodenal fistula, 501
Arterioenteric fistula, 1005-1006
  gastrointestinal endoscopy in, 976, 977, 978
Arteriography; see also Angiography
  in abdominal trauma with therapeutic
        embolization, 2143-2154; see also
        Abdominal trauma, arteriography and
        therapeutic embolization in
  of hepatic vessels, 1605, 1606
    in hepatocellular carcinoma, 1690
    preembolization, 1725
  iliac, 2144, 2151
  in islet cell tumors, 1182-1187, 1189, 1193
    venous sampling and, 1188
  pelvic, in trauma, 2144, 2150-2152
  of small bowel vessels
    in arteriovenous malformation, 657
    in lymphoma, 639
    in sarcoma, 642
Arterioportal communications, 1572-1574,
        1610
  in cirrhosis, 1619, 1620
  in hemangioma, 1642
  in hepatocellular carcinoma, 1671, 1672,
        1673
Arteriosclerosis
  hepatic artery, 1614, 1615
  pancreatic artery, 1124
Arteriovenous fistula
  after transplantation
    of liver, 1746
    of pancreas, 1198, 1217
  in liver, 1616, 1617-1618
  transcatheter embolization and, 2146, 2148
Arteriovenous iodine difference, 1456, 1457
Arteriovenous malformations
  portal hypertension and, 1596, 1597, 1598
  of small bowel vessels, 657
Arteriovenous shunt in liver
  Doppler analysis in, 1480
  in hepatocellular carcinoma, 1677
Arteritis, hepatic artery, 1616
Arthritis
  in Crohn's disease, 588, 1892
  Forestier's, 101, 102
  ossification of neck in, 123
  rheumatoid
    hepatic macroregenerative nodule and
        nodular regenerative hyperplasia and,
        1655
    small intestinal vascular disorders and,
        655
  in ulcerative colitis, 575
Artifacts
  barium as, 286, 287
  colon neoplastic lesions versus, 771-772,
        773
  in esophageal fluoroscopy, 168, 177, 180
  in gastric and duodenal magnetic resonance
        imaging, 307

Artifacts—cont'd
  in gastric endoscopy, 314
  ghosting, 1487
  in hepatic magnetic resonance imaging,
        1487-1489, 1490
  kissing, 288, 289
  in percutaneous abscess drainage, 1998
  in rectal endosonography, 815
  ring-down, 1998
  in small bowel fine-needle aspiration
        cytology
    fixation, 558, 559
    smearing, 560
  in spleen
    in computed tomography, 1757, 1758,
        1759
    in radionuclide studies, 1755-1757
    in ultrasonography, 1753, 1754
Aryepiglottic folds, 106
ASA; see Acetylsalicylic acid
ASAP needle, 1988
Ascariasis, 926-930
  cholangitis in, 1312, 1313, 1314
    recurrent pyogenic, 1303, 1312
    sonography of, 2112
  in intrahepatic stones, 1350
  ulcerative colitis versus, 604
  whipworm and, 935-937, 938
Ascites
  in cirrhosis, 1537, 1538
  as contraindication to percutaneous
        intervention in malignant biliary tract
        disease, 1400
  in hepatocellular carcinoma, 1665
  in ovarian carcinoma, 1822
  peritoneal, 1801
    in carcinomatosis, 1118, 1119
    in peritonitis, 2080
  physiology of, 87
  plain films and contrast studies in,
        2028-2029
  in recurrent gastric cancer, 423
  in small bowel examinations, 526
  in transplantation rejection
    of liver, 1739
    of pancreas, 1198, 1214
  ultrasonography of, 1470, 1472
Ascorbic acid
  in esophageal ring strictures, 235
  esophagitis from, 231
Asialo glycoprotein receptors, 1502
Aspergillus
  hepatocellular carcinoma and, 1663
  in pediatric fungal abscess, 1937
Aspiration
  after percutaneous fluoroscopically guided
        gastrostomy, 2018
  fine-needle; see Fine-needle aspiration
        cytology
  in pancreatic transplantation, 1205,
        1217-1221
  in percutaneous interventional radiology in
        abdominal masses, 1988
Aspirin; see Acetylsalicylic acid
Asplenia
  in child, 1933-1934
  functional, 1766-1769
Atherosclerosis; see Arteriosclerosis
Atony, gastric, 361-362
  reflux, in enteroclysis, 535
Atresia
  biliary, 1981-1982
    in child, 1981-1982
    liver transplantation technique and, 1737
  duodenal, 1884, 1885

Atresia—cont'd
  esophageal, 212, 213, 1839-1842
    tracheoesophageal fistula and, 205
  gastric, 1865, 1866
  ileal, 1885, 1886
  jejunal, 1885, 1886
  in large bowel, 1908, 1909
  rectal, 719
Atrophic gastritis, 330
Atropine
  before barium enema, 701
  in esophageal fluoroscopy, 181, 199-201
    foreign bodies and, 216
    in motility disorders, 210
  in toxic dilatation of colon, 565
Attenuation in pancreatic adenocarcinoma,
        1112-1113, 1117
Auerbach's plexus
  absence or impairment of, 202
  gastric neurofibromas and, 381
Autocrine substances, 67
Autoimmune disease in hemobilia, 976, 977
Autologous blood clot in splenic artery
        embolization, 1791
Avascular necrosis in pancreatic
        transplantation, 1203
Averaging, signal, 1487-1488
Axillary artery, 1604
Azathioprine, 1592
Azygoesophageal recess, 173
Azygos vein, 32

B

B cell, 87, 1167
  in gastrointestinal physiology, 82
  proliferation of, after liver transplantation,
        1748
B cell tumors
  of colon, 791-792, 793, 794
  of small bowel, 635
    lymphomatous, in acquired
        immunodeficiency syndrome, 673,
        674
B-mode ultrasound, history of, 16
B ring in hiatus hernia, 219
Bacillary dysentery, 898-900
  toxic megacolon in, 603
Backwash ileitis, 577, 580
Bacteremia after barium enema, 565, 714
Bacterial infections, 888-904; see also
        Infections and infestations
  in acquired immunodeficiency syndrome,
        958-959
  cholangitis and, 1303-1306
  gastritis and, 333
  peritonitis and, 1802
Bacteroides, 901
Balanced electrolyte solutions
  bowel preparation and, 90
  in distal intestinal obstruction syndrome in
        child, 1897
Balloon
  in endoscopic retrograde
        cholangiopancreatography,
        1241-1242
  in endoscopic sphincterotomy, 1346
  in enteroclysis, 514
  in hepatic artery embolization, 1726
  Lahr, 844
  latex
    in rectal endosonography, 813-814
    sensitivity to, 715
  in magnetic resonance imaging of colorectal
        carcinoma, 807
  in minicholecystostomy, 1374

Ballon—cont'd
  in percutaneous choledocholithotomy, 1371
  in percutaneous fluoroscopically guided
      gastrostomy, 2015
  in percutaneous intervention in malignant
      biliary tract disease, 1407
  in proctography, 844
  in rectal endosonography, 813-814
  for stone extraction in chronic pancreatitis,
      1094
Balloon angioplasty, percutaneous
    transluminal, 1628
Balloon expulsion test, 844
Barclay, AE, 4
Bard Biopsy gun, 1988
Barium
  acid, in esophageal fluoroscopy, 181
  as artifact
    in colon, 772
    in computed tomography, 286, 287
  bubbly, 289
  as contrast agent for colon, 699-700
  in defecography, 842, 844, 849
  flocculation of, in celiac disease, 664-665
  low-density, in computed tomography, 305
Barium examination; see also specific organ
  in acquired immunodeficiency syndrome,
      954
  after laryngopharyngectomy with jejunal
      interposition, 162
  in anisakiasis, 935
  antigravity swallow in, 289
  in biliary-enteric fistula, 1316
  biphasic, 289
    in enteroclysis with methylcellulose; see
        Enteroclysis, biphasic, with
        methylcellulose
    in gastric cancer, 387
  of choledochal cysts, in child, 1976, 1977
  in cirrhosis with portal hypertension, 1575,
      1576
  diagnostic accuracy of, 299
  history of use of, 2-8, 9, 10
  patient position in, 290-206
  in pediatric hemolytic uremic syndrome,
      1924
  in subphrenic and subhepatic abscess, 2037
Barium tablet, 177
Barosperse, 514-515
Barrett's esophagus, 224-226
  in child, 1863
  strictures in, 236
Basket
  in biliary stent exchange, 1431
  in percutaneous choledocholithotomy, 1367,
      1368, 1369
  in percutaneous endoscopy of biliary tract,
      1426
Beaded duct appearance in cholangitis, 1307,
    1308
Beef tapeworm, 939-943
Behçet's syndrome, 655
  in child, 1894, 1924
  in Crohn's disease, 587-588
  esophagitis in, 232
  in toxic megacolon, 603
  ulcerative colitis in, 581
Belching, 77
Belsey procedure, 220
Bender, MA, 14
Benzodiazepines
  antagonists to, 302
  in colonic endosonography, 726
  in duodenal endoscopy, 316
  in esophageal endosonography, 190

Benzodiazepines—cont'd
  in gastric endoscopy, 302, 314
Beta-adrenergic blockers before barium enema,
    701
Beta cells, 1167
Beta-melanocyte–stimulating hormone, 384
Bezoar, 365, 366-368
  in bowel obstruction, 2107
  in child, 1873-1874
  esophageal tumors and, 242
Bias intervals, 830-831
Bicarbonate, mucous cells and, 76-77
Bifurcation of bile ducts
  in percutaneous intervention in malignant
      biliary tract disease, 1402-1403
  tumors of, biliary stent palliative drainage
      in, 1434, 1435, 1436
Biguanides, 684-685
Bilbao-Dotter tube, 297
Bile
  aspiration of, before occlusion
      cholangiography, 1344
  flow of, 86
  inspissated, after liver transplantation, 1743
  leakage of
    abdominal masses and, 1995
    biliary duct malignant disease and, 1418,
        1420
    disparate sulfur colloids and iminodiacetic
        acid scintigraphic images in, 1523,
        1524, 1525
    in percutaneous interventional radiology,
        1418, 1420, 1995
    in percutaneous transhepatic
        cholangiography, 1240
    in posttraumatic strictures, 1314
  reflux of, in stomach after obesity surgery,
      464
Bile acids, 80
  deficiency of, 80
  oral, in extracorporeal shock wave
      lithotripsy, 1359
  synthesis of, 84
Bile canaliculi, 83-84, 85
Bile duct; see also Biliary tract
  accessory, 1256-1257
  anatomy of, 28, 33-34, 1446
  anomalies of, 1446
  in ascariasis, 2112
  atresia of; see Biliary atresia
  bifurcation of
    biliary stent palliative drainage in, 1434,
        1435, 1436
    in percutaneous intervention in malignant
        biliary tract disease, 1402-1403
  biopsy of, 1336
  blood supply of, 1608-1610
  calculi in; see Choledocholithiasis
    endoscopy of, 1344-1354; see also
        Calculus disease, endoscopic
        intervention in
  carcinoma of
    percutaneous biliary dilation of strictures
        in, 1383
    primary; see Cholangiocarcinoma
    in ulcerative colitis, 574
  common; see Common bile duct
  common channel for pancreatic duct and,
      1262, 1263
  computed tomography of, 1233
  conjugated contrast in, 1228, 1229
  constriction of, 1108, 1122
  cystadenoma of, 1476
  cystic duct insertion into, 1259, 1260, 1261
  cysts of, from liver infarcts, 1319

Bile duct—cont'd
  debris after transplantation and, 1743
  dilatation of
    endosonography of, 1131
    in primary sclerosing cholangitis, 1308,
        1309, 1310
    ultrasonography of, 1296, 1297, 1298,
        1299
  drainage catheter internalization for, 1426
  duplications of, 1271-1272
  embryology of, 1251
    choledochal cyst and, 1265
  in endoscopic retrograde
      cholangiopancreatography, 1241
  endoscopy of; see also Biliary tract,
      percutaneous endoscopy of;
      Percutaneous interventional radiology
    in calculi, 1344-1354
    in dilatation, 1131
    drainage catheter internalization in, 1426
    entry and technical approach to, in
        percutaneous intervention in
        malignant biliary tract disease,
        1401-1403
  extrahepatic; see Extrahepatic bile duct
  gallbladder carcinoma spread into, 1326
  gas in, sonography of, 2100
  hepatocellular carcinoma in, 1665, 1673
  intrahepatic, anatomy of, 1223-1224, 1256
  intraoperative guidewire in, for percutaneous
      biliary stricture dilation, 1383
  leakage from
    after liver transplantation, 1738,
        1739-1740
    anastomotic, 1739-1740
    in hemobilia, 1321
    nonanastomotic, after transplantation,
        1739-1740
    T-tube site, 1739, 1740
  liver diseases affecting, 1318
  liver transplantation and, 1737, 1739-1740
  lymph nodes in external compression of,
      chemotherapy-induced cholangitis
      versus, 1311
  magnetic resonance imaging of, 1236
  necrosis of, liver infarcts in, 1319
  nonneoplastic disease of, 1294-1324
    acquired immunodeficiency syndrome in
        cholangitis as; see Acquired
        immunodeficiency syndrome
    Alagille's syndrome in, 1320
    ampullary stenosis in, 1318-1319
    bacterial cholangitis in, 1303-1306
    benign strictures in, 1314-1316
    chemotherapy-induced cholangitis in,
        1311
    choledochal varices in, 1319
    choledocholithiasis in, 1294-1302, 1303;
        see also Choledocholithiasis
    cystic fibrosis in, 1320
    cysts from liver infarcts in, 1319
    eosinophilic cholangitis in, 1312
    fistulas in, 1316-1318
    graft versus host disease in, 1320
    hemobilia in, 1321
    hepatic hilar cysts in, 1319, 1320
    histiocytosis in, 1320
    liver diseases and, 1318
    parasitic, 1312-1314
    primary sclerosing cholangitis in,
        1306-1310, 1311
    rare infections in cholangitis as,
        1311-1312
    recurrent pyogenic cholangitis in,
        1302-1303, 1304

Bile duct—cont'd
 nonneoplastic disease of—cont'd
  scolicidal-agent cholangitis in, 1312
  scolicidal cholangitis in, 1312
  tuberculosis in, 1311
 obstruction of
  after liver transplantation, 1739,
   1740-1744
  anastomotic strictures in, 1740, 1741
  appearances of, 1432, 1433
  in child, 1978-1980
  in cholangiocarcinoma, 1334
  choledocholithiasis in, 1296-1298
  endoscopic intervention for, 1426, 1429,
   1432
  endoscopic sphincterotomy for cholangitis
   with, 1347
  endoscopic therapy for, 1098
  hepatic hilar cysts in, 1319
  imaging in, 1978-1980
  as lithotripsy contraindication, 1359
  nonanastomotic strictures in, 1740-1743
  pediatric, 1978-1980
  percutaneous intervention in malignant
   disease causing, 1399; see also
   Percutaneous interventional
   radiology, in malignant biliary tract
   disease
 plain films and contrast studies of, 2031
 in pancreatic adenocarcinoma, 1108, 1122
 pancreatic duct union with, 1261,
  1262-1263
 percutaneous interventional radiology in,
  1367-1439; see also Percutaneous
  interventional radiology
 percutaneous transhepatic cholangiography
  of, 1240
 spontaneous perforation of, in child,
  1977-1978
 stones in; see Choledocholithiasis
 strictures of
  after liver transplantation, 1738,
   1740-1743
  benign, 1314-1316
  in child, 1978
  cholangiocarcinoma versus, 1336
  endoscopy in, 1434, 1435
  intrahepatic stones in, 1350, 1351
  percutaneous balloon dilation of,
   1383-1396; see also Percutaneous
   biliary stricture dilation
 ultrasonography of
  in acute abdomen, 2108-2112
  in calculi, 1296-1298, 2111-2112
  in cystadenoma, 1476
  in dilatation, 1131, 1296, 1297, 1298,
   1299
  in obstruction, 1296-1298
 variants and anomalies of, 1256-1272
  aberrant ducts in, 1256-1258, 1259
  Caroli's disease in, 1270-1271
  choledochal cyst in, 1263-1268
  choledochocele in, 1268-1270
  common hepatic and common bile ducts
   in, 1258-1259, 1260
  cystic duct in, 1259-1262
  drainage, 1261
  duplications in, 1271-1272
  intrahepatic and hepatic duct, 1256, 1257
  major papilla site in, 1262
  pancreaticobiliary duct union in, 1261,
   1262-1263
Bile salts
 in acute cholecystitis, 1275
 contrast absorption and, 1228

Bilharziasis, 944-946
Biliary access for percutaneous biliary stricture
  dilation, 1383
Biliary atresia, 1981-1982
 liver transplantation technique and, 1737
Biliary calculi; see Choledocholithiasis
Biliary casts, cholangitis and, 1312
Biliary cirrhosis in posttraumatic strictures,
  1314, 1318
Biliary colic, 1275
 after extracorporeal shock wave lithotripsy,
  1360
 in bile duct obstruction, 2032
 ultrasonography of, 2111-2112
Biliary-cutaneous fistula, 1317, 1318
Biliary-enteric fistula, 1316
Biliary juice reflux as carcinogen, 1325
Biliary mud, 1340
Biliary sludge, 1981
Biliary sphincter, spasms of, 1295, 1296
Biliary stents in obstruction, 1098
Biliary tract; see also Bile duct; Gallbladder
 in acquired immunodeficiency syndrome,
  961
 in acute abdomen, 2108-2112
 anatomy of, 83-84, 85, 1223-1227
 calculi in; see Choledocholithiasis
 cholecystography of, 1227-1230, 1231; see
  also Cholecystography
 choledochal cyst and, 961
 cholescintigraphy of; see Cholescintigraphy
 computed tomography of, 1230-1233
  barium examination with, 1231
  dynamic versus nondynamic, 1231-1232
  pediatric, 1978-1980
  techniques for, 1230-1233
 congenital anomalies of, 1976-1977
 decompression of
  after liver transplantation, 1740
  in cholangiocarcinoma, 1340
  versus interventional percutaneous
   endoscopy in malignant disease,
   1399-1400
  palliative, in malignant disease, 1399,
   1400
 embryology of, 1251, 1252
 endoprosthesis for, 1430; see also Biliary
  tract, percutaneous endoscopy of
  clogged, 1431
 endoscopic retrograde
  cholangiopancreatography of; see
  Endoscopic retrograde
  cholangiopancreatography
 endoscopy of; see Biliary tract, percutaneous
  endoscopy of
 extracorporeal shock wave lithotripsy and;
  see Extracorporeal shock wave
  lithotripsy
 function of, 83-84, 85
 gallbladder agenesis and, 1251
 gas in, 2051
  after sphincterotomy, 2055
  causes of, 2053
  plain films and contrast studies in, 2032,
   2033, 2053, 2055
 hepatocellular carcinoma in, 1673
 history of radiology of, 10-13
 in liver transplantation complications,
  1738-1740
 magnetic resonance imaging in, 1235-1236
 neoplasms of, 1325-1343
  carcinoma in, 1325-1333; see also
   Carcinoma, of biliary tract
  cholangiocarcinoma in, 1333-1342; see
   also Cholangiocarcinoma

Biliary tract—cont'd
 neoplasms of—cont'd
  choledochal cyst and, 1265-1266, 1267
  endoscopic intervention in, 1430-1439
  endoscopy in; see Biliary tract,
   percutaneous endoscopy of
  pediatric, 1978
 nonneoplastic diseases of; see Bile duct,
  nonneoplastic disease of
 obstruction of; see Bile duct, obstruction of
 parasites in, 2112
 pediatric, 1975-1985
  biliary atresia and neonatal hepatitis in,
   1981-1982
  congenital anomalies of, 1976-1977
  gallbladder and, 1980-1981
  obstruction in, 1978-1980
  pancreatitis and, 1980
  rhabdomyosarcoma in, 1978-1980
  spontaneous perforation in, 1977-1978
 percutaneous endoscopy of, 1423-1429
  complications of, 1434-1436
  endoscopes in, 1423-1424
  endoscopy versus, 1437
  indications for, 1425-1426, 1427, 1428
  indications for stent placement in,
   1432-1434, 1435, 1436
  metallic expanding stents in, 1436-1437
  palliative endoscopic stent placement
   versus, 1437
  radiologic procedures combined with,
   1431
  rendezvous procedure in, 1431
  results and complications of, 1426-1429
  selection of approach in, 1400
  stents versus other palliative treatment in,
   1437-1438
  techniques for, 1424-1425, 1426,
   1430-1431
 percutaneous interventional radiology for,
  1367-1398; see also Percutaneous
  interventional radiology
 percutaneous transhepatic cholangiography
  of; see Percutaneous transhepatic
  cholangiography
 physiology of, 83-87
 preoperative drainage of, 1432
 scintigraphy of; see Cholescintigraphy
  in bacterial cholangitis, 1306
  in choledochoceles, 1269
 secretions of, 84-86
 stenoses of
  ampullary, 1318-1319
  in chronic calcific pancreatitis, 1098
  endoscopic therapy in, 1098
 stents in; see Stent
 strictures of, percutaneous interventional
  radiology for, 1383-1396; see also
  Percutaneous biliary stricture dilation
 synthesis in, 84
 tuberculosis of, 1311
 ultrasonography of, 2108-2112
  in bacterial cholangitis, 1305-1306
  in Caroli's disease, 1271
  in cholangiocarcinoma, 1334, 1335
  in cholecystitis; see Cholecystitis,
   ultrasonography of
  in choledochal cyst, 1266
  in choledochoceles, 1269
  in choledocholithiasis, 1296-1298
  in cholesterolosis, 1291
  before extracorporeal shock wave
   lithotripsy, 1359
  in hyperplastic cholesteroses, 1289, 1290,
   1291

Biliary tract—cont'd
  ultrasonography of—cont'd
    in obstruction, 1978-1980
    in percutaneous cholecystostomy, 1381,
      1416
    in percutaneous intervention in malignant
      biliary tract disease, 1404
    in primary sclerosing cholangitis,
      1308-1310, 1311
    in recurrent pyogenic cholangitis, 1303
    sequence for, in biliary tract stone
      disease, 1302
    in transperitoneal approach for
      percutaneous cholecystolithotomy,
      1378
  variants and anomalies of, 1256-1272; see
    also Bile duct, variants and
    anomalies of
Biliary-vascular fistula, 1316
Bilirubin, serum, 1325, 1334
Billroth II gastrectomy
  postoperative studies after, 298
  prior to endoscopic intervention in calculus
    disease, 1348
  recurrent gastric cancer after, 423
Biloma, 1259
  after liver transplantation, 1737, 1739,
    1740, 1748
    percutaneous drainage of, 1740
  in child, 1975
  in cholescintigraphy, 1235
  percutaneous drainage of, 1420, 2002
Bilopaque; see Sodium tyropanoate
Biochemistry, intestinal, 683-684
Biopsy
  in abdominal masses, 1987-1997; see also
    Percutaneous biopsy, in abdominal
    masses
  of bile duct
    in cholangiocarcinoma, 1336
    in primary sclerosing cholangitis, 1307
  of colon
    in colorectal carcinoma, 779, 809
    in Crohn's disease, 602
    in familial multiple polyposis, 780
    radiologic caveats and, 795
  of duodenum
    in cytomegalovirus disease, 477
    in heterotopic gastric mucosa, 477
    in nonspecific duodenitis, 473
  of esophagus in strictures, 211
  fine-needle aspiration; see Fine-needle
    aspiration cytology
  of gallbladder
    in carcinoma staging, 1333
    percutaneous aspiration, 1382
  liver
    in abdominal masses, 1991
    arteriovenous fistulas after, 1617
    in hemangioma, 1642-1643
    in hemochromatosis, 1561-1562
    imaging-guided, in metastases, 1708,
      1715
    before transplantation, 1736
  of pancreas, 1128
    in adenocarcinoma, 1110, 1125
    in cystic neoplasm, 1152
    endoscopically guided, 1128-1129
    in lymphoma, 1162
    in plasmacytoma, 1163
    in transplantation with abnormal fluid
      collections, 1218
  percutaneous; see Percutaneous biopsy
  in polyarteritis nodosa, 1616
  of rectum, 820, 821

Biopsy—cont'd
  of rectum—cont'd
    in inflammatory bowel disease, 570
  renal
    in abdominal masses, 1994
    in pancreatic transplantation, 1197
    in Ruvalcaba-Myhre-Smith syndrome, 785
  small bowel
    in celiac disease, 665, 666
    in Crohn's disease, 602
    in giardiasis, 670
    in inflammatory bowel disease, 608
    jejunal, in intestinal lactase deficiency,
      684
    peroral, 552-555, 653, 661
    in systemic sclerosis, 653
    ulcerative colitis in, 581
    in Whipple's disease, 680
  of stomach
    in carcinoma, 397
    in leiomyosarcoma, 432
    in peptic ulcer disease, 478
Biopsy-Cut needle, 1988
Biopsy transducer, in percutaneous
    interventional radiology in abdominal
    masses, 1990
Biosponder needle, 1990-1991
Biphasic enteroclysis with methylcellulose; see
    Enteroclysis, biphasic, with
    methylcellulose
Bird-beak configuration, 203, 211
Bird-of-prey sign, 2063
Bisacodyl, 90
  in cathartic colon, 583
  in double-contrast large bowel examination,
    565
  in pneumocolon for small bowel
    examination, 516
Bismuth
  hilar tumor with palliation endoprosthesis
    and, 1435, 1436
  history of use of, 5
Bismuth subnitrate, 88
Bismuth subsalicylate, 903
BL; see Burkitt's lymphoma
Bladder
  colon fistula to, 793
  computed tomography of, 2136-2138
  in pancreatic transplantation rejection, 1197,
    1214
  pelvic spaces and, 1799
  retroperitoneal fibrosis in tumors of, 1815
  trauma to, 2136-2138
Blastomyces dermatidis, 1312
Blau, M, 14
Bleeding; see also Hemorrhage
  in biphasic enteroclysis with
    methylcellulose, 545-546
  into duodenum, 502, 503-506
  endoscopy in, 967-982; see also Endoscopy
  fecal occult-blood test for, 831
  in leiomyomas of small bowel, 628
  lower tract
    endoscopy in, 976-978
    scintigraphy in, 983
  occult, 977-978
  peptic ulcer, gastrointestinal endoscopy in,
    970-972
  rectal
    in colonic neoplasia, 765
    in inflammatory bowel disease, 586
    in juvenile polyposis, 788
  scintigraphy in, 983-993; see also
    Scintigraphy
  in ulcerative colitis, 573

Bleeding—cont'd
  upper tract, 298; see Upper gastrointestinal
    bleeding
Bleeding diatheses, 1400
Bleeding diathesis, 1987
Bloch, F, 19, 20
Blood clot
  in hemobilia, 1321
  in splenic artery embolization, 1791
Blood vessels
  in hepatic magnetic resonance imaging,
    1503-1505
  tortuous, pharyngeal, 120, 123
  in trauma
    computed tomography and, 2139
    to kidney, 2149
    to liver, 2147-2148
Blooming in cholescintigraphy, 1234
Blue rubber-bleb nevus syndrome, 630
Blunt abdominal trauma
  algorithm for management of, 2152
  mechanism and pattern of injury in, 2120
BMT; see Bone marrow transplant, allogeneic
Bochdalek's foramen hernia, 255
  in child, 1853-1856
Boerhaave's syndrome, 217
Bolus, 127, 128
  in child, 1827, 1828
  in esophagus, 168, 177
  in pharynx, 1827
Bone, pharyngeal malignancy extending to,
    142, 147-150
Bone marrow transplant, allogeneic, 674, 675,
    676
Borman classification of gastric carcinoma,
    416-422
Bowel
  colon fistula to adjacent, 793
  enemas after resection of, 713
  inflammatory disease of; see Inflammatory
    bowel disease
  irritable, prostaglandins and, 72
  ischemia of; see Ischemia, intestinal
  large; see Colon; Large bowel
  obstruction of
    in colorectal carcinoma, 805
    in Gardner's syndrome, 781
    percutaneous abscess drainage and, 1998
    secondary neoplasms and, 643
    ultrasonography of mechanical, 2101,
      2106-2108
  pancreatic pseudocysts and, 1035
  small; see Small bowel
  trauma to, 2153
Bowel habit training, 1915
Bowel preparation
  for biphasic enteroclysis with
    methylcellulose, 534
  for colon imaging, 697
    computed tomography and, 802
    inadequate, 710
    magnetic resonance imaging and, 719
  for colonoscopy, 716
  in defecography, 844
  physiology of, 90
Bowel wall
  in bowel obstruction, sonography of, 2106
  gas in, in acute abdomen, 2099-2100
  interstitial emphysema of, 2069
  metastases to, 802
  thickening of
    in chronic radiation enteritis, 651
    in diverticulitis, 2104-2105
  thinning of, in sprue, 912
Boyd, DP, 19

Brachial artery, 1604
Brachial cyst, 1829, 1830
Brachial fistula, 1829, 1830
Brachial sinus, 1829, 1830
Brachytherapy in biliary tract malignancy,
    1403
Brain
    hypoglycemia and, 1169
    tumors of, in Turcot's syndrome, 786
Brainstem lesions, 134
Branchial arch anomalies, 1829, 1830
Branchial cleft anomalies, 120, 121
Breast carcinoma
    in gastric metastasis, 433
    in hepatic metastases, 1710, 1724
    in hereditary nonpolyposis colon cancer, 825
    laser heat ablation in metastases from, 1719
    retroperitoneal fibrosis in, 1815
    in small bowel metastasis, 646
Breath-holding in hepatic magnetic resonance
    imaging, 1488-1489
Bronchobiliary fistula, 1316, 1317
Bronchoesophageal fistula, congenital, 212
Bronchogenic carcinoma; *see* Lung, carcinoma
    of
Bronchogenic cyst, 270
Bronchoscope, pediatric, 1423
Bronchus
    esophageal, in child, 1843
    esophageal carcinoma invasion of, 273, 277,
        279
Brown pigment stones, endoscopic intervention
    in; *see* Calculus disease, endoscopic
    intervention in
Brüel & Kjær rectal endoprobe, 813, 814
Brunneroma, giant, 500-501
Brunner's gland
    adenoma of, 488
    hyperplasia of, 377, 498-501
Bruton's X-linked hypogammaglobulinemia,
    676
Buccal mucosa, 146
Budd-Chiari syndrome
    ascites and, 87
    in child, 1973
    hepatic vein in, 1625, 1626-1628
        drainage of, 1446
    liver transplantation and, 1746
    portal vein in, 1611
    scintigraphy of, 1519, 1522, 1523, 1524
        technetium 99m sulfur colloid, 1519,
            1522, 1523
    ultrasonography of, 1472
Bulbarduodenitis, nonspecific, 473
Bullous dermatoses
    in esophageal strictures, 235, 236, 238
    in esophagitis, 232
Bull's-eye lesions
    in colon, 774
    in Crohn's disease, 615
    in duodenum, 508
    in liver, 1478
    in small bowel, 643
    in stomach, 434
Bupivacaine, 1386
Burckardt, H, 13
Burhenne, J, 10, 23
Burhenne technique for common duct stone
    removal, 23
Burkitt's lymphoma
    in pancreas, 1162
    in small bowel, 639
        in child, 1895
Bursa, omental
    anatomy of, 1797

Bursa, omental—cont'd
    gas in, from misplaced needle, 1821
Buscopan; *see* Hyoscine-*N*-butyl bromide
N-Butylscopolammonium bromide; *see*
    Hyoscine-*N*-butyl bromide
Byler's disease, 1977
Bypass
    gastric, 455, 456; *see also* Obesity, gastric
        surgery for
        Crohn's enteritis after, 829
    surgical, versus percutaneous intervention in
        malignant disease, 1399

C

C-peptide, 1169
CA 19-9, pancreatic, 1132, 1134, 1146
    of acinar cell carcinoma, 1154
    in mucinous adenoma, 1149
Calcification
    in acute abdomen, 2022, 2023, 2073
    bile duct
        in child, 1978
        in cystadenocarcinoma, 1682
        difficulty in extraction of, 1348-1350,
            1351, 1352
        endoscopy for, 1344-1354, 1425-1427,
            1428; *see also* Calculus disease,
            endoscopic intervention in
        extracorporeal shock wave lithotripsy for,
            1355-1366; *see also* Extracorporeal
            shock wave lithotripsy
        large, 1348-1350
        in obstruction, 1978
        percutaneous endoscopy for, 1425-1427,
            1428
        sonography of, 2111-2112
    common bile duct, 1426-1427
    endoscopic intervention in; *see also* Calculus
        disease, endoscopic intervention in
    gallbladder; *see* Cholelithiasis
    intestinal, 893-894
        in duodenal wall cysts, 471
        in meconium peritonitis, 1891
    intrahepatic duct, 1350, 1351, 1352
        percutaneous endoscopy for, 1427-1429
    in liver
        in hemangioma, 1631
        in hepatocellular carcinoma, 1669, 1671,
            1699
        magnetic resonance imaging of, 1493
        in metastases, 1714
        in portal vein thrombosis, 1622
    in pancreas
        choledocholithiasis versus, 1300
        head of, in gallbladder ultrasonography,
            1250
        in lymphangioma, 1160
        in serous adenoma, 1141, 1142
    pancreatic duct
        extracorporeal shock wave lithotripsy of,
            1101-1106
        sphincterotomy for, 1091-1094
    in peritoneum, Armillifer and, 946
    in pharyngeal benign structural diseases, 26
    punctate, in pediatric granulomatous
        infection, 1937
    in spleen, 1772-1774
    in stomach
        in smooth muscle tumor, 378
        in vascular tumor, 383
    transcatheter dissolution of, in
        extracorporeal shock wave
        lithotripsy, 1361
    urinary, 80
        in malabsorption, 80

Calcification—cont'd
    urinary—cont'd
        in ulcerative colitis, 575
Calcium
    in biliary sludge, 1981
    in choledocholithiasis, 1299
    islet cell tumor hormone and, 1188
Calculous cholecystitis, acute, 1279-1281,
    1282, 1283
    pathophysiology of, 1275
Calculus disease, endoscopic intervention in,
    1344-1354; *see also* Calcification
    choledochoscopy in, 1350-1351, 1353
    diagnostic endoscopic retrograde
        cholangiopancreatography in,
        1344-1345, 1346
    difficulties of sphincterotomy and stone
        extraction in, 1348-1350, 1351, 1352
    duct stones in, 1345-1350, 1351, 1352
    for gallbladder stones, 1351, 1353
    indications for, 1347-1348
    for intrahepatic stones, 1350
    pancreatic duct, 1091-1094
    success rates and complications of,
        1346-1347
    techniques for, 1345-1346
CAMECO Syringe Pistol, 558
Campylobacter
    acquired immunodeficiency syndrome and,
        959
    in dysentery, 900-901
    in gastritis, 326-327
        in child, 1869
    in ileitis versus appendicitis, 716
    in primary immunodeficiency syndromes,
        676
    in small bowel inflammatory changes, 677
    toxic megacolon in, 603
    ulcerative colitis versus, 604
Canaliculi, bile, 83-84, 85
Cancer family syndrome, 825-827
    screening guidelines for, 835-836
Candidiasis, 908-909, 910
    in acquired immunodeficiency syndrome,
        954-955
        small bowel enteropathy in, 673
    cholangitis in, 1312
    computed tomography of, 2083
    in duodenal disease, 476, 477
    in esophagitis, 226-228
        in child, 1846
    pediatric, 1846, 1937, 1960
    of pharynx, 114
    in splenic infection, 1780
        percutaneous abscess drainage of, 2004
    ulcerative colitis versus, 604
Cannon, WB, 4, 5, 88
Capillariasis, intestinal, 937-938
Capillary hemangioma
    small bowel vessels in, 657
    technetium 99m-red blood cell imaging in,
        1527-1528
Capillary plexus in liver, 1610
Carbohydrate digestion, 79
Carbon dioxide contrast
    in angiography in hepatocellular carcinoma,
        1688, 1689
    in colon, 700, 708
    equipment for administering, 700
    in hepatic ultrasonography, 1473
    in intussusception imaging, 1901-1902
    in small bowel, 517, 545
        in child, 1901-1902
        with ostomy stomal dysfunction, 524

Carcinoembryonic antigen
  in cholangiocarcinoma, 1333
  in colorectal cancer screening, 801, 809, 831
  in hepatic metastases, 1715
  in pancreatic tumors, 1132, 1134, 1146, 1154
Carcinoid
  cholangiocarcinoma as, 1333
  of colon, 778
    classification of epithelial, 762
    morphology of, 774
  duodenal, 492, 495
  esophageal submucosal, 270
  humeral activity of, 1725
  in islet cell tumors, 1172
  in liver
    clinical features of, 632
    embolization in, 1727
    metastatic, 634, 635, 1473, 1479, 1723, 1727
    ultrasonography of, 634, 635, 1473, 1479
  in mesentery
    portal hypertension and, 1596
    of small bowel, 1823
  in small bowel, 632-634, 635, 1823
  somatostatin analogue in, 71
  in stomach, 434
    benign, 383, 384
  transcatheter embolization in, 1725, 1727, 1732
Carcinoma
  adenoid cystic; see Adenoid cystic carcinoma
  of ampulla of Vater
    cholangiocarcinoma versus, 1336
    papillary, 1432
  of biliary tract, 1325-1333
    adenocarcinoma in, 1266, 1267
    cholangiocarcinoma as, 1333-1342; see also Cholangiocarcinoma
    diagnostic imaging in, 1327-1333
    mode of spread in, 1326-1327
    pathogenesis in, 1325
    pathology of, 1325-1326
    percutaneous biliary dilation of strictures in, 1383
    percutaneous endoscopy in, 1423-1429
    presentation of, 1325
    prognosis and treatment in, 1333
    staging of, 1327
    stent drainage in, 1432-1434, 1435, 1436, 1437-1438
    surgical bypass versus endoscopic stent in, 1437-1438
    in ulcerative colitis, 574
  of breast; see Breast carcinoma
  of cecum, periappendiceal abscess versus, 2007
  cholangiocellular, versus fatty liver, 1553-1554
  of colon; see also Colorectal carcinoma
    cancer family syndrome and, 825, 827, 835-836
    carcinogenesis of, 764-765
    cloacogenic, 791
    complications in, 793-795
    computed tomography angiography of, 1460
    Crohn's disease and, 601
    diverticulitis versus, 756, 757, 758, 759
    doubling time of, 776-777
    Dukes classification of, 805
    in familial multiple polyposis, 780
    in Gardner's syndrome, 783

Carcinoma—cont'd
  of colon—cont'd
    growth rate determination of, 776
    in hepatic metastases, 1710, 1712-1715, 1718, 1719, 1724
    hereditary nonpolyposis, 788-790, 825, 827
    laser heat ablation in metastases from, 1719
    liver metastasis in, 1706; see Metastases, to liver
    metastatic, to liver, 1493
    in obstruction, 2058, 2059
    origin of, 764-765
    radiologic findings in, 790-791
    radiology caveats in, 795-797
    resection in, 805
    sessile, 771
    splenic invasion of, dynamic incremental computed tomography of, 1463
    surgical resection in metastases from, 1720
    ulcerative colitis and, 583, 584, 791
  colorectal; see Colorectal carcinoma
  in Crohn's disease, 601-602
  endocrine, in hepatic metastases, 1711
  esophageal, 242-249
    computed tomography of, 240, 241, 272-278
    endoscopy in, 265-269, 271, 973
    endosonography of, 265-269
    intrathoracic, 277
    laser-photocoagulation in, 271
    magnetic resonance imaging of, 272, 278-281
    metastasis of; see Metastases, from esophagus
    motility disorders in, 210
    oat cell, 243
    polypoid, endosonography of, 265-269
    staging of, 265-269, 272-281
    strictures and, 238
    ultrasonography of, 265-269
    varices and, 240, 241
    webs and, 236
  of gallbladder, 1325-1333
    abscess formation in, 1331
    adenosquamous, 1326
    biliary stent drainage in papillary, 1433-1434, 1435
    cholecystectomy in, 1333
    classification in, 1327
    diagnostic imaging in, 1327-1333
    diffuse calcification with, 1325
    endoscopic management of common duct obstruction in, 1433
    hematogenous spread of, 1326
    infiltrating and fungating, 1325
    magnetic resonance imaging in, 1327
    metastases from, 1328
    mode of spread in, 1326-1327
    multiple stones in, 1327, 1328
    oat cell, 1331
    pathogenesis in, 1325
    pathology of, 1325-1326
    percutaneous aspiration biopsy in, 1382
    porcelain, 1325, 1329, 1332
    presentation of, 1325
    prognosis and treatment in, 1333
    scirrhous, 1326
    squamous cell, 1326
    staging of, 1327
    wall thickening in, 1328, 1329
  of genital tract, 651
  hepatocellular; see Hepatocellular carcinoma

Carcinoma—cont'd
  of large bowel; see Carcinoma, of colon; Colorectal carcinoma
  of liver; see Liver, primary malignant neoplasms of
  of lung
    metastatic, 1710
    oat cell, 645
    retroperitoneal fibrosis in, 1815
  of mouth, 142, 143
  of ovaries, 1804
    duodenal metastasis of, 508
    greater omentum pathology and, 1822
    peritoneography of, 1799
  of pancreas
    biliary stent palliative drainage in, 1432-1433, 1435, 1436
    biopsy of, 1037
    cholangiocarcinoma versus, 1336
    in cirrhosis with portal hypertension, 1593, 1594
    gastric metastasis of, 433
    involving only common bile duct, percutaneous intervention in, 1400
    laser heat ablation in metastases from, 1719
    liver metastasis of, 1706, 1710, 1711, 1712
    percutaneous interventional radiology in abdominal masses and, 1992, 1993
    percutaneous transhepatic cholangiography of, 1021, 1022
    in splenic vein obstruction, 1593, 1594
    in papilla of Vater, palliation in, 1432, 1433
    in Peutz-Jeghers syndrome, 785, 786
    in pharynx
      esophageal webs and, 236
      squamous cell; see Squamous cell carcinoma, of pharynx
    of rectum in hereditary nonpolyposis colorectal cancer, 788; see also Colorectal carcinoma
    renal cell, in retroperitoneum, 1815
    of salivary glands, 139
    small bowel, 639-640, 641
      metastatic spread of, 645, 646
    squamous cell; see Squamous cell carcinoma
    of stomach; see Gastric carcinoma
Carcinomatosis
  percutaneous fluoroscopically guided gastrostomy in, 2011
  peritoneal, 1803
    in pancreatic adenocarcinoma, 1118
    in small bowel mesentery, 1823
Carcinosarcoma, esophageal, 240, 241, 249
Cardia, 282
  anatomy of, 311
  in computed tomography, 211
  in endosonography, 187
  in esophageal motility disorders, 210, 211
  intraluminal bulge at, 306
  progressive relaxation of, 170
Cardiac agents, barium enema and, 701
Carina
  enlarged node of, in esophageal displacement, 254
  in esophageal endosonography, 188, 189
Carman, RD, 7, 8, 10
Carney's triad, 379
Caroli's disease, 1270-1271
  in child, 1976-1977
  choledochal cyst in, 1263
Carotid artery
  hypoglossal tumors and, 158
  tortuous, 120, 123

Cary-Coons endoprosthesis, 1407, 1409
Case, JT, 4
Castor oil
  in cathartic colon, 583
  before colon imaging, 697
Casts
  biliary, 1312
  in small bowel, 1903, 1904
Catecholamines, excess of, 1169
Cathartics
  abnormal contractions from
    colonic strictures versus, 583
    ulcerative colitis versus, 604
  before colon imaging, 697
Catheter
  balloon
    in endoscopic retrograde
      cholangiopancreatography,
      1241-1242
    enteroclysis, 542
    in percutaneous intervention in malignant
      biliary tract disease, 1407
  biliary drainage
    blockage of, 1419-1420
    displacement of, 1413-1414
    in endoscopy, 1426, 1430-1431
    in percutaneous interventional radiology;
      see Catheter, in percutaneous
      intervention in malignant biliary tract
      disease
  Cope, 1377
  echoprobe, 264, 265
  enteroclysis
    balloon, 542
    types of, 543
  Fink, 2144
  Fogarty balloon
    in minicholecystostomy, 1374
    in percutaneous choledocholithotomy,
      1371
  Foley, in defecography, 842
  gastrostomy, 2012, 2014, 2016, 2017
    blockage of, 2018
    leakage around, 2017
    in transgastric jejunostomy, 2012-2013,
      2016, 2017
  in hepatic artery spasm, 1311, 1313
  McGahan, 1416
  nasobiliary, in percutaneous intervention,
    1413, 1414
  nasocystic, in endoscopic retrograde
    cholangiopancreatography, 1351
  Neff, 1406
  in percutaneous abscess drainage, 2000
  in percutaneous choledocholithotomy, 1367,
    1368
  in percutaneous intervention in malignant
    biliary tract disease, 1406; *see also*
    Percutaneous interventional
    radiology, in malignant biliary tract
    disease
    balloon, 1407
    characteristics of, 1413-1414
    displacement in, 1413-1414
    internalization of, 1426
    point of entry for, 1404-1405
    size of, 1413
  percutaneous pancreatic drainage, 1025
  pigtail flush, in aorta, 2144
Catheterization
  of hepatic vein, 1607-1608
  in liver angiography, 1604-1605
  of portal vein, 1187-1188, 1189, 1607-1608
Caudate hepatic veins, 29

Caudate lobe of liver
  anatomy of, 29, 33
  papillary process of, 29, 30, 33
Cauliflower appearance
  of duodenal adenoma, 488
  in gallbladder carcinoma, 1325
Caulking gun in defecography, 841
Caustic esophagitis, 229-230
  in child, 1847, 1848
Caustic infection, duodenum and, 476
Cavernoma, portal, 1972
Cavernous hemangioma; *see* Hemangiomas,
  cavernous
Cavernous lymphangioma of pancreas, 1160,
  1161
Cavernous transformation of portal vein in
  child, 1972
CBD; *see* Common bile duct
CCK; *see* Cholecystokinin
Cecostomy in percutaneous abscess drainage,
  2009
Cecum
  amebiasis and, 917
  anatomy of, 692, 725
  angiodysplasia in, 977
  barium examination of, 711
  carcinoma of
    intussusception and, 2055
    local adenopathy in, 804
  congenital mobile, 1882-1883
  in Crohn's disease, 595, 611
  diverticulitis of, 2083
  inflammatory reaction around, in
    appendicitis, 2085
  polypoid tumor of, 803
  tuberculosis of, 891-893
  vascular ectasia of, 1598, 1599
  volvulus of, 2061-2063
    gastric dilation and, 2043
Cefamandole, 1236
Celiac angiography
  after liver transplantation, 1745
  in cirrhosis, 1545
  in hepatocellular carcinoma, 1677
  in liver metastasis of small bowel carcinoid,
    635
  technique for, 1605-1606
Celiac artery stenosis, 1611, 1613
Celiac axis, 28
  in pancreatic adenocarcinoma, 1108
  of stomach, 311, 312
Celiac disease, 1898
  abetalipoproteinemia in, 668
  aspiration cytology and peroral biopsy of
    small bowel in, 552, 553
  barium examination in, 1898
  chronic ulcerative jejunoileitis in, 665-666
  collagenous sprue in, 553, 554, 666
  complications of, 553, 554, 665-668
  cow's milk protein allergy in, 666, 668
  duodenum in, 505, 506
  flocculation in, 664-665, 666
  hypersecretion in, 664, 665
  intestinal lymphangiectasia in, 666-668, 669
  intestinal permeability in, 82
  intussusception in, 665
  lymphoma of small bowel with, 659, 665
  in malabsorption, 80
  moulage sign in, 665
  radiology of, 663-665, 666
  refractory, 663
  small bowel adenocarcinomas and, 640
  small bowel dilatation in, 663
  small bowel lymphoma in, 635, 636
  small bowel narrowing and, 661

Celiac disease—cont'd
  soy protein allergy in—cont'd
    unclassified, 663
  valvulae conniventes in, 559, 562, 664, 665
Celiac ganglion, 28
Celiac lymph nodes, 29
  metastasis in, 270
Cellulose suspensions in ultrasonography, 717
Central anlage, embryologic, of pancreas,
  467-468
Central dot sign in Caroli's disease, 1271
Central nervous system
  in esophageal motility disorders, 209
  tumors of, in Turcot's syndrome, 786
Central vein, 61
Centroacinar cell serous adenoma, 1138
Ceruletide, 524
Cervical esophagogastric anastomosis, 277
Cervical sinus, 1829
Cervical spine, osteophytes of, 101, 120, 123
Cestodes, 939-943
CF; *see* Cystic fibrosis
Chagas' disease, 209-210, 211
  infections and infestations in, 918-923, 924,
    925
Chalasia, 205-206
Chandelier sign, 1248
Channel obstruction after obesity surgery, 461,
  463, 464
Charcot's triad, 1303
Chemical shift imaging in fatty liver,
  1551-1553
Chemolithiasis
  with extracorporeal shock wave lithotripsy,
    1359
  percutaneous, 1378-1379
Chemotherapy
  in cholangiocarcinoma, 1342
  cholangitis induced by, 1311
  in esophageal carcinoma
    esophageal-fat interface and, 275, 276
    in recurrences, 278
  in esophageal sarcoma, 249
  in esophagitis in child, 1848
  in gallbladder carcinoma, 1333
  in gastric lymphoma, 431
  in hepatic artery, 1611, 1613
    catheters for, 1531
  ischemic bowel from, 614
  in liver neoplasms
    in hepatocellular carcinoma, 1677
    portal infusion of, 1729
    in transcatheter embolization, 1717-1718,
      1729
    ultrasonography of metastatic tumor in,
      1479-1480
  small bowel lymphoma in, 635
Chest pain of esophageal origin, 181
Chest radiography
  in acute abdomen, 2077
  in diaphragmatic hiatus hernia, 256
  in duodenal tuberculosis, 476
  in esophageal perforation, 217
  techniques for, 2020-2021
Chiba needle
  in percutaneous intervention
    in abdominal masses, 1988
    in abscess drainage, 1999
    in malignant biliary tract disease, 1404
  in percutaneous transhepatic
    cholangiography, 1236, 1237, 1240
Chilaiditi's syndrome, 2027
Child; *see* Pediatrics
Chlamydia
  in lymphogranuloma venereum, 904-908

Chlamydia—cont'd
  ulcerative colitis versus, 604
Chloramphenicol, 901
Chloroquine, 2001
Chlortetracycline, 901
Cholangiocarcinoma, 1333-1342
  anomalous pancreaticobiliary duct union
      and, 1262-1263
  in Caroli's disease, 1270
  common duct obstruction in, 1433
  computed tomography of, 1232
  conditions predisposing to, 1333
  diagnostic imaging in, 1334-1336,
      1337-1341
  differential diagnosis of, 1336-1340, 1342
  fluoroscopically guided biopsy of, 1989
  hemochromatosis and, 1561
  history of, 1333
  intrahepatic, 1680-1681
  location of, 1334
  management in, 1340-1342
  palliation in, 1340
  pathology of, 1333-1334
  peripheral, 1680-1681
  in portal vein, 1461, 1592
  presentation of, 1334
  pretransplant imaging and, 1736
  in primary sclerosing cholangitis, 1307,
      1308
  resectability of, 1340
  sclerosing, nodular or papillary, 1333-1334
  site of occurrence of, 1333, 1334
  ultrasonography of, 1478
Cholangiocellular carcinoma, fatty liver
    versus, 1553-1554; *see also*
    Cholangiocarcinoma
Cholangiography
  air, in bifurcation tumors with palliation
      endoprosthesis, 1435
  in bacterial cholangitis, 1304-1305
  in biliary tract stone disease sequence,
      1302
  in Caroli's disease, 1271
  in choledochal cyst, 1266, 1267
  in choledochoceles, 1269
  in choledocholithiasis, 1294-1296
    incomplete filling of contrast around
        stones in, 1295
  of common channel for bile and pancreatic
      ducts, 1262
  gallbladder ultrasonography and, 1249
  in hemobilia, 1321
    after percutaneous interventional
        radiology, 1418, 1419
  of hepatic artery thrombosis after
      transplantation, 1745
  in hepatic hilar cysts, 1319
  history of, 13
  of intrahepatic and hepatic ducts, 1223,
      1256, 1257
  occlusion, 1344, 1345
    in intrahepatic stones, 1350
  in percutaneous choledocholithotomy, 1367,
      1370-1371
  percutaneous transhepatic; *see* Percutaneous
      transhepatic cholangiography
  in postinflammatory strictures, 1316
  in postoperative liver transplantation
      imaging, 1738, 1739
  predrainage, 1403-1405
  for pretransplant liver imaging, 1736
  in primary sclerosing cholangitis,
      1307-1308, 1310
  in recurrent pyogenic cholangitis, 1303

Cholangiopancreatography, retrograde
    endoscopic; *see* Endoscopic
    retrograde cholangiopancreatography
Cholangitis
  acute, 1303
  after percutaneous interventional radiology
      for biliary duct malignant disease,
      1417, 1419-1420
  ascending, 1303, 1306
  bacterial, 1303-1306
  biliary tree gas and, 2053
  chemotherapy-induced, 1311
  cholangiocarcinoma versus, 1336, 1337,
      1342
  in choledochal varices, 1319
  computed tomography of, 1232, 1305-1306
  endoscopic sphincterotomy for obstructive,
      1347
  eosinophilic, 1312
  in intrahepatic abscess, 2039
  as lithotripsy contraindication, 1359, 1361
  oriental, cholangiocarcinoma versus, 1337,
      1342
  percutaneous biliary stricture dilation in,
      1383, 1384
    transhepatic route for, 1236, 1384
  percutaneous transhepatic cholangiography
      of, 1236
  primary sclerosing, 1306-1310, 1311
    liver transplantation rejection and, 1742,
        1743
  rare infections in, 1311-1312
  recurrent pyogenic, 1302-1303, 1304
  sclerosing
    primary, 1736, 1737
    transjugular intrahepatic portographic
        shunting in, 1011
    in ulcerative colitis, 574
  scolicidal, 1312
  stenting after percutaneous balloon repair of
      strictures in, 1394
Cholecystectomy
  in choledocholithiasis, 1294
  in gallbladder carcinoma, 1333
  in hemorrhagic cholecystitis, 1285
  laparoscopic
    choledochoscopy and, 1350
    endoscopic sphincterotomy and, 1348
  in liver transplantation, 1736-1737
  in pericholecystic abscess, 1286
  strictures of biliary tree after, 1314-1315
Cholecystitis, 1275-1286
  acalculous, 1279-1281, 1282, 1283
    fine needle aspiration in, 1380
    sonography of, 2110-2111
  accuracy of studies in, 1279
  acute, 1275-1291
    acalculous, 1279-1281, 1282, 1283
    accuracy of studies of, 1279
    aspiration and drainage in, 1281
    calculous, 1275-1279; *see also*
        Cholelithiasis
    in child, 1980-1981
    cholescintigraphy of, 1279, 1280
    cholesterolosis and, 1291
    clinical features of, 1275
    complications of, 1281-1291
    computed tomography of, 1281, 1283,
        1284, 2089, 2090
    emphysematous, 1286, 1288
    empyema and, 1287-1289
    with gallbladder carcinoma, 1325
    gangrenous, 1281-1284
    Gram's stain for fluid in, 1281
    hemorrhagic, 1284-1285

Cholecystitis—cont'd
  acute—cont'd
    hepatic scintigraphy in, 1523
    hyperplastic cholesterosis and, 1289,
        1290, 1291
    imaging studies of, 1275-1276
    pathophysiology of calculus, 1275
    percutaneous interventional radiology in,
        1380-1383
    perforation and pericholecystic abscess in,
        1285-1286, 1287
    plain films and contrast studies of, 2031
    torsion in, 1286-1287, 1288
    ultrasonography of, 1330, 2109-2111
    uncomplicated, 1276-1279, 1280
    xanthomatous, 1289
  after extracorporeal shock wave lithotripsy,
      1360
  in child, 1980
  cholescintigraphy in, 1275-1279
  chronic
    acalculous, cholescintigraphy in, 1234
    with carcinoma of gallbladder, 1325
    in child, 1981
  clinical features of, 1275
  computed tomography of
    acute inflammation in, 1281, 1283, 1284,
        2089, 2090
    in child, 1980
    in emphysematous gallbladder, 2087,
        2088
    with gallbladder wall thickening, 1286,
        1287
    in gangrenous gallbladder, 2087
  emphysematous
    biliary tree gas and, 2053
    computed tomography of, 2087, 2088
    plain films and contrast studies of, 2031,
        2070
    sonography of, 2110, 2111
  extracorporeal shock wave lithotripsy in,
      1355-1361, 1362
  gangrenous, 1277, 1279
    computed tomography of, 2087
    scintigraphy of, 1523
    sonography of, 2111
  hemorrhagic, 1284-1285
  imaging studies of, 1275-1279, 1280
  as lithotripsy contraindication, 1359
  pathophysiology of, 1275
  ultrasonography of, 1248, 1281, 1282,
      1283, 1284
    accuracy of, 1279
    in acute cholecystitis, 1275, 1276-1279
    in child, 1980
    in fine needle aspiration, 1380
  xanthogranulomatous, 1289, 1327, 1331
Cholecystography
  conjugated contrast in bile duct and intestine
      in, 1228, 1229
  failure to opacity during, 1228
  in gallbladder duplications, 1253
  history of, 11-13
  multiseptated gallbladder in, 1255
  oral, 1227-1230, 1231
    before extracorporeal shock wave
        lithotripsy, 1359
Cholecystokinin, 1229
  in acute cholecystitis, 1276
  in cholescintigraphy, 1234
  discovery of, 67
  in gastric motility, 77
  liver function tests and, 84-86
  mechanism of action of, 68
  in sphincter of Oddi pressure, 1318

Cholecystolithotomy, percutaneous, 1375
  large tract, 1376-1378
Cholecystostomy, percutaneous
  in abscess drainage, 2009
  in cholecystitis, 1281
  in percutaneous intervention in malignant
      biliary tract disease, 1416
Choledochal cyst, 1263-1268
  anomalous pancreaticobiliary duct union
      and, 1263, 1265
  in biliary tract neoplasia, 1265-1266, 1267
  in child, 1976, 1977
  classification of, 1263, 1264
  clinical features of, 1265-1266
  computed tomography of, 1976, 1977
  in neonate, 1265
  pathogenesis of, 1263-1265
  radiologic features of, 1266-1268
  ultrasonography of, 1976, 1977
Choledochal varices, 1319
Choledochocele, 1263, 1268-1270
  in child, 1976, 1977
Choledochocholedochostomy in liver
      transplantation, 1737, 1739-1740
Choledochocolonic fistula, 1316, 1317
Choledochocutaneous fistula, 1317
Choledochoduodenal fistula, 1316
Choledochoduodenal junction, 1227
Choledochoenteric anastomosis, percutaneous
      endoscopy and, 1426
Choledochojejunal anastomoses, strictures at,
      1384, 1387, 1388-1389
Choledochojejunostomy in liver
      transplantation, 1737, 1739-1740
Choledocholithiasis, 1294-1302, 1303
  after biliary surgery, endoscopic
      sphincterotomy for, 1347
  in child, 1978
  cholangiocarcinoma versus, 1336
  cholangiography of, 1294-1296
  cholesterol stones in, 1298
  computed tomography of, 1298-1300,
      1301-1303
  dissolution of, 1375
  endoscopic intervention in, 1344-1354; see
      also Calculus disease, endoscopic
      intervention in
  extracorporeal shock wave lithotripsy of,
      1102, 1355-1366; see Extracorporeal
      shock wave lithotripsy
  in gallbladder agenesis, 1251
  imaging approach to, 1300-1302
  impacted
    in cystic duct, 1372
    in intrahepatic radicles, 1371
    as lithotripsy contraindication, 1359
  magnetic resonance imaging in, 1300, 1303
  pancreatitis and, endoscopic sphincterotomy
      for, 1347
  percutaneous cholecystolithotomy for, 1375
  percutaneous choledocholithotomy for,
      1367-1373
  percutaneous endoscopy for, 1425-1426,
      1427, 1428
  percutaneous transhepatic cholangiography
      of, 1240
  in postinflammatory strictures, 1316
  in recurrent pyogenic cholangitis, 1303
  stenting after percutaneous balloon stricture
      repair and, 1392
  strictures of biliary tree after, 1315-1316
  treatment of, 1361-1364
    results of lithotripsy in, 1361
  ultrasonography of, 1296-1298, 2111-2112

Choledocholithotomy, percutaneous,
      1367-1373
  results and complications of, 1427-1429
Choledochoscope
  in hepatic duct, 1375
  in percutaneous endoscopy of biliary tract,
      1423, 1424, 1426
Choledochoscopy
  in endoscopic intervention, 1350-1351, 1353
  percutaneous, 1367-1373
    results and complications of, 1427-1429
  peroral, in percutaneous endoscopy of
      biliary tract, 1423
Cholelithiasis, 1275-1291
  in acute cholecystitis, 1275
    ultrasonography of, 2109
  in ampullary pouch, 1227
  in ampullary stenosis, 1318
  with carcinoma of gallbladder, 1325
  in choledochoceles, 1269
  computed tomography of, in child, 1981
  congenital gallbladder septa and, 1255
  endoscopic intervention of, 1344-1354,
      1425-1427, 1428; see also Calculus
      disease, endoscopic intervention in
  endoscopic retrograde
      cholangiopancreatography of, 1242
  extracorporeal shock wave lithotripsy for,
      1102, 1355-1366; see also
      Extracorporeal shock wave lithotripsy
  floating, 1229, 1230
  in gallbladder sonography, 1246, 1247
  large stones in, 1348-1350
  percutaneous cholecystolithotomy in, 1375
  percutaneous endoscopy for, 1425-1426,
      1427, 1428
  percutaneous procedures for, 1375-1379
  recurrent, after lithotripsy, 1361
  stenting after percutaneous balloon stricture
      repair and, 1392
  ultrasonography of, in child, 1981
Cholera
  pancreatic, 1171
  toxic megacolon in, 603
Cholescintigraphy, 1275-1279
  in acute cholecystitis, 1275, 1279
    accuracy of, 1279
    nonvisualization in, 1281
  in pericholecystic abscess, 1286
  reflux of tracer in, 1235
  techniques for, 1233-1235
Cholestasis
  in acalculous cholecystitis, 1280
  technetium 99m-iminodiacetic acid
      retention in, 1523
Cholesterol
  abnormal deposits of, 1289, 1291
  in biliary sludge, 1981
  in cholecystitis, 1277
  in choledocholithiasis, 1298
    endoscopic intervention in, 1344-1354
  in gallbladder polyp, 1329
  liver and, 84
  in pancreatic cystic neoplasms, 1150
Cholesterolosis, 1291
  in hyperplastic cholesterosis, 1289
Cholesterosis, hyperplastic, 1289, 1290, 1291
Cholestyramine, 684-685
Chondrosarcoma of esophagus, 249
Choriocarcinoma, 1714
Chorionic gonadotropin, human; see Human
      chorionic gonadotropin
Chromium 51-EDTA, 82
Chromosome 5, 824

Chronic pain in chronic pancreatitis,
      1091-1098
Chronic pancreatitis; see Pancreatitis, chronic
Churchman, JW, 11
Chylous fluid in pancreatic lymphangioma,
      1162
Chymotrypsin
  in acinar cell carcinoma, 1154
  in pancreatoblastoma, 1156
Cicatrization after corrosive gastropathy, 357
Cimetidine
  in barium meal preparation, 286
  esophagitis from, 231
  in Meckel's diverticulum, 1890
Cinefluorography
  history of use of, 10
  of pharyngeal function, 97, 101, 107-109
Cineradiography
  in defecography, 842, 843
  in dysphagia, 165, 167
Cirrhosis, 1534-1546
  alcoholic, 1549
  alpha$_1$-antitrypsin deficient, 1534
  angiography in, 1545
  caudate lobe-right lobe ratio in, 1540
  in child, 1970-1971
  computed tomography of, 1539-1541, 1542
  diagnosis of, 1534-1545
  disparate sulfur colloids and iminodiacetic
      acid scintigraphic images in, 1523
  in esophageal varices, 238
  fatty liver in, 1553
    focal infiltration and, 1519
  in hemochromatosis, 1534, 1560, 1561,
      1562
  hepatic sinusoidal and arterial changes in,
      1619, 1620
  hepatic vein changes in, 1628
  in hepatocellular carcinoma, 1536,
      1662-1663, 1674, 1675-1676
  hilar cysts in, 1319
  intrahepatic vascular changes in, 1628
  Laënnec's, 1534
  liver and organ changes in, 1536-1537
  macronodular, 1534
    mixed micronodular and, 1534
    ultrasonography of, 1538
  magnetic resonance imaging of, 1493, 1498,
      1502, 1541-1544
  malignant neoplasms with, 1477
  micronodular, 1534, 1549
    computed tomography of, 1540, 1541
    mixed macronodular and, 1534
    ultrasonography of, 1537
  nodular lesions in
    ascites and, 1538
    differential diagnosis of, 1701-1702
    hepatocellular carcinoma and, 1692,
        1701-1702
    histology of, 1692
    magnetic resonance imaging of, 1542,
        1543
    regenerating, 1542-1543, 1544, 1545,
        1655-1656, 1674, 1675-1676
  nutritional, 1534
  percutaneous intervention in malignant
      biliary tract disease contraindicated
      in, 1400
  portal, 1534
  portal hypertension and, 1566-1603; see also
      Portal hypertension
    venous obstruction in, 1591-1592
  portal vein changes in, 1628
  posthepatic, 1534
  postnecrotic, 1534

Cirrhosis—cont'd
  postsinusoidal portal hypertension in, 1574
  in posttraumatic strictures, 1314, 1318
  primary, or secondary, 1534
  radionuclide study of, 1544-1545
  scintigraphy in, 1510, 1516, 1517
  single-photon-emission computed
      tomography of, 1519
  sinusoidal and arterial changes in, 1619,
      1620
  small bowel fine-needle aspiration cytology
      hazards and, 561
  technetium 99m sulfur colloid scintigraphy
      in, 1516, 1517
  transjugular intrahepatic portographic
      shunting in, 1010, 1013
  ultrasonography of, 1470, 1537-1539
    laparoscopic biopsy guided by, 1534-1535
  venography of, 1586
  venous outflow obstructive, 1534
Cisapride
  in intestinal pseudoobstruction, 669
  in small bowel studies, 524, 670
Cisplatin with Lipiodol, 1717-1718
Citro-Mag; see Magnesium citrate
Clay minerals as contrast, 308
Cleft, laryngotracheoesophageal, 212, 1829
Clindamycin, 231
Clinitest tablets, 235
Clonidine, 661
Clonorchis sinensis, 943
  cholangiocarcinoma from, 1680
  cholangitis in, 1312
    recurrent pyogenic, 1303, 1312
  in intrahepatic stones, 1350, 1351
Closed swallow, term, 129
Clostridium
  acquired immunodeficiency syndrome and,
      959
  in emphysematous cholecystitis, 2031
  in gas-forming infections, 2070
  in phlegmonous gastritis, 333, 334
  in pseudomembranous colitis, 2067
    plain films and contrast studies in, 2067
  ulcerative colitis versus, 604
Clotted blood; see Coagulation
Club appearance in congenital colonic atresia,
    1909
CMV; see Cytomegalovirus
CNR; see Contrast-to-noise ratio
Coagulation
  in corrosive gastropathy, 357
  disorders of, as contraindication to
      percutaneous transhepatic
      cholangiography, 1236, 1359, 1364
  in hemobilia, 1321
  in malabsorption, 80
Coaxial microcatheters, 2144
Cobalamin, 77
Cobblestone pattern
  in benign lymphoid hyperplasia of
      duodenum, 501
  in Crohn's disease, 475, 587, 591, 592, 599
  in esophagitis, 909
  in ulcerative colitis, 577
Cobra-head appearance in congenital colonic
    atresia, 1909
Coccidioides immitis, 1819
Cogan's syndrome, 656
Cogwheel appearance in sprue, 912, 913
Coil
  Gianturco, 2144, 2148
  in magnetic resonance imaging of colon,
      719

Coil embolization, 2144
  of hepatic artery, 1726
  of liver, 2148
  of renal vessels, 2149
Coiled-spring pattern of duodenum
  in intramural hematoma or bleeding, 503
  in intussusception, 472
Colchicine
  in Mediterranean fever, 678
  in small bowel malabsorption, 684-685
Cole LG, 7
Cole WH, 10, 11
Colectomy
  in familial multiple polyposis, 781
  in Gardner's syndrome, 783
  total, in ulcerative colitis, 584-585
Colic
  biliary, 1275
    after extracorporeal shock wave
        lithotripsy, 1360
    ultrasonography of, 2111-2112
  renal, 2070-2071
Colic vein, 30, 694, 1566
Colitis; see also Inflammatory bowel disease,
      idiopathic
  acute
    necrotizing, 2086-2087
    plain films and contrast studies in,
        2065-2068
    ulcerative, 2065
  amebic, 2067-2068
  in cow's milk allergy, 1925
  Crohn's; see Crohn's disease
  extensive, 580
  granulomatous; see Granulomatous colitis
  Hirschsprung's, 1925
  histologic, 580
  indeterminate or cross-over, 581, 582
  infectious, 1924
    Clostridium difficile in; see
        Pseudomembranous colitis
    Strongyloides in, 931-933
    tuberculosis in, 893
    Yersinia in, 1924-1925
  ischemic
    in carcinoma, 795
    computed tomography of, 613
    plain films and contrast studies in, 2068
    ultrasonography of, 615
  neutropenic
    in child, 1918, 1919
    computed tomography in, 2086
  in obstruction and carcinoma, 793-795
  pseudomembranous; see Pseudomembranous
      colitis
  radiographic features of types of, 581
  ulcerative; see Ulcerative colitis
Collapsible large-caliber metal endoprostheses,
    1407-1411
Collar button sign
  in peptic ulcer, 341, 342
  in ulcerative colitis, 576
Collimation in acute abdomen computed
    tomography, 2077
Colloid carcinoma of pancreas, 1152
Coloduodenal fistula, 475
Colon
  absorption in, 89
  aganglionosis of, total, 1914-1915
  amebiasis and, 917
  anatomy of, 725-726
    ascending, 28
    descending, 29
    models of, 692-696
    transverse, 32, 35

Colon—cont'd
  arteriovenous malformations of, portal
      hypertension and, 1598
  in Chagas' disease, 920-923
  cirrhosis with portal hypertension and,
      1598-1599, 1600
  colitis and; see Colitis
  in Crohn's disease, 600
    biopsy and, 602
  decompression of, in toxic dilatation, 712
  diverticula of; see Diverticula
  endometriosis in, 778-779
  endoscopy of, 715-716
    in carcinoma follow-up, 832
    in carcinoma screening, 835
  endosonography of, 725-727
    patient tolerance of, 727
  granulomatous colitis and; see
      Granulomatous colitis
  haustral pattern in, 1907
  hepatic flexure of, 29
  inflammation of; see Colitis
  inflammatory diseases of; see Inflammatory
      bowel disease, idiopathic
  intussusception in
    in carcinoma, 795, 796
    in child, 1900, 1902
  metastases in; see Metastases
  obstruction in; see Intestinal obstruction
  polyps in; see Polyp, colon
  pseudomembranous colitis in, 901-903; see
      also Pseudomembranous colitis
  reanastomosis of, with rectum, 752
  resection of
    in diverticulitis, 750
    in polyposis syndromes, 779
  sigmoid; see Sigmoid colon
  splenic flexure of, 31
  thumbprinting in, 901
  transit time in, 88
  transverse
    anatomy of, 32, 35
    bleeding in, 987, 990
  tuberculosis and strictures of, 893
  ulcerative colitis of; see Ulcerative colitis
  volvulus in; see Volvulus
Colon cutoff sign, 2034
Colonoscope, ultrasound, 716
Colonoscopy, 696-697, 698, 767-770, 976-978
  after abdominoperineal resection, 712
  bowel preparation for, 716
  in carcinoma therapy, 779
  before endosonography, 726
  flexible, in diverticulitis for differential
      diagnosis, 755-757
  flexible sigmoidoscopy before, 832
  in hereditary nonpolyposis colon cancer,
      836
  in inflammatory bowel disease, 608-609
  in neoplasia, 765-767, 768
  pain after, 700
  in pediatric ulcerative colitis, 1921
  resection after, 832
  in screening, 829, 832
    bias and, 831
  in strictures, 583
  therapeutic, 832
Color-flow imaging of liver, 1971
Colorectal carcinoma, 824-839; see also
      Carcinoma, of colon
  in average-risk individual, 835
  biopsy in, 809
  carcinogenesis of, 764-765
  compliance in, 829-830

Colorectal carcinoma—cont'd
  computed tomography of, 801-806,
        809-810; see also Large bowel,
        computed tomography of
    accuracy of, 805
    baseline, 809
    colon preparation and rectal contrast
        material in, 802
    complications and, 805-806
    distant metastases and, 804-805
    goals of imaging and, 801
    intravenous contrast in, 802-803
    lymph node metastases and, 803-804
    patient positioning and techniques of, 802
    primary carcinoma in, 803
    soft tissue stranding and, 809
    staging and, 809
    techniques for, 801-802
  costs of screening for, 834
  depth of tumor penetration in, 801
  diagnostic follow-up in, 832-833
  fine-needle aspiration cytology of, 809, 810
  first-degree relatives in, 836
  ^{18}F-Fluorodeoxyglucose uptake in, 810
  follow-up imaging of, 809-810
  goals of imaging studies of, 801
  hereditary nonpolyposis, 788-790
  immunoscintigraphy in, 811
  incidence of, 825
  magnetic resonance imaging in, 801, 806-810
    goals of, 801
  metastases of, 801
  monoclonal antibodies in, 810
  in obstruction, 2057
  pericolic changes in, 802
  in Peutz-Jeghers syndrome, 785, 786
  positron emission tomography of, 810
  prevention in, 829-836
  previous, 835
  rectosigmoid lesions in, 802
  recurrent, 809, 810
  in right colon, 802
  risk factors for, 765, 824-829
  screening for
    guidelines in, 835-836
    methodology in, 831-832
    principles of, 829-831
    results of, 833-835
  single-photon-emission computed
        tomography of, 811
  staging of, computed tomography of, 805
  ulcerated, computed tomography of, 803
  ulcerative colitis and, 583, 584
Colostomy
  in anorectal malformation, 1912
  enemas in, 712-713
  retrograde small bowel examination in, 524
Colovaginal fistula, 712, 793
Combined transhepatic-endoscopic approach in
        percutaneous interventional
        radiology, 1411-1414
Comet tail sign
  in focal nodular hyperplasia of liver, 1651
  in hyperplastic cholesterosis, 1289, 1291
Commode for defecography, 841, 842
Common bile duct
  absence of, 1259
  anatomy of, 28, 33-34, 47, 1225-1227
  calculi in; see also Choledocholithiasis
    in child, 1978
    cholangiocarcinoma versus, 1336
    cholangiography of, 1294-1296
    computed tomography of, 1298-1300
    extracorporeal shock wave lithotripsy for,
        1361

Common bile duct—cont'd
  calculi in—cont'd
    percutaneous endoscopy for, 1426-1427
    percutaneous transhepatic cholangiography
        of, 1240
    ultrasonography of, 1296-1298
  cholangiocarcinoma in, 1334
  cholecystography of evaluation of, 1229,
        1231
  choledochal cyst in, 1263
  computed tomography of, 1227
  diverticulum of, 1976, 1977
  draining into gallbladder, 1259
  for extraction of bile duct stones, 1367-1373
  in gallbladder ultrasonography, 1250
  low union of, with cystic and hepatic ducts,
        1258, 1259, 1260
  in pancreatic adenocarcinoma, 1108, 1122
  spontaneous perforation of, 1977-1978
  stenosis of, 1315-1316
  stenting of
    after percutaneous balloon repair,
        1394-1395
    palliative, 1433
  strictures of, 1315-1316
    in chronic calcific pancreatitis, 1098
    percutaneous dilation in; see Percutaneous
        biliary stricture dilation
  thickening of wall of, 1299, 1301
  variants and anomalies of, 1258-1259, 1260
Common hepatic artery, 28
Common hepatic duct
  anatomy of, 1225
  bifurcation of, 1223, 1224
    endoscopic palliation in tumors at, 1434,
        1435
  chemotherapy-induced strictures of, 1311
  cholangiocarcinoma in, 1334
  cholecystography of, 1229, 1231
  computed tomography of, 1232
  entry and technical approach to, 1402-1403
  for extraction of bile duct stones, 1367-1373
  fistulas of, 1316
  magnetic resonance imaging of, 1236
  in pancreatic carcinoma with strictures, 1435
  percutaneous biliary stricture dilation in; see
        Percutaneous biliary stricture dilation
  trifurcation of, 1256, 1257
  ultrasonography of, 1229, 1249
  variants and anomalies of, 1258-1259, 1260
Common iliac artery, 29, 30, 31
Common iliac vein, 29
Common variable hypoglobulinemic states,
        676
Compartments
  intraperitoneal, 35, 54
  prestyloid and poststyloid, 106, 110
  retroperitoneal, 63
Compliance
  in colorectal cancer screening, 829-830
  rectal, 841
Compression radiography
  in biphasic enteroclysis with
        methylcellulose, 533, 541
  in dedicated small bowel follow-through
        examination, 566
  for small bowel barium examination, 514,
        517
  sonographic schematic for, 2102
Computed tomography; see also specific organ
  of acute abdomen, 2076-2098; see also
        Acute abdomen, computed
        tomography of
  after pull-through surgery in anorectal
        malformation, 1912

Computed tomography—cont'd
  in appendicitis, 2031
    versus graded-compression sonography,
        2085
  in bacterial cholangitis, 1305-1306
  in Bochdalek's hernia, 255
  in Caroli's disease, 1271
  in cholangiocarcinoma, 1334, 1336-1338
  in cholecystitis, 1281, 1283, 1284
    with gallbladder wall thickening, 1286,
        1287
  in choledochal cyst, 1266, 1267
  in choledochoceles, 1269
  in choledocholithiasis, 1298-1300,
        1301-1303
  in cirrhosis, 1539-1541, 1542
  in Crohn's disease in child, 1924
  in diverticulitis, 2034
  dual-energy, in hemochromatosis, 1563
  dynamic
    in hepatic metastases, 1706, 1715
    in hepatocellular carcinoma, 1669, 1673
    incremental bolus; see Incremental
        dynamic bolus computed tomography
        of liver
    of liver, 1455, 1456
    liver transplantation and, 1736,
        1737-1738
    of portal and hepatic veins, 1446-1447
  in graft infection in aortoduodenal fistula
        repair, 501
  in hemobilia, 1321
  in hemochromatosis, 1563
  history of, 17-19
  in intussusception, 2054
  of oral cavity malignancy, 148, 149, 151
  in percutaneous biliary dilation of strictures,
        1383
  in percutaneous chemolithiasis, 1378, 1379
  in percutaneous cholecystolithotomy,
        1376-1378
  in pericholecystic abscess, 1286
  of porta hepatis, 53, 1225
  of portal and hepatic veins, delayed, 1447
  in primary sclerosing cholangitis,
        1308-1310, 1311
  in sequence of biliary tract stone disease,
        1302
  single-energy, in hemochromatosis, 1563
  in subphrenic and subhepatic abscess, 2037
  ultrafast, 1453
Computed tomography angiography,
        1459-1463
  contrast in, 1459
  in hepatocellular carcinoma, 1688-1690
  of liver, number of hepatic tumor nodules
        in, 1463, 1464
  in liver metastases, 1706
  perfusion abnormalities with, 1460-1462
  two-scan cluster technique in, 1459
Computed tomography arterial portography,
        1460-1463
  in cirrhosis, 1540
  in hepatic metastases, 1715
  of hepatic vein, 1447-1448
  in hepatocellular carcinoma, 1688-1690
  of liver, number of hepatic tumor nodules
        in, 1463, 1464
  in liver metastases, 1706-1707
  perfusion abnormalities in, 1461, 1462-1463
  in portal hypertension, 1462
  of portal vein, 1447-1449
    in obstruction, 1461
  relative contrast attenuation in, 1458
  three-dimensional, 1448-1449

Computed tomography arterial
    portography—cont'd
  through superior mesenteric artery, 1462
Condemned mucosa theory, 144
Congenital abnormalities; *see also* Vascular
    abnormalities
  absence of diaphragm in, 255
  of amino acid transport, 79-80
  of biliary tract, 1976-1977
  of diaphragm and esophagogastric junction
      in child, 1853-1858
  of duodenum, 467-473; *see also* Duodenum,
      congenital abnormalities of
  of esophagus, of child, 1839-1844
  of gallbladder, 1251-1255
  hepatic arteriovenous fistulas in, 1617
  with hernias in child, 1853-1858
  of large bowel, 1908, 1909-1912
  of pancreas, 1039-1051, 1946-1950; *see
      also* Pancreas, congenital
      abnormalities of
  of pharynx, 1829-1831
  in polycystic liver disease, 1658
  of portal vein, 1622
  of small bowel, 1878-1891; *see also* Small
      bowel, congenital anomalies of
  of stomach, 318-325, 1865-1866; *see also*
      Stomach, congenital abnormalities of
  of vena cava, 1819-1820
Congenital arterioportal fistula, 1574
Congenital colonic atresia, 1908-1909
Congenital heart defects, 1766, 1767
Congenital hepatic cysts, 1967-1968, 1969
Congenital hepatic fibrosis, 1270
  presinusoidal portal hypertension in, 1574
Congenital short pancreas, 1947
Congenital splenic cyst, 1938-1939
Congestive heart failure
  dynamic computed tomography of, 1446
  technetium 99m sulfur colloid hepatic
      scintigraphy of, 1522
Congo red solution, 498, 499
Connective tissue
  of colon, cystlike stoma of, 787
  esophageal motility and, 206-207
Constipation
  colon studies in, 713
  in diverticulitis, 751
  in inspissation after barium enema, 714
  iron in, 90
  pediatric, 1915, 1916
Constrictor muscles, pharyngeal
  in functional abnormalities of swallowing,
      130-133
  tongue and, 154-156, 157
Contained stone sign in gallbladder imaging,
      1327, 1328
Continent ileostomy, 585
Contrast agents
  for acute abdomen, 2020-2075; *see also*
      Acute abdomen, plain films and
      contrast studies in
  adverse reactions to, 287
  in barium meal, volume of, 287
  barium sulfate in; *see* Barium; Barium
      examination
  in biphasic enteroclysis with
      methylcellulose, 534
  for brachial arch anomalies, 1829, 1830
  for colon, 697, 699-703
    negative, in computed tomography, 802
    radiologic caveats and, 795
  in computed tomography
    of biliary tract, 1231
    of colon, 718, 802, 803

Contrast agents—cont'd
  in computed tomography—cont'd
    of colorectal carcinoma, 802-803
    for diverticular abscess, 755
    of diverticulitis, 753-754
    of esophagus, 270
    of inflammatory bowel disease, 610
    of rectum, 802
    of small bowel, 530
  in computed tomography angiography, 1459
  for Crohn's disease, 1892
  in defecography, 842, 844
  for diaphragm and esophagogastric junction,
      1860
  in diverticulitis, 755-759
  in duodenal diverticula, 469
  in duodenal perforation, 297
  in duodenal trauma study, 502
  in duodenal wall in endoscopic retrograde
      cholangiopancreatography, 1241
  in esophageal atresia, 1840
  in esophageal perforation, 1850
  in esophageal varices, 241
  in esophagography, 192
  in hepatic angiography, 1605
  in intussusception imaging, 1902
  in islet cell tumors, 1177
  in jejunal or ileal atresia or stenosis, 1885
  in liver angiography, 1604
  in magnetic resonance imaging
    of liver, 1496-1503
    of stomach and duodenum, 307
  in meconium ileus, 1886
  in pancreatic adenocarcinoma imaging,
      1112-1113, 1114
  in pancreatic transplantation rejection, 1207
  percutaneous injection of, through anal
      dimple, 1912
  in percutaneous intervention in malignant
      biliary tract disease, 1405
  in postoperative studies of stomach and
      duodenum, 297-298
  in radiographs before obesity surgery, 458,
      460
  in small bowel, 530, 638, 690, 1881, 1885
  for small bowel congenital anomalies, 1881
  in small bowel lymphoma, 638
  for spleen in bolus administration for child,
      1932
  stalactite phenomenon of, 287
  superparamagnetic iron oxide; *see* Iron oxide
      contrast agents
  water-soluble, 288, 306
    for biliary tract, 1231
    for colon, 700, 711-712, 718, 802
    in defecography, 842
    for duodenum, 297
    for gastrointestinal perforation, 297, 2077
    in Hirschsprung's disease, 1914
    in meconium plug/small left hemicolon
        syndrome, 1915
    radiologic caveats and, 795
Contrast enema
  in colonic neoplasms, 765-767, 768
  in colonic polyps, 765-767, 768
  in diverticulitis, computed tomography
      versus, 757-759
  in Hirschsprung's disease, 1914
  in meconium plug/small left hemicolon
      syndrome, 1915, 1916
  in milk curd syndrome, 1915
  in stricture, in neonatal necrotizing
      enterocolitis, 1918
  water-soluble, 711-712
Contrast-to-noise ratio, 1486, 1487

Contrast tracer studies in small bowel
    obstruction, 2047
Cook catheter, 1407, 1408
Cook ureteral stone basket, 1367, 1368
Cope catheter, 1377, 1407, 1408
Cope loop, 2014
Copper, accumulation of, 1492, 1699-1700
Corkscrew appearance of hepatic artery, 1545,
    1619, 1620
Cormack, AM, 18, 19
Corn oil emulsion, 306, 530
Coronary ligament, 30, 31
Coronary vein, 30
Coronocaval shunt, 1588, 1589
Corrected sinusoidal pressure, 1583
  hepatic vein catheterization and, 1607
Corrosive esophagitis, 1847
Corrosive gastritis in child, 1870
Corrosive gastropathy, 357, 359
Corticosteroids; *see* Steroids
Corticotropinoma, 1172
Costs
  of colorectal cancer screening, 834
  of endoscopy of stomach and duodenum,
      300-301
  of gastric cancer screening, 427
Cotrimoxazole, 903
Cotte, G, 13
Couinaud nomenclature of liver segments,
      1440-1444
  hepatic resection and, 1469
Coumadin, 2092
Cowden's disease, 786-787, 1926
  polyp distribution and malignancy risk in,
      1928
Cow's milk allergy, 1925
  in celiac disease, 666, 668
Coxsackievirus, 228
Cranial nerves in swallowing, 98-101
Creatine in pancreatic transplantation, 1197
Creatinine in Brunner's gland hyperplasia, 499
Creeping fat, 597
Crescent sign, 341, 342-345
Cricopharyngeal achalasia, 1828
Cricopharyngeal bar, 74
Cricopharyngeal impression in barium
      examination, 1829
Cricopharyngeal muscle, 133, 187
  abnormalities of, 74
  hypoglossal tumors and, 158
Cricopharyngeal myotomy, 133
Cricopharyngeal web, 120
Crohn's disease, 330, 332, 333, 585-603,
    1920-1924; *see also* Granulomatous
      colitis; Granulomatous enterocolitis
  accuracy of radiographic examination in,
      600-603
  barium examination of, 1892
  basic pattern in, 596-599
  in child, 1892, 1921-1924
  classification of, 594-595
  clinical features of, 585-587
  cobblestoning in, 571
  colonoscopy in, 609
  colorectal carcinoma and, 829
  complications of, 601-603
  contrast media for, 1892
  differential diagnosis in, 603-608
  diverticula in, small bowel stasis and, 669
  double-contrast enteroclysis with air in, 549,
      551
  duodenitis in, 473-475
  endoscopy of, 585-588
  esophagitis in, 232
  extraintestinal manifestations of, 588-589

Crohn's disease—cont'd
  gastritis in, 1869, 1870, 1872
  granulomas in, 553, 554
  intestinal permeability in, 82
  linear ulcers in, 572
  magnetic resonance imaging of, 617, 618
  malabsorption in, 80
  mesenteric pathology in, 1821
  percutaneous abscess drainage in, 2005
  portal hypertension in, 1599
  primary sclerosing cholangitis in, 1307
  radiographic features of, 589-600, 601, 602
    advanced disease in, 590-591, 592, 593
    early disease in, 589-590
    esophageal, gastric, and duodenal,
        599-600
    intermediate disease in, 590
    large bowel, 589-594
    small bowel, 595-599
  recurrence of, 593-594
  retroperitoneal inflammation in, 1818
  reversibility of, 593
  severity of disease in, 594-595
  small bowel follow-through study of, 1892,
      1893
  small bowel lymphoma in, 635
  small bowel meal with pneumocolon in,
      519, 521
  small bowel mesentery in, 1822
  small bowel obstruction in, 2048
  in small bowel other than terminal ileum,
      599
  surgery in, 609
  ulcerative colitis versus, 603-608
  ulceronodular form of, 599-600, 601, 602
  ultrasonography of, 526, 527, 528, 615, 616
    abscess in, 2100
    pediatric, 1892, 1894
Cronkhite-Canada syndrome, 787
  polyp distribution and malignancy risk in,
      1928
  in small bowel neoplasms, 632
  in stomach tumors, 376-377
Crooks, LE, 21
Crosby-Kugler capsule, 552, 553
Cross-sectional imaging, history of, 16-22; *see
      also* specific technique
Crura of diaphragm, 32
  in esophageal endosonography, 189, 190
Crural margin of esophageal hiatus, 29
Cryoglobulinemia, 656
Cryosurgery in liver neoplasms, 1720
Crypt abscesses, 573
Cryptitis, 573
Cryptococcosis, 1311-1312
Cryptosporidiosis
  in acquired immunodeficiency syndrome,
      671, 673, 955-957
  in duodenal disease, 476, 477
  in gastritis, 333
  in primary immunodeficiency syndromes,
      676
  in small bowel inflammatory changes, 677
  ulcerative colitis versus colitis from, 604
Crypts of Lieberkühn
  abscesses of, 573
  adenoma of, 488
  benign gastric carcinoid and, 384
CSP; *see* Corrected sinusoidal pressure
CT; *see* Computed tomography
Cushing's syndrome, 1180
Cut-film technique in therapeutic embolization,
      2149
Cutaneous jejunostomy, 1383
Cyatic artery, 1608, 1609

Cyclic adenosine monophosphate, 90
Cyclooxygenase, 72
Cyclosporine
  after liver transplantation, 1735, 1739, 1748
  in rare focal liver lesion increase, 1480
Cylindroma, esophageal, 243
Cyst
  brachial, 1829, 1830
  bronchogenic, 270
  choledochal; *see* Choledochal cyst
  duplication
    of duodenum, 471
    enteric, 1888-1889
    of stomach, 318, 319
  embryonal, 318
  enterogenic, 471
  epidermoid splenic
    in child, 1938
    ultrasonography of, 2115, 2116
  esophageal, 252
  foregut, 1843-1844
  gastroenteric, 1843
  in giant cell carcinoma of pancreas, 1153
  glandular, of fundus, 376
  hepatic; *see* Liver, cysts of
  hydatid, 1657, 1776
  inclusion, 781
  as lithotripsy contraindication, 1359, 1361
  in meconium peritonitis, 1891
  mesenteric
    in child, 1888-1889
    ultrasonography of, 1888, 1889
  neurenteric, 1843
  omental
    in child, 1888-1889
    ultrasonography of, 1888, 1889
  of omphalomesenteric duct, 1889
  pancreatic; *see* Pancreas, cysts of
  in peritoneal cavity mesothelioma, 1803
  pharyngeal, congenital, 1832
  pseudocysts and
    ectopic, 1034
    false-positive, 1035
  sebaceous, in Gardner's syndrome, 781
  splenic; *see* Spleen, cysts of
  thyroglossal duct, 126
  in valleculae, 114, 115
Cystadenocarcinoma
  biliary, 1681-1682
  pancreatic, 1036, 1133, 1134
    imaging procedures in, 1146-1149
    macrocystic, 1136, 1141-1149
    microcystic, 1136, 1138-1141
    microcystic and macrocystic, 1136
Cystadenoma
  biliary, 1681-1682
    ultrasonography of, 1476
  glycogen-rich, term, 1138
  pancreatic, 1036
    ductectatic mucinous, 1133, 1136, 1137,
        1138, 1146
    endoscopic retrograde
        cholangiopancreatography of, 1127,
        1128
Cystic adenomatous malformation of lung,
      1856
Cystic dilatation of intrahepatic bile ducts,
      1270-1271, 1976
Cystic disease of kidney in Caroli's disease,
      1270
Cystic duct
  ablation of, percutaneous, 1382-1383
  absence of, 1262
  after liver transplantation, occlusion of,
      1743-1744

Cystic duct—cont'd
  anatomy of, 29, 34, 1225, 1226
  anomalous ducts draining into, 1258, 1259
  in bile duct variants and anomalies,
      1259-1262
  in biliary tract and gallbladder computed
      tomography, 1232-1233
  calculi in
    in acute cholecystitis, 1275, 1276, 1279
    endoscopic retrograde
        cholangiopancreatography of, 1351,
        1353
    extracorporeal shock wave lithotripsy in,
        1362-1364
    impacted, 1372
    transcholecystic extraction of, 1373-1374
  double, 1260-1262
  low union of, with hepatic and common bile
      ducts, 1258, 1259, 1260
  variations in insertion of, 1260, 1261
Cystic fibrosis
  barium examination in, 1897
  bile ducts in, 1320
  cholelithiasis in, in child, 1981
  inspissation in, 713
  large bowel in, 1930
  meconium peritonitis in, 1891
  in pancreas, 1157
  small bowel in, 684, 1896-1897
    duodenal, 506
Cystic islet cell tumors, 1157-1158
Cystic lesions in von Hipple–Lindau disease,
      1954
Cystic mesenchymal hamartoma of liver,
      1966, 1968
Cystic mesothelioma in peritoneal cavity, 1803
Cystic pneumatosis, 2068-2069; *see also*
      Pneumatosis, intramural
Cystic teratoma, 1158, 1160
Cystic tumors of pancreas
  in child, 1954, 1955
  mucinous, 1141-1149
  papillary, 1134-1135, 1149-1152, 1954,
      1955
Cystitis, emphysematous, 2070
Cystoduodenostomy, 1097
Cystogastrostomy, 1096, 1097
Cystography in pancreatic transplantation,
      1214, 1221
Cystohepatic ducts, 1257, 1258
Cystoscintigraphy after pancreatic
      transplantation, 1221
Cystourethrography after pancreatic
      transplantation, 1221
Cytology, aspiration
  fine-needle; *see* Fine-needle aspiration
      cytology
  in pancreatic mucinous adenomas, 1149
Cytology brush in biliary endoscopy, 1430
Cytomegalovirus
  in acquired immunodeficiency syndrome,
      553, 554
    small bowel enteropathy in, 671, 675
  in duodenal disease, 476, 477
  in esophageal infection, 183, 228-229
    in acquired immunodeficiency syndrome,
        955, 956
  in gastritis, 333
  in typhlitis, 2104
  ulcerative colitis versus, 604
Cytoprotection, 72

D

D cells, 69, 87, 1167
Dally, C, 3

Damadian, R, 19-21
Dapsone, 663
Debridement of pancreas, 2003
Decompensation in pharyngeal imaging, 106, 107-109, 133-137
Decompression
 biliary, 1399, 1400; *see also* Percutaneous interventional radiology, in malignant biliary tract disease
 of small bowel, 2011
 of stomach, 2011
Dedicated small bowel study, 514-515, 516, 517
 in inflammatory bowel disease, 566-567
 in irritable bowel syndrome, 686
Defecation, defecography of; *see* Defecography
Defecography
 anal canal in, 845, 846, 847
 anatomy and physiology in, 840-841
 anorectal angle in, 845-847, 848
 anorectal junction level in, 845, 847
 changes during, 847-850
 commode for, 842
 in defecation changes, 849
 equipment for, 841
 examination procedure for, 841-845
 history of use of, 10
 normal appearances in, 845-850
 in pelvic floor descent on defecation, 849
 recording of rectal evacuation in, 842-844
 rectal wall configuration in, 849-850
 rectovaginal septum in, 847
 in straining, 849
 techniques of, 841-844
 vaginal opacification in, 841-842
Deficiency states, immunoglobulin, 671-677
Deglutition; *see* Swallowing
Dehiscence, staple line, 460-461, 462, 464
Delayed computed tomography of portal and hepatic veins, 1447
Delayed iodine scan
 in colon imaging, 1458-1459
  in metastasis, 1461
 in liver imaging, 1461, 1462, 1464
  in metastasis, 1706, 1707
Delta cells, 1167
Dermatologic disease
 in Crohn's disease, 589
 in ulcerative colitis, 574
Dermatomyositis, 1904
Dermatoses, bullous
 in esophageal strictures, 235, 236, 238
 in esophagitis, 232
DES; *see* Diffuse esophageal spasm
Descending colon, 29
Descending duodenum, 29
Desmin, antibodies against, 555
Desmoid
 in mesentery, 1824
 in retroperitoneum, 1813, 1814
Developmental anomalies; *see also* Congenital abnormalities
 of diaphragm and esophagogastric junction, 1853-1858
 of large bowel, 1908, 1909-1912
 of pancreas, 1946-1947
 of stomach, 1865-1866
Dextran, 1499
Dextrocardia, 1865
Diabetes
 dysphagia in, 136
 esophageal motor function and, 209
 gastric atony and, 362
 in hemochromatosis, 1560

Diabetes—cont'd
 pancreatic transplant in, 1197; *see also* Pancreatic transplantation
 pericholecystic abscess and, 1285
 pneumocolon for small bowel examination for, 516
 in somatostatinoma, 1172
Diamagnetic agents in magnetic resonance imaging, 308
Diaphragm, 255-256
 anatomy of, 29, 32
 antral, 320-322, 323
 congenital absence of, 255
 crura of, 30, 31, 32
  in esophageal endosonography, 189, 190
 in duodenum, congenital, 467
 and esophagogastric junction in child, 1853-1864
  barium examination of, 1860
  Bochdalek's hernia versus eventration in, 1856
  congenital and developmental anomalies of, 1853-1858
  contrast study of, 1860
  eventration in, 1856, 1857
  fluoroscopy of, 1859
  in gastroesophageal reflux, 1859-1863
  hiatus hernia in, 1859-1863
  paralysis of, 1858-1863
  scintigraphy of, 1860-1861
  total absence of diaphragm in, 1858
  ultrasonography of, 1859, 1860
 rupture of, in trauma, 2153
 screening for subphrenic and subhepatic abscess in, 2036
 sliding hiatus hernia of, 256
 ultrasonography of, 256
 unilateral elevation of, 256
Diaphragmatic fibers, costal, 32
Diaphragmatic hiatus, esophageal, 219
Diarrhea, 89-90
 from contrast agents, 1230
 in Cronkhite-Canada syndrome, 787
 in diverticulitis, 751
 in ulcerative colitis, 573
 in VIPoma, 1171
Diathermy
 in bleeding ulcer hemostasis, 972
 in endoscopic sphincterotomy, 1346
Diathesis, bleeding, 1400, 1987
Diatrizoate meglumine, 1718
 in colon studies, 700, 711-712, 718
  for constipation, 713
 in gastric and duodenal studies, 305
 in small bowel studies, 530
 in suspected duodenal perforation, 297
Diazemul; *see* Diazepam
Diazepam
 in biphasic enteroclysis with methylcellulose, 534
 before esophageal endosonography, 264
 before gastric endoscopy, 302
 in percutaneous biliary tract intervention, 1401
 in percutaneous cholangioscopy, 1424
Diet
 colon imaging and, 697
 in diverticulitis, 750
Dieulafoy lesion, 974-975, 977
Diffuse endocrine system, 67
Diffuse esophageal spasm, 204, 211
Diffuse familial polyposis, 780; *see also* Familial multiple polyposis
Diffuse hepatic parenchymal disease, 1469-1471

Diffuse primary small bowel lymphoma, 677
Diffuse pyloric hypertrophy, 324-325
Digestion
 in duodenum and small bowel, 79-83; *see also* Gastrointestinal tract, physiology of
 esophagus and, 73-75
 in stomach, 75-79
Digestive enzymes in esophageal perforation, 216
Digital subtraction angiography
 in hepatic angiography, 1605-1606
 in hepatic vein catheterization, 1607
 in pancreatic transplantation, 1202
Digitization of fluoroscopic image, 844
Dilatation
 balloon; *see* Balloon
 esophageal, 210-211
Dilation
 gastric, in intestinal obstruction, 2042-2043, 2044, 2045
 of intrahepatic bile ducts in Caroli's disease, 1976
2,6-Dimethylphenylcarbamoylethyl iminodiacetic acid, 1233
Diphtheria, 136
Diphyllobothrium latum, 931-933
DIS; *see* Delayed iodine scan
Disaccharides, 79
Disease
 Alzheimer's, 133
 Behçet's; *see* Behçet's syndrome
 Byler's, 1977
 Caroli's; *see* Caroli's disease
 Chagas'; *see* Chagas' disease
 Cowden's; *see* Cowden's disease
 Crohn's; *see* Crohn's disease
 Duhring's, 663
 Hirschsprung's, 1913-1914, 1925
 Hodgkin's; *see* Hodgkin's disease
 Kawasaki; *see* Kawasaki disease
 Ménétrier's; *see* Ménétrier's disease
 Osler-Weber-Rendu; *see* Hereditary hemorrhagic telangiectasia
 Parkinson's, 133
 von Hippel–Lindau; *see* von Hippel–Lindau disease
 von Recklinghausen's; *see* von Recklinghausen's disease
 Weber-Christian, 1823
 Whipple's; *see* Whipple's disease
 Wilson's, 133, 1663
Dissection of hepatic artery, 1611, 1613
Disse's space, 84, 85
Diverticula
 abscess around, percutaneous drainage of, 2005-2006
 of colon, 730-749
  air- or stool-filled, as artifact, 772
  barium enema in, 709
  classification of, 747
  complications of, 744-745
  differential diagnosis of, 742-744
  diseases coexisting with, 745-747
  diverticulitis as, 739-742
  incidence of, 731-732
  method of examination of, 730-731
  muscular abnormality in, 737-739
  pathogenesis of, 732-737
  ultrasonography of, 716-717
 of common bile duct, 1976, 1977
 of duodenum, 468-469
  fluid-filled, 469
  intraluminal, 469-471

Diverticula—cont'd
  of duodenum—cont'd
    periampullary, choledocholithiasis versus,
      1300
    pulsion, 469
  esophageal, 214-216
    intramural, 215, 216
  of gallbladder, 1255
  gastric, 318, 319, 320
    partial, 318
  gastrointestinal physiology and, 88
  inflamed, sonography of, 2105
  intrahepatic duct, outpouchings of, 1307,
    1309
  Killian-Jamieson's, 118, 119
  Meckel's; see Meckel's diverticulum
  perforation of, in acute diverticulitis, 2034
  of pharynx, 1831-1832
  small bowel, in stasis, 669
  Zenker's; see Zenker's diverticulum
    pharyngeal perforation in, 115
Diverticular abscess, 752-753, 759
  formation of, 755
  paracolic, percutaneous drainage of, 752
Diverticulitis
  acute, 2034, 2035
    computed tomography of, 2085-2086
    ultrasonography of, 2104-2106
  cecal, 2083
  of colon
    in carcinoma, 793, 806
    computed tomography of, 613
    peritonitis and, 2078
    resection and, 750
  computed tomography of, 753-759,
    2085-2086
    in cecum, 2083
    in colon, 613
    contrast enema study versus, 757-759
    differential diagnosis in, 754-757, 758
    indications for, 759
    technique for, 753-754
  contrast enema in, versus computed
    tomography, 757-759
  cross-sectional imaging of, 750-761
    clinical presentation in, 751
    computed tomography in, 753-759
    pathophysiology in, 750-751
    right-sided, 759-760
    sonography in, 760
    treatment and, 751-753
  diet and, 750
  duodenal, 469
  epidemiology of, 750
  muscular hypertrophy in, 751
  perforation in, 751
  plain films and contrast studies in, 2034,
    2035
  segmentation in, 750
  of sigmoid colon
    computed tomography of, 613
    peritonitis and, 2078
  of small bowel mesentery, 1822-1823
  ultrasonography of, 615-616, 2104-2106
Diverticulosis
  in Crohn's disease, 601-602
  gastrointestinal bleeding in, 983
DNA analysis, flow cytometry, 829
Doppler ultrasonography; see also Duplex
    Doppler imaging
  of duodenal varices, 501
  history of use of, 17
  of liver and biliary tract, 1246, 1480-1481
    in focal nodular hyperplasia, 1651

Doppler ultrasonography—cont'd
  of liver and biliary tract—cont'd
    in hepatic artery thrombosis after
      transplantation, 1744
    in portal venous shunts, 1575-1577
    in primary malignant neoplasms, 1477,
      1478
  of mesenteric blood vessels, 526
  in pancreatic transplantation, 1203
  in vascular complications, 1214
Dormia ureteral stone basket
  in biliary stent exchange, 1431
  in percutaneous choledocholithotomy, 1367,
    1367
Dotted-line sign, 1537-1538
Double-arc shadow sign, 1248
Double-barrel shotgun sign, 1249
Double-bubble sign, 468, 2044
  in pediatric annular pancreas, 1946
  in pediatric duodenal atresia and stenosis,
    1884
Double-bulb effect in antral diaphragm or web,
    322
Double-channel esophagus, 218
Double-contrast barium enema, 704-711; see
    also Double-contrast examination
  choice of, versus single-contrast enema, 711
  contraindications to, 701
  in Crohn's disease, 1921, 1922
  in generalized juvenile gastrointestinal
    polyposis, 1929
  in growth rate determination of colonic
    neoplasia, 776
  instant, 712
  in juvenile polyposis coli, 1929
  in neoplasia, 765-767, 768-770
    colonoscopy in, 768, 769, 770
  in neoplasia screening, 835
  in pediatric lymphoid hyperplasia, 1907
  problem solving in, 710
  sigmoid flush after, 709
  sigmoid loop and, 692
  in toxic dilatation of colon, 565
  in trichuriasis, 938
  in ulcerative colitis, 1920, 1921
  variations of, 707-710
Double-contrast enteroclysis with air, 548-551
  problems in, 550, 551
  technique for, 548-550
Double-contrast examination
  in amyloidosis, 681, 682
  in biphasic enteroclysis with
    methylcellulose, 534, 535-539, 540,
    541
  of colon; see Double-contrast barium enema
  in Crohn's disease, 589
    with reflux from cecum, 595
  in dedicated small bowel follow-through
    examination, 566
  of duodenum, 467
    in adenomas, 492
    hypotonic; see Hypotonic duodenography
    in nonepithelial tumors, 496
  of esophagus, 171, 172, 176-177
    in Barrett's esophagitis, 226
    in carcinoma, 249
    in reflux esophagitis, 222
  in familial multiple polyposis, 780
  history of use of, 8, 10
  in juvenile polyps, 1926
  morbidity for, 832
  nontube, 522-524
  in peptic ulcer disease, 478
  in pharyngography, 103-106

Double-contrast examination—cont'd
  in pneumocolon for small bowel
    examination, 517, 518-523
  and small bowel barium examination, biopsy
    and, 555, 557
  of small bowel with oral effervescent agent,
    522-524
  in ulcerative colitis, 579, 580, 581
Double-contrast pharyngography, 103-106
Double-contrast small bowel radiography; see
    Enteroclysis, biphasic, with
    methylcellulose
Double-duct sign in pancreas, 1434
Double-halo sign in intestinal ischemia, 2090
Double-loop ileostomy, 567
Double-target sign, 1959, 1960
Douglas, pouch of, 1799-1800
Dournier lithotriptor, 1094, 1101
Doxorubicin
  radiation esophagitis and, 232
  in transcatheter embolization of liver
    neoplasm, 1717-1718
Doxycycline
  in esophageal ring strictures, 235
  esophagitis from, 230, 231
DP 2.5, 827
Dracunculus medinensis, 934, 937
Dromedary hump of kidney, 29, 63
DTPA; see Gadolinium-diethylenetriamine
    pentaacetic acid
Duct; see also Bile duct; Common bile duct;
    Common hepatic duct; Hepatic duct;
    Pancreatic duct
  of Santorini; see Santorini, duct of
  of Wirsung
    calculi in, 1101
    embryology of, 1039
    pediatric, 1946
    variations in, 1040, 1041
Ductectatic mucinous cystadenoma in
    pancreas, 1133
  endoscopic retrograde
    cholangiopancreatography of, 1136,
    1137, 1138, 1146
Duhring's disease, 663
Dukes classification
  of colon carcinoma, 805
    fecal occult-blood test and, 831
    uncontrolled trials in screening procedures
      and, 834
  of rectal carcinoma, 813
Dulcolax; see Bisacodyl
Dumbbell tumors of duodenum, 496
Dumping syndrome, 455
Duodenal atresia and stenosis
  antenatal ultrasonography and, 1884
  in child, 1884, 1885
Duodenal bulb, 284
  pedunculated polyp in, 489
  sessile adenoma at, 490
  ulcer disease of, 483, 484
Duodenal cap, 284
Duodenal ulcer; see Peptic ulcer disease
Duodenal wall
  cysts of, 471
  perforation of, in endoscopic retrograde
    cholangiopancreatography, 1241
Duodenectomy, partial, 496
Duodenitis; see Duodenum, inflammations in
Duodenobiliary fistula, 475
Duodenocholecystic fistula, 487
Duodenocholedochal fistula, 487
Duodenocolic fistula, 475, 487
Duodenoenterocutaneous fistula, 475
Duodenography, hypotonic, 296

Duodenojejunal flexure, 29, 469
Duodenoscope
  in biliary endoscopy, 1430
  in biliary stent exchange, 1430
  with diathermy sphincterotome, 1345
Duodenum, 467-511
  ampulla of; *see* Ampulla, duodenal
  amyloidosis in, 508
  anatomy of, 35, 284-285, 306-307
    ascending portion, 29
    descending portion, 29
    duodenal bulb in, 29
    duodenal papilla in, 284-285; *see also*
      Ampulla, duodenal
    in endosonography, 314-316
    mucosal pattern in, 284
    transverse portion, 29
      sections through, 60
    variants in, 285-286
  arteriovenous malformations of, 1596
  barium examination of, 286-297
    biphasic, 296
    in bleeding, 298
    Buscopan in, 288
    in congenital abnormalities, 467, 469
    contraindications to, 286
    contrast media in, 287-288
    in Crohn's disease, 475
    in cryptosporidiosis, 477
    in cytomegalovirus disease, 477
    double-contrast, 289-296
    in duodenal wall cysts, 471
    gas-producing agents in, 288-289
    glucagon in, 288
    historical perspective of, 286
    hypotonic duodenography in, 296-297
    indications for, 286
    in intraluminal diverticula, 471
    modified postoperative, 297-298
    in nonepithelial tumors, 496
    paralysis of peristalsis in, 288
    patient preparation for, 286-287
    roles of, 298-301
    single-contrast, 289
    in superior mesenteric artery compression
      syndrome, 506
    in suspected perforation, 297
    techniques for, 289
  benign diseases of, 467-488, 489-492,
    498-508
    adenoma in, 488, 489-492
    celiac disease in, 506
    congenital and miscellaneous, 467-473;
      see also Duodenum, congenital
      abnormalities of
    cystic fibrosis in, 506
    gastrinoma in, 1170
    inflammations in, 473-477; *see also*
      Duodenum, inflammations in
    as part of extensive disease, 506-508
    peptic disease in, 477-488; *see also* Peptic
      ulcer disease, duodenal
    somatostatinoma in, 1171-1172
    tumorlike lesions in, 498-501
    vascular abnormalities in, 501-506
    venous congestion in, 508
    in Whipple's disease, 506
  biopsy of
    in cytomegalovirus disease, 477
    in heterotopic gastric mucosa, 477
    in nonspecific duodenitis, 473
  cirrhosis with portal hypertension and,
    1596-1598
  computed tomography of, 305, 306-307
    in adenoma, 492

Duodenum—cont'd
  computed tomography of—cont'd
    in carcinoid, 492
    in carcinoma, 493
    in Crohn's disease, 475
    in cytomegalovirus disease, 477
    diagnostic accuracy in, 305
    in diverticulitis, 469
    in duodenal wall cysts, 471
    gas-contrast technique in, 306
    hematoma in, 1896, 1897
    in intramural hematoma or bleeding, 504
    in lipoma, 496
    in non-Hodgkin's lymphoma, 496
    in nonepithelial tumors, 496, 4979
    in perforation of ulcer, 487
    periampullary region of, 1110
    pseudotumor in, 306
    transverse, 61
    in trauma, 502, 1896, 2133-2134
    in Whipple's disease, 506
  congenital abnormalities of, 467-473
    annular pancreas in, 467-468
    antral mucosal prolapse in, 471, 472
    atresia and stenosis in, 1884, 1885
    diaphragm in, 467
    dilatation in, 467, 661
    diverticulum in, 468-469
      intraluminal, 469-471
    intussusception in, 472-473
    Ladd's band in, 467
    malrotation in, 1882
    paraduodenal hernias in, 473
    periampullary diverticulum of, versus
      choledocholithiasis, 1300
    positional anomalies in, 467
    wall cysts in, 471
    webs in, 1884, 1885
  ectopic pancreas and, 1048
  endoscopy of, 301-308
    of adenoma, 488
    aftercare for, 304
    alternative imaging modalities to, 305
    in benign lymphoid hyperplasia, 501
    in candidiasis, 477
    of carcinoma, 493
    complications of, 304-305
    computed tomography in, 305; *see also*
      Duodenum, computed tomography of
    in Crohn's disease, 475, 587-588, 1921
    difficulties and pitfalls in, 316-317
    in diverticula, 469
    duodenal cap or bulb, 304, 315
    gallbladder in, 315
    in histoplasmosis, 477
    intubation in, 302-304
    in Kaposi's sarcoma, 492
    in lipoma, 496
    lymphatic drainage, 315
    magnetic resonance imaging in, 307-308
    in mucosal folds thickening, 476
    normal, 304, 306-307
    patient preference in, 300
    patient preparation in, 301-302
    in peptic ulcer, versus radiography, 488
    radiologists performing, 305
    roles of, 298-301
    sedation for, 302
    technique for, 301, 305-306
    in tuberculosis, 476
    in ulcer hemorrhage, 486
    of villous adenoma, 491
  endosonography of, 314-317
    in carcinoma, 493
    in periampullary region, 1127, 1128

Duodenum—cont'd
  endosonography of—cont'd
    of villous adenoma, 491
  enteroclysis reflux into, 541
  erosions of, 473
  in extensive disease, 506-508
  fistulization through, for pancreatic
    pseudocyst drainage, 1097
  heterotopic gastric mucosa in, 284
  in hypoproteinemia, 508
  inflammations in, 473-477
    Chagas' disease in, 920, 921
    Crohn's disease, 473-475, 599-600, 601
    eosinophilic gastroduodenitis in, 475-476
    giardiasis and, 924, 926
    infective, 476-477
    nonspecific, 473
    radiation ischemic, 476
    in tuberculosis, 476, 477
  intubation study of, 296-297
  liquefactive necrosis of, in nonepithelial
    tumors, 496
  magnetic resonance imaging of, 307-308
    in intramural hematoma or bleeding, 503,
      504
    in nonepithelial tumors, 496
  malignant diseases of, 488-498, 508
    metaplastic gastric epithelium in, 498
  metastases to, 508
    adenocarcinoma in, 488-492, 493, 495
    pancreatic adenocarcinoma in, 1108
  mucosal prolapse of, 471, 472
  obstruction of
    in annular pancreas, 468
    from cytomegalovirus disease, 477
    plain films and contrast studies in,
      2044-2045
  peptic disease of; *see* Peptic ulcer disease,
    duodenal
  perforation of
    in cytomegalovirus disease, 477
    in percutaneous cholecystostomy of
      cholecystitis, 1381
    in ulcer disease, 486-487
  physiology of, 79-83
  polypoid lesions of, 508
  postoperative studies of, 297-298, 300
  in progressive systemic sclerosis, 506
  in scleroderma, 661
  strictures of
    in Crohn's disease, 474
    iatrogenic postischemic, 476
  trauma to, 502
    computed tomography of, 1896,
      2133-2134
  tumorlike lesions of, 498-501
  tumors of, 488-501
    adenocarcinomatous, 488-492
    adenomatous, 488
    carcinoid, 492, 495
    intussusception and, 472
    Kaposi's sarcoma in, 492, 494
    nonepithelial, 496-498
  ultrasonography of, 314-317
    in adenoma, 492
    in carcinoma, 493
    in diverticulitis, 469
    in duodenal wall cysts, 471
    in intramural hematoma or bleeding, 503
    in nonepithelial tumors, 496
    in peptic ulcer disease, 484, 485
    in perforation of ulcer, 487
  varices of, 501
  venous congestion in, 508
  wall cysts of, 471

Duodenum—cont'd
in Zollinger-Ellison syndrome, 508
Duplex Doppler imaging; *see also* Doppler
ultrasonography
of duodenal varices, 501
of liver
in focal lesions, 1480
in portal hypertension, 1971, 1972
in transplantation, 1735-1736, 1737,
1738, 1975
in pancreatic transplantation, 1203
in rejection, 1212
Duplication
of bile ducts, 1271-1272
extrahepatic, 1259, 1260
esophageal, 212
in child, 1843, 1844
gallbladder, 1252, 1253
gastric, 318, 319
in child, 1865
scintigraphy in, 1865
ultrasonography of, 1865
hepatic artery cirrhotic changes versus, 1620
of inferior vena cava, 1819-1820
of pancreas, 1049
Duplication cyst
of duodenum, 471
enteric, 1888-1889
of stomach, 318, 319
Dynamic, computed tomography; *see*
Computed tomography, dynamic
Dysentery
amebic, 915-919, 920
bacillary, 898-900
toxic megacolon in, 603
inflammatory bowel disease toxic, 568
Dysgammaglobulinemia
in child, 1898
giardiasis in, 926
Dysphagia, 165-167
in candidiasis, 908
multidisciplinary approach to, 165-167
psychogenic, 165-167
triage evaluation of, 165-167
Dysphagia aortica, 252, 253
Dysphagia lusoria, 254
Dysplasia in colon
colonoscopy in, 608, 609
neuronal, 1915
screening for, 827-829
in ulcerative colitis, 583

E

E ring, 168
Echinococcal organisms, 940-943
Echinococcus
in pediatric hydatid disease, 1961
percutaneous abscess drainage in, 2002
Echinostoma ilocanum, 946
Echo texture in ultrasonography, 1119
Echoprobe, catheter, 264, 265
Ectasia, vascular, 983
portal hypertension and, 1598, 1599
Ectodermal changes in Cronkhite-Canada
syndrome, 631, 787
Ectopic esophageal tissue, 252
Ectopic hormones in islet cell tumors, 1172;
see also Islet cell tumor
Ectopic pancreas, 318-320, 321, 1048-1049
in child, 1947, 1948
in duodenum, 498
endosonography of, 450
in gallbladder, 1255
in small bowel, 630
in stomach, 318-320, 321, 377, 378, 1048

Ectopic pancreas—cont'd
in stomach—cont'd
in child, 1866, 1867
endosonography of, 450
Ectopic pregnancy, ruptured, 2073
Ectopic pseudocysts of pancreas, 1034
Ectopic spleen, 1768, 1769
technetium 99m heat-damaged red blood
cells scintigraphy in, 1528
Ectopic tumors, gastrinoma as, 1170
Edema
in Crohn's disease, 593
small bowel, 684, 685
mesenteric, 1823
Edison, TE, 1
Edrophonium chloride, 181, 209
Effusions after pancreatic transplantation, 1198
Ehlers-Danlos syndrome, 655
Electrohydraulic lithotriptor, 1356
in choledocholithiasis, 1361, 1362
in percutaneous biliary endoscopy, 1425
repeat lithotripsy with, 1360
Electrolyte imbalance in esophageal motility
disorders, 209
Electrolyte solutions, balanced, 90
Electromagnetic lithotriptor, 1356
repeat lithotripsy with, 1360
Electron-beam scanners, 1453
Electron microscopy
in acinar cell cystadenocarcinoma, 1155
in pancreatic cystic neoplasms, 1151
in small bowel fine-needle aspiration
cytology, 559
Embolism; *see* Embolus
Embolization
in acute arterial hemorrhage, 997-999
hepatic
Gelfoam, 1728
inadvertent, arterial, 1729
selective arterial, in vascular diseases,
1628
silicone, 1728
transcatheter, 1717-1718, 1722-1734; *see
also* Hepatocellular carcinoma,
transcatheter embolization of
in iliac artery, failure of, 2145
splenic artery, 1791
therapeutic, history of development of, 24
transhepatic, of gastroesophageal varices,
1006-1007
Embolus
of barium to lungs, 287
in Crohn's disease, 589
mesenteric, small bowel infarction and,
2056
septic, 2082
Embryo, 3-week-old, 1795
Embryology
of gallbladder and biliary tract, 1251, 1252
of large bowel, 1907
of liver, 1796
of pancreas, 1039, 1040
central anlage in, 467-468
of peritoneum, 1795-1797
of retroperitoneum and mesentery, 1807
secondary ligament formation in, 1796
of spleen, 1761-1762
Embryonal cyst of stomach, 318
Embryonal sarcoma of liver, 1480
Emergency, esophageal fluoroscopy in, 168,
183
Emperonium, 231
Emphysema
of gallbladder, 1286, 1288; *see also*
Emphysematous cholecystitis

Emphysema—cont'd
interstitial bowel wall, 1870, 2069, 2070
interstitial gastric, 334-336
Emphysematous cholecystitis, 2032, 2033
biliary tree gas and, 2053
computed tomography and, 2087, 2088
plain films and contrast studies in, 2031,
2070
sonography of, 2110, 2111
Emphysematous cystitis, 2070, 2071
Emphysematous enterocolitis, 2069, 2070
Emphysematous gastritis, 334-336
in child, 1870
plain films and contrast studies in, 2070
Emphysematous pancreatitis, 2034
Emphysematous pyelonephritis, 2070, 2071
Empyema
in cholecystitis, 1287-1289
of gallbladder
after extracorporeal shock wave
lithotripsy, 1364
in carcinoma, 1327
plain films and contrast studies of, 2031
Encephalopathy, portohepatic venous shunt in,
1625
Encopresis, 1915
Endarteritis, reactive obliterative, 685
Endocrine pancreas, 87
Endocrine substances, 67
Endocrine system
disorders of
esophageal motility and, 209
multiple endocrine neoplasia in; *see*
Multiple endocrine neoplasia
gastroenteropancreatic tumors in; *see* Islet
cell tumor
gut physiology and, 67; *see also*
Gastrointestinal tract, physiology of
Endodermal web, 1251
Endometriosis
in colon, 778-779
in peritoneal cavity, 1804
Endoprobe
for colonic sonography, 726
for rectal sonography, 727, 813, 814
Endoprostheses, biliary, 1407-1411
blocked, 1419-1420
in chronic pancreatitis with stones,
1094-1097
collapsible large-caliber metal, 1407-1411
management after, 1417-1418
Endoprosthesis, biliary, 1430
blocked, 1431
Endoscope, 264, 265
in combined transhepatic-endoscopic
approach, 1411-1412
in percutaneous endoscopy of biliary tract,
1423-1424
sterilization of, 1424
Endoscopic intervention
in balloon dilatation of stomach after obesity
surgery, 461, 464
in biliary tract neoplasm, 1430-1439
combined with transhepatic approach,
1411-1414
in calculus disease, 1344-1354; *see also*
Calculus disease, endoscopic
intervention in
in chronic pancreatitis, 1091-1100
abandoned, 1099
in biliary obstruction, 1098
in calculus extraction, 1091-1094
in chronic pain, 1091-1098
in prosthesis placement, 1094-1097
in pseudocyst drainage, 1097-1098

Endoscopic intervention—cont'd
  in chronic pancreatitis—cont'd
    in relapsing pancreatitis, 1091-1098
    in sphincterotomy, 1091, 1092
Endoscopic retrograde cholangiography of bile
    duct stones, 1361; *see also*
    Endoscopic retrograde
    cholangiopancreatography
Endoscopic retrograde
    cholangiopancreatography,
    1240-1243
  in acquired immunodeficiency syndrome,
    961
  alcohol-prolamin solution hazards in, 1099
  of annular pancreas, 468
  of anomalous hepatic ducts, 1259
  of anomalous pancreaticobiliary duct union,
    1262
  of cholangiocarcinoma, 1334, 1339, 1340
  of choledochal cyst, 1266
  of chronic pancreatitis, 1094
    with stones, 1094, 1095
  complications of, 1243
  delayed films in, 1344
  diagnostic uses of, 1344
  of emphysematous cholecystitis, 1286
  before endoscopic intervention in calculus
    disease, 1344-1345, 1346
  free cannulation in, 1243
  gallbladder ultrasonography and, 1249
  in liver pretransplant imaging, 1736
  of pancreas, 1020-1022
  of pancreas divisum, 1042-1043
  of pancreatic duct
    accuracy of, in stone detection, 1344
    in adenocarcinoma, 1110, 1122-1123,
      1127, 1128
    in rare tumors, 1135-1136, 1147-1149
    risks of, 1344-1345
  before percutaneous intervention in
    malignant biliary tract disease, 1401
  in sequence of biliary tract stone disease,
    1302
  in ulcerative colitis, 574
Endoscopic sphincterotomy; *see*
    Sphincterotomy, endoscopic
Endoscopic ultrasonography; *see*
    Endosonography
Endoscopy, 967-982
  of annular pancreas, 468
  in arterioenteric fistula, 976
  for biopsy
    of colon, radiologic caveats and, 795
    in colorectal carcinoma, 779
  in bleeding
    in lower tract, 976-979
    in peptic ulcer, 970-972
    scintigraphy versus, 984
  in celiac disease, 506
  clinical aspects of, 967, 968
  in Crohn's disease, 475, 587-588, 1921
  defecography and, 840; *see also*
    Defecography
  diagnostic accuracy of, 299
  in Dieulafoy lesion, 974-975, 977
  in esophageal and gastric tumors, 973
  in esophageal varices, 968-969
  in esophagitis, 972
  in gallbladder and bile duct stone disease,
    1344-1354; *see also* Calculus
    disease, endoscopic intervention in
  in gastric carcinoma, 397
  in gastric varices, 969-970
  in gastritis, 974
  in giardiasis, 670

Endoscopy—cont'd
  in hemobilia, 976
  in hemostasis, 971
  in heterotopic gastric mucosa in duodenum,
    498, 499
  in hyperplasia of Brunner's glands, 499
  in inflammatory bowel disease, 608
  interventional; *see* Endoscopic intervention
  in laser-photocoagulation of esophageal
    carcinoma, 271
  in Mallory-Weiss tear, 972-973
  mother and baby, in choledochoscopy,
    1351, 1353
  of nonspecific duodenitis, 473
  in odynophagia, 183
  of pancreas, abandoned, 1099
  in peptic ulcer disease, 478
  percutaneous, of biliary tract; *see* Biliary
    tract, percutaneous endoscopy of
  pharyngeal perforation in, 115
  as primary investigation, 299-300
  repeat enema versus, 712
  in staging of rectal cancer; *see* Rectal
    carcinoma, endosonographic staging
    of
  technique of, 968
  in telangiectasia, 973, 975-976
  timing of, 967-969
  in ulcerative colitis, 573, 574, 575, 577,
    580
  upper gastrointestinal
    in bleeding, 298, 299-300
    normal, 303
    in postoperative studies, 297-298, 300
  in watermelon stomach, 975-976
Endosonographic scope, 314
  in colonic endosonography, 726
  in rectal endosonography, 727, 813
Endosonography
  in aspiration cytology, 264-265
  of colon; *see* Colon, endosonography of
  in gastric cancer, 389
  of gastrointestinal wall, 186-187
  in linitis plastica studies, 397
  of pancreas
    in carcinoma, 1127-1131
    in islet cell tumors, 1189-1190, 1191,
      1192-1193
    in pancreatic mucinous tumors, 1146
    in rare pancreatic tumors, 1135
    in serous adenoma, 1141
  of rectum, 727-729
    in cancer staging; *see* Rectal carcinoma,
      endosonographic staging of
  history of use of, 17
  vaginal, in rectal carcinoma, 820
Enema
  barium; *see* Barium examination
    double-contrast; *see* Double-contrast
      barium enema
    repeat, endoscopy versus, 712
  bowel preparation and, 90
  cleansing
    before colon imaging, 698-699
    fluoroscopically controlled, during barium
      enema study, 710
  colostomy, 712-713
  enteroclysis; *see* Enteroclysis
  gas, 712
  gas or carbon dioxide, in pediatric small
    bowel, 1901-1902; *see also* Carbon
    dioxide contrast
  hydrostatic, 1900-1901
  instant, 565, 712
  in intussusception imaging, 1900-1902

Enema—cont'd
  pediatric tip for, 517
  Phosphosoda, 715-716
  postresection, 713
  single-contrast; *see* Single-contrast
    examination
  water-soluble contrast, 711-712
Enprostil; *see* Prostaglandin analogue
Ensure, 516
Entamoeba coli
  in colitis, ulcerative colitis versus, 604
  in recurrent pyogenic cholangitis, 1303
Entamoeba histolytica
  in acquired immunodeficiency syndrome,
    958
  in acute gastroenteritis, 903
  in amebic colitis, 2067
    in child, 1961
Enteric duplication cyst, 1888-1889
Enteric hormones, 67-73
Enteric neuropeptides, 67-73
Enteric pathogens in acquired
    immunodeficiency syndrome,
    954-959
Enteritis
  acute necrotizing, 2086-2087
  Crohn's; *see* Crohn's disease
  granulomatous; *see* Granulomatous enteritis
  ischemic, 685, 686
    small intestinal, 685, 686
  nonsteroidal antiinflammatory drug-induced,
    656-657
  pseudomembranous; *see* Pseudomembranous
    enterocolitis
  radiation, 651-652, 653, 685-686
  regional, 639, 640
Enterocele, 841
Enteroclysis, 514-515
  advantages of, 525-526, 659, 691
  barium in, 515
    bleeding and, 546
    complications of, 546
    inappropriate amount of, 541
    in obstruction, 2047
    in partial obstruction, 543
  biphasic, with methylcellulose, 533-547,
    689-690
    barium in, 534, 535, 541, 543, 546
    colon radiography after, 541
    contrast materials in, 534
    end-stage renal disease bleeding and, 690
    enteroscopy combined with, 545
    faint opacification of terminal ileum in,
      542
    fecal material in terminal ileum in,
      541-542
    filming sequence in, 536-537
    fluoroscopy and filming sequence in,
      534-535, 536, 537
    gastrointestinal bleeding in, 545-546
    ileostomy, 542-543
    inappropriate amount of barium in, 541
    incomplete distention of small bowel in,
      541
    infusion rates in, 535-539
    intubation in, 534
    modifications of technique in, 542-545
    overview of, 689
    patient preparation for, 534
    poor coating in, 538
    poorly distended terminal ileum in, 541
    prolapse of small bowel into pelvis in,
      541
    prolonged examination in, 539-541
    rate of flow in, 535, 539, 540, 541, 542

Enteroclysis—cont'd
  biphasic, with methylcellulose—cont'd
    reflux into duodenum and stomach in, 541
    small bowel obstruction and, 543-545
    speed of infusion in, 540
    technique-related problems in, 539-542
  catheter for
    balloon, 542
    in biphasic procedure with
        methylcellulose, 534
    types of, 543
  in celiac disease, 664, 665
  in chronic radiation enteritis, 651
  in Crohn's disease, 595, 601
    in child, 1892
  double-contrast, with air, 548-551, 690
    barium in, 548
    problems in, 550, 551
    technique for, 548-550
  endoscopy with, 545
  history of use of, 8
  indications for, 567
  inflammatory disease and, 566-567
    Crohn's, 595, 601, 1892
    idiopathic, 514-515
    in ulcerative colitis, 580
  in neoplasms, 627
    in adenocarcinoma, 640
    in jejunal lymphoma, 637
    in lymphoma, 637, 638
    in metastases, 643
  pump for, 689
  single-contrast retrograde, 524
Enterococci in bacterial cholangitis, 1304
Enterocolitis
  emphysematous, 1870, 2069, 2070
  granulomatous; see Crohn's disease;
        Granulomatous enteritis
  in infant, 666
  milk allergy, pneumocolon in, 522, 523
  neonatal necrotizing, 1916-1919
  pseudomembranous; see Pseudomembranous
        enterocolitis
Enterocolonopathy, functional, 686
Enterocystoma of stomach, 318
Enterogenous cyst
  of duodenum, 471
  of stomach, 318
Enteroglucagon, 68, 69
Enteroliths, 893-894
Enteropathic immunoglobulin deficiency states,
        671-677
Enteropathy
  acquired immunodeficiency syndrome and,
        959-960
  gluten-induced, 663
  necrotizing, in child, 1918, 1919
Enteroscopy
  with enteroclysis, 545
  scope in, 691
  Sonde-type, 978
Entrocel, 534
Enzymes
  digestive, in esophageal perforation, 216
  pancreatic, in pancreatic tumors, 1132
  proteolytic, in esophageal foreign bodies,
        216
Eosinophilia in cholangitis, 1312
Eosinophilic gastritis, 325, 330
  in child, 1869, 1870
Eosinophilic gastroduodenitis, 475-476
Eosinophilic gastroenteritis, 359, 683-684
  in child, 1869, 1892-1894, 1924
  in esophagitis, 1848
Eosinophilic gastropathy, 359-360

Eosinophilic granuloma
  esophageal, 251
  of stomach, 326, 359, 360
Epicholedochal plexus, 1319
Epidemic gastroenteritis, 903-904
Epidermal growth factor, 68
Epidermal neurolysis, toxic, 232
Epidermoid cyst of spleen
  in child, 1938-1939
  ultrasonography of, 2115, 2116
Epidermolysis bullosa dystrophica, 232
  in esophageal strictures and webs, 235
  in esophagitis, 1848
Epigastric pain in gastrinoma, 1170
Epigastric vein, inferior, 1472
Epiglottis, functional abnormalities of,
        129-130
Epiglottitis, pharyngeal, 1835, 1836
Epinephrine
  carcinoid and
    gastric, 384
      small bowel angiography of, 634
  in gastric ulcer, 971, 972
Epiphrenic diverticulum, esophageal, 214
Epiploic foramen, 29, 34, 35
Epithelial dysplasia
  colonoscopy in, 608, 609
  in ulcerative colitis, 583
Epithelial lesions of liver, 1967
Epithelial polyps and tumors in stomach,
        373-377
Epithelioid hemangioendothelioma of liver,
        1480, 1682-1683
Epithelioid variant in gastric benign tumors,
        377-379
Epithelium
  colonic, dysplastic, 827-829
  gastric, atypical, 406
  of small bowel, 513
Epstein-Barr virus, 1748
Equilibrium phase of computed tomography,
        1456
ERCP; see Endoscopic retrograde
        cholangiopancreatography
Ergot toxicity, 1311
Ernst, 19
Erosion, gastric, 329, 336
  in child, 1870, 1872
  in peptic ulcer disease, 336
Erythema nodosum, 575
Erythromycin, 79
Escape phenomenon in esophageal peristalsis,
        198
Escherichia coli
  in acalculous cholecystitis, 1281
  in acute gastroenteritis, 903
  in bacterial cholangitis, 1303, 1305
  in emphysematous cholecystitis, 1286
  in emphysematous cystitis, 2070
  in gas-forming infections, 2070
  in hemolytic uremic syndrome, 1924
  in phlegmonous gastritis, 333, 334
  in pseudomembranous enterocolitis, 901
  in recurrent pyogenic cholangitis, 1303
  in small bowel stasis, 669
  in splenectomy infections, 1790
  ulcerative colitis versus infections from, 604
Esophageal bronchus, 1843
Esophageal rosette, 282
Esophageal sphincter
  lower, 75, 168, 190
    abnormal, 168, 201-202, 211
    in gastric carcinoma, 204
    radiologic appearance of, 197
  upper, 73, 94, 168, 188, 189

Esophageal sphincter—cont'd
  upper—cont'd
    abnormal, 201
    radiologic appearance of, 196
    in swallowing, 106
Esophageal varices; see Esophagus, varices of
  gastrointestinal endoscopy in, 968-969
Esophagectomy, 277, 278
  tumor recurrence after, 279
Esophagitis, 220-232
  in acquired immunodeficiency syndrome,
        954, 955, 957
  in Barrett's esophagus, 224-226
  caustic, 229-230
    in child, 1847, 1848
  in child, 1845, 1846-1848, 1861-1863
  in Crohn's disease, 599-600
  diffuse esophageal spasm in, 204, 211
  drug-induced, 230, 231
    in child, 1847-1848
    strictures in, 236
  gastrointestinal endoscopy in, 972
  infectious, 226-229
    in child, 1846-1847
  reflux, 207-208, 211, 220-223
    in child, 1845, 1846
    esophageal manometry in, 200
    in stroke, 135
  with systemic disease, 1848
  in tuberculosis, 229
Esophagitis cystica, 252
Esophagogastric anastomosis, cervical, 228,
        277
Esophagogastric junction, 1853-1864; see also
        Diaphragm, and esophagogastric
        junction
  hiatus hernia at, 219
Esophagogastric varices; see Esophagus,
        varices of
Esophagography, 192, 193
  in carcinoma, 243, 244, 245, 246
  in caustic esophagitis, 230
  fluoroscopy in, 192
  in hiatus hernia, 219
  indentations and, 254
  in leiomyoma, 250
  overhead, 192
  perforation and, 216-218
  postvagotomy syndrome and, 208
  pseudodiverticulosis and, 216
Esophagoscopy in lower sphincter opening
        abnormalities, 211
Esophagotrachea, 1829
Esophagram; see Esophagography
Esophagus, 168-281
  abdominal, 28
  anastomosis of
    esophagogastric, 228, 277
    in tracheoesophageal fistula and atresia,
        212
  anatomy of, 168-176
    body of esophagus in, 193
    in child, 1836-1838
    cross-sectional, 173-176
    distal, 168, 190
    endosonography and, 187-190
    general radiographic, 168-173
    imaging techniques and, 193-194
    pediatric, 1836-1838
    squamocolumnar junction in distal, 168,
        169
    upper segment in, 73, 94, 168, 188, 189
    vestibule in, 168
    wall thickness in, 173
  in ascariasis, 929

Esophagus—cont'd
  barium examination of
    versus endosonography in carcinoma
      staging, 268
    in esophagography, 176-184, 192
    in varices, 241
  Barrett's, 224-226, 1863
    strictures in, 236
  in Chagas' disease, 920, 921
  of child, 1836-1852, 1923
  computed tomography of, 168, 174, 176,
      184, 272-278
    in carcinoma, 184, 243, 248, 268,
      272-278
    in deviations, 255
    diaphragm and, 255
    in endosonography, 264
    versus endosonography in carcinoma
      staging, 268
    lymph nodes in, 275
    metastases in, 276
    nasogastric tube and, 184
    normal, 272
    pediatric, 1837
    with phosphor technology, 184
    predicting resectability of tumor in,
      276-278
    primary tumor in, 273-275
    recurrent tumor in, 278
  congenital abnormalities of, 212-213
    atresia and tracheoesophageal fistula in,
      212, 213, 1839-1842
    in child, 1839-1844
    esophageal bronchus in, 1843
  diaphragm and, 255-256
  displacements of, 254-255
  distention of, 210-211
    abrupt, 218
  diverticula of, 214-216
  double-channel, 218
  in duodenal endoscopy, 304
  duplications of, 212
    in child, 1843, 1844
  endoscopy of
    with foreign bodies, 183
    rings of, 234
  endosonography of, 186-191, 264-271
    anatomy in, 187-190
    axial resolution in, 187
    bony spurs in, 188
    cancer staging in, 265-269
    common errors in, 190-191
    focal zone in, 187
    fundamentals of, 186
    gastrointestinal wall in, 186-187
    image interpretation in, 265, 266
    instrumentation in, 264, 265
    lymph nodes and, 265
    mediastinum in, 270
    preparation for, 190
    procedure in, 190-191
    scattering, penetration and frequency in,
      187
    submucosal lesion in, 269-270
    technique for, 264-265
    transcutaneous cervical sonography in,
      264
    tumor recurrences in, 269
  esophagitis and; see Esophagitis
  examination techniques for, 176-185
  feline, 172
  fistula of, 1839-1842
  fluoroscopy of, 168, 176-184
    additional gas in, 168, 177-181
    artifacts in, 168, 177, 180

Esophagus—cont'd
  fluoroscopy of—cont'd
    diverticula in, 214
    drug enhancement in, 168, 181-184
    drugs in, 168, 181-184
    emergency, 168, 183
    equipment in, 168, 183-184
    foreign body in, 168, 183
    gastroesophageal junction in, 168,
      182-183
    indentations in, 254
    indications for, 176
    leaks in, 168, 183
    multiphasic, 168, 176-177
    pediatric, 1838
    plain x-ray film in, 168, 176
    prone-oblique position for, 177, 179
    radiologic equipment in, 168, 183-184
    in reflux esophagitis, 208, 220
    rings in, 133, 234
    routine multiphasic examination in, 168,
      176-177
    solid bolus in, 168, 177
    tailored examination in, 168, 183
  foreign bodies in, 183, 216
    in child, 1849, 1850
  in gastric endoscopy, 304
  glycogenic acanthosis of, 171, 172
  hiatus hernia in, 29, 218-220
  image intensifier in examination of, 183
    digital fluoroscopy in, 183
    laser camera in, 183
    video recorder in, 183
  imaging techniques for, 176-185, 192-263
    in abnormal peristalsis, 211
    anatomy in, 168-173, 193-194
    barium examination in, 1840
    choice of method and, 176
    cross-sectional, 168, 173-176, 184
    double-contrast, 171, 172
    endosonographic; see Esophagus,
      endosonography of
    examination in, 192, 193
    fluoroscopy in; see Esophagus,
      fluoroscopy of
    magnetic resonance imaging in; see
      Esophagus, magnetic resonance
      imaging of
    performance of examination in, 192-193
    physiology in, 194-198
    scintigraphy in, 168, 184
    spot films in, 192, 193
  impressions and indentations on, 172,
    252-254
  laryngotracheal cleft in, 212
  lymphatic drainage of, 173, 265
  magnetic resonance imaging of, 168, 175,
    176, 184, 278-281
    staging of tumors in, 272, 278-281
  manometry of, 194, 195, 198-202
    in achalasia, 202
    in diffuse esophageal spasm, 204
    in gastroesophageal reflux, 208
    in lower esophageal sphincter
      incompetence, 208
    in motility disorders, 202-206
    in postvagotomy syndrome, 209
    in presbyesophagus, 205
    in reflux esophagitis, 207-208
    in tracheoesophageal fistula, 205
  mediastinal, 30
  middle, 188-190
  motility disorders of, 198-202
    abnormal peristalsis in, 211
    achalasia as, 202-204

Esophagus—cont'd
  motility disorders of—cont'd
    chalasia as, 205-206
    classification of, 198
    connective tissue disorders in, 206-207
    curling or corkscrew contractions in, 199,
      200
    differential diagnosis in, 210-211
    diffuse esophageal spasm as, 204
    dilatation in, 210-211
    gastroesophageal reflux in, 211
    hypertensive peristalsis as, 204-205
    idiopathic intestinal pseudoobstruction as,
      205
    lower sphincter opening abnormalities in,
      211
    metabolic and endocrine disorders in, 209
    neuromuscular disease in, 209
    nonpropulsive contractions in, 199, 200,
      211
    pediatric, 1838-1839
    pharyngeal function and, 134-135
    postvagotomy syndrome in, 208-209
    presbyesophagus as, 205
    primary, 202-206
    radiographic and manometric features in,
      198-202
    reflux esophagitis in, 207-208
    scleroderma in, 206, 211
    secondary, 206-210
    tertiary contractions in, 199
    tracheoesophageal fistula and, 205
  mucosa of, 172, 173
  multiphasic examination of, 168, 176-177
  myotomy of, 1841
  nerve fibers to, 194
  obstruction of, versus brainstem lesion, 183
  pediatric, 1836-1852, 1923
    anatomy of, 1836-1838
    atresia in, 1839-1842
    columnar-lined, 1863
    congenital abnormalities of, 1839-1844
    esophagitis and, 1846-1848
    motility in, 1838-1839
    neoplasms of, 1844
    stenosis in, 1842-1843
    strictures in, 1861-1863
    technique for, 1923
    trauma to, 1850
    varices of, 1848-1850
    vascular anomalies in, 1844-1846
  percutaneous abscess drainage of, 2009
  perforation of, 183, 216-218
  peristalsis in, 194, 195, 196
  phrenic ampulla of, 30
  phrenicoesophageal membranes in, 218
  physiology of, 73-75
    resting conditions in, 194
  postoperative stricture after repair of, 1842
  rings, webs, and strictures in, 212, 233-238,
    239
    food bolus and, 177
    pediatric, 1846, 1861-1863
  rupture of, 216-218
    anatomy and, 168
    frank, 218
  stenosis of, 212, 1842-1843
  subserosa of, 265
  tears of, 218
  transhiatal dissection of, 277
  transit in, 73-75
  trauma to, 216-218
    pediatric, 1850
  tuberculosis of, 889
  tumors of, 242-252

Esophagus—cont'd
  tumors of—cont'd
    benign, 250-252
    carcinoma in; see Carcinoma, esophageal
    endoscopy in, 973; see also Esophagus,
        endosonography of
    malignant, 242-249; see Carcinoma,
        esophageal
    metastatic; see Metastases, from
        esophagus
    pediatric, 1844
    recurrent, 269, 278
    sarcoma in, 249
  ultrasonography of, 186-191
  varices of, 238-242
    in child, 1848-1850
    computed tomography arterial portography
        of, 1462, 1586
    gastrointestinal endoscopy in, 968-969
    portal hypertension and, 1577-1579
    prophylactic injection of, 970
    solitary, 252
    transhepatic embolization in, 1006-1007
    transjugular intrahepatic portographic
        shunting in, 1010, 1013
  vascular anomalies of, 1844-1846
  venous drainage of, 172-173
  wandering, 254-255
Estrogens
  adenoma of liver and, 1511
  focal nodular hyperplasia of liver and, 1508
  in hepatocellular adenoma, 1645
ESWL; see Extracorporeal shock wave
    lithotripsy
Ethanol; see also Alcohol
  in fixation of stain, 558, 559
  injections of
    in ablation of gallbladder and cystic duct,
        1383
    in hepatocellular carcinoma, 1667, 1668,
        1701, 1702
    in liver neoplasms, 1667, 1668, 1701,
        1702, 1718-1719, 1728, 1729
  in small bowel malabsorption, 684-685
Ethiodized oil, 1453
Ethiodol; see Ethiodized oil
Europe, gastric cancer in; see Gastric
    carcinoma, in Europe
EUS; see Endosonography
Evacuation proctography, 840; see also
    Defecography
Eventration, diaphragmatic, 1856, 1857
  Bochdalek's hernia versus, 1856
Excretory urography, 1751, 1752
Exocrine pancreas, 87-88
  pediatric, tumors in, 1954
Exposure, radiation; see Radiation effects
External anal sphincter, voluntary, 840
Extracorporeal shock wave lithotripsy,
    1355-1366
  in bile duct stones, 1361-1364, 1373, 1374
  in choledochoscopy, 1350
  in chronic pancreatitis with stones, 1094
  clearance of fragments after, 1357, 1358
  in endoscopic sphincterotomy for large
      stones, 1348-1350
  follow-up algorithm after, 1360
  in gallbladder stones, 1355-1361, 1362
    complications of, 1360
    contraindications to, 1359
    follow-up for, 1360
    long-term risks of gallbladder
        conservation in, 1360-1361
    oral bile acids and, 1359
    patient selection for, 1355-1359

Extracorporeal shock wave lithotripsy—cont'd
  in gallbladder stones—cont'd
    preliminary investigations to, 1359
    procedure for, 1359-1360
    results of, 1357, 1358, 1359
    symptoms after, 1360
    transcatheter stone dissolution in, 1361
    ultrasonography and, 1248
  of pancreatic duct calculi, 1101-1106
    adverse effects of, 1102-1105, 1106
    indications for, 1102
    principles of, 1101-1102
    procedure for, 1102
    results in, 1102-1105, 1106
  in percutaneous biliary tract endoscopy,
      1425
  principles of, 1355, 1356
  shock wave generation in, 1356
Extrahepatic bile duct
  agenesis of, 1259
  anastomosis of, to intestine, 1981
  anatomy of, 1225-1227, 1256
  in cirrhosis with portal hypertension,
      1591-1592
  computed tomography of, 1309, 1311
  dilation of, in child, 1978
  drainage patterns of, 1256, 1257
  duplications of, 1259, 1260
  in gallbladder ultrasonography, 1249-1250
  in primary sclerosing cholangitis, 1307,
      1308, 1309, 1311
  strictures of, 1307, 1308
  trifurcation of, 1256, 1257
  ultrasonography of, 1309, 1311
Extrahepatic veins, pancreatic tumors invasion
    of, 1593
Extraluminal fluid, abdominal, 2100
Extramedullary hematopoiesis, intrahepatic,
    1480
Extrapancreatic masses, pancreatic
    adenocarcinoma versus, 1121
Extraperitoneal air, 2078-2079
Extraperitoneal compartments, perirenal, 62
Extrapleural fat, 29
Extrapyramidal nervous system, 209
Extrasystole after lithotripsy, 1364
Eye
  in Crohn's disease, 589
  in ulcerative colitis, 574

F

F iodized oil emulsion, 1757
F spoon, 514
Factor XII, 1280-1281
Falciform artery, 1608
Falciform ligament, 29, 2024
False-positive pseudocysts, 1035
Familial adenomatous polyposis, 780-783,
    784, 785
  chromosome 5 in, 824
  screening for, 824
Familial Mediterranean fever, 678
Familial multiple polyposis, 780-781, 782-783
Familial paroxysmal polyserositis, 678
Familial polyposis coli
  in child, 1873
  polyp distribution and malignancy risk in,
      1928
  screening in, 827
  small bowel and, 631
Fascia
  lateroconal, 28
  renal, 29, 30, 31
    computed tomography of, 63
  thoracolumbar, 32

Fascia—cont'd
  transversalis, 32, 1807
Fasciola hepatica, 943
Fasting
  duodenal and small intestinal physiology
      and, 81
  gastric motility in, 77-79
Fat
  digestion of, 79-80
  extrapleural, 29
  intraperitoneal, 2022
  malabsorption of, 80
  pericardial, 30
  perirenal, 30, 63
  renal sinus, 63
  right sinus, 31
  subdiaphragmatic, 31
Fat necrotic metastases in pancreatic
    carcinoma, 1154
Fatty infiltration of liver; see Liver, fatty
    infiltration of
Fatty meal in cholecystography, 1229, 1230
Fatty pancreas in cystic fibrosis, 1948
FDG; see
    Fluorine-18-2-fluoro-2-deoxy-D-glucose
Fecal occult-blood tests in colorectal cancer
    screening, 831-832
  in average-risk person, 835
  clinical trials with, 833-834
Fecal retention in cystic fibrosis, 1930
Fecaloma, 1930
Feces
  in colon as artifacts, 772
  in terminal ileum in enteroclysis, 541-542
Fed state, 81-82
Felinization in esophagus, 172, 220, 221
Femoral vein, 1605
Fentanyl
  in hepatic arterial embolization, 1725
  in percutaneous intervention in malignant
      biliary tract disease, 1401
Ferric ammonium citrate as contrast, 307
Ferrites, 1501
Ferritin
  in hemochromatosis, 1561
  in hepatocellular adenoma, 1649
Ferrous sulfate, esophagitis from, 231
Fetal circulation, persistent, 1856
Fetus, small bowel of, 526
Fiberoptic colonoscopy, 767-770
  in inflammatory bowel disease, 608
Fibroid polyp, inflammatory
  gastric, 360, 381-383
  small bowel, 630
    peroral biopsy in, 553, 554
Fibrolamellar hepatocarcinoma, 1678-1680
  in child, 1964, 1965
  necrosis in, 1679
  ultrasonography of, 1478
Fibrolipoma of esophagus, 251
Fibroma
  of esophagus, 251
  of stomach in child, 1873
Fibrosarcoma
  of esophagus, 249
  of liver, 1684
  of mesentery, 1824
  of pancreas, 1155
  of retroperitoneum, 1813
Fibrosis
  in ampullary stenosis, 1318
  in colorectal carcinoma, 809
  cystic; see Cystic fibrosis
  of liver

Fibrosis—cont'd
  of liver—cont'd
    congenital, presinusoidal portal
      hypertension in, 1574
    in hemochromatosis, 1561
  of retroperitoneum, 1815-1816
Fibrous histiocytoma, malignant; *see*
  Malignant fibrous histiocytoma
Fibrous polyp, esophageal, 251
Fibrous tissue in Gardner's syndrome, 781
Fibrovascular polyp, esophageal, 251
Filiform polyp
  in Crohn's disease, 591, 1923
  in inflammatory bowel disease, 570, 571
  in ulcerative colitis, 574, 577, 579
Filiform surface pattern of colonic lesions, 774
Fine-needle aspiration cytology
  of colon, 809, 810
  complications of, 562
  of esophagus, 264-265
  in fibrolamellar hepatic carcinoma, 1680
  of gallbladder
    in carcinoma staging, 1333
    transcholecystic, 1380-1381
  of liver
    in hepatocellular carcinoma, 1480
    ultrasonography-guided, 1476
  of pancreas, 1025
    in giant cell tumor, 1153
    in lymphoma, 1162
    in mucinous adenomas, 1149
    in plasmacytoma, 1163
    in transplantation, 1205, 1218
  in percutaneous interventional radiology,
    1988
  of small bowel, 555-561
    complications of, 562
  transcholecystic, 1380-1381
Fink catheter, 2144
Firestone, FA, 16
First lumbar vertebra, 29
Fischer, AW, 10
Fissures
  for gallbladder, 29
  ligamentum teres hepatis, 29
  ligamentum venosum, 29
  of liver, 32
Fistula
  in anorectal malformations, 1909-1912
  aortoduodenal, 501
  aortoenteric, 1005-1006
  arterioduodenal, 501
  arterioenteric, 1005-1006
    gastrointestinal endoscopy in, 976
  arterioportal; *see* Arterioportal
    communications
  arteriovenous, transcatheter embolization
    and, 2146, 2148; *see also*
    Arteriovenous malformations
  bile duct, 1316-1318
  biliary-cutaneous, 1317, 1318
  biliary-enteric, 1316
  biliary-vascular, 1316
  brachial, pediatric, 1829, 1830
  bronchobiliary, 1316, 1317
  bronchoesophageal, congenital, 212
  choledochocolonic, 1316, 1317
  choledochocutaneous, 1317
  choledochoduodenal, 1316
  in chronic radiation enteritis, 652
  coloduodenal, 475
  of colon
    in carcinoma, 793
    to vagina, 712, 793
    water-soluble contrast enema in, 711-712

Fistula—cont'd
  colovaginal, 712, 793
  in Crohn's disease, 526, 597-603
  duodenobiliary, 475
  duodenocholecystic, 487
  duodenocholedochal, 487
  duodenocolic, 475, 487
  duodenoenterocutaneous, 475
  of esophagus, 1839-1842
  ileojejunal, 597
  intramural, in inflammatory bowel disease,
    617-618, 619
  omphalomesenteric duct, 1889
  perineal, 597
  short bowel syndrome with, 684
  subcutaneous, in Crohn's disease, 612
  tracheoesophageal; *see* Tracheoesophageal
    fistula
Fistulization of pancreatic pseudocyst for
  drainage, 1097
Fixation of midgut, 1878-1884
Fixation artifacts in fine-needle aspiration
  cytology, 558, 559
Flank overlap sign, 2062
Flaps in pharyngeal reconstruction, 160-163
Flexible choledochoscope, 1423, 1424, 1426
Flexible colonoscopy, 755-757
Flexible endoscope
  in pancreatic endosonography, 1127
  in rectal endosonography, 727, 729
Flexible fiberoptic instruments
  advantages of, 301
  rigid gastroscope versus, 298
Flexible sigmoidoscopy, 715-716
  before barium enema, 709, 832
  in colorectal cancer screening, 832, 834,
    835
    mortality rates, 833
  in diverticulitis, 755-757
  with double-contrast examination, 832
  in hereditary nonpolyposis colon cancer, 836
  perforation in, 832
Flow cytometry DNA analysis, 829
Floxuridine, 1311
Fluid collection
  in abdomen
    normal appearance of, 2022
    sonography of, 2100-2101
  in acute pancreatitis, sonography of, 2113
  after liver transplantation, 1747-1748, 1749
  after pancreatic transplantation, 1198,
    1217-1221
  pancreatic percutaneous abscess drainage of,
    2002-2004
  in peritoneal cavity, 1801-1802, 2028-2029
  in retroperitoneum, 1816-1818
  subphrenic, after percutaneous intervention,
    1421
Fluid-filled bowel
  false-positive pseudocysts and, 1035
  in small bowel obstruction, 2046
Flukes, 604
Flumazenil, 302
Fluorine-18-2-fluoro-2-deoxy-D-glucose, 720
5-Fluoro-2-deoxyuridine-C8, 1717-1718
[18]F-Fluorodeoxyglucose uptake, 810
Fluoroscopy; *see also* Single-contrast
    examination; Videofluoroscopy
  after pharyngeal reconstruction, 163
  in biphasic enteroclysis with
    methylcellulose, 533, 534, 535
  in cholangiography for choledocholithiasis,
    1296
  in dedicated small bowel follow-through
    examination, 566

Fluoroscopy—cont'd
  diaphragmatic movement and, 256
  digital, in esophageal examination, 183
  digitization in, 844
  in double-contrast examination, 289-290
    in enteroclysis, 548
  in endoscopic retrograde
    cholangiopancreatography for
    sphincterotomy, 1345
  in enteroclysis for small bowel examination,
    515, 548
  in esophagitis, 220
  esophagus and
    diverticula in, 214
    indentations in, 254
    reflux esophagitis in, 208
    rings in, 133, 234
  and filming sequence in biphasic
    enteroclysis with methylcellulose,
    534-535, 536, 537
  for guidance in Roux-en-[/e3]Y[/e3]
    anastomosis biliary access,
    1414-1416
  history of use of, 2, 9
  in inflammatory bowel disease, 564-568
  in percutaneous cholecystostomy, for
    percutaneous intervention in
    malignant biliary tract disease, 1416
  in percutaneous endoscopy of biliary tract,
    1424, 1425
  in percutaneous intervention in malignant
    biliary tract disease, 1405
  in percutaneous transhepatic
    cholangiography, 1236
  of pneumocolon examination in colonic
    neoplasia, 763
  in postoperative studies, 298
Fluorouracil, 231
  in hepatic ultrasonography, 1473
Flying bat pattern, 1544
FNAC; *see* Fine-needle aspiration cytology
FNH; *see* Focal nodular hyperplasia
FOBT in colorectal cancer screening; *see* Fecal
    occult-blood tests in colorectal cancer
    screening
Focal liver lesions; *see* Liver, focal lesions in
Focal nodular hyperplasia, 1651-1654, 1655;
    see also Liver, focal lesions in
  angiography of, 1654
  in child, 1967
  clinical background in, 1651
  computed tomography of, 1651, 1652,
    1653, 1654-1655
  fatty infiltration in
    intratumoral secretions versus, 1492
    iron accumulation versus, 1492
    magnetic resonance imaging and, 1492
  hepatic scintigraphy in, 1508-1511
    technetium 99m–sulfur colloid,
      1508-1511, 1512, 1513
    technetium 99m–iminodiacetic acid, 1523
  hepatocellular carcinoma versus, 1696-1697
  hormonal influence in, 1651
  magnetic resonance imaging in, 1492, 1494,
    1652, 1653, 1655
  pathology of, 1651, 1652
  radiology in, 1651-1654, 1655
  scintigraphy of, 1508-1511, 1651-1653
  ultrasonography of, 1476, 1651
Focal splenic lesions, 1774-1788; *see also*
    Spleen, focal mass lesions in
Fogarty balloon catheter
  in minicholecystostomy, 1374
  in percutaneous choledocholithotomy, 1371
Folds, Kerckring's, 467

Foley catheter, 842
Folic acid in tropical sprue, 663
Folic acid antagonists, 614
Follow-up examination
    of colorectal carcinoma, 809-810, 832-833
    in inflammatory bowel disease, 609
Food bolus, 1827, 1828
Food poisoning, 895
Food residue, abdominal, 2022
Football sign, 2025
Foramen
    palatine, perineural extension into, 150, 151
    Winslow, 34, 35
Foregut cysts, 1843-1844
Foreign bodies
    in esophagus, 216
        of child, 1849, 1850
        fluoroscopy of, 168, 183
    in perforation of gastrointestinal tract, 2079
        diverticulitis versus, 756
    in peritonitis, 1803
    in pharynx, 114, 115, 1836
Forestier's arthritis, 101, 102
Formaldehyde, cholangitis from, 1312
Forssell, G, 6, 7
Fossa
    pterygopalatine, 150, 151
    tonsillar, 118
    uterovesical, 1800
Fractures
    of liver, 1974
    of spine, 2139, 2140
Fragmentation of barium in celiac disease, 665
Free flaps in pharyngeal reconstruction, 160,
        161
Free portal vein pressure, 1607
Freezing in cryosurgery, 1720
Functional asplenia, 1766-1769
Functional constipation, 1915
Functional enterocolonopathy, 686
Functional metabolic imaging of colon, 720
Functional motility disorders in large bowel in
        child, 1912-1916
Fundic gland polyp in stomach, 376
Fundoplication, 220, 238
Fundus, gastric, 282
    air shadow from, pseudopneumoperitoneum
        versus, 2028
    anatomy of, 34, 311
    glandular cysts of, 376
    lipoma of, 382
    relaxation of, 77-79
    varices at, 969-970
Fungal disease
    in abscess
        in child, 1937, 1960-1961
        percutaneous drainage of, 1999
        of spleen, 1937
    in acquired immunodeficiency syndrome,
        954
    in gastritis, 333
    in spleen, 1780, 1782, 1937
    splenic calcifications and, 1772
    ulcerative colitis versus, 604
Fusion
    in pancreatic anomalies, 1042-1045
    splenogonadal, 1765-1766
    splenorenal, 1765-1766

G

G cells, 67
^{67}Ga citrate; *see* Gallium 67 citrate
Gadolinium
    in biliary tract, 1235
    in liver, 1499-1503, 1510, 1674

Gadolinium—cont'd
    in stomach and duodenum, 307
Gadolinium chelates; *see*
        Gadolinium-diethylenetriamine
        pentaacetic acid
Gadolinium-diethylenetriamine pentaacetic acid
    in colorectal carcinoma, 807
    in gastrointestinal bleeding, 984, 987
    in liver imaging, 1528
        in adenoma, 1649
        in hemangioma, 1637-1638
        in magnetic resonance imaging,
            1499-1503
        in pediatric angiomas, 1966
    in magnetic resonance imaging of colorectal
        carcinoma, 807
    in pancreatic transplantation rejection, 1207
Gadolinium dimeglumine, 1178
    in gastric carcinoma, 446
    in pancreatic transplantation, 1201, 1202
Galambos classification of cirrhosis, 1535
Gallbladder
    accessory, 1252-1254
    agenesis of, 1251-1254
    ampullary pouch of, 1226, 1227
    anatomy of, 29, 34, 1223, 1225-1227
    biopsy of
        in carcinoma staging, 1333
        percutaneous aspiration, 1382
    calculi in; *see* Cholelithiasis
    carcinoma of; *see* Carcinoma, of gallbladder
    cholangiocarcinoma of bile ducts and,
            1333-1342; *see also*
            Cholangiocarcinoma
    cholecystitis and; *see* Cholecystitis
    cholecystography of; *see* Cholecystography
    cholelithiasis and; *see* Cholelithiasis
    cholescintigraphy of; *see* Cholescintigraphy
    cholesterolosis in, 1291
    in cirrhosis, 1537
    computed tomography of, 1230-1233, 2095,
        2096
        in carcinoma, 1327
    diverticula of, 1255
    in duodenal endoscopy, 315
    duplications of, 1252, 1253
    effervescent, 1286
    embryology of, 1251, 1252
    emphysematous, 1286, 1288
    empyema of, 1287-1289
        after extracorporeal shock wave
            lithotripsy, 1364
        plain films and contrast studies of, 2031
    endoscopic retrograde
            cholangiopancreatography of,
            1240-1243
    erosion of mucosal surface of, 1275
    failure to opacify, 1228
    fissure for, 29
    folds of, 1255
    gangrene of, 1277, 1279, 1281-1284
    heterotopic pancreatic or gastric tissue in,
        1255
    history of radiology of, 10-13
    hydrops of, 1275
    hyperplastic cholesteroses in, 1289
    imaging studies of, 1275-1279, 1280
        accuracy of, 1279
    inflammatory and nonneoplastic diseases of,
            1275-1293; *see also* Cholecystitis
        clinical features of, 1275
        percutaneous intervention in, 1367-1398;
            see also Percutaneous interventional
            radiology, in gallbladder and biliary
            duct benign disease

Gallbladder—cont'd
    intrahepatic, 1254
    laceration of, 2095, 2096
    left-sided, 1254
    leukemic infiltration of, 1330
    magnetic resonance imaging of, 1235-1236
    malposition of, in cirrhosis, 1541, 1542
    mobile, wandering, or floating, 1254
    mucocele of, 2031
    multiseptated, 1255
    neoplasms of, 1325-1343
        carcinoma in, 1325-1333; *see also*
            Carcinoma, of gallbladder
        percutaneous interventional radiology for;
            see Percutaneous interventional
            radiology, in malignant biliary tract
            disease
    number variants in, 1251-1254
    oral cholecystography of, 1227-1230, 1231
    pediatric, 1980-1981
    percutaneous ablation of, 1382-1383
    percutaneous transhepatic cholangiography
        of, 1236-1240
    perforation of, in pericholecystic abscess,
        1286
    polypoid or fungating mass in, 1328, 1329
    porcelain, 1325, 1329, 1332
    scintigraphy of; *see* Cholescintigraphy
    septa of, 1255
    shape of, 1255
    in somatostatinoma, 1172
    sonography of; *see* Gallbladder,
        ultrasonography of
    strawberry, 1291
    suprahepatic, 1254
    torsion of, 1286-1287
    transverse septa of, 1255
    ultrasonography of, 1246-1250, 1275-1279
        bile-filled, 1247
        in carcinoma, 1327
        in cholelithiasis, 1246, 1247
        distention in, in cholecystitis, 2110
        equipment for, 1246
        examination in, 1246-1250
        fossa in, 1248, 1468
        gallbladder neck in, 1247
        in inflammatory diseases, 1275-1279
        longitudinal axis in, 1247
        neck in, 1247
        preparation for, 1246
    variants and anomalies of, 1251-1255
    wall of; *see* Gallbladder wall
Gallbladder hydrops
    in carcinoma, 1328
    in child, 1980
Gallbladder neck, 29, 1247
Gallbladder wall
    asymmetric irregularities of, 1278
    direct extension of carcinoma into, 1326
    edema of, 1279, 1281, 1283
        in hepatitis, 2114
    necrosis of, 1286
    striated pattern of, 1278
    thickening of, 1277-1278, 1283, 1284
        in cholecystitis, 2109-2110
        focal, 1289, 1291
    xanthogranulomata of, 1289
Gallium 67 citrate
    in hepatic scintigraphy, 1531
    before obesity surgery, 460
    pitfalls with, 1755-1756
    in splenic infection, 1780
    in splenic tumors, 1782
Gallstone ileus, 2051-2053, 2054
Gallstones; *see* Cholelithiasis

Gamma globulins, 82; *see also*
  Hypogammaglobulinemia
Gamma glutamyltranspeptidase, 1334
Gamna-Gandy bodies, 1542
Ganglia, celiac, 28
Ganglioneuroblastoma, 1833
Ganglioneuroma
  in child, 1833-1834
  in stomach, 379-381
Gangrenous cholecystitis, 1277, 1279,
    1281-1284
  computed tomography of, 2087
  scintigraphy of, 1523
  sonography of, 2111
Gardner's syndrome, 781-783, 784, 785
  desmoid tumor in retroperitoneum and, 1813
  fundic gland polyps in, 376
  gastric tumors in child in, 1873
  polyp distribution and malignancy risk in,
    1928
  screening in, 827
  small bowel and, 631
Gas
  abdominal
    in Bochdalek's hernia, 1853
    intramural, plain films and contrast
      studies in, 2068-2070
    normal appearance of, 2022
    signs of free, in supine radiograph, 2025
  in biliary tree, 2050, 2053
    after sphincterotomy, 2055
    causes of, 2053
    plain films and contrast studies in, 2032,
      2033, 2053, 2055
  in bowel wall in acute abdomen, 2099-2100
  in colon as artifact, 772
  as contrast agent for colon, 700-701
  in duodenum from trauma, 502
  in esophageal fluoroscopy, 168, 177-181
  extraluminal, in peritoneum, 1802
  from infections in large bowel, 2070
  intrahepatic, arterial embolization and,
    1730-1731
  in intrahepatic ducts, 1304, 1305
    as lithotripsy contraindication, 1364
  intraperitoneal, in acute abdomen, 2099
  intrathoracic, in Bochdalek's hernia, 1853
  in portal vein, 2051
  portal vein, in neonate, 1917
  typhoid fever and, 897
Gas-contrast technique in computed
    tomography, 306; *see also* Carbon
    dioxide contrast; Peroral
    pneumocolon
Gas enema in pediatric small bowel,
    1901-1902; *see also* Double-contrast
    examination
Gasless colon, 2065
Gastrectomy
  bile duct strictures after, 1314
  Billroth II, previous, 1348
  carcinoma in stump after, 423-424
  for obesity; *see* Obesity, gastric surgery for
  postoperative studies after, 298
Gastric accommodation, 77; *see also* Stomach
Gastric acid, 75-76
  hypersecretion of, 352
Gastric angulus, 304
Gastric antrum, 282, 283
  adenoma of, 406
  anatomy of, 29, 35, 313-314
  chronic granulomatous reaction of, 1869
  diaphragm or web in, 320-322, 323
  in esophageal fluoroscopy, 177
  lipoma of, 381

Gastric antrum—cont'd
  mucosal prolapse of, 471, 472
  in radiation antritis, 359
  telangiectasia of, 975-976
  tuberculous gastritis in, 890
Gastric artery
  anatomy of, 1608, 1609
  arteriography of, 1585, 1586
  left, 30, 311
Gastric atony, 361-362
  reflux, in enteroclysis, 535
Gastric bezoar; *see* Bezoar
Gastric bypass, 455, 456; *see also* Obesity,
    gastric surgery for
  Crohn's enteritis after, 829
Gastric carcinoma
  adenocarcinoma in; *see* Adenocarcinoma, in
    stomach
  adenoma and, 406-407
  adenopathy in, 442, 443
  advanced, 416-421
    Bormann types 1 and 2, 416, 420
    Bormann type 3, 416-419
    Bormann type 4, 419, 422
    classification of, 416
    definition and classification of, 404-405
    linitis plastica–type of, 420
    radiology in, 394
    simulating type IIc, 421
  anastomotic recurrence of, 453-454
  anatomy and, 438-439
  barium examination in, 387-389
    endoscopy versus, 392-394
  in child, 1873
  classification of, 404-405, 411-421
  computed tomography of, 305
    staging, 441-445, 446
  depressed, 410-416
    histologic type and, 410-412
    smaller than 1 cm, 413-414, 415
    superficial spreading, 415-416
    type IIb-like lesion in, 414-415
    types IIc, IIc + III, and III, 412-413
  depth of invasion of, 404, 411, 421, 440
  diagnosis of, 394-397
    accuracy in, 299
    radiographic, 412-421
  diffuse, 419
  early, 396, 437
    depressed, 410-416
    histologic type of, 410-412
    polypoid, 406-409
    radiology in, 394
    types I and IIa, 407, 408, 409
    types IIa + IIc and IIc + IIa, 407, 409,
      410
  endoscopy in, 973
  endosonography in recurrences of, 453-454
  esophageal invasion by, 422
  in Europe, 387-398
    barium examination for, 387-389,
      392-394
    cross-sectional techniques for, 389-392
    Dutch general hospital experience and,
      397
    early and advanced, 394-397
    endoscopy in, 392-394
    excavated, 395, 404
  in gastrectomy stump, 399, 423-424
  gastrohepatic ligament extension of, 440
  grading system of, 404
  histology of, 410-412
  imaging techniques for
    barium examination in, 387-389, 392-394
    computed digital radiography in, 402

Gastric carcinoma—cont'd
  imaging techniques for—cont'd
    computed tomography in; *see* Gastric
      carcinoma, computed tomography of
    cross-sectional, 389-392
    double-contrast, 289, 402, 408
    endosonography in, 403, 404, 451-454
    magnetic resonance imaging in, 445-446
  incidence of, 399
  infiltrative, 419
  intraperitoneal spread of, 644
  in Japan, 399-428
    advanced, 416-421
    diagnosis of, 402-404
    early, 404-405
    early depressed, 410-416
    early polypoid, 406-409
    esophageal invasion of, 422
    in gastric stump after gastrectomy,
      423-424
    linitis plastica–type of, 420
    mass screening program for, 399-402,
      424-427
    radiographic correlation with endoscopy
      in, 405-406
    radiographic technique in, 399-402
  linitis plastica and, 395-397, 420
  lymphadenopathy in, 442, 443
  macroscopic types of, 394, 396
  metastases from, 441
    direct spread in, 438
    endosonography of, 453
  mortality rates in, 399
  pancreatic invasion in, 443, 444
  pathology of, 437-439
  peritoneal metastases in, 438
  polypoid, 404, 406-410, 437
  prognosis in, 387
  protruded type of, 394-395, 396
  regional lymph nodes in, 440
  scirrhous, 437
  screening program for, 424-427
  staging of, 438-441, 445-446
    computed tomography in, 441-445
    magnetic resonance imaging in, 445-446
    tumor, nodal, and metastasis, 443-445
  superficial, 395, 404
  tuberculosis and, 895
  type IIb–like lesion in, 405
  ulcerative, 437
Gastric folds; *see* Rugae
Gastric fundus; *see* Fundus, gastric
Gastric incisura, 304, 313
Gastric motility, 77-79
Gastric mucosa
  in antral diaphragm or web, 320
  erosion of, 336
  folds in; *see* Rugae
  heterotopic, in duodenum, 498
Gastric outlet obstruction
  after surgery for obesity, 465
  barium examination in, 286
  in child
    acquired, 1866-1869
    in gastroesophageal reflux, 1859
  hepatic venous gas in, 336
  pedunculated fibroid polyps in, 382
Gastric polyps; *see* Polyp, gastric
Gastric pouch, 455, 458
Gastric pull-through operation
  in esophageal carcinoma, 278, 279
  in pharyngeal reconstruction, 163
Gastric remnant, cancer in, 423-424
Gastric ulcer; *see* Peptic ulcer disease
Gastric varices; *see* Stomach, varices of

Gastric vein, 30
  anatomy of, 1566
  in ultrasonography, 1575, 1577
Gastric wall
  cancer of, 387-392
  lymphoma of, 431
  normal, 311, 312
  thickening of, differential diagnosis in, 397
Gastrin
  benign gastric carcinoid and, 384
  discovery of, 67
  gastric acid secretion and, 75
  in gastrointestinal physiology, 67-69
  in islet cell tumors, 1168
  mechanism of action of, 68
  in pancreatic tumors, 1132, 1146
Gastrin-releasing polypeptide, 67
Gastrin-secreting tumors in small bowel, 683
Gastrinoma, 352, 1170-1171
  epidemiology in, 1167
  hepatic metastasis from, 1177, 1178
  imaging in, 1173, 1185, 1186, 1187
    intraoperative, 1191
    localization procedures and, 1192-1193
  in multiple endocrine neoplasia, 1169
  portal vein sampling in, 1188
  in Zollinger-Ellison syndrome, 683
Gastrinoma triangle, 508
Gastritis, 325-336
  after surgery for obesity, 464, 465
  atrophic, 77, 330
  in child, 1869-1873
  chronic, 330
  chronic lymphoid, 354
  corrosive, 1870
  Crohn's, 325
  emphysematous, 334-336
    in child, 1870
    plain films and contrast studies in, 2070
  endoscopy in, 974
  endosonography of, 448
  eosinophilic; *see* Eosinophilic gastritis
  erosive, 329
    in child, 1869, 1870, 1872
    incomplete or complete, 327, 329
  granulomatous, 330-331; *see also*
    Granulomatous disease
    in child, 1869, 1871
  Helicobacter pylori, 330, 478
  hemorrhagic, in portal hypertension, 1582
  infective, 333
  interstitial emphysema in, 334-336
  pediatric, 1869-1873
  phlegmonous, 333-334
  radiographic signs of, 327-329
  radiologic manifestations of, 331
  term of, 326
  type B, 330
  varioliform, 325, 327, 328, 330
    in child, 1870, 1871
Gastrocolic reflex, 88
Gastrocolic trunk dilatation, 1117
Gastrodiscoides hominis, 946
Gastroduodenal artery
  anatomy of, 29, 1610
  in gallbladder ultrasonography, 1250
Gastroduodenitis, eosinophilic, 475-476
Gastroenteric cyst, 1843
Gastroenteritis
  in child, 1891
  eosinophilic; *see* Eosinophilic gastroenteritis
  in infections and infestations, 903-904
Gastroenteropancreatic endocrine tumors; *see*
  Islet cell tumor
Gastroenterostomy, percutaneous, 2009

Gastroepiploic vein
  anatomy of, 1566
  right, 31
Gastroesophageal junction
  fluoroscopy of, 168, 182-183
  normal
    in barium examination, 283
    in endoscopy, 304
Gastroesophageal reflux; *see also* Reflux
    esophagitis
  in child, 1859-1863
  esophagitis and, 207-208
  inducement of, in fluoroscopy, 181-182
  lower esophageal sphincter function in, 202,
    211
  pharyngeal function and, 135
  sphincter relaxation in, 77
Gastroesophageal varices; *see* Esophagus,
    varices of; Stomach, varices of
Gastrogastrostomy, 455
Gastrografin; *see* Diatrizoate meglumine
Gastrohepatic space, 29
Gastrointestinal tract
  acquired immunodeficiency syndrome and,
    952-966; *see also* Acquired
    immunodeficiency syndrome
  angiography of; *see* Angiography
  bacillary dysentery in, 898-900
  barium examinations of; *see* Barium
    examination
  bleeding from; *see* Bleeding
  Campylobacter infection in, 900-901
  candidiasis in, 908-909, 910
  chlamydial infections in, 904-908
  cirrhosis with portal hypertension and,
    1596-1603
  double-contrast examination of; *see*
    Double-contrast examination
  endoscopy of; *see* Endoscopy
  fungal infections in, 908-910
  gastroenteritis in, acute, 903-904
  histoplasmosis of, 909-910
  history of radiology of, 1-10
  infections of unknown etiology in, 910-913,
    914
  inflammatory lesions of, computed
    tomography of, 2084-2087
  negative percutaneous abscess drainage and,
    2007
  obstruction of; *see* Obstruction
  pancreatitis and; *see* Pancreatitis
  parasitic diseases of, 913-946; *see also*
    Parasites
  percutaneous abscess drainage of,
    1998-2010; *see also* Abscess,
    percutaneous drainage of
  perforation of; *see also* Perforation
    computed tomography of, 2077-2081
    sealed-off, 2080
    site and etiology of, 2079-2080
  physiology of, 67-93
    anatomy and, 67
    biliary system and liver in, 83-87
    clinical implications of, 69-72
    colon in, 88-91
    distal intestinal, 69, 70
    duodenum and small bowel in, 79-83
    enteric neuropeptides and enteric
      hormones in, 67-73
    gastrin and, 67-69
    glucagon and, 69
    insulin and, 69
    mechanism of peptide and hormone action
      in, 68
    oropharynx and swallowing in, 73-75

Gastrointestinal tract—cont'd
  physiology of—cont'd
    pancreas in, 87-88
    prostaglandins and, 72
    proton pump inhibitors and, 72-73, 76
    regulatory pathways of, 68
    secretin and, 69
    somatostatin and, 69
    stomach in, 75-79
    vasoactive intestinal polypeptide and, 69
  polyposis of; *see* Polyposis
  pseudomembranous enterocolitis in, 901-903
  Salmonella infections in, 895, 896, 897
  single-contrast examination in; *see*
    Single-contrast examination
  tropical sprue in, 910-913, 914
  tuberculosis of, 888-895
  typhoid fever in, 895-898, 899
  ultrasonography of; *see* Ultrasonography
Gastrojejunostomy, loop, 456
Gastroparesis diabeticorum, 361
Gastropathy
  corrosive, 357, 359
  eosinophilic, 359-360
  hypertrophic, 326
  injury, 357
Gastropexy, 2015-2016
Gastrophrenic ligament, 29
Gastroplasty for obesity, 455-458; *see also*
  Obesity, gastric surgery for
Gastroschisis, 1890
Gastroscope; *see also* Endoscopy;
  Endosonography
  advantages of, 301
  rigid, 298
  technique and use of, 301
  types of, 301
Gastrosplenic ligament, 29, 34
Gastrosplenic space, 29
Gastrostomy, percutaneous fluoroscopically
  guided, 2011-2019; *see also*
  Percutaneous fluoroscopically guided
  gastrostomy
Gastrostomy tube
  in obesity surgery, 458
  in percutaneous fluoroscopically guided
    gastrostomy, 2012, 2014, 2016,
    2017
  inadvertent removal of, 2016
Gating, respiratory, in hepatic magnetic
  resonance imaging, 1489
Gaucher's disease
  pediatric splenomegaly and, 1935
  spleen and, 1787-1788
Gd-BOPTA in hepatic magnetic resonance
  imaging, 1503
Gd-DTPA; *see* Gadolinium-diethylenetriamine
  pentaacetic acid
Gelatin sponge embolization
  of hepatic artery, 1717, 1728, 1729, 2148
  of iliac artery, 2145
  of renal vessels, 2149
  in splenic artery, 1791, 2147
Gelatinous carcinoma of pancreas, 1152
Gelfand and Ott method for barium enema,
  707
Gelfoam embolization; *see* Gelatin sponge
  embolization
Genital tract
  carcinoma of, 651
  in Crohn's disease, 589
  in Ruvalcaba-Myhre-Smith syndrome, 785
Gentamicin, 1236
GER; *see* Gastroesophageal reflux
Germ cell tumors, 645

Ghosting artifacts, 1487
GI tract; *see* Gastrointestinal tract
Giant Brunneroma, 500-501
Giant cell carcinoma of pancreas, 1152-1153
    with osteoclast-type cells, 1153
Giant hypertrophic gastropathy, 1870; *see also*
    Ménétrier's disease
Giant migrating contractions, 81
Giant rugal hypertrophy, 429
Gianturco steel coil, 2144, 2148
Gianturco [/e3]Z[/e3]-stent, 1407, 1409, 1410
Giardiasis
    in acquired immunodeficiency syndrome,
        957-958
    in acute gastroenteritis, 903
    infections and infestations and, 923-926,
        927
    in kwashiorkor, 553, 554
    malabsorption patterns in, 669-670, 910
    nodular lymphoid hyperplasia in, 676
    in primary immunodeficiency syndromes,
        676
    small bowel changes in, 677
    thickened valvulae conniventes in, 660, 661
Giemsa staining, 1149
Gingiva, 146
    tumors of, 147
Glandular cysts of fundus, 376
Glaucoma, 701
Glisson's sheath, 1543
Globus hystericus, 165, 220
Glomus tumor in stomach, 383
Glossopharyngeal nerve, 150
    esophagus and, 194
    tumors of tongue base and, 157
Glucagon
    in absence of peristalsis, 288
    in colon imaging, 565, 695, 718, 719, 802
        before barium enema, 701, 702, 705, 707
        for inflammatory bowel disease, 616
        for neoplasia detection, 771
    contraindications to, 288
    in enteroclysis, 541, 543, 690
    in esophageal imaging
        for foreign bodies, 216
        for motility studies, 181, 210
        for varices, 242
    in gastrointestinal physiology, 69
    in glucagonoma, 1171
    in hepatic angiography, 1604
    in linitis plastica studies, 395
    mechanism of action of, 68
    in pancreatic tumors, 1132
        of islet cells, 1167, 1168
    in peroral pneumocolon, 567
    in postoperative studies, 297-298
    in single-contrast retrograde examination,
        524
    in small bowel studies, 524, 525
        in pneumocolon, 517
    in sphincter of Oddi pressure, 1318
    in stomach and duodenal imaging, 282, 306,
        307, 316, 317
        for gastric cancer, 389, 392, 397
        heterotopic gastric mucosa in, 498, 499
        for percutaneous fluoroscopically guided
            gastrostomy, 2012
Glucagonoma, 70, 1171, 1183-1184
Glucose-dependent insulinotropic peptide, 68
Glucose intolerance in glucagonoma, 1171
Glutaraldehyde, 555
Gluten, intolerance to, 663, 676, 1898
Gluten-induced enteropathy, 663
    malabsorption pattern in, 676
Glycerin suppository, 814

Glycogen in pancreatic serous adenomas,
    1138, 1140
Glycogen-rich cystadenoma, term, 1138
Glycogen storage disease
    in child, 1970
    in hepatocellular adenoma, 1645, 1663
Glycogenic acanthosis, 171, 172
GMCs; *see* Giant migrating contractions
Gold radioisotopes, history of, 14, 15
Gold therapy, 270
Goldstein and Miller technique for colostomy
    enema studies, 713
Golytely, 81
    in cystic fibrosis, 1930
    in pediatric intestinal obstruction, 1897
Gonadal vein, 30, 31
Gonadotropin, human chorionic, 1168
Gonorrhea, 604, 607
Gout, 1230
Graded compression sonography in
        appendicitis, 2031, 2102
    in child, 1926
    computed tomography versus, 2085
    in women of child bearing age, 2031
Gradients, motion compensating, 1489
Graft-versus-host disease
    in bile ducts, 1320
    in child, 1898
    in esophageal webs, 235
    in esophagitis, 232, 1848
    small bowel enteropathy in, 674-675, 676
    small bowel functional diseases in, 674-675,
        676
    small bowel pneumocolon in, 522, 523
Graham, EA, 10, 11
Gram's stain
    for cholecystitis fluid, 1281
    in percutaneous abscess drainage, 1999
Granular cell tumor
    of esophagus, 251
    of stomach, benign, 384
Granular pattern in Crohn's disease, 596
Granulocytes, indium 111-labeled, 1529-1531;
        see also Indium 111–labeled
        leukocytes
Granuloma
    cholesterol, 1150
    in Crohn's disease, 553, 554, 589-590
    eosinophilic esophageal, 251
    in gastritis, 330-331
    in helminthoma, 933
    in histoplasmosis, 910
    in ileocecal tuberculosis, 892
    rectal, 820
    in ulcerative colitis, 575-576, 577
Granulomatous colitis
    computed tomography of, 610-615
    in Crohn's disease, 585, 589, 602-603
    filiform polyposis in, 571
    fissure in muscularis mucosa in, 572
    lymphogranuloma venereum versus, 907
    portal hypertension and, 1599
    radiographic features of, 581
    tuberculosis and, 895
Granulomatous disease
    chronic pediatric, 1961
        in esophagitis, 1846
        in stomach, 1869, 1871
    peritonitis in, 1803
    of spleen
        calcifications in, 1772, 1773-1774
        in child, 1937
    in stomach, 330-331
    of child, 1869, 1871

Granulomatous enteritis, 1818
    in primary retroperitoneal inflammation,
        1818
Granulomatous enterocolitis; *see also* Crohn's
        disease
    of small bowel mesentery, 1822
Gray scale examination of pancreas, static,
        1028
Great vessels
    anatomy of, 65
    in retroperitoneum, 1811-1812
    vascular conditions of, 1819-1820
Greater omentum, 29
Greenen cytology brush, 1430
GRF; *see* Growth hormone-releasing hormone
GRFoma, 1172
Growth factor, epidermal, 68
Growth hormone-releasing hormone, 1168,
        1172
GRP; *see* Gastrin-releasing polypeptide
Grüntzig, A, 23
Guaiac test, 831
Guanidine, 230
Guided percutaneous drainage; *see also*
        Percutaneous entries
Guidewire
    in biliary endoscopy, 1430
    intraoperative, for percutaneous biliary
        stricture dilation, 1383
    in percutaneous cholangioscopy, 1424
    in percutaneous intervention in malignant
        biliary tract disease, 1405, 1406,
        1407
Guinea worm infestation, 934, 937
Gut, physiology of; *see* Gastrointestinal tract,
        physiology of
Gut peptides, 69-72
GVHD; *see* Graft-versus-host disease
Gynecologic disorders, 2073

H

Haemophilus influenzae
    in epiglottitis in child, 1836
    in splenectomy infections, 1790
Haenisch GF, 3, 8, 9
Hageman factor, 1280-1281
Halo pattern in hepatic metastases, 1712
Halothane, 1311
Hamartoma
    in Cowden's disease, 1926
    of esophagus, 252
    of liver
        mesenchymal, 1480, 1966, 1968
        scintigraphy in, 1510
    mesenchymal, 1480, 1966, 1968
    pancreatic, 1160
    of small bowel, 630
    of spleen, 1780
        in child, 1937
    of stomach in child, 1873
Hamartomatous polyps in stomach, 375
Hampton's line, 341, 342
Harrington rod, 1903
Hartmann's pouch, 1226, 1227
Hartmann's procedure, 752
Hat sign in colonic neoplasia, 763
Haudek, M, 6, 7
Haustral pattern in large intestine, 694
    in acute inflammatory colitis, 2065
    in cecal volvulus, 2061
    in large bowel dilatation, 2044
    in normal pediatric anatomy, 1907
    in ulcerative colitis, 1920
Heart, congenital defects of, 1766, 1767

Heart failure, congestive
  dynamic computed tomography of, 1446
  technetium 99m sulfur colloid hepatic
    scintigraphy of, 1522
Heimlich maneuver, 369
Heister, spiral valves of, 1227
Helicobacter pylori, 904
  in gastritis, 326, 330, 333, 478
    in child, 1869
  in peptic ulceration, 478, 1872
Heller's myotomy, 204
Helminthic infections, 926-946
  ancylostomiasis in, 930-931
  angiostrongyliasis as, 939
  anisakiasis in, 934-935
  helminthoma in, 933-934
  hookworm disease and, 930-931
  oesophagostomiasis in, 933-934
  strongyloidiasis and, 931-933
  trichuriasis in, 935-937, 938
  ulcerative colitis versus, 604
Helminthoma, 933-934
Hemangioendothelioma
  in child, 1966
  in liver, epithelioid, 1480, 1682-1683
  in pancreas, 1155
  in stomach, 383-384
Hemangiomas
  cavernous
    angiography of, 1640, 1641
    in child, 1966
    computed tomography of, 1634
    fatty liver versus, 1557, 1558
    giant subcapsular, interventional radiology
      in, 1992
    hepatic angiosarcoma versus, 1684
    hepatic metastases versus, 1712, 1713
    hepatocellular carcinoma versus,
      1694-1696
    imaging features of, 1630-1642; *see also*
      Liver, benign tumors of
    incidence of, 1630
    magnetic resonance imaging of, 1635
    percutaneous biopsy in, 1642
    of pharynx in child, 1833
    scintigraphy in, 1509, 1527
    ultrasonography of, 1476
  gastric, 383-384
    in child, 1873
  liver, 1630-1645; *see also* Liver, benign
      tumors of
    approach to imaging of, 1642-1643
    capillary, technetium 99m–red blood cell
      imaging in, 1527-1528
    cavernous; *see* Hemangiomas, cavernous
    clinical background and pathology in,
      1658
    differential diagnosis in, 1630, 1631,
      1636-1637
    with fibrocollagenous scar, 1631, 1634
    imaging features of, 1630-1642; *see also*
      Liver, benign tumors of
    incidence of, 1630
    indium 111-labeled platelets in
      scintigraphy of, 1532
    infantile, 1480
    magnetic resonance imaging of, 1488,
      1490, 1493, 1494, 1498
    mesodermal origin of, 1630
    multiple suspected, 1642
    pre-test probability of, 1642
    scintigraphy in, 1522, 1526, 1527-1528,
      1532
    technetium 99m sulfur colloid
      scintigraphy of, 1522

Hemangiomas—cont'd
  liver—cont'd
    technetium 99m–red blood cell scan in,
      1463, 1526, 1527-1528
    technetium 99m–sulfur colloid
      scintigraphy in, 1522
  pancreatic, 1158-1160, 1161
  of pharynx, 114
    in child, 1832-1833
  of small bowel, 629-630, 657
  of spleen, 1780-1783
    abdominal film and, 1752
    in child, 1937, 1938
    in esophageal varices, 238
Hemangiopericytoma
  of pancreas, 1155
  in retroperitoneum, 1814
  in stomach, 383-384
Hematemesis, 983
Hematochezia, 983
Hematoma
  after extracorporeal shock wave lithotripsy,
    1360, 1364
  after hemithyroidectomy, 115, 117
  after liver transplantation, 1737, 1747-1748,
    1749
  after pancreatic transplantation, 1198
  duodenal
    computed tomography of, 1896, 1897
    intramural, 502, 503-506
  esophageal, 211, 218, 252
    intramural, after sclerotherapy, 238
    strictures and, 238
  hepatic
    in child, 1974
    subcapsular, in peliosis hepatis, 1619
    subcapsular, technetium 99m
      heat-damaged red blood cells
      scintigraphy in, 1530
    trauma and, 1475
  in mesentery, 2096, 2097
  in pancreatic transplantation rejection, 1207
  in perirenal space, 1810
  in retroperitoneum, 1817
    abdominal aortography of, 2145
  of spleen, 1777-1778, 1779
    intraparenchymal, in pediatric trauma,
      1939, 1940
    percutaneous abscess drainage of, 2004
  subdiaphragmatic, 2114, 2115
Hematopoiesis, intrahepatic extramedullary,
    1480
Hematoxylin-eosin–Harris stain, 558
Hematoxylin-erythrosin stain, 558
Hematuria
  percutaneous interventional radiology in
    abdominal masses and, 1995
  transient, after extracorporeal shock wave
    lithotripsy, 1360, 1364
Heme-porphyrin tests, 831
Hemiazygos vein, 29
Hemidiaphragm, 256
Hemithyroidectomy, 115, 117
Hemobilia
  after extracorporeal shock wave lithotripsy,
    1364
  bile ducts in, 1321
    after percutaneous interventional radiology
      for malignant disease, 1418, 1419
  gastrointestinal, 1004, 1005
    endoscopy in, 976
  hepatic artery pseudoaneurysm in, 1615
  ultrasonography of, 2112, 2113
Hemoccult test, 831
  sensitivity of, 833

Hemochromatosis, 1560-1565
  clinical presentation in, 1561
  computed tomography of, 1562-1564, 1563
  diagnosis of, 1561-1562
  hepatic
    angiosarcoma and, 1683
    complications of, 1561
    hepatocellular carcinoma and, 1663
    magnetic resonance imaging in, 1496,
      1563-1564
    noninvasive evaluation in, 1562-1564
    pediatric, 1969, 1970
    scintigraphy in, 1528
    ultrasonography of, 1477
  splenic lesions in, 1787-1788
  superconducting quantum-interference-device
    in, 1564
  term of, 1560
  treatment of, 1564
Hemodialysis, 1560
Hemolytic uremic syndrome, 1924
Hemoperitoneum
  in child, 1974
  from liver laceration, 1475
Hemoquant test, 831
Hemorrhage; *see also* Bleeding
  abdominal
    computed tomography of, 2087-2089
    intramural, 2089-2091
    spontaneous, 2088
  of adrenal gland after liver transplantation,
    1748
  after pancreatic transplantation, 1197
  after percutaneous interventional radiology
    for biliary duct malignant disease,
    1418, 1419, 1420
  arterial
    angiography of, 994-999
    chronic, 999-1004
  in cholecystitis, 1284-1285
  in colon carcinoma ulceration, 793
  in Crohn's disease, 602, 603
  in duodenum, 502, 503-506
    in ulcer, 486
  in gastritis, 330
  in hepatic angiosarcoma, 1684
  in hepatocellular carcinoma, 1665, 1669
  intramural intestinal, 650-651
    computed tomography in, 2091
  in pancreatic cystic neoplasms, 1151
  in pancreatic serous adenomas, 1138
  in peritoneal space, 1801
  in polycystic liver disease, 1658
  in portal hypertension from gastritis, 1582
  in retroperitoneum, 1817
  small bowel
    fine-needle aspiration cytology and, 561
    pediatric, 1896
  ultrasonography of, 2101
  upper gastrointestinal, 298
Hemorrhagic cholecystitis, 1284-1285
Hemorrhagic cysts, 1153
Hemorrhagic telangiectasia; *see* Hereditary
    hemorrhagic telangiectasia
Hemorrhoidal arteries, 694
Hemosiderin
  in hepatic magnetic resonance imaging,
    1496
  in hepatocellular adenoma, 1649
  in pancreatic serous adenomas, 1138
  in pancreatic transplantation rejection, 1207
  in splenic hematoma, 1778
Hemosiderosis, 1560
Hemostasis, endoscopic, 971
Hemselect test, 832

Henoch-Schönlein purpura, 653, 655, 1896
Hepatectomy, types of, 1451
Hepatic abscess; *see* Abscess, hepatic
Hepatic arteriography; *see* Liver, angiography of
Hepatic artery, 29, 1608-1610
  aberrant, 1605, 1606, 1608
  after liver transplantation, 1737
  anatomy of, 1225, 1446
  aneurysm of, 1615-1616
  angiography of, 1606, 1611-1619, 1620; *see also* Liver, angiography of
    in liver transplantation, 1744
  anomalies of, 1446
  arteriosclerosis in, 1614, 1615
  arteritis in, 1616
  chemotherapy in, 1611, 1613
  in cholangiography for choledocholithiasis, 1295
  cirrhotic changes versus duplications of, 1620
  collaterals for, 1614, 1615
  common, 28
  diseases of, 1611-1619, 1620
    in child, 1971-1973, 1974
  extraparenchymal branches of, 1608, 1609
  hepatocellular carcinoma in, 1665
  infarction in, 1616-1617
  in liver transplantation complications, 1740, 1741, 1744-1746
  in magnetic resonance imaging of biliary tract, 1236
  physiology of, 1611
  pseudoaneurysm of, 1615
    stenting after percutaneous stricture repair and, 1394-1395
  replaced, in computed tomography abnormalities, 1460
  right, 31
  spasm and dissection of, 1611, 1613
  thrombosis of, after transplantation, 1740, 1741, 1744-1746
  transcatheter embolization of, 1722-1734; *see also* Transcatheter hepatic embolization
  ultrasonography of, 1471
  vascular anatomy and, 1608-1610
Hepatic carcinoma; *see* Hepatocellular carcinoma; Liver, primary malignant neoplasms of
Hepatic cirrhosis; *see* Cirrhosis
Hepatic cysts; *see* Liver, cysts of
Hepatic duct
  bifurcation of
    cholangiocarcinoma in, 1334
    tumors of, endoscopic palliation in, 1434, 1435
  common; *see* Common hepatic duct
  low union of, with cystic and common bile ducts, 1258, 1259, 1260
  normal, 1224
  percutaneous biliary stricture dilation in; *see* Percutaneous biliary stricture dilation
  percutaneous entry and technical approach to, 1402-1403
  strictures of, stenting after percutaneous repair of, 1393
  trifurcation of, 1256, 1257
  variants and anomalies of, 1256, 1257
Hepatic embolization, transcatheter, 1722-1734; *see also* Transcatheter hepatic embolization
Hepatic flexure of colon
  anatomy of, 29, 692, 725
  bleeding at, 986

Hepatic imaging; *see* Liver
Hepatic lobes; *see* Liver, lobes of
Hepatic lobules, term, 1611; *see also* Sinusoids
Hepatic scintigraphy; *see* Liver, scintigraphy of
Hepatic sinusoids; *see* Sinusoids
Hepatic ultrasound; *see* Liver, ultrasonography of
Hepatic vein
  anatomy of, 29, 30, 31, 33, 1444-1446
  angiography of, 1625-1628
    catheterization in, 1607-1608
    technique of, 1605-1606
    vascular anatomy and, 1610-1611
  anomalies of, 1444-1446
  in Budd-Chiari syndrome, 1625, 1626-1628
  catheterization of, 1607-1608
  in cirrhosis, intrahepatic vascular changes in, 1628
  diseases of, 1625-1628
    in child, 1971-1973, 1974
  duplex ultrasonography of, liver transplantation and, 1736
  gas in, in gastric outlet obstruction, 336
  hepatocellular carcinoma in, 1671, 1672
  obstruction of, 1625, 1626-1628; *see also* Hepatic venoocclusive disease
    in cirrhosis with portal hypertension, 1591-1592
    hepatic scintigraphy in, 1519
    postoperative, 1592
    ultrasonography of, 1472
    unilobar, 1627
  in red blood cell scintigraphy for hemangioma, 1640
  ultrasonography of, 1468
  venography and; *see* Hepatic venography of cirrhosis
Hepatic venography of cirrhosis, 1545
  portal hypertension and, 1583
  sinusoid alterations and, 1619
Hepatic venoocclusive disease; *see also* Hepatic vein, obstruction of
  in child, 1973
  scintigraphy in, 1519
  ultrasonography of, 1472
Hepatic venules, 83
Hepaticojejunobiliary anastomosis, 689, 690
Hepatitis
  alcoholic, 1549
  in child, 1958-1961
  disparate sulfur colloids and iminodiacetic acid scintigraphic images in, 1523
  in fatty liver, 1553
  magnetic resonance imaging of, 1502
  malignant hepatic neoplasms with, 1477, 1663
  neonatal, 1981-1982
    liver and biliary tract imaging in, 1981-1982
  pediatric, 1958-1961
  radiation, 1975
  technetium 99m sulfur colloid scintigraphy in, 1517
  transjugular intrahepatic portographic shunting in, 1011
  ultrasonography of, 1471, 2114-2115
  viral
    in child, 1958-1959
    in cirrhosis, 1534, 1538
Hepatitis B, 1663
Hepatitis C, 1663
Hepatobiliary cystadenoma, 1681-1682
Hepatoblastoma, 1961-1964

Hepatocarcinoma; *see* Hepatocellular carcinoma
Hepatocellular adenoma, 1645-1651; *see also* Adenoma, of liver
  angiography of, 1649
  classification of, 1645
  clinical background of, 1645
  computed tomography of, 1646-1649
  fatty infiltration in, 1492
  hepatocellular carcinoma versus, 1677, 1696-1697
  intratumoral bleeding in, 1649
  magnetic resonance imaging of, 1492, 1646, 1648, 1649, 1650
  multiple, 1649-1650
  pathology of, 1645, 1646
  radiology of, 1645-1649
  scintigraphy in, 1509, 1510, 1511-1514, 1515, 1647-1648, 1649
  technetium 99m sulfur colloid studies of, 1511-1514, 1515
  ultrasonography of, 1645-1646, 1647
Hepatocellular carcinoma, 1662-1678
  alcoholism and, 1663
  alpha fetoproteins in, 1665, 1666
  arterial vascularity of, 1693-1694
  calcifications in, 1669, 1671
  in child, 1961-1964
  cholangiocarcinoma versus, 1336
  in cholangiography for choledocholithiasis, 1295
  cirrhosis in, 1536, 1537, 1662-1663
  classical, with atypical histologic features, 1698-1701
  clinical presentation of, 1663-1665
  collagenous scar tissue in, 1671
  computed tomography of, 1463, 1669-1674
    contrast for, 1453
    noncontrast, 1455
  computed tomography angiography of, 1460
  computed tomography arterial portography of, 1462
  diagnostic imaging in, 1666
  differential diagnosis in, 1667
  Doppler analysis of, 1480
  early, 1676; *see also* Hepatocellular carcinoma, small
  encapsulation of, 1665-1666, 1673, 1674
  epidemiology of, 1662, 1688
  ethanol injections in, 1718-1719
  fatty infiltration in, 1492
  fatty infiltration versus, 1553-1554
  fibrolamellar
    in child, 1964, 1965
    ultrasonography of, 1478
  hemangiomas versus, 1637
  hemochromatosis and, 1561
  hepatitis B and, 1663
  hepatitis C and, 1663
  Japanese experience with, 1688-1705
  liver transplantation in, 1666, 1667
  magnetic resonance imaging of, 1490-1491, 1492, 1495, 1496, 1542, 1543, 1674-1676
    cirrhosis with, 1498
    contrast-enhanced, 1500-1503, 1504
  morbid anatomy in, 1665-1666
  mosaic pattern of, 1665, 1671, 1674
  necrosis of liver in, 1667, 1671, 1672
  nodular lesions with cirrhosis in differential diagnosis in, 1701-1702
    histology of, 1692
  portal vein invasion in, 1592
  portal vein occlusion in, 1623, 1624
  pretransplant imaging and, 1736

Hepatocellular carcinoma—cont'd
  primary, transcatheter embolization in,
      1723-1724
  radiologic imaging in
    angiographic, 1677
    combined computed tomographic and
        angiographic, 1678
    computed tomographic; see Hepatocellular
        carcinoma, computed tomography of
    diagnostic, 1666
    in differential diagnosis, 1676-1677
    interventional, 1667
    magnetic resonance, 1490-1491, 1492,
        1495, 1496, 1674-1676
    rationale and general considerations for,
        1666-1667
    scintigraphy in; see Hepatocellular
        carcinoma, scintigraphy of
    screening, 1666
    sonographic, 1471-1472, 1473,
        1477-1478, 1664, 1667-1669, 2115
    staging, 1666-1667
  resectability of, 1477-1478, 1665-1666,
      1674
  metastases and, 1715-1716
  radiologically-guided percutaneous
      procedures and, 1719
  results of, 1732
  risk factors for, 1662-1663
  rupture of, 1475
  scintigraphy of, 1509, 1510, 1514, 1515,
      1531
    gallium 67, 1531
    technetium 99m–iminodiacetic acid, 1523
  screening in, 1666
  skeletal metastasis of, 1674
  small
    angiography of, 1692-1698
    computed tomography of, 1692, 1693
    findings and differential diagnosis of,
        1692-1698
    imaging methods for, 1689-1692
    interventional radiology in, 1702, 1703
    magnetic resonance imaging of, 1692,
        1694
    screening for, 1688-1692
    ultrasound in, 1692, 1693
  staging of, 1666-1667
  transcatheter embolization of, 1722-1734;
      see also Transcatheter hepatic
      embolization
  ultrasonography of, 1471-1472, 1477-1478,
      1664, 1667-1669, 2115
    carbon dioxide microbubble enhancement
        of, 1473
  unresectable, cryosurgery in, 1720
  vascular invasion of, 1676
Hepatocyte
  in hepatocellular adenoma, 1645
  hyperplasia of, 1651; see also Focal nodular
      hyperplasia
  metabolic function of, 84, 85, 1486
Hepatoduodenal ligament, 1224, 1225
  hematoma and, 1821
Hepatofugal flow
  in evaluation for shunt surgery, 1588
  portal hypertension and, 1574, 1578
  vascular anatomy of, 1610
Hepatofugal or hepatopetal varices, 241
Hepatoma; see Hepatocellular carcinoma
Hepatomegaly
  in cholangiocarcinoma, 1334
  in ulcerative colitis, 574
  ultrasonography of, 1469
  volumetric analysis in, 1469

Hepatoportoenterostomy, 1981
Hepatorenal space, 35
Hepatovenoocclusive disease, 1607
Hereditary hemorrhagic telangiectasia, 1618
  congenital arterioportal fistula in, 1574
  small bowel hemangioma in, 630
  small bowel vessels in, 657
Hereditary nonpolyposis colon cancer,
    788-790, 825, 827
  screening guidelines for, 836
Hereditary pancreatitis, 1952, 1953
Hereditary polyposis syndromes, 827
  screening guidelines for, 836
Herlinger methylcellulose small bowel enema,
    533; see also Enteroclysis, biphasic,
    with methylcellulose
Hernia
  Bochdalek's, 255
    in child, 1853-1856
  in bowel obstruction, 2050, 2106
  diaphragmatic, 256
  in diaphragmatic eventration, 1856
  hiatal; see Hiatal hernia
  in intestinal ischemia, 2092-2093
  Morgagni's, 255
    in child, 1856-1858
  of omentum, 1857-1858
  paraduodenal, 473
  peritoneopericardial, 1858
  pleuroperitoneal, 1853-1856
  retrosternal, 1856-1858
  small bowel, 2045, 2048, 2050, 2053, 2106
  strangulated, 2048
    in ischemic intestinal strictures, 650
    small bowel obstruction and, 2045
  traumatic, in child, 1856-1858
  ventral, 2053
Herpes colitis, 604
Herpesvirus
  in colitis, 604
  in esophageal infection, 183, 227
  in gastritis, 333
Herpetiform dermatitis, 663
Heterotopic gastric mucosa in duodenum, 498
Heterotopic pancreatic or gastric tissue in
    gallbladder, 1255; see also Ectopic
    pancreas
Heterotopic pancreatic rests, 1866, 1948
Heterotopic polyps in stomach, 377, 378
Heterotopic rests in liver, 1658-1660
Hexabrix; see Ioxaglate meglumine-sodium
Hiatal hernia, 218-220
  anatomy of, 29
  chalasia and, 206
  in child, 1859-1863
  diaphragmatic, 256
  esophageal computed tomography of, 272,
      273
  esophageal muscle fibers and, 168, 169, 211
  strictures in, 236
HIDA; see Technetium-99m HIDA
Hidebound appearance
  in scleroderma, 679
  in small bowel systemic sclerosis, 653
High-density contrast in percutaneous biliary
    tract intervention, 1405
Hilal platinum microcoils, 2144
Hilar cysts, hepatic, 1319, 1320
Hilar tumors, bifurcation, 1435, 1436
Hip spica, 1903
Hippel–Lindau disease; see von
    Hippel–Lindau disease
Hirschsprung's disease, 1913-1914, 1925
Histamine
  benign gastric carcinoid and, 384

Histamine—cont'd
  gastric acid secretion and, 75-76
Histamine H_2 blockers, 76, 226
  in Meckel's diverticulum, 1890
Histiocytes, protein-laden, 556
Histiocytoma, malignant fibrous; see Malignant
    fibrous histiocytoma
Histiocytosis
  in bile ducts, 1320
  in celiac disease, 665
  of small bowel, 636, 637
Histocompatibility antigens, 1560, 1561-1562
Histologic colitis, 580
Histoplasmosis, 330, 909-910
  in duodenal disease, 476, 477
  in esophagitis, 1846-1847
  in gastritis, 333
  in small bowel, 682-683
  ulcerative colitis versus, 604
History of alimentary tract radiology, 1-27
  cross-sectional imaging in, 16-22
    computed tomographic, 17-19
    magnetic resonance, 19-22
    sonographic, 16-17
  of gallbladder and biliary system, 10-13
  of gastrointestinal tract, 1-10
    colon in, 8-10
    small bowel in, 8
    upper gastrointestinal study in, 2-8, 9
  interventional radiology and, 23-24
  of liver, spleen, and pancreas, 13-15
HIV; see Human immunodeficiency virus
HLA; see Histocompatibility antigens
HNPCC; see Hereditary nonpolyposis colon
    cancer
Hodgkin's disease
  intestinal lymphomas and, 635
  of rectum, 792
  of small bowel, 639
  of spleen, 1786, 1937
Hollow viscera in acute abdomen, 661, 669,
    2101-2108
Holzknecht, G, 3, 8
Hookworm disease, 930-931
Hopff, H, 23
Hormones
  physiology of enteric, 67-73
  production of
    in hepatocellular adenoma, 1663
    in islet cell tumor, 1188
Hounsfield, GN, 18, 19
Houston, transverse folds of, 727
Howry, D, 16
HPS; see Hypertrophic pyloric stenosis
Human chorionic gonadotropin, 1168
Human immunodeficiency virus infection
  clinical presentation and staging of, 952-953
  enteropathy in, 959-960
  imaging of patient with, 954
Human pancreatic polypeptide, 70
Humeral activity, transcatheter embolization
    and, 1725
HUS; see Hemolytic-uremic syndrome
Hutson loop, 1414
Hydatid disease, 940-943, 1350
  in child, 1961
  of liver, 1657
  of pancreas, 1158, 1159
  of spleen, 1776
Hydrogen breath test, 684
Hydrops, gallbladder, 1275
  in carcinoma, 1328
  in child, 1980
Hydrostatic enema in pediatric imaging,
    1900-1901

Hydroxypropyl methylcellulose, 534
5-Hydroxytryptamine, benign carcinoid and, 384
5-Hydroxytryptophan
    benign carcinoid and, 384
    malignant carcinoid and, 434
Hyoid bone
    abnormal anterior movement of, 128, 134
    in swallowing abnormalities, 129
Hyoscine-*N*-butyl bromide, 181, 517
    in absence of peristalsis, 288
    anticholinergic effects of, 288
    before barium enema, 701, 702
    in computed tomography of colon, 718
    in double-contrast barium enema, 565, 705
    in gastric imaging, 282
    in percutaneous fluoroscopically guided gastrostomy, 2012
    in peroral pneumocolon, 567
    in single-contrast retrograde examination, 524
    in small bowel studies, 524, 525
Hypaque; *see* Diatrizoate meglumine
Hyperbilirubinemia, 1315-1316
Hypercalcemia
    esophageal motor function and, 209
    in sclerosing hepatic carcinoma, 1680
Hypergastrinemia, 1170
Hyperinsulinism
    in glucagonoma, 1171
    in insulinoma, 1169, 1170
Hyperkinetic portal hypertension, 1572-1574
Hyperoxaluria, 80
Hyperparathyroidism
    in chronic pancreatitis, 1091
    in multiple endocrine neoplasia, 1169
Hyperperistalsis in enteroclysis, 539, 540
Hyperplasia
    Brunner's gland
        in duodenum, 498-501
        in stomach, 377
    cholesterotic, in cholecystitis, 1289, 1290, 1291
    focal nodular; *see* Focal nodular hyperplasia
    lymphoid
        benign, of duodenum, 501
        in Crohn's disease, 596
        nodular; *see* Nodular lymphoid hyperplasia
        reactive, 354
        in stomach, 384
        ulcerative colitis versus, 605
    mucosal, in ampullary stenosis, 1318
    nodular regenerative, 1542-1543, 1544, 1545, 1655-1656
    torus, 322, 324
Hyperplastic gastric polyps, 374, 375
    in familial multiple polyposis, 780
Hyperrugosity, 347, 351, 352, 353
Hypersecretion, gastric, 448
Hypersplenism, 1772
Hypertension, portal; *see* Portal hypertension
Hypertensive peristalsis, esophageal, 204
Hyperthyroidism, 209
Hypertrophic gastropathy; *see* Stomach, hypertrophic gastropathy of
Hypertrophic pyloric stenosis; *see also* Hypertrophy, pyloric
    in child, 1868-1869
    conditions mimicking, 1869
Hypertrophy
    muscular; *see* Muscular hypertrophy
    pyloric; *see also* Hypertrophic pyloric stenosis
        in adult, 322-325

Hypertrophy—cont'd
    pyloric—cont'd
        in child, 1868-1869
    of renal cortical column, 63
Hypnovel; *see* Midazolam
Hypogammaglobulinemia, 1898
    in gastrointestinal physiology, 82
    in nodular lymphoid hyperplasia of small bowel, 661
    with small bowel enteropathy, 676
Hypoglossal nerve, 150
    tumors of tongue base and, 157
Hypoglycemia
    brain and, 1169
    nesidioblastosis and, 1950
Hypomotility, esophageal; *see* Esophagus, motility disorders of
Hypopharyngeal ears, 118
Hypopharynx
    in child, 1826
        diverticula of, 1831
        trauma to, 1836
        webs in, 1831, 1832
    in esophageal radiology, 193
    malignant diseases of, 157-160
        direct extension in, 158, 159, 160
        perineural and lymphatic spread of, 158
        wall in, 143
    oropharyngeal malignancies and, 150-157
    outpouchings of, 118
Hypoplasia
    of lung
        in Bochdalek's hernia, 1856
        in diaphragmatic eventration, 1856
    of pancreas, 1045-1046
Hypoproteinemia
    duodenum in, 508
    small bowel mesentery and, 1823
Hypothrombinemia, 574
Hypotonic agents, computed tomography and, 306; *see also* Hypotonic duodenography
Hypotonic duodenography, 296
    in heterotopic gastric mucosa in duodenum, 498, 499
    in nonepithelial duodenal tumors, 497
    in postbulbar duodenal ulcer, 486
    in superior mesenteric artery compression syndrome, 506
    in villous duodenal adenoma, 491

I
I cells, 69
[131]I-meta-iodobenzylguanidine, 87
Iatrogenic disease
    hemobilia and, 1321
    strictures and
        percutaneous biliary dilation of, 1383, 1384, 1386
        postischemic duodenal, 476
IDA; *see* Technetium 99m–labeled iminodiacetic acid
IDBCT; *see* Incremental dynamic bolus computed tomography
Idiopathic inflammatory bowel disease; *see* Inflammatory bowel disease, idiopathic
Idiopathic intestinal pseudoobstruction, 2059, 2060
IgA
    deficiency of, in child, 1898
        malabsorption pattern in, 676
        with small bowel enteropathy, 676
    secretory, 82
        in Mediterranean lymphoma, 677

IgG, 82; *see also* Hypogammaglobulinemia
IgM, 681-682
Ileal brake concept, 69, 70
Ileal loops, pelvic, 517, 522
Ileal pouch, 585, 586
Ilealisution, 506
Ileitis
    backwash, 577, 580
    Campylobacter, appendicitis versus, 716
    terminal
        in acute abdomen, 2104
        ulcerative colitis versus, 605
        Yersinia in, 615
Ileoanal anastomosis, 585
    retrograde study of, 567
Ileoanal pouch, 585, 586
    computed tomography of, 614
    in inflammatory bowel disease, 567
Ileocecal anastomosis, 596
Ileocecal junction, 695
Ileocecal tuberculosis, 891-893
Ileocecal valve
    anatomy of, 725
    fat artifact in, 772
    gaping, 891
    incompetent, 541
Ileocolic anastomosis, 593
Ileocolic artery, 694
Ileocolic intussusception, 2055
    in child, 1900, 1902
Ileocolic vein, 29
Ileocolitis, 589
Ileojejunal fistula, 597
Ileorectal anastomosis
    in familial multiple polyposis, 781
    in ulcerative colitis, 584-585
Ileosigmoid knot, 2063
Ileostomy
    barium examination of, 524, 567
        in inflammatory bowel disease, 567
    continent, 585
    double-loop, 567
    dysfunction of, 567
    enteroclysis in, 542-543
    permanent, 567
    postoperative radiographs of, 567
    retrograde small bowel examination in, 524
Ileum
    in amyloidosis, 681, 682
    anatomy of, 512, 513
    in ascariasis, 929
    atresia or stenosis of, 1885, 1886
    in Crohn's disease, 600
        abscess of, 1893, 1894
        computed tomography of, 611, 612
        terminal ileum in, 595-599
    diverticulum of; *see* Meckel's diverticulum
    ectopic pancreas in, 1048
    enteroclysis in
        distal, 515, 549
        double-contrast, with air, 549
        faint opacification of terminal ileum in, 542
        poorly distended terminal ileum in, 541
    in Gardner's syndrome, 783
    in giardiasis, 924, 926
    intussusception in, 1900, 1902
    lipoma in, 630
    pneumocolon in
        of pelvic loops, 517, 522
        peroral, 566
        terminal ileum in, 515-522
    in tuberculosis, 890-891
    in ulcerative colitis, 580

Ileus
  adynamic or paralytic
    causes of, 2064
    in large bowel obstruction, 2057
    plain films and contrast studies of, 2028, 2063, 2064
  gallstone, in small bowel obstruction, 2051-2053, 2054
  meconium, 1886-1888
Iliac artery
  anatomy of, 29, 30, 31
  transcatheter embolization of, 2145
    in pelvic injury, 2151
Iliac fossa soft tissue mass in neutropenic colitis, 1919
Iliac vein, 29
Iliacus muscle, 29
Iminodiacetic acid
  in bacterial cholangitis, 1306
  in cholescintigraphy, 1233
  in cystic fibrosis imaging, 1320
  derivatives of; see Technetium 99m–labeled iminodiacetic acid
  technetium 99m labeled; see Technetium 99m–labeled iminodiacetic acid
Imipenem, 1725
Immobile patient, barium enema in, 710-711
Immune system, impairment of, 671; see also Immunodeficiency disorders
  in diverticulitis, 751
Immunochemical tests in colorectal carcinoma, 832
Immunodeficiency disorders, 1898
  acquired immunodeficiency syndrome and; see Acquired immunodeficiency syndrome
  duodenum and, 476
  enteropathic malabsorption states in, 671-677
  intestinal physiology and, 82
  small bowel and, 659-688; see also Small bowel, functional diseases of
  primary syndromes in, 676-677
Immunoglobulins, physiology of, 82
Immunoproliferative small intestinal disease, 677
Immunoscintigraphy in colorectal studies, 720, 811
Immunosuppressives
  in pancreatic transplantation, 1198
  in small bowel lymphoma, 635
  in splenic infections, 1780, 1782
  in strongyloidiasis, 931
Implantation radiotherapy in malignant biliary tract disease, 1403
Implants
  endometrial, 778-779
  peritoneal, 792
111In-labeled leukocytes; see Indium 111–labeled leukocytes
Inborn error of metabolism, 1560
Incisura, gastric, 304, 313
Inclusion bodies in esophagitis, 228
Inclusion cysts, 781
Incontinence, fecal
  in barium examination of colon, 710
  defecography of, 845
Incremental dynamic bolus computed tomography of liver, 1455-1458
  in hepatocellular carcinoma, 1463
  in metastases, 1463-1464
  in multimodality approach, 1464
  number of hepatic tumor nodules in, 1458
Indentations, esophageal, 252-254
Indigo-carmine dye, 506

Indium 111–labeled leukocytes
  in excretion test, 82
  in hepatic scintigraphy, 1529-1531
  in inflammatory bowel disease scintigraphy, 609-610
  in intraabdominal abscesses, 1998-1999, 2035
  in obesity surgery radiography, 460
  in percutaneous abscess drainage, 1998-1999
  pitfalls with, 1755
  in splenic infection, 1780
Indium 111–labeled platelets
  in hepatic scintigraphy, 1532
  in pancreatic transplantation, 1203
Indomethacin
  bowel preparation and, 90
  esophagitis from, 231
  mucus secretion and, 77
  prostaglandins and, 72
Infant; see also Pediatrics
  enterocolitis in, 666
  percutaneous fluoroscopically guided gastrostomy in, 2018
  superior mesenteric vein of, 526
Infantile hepatic hemangioma, 1480
Infarction
  after pancreatic transplantation, 1198, 1217, 1220
  extrahepatic, hepatic arterial embolization and, 1729
  hepatic, 1480
    bile duct cysts and, 1319
    in child, 1973
    fatty liver versus, 1554
  in hepatic artery, 1616-1617
  intestinal ischemia in, 2092
  of intrahepatic bile ducts, 1270
  mesenteric, 649-650
    embolus in, 2056
  in small bowel obstruction, 2054-2057
  of spleen, 1776-1777, 1778, 1779
    in child, 1941-1932
    ultrasonography of, 2115
Infections and infestations, 888-951; see also Sepsis
  acquired immunodeficiency syndrome and, 952-966
  in acute gastroenteritis, 903-904
  after endoscopic retrograde cholangiopancreatography, 1344-1345
  after splenectomy, 1790
  amebiasis in, 915-918, 919, 920
  ancylostomiasis in, 930-931
  angiostrongyliasis in, 938
  anisakiasis in, 934-935
  Armillifer in, 946
  bacillary dysentery in, 898-900
  bacterial, 888-904
  Campylobacter, 900-901
  candidiasis in, 908-909, 910
  cestodes in, 939-943
  in Chagas' disease, 918-923, 924, 925
  chlamydial, 904-908
  in cholangitis, 1303
    rare, 1311-1312
  in colitis; see also specific disease
    in child, 1924
    radiographic features of, 581
  differential diagnosis of, 895
  Dracunculus medinensis in, 937, 938
  in duodenitis, 476-477
  echinococcosis in, 940-943
  in esophagitis, 226-229
    in child, 1846-1847

Infections and infestations—cont'd
  fungal, 908-910; see also specific disease
  in gastritis, 333
  giardiasis in, 923-926, 927
  guinea worm in, 937
  helminthic, 926-946; see also Helminthic infections
  helminthomas in, 933-934
  histoplasmosis in, 909-910
  hookworm disease in, 930-931
  hydatid disease and, 940-943
  intestinal capillariasis in, 937-938
  large bowel
    in child, 1916-1926
    gas-forming, plain films and contrast studies in, 2070
  liver flukes and, 943-946
  lymphogranuloma venereum in, 904-908
  nematodes in, 926-930
  oesophagostomiasis in, 933-934
  in pancreatic transplantation, 1198, 1217-1221
  parasitic, 913-946; see also specific disease
  pentastomida in, 946
  in pseudomembranous enterocolitis, 901-903
  Salmonella in, 895, 896, 897
  in small bowel
    of child, 1891-1894
    with malabsorption patterns, 669-671
  of spleen, 1780, 1781, 1782
  in stomach after obesity surgery, 458-459
  strongyloidiasis in, 931-933
  tapeworms in, 939-943
  trematodes in, 943-946
  trichuriasis in, 935-937, 938
  in tropical sprue, 910-913, 914
  tuberculosis in, 888-895
  typhoid fever in, 895-898, 899
  of unknown etiology, 910-913, 914
  whipworm in, 935-937, 938
Infectious mononucleosis, 1939, 1940
Inferior vena cava; see Vena cava, superior
Inferior venacavography, 1746
Infestations; see Infections and infestations
Inflammation
  in acute abdomen
    computed tomography of, 2084-2087
    plain films and contrast studies in, 2029-2032, 2065-2068
  of biliary tract, strictures after, 1315-1316
  bowel mucosa in, 568, 569
  in child
    in large bowel, 1916-1926
    in pharynx, 1834-1835
    in small bowel, 1891-1894
    in spleen, 1936-1937
  of colon; see Colitis
  in duodenum, 473-477
  of esophagus; see Esophagitis
  of gallbladder, 1275-1293; see also Cholecystitis
  in gastrointestinal perforation, 2079
  idiopathic, of bowel; see Inflammatory bowel disease, idiopathic
  injury to colon in, 568
  of liver; see Hepatitis
  in mesentery, 1822-1823
  in paracolic fat, 754-755
  of pericolic fat, 2105
  in retroperitoneum, primary, 1818-1819
  of small bowel; see Enterocolitis
  of stomach, 325-336; see Gastritis; Stomach, inflammatory diseases of

Inflammatory bowel disease, idiopathic, 564-626
  barium examination in, 565-568
  carcinoma in, 795
  in child, 1919-1925
  colitis in; *see* Colitis
  colonoscopy in, 608-609; *see also* Colonoscopy
  computed tomography for, 610-615
  Crohn's disease in, 585-603; *see also* Crohn's disease
  differential diagnosis of, 603-608
  diverticula in; *see* Diverticula
  double-contrast enema in; *see* Double-contrast examination
  evaluation of therapy for, 609
  fluoroscopy in, 564-568
  imaging techniques for, 564-568
  intestinal permeability in, 83
  magnetic resonance imaging of, 616-619
  pathology of, 568-573
  plain films of, 564-565
  portal hypertension and, 1596, 1597, 1598
  primary sclerosing cholangitis in, 1306-1307
  radiologic follow-up in, 609
  scintigraphy in, 609-610
  single-contrast barium enema in; *see* Single-contrast examination
  small bowel meal with pneumocolon in, 517, 519, 521
  ulcerative colitis in, 573-585, 1919-1921; *see also* Ulcerative colitis
  ultrasonography of, 615-616
Inflammatory lymph nodes, sonography of, 2101
Inflammatory polyps; *see also* Polyp
  in Crohn's disease, 591, 593
  fibroid
    gastric, 360
    peroral biopsy in, 553, 554
    small bowel, 553, 554, 630
  in juvenile polyposis of colon, 787
  in large bowel inflammatory disease, 576
Inflammatory pseudotumor
  of small bowel, 630
  of stomach, 359
Inframesocolic spaces, 1797, 1800
Infusion rates in biphasic enteroclysis, 535-539
Inhibitors, proton pump, 72-73, 76
Inhibitory reflex, rectoanal, 840, 845
Ink as dye in gastric endoscopy, 304
Inspissated bile and debris after liver transplantation, 1743
Inspissated milk or milk curd syndrome, 1915
Insulin
  in gastrointestinal physiology, 69
  in glucagonoma, 1171
  in insulinoma, 1169
  in islet cell tumors, 1168
  mechanism of action of, 68
  in pancreatic tumors, 1132
Insulin antibodies, serum, 1169
Insulinoma, 69, 70, 1169-1170
  epidemiology in, 1167
  in hepatic metastases, 1711
  imaging of, 1173, 1174, 1175
    intraoperative, 1191
    localization procedures and, 1192
    magnetic resonance, 1181
  pancreatic ultrasonography of, 1028, 1029
  portal vein sampling in, 1188
Interlobar vessel, 29
Internal anal sphincter, 840
Interstitial compartment of liver, 1709-1713, 1714

Interstitial emphysema
  bowel wall, 2069
  gastric, 334-336
Interval cancers, 830
Interventional radiology
  in hepatocellular carcinoma, 1667, 1702, 1703
  history of, 23-24
  percutaneous; *see* Percutaneous interventional radiology
Intestinal atresia; *see* Atresia
Intestinal calculi, 893-894
Intestinal capillariasis, 937-938
Intestinal dysplasia, neuronal, 1915
  in child, 1915
Intestinal hurry, 661
Intestinal lactase deficiency, 684
Intestinal lipodystrophy, 679
Intestinal lymphangiectasia
  in celiac disease, 666-668, 669
  in child, 1898, 1899
  thickened valvulae conniventes in, 660
  Whipple's disease versus, 506
Intestinal metaplasia, 330
Intestinal obstruction; *see also* Large bowel, obstruction of; Small bowel, obstruction of
  afferent loop, 2107-2108
  anal sphincter, 845
  channel, after obesity surgery, 461, 463, 464
  in child, 1897, 1899-1902
  closed loop, 2092
    computed tomography and, 2093
    sonography of, 2107
  of colon
    in carcinoma and colitis, 793-795
    in colorectal carcinoma, 805
    radiologic caveats in, 795, 797
    single-contrast barium enema in, 704
    water-soluble contrast enema in, 712
  duodenal
    in annular pancreas, 468
    from cytomegalovirus disease, 477
    plain films and contrast studies in, 2044-2045
    tuberculosis and, 891
  in Gardner's syndrome, 781
  gastric outlet; *see* Gastric outlet obstruction
  mechanical, 2101
  percutaneous abscess drainage and, 1998
  plain films and contrast studies in, 2042-2063
    in biliary tree gas, 2032, 2033, 2053, 2055
    in cecal volvulus, 2061-2063
    in confirming diagnosis, 2047, 2050
    distinction between small and large bowel dilatation in, 2044-2045
    in duodenum, 2044-2045
    in gallstone ileus, 2051-2053, 2054
    in gastric dilation, 2042-2043, 2044, 2045
    in hernias, 2048, 2053
    in infarction of small bowel, 2054-2057
    in intussusception, 2054, 2055
    in large bowel, 2057-2063
    in mesenteric thrombosis, 2054-2057
    in pseudoobstruction, 2059, 2060
    in small bowel, 2045-2057
    in strangulation, 2047-2048
    in volvulus of large bowel, 2059, 2060
    in volvulus of small bowel, 2048, 2052
  small bowel; *see* Small bowel, obstruction of
  in stomach, 361

Intestinal obstruction—cont'd
  ultrasonography of, 2106-2108
Intestinal parasites; *see* Parasites
Intestinal peptides; *see also* Vasoactive intestinal peptides
  clinical implications of, 69-72
  physiology of, 68, 69, 70
Intestinal pseudoobstruction; *see* Pseudoobstruction, intestinal
Intestinal tuberculosis; *see* Tuberculosis
Intestinal vein catheterization, 1608
Intestinal walls; *see* Bowel wall
Intestine; *see also* Bowel; Colon; Small bowel
  anastomosis of extrahepatic duct to, 1981
  bowel preparation of, 90
  conjugated contrast in, 1228, 1229
  gas in, in liver ultrasonography, 1466
  hypomotility syndrome of, in neonate, 1902-1903
  ischemia of; *see* Ischemia, intestinal
  obstruction of; *see* Intestinal obstruction
  permeability of, 82, 83
  radioactive tracer reflux into, 1235
  in Ruvalcaba-Myhre-Smith syndrome, 785
  somatostatinoma in, 1171-1172
Intraabdominal abscesses, 2035-2042; *see also* Abscess
Intraarterial digital subtraction angiography, 1605-1606
Intraarterial vasopressin; *see* Vasopressin
Intracorporeal shock wave lithotripsy, 1426
Intrahepatic bile duct
  after liver transplantation, 1738
  calculi in, 1350, 1351, 1352
    extracorporeal shock wave lithotripsy for, 1361-1362
    percutaneous endoscopy for, 1427-1429
  in cirrhosis with portal hypertension, 1574
  computed tomography of, 1232
  dilatation of
    in Caroli's disease, 1976
    cystic, 1270-1271, 1976
    in primary sclerosing cholangitis, 1308, 1309, 1310
    in recurrent pyogenic cholangitis, 1303
  diverticular outpouchings of, 1307, 1309
  drainage patterns of, 1256, 1257
  embryology of, 1270
  gas in, 1304, 1305
  infarction of, 1270
  ischemia of, 1270
  leaks from, disparate sulfur colloids and iminodiacetic acid scintigraphic images in, 1523, 1524, 1525
  magnetic resonance imaging of, 1236
  percutaneous transhepatic cholangiography of, 1238-1239
  strictures of
    in primary sclerosing cholangitis, 1307, 1308
    in recurrent pyogenic cholangitis, 1303
  trifurcation of, 1256, 1257
  tumor extension beyond, percutaneous intervention and, 1403
  variants and anomalies of, 1256, 1257
Intramural hemorrhage
  abdominal, 2089-2091
  intestinal, 650-651, 2091
Intramural pneumatosis; *see* Pneumatosis, intramural
Intramural pseudodiverticulosis, esophageal, 216, 226
  strictures in, 238
Intraoperative guidewire for percutaneous biliary stricture dilation, 1383

Intravascular intervention; *see* Interventional radiology
Intravenous contrast media; *see* Contrast agents
Intravenous pyelography, 1751, 1752, 1763
Intravenous urography, 2071
Intrinsic factor, 77
Intubation of stomach and duodenum, 296-297
    in endoscopy, 302-304
Intussusception, 2054
    of anus, defecography of, 845, 849
    barium examination in, 1900-1902
    in celiac disease, 665
    in child, 1899-1902
    of colon, 714
        in carcinoma, 795, 796, 805-806
    in cystic fibrosis, 1930
    of duodenum, 472-473
    in gastric pedunculated fibroid polyps, 382
    ileocolic
        in child, 1902
        in small bowel obstruction, 2055
    of rectum
        in carcinoma, 805-806
        defecography of, 845, 849
    of small bowel
        in carcinoid tumor, 633
        in neoplasms, 627, 628
        in obstruction, 527, 530, 2054, 2055
        in perforation in child, 1902
        in Peutz-Jeghers syndrome, 1895
    ultrasonography of, 1900, 2106
Iodinated contrast media; *see also* specific agent
    in computed tomography arterial portography, 1460
    in liver, 1453
        in hemangioma, 1634
        in hepatocellular carcinoma, 1678
        in metastases, 1709, 1712
    in small bowel, 530
Iodine 131 anti-CEA, 1333
Iodine 131 as radioactive tracer, 87
Iodine 131 metaiodobenzylguanidine, 634
Iodine-labeled meta-iodobenzylguanidine, 87
Iodine-labeled rose bengal, 1233
    history of use of, 15
Iodipamide, history of use of, 13
Iodipamidol, 288
Iodized oil in transcatheter embolization; *see* Lipiodol
Iohexol
    in hepatic angiography, 1604
    in hepatic computed tomography, 1458
Iopamidol
    in hepatic angiography, 1604
    in hepatic computed tomography, 1458
Iopanoic acid, 1227, 1228
Iothalamate meglumine, 1458
Ioversol, 1604
Ioxaglate meglumine-sodium
    as esophageal contrast, 183
    in hepatic angiography, 1604
Ioxaglic acid; *see* Ioxaglate meglumine-sodium
IPSID; *see* Immunoproliferative small intestinal disease
Iron
    in constipation, 90
    in liver
        fatty infiltration versus, 1492
        in hemochromatosis, 1560-1565
        magnetic resonance imaging of, 1492, 1496, 1542-1543
        ultrasonography of, 1477
    serum, in hemochromatosis, 1561

Iron oxide contrast agents
    in hepatic imaging, 1501, 1502
        of hemangioma, 1638
        in metastases, 1708
    in stomach and duodenal imaging, 308
Iron sulfate in esophagitis, 1847
Irradiation damage; *see* Radiation
Irritable bowel syndrome, 686
    diagnostic studies in, 701-702
    prostaglandins and, 72
Irritant cathartics before colon imaging, 697
Irritant drugs in esophageal ring strictures, 235
Ischemia
    of gallbladder, 1280
    in hepatic infarction, 1616-1617
    intestinal, 685, 686; *see also* Ischemic colitis
        computed tomography of, 2089-2091
        Crohn's disease versus, 603, 605, 606
        mesenteric, 649-650
        strictures and, 650
        toxic megacolon in, 603
        ultrasonography of, 2108, 2109
    of intrahepatic bile ducts, 1270
Ischemic colitis; *see also* Colitis; Ischemia
    in carcinoma, 795
    computed tomography of, 613
    plain films and contrast studies in, 2068
    ultrasonography of, 615
Ischemic duodenitis, radiation, 476
Ischemic enteritis, 685, 686
Ischial tuberosity in defecography, 845
Islet cell abnormality in nesidioblastosis, 1950
Islet cell tumor, 1167-1196
    adenocarcinoma versus, 1122, 1177
    arterial stimulation and venous sampling in, 1188-1189
    carcinoid tumors in, 1172
    in child, 1952-1953
    corticotropinoma in, 1172
    cystic, 1157-1158
    ectopic hormones and, 1172
    endosonography of, 1189-1190, 1191
    epidemiology of, 1167
    gastrinoma in, 1170-1171
    glucagonoma in, 1171
    GRFoma in, 1172
    in hepatic metastases, 1711
    insulinoma in, 1169-1170
    localization of, 1173-1193
        arterial stimulation and venous sampling in, 1188-1189
        arteriography in, 1182-1187, 1189
        choice of method in, 1191-1193
        computed tomography in, 1174-1177, 1178-1187
        endosonography in, 1189-1190, 1191
        gastrinoma in, 1192-1193
        insulinoma in, 1192
        intraoperative ultrasound in, 1190-1191
        magnetic resonance imaging in, 1178-1182, 1183
        portal venous sampling in, 1187-1188, 1189
        somatostatin receptor imaging in, 1191
        specific procedures for, 1173-1191
        ultrasonography in, 1173-1174, 1175
    multiple endocrine neoplasia in, 1168-1169
    neurotensinoma and, 1172
    nonfunctioning, 1172-1173
    pancreatic, hepatic magnetic resonance imaging and, 1495
    pancreatic islet in, 1167
    parathyrinoma in, 1172
    pathology of, 1167-1168

Islet cell tumor—cont'd
    pediatric, 1952, 1953
    PPomas in, 1172
    small or large, 1173
    small primary tumors, 1177, 1179
        imaging in, 1187, 1192
    somatostatinoma in, 1171-1172
    VIPoma in, 1171
Isospora belli, 957
Isotopes
    in intestinal permeability, 82
    in obesity surgery radiographs, 460
    in pancreatic transplantation, 1202, 1203
Isovue; *see* Iopamidol
Ito cell, 85
IVC; *see* Vena cava, inferior

J

J maneuver, 304
J-pouch, 585
J-tipped guidewire, 1424
Japanese experience
    in gastric carcinoma; *see* Gastric carcinoma, in Japan
    in hepatocellular carcinoma, 1688-1705; *see also* Hepatocellular carcinoma
Jaundice
    in bile duct obstruction, from hepatic hilar cysts, 1319
    in biliary tract obstruction, percutaneous endoscopy for, 1429
    in child, 1975-1976
    in cholangiocarcinoma, 1334
    in hepatocellular carcinoma, 1665
    obstructive
        endoscopic intervention for, 1426, 1429, 1433
        with gallbladder carcinoma, 1325
        as indication for stent placement, 1432
        in pancreatic adenocarcinoma, 1107
Jejunal anastomosis, biliary access through, 1414
Jejunal atresia or stenosis, 1885, 1886
Jejunal capsule biopsy, peroral, 552
Jejunal folds of small bowel, 513
Jejunal interposition, 162, 163
Jejunal loop, Roux-en-Y, 689, 690
Jejunal tube in duodenal compression, 1903
Jejunization of ileum, 681, 682
Jejunobiliary anastomosis, 689, 690
Jejunoileitis, ulcerative, 665-666
Jejunostomy
    in abscess drainage, 2009
    for percutaneous biliary stricture dilation, 1383
    in percutaneous fluoroscopically guided gastrostomy, 2012-2013, 2016, 2017
Jejunum
    adenocarcinoma of, 641
    anatomy of, 29, 512, 513
    in ascariasis, 929
    in biphasic enteroclysis with methylcellulose, 535
    in celiac disease, 664
    in Chagas' disease, 921, 922
    in Crohn's disease, 600, 601
        ultrasonography of, 616
    in double-contrast enteroclysis with air, 549
    ectopic pancreas and, 1048
    in giardiasis, 924, 926
    in intestinal lactase deficiency, 684
    lymphoma of
        enteroclysis in, 637
        moulage phenomenon in, 638
        small bowel, 637, 638

Jejunum—cont'd
  metastatic melanoma to, 646
Jugular vein in hepatic angiography, 1605
Jugulodigastric area, 142, 143
Juvenile polyposis
  of colon, 787-788, 1926, 1927, 1928
  generalized, 1926, 1927, 1928, 1929
  of infancy, 1926, 1927, 1928
  small bowel and, 631
  of stomach, 376
Juvenile polyps in large bowel, 778, 1926,
    1927
  in large bowel, 1926, 1927, 1928, 1929
Juxta-Vaterian diverticulum, 469

K

Kajitani classification of gastric carcinoma,
    416
Kaposi's sarcoma
  in colon, 792-793, 795
  in duodenum, 492, 494
  in gastrointestinal bleeding, 961-962, 963
  in retroperitoneum, 1814
  in small bowel, 645, 673, 674
  in spleen, 1787
  in stomach, 435
Kasai procedure, 1981
Kawasaki disease, 1980
Keloids, 781
Keratoacanthoma in Muir-Torre syndrome, 786
Kerckring's folds, 467
Kidney
  anatomy of, 30, 31, 61-63
  biopsy of, 1197
  blood vessel trauma in, 2149
  calculi in, extracorporeal shock wave
      lithotripsy in, 1102
  computed tomography of, 63
    of midkidneys, 63
    of renal fascia, 63
    of renal poles, 63
    in trauma, 2135, 2136
  cystic disease of, 1270
  dromedary hump of, 29, 63
  in hepatic ultrasonography, 1469
  left, 30
    magnetic resonance imaging of midplane
        in, 47
    sagittal anatomic section of, 46
  magnetic resonance imaging of, 47
  metastases to, 1992-1993
  percutaneous interventional radiology and,
      1992-1994
  polycystic disease of, 1156
  in red blood cell scintigraphy, 1640
  right, 31
  trauma to, 2135, 2136
  ulcerative colitis and, 574
Killian-Jamieson's diverticulum, 118, 119
Killian's triangle, 73
Kinin peptides, 632
Kissing artifact, 288, 289
Kissing ulcers, 478, 481
  linear ulcer with, 484
Klatskin's tumor, 1339
Klebsiella
  in bacterial cholangitis, 1304
  in emphysematous cholecystitis, 1286
  in emphysematous cystitis, 2070
  in gas-forming infections, 2070
Koch pouch, 585
Kocher maneuver, 1190
Krukenberg tumor, 438, 1326
Kulchitsky cells, 384, 434, 778

Kupffer cells, 1486
  in hemochromatosis, 1562
  in hepatocellular carcinoma, 1511
  in magnetic resonance imaging, 1502
  in scintigraphy of cirrhosis, 1544
Kwashiorkor, 553, 554
  liver in, 1547-1548
Kyphosis, 120, 123

L

Laceration
  of liver
    scintigraphy in, 1515
    ultrasonography of, 1475
  of spleen, scintigraphy in, 1515-1517
Lactase deficiency, 79, 684
Lactobezoar
  in child, 1873
  in milk curd syndrome, 1915
Lactose in barium examination, 684
Lactulose
  in bowel preparation, 90
  in enteroclysis for small bowel examination,
      515
  in inspissation after barium enema, 714
  in intestinal permeability, 82
Ladd's band, 467
  in child, 1883
Laënnec's cirrhosis, 1534
Lahr balloon, 844
Laimer's triangle, 118
Lamina propria, 82
  of gastrointestinal wall, 187
  of small bowel, 513
Laminar retroperitoneum, 1807-1808
Laparoscopy in pancreatic adenocarcinoma,
    1110
Laparotomy
  adhesions after, 2028
  in colorectal carcinoma, 779
Laplace's law, 750
Large bowel; *see also* Colon
  assessment of function of, 88-89
  atresia of
    congenital, 1908, 1909
    imaging in, 1909
  barium examination of, 565-566, 696
    air lock in, 710
    in cancer screening, 829, 832-833, 835
    in carcinoma follow-up, 832
    cleansing enema before, 698
    colonoscopy versus, 608
    with computed tomography for
        diverticulitis, 753
    contraindications to, 701
    in defecography, 841, 844, 845
    in endometriosis, 778
    failure in filling of cecum in, 711
    in familial multiple polyposis, 782, 783
    flexible sigmoidoscopy before, 832
    in functional constipation, 1915
    in hereditary nonpolyposis colon cancer,
        836
    for immobile patient, 710-711
    inadequate bowel preparation in, 710
    indications for, 567-568
    in inflammatory bowel disease, 608
    in ischemic colitis, 2068
    in juvenile polyps, 778
    in neoplasia, morphology and, 763
    perforation in, 714
    in polyps, 765-767, 768
    radiologic caveats in, 795, 797
    single-contrast enema in, 703-704
    spasm and incontinence in, 710

Large bowel—cont'd
  barium examination of—cont'd
    in sprue, 912, 913
    in ulcerative colitis, 1920
  computed tomography of, 696, 697,
      717-719
    in carcinoma staging, 795
    in colorectal carcinoma; *see* Colorectal
        carcinoma, computed tomography of
    in Crohn's disease, 611
    in diverticulitis, 753-759; *see also*
        Diverticulitis, computed tomography
        of
    in familial multiple polyposis, 783
    preparation for, 802
    rectal contrast material in, 802
    techniques for, 717-719
    thickening of descending colon in, 610
  congenital anomalies of, 1908, 1909-1912
    anorectal malformations in, 1909-1912
    atresia in, 1908-1909
  Crohn's disease in, 589-594; *see also*
      Crohn's disease
  cystic fibrosis in, 1930
  developmental anomalies of, 1908,
      1909-1912
  diarrhea and, 89-90
  dilation of, small bowel dilatation versus,
      2044-2045
  double-contrast barium enema in, 704-711
  endoscopy of, 715-716
  endosonography of, 725-727
  history of radiology of, 8-10
  ileus and, 2059
  infection and inflammation in, 1916-1919
    appendicitis as, 1925-1926
    Behçet disease as, 1924
    in child, 1916-1926
    cow's milk allergy colitis as, 1925
    Crohn's colitis as, 1921-1924
    eosinophilic gastroenteritis as, 1924
    hemolytic uremic syndrome and, 1924
    Hirschsprung's colitis as, 1925
    idiopathic inflammatory bowel disease in,
        1919-1925
    infectious colitis as, 1924
    neonatal necrotizing enterocolitis in,
        1916-1919
    neutropenic colitis in, 1918, 1919
    typhlitis in, 1918, 1919
    ulcerative colitis as, 1919-1921
    Yersinia colitis as, 1924-1925
  inflammatory disease of
    granularity in, 575-576
    idiopathic, 564-626; *see also*
        Inflammatory bowel disease,
        idiopathic
    plain films in, 564-565
    ulceration in; *see* Ulcerative colitis
  magnetic resonance imaging of, 697,
      719-720
    in colorectal carcinoma; *see* Colorectal
        carcinoma, magnetic resonance
        imaging in
  neoplasms of, 762-800
    adenomas in; *see* Adenoma, of colon
    artifacts versus, 771-772, 773
    benign, 1926-1927, 1928, 1929
    carcinoid in, 778
    characteristic features of, 789
    clinical symptoms of, 765
    colonoscopy in, 767-770
    complications of, 793-795
    confidence level for detection of, 770-771
    contrast enema in, 765-767, 768

Large bowel—cont'd
neoplasms of—cont'd
Cowden's disease in, 786-787, 1926
Cronkhite-Canada syndrome in, 787
detection of, 765-771
differential diagnosis in filling defects in, 788
distribution of, 763-764
endometriosis in, 778-779
familial multiple polyposis in, 780-781, 782-783
Gardner's syndrome in, 781-783, 784, 785
hereditary nonpolyposis colorectal carcinoma in, 788-790
high-risk groups for, 765
histology of, 762-763
juvenile polyposis syndrome in, 778, 779-788, 1926, 1927, 1928, 1929
lipomas in, 777-778
location of, 776-777
malignant, 790-796, 1927
management of, 779
morphologic findings in, 772-774
morphology of, 763
Muir-Torre syndrome in, 786
multiple hamartoma in, 786-787
origin of, 764-765
pathology of, 762-765
pediatric, 1926-1927, 1928, 1929
pedunculation of, 774
peritoneal implants and, 792
Peutz-Jeghers syndrome in, 783-785
polypoid, specific, 777-779
polyposis syndromes in, 779-788, 1926, 1928, 1929
radiologic features of, 771-777
radiology caveats in carcinoma and, 795-797
rare benign, 779
reticular or filiform surface pattern of, 774, 775
Ruvalcaba-Myhre-Smith syndrome in, 785
secondary, 792
size of, 774
surface contour in, 774-776, 777
Turcot syndrome in, 786
obstruction of; see also Intestinal obstruction
cecal volvulus in, 2061-2063
in colorectal carcinoma, 805
in Gardner's syndrome, 781
plain films and contrast studies in, 2057-2063
radiologic caveats in, 795, 797
single-contrast barium enema in, 704
types of, 2056, 2057
volvulus in, 2059, 2060
pediatric, 1907-1931
anatomy of, 1907
cystic fibrosis and, 1930
developmental and congenital anomalies of, 1908, 1909-1912
embryology and, 1907
functional immaturity of, 1915
functional motility disorders of, 1912-1915, 1916
infection and inflammation in, 1916-1926
neoplasms of, 1926-1927, 1928, 1929
normal appearance of, 1907
trauma in, 1927
perforation of
after liver transplantation, 1748
in barium enema, 714, 715
in carcinoma, 793
by colon carcinoma, 756

Large bowel—cont'd
perforation of—cont'd
in colorectal carcinoma, 805
in percutaneous cholecystostomy of cholecystitis, 1381
retroperitoneal abscess and, 2039
peroral pneumocolon in, 713
physiology of, 88-91
polypoid lesions of, in inflammatory bowel disease, 576
polyps of, juvenile, 778, 779-788, 1926, 1927, 1928, 1929
potential for malignancy of, 774-777
rare benign neoplasms of, 779
reporting of examination of, 715
single-contrast barium enema of, 703-704
surveillance of tumor-prone, 779
techniques for, 696-720
choice of double versus single contrast in, 711
colostomy enemas in, 712-713
complications of, 714-715
contrast agents and, 699-703
equipment and, 697
errors in, 699
in functional metabolic imaging, 720
instant and gas enemas in, 712
integration of endoscopy and radiology in, 716
postresection enemas in, 713
preliminaries and, 697-699
in radiographic contrast examinations, 697
repeat enema versus endoscopy in, 712
in therapeutic examinations, 713
transit studies of, 88
trauma to
in child, 1927
computed tomography of, 2138-2139
ultrasonography of, 697, 716-717
transabdominal, 716-717
varices of, 977
portal hypertension and, 1599, 1600
vascular supply of, 694, 695
wall thickening in, diverticulitis differential diagnosis and, 754
water-soluble contrast enema in, 711-712
Large cell carcinoma of pancreas, 1152-1153
Laryngeal muscles, 106
Laryngeal nerve, paresis of, 130
Laryngeal vestibule of pharynx, 127, 130, 131
Laryngectomy
in pharyngeal reconstruction, 160
supraglottic partial, 158
Laryngocele, 120, 122
Laryngotracheal complex, 94
Laryngotracheoesophageal cleft, 212, 1829
Larynx
elevation of, epiglottic mobility and, 130
hypoglossal tumors and, 157, 158, 159
vestibule of, 127
in functional abnormalities of swallowing, 130, 131
Laser
in bleeding gastric ulcer hemostasis, 971-972
in heat ablation of liver neoplasms, 1719
in lithotripsy and endoscopic sphincterotomy for large stones, 1348-1350
magnetic resonance imaging in necrosis from, 1499
in probes for hepatic duct, 1375
Lateral abdominal view, 2021-2022
Lateral decubitus view in pneumoperitoneum, 2022
Lateroconal fascia, 28

Latex, sensitivity to, 715
Latex balloon in rectal endosonography, 813-814
Laurell, 10
Lauterbur, P, 20, 21
Law, Laplace's, 750
Laxatives
in bowel preparation, 90
for colon studies, 565
in constipation, 713
for enteroclysis, 515, 548
for inspissation after barium enema, 714
Lead time bias, 830
Leak
of abdominal aortic aneurysm, 2071-2073
anastomotic
after obesity surgery, 459-460
after pancreatic transplantation, 1198, 1221
bile duct
in liver transplantation complications, 1739-1740
of T-tube site, 1739, 1740
in esophageal fluoroscopy, 168, 183
exocrine pancreatic, after transplantation, 1198, 1221
Leather bottle structure in gastric radiology, 420
Lecithins, 84
Left lateral decubitus position, 2021
Leioblastoma, gastric, 453
Leiomyoblastoma
esophageal, 269-270
gastric, 377
of small bowel, 628
Leiomyoma
of duodenum, 496
ectopic pancreas and, 1048
esophageal, 250-251, 269-270
diffuse, 251
gastric, 377-379
bleeding, 973
in child, 1873
endosonography of, 450, 453
small bowel, 627-628
portal hypertension and, 1596
Leiomyosarcoma
of duodenum, 496, 497
ectopic pancreas and, 1048
esophageal, 269-270
gastric, 432-433, 450, 453
in greater omentum, 1822
of liver, 1684
in metastases, 1713
of pancreas, 1155
in peritoneal cavity, 1804
small bowel, 642
biopsy in, 557
portal hypertension and, 1596
Length time bias, 830
Leonard, CL, 5
Lesser omentum, 30, 35
computed tomography of, 306
Lesser sac of pancreas
abscess of, 2040
plain films and contrast studies of, 2037-2039
anatomy of, 30, 1797
gas in, from misplaced needle, 1821
superior recess of, 31
Leukemia
gallbladder infiltration in, 1330
spleen in
infarct of, 1777, 1779, 1781
pediatric, 1938

Leukemia—cont'd
  stomach in, 435
Leukocytes
  indium-labeled; *see* Indium 111–labeled
      leukocytes
  in pancreatic transplantation, 1202
  in rejection, 1207, 1213
Leukotrienes, 72
Levator ani muscle, 841
  contraction of, 847
  in straining, 849
Levocardia, 1865
LGV; *see* Lymphogranuloma venereum
Lidocaine
  in hepatic angiography, 1604
  for percutaneous biliary dilation of
      strictures, 1386
  in percutaneous transhepatic
      cholangiography, 1237
Lieberkühn, crypts of; *see* Crypts of
      Lieberkühn
Lienorenal ligament, 30
Ligament
  in abdomen, 1808
  hepatoduodenal, 1224, 1225
      hematoma and, 1821
  of Treitz, 32, 284
Ligamentum teres hepatis, 29, 31
Ligamentum venosum, 29
Light-bulb sign
  in hemangiomas, 1636
  in hepatic metastases, 1712, 1713
Lincomycin, 901
  esophagitis from, 231
Linear ulcers in Crohn's disease, 572
Lingual nerve, 150
Linitis plastica, 394
  carcinoma and, 395-397, 419, 420
  cross-sectional studies of, 397
  endoscopy and, 406
  endosonography of, 449, 450, 453
Lip
  papillomas of, in Cowden's disease,
      786-787
  tumors of, 147
Lipase
  in acinar cell carcinoma, 1154
  in pancreatoblastoma, 1156
Lipiodol
  in hepatocellular carcinoma computed
      tomography, 1678
  history of use of, 13
  in transcatheter embolization, 1717-1718,
      1728-1729
Lipodystrophy, intestinal, 679
Lipoma
  of colon, 777-778
      primary, 791-792, 793, 794
      surface contour of, 776
  of duodenum, 496
      intussusception and, 472
  of esophagus, 251, 270
  hepatic, 1480
      clinical background and pathology in,
          1658
      hepatocellular carcinoma versus,
          1697-1698
  of pancreas in Shwachman-Diamond
      syndrome, 1948-1949
  pleomorphic, in retroperitoneum, 1812
  small bowel, 628-629, 630
  in stomach, 381
      of child, 1873
Liposarcoma
  of esophagus, 249

Liposarcoma—cont'd
  of mesentery, 1824
  of pancreas, 1155
  in retroperitoneum, 1812-1813
Liquefaction necrosis
  of duodenum in nonepithelial tumors, 496
  of liver
      in hepatocellular carcinoma, 1667
      magnetic resonance imaging in, 1496
      ultrasonography of, 1476
Lithostar lithotriptor, 1094
Lithotripsy
  in bile duct stones, 1373, 1374
  in choledochoscopy, 1350
  in chronic pancreatitis, 1094
  clearance of fragments after, 1105, 1357,
      1358
  in endoscopic sphincterotomy, 1346
      for large stones, 1348-1350
  extracorporeal shock wave; *see*
      Extracorporeal shock wave lithotripsy
  history of development of, 24
  noncalcified pancreatic duct stone fragments
      after, 1105
  with percutaneous endoscopy of biliary
      tract, 1426
Lithotriptor
  electrohydraulic, 1356
      in choledocholithiasis, 1361, 1362
      in percutaneous endoscopy, 1425
      repeat lithotripsy with, 1360
  electromagnetic, 1356
      repeat lithotripsy with, 1360
  piezoelectric, 1359
      repeat lithotripsy with, 1360
  Soehendra, 1347
  types of, 1101-1102
  ultrasound, in choledocholithiasis, 1375
Liver
  abscess of; *see* Abscess, hepatic
  acinus of, 83
  in acquired immunodeficiency syndrome,
      960-961
  alcoholism and, 1548-1549; *see also*
      Alcohol abuse
  anatomy of, 32-33, 36-53, 1440-1452
      in angiography, 1608-1611, 1612, 1613
      bile ducts in, 1446
      in computed tomography during arterial
          portography, 1447-1448
      in delayed computed tomography, 1447
      in dynamic computed tomography,
          1446-1447
      hepatic arteries in, 1446
      hepatic veins in, 1444-1446, 1445
      in hepatocellular carcinoma, 1665-1666
      in magnetic resonance imaging,
          1449-1451
      portal veins in, 1444, 1445
      right lobe in, 31, 32-33
      segmental, 1440-1444
      surgical implications of, 1451
      in three-dimensional computed
          tomography during arterial
          portography, 1448-1449
      in transcatheter embolization, 1722-1723
      in transhepatic percutaneous
          cholecystolithotomy, 1376
      in ultrasonography, 1449, 1450,
          1468-1469
  aneurysm of, in child, 1975
  angiography of, 1608-1610, 1611-1619,
      1620
      anatomy in, 1608-1611, 1612, 1613
      arterial portography in, 1545, 1606-1607

Liver—cont'd
  angiography of—cont'd
      carbon dioxide, in carcinoma, 1688, 1689
      catheterization technique for, 1604-1605
      in cirrhosis, 1545, 1582-1583,
          1584-1586, 1596
      complications of, 1605
      computed tomography with, 1678
      contraindications to, 1605
      contrast medium in, 1604
      digital subtraction techniques in, 1604
      equipment and technique for, 1604
      glucagon in, 1604
      in hemangiomas, 1640-1642
      in hepatic artery diseases, 1608-1610,
          1611-1619, 1620
      in hepatic vein disease, 1607-1608,
          1610-1611, 1625-1628
      in hepatocellular carcinoma, 1677, 1688,
          1689, 1692-1698
      magnetic resonance imaging and, 1502,
          1503-1505
      in metastases, 635, 1706
      in multimodality approach to neoplasia,
          1464
      in pancreatic lymphangioma, 1161
      portal catheterization in, 1607-1608
      in portal hypertension, 1582-1583,
          1584-1586, 1596
      in portal vein diseases, 1610, 1619-1625
      for pretransplant imaging, 1736
      selective, in pancreatic lymphangioma,
          1161
      of sinusoids, 1611, 1612
      technical considerations in, 1604-1605
      technique for, 1605-1609
      transaxillary or transbrachial approach in,
          1604
      in transcatheter therapy, 1628
      in transplantation, 1736, 1744
  arterial disease of
      in child, 1973, 1974
      in cirrhosis, 1619, 1620
  in arteriosclerosis, 1614, 1615
  arteriovenous fistulas in, 1616, 1617-1618
  bare area of, 28
  benign tumors of, 1476-1477, 1630-1661
      adenoma in; *see* Adenoma, of liver;
          Hepatocellular adenoma
      angiography of, 1640-1642
      in child, 1966-1967, 1968
      computed tomography of, 1632-1635
      cysts in; *see* Liver, cysts of
      fatty infiltration versus, 1553-1554
      focal nodular hyperplasia in, 1651-1654,
          1655
      hemangiomas in; *see* Hemangiomas, liver
      heterotopic rests in, 1658-1660
      imaging features of, 1630-1642
      magnetic resonance imaging in,
          1635-1639
      mesenchymal tumors in, 1658-1660
      nodular regenerative hyperplasia in,
          1542-1543, 1544, 1545, 1655-1656;
          see also Liver, macroregenerative
          nodule in
      percutaneous biopsy in, 1642-1643
      plain films in, 1630-1631
      polycystic disease in, 1658, 1659
      in portal vein occlusion, 1623, 1624
      red blood cell scintigraphy in, 1639-1640
      technetium 99m sulfur colloid hepatic
          scintigraphy in, 1508-1514, 1515
      ultrasonography of, 1476-1477,
          1631-1632

Liver—cont'd
bile duct pathology and, 1318
biopsy of
arteriovenous fistulas after, 1617
hemobilia from, 976
in hemochromatosis, 1561-1562
imaging-guided, in metastases, 1708
percutaneous interventional radiology in
abdominal masses and, 1991
carcinoma of
metastatic; *see* Metastases, to liver
primary; *see* Hepatocellular carcinoma;
Liver, primary malignant neoplasms
of
caudad lobe of, 1441
caudate lobe of, 29, 33, 1441
papillary process of, 30, 34
caudate process of, 29
cirrhosis of; *see* Cirrhosis
computed tomography of, 1669-1674
in amebic abscess, 1961
anatomy and, 1441-1450
angiography combined with, 1678
arteriovenous iodine difference in, 1456,
1457
biphasic injection in, 1457
in cirrhosis with portal hypertension,
1577-1582, 1583, 1594-1596
contrast media in, rate of injection of,
1457
delayed, 1447, 1458-1459
dynamic; *see* Computed tomography,
dynamic; Incremental dynamic bolus
computed tomography of liver
equilibrium phase of, 1456
in fatty liver, 1551
findings in, 1669-1674
in hemangiomas, 1632-1635
in hepatic abscess aspiration, 2083
in hepatocellular carcinoma, 1689
hypervascular tumors in, 1460-1462
incremental dynamic bolus, 1458
maximal hepatic parenchymal contrast
enhancement in, 1456
maximal relative lesion contrast
attenuation in, 1456
in multimodality approach to liver
neoplasia, 1464
noncontrast, 1453-1454, 1456
followed by contrast, 1455, 1456
number of tumor nodules in, 1458, 1463,
1464
pediatric; *see* Liver, pediatric
in posttransplant imaging, 1737-1738,
1739
in pretransplant imaging, 1736
rate of contrast injection in, 1457
survey in, 1463-1464
techniques of, 1669
three-dimensional, 1448-1449
in trauma, 2123-2130
ultrasonography compared to, 1480
uniphase injection in, 1457
computed tomography angiography of,
1463, 1464
computed tomography arterial portography
of, 1447-1449, 1463, 1464
conjugation of contrast agents in, 1227-1228
in Crohn's disease, 589
cysts of, 1656-1658
anechoic, 1474, 1475
angiography of, 1657
in appendicitis, 2114
aspiration of, 1658
in child, 1967-1968, 1969

Liver—cont'd
cysts of—cont'd
clinical background and pathology of,
1656-1657
computed tomography of, 1657
hilar, 1319, 1320
hydatid, 1657
magnetic resonance imaging in, 1493,
1494, 1657
in mesenchymal hamartoma, 1966, 1968
in peliosis hepatis, 1618-1619
in polycystic disease, 1656-1658
radiology in, 1657-1658
scintigraphy in, 1657
ultrasonography of, 1474-1475
diffuse parenchymal disease of
magnetic resonance imaging in, 1496,
1500
ultrasonography of, 1469-1471
Doppler analysis of lesions of, 1480-1481
duplex Doppler imaging of
in pediatric liver transplantation, 1975
in pediatric portal hypertension, 1971,
1972
embryology of, 1251, 1796
endoscopic retrograde
cholangiopancreatography of; *see*
Endoscopic retrograde
cholangiopancreatography
enlarged; *see* Hepatomegaly
epithelial lesions of, 1967
fatty infiltration of, 1547-1559
alcoholic liver diseases in, 1548-1549
in child, 1969, 1970
in cirrhosis, 1541, 1553, 1563
classification of, 1547, 1549-1553
computed tomography of, 1551
differential diagnosis in, 1553-1554
dynamic computed tomography of, 1446
focally spared liver in, 1554-1556, 1557
hepatic masses versus, 1553-1554
in hepatitis, 1553
in hepatocellular carcinoma, 1667, 1669
hepatocellular carcinoma versus,
1697-1698
in kwashiorkor, 1547-1548
macrovesicular, 1547
magnetic resonance imaging of, 1492,
1496, 1500, 1551-1553
versus masses, 1553-1554
microvesicular, 1547
pathophysiology of, 1547-1549
pitfalls in evaluation of, 1556-1557, 1558
in pregnancy, 1549
prolonged parenteral nutrition in, 1548
radiology in, 1549-1558
Reye's syndrome in, 1549
round, 1554, 1555, 1556
round multifocal, 1556
scintigraphy of, 1509, 1517-1519, 1520,
1521, 1551-1553
technetium 99m sulfur colloid
scintigraphy of, 1517-1519, 1520,
1521
in ulcerative colitis, 574
ultrasonography of, 1470, 1549-1551
fibrosis of
in Caroli's disease, 1270
congenital, 1270, 1574
in hemochromatosis, 1561
presinusoidal portal hypertension in, 1574
fissures of, 32
computed tomography of, 1469
ultrasonography of, 1468-1469
focal lesions in, 1473-1481

Liver—cont'd
focal lesions in—cont'd
abscesses as, 1475, 1476
computed tomography of, 1448, 1449
cysts as, 1474-1475
Doppler analysis of, 1480-1481
magnetic resonance imaging of,
1491-1496, 1497-1499
metastases as, 1478-1480
primary benign hepatic neoplasms as,
1476-1477
primary malignant hepatic neoplasms as,
1477-1478
rare, 1480
trauma as, 1475
ultrasonography of, 1473-1481
focal nodular hyperplasia of; *see* Focal
nodular hyperplasia
fractures of, in child, 1974
gadolinium DTPA of, in angioma, 1966
hemangiomas of; *see* Hemangiomas
hematoma in
after extracorporeal shock wave
lithotripsy, 1360
in child, 1974
hemochromatosis and, 1561, 1969, 1970
hepatic artery and, 1608-1610
aneurysm of, 1615-1616
arteriosclerosis in, 1614, 1615
arteritis of, 1616
diseases of, 1611-1619, 1620, 1971-1973,
1974
infarction in, 1616-1617
spasm and dissection of, 1611, 1613
thrombosis of, after liver transplantation,
1744-1746
hepatic lobe of, 1441-1444
hepatic vein of
Budd-Chiari syndrome and, 1625,
1626-1628
cirrhosis and, 1628
diseases of, 1625-1628, 1971-1973, 1974
obstruction of, 1625, 1626-1628
portohepatic shunt and, 1625
hepatitis and; *see* Hepatitis
hepatocellular carcinoma of; *see*
Hepatocellular carcinoma
in hereditary hemorrhagic telangiectasia,
1618
herniations in, in diaphragmatic eventration,
1856
history of radiology of, 13-15
infarcts of, 1480
after transplantation, 1745
bile duct cysts and, 1319
in child, 1973
fatty liver versus, 1554
inflammation of; *see* Hepatitis
interstitial compartment size in, 1709-1713,
1714
interventional radiology for, 1667
intratumoral secretions in, fatty infiltration
versus, 1492
intratumoral vessels in, magnetic resonance
imaging of, 1496, 1504
laceration of
computed tomography of, 2095
scintigraphy of, 1515
ultrasonography of, 1475
left lobe of, 30, 31, 32-33
liquefaction necrosis of
magnetic resonance imaging in, 1496
ultrasonography of, 1476
lobectomy of, 1469
lobes of

Liver—cont'd
  lobes of—cont'd
    nomenclature of, 1440-1444
    normal segmental ducts of, 1224
    resection of, 1469
    ultrasonography of, 1468, 1469, 1471
  lymphatics of, in percutaneous transhepatic
      cholangiography, 1238
  macroregenerative nodule in, 1542-1543,
      1544, 1545, 1655-1656
    hepatocellular carcinoma and, 1674,
        1675-1676
  macrovesicular fatty infiltration of, 1547
  magnetic resonance imaging of, 1449-1451,
      1486-1507, 1674-1676
    acquisition time sequences in, 1488-1489
    angiography with, 1502, 1503-1505
    during arterial portography, 1499
    breath-holding in, 1488-1489
    in cirrhosis, 1541-1544, 1577-1582,
        1583, 1594-1596
    contrast-enhanced, 1496-1503
    contrast-to-noise ratio in, 1486, 1487
    in differential diagnosis, 1676-1677
    in diffuse disease, 1496, 1500
    in fatty liver, 1551-1553
    focal lesions in, 1491-1496, 1497-1499
    in hemangiomas, 1635-1639
    in hepatocellular carcinoma, 1692, 1694
    hypervascular tumors, 1545
    imaging strategies for, 1487
    intratumoral vessels in, 1496, 1504
    magnetic field in, 1489-1490
    modulation transfer function in, 1486
    motion-induced artifacts in, 1487-1489,
        1490
    in neoplasms, 1450, 1464
    pediatric; see Liver, pediatric
    in portal hypertension, 1577-1582, 1583,
        1594-1596
    proton density in, 1487, 1490
    respiratory gating in, 1489
    short-acquisition time in, 1488
    signal averaging in, 1487-1488
    spatial resolution in, 1486, 1487
    spatial saturation pulses in, 1489
    technical considerations in, 1486-1490
    techniques of, 1674
    tissue characterization in, 1490-1496,
        1497-1500
    vascular, 1503-1505
  metastases to; see Metastases, to liver
  neoplasms of
    benign; see Liver, benign tumors of
    fatty infiltration versus, 1553-1554
    metastatic; see Metastases, to liver
    multimodality approach to, 1464
    pediatric, 1961-1967
    portal hypertension from, 1575
    in portal vein occlusion, 1623, 1624
    primary malignant, 1662-1687; see also
        Liver, primary malignant neoplasms
        of
    rupture of, 1475
    ultrasonography of, 1476-1478, 1575
  parasites in, 915-918, 919, 920
  parenchyma of
    after transplantation, 1197, 1737, 1745
    computed tomography arterial portography
        of, 1460
    diffuse, 1469-1471, 1496, 1500
    hepatocellular carcinoma in, 1523
    magnetic resonance imaging of, 1496,
        1500
    metastases in, 1400, 1708

Liver—cont'd
  parenchyma of—cont'd
    nontumorous conditions in, 1523
    in percutaneous transhepatic
        cholangiography, 1238
    physiology of, 83-84
    primary tumor in, 1523
    technetium 99m—iminodiacetic acid
        scintigraphy of, 1522-1523, 1523,
        1525
    ultrasonography of, 1467, 1469-1471
  pediatric, 1958-1975, 1982-1985; see also
      Pediatrics, liver and biliary tract
      imaging in
  in peliosis hepatis, 1618-1619
  percutaneous interventional radiology in,
      1991-1992
  percutaneous needle aspiration of
    in pediatric hydatid disease, 1961
    in pediatric pyogenic abscess, 1959
  percutaneous transhepatic cholangiography
      in, 1238
  physiology of, 83-87
  portal vein of
    abnormalities of, after liver
        transplantation, 1747
    aneurysm of, 1623, 1624
    congenital anomalies of, 1622
    diseases of, 1619-1625
    intrahepatic vascular changes in cirrhosis
        and, 1628
    neoplastic occlusion of, 1623, 1624
    portohepatic shunt and, 1625
    thrombosis in, 1621, 1622-1623
  primary malignant neoplasms of
    alpha fetoproteins in, 1463, 1478, 1678
    angiosarcoma in, 1683-1684
    biliary cystadenocarcinoma in, 1681-1682
    computed tomography of, 1463
    epithelioid hemangioendothelioma in,
        1682-1683
    fibrolamellar, 1678-1680
    fibrosarcoma in, 1684
    hepatocellular carcinoma in, 1662-1678;
        see also Hepatocellular carcinoma
    intrahepatic cholangiocarcinoma in,
        1680-1681
    leiomyosarcoma in, 1684
    lymphoma in, 1684-1685
    malignant fibrous histiocytoma in, 1684
    neurofibrosarcoma in, 1684
    primary hepatic sarcomas in, 1684
    sclerosing, 1680
  quadrate lobe of, 31
  radiation effects on, 1975
  radiologically guided percutaneous
      procedures for, 1717-1721
    cryosurgery in, 1720
    ethanol injections in, 1718-1719
    intraoperative treatment in, 1719-1720
    laser heat ablation in, 1719
    percutaneous treatment in, 1717-1719
    resection in, 1719-1720
    transcatheter embolization in, 1717-1718
  rare focal lesions of, ultrasonography of,
      1480
  resection of
    anatomy and, 1451
    bile duct strictures after, 1314
    in cirrhosis, 1719
    hemobilia from, 976
    in hepatocellular carcinoma; see
        Hepatocellular carcinoma,
        resectability of
    segmental anatomy and, 1469

Liver—cont'd
  resection of—cont'd
    types of, 1451
  scintigraphy of, 1508-1533
    in abscess, 1519, 1531
    in acute cholecystitis, 1523
    in adenoma, 1511-1514, 1515
    in bacterial cholangitis, 1306
    in benign tumors, 1508-1514, 1515
    in Budd-Chiari syndrome, 1519, 1522,
        1523, 1524
    in choledochoceles, 1269
    in cirrhosis, 1516, 1517
    in congestive heart failure, 1522
    delayed iodine, in neoplasia, 1464
    disparate sulfur colloids and iminodiacetic
        acid images in, 1523, 1525
    in fatty liver, 1517-1519, 1520, 1521
    in focal nodular hyperplasia, 1508-1511,
        1523
    with gallium 67, 1531
    in hemangioma, 1522, 1526, 1527-1528
    in hepatitis, 1517
    in hepatocellular carcinoma, 1514, 1523,
        1531
    imaging techniques in, 1509
    with indium 111-labeled platelets, 1532
    with indium 111-labeled white blood
        cells, 1529-1530
    in malignant tumors, 1514, 1515
    in metastases, 1514, 1515
    in nontumorous disorders, 1514-1522,
        1523, 1524
    in pediatric angioma, 1966
    in primary tumor, 1508-1514, 1515, 1523
    rim sign in, 1523
    in secondary tumors, 1514, 1515
    with technetium 99m heat-damaged red
        blood cells, 1528-1529, 1530
    with technetium 99m—labeled white blood
        cells, 1531
    with technetium 99m microspheres, 1531
    with technetium 99m phosphate, 1531
    technetium 99m phosphate accumulation
        in, 1531
    with technetium 99m sulfur colloids,
        1508-1522, 1523, 1524
    with technetium 99m—iminodiacetic acid,
        1522-1523, 1525
    with technetium 99m—red blood cells,
        1526, 1527-1528
    in trauma, 1514-1517
    in vascular disorders, 1519-1523
    in wandering spleen, 1770
    with xenon 133, 1531
  segmentectomy of, 1469
  septal thickenings in, in biliary
      cystadenocarcinoma, 1682
  sinusoids of; see Sinusoids
  transplantation of; see Liver transplantation
  transverse anatomic section of upper, 48
  trauma to
    in child, 1974-1975
    computed tomography of, 1475,
        2123-2130
    technetium 99m sulfur colloid
        scintigraphy in, 1514-1517
  trisegmentectomy of, 1469
  tuberculosis of, 1311
  in ulcerative colitis, 574
  ultrasonography of, 1449, 1450, 1466-1485,
      1664, 1667-1669
    in acute abdomen, 2114-2115
    altered echogenicity in, 1470
    amplification in, 1466

Liver—cont'd
  ultrasonography of—cont'd
    anatomy and, 1468-1469
    in appendicitis, 2114
    architectural pattern in, 1471
    beam attenuation in, 1470
    bony structures in, 1466
    in calcifications, 1478
    in cirrhosis, 1470, 1537-1539,
      1575-1577, 1578, 1594-1596
    color-flow, in pediatric portal
      hypertension, 1971
    computed tomography compared to, 1480
    computer analysis of, 1470
    contrast-enhanced, 1473, 1478
    in debilitated patient, 1467
    diffuse parenchymal disease in,
      1469-1471
    echo texture in, 1466
    in fatty liver, 1549-1551
    focal lesions in, 1473-1481
    frequency-modulated imaging in, 1470
    in hemangiomas, 1631-1632
    hepatic vascular system in, 1471-1473
    in hepatitis, 1471
    in hepatocellular carcinoma, 1689
    intestinal gas in, 1466
    intraoperative, 1481-1482, 1715
    in malignant neoplasms, 1477-1478
    parenchyma in, 1467
    pediatric
      in amebic abscess, 1961
      in angiomatous lesions, 1966
      in cirrhosis, 1970, 1971
      in cysts, 1968, 1969
      in epithelial lesions, 1967
      in fibrolamellar hepatocarcinoma, 1964,
        1965
      in fungal abscess, 1960
      in granulomatous disease, 1961
      in hepatic arterial disease, 1973
      in hepatic trauma, 1974
      in hepatoblastoma, 1962, 1963
      in hydatid disease, 1961
      in liver transplantation, 1975
      in mesenchymal hamartoma, 1966
      in neoplasms, 1961
      in portal hypertension, 1971, 1972
      in portal vein thrombosis, 1972, 1973
      in pyogenic abscess, 1959, 1960
      in venoocclusive disease, 1973
      in viral hepatitis, 1959
    in pediatric metastases, 1965
    in portal hypertension, 1575-1577, 1578,
      1594-1596
    pseudotumor in, 1471
    refraction phenomenon in, 1474
    sensitivity of, 1470
    serial, in pediatric portal vein thrombosis,
      1972, 1973
    signal amplitude in, 1470
    spectral analysis in, 1470
    technical considerations in, 1466-1468
    time, gain, compensation settings in,
      1470
    transverse, 49
    tumefactions in, 1471
    upper, 49
    venous waveforms in, 1471
  vascular diseases of, 1486, 1604-1629
    anatomy and, 1608-1611, 1612, 1613
    angiography of; see Liver, angiography of
    hepatic artery, 1611-1619, 1620
    hepatic vein, 1625-1628
    portal vein, 1619-1625

Liver—cont'd
  vascular diseases of—cont'd
    technetium 99m sulfur colloid
      scintigraphy of, 1519-1523
    transcatheter therapy in, 1628
    ultrasonography of, 1471-1473
    vascular system of, 1486, 1608-1611; see
      also Hepatic artery; Hepatic vein
    trauma to, arteriography and therapeutic
      embolization in, 2147-2148
    ultrasonography of, 1471-1473
Liver cell adenoma, sonography of, 1476,
  2114, 2115; see also Adenoma, of
  liver; Hepatocellular adenoma
Liver flukes, 943-946, 1260-1261
  Clonorchis sinensis and, 943
  opisthorchiasis and, 943
  schistosomiasis and, 944-946
Liver function tests
  in gallbladder carcinoma, 1325
  in impairment, 1724
  in posttraumatic strictures, 1314
Liver overlap sign in volvulus, 2062
Liver transplantation, 1735-1750
  abdominal complications after, 1747-1748,
    1749
  angiography of, 1736, 1744
  biliary complications of, 1738-1744
  in child, 1975
  in cholangiocarcinoma, 1342
  cholangiography of, 1736
  in hepatic vein occlusion, 1628
  in hepatocellular carcinoma, 1666, 1667
  malignancy after, 1748-1749
  orthotopic, 1736-1737
  postoperative imaging in, 1738-1749
    bile duct leaks and, 1739-1740
    biliary complications and, 1738-1740
    normal, 1737-1738, 1739
    vascular complications and, 1744-1747
  pretransplant imaging in, 1735-1736
  primary sclerosing cholangitis in, 1307
  procedure for, 1736-1737
  ultrasonography of, 1470
  vascular complications after, 1744-1747
    hepatic artery thrombosis in, 1744-1746
    pseudoaneurysm in, 1746
Loop gastrojejunostomy, 456
Loopogram after colostomy, 1912
Lorazepam, 1725
Lower esophageal ring, 233
Lower esophageal sphincter; see Esophageal
  sphincter, lower
Lower motor neuron disease, 133
Lower renal poles, 63
Lumbar artery and vein, 30
  trauma to, therapeutic embolization in,
    2153
Lumbar vertebrae, 29
Lung
  anatomy of, 30
  carcinoma of
    esophageal endosonography of, 270
    esophageal submucosal spread of, 270
    oat cell, 645
  cystic adenomatous malformation of,
    Bochdalek's hernia versus, 1856
  embolus of barium to, 287
  hypoplasia of
    in Bochdalek's hernia, 1856
    in diaphragmatic eventration, 1856
  metastases to, from colon carcinoma,
    804
Lupus erythematosus, 656

Lymph nodes
  calcified
    in pharyngeal benign structural diseases,
      26
    in tuberculosis, 893-894, 894-895
  celiac, 29
    esophageal endosonography of metastases
      to, 270
    conglomerates of, in esophageal
      endosonography, 270
    dissection of, in gallbladder carcinoma,
      1333
  esophageal
    drainage from, 188
    endosonography of, 265, 266
    metastases in, 265, 266, 270
  in external compression of bile ducts,
    chemotherapy-induced cholangitis
    versus, 1311
  in gastric carcinoma, 438-441
    false-negative, 445
  mesenteric, 526
  in mesorectum, 818
  metastases to
    colorectal carcinoma, 803-804
    esophageal cancer, 265, 266, 270
    from pancreatic adenocarcinoma,
      1117-1118, 1121, 1158
    pharyngeal malignancy, 142, 150, 152,
      157
    rectal cancer, 818-820
  periintestinal, 265, 266
  peripancreatic, 1158
  portacaval, 34
  posterior triangle of, 144
  in reactive hyperplasia of colon, 804
  in rectal carcinoma, 813
  regional, in gastric carcinoma, 440
  retroportal, 34
  spinal accessory chain of, 144
Lymphadenopathy
  in esophageal cancer, 277, 280
  in gastric carcinoma, 442, 443
  in giant cell carcinoma of pancreas, 1153
  metastatic, in jugulodigastric area, 142, 143
  perigastric, in gastric lymphoma, 431
  in tuberculosis, 891
    of cecum and colon, 893
  in Whipple's disease, 680
Lymphangiectasia, intestinal, 1898
  in celiac disease, 666-668, 669
  thickened valvulae conniventes in, 660
  Whipple's disease versus, 506
Lymphangioma
  cavernous, 1160, 1161
  duodenal, 501
  gastric, 383-384
  pancreatic, 1160-1162
    calcifications in, 1160
    pediatric, 1954
    serous, 1138
  of pharynx in child, 1832, 1833
  in retroperitoneum, 1814
  of spleen, 1780
    in child, 1937
Lymphatics
  of colon, 804
  in duodenal endoscopy, 315
  of esophagus, 173, 188
  of gallbladder, 1326
  in gastrointestinal physiology, 82
  hepatic, in percutaneous transhepatic
    cholangiography, 1238
  of pancreas, 1108, 1117-1118, 1121
  of pharynx, 142, 152

Lymphatics—cont'd
  of stomach, 311, 312, 313, 314, 438
    endosonography of, 451-453
Lymphocytes, 82
  IgA-secreting, 677
Lymphocytic lymphoma of liver, 1684
Lymphogranuloma venereum, 904-908
  Crohn's disease versus, 603, 607
  ulcerative colitis versus, 604
Lymphoid gastritis, chronic, 354
Lymphoid hyperplasia
  benign
    of duodenum, 501
    of stomach in child, 1873
  in Crohn's disease, 596
  in Gardner's syndrome, 783
  nodular; see Nodular lymphoid hyperplasia
  reactive, 354
  of small bowel in giardiasis, 670, 671
  in stomach, 384
  ulcerative colitis versus, 605
Lymphoma
  Burkitt's; see Burkitt's lymphoma
  clinical features of, 634-635
  of colon, primary, 791-792, 793, 794
  conditions associated with, 635, 636
  differential diagnosis in, 639
  of esophagus, 249
  gastric
    acquired immunodeficiency syndrome
      and, 962-963, 964
    endosonography of, 449, 453
    tuberculosis and, 895
  in liver, 1684-1685
    after transplantation, 1748-1749
    in metastases in child, 1964, 1965
    secondary, 1685
  Mediterranean, 639, 677-678
  negative percutaneous abscess drainage and,
    2007
  non-Hodgkin's; see Non-Hodgkin's
    lymphoma
  of pancreas, 1162-1163
    adenocarcinoma versus, 1122
    in child, 1954
  pediatric, 1927, 1954
    in small bowel, 1895
    in spleen, 1935-1938
  in peritoneal cavity, 1804
  of pharynx, 139
    in child, 1834
    spread of, 142, 154
  primary, cholangiocarcinomas as, 1333
  radiographic features of, 635-639
  retroperitoneal, percutaneous interventional
    radiology in, 1994
  small bowel, 634-639, 1895
    biopsy in, 557
    celiac disease with, 659
    clinical features of, 634-635
    differential diagnosis of, 639
    diffuse primary, 677
    enteroclysis in, 659
    Mediterranean, 677-678
    mesentery and, 1824
    in nodular lymphoid hyperplasia, 635,
      636, 638, 661
    nodules in, 635, 636, 638
    in obstruction, 2050
    radiographic features of, 635
    variants in, 639
  of spleen, 1785, 1786
    in child, 1935-1938
  in stomach, 429-431, 453

Lymphoma—cont'd
  of tongue base and lingual tonsil, 154
  variants of, 639
Lymphoproliferative disease after liver
    transplantation, 1748
Lymphoreticular hyperplasia, 354
Lynch syndromes, 788, 825, 836
Lyophilized milk, 530
Lysine chains, 1499

M

Macroglobulinemia, Waldenström's, 681-682,
    683
  peroral biopsy in, 555, 556
Macrophages, 82
Macroregenerative nodule in liver, 1542-1543,
    1544, 1545, 1655-1656
Macrovesicular fatty liver, 1547, 1548
Maglinte biphasic enteroclysis with
    methylcellulose, 533
Magnesium citrate, 90
  for biphasic enteroclysis with
    methylcellulose, 534
  before colon imaging, 697
  in pneumocolon for small bowel
    examination, 515
Magnesium salts; see Magnesium citrate
Magnetic field, 1489-1490
Magnetic resonance imaging; see also specific
    organ
  of adrenal gland
    left sagittal, 45
    transverse, 53
  after pull-through surgery, 1912
  of anorectum, 696, 1912
  in Budd-Chiari syndrome, 1446
  in choledochal cyst, 1266
  in choledocholithiasis, 1300, 1303
  in cystic teratoma, 1158
  in glucagonoma, 1183-1184
  in hemochromatosis, 1563-1564
  history of, 19-22
  in islet cell tumors, 1178-1182, 1183
    in localization procedures, 1192
  in pediatric accessory spleen, 1933
  in pediatric lymphoma, 1938
  in pediatric pancreas, 1945-1946
  in splenomegaly, 1935
Mal du turista, 903
Malabsorption
  diagnosis of, 659
  duodenum in
    nonepithelial tumors of, 498
    physiology of, 80-81
  in giardiasis, 669-670, 923, 925
  small bowel in, 910-913
    aspiration cytology and peroral biopsy of,
      552
    in child, 1898, 1899
    functional diseases of, 659-688; see also
      Small bowel, functional diseases of
    infestations of, 669-671
    mucosal disease of, 1896-1898
    physiology of, 80-81
  in strongyloidiasis, 932
  term of, 661
Malacoplakia, 555, 556
Malecot catheter, 2014
Malformations; see Congenital abnormalities
Malignancy; see specific neoplasm or organ
Malignant colonic strictures, 583
Malignant fibrous histiocytoma
  in liver, 1684
  of pancreas, 1155
  in retroperitoneum, 1813

Malignant hemangiopericytoma; see
    Hemangiopericytoma
Malignant histiocytosis, 665
Malignant lymphoma polyposis, 791-792
Malignant schwannomas, in retroperitoneum,
    1813-1814
Mallory-Weiss tear, 218, 241
  gastrointestinal endoscopy in, 972-973
  in portal hypertension, 1582
Malmo technique for small bowel examination,
    514
Malnutrition in pancreatitis, 1091
Malrotation, small bowel, 1878-1884
  in neonatal megacystis-microcolon-intestinal-
    hypomotility syndrome, 1902-1903
  types of, 1881-1882, 1883
MALT; see Mucosa-associated lymphoid tissue
Mandible, tumors of, 147, 148, 150
Mandibular nerve, 150
Manganese-dipyridoxyl-5-diphosphate
  in focal nodular hyperplasia of liver, 1654
  in hepatic metastases, 1708
Mannitol, 90
  in intestinal permeability, 82
  in magnetic resonance imaging, 308
Manometry
  in defecography, 845
  esophageal; see Esophagus, manometry of
  hepatic
    angiography in, 1605-1606
    in cirrhosis with portal hypertension, 1583
    hepatic vein catheterization in, 1607
Marcaine; see Bupivacaine
Mass, defined, 762
Mast cell, 76, 82
Masticator space, 106, 110
Mastocytosis, 496-498, 682
Maxilla, tumors of, 147, 149
May-Grünwald-Giemsa stain, 558
Mayo spoon, 514
Mazzariello forceps, 1374
McGahan catheter, 1416
MDEC-1400 enteroclysis catheter, 543
Mechanical bowel obstruction, 2106-2108; see
    also Intestinal obstruction
Mecholyl test of esophagus, 181, 199-201
  in achalasia, 202
  in Chagas' disease, 210
  in diffuse spasm, 204
Meckel's diverticulum
  anatomy and, 512, 514
  angiography of, 1004
  in child, 1889-1892
  ectopic pancreas and, 1048
  scintigraphy in, 989-992
Meconium ileus
  barium examination of, 1886
  in child, 1886-1888
Meconium ileus equivalent, 1897
Meconium peritonitis
  antenatal ultrasonography of, 1891
  in child, 1891, 1892
Meconium plug, 1885, 1915
Mediastinal esophagus, 30
Mediastinum
  abscess of
    parapharyngeal, 120
    percutaneous abscess drainage of, 2009
  in esophageal computed tomography, 270
  in esophageal displacements, 254
  in esophageal endosonography, 188, 189,
    270
Mediterranean fever
  familial, 678

Mediterranean fever—cont'd
  small bowel in, 678
Mediterranean lymphoma, 639, 677-678
Megacolon
  in Chagas' disease, 921, 922-923
  idiopathic intestinal pseudoobstruction and,
      205
  in plain films and contrast studies, 2022,
      2065-2066, 2067
  toxic, 581-582, 712
    barium examination in, 565
    computed tomography in, 2086
    in Crohn's disease, 602
    in ulcerative colitis, 574, 581-582, 2067
Megacystis-microcolon-intestinal-hypomotility
    syndrome, 1902-1903
Megaduodenum
  in Chagas' disease, 921, 922
  congenital, 467
  idiopathic intestinal pseudoobstruction and,
      204
Megaesophagus, 203, 210
  achalasia and, 203
  in Chagas' disease, 921, 922
Megajejunum, 921, 922
Meglumine diatrizoate
  in double-contrast examination of small
      bowel, 524
  in percutaneous cholangioscopy, 1424
  in pharyngeal reconstruction imaging, 163
  in vaginography, 712
  as water-soluble contrast medium, 288
Meglumine sodium, 712
Meissner's plexus neurofibroma, 381
Melanocyte–stimulating hormone, 384
Melanoma metastasis
  to duodenum, 508
  to esophagus, 249
  to liver, 1712
  to small bowel, 643-645, 646
  to stomach, 432
Melena
  colonoscopy and, 696
  in small bowel leiomyosarcoma, 642
Membranes
  in duodenum as congenital abnormality, 467
  phrenicoesophageal, 218
MEN; see Multiple endocrine neoplasia
Ménétrier's disease, 351, 352, 353
  gastritis in, 326, 1870
Meperidine
  in biphasic enteroclysis with
      methylcellulose, 543
  in colonic endosonography, 726
  in duodenal endoscopy, 316
  in esophageal endosonography, 190
  in gastric endoscopy, 314
  in percutaneous cholangioscopy, 1424
Mesenchymal hamartoma of liver, 1480
  in child, 1966, 1968
Mesenchymal tumor
  in Gardner's syndrome, 781
  in liver, 1658-1660
  of mesentery, 1824
Mesenteric angiography
  in intestinal varices, 657
  in liver metastases, 1706
  in rectal bleeding, 978
  in small bowel lymphoma, 639
  technique of, 1605-1606
Mesenteric artery
  angiography of; see Mesenteric angiography
  inferior, 29, 694
  superior, 31
    accidental ligation of, 476

Mesenteric artery—cont'd
  superior—cont'd
    compression syndrome of, 506, 1903,
        1904
    computed tomography arterial portography
        through, 1462, 1585
    hepatic angiography technique and,
        1605-1606
    in pancreatic adenocarcinoma, 1108
Mesenteric artery syndromes, superior, 506,
    1903, 1904
Mesenteric bands, congenital, 467
Mesenteric blood vessels, 526
  ischemia and infarction of, 649-650
Mesenteric cysts, 1888-1889
Mesenteric fat
  in cirrhosis, 1541, 1542
  creeping, sonography of, 2101
Mesenteric lymph nodes, 526
  in terminal ileitis, 2104
Mesenteric panniculitis, 1823, 1824
Mesenteric thrombosis, 2054-2057
  plain films and contrast studies in,
      2054-2057
  small bowel infarction and, 2056
Mesenteric vein
  anatomy of, 1566
  cirrhosis with portal hypertension and,
      1596-1603
  inferior, 29, 30
  occlusion of, portal hypertension and,
      1596-1598
  portography of, 1590, 1591
  superior, 30, 31
    in gallbladder ultrasonography, 1249-1250
    in infant, 526
    in pancreatic adenocarcinoma, 1117
    thrombosis or tumor invasion of, 1594
  thrombosis of, 1594, 1824
Mesenteritis, refractile, ulcerative colitis
    versus, 604
Mesenteroaxial volvulus, 365
  in child, 1874-1876, 1877
  gastric dilation and, 2043
Mesentery, 1820-1824
  anatomy of, 512, 1820-1822
  embolus in, small bowel infarction and,
      2056
  gallbladder position and, 1254, 1287
  ischemia or infarction of, 649-650
  pathology of, 1822-1825
    adhesions in, 1599, 1600
    hematoma in, 2096, 2097
    inflammation in, 1822-1823
    primary tumors in, 1823
  thickening and retraction of
    in Crohn's disease, 597
    ulcerative colitis versus, 608
  trauma to, 2138-2139
    computed tomography in, 2138-2139
  varices of, portal hypertension and, 1599,
      1600
Mesocaval shunt
  in hepatic vein occlusion, 1627
  postoperative stenosis of, 1591
  spontaneous, 1582
Mesocolon
  anatomy of, 692
  transverse, 30, 35
Mesorectum, 818
Mesothelioma, 1803
Metaanalysis of controlled trials, 834
Metabolic disorders in esophageal motility,
    209
Metabolic imaging of colon, 720

Metagonimus yokogawai, 946
Metal endoprostheses, collapsible large-caliber,
    1407-1411
Metal stent; see Stent
Metaplasia, epithelial
  of colon, 762
  in duodenum, 498
  intestinal, 330
Metastases
  to adrenal glands, 1992-1993
    from fibrolamellar hepatic carcinoma,
        1679
  from breast; see Breast carcinoma
  from colon, 803-805
    to bowel wall, 802
    to liver, 804, 1479, 1481, 1502
  to colon
    computed tomography angiography of,
        1460, 1461
    hematogenous, 792
  to duodenum, 508
    of nonepithelial tumors, 496
  from esophagus, 249, 274, 275, 276, 1497
    computed tomography of, 276
    endosonography of, 266
    to liver, 1497
    sarcomatous, 249
    to tracheobronchial tissue, 273, 277
  from gallbladder, 1328
  to kidney, 1992-1993
  from liver, 1665
    to bone, 1674
  to liver, 1706-1716
    adenocarcinomatous, 1496
    from breast carcinoma, 1724
    calcification in, 1714
    carcinoid tumor in, 634, 635, 1473,
        1479, 1723
    in child, 1964-1966
    cholangiocarcinoma versus, 1336
    from colon, 804, 1479, 1481, 1493, 1502
    computed tomography of, 1463-1464,
        1706-1707, 1708
    computed tomography arterial portography
        of, 1460
    cystic, 1478, 1479
    from endocrine carcinoma, 1711
    from esophagus, 1497
    fatty liver and, 1557, 1558
    from gallbladder, 1326
    hemangiomas versus, 1636-1637
    hepatocellular carcinoma versus,
        1694-1696
    histology of, 1708-1709
    hypervascular, 1711-1713, 1714
    hypovascular, 1710-1711
    imaging methods in, 1706-1708
    incremental dynamic bolus computed
        tomography in, 1459
    interstitial compartment size in,
        1709-1713, 1714
    intraoperative ultrasonography of, 1481
    islet cell tumors in, 1174, 1177, 1178,
        1187
    lymphomatous, 1964, 1965
    magnetic resonance imaging of, 1490,
        1707-1708, 1709, 1710
    from multiple endocrine neoplasia, 1182
    necrosis in, 1713-1714
    negative percutaneous abscess drainage
        and, 2007
    neuroblastoma in, 1964-1965
    noncontrast computed tomography of,
        1455

Metastases—cont'd
  to liver—cont'd
    from pancreatic adenocarcinoma, 1117, 1119
    from pancreatic cystic neoplasms, 1150
    from pancreatic islet cell tumor, 1495
    parenchyma and, 1400, 1708
    percutaneous intervention contraindicated in, 1400
    percutaneous interventional radiology in, 1992
    scintigraphy in, 1509, 1514, 1515
    size of, 1714-1715
    surgical resection of, 1715-1716
    transcatheter embolization in, 1723
    tumor-related factors in detection of, 1708-1715
    ultrasonography of, 1478-1480, 1481
    vascular size in, 1709-1710
    vascularity of, 1187, 1710-1713, 1714
    from Wilms' tumor, 1964
  to lymph nodes, 1964, 1965
    from colorectal carcinoma, 803-804
    from esophageal tumor, 265, 266, 270
  from pancreas, 1145
    adenocarcinomatous, 1108
    computed tomography of, 1117-1118
    of cystic neoplasms, 1150
    to gastrointestinal tract, 1124-1125
    ultrasonography of, 1119
  to pancreas, 1154
    from gastric carcinoma, 443, 444
  to peritoneum
    carcinomatosis in, 1118
    from gallbladder carcinoma, 1326
    from gastric cancer, 423
    from pancreatic adenocarcinoma, 1118
  from pharyngeal malignancy, 142-144, 150
  to porta hepatis region, cholangiocarcinoma versus, 1336
  from rectum, 803-805
    to lymph nodes, 813, 818-820
  to rectum, 804, 806
  to retroperitoneum, 1815
  to small bowel, 643-646
    general features of, 643, 644, 645
    Kaposi's sarcoma and, 645
    lymphoma versus melanomatous, 639
    melanoma in, 643-645, 646
    route of spread of, 643, 644
  to spleen, 1783-1785
    in child, 1937-1938
  from stomach, 441
    endosonography of, 453
  to stomach, 433-434
    from esophageal tumor, 432
    from pancreatic carcinoma, 1130
  unresectable, percutaneous interventional radiology in, 1987
Meteorism, 2022
Methacholine test, 181, 199-201
  for child, 1838-1839
  historical aspects of, 181
Methemoglobin, 1649
Methotrexate, 685
Methyl tert butyl ether
  adverse effects of, 1378-1379
  in choledocholithiasis, 1375, 1378
  in endoscopic retrograde cholangiopancreatography for gallbladder stones, 1351, 1361
  equipment for delivery of, 1379
  with percutaneous endoscopy of biliary tract, 1426

Methylcellulose, in biphasic enteroclysis of small bowel; see Enteroclysis, biphasic, with methylcellulose
Methyldopa, 685
Methylene blue
  in colon imaging, 696
  in duodenum imaging, 506
  in gastric endoscopy, 304
Methysergide, 1815
Metoclopramide, 90
  in barium meal preparation, 286
  in biphasic enteroclysis with methylcellulose, 534, 535, 541
    in prolonged examination, 539, 542
  in computed tomography
    of acute abdomen, 2076
    of colon, 718
    of diverticulitis, 753
  in endoscopy for esophageal varices, 969
  in small bowel studies, 524
Metricide, 1424
Metronidazole, 2001
MI; see Meconium ileus
MIBG; see 131I-meta-iodobenzylguanidine
Micelles, 80
Michaelis-Gutmann bodies, 556
Microabscesses in cholangitis, 1312
Microcarcinoma, gastric, 414
Microcatheters, coaxial, 2144
Microcoils, platinum, 2144
  in hepatic therapeutic embolization, 2148
Microcolon
  meconium ileus in, 1886, 1887
  in neonatal megacystis-microcolon-intestinal hypomotility syndrome, 1902-1903
Microcystic adenoma of pancreas, 1036
Microcystic pancreas, 1138-1141
Microgastria, 1865
Micronodular cirrhosis, 1549
Microperforation of intestine, 2105
Microvesicular fatty liver, 1547, 1548
Midazolam
  in biphasic enteroclysis with methylcellulose, 534
  in esophageal endosonography, 264
  in extracorporeal shock wave lithotripsy, 1359
  in gastric endoscopy, 302
  in hepatic arterial embolization, 1725
  in percutaneous biliary tract intervention, 1401
Middle hepatic vein, 30, 33
Midgut
  fixation of, 1878-1884
  volvulus of, 2052
Midkidney
  anatomic section of, 46
  computed tomography of, 63
  magnetic resonance imaging of, 47
Migrating myoelectric complex, 78, 79, 81
Migratory monoarthritis, 588
Milk, lyophilized, 530
Milk allergy, 1925
  in celiac disease, 666, 668
  small bowel pneumocolon in, 522, 523
Milk curd syndrome, 1915
Miller and Maglinte method for barium enema, 707
Mineral oil
  in double-contrast examination of large bowel, 565
  in gallbladder ultrasonography, 1246
Minicholecystostomy, 1374-1375
Minnesota tube, 969
Mirizzi syndrome, 1294
Mitomycin C, 1717-1718

MMC; see Migrating myoelectric complex
Mn-DPDP
  in hepatic magnetic resonance imaging, 1503
  in pancreatic diagnosis, 1019, 1021
Mobile cecum, congenital, 1882-1883
Modulation transfer function, 1486
Molage sign, 553
Molnar, W, 23
Molnar retention disc, 1418
Moniliasis, 908-909, 910
  in esophageal motility disorders, 210
  in esophageal strictures, 238
  in esophagitis, 226-228
  in necrotizing enteritis, 2087
  in pseudodiverticulosis, 216
Monoclonal antibodies
  in colorectal carcinoma, 810
  in small bowel fine-needle aspiration cytology, 559
Monoctanoin, 1375
Morgagni's hernia, 255
  in child, 1856-1858
Morphine
  in acalculous cholecystitis, 1280
  in acute cholecystitis, 1276
  in cholescintigraphy, 1234
  in toxic dilatation of colon, 565
Motilin, 68
Motility disorders
  duodenum and small bowel physiology and, 81-83
  of esophagus, 198-211; see also Esophagus
    in child, 1838-1839
    differential diagnosis in, 210
    studies of, 1838
  of large bowel in child, 1912-1916
  of pharynx in child, 1828-1829
Motion-compensating gradients in magnetic resonance imaging, 1489
Motion-induced artifacts, 1487-1489, 1490
Motor neuron disease, 133
Moulage phenomenon
  in celiac disease, 665
  in jejunal lymphoma, 638
  in small bowel peroral biopsy, 553
  in sprue, 912
Mouth, carcinoma of, 142, 143, 144-150; see also Oral cavity, malignant diseases of
  nodal metastasis of, 150
MRI; see Magnetic resonance imaging
MTBE; see Methyl tert butyl ether
Mucin production in cholangiocarcinoma, 1680
Mucinous tumors of pancreas, 1134, 1152
  biliary cystadenocarcinoma versus, 1682
  carcinoma in, 1134-1135, 1152
  cystic tumors in, 1134-1135, 1141-1149
  ductectatic cystadenoma in, 1133, 1134-1135, 1136, 1137, 1138, 1146
  histologic types of, 1144
Mucocele
  after liver transplantation, 1743-1744
  of gallbladder, 2031
Mucoepidermoid carcinoma
  of pancreas, 1152
  of salivary glands, 139
Mucomyst; see Acetylcysteine
Mucormycosis, 604
Mucosa
  anal, 841
  anatomy of, 30
  buccal, 146
  of colon, 695
    in inflammatory bowel disease, 568, 569

Mucosa—cont'd
  of duodenum, 498
  of esophagus, 172, 173
    in endosonography, 265
  of gastrointestinal wall, 187
  hyperplasia of, in ampullary stenosis, 1318
  of pharynx, 114
  of small bowel in child, 1896-1898
  of stomach, heterotopic, 498
  tumor spread and, 142
Mucosa-associated lymphoid tissue, 635
Mucosal folds
  of duodenum, 284, 285
    double-contrast examination in, 289
    thickening of, 476, 596, 602
  of rectum in defecography, 849
  of small bowel, 513
    in Crohn's disease, 596
  of stomach, 282
Mucosal islands in inflammatory colitis, 2065, 2066
Mucosal patterns in ulcerative colitis, 580
Mucosal retention cysts, 899
Mucosal rings in hiatus hernia, 219
Mucosal tacking in radiation enteritis, 651, 652
Mucosal ulcers in ulcerative colitis, 576, 577
Mucus
  gastric, 284
  physiology of, 76-77
Muir-Torre syndrome, 786
  screening in, 827
Muller, W, 13
Multidisciplinary approach in swallowing impairment, 165-167
Multiple endocrine neoplasia, 1168-1169, 1915
  endocrine-secreting tumors in, 71
  gastrinoma in, 1170
  imaging in, 1182, 1186
  small bowel polyps in, 632
  type I, 1168-1169
  type II, 1915
    in child, 1915
Multiple hamartoma syndrome, 1926
Multiple sclerosis, 133
Multiseptated gallbladder, 1255
Murphy's sign, 1248, 1275, 1276, 1277, 1281, 1283
  sonography and, 2109, 2110
Muscle disorders in dysphagia, 134
Muscle rings in hiatus hernia, 219
Muscular dystrophy, 209, 211
Muscular hypertrophy
  in diverticulitis, 751
  esophageal, 212
Muscularis mucosae, 30, 35
  contractions of, 172, 173
  of esophagus
    anatomy of, 193-194
    in endosonography, 265
  of small bowel, 513
Muscularis propria, 30, 35
  of esophagus
    anatomy of, 193-194
    in endosonography, 265
    in leiomyoma and leiomyosarcoma, 269-270
  gastric, in advanced cancer, 416
  of gastrointestinal wall, 187
  in rectal carcinoma, 813, 814, 816, 818
  in scleroderma, 679
Musculoskeletal system
  in Crohn's disease, 588
  in ulcerative colitis, 574

Myasthenia gravis, 209, 211
  dysphagia in, 134
Mycobacteria, 553, 671, 958-959
  percutaneous abscess drainage and, 1999, 2004
  in retroperitoneal inflammation, 1819
  in splenic abscess, 1780, 2004
Mycosporidium, 673
Mycostatin; *see* Nystatin
Mycotic infection; *see* Fungal disease
Myelofibroma of esophagus, 251
Myelolipoma, hepatic, 1658, 1659
Myenteric plexus, 1912-1915
Mylohyoid, carcinoma spread and, 142, 143
Myoblastoma in stomach, 384
Myochosis, 88
Myocutaneous flaps, 160, 161
Myoepithelial hamartoma, 630
Myopathy, hollow visceral, 669
  small bowel motility in, 661
Myosarcoma of esophagus, 249
Myotomy, esophageal, 1841
  Heller's, 204
Myotonia, 209, 211
Myxedema, 209
Myxofibroma of esophagus, 251
Myxoid sarcoma, 1812-1813

N

Nacleiro sign, 217
Nakamura's type III adenoma, 406
Naproxen, 72
Nasal intubation in duodenography, 296-297
Nasobiliary catheter in percutaneous biliary intervention, 1413, 1414
Nasobiliary drain in endoscopic sphincterotomy, 1346, 1347, 1348
Nasogastric-nasoenteric decompression enteroclysis tube, 543
Nasopharynx
  adenoids of, 139
  carcinoma in, 160, 161
    in oropharyngeal malignancies, 150-157, 160
  reflux in, 1828
NEC; *see* Necrotizing enterocolitis
Necator americanus, 930
Neck
  abscess in, 1834
    computed tomography of, 1835
  trauma to, 115, 116, 117
Necrolytic migratory erythema, 1171
Necrosectomy, 2003
Necrosis
  of bile ducts in liver infarcts, 1319
  bowel; *see* Necrotizing enterocolitis
  coagulation, in corrosive gastropathy, 357
  of duodenum, liquefactive, 496
  of gallbladder wall, 1286
  hepatic
    in angiosarcoma, 1684
    in fibrolamellar carcinoma, 1679
    in hepatocellular carcinoma, 1667, 1671
    versus hepatocellular carcinoma, 1699-1700
    in infarction, 1616-1617
    laser-induced, 1499
    liquefactive, 1476, 1496
    in metastases, 1713-1714
  of pancreas, 2003, 2004
  in pancreatic transplantation, 1203
  tumor, percutaneous abscess drainage and, 1999, 2003, 2004
Necrotizing colitis, 2086-2087
Necrotizing enteritis, 2086-2087

Necrotizing enterocolitis, neonatal, 1916-1919
Necrotizing enteropathy
  computed tomography of, 614
  in large bowel in child, 1918, 1919
Necrotizing vasculitis in child, 1904
Needle
  nonvisualization of, 1990-1991
  in percutaneous fluoroscopically guided gastrostomy, 2012
  in percutaneous interventional radiology, 1987-1988
Needle aspiration; *see* Fine-needle aspiration cytology
  in percutaneous interventional radiology, 1988
Needle guide attachments in percutaneous interventional radiology, 1990
Needle knife in endoscopic sphincterotomy, 1346
Needle-track seeding, 1995-1996
Needle-tract seeding, 561
Neff catheter, 1406
Negative contrast agent for computed tomography of colon, 802
Neisseria gonorrhoeae, 604, 607
Neisseria meningitidis, 1790
Nematodes, 926-930
  in angiostrongyliasis, 939
  in colitis, ulcerative colitis versus, 604
Nembutal, 1902
Neodymium:yttrium-aluminum-garnet laser, 1719
Neomycin, 684-685
Neonatal necrotizing enterocolitis, 1916-1919
Neonate; *see also* Pediatrics
  choledochal cyst in, 1265
  functional immaturity of large bowel in, 1915
  hepatitis in, 1981-1982
  necrotizing enterocolitis in, 1916-1919
  nesidioblastosis in, 1950
Neoplasm; *see also* specific organ or tumor type
  in acquired immunodeficiency syndrome, 961-963
  metachronous, 144
  in multiple endocrine neoplasia; *see* Multiple endocrine neoplasia
  synchronous, 144
Neostigmine, 524
Nephrolithiasis, 575
Nephroscope, rigid, 1423
  in percutaneous cholecystolithotomy, 1377
  in percutaneous cholecystostomy, 1427
Nesidioblastosis, 1167, 1170
  in child, 1950
Neurenteric cyst, 1843
Neurilemoma, gastric, 450
Neuroblastoma in child, 1827, 1833
  hepatic metastases and, 1964-1965
Neurocrine substances, 67
Neuroendocrine tumors, transcatheter embolization in, 1723-1724, 1725
Neuroenteric cysts, esophageal, 212
Neurofibroma
  of esophagus, 251
  of retroperitoneum, 1813-1814
  of small bowel, 630
  of stomach, 379-381
Neurofibrosarcoma of liver, 1684
Neurogenic tumor
  gastric, 379-381, 1873
  pharyngeal, 1832, 1833-1834
Neurohumoral mechanisms of fed state, 81-82
Neuromuscular disorders, esophageal, 209

Neuron-specific enolase, 1132, 1150
Neuronal intestinal dysplasia, 1915
Neuropeptides, enteric, 67-73
Neurotensin
    in islet cell tumors, 1168
    mechanism of action of, 68
Neurotensinoma, 1172
Neutralization of acid in esophagus, 73-75
Neutropenic colitis
    in child, 1918, 1919
    computed tomography of, 614, 2086
Newborn; *see* Neonate
Nifedipine, 1605
Niopam; *see* Iodipamidol
Nissen fundoplication, 220, 238
Nitroglycerin, 1605
Node of Rouviere, metastatic, 143, 144, 157
Nodular hyperplasia, focal; *see* Focal nodular
        hyperplasia
Nodular lymphoid hyperplasia
    primary immunodeficiency syndromes with,
            676-677
    of small bowel, 661
Nodular pattern in Crohn's disease, 596
Nodule
    hepatic
        adenomatous hyperplastic, 1480
        with cirrhosis in hepatocellular carcinoma,
                1692, 1701-1702
        focal hyperplastic; *see* Focal nodular
                hyperplasia
        in hepatocellular carcinoma, 1694
        macroregenerative, 1542-1543, 1544,
                1545, 1655-1656
        regenerative hyperplasia and, 1542-1543,
                1544, 1545, 1655-1656
    in malignant intestinal lymphoma, 635
Non-Hodgkin's lymphoma, 1895
    in acquired immunodeficiency syndrome,
            673, 674
    of duodenum, 496
    of liver, 1684
        after transplantation, 1748
    pediatric spleen and, 1937-1938
    small bowel mesentery and, 1824
Nonepithelial benign tumors of stomach,
        377-386
Nonionic contrast enema, 1914
Nonpolyposis colon cancer, hereditary; *see*
        Hereditary nonpolyposis colon cancer
Nonsteroidal anti-inflammatory agents
    in cholecystitis, 1275
    endoscopic sphincterotomy hazards of, 1345
    in enteritis, 656-657
    in gastritis, 327, 329, 1869
    as hazard in percutaneous transhepatic
            cholangiography, 1236
    in injury gastropathy, 357
    as lithotripsy contraindication, 1359
    in peptic ulcer disease, 336, 345
    prostaglandins and, 72
NSAIDs; *see* Nonsteroidal anti-inflammatory
        agents
Nuclear medicine; *see also* Scintigraphy
    in bacterial cholangitis, 1306
    in percutaneous biliary dilation of strictures,
            1383
Nucleus tractus solitarii, 98, 100
Nutcracker esophagus, 181, 204
Nutcracker syndrome, 506
Nutrients, deficiency of, 661; *see also*
        Malabsorption
Nystatin, 228

O
Oat cell carcinoma
    esophageal, 243
    of gallbladder, 1331
    of lung, 645
Obesity, gastric surgery for, 455-466
    delayed complications of, 461-466
    gastroplasty in, 455-458
    immediate complications of, 459-461
    pouch volumes in, 455
    radiology in, 458-459
    staple-line geometry in, 458
    vertical banded, 457
    weight control and, 458
Oblique fissure of liver, 32
Obstruction
    bile duct; *see also* Bile duct, obstruction of
        after transplantation, 1739, 1740-1744
        appearances of, 1432, 1433
        in child, 1978-1980
        in cholangiocarcinoma, 1334
        choledocholithiasis in, ultrasonography of,
                1296-1298
        endoscopic intervention for, 1426, 1429,
                1432
        endoscopic sphincterotomy for cholangitis
                with, 1347
        hepatic hilar cysts in, 1319
        as lithotripsy contraindication, 1359
        liver and biliary tract imaging of,
                1978-1980
        percutaneous intervention in malignant
                disease causing, 1399; *see also*
                Percutaneous interventional
                radiology, in malignant biliary tract
                disease
        plain films and contrast studies of, 2031
    of biliary drainage catheter, 1417
    of bladder, 1197, 1214
    of esophagus, foreign bodies in, 216
    of hepatic vein, 1625, 1626-1628
        in cirrhosis with portal hypertension,
                1591-1592
    of pancreatic duct in pancreatic
            adenocarcinoma, 1107, 1109,
            1113-1115, 1118, 1119
    of portal vein, 1461
    of splenic vein
        in cirrhosis, 1593-1594
        duodenal varices in, 501
Obstructive jaundice
    endoscopic stent placement in, 1432-1434,
            1435, 1436
    endoscopic therapy in, 1426, 1429
    in gallbladder carcinoma, 1325
Occlusion
    after pancreatic transplantation, 1198, 1216,
            1217, 1219
    of hepatic vein
        postoperative, 1592
        scintigraphy of, 1519
        ultrasonography of, 1472
    of mesenteric vein, 1596-1598
        in postoperative evaluation, 1590, 1591
    of portal vein; *see* Portal vein, occlusion of
    of Z-stent in percutaneous intervention,
            1414
Occult blood tests, fecal; *see* Fecal
        occult-blood tests in colorectal cancer
        screening
Octreotide; *see also* Somatostatin analogue
Ocular disease
    in Crohn's disease, 589
    in ulcerative colitis, 574

Oculopharyngeal dystrophy, 209
Oddi's sphincter, 86, 88, 1262
    morphine and, 1234
    stenosis of, 1318
Odynophagia, 202
    endoscopy in, 183
    in esophagitis, 226, 228
Oesophagostomiasis, 933-934
Ogilvie's syndrome, 2008, 2009, 2059; *see
        also* Pseudoobstruction, intestinal
Oil emulsions as contrast, 307
Oki, 13
Olympus scope in endosonography
    of colon, 726
    of esophagus, 265
    of pancreas, 1127
    of stomach and duodenum, 314
Omega sign in Crohn's disease, 597, 598
Omental bursa
    anatomy of, 1797
    gas in, from misplaced needle, 1821
Omental cake in peritonitis, 2080
Omental cysts, 1888-1889
Omental tuberosity, 30
Omentum
    gastric carcinoma spread into, 438
    herniation of, 1857-1858
    lesser, 30, 31
        computed tomography of, 306
Omeprazole, 72-73, 76
    in *Helicobacter pylori* disease, 478
    in Zollinger-Ellison syndrome, 73
Omnipaque; *see* Iohexol
Omnopon, 1725
Omphalocele, 1890
Omphalomesenteric duct anomalies, 1889-1890
Open swallow, defined, 129
Opisthorchiasis, 943-944
Opportunistic infections in acquired
            immunodeficiency syndrome,
            954-961
Optiray; *see* Ioversol
Oral cavity
    anatomy of, 144-146
    malignant diseases of, 144-150
        anatomy and, 144-146
        direct extension in, 147-150
        lymphatic spread in, 150
        magnetic resonance imaging of, 145, 147,
                148
        perineural extension of, 150, 151-153
Oral cholecystography
    before extracorporeal shock wave
            lithotripsy, 1359
    techniques for, 1227-1230, 1231
Oral contraceptives
    benign hepatic neoplasms and, 1476, 1510,
            1511
    Budd-Chiari syndrome and, 1626
    in focal nodular hyperplasia of liver, 1651
    in hepatic vein occlusion, 1592
    in hepatocellular adenoma, 1645
    in hepatocellular carcinoma, 1663, 1677
Oral contrast media; *see* Contrast agents
Organoaxial volvulus, 365
    in child, 1874-1876, 1877
    gastric dilation and, 2043, 2044
    of stomach, 2044
Oriental cholangitis, 1302
    cholangiocarcinoma versus, 1337, 1342
Oropharynx
    axial section of, 109, 110
    in child, 1826
    functional abnormalities of, 127-129
    in gastrointestinal physiology, 73-75

Oropharynx—cont'd
malignant diseases of, 150-157
direct extension of, 150-156
lymphatic spread of, 157
perineural spread of, 157
ultrasonography of, 111, 112
Osler-Weber-Rendu disease; *see* Hereditary
hemorrhagic telangiectasia
Osmotic agents, 90
in magnetic resonance imaging, 308
Osmotic diarrhea, 89-90
Osteoarthritis, 101
Osteoclast-type cells in pancreatic carcinoma,
1153
Osteoma, 783
Osteomalacia, 80
Osteonectin, 1153
Osteophytes, cervical spine, 120, 123
Outlet obstruction of stomach; *see* Gastric
outlet obstruction
Ovarian vein catheterization, 658
Ovaries
carcinoma of, 1804
ascites in, 2029
greater omentum pathology and, 1822
intraperitoneal spread of, 643, 644
metastasis of, to duodenum, 508
peritoneography of, 1799
cystic torsion of, 2073
Krukenberg tumors of, 1326
metastases to
from colon carcinoma, 804
from gallbladder carcinoma, 1326
Overhead films in enteroclysis, 515
Oxygen in colonic endosonography, 726
Oxyntic cells, 75

P
PAD; *see* Abscess, percutaneous drainage of
Pain
chest, of esophageal origin, 181
in cholangiocarcinoma, 1334
in chronic pancreatitis, 1091-1098
in esophageal fluoroscopy, 181
in gastrinoma, 1170
in pancreatic adenocarcinoma, 1107
percutaneous interventional radiology in
abdominal masses and, 1995
Palatal constrictors in swallowing, 106
paresis of, 129
Palate
hard, tumors of, 147, 149
soft, paresis of, 129
Palatine foramen, perineural extension into,
150, 151
Palatoglossus muscle, 156
Pale cells in pancreatic neoplasms, 1151
Pancoast, HK, 4
Pancolitis, peroral pneumocolon in, 565
Pancreas
aberrant, in duodenum, 498
abscess of; *see* Abscess, pancreatic
acini of, in cystic fibrosis, 1157
adenocarcinoma of; *see* Pancreatic
adenocarcinoma
agenesis of, 1946, 1947
anatomy of, 47-61
adenocarcinoma and, 1107-1109
angiography and, 1023-1025
in child, 1944
endoscopic retrograde
cholangiopancreatography and, 1020
lesser sac in, 30
magnetic resonance imaging and, 1018

Pancreas—cont'd
anatomy of—cont'd
percutaneous transhepatic
cholangiography, 1022
angiography of, 1023, 1024
annular, 1046-1048
in child, 1946, 1947
in small bowel of child, 1884-1885
barium examination of
in adenocarcinoma, 1110, 1124
in child, 1944
in mucinous tumors, 1146
in pancreatoblastoma, 1156
in pediatric annular pancreas, 1946
biopsy of, 1037, 1128
endoscopically-guided, 1128-1129
body of, 1030
adenocarcinoma of, 1115, 1116, 1125
anatomy of, 30, 47
omental tuberosity of, 30
calcifications of; *see* Calcification,
pancreatic
carcinoma of; *see* Carcinoma, of pancreas
cell function in, 88
cellular ultrastructure of, 1133
central embryologic anlage of, 467-468
clinically silent or minimally functioning,
1168, 1172-1173
computed tomography of, 1017-1018
in abscess, 2039
in acinar cell carcinoma, 1154
in adenocarcinoma, 1110-1120
in cystic fibrosis, 1157
in cystic islet cell tumors, 1157
in cystic neoplasms, 1151
in cystic teratoma, 1158
in giant cell carcinoma, 1153
in glucagonoma, 1183-1184
in hemangioma, 1160
inferior pancreatic head and, 61
in insulinoma, 1173, 1174, 1175
in islet cell tumors, 1174-1177,
1178-1187, 1192
in lymphangioma, 1160, 1161
in lymphoma, 1162
in metastases, 1158
in mucinous tumor, 1146, 1148, 1149
in multiple true cysts, 1156
in nontumoral true cysts, 1156
in pancreas divisum, 1043-1044
pancreatic tail in, 51, 55
in pancreatoblastoma, 1156
pediatric, 1944
in acute pancreatitis, 1950, 1951
in agenesis, 1946, 1947
in annular pancreas, 1946
in fatty pancreas, 1948, 1949
in hereditary pancreatitis, 1952, 1953
in malignant tumors, 1954
in nesidioblastosis, 1950
in pancreatitis, 1950-1951, 1952
in papillary epithelial neoplasm, 1954
in phlegmon, 1950
in pseudoaneurysm, 1952
in Shwachman-Diamond syndrome,
1949
in trauma, 1955
in serous adenoma, 1141, 1143
in small primary tumors, 1177, 1179
transplantation and, 1205-1206, 1212,
1217
in trauma, 1955, 2133
ultrasonography complementing,
1119-1120
ultrasonography versus, 1027

Pancreas—cont'd
pediatric—cont'd
in von Hippel–Lindau disease,
1156-1157, 1949
congenital abnormalities of, 1039-1051
agenesis of, 1045-1046
annular pancreas in; *see* Pancreas, annular
anomalous ducts producing pseudomasses
in, 1049
duplication, 1049
ectopic pancreas in, 1048-1049
fusion anomalies in, 1042-1045
hypoplasia of, 1045-1046
short pancreas in, 1947
variations of duct drainage in, 1039-1042
cysts of, 1034-1035
congenital, 1035-1036
endoscopic retrograde
cholangiopancreatography of, 1127,
1128
multiloculated, 1153
multiple true, 1156
nontumoral true, 1156-1163
ultrasonography of, 1033
in von Hippel–Lindau disease, 1949
diagnostic and interventional techniques for,
1017-1026
digestion and, 88
duct of; *see* Pancreatic duct
in duodenal examination, 296, 316
ectopic; *see* Ectopic pancreas
embryology of, 1039, 1040, 1251
endocrine, 87
endoscopic retrograde
cholangiopancreatography of,
1020-1022
endosonography of, 1028, 1127-1131
in adenocarcinoma, 1110
in islet cell tumors; *see* Islet cell tumor,
endosonography of
in pancreatic mucinous tumors, 1146
in rare pancreatic tumors, 1135,
1146-1147
role of, 1131
exocrine, 87-88
exocrine leak from, after transplantation,
1198, 1221
fluid collections in
after transplantation, 1198, 1217-1221
percutaneous abscess drainage of,
2002-2004
function tests for, 88
gastric carcinoma in, 443, 444
head of, 1029, 1030
adenocarcinoma in, 1117
anatomy of, 30
calcification of, in gallbladder
ultrasonography, 1250
computed tomography of, 61
sagittal sonogram of, 41
transverse scans of, 56-59
hemorrhage of, 1004, 1007
history of radiology of, 13-15, 17
hydatid disease of, 1158, 1159
islet cell tumors of; *see* Islet cell tumor
lacerations of, pediatric, 1955
lesser sac of; *see* Lesser sac of pancreas
magnetic resonance imaging of, 1018-1020,
1021
in adenocarcinoma, 1110, 1120, 1121
in mucinous tumors, 1146, 1148
in serous adenomas, 1141, 1142
in transplant rejection, 1206, 1208-1211
in transplantation, 1199-1202

Pancreas—cont'd
  magnetic resonance imaging of—cont'd
    masses near, pancreatic adenocarcinoma
        versus, 1121
    masses of
      computed tomography of biliary tract and
          gallbladder in, 1232
      in duodenal impressions, 285-286
    metastases to, 1158
      from gastric carcinoma, 443, 444
    neck of, 30, 47
      adenocarcinoma in, 1113
    neoplasms of; see also Pancreas, tumors of
      adenocarcinoma in; see Pancreatic
          adenocarcinoma
      carcinomas in; see Carcinoma, of
          pancreas
      metastatic; see Pancreas, metastases to
      mucinous, 1136, 1138, 1141-1149
      pediatric, 1952-1954
      serous, 1136
    normal structures around, 1120
    pancreatitis and; see Pancreatitis
    papillary cystic neoplasm and, 1139
    parenchyma of, 61
      after transplantation, 1197, 1206-1214,
          1215
    pediatric, 1944-1957
      anatomy of, 1944
      congenital anomalies of, 1946-1947
      congenital diseases of, 1947-1950
      developmental variants of, 1946-1947
      imaging features of, 1944-1946
      imaging technique for, 1944, 1945
      neoplasms of, 1952-1954
      pancreatitis in, 1950-1952, 1953
      trauma in, 1954-1955
    percutaneous interventional radiology in
        abdominal masses in, 1992
    physiology of, 87-88
    pseudocyst of; see Pseudocyst, of pancreas
    rare tumors of, 1132-1166
      acinar cell carcinoma in, 1153-1154
      acinar cell cystadenocarcinoma in, 1155
      adult polycystic kidney disease, 1156
      cystic fibrosis in, 1157; see also Cystic
          fibrosis
      cystic islet cell tumors in, 1157-1158; see
          also Islet cell tumor
      cystic teratoma in, 1158, 1160
      intraductal, 1132-1138
      metastases in, 1158
      microcystic, 1138-1141
      mucinous cystic, 1141-1149
      nontumoral true cysts of pancreas in,
          1156-1163
      pancreatic hemangioma in, 1158-1160,
          1161
      pancreatic lymphangioma in, 1160-1162
      pancreatoblastoma in, 1155-1156
      papillary cystic, 1134-1135, 1149-1152
      plasmacytoma in, 1163
      primary hydatid disease of, 1158, 1159
      sarcomas in, 1155
      serous, 1138-1141, 1142, 1143
      subtypes of ductal adenocarcinoma in,
          1152-1153
      von Hippel–Lindau disease in, 1156-1157
    sagittal scan of, 1029, 1030
    size of, 1031
    tail of, 30, 47, 1029
      adenocarcinoma of, 1112, 1125
      anatomy of, 47
      computed tomography of, 51
      morphology of, 55
      transverse sections through, 50, 52, 54

Pancreas—cont'd
  texture of, 1031, 1032
  transplantation of; see Pancreatic
      transplantation
  transverse scan of, 1029, 1030
  trauma to
    arteriography and therapeutic embolization
        in, 2153
    in child, 1954-1955
    computed tomography of, 2133
  tumors of; see also Pancreas, neoplasms of
    classification of, according to histogenetic
        deviation, 1132
    ductectatic mucinous cystadenoma in,
        1136, 1138, 1141-1149
    enzymes in, 1132
    epithelial, 1132, 1133
    intraductal; see Pancreatic duct, tumors of
    metastatic, 1145
    nonfunctioning, 1168, 1172-1173
  ultrasonography of, 1027-1038
    in acinar cell carcinoma, 1154
    in acute abdomen, 2112-2113
    in acute pancreatitis, 2113
    in adenocarcinoma, 1110, 1118-1120
    after transplantation, 1203-1205
    anatomy in, 1029-1031
    assessment in, 1027
    computed tomography with, 1119-1120
    conduct of examination in, 1027-1029
    in cystic fibrosis, 1157
    in cystic neoplasms, 1151
    in cystic teratoma, 1158
    cysts and, 1033, 1035-1036
    endoscopic, 1028
    in giant cell carcinoma, 1153
    in insulinoma, 1173, 1174, 1175
    in islet cell tumors, 1157, 1173-1174,
        1175
      intraoperative, 1190-1191
      in localization procedures, 1192
    in lymphangioma, 1160
    in lymphoma, 1162
    in metastases, 1158
    in mucinous tumors, 1146
    in multiple true cysts, 1156
    in nontumoral true cysts, 1156
    of pancreatic head, 41
    in pancreatoblastoma, 1156
    pathology in, 1031-1037
    patient preparation in, 1027
    pediatric, 1944-1957
      in acute pancreatitis, 1950-1951, 1952
      in agenesis, 1946, 1947
      in fatty pancreas, 1948
      in hereditary pancreatitis, 1952, 1953
      in malignant tumors, 1954
      in pancreatitis, 1950, 1951
      in papillary epithelial neoplasm, 1954
      in trauma, 1955
    pseudocysts in, 1033, 1034
    in serous adenoma, 1141
    in transplantation; see Pancreatic
        transplantation, ultrasonography of
    upper, 57
  uncinate process of
    adenocarcinoma of, 1111, 1112, 1117
    cystadenoma and cystadenocarcinoma in,
        1134, 1135
  veins of, 1188
    adenocarcinoma and, 1108, 1117
  vessels in, 30; see also Pancreas, veins of
Pancreas divisum, 88, 1042-1044
  in child, 1946
  incomplete, 1044-1045

Pancreas divisum—cont'd
  pancreatitis and, 1091, 1095
Pancreatic adenocarcinoma, 1036, 1107-1126
  angiography of, 1123-1124
  in child, 1954
  clinical manifestations of, 1107
  computed tomography of, 1110-1118
    altered attenuation in, 1112-1113, 1117
    ductal obstruction in, 1113-1115, 1118
    interpretation of, 1112-1118
    local pancreatic extension in, 1115-1117
    mass effect in, 1112, 1113-1116
    metastases in, 1117-1118
    technical considerations for, 1110-1111
    ultrasonography complementing,
        1119-1120
  detection rate for, 1128
  diagnostic imaging of, 1109-1110
    choice of methods in, 1110
  differential diagnosis in, 1120-1122, 1129
    carcinoma versus pancreatitis in, 1121
    extrapancreatic masses and, 1121
  direct invasion of, 1129, 1130
  endoscopic retrograde
      cholangiopancreatography of,
      1122-1123, 1127, 1128
  endosonography of, 1127-1131
  gastrointestinal examinations in, 1124-1125
  in hepatic metastases, 1712
  islet cell tumors versus, 1177
  local extension of, 1115-1117
  magnetic resonance imaging of, 1120, 1121
  metastatic to gastrointestinal tract,
      1124-1125
  pancreatic endosonography of, 1127, 1128
  pathologic anatomy and biologic behavior
      of, 1107-1109
  percutaneous biopsy in, 1125
  percutaneous transhepatic cholangiography
      of, 1123
  resectability of, 1109
  seeding of tumor cells in, 1125
  staging of, 1109-1110
    endosonography in, 1129-1131
  ultrasonography of, 1118-1120
    computed tomography complementing,
        1119-1120
    ductal obstruction in, 1119
    echo texture in, 1119
    metastases in, 1119
    vascular involvement in, 1119
Pancreatic cell function tests, 88
Pancreatic cholera, 1171
Pancreatic cytosis, pediatric, 1948
Pancreatic duct
  absence of, 1261
  adenocarcinoma in, subtypes of, 1152-1153
  anatomy of, 30, 61
    variations in, 1039-1042
  anomalous, producing pseudomasses, 1049
  biliary duct union with, 1261, 1262-1263
  calculi in
    clearance of fragments of, 1105-1106
    endoscopic therapy in extraction of,
        1091-1094
    extracorporeal shock wave lithotripsy in,
        1101-1106
    location of, 1101
    sphincterotomy for, in chronic
        pancreatitis, 1091-1094
  categories of drainage of, 1041
  common channel for bile ducts and, 1262,
      1263
  communicating, drainage from, 1041
  in cystic fibrosis, 1157

Pancreatic duct—cont'd
dilated
on endosonography, 1131
percutaneous transhepatic cholangiography
of, 1123
sticky mucin in, 1134
endoprosthesis in
endoscopic therapy in placement of,
1094-1097
major papillary, 1094-1095
minor papillary, 1095-1097
in endoscopic retrograde
cholangiopancreatography, 1241
epithelium of
hyperplastic, 1134
papillary growth of, 1134
fusion anomalies of, 1042-1045
obstruction of, in pancreatic
adenocarcinoma, 1107, 1109,
1113-1115, 1118, 1119
papillary projections in, 1134
in primary sclerosing cholangitis, 1308
single, drainage from, 1041
sphincterotomy of
in chronic pancreatitis, 1091, 1092
endoscopic therapy in, 1091, 1092
stenosis of, 1045, 1091
tumors of, 1132-1138
adenomas in, 1133, 1134-1135
carcinomas in, 1132
mucin-hypersecreting, 1133
papilloma in, 1133, 1134
variations in drainage of, 1039-1042, 1261
Pancreatic ductography, 1122
Pancreatic endocrine tumors; see Islet cell
tumor
Pancreatic enzymes, 1132
Pancreatic fracture, pediatric, 1955
Pancreatic juice, reflux of, as carcinogen, 1325
Pancreatic polypeptide, 69
human, 70
in islet cell tumors, 1168
mechanism of action of, 68
in polypeptide cells, 1167
in tumors, 1132, 1146
Pancreatic polypeptide cells, 1167
Pancreatic pseudocyst; see Pseudocyst, of
pancreas
Pancreatic remnants, 1123
Pancreatic rests, 1866, 1948
Pancreatic transplantation, 1197-1222
complications of, 1197-1198
arteriovenous fistulas in, 1198
infarction in, 1198
radiologic diagnosis of, 1198-1221; see
also Pancreatic transplantation,
radiologic diagnosis after
imaging complications in, 1206-1221
abnormal fluid collections and, 1217-1221
parenchymal, 1206-1214, 1215
vascular, 1214-1217, 1218-1220
radiologic diagnosis after, 1198-1221
computed tomography in, 1205-1206
imaging complications in, 1206-1221; see
also Pancreatic transplantation,
imaging complications in
imaging techniques in, 1199-1206, 1207
magnetic resonance imaging in,
1199-1202
normal findings in, 1199-1206, 1207
scintigraphy in, 1202-1203
sonography in, 1203-1205
ultrasonography of, 1203, 1214, 1217, 1218
in follow-up, 1203-1205
in rejection, 1206, 1212, 1213

Pancreatic transplantation—cont'd
vascular abnormalities in, 1198
from imaging complications, 1214-1217,
1218-1220
Pancreatic venous sampling, 1187-1188, 1189
Pancreaticobiliary duct union, 1261,
1262-1263
anomalous, 1262, 1263
gallbladder carcinoma and, 1325
Pancreaticoblastoma, pediatric, 1954
Pancreaticocholangiography, endoscopic
retrograde; see Endoscopic retrograde
cholangiopancreatography
Pancreaticocutaneous fistula, calculus in, 1093
Pancreaticoduodenal space, 1807, 1811
Pancreaticoduodenal vein, 40, 1566
Pancreaticoduodenal vessels, 30
Pancreaticoduodenectomy, radical, 488
Pancreatitis
acute
after liver transplantation, 1748
in child, 1950-1952
computed tomography of, 2088, 2089
plain films and contrast studies in,
2032-2034
signs of, 2033
ultrasonography of, 2112-2113
adenocarcinoma versus, 1121, 1127-1129
after endoscopic retrograde
cholangiopancreatography,
1344-1345
after extracorporeal shock wave lithotripsy,
1360
after transplantation, 1197, 1214, 1215
viral, 1213
in ampullary stenosis, 1318
biliary strictures after, 1315-1316
in child, 1950-1952, 1953
chronic
in child, 1952, 1953
endoscopic therapy in, 1091-1100; see
Endoscopic intervention, in chronic
pancreatitis
extracorporeal shock wave lithotripsy in
calcific, 1101-1106
relapsing, duodenal wall cysts and, 471
small bowel in, 684
in cirrhosis with portal hypertension, 1593,
1594
in endoscopic retrograde
cholangiopancreatography, 1243
gallstone-induced, 1262
endoscopic sphincterotomy for, 1347
hereditary, 1952, 1953
kidney and, 1810
as lithotripsy contraindication, 1359
percutaneous interventional radiology and,
1995
percutaneous transhepatic cholangiography
and, 1021-1022
relapsing, endoscopic therapy in, 1091-1098
in retroperitoneum, 1816-1817, 1823
in splenic vein obstruction, 1593, 1594
texture in, 1031, 1032
transverse scan in, 1032
ultrasonography of, 1031-1037
Pancreatoblastoma, 1155-1156
Pancreozymin, 67
Panhepatic angiography, 1607
Panniculitis, mesenteric, 1823, 1824
Papain, 216
Papanicolaou stain, 558, 1149
Papaverine, 1596
Papilla; see also Ampulla, duodenal
accessory, 285

Papilla—cont'd
anatomy of, 1227
carcinoma of, 1432, 1433
palliative drainage of, 1432, 1433
in child, 1946
endoprosthesis in, 1094-1097
in normal endoscopy, 304
pancreatic endosonography of, 1127, 1128
stenosis of, in chronic pancreatitis, 1091
stones in, endoscopic intervention in,
1344-1354
variants and anomalies of site of, 1262
Papillary adenoma
of duodenum, 488
of stomach, 374, 376
Papillary cystic neoplasms of pancreas,
1134-1135, 1139, 1149-1152
Papillary epithelial neoplasm in child, 1954,
1955
Papillary mesothelioma, 1803
Papillary tumor
of duodenum, 488
of esophagus, 251-252
of lips in Cowden's disease, 786-787
of pancreas, 1134-1135, 1139, 1149-1152
in pancreatic duct, 1133, 1134
Papilloma; see Papillary tumor
Papillotubular adenoma of stomach, 374
Paraaminosalicylic acid, 684-685
Paracolic abscess, 2039
diverticular, percutaneous drainage of, 752
plain films and contrast studies of, 2035,
2039
Paracolic fat inflammatory changes, 754-755
Paracrine substances, 67
Paraduodenal hernia, 473
Paraesophageal hernia, 218, 219
spurious, 220
Paraganglioma in stomach, 379-381
Parallel channels sign in gallbladder, 1249
Paralysis, diaphragmatic, 1858-1859
Paralytic ileus
causes of, 2064
gastric dilation and, 2043
in large bowel obstruction, 2057
plain films and contrast studies of, 2028,
2063, 2064
in postoperative abdomen, 2063-2064
Paramagnetic agents
in focal nodular hyperplasia of liver, 1654
iron oxide; see Iron oxide contrast agents
in stomach and duodenum, 307
Parapharyngeal region
abscess of, 120
benign abnormalities of, 120-126
fat in, 111
neoplasms in, 125, 126
Parapharyngeal space, 106, 110
Pararenal fat, posterior, 30
Pararenal space, 1807-1808, 1809-1811
abscess in, 1818
anterior, 63
posterior, 63, 1809-1810
Parasites, 913-946
in amebiasis, 915-918, 919, 920
in ancylostomiasis, 930-931
in angiostrongyliasis, 939
in anisakiasis in, 934-935
Armillifer as, 946
in ascariasis in, 926-930
in bile ducts, 1312-1314
ultrasonography of, 2112
in capillariasis in, 937-938
cestodes in, 939-943
in Chagas' disease, 918-923, 924, 925

Parasites—cont'd
in colitis, ulcerative colitis versus, 604
Dracunculus medinensis in, 937
in duodenum, 476
in echinococcosis, 940-943
in gastritis, 333
in giardiasis, 923-926, 927
in guinea worm infestations, 937
helminthic, 926-946
helminthomas and, 933-934
in hookworm disease, 930-931
in hydatid disease, 940-943
in intrahepatic stones, 1350, 1351
liver flukes in, 943-946
nematodes in, 926-939
in oesophagostomiasis, 933-934
in pediatric spleen, cyst and, 1938
in pentastomidiasis, 946
protozoal, 915-918, 919, 920
roundworms as, 926-930
in strongyloidiasis, 931-933
tapeworms in, 939-943
trematodes in, 943-946
in trichuriasis, 935-937, 938
whipworm infection in, 935-937, 938
Parasplenic abnormalities, 1788-1789, 1790
calcifications in, 1772-1774
varices in, 1788-1789
Parathyrinoma, 1168, 1172
imaging of, 1176, 1177
Parathyroid hormone in islet cell tumors,
1168, 1172
imaging and, 1176, 1177
Parathyroid hormone-like substance in islet cell
tumors, 1168, 1172
Paratyphoid fevers, 898
Paraumbilical vein, 1575, 1577, 1581
dilated, 1580, 1581
Parenchyma of liver; *see* Liver, parenchyma of
Parenteral nutrition in fatty liver, 1548
Parietal cells, 75-76
Parkinsonism
in dysphagia, 133
in esophageal motility disorders, 209
Parotid gland, malignancies of, 139
Particulate superparamagnetic iron oxide
contrast agents; *see* Iron oxide
contrast agents
PAS mucin staining; *see* Periodic acid-Schiff
mucin staining
Passavant's cushion or ridge, 107, 129
Pediatric bronchoscope, 1423
Pediatric enema tip, 517
Pediatrics
biliary tract imaging in; *see* Pediatrics, liver
and biliary tract imaging in
diaphragm and esophagogastric junction
studies in, 1853-1864; *see also*
Diaphragm, and esophagogastric
junction in child
esophagogastric junction study in,
1853-1864; *see also* Diaphragm, and
esophagogastric junction
liver and biliary tract imaging in,
1958-1975, 1982-1985
in angiomatous lesions, 1966
in arterial disease, 1973, 1974
in biliary atresia, 1981-1982
in biliary tract obstruction, 1978-1980
in cirrhosis, 1971
computed tomography in, 1958-1959
in congenital biliary tree anomalies,
1976-1977
in cysts, 1967-1968, 1969
in diffuse diseases, 1969-1971

Pediatrics—cont'd
liver and biliary tract imaging in—cont'd
in epithelial lesions, 1967
in fatty infiltration, 1969, 1970
in fibrolamellar hepatocarcinoma, 1964,
1965
in fungal abscess, 1960, 1961
of gallbladder, 1980-1981
in glycogen storage disease, 1970
in granulomatous disease, 1961
in hemochromatosis, 1969, 1970
in hepatic vessel disorders, 1971-1973,
1974
in hepatoblastoma and hepatocellular
carcinoma, 1962, 1963-1964
in hydatid disease, 1961
in inflammatory lesions, 1958-1961
in jaundice, 1975-1976
in mesenchymal hamartoma, 1966-, 1966,
1968
in metastases, 1965-1966, 1966
in neonatal hepatitis, 1981-1982
in neoplasms, 1961-1967
in portal hypertension, 1971
in portal vein thrombosis, 1972
in pyogenic abscess, 1959, 1960
in radiation effects, 1975
in spontaneous common bile duct
perforation, 1977-1978
in transplantations, 1975
in trauma, 1974-1975
in venoocclusive disease, 1973
in viral hepatitis, 1959
lymphangioma and, 1954
milk allergy enterocolitis and, 522, 523
small bowel studies in, 1878-1906; *see also*
Small bowel, pediatric
ultrasonography in
of appendix, 1926
in Crohn's disease, 1921-1924
in neonatal necrotizing enterocolitis, 1917
in nesidioblastosis, 1950
in neutropenic colitis, 1919
in phlegmon, 1950
in pseudoaneurysm, 1951-1952
in pyogenic splenic abscess, 1936-1937
in Shwachman-Diamond syndrome, 1949
of spleen, 1932
in infarction, 1941
in splenomegaly, 1935
in trauma, 1939-1940
in visceroatrial anomalies, 1934
in wandering spleen, 1933
in Von Hippel–Lindau disease, 1949
in *Yersinia* colitis, 1925
Pedunculated lesions
of colon
in fluoroscopy with pneumocolon
examination, 773
morphology of, 763
sessile, potential for malignancy of, 774
in duodenal bulb polyps, 489
of esophagus, 251
Peliosis hepatis, 1618-1619
Pelvic abscess, 1801-1803, 2035
after surgery, 1801-1802
appendicitis with, 1802
percutaneous drainage of, 2006
plain films and contrast studies of, 2039,
2041
Pelvic arteriography, 2150-2152
in trauma, 2144
Pelvic floor, relaxation of, 849
Pelvic inflammatory disease, 2041
Pelvic loops, pneumocolon in, 517, 522

Pelvic small bowel, prior opacification of, 849
Pelvic spaces, 1799-1800
Pelvis
adhesions in, 533
arteriography of, 2150-2152
in trauma, 2144
computed tomography of
in Crohn's disease, 612
in trauma, 2140
in magnetic resonance imaging of colon,
719, 720
percutaneous interventional radiology and,
1992-1994
prolapse of small bowel into, 541
trauma to
arteriography in, 2144, 2150-2152
computed tomography of, 2140
therapeutic embolization in, 2150-2152
Pemphigus, 235
Penetrating abdominal trauma, 2140-2141
Penicillin
pseudomembranous colitis and, 901
ulcerative colitis versus, 604
in Whipple's disease, 679
Pentastomiasis, 946
Pepsin, 76
Pepsinogen, 75
Peptic esophagitis, 207-208
Peptic stricture, pediatric, 1846
Peptic ulcer disease
antral diaphragm or web with, 322, 323
bleeding
endoscopy in, 968, 970-972
pathophysiology of, 970
ultrasonography of, 2108
in child, 1872, 1903-1904
double-contrast examination in, 1872
endoscopy in, 1872
complications of, 347, 350
definitions and location of, 336-337
diagnostic accuracy in, 299
differential diagnosis of, 347
diverticulitis versus, 760
duodenal, 477-488
baseline tenting in, 484
in child, 1903-1904
complications of, 486-487
differential diagnosis and pitfalls in
imaging of, 487-488
giant, 484, 486
linear, 484, 486
as lithotripsy contraindication, 1359
from methyl tert butyl ether, 1379
nonepithelial tumors and, 498
perforation of, 486-487, 2026
postbulbar, 486, 487
of posterior wall, 478, 479
radiologic features of, 478-484, 485
x-ray versus endoscopy of, 488
duodenitis in, 473
endoscopy in, 970-972
endosonography of, 449
epidemiology of, 336
fulminating diathesis in, 352
gastric
barium contrast examination of, 337, 339
biopsy in, 478
in child, 1872
complications of, 347, 350
definitions and location of, 336-337
differential diagnosis of, 347
epidemiology of, 336
healing of, 347, 348, 349
lesser sac and, 1800
as lithotripsy contraindication, 1359

Peptic ulcer disease—cont'd
  gastric—cont'd
    pediatric, 1872
    plain film evaluation of, 337, 338-339
    pyloric hypertrophy with, 325
    radiographic signs of benign, 339-346
  in gastrinoma, 1170
  in gastritis, 329
  healing of, 347, 348, 349
  lesser sac and, 1800
  as lithotripsy contraindication, 1359
  multiphasic double-contrast examination in,
      478
  plain film evaluation of, 337, 338-339
  radiographic signs of, 339-346
    penetration in, 341
    radiating fold pattern in, 341-342
    signs of undermining in, 342-346
  terms defined in, 336
  ulcer crater in, 2108, 2109
  Zollinger-Ellison syndrome in, 508
Peptide YY, 69
  mechanism of action of, 68
Peptides, intestinal; *see also* Vasoactive
      intestinal peptides
  clinical implications of, 69-72
  physiology of, 69, 70
Percutaneous biliary stricture dilation,
      1383-1396
  access in, 1384, 1385, 1386, 1387
  analgesia in, 1386
  antibiotics in, 1386
  imaging of, 1383-1385
  metallic stents in, 1394-1395, 1396
  morbidity and mortality in, 1396
  number of dilations in, 1386-1389,
      1390-1391
  patient selection in, 1383
  pressure measurements after, 1390-1391
  results of, 1390-1396
  role of stenting in, 1389-1390, 1392
  technique for, 1384, 1385-1386, 1387
Percutaneous biopsy
  of abdominal masses, 1987-1997
    biopsy sites in, 1991-1995
    complications of, 1995-1996
    computed tomography in, 1989, 1991
    fluoroscopy in, 1989
    guidance systems in, 1988-1991
    indications and contraindications for,
        1987
    needle selection in, 1987-1988
    patient preparation in, 1988
    ultrasonography in, 1989-1991, 1991
  of gallbladder, 1382
  of liver in hemangioma, 1642-1643
  of pancreas
    in adenocarcinoma, 1110, 1125
    in cystic neoplasms, 1152
Percutaneous catheter drainage before obesity
      surgery, 460
Percutaneous chemolithiasis, 1378-1379
Percutaneous cholangioscopy, nephroscopes
      for, 1423
Percutaneous cholecystolithotomy, 1375
  large tract, 1376-1378
  results and complications of, 1426-1427
  small tract, 1378
Percutaneous cholecystostomy
  in abscess drainage, 1381-1382
  in cholecystitis, 1281, 1380, 1381
  in malignant biliary tract disease, 1416
Percutaneous choledocholithotomy, 1367-1373
  results and complications of, 1427-1429

Percutaneous choledochoscopy, 1367-1373
  results and complications of, 1427-1429
Percutaneous drainage
  of abscesses, 1998-2010; *see also* Abscess,
      percutaneous drainage of
  biliary; *see also* Percutaneous biliary
      stricture dilation
    after liver transplantation, 1740, 1748
    hemobilia from, 976
  of biloma, 1420
  guided aspiration
    after liver transplantation, 1748
    after pancreatic transplantation,
        1217-1221
  of pancreas, 1025
  of paracolic diverticular abscess, 752
Percutaneous endoscopy of biliary tract,
      1423-1429; *see also* Biliary tract,
      percutaneous endoscopy of
Percutaneous ethanol injection in
      hepatocellular carcinoma, 1701,
      1702; *see also* Alcohol
Percutaneous fine-needle aspiration cytology;
      see Fine-needle aspiration cytology
Percutaneous fluoroscopically guided
      gastrostomy, 2011-2019
  antegrade, in infant, 2018
  comparison of, with other gastrostomy,
      2018
  contraindications to, 2011-2012
  decompression of stomach and small bowel
      in, 2011
  history of, 2011
  indications for, 2011
  in infant, 2018
  long-term management of catheters after,
      2016
  modifications of, 2015-2016
  mortality and morbidity rates in, 2017
  needle in, 2012
  nutritional support and, 2011
  puncture site in, 2012
  results and complications of, 2016-2018
  technique for, 2012-2014, 2015
Percutaneous injection of contrast media
      through anal dimple, 1912
Percutaneous interventional radiology
  in antegrade transhepatic sphincterotomy,
      1426
  in biliary stricture dilation; *see* Percutaneous
      biliary stricture dilation
  biliary tract drainage catheter in, 1417, 1426
    endoscopy for internalization of, 1426
    palliative, 1432-1434, 1435, 1436
  endoscopy in, 1426
  in gallbladder and biliary duct benign
      disease, 1367-1398
    for acute cholecystitis, 1380-1383
    balloon dilation of strictures in,
        1383-1396; *see also* Percutaneous
        biliary stricture dilation
    bile ducts in, 1367-1374
    gallbladder in, 1375-1379
    stricture dilation and, 1383
  in hepatic neoplasm, 1717-1719
  in malignant biliary tract disease, 1399-1422
    alternate access routes in, 1414-1417
    approach to, 1401-1403
    catheter changes after, 1417
    catheter insertion in, 1405-1407
    catheter management after drainage in,
        1417-1418
    catheter selection in, 1407-1411
    combined transhepatic-endoscopic
        approach in, 1411-1414

Percutaneous interventional radiology—cont'd
  in malignant biliary tract disease—cont'd
    complications of, 1418-1420, 1421
    contraindications to, 1400
    equipment for, 1401
    indications for, 1399-1400
    with no relief of symptoms, 1417-1418
    patient management after drainage in,
        1417-1418
    point of entry for catheter in, 1404-1405
    predrainage cholangiography in,
        1403-1405
    rendezvous procedure in, 1411-1414
    results of, 1420-1421
    technique for, 1400-1417
  in unresectable malignancy, 1987
Percutaneous needle aspiration in
      interventional radiology in abdominal
      masses, 1987-1997; *see also*
      Percutaneous biopsy, in abdominal
      masses
Percutaneous pancreatography in pancreatic
      fluid aspiration, 1025
Percutaneous transhepatic cholangiography,
      1236-1240
  in cholangiocarcinoma, 1334
  in choledochal cyst, 1266
  complications of, 1240
  historical review of, 24
  pancreas in, 1021-1022
    adenocarcinoma of, 1123
  in percutaneous intervention in malignancy,
      1401, 1405
Percutaneous transhepatic portography of
      cirrhosis, 1545
Percutaneous transjugular intrahepatic
      portosystemic shunt, 1472-1473; *see
      also* Portosystemic shunt,
      transjugular intrahepatic
Percutaneous transluminal angioplasty, 1628
Perfluorochemicals, 1473
Perfluorooctal bromide, 1757
Perforation
  in acute appendicitis, 2102-2103
  of bile duct in child, 1977-1978
  of colon
    after liver transplantation, 1748
    in barium enema, 714, 715
    in carcinoma, 756, 793, 805
    in flexible sigmoidoscopy, 832
    in percutaneous cholecystostomy of
        cholecystitis, 1381
    plain films and contrast studies in, 2066
    in typhoid fever, 898
  computed tomography of, 2077-2081
    limitations to, 2080-2081
  in Crohn's disease, 601-602
  in diverticulitis, 751
  of duodenum
    from cytomegalovirus disease, 477
    in endoscopic retrograde
        cholangiopancreatography, 1241
    in percutaneous cholecystostomy of
        cholecystitis, 1381
    suspected, 297
    in ulcer, 486-487, 2026
  in endoscopic retrograde
      cholangiopancreatography, 1241
  in endoscopic sphincterotomy, 1318, 1347
  of esophagus, 183, 216-218
  by foreign body, diverticulitis versus, 756
  of gallbladder
    in cholecystitis, 1285-1286, 1287
    in pericholecystic abscess, 1286

Perforation—cont'd
  gastric; *see also* Peptic ulcer disease
    after endoscopy, 304-305
    of pouch after obesity surgery, 460, 461
    suspected, 297
  in intussusception, 1902
    in child, 1902
  in percutaneous cholecystostomy of
      cholecystitis, 1381
  of pharynx, 115, 116, 117
    in child, 1835
  sealed-off, 2080
  site and etiology of, 2079-2080
  suspected, 297
    plain films and contrast studies in, 2026,
        2034
  suspected duodenal, contrast medium in,
      297
  in ulcerative colitis, 582
Perfusion–blood-pool mismatch in red blood
      cell scintigraphy, 1640
Periampullary region of duodenum
  computed tomography of, 1110; *see also*
      Ampulla
  diverticulum of, choledocholithiasis versus,
      1300
  pancreatic endosonography of, 1127, 1128
Periappendiceal abscess; *see also* Appendix
  drainage of, 2006-2007
Periappendiceal fat, 1926
Periappendiceal inflammatory reaction, 2085
Periarteritis nodosa, 2089, 2090
Peribiliary venous plexus, 1610
Pericardium, 30
  in esophageal endosonography, 190
  esophageal tumor spread to, 273
  fat around, 30
Pericholangitis, 1307
  in ulcerative colitis, 574
Pericholecystic abscess, 1285-1286, 1287
  drainage of, 1381-1382
Pericholecystic fat, 1281, 1283
Pericholecystic fluid, 1277-1278, 1283, 1284
Pericholecystic inflammation in gangrenous
      cholecystitis, 2087, 2088
Pericholecystic lymph node involvement,
      1382
Pericolic fat, inflammation of, 2105
Pericolonic space, 1811
  abscess in, 618
Peridiverticular abscess, 2005-2006
Perienteric fat, edema of, 2101
Perigastric lymphadenopathy, 431
Perihepatic space, ascites in, 1801
Perineal fistula, 597
Perinephric abscess, 2036
Perineural spread
  of nasopharyngeal malignancy, 161
  of pharyngeal malignancy, 142
Periodic acid-Schiff mucin staining, 1134,
      1145, 1150
Peripancreatic vessels, 30
Peripheral joint disease, 588
Peripheral nerves in swallowing, 98-101
Periportal cuffing, 2114
Periportal trucking, 1974
Perirectal infiltration, 822
Perirenal fat, 30, 63
Perirenal space, 62, 63, 1810
  abscess in, 1810, 1818
  anterior, 1810-1811
  hematoma in, 1810
Perisigmoid abscess, 2059
Perisplenic space, ascites in, 1801

Peristalsis
  esophageal, 181, 194, 195, 196
    abnormalities of, 182, 211
    absent, in tracheoesophageal fistula and
        atresia, 212
    in achalasia, 202-203
    in diffuse esophageal spasm, 204
    hypertensive, 204
    primary, 196, 197
    secondary, 198
    variable, in tropical sprue, 912
Peritoneal bands, 467
  in child, 1883
Peritoneal cavity, 35; *see also* Peritoneum
  fluid collections in, 1801-1802
  pathology of, 1801-1804
  tumors in, 1803-1804
Peritoneal lavage, diagnostic, 2120-2121
  high false-positive rates with, 2150
Peritoneal spaces, 1798, 1799, 1800
Peritoneography, 1799
Peritoneopericardial hernia, 1858
Peritoneum; *see also* Peritoneal cavity
  abscess in, 1801-1802
    computed tomography of, 2081-2084
  air in
    in appendicitis, 2078
    computed tomography of, 2077-2078
    free, 297
    in typhoid fever, 897
    ultrasonography of, 2099
  anatomy of, 30, 1795-1800
  Armillifer armillatus in, 946
  barium examination of, 1802
  calcifications of, 946
  in cholecystitis, 1275
  compartments of, 35, 54
  computed tomography of, 1801
  cross-sectional imaging of, 1802
  dissemination of cancer in; *see* Metastases,
      to peritoneum
  embryology of, 1795-1797
  fat in, 2022
  fluid collections in
    in abdominal trauma, 2120-2121
    computed tomography versus diagnostic
        peritoneal lavage in, 2120-2121
    plain films and contrast studies in,
        2028-2029
  free gas within, 297
  gallbladder position and, 1254
  Gardner's syndrome and, 781
  hemorrhage in, 1801
  implants in, 792
  inflammation of; *see* Peritonitis
  in mesenteric pathology, 1823
  in pelvic abscess, 1802
  plain films of, 1802
  tuberculosis of, 894-895
  tumor seeding in, 1326
Peritonism after percutaneous fluoroscopically
      guided gastrostomy, 2017
Peritonitis, 1802-1803
  after percutaneous fluoroscopically guided
      gastrostomy, 2016-2017
  aseptic, 1802-1803
  computed tomography of, 2077-2081
    limitations of, 2080-2081
  in duodenal ulcer perforation, 487
  meconium, 1891, 1892
    antenatal ultrasonography of, 1891
  pelvic abscess and, 2035
  percutaneous interventional radiology in,
      1995
  in pericholecystic abscess, 1286

Peritonitis—cont'd
  tuberculous, 894
  ultrasonography of, 2100
Perivascular space, 1812
Permeability of intestines, 82
Pernicious anemia, 77
  in gastritis, 330
Peroral biopsy
  jejunal, in small bowel vascular occlusion,
      653
  of small bowel, 552-555
Peroral choledochoscopy, 1423
Peroral pneumocolon, 565, 713
  for cecal filling, 711
  in Crohn's disease, 594, 595
    in child, 1892, 1893
  in idiopathic inflammatory disease, 566-567
  in neoplasia, 765-767, 768, 770
    morphology and, 773
  in ulcerative colitis, 580
Peroral small bowel examination, 515-522
  in Crohn's disease, 594, 595
    in child, 1892, 1893
  in idiopathic inflammatory disease, 566-567
  in inflammatory bowel disease, 566-567
  with small bowel follow-through method,
      689
  small bowel meal with, 515-522, 523
  in ulcerative colitis, 580
Persistent fetal circulation, 1856
PET; *see* Positron emission tomography
Petechiae after lithotripsy, 1364
Pethidine, 1725
Petroleum jelly, barium-impregnated, 844
Peutz-Jeghers syndrome, 783-785
  gastric polyps in, 375
  gastric tumors in, 1873
  polyp distribution and malignancy risk in,
      1928
  small bowel intussusception in, 1895
  small bowel neoplasms and, 631
Peyer's patches, 82
  tuberculosis and, 890
  typhoid fever and, 896
Pfahler, GE, 3
PFOB; *see* Perfluorooctal bromide
PGE$_2$; *see* Prostacyclin
Pharmacoangiography, 994-995
Pharyngeal constrictors in swallowing, 106
  functional abnormalities of, 130-133
Pharyngeal inlet, 94
Pharyngeal outpouchings, lateral, 115-118
Pharyngeal space, 110
Pharyngoesophageal segment
  dysfunction of, 133
  structural disease of, 118-120
Pharynx
  adaptation in, 106, 107-109
    functional abnormalities of, 106, 107-109,
        133-137
  imaging of, 106
  anatomy of, 94-98
    in functional phases of swallowing, 96-98
    landmarks in, 94
    pediatric, 1826-1828
    sagittal, 94
    zones in, 96
  benign structural disease of, 114-126
    branchial cleft anomalies in, 120, 121
    in child, 1829-1833
    diverticula in, 1831-1832
    foreign bodies in, 114, 115
    lateral outpouchings in, 115-118
    mucosal abnormalities in, 114
    neoplasms in, 114, 115

Pharynx—cont'd
  benign structural disease of—cont'd
    parapharyngeal abnormalities in, 120-126
    pharyngoesophageal segment, 118-120
    tonsillar enlargement in, 120, 121
    trauma in, 115, 116, 117
    webs in, 1831-1832
  computed tomography of, 111
    in child, 1829, 1830, 1982-1833
  dynamic recording of, 103
  functional abnormalities of, 127-138
    adaptation, compensation, and
      decompensation, 133-137
    cause of dysfunction in, 133-135, 136
    multidisciplinary approach to, 165-167
    oral stage, 127-129
    pediatric neurogenic tumor in, 1834
    pharyngeal stage, 129-133
    pharyngoesophageal segment dysfunction
      in, 133
    solitary, 137
    treatment planning in, 137
  imaging techniques for, 94-113
    adaptation, compensation, and
      decompensation in, 106
    anatomy and, 94-98
    axial studies in, 106-111
    barium studies in, 101-103, 130-133, 160
    choice of studies in, 101
    compensation in, 106, 107-109, 133-137
    computed tomography in, 106-111,
      140-142; see also Pharynx, computed
      tomography of
    double-contrast pharyngography of,
      103-106
    dynamic recording in, 103
    frontal view, during swallowing, 103, 105
    future directions in, 112
    insufflation in, 103, 105
    lateral view, during swallowing, 103, 104
    magnetic resonance imaging in; see
      Pharynx, magnetic resonance
      imaging of
    neural control of pharyngeal phase and,
      98-101
    pediatric, 1923
    pharyngeal swallowing phase in, 98
    in piriform sinus tumor, 160
    plain radiography of, 101, 102
    tailored examination in, 101-103
    ultrasonography in, 106, 111-112, 1832,
      1833
  magnetic resonance imaging of, 111
    in adenoid cystic carcinoma, 152-153
    in child, 1829, 1830, 1832, 1833
    in malignancy, 140-142
    in swallowing, 100, 106-111
  malignant diseases of, 139-164
    brainstem lesions in, esophageal
      obstruction versus, 183
    direct encroachment in, 142, 147-150
    esophageal webs and, 236
    hematogenous metastasis in, 144
    hypopharyngeal, 157-160
    imaging in staging of, 140-142
    lymphatic spread in, 142-144, 150, 152,
      157, 158
    metastasis from, 142-144, 150
    nasopharyngeal, 160
    oral cavity, 144-150
    oropharyngeal, 150-157
    pathology of, 139
    perineural spread of, 142, 150, 151-153,
      152, 158
    positive nodes in, 144

Pharynx—cont'd
  malignant diseases of—cont'd
    postoperative evaluation of, 160-163
    reconstruction in, 160-163
    second primary, 144
    staging of, 139-144
    tumor spread estimation in, 142-144
    unknown primary, 144
  pediatric, 1826-1836
    anatomy of, 1826-1828
    bolus formation in, 1827
    congenital anomalies of, 1829-1831
    deglutition in, 1827
    diverticula and webs in, 1831-1832
    masses in, 1832-1835
    motility disturbances in, 1828-1829
    sucking and, 1827
    swallowing and, 1827-1828
    technique for, 1923
    trauma in, 1835-1836
  perforation of, 115, 116, 117
    in child, 1835
  swallowing in; see Swallowing, pharyngeal
  trauma to
    in child, 1835-1836
    foreign body in, 1836
Phenergan; see Promethazine
Phenolphthalein, 11
  in bowel preparation, 90
Phenomenon
  escape, in esophageal peristalsis, 198
  moulage; see Moulage phenomenon
  refraction, 1474
  siphoning, 1460, 1461
Phenylbutazone, 231
Pheochromocytoma, 71
  inadvertent biopsy of, 1993
  in multiple endocrine neoplasia, 1169
Phlebolith
  calcified, in hepatic hemangioma, 1631
  in splenic tumors, 1780
Phlebotomy, 1562
Phlegmon
  in appendicitis, 2085
  in colorectal carcinoma, 806
  in diverticulitis, 2105
  in gangrenous cholecystitis, 2087
  in gastritis, 333-334
  in hollow gut disease, 2101-2102
  in pancreatitis, 1950
Phospholipids, 80
  liver and, 84
Phosphosoda enema, 715-716
Photofluorography in mass screening, 425
Phrenic ampulla, 168, 196
Phrenic artery, 29
Phrenic nerve, damage to, 1858-1859
Phrenicoesophageal membranes, 218
Phrenicosplenic ligament, 30
Phrygian cap of gallbladder, 1227
  abnormalities of, 1255
Physiology, gastrointestinal; see
    Gastrointestinal tract, physiology of
Phytobezoar, 365
  in child, 1874
Picket fence appearance
  in intramural hematoma or bleeding, 503
  in ischemic enteritis, 685
Piezoelectric lithotriptor, 1359, 1360
Pigmented lesions
  in hemochromatosis, 1560
  in Peutz-Jeghers syndrome, 784
Pigtail flush catheter
  in aorta, 2144
  in pelvic arteriography, 2150

Pipe-stem stenosis, 671
Piriform sinus
  barium retention in, 132
  squamous carcinoma of, 159
  weblike structures of, 120
Pitfalls
  in splenic radionuclide studies, 1755-1757
  in splenic ultrasound, 1753, 1754; see also
    Artifacts
Pitressin; see Vasopressin
Plain films
  of acute abdomen, 2020-2075; see also
    Acute abdomen, plain films and
    contrast studies in
  in appendicitis, 2029
  in bacterial cholangitis, 1304, 1305
  in cholangiocarcinoma, 1334
  in cholecystitis, 2031
  in congenital anomalies of small bowel,
    1881
  in congenital anorectal malformations,
    1910-1912
  in dedicated small bowel follow-through
    examination, 566
  of esophagus, 168, 176
  in functional constipation, 1915
  in graft-versus-host disease, 675, 676
  in hepatic hemangiomas, 1630-1631
  in inflammatory bowel disease, 564-565,
    2065
  in intestinal pseudoobstruction, 669
  in intraabdominal abscesses, 2035
  in intussusception, 2054
  in ischemia and infarction of mesenteric
    blood vessels, 649
  in large bowel obstruction, 2057
  in leaking abdominal aortic aneurysm, 2071
  in Mediterranean fever, 678
  in neonatal necrotizing enterocolitis, 1916
  in neutropenic colitis, 1919
  in obesity surgery, 458
  in obstruction of small bowel, 2045
  in pancreatic mucinous tumors, 1146
  in pancreatoblastoma, 1156
  in pediatric annular pancreas, 1946
  in pediatric pyogenic splenic abscess, 1936
  in pediatric splenic cyst, 1938
  in pelvic abscess, 2039
  in peptic ulcer disease, 337, 338-339
  of pharynx, 101, 102
  in renal colic, 2070-2071
  in subphrenic and subhepatic abscess, 2036
  in toxic megacolon in ulcerative colitis, 581,
    582
  in wandering pediatric spleen, 1933
Plaque, sessile, of colon, 763
Plasmacytoma
  in pancreas, 1163
  in stomach, 384-385
Platelets, indium 111–labeled
  in hepatic scintigraphy, 1532
  in pancreatic transplantation, 1202-1203
Platinum microcoils, 2144
  in therapeutic embolization of liver, 2148
Pleating appearance in scleroderma, 679
Pleomorphic carcinoma of pancreas,
  1152-1153
Pleomorphic lipoma in retroperitoneum, 1812
Pleomorphic sarcoma of pancreas, 1155
Pleural space, trauma and, 2153
Pleuroperitoneal hernia, 1853-1856
Plexus
  Auerbach's, 202
  epicholedochal, 1319
  myenteric, 1912-1915

Plummer-Vinson syndrome, 120
   esophageal webs in, 235
PN; *see* Polyarteritis nodosa
Pneumatosis, intramural, 2068, 2069
   after liver transplantation, 1748
   of colon in neutropenic colitis, 1919
   plain films and contrast studies in,
         2068-2069
   of small bowel
      computed tomography of, 614
      in enteropathy, 675
      in neonatal necrotizing enterocolitis, 1917
      in scleroderma, 679
   of stomach, 334
      in volvulus, 364
   ultrasonography of, 2100
Pneumatosis cystoides; *see* Pneumatosis,
         intramural
Pneumobilia, 1305
Pneumococcus
   in phlegmonous gastritis, 333
   in splenectomy infections, 1790
Pneumocolon, peroral; *see* Peroral
         pneumocolon
Pneumocystis carinii
   in acquired immunodeficiency syndrome,
         with small bowel lesions, 553
   splenic calcifications and, 1772
Pneumonia
   ascariasis and, 930
   streptococcal, Bochdalek's hernia versus,
         1856
   strongyloidiasis in, 930
   in tracheoesophageal fistula and atresia, 212
Pneumoperitoneum
   after liver transplantation, 1749
   after percutaneous fluoroscopically guided
         gastrostomy, 2017
   in child, 1874, 1875
   conditions simulating, 2027-2028
   in gastric rupture, 369
   plain films and contrast studies in,
         2023-2028
   in scleroderma, 679
   ultrasonography of, 2099
   without peritonitis, 2026-2027
Pneumothorax, 1995
Podophyllum, 583
Polidicanol, 972
Poliomyelitis, 132, 134
Polya-type gastrectomy, 298
Polyarteritis nodosa
   hepatic artery and, 1616
   hepatic macroregenerative nodule and
         nodular regenerative hyperplasia and,
         1655
   in small bowel, 653-655
Polycystic disease
   in kidney, 1156
   in liver, 1658, 1659
Polyethylene glycol
   before colon imaging, 698, 699
   in intestinal permeability, 82
Polyethylene stent, Wallstent versus, 1436
Polylysine, 1499
Polymyositis, 129
Polyp; *see also* Polypoid lesions; Polyposis
   cholesterol, in gallbladder, 1329
   of colon
      barium-coated, as artifact, 772
      in Cowden's disease, 786-787
      in Cronkhite-Canada syndrome, 632
      in inflammatory disease, 576-578
      juvenile, 778, 779-788, 1926, 1927,
            1928, 1929

Polyp—cont'd
   of colon—cont'd
      in Peutz-Jeghers syndrome, 631
      postinflammatory, 576-578
   in Cowden's disease, 786-787
   defined, 762
   distribution and malignancy risk of, 1928
   esophageal
      inflammatory, 251
      sessile, 247, 249
   extracolonic, in Gardner's syndrome, 783
   in familial multiple polyposis, 780-781,
         782-783
   filiform
      in Crohn's disease, 591, 1923
      in inflammatory bowel disease, 570, 571
      in ulcerative colitis, 574, 577, 579
   gastric
      cancer and, 395
      in Cronkhite-Canada syndrome, 631
      cross-sectional imaging of, 373
      endosonography of, 451
      epithelial, 373-377
      fundic gland, 376
      hamartomatous, 375
      heterotopic, 377
      hyperplastic, 374, 375
         in familial multiple polyposis, 780
      inflammatory fibroid, 360, 381-383
      in Peutz-Jeghers syndrome, 631
      regenerative, 374, 375
      retention, 376-377
      sessile, 374, 406
   inflammatory
      in Crohn's disease, 591, 593
      in large bowel, 576
      in small bowel, fibroid, 630
   pedunculated
      in duodenal bulb, 489
      in fluoroscopy with pneumocolon
            examination, 773
   peroral biopsy of small bowel and, 553, 554
   in Peutz-Jeghers syndrome, 785, 786
   single-contrast barium enema in, 703
   umbilical, 1889
Polypectomy combined with screening
         procedures, 833
Polypeptides
   pancreatic, 1132, 1146
   vasoactive intestinal; *see* Vasoactive
         intestinal peptides
Polypoid lesions; *see also* Polyp; Polyposis
   in cecal tumors, 803
   of colon, 777-779
      artifacts versus, 771-772
      classification of, 762
      confidence level in diagnosis of, 771
      diminutive, 767
      familial multiple, 780-781, 782-783
      juvenile benign, 778
      malignant potential of, 763, 771, 774
      morphology of, 763
      sessile, 774
   of duodenum, 498
      in benign lymphoid hyperplasia, 501
      in Brunner's gland hyperplasia, 501
      in Zollinger-Ellison syndrome, 508
   in esophageal carcinosarcoma, 249
   in gastric cancer, 395, 437
   in gastric lymphoma, 429
Polyposis, 1926; *see also* Polyp; Polypoid
         lesions
   cancer family syndrome and, 827, 836

Polyposis—cont'd
   of colon, 763, 779-788
      characteristic features of, 789
      in child, 1926, 1928, 1929
      in Cronkhite-Canada syndrome, 787
      differential diagnosis in, 788, 790
      familial adenomatous; *see* Familial
            adenomatous polyposis
      in Gardner's syndrome, 783
      juvenile, 787-788
      malignant lymphomatous, 791-792
      screening in, 790, 825
      in Turcot's syndrome, 786
   with gastric involvement, 373-374
   gastric tumors in child in, 1873
   hereditary or nonhereditary, 780
   juvenile, in stomach, 376
   Peutz-Jeghers syndrome and; *see*
         Peutz-Jeghers syndrome
   of small bowel, 631-632
      metastatic tumors in, 645
Polysaccharides, 79
Polysplenia, 1934, 1935
   in pancreatic agenesis, 1946
   syndromes of, 1766, 1767
Polyvinyl alcohol, 1728, 1729
Pool-of-barium appearance, 652, 653
Porcelain gallbladder, 1325, 1329, 1332
Porta hepatis
   anatomy of, 1224-1225
      coronal, 64
      sagittal, 38
   computed tomography of, 53, 1232, 1233
   in endoscopy of stomach, 314
   magnetic resonance imaging of, 65
   ultrasonography of, 39, 53
      gallbladder, 1249
      right anterior oblique, 39
      transverse, 53
Portacaval nodes, 34
Portacaval shunt; *see also* Portosystemic shunt
   in hepatic vein occlusion, 1627
   postoperative evaluation of, 1589-1591
   transjugular intrahepatic, 1567
      in cirrhosis with portal hypertension, 1587
Portacaval space, 34
Portal cavernoma, 1972
Portal cavernomatous transformation, 1610
Portal fissure, 1224
Portal hypertension, 1566-1603; *see also* Portal
         vein
   after liver transplantation, 1747
   angiography of, 1582-1583, 1584-1586,
         1596
   arterial portography of, 1606
   ascites and, 87
   in child, 1848-1850, 1971, 1972
   in cholangiocarcinoma, 1342
   choledochal cyst and, 1266
   cirrhosis versus, hepatic angiography of,
         1545
   colon in, 1598-1599, 1600
   computed tomography of, 1577-1582, 1583,
         1594-1596
   computed tomography arterial portography
         of, 1462
   direct tumor invasion of portal vein in, 1592
   duodenum in, 1596-1598
   in esophageal varices, 238
   extrahepatic, 1591-1592
   gastrointestinal tract and, 1596-1603
   hepatic arteriovenous fistulas in, 1617
   hepatic vein catheterization in, 1607
   hepatic venography of, 1583

Portal hypertension—cont'd
  hepatic venous obstruction in, 1591-1592
  hyperkinetic, 1572-1574
  intrahepatic, 1574-1584
    angiography of, 1582-1583, 1584-1586
    barium examination in, 1575, 1576
    computed tomography of, 1577-1582,
      1583
    magnetic resonance imaging in,
      1577-1582, 1583
    manometry in, 1583
    portal venography of, 1583-1584,
      1587-1589
    splenoportography of, 1583
    ultrasonography of, 1575-1577, 1578
    venography of, 1566-1572
  magnetic resonance imaging of, 1577-1582,
    1583, 1594-1596
  mesenteric venous diseases in, 1596-1603
  pancreatic carcinoma in, 1593, 1594
  pancreatitis in, 1593, 1594
  in parasplenic neoplasms, 1788-1789
  portal venous resistance increase in, 1574
  posthepatic, 1591
  postsinusoidal, 1574
  prehepatic, 1592, 1594
  preoperative and postoperative portosystemic
    shunt evaluation in, 1584-1591
  presinusoidal, 1574
  radiologic evaluation of, 1574-1584,
    1585-1589
  regional, 1594
  selective shunts in, 1588
  small bowel and, 1596-1598
  splenic vein obstruction in, 1593-1594
  stomach and, 1596
  total shunts in, 1588
  ultrasonography of, 1575-1577, 1578,
    1594-1596
  venography of, 1596
  venous obstruction in, 1591-1592
Portal vein; see also Portal hypertension
  abnormalities of, 1444, 1445
    congenital, 1622, 1885
    liver transplantation and, 1735-1736,
      1737, 1747
  absence of, 1622
  anatomy of, 30, 31, 33, 35
    angiography and, 1610
    dorsal right, 29
    left, 30, 31, 33
    radiographic, 1225, 1444, 1445, 1566
  aneurysm of, 1623, 1624
  angiography of, 1619-1625
    technique in, 1605-1606
  catheterization of, 1187-1188, 1189,
    1607-1608
    in localization procedures, 1192-1193
  cavernous transformation of, 1594-1596
    in child, 1972
  chemotherapy infusion in, 1729
  in cirrhosis, 1628
  collateral channels of, 1596, 1735-1736
    arterial portography of, 1606
    in Budd-Chiari syndrome, 1626, 1627
  congenital absence of, 1566
  double, 1622
  dynamic computed tomography of, 1568
  in endoscopy, 314
  gas in, 2051
    in neonatal necrotizing enterocolitis, 1917
    ultrasonography of, 2100
  in intrahepatic portohepatic shunt, 1625
  in islet cell tumors, 1187-1188, 1189

Portal vein—cont'd
  magnetic resonance imaging of, 1235, 1569
  occlusion of, 1594, 1724
    cholangiocarcinoma in, 1341, 1461
    extrahepatic, 1596
    hepatic vein catheterization in, 1607
    in hepatocellular carcinoma, 1699
    neoplastic, 1623, 1624
    postoperative, 1592
  physiology of, 1611
    Budd-Chiari syndrome and, 1611
  preduodenal, in small bowel of child, 1885
  pressure in, 1583, 1607
  sampling from, in tumor localization
    procedures, 1192-1193
  stenosis of, after liver transplantation, 1747,
    1975
  thrombosis of, 1594, 1621, 1622-1623
    after liver transplantation, 1735, 1747,
      1975
    calcification in, 1622
    in child, 1972-1973, 1973
    extrahepatic, 1622
    intrahepatic, 1622, 1623
    postoperative, 1592
    ultrasonography of, 1471
  transcatheter hepatic embolization in,
    1729-1732
  tumor invasion of, 1594, 1706
    arterial portography of, 1606
    cirrhosis and, 1592
    hepatocellular carcinoma in, 1665, 1671,
      1672
  ultrasonography of, 1468, 1471, 1567
    Duplex, 1735-1736
    gallbladder, 1249
  venous resistance in, 1574
  ventral, 1622
Portal venography, 1566-1572
  in cirrhosis, 1545, 1583-1584, 1587-1589,
    1596
  with portal hypertension, 1566-1567,
    1570, 1583-1584, 1587-1589
  before liver transplantation, 1736
Portography
  arterial, 1567-1572
    in cirrhosis with portal hypertension,
      1567-1572
    computed tomography in; see Computed
      tomography arterial portography
    of liver, 1606-1607
  in cirrhosis, 1545, 1566-1567, 1569, 1572,
    1583
  in hepatocellular carcinoma, 1688-1690
  transhepatic, 1545, 1566-1567, 1570
    in pancreatic tumoral invasion, 1593
  transjugular, 1567
  umbilical, 1572
    in cirrhosis, 1572
Portohepatic shunt, intrahepatic, 1625
Portosystemic shunt, 1584; see also Portacaval
    shunt
  angiography of, 1583
  postoperative evaluation of, 1589-1591
  postsinusoidal portal hypertension and, 1574
  preoperative evaluation of, 1584-1589
  previous, liver transplantation and, 1735
  transjugular intrahepatic, 1007-1014,
    1472-1473, 1628
    in cirrhosis with portal hypertension, 1587
    in hepatic vascular diseases, 1628
  ultrasonography of, 1575
Portovenous shunt, intrahepatic, 1575
Positron emission tomography, 720, 810

Postcricoid region, 158
Postembolization syndrome, hepatic arterial
    embolization and, 1729
Posterior anorectal angle, 847
Posthepatic portal hypertension, 1591
Postinflammatory polyps, 576-578
Postinflammatory pseudopolyps, 779
Postinflammatory strictures of biliary tree,
    1315-1316
Postoperative abdomen, 2028, 2063-2065
Postoperative effusions, 1198
Postoperative imaging after liver
    transplantation, 1737-1738, 1739
  in complications, 1738-1749
Postoperative pneumoperitoneum, 2063
Postpolio syndrome, 132
Postradiation lesions; see Radiation
Postsinusoidal portal hypertension, 1574
Potassium
  enteric-coated, 650
  in esophagitis, 230, 231, 1847
Pouch
  after obesity surgery
    decompression of, 461
    dilatation of, 463-464
    perforation of, 460, 461
    rate of emptying of, 458
  of Douglas, 693, 1799-1800
  ileal, 585, 586
  ileoanal, 585, 586
    computed tomography of, 614
    in inflammatory bowel disease, 567
  Koch, 585
Pouchitis, 585, 588
Pouchogram, 567
Povidone-iodine, 1237
PP cells; see Pancreatic polypeptide cells
PPoma, 1168, 1172
Precut techniques in endoscopic
    sphincterotomy, 1345
Prednisolone, 1231
Predrainage cholangiography, 1403-1405
Preduodenal portal vein in child, 1885
Preembolization arteriography, transcatheter
    hepatic, 1725
Pregnancy
  fatty infiltration of liver in, 1549
  as lithotripsy contraindication, 1359, 1364
  ruptured ectopic, 2073
  varices and, 970
Prehepatic portal hypertension, 1592, 1594
Premedication
  for gastric endoscopy, 302
  for transcatheter hepatic embolization,
    1724-1725
Presacral space, 579
Presbyesophagus, 205, 211
Presinusoidal portal hypertension, 1574
Prestyloid and poststyloid compartments, 106,
    110
Pretransplant imaging in liver transplantation,
    1735-1736
Prevertebral muscles, 158
Prevertebral space, 106, 110
Primary immunodeficiency syndromes
  radiology in, 676-677
    in small bowel enteropathy, 676
    in small bowel functional diseases, 676-677
Primary sclerosing cholangitis; see Cholangitis
Priscoline; see Tolazoline
Probes of intestinal permeability, 82
Proctitis
  double-contrast examination in, 566
  gonorrheal, 604, 607
  ulcerative, 904, 905

Proctography, 840, 844; *see also*
  Defecography
Proctoscopy
  in colonic neoplasia detection, 767
  in ulcerative colitis, 581
Proctosigmoidoscopy
  in follow-up, 832
  in neoplasia detection, 767
Progressive systemic sclerosis
  duodenum in, 506
  small bowel in, 678-679, 680
Proinsulin, 1169
Prolapse
  antral mucosal, of duodenum, 471, 472
  of small bowel, 841
    into pelvis in enteroclysis, 541
Promethazine, 1424
Prone mucosal relief film in mass screening,
  425
Prostacyclin, 72
Prostaglandin analogue, 72
Prostaglandins
  gastric acid secretion and, 76
  irritable bowel and, 72
  mucus secretion and, 77
  physiology of, 72
Prostate
  anatomy of, 727, 728
  rectal carcinoma infiltration of, 818
  retroperitoneal fibrosis in, 1815
Prosthesis, pancreatic, 1094-1097
Prostigmin; *see* Neostigmine
Protein allergy, 666, 668
Protein digestion, 79-80
Protein synthesis, 84
Proteolytic agents, 216
Proteus
  in bacterial cholangitis, 1304
  in phlegmonous gastritis, 333
  in pseudomembranous enterocolitis, 901
Proton pump inhibitors, 72-73, 76
Proton spectroscopic imaging, 1551-1553
Protozoal disease, 915-918, 919, 920
  in acquired immunodeficiency syndrome
    patient, 955-958
Pruned tree appearance, 1308, 1309
Pseudo-Billroth I appearance, 333, 475
Pseudo-Billroth II appearance, 599
Pseudoachalasia
  amyl nitrite test in, 181, 204
  in sphincter opening abnormalities, 211
Pseudoaneurysm
  after liver transplantation, 1746
  after pancreatic transplantation, 1198, 1216,
    1217
  computed tomography of infected, 2088
  of hepatic artery, 1615
    stenting after stricture repair and,
      1394-1395
  in pediatric acute pancreatitis, 1951-1952
  splenic artery embolization in, 1791
  transcatheter embolization and, 2146, 2148,
    2149
Pseudoappendicitis versus Crohn's disease,
  1921-1924
Pseudo–Budd-Chiari syndrome, 1519
Pseudocyst
  in esophageal strictures, 238
  in meconium peritonitis, 1891
  of pancreas
    in acute pancreatitis, 1950-1951, 1952
    after transplantation, 1198, 1220
    drainage of, 1034
    ectopic, 1034

Pseudocyst—cont'd
  of pancreas—cont'd
    endoscopic therapy in drainage of,
      1097-1098
    false-positive, 1035
    history of radiography of, 17
    in mucinous cystic neoplasms, 1144
    percutaneous abscess drainage and, 1999,
      2002-2003, 2004
    retroperitoneal fluid collections in, 1816,
      1817
    sonography of, 1033
    sphincterotomy for, in chronic
      pancreatitis, 1091
    temporal relationships of, 1034-1035
    ultrasonography of, 1033-1034
  in spleen, 1775
Pseudodiverticula
  of duodenum, 469
    in Crohn's disease, 475
    intraluminal, 470
  esophageal, 215, 216, 238
    in moniliasis, 226
  in pediatric Crohn's disease, 1923
  in peptic ulcer disease, 478, 482
  in small bowel systemic sclerosis, 653
Pseudolesions, Doppler sonography and, 1753
Pseudolymphoma, 326, 354-357, 384
Pseudomasses in pancreas from anomalous
  ducts, 1049
Pseudomembranous colitis
  after liver transplantation, 1748
  appendicitis versus, 716
  computed tomography of, 2086
  in differential diagnosis, 603, 604
  plain films and contrast studies in, 2067
  thumbprinting in, 564
  toxic megacolon in, 603
  ulcerative colitis versus, 603, 604
Pseudomembranous enterocolitis, 901-903
Pseudomonas
  in bacterial cholangitis, 1304
  in emphysematous cholecystitis, 1286
Pseudomyxoma peritonei, 1803-1804
Pseudoneoplasm; *see* Pseudotumor
Pseudoobstruction, intestinal
  in child, 1902-1903
  idiopathic, 2060
    esophageal motility disorders and, 205,
      211
    percutaneous abscess drainage in, 2008,
      2009
    plain films and contrast studies in, 1903,
      2059, 2060
    small bowel motility in, 661, 669,
      1902-1903
    ultrasonography of, 1903
Pseudopneumoperitoneum, plain films and
  contrast studies in, 2027-2028
Pseudopolyps
  in acute inflammatory colitis, 2065, 2066
  in Crohn's disease, 591, 592
  duodenal, in tuberculosis, 476
  in inflammatory bowel disease, 569
  postinflammatory, in colon, 779
  in ulcerative colitis, 573, 577, 606
Pseudosacculations, 591, 592
Pseudosarcoma, esophageal, 249
Pseudostalk of polypoid lesions, 763
Pseudotumor
  after hiatal hernia repair, 220
  in colon as artifact, 772
  gastric, 283
    computed tomography of, 306
    lymphoma in, 326, 354-357, 384

Pseudoulcer in duodenum, 480
Psoas muscle, 30
  in retroperitoneum, 1809
Psoas space, 1809
  abscess in, 1818
Psychotropics, xerostomia and, 73
PTC; *see* Percutaneous transhepatic
  cholangiography
Pterygopalatine fossa, 150, 151
PTH; *see* Parathyroid hormone
Pubococcygeal line, 845
Puborectalis muscle, 840, 841
  in straining, 849
Pudendal nerve, 840-841
Pulmonary sling, 1844
Pulse-spray thrombolysis, 1628
Pulses, spatial saturation, 1489
Pulsion diverticula
  of duodenum, 469
  of esophagus, 214
Pump inhibitors, 72-73, 76
Purcell, EM, 19, 20
Purgatives
  bowel preparation and, 90
  in small bowel malabsorption, 684-685
Purpura, Henoch-Schönlein, 653, 655, 1896
Purulent exudate, sonography of, 2101
PVA; *see* Polyvinyl alcohol
PVE; *see* Portal vein, transcatheter hepatic
  embolization in
Pyelography, intravenous, 1751, 1752
Pyelonephritis, 575
Pylephlebitis with liver abscess, 2083
Pylethrombophlebitis, 1622
Pyloric antrum; *see* Gastric antrum
Pyloric canal, 31
Pyloric hypertrophy
  in adult, 322-325
  diffuse, 324-325
Pyloric sphincter, 31, 35
  hypertrophic stenosis of
    in child, 1868-1869
    conditions mimicking, 1869
Pylorospasm, 1869, 1870, 1871
Pylorus, 282
  in endoscopy, 314
  musculature of, 323
  in normal endoscopy, 304
  ulcer of, 483
Pyoderma gangrenosum, 575
Pyogenic abscess
  in child, 1959
  computed tomography of, 2082
  of liver, 2001
    ultrasonography of, 1475
  of spleen in child, 1936-1937
Pyogenic cholangitis; *see* Cholangitis
Pyramids, renal medullary, 31, 61-63
Pyridoxylidene glutamate, 2031
Pyrrolizidine alkaloids, 1592

Q

Quadrate lobe of liver, 31
Quadratus lumborum muscle, 31
Quinacrine hydrochloride, 925
Quinidine
  esophageal rings and, 235
  esophagitis from, 230, 231

R

Radial forearm flap, 163
Radiating fold pattern
  in gastric carcinoma, 412
  in peptic ulcer, 341-342

Radiation effects; *see also* Radiation therapy
  in colitis, ulcerative colitis versus, 604, 608
  in enteritis, 651, 685-686
    chronic, small intestinal, 651-652, 653
    portal hypertension and, 1597
  in esophageal strictures, 236, 237
  in esophagitis, 1848
  in ischemic duodenitis, 476
  in liver in child, 1975
  in rectal wall changes, 818, 819
  in stomach, 359
Radiation therapy
  in cholangiocarcinoma, 1342
  in esophageal carcinoma, 243
    esophageal-fat interface and, 275, 276
    in recurrences, 278
  in esophageal sarcoma, 249
  in gallbladder carcinoma, 1333
  in gastric lymphoma, 431
  in hepatocellular carcinoma, 1677
  implantation, in percutaneous intervention in
    malignant biliary tract disease, 1403
Radiographic contrast agents; *see* Contrast
    agents
Radiographic voltage, 2022
Radioiodine; *see* Iodinated contrast media
Radioisotopes; *see* Radionuclides
Radiolucent commode, 841, 842
Radiomanometry; *see also* Esophagus,
    manometry of
Radionuclides; *see also* Scintigraphy
  in cirrhosis of liver, 1544-1545
  in colonic function tests, 88-89
  in gastroesophageal reflux in child,
    1860-1861
  in liver angiomatous lesions, 1966
  in obesity surgery studies, 460
  in percutaneous biliary stricture dilation,
    1383
  in small bowel carcinoid tumors, 634
  in spleen, 1753-1757
    in infection, 1780
    in tumors, 1782
Radiotelemetry, 89
Radiotherapy; *see* Radiation therapy
Radiplast, 1988
Radium exposure, 1528, 1640
Radt, P, 13
Ram's horn sign, 333, 475, 599, 600
Rapid acquisition spin-echo, 1759
Rare tumors of pancreas, 1132-1166; *see also*
    Pancreas, rare tumors of
Reactive lymphoid hyperplasia, 354
Real-time ultrasonography of pancreas, 1028;
    see also Ultrasonography
Receptor, somatostatin, 1191
Recess, azygoesophageal, 173
Rectal carcinoma; *see also* Colorectal
    carcinoma
  computed tomography of, 807, 808
    invasive lesions in, 803, 804
  detection of, 768
  endosonographic staging of, 813-823
    depth of tumor penetration in, 815-818,
      819
    local recurrence in, 820-821, 822
    lymph node involvement in, 818-820
    in perirectal infiltration, 822
    rectal wall anatomy in, 814-815
    role of, 821-822
    technique and apparatus for, 813-814
  hepatic metastases from, 1724
  in hereditary nonpolyposis colorectal cancer,
    788
  infiltration by, 817-818

Rectal carcinoma—cont'd
  magnetic resonance imaging of, 807, 808
  metastatic, 813
  prognosis in, 822
  recurrence of, 818, 819, 820-821, 822
  thickness of tumor in, 816
Rectal evacuation
  quantification of, 844
  recording of, 842-844
Rectal sphincters, 728
Rectal thermometer, trauma from, 1927
Rectal wall
  in defecography, 849-850
  in endosonography, 814-815
Rectoanal inhibitory reflex, 840, 845
Rectocele, 849
Rectocloacal fistula, 1912
Rectodynamics, 844
Rectosigmoid colon
  anatomy of, 695
  strictures of, lymphogranuloma venereum
    and, 905
Rectourethral fistula, 1912
Rectovaginal fistula, 1912
Rectovaginal separation, 849
Rectovaginal septum, 847
Rectovesical fistula, 1912
Rectovesical pouch, 693
Rectovestibular fistula, 1912
Rectum
  anatomy of, 693, 727-728
  in ascariasis, 929
  biopsy of, 820
    after endosonographic staging, 821
    in inflammatory bowel disease, 570
  bleeding from, 987
    in colonic neoplasia, 765
    in inflammatory bowel disease, 586
    in juvenile polyposis of colon, 788
    in Meckel's diverticulum, 1890
    in trichuriasis, 936
  carcinoid tumors in, 778
  carcinoma of; *see* Rectal carcinoma
  compliance of, 841
  computed tomography of
    abscess in, 614
    after endosonographic staging, 821
  congenital malformations of, 1909-1912
  in Crohn's disease, 591, 617-618
  curative resection in tumors of, 821
  distension of, 841
    in defecography, 849
  endosonography of, 727-729
    history of use of, 17
    in staging, 821
  filling defects in low, malignant potential of,
    776
  magnetic resonance imaging of
    in atresia, 719
    in Crohn's disease, 617-618
  percutaneous abscess drainage and, 2008,
    2009
  reanastomosis of colon with, 752
  Schistosoma mansoni and, 944-946
  sessile neoplasia of, malignant potential of,
    776
  ulcerative colitis in, 581
  volume of, 845
Rectus abdominis flap, 163
Rectus abdominis muscle, 31
Recurrent laryngeal nerve paresis, 130
Recurrent neoplasms
  of gastric stump, 423-424
  pancreatic cystic, 1150

Red blood cell scintigraphy
  in functional asplenia, 1769
  in gastrointestinal bleeding, 987-989,
    990-992
  in hepatic hemangiomas, 1639-1640
  in hepatic metastases, 1708
  in leiomyoma of small bowel, 628
  of liver, 1526, 1527-1528
    in hemangioma, 1463
    in pediatric angiomatous lesions, 1966
    in pediatric visceroatrial anomalies, 1934,
      1935
Red pulp, 31, 34
Reflectoscope, history of use of, 16
Reflex
  gastrocolic, 88
  rectoanal inhibitory, 840, 845
Reflux
  from cecum in Crohn's disease, 595
  in cholescintigraphy, 1235
  in duodenum in enteroclysis, 535, 541, 546
  gastroesophageal; *see* Gastroesophageal
    reflux; Reflux esophagitis
  nasopharyngeal, 1828
  of pancreatic and biliary juice as carcinogen,
    1325
  in stomach in enteroclysis, 535, 541, 546
  urinary, 1197, 1214, 1221
Reflux atony in enteroclysis, 535, 541, 546
Reflux esophagitis, 207-208; *see also*
    Gastroesophageal reflux
  in child, 1845, 1846
  esophageal manometry in, 200
  in hiatus hernia, 218-220
  in stroke, 135
Refractile mesenteritis, 604
Refraction phenomenon, 1474
Regenerative hyperplasia in liver, 1542-1543,
    1544, 1545, 1655-1656
Regenerative polyps in stomach, 374, 375
Regional lymph nodes; *see* Lymph nodes
Reglan; *see* Metoclopramide
Regurgitation; *see* Reflux
Rejection
  after liver transplantation, 1747
  after pancreatic transplantation, 1197,
    1206-1221; *see also* Pancreatic
    transplantation
Relapsing pancreatitis, 1091-1098
Relaxants
  before barium enema, 707
    in colostomy, 713
  in small bowel studies, 525
Remnants
  pancreatic, 1123
  tracheobronchial, 1842
Renal artery, 30, 31
Renal biopsy
  in pancreatic transplantation, 1197
  percutaneous interventional radiology and,
    1994
Renal cell carcinoma, 1815
Renal colic, 2070-2071, 2072
Renal cortex, 29, 63
Renal dromedary hump, 29, 63
Renal fascia, 29, 31
  computed tomography of, 63
Renal hilus, 30, 31
Renal medulla, 31, 63
Renal pelvis, 30, 31
Renal poles, 63
Renal sinus fat, 63
Renal tubular ectasia, 1976
Renal vascular injury, 2149
Renal vein, 30, 31

Rendezvous procedure
  in endoscopic intervention, 1431
  in percutaneous interventional radiology,
    1411-1414
Resectability of tumor
  of cholangiocarcinoma, 1340
  percutaneous interventional radiology and,
    1987
Resection
  bowel
    in diverticulitis, 750, 751
    enemas after, 713
  of liver neoplasms, 1719-1720
Residual cancer of gastric stump, 423-424
Resolution, spatial, 1487
Respiratory distress in Bochdalek's hernia,
    1853
Respiratory gating, 1489
Rests
  hepatic, 1658-1660
  pancreatic, 1866, 1948
Retention cyst
  esophageal, 252
  mucosal, *Shigella* bacilli and, 899
  in valleculae, 114, 115
Retention polyps
  in colon, 787
  in stomach, 376-377
Reticular surface pattern of colon, 774, 775
Retinal pigment epithelium hypertrophy, 827
Retinitis pigmentosa, 668
Retroaortic left renal vein, 31
Retrocecal appendicitis, 2030
Retrograde cholangiopancreatography,
    endoscopic; *see* Endoscopic
    retrograde cholangiopancreatography
Retrograde small bowel examination, 524
  in idiopathic inflammatory disease, 566, 568
  in ileostomy, 567, 588
Retromolar trigone, 146
  tumor of, 149
Retropancreatic recess, 31
Retroperitoneum, 1807-1825
  abdominal aortography of, 2145
  abscess in, 1818-1819, 2039-2042
  adenopathy and, 1819
  anatomy of, 63, 1807-1812
  computed tomography of, 2078-2079
  desmoids in, 1814
  extraperitoneal air in, 2078-2079
  fibrosarcoma in, 1813
  fibrosis of, 1815-1816
  fluid collections in, 1816-1818
  hemangiopericytomas in, 1814
  hematoma in, 2145
  hemorrhage in, 1817
  inflammation in, 1818-1819
  Kaposi's sarcoma in, 1814
  laminar, 1807-1808
  liposarcoma in, 1812-1813
  lymphangioma in, 1160, 1814
  magnetic resonance imaging of, 1816
  malignant fibrous histiocytoma in, 1813
  malignant schwannomas in, 1813-1814
  mesentery and, 1807, 1820-1824
  neoplasms of
    metastatic, 1815
    primary benign, 1814
    primary malignant, 1121, 1812-1814
  pancreatitis and, 1816-1817
  percutaneous interventional radiology in,
    1992-1994
  perforation of, 2078-2079
  peritoneal cavity and; *see* Peritoneal cavity;
    Peritoneum

Retroperitoneum—cont'd
  psoas muscle in, 1809
  spaces of, 63
    anterior perirenal, 1810-1811
    great vessel, 1811-1812
    posterior perirenal, 1809-1810
  teratomas in, 1814
  urinomas in, 1817-1818
  vascular conditions in, 1819-1822
Retropharyngeal soft tissues in child, 1826,
    1827
Retropharyngeal spaces, 106, 110
Retropharyngeal tendinitis, 124, 126
Retropharyngeum, abscess in, 1834
Retroportal lymph nodes, 34
Retrosternal hernia, 1856-1858
Retrovirus, 228
Reversed malrotation of small bowel, 1882
Reye's syndrome, 1549
Rhabdomyoma of pharynx, 124
Rhabdomyosarcoma
  of biliary tract, 1978-1980
  of pancreas, 1155
  of pharynx in child, 1832, 1834
Rheumatoid arthritis
  hepatic nodules and, 1655
  small intestinal vascular disorders and, 655
Rib, anatomy of, 31
Ricinoleic acid, 90
Rieder, H, 3
Rieder meal, 3
Rigid picket fence appearance, 685
Rigler, LG, 286
Rigler's sign, 2023, 2024
Rim sign
  in hepatic scintigraphy of cholecystitis, 1523
  in splenic calcifications or cysts, 1775
Ring, esophageal, 212, 233-235
Ring catheter in percutaneous intervention,
    1407, 1408
Ring-down artifact, 1998
Ring sign
  in duodenal intramural hematoma or
    bleeding, 503
  in peptic ulcer disease, 339, 340
  in small bowel computed tomography, 529
Risk factors for colorectal cancer, 765,
    824-829
Rod, orthopedic, 1903
Roentgen, WC, 1
Rokitansky-Aschoff sinuses, 1230, 1231
  in hyperplastic cholesteroses, 1289
Rolling-stone sign, 1247
Rose bengal, iodine-labeled, 1233
  history of use of, 15
Rotating gantry scanners, 1453, 1454
Rotation of small bowel, abnormal,
    1878-1884; *see also* Malrotation,
    small bowel
Rotavirus colitis, 604
Roundworms, 926-930
Rouviere node, metastatic, 143, 144, 157
Roux-en-Y anastomosis
  in biphasic enteroclysis with
    methylcellulose, 689, 690
  in obesity surgery, 455, 456
  in percutaneous intervention, 1414-1416
Rugae, 282, 283
  absent, 330
  in child, 1860, 1861
  double-contast examination of, 289
  in endoscopy, 313
  enlarged, 347-351
  excessive, 351, 352, 353
  large, endosonography of, 449

Rugae—cont'd
  lymphoma in, 429
  normal appearance of, 2022
Rupture
  of diaphragm, 2153
  of hepatic neoplasm, 1475
  of spleen
    in trauma, 2146
    ultrasonography of, 2115
  of stomach, 369
    in child, 1874, 1875
    plain films and contrast studies of, 2025,
      2026
Ruvalcaba-Myhre-Smith syndrome, 632, 785
Ruzicka, FF, 286

S

S-100 protein antibodies, 555
S cells, 69
S-pouch, 586, 588
Sacroileitis
  in Crohn's disease, 588
  in ulcerative colitis, 575
Sacrum, deficient, 1910
Sagittal fissure of liver, 32
Sagittal section
  of aorta, 42
  of inferior vena cava, 40
  of left adrenal gland, 44, 45
  of left kidney midplane, 46, 47
  of right upper quadrant, 36
  through inferior vena cava, 40
  through porta hepatis, 38
Sagittal sonogram
  of aorta, 43
  of oropharynx, 111, 112
  of pancreatic head, 41
  of right upper quadrant, 37
Salicylates, 79
Salicylazosulfapyridine, 579
Saline cathartics, 697
Saline injections, cholangitis from, 1312
Saliva, 73
Salivary glands, tumors of, 139
Salmonella, 895, 896, 897, 898
  acquired immunodeficiency syndrome and,
    895
  in pediatric splenic abscess, 1936
  toxic megacolon in, 603
  ulcerative colitis and, 581, 608
Salpingitis, 2073
Sampling zone in defecography, 845
Sandostatin; *see* Somatostatin analogue
Santorini, duct of, 285, 1047; *see also* Papilla
  accessory, 285
  in child, 1946
  embryology of, 1039
  variations in, 1040, 1041
Sarcoidosis
  gastric, 333
  mediastinal, 270
  in primary retroperitoneal inflammation,
    1818
  of spleen, 1787-1788
Sarcoma
  cholangiocarcinoma as, 1333
  of colon, classification of, 762
  in Gardner's syndrome, 781
  Kaposi's; *see* Kaposi's sarcoma
  of liver, 1480, 1684
    in metastases, 1713
  negative percutaneous abscess drainage and,
    2007
  of pancreas, 1155
  in retroperitoneum, 1812-1813

Sarcoma—cont'd
   of small bowel, 640-643
Sarcomatoid carcinoma of pancreas,
      1152-1153
SBFT; *see* Small bowel follow-through
      examination
Scalloping sign of duodenal mucosal folds,
      476
Scanners, 1453, 1454
Scanning transmission electron microscopy,
      555
Scattering of barium, 665
Schatzki ring, 233-234
Schistosomiasis
   lymphogranuloma venereum versus, 907
   presinusoidal portal hypertension in, 1574
   ulcerative colitis versus, 604
Schönlein-Henoch purpura; *see*
      Henoch-Schönlein purpura
Schüle, A, 8
Schwannoma
   of pharynx, 125
   in retroperitoneum, 1813-1814
   in stomach, 379-381
Schwartz, G, 8
Scintigraphy; *see also* Nuclear medicine;
      Radionuclides
   after pancreatic transplantation, 1202-1203
   balloon proctography and, 844
   biliary
      in acute cholecystitis, 1275, 1279
      in pericholecystic abscess, 1286
   in Caroli's disease, 1271
   of choledochal cysts, 1976, 1977
   of esophagus, 168, 184
   in fatty liver, 1551-1553
   in gastrointestinal bleeding, 983-993
      albumin, heat-damaged red blood cells,
         and DTPA in, 987
      causes of bleeding and, 983
      extent of problem and, 983
      labeled red blood cells in, 987-989,
         990-992
      Meckel's scans and, 989-992
      nonscintigraphic evaluation versus, 984
      sulfur colloids in, 984-986, 987
      surgery and, 983-984
   hepatobiliary
      in bacterial cholangitis, 1306
      in choledochoceles, 1269
   history of, 13
   for inflammatory bowel disease, 609-610
   of liver, 1508-1533; *see also* Liver,
      scintigraphy of
   in pediatric visceroatrial anomalies, 1934
   in radiographs before obesity surgery, 460
   red blood cell; *see* Red blood cell
      scintigraphy
   technetium 99m in; *see* Technetium 99m
   xenon 133-enhanced, 1517, 1521, 1531,
      1554
Scirrhous carcinoma
   of gallbladder, 1326
   of stomach, 437
Scleroderma
   in Crohn's disease, 591
   duodenum in, 506
      dilatation of, 661
   esophageal motility disorders in, 206, 211
   small bowel in, 678-679, 680
      motility of, 661
      vascular occlusion of, 653
Sclerosing cholangitis
   cholangiocarcinoma versus, 1336, 1337,
      1342

Sclerosing cholangitis—cont'd
   computed tomography of biliary tract and
      gallbladder in, 1232
   as lithotripsy contraindication, 1359
   percutaneous biliary dilation of strictures in,
      1383
   primary, 1306-1310, 1311
   secondary, 1306
   stenting after percutaneous balloon repair of
      strictures in, 1394
   transjugular intrahepatic portographic
      shunting in, 1011
   in ulcerative colitis, 574
Sclerosing hepatic carcinoma, 1680
Sclerosis
   in cholangitis; *see* Cholangitis
   systemic; *see* Systemic sclerosis
Sclerotherapy
   complications of, 969
   in *Echinococcus* hepatic abscess drainage,
      2002
   in esophageal strictures, 238
   in esophageal varices, 239, 969, 970
Scolicides, 1312
Scout films before computed tomography of
      colon, 718
Screening
   for colorectal cancer, 765, 824-839; *see also*
         Colorectal carcinoma, screening for
      intervals in, 831
      selection bias in, 830
   computer-based preliminary, 299
   in gastritis, 299
   for hepatocellular carcinoma, 1666,
      1688-1692
   nonresponders in, 830
   in peptic ulcers, 299
   in polyposis syndrome of colon, 790
SE; *see* Spin echo pulse sequences
Sebaceous cysts, 781
Sebaceous gland neoplasms, 786
Secretagogue, 1188
Secretin, 87
   discovery of, 67
   in gastrinoma, 1170
   islet cell tumor hormone production and,
      1188
   mechanism of action of, 68
   physiology of, 69
   in Zollinger-Ellison syndrome, 683
Secretory diarrhea, 89-90
Secretory IgA, 82
Sedation
   before barium enema, 701
   in biphasic enteroclysis with
         methylcellulose, 535, 541
   in colonic endosonography, 726
   before extracorporeal shock wave
         lithotripsy, 1359
   in intussusception imaging, 1902
   in percutaneous interventional radiology in
         abdominal masses, 1987, 1988
   for stomach and duodenal endoscopy, 302
Seeding of tumor
   intraperitoneal, in gallbladder carcinoma,
      1326
   in percutaneous radiology, 1995-1996
      in small bowel, 561
Segmentation
   in diverticulitis, 750
   in sprue, 912, 913
Seldinger, SI, 15
Seldinger technique, 24
   in hepatic angiography, 1604

Seldinger technique—cont'd
   in percutaneous abscess drainage, 2000,
      2008
   in percutaneous cholecystostomy, 1381
   in percutaneous fluoroscopically guided
      gastrostomy, 2012
Selection bias, 830
Selective angiography
   of duodenum, 496, 497
   of liver, 1161
Selective arterial embolization in hepatic
      diseases, 1628
Seminal vesicles, 727
Seminoma, 1815
Senna, 90, 583
Sentinel clot sign, 1801
Sentinel loop sign, 1823
Sepsis; *see also* Infections and infestations
   in bile duct obstruction from malignant
         disease, 1399; *see also* Percutaneous
         interventional radiology, in malignant
         biliary tract disease
   in cholecystitis, 1275, 1280
   in percutaneous biliary stricture dilation,
      1384
   in percutaneous biliary tract interventional
         radiology, 1418
   in percutaneous transhepatic
         cholangiography, 1240
   in portal vein, 2082
Serial sonography of liver, 1972, 1973
Serology, 1561-1562
Seroma, 1748
Serosa, 187
   anatomy of, 31
   in endosonography, 265
Serotonin
   in islet cell tumors, 1168, 1172
   in small bowel carcinoid tumors, 632
Serous tumors of pancreas, 1138-1141, 1142,
      1143
Serum alkaline phosphatase, 1325
Serum amylase, 1105
Serum bilirubin, 1325, 1334
Serum ferritin, 1561
Serum insulin antibodies, 1169
Serum iron, 1561
Sessile adenoma of duodenum, 490
Sessile carcinoma of colon, 771
   morphology of, 772-773
   surface contour of, 775, 776
Sessile hemispheres of colon, 763
Sessile lesions of colon
   morphology of, 763
   potential for malignancy of, 774
Sessile polyp of colon, 763
Shigellosis, 898-900
   in acquired immunodeficiency syndrome,
      959
   in gastroenteritis, 903
   in hemolytic uremic syndrome, 1924
   ulcerative colitis versus, 604, 605, 607-608
Shock wave lithotripsy
   in bile duct stones, 1373, 1374
   extracorporeal; *see* Extracorporeal shock
         wave lithotripsy
   with percutaneous endoscopy of biliary
         tract, 1426
Short bowel syndrome, 684, 685
   in child, 1898-1899
Shunt
   arterioportal; *see* Arterioportal
         communications
   arteriovenous, in liver, 677, 1480
   coronocaval, 1588, 1589

Shunt—cont'd
    mesocaval
        in hepatic vein occlusion, 1627
        postoperative stenosis of, 1591
        spontaneous, 1582
    portacaval; *see* Portacaval shunt
    portal, in ultrasonography, 1575, 1577,
        1579-1582
    portohepatic, 1625
    portosystemic; *see* Portosystemic shunt
    splenorenal; *see* Splenorenal shunt
Shwachman syndrome, 1897-1898, 1948-1949
Sickle cell disease
    bone scan in, 1756
    in pediatric splenic infarction, 1941
Sideroblastic anemia, 1560
Sigmoid colon; *see also* Colon
    abscess around, 2059
    anatomy of, 692, 725, 726
    annular carcinoma of, 803
    bleeding in, 987, 990
    diverticulitis of, 613
        computed tomography of, 753
        differential diagnosis in, 755-756
        peritonitis and, 2078
    Schistosoma mansoni and, 944-946
    single-contrast examination of, 770
    volvulus in, 2062-2063
        Chagas' disease and, 923
        identification of loop in, 2062
Sigmoid loop, 692, 694
Sigmoid overlap, 524
Sigmoidectomy, 753
Sigmoidoscope, 715
    neoplasia beyond reach of, 763-764
Sigmoidoscopy
    in Crohn's disease, 587
    flexible, 715-716
        in average-risk person, 835
        before barium examination or
            colonoscopy, 832
        in colorectal cancer screening, 832
        in controlled trials in screening, 834
        in diverticulitis, 755-757
        in double-contrast examination, 832
        in hereditary nonpolyposis cancer, 836
        mortality rates after screening with, 833
        perforation in, 832
    in infant with enterocolitis, 666
    in polyps, 765
Sign
    air-dome, 2025
    bull's eye; *see* Bull's-eye lesions
    central dot, 1271
    chandelier, 1248
    collar button, 341, 342
    comet tail
        in focal nodular hyperplasia of liver, 1651
        in hyperplastic cholesteroses, 1289, 1291
    contained stone, in gallbladder, 1327, 1328
    crescent, 341, 342-345
    dotted-line, 1537-1538
    double-arc shadow, 1248
    double-barrel shotgun, 1249
    double-bubble; *see* Double-bubble sign
    double-duct, 1434
    double-target, 1959, 1960
    football, 2025
    Hampton's line, 341, 342
    hat, 763
    light-bulb, 1636
    moulage; *see* Moulage phenomenon
    Murphy's, 1248, 1275, 1276, 1277, 1281,
        1283
    Nacleiro, 217

Sign—cont'd
    parallel channels, 1249
    pseudo-Billroth I, 333, 475
    pseudo-Billroth II, 599
    ram's horn, 333, 475, 599, 600
    Rigler's, 2023, 2024
    rim, 1523, 1775
    ring
        of duodenum in intramural hematoma or
            bleeding, 503
        in peptic ulcer disease, 339, 340
        in small bowel computed tomography,
            529
    rolling-stone, 1247
    scalloping, 476
    sentinel clot, 1801
    sentinel loop, 1823
    Stierlin's, 891
    straight line, 341, 342
    string, 591, 596, 1869
    target; *see* Target lesions
    thread-and-streaks, 1185, 1592, 1622, 1624
    too-many-tubes, 1249
    ulcer collar, 341, 342
    WES, 1248
Signal averaging, 1487-1488
Silicone in embolization, 1728, 1729
Simethicone, 289, 548
    as colon artifact, 772
Similac with Iron, 531
Sincalide, 1229
Single-contrast examination, 703-704
    after double-contrast barium enema, 709
    in biphasic enteroclysis with
        methylcellulose, 533, 534, 535
        opacification of terminal ileum and, 542
    choice of, versus double-contrast enema,
        711
    in colon neoplasia, 765-767, 768, 773
        for polypoid lesions, 771
    contraindications to, 701
    of esophagus, 177, 179
    in gastric cancer, 388
    in idiopathic inflammatory bowel disease,
        565, 566
        in Crohn's disease, 589, 590, 602
        in toxic dilatation of colon, 565
        in ulcerative colitis, 565, 566
    retrograde, 524
    techniques for, 703-704
    tips and administration sets for, 702-703
    in ulcerative colitis, 579, 580, 581
Single-photon emission computed tomography
    of colon
        in colorectal carcinoma, 811
        in metabolic imaging, 720
    of liver
        sulfur colloid technetium 99m imaging
            and, 1508, 1519, 1520
        technetium 99m–red blood cell imaging
            and, 1527
    in pancreatic transplantation imaging, 1202
    in red blood cell scintigraphy, 1639, 1640
Sinus
    brachial, pediatric, 1829, 1830
    cervical, 1829
    in chronic radiation enteritis, 652
    in Crohn's disease, 590, 597
    of omphalomesenteric duct, 1889
    piriform, weblike structures of, 120
    Rokitansky-Aschoff, 1230, 1231
        in hyperplastic cholesteroses, 1289
Sinusoids, 83, 84, 85
    angiography of, 1611, 1612
        hemangioma and, 1640

Sinusoids—cont'd
    in cirrhosis, 1612, 1619, 1620
    corrected pressure in, 1583
        hepatic vein catheterization and, 1607
    in hepatic angiosarcoma, 1684
    physiology of, 84
    vascular anatomy of, 1611, 1612
Siphoning phenomenon in computed
        tomography angiography, 1460, 1461
Situs of stomach in child, 1865
Situs ambiguus, 1865
Situs inversus, 1865, 1934
Sjögren's syndrome, 134
Skeletal radiographs, 1154
Skin
    in Cowden's disease, 786-787
    in Crohn's disease, 589
    in hemochromatosis, 1560
    in Ruvalcaba-Myhre-Smith syndrome, 785
    ulcerative colitis and, 574
Skip areas
    in Crohn's disease, 475, 587, 590, 592,
        597, 598
    in lymphogranuloma venereum, 906
    in primary sclerosing cholangitis, 1308
Skull base, 100, 106
Sliding hiatal hernia, 218, 256
Slow-K; *see* Potassium, enteric coated
Sludge, biliary, 1981
    in acalculous cholecystitis, 1280
Small bowel, 512-688, 689-691
    anatomy of, 512-514
    arteriovenous malformations of, 1596, 1597
    in ascariasis, 929
    barium examination of, 514-525
        in adenocarcinoma, 642, 643
        in amyloidosis, 681, 682
        barium meal and follow-through, 514,
            515
        in celiac disease, 663-665, 666
        computed tomography with, 530, 610
        in cystic fibrosis, 684
        dedicated small bowel meal in, 514-515,
            516, 517
        double-contrast study with oral
            effervescent agent in, 522-524
        drug assistance in, 524-525
        in drug-induced enteritis, 656-656
        in edema, 684, 685
        in eosinophilic gastroenteritis, 683
        fine-needle aspiration cytology and, 555,
            557
        in follow-through examination, 514, 515,
            566
        in giardiasis, 670
        ileostomy, 524
        indications for, 567-568
        in inflammatory bowel disease, 565-568,
            610
        in intramural hemorrhage, 651
        in irritable bowel syndrome, 686
        in ischemia and infarction of mesenteric
            blood vessels, 649, 650
        in ischemic intestinal strictures, 650
        in lipoma, 629, 630
        in lupus vasculitis, 656
        motility and, 661
        in neoplasms, 627, 630, 642, 643
        nodular lymphoid hyperplasia in, 677
        in obstruction, 2047
        in ostomy stomal dysfunction, 524
        peroral pneumocolon and, 567
        pneumocolon in, 516
        in pseudoobstruction, 669
        in radiation enteritis, 685

Small bowel—cont'd
  barium examination of—cont'd
    retrograde, 524
    in scleroderma, 679
    small bowel meal with pneumocolon in,
      515-522, 523
    in strongyloides stercoralis infection, 671
    in uncommon tumors, 630
    in varices, 658
    in Whipple's disease, 680, 681
  biopsy of
    in Crohn's disease, 602
    in ulcerative colitis, 581
  biphasic enteroclysis with methylcellulose
    for; see Enteroclysis, biphasic, with
    methylcellulose
  in celiac disease; see Celiac disease
  cirrhosis with portal hypertension and,
    1596-1598
  computed tomography of, 527, 530, 627
    in adenocarcinoma, 640
    in carcinoid tumors, 634
    in celiac disease, 664, 665
    in Crohn's disease, 602
    in inflammatory bowel disease, 610-615
    in ischemia and infarction of mesenteric
      blood vessels, 649
    lumen measurement in, 305
    in lymphoma, 637, 638
    in Mediterranean lymphoma, 678
    mesenteric lymph nodes and, 526
    in sarcomas, 642
    in trauma, 2138-2139
    in Waldenstrom's macroglobulinemia,
      681-682
    for wall measurement, 305
    in Whipple's disease, 680
  congenital anomalies of, 1878-1891
    abnormal rotation in, 1878-1884
    clinical features of, 1879-1881
    contrast examination in, 1881
    cross-sectional imaging of, 1881
    duodenal malrotation in, 1882
    fixation of midgut in, 1878-1884
    imaging of, 1881-1884
    malfixation in, 1878-1884
    malrotation in; see Small bowel,
      malrotation of
    mobile cecum in, 1882-1883
    nonrotation, 1881-1882
    plain films in, 1881
    reversed malrotation in, 1882
    unusual variants in, 1883-1884
  decompression of, in percutaneous
    fluoroscopically guided gastrostomy,
    2011
  dilatation of, 660
    large bowel dilatation versus, 2044-2045
  edema of, 684, 685
  enteroclysis in; see Enteroclysis
  fixation of midgut in, 1878-1884
  fluid level variations in, 661, 2021
  fluoroscopy of
    in barium examination, 514, 515
    fine-needle aspiration cytology and, 555
    with follow-through method, 689
    in neoplasms, 627
    in ostomy stomal dysfunction, 524
  functional diseases of, 659-688
    celiac disease complications in, 665-668
    cystic fibrosis in, 684
    enteropathic immunoglobulin deficiency
      states in, 671-677
    eosinophilic gastroenteritis in, 683-684

Small bowel—cont'd
  functional diseases of—cont'd
    infestations with malabsorption patterns
      in, 669-671
    inflammatory, 684
    intestinal lactase deficiency in, 684
    irritable bowel syndrome in, 72, 685-686
    ischemic enteritis in, 685, 686
    pancreatitis in, 684
    pathology and biochemical changes in,
      683-684
    primary, 661-665
    radiation enteritis in, 685-686
    radiologic findings in, 659-661
    secondary, 684-685
    stasis in, 669, 670
    systemic diseases and, 677-683; see also
      Small bowel, systemic diseases and
    Zollinger-Ellison syndrome in, 683
  herpetiform dermatitis and, 663
  history of radiology of, 8
  immunodeficiency disorders of, 659-688; see
    also Small bowel, functional diseases
    of
  infarction of, 2054-2057
    mesenteric thrombus or embolus in, 2056
  inflammatory diseases of, 564-626; see also
    Inflammatory bowel disease,
    idiopathic
  intussusception of, 472-473
    in Peutz-Jeghers syndrome, 1895
  irritable, 685-686
    prostaglandins and, 72
  ischemic strictures of, 650
  magnetic resonance imaging of, 530-531
    in inflammatory bowel disease, 616-619
  malabsorption in, 659-688; see also Small
    bowel, functional diseases of
    in child, 1898, 1899
    drugs and, 684-685
  malrotation of, 1878-1884
    barium examination in, 1881, 1882, 1883
    computed tomography of, 1881
    imaging of, 1881-1884
    reversed, 1882
    ultrasonography of, 1881
  mesentery of; see Mesentery
  motility changes in, 661
  narrowing of, 661, 662
  neoplasms of, 627-648
    adenocarcinomas in, 639-640, 641
    barium examination in, 1895
    benign, 627-630, 1894-1895
    carcinoid in, 632-634
    in child, 1894-1896
    computed tomography of, 527, 529,
      627-628, 1895
    Crohn's disease with, 601
    fine-needle aspiration cytology
      differentiating, 559, 561
    leiomyomas in, 627-628
    lymphomas in, 634-640, 641
    metastatic, 643-646
    polyposis syndromes in, 631-632
    portal hypertension and, 1596
    radiographic detection of, 627
    sarcomas in, 640-643
    small-bowel follow-through study in,
      1895
    uncommon, 630
  nodulation of, 661
  nontube examinations of, 514-531
    barium; see Small bowel, barium
      examination of

Small bowel—cont'd
  nontube examinations of—cont'd
    computed tomography in; see Small
      bowel, computed tomography of
    magnetic resonance imaging in; see Small
      bowel, magnetic resonance imaging
      of
    ultrasonography in; see Small bowel,
      ultrasonography of
  obstruction of; see also Intestinal obstruction
    adhesions and, 2049, 2051
    cecal carcinoma in, 2055
    in child, 1860, 1899-1902
    in Crohn's disease, 527
    enteroclysis in, 543-545
    fluid-filled intestinal loop in, 2046
    gallstone ileus in, 2051-2053, 2054
    hernias in, 2048, 2053
    ileocolic intussusception and, 2055
    infarction in, 2054-2057
    internal hernia and, 2050
    intraluminal gas and fluid ratio in, 2048
    in intussusception, 527, 530, 2054, 2055
    lymphoma and, 2050
    mesenteric thrombosis in, 2054-2057
    in neutropenic colitis, 1919
    plain films and contrast studies in, 1919,
      2045-2057
    secondary neoplasms in, 643
    strangulating, 650, 2045, 2047-2048,
      2091-2094
    tuberculosis in, 891
    ventral hernia in, 2052
    volvulus in, 2048, 2052
  pediatric, 1878-1906
    annular pancreas in, 1884-1885
    anterior abdominal wall defects in,
      1890-1891
    barium examination in, 1895
    cast syndromes in, 1903, 1904
    computed tomography of, 1895, 1896
    congenital anomalies of, 1878-1891; see
      also Small bowel, congenital
      anomalies of
    contrast examination in, 1881
    cross-sectional imaging of, 1881
    dermatomyositis in, 1904
    duodenal atresia and stenosis in, 1884,
      1885
    duodenal ulcer in, 1903-1904
    hemorrhage in, 1896
    ileal atresia or stenosis in, 1885, 1886
    infection and inflammation in, 1891-1894
    intussusception in, 1899-1902
    jejunal atresia or stenosis in, 1885, 1886
    malabsorption in, 1896-1898
    meconium ileus in, 1886-1888
    mesenteric cysts in, 1888-1889
    mucosal disease in, 1896-1898
    neoplasms of, 1894-1896
    obstruction in, 1860, 1899-1902
    omental cysts in, 1888-1889
    omphalomesenteric duct anomalies in,
      1889-1890
    plain films in, 1881, 1896
    preduodenal portal vein in, 1885
    pseudoobstruction in, 1902-1903
    short gut syndrome in, 1898-1899
    small-bowel follow-through study of,
      1895
    superior mesenteric artery syndromes in,
      1903, 1904
    trauma in, 1896
    ultrasonography of, 1895

Small bowel—cont'd
percutaneous fine-needle aspiration cytology
of, 555-561
complications of, 562
technique in, 555-561
peroral biopsy of, 552-555
physiology of, 79-83
plain films of
in congenital anomalies, 1881, 1896
in inflammatory bowel disease, 565
in obstruction, 1919, 2045-2057
primary disease of, 661-665
prolapse of, 841
in enteroclysis, 541
pseudomembranous colitis in, 901-903
rotation of, abnormal; *see* Small bowel,
malrotation of
secondary changes in, 684-685
drugs and, 684-685
edema and, 684
short bowel syndrome and, 684
stasis in, 669, 670
syndromes rarely affecting, 632
systemic diseases and, 677-683
alpha-chain in, 677-678
amyloidosis in, 678-679
histoplasmosis in, 682-683
mastocytosis in, 682
Mediterranean fever in, 678
Mediterranean lymphoma in, 677-678
scleroderma in, 678-679
Waldenstrom's macroglobulinemia in,
681-682, 683
Whipple's disease in, 678-679, 679-681
trauma to
computed tomography of, 1896,
2138-2139
plain films in, 1896
in tropical sprue, 663
tuberculosis of, 891-892
in ulcerative colitis, 580
ultrasonography of, 526-527, 528
in celiac disease, 665
in diverticulitis, 760
in eosinophilic gastroenteritis, 684
in inflammatory bowel disease, 615-616
in lymphoma, 639, 678
in Mediterranean lymphoma, 678
mesenteric lymph nodes in, 526
mesenteric vessels in, 526
in obstruction, 2047
in Whipple's disease, 680
valvulae conniventes in; *see* Valvulae
conniventes
varices of, 657-658
vascular disorders of, 649-658
Behçet's disease in, 655
chronic radiation enteritis in, 651-652,
653
Cogan's syndrome in, 656
cryoglobulinemia in, 656
Ehlers-Danlos syndrome in, 655
Henoch-Schönlein purpura in, 653, 655
intramural hemorrhage in, 650-651
ischemic strictures in, 650
malformations in, 657
mesenteric ischemia and infarction in,
649-650
nonsteroidal antiinflammatory
drug-induced enteritis in, 656-657
polyarteritis nodosa in, 653-655
rheumatoid arthritis and, 655
systemic lupus erythematosus in, 656
systemic sclerosis in, 653, 654
thromboangiitis obliterans in, 655-656

Small bowel—cont'd
vascular disorders of—cont'd
varices in, 657-658
vasculitis in, 653-656
Small bowel enema; *see* Enteroclysis
Small bowel follow-through examination, 689
in child
in Crohn's disease, 1892, 1893
in malignant tumors, 1895
dedicated
in inflammatory bowel disease, 566-567
in irritable bowel syndrome, 686
Small bowel meal
dedicated, 514-515, 516, 517
with pneumocolon, 515-522, 523
normal films in, 518, 520
Small duct primary sclerosing cholangitis,
1307
Small field-of-view imaging, magnetic
resonance, 807
Small left hemicolon/meconium plug
syndrome, 1915
Smearing technique in aspiration cytology,
558, 560
Smooth muscle
in benign tumors of stomach, 377-386
esophageal, 194
tumors of, 269-270
physiology of, 75
Soap bubble appearance of duodenal adenoma,
488, 491
Sodium picosulfate, 697
Sodium tetradecyl sulfate
in ablation of gallbladder and cystic duct,
1383
in arterial hemorrhage from gastric ulcer,
971
in sclerotherapy, 969
Sodium tyropanoate, 1227, 1228
Soehendra lithotriptor, 1347
Soehendra retriever, 1431
Soft tissue malignancy from pharynx, 142,
147-150
Solid and cystic neoplasm of pancreas,
1134-1135, 1139, 1149-1152
Solid and papillary neoplasm of pancreas,
1134-1135, 1139, 1149-1152
Somatostatin
in gastrointestinal physiology, 69
in hepatic arterial embolization, 1725
in islet cells, 1167, 1168
mechanism of action of, 68
in pancreatic tumors, 1132, 1146
Somatostatin analogue, 71-72, 1191
Somatostatin cell, 76
Somatostatin receptor imaging, 1191
Somatostatinoma, 1170, 1171-1172
Sonde-type enteroscopy, 978
Sonography; *see* Ultrasonography
Sorbitol, 90
Sosman, MC, 11, 12
Soy protein allergy, 666, 668
Space
anterior fusion, 1812
pancreaticoduodenal, 1807, 1811
pararenal, 1807-1808, 1809-1811
abscess in, 1818
pelvic, 1799-1800
pericolonic, 1811
perihepatic, ascites in, 1801
perirenal
abscess in, 1810, 1818
hematoma in, 1810
perisplenic, ascites in, 1801
peritoneal, 1798, 1799, 1800

Space—cont'd
perivascular, 1812
psoas, 1809
abscess in, 1818
Spasm
in barium examination of colon, 710
of biliary sphincter, 1295, 1296
in Crohn's disease, 591
of hepatic artery, 1611, 1613
in postbulbar duodenal ulcer, 486
Spatial resolution
in hepatic magnetic resonance imaging,
1487, 1489
in liver magnetic resonance imaging, 1486,
1487, 1489
Spatial saturation pulses, 1489
SPECT; *see* Single photon-emission computed
tomography
Sphincter
anal, 840
biliary, spasms of, 1295, 1296
esophageal
lower, 168
upper, 73, 94, 106
Oddi's; *see* Oddi's sphincter
rectal, 728
Sphincterotome, 1345
Sphincterotomy
endoscopic, 1345-1350, 1351, 1352; *see
also* Calculus disease, endoscopic
intervention in
after liver transplantation, 1739, 1748
in ampullary stenosis, 1318
failed clearance of large stones in, 1428
indications for, 1347-1348
in intrahepatic stones, 1348-1350, 1351,
1352
in large stones, 1348-1350
pancreatic duct, 1091, 1092
percutaneous endoscopy of biliary tract
and, 1426
perforation in, 1318, 1347
prior Billroth II gastrectomy and, 1348
risks of, 1346-1347
success rates and complications of,
1346-1347
technical difficulties of, 1348-1350, 1351,
1352
techniques of, 1345-1346
transhepatic antegrade, percutaneous
interventional radiology in, 1426
Spica cast of hip, 1903
Spiculation
in Crohn's disease, 599
in intramural hematoma or bleeding, 503
Spider-web collaterals, 1626
Spigelian hernia, 2092, 2093
Spin-echo pulse sequences, 1757, 1759
Spinal fracture, 2139, 2140
Spindle cell leiomyoma of stomach, 377-379
Spine, computed tomography of, 2139, 2140
Spiral scanners, 1453, 1455
Spiral valves of Heister, 1227
Splanchnic arteries, 1117
Spleen
abscess of, 1780, 1781, 1782
computed tomography of, 2083
fungal, 1937
percutaneous drainage of, 2004-2005
pyogenic, in child, 1936-1937
technetium 99m heat-damaged red blood
cells scintigraphy in, 1530
technetium 99m-labeled sulfur colloids
in, 1530
absence of, 1766, 1767

Spleen—cont'd
  accessory, 988, 1763-1764
    anatomy of, 28
    in child, 1933, 1934, 1935
  in acute abdomen, 2115, 2116
  anatomy of, 31, 34
    in child, 1932
    variants in, 1763-1771
  angiography of, 1759-1760, 1761
  calcifications of, 1772-1774
  in cirrhosis, 1536
  computed tomography of, 1757, 1758, 1759
    in ectopic spleen, 1768, 1769
    in infarct, 1777
    in infections and abscess, 1780, 1781,
      1782
    pediatric, 1932
      in accessory spleen, 1933
      in angiosarcoma, 1937
      in candidiasis, 1937
      in cyst, 1938-1939
      in granulomatous infection, 1937
      in infarction, 1941-1942
      in leukemia, 1938
      in lymphoma, 1938
      in pyogenic abscess, 1937
      in splenomegaly, 1935
      in trauma, 1939
      in visceroatrial anomalies, 1934
      in wandering spleen, 1933
    in trauma, 2094, 2130-2133
  cysts of, 1774-1776
    in child, 1938-1939
    congenital, 1938
    parasitic, 1938
    percutaneous drainage of, 2004-2005
    posttraumatic, 1938
  diseases of, 1763-1794
    anatomic variants and, 1763-1771
    calcifications in, 1772-1774
    focal mass lesions in, 1774-1788; see also
      Spleen, focal mass lesions in
      splenomegaly in, 1771-1772
  ectopic, 1768, 1769
    technetium 99m heat-damaged red blood
      cells scintigraphy in, 1528
  embryology of, 1761-1762
    splenorenal fusion and, 1766
  enlarged; see Splenomegaly
  focal mass lesions in, 1774-1788
    cysts as, 1774-1776
    hematoma as, 1777-1778, 1779
    infarcts as, 1776-1777, 1778, 1779
    infections and abscess as, 1780, 1781,
      1782
    tumors as, 1780-1788
  fracture of
    angiography and, 1761
    in child, 1939, 1940
  functional absence of, 1766-1769
  functions of, 1762
  fusion abnormalities of, 1765-1766
  granulomatous infection of, in child, 1937
  hemangiomas of, 238
  herniations in, 1856
  histology of, 1760-1761
  history of radiology of, 13-15
  infarction of
    in child, 1941-1932, 1941-1942
    ultrasonography of, 2115
  infections in, 1780, 1781, 1782
  interventional procedures for, 1791
  lobulation and clefts in, 1765
  lymphoma of, 431, 1785, 1786
  magnetic resonance imaging of, 1784, 1785

Spleen—cont'd
  multiple, 1766, 1767
  in pancreatic adenocarcinoma, 1108
  parasplenic abnormalities and, 1788-1789,
    1790
  parenchyma of
    hematoma of, 1939, 1940
    intravenous contrast medium and, 1932
  pediatric, 1932-1943
    anatomy in, 1932
    candidiasis in, 1937
    congenital anomalies in, 1932-1934, 1935
    infarction in, 1941-1932
    inflammatory disease in, 1936-1937
    laceration of, 1939
    neoplasm of, 1937-1939
    normal variants in, 1932-1934, 1935
    splenomegaly in, 1935-1936
    trauma in, 1939-1941
  plain films of, 1751, 1752
  radionuclide studies of, 1508-1533,
    1753-1757; see also Liver,
    scintigraphy of
    radiopharmaceutic uptake in, 1544
    technetium 99m phosphate accumulation
      in, 1531
    in trauma, 1515-1517
    in wandering spleen, 1770
  rupture of
    in trauma, 2146
    ultrasonography of, 2115
    splenectomy and, 1789-1790
    splenic artery embolization and, 1791
  trauma to
    arteriography and therapeutic embolization
      in, 2146-2147
    in child, 1939-1941
    computed tomography of, 2094,
      2130-2133
    lacerations in, 2095
    scintigraphy in, 1515-1517
    technetium 99m heat-damaged red blood
      cells scintigraphy in, 1528
  tumors of, 1780-1788
    in child, 1937-1939
    malignant, 1783-1787
    metastases in, 1783-1785
    percutaneous abscess drainage of,
      2004-2005
  ultrasonography of, 1751-1753, 1754
    in accessory spleen, 1933
    in angiosarcoma, 1937
    in epidermoid cyst, 2115, 2116
    in torsion, 2115
    in tumors, 1784, 1785
  varices of, 1753
  wandering, 1769-1771
    in child, 1933, 1934
    in splenic vein obstruction, 1594
Splenculi, 1766, 1767
Splenectomy, 1789-1790
  in thrombocytopenia, 1532
Splenic artery
  anatomy of, 31, 34
  angiography of, in islet cell tumors, 1179
  embolization of, 1791
  percutaneous transcatheter coil occlusion of,
    2147
Splenic flexure, 31
  anatomy of, 692, 725, 726
  in carcinoma screening, 828
  in Crohn's disease, 592
  filling defects in, 776
Splenic index, 1538-1539, 1771

Splenic vein, 31
  anatomy of, 31, 1566
  collaterals for, 1582, 1583
  duplex examination of, in pancreatic
    transplantation, 1203
  in endoscopy, 314
  obstruction of
    in cirrhosis with portal hypertension,
      1593-1594
    duodenal varices in, 501
    in portal hypertension, 1596
  pancreatic tumor invasion of, 1130, 1593
  thrombosis of, 1789, 1790
    in pancreatic transplantation
      complications, 1214
    splenic rupture and, 2115
Splenogonadal fusion, 1765-1766
Splenomegaly, 1771-1772
  in abdominal films, 1752
  in child, 1935-1936, 1937
    in lymphoma, 1938
  in cholangiocarcinoma, 1334
  in cirrhosis, 1541
  in esophageal varices, 241
  ultrasonography of, 1472, 1538
    in portal hypertension, 1575
Splenoportography in cirrhosis, 1566, 1569
  with portal hypertension, 1566-1567, 1569,
    1583
Splenorenal fusion, 1765-1766
Splenorenal ligament, 34
Splenorenal shunt
  magnetic resonance imaging of, 1589
  parasplenic abnormalities and, 1788-1789
  postoperative evaluation of, 1591
  preoperative evaluation for, 1588, 1589
  ultrasonography of, 1575, 1578, 1579-1580
Splenorenal space, 31, 35
Splenoretroperitoneal shunt, 1575, 1579-1580
Splenosis
  intrathoracic, 1768, 1769
  technetium 99m heat-damaged red blood
    cells scintigraphy in, 1528
Spoke-wheel pattern in liver, 1654
Spondylitis, ankylosing
  in Crohn's disease, 588, 1892
  in ulcerative colitis, 575
Spondyloarthritis, 123
Spontaneous common bile duct perforation in
  child, 1977-1978
Spontaneous rupture of stomach, 1874, 1875
Spot films
  in double-contrast barium enema, 705, 707
  duodenal, of adenoma, 488
  of esophagus
    in reflux esophagitis, 220
    in varices, 241
  in percutaneous transhepatic
    cholangiography, 1239
  in single-contrast barium enema, 703
Sprue
  collagenous, 553, 554, 666
  nontropical, 553, 554
  tropical, 663, 910-913, 914
Spurs, cervical spine, 120, 123
Squamous cell carcinoma
  of anal canal, 803
  of esophagus, 243, 248, 276, 279
  of gallbladder, 1326, 1333
  of nasopharynx, 160
  of pancreas, 1152
  of pharynx, 139, 1832
    lymphatic spread of, 142-144, 156
    magnetic resonance imaging of, 140, 141
    pediatric, 1832

Squamous cell carcinoma—cont'd
  of piriform sinus, 159
  of skin after liver transplantation, 1748
Squamous mucous membranes of esophagus,
  232
Stacked coin appearance
  of duodenum, 503
  of small bowel in ischemic enteritis, 685
Staging
  of esophageal neoplasms
    esophageal endosonography in, 265-269
    lymph node metastasis and, 266
    magnetic resonance imaging in, 279-280
  of gallbladder carcinoma, 1327
  of gastric carcinoma, 438-441
  of hepatocellular carcinoma, 1666-1667
  of pancreatic adenocarcinoma, 1109-1110
    endosonography in, 1129-1131
  of rectal cancer; see Rectal carcinoma,
    endosonographic staging of
Stalactite phenomenon of contrast medium,
  287
Staphylococci
  Bochdalek's hernia infection versus, 1856
  in phlegmonous gastritis, 333
  in pseudomembranous enterocolitis, 901
  ulcerative colitis versus, 604
Staphylococcus aureus
  in child
    in granulomatous disease, 1961
    in pyogenic abscess, 1936, 1959
    in retroperitoneal abscesses, 1818
Staple line dehiscence, 460-461, 462, 464
Stasis
  in duodenum, 506
  in small bowel, 669, 670
Static gray scale examination, 1028
Steatonecrosis, 1547
Steatorrhea, 1172
Steatosis, alcoholic, 1548
Steel coils
  in arteriography and therapeutic
    embolization, 2149
  Gianturco, 2144
  in splenic artery embolization, 1791
Steerable catheter in percutaneous
    choledocholithotomy, 1367, 1368
Stellate pattern in duodenum, 492
Stenosis
  biliary tract; see Biliary tract, stenoses of
  in double-contrast enteroclysis with air, 550
  duodenal, in child, 1884, 1885
  esophageal, 1842-1843
  hypertrophic pyloric
    in child, 1868-1869
    conditions mimicking, 1869
  ileal
    barium examination in, 1885
    pediatric, 1885, 1886
  jejunal
    barium examination in, 1885
    in child, 1885, 1886
  papillary, 1091
  pipe-stem, 671
  of portal vein in liver transplantation, 1975
Stent
  biliary
    after endoscopic sphincterotomy for large
      stones, 1348
    after liver transplantation, 1742, 1743
    after percutaneous dilation of strictures,
      1389-1390, 1392, 1396
    Amsterdam, 1430
    in chronic calcific pancreatitis, 1098
    complications of, 1436

Stent—cont'd
  biliary—cont'd
    exchange of, 1431
    indications for, 1432-1434, 1435, 1436
    malfunction of, 1417
    management after, 1417-1418
    metallic expanding, 1436-1437
    migration of, 1417
    versus other palliative treatments for
      malignancy, 1437-1438
  Cary-Coons, 1407, 1409
  Gianturco, 1407, 1409, 1410
    occluded, 1414
  in pancreatitis with stones, 1094-1097
  transjugular intrahepatic portosystemic, 1628
Sterilization of endoscopes, 1424
Steroids
  in biliary tract computed tomography, 1231
  in diverticulitis, 751
  in eosinophilic gastroenteritis, 683
  in gastritis, 329, 330
    in child, 1869
  in hepatic angiography, 1605
  in hepatocellular adenoma, 1645
  in injury gastropathy, 357
  in ischemic bowel, 614
  in lupus gastrointestinal vasculitis, 656
  in peptic ulcer disease, 478
Stevens-Johnson syndrome, 232
Stierlin's sign, 891
Stockum, AE, 23
Stomach; see also Gastric entries
  anatomy of, 31, 34-35, 282-284
    celiac axis in, 311, 312
    computed tomography and, 306-307
    endosonography and, 311
    gastric body in, 34-35, 282, 313
    gastric carcinoma and, 438-439
    hepatic lobe and lateral fundal segment
      in, 311, 312
    mucosal folds in; see Rugae
    variants in, 285
    wall of stomach in, 35, 311, 312; see
      also Stomach, wall of
  antrum of; see Gastric antrum
  barium examination of, 286-297
    after obesity surgery, 461
    in atony, 362
    biphasic, 296
    in bleeding, 298, 984
    Buscopan in, 288
    in cancer, 387-389, 390, 392-394, 397,
      399, 419
    contraindications to, 286
    contrast media in, 287-288
    diagnostic role of, 298-301
    double-contrast, 289-296; see also
      Stomach, double-contrast
      examination of
    endoscopy compared to, 392-394
    gas-producing agents in, 288-289
    glucagon in, 288
    historical perspective of, 286
    hypotonic duodenography in; see
      Hypotonic duodenography
    indications for, 286
    limitations of, 387-389
    in linitis plastica, 395
    in lymphoma, 429, 430, 431
    magnetic resonance imaging with, 308
    modified postoperative, 297-298
    in obesity surgery, 458
    paralysis of peristalsis in, 288
    patient preparation for, 286-287
    roles of, 298-301

Stomach—cont'd
  barium examination of—cont'd
    scintigraphy versus, 984
    single-contrast, 289, 419
    in suspected perforation, 297
    techniques for, 289
    in ulcers, 337, 338, 339-346, 478
  benign tumors of, 373-386; see also Polyp,
    gastric
    adenoma in; see Adenoma, gastric
    adenomyoma in, 377
    Brunner's gland hyperplasia in, 377
    carcinoid in, 383, 384
    Cronkhite-Canada syndrome in, 376-377
    cross-sectional imaging of, 373
    ectopic pancreas in, 377
    epithelial polyps and tumors in, 373-377
    epithelioid variant in, 377-379
    fundic gland polyp in, 376
    ganglioneuroma in, 379-381
    glomus tumor in, 383
    granular cell, 384
    hamartomatous polyps in, 375
    hemangioendothelioma in, 383-384
    hemangioma in, 383-384
    hemangiopericytoma in, 383-384
    heterotopic polyps in, 377, 378
    inflammatory fibroid polyp in, 381-383
    juvenile polyposis syndrome in, 376
    leiomyoma in, 377-379
    lipoma in, 379-381
    lymphangioma in, 383-384
    lymphoid hyperplasia in, 384
    myoblastoma in, 384
    neurofibroma in, 379-381
    neurogenic tumors in, 379-381
    nonepithelial, 377-386
    paraganglioma in, 379-381
    pediatric endoscopy in, 1873
    Peutz-Jeghers syndrome in, 375
    plasmacytoma in, 384-385
    pseudolymphoma in, 384
    radiologic evaluation of, 373
    regenerative polyps in, 374, 375
    retention polyps in, 376-377
    schwannoma in, 379-381
    smooth muscle, 377-386
    spindle cell leiomyoma in, 377-379
    teratoma in, 377
    vascular tumors in, 383-384
  cascade, 285
  cirrhosis with portal hypertension and, 1596
  computed tomography of, 305
    in acquired immunodeficiency syndrome,
      954
    anatomy in, 306-307
    in benign polyps, 373
    in cancer, 390
    in carcinoma, 402, 403, 404, 441-445,
      446
    contrast media in, 306
    diagnostic accuracy in, 305
    in duplications, 318
    endosonography versus, 451-454
    in gastrinoma, 1185, 1186, 1187
    in leiomyosarcoma, 431, 432, 433
    in lipomas, 381
    in lymphoma, 429-431
    in metastases, 432-433
    obesity surgery and, 458
    in smooth muscle tumors, 378-379
    in staging, 441-445
  congenital abnormalities of, 318-325
    adenomyosis in, 318
    adult pyloric hypertrophy in, 322-325

Stomach—cont'd
  congenital abnormalities of—cont'd
    antral diaphragm in, 320-322, 323
    atresia in, 1865, 1866
    diverticula in, 318, 319, 320
    duplications in, 318, 319, 1865
    ectopic pancreas in, 318-320, 321, 377,
      450, 1866, 1867; *see also* Ectopic
      pancreas
    situs in, 1865
    webs in, 320-322, 323, 1865, 1866
  cup-and-spill, 285
  decompression of, in percutaneous
    fluoroscopically guided gastrostomy,
    2011
  dilation of
    acute retention in, 361-362
    causes of, 2042
    in intestinal obstruction, 2042-2043,
      2044, 2045
    plain films and contrast studies of,
      2042-2043
    in volvulus, 2043
  double-contrast examination of, 289-296
    in advanced cancer, 417, 420-421
    in anisakiasis, 935
    availability and cost of, 300-301
    capabilities and limitations in, 388
    in carcinoma, 402, 403, 408, 413-415,
      417, 420-421
    complications of, 300
    diagnostic accuracy of, 299
    in hemorrhagic gastritis, 330
    history of use of, 286
    in Japan, 399
    in leiomyosarcoma, 432-433
    in mass screening, 425
    in metastases, 432, 433
    mortality rate in, 300
  emptying of, after gastric surgery, 458, 460
  endoscopy of, 301-308; *see also* Stomach,
      endosonography of
    in adenoma resection, 407
    after obesity surgery, 461, 464
    aftercare for, 304
    alternative imaging modalities to, 305
    artifacts in, 314
    barium examination compared to, 392-394
    in carcinoma, 392-394, 397, 402, 403,
      404, 405-406
    complications of, 304-305
    computed tomography in, 305
    intubation in, 302-304
    in linitis plastica, 397
    magnetic resonance imaging in, 307-308
    normal appearances of, 304
    patient preference in, 300
    patient preparation in, 301-302
    pitfalls in, 314
    radiologists performing, 305
    roles of, 298-301
    sedation for, 302
    technique for, 301, 305-306
    in tumors, 973
  endosonography of, 311-314, 448-454; *see
      also* Stomach, endoscopy of;
      Stomach, ultrasonography of
    benign processes in, 448-451
    in carcinoma, 403, 404, 451-454
    in gastric lymphoma, 429
    in linitis plastica, 449, 450, 453
    in lymphoma, 449, 451-453
    malignant tumors in, 451-454
    in submucosal tumors, 449, 450
  enteroclysis reflux into, 541, 546

Stomach—cont'd
  fistulization through, for pancreatic
      pseudocyst drainage, 1096, 1097
  fluoroscopy of, after obesity surgery, 458,
      461
  function abnormalities of, 361-365, 366-369
    agastria in pediatric, 1865
    atony in, 361-362
    bezoar in, 365, 366-368
    obstruction in, 361
    rupture in, 369
    varices in, 365, 368-369
    volvulus in, 362, 364-365
  fundus of; *see* Fundus, gastric
  heterotopic tissue of, in gallbladder, 1255
  hypersecretion in, 352
  hypertrophic gastropathy of, 347-351
    in child, 351, 352, 353, 1870
    corrosive, 357, 359
    gastric radiation injury in, 359
    hyperrugosity in, 351, 352, 353
    injury, 357
    Ménétrier's disease in, 351, 352, 353,
      1870
    pseudolymphoma in, 354-357
    tuberculosis and, 326, 347-359, 892
    Zollinger-Ellison syndrome in, 351-354
  hypertrophic pyloric stenosis of
    in child, 1868-1869
    conditions mimicking, 1869
  hypotonic duodenography of; *see* Hypotonic
      duodenography
  inflammatory diseases of, 325-336
    after surgery for obesity, 464
    anisakiasis and, 935
    atrophic, 330
    chronic, 330
    Crohn's disease in, 332, 333, 599-600
    endosonography of, 448-449
    eosinophilic gastroduodenitis in, 475-476
    erosive, 329
    gastritis in; *see* Gastritis
    granulomatous, 330-331, 1869, 1871
    Helicobacter pylori in, 330
    hemorrhagic, 330
    infective, 333
    interstitial gastritis emphysema in,
      334-336
    phlegmonous, 333-334
    radiographic signs of, 327-329
    sarcoidosis in, 333
    syphilis in, 331
    tuberculosis in, 889, 890
  intubation study of, 296-297
  lymphatics of, 311, 312, 313, 314, 438
    endosonography and, 451-453
  magnetic resonance imaging of, 307-308
    in benign polyps, 373
    in carcinoma, 445-446
    in gastric cancer, 402
    in staging, 445-446
  malignant tumors of, 429-447
    carcinoid in, 434
    carcinoma in; *see* Adenocarcinoma, of
      stomach; Gastric carcinoma
    Kaposi's sarcoma in, 435
    leiomyosarcoma in, 432-433
    leukemia and, 435
    lymphoma in, 429-431
    metastases in, 432, 433-434, 1130
    pediatric, 1873
    sarcoidosis in, 333
    villous adenoma in, 435
  microgastria of, 1865
  mucosal folds of; *see* Rugae

Stomach—cont'd
  nonneoplastic diseases of, 318-372
    amyloidosis in, 360
    bezoar in; *see* Bezoar
    congenital lesions in, 318-325; *see also*
      Stomach, congenital abnormalities of
    eosinophilic gastropathy in, 359-360
    function abnormalities in, 361-365,
      366-369; *see also* Stomach, function
      abnormalities of
    hypertrophic gastropathy in, 347-351; *see
      also* Stomach, hypertrophic
      gastropathy of
    inflammatory diseases in, 325-336; *see
      also* Stomach, inflammatory diseases
      of
    Ménétrier's, 351
    peptic ulcer disease in, 336-347; *see also*
      Peptic ulcer disease
  obesity surgery of, 455-466; *see also*
      Obesity, gastric surgery for
  outlet obstruction of; *see* Gastric outlet
      obstruction
  pediatric, 1865-1877
    acquired abnormalities of, 1869-1876
    acquired outlet obstruction of, 1866-1869
    developmental and congenital anomalies
      of, 1865-1866
  peptic ulcer disease of, 336-347; *see also*
      Peptic ulcer disease
  physiology of, 75-79
    gastric motility in, 77-79
    receptive relaxation in, 77
    secretion in, 75
  pneumoperitoneum in, 1874, 1875
  postoperative studies of, 297-298, 300
  pseudotumor in
    computed tomography of, 306
    pseudolymphoma as, 354
  pylorospasm of, 1869, 1870, 1871
  radiation injury to, 359
  resection of; *see* Gastrectomy
  rupture of, 369
    plain films and contrast studies of, 2025,
      2026
    spontaneous, 1874, 1875
  tumors of
    benign, 373-386; *see also* Stomach,
      benign tumors of
    in child, 1873
    epithelial, 373-377
    malignant, 429-447; *see also* Stomach,
      malignant tumors of
  ulcers in; *see* Peptic ulcer disease, gastric
  ultrasonography of, 311-314; *see also*
      Stomach, endosonography of
    in benign polyps, 373
    in cancer, 402, 403, 404
    in leiomyosarcoma, 432, 433
    in linitis plastica, 397
    in lymphoma, 429
    before obesity surgery, 458
    in schwannoma, 380
    transabdominal, 389-392
  upside-down, 362
  varices of, 365-369
    arterial portography of, 1586
    computed tomography arterial portography
      of, 1462
    endosonography of, 449, 450
    portal hypertension and, 1596
    radiographic appearance of, 368
    transhepatic embolization in, 1006-1007
    transjugular intrahepatic portographic
      shunting in, 1010, 1013

Stomach—cont'd
  veins of, in portal hypertension, 1596
  volvulus of, 362-365
    in child, 1874-1877
    gastric dilation and, 2043
  wall of
    anatomy of, 35, 311, 312
    differential diagnosis in thickening of,
      397
    in gastric cancer, 387-390
Stone basket
  in biliary stent exchange, 1431
  in chronic pancreatitis, 1094
  in percutaneous choledocholithotomy, 1367,
    1368, 1369
  in percutaneous endoscopy of biliary tract,
    1426
Stones; see Calcification
Straight line sign, 342
Straining, defecography of, 849
Strangulated hernia, 650, 2045, 2048
Strangulation of small bowel; see also
      Strangulated hernia
  computed tomography of, 2091-2094
  plain films and contrast studies of,
    2047-2048
Strawberry gallbladder, 1291
Streptococcal pneumonia, 1856
Streptomycin, 901
  in Whipple's disease, 679
Stress test of small bowel, 689
Striated muscle
  of esophagus, 194
  in peristalsis, 73-75
Strictures
  bile duct
    posttraumatic, 1314-1315
    in primary sclerosing cholangitis, 1307,
      1308
    in recurrent pyogenic cholangitis, 1303
  of colon
    in amebiasis, 916, 917
    colonoscopy in, 609
    malignant, 583
    in tuberculosis, 893
  in Crohn's disease, 474, 591, 593, 602,
    1923
  of duodenum
    in Crohn's disease, 474
    iatrogenic postischemic, 476
    postbulbar radiation-induced, 476
  of esophagus, 211
    in child, 1846, 1861-1863
  in neonatal necrotizing enterocolitis,
    1918-1919
  rectosigmoid, in lymphogranuloma
    venereum, 905
  of small bowel
    in ileocecal tuberculosis, 891-892
    ischemic, 650
  in ulcerative colitis, 574, 582-583
String-of-beads sign, 2046
String sign
  in Crohn's disease, 591, 596
  in hypertrophic pyloric stenosis, 1869
Stroke, dysphagia in, 133, 135
Stroma
  in pancreas
    infiltration of, by mucinous tumors, 1145
    in serous adenomas, 1138
  of small bowel, malignant tumors of, 555
Strongyloidiasis, 931-933
  in acquired immunodeficiency syndrome,
    673, 959
  in colitis, ulcerative colitis versus, 604

Strongyloidiasis—cont'd
  malabsorption patterns in, 670, 672
  in primary immunodeficiency syndromes,
    676
  in progressive systemic sclerosis, 506
  small bowel inflammatory changes in, 677
Stump
  appendiceal, 772
  gastric, 423-424
Sturge-Weber syndrome, 629-630
Subcapsular cavernous hemangioma, 1992
Subcapsular hematoma
  in peliosis hepatis, 1619
  technetium 99m heat-damaged red blood
    cells scintigraphy in, 1530
Subclavian artery, abberant left, 1845
Subdiaphragmatic fat, 31
Subdiaphragmatic hematoma, 2114, 2115
Subhepatic abscess, 2036-2037
Subhepatic space, 35
Sublingual gland, 139
Submandibular gland, 139
Submucosa, 31
  in Crohn's disease, 593
  of esophagus, 265, 269-270
  of gastrointestinal wall, 187
  of stomach, 449-450
Subphrenic abscess, 2038
  plain films and contrast studies of,
    2036-2037
Subphrenic space, 35
  anterior, 1797, 1799
  fluid collection in, after percutaneous
    intervention, 1421
Subvesicle ducts, 1258
Sucking in child, 1827
Sulfamethoxazole, 904
Sulfonylurea, 1169
Sulfur colloid, technetium 99m–labeled; see
      Technetium 99m–labeled sulfur
      colloid
Sump syndrome, 690
Sunburst pattern in islet cell tumors, 1177
Superconducting quantum-interference-device,
    1564
Superior vena cava; see Vena cava, superior
Supernumerary stomach, 318
Superparamagnetic agents, 308
  iron oxide as; see Iron oxide contrast agents
Superselective renal arteriography and
      therapeutic embolization, 2149
Suppurative cholangitis, 1304, 1305
Supramesocolic spaces, 1797, 1798-1800
Surecut needle, 1988
Surgery
  in diverticulitis, 750, 751
  in gastrointestinal bleeding, 983-984
  in liver metastases, 1715-1716
    radiologically guided, 1719-1720
  in ulcerative colitis, 584-585
Surgical bypass
  Crohn's enteritis after, 829
  in malignant disease
    versus biliary tract endoscopic stent,
      1437-1438
    versus biliary tract percutaneous
      intervention, 1399
Suture anchors, 2016
Suture-line recurrences of colorectal
      carcinoma, 810
Swallowing, 73-75
  anatomy and, 96-98, 127
  in child, 1827-1828
    disorders of, 1828-1829
  esophageal, 98-99

Swallowing—cont'd
  multidisciplinary approach to impairment of,
    165-167
  oral, abnormalities in, 127-129
  pharyngeal, 98
    abnormalities of, 106, 129-133
    in child, 1827-1828
    dissociation between oral and, 128, 129
    imaging techniques for, 98
    neural control of, 98-101
Sweat test, 684
Syndrome
  Alagille's, 1320
  Behçet's; see Behçet's syndrome
  Boerhaave's, 217
  Budd-Chiari; see Budd-Chiari syndrome
  Caroli; see Caroli's disease
  Chilaiditi's, 2027
  Cogan's, 656
  Cowden's; see Cowden's disease
  Cronkhite-Canada; see Cronkhite-Canada
      syndrome
  Ehlers-Danlos, 655
  Gardner's; see Gardner's syndrome
  Mallory-Weiss; see Mallory-Weiss tear
  Mirizzi, 1294
  Muir-Torre, 786
  Ogilvie's, 2008, 2009; see also
      Pseudoobstruction, intestinal
  Peutz-Jeghers; see Peutz-Jeghers syndrome
  Plummer-Vinson, 120, 235
  Reye's, 1549
  Ruvalcaba-Myhre-Smith, 632, 785
  Shwachman, 1897-1898, 1948-1949
  Stevens-Johnson, 232
  Turner's, 629
  Verner-Morrison, 69, 70, 1171
  Werner's, 1169
  Zollinger-Ellison; see Zollinger-Ellison
      syndrome
Syphilis, gastric, 330, 331
  tuberculosis and, 895
Systemic lupus erythematosus, 656
Systemic sclerosis
  esophageal motility disorders in, 206
  progressive, 506, 678-680
    duodenum in, 506
    small bowel and, 653, 654

T

T cells, 82
T-tube
  in choledochoscopy, 1351
  in endoscopic sphincterotomy for stones,
    1347
  in liver transplantation, 1739, 1740
    malpositioning of, 1743
    percutaneous dilation of thrombosed
      artery through, 1742
    as site of bile duct leaks, 1739, 1740
  in minicholecystomy, 1374
  in percutaneous biliary stricture dilation,
    1383, 1385
  in percutaneous biliary tract endoscopy,
    1423
  in percutaneous biliary tract intervention,
    1414
  in percutaneous choledocholithotomy, 1367,
    1368, 1369, 1370-1371
Tabes dorsalis, 133
Tachycardia after lithotripsy, 1364
Taeniae, 694, 939-943
Tamoxifen, 1150
Tampon soaked in contrast material, 842
Tantalum paste, 241

Tapeworms, 939-943, 1961
Target lesions
  in Crohn's disease, 589, 615
  in hepatic epithelioid
      hemangioendothelioma, 1683
  in hepatic metastases, 1478, 1712
  in intestinal ischemia, 2090
  of intestinal metastases, 643
  in intestinal neoplasia, 774
  in trichuriasis, 937
[99m]Tc radioscintigraphy; *see* Technetium 99m
    entries
Tears, esophageal, 218, 241
Technetium 99m–labeled macroaggregated
    albumin, 1519
Technetium 99m-angioscintigraphy
  for gastrointestinal bleeding, 984-986,
      987-988
  in pancreatic transplantation imaging, 1214
Technetium 99m-DISIDA; *see* Technetium
    99m–labeled iminodiacetic acid
Technetium 99m-DTPA; *see* Technetium
    99m–labeled
    gadolinium-diethylenetriamine
    pentaacetic acid
Technetium 99m–heat-damaged red blood
    cells, 1528-1529, 1530; *see also* Red
    blood cell scintigraphy
Technetium 99m-HIDA; *see also* Technetium
    99m–labeled iminodiacetic acid
  in cholescintigraphy, 1233
  in hemobilia or hemorrhage after
      percutaneous interventional
      radiology, 1418
  of obstructed biliary drainage catheter,
      1417, 1418
Technetium 99m-HIPDM; *see* Technetium
    99m–*N*-pyridoxyl-5-methyltryptophan
Technetium 99m-HMPAO, 1202
Technetium 99m-IDA; *see* Technetium
    99m–labeled iminodiacetic acid
Technetium 99m–labeled colloids; *see*
    Technetium 99m–labeled sulfur
    colloids
Technetium-99m–labeled derivatives of
    aminodiacytic acid, 2031; *see also*
    Technetium 99m–labeled
    iminodiacetic acid
Technetium 99m–labeled
    gadolinium-diethylenetriamine
    pentaacetic acid
  in pancreatic transplantation, 1202, 1203
  in rejection, 1206, 1212, 1213
Technetium 99m–labeled glucoheptonate,
    1202
Technetium 99m–labeled iminodiacetic acid;
    see also Technetium 99m-HIDA
  in acute cholecystitis, 1279
  in Caroli's disease, 1271
  in choledochal cyst, 1266
  in cholescintigraphy, 1233, 1234
  in focal nodular hyperplasia of liver, 1510
  in hepatic parenchyma scintigraphy,
      1522-1523, 1525
    disparate sulfur colloids and iminodiacetic
        acid images in, 1523, 1525
  in hepatoblastoma, 1510
  in hepatocellular carcinoma, 1510, 1514
Technetium 99m–labeled mebrofenin, 1233,
    1235
Technetium 99m–labeled pertechnetate
  in Meckel's diverticulum, 1890
  in leiomyoma, 628
  in pancreatic transplantation imaging, 1202
Technetium 99m–labeled phosphate, 1531

Technetium 99m–labeled phytate, 1544
Technetium 99m–labeled sulfur colloids
  in accessory spleen, 1764
  in child
    in Bochdalek's hernia, 1854
    in gastroesophageal reflux, 1860-1861
  in gastric duplications, 1865
  in gastrointestinal bleeding, 984-986, 987
  in hepatic scintigraphy, 1508-1522, 1523,
      1524, 1754, 1755
    in abscess, 1519
    in adenoma, 1511-1514, 1515, 1649
    in benign tumors, 1508-1514, 1515
    in Budd-Chiari syndrome, 1519, 1522,
        1523, 1524
    in cirrhosis, 1516, 1517, 1544
    in congestive heart failure, 1522
    in fatty liver, 1517-1519, 1520, 1521,
        1553
    in fibrolamellar carcinoma, 1680
    in focal nodular hyperplasia, 1508-1511,
        1512, 1513, 1651
    in hemangioma, 1522
    in hepatitis, 1517
    in hepatocellular adenoma, 1649
    in hepatocellular carcinoma, 1531
    in malignant tumors, 1514, 1515, 1531,
        1708
    in metastases, 1514, 1515, 1708
    in nontumor disorders, 1514-1522, 1523,
        1524
    in primary tumor, 1508-1514, 1515
    in secondary tumors, 1514, 1515
    in trauma, 1514-1517
    in vascular disorders, 1519-1523
  mechanism of uptake of, 1508
  in pancreatic transplantation, 1202, 1203
    with pancreatitis, 1214
    in rejection, 1207
  in planar imaging, 1508
  in single-photon-emission tomography,
      1508, 1519
  in splenic scan, 1754, 1755
    in infarct, 1777
    in infection, 1780
    in tumors, 1782
Technetium 99m–labeled white blood cells
  in hepatic scintigraphy, 1531
  in pancreatic transplantation, 1213
Technetium 99m microspheres in hepatic
    scintigraphy, 1531
Technetium 99m radioscintigraphy in small
    bowel sarcoma, 643
Technetium 99m-red blood cell scintigraphy;
    see Red blood cell scintigraphy
Technetium 99m–labeled derivatives of
    iminodiacetic acid, 2031
Technetium
    99m–*N*-pyridoxyl-5-methyltryptophan,
    1202, 1523
TEF; *see* Tracheoesophageal fistula
Teflon catheter in biliary endoscopy,
    1430-1431
Telangiectasia
  gastrointestinal endoscopy in, 973, 975-976
  hereditary hemorrhagic; *see* Hereditary
      hemorrhagic telangiectasia
Telebrix, 530
Telepaque; *see* Iopanoic acid
Tendinitis, retropharyngeal, 124, 126
Tensilon; *see* Edrophonium chloride
Teratoma
  cystic, in pancreas, 1158, 1160
  in pharynx in child, 1832, 1833
  in retroperitoneum, 1814

Teratoma—cont'd
  in stomach, 377
  in child, 1873
Terminal ileitis; *see also* Ileum
  in acute abdomen, 2104
  ultrasonography of, 615, 2104
  Yersinia in, 615
Testes, germ cell tumors of, 645
Tetrabromophenolphthalein, 1227
Tetracyclines
  in esophagitis, 230, 231, 1847
  in tropical sprue, 663
Tetraiodophenolphthalein, 11, 12
Thalassemia
  hemochromatosis in, 1560, 1561
  spleen in, 1752, 1941
Thallium 201 in pancreatic transplantation,
    1202
  in rejection, 1207
Therapeutic embolization, in abdominal
    trauma, 2143-2154; *see also*
    Abdominal trauma, arteriography and
    therapeutic embolization in
Thoracic duct, 32, 188, 189, 190
Thoracic inlet, 188, 189
Thoracic vertebrae, 31
Thoracolumbar fascia, 32
Thorax, bowel gas in, 1853, 1854
Thorium
  exposure to
    cholangiocarcinoma from, 1680
    hepatic angiosarcoma from, 1683
    hepatic scintigraphy in, 1528, 1640
    hepatocellular carcinoma and, 1663
  history of use of, 13-15
Thorotrast; *see* Thorium
Thread-and-streaks sign, 1185, 1592, 1622,
    1624
Thromboangiitis obliterans, 655-656
Thrombocytopenia, 1532
Thromboembolic disease
  in Crohn's disease, 589
  in ulcerative colitis, 574
Thrombolysis, 1628
Thrombosis
  in Crohn's disease, 589
  in hemangioma, 1642
  in hepatic angiosarcoma, 1684
  in hepatic vessels
    after liver transplantation, 1740, 1741,
        1742, 1744-1746
    magnetic resonance imaging of, 1471
    ultrasonography of, 1471
  in mesenteric vessels, 1824
    portal hypertension and, 1596-1598
    in small bowel infarction, 2056
    in small bowel obstruction, 2054-2057
  in pancreatic transplantation, 1198, 1202,
      1207, 1214, 1216, 1217
  of portal vein; *see* Portal vein, thrombosis of
  of portosystemic shunt, 1591
  in small intestinal vascular disorders, 649,
      650
  in splenic vein, 1789, 1790
  in pancreatic transplantation, 1214
Thrombotic index, 1202, 1214
Thromboxane, 72
Thumbprinting
  in amebiasis, 917
  of duodenal mucosal folds, 476
  in ischemic colitis, 2068
  in ischemic enteritis, 685
  in pseudomembranous colitis, 564, 605, 901
  in radiation enteritis, 685
Thyroglossal duct cyst, 126

Thyroid gland
    aberrant, 122
    benign structural disease of, 120, 122
Thyrotoxicosis, 120, 209
Tinnitus, 120, 123
TIPS; *see* Portosystemic shunt
Tissues, homogenous, 186-187
TNM staging; *see* Tumor, nodal, and
        metastasis staging
Tobacco in pharyngeal malignancies, 139
Tolazoline
    in arterial portography, 1567, 1607
    in portal hypertension, 1583, 1586
    in portal vein venography or angiography,
        1596
Tongue
    food bolus on, 127, 128
    muscles of, 106
    tumors of, 147
        at base of tongue, 150, 154, 155
        glossectomy in, 154
        nodal metastasis in, 150
Tongue thrust, 128
Tonsil
    in child, 1827
    enlargement of, 120, 121
Tonsillar fossa, 154-156
Tonsillar pillars, 103
    tumors of, 146, 147, 149, 157
Tonsillar ring of Waldeyer, 139
Tonsillectomy, outpouchings after, 118
Too-many-tubes sign, 1249
Tooth in pharyngoesophageal segment, 115
Torsion
    in cholecystitis, 1286-1287, 1288
    of spleen, 2115
Tortuous vessels in pharynx, 120, 123
Torus, 322, 324
Total iron-binding capacity, 1561
Toxic megacolon, 581-582, 712
    barium examination in, 565
    computed tomography in, 2086
    in Crohn's disease, 602
    in plain films and contrast studies, 2022,
        2065-2066, 2067
    in ulcerative colitis, 574, 581-582, 2067
Toxin, dysentery, 568
Trachea
    esophageal carcinoma invasion of, 273, 277,
        279
    in esophageal endosonography, 188, 189
Tracheal stripe, 176
Tracheobronchial remnant, 1842
Tracheoesophageal fistula
    congenital, 205, 212, 213, 1839-1842
        strictures and, 238
    esophageal atresia and, 205
    in esophageal carcinoma, 248, 273
    motility disorders and, 205, 211
Tracheostomy, 160
Tracker coaxial microcatheter, 2144
Transabdominal ultrasonography, 389-392
    of colon, 716-717
Transcatheter hepatic embolization, 1722-1734
    arterial, 1723-1729
        adjuvant therapy in, 1728-1729
        agents in, 1726-1728
        complications of, 1729, 1730-1731
        contraindications to, 1724
        in hepatocellular carcinoma, 1701, 1702
        indications for, 1723-1724
        preembolization arteriography in, 1725
        premedication for, 1724-1725
        technique for, 1724-1728
    of gastroesophageal varices, 1006-1007

Transcatheter hepatic embolization—cont'd
    of liver neoplasms, 1701, 1702, 1717-1718
    portal vein in, 1729-1732
    results of, 1732
    vascular anatomy in, 1722-1723
Transcatheter therapy
    in hepatic vascular diseases, 1628
    in lithotripsy stone dissolution, 1361
Transcholecystic extraction of bile duct stones,
        1373-1374
Transducer
    biopsy, in percutaneous interventional
        radiology, 1990
    in gallbladder ultrasonography, 1246
    in graded compression ultrasonography of
        acute appendicitis, 2102
    in hepatic ultrasonography, 1466
    in percutaneous biliary tract intervention,
        1404
Transesophageal ultrasound, 270; *see also*
        Esophagus, endosonography of
Transferrin iron saturation, 1561
Transgastric jejunostomy tube, 2012-2013,
        2016, 2017
Transhepatic approach in percutaneous
        interventional radiology combined
        with endoscopy, 1411-1414
Transhepatic cholangiography
    in pancreatic adenocarcinoma, 1110
    percutaneous; *see* Percutaneous transhepatic
        cholangiography
Transhepatic embolization; *see* Transcatheter
        hepatic embolization
Transhepatic-endoscopic approach, combined,
        1411-1414
Transhepatic portal vein catheterization,
        techniques for, 1608
Transhepatic portography, 1566-1567, 1570
    in cirrhosis, 1545, 1588
        with portal hypertension, 1566-1567,
            1570, 1583-1584, 1587-1589
    in pancreatic tumor invasion, 1593
Transhepatic route
    for percutaneous cholecystolithotomy,
        1376-1378
    for percutaneous dilation, 1383, 1384, 1747
    for percutaneous endoprosthesis, 1407
Transhepatic sphincterotomy, antegrade, 1426
Transhepatic venous sampling, 1187-1188,
        1189
Transit
    colonic, 88
    esophageal, 73-75
Transjugular intrahepatic portosystemic shunt;
        see Portosystemic shunt
Transjugular portography, 1567
    in cirrhosis with portal hypertension, 1567,
        1583-1584, 1587-1589
    uses of, 1608
Transluminal angioplasty, percutaneous, 1628
Transmission electron microscopy, 555
Transoral biopsy, 661
Transpapillary endoprostheses, 1094-1097
Transplantation
    bone marrow, 674, 675, 676
    liver, 1735-1750; *see also* Liver
        transplantation
    of pancreas; *see also* Pancreatic
        transplantation
Transrectal approach in abscess drainage,
        2008, 2009
Transvaginal approach in abscess drainage,
        2008, 2009
Transversalis fascia, 32, 1807

Transverse anatomic section
    of extraperitoneal perirenal compartments,
        62
    of pancreatic head, 56-59
    of pancreatic tail, 50, 52, 54
    of transverse duodenum, 60
    of upper liver, 48
Transverse colon
    anatomy of, 32, 35
    volvulus of, 2060
Transverse duodenum, 29
Transverse folds of Houston, 727
Transverse mesocolon, 30, 35
Transverse process of vertebra, 31
Transverse sonogram
    of porta hepatis, 53
    of upper liver, 49
    of upper pancreatic head, 57
Transversus abdominis muscle, 32
Trauma
    in acute abdomen, 2094-2097
    arteriography and therapeutic embolization
        in, 2143-2154
    bile duct strictures after, 1314-1315
    to bladder, 2136-2138
    blunt, 2120
    to diaphragm
        arteriography and therapeutic embolization
            in, 2153
        computed tomography of, 2141
        rupture in, 256
    to duodenum, 502
        computed tomography of, 1896,
            2133-2134
    to esophagus, 216-218
        in abdomen, 216-218
    hemobilia from, 976
    hernia in child from, 1856-1858
    imaging in, 2120-2142
    to kidney, 2135, 2136
    to large bowel
        arteriography and therapeutic embolization
            in, 2153
        in child, 1896, 1927
        computed tomography of, 2138-2139
    to liver
        of child, 1974-1975
        computed tomography of, 1475,
            2123-2130
        hepatic blood vessels and, 2147-2148
        scintigraphy in, 1514-1517
        technetium 99m sulfur colloid
            scintigraphy in, 1514-1517
        ultrasonography in, 1475
    to lumbar arteries, 2153
    to mesentery, 2138-2139
    to pancreas
        arteriography and therapeutic embolization
            in, 2153
        in child, 1954-1955
        computed tomography of, 2133
        pancreatitis and, 1091, 1955
    to pelvis
        arteriography and therapeutic embolization
            in, 2150-2152
        computed tomography of, 2140
    penetrating, 2140-2141
    to pharynx, 115, 116, 117
        in child, 1835-1836
    to pleural space, 2153
    to renal blood vessels, 2149
    to small bowel
        arteriography and therapeutic embolization
            in, 2153
        in child, 1896, 1927

Trauma—cont'd
  to small bowel—cont'd
    computed tomography of, 2138-2139
    strictures after, 650
  to spine, 2139, 2140
  to spleen
    arteriography and therapeutic embolization
        in, 2146-2147
    in child, 1939-1941
    computed tomography of, 2130-2133
    cyst after, 1938-1939
  to stomach
    in gastropathy, 357
    from radiation, 359
    rupture and, 369
  strictures after, 650
    bile duct, 1314-1315
  vascular, 2139
    hepatic, 2147-2148
Traveler's diarrhea, 903
Treitz ligament, 32, 284
Trematodes, 943-946
  ulcerative colitis versus, 604
Trendelenburg position, 522
  in endoscopic retrograde
        cholangiopancreatography,
        1241-1242
  negative, 290
Triangle chain, posterior, 144
Tribromo iminodiacetic acid, 1523
Trichobezoar, 365, 366-367
  in child, 1873-1874
Trichosporon, 1312
Trichotillomania, 365
Trichuriasis, 935-937, 938
Tricyclic antidepressants, 73, 661
Trigeminal nerve, 150
Triglycerides, 80
Trigone, retromolar, 146
  tumor of, 149
Triiodinated benzene ring, 1227, 1228
Trimethoprim and sulfamethoxazole, 679
Tropical sprue, 663, 910-913, 914
Tru-Cut needle, 1988
Trypanosomiasis, 209, 918-923, 924, 925
Trypsin
  in acinar cell carcinoma, 1154
  in pancreatoblastoma, 1156
Tubeless hypotonic duodenography, 296
Tuberculosis, 888-895
  cholangitis in, 1311
  colitis in, 893
    radiologic follow-up in, 609
    ulcerative, 581
      Crohn's disease and, 599
  differential diagnosis in, 895
  duodenal, 476, 477, 890-891
  of esophagus, 229, 889
    in child, 1846
    in strictures, 238
  gastric, 330, 333, 889, 890
  ileocecal, 891-893
  lymphogranuloma venereum versus, 907
  percutaneous abscess drainage in, 1999
  peritoneal, 894, 1802
  rectal, 893
  retroperitoneal, 1818
  of small bowel, 890-891
    enteroliths in, 893-894
  splenic, 1780
d-Tubocurare, 210
Tubular adenoma
  of colon, 763
  of duodenum, 488, 492, 495
  of small bowel, 629

Tubular adenoma—cont'd
  of stomach, 374
Tubular colon, 578, 579
Tubular ectasia, renal, 1976
Tubulovillous adenoma of duodenum, 488
Tumor; *see also* specific tumor or organ
  defined, 762
  dysphagia in, 133, 134
  enteric, negative percutaneous abscess
      drainage and, 2007
  extension of, in percutaneous intervention
      techniques, 1403
  resectability of
    of cholangiocarcinoma, 1340
      percutaneous interventional radiology and,
          1987
  resection of; *see* Resection
  seeding of, percutaneous interventional
      radiology in, 1995-1996
  tumorlike lesions in, 498-501
Tumor, nodal, and metastasis staging
  of esophageal cancer, 274, 276, 277
  of gallbladder carcinoma, 1327
  in gastric carcinoma, 439-441, 443-445
  of pharyngeal tumor, 140
  of rectal carcinoma, 815-818
Tungsten, history of use of, 19
Turcot syndrome, 1928
Turner's syndrome, 629
Two-scan cluster technique in computed
      tomography angiography, 1459
Typhilitis, 1918-1919
Typhlitis
  computed tomography of, 614
  in large bowel in child, 1918, 1919
  ultrasonography of, 2104
Typhoid fever, 895-898, 899
  toxic megacolon in, 603
Tyropanoate sodium, 1227, 1228

U
Ulcer; *see also* Peptic ulcer disease; Ulcerative
      colitis
  after obesity surgery, 464-466
  in amebiasis, 917
  in anisakiasis, 935
  aphthous
    in child, 1921
    in Crohn's disease, 587, 589, 594, 599,
        600, 1921
    in gastritis, 327, 333
    small bowel, 517, 522, 550
    in ulcerative colitis, 575
  bleeding
    endoscopy for, 968, 970-972
    pathophysiology of, 970
  collar-button, 341, 342, 576
  of colon, 803; *see also* Ulcerative colitis
    aneurysmal, 792
    in inflammatory disease, 576
  in Crohn's disease, 572, 597
  in esophagus, 1845
  in gastric lymphoma, 429
  malignant, endosonography of, 449
  peptic; *see* Peptic ulcer disease
  sealed-off, 2080
  in strongyloidiasis, 931
  tuberculous, 889
Ulcer crater, 2108, 2109
Ulcer mound, 345, 346, 478
  endosonography of, 449
Ulcer niche, 478, 480
  first use of term of, 6, 7
Ulcer-within-an-ulcer appearance in
      duodenum, 486

Ulcerative colitis, 573-585
  accuracy of examination in, 580-581
  in acute abdomen, 2065, 2066
  in child, 1919-1921
  clinical features of, 573-574
  complications of, 581-584
  computed tomography of, 610
  Crohn's disease versus, 603-608
  differential diagnosis of, 603-608
  diffuse, 573
  endoscopy in, 574
  esophagitis in, 232
  extraintestinal manifestations of, 574-575
  hematology and, 574
  instant double-contrast barium enema in,
      565, 712
  lymphogranuloma venereum versus, 907
  malignancy in, 583-584
    colon, 791, 827-829
    gallbladder, 1325
    rectal, 827-829
    screening for, 829
  perforation in, 582
  polyps in, 574
  portal hypertension and, 1599
  primary sclerosing cholangitis in, 1307
  radiographic features of, 575-580, 581
  secondary changes in large bowel in,
      579-580
  severe or fulminant, 574
    surgery in, 609
  strictures in, 582-583
  surgery in, 584-585, 609
  toxic megacolon and, 2067
  tuberculosis and, 895
  tubular colon in, 578, 579
Ulcerative enteritis in histoplasmosis, 682-683
Ulcerative gastric carcinoma, 437
Ulcerative jejunoileitis, 665-666
Ulcerative proctitis, 904, 905
Ulceronodular pattern in Crohn's disease, 596
Ultrafast computed tomography, 1453
Ultrasonography; *see also* specific organ
  of acute abdomen, 2099-2117; *see also*
      Acute abdomen, ultrasonography of
  compression, schematic of, 2102
  defined, 186
  in diaphragmatic movement, 256
  Doppler; *see* Doppler ultrasonography
  duplex Doppler imaging; *see* Duplex
      Doppler imaging
  graded compression, in appendicitis, 2031,
      2102
  history of use of, 16-17
  pediatrics and; *see* Pediatrics,
      ultrasonography in
  right upper quadrant, 37
Ultrasound colonoscope, 716
Ultrasound lithotriptor, 1375
Umbilical polyp in child, 1889
Umbilical portography, 1572
  in cirrhosis with portal hypertension, 1572
  uses of, 1608
Umbilical vein, 1472
Uncinate process, 32, 47
Upper esophageal sphincter, 73, 94
  in swallowing, 106
Upper gastrointestinal bleeding, 298
  barium examination in, 298
  endoscopy in, 298, 299-300
  fecal occult-blood test for, 831
  scintigraphy in, 983
Upper gastrointestinal endoscopy, 967-982; *see*
      also Endoscopy

Upper gastrointestinal series
  in aortoduodenal fistula, 501
  in choledochoceles, 1269
  in duodenal diverticulitis, 469
  in duodenal strictures, 486
  in duodenal trauma, 502
  in duodenal ulcer in young person, 488
  of esophagus, 192
  history of, 2-8, 9
  in superior mesenteric artery compression
      syndrome, 506
Upper motor neuron disease, 133
Urea
  in hyperplasia of Brunner's glands, 499
  liver and, 84
Uremic syndrome, hemolytic, 1924
Ureter, 32
Urinary bladder; see Bladder
Urinary calculi
  in malabsorption, 80
  in ulcerative colitis, 575
Urinary reflux, 1197, 1214
Urinary system in Crohn's disease, 589
Urinoma, 2071
  after pancreatic transplantation, 1198, 1221
  in renal colic, 2072
  in retroperitoneum, 1817-1818
Urogastrone, 68
Urography, excretory, 1751, 1752
Urokinase, 1628
Urolithiasis
  in malabsorption, 80
  in ulcerative colitis, 575
Ursodeoxycholic acid, 1359
Urticaria pigmentosa, 682
Urticarial colitis, 795
US; see Ultrasonography
Uterovesical fossa, 1800
Uterus
  in pelvic space, 1800
  rectal endosonography and, 728

V
V-shaped radiolucency of Nagleiro, 217
Vagina
  in colovaginal fistula, 712, 793
  in defecography, 841-842
  percutaneous abscess drainage and, 2008,
      2009
  in rectal carcinoma, 820
Vaginography, 712
Vagotomy, 77, 79
  functional changes after, 208-209
Vagus nerve, 194
  neuropathy with, 209
Valium; see Diazepam
Valleculae, 103-106
  barium retention in, 132
  cysts in, 114, 115
Valproic acid, 1547
Valsalva maneuver, modified, 101
Valvulae conniventes, 284, 467, 513
  atrophy of, 506, 507
  in celiac disease, 559, 662, 664, 665
  in giardiasis, 925
  in jejunum, 527
  in mesenteric thrombosis, 2054
  in small bowel dilation, 2045
  in sprue, 912, 913
  thickened, 660
    in ischemia and infarction of mesenteric
        blood vessels, 649, 650
    in radiation enteritis, 651
    in Whipple's disease, 680
Vancomycin, 902

Varices
  choledochal, 1319
  of colon, 977
    portal hypertension and, 1599, 1600
  of duodenum, 501
  of esophagus; see Esophagus, varices of
  gastric; see Stomach, varices of
  hepatofugal or hepatopetal, 241
  mesenteric, 1599, 1600
  parasplenic, 1788-1789
  in portal hypertension, 1575, 1576, 1577
  in pregnancy, 970
  in small intestinal vessels, 657-658
  splenic, 1753
  transhepatic portal vein catheterization for,
      1608
Vascular abnormalities; see also Congenital
      abnormalities
  after liver transplantation, 1744-1747
  after pancreatic transplantation, 1198, 1214
    from imaging complications, 1214-1217,
        1218-1220
  of duodenum, 501-506
  of esophagus of child, 1844
  of retroperitoneum, 1819-1822
  of small bowel, 657
Vascular anatomy of liver, 1471-1473; see
      also Liver
  in angiography, 1608-1611, 1612, 1613
  in magnetic resonance imaging, 1503-1505
  in transcatheter hepatic embolization,
      1722-1723
Vascular congestion, small bowel mesentery
      and, 1823
Vascular disease
  angiography and; see Angiography
  of liver, 1604-1629; see also Liver, vascular
      diseases of
    technetium 99m sulfur colloid
        scintigraphy of, 1519-1523
  of small bowel, 649-658; see also Small
      bowel, vascular disorders of
Vascular ectasia, 983
  portal hypertension and, 1598, 1599
Vascular flukes, 944-946
Vascular injury
  arteriography and therapeutic embolization
      in
    hepatic, 2147-2148
    renal, 2149
  computed tomography of, 2139
Vascular invasion
  in gallbladder carcinoma, 1326
  in pancreatic adenocarcinoma, 1124
Vascular tumor
  cryosurgery in, 1720
  in pancreatic serous adenomas, 1141
  in stomach, 383-384
Vasculitis
  lupus gastrointestinal, 656
  necrotizing, 1904
  in pancreatic transplantation, 1198, 1202
  small bowel, 653-656
    in rheumatoid arthritis, 655
Vasoactive intestinal peptides
  hepatic arterial embolization and, 1729
  in pancreatic tumors, 1132, 1146
    in islet cell tumors, 1168
  physiology of, 69, 70
  in VIPoma, 1171
Vasoconstrictive infusion therapy, 995-997
Vasodilators, 1583
Vasopressin
  in angiography, 1006
  in Mallory-Weiss syndrome, 218

Vasovagal reaction
  in percutaneous cholecystostomy, 1381
  in percutaneous interventional radiology,
      1995
Vater
  ampulla of; see Ampulla, duodenal
  papilla of; see Papilla
VATER association, 1910
Vater's papilla; see Ampulla, duodenal
Velopharyngeal incompetence, 129, 1829
Vena cava
  anomalies of
    congenital, 1819-1820
    liver transplantation and, 1735
  inferior
    after liver transplantation, 1736,
        1746-1747
    anatomy of, 32, 40
    congenital anomalies of, 1819-1820
    in duodenal endoscopy, 314
    duplications of, 1819-1820
    in gallbladder ultrasonography, 1250
    in gastric endoscopy, 311
    in hepatic angiography, 1605-1606
    hepatic vein drainage into, 1444-1446
    intrahepatic, 1468
    obstruction of, 1519, 1522
    retroperitoneal diseases and, 1819-1820
    ultrasonography of, 40
  superior
    in esophageal endosonography, 188
    obstruction of, hepatic scintigraphy in,
        1519, 1521
Venacavography, inferior, 1746
Venography, portal; see Portal venography
Venoocclusive disease in child, 1973
Venous drainage, rectal, 728
Venous infarct in pancreatic transplantation,
      1216-1217
Venous plexus, peribiliary, 1610
Venous thrombosis; see Thrombosis
Ventral hernia, small bowel, 2053, 2107
Ventral veins, manometry of, 1583
Ventricles, 30, 31
Venules, hepatic, 83
Verner-Morrison syndrome, 69, 70, 1171
Verrucose skin lesions, 786-787
Verrucous squamous cell carcinoma of
      esophagus, 243, 248
Vertebra, 29
  transverse process of, 32
Vertebral body, 32
  in esophageal endosonography, 189, 190
Vertical gastroplasty; see Obesity, gastric
      surgery for
Vestibule
  of esophagus, 168
  of larynx, 127
    in swallowing abnormalities, 130, 131
Videoendoscope, 715
Videofluoroscopy; see also Fluoroscopy
  in defecography, 844
  in dysphagia, 165, 167
  of esophagus, 192
  of pharyngeal function, 97, 101
Villi
  of colon in Cronkhite-Canada syndrome,
      787
  of small bowel, 514
    in celiac disease, 553
    in Crohn's disease, 595, 596
Villous adenoma
  colon, 777
    origin of, 764
    screening in, 826

Villous adenoma—cont'd
  of duodenum, 488, 491
  of small bowel, 629, 631
  of stomach, 374, 376, 435
Vimentin
  antibodies against, 555
  in giant cell tumor of pancreas, 1153
Vinyl chloride exposure
  in hepatic angiosarcoma, 1683
  hepatic scintigraphy in, 1528, 1640
VIP; *see* Vasoactive intestinal peptides
VIPoma, 69-70, 71, 1171
Viral disease
  in acquired immunodeficiency syndrome,
    955
  in esophagitis, 228-229
  in gastritis, 333
  in hepatitis
    in child, 1958-1959
    in cirrhosis, 1534, 1538
  in pancreatitis after transplantation, 1213
  ulcerative colitis versus, 604
Viscera, hollow, 661, 669, 2101-2108
Visceroatrial anomalies, 1933-1934, 1935
Vitamin B_{12}, 77
Vitamin E, 668
Voltage in radiographic contrast, 2022
Voluntary external anal sphincter, 840
Volvulus
  in Bochdalek's hernia, 1854-1855
  in cecum, 2061
    gastric dilation and, 2043
    plain films and contrast studies in,
      2061-2063
  in Chagas' disease, 923
  of colon
    plain films and contrast studies in, 2059,
      2060
    sigmoid, 2062
    transverse, 2060
  mesenteroaxial, 365
    in child, 1877
    gastric dilation and, 2043
    of stomach, 2045
  midgut, 2052
  organoaxial, 365
    in child, 1877
    gastric dilation and, 2043
    of stomach, 2044
  of small bowel, 2048, 2052
  of stomach, 362-365
    in child, 1874-1877
    dilation and, 2043
    mesenteroaxial, 2045
    true, 362
von Hippel–Lindau disease, 1156-1157
  in child, 1949, 1950
  cystic lesions in, 1954
von Recklinghausen's disease
  gastric neurofibromas and, 379-381

von Recklinghausen's disease—cont'd
  schwannomas and, 1813-1814
  small bowel tumors in, 630

W

Waldenström's macroglobulinemia, 681-682,
    683
  peroral biopsy in, 555, 556
Waldeyer's tonsillar ring, 139
Wallstent
  in chronic pancreatitis with stones, 1094
  in malignant biliary tract disease, 1407,
    1409, 1410
  polyethylene stent versus, 1436
  in transjugular intrahepatic portacaval shunt,
    1587
Wandering esophagus, 254-255
Wandering spleen, 1769-1771
  in child, 1933, 1934
  in splenic vein obstruction, 1594
Warfarin sodium, 2092
Water as contrast agent; *see* Contrast agents,
    water-soluble
Water siphon test, 182, 220
Water-soluble contrast media; *see* Contrast
    agents, water-soluble
Watermelon stomach, 975-976
WDHA syndrome, 1171
Web
  of duodenum, 467, 1884, 1885
  endodermal, 1251
  of esophagus, 212
  of gastric antrum, 320-322, 323
  of pharynx, 118-120, 1831-1832
    in child, 1831-1832
  of stomach, 1865, 1866
Weber-Christian disease, 1823
Weeping willow tree appearance in liver, 1545
Weight
  after obesity surgery, 458
  in pancreatic adenocarcinoma, 1107
Werner's syndrome, 1169
WES sign, 1248
Wet bowel, 661
Wetting agents in colon as artifact, 772
Wheels-within-wheel appearance in spleen,
    1780
Whipple's disease
  in duodenum, 506
  endoscopic biopsy in, 680
  in mesentery, 1823
  in small bowel, 679-681, 1823
    peroral biopsy in, 555
Whipple's triad, 1169
Whipworm, 935-937, 938
White blood cell scanning
  indium-labeled; *see* Indium 111–labeled
    leukocytes
  of liver, 1531
  in pancreatic transplantation, 1213

White pulp, 32, 34
Wild, J, 16
Williams, FH, 4, 5, 10
Wilms' tumor, 1964
Wilson's disease
  dysphagia in, 133
  hepatocellular carcinoma and, 1663
Windsock appearance in colon, 1909
Winslow foramen, 34, 35
Wire-spring appearance in small bowel, 653
Wirsung, duct of
  calculi in, 1101
  embryology of, 1039
  pediatric, 1946
  variations in, 1040, 1041

X

X-ray diffraction analysis, 555, 557
Xanthoma
  in cholecystitis, 1289, 1327, 1331
  small bowel peroral biopsy and, 555
Xenon 133 scintigraphy, 1531
  in fatty liver, 1517, 1521
    versus carcinoma, 1554
Xenon detectors, 19
Xerostomia, 73
Xylocaine
  in biphasic enteroclysis with
    methylcellulose, 534
  in percutaneous biliary tract intervention,
    1401

Y

Yersinia
  in colitis
    in child, 1924-1925
    ulcerative colitis versus, 604, 605
  in terminal ileitis, 615, 2104
  in ulcerative colitis, 580, 581, 589

Z

Z line, 304
Zenker's diverticulum, 73, 74, 118, 119, 214
  in child, 1831
  pharyngeal perforation in, 115
Zollinger-Ellison syndrome, 69, 351-354, 355
  APUD system and, 67
  duodenum in, 508
  of esophagus
    in esophagitis, 223
    perforation in, 216
  gastrinoma in, 1170, 1180
    imaging of, 1186, 1192
  gastritis in, 326
  small bowel in, 683
Zymogen granules
  in acinar cell cystadenocarcinoma, 1155
  in pancreatoblastoma, 1155